CLINICAL Gastroenterology AND Hepatology

Commissioning Editor: **Karen Bowler**
Project Development Manager: **Hilary Hewitt**
Project Manager: **Glenys Norquay**
Illustration Manager: **Mick Ruddy**
Designer: **Andy Chapman**
Illustrators: **Designers Collective**

CLINICAL Gastroenterology AND Hepatology

Editors

Wilfred M Weinstein MD
Professor of Medicine
Digestive Diseases
David Geffen School of Medicine at UCLA
Los Angeles, CA, USA

C J Hawkey DM FRCP
Professor of Gastroenterology
Wolfson Digestive Diseases Centre
University Hospital
Nottingham, UK

Jaime Bosch MD
Professor of Medicine
Liver Unit, Institut de Malalties Digestives i Metaboliques
Hospital Clínic
University of Barcelona
Barcelona, Spain

Associate Editors

Guadalupe Garcia-Tsao MD
Professor of Medicine
Department of Internal Medicine
Yale University School of Medicine
New Haven, CT, USA

Paul J Fortun BM MRCP FRACP
Clinical Lecturer in Gastroenterology
Wolfson Digestive Diseases Centre
University Hospital
Nottingham, UK

Kirsten Tillisch MD
Clinical Instructor
David Geffen School of Medicine at UCLA
Los Angeles, CA, USA

ELSEVIER
MOSBY

ELSEVIER
MOSBY

Mosby is an affiliate of Elsevier Inc.

First published 2005

ISBN 0 323 02751 2

This book is also available as an edition package, including access to online updates:
ISBN 0 323 03596 5

An online version of this book, with updates, is also available:
ISBN 0 323 03595 7

British Library Cataloguing in Publication Data
A catalogue record for this book is available from the British Library

Library of Congress Cataloging in Publication Data
A catalog record for this book is available from the Library of Congress

Notice

Medical knowledge is constantly changing. Standard safety precautions must be followed, but as new research and clinical experience broaden our knowledge, changes in treatment and drug therapy may become necessary or appropriate. Readers are advised to check the most current product information provided by the manufacturer of each drug to be administered to verify the recommended dose, the method and duration of administration, and contraindications. It is the responsibility of the practitioner, relying on experience and knowledge of the patient, to determine dosages and the best treatment for each individual patient. Neither the Publisher nor the editors/contributors assume any liability for any injury and/or damage to persons or property arising from this publication.

The Publisher

Printed in Spain
Last digit is the print number : 9 8 7 6 5 4 3 2 1

The Publisher's policy is to use **paper manufactured from sustainable forests**

Contents

Contributors

Samuel N Adler MD
Medical Doctor
Jerusalem, Israel

Dennis Ahnen MD
Professor of Medicine
Denver VAMC
Denver, CO, USA

Bhupinder S Anand MD DPhil
Professor of Medicine
Baylor College of Medicine
Staff Physician
Michael E DeBakey VA Medical Center
Houston, TX, USA

Åke Andrén-Sandberg MD PhD
Professor of Surgery
Department of Surgery
Rogaland Central Hospital
University of Bergen
Stavanger, Norway

Miguel R Arguedas MD MPH
Assistant Professor of Medicine
Department of Medicine and Liver Center
University of Alabama at Birmingham
Birmingham, AL, USA

Vicente Arroyo MD
Director, Institute of Digestive Medicine
Head of Liver Unit
Hospital Clinic
Barcelona, Spain

Tarik Asselah MD
Service d' Hepatologie
Hôpital Beaujon
Clichy, France

John C Atherton MRCP
Professor of Gastroenterology
MRC Senior Clinical Fellow
Wolfson Digestive Diseases Centre and Institute of Infection, Immunity and Inflammation
University of Nottingham
Nottingham, UK

Matthew R Banks BSc PhD MRCP
Advanced Trainee
Department of Gastroenterology
Concord Repatriation General Hospital
Concord, NSW, Australia

Heike Bantel MD
Assistant Professor of Molecular Medicine
Department of Gastroenterology, Hepatology and Endocrinology
Hannover Medical School
Hannover, Germany

John A Baron MD MS MSc
Professor of Medicine and of Community and Family Medicine
Dartmouth Medical School
Lebanon, NH, USA

Malcolm C Bateson MD FRCP FRCP(Edin)
Consultant Physician and Specialist in Gastroenterology
Bishop Auckland General Hospital
Bishop Auckland, UK

Pascal O Berberat MD
Department of General Surgery
University of Heidelberg
Heidelberg, Germany

Marina Berenguer MD
Adjunct Professor
Servicio de Gastroenterología y Hepatología
Hospital Universitario La FE
Valencia, Spain

Nora V Bergasa MD
Professor of Medicine
Division of Hepatology
State University of New York at Downstate
Brooklyn, NY, USA

R Bhardwaj MBChB FRCS FRCS(Ed) MD
Registrar in General Surgery
Department of Surgery
Darent Valley Hospital
Dartford, UK

Juliane Bingener MD
Assistant Professor of Surgery
Department of Surgery
University of Texas Health Sciences Center
San Antonio, TX, USA

Ingvar Bjarnason MD MSc FRCPath FRCP DSc
Professor of Digestive Diseases
Department of Medicine
GKT Medical School
London, UK

Andres T Blei MD
Professor of Medicine
Northwestern University Feinberg School of Medicine;
Medical Director of Hepatology at NMH
Attending Physician
Northwestern Memorial Hospital
Chicago, IL, USA

Hubert E Blum MD
Professor of Medicine
Department of Medicine
University Hospital Freiburg
Freiburg, Germany

John H Bond MD
Chief, Gastroenterology Section
Minneapolis Veterans Affairs Medical Center
Professor of Medicine
University of Minnesota
Minneapolis, MN, USA

John A Bonino MD
Chief Resident
Department of Internal Medicine
University of Kansas School of Medicine
Kansas City, MO, USA

Jaime Bosch MD
Professor of Medicine
Liver Unit, Institut de Malalties Digestives i Metaboliques
Hospital Clínic
University of Barcelona
Barcelona, Spain

James B Bourke FRCS MBBCh
Division of Surgery
University Hospital
Nottingham, UK

Timothy E Bowling MBBS MD FRCP
Consultant in Gastroenterology and Clinical Nutrition
Clinical Nutrition Unit
Queens Medical Centre
University Hospital
Nottingham, UK

H Worth Boyce MD MS MACG
Professor of Medicine and Director
Joy McCann Culverhouse Center for Swallowing Disorders
University of South Florida College of Medicine
Tampa, FL, USA

Nathalie Boyer MD
Service d' Hepatologie
Hôpital Beaujon
Clichy, France

Elizabeth Broussard MD
Senior Fellow
Division of Gastroenterology
University of Washington School of Medicine
Seattle, WA, USA

William R Brugge MD
Director of Clinical Endoscopy
GI Unit
Massachusetts General Hospital
Boston, MA, USA

Miguel Bruguera Cortada MD
Professor of Medicine
University of Barcelona
Liver Unit
Hospital Clinic
Barcelona, Spain

Jordi Bruix MD
Professor of Medicine
Liver Unit – BCLC Group
Hospital Clínico
Barcelona, Spain

Markus W Büchler MD
Professor of Surgery
Chairman
Department of Surgery
University of Heidelberg
Heidelberg, Germany

Andrés Cárdenas MD MMSc
Instructor in Medicine
Division of Gastroenterology and Hepatology
Beth Israel Deaconess Medical Center
Harvard Medical School
Boston, MA, USA

Elizabeth J Carey MD
Fellow
Gastroenterology and Hepatology
Mayo Clinic
Scottsdale, AZ, USA

Anna Casburn-Jones BSc MB MRCP
Specialist Registrar
Department of Gastroenterology
Barking, Havering and Redbridge Hospitals Trust
London, UK

Dean Cekic MD PhD
Postdoctoral Fellow
Centro Studi Fegato
Trieste, Italy

Natascha Celli MD
Department of Internal Medicine and Gastroenterology
University of Bologna
Bologna, Italy

Francis K L Chan MD FRCP FACG
Reader in Medicine
Department of Medicine and Therapeutics
Prince of Wales Hospital
The Chinese University of Hong Kong
Hong Kong SAR, China

Kenneth J Chang MD
Executive Director
Comprehensive Digestive Diseases Center
UCI Medical Center
Orange, CA, USA

Daniel Cherqui MD
Professor of Medicine
Service de Chirurgie Digestive
Hôpital Henri Mondor
Créteil, France

Victor Ching BSc
Graduate Student
Toronto, ON, Canada

Vicky Chudleigh BA(Hons) PGDip SRD
Gastroenterology Research Dietician
Gastroenterology Research Unit
Addenbrookes Hospital
Cambridge, UK

S C Sydney Chung MD
Professor of Surgery and Dean
Faculty of Medicine
The Chinese University of Hong Kong
Hong Kong, China

Kevin M Comar MD
House Staff
Department of Internal Medicine
Virginia Commonwealth University
Richmond, VA, USA

Robert N Cunliffe BSc BM BCh DM MRCP
Specialist Registrar in Gastroenterology
Wolfson Digestive Disease Center
Queens Medical Centre
University Hospital
Nottingham, UK

Abraham H Dachman MD FACR
Professor of Radiology
Director of CT
Department of Radiology
The University of Chicago
Chicago, IL, USA

Z Dambrauskas MD
University of Heidelberg
Heidelberg, Germany

Gennaro D'Amico MD
Chief of Gastroenterology
Department of Gastroenterology
Ospedale V Cervello
Palermo, Italy

Michael Darcy MD
Professor of Radiology and Surgery
Chief, Interventional Radiology
Mallinckrodt Institute of Radiology
Washington University School of Medicine
St Louis, MO, USA

Giovanna M da Silva MD
Research Fellow
Department of Colorectal Surgery
Cleveland Clinic Florida
Weston, FL, USA

Mark Davenport ChM FRCS(Paeds) FRCS(Eng) FRCPS(Glas)
Consultant Paediatric Hepatobiliary Surgeon
Department of Paediatric Surgery
King's College Hospital
London, UK

Raquel E Davila MD
Assistant Professor of Medicine
Department of Gastroenterology
Oregon Health & Science University
Portland, OR, USA

Vincent P De Rosa MD
Chief Medical Resident
VA Greater Los Angeles Healthcare System
Clinical Instructor
Department of Internal Medicine
David Geffen School of Medicine at UCLA
Los Angeles, CA, USA

Jean-Charles Deybach MD PhD
Professor of Medicine
Head of Department of Biochemistry and Molecular Genetics
Centre Français des Porphyries
Hôpital Louis Mourier
Colombes, France

Daniel Dhumeaux MD
Professor of Medicine
Service d'Hépatologie et de Gastroentérologie
Hôpital Henri Mondor
Créteil, France

Ahmet Dogan MD PhD MRCPath
Professor of Pathology
Division of Anatomic Pathology
Mayo Clinic
Rochester, MN, USA

Gareth S Dulai MD MSHS
Assistant Professor in Medicine
Co-Director, Center for the Study of Digestive Healthcare Quality and Outcomes
Greater Los Angeles VA Healthcare System
David Geffen School of Medicine at UCLA
Los Angeles, CA, USA

Franz Ludwig Dumoulin MD
Assistant Professor of Medicine
Department of Medicine I
University of Bonn
Bonn, Germany

Andrew W DuPont MD
Assistant Professor
University of Texas Medical Branch
Galveston, TX, USA

Herbert L DuPont MD
Clinical Professor
Chief of Internal Medicine
St Luke's Episcopal Hospital
Houston, TX, USA

Emad M El-Omar BSc (Hons) MB ChB MD FRCP (Edin)
Chair in Gastroenterology
Department of Medicine and Therapeutics
University of Aberdeen
Aberdeen, UK

Joel B Epstein DMD MSD
Department Head
Oral Medicine and Diagnostic Sciences
University of Illinois at Chicago
Chicago, IL, USA

Douglas O Faigel MD
Associate Professor of Medicine
Department of Gastroenterology
Oregon Health & Science University
Portland, OR, USA

Michael B Fallon MD
Associate Professor of Medicine
Department of Medicine and Liver Center
University of Alabama at Birmingham
Birmingham, AL, USA

Patrizia Farci MD
Professor of Medicine
Department of Medical Sciences
University of Cagliari
Cagliari, Italy

Michael J G Farthing MD FRCP
Principal and Professor of Medicine
St Georges Hospital Medical School
London, UK

Ronnie Fass MD FACP FACG
Associate Professor of Medicine
Department of Medicine
University of Arizona
Tucson, AZ, USA

Peter Ferenci MD
Professor of Medicine
Department of Internal Medicine
Gastroenterology and Hepatology
Medical University of Vienna
Vienna, Austria

David E Fleischer MD
Professor of Medicine
Mayo College of Medicine
Chair, Division of Gastroenterology and Hepatology
Mayo Clinic
Scottsdale, AZ, USA

Evan L Fogel MD
Associate Professor of Clinical Medicine
Division of Gastroenterology/Hepatology
Indiana University Hospital
Indianapolis, IN, USA

Alexander C Ford MRCP
Lecturer in Medicine
Honorary Specialist Registrar in Gastroenterology
Department of Academic Medicine
St James's University Hospital
Leeds, UK

Xavier Forns MD
Specialist in Hepatology
Liver Unit
IDIBAPS
Hospital Clinic
Barcelona, Spain

Paul J Fortun BM MRCP FRACP
Clinical Lecturer in Gastroenterology
Wolfson Digestive Diseases Center
University Hospital
Nottingham, UK

Bruce M Fox MRCP FRCR PG Cert
Consultant GI Radiologist
Honorary University Fellow
Derriford Hospital
Plymouth, UK

H Friess MD
Professor of Surgery
Department of General Surgery
University of Heidelberg
Heidelberg, Germany

Simon M Gabe MD MSc BSc (Hons) MBBS FRCP
Senior Lecturer and Honorary Consultant Gastroenterologist
Department of Gastroenterology
St Mark's Hospital
Harrow, UK

Juan Carlos Garcia-Pagán MD
Consultant in Hepatology
Hepatic Hemodynamic Laboratory
Liver Unit
Hospital Clinic
Barcelona, Spain

Guadalupe Garcia-Tsao MD
Professor of Medicine
Department of Internal Medicine
Yale University School of Medicine
New Haven, CT, USA

Robert H Geelkerken MD PhD
Consultant Vascular Surgeon
Department of Vascular Surgery
Medisch Spectrum Twente
Enschede, The Netherlands

Robert M Genta MD FACG
Professor and Chair
Division of Anatomic Pathology
Geneva University Hospital
Geneva, Switzerland;
Adjunct Professor of Pathology and Medicine
Baylor College of Medicine
Houston, TX, USA

Paula Ghaneh FRCS MD
Senior Lecturer in Surgery
Department of Surgery
University of Liverpool
Liverpool, UK

Fathia Gibril MD
Senior Clinical Investigator
Digestive Diseases Branch
National Institute of Diabetes and Digestive and Kidney Diseases
National Institutes of Health
Bethesda, MA, USA

Alexander Gimson MB FRCP
Consultant Physician and Hepatologist
Liver Transplant Unit
Addenbrookes Hospital
Cambridge, UK

Pere Ginès MD
Consultant Hepatologist
Liver Unit
Hospital Clinic
Barcelona, Spain

Gregory G Ginsberg MD
Associate Professor of Medicine
Director of Endoscopic Services
Division of Gastroenterology
Hospital of the University of Pennsylvania
Philadelphia, PA, USA

Gregory J Gores MD
Reuben R Eisenberg Professor of Medicine
Mayo Medical Clinic
Rochester, MN, USA

Norman D Grace MD
Professor of Medicine
Tufts University School of Medicine
Lecturer on Medicine
Harvard Medical School
Director of Clinical Hepatology
Brigham and Women's Hospital
Boston, MA, USA

Roberto J Groszmann MD FRCP
Professor of Medicine
Chief, Section of Digestive Diseases
VA Connecticut Healthcare System
Department of Internal Medicine
Yale University School of Medicine
New Haven, CT, USA

Miriam Grushka DDS MSc PhD MEd
Clinical Instructor
Yale University (ENT)
New Haven, CT, USA

Sushovan Guha MD MPhil PhD
Assistant Professor in Residence
Division of Digestive Diseases
Department of Medicine
David Geffen School of Medicine at UCLA
Los Angeles, CA, USA

Nedim Hadžić MD MSc
Consultant and Senior Lecturer in Paediatric Hepatology
Department of Child Health and Institute of Liver Studies
King's College Hospital
London, UK

I M Harkema MD
Trainee in Gastroenterology
Department Gastroenterology
Medical Spectre Twente Hospital
Enschede, The Netherlands

C J Hawkey DM FRCP
Professor of Gastroenterology
Wolfson Digestive Diseases Centre
University Hospital
Nottingham, UK

Philip N Hawkins PhD FRCP FRCPath FMedSci
Professor of Medicine
National Amyloidosis Centre
Royal Free Hospital
London, UK

J Eileen Hay MBChB FRCP
Professor of Medicine
Consultant in Gastroenterology and Hepatology
Mayo Medical School
Rochester, MN, USA

J Michael Henderson MB ChB
Professor of Surgery
Division of Surgery
The Cleveland Clinic Foundation
Cleveland, OH, USA

Paula Hidalgo MD
Research Fellow, Abdominal Imaging
Department of Radiology
Brigham and Women's Hospital
Boston, MA, USA

John Hunter MA MD BChir FRCP FACG
Consultant Physician
Gastroenterology Research Unit
Addenbrookes Hospital
Cambridge, UK

Clement W Imrie BSc MB ChB FRCS
Professor of Upper Gastrointestinal Surgery
Consultant Surgeon
Lister Department of Surgery
Royal Infirmary
Glasgow, UK

Haruhiro Inoue MD PhD
Chief of Upper GI Endoscopy and Surgery
Associate Professor
Digestive Disease Center
Showa University
Northern Yokohama Hospital
Yokohama, Japan

Simon A Jackson MBBS FRCS FRCR
Consultant GI Radiologist
Imaging Directorate
Derriford Hospital
Plymouth, UK

Vaman S Jakribettuu MD
Assistant Professor of Medicine
Division of Gastroenterology/Hepatology
University of Colorado School of Medicine
Denver, CO, USA

Rajiv Jalan MD FRCPE FRCP
Senior Lecturer in Hepatology
Institute of Hepatology
Division of Medicine
Royal Free and University College Medical School
London, UK

Dennis M Jensen MD
Professor of Medicine
David Geffen School of Medicine at UCLA
Division of Digestive Diseases
UCLA Center for the Health Sciences and
VA Greater Los Angeles Healthcare System;
Associate Director
CURE Digestive Diseases Research Center
Los Angeles, CA, USA

Robert T Jensen MD
Chief, Cell Biology Section
Digestive Diseases Branch
National Institute of Diabetes and Digestive and Kidney Diseases
National Institutes of Health
Bethesda, MA, USA

Peter J Kahrilas MD
Gilbert H Marquardt Professor of Medicine
Chief, Division of Gastroenterology
Northwestern University Medical School
Chicago, IL, USA

Anthony Kalloo MD
Associate Professor of Medicine
Division of Gastroenterology
The Johns Hopkins University - School of Medicine
Baltimore, MD, USA

Patrick S Kamath MD
Professor of Medicine
Mayo Clinic College of Medicine
Consultant and Vice Chair (Education)
Division of Gastroenterology and Hepatology
Mayo Clinic
Rochester, MN, USA

John M Kauffman MD
Instructor in Medicine
Harvard Vanguard Medical Associates
West Roxbury, MA, USA

David J Kearney MD
Associate Professor of Medicine
Division of Gastroenterology
University of Washington School of Medicine;
Staff Physician
VA Puget Sound Health Care System
Seattle, WA, USA

Ciarán P Kelly MD
Associate Professor of Medicine
Division of Gastroenterology and Hepatology
Beth Israel Deaconess Medical Center
Harvard Medical School
Boston, MA, USA

Paul Kelly MA MD FRCP
Reader and Wellcome Trust Senior Fellow
Department of Adult and Paediatric Gastroenterology
Barts and the London School of Medicine
London, UK

David J Kerr CBE MA MD DSc FRCP (Glas & Lon) FMedSci
Rhodes Professor of Clinical Pharmacology and Cancer Therapeutics
Director, National Translation Cancer Research Network
Department of Clinical Pharmacology
University of Oxford
Radcliffe Infirmary
Oxford, UK

Michael S Kipper MD
Associate Clinical Professor of Radiology
University of California
Director of Imaging
Pacific Imaging and Treatment Center
San Diego, CA, USA

Jason B Klapman MD
Clinical Instructor
Comprehensive Digestive Diseases Center
UCI Medical Center
Orange, CA, USA

Jeroen J Kolkman MD PhD
Gastroenterologist
Department of Gastroenterology
Medisch Spectrum Twente
Enschede, The Netherlands

Hartvig Körner MD
Department of Surgery
Rogaland Central Hospital
University of Bergen
Stavanger, Norway

Ayman Koteish MD
Assistant Professor of Medicine
Division of Gastroenterology
The Johns Hopkins University – School of Medicine
Baltimore, MD, USA

Thomas O G Kovacs MD
Professor of Medicine
Cure Digestive Disease Research Center
David Geffen School of Medicine at UCLA
Los Angeles, USA

Maria Eliana Lai MD
Associate Professor of Medicine
Department of Medical Sciences
University of Cagliari
Cagliari, Italy

James Y W Lau MD
Consultant Surgeon
Prince of Wales Hospital;
Honorary Associate Professor
Department of Surgery
The Chinese University of Hong Kong
Hong Kong, China

Konstantinos N Lazaridis MD
Assistant Professor of Medicine
Mayo Clinic
Rochester, MN, USA

Sum P Lee MD PhD
Professor and Head
Division of Gastroenterology
Department of Medicine
University of Washington
Seattle, WA, USA

William Lees MBBS FRCR FRACR FRCS
Professor of Medical Imaging
Department of Imaging
The Middlesex Hospital
London, UK

Joel S Levine MD
Professor of Medicine
Division of Gastroenterology/Hepatology
University of Colorado Health Sciences Center
Denver, CO, USA

George Thomas Lewith MA DM FRCP MRCGP
Senior Research Fellow
Primary Medical Care
Complementary Medicine Research Unit
University of Southampton
Southampton, UK

Keith D Lindor MD
Professor of Medicine
Division of Gastroenterology and Hepatology
Mayo Clinic
Rochester, MN, USA

Dileep N Lobo DM FRCS
Senior Lecturer in Gastrointestinal Surgery
Honorary Consultant Hepatopancreaticobiliary Surgeon
Section of Surgery
University Hospital
Queen's Medical Centre
Nottingham, UK

Alain Luciani MD
Doctor of Medicine
Service de Radiologie
Hôpital Henri Mondor
Créteil, France

Ryan D Madanick MD
Assistant Professor of Medicine
Division of Gastroenterology
University of Miami School of Medicine
Miami, FL, USA

Laurence Maiden MRCP
Research Fellow
GKT Medical School
London, UK

Peter Malfertheiner MD
Director
Klinik für Gastroenterologie, Hepatologie und Infektiologie
Otto-von-Guericke-Universität
Magdeburg, Germany

Giuseppe Malizia MD
Consultant in Gastroenterology
Department of Gastroenterology
Ospedale V Cervello
Palermo, Italy

Michael P Manns MD
Professor and Chairman
Department of Gastroenterology, Hepatology and Endocrinology
Hannover Medical School
Hannover, Germany

Patrick Marcellin MD PhD
Professor of Medicine
Service d' Hepatologie
Hôpital Beaujon
Clichy, France

Arthur J McCullough MD
Director of Gastroenterology, Metro Health Medical Center
Professor of Medicine, Case Western Reserve University
Gastroenterology Unit
Metro Health Medical Center
Cleveland, OH, USA

George B McDonald MD
Professor of Medicine
University of Washington School of Medicine
Seattle, WA, USA

Dermot P B McGovern MBBS MRCP
Specialist Registrar - Gastroenterology
University of Oxford
Oxford, UK

Alastair W McKinlay BSc (Hons) MB ChB FRCP (Edin & Glas)
Consultant Gastroenterologist
Aberdeen Royal Infirmary
Honorary Senior Lecturer
University of Aberdeen
Aberdeen, UK

J W R Meijer MD PhD
Department of Pathology
Rijnstate Hospital
Arnhem, The Netherlands

Flavia D Mendes MD
Instructor in Medicine
Mayo Clinic
Rochester, MN, USA

Arend E H Merrie MB ChB PhD FRACS
Senior Lecturer and Consultant Colorectal Surgeon
Department of Surgery
Auckland Hospital
Auckland, New Zealand

Rachel S Midgley MD
DoH Clinician Scientist in Medical Oncology
Department of Clinical Pharmacology
University of Oxford
Oxford, UK

Giorgina Mieli-Vergani MD PhD
Alex Mowat Professor of Paediatric Hepatology
Department of Child Health and Institute of Liver Studies
King's College Hospital
London, UK

Vivek Mittal MD
Resident
Department of Internal Medicine
Emory University
Atlanta, GA, USA

Paul Moayyedi MB ChB PhD MPH FRCP
Professor of Gastroenterology
Department of Medicine
McMaster University
Hamilton, ON, Canada

Rajeshwar P Mookerjee BSc MRCP
Specialist Registrar in Hepatology
Institute of Hepatology
Division of Medicine
Royal Free and University College Medical School
London, UK

Koenraad J Mortele MD
Assistant Professor of Radiology
Harvard Medical School
Associate Director
Division of Abdominal Imaging and Intervention
Director, Abdominal and Pelvic MRI
Director, CME
Department of Radiology
Brigham and Women's Hospital
Boston, MA, USA

Neil J Mortensen MD FRCS
Professor of Colorectal Surgery
Department of Colorectal Surgery
John Radcliffe Hospital
Oxford, UK

Ulf Müller-Ladner MD
Professor of Internal Medicine/Rheumatology
Department of Rheumatology
University of Giessen
Bad Nauheim, Germany

C J J Mulder MD PhD
Head of Gastroenterology
Department of Gastroenterology
VU University Medical Center
Amsterdam, The Netherlands

Simon Murch PhD FRCP FRCPCH
Professor of Paediatrics and Child Health
Warwick Medical School
University of Warwick
Coventry, UK

Bommayya Narayanaswamy MS FRCS(Edin)
Specialist Registrar in Paediatric Surgery
Department of Paediatric Surgery
King's College Hospital
London, UK

John P Neoptolemos MA MD FRCS
Professor of Surgery
Department of Surgery
University of Liverpool
Liverpool, UK

James Neuberger DM FRCP
Consultant Physician and Honorary Professor of Medicine
Liver Unit
Queen Elizabeth Hospital
Birmingham, UK

Julia L Newton MBBS FRCP PhD
Senior Lecturer in General and Geriatric Medicine
Institute for Ageing and Health
University of Newcastle
Newcastle, UK

Kjell Öberg MD PhD
Dean of the Medical Faculty
Department of Medical Sciences
Uppsala University Hospital
Uppsala, Sweden

John G O'Grady MD FRCPI
Consultant Hepatologist
Institute of Liver Studies
King's College School of Medicine
London, UK

M Raquel Oliva MD
Fellow in Abdominal Imaging and Intervention
Department of Radiology
Brigham and Women's Hospital
Harvard Medical School
Boston, MA, USA

Harry T Papaconstantinou MD MMS
Assistant Professor
Department of Surgery
University of Texas Southwestern Medical Center
Dallas, TX, USA

Konstantinos A Papadakis MD
Assistant Professor of Medicine
Division of Gastroenterology
IBD Center
Cedars-Sinai Medical Center
Los Angeles, LA, USA

Michael C Parker BSc MS FRCS FRCS (Ed)
Consultant Surgeon
Department of Surgery
Darent Valley Hospital
Dartford, Kent, UK

David Patch MB BS FRCP
Consultant Hepatologist
Department of Hepatobiliary Medicine and Liver Transplantation
Royal Free Hospital
London, UK

Sandeep C Patel MD
Gastroenterology Fellow
Department of Gastroenterology and Hepatology
Cleveland Clinic Foundation
Cleveland, OH, USA

Sonal Patel MD
Clinical Fellow
Division of Gastroenterology and Hepatology
Beth Israel Deaconess Medical Center
Harvard Medical School
Boston, MA, USA

Stephen P Pereira PhD FRCP
Senior Lecturer in Hepatology and Gastroenterology
Institute of Hepatology
University College London Medical School
London, UK

Patrick R Pfau MD
Assistant Professor of Medicine
Director of Endoscopy
Section of Gastroenterology and Hepatology
University of Wisconsin Medical School
Madison, WI, USA

Erik Pieramici MD JD
Fellow
Division of Gastroenterology and Hepatology
University of Colorado Health Science Center
Denver, CO, USA

Jeffrey L Ponsky MD
Oliver H Payne Professor and Chairman
Department of Surgery
Case Western Reserve University School of Medicine
Cleveland, OH, USA

Todd A Ponsky MD
Resident in Surgery
George Washington University Medical Center
Washington, DC, USA

John J Poterucha MD
Associate Professor of Medicine
Division of Gastroenterology and Hepatology
Mayo Clinic
Rochester, MN, USA

Hervé Puy MD PhD
Professor of Medicine
Centre Français des Porphyries
Hôpital Louis Mourier
Colombes, France

Rodrigo M Quera MD
Staff Gastroenterologist
Department of Medicine
University of Chile
Santiago, Chile

Eamonn M M Quigley MD FRCP FACP FACG FRCPI
Professor of Medicine and Human Physiology
Head of Medical School
Department of Medicine
Cork University Hospital
Cork, Ireland

Krish Ragunath MD DNB MRCP
Consultant Gastroenterologist
Queen's Medical Centre
Division of Gastroenterology
Wolfson Digestive Diseases Centre
Nottingham University Hospital
Nottingham, UK

Satish S C Rao MD PhD FRCP (Lon)
Professor of Medicine
Director of Internal Medicine
Division of Gastroenterology
University of Iowa
Iowa City, IA, USA

Jürg Reichen MD
Professor of Medicine
Chairman, Department of Clinical Pharmacology
University of Berne
Berne, Switzerland

Carol M Reife MD
Assistant Professor of Medicine
Division of Internal Medicine
Jefferson Medical College
Philadelphia, PA, USA

Adrian Reuben MBBS FRCP
Professor of Medicine
Director of Liver Service
Medical University of South Carolina
Charleston, SC, USA

Melanie L Richards MD
Associate Professor and Program Director
Department of Surgery
University of Texas Health Sciences Center
San Antonio, TX, USA

Igino Rigato MD
Postdoctoral Fellow
Centro Studi Fegat
Trieste, Italy

Douglas J Robertson MD MPH
Assistant Professor of Medicine
Dartmouth Medical School;
Chief, Section of Gastroenterology
White River Junction VAMC
White River Junction, VT, USA

Arvey I Rogers MD
Professor Emeritus
Internal Medicine and Gastroenterology
University of Miami School of Medicine
Miami, FL, USA

Pablo R Ros MD MPH FACR
Professor of Radiology
Harvard Medical School
Executive Vice Chair and Associate Radiologist-in-Chief
Department of Radiology
Brigham and Women's Hospital
Boston, MA, USA

Martin Rössle MD
Consultant
University Hospital, Freiburg
Professor of Medicine
Praxiszentrum für Gastroenterologie und Endokrinologie
Freiburg, Germany

Laura Rubbia-Brandt MD PhD
Unité de Pathologie Gastro-entérologique et Hépatique
Service de Pathologie Clinique
Hôpital Universitaire de Geneve
Geneva, Switzerland

Stefan Russmann MD
Boston Collaborative Drug Surveillance Program
Boston University
Lexington, MA, USA;
Department of Clinical Pharmacology
University of Berne
Bern, Switzerland

Paul Rutgeerts MD PhD FRCP
Professor of Medicine
Department of Gastroenterology
University Hospital Gasthuisberg
Leuven, Belgium

Margarita Sala MD
Liver Unit – BCLC Group
Hospital Clínico
Barcelona, Spain

Jose M Sánchez-Tapias MD
Senior Consultant in Hepatology
Liver Unit
IDIBAPS
Hospital Clinic
Barcelona, Spain

Arun J Sanyal MBBS MD
Charles Caravati Professor of Medicine
Chairman, Division of Gastroenterology, Hepatology and Internal Medicine
Virginia Commonwealth University
Richmond, VA, USA

Tilman Sauerbruch MD
Professor of Medicine and Director
Department of Medicine I
University of Bonn
Bonn, Germany

Drew Schembre MD
Assistant Clinical Professor of Medicine
University of Washington
Seattle, WA, USA

Jürgen Schölmerich MD
Professor of Medicine
Department of Internal Medicine I
University of Regensburg
Regensburg, Germany

Fergus Shanahan MD
Professor and Chair, Department of Medicine
Director, Alimentary Pharmabiotic Center
University College Cork, National University Ireland
Cork University Hospital
Cork, Ireland

Prateek Sharma MD
Associate Professor of Medicine
Director of Gastroenterology Fellowship
Department of Gastroenterology
University of Kansas School of Medicine and VA Medical Center
Kansas City, MO, USA

Maria Sheridan MRCP FRCR
Consultant GI Radiologist
Department of Radiology
St James's University Hospital
Leeds, UK

Stuart Sherman MD
Professor of Medicine and Radiology
Division of Gastroenterology/Hepatology
Indiana University Hospital
Indianapolis, IN, USA

Tomas J Silber MD MASS
Senior Attending
Division of Adolescent and Young Adult Medicine
Children's National Medical Center
Professor of Pediatrics
George Washington University School of Medicine and Health Sciences
Washington, DC, USA

David B A Silk MD FRCP
Consultant
Department of Surgical Oncology and Technology
Imperial College London
St Mary's Hospital
London, UK

Clifford L Simmang MD MS
Associate Professor of Surgery
Department of Surgery
University of Texas Southwestern Medical Center
Dallas, TX, USA

Kenneth R Sirinek MD PhD
Professor and Division Head
General and Laparoscopic Surgery
Department of Surgery
University of Texas Health Sciences Center
San Antonio, TX, USA

Hans Christian Spangenberg MD
Department of Medicine
University Hospital Freiburg
Freiburg, Germany

Robin Spiller MB BChir MD (Cantab) FRCP
Professor of Gastroenterology
Wolfson Digestive Diseases Centre
University Hospital
Nottingham, UK

Robert J C Steele MD FRCS
Professor of Surgery
Department of Surgery and Molecular Oncology
Ninewells Hospital
Dundee, UK

Matthias Stelzner MD FACS
Professor and Vice-Chairman
Department of Surgery
University of California at Los Angeles
Los Angeles, CA, USA

Christian P Strassburg MD
Associate Professor of Experimental Gastroenterology (Privatdozent)
Department of Gastroenterology, Hepatology and Endocrinology
Hannover Medical School
Hannover, Germany

Lisa Strate MD MPH
Instructor in Medicine
Harvard Medical School
Division of Gastroenterology
Brigham and Women's Hospital
Boston, MA, USA

Christina Surawicz MD
Professor of Medicine
University of Washington School of Medicine
Seattle, WA, USA

C Paul Swain MD
Professor
Academic Department of Surgery
Imperial College
St Mary's Hospital
London, UK

Jan Tack MD PhD
Professor of Medicine and Head of Clinic
Department of Gastroenterology
University Hospitals Leuven
Leuven, Belgium

Ken Takeuchi MD PhD
Consultant Gastroenterologist
GKT Medical School
London, UK

Stephan R Targan MD
Director, Division of Gastroenterology
Inflammatory Bowel Disease Center
Professor of Medicine, UCLA School of Medicine
Cedars Sinai Medical Center
Los Angeles, CA, USA

Robert Thimme MD
Department of Medicine
University Hospital Freiburg
Freiburg, Germany

Richard Thompson MFCP MRCPCH
Senior Lecturer
Department of Liver Studies and Transplantation
King's College Hospital
London, UK

Eva Tiensuu Janson MD PhD
Associate Professor of Medicine
Department of Medical Sciences
Uppsala University Hospital
Uppsala, Sweden

Claudio Tiribelli MD PhD
Director and Professor of Medicine
Centro Studi Fegato
Trieste, Italy

George Triadafilopoulos MD
Clinical Professor of Medicine
Division of Gastroenterology and Hepatology
Stanford University School of Medicine
Stanford, CA, USA

Juan Turnes MD
Clinical Research Associate
Hepatic Hemodynamic Laboratory
Liver Unit
Hospital Clinic
Barcelona, Spain

Dominique-Charles Valla MD
Professor of Medicine
Service d'Hépatologie
Hôpital Beaujon
Clichy, France

J Hajo van Bockel MD PhD
Professor of Surgery
Department of Surgery
Leiden University Medical Center
Leiden, The Netherlands

Jon A Vanderhoof MD
Chief, Pediatric Gastroenterology and Nutrition
University of Nebraska Medical Center
Omaha, NE, USA

María Varela MD
Liver Unit – BCLC Group
Hospital Clínico
Barcelona, Spain

John J Vargo MD MPH
Staff Gastroenterologist
Section of Therapeutic and Hepatobiliary Endoscopy
Department of Gastroenterology and Hepatology
Cleveland Clinic Foundation
Cleveland, OH, USA

Severine Vermeire MD PhD
Department of Gastroenterology
University Hospital Gasthuisberg
Leuven, Belgium

Arnold Wald MD
Professor of Medicine
Division of Gastroenterology, Hepatology and Nutrition
University of Pittsburgh Medical Center
Pittsburgh, PA, USA

Kenneth K Wang MD
Associate Professor of Medicine
Mayo Clinic College of Medicine
Rochester, MN, USA

Jerome D Waye MD
Director of Endoscopic Education
Mount Sinai Medical Center
New York, NY, USA

George J M Webster BSc MRCP MD
Consultant Gastroenterologist
Department of Gastroenterology
University College London Hospitals
London, UK

Wilfred M Weinstein MD
Professor of Medicine
Digestive Diseases
David Geffen School of Medicine at UCLA
Los Angeles, CA, USA

Julia Wendon MB ChB FRCP
Senior Lecturer and Consultant in Liver Intensive Care
Institute of Liver Studies
King's College Hospital
London, UK

Steven D Wexner MD
Chairman
Department of Colorectal Surgery
Chief of Staff
Cleveland Clinic Florida
Weston, FL, USA

C Mel Wilcox MD
Professor of Medicine
Division of Gastroenterology and Hepatology
University of Alabama
Birmingham, AL, USA

Wai-Man Wong MD MRCP FACG
Visiting Scholar/RGC Clinical Research Fellow
Department of Medicine
University of Hong Kong
Queen Mary Hospital
Hong Kong

Andrew C Wotherspoon MD MRCPath
Consultant Histopathologist
Department of Histopathology
Royal Marsden Hospital
London, UK

Teresa L Wright MD
Professor of Medicine
University of California San Francisco
Chief, Division of Gastroenterology
Veterans' Affairs Medical Center
San Francisco, CA, USA

Neville D Yeomans MD FRACP FACG
Dean of Medical School
University of Western Sydney
Sydney, NSW, Australia

Hiroyuki Yoshida MSc PhD
Associate Professor of Radiology
Department of Radiology
The University of Chicago
Chicago, IL, USA

Rosemary J Young MS RN
Pediatric Gastroenterology Clinical Nurse Specialist
University of Nebraska Medical Center
Omaha, NE, USA

Elie Serge Zafrani MD
Professor of Medicine
Service d'Anatomie et de Cytologie Pathologique
Hôpital Henri Mondor
Créteil, France

Preface

Mark Twain once said 'If I'd had more time I would have written a shorter letter'. That is the principle underlying this brand new textbook of gastroenterology. We wanted it to be:

Concise but comprehensive. We asked authors to achieve short, crisp text by avoiding waffle.

Up to date. Many textbooks still bear the watermarks of the last-edition-but-three written in the 1970s. We asked authors to look at their topic from a modern standpoint and avoid discussion of issues which were once, but are no longer, important.

Clinically focused. This book tells you how to respond to specific symptoms and scenarios, describes diagnosis and management of all important gastrointestinal diseases, includes primers of diagnosis and treatment and is full of practical 'how to do it' descriptions and algorithms.

Technologically advanced. Elsevier are known for the attractiveness of their illustrations. We wanted to go further and offer video footage too, as this better replicates the diagnostic and therapeutic situation in gastroenterology. Access to illustrations and video sequences online is included as part of the electronic **edition** package.

Available when you need it. An abbreviated PDA downloadable version is also available allowing ward round access to key facts.

International. We have been careful to assemble a representative authorship and have asked authors to cover international differences in presentation and management.

Fresh and forward looking. In choosing our authors we have looked to rising stars who are the authorities of the future rather than the past.

Wilfred M Weinstein MD
C J Hawkey DM FRCP
Jaime Bosch MD
2005

Abbreviations

AC	adenylate cyclase
ACA	adenocarcinoma
ACTH	adrenocorticotropic hormone
ADA	adenosine deaminase
AFP	alfa-fetoprotein
AH	alcoholic hepatitis
ALF	acute liver failure
ALT	alanine aminotransferase
APTT	activated partial thromboplastin time
5-ASA	5-acetylsalicyclic acid
ASCA	anti-*Saccharomyces cerevisiae* antibody
AST	aspartate aminotransferase
ATI	antibodies to infliximab
ATP	adenosine triphosphate
ATPase	adenosine triphosphatase
AZA	azathioprine
BCAA	branched-chain amino acid
BEE	basal energy expenditure
BIS	bispectral
BMI	body mass index
BSEP	bile salt export pump
BUN	blood urea nitrogen
CAM	complementary and alternative medicine
cAMP	cyclic adenosine monophosphate
CARD	caspase activation and recruitment domain
CCD	charged coupled device
CCK	cholecystokinin
CD	Crohn's disease
CDEIS	Crohn's Disease Endoscopic Index of Severity
cfu	colony-forming units
CI	confidence interval
CIN	chromosomal instability
CLD	chronic liver disease
cMOAT	canalicular multispecific organic anion transporter
CMV	cytomegalovirus
CRC	colorectal cancer
COX	cyclo-oxygenase
CT	computed tomography *or* cholera toxin
DCBE	double-contrast barium enema
DIC	disseminated intravascular coagulation
DOT	directly observed therapy
DPD	dihydropyrimidine dehydrogenase
EAEC	enteroaggregative *Escherichia coli*
EAST-1	enteroaggregative *E. coli* heat-stable toxin 1
EBL	endoscopic banding ligation
EBV	Epstein-Barr virus
EBV-LPD	Epstein-Barr virus–lymphoproliferative disease
ECL	enterochromaffin-like (cell)
EGD	esophagogastroduodenoscopy
EGF	epidermal growth factor
EGJ	esophagogastric junction
EHEC	enterohemorrhagic *Escherichia coli*
EIA	enzyme immunoassay
EMA	endomysial antibody
EMR	endoscopic mucosal resection
ENS	enteric nervous system
EPEC	enteropathogenic *Escherichia coli*
ERC	endoscopic retrograde cholangiography
ERCP	endoscopic retrograde cholangiopancreatography
ESD	endoscopic submucosal dissection
ESR	erythrocyte sedimentation rate
ETEC	enterotoxigenic *Escherichia coli*
FAP	familial adenomatous polyposis
FAPS	functional abdominal pain syndrome
FdUMP	fluorodeoxyuridine monophosphate
FNA	fine-needle aspiration
FNH	focal nodular hyperplasia
FOB	fecal occult blood
FOBT	fecal occult blood test
5-FU	5-fluorouracil
GABA	gamma-aminobutyric acid
GALT	gut-associated lymphoid tissue
GER	gastroesophageal reflux
GH	growth hormone
GI	gastrointestinal
GIST	gastrointestinal stromal tumor
GLP	glucagon-like peptide
GRE	gradient echo
GSH	glutathione
GERD	gastroesophageal reflux disease
GvHD	graft-versus-host disease
HASTE	half-Fourier acquisition single-shot turbo spin echo
HBc	hepatitis B core
HBeAg	hepatitis B e antigen
HBIg	hepatitis B immunoglobulin
HBsAg	hepatitis B surface antigen
HBV	hepatitis B virus
HCC	hepatocellular carcinoma
HCV	hepatitis C virus
HDAg	hepatitis delta antigen
HE	hepatic encephalopathy
HII	hepatic iron index
HIV	human immunodeficiency virus
HLA	human leukocyte antigen
HNPCC	hereditary nonpolyposis colorectal cancer
HPN	home parenteral nutrition
HPV	human papilloma virus
H2RA	H_2 receptor antagonist
HRS	hepatorenal syndrome
5-HT	5-hydroxytryptamine
HVPG	hepatic venous pressure gradient
IBD	inflammatory bowel disease
IBS	irritable bowel syndrome
IC	indeterminate colitis
IDUS	intraductal ultrasonography
Ig	immunoglobulin
IL	interleukin
INR	international normalized ratio
IPAA	ileal pouch–anal anastomosis
IU	international units
kbp	kilobase pair
L	litre
LES	lower esophageal sphincter
LFTs	liver function tests
LGI	lower gastrointestinal
LT	heat-labile toxin
MAC	mid upper arm circumference
MALT	mucosa-associated lymphoid tissue
MAMC	mean arm muscle circumference
MAP	MYH-associated polyposis
MARS	molecular adsorbent recirculating system
MDP	muramyl dipeptide
MELD	model for end-stage liver disease
MEN1	Multiple endocrine neoplasia type 1
MHC	major histocompatibility complex
MMC	migrating motor complex
MMP	matrix metalloproteinase
MODS	multiorgan dysfunction syndrome
6-MP	6-mercaptopurine
MRA	magnetic resonance angiography
MRCP	magnetic resonance cholangiopancreatography
MRI	magnetic resonance imaging
MRP	multidrug resistance protein
MYH	MutY homolog
NAFLD	nonalcoholic fatty liver disease
NAPQI	*N*-acetyl-benzoquinone-imide
NCCP	noncardiac chest pain
NERD	nonerosive reflux disease
NG	nasogastric (tube)
NHL	non-Hodgkin lymphoma
NJ	nasojejunal (tube)
NSAID	nonsteroidal anti-inflammatory drug
NUD	nonulcer dyspepsia
OATP	organic anion-transporting polypeptide
OR	odds ratio
OTC	over-the-counter
P-ANCA	perinuclear antineutrophil cytoplasmic antibody
PBC	primary sclerosing cholangitis *or* primary biliary cirrhosis
PBMC	peripheral blood monocyte cell
PCR	polymerase chain reaction
PDGF	platelet-derived growth factor
PDT	photodynamic therapy
PEG	percutaneous endoscopic gastrostomy
PEGJ	percutaneous endoscopic gastrojejunostomy
PEJ	percutaneous endoscopic jejunostomy
PEPT1	peptide transporter 1
PFIC	progressive familial intrahepatic cholestasis
PHG	portal hypertensive gastropathy
PMN	polymorphonuclear
PPI	proton pump inhibitor
ppm	parts per million
PTBD	percutaneous transhepatic biliary drainage
PTC	percutaneous transhepatic cholangiography
PTFE	polytetrafluoroethylene
PVT	portal vein thrombosis
RARE	rapid acquisition with relaxation enhancement
RBC	red blood cell
REE	resting energy expenditure
RES	reticuloendothelial system
RR	relative risk
SBBO	small bowel bacterial overgrowth
SBFT	small-bowel follow-through
SBP	spontaneous bacterial peritonitis
SBS	short bowel syndrome
SCC	squamous cell carcinoma
SE	spin echo
SEC	sustained esophageal contraction
SeHCAT	[^{75}Se]homocholic acid–taurine
SEMS	self-expanding metal stent
SIRS	systemic inflammatory response syndrome
SNP	single nucleotide polymorphism
SPIO	superparamagnetic iron oxide particle
SPGP	sister of P-glycoprotein
SSRI	selective serotonin reuptake inhibitor
ST	heat-stable toxin
T1W	T1-weighted (image)
T2W	T2-weighted (image)
TFA	trifluoroacetylated
TGF	transforming growth factor
TIMP	tissue inhibitor of matrix metalloproteinase
TIPS	transjugular intrahepatic portosystemic shunt
TLESR	transient lower esophageal sphincter relaxation
TME	total mesorectal excision
TMPT	thiopurine methyltransferase
TMP-SMX	trimethoprim–sulfamethoxazole
TNFα	tumor necrosis factor alfa
TPN	total parenteral nutrition
TSF	triceps skinfold thickness
UC	ulcerative colitis
UDCA	ursodeoxycholic acid
UDPGA	uridine diphosphoglucuronic acid
UGI	upper gastrointestinal
UGT	uridine diphosphoglucuronosyltransferase
UNOS	United Network of Organ Sharing
US	ultrasonography
VC	virtual colography
VIP	vasoactive intestinal peptide
WCE	wireless capsule endoscopy

Chapter 1

Burning mouth syndrome: differential diagnosis and management

Miriam Grushka, Victor Ching, and Joel B Epstein

INTRODUCTION AND DEFINITION

Over the last 10 years there has been increasing interest in burning mouth syndrome (BMS, or syndrome of oral complaints or glossodynia, when only the tongue is affected). The current working definition of BMS is a condition in which individuals experience an oral burning sensation at one or more sites without relevant clinical signs or laboratory findings.

HOW COMMON IS IT?

BMS is surprisingly common, with a reported prevalence rate of between 0.7% and 2.6%, and a National Institute of Health (NIH) survey estimating close to 1 million burning mouth sufferers in the US. The majority of burning mouth sufferers are peri/postmenopausal women aged 50–60 years (see review in References)[1] but men and women of any age can be affected.[2]

PATHOPHYSIOLOGY

Burning mouth syndrome is a neuropathic pain disorder but there is speculation regarding the etiology. BMS is almost always associated with a specific pattern of taste loss leading to the suggestion that the burning is maintained by a defect in a central inhibitory mechanism related to the taste pathways.[1]

CAUSES/DIFFERENTIAL DIAGNOSIS

Systemic and peripheral etiology for the burning pain should be ruled out before a diagnosis of BMS is entertained. Psychological changes including anxiety and depression are currently believed to be a consequence, rather than a cause of BMS. Conditions in the oral cavity may give rise to burning pain, including candidiasis in susceptible patients and painful lesions in the mucosa. Systemic autoimmune disorder including systemic lupus and Sjögren's syndrome need consideration although low salivary flow can coexist with BMS and exacerbate the pain. ACE inhibitors have been reported to cause burning pain. Clinical features that help to diagnose BMS are listed in Table 1.1.

SYMPTOM COMPLEXES

Most individuals with BMS report oral burning on the tongue tip, lateral borders of the tongue, anterior palate, mucosal lower and upper lip, attached gingival tissue, and other areas within the oral mucosa. The burning generally becomes progressively worse over the course of a day, and is frequently relieved by eating. The oral mucosa is often clinically normal, although there is an association with geographic tongue.[3]

Other reported sensations include feelings of 'roughness,' 'sandiness,' dry mucosa, and phantom taste sensations. Patients often report dry mouth even in cases where salivary flow is observed to be normal. The taste loss common in BMS can be quantified by spatial taste testing but is rarely perceived by the patients. Phantom taste sensations are often bitter, metallic, and foul in nature, and when sufficiently intense, can be associated with nausea, which can be very distressing. In BMS, burning and other sensory disturbances usually respond in tandem to efficacious medical management, often with GABAergic medications including clonazepam,[3] although randomized controlled trials of these medications and others are still needed.[4]

TABLE 1.1 CLINICAL FEATURES TO HELP DIAGNOSIS OF BMS
Pain that gets worse over the day
Decreased pain on eating
Decreased pain with sleep
Lack of clinical findings
Phantom tastes, especially bitter and metallic
Dry mouth
Other sensory disturbances including oral tactile changes, e.g., roughness, sandpaper
Unilateral or bilateral burning pain localized to tongue, palate, lips, and gingival

CAUSES/DIFFERENTIAL DIAGNOSIS

- Nutritional deficiency – B vitamins, iron, zinc
- Allergy – food or dental materials
- Dry mouth secondary to autoimmune disorders
- Oral candidiasis infection
- Oral vesiculobullous conditions, including lichen planus
- Esophageal reflux
- Oral viral infection (herpes simplex, herpes zoster)
- Uncontrolled diabetes
- Neurodegenerative disease

DIAGNOSIS

History taking is the key to diagnosis of BMS. BMS usually begins suddenly with either intermittent or constant pain. Usually the pain remits during sleep and increases from mild morning pain to a maximal level in the evening. Eating often reduces the pain although specific foods may exacerbate it. Important clinical questions are shown in Table 1.1. Dental referral to rule out oral mucosal disease can be useful when the clinical history and negative laboratory findings suggest BMS, whilst neurological investigation for neurodegenerative disorders such as multiple sclerosis, Parkinson's disease, and stroke should be considered when the symptom array is more complex and includes both sensory and motor changes.

DIAGNOSTIC METHODS

- Blood tests – fbc, glucose, nutritional factors, autoimmune screen
- Oral cultures for fungal, viral or bacterial infection if suspected
- MRI to rule out central changes, especially if pain is unilateral, atypical or does not respond to medication
- Salivary flows for unstimulated and stimulated whole saliva (<1.5 ml/5 min unstimulated; < 4.5 ml/5 min stimulated)
- Salivary uptake scan if low salivary flows and Sjögren's syndrome suspected
- Allergy testing, especially to dental panel of allergens
- Removal of possible offending medication including ACE inhibitors

SOURCES OF INFORMATION FOR PATIENTS AND DOCTORS

http://dermnetnz.org/site-age-specific/aphthae.html

REFERENCES

1. Grushka M, Epstein JB, Gorsky, M. Burning mouth syndrome. Am Fam Physician 2002; 65:615–620.
2. Ship JA, Grushka M, Lipton JA et al. Burning mouth syndrome: an update. J Am Dent Assoc 1995; 126:842–853.
3. Grushka M, Epstein J, Mott A. An open-label, dose escalation pilot study of the effect of clonazepam in burning mouth syndrome. Oral Surg Oral Med Oral Pathol Oral Radiol Endod 1998; 86:557–561.
4. Zakrzewska JM, Forssell H, Glenny AM. Interventions for the treatment of burning mouth syndrome: a systematic review. J Orofac Pain 2003; 17:293-300.

Chapter 2

Heartburn and noncardiac chest pain

Wai-Man Wong and Ronnie Fass

INTRODUCTION

In this chapter heartburn and noncardiac chest pain are discussed in tandem for each subsection. The objective is to provide comparisons and contrasts in each category discussed. Noncardiac chest pain (NCCP) is a different symptom complex from heartburn, yet, as discussed subsequently, gastroesophageal reflux is the most common cause of NCCP. In other words, reflux may result in typical heartburn or, in more atypical discomfort, NCCP.

Heartburn is the cardinal symptom of patients with gastroesophageal reflux disease (GERD). In patients with heartburn as the predominant symptom, GERD is the likely cause in at least 75% of individuals.[1] In a US population-based study, the prevalence of at least one episode of heartburn over 1 year was 42% and weekly episodes (=1) of heartburn was 20%.[2] However, the majority of patients with heartburn will never seek medical attention and treat their symptom with over-the-counter medications.

NCCP is defined as recurrent episodes of retrosternal angina-like pain in patients without cardiac abnormality. Sir William Osler, in 1892, described 'esophagismus,' or pain secondary to spasms of the esophagus, which may have initiated the clinical concept that esophageal pain can mimic cardiac pain. It has been estimated that the US prevalence of NCCP is 23%.[2] Patients with chest pain fall under the category of NCCP following a negative cardiac workup. The extent of cardiac workup is individually determined and may not include cardiac angiography in all subjects. NCCP is a benign condition, although the associated morbidity and economic burden, as a result of inability to work and healthcare utilization, are significant.

WHAT IS IT?

The definition of GERD is hampered by the fact that the word 'heartburn' is interpreted variably by patients.[1] It is important in history-taking to establish whether the patient and physician understand the term similarly. One can prompt patients to determine whether the symptom they are describing as heartburn refers to a burning sensation behind the breastbone rising up from the pit of the stomach or from the lower part of the breastbone towards the throat or neck. Heartburn may be associated with a sour or bitter taste in the mouth, commonly occurring within 2 h after a meal. A large-volume or fatty meal is more likely to precipitate heartburn. Additionally, heartburn often disturbs the sleep of affected individuals and significantly impairs patients' quality of life.

NCCP is a complex and heterogeneous disorder. Several etiologic mechanisms have been suggested, including gastroesophageal reflux, esophageal dysmotility, and visceral hyperalgesia (heightened perception of esophageal stimuli). The latter group has been termed as functional chest pain of presumed esophageal origin.[3] These patients report a midline chest pain or discomfort that is not of burning quality in the absence of pathologic gastroesophageal reflux, achalasia, or other motility disorder.

Patients who later are designated as having NCCP often have initial evaluations for heart disease. Their symptoms are commonly described as squeezing or burning substernal chest pain, which may radiate to the back, neck, arms, and jaws. Taking a history for the typical features is the first step in distinguishing angina from NCCP.[4]

HOW COMMON IS IT?

GERD: In Western developed countries, it is estimated that around 10–30% of the adult population is affected by GERD.[1,2] All phenotypic presentations of GERD appear to affect caucasians more often than African Americans or Native Americans. In the Asia Pacific region, the prevalence of GERD in the general population is around 2–5%.[5] GERD without esophageal mucosal damage (nonerosive reflux disease) is more common in females, in contrast to erosive esophagitis, peptic stricture, and Barrett's esophagus which are more common in males. The prevalence of GERD increases with age and several risk factors for GERD have been identified (Table 2.1).

NCCP: The incidence and prevalence of NCCP have not been studied so well. Based on recent population studies, the prevalence of NCCP (defined as chest pain but not including heartburn or history of ischemic heart disease) is 20–25%.[2,6] It appears that NCCP is a very common condition, regardless of sex or ethnic background. While most tertiary referral-based studies report a female predominance, a population-based study showed no sex difference.[2] However, females appear more likely to seek medical care for NCCP. Information about risk factors that are associated with NCCP is scarce. Patients with GERD-related NCCP are likely to share the same risk factors as the general GERD population (Table 2.1). Otherwise, psychologic factors such as anxiety, panic disorder, major depression, and somatoform disorders have been demonstrated to be closely associated with NCCP.

PATHOPHYSIOLOGY

Pathophysiology of heartburn

The mechanisms responsible for the development of heartburn remain poorly understood. It is postulated that sensitization of esophageal chemoreceptors, either directly by exposure to acid

TABLE 2.1 RISK FACTORS FOR GASTROESOPHAGEAL REFLUX DISEASE

Risk factor	Underlying mechanisms
Smoking	Decreases LES pressure and alters esophageal defense mechanisms
Alcohol	Direct mucosal damage
Obesity	Increases intra-abdominal pressure
High-fat diet	Decreases LES pressure, increases TLESR, increases esophageal sensitivity to acid, and delays gastric emptying
Chocolate, peppermint, caffeine	Decrease LES pressure
Drugs (calcium channel blockers, tricyclics, nitrates, benzodiazepines, aspirin, NSAIDs, etc.)	Decrease LES pressure or cause direct mucosal damage
Abdominal trauma	Disrupts diaphragmatic sphincter function
Nasogastric tubes	Direct trauma to the esophageal mucosa and LES interruption
Exercise	Increases intra-abdominal pressure
Systemic disorders (e.g., scleroderma, diabetes mellitus)	Scleroderma – decreased or absent LES pressure, decreases esophageal peristalsis Diabetes mellitus – autonomic neuropathy and reduced esophageal peristalsis
Asthma	Increased pressure gradient between thorax and abdomen, higher incidence of hiatus hernia, and effects of medications used to treat asthma
Sleep apnea	Large negative intrapleural pressure during apnea
Stress	Increase perception of intraesophageal stimuli

LES, lower esophageal sphincter; NSAID, nonsteroidal anti-inflammatory drug; TLSER, transient lower esophageal sphincter relaxation.

reflux or indirectly through release of inflammatory mediators, is responsible for the generation of heartburn.[7] Both animal models and human studies have demonstrated dilatation of intercellular spaces in acid exposed tissues, and this might permit an increase in paracellular permeability, permitting acid to reach sensory nerve endings located within the mucosa. However, this prevailing hypothesis does not fully explain symptoms in patients with heartburn, primarily because more than 90% of acid reflux events are never perceived by patients with GERD.

Triggers: Physiologically, the most common trigger for GERD symptoms is a meal, particularly if it contains a large amount of fat. However, the mechanisms by which luminal fat and possibly other nutrients modulate the perception of esophageal stimuli remain to be elucidated. Fat has been shown to cause a reduction in lower esophageal sphincter basal pressure and delay in gastric emptying. However, fat may also exacerbate the symptoms of GERD by heightening perception of intra-esophageal acid. Enteric hormones such as cholecystokinin or other gut neurotransmitters and enzymes are believed to mediate the effect of fat on the lower esophageal sphincter and sensory afferents. Furthermore, nonacid-related intraesophageal stimuli may also lead to the development of heartburn. For example, esophageal balloon distention induced heartburn symptoms in a subset of normal subjects and reproduced typical heartburn in half of the patients with GERD,[8] suggesting that mechanical stimuli may also be perceived as heartburn by some patients, even in the absence of actual acid reflux. This suggests that heartburn is not stimulus specific, and that nonacid-related intraesophageal events may lead to this type of symptom as well. Simultaneous intraesophageal impedance and pH measurements can demonstrate that nonacidic reflux (pure liquid or mixture of gas and liquid) may also play a role in the pathophysiology of heartburn. Other than intraesophageal stimuli, one should bear in mind that central factors could modulate esophageal perception (Fig. 2.1). Psychologic co-morbidity (anxiety, depression, etc.), stress, and possibly poor sleep may cause patients to perceive low-intensity esophageal stimuli as being painful.

PATHOPHYSIOLOGY OF NCCP

GERD is the most common esophageal cause of NCCP as abnormal 24-h esophageal pH monitoring and/or positive endoscopic findings are present in up to 60% of the patients.[4,9] This is further supported by the efficacy of acid suppressive therapy

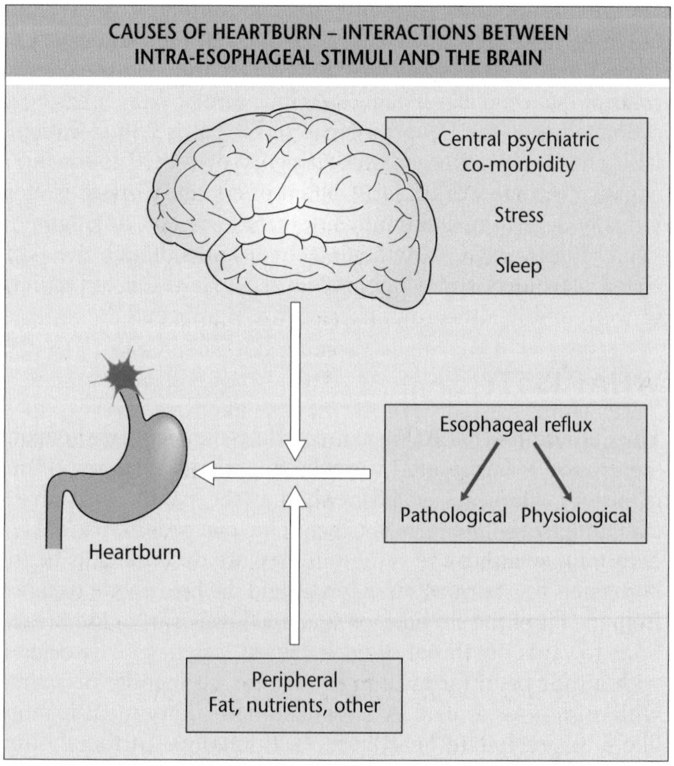

Fig. 2.1 Causes of heartburn. Proposed causes of heartburn – interactions between intraesophageal stimuli and the brain. (Adapted from Fass R, Tougas G. Functional heartburn – the stimulus, the pain and the brain. Gut 2002; 51:885–892, with permission.)

in relieving patients' symptoms and the reproducibility of chest pain by esophageal acid perfusion studies. Acid perfusion into the distal esophagus has been demonstrated to alter the perception of painful stimuli in the distal portion of the esophagus (primary hyperalgesia) as well as the proximal portion of the esophagus (secondary hyperalgesia) in patients with NCCP.

Motility: The increased prevalence of esophageal motility disorders in patients with NCCP suggests that chest pain may also result from stimulation of mechanoreceptors within the esophageal wall. Approximately 30% of patients with non-GERD-related NCCP demonstrate some type of esophageal dysmotility. The motility abnormalities include diffuse esophageal spasm, nutcracker esophagus, achalasia, long-duration contractions, multi-peaked waves, and hypertensive lower esophageal sphincter. However, there is a poor temporal correlation between esophageal motility disorders and episodes of chest pain, suggesting that the presence of esophageal dysmotility during esophageal manometry may be a marker for an underlying motor disorder responsible for the patient's symptoms. High-frequency intraesophageal ultrasonography has revealed a strong correlation between spontaneous and edrophonium-induced chest pain and sustained esophageal contractions (SECs). These contractions are caused by shortening of the longitudinal muscle of the esophagus and thus are not readily detected by traditional esophageal manometry. SECs have been suggested to be the motor corollary of esophageal chest pain. However, it is unclear whether SECs are the direct cause of chest pain or simply an epiphenomenon.[9]

Visceral sensitivity: Cerebral-evoked potential studies in patients with NCCP using esophageal balloon distention protocols demonstrated abnormal cerebral processing of esophageal stimuli. The recorded cerebral-evoked potentials (marker of central nociceptive processing) were of lower quality and amplitude compared with those of control subjects. Peripheral and central sensitization of esophageal sensory afferents and spinal cord neurons has been suggested to cause increased responses to innocuous and noxious intraesophageal stimuli.[4] It has been postulated that inflammation or other injuries to the esophageal mucosa set off a cascade of events that leads to the upregulation of receptors and induces the development of visceral hypersensitivity through peripheral and central sensitization. Patients with NCCP appear to have a decreased threshold for esophageal stimulation, similar to that documented in patients with irritable bowel syndrome.

Psychologic factors: An increased association with psychiatric disorders, including anxiety, somatization, depression, and panic disorder, has been seen in patients with NCCP. These patients often report chest pain or tightness under stress, possibly due to sympathetic nervous system arousal. Previous experimental studies have shown that patients with NCCP are more sensitive than those with coronary artery disease to both cardiovascular and noncardiovascular painful stimuli. Body awareness is also greater in patients with NCCP. Thus, for many patients with NCCP, psychologic co-morbidity may contribute to the emergence of chest pain by amplifying the perception of intraesophageal events.[4,9]

CAUSES/DIFFERENTIAL DIAGNOSIS

In addition to GERD and functional heartburn, peptic ulcer disease or upper gastrointestinal malignancy can lead to heartburn symptoms.[10] Furthermore, a sudden and isolated attack of heartburn may be caused by pill-induced injury, or even caustic injury to the esophageal mucosa.

Empiric treatment with potent acid suppressive agents has been proposed as an initial diagnostic tool for patients presenting with heartburn. However, in patients with alarm symptoms in addition to heartburn, such as weight loss, anorexia, dysphagia, odynophagia, hematemesis, or anemia, prompt upper endoscopy is warranted. The most important diagnosis to be excluded during the evaluation of a patient with chest pain is ischemic heart disease. The potential causes of NCCP (besides esophageal disorders) include gastric and gallbladder disorders, musculoskeletal abnormalities, pulmonary and pericardial disorders, and psychiatric abnormalities – primarily panic disorder.

CAUSES AND DIFFERENTIAL DIAGNOSIS

COMMON CAUSES OF NONCARDIAC CHEST PAIN

GASTROINTESTINAL
- Gastroesophageal reflux disease
- Esophageal dysmotility
- Peptic ulcer disease
- Biliary disease
- Hepatitis
- Pancreatitis

MUSCULOSKELETAL CAUSES
- Costochondritis
- Fibromyalgia
- Xyphoditis
- Thoracic outlet syndrome
- Cervical or thoracic spinal disease

PULMONARY OR INTRATHORACIC CAUSES
- Pleurisy
- Pneumonia
- Pneumothorax
- Pulmonary embolism
- Mediastinitis
- Aortic aneurysm

PSYCHIATRIC CAUSES
- Panic disorder
- Anxiety
- Depression
- Somatization
- Hypochondriasis
- Munchausen's syndrome

SYMPTOM COMPLEXES

Heartburn, as the predominant symptom, is highly specific for the diagnosis of GERD. However, other symptoms are also commonly found in patients with GERD and are outlined below.

Regurgitation

Regurgitation is defined as an effortless return of a bitter- or sour-tasting fluid into the throat and is commonly associated with heartburn. Although regurgitation is less prevalent than heartburn in patients with GERD, in some it may be the sole presentation of the disorder. Regurgitation is particularly severe at night, when patients are recumbent, or when bending over.

In general, regurgitation appears to be more difficult to control medically. It should be emphasized that regurgitation may also be a presentation of a pharyngeal pouch, esophageal obstruction, or gastric outlet obstruction.

Waterbrash

Waterbrash is the sudden filling of the mouth with clear, slightly salty fluid due to secretions of the salivary glands in response to intraesophageal acid exposure.

Globus sensation

Globus is the constant sensation of a lump or fullness in the throat, which improves transiently during swallowing. Globus usually occurs in the absence of dysphagia.

Dysphagia

The term dysphagia refers to the sensation that food is being hindered in its normal passage from the oral cavity to the stomach. In patients with GERD, sensation of dysphagia may be perceived below the breast bone anywhere up to the sternal notch. The latter is commonly referred sensation from a lesion in the distal part of the esophagus. Dysphagia may be referred cephalad to the site of the obstruction, but never caudad. Dysphagia in a patient with heartburn may suggest the presence of erosive esophagitis, peptic stricture, or adenocarcinoma of the esophagus.

Atypical manifestations of GERD

Atypical symptoms may occur in patients with GERD, which may – or more commonly may not – be associated with heartburn. These atypical presentations of GERD include the extraesophageal manifestations such as asthma, chronic cough, hoarseness, throat clearing, and sleep disorders.

Dyspepsia

Many patients with predominantly heartburn symptoms may also complain of dyspeptic symptoms, such as epigastric pain or discomfort, bloating, nausea, and even vomiting. These symptoms are reported by patients with or without esophageal mucosal injury. It is unclear whether these symptoms represent an overlap with functional dyspepsia or are part of the GERD symptom complex.

Odynophagia

Odynophagia is pain during swallowing. It occurs in up to 50% of patients with GERD and is characteristically associated with erosive esophagitis, infection, or corrosive (pills) induced injury. A milder variant without pain is a sensation that the patient can feel solids and liquids passing down the esophagus.

DIAGNOSIS

Patient reports of heartburn and/or acid regurgitation are commonly interpreted as diagnostic of GERD. Symptom response to antireflux treatment may further cement the diagnosis.[1] Other diagnostic tools that are currently available include barium esophagraphy, upper endoscopy, ambulatory 24-h esophageal pH monitoring, multichannel intraluminal impedance with pH sensor, and the proton pump inhibitor (PPI) test.[1]

In contrast, clinical history does not always help to distinguish esophageal from cardiac chest pain. Both esophageal and cardiac chest pain can produce a pressure-like squeezing or burning substernal chest pain. Both may improve with nitrates or calcium channel blockers. Additionally, both may be exertional in nature. The presence of regurgitation, and pain relieved with antacids, may suggest an esophageal etiology in patients with NCCP.[10]

Barium esophagraphy

Barium esophagraphy should not serve as the primary test for the evaluation of patients with heartburn. The test has a very low sensitivity and specificity for the diagnosis of GERD. The presence of barium reflux does not necessarily denote GERD, as 20% of normal subjects may demonstrate similar abnormality during esophagraphy. Barium esophagraphy may be helpful and should be considered as the first diagnostic tool in patients with GERD who develop dysphagia.

Upper endoscopy

GERD: Upper endoscopy has a relatively low sensitivity for the diagnosis of GERD. Between 50% and 70% of patients do not demonstrate any evidence of esophageal mucosal injury on endoscopy. Endoscopy is the gold standard for diagnosing erosive esophagitis, Barrett's esophagus, peptic stricture, and adenocarcinoma of the esophagus. Furthermore, the test allows assessment of the degree of esophageal mucosal injury and provides an opportunity for histopathologic diagnosis.

Ultrathin endoscopy has been recently introduced as a rapid, ambulatory, and easily tolerated method to examine the esophageal mucosa. However, the technique is limited by lack of biopsy channel.

NCCP: Upper endoscopy in the absence of alarm symptoms, while commonly performed in clinical practice, has been shown to provide little useful information in the initial evaluation of NCCP. Studies have demonstrated that less than 10–25% of patients demonstrate some type of esophageal mucosal injury.

24-hour esophageal pH monitoring

GERD: Twenty-four-hour esophageal pH monitoring of distal esophageal acid exposure is a sensitive test for the diagnosis of GERD but should not be considered as the gold standard. Presently, usage of pH monitoring is limited to patients who have not responded to at least a double dose of PPI, patients with normal endoscopy who are candidates for antireflux surgery, and patients who have had antireflux surgery but report recurrence of GERD symptoms. In patients with atypical or extraesophageal manifestations of GERD, pH monitoring should be performed in patients who have failed treatment with at least double-dose PPI (the test is done on treatment).[1] This procedure is commonly uncomfortable to patients, costly, and may not be readily available to community-based physicians.

NCCP: The use of 24-h esophageal pH monitoring in NCCP has been transformed in the past decade, primarily owing to increased usage of empiric PPI therapy or the PPI test. Presently, the test is recommended only in patients who have failed PPI treatment (on therapy). The sensitivity of the test in NCCP is unknown, but approximately 50–60% of patients with untreated NCCP demonstrate increased distal esophageal acid exposure and/or a positive symptom index alone.

Multichannel intraluminal impedance

The combination of an impedance catheter and a pH sensor provides a unique opportunity to study physiologic events within the esophagus and their relationship to symptoms. In addition, the recording assembly can disclose the characteristics of the gastric refluxate (acid, nonacid, gas, and mixed gas and liquid). The value of this technique has been demonstrated by recent studies showing that nonacidic reflux is not uncommon in patients with GERD, and may lead to classic heartburn symptoms as well. However, its role in clinical practice remains to be elucidated.

Esophageal manometry

Esophageal manometry has no role in diagnosing GERD. Abnormalities in esophageal motility have been identified in 25–30% of the patients with non-GERD-related NCCP during esophageal manometry. The most common motility abnormalities identified are nutcracker esophagus, nonspecific esophageal motility disorders, and diffuse esophageal spasm. The presence of a motility abnormality during esophageal manometry is rarely associated with reports of chest pain, raising a question about the exact relationship between these motility findings and chest pain.

Provocative tests

The commonly used provocative tests include the Bernstein or acid perfusion test (reproducing chest pain by infusing acid into the mid-esophagus), the Tensilon test (reproducing chest pain by inducing augmented esophageal contractions using intravenous edrophonium, an acetylcholine esterase antagonist), and the balloon distention test (reproducing chest pain by using graded esophageal balloon distentions). These provocative tests are rarely used clinically as the sensitivity is low (0–50%).

The proton pump inhibitor (PPI) test

The PPI test is a short course of high-dose PPI (e.g., single- or double-dose PPI in the morning before breakfast and a single dose before dinner for 7 days). It provides high accuracy in the diagnosis of GERD-related NCCP (Fig. 2.2).[4,9,12] It is a simple, cost-effective, and noninvasive diagnostic tool.[11–13] Although there is no consensus regarding the objective measurement of symptom response, optimal dose, frequency, and duration of the PPI test, thus far several studies of GERD-related NCCP have demonstrated a high sensitivity, specificity, and positive predictive value.[4]

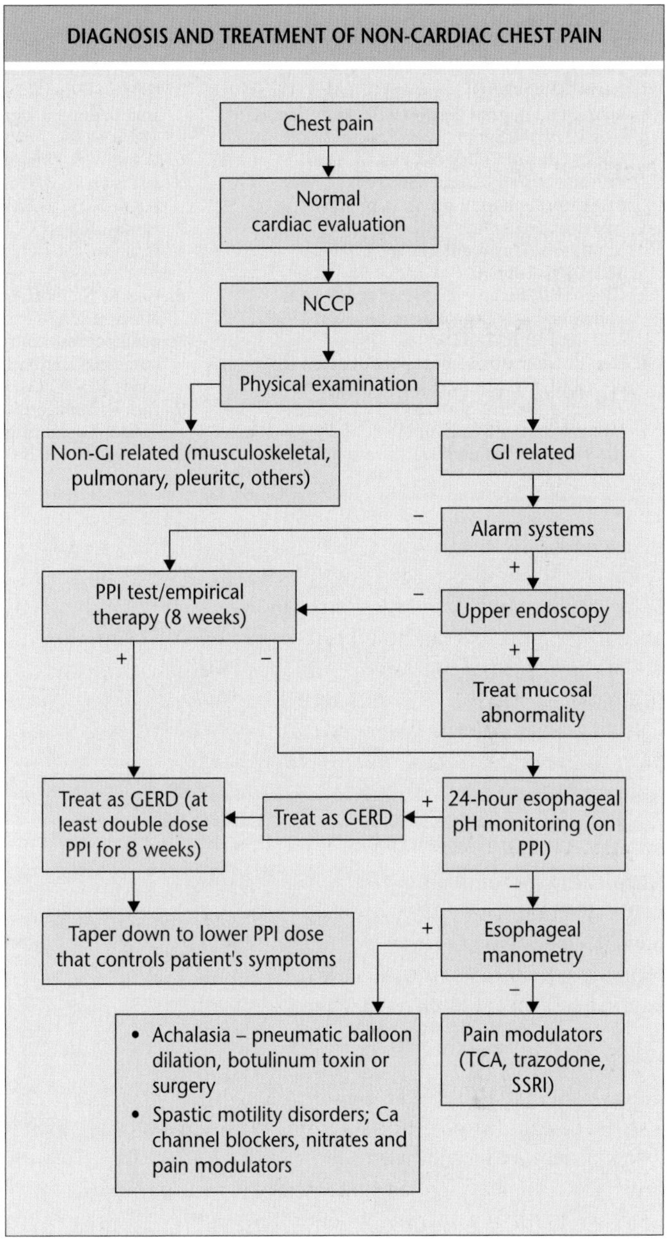

Fig. 2.2 Diagnosis and treatment of noncardiac chest pain. Suggested algorithm for the diagnosis and treatment of patients with noncardiac chest pain (NCCP). GERD, gastroesophageal reflux disease; GI, gastrointestinal; PPI, proton pump inhibitor; SSRI, selective serotonin reuptake inhibitor; TCA, tricyclic antidepressant.

FUTURE DIRECTIONS

Despite current advances in understanding the pathophysiology, diagnosis, and treatment of patients with heartburn and NCCP, the exact underlying mechanisms for these symptoms remain poorly understood. The lack of association between symptom severity or anatomic or pathophysiologic findings remains perplexing. Future investigation should bring further understanding of the peripheral and central factors that may modulate perception of heartburn or NCCP. The development of new visceral analgesics will likely revolutionize the treatment in non-GERD-related NCCP and patients with heartburn who have failed PPI therapy. Improved PPIs or the introduction of acid pump antagonists (rapid onset of action) will be tested as empiric tools for diagnosing GERD-related NCCP. The value of new diagnostic techniques, such as the multichannel intraluminal impedance, will be assessed in special GERD groups and pateints with NCCP.

SOURCES OF INFORMATION FOR PATIENTS AND DOCTORS

http://www.patient.co.uk/showdoc/345/

REFERENCES

1. Dent J, Brun J, Fendrick AM et al. An evidence-based appraisal of reflux disease management – the Genval Workshop Report. Gut 1999; 44(Suppl 2):S1–S16.
2. Locke GR 3rd, Talley NJ, Fett SL et al. Prevalence and clinical spectrum of gastroesophageal reflux: a population-based study in Olmsted County, Minnesota. Gastroenterology 1997; 112:1448–1456.
3. Clouse RE, Richter JE, Heading RC et al. Functional esophageal disorders. Gut 1999; 45(Suppl II):II31–II36.
4. Fass R. Noncardiac chest pain. In: Fass R, ed. GERD/dyspepsia, 1st edn. Philadelphia: Hanley & Belfus, 2004:183–196.
5. Wong WM, Lai KC, Lam KF et al. Prevalence, clinical spectrum and health care utilisation of gastro-oesophageal reflux disease in Chinese population: a population-based study. Aliment Pharmacol Ther 2003; 18:595–604.
6. Wong WM, Wong BC. Noncardiac chest pain: an Asian view. Gastroenterol Clin North Am 2004; 33:125–133.
7. Fass R, Tougas G. Functional heartburn: the stimulus, the pain and the brain. Gut 2002; 51:885–895.
8. Fass R, Naliboff B, Higa L et al. Differential effect of long-term esophageal exposure on mechanosensitivity and chemosensitivity in humans. Gastroenterology 1998; 115:1363–1373.
9. Fass R, Malagon I, Schmulson M. Chest pain of esophageal origin. Curr Opin Gastroenterol 2001; 17:376–380.
10. Castell DO, Richter JE, eds. The esophagus, 3rd edn. Philadelphia: Lippincott Williams & Wilkins, Brown, 1999.
11. Fass R, Ofman JJ, Gralnek IM et al. Clinical and economic assessment of the omeprazole test in patients with symptoms suggestive of gastroesophageal reflux disease. Arch Intern Med 1999; 159:2161–2168.
12. Fass R, Fennerty MB, Ofman JJ et al. The clinical and economic value of a short course of omeprazole in patients with noncardiac chest pain. Gastroenterology 1998; 115:42–49.
13. Juul-Hansen P, Rydning A, Jacobsen CD, Hansen T. High-dose proton-pump inhibitors as a diagnostic test of gastro-oesophageal reflux disease in endoscopic-negative patients. Scand J Gastroenterol 2001; 36:806–810.

Chapter 3

Dysphagia and odynophagia

H Worth Boyce

INTRODUCTION

Dysphagia and odynophagia are the most important symptoms related to disorders of swallowing. They may occur together and be perceived by the patient at any level during the passage of a food bolus from mouth to stomach. Dysphagia and/or odynophagia are sensed within seconds when neuromotor malfunction of mouth, pharynx, or esophagus occurs, with obstruction of the orogastric lumen pathway, or in the presence of an inflammatory or ulcerative lesion. The processes of preparation and passage of food and swallowing are seemingly so simple that they occur as relatively unrecognized conscious acts. The average person swallows over 600 times a day, and for most between-meal swallows is unaware of the function. The approximate rate of swallows during a meal is about 170/h. During sleep, the rate is markedly diminished to less than 7 times per hour. It is remarkable indeed that so few swallows result in any significant related event in normal persons.

WHAT IS IT?

Dysphagia

A useful clinical definition for dysphagia is as follows: difficulty or delay in the preparation and/or passage of a liquid or solid food bolus that is sensed by the patient within 10 s of the initiation of a swallow attempt. The definition comprises two distinct symptoms – difficulty in the initiation of swallowing (usually neuromuscular) and obstructive dysphagia (see below). Dysphagia by this definition is never psychogenic.

Dysphagia is often confused with the globus sensation, originally called 'globus hystericus.' The former term is preferred since there is no evidence to support the occurrence of hysteria with this condition. The globus sensation is a constant or intermittent sensation of a lump, fullness, or pressure in the throat or neck. It is neither directly related to, nor induced by, the act of swallowing, typically is intermittent, and may disappear or transiently lessen during swallowing. The clinical features of globus sensation may occur with organic disease in the neck, pharynx, or cervical esophagus, hence this diagnosis should only be made after a complete evaluation. There is no evidence to support acid reflux as a cause of globus sensation but increased afferent sensation and elevated upper esophageal sphincter pressure are possible etiologies.[1]

Odynophagia

Odynophagia refers to a pain or burning sensation directly associated with swallowing, especially acidic and spicy foods or those at temperature extremes. The symptoms of burning and pain are precise indicators for the presence of an acute inflammatory or ulcerative process. Less acute swallowing-related pain may be associated with obstructive disorders and is described clinically as impact pain that is caused by bolus impaction with resulting esophageal wall contraction or distention proximal to the site of obstruction.

HOW COMMON IS IT?

Approximately 8 million people in the USA report some degree of dysphagia annually.[2] Prevalence increases with age since more dysphagia-related conditions occur in the elderly. The growth of the 65 and older population ensures increasing diagnostic challenges for both dysphagia and odynophagia. Dysphagia related to cerebrovascular accidents, Parkinson's disease, and other neurologic disorders is reported to be present in 30–70% of patients in nursing homes.[3] Approximately 10% of patients evaluated for gastroesophageal acid reflux disease present with dysphagia.

PATHOPHYSIOLOGY

Intake and preparation of a bolus are the first voluntary actions in the swallowing sequence. A conscious decision is made regarding a tolerable bolus size and consistency prior to initiation of a swallow. The comfort level for drinking, chewing, and swallowing pace is variable from person to person with much of this action being related to habits developed early in life. Unintended or involuntary variations in these parameters can lead to either oropharyngeal or esophageal dysphagia, even in those with no neuromuscular or obstructive disorder.

The primary oropharyngeal function is preparation and transfer of a properly prepared bolus from mouth through pharynx and upper esophageal sphincter to the esophagus. During this process, the patent aerodigestive pathway is altered by closure of the nasopharynx and vocal cords, opening of the upper esophageal sphincter related to laryngeal elevation downward movement, and further closure of the airway by the epiglottis followed by peristaltic contraction of the pharyngeal muscles. All of these events occur in less than 1 s after initiation of a swallow. Mild functional deviations from normal in these highly coordinated actions may have symptomatic consequences of which dysphagia is only one.

Oropharyngeal dysphagia results from either neuromotor deficits, myopathy with weakness and atrophy of muscle, a combination of the two, or an obstructing lesion (Fig. 3.1). Neural deficits usually produce alterations in the highly integrated neuromotor phenomena that are controlled via the swallowing center in the brainstem. Myopathic disorders produce dysphagia as a consequence of muscle disease or weakness of skeletal muscle contractility. Pharyngeal inflammation and neoplasms produce both dysphagia and odynophagia.

Esophageal dysphagia: The efficient transport of a bolus through the esophagus is dependent upon intact neuromotor function and a patent lumen. There are many conditions that may alter the transport phase. A swallow initiates a primary esophageal peristaltic wave that propels the bolus through the esophagus at a speed of 3–4 cm/s. This transport time to stomach through the average 25-cm length of the adult esophagus requires 6–8 s. Gravity enhances passage of liquids, but solids pass more slowly and thereby may provoke secondary peristalsis that normally ensures complete bolus clearance. Esophageal neuromotor disorders may produce both solid and liquid bolus delay. Classic achalasia is characterized by aperistalsis in the esophageal body, elevated pressure, and incomplete relaxation of the lower esophageal sphincter (LES) with the sensation of delayed transport for both solids and liquids.

Dysphagia with solids is the typical initial presentation of obstructing lesions. Obstructive dysphagia occurs consistently with an attempt to eat a normal diet when either the pharyngeal or esophageal lumen is narrowed. Dysphagia with lesser degrees of obstruction may become manifest with a faster pace of eating, larger bolus size, solid bolus consistency, and recumbent position. Patients modify one or several of these variables to reduce or eliminate the sensation of hang-up and, as a consequence, may provide unintentional and inaccurate historical information related to the duration and severity of dysphagia.

CAUSES

CAUSES OF OROPHARYNGEAL DYSPHAGIA

NEUROMOTOR DYSPHAGIA (CNS)
- Cardiovascular accidents (strokes)*
- Parkinson's disease*
- Myasthenia gravis
- Multiple sclerosis
- Amyotrophic lateral sclerosis
- Wilson's disease
- Huntington's disease
- Laryngeal nerve injury
- Bulbar poliomyelitis
- Peripheral neuropathy
  Diphtheria
  Rabies
  Botulism
- Myopathies
  Primary myositis
  Dermato- or polymyositis
  Amyloidosis
  Metabolic myopathy
  Oculopharyngeal muscular dystrophy

OBSTRUCTIVE DYSPHAGIA
- Inflammation*
  Pharyngitis/abscess
- Structural
  Neoplasms*
  Radiation stricture*
  Pharyngeal webs
  Surgical resection
  Extrinsic compression
  Cervical spine osteophytes

*Most common causes

SYMPTOM COMPLEXES

The most common symptoms related to oropharyngeal dysphagia are cough and/or choking due to laryngeal penetration or aspiration of a liquid food bolus or saliva, less often due to a solid bolus. These sequelae may result from premature leakage of material from the oral cavity prior to swallow initiation with retention in the valleculae or piriform sinuses after an ineffective swallow. Overflow or spillage into the larynx occurs during or between swallows. When palatal closure is incomplete, nasal regurgitation occurs. Nasal speech, hoarseness, or dysphonia is subtle to severe, at times being more obvious than the associated swallowing disorder. Patients with oropharyngeal dysmotility typically are able to tolerate soft to solid consistencies with less problems than they have with liquids.

Oropharyngeal myopathy with intact neural function may present first with a complaint of solid bolus dysphagia due to muscle weakness. The striated muscles responsible for oropharyngeal bolus transfer are weakened and fatigued with use, so dysphagia is more noticeable later in the day. Associated skeletal muscle weakness such as eyelid ptosis, nasal twang, dysphonia, or extremity muscle weakness provide clues to the dysphagia etiology.

With the exception of acute cerebrovascular accidents, or ingestion of foreign bodies, the onset of dysphagia is typically gradual and described as the sensation of food hangup or sticking. A lower esophageal (Schatzki) ring or peptic stricture may become manifest abruptly, but a good history usually reveals transient solid impaction episodes prior to the first one that requires endoscopic removal. The combination of esophageal dysphagia with solids and liquids, regurgitation of unaltered food, and hypersalivation or sialorrhea is typical for classic achalasia.

When there is pharyngitis or esophagitis, the resulting odynophagia can be so severe as to lead to aphagia, i.e., the loss of ability or refusal to swallow. Likewise, hangup of a solid bolus produces impact pain and fear of swallowing.

DIAGNOSIS

Medical history

The history provides a presumptive diagnosis in at least 80% of patients who have dysphagia.[4,5,6] Detailed questioning about associated illnesses or symptoms involving other body systems, a complete physical examination, and objective tests are needed to establish etiology (Fig. 3.1).

A caveat regarding proper history for localizing dysphagia is necessary. The patient with dysphagia may think of swallowing as the act of initiating a swallow at the oropharyngeal level. If the question is 'do you have trouble swallowing?' and the answer is 'no,' the examiner must ask the question 'does solid or liquid food stick or hang up during a swallow?'

If there is trouble with liquids, but solids pass without delay, the typical problem is pharyngeal transfer. Coughing or 'choking' indicate aspiration and an oropharyngeal neuromotor disorder.

CAUSES
CAUSES OF ESOPHAGEAL DYSPHAGIA
NEUROMUSCULAR DYSPHAGIA • Upper esophageal sphincter Hypertensive, incomplete or delayed relaxation • Esophageal Achalasia* Scleroderma* Diffuse spasm Nutcracker esophagus **OBSTRUCTIVE DYSPHAGIA** • Systemic diseases Epidermolysis bullosa Lichen planus Stevens-Johnson syndrome Graft-versus-host disease Tylosis (squamous carcinoma) Crohn's disease Amyloid disease Plummer-Vinson syndrome • Inflammation (esophagitis) Acid reflux* Herpetic* Candida* Radiation* Cytomegalovirus Eosinophilic ('ringed' esophagus) Drug-induced Photodynamic laser therapy (PDT) • Neoplasm Carcinoma – primary* Carcinoma – metastatic Submucosal benign tumors, cysts • Structural Strictures* (peptic,* radiation, caustic, anastomotic, drug-induced, etc.) Webs* Schatzki ring Congenital atresia • Compression Vascular anomalies Vertebral osteophytes Mediastinal lesions • Foreign bodies

*Most common causes

If solids but not liquids cause dysphagia, either pharyngeal or esophageal obstruction or, rarely, oropharyngeal myopathy are causative. When dysphagia occurs with liquids and solids starting at about the same time, the problem is related to altered esophageal transport, usually achalasia, until proven otherwise.

The duration of dysphagia is predictably longer than that reported by the patient, especially for solid food-related esophageal dysphagia. Often there is a dragging or sticking sensation for months before the patient seeks help. Dysphagia due to malignancy is constant and progressive compared to benign strictures that produce an intermittent and stable degree of dysphagia. A more precise date of onset can be determined by referring to meal content at the time of special life events such as a birthdays, anniversaries, and religious or other holidays.

Compensation for dysphagia is achieved by modifying food consistency and increasing eating time. With benign disease, patients are able to maintain regular caloric intake by extending eating time plus diet modifications. Foods that accentuate solid food dysphagia include bread, beef or pork, white meat of chicken or turkey, and apple. Questions should be specific regarding food preparation when discussing food tolerances and swallowing. Difficult to eat foods may be avoided or cut into small pieces to reduce dysphagia.

If dysphagia/hang-up sensation is localized to the mid to lower retrosternal area, the esophageal obstruction site correlates with the level the patient senses.[7] If this sensation onset is timed, it is known that it takes 6–8 s after swallowing a bolus before the patient feels the sensation of dysphagia due to a distal lesion, sooner (2–4 s) if more proximal. When food hang-up is sensed at the level of the jugular notch, at least 30% of the time the actual level of obstruction will be more distal.

Some strictures are primarily due to acid reflux but are associated with and enhanced by prior nasogastric intubation or impacted pills. Detection of aggravating factors requires careful, specific questioning. Such atypical strictures may be extremely difficult to treat.

Odynophagia is variable in severity and usually indicative of mucosal disease. Acute injury such as pill esophagitis, viral or candida esophagitis, or acid reflux are the most common causes of odynophagia. Iatrogenic etiologies include mucosal injury following chemotherapy, irradiation, or photodynamic therapy (PDT). About one-third of patients with acquired immunodeficiency syndrome (AIDS) are reported to suffer from odynophagia at some time during their illness.[8] Sialorrhea is commonly associated with odynophagia, achalasia, and severe obstructive dysphagia.

Physical examination

Visual inspection of the oropharynx and neck palpation during physical examination and having the patient perform motor functions of the tongue, lips, or jaw and head during complete neurological examination, are diagnostic essentials for oropharyngeal dysphagia, especially with acute esophageal foreign body impaction. During the neurological examination the patient may be asked to swallow sips of water. Direct observation of posturing, or learned compensatory maneuvers, development of cough, or nasal regurgitation provide helpful information.

Diagnostic testing

Combined endoscopic and radiographic approaches are often necessary in the diagnosis of dysphagia/odynophagia (Fig. 3.1). Properly performed barium radiography with boluses and motion recording plus endoscopy, and in some cases esophageal manometry, will provide an accurate diagnosis for virtually all etiologies of esophageal dysphagia and odynophagia.

Barium radiography

With new onset dysphagia especially, barium radiography provides an important roadmap to what will be encountered at endoscopy. This section details the different kinds of radiography that are most useful in different clinical settings.

Modified barium swallow

Patients with neuromotor abnormalities, especially oropharyngeal, should have a modified barium swallow or a dynamic

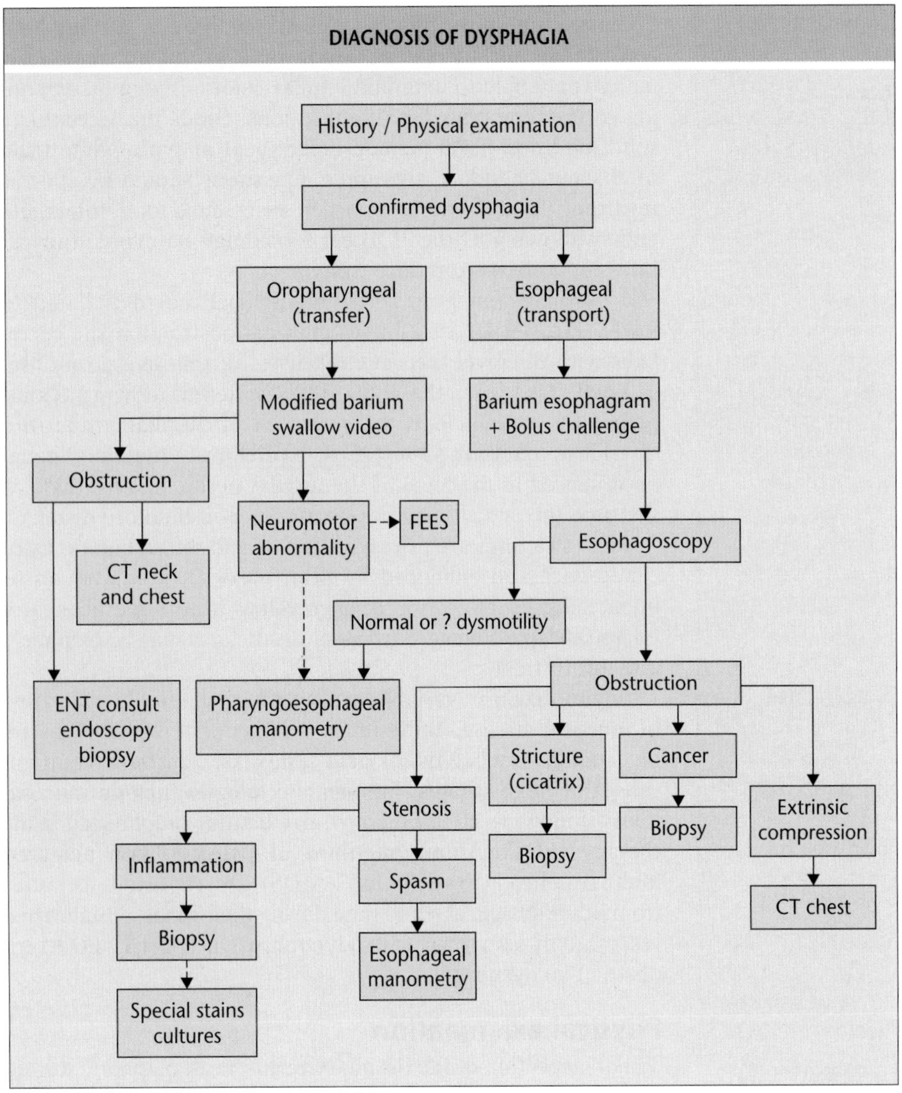

Fig. 3.1 Diagnosis of dysphagia. Broken line indicates diagnostic option.

video pharyngo-esophagram.[9] Radiographic evaluation is best performed using various bolus consistencies including thin liquid barium, thick barium, pudding with barium, crackers with barium, and a barium pill (12.5-mm diameter). If the patient has noted a problem with specific solid foods, a mixture of barium paste plus the offending food, often a sandwich or meat, may provide definitive information.

Odynophagia suspected to be due to acute inflammation or erosive esophagitis is best evaluated radiographically by a double-contrast barium esophagram that is most sensitive for study of mucosal detail.[10]

Not uncommonly in patients with odynophagia, clinicians will elect to bypass radiography and proceed directly to endoscopy. It should be done with care in cases where the odynophagia may also herald or be accompanied by a deep penetrating esophageal ulceration as in the immunocompromised patient.

Standard barium esophagram

The barium esophagram is highly accurate when properly performed. Stricture diagnosis may be missed with a routine full-column barium swallow alone, thus a negative standard barium swallow should not be accepted as the only study. The patient may report trouble in swallowing solids such as steak or bread, but the test often used is the barium mixture of milk-shake consistency. The esophagus must be challenged by a solid bolus during fluoroscopy in order to be absolutely certain not to miss a significant lesion. Videoesophagography is helpful for diagnosis of nonobstructive esophageal dysphagia.[11]

Bolus challenge esophagram

The bolus challenge identifies the significant obstructive problems in the esophagus when the standard liquid barium study is negative or equivocal. The bolus challenge allows detection of stenosis at an earlier stage. The initial challenge is provided by having the patient swallow a 12.5-mm barium pill with a sip of water.[12] If this diameter pill passes to the stomach in less than 20 s, a larger bolus challenge is appropriate. For this purpose, a standard marshmallow (3×3×3 cm) is used.[13] The patient is instructed to soften the entire marshmallow by compressing (not chewing!) it between the tongue and hard palate. When the consistency is comfortable to the patient, this bolus is swallowed with a sip of liquid barium. The marshmallow bolus has the appearance of a small air-filled balloon, capped by the barium traversing and distending the esophagus. Both the barium pill and marshmallow will be delayed briefly at the level of the aortic arch but normally pass with peristalsis to the stomach in less than 20 s. When there is stenosis of the esophagus to a diameter between 14 mm and the normal 25 mm, the marshmallow impacts and often precisely reproduces the hang-up sensation and location the patient had noticed with food. Both the pill and marshmallow soften and dissolve in about 30 min and do not pose a threat for prolonged obstruction.

Timed barium emptying study

A simple test for esophageal emptying can be made by using a timed barium emptying study, which is especially useful for patients with achalasia. This method is performed in the upright position by having the patient ingest 240 mL of barium as rapidly as possible. Retention is determined by measuring the height of the residual column of barium immediately after ingestion and at 5 and 15 min. A small amount of barium may be noted in the immediate film but the normal esophagus should be completely empty at 5 and 15 min. This technique is excellent for initial diagnosis and for evaluating response to therapy for achalasia.

Endoscopy

Videoendoscopy permits direct visual inspection and also biopsy and/or cytology. Subtle mucosal abnormalities of esophagitis or cancer may be recognized only by endoscopy. A consensus panel evaluating the final diagnosis in patients with dysphagia found that endoscopy was more sensitive (92% vs. 54%) and more specific (100% vs. 91%) than double-contrast radiography.[10]

An important diagnostic caveat relates to the accuracy of endoscopic diagnosis in patients with dysphagia who have subtle lumen stenosis without other intraluminal signs of disease. If endoscopy as the initial examination is negative and/or a standard column esophagram is negative, a bolus challenge of lumen patency as described above should be done. Neither a negative standard column barium esophagram nor a negative endoscopy will rule out esophageal obstruction.

Fiberoptic endoscopic evaluation of swallowing (FEES) with a small-diameter endoscope via the nares permits direct examination of the pharyngeal phase of swallowing and related abnormalities such as residue in the valleculae, hypopharynx as well as laryngeal penetration and aspiration.[2] This method is not a substitute for a modified barium swallowing study, but may be complementary.

Esophageal manometry

If no obstructing lesion is identified by endoscopy or bolus challenge, an esophageal manometry should be done to complete the dysphagia evaluation. Esophageal manometry provides unique objective data on the motility of the pharynx and esophagus, including upper and lower esophageal sphincters. Documentation of dysphagia due to achalasia, scleroderma, diffuse esophageal spasm, nutcracker esophagus, or other disorders is possible only with manometry.

CONCLUSION

A complete history will confirm the existence of dysphagia and odynophagia, and suggest the etiology in most patients. Every patient with documented dysphagia and/or odynophagia should be examined by radiographic and endoscopic methods. A complete examination should include both methods since they are not mutually exclusive. Esophageal manometry is needed to identify motility disorders.

SOURCES OF INFORMATION FOR PATIENTS AND DOCTORS

http://www.patient.co.uk/showdoc/40024630/

REFERENCES

1. Corso MJ, Pursnani KG, Mohiuddin MA et al. Globus sensation is associated with hypertensive upper esophageal sphincter but not with gastroesophageal reflux. Dig Dis Sci 1998; 43:1513–1517.
2. Hiss SG, Postma GN. Fiberoptic endoscopic examination of swallowing. Laryngoscope 2003; 113:1386–1393.
3. Dray TG, Hillel AD, Miller RM. Dysphagia caused by neurologic deficits. Otolaryngol Clin North Am 1998; 31:507–524.
4. Edwards DAW. Discriminatory value of symptoms in the differential diagnosis of dysphagia. Clin Gastroenterol 1976; 5:49–57.
5. Castell DO, Katz PO. Approach to the patient with dysphagia and odynophagia. In: Yamada T, Alpers DH, Laine L, Owyang C, Powell DW, eds. Textbook of gastroenterology, 4th edn. Philadelphia: Lippincott, Williams & Wilkins; 2003:683–693.
6. Kim CH, Weaver AL, Hsu JJ et al. Discriminate value of esophageal symptoms: a study of the initial clinical findings in 499 patients with dysphagia of various causes. Mayo Clin Proc 1993; 68:948–954.
7. Wilcox CM, Alexander LN, Clark WS. Localization of an obstructing esophageal lesion. Is the patient accurate? Dig Dis Sci 1995; 40:2192–2196.
8. Connolly GM, Hawkins D, Harcourt-Webster et al. Oesophageal symptoms, their causes, treatment, and prognosis in patients with the acquired immunodeficiency syndrome. Gut 1989; 30:1033–1039.
9. Sonies BC, Baum BJ. Evaluation of swallowing pathophysiology. Otolaryngol Clin North Am 1988; 21:637–648.
10. Dooley CP, Larson AW, Stace NH et al. Double-contrast barium meal and upper gastrointestinal endoscopy. A comparative study. Ann Intern Med 1984; 101:538–545.
11. Parkman HP, Maurer AH, Caroline DF et al. Optimal evaluation of patients with non-obstructive esophageal dysphagia. Dig Dis Sci 1996; 41:1355–1368.
12. Wolf BS. Use of a half-inch barium tablet to detect minimal esophageal strictures. J Mt Sinai Hosp, New York 1961; 28:80–82.
13. Kelly JE. The marshmallow as an aid to radiologic examination of the esophagus. New Engl J Med 1961; 265:1306–1307.

Chapter 4

Chronic or recurrent abdominal pain

Ayman Koteish and Anthony Kalloo

INTRODUCTION

Whether acute or chronic, abdominal pain remains the most common chief complaint in gastroenterology and family medicine practices. The reporting of pain by patients, however, is highly subjective. Moreover, numerous psychosocial, neurophysiologic, anatomic, and pathologic factors influence the patient's presentation, thus accounting for a wide range of variability in the perception and reporting of pain.[1] See Chapter 22 for a discussion of acute abdominal pain.

WHAT IS IT?

When referring to abdominal pain or discomfort, several terminologies are worth defining as they are widely used and may have different implications.

Recurrent abdominal pain (or chronic intermittent abdominal pain) refers to situations where the patient has episodic attacks of pain and is entirely asymptomatic between attacks.

Chronic persistent abdominal pain can be attributed to conditions that can be positively diagnosed and to others where the diagnosis is one of exclusion. The latter includes **chronic intractable pain**, defined as undiagnosed abdominal pain of at least 6 months' duration despite adequate medical evaluation. Most of this chapter is focused on diagnosable causes of abdominal pain.

Dyspepsia is one of the most commonly reported symptoms, yet is nonspecific. In fact, dyspepsia is better considered as a symptom complex, because it encompasses a wide spectrum of individual symptoms, namely indigestion, heartburn, pain, or generalized abdominal discomfort. When reported as a symptom, dyspepsia refers to **persistent or recurrent abdominal pain** or **discomfort located in the upper abdomen**. Dyspepsia can be caused by a variety of disorders, and has been defined by several international and national expert committees (e.g., Rome II and the American Gastroenterology Association (AGA) guidelines). See Chapter 5 for a more detailed discussion of dyspepsia.

PATHOPHYSIOLOGY

Neurologic basis of pain[2]

Two types of nerve fiber are involved in mediating pain (i.e., nociception): unmyelinated C fibers and myelinated A-δ fibers. The majority of fibers are C fibers, located within the mucosa and muscularis of the gastrointestinal tract, on the serosal surface, and in the mesentery, that mediate mechanical, chemical, and thermal stimuli. C fibers transmit most of the painful stimuli from abdominal viscera, and relay sensation that is poorly localized, dull, gradual in onset, and longer in duration. The other group of fibers consists of A-δ fibers, which are mainly located in the mucosa (as well as skin and muscle, and respond to mechanical and heat stimuli (hence the name A-mechano-heat). These fibers relay sharp, sudden, and localized pain after an acute injury.

Cell bodies of these first-order C or A-δ neurons lie in the dorsal ganglia. **Second-order** neurons transmit information from the dorsal horn via the contralateral spinothalamic tract up to the thalamic nuclei, and to the reticular formation in the pons and medulla. **Third-order** neurons project from the pons to the somatosensory cortex, and from the medulla to the limbic system and frontal cortex (Fig. 4.1).

Anatomic basis of pain (localization of pain)

Localization of abdominal pain may be quite frustrating to patients. The difficulty is due to the fact that relatively few visceral sensory afferents enter the spinal cord at a given level. Moreover, one splanchnic afferent neuron may originate from multiple sites in the viscera. More importantly, however, a single first-order afferent may activate a large number of second-order neurons at the level of the dorsal horn, hence activating a large number of spinothalamic tract neurons and resulting in poor pain localization. Despite the imprecise location of visceral pain, a few facts are worth highlighting when evaluating a patient at the bedside:

- Because of the bilateral symmetric innervation of the gastrointestinal tract, visceral pain is most commonly located to the midline. When felt laterally, the ipsilateral kidney, ureter, ovary, or somatic structures may be the source, as they have unilateral sensory innervation.
- The site of perceived visceral pain corresponds to the spinal level of entry of the visceral afferent into the spinal cord. For example, afferents from the liver, biliary tree, pancreas, distal esophagus, stomach, and proximal duodenum enter the spinal cord between segments T5–T6 and T8–T11, resulting in pain between the xiphoid and the umbilicus.[2–5]

Somatoparietal pain

Contrary to visceral pain, which is dull and vague, **somatoparietal pain** is more intense and more precisely located, in part because innervation of different parts of the parietal peritoneum is unilateral. This type of pain is aggravated by movement and is caused by noxious stimuli to the parietal peritoneum. An example of the difference between the two types of pain is appendicitis pain. At first this tends to be vague and

NEURONAL VISCERAL SENSORY PATHWAY

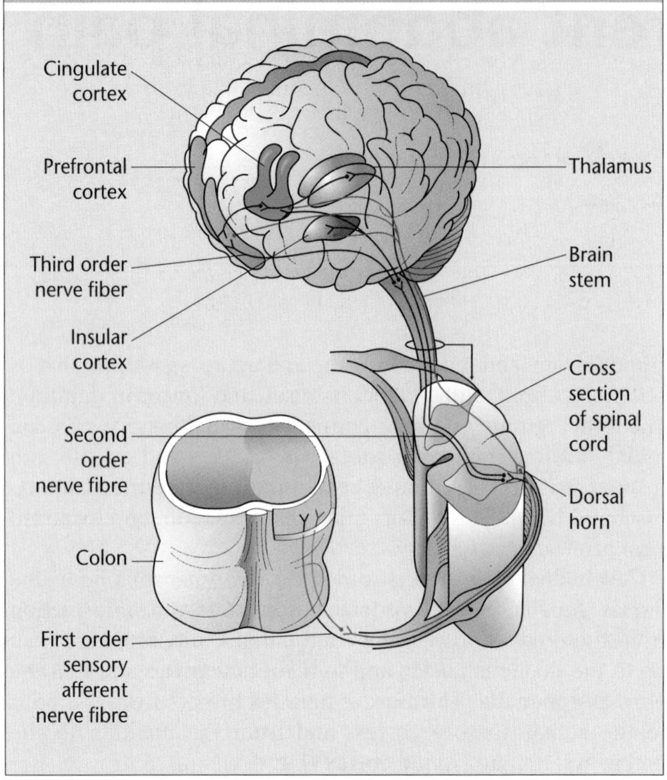

Fig. 4.1 Neuronal visceral sensory pathway. Schematic representation of first-, second-, and third-order neurons. Reproduced with permission from www.hopkins-gi.org.

periumbilical as a result of visceral inflammation, but is followed by a more intense pain, localized at McBurney's point, as a result of the inflammation extending to the overlying peritoneum.

Referred pain

Not only is abdominal pain poorly localized, it may also tend to be reported at sites far distant from the affected organ, thus giving rise to the concept of **referred pain** (Fig. 4.2). Referred visceral pain most commonly involves cutaneous dermatomes that share the same spinal entry level as the sensory visceral afferents. For example, gallbladder nociceptive stimuli enter the cord between T5 and T10; hence, cholecystitis pain may be perceived in the back, right shoulder, or right scapula.

CAUSES/DIFFERENTIAL DIAGNOSIS

The differential diagnosis pertaining to chronic abdominal pain is wide. One must therefore start by taking a good history and review of systems as well as performing a complete physical examination in order to identify the correct diagnosis. Categorization of chronic abdominal pain as intermittent or recurrent, or as persistent helps to orient the clinical investigation. These categories are not mutually exclusive as many entities or conditions may present differently depending on severity or stage of the illness (e.g., vasculitides, inflammatory bowel disease, early versus late malignancy).[6,7] Not uncommonly, however, the physician may fail to define an organic etiology for the pain despite adequate and extensive testing; this, in fact, characterizes functional disorders.

Chronic recurrent abdominal pain

CAUSES AND DIFFERENTIAL DIAGNOSIS
CAUSES OF CHRONIC RECURRENT ABDOMINAL PAIN
Irritable bowel syndrome (IBS)
Nonulcer dyspepsia (NUD)
Acute relapsing pancreatitis
Sphincter of Oddi dysfunction
Cholelithiasis
Diabetic gastroparesis
Radiculopathy
Intermittent intestinal obstruction
Inflammatory bowel disease
Chronic mesenteric ischemia
Musculoskeletal syndromes
Endometriosis
Familial Mediterranean fever
Acute intermittent porphyria
Nerve entrapment syndromes
Functional abdominal pain syndromes (FAPS)
CAUSES OF CHRONIC PERSISTENT DIAGNOSABLE ABDOMINAL PAIN
Chronic pancreatitis
Malignancy
Intra-abdominal abscess(es)
Somatoform disorders
CAUSES OF CHRONIC PERSISTENT UNDIAGNOSABLE ABDOMINAL PAIN
Irritable bowel syndrome (IBS)
Nonulcer dyspepsia (NUD)
Functional abdominal pain syndromes (FAPS)

Chronic persistent abdominal pain

Certain conditions can cause persistent abdominal pain for several months or more. The most common causes are malignancies, neuromuscular degenerative disorders, autoimmune or connective tissue diseases, infiltrative disorders, chronic pancreatitis, severe inflammatory bowel disease, history of abdominal trauma, and iatrogenic postsurgical complications.[8,9] In many patients the underlying cause of the pain is not curable. Treatment should therefore be aimed at decreasing the patient's suffering.[10] To improve patient survival, it is important, however, to make the distinction between malignant and nonmalignant processes.

Chronic undiagnosed abdominal pain: the functional abdominal pain syndrome (FAPS) (see also Chapter 1)

This entity is also referred to as chronic intractable abdominal pain. The International Working Team Committee has recently defined criteria to help diagnose FAPS. There is overlap between the definition of FAPS and that of irritable bowel syndrome (IBS) and nonulcer dyspepsia (NUD).[11–15] (See also Chapters 5, 13 and 64.) In fact, these entities may coexist in the same patient. It is important to note, however, that in contrast to the pain of IBS and NUD, which is intermittent, the pain of FAPS is constant and persistent. Although FAPS may occur in bouts lasting for hours to days to weeks, it is characterized by persistent residual pain between attacks. Patients do appear to have a higher prevalence of psychosocial disturbance, and frequently

BASIS OF REFERRED PAIN

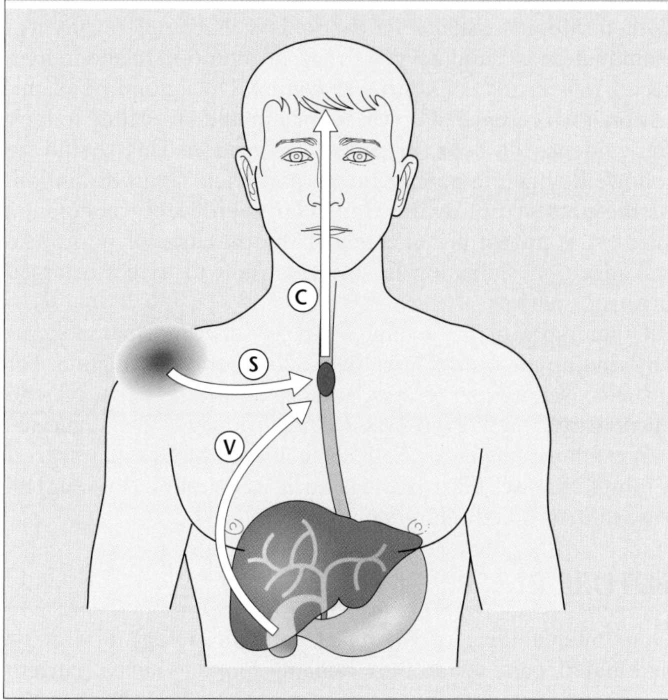

Fig. 4.2 Basis of referred pain. This figure illustrates the example of cholecystitis: visceral (first order) neuron afferents synapse with second-order neurons in the spinal cord at the same level as somatic afferent neurons from the shoulder (C3–C5). The cortex perceives the pain as if originating from the right shoulder. V, visceral first-order neuron afferents; C, second-order neurons in the spinal cord; S, somatic afferent neurons. Reproduced with permission from www.hopkins-gi.org.

emotional disturbance. Pain is a central feature of the patients' lives and is usually described in vague, nonspecific terms. It tends to be exacerbated by psychologic or social stressors, and is associated with a multitude of somatic complaints. FAPS does appear to be less common than IBS, but is nevertheless important to consider, as these patients utilize significant medical resources, are unresponsive to standard medical therapy, and have a high morbidity. Women constitute 70% of this patient population, and a history of physical and sexual abuse is not uncommon. Lack of weight loss and fever, in the absence of major or significant depression, is supportive of a diagnosis of FAPS. Table 4.1 gives management guidelines for patients with FAPS.

TABLE 4.1 MANAGEMENT GUIDELINES IN FUNCTIONAL ABDOMINAL PAIN SYNDROMES

- Gain the patient's trust
- Frequent visits
- Acknowledge existence of real disorder
- Minimize testing and focus on therapy
- Set goals of therapy
- Absence of cure
- Symptomatic therapy
- Encourage patient to cope and get back to functional social life
- Consider consultatory help from psychiatry, physical therapy, pain management clinic

Extra-abdominal causes of abdominal pain

This subgroup is more relevant to acute abdominal pain, which is covered in detail in Chapter 22. An example would be a herpes zoster attack[16] involving lower thoracic dermatomes that may be confounded with an acute cholecystitis attack.

DIAGNOSIS

History

The history is the most important clue to the etiology of abdominal pain. Consequently, several features of the pain are worth identifying to home in on the diagnosis.

Location

In chronic pain disorders, location tends to be less well characterized except in defined pathologies, e.g., sphincter of Oddi dysfunction. Examples of diseases according to the location of the pain are, for **right upper quadrant syndromes**, biliary disease (e.g., cholelithiasis, sphincter of Oddi dysfunction, cholecystitis, cholangitis, and gallstone pancreatitis); similarly, diaphragmatic, pulmonary (e.g., right lower lobe pneumonia), gastric, pancreatic, and intestinal disorders may also present with right upper quadrant pain. **Left upper quadrant pain** may indicate peptic ulcer disease, splenic rupture (more acute than chronic) or abscess (Table 4.2).

Pain quality

Certain conditions are associated with rather specific pain qualities. Whereas 'sharp or cutting' pain is characteristic of pancreatitis, 'crampy or rhythmically squeezing pain' is more typical of intestinal obstruction. Although renal and biliary

TABLE 4.2 LOCALIZATION OF ABDOMINAL PAIN

- **Right upper quadrant**
  Biliary colic
  Slipping rib syndrome
- **Left upper quadrant**
  Splenic abscess or infarct
- **Right lower quadrant**
  Ileitis
  Renal disorders
  Sacroileitis
  Iliopsoas syndrome
- **Left lower quadrant**
  Tubo-ovarian disorders
  Colitis
  Sacroileitis
  Iliopsoas syndrome
- **Epigastric**
  Peptic ulcer disease
  Pancreatitis
- **Diffuse**
  Inflammatory bowel disease
  Familial Mediterranean fever
  Acute intermittent porphyria
  Irritable bowel syndrome
  Nonulcer dyspepsia
  Functional abdominal pain syndromes

pain is described as typically colicky, obstruction of either organ may yield a rather constant pain. the pain of appendicitis, on the other hand, may be gnawing and dull.

Pain severity

It is easy to classify acute abdominal pain as severe, moderate, or mild. Chronic pain, on the other hand, is much more difficult to assess, as psychological factors play an important role in modifying pain perception. One must therefore resort to an indirect assessment of pain severity, i.e., whether the pain interferes with sleep or daily activities.

Aggravating and alleviating factors

The identification of pain-modifying factors may further help in the diagnosis and management of abdominal pain. For example, pain relieved by acid suppression points to reflux esophagitis, or peptic ulcer disease. Pain from pancreatitis, intestinal obstruction, mesenteric ischemia, and gastric ulcer is almost always exacerbated by food intake. Meal intake, on the other hand, may relieve duodenal ulcer pain. Body position may also impact abdominal pain: spinal hyperextension relieves irritable bowel pain, but exacerbates pancreatic pain, which is relieved by leaning forward in the sitting position. Moreover, the supine position exacerbates heartburn, which is relieved by an upright position.

Pain chronology

Changes in the nature of the pain (e.g., from intermittent to constant), in the time to reach peak intensity, as well as diurnal variation, provide valuable information that may assist in reaching a diagnosis. For example, pelvic pain at regular monthly intervals suggests endometriosis.

Associated symptoms

Nausea and/or vomiting commonly accompany abdominal pain. The temporal relation to pain may hint to the etiology: pain precedes nausea in patients with a disorder requiring surgery, but tends to follow nausea in nonsurgical disorders. When occurring early in the disease course, a fever may suggest cholangitis or a urinary infection. On the other hand, fevers that develop late in the disease course may implicate diverticulitis, cholecystitis, or appendicitis. Patients with familial Mediterranean fever, and those with connective tissue diseases, may have arthritis and/or pleuritis. Accompanying jaundice should suggest pancreatobiliary disorders. If anorexia and weight loss are prominent, one should suspect a malignant process. Fever may suggest intra-abdominal abscesses, autoimmune disorders, or malignancies such as lymphoma.

Physical examination

The examination should start by noting the general appearance and well-being of the patient. Severe pain is invariably reflected in the face, although this may be less apparent or nonexistent in patients with chronic pain. Moreover, restlessness with diaphoresis point to a more severe illness. Patients with peritonitis usually lie motionless. A complete physical examination is mandatory with special attention to abdominal, rectal, pelvic, and genitourinary regions. On abdominal examination, the presence of bowel sounds should be elicited to look for evidence of ileus, or bowel obstruction. This should be followed by gentle percussion for peritoneal signs, distention, or the presence of ascites. Muscular guarding (or abdominal rigidity) is an early indication of the presence of peritoneal inflammation. Palpation is also important to detect enlarged organs or masses.

Other parts of the examination are also indispensable, as any finding may provide valuable diagnostic information. For instance, scleral icterus and jaundice suggest hepatic, pancreaticobiliary, or hemolytic disease. Adenopathy with hepatomegaly may point to malignancy. Perianal fissures or fistulae may suggest Crohn's disease. Skin findings such as purpura may suggest vasculitis or an autoimmune process.

FUTURE PERSPECTIVES

Our understanding of the exact pathophysiology of chronic abdominal pain syndromes remains limited; hence, current therapeutic interventions remain modest at best. Despite the fact that our approach to these disorders should remain multidisciplinary, the ongoing trials for the development of drugs with multiple yet more specific sites of action in the pain pathway are quite promising. Newer drugs have been studied for the treatment of IBS, the newest being 5-HT_3 antagonists and 5-HT_4 agonists. These drugs have been shown effective in decreasing visceral sensitivity and pain. One would speculate that expansion of this work to target specific receptor types at one or multiple synapse levels (primary, secondary, or tertiary neurons, and/or centrally) may yield more pain relief with minimal side effects (e.g., alteration in bowel motility, or sedation, in the case of centrally acting drugs). On a different level, alternative therapies are gaining more attention. For example, hypnotism has been shown in randomized controlled trials to enhance coping mechanisms and reduce pain in patients with IBS. Therefore, an integrated multidisciplinary approach to manage chronic abdominal pain syndromes seems indispensable, and should inform the development of future therapeutic strategies.

SOURCES OF INFORMATION FOR PATIENTS AND DOCTORS

http://www.nlm.nih.gov/medlineplus/abdominalpain.html
http://unthsc-dl.slis.ua.edu/patientinfo/gastroenterology/symptoms/abdominal-pain.htm

Children:
http://www.aafp.org/afp/990401ap/1823.html

REFERENCES

1. Melzack R, Wall PD. Pain mechanisms: a new theory. Science 1965; 150:971–979.
2. Kalloo AN. Overview of differential diagnoses of abdominal pain. Gastrointest Endosc 2002; 56:675–680.
3. Leek B. Abdominal visceral receptors. In: Neil E, ed. Enteroceptors: handbook of sensory physiology, vol. 3. New York: Springer; 1972:113.
4. Yamamoto W, Kono H, Maekawa H, Fukui T. The relationship between abdominal pain regions and specific diseases: an epidemiologic approach to clinical practice. J Epidemiol 1997; 7:27–32.
5. Fields H. Pain. New York: McGraw-Hill, 1987.
6. Moawad J, Gewertz BL. Chronic mesenteric ischemia. Clinical presentation and diagnosis. Surg Clin North Am 1997; 77:357–369.
7. Poole JW, Sammartano RJ, Boley SJ. Hemodynamic basis of the pain of chronic mesenteric ischemia. Am J Surg 1987; 153:171–176.
8. Lankisch PG. The problem of diagnosing chronic pancreatitis. Dig Liver Dis. 2003; 35:131–134.
9. Evans JP, Cooper J, Roediger WE. Diverticular colitis—therapeutic and etiological considerations. Colorectal Dis 2002; 4:208–212.
10. Chambers PC. Coeliac plexus block for upper abdominal cancer pain. Br J Nursing 2003; 12:838–844.
11. Schwetz I, Bradesi S, Mayer EA. Current insights into the pathophysiology of irritable bowel syndrome. Curr Gastroenterol Rep 2003; 5:331–336.
12. Hoogerwerf WA, Pasricha PJ, Kalloo AN, et al. Pain: the overlooked symptom in gastroparesis. Am J Gastroenterol 1999; 94:1029–1033.
13. Vakil N. Epigastric pain in dyspepsia and reflux disease. Rev Gastroenterol Disord. 2003; 3(Suppl 4):S16–21.
14. Kurata JH, Nogawa AN, Everhart JE. A prospective study of dyspepsia in primary care. Dig Dis Sci 2002; 47:797–803.
15. Westbrook JI, McIntosh JH, Duggan JM. Accuracy of provisional diagnoses of dyspepsia in patients undergoing first endoscopy. Gastrointes Endosc 2001; 53:283–288.
16. Au WY, Ma SY, Cheng VC, et al. Disseminated zoster, hyponatremia, severe abdominal pain and leukemia relapse: recognition of a new clinical quartet after bone marrow transplantation. Br J Dermatol 2003; 149:862–865.

Chapter 5

Dyspepsia: ulcer and nonulcer

Paul Moayyedi

KEY POINTS*

- A noninvasive *H. pylori* test and treat strategy is as effective as endoscopy in the initial management of patients with uncomplicated dyspepsia who are less than 55 years old (A)
- A noninvasive *H. pylori* test and treat policy may be as appropriate as early endoscopy for the initial investigation and management of patients over the age of 55 years presenting with uncomplicated dyspepsia (C)
- Referral for assessment should be considered for those patients over 55 years old with uncomplicated dyspepsia whose symptoms persist after initial management with the *H. pylori* test and treat strategy (√)

*Based on SIGN Dyspepsia Guidelines[1]
Levels of evidence:
A: systematic review of randomized controlled trials (RCTs)
C: includes 2 RCTs
√: recommended best practice based on clinical experience of the guideline development group.
For full details relating to SIGN levels of evidence and grades of recommendation, please visit www.sign.ac.uk

INTRODUCTION

Dyspepsia is a hybrid word, derived from Latin and Greek meaning bad (*dys*) digestion (*pepsis*). The word was coined only a few centuries ago but references to dyspepsia have occurred since written records began. Diagnosis and treatment, however, remained empirical until the advent of radiology in the early twentieth century when it was discovered that ulcers were often not present on a barium meal or operation despite 'typical' ulcer symptoms. This led to the concept of X-ray negative dyspepsia or nonulcer dyspepsia and a new disease was born.

WHAT IS IT?

The definition of dyspepsia is controversial. Some definitions include all symptoms referable to the upper gastrointestinal tract including heartburn[2] whilst others specifically exclude patients with predominant heartburn.[3] The best example of the latter is the ROME-II definition (see Chapter 13),[3] which states that patients with dyspepsia have pain or discomfort centered in the upper abdomen for at least 12 weeks (although not necessarily consecutive) in the previous 12 months. In addition, there must be no evidence that dyspepsia is exclusively related to defecation or associated with change of frequency or form of the stool. Patients that have a normal endoscopy with pain centered in the upper abdomen are defined as having functional or nonulcer dyspepsia. This definition of nonulcer dyspepsia (NUD) is very useful for research purposes as it excludes patients with predominant heartburn and a normal endoscopy. Many of these patients have endoscopy-negative reflux disease and should not be included in NUD trials.

Definitions that include predominant heartburn should not be used to define NUD but can be helpful in undiagnosed dyspepsia. In this setting, patients often find it difficult to distinguish their predominant symptom and all-inclusive definitions can still be useful in clinical practice in the undiagnosed dyspepsia patient. In addition, they have a further advantage in that they allow guidelines to outline the management of all upper gastrointestinal disease rather than specific subgroups.

HOW COMMON IS IT?

Epidemiology

A review of the literature identified 14 studies reporting the prevalence of dyspepsia.[4] The reported prevalence varied between 13% and 48% but much of the variation was due to the definition of dyspepsia used. When Rome definitions were used the prevalence ranged from 13% to 28% with a mean of 21% (Fig. 5.1).

England and Wales Hospital Episode Statistics[5] suggest that of all patients presenting with upper GI disease in secondary care approximately 16% will have peptic ulcer disease with the remainder having either nonulcer dyspepsia or gastroesophageal reflux disease in about equal proportions (Fig. 5.2). The proportion of patients with peptic ulcer in primary care is likely to be lower as selection bias will inflate secondary care figures.

PATHOPHYSIOLOGY

Peptic ulcer disease

Peptic ulcers arise from damage caused by acid and pepsin on a compromised mucosal defense (see Chapter 35). An adherent mucous gel traps mucosal bicarbonate secretion to create a pH gradient between the lumen and epithelial cell. The apical membrane and paracellular junctions between gastric mucosal cells act as a specialized barrier to hydrogen ion diffusion. Furthermore, epithelial cells have basolateral transport systems that can remove excess hydrogen ions. The integrity of these defense mechanisms depends on mucosal blood flow and the impairment of this is thought to be of primary importance in acute stress ulceration.

The two main agents that compromise mucosal defense are *Helicobacter pylori* (see Chapter 34) and nonsteroidal anti-inflammatory drugs (see Chapter 25). *Helicobacter pylori* is

PREVALENCE OF DYSPEPSIA ACCORDING TO DYSPEPSIA DEFINITION

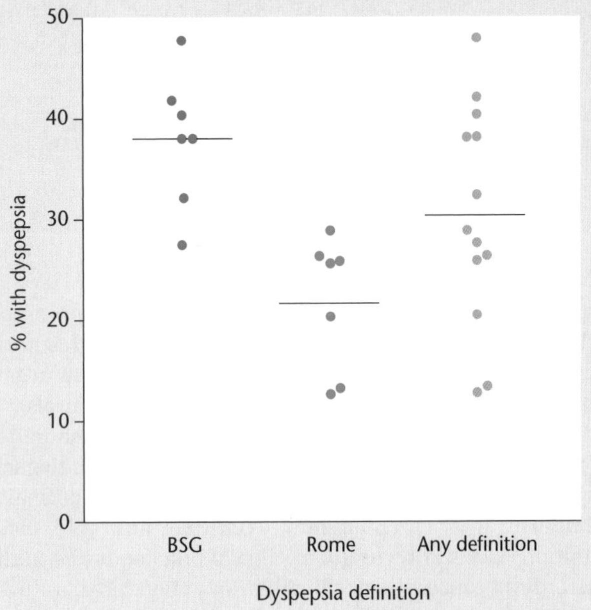

Fig. 5.1 Prevalence of dyspepsia. Prevalence of dyspepsia according to dyspepsia definition.

NON-MALIGNANT UPPER GI DIAGNOSES IN ENGLAND AND WALES

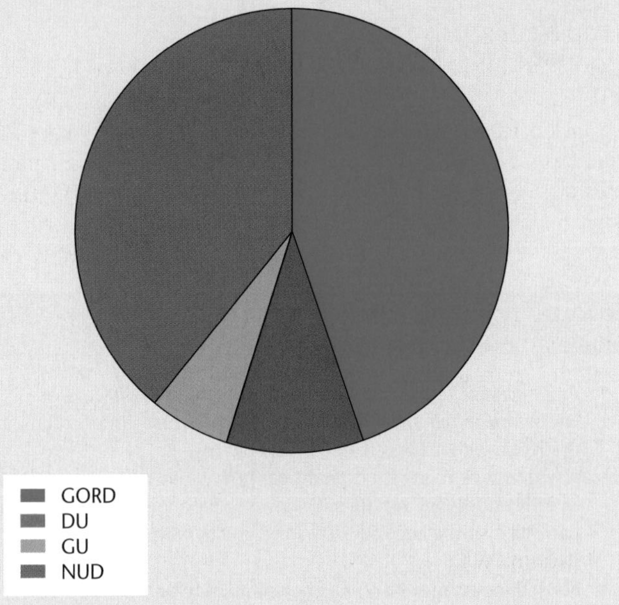

Fig. 5.2 Nonmalignant upper gastrointestinal diagnoses. Proportion of nonmalignant upper gastrointestinal diagnoses made in England and Wales 2002–2003. GORD, gastroesophageal reflux disease; DU, duodenal ulcer; GU, gastric ulcer; NUD, nonulcer dyspepsia.

most likely to cause duodenal ulceration when there is an antral predominant infection (Fig. 5.3). The antral inflammation causes a decrease in somatostatin production, which reduces the negative inhibitory effect on gastrin production. This leads to an increased gastrin production that increases parietal cell mass and acid output. The excess acid entering the duodenum causes the mucosa to undergo gastric metaplasia that can in turn be infected with *H. pylori*. The organism then causes inflammation, epithelial injury, and reduces duodenal bicarbonate excretion. This compromise to duodenal mucosal defense predisposes to ulcer formation. *Helicobacter pylori* is more likely to cause gastric ulceration if the infection is more evenly spread throughout the stomach. The pangastritis that results will cause inflammation of parietal cells and overall gastric acid secretion will be reduced. The inflammation will also impair mucosal defense and this can result in gastric ulceration even in a relatively hypochlorhydric environment.[6]

The distribution of *H. pylori* is predicted by environmental factors. When *H. pylori* is acquired soon after birth (particularly in the presence of poor nutrition) this will lead to the infection occurring throughout the stomach and predispose the subject to gastric ulceration. If the infection is acquired later in childhood when acid secretion is higher, *H. pylori* will reside preferentially in the antrum where less acid is produced. This will lead to an antral predominant infection and the subject will be at risk of developing duodenal ulceration. In addition, there are more pathogenic *H. pylori* such as cytotoxin-associated protein A (cagA) or vacuolation (VacA) toxin-producing strains that are more likely to cause peptic ulceration.

Nonsteroidal anti-inflammatory drugs (NSAIDs) (see Chapter 25) impair mucosal defenses primarily through inhibition of gastric and duodenal prostaglandin production. Prostaglandins protect the gastroduodenal mucosa by stimulating mucus production, increasing mucosal blood flow, accelerating cell proliferation, and enhancing cellular ion transport mechanisms.[7]

MECHANISM BY WHICH ANTRAL *H. PYLORI* INFECTION PREDISPOSES TO ULCERATION

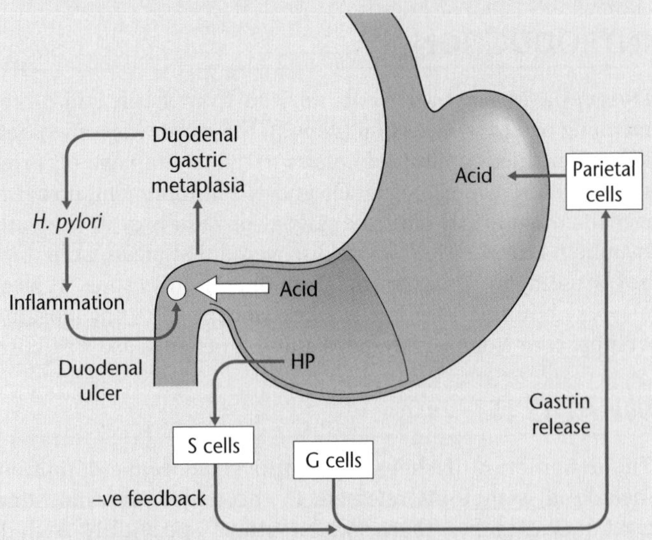

Fig. 5.3 Mechanism of *H. pylori* infection. Mechanism by which antral predominant *H. pylori* infection predisposes to duodenal ulceration. S cells, somatostatin cells; G cells, antral G cells

Rarely, excessive acid secretion alone can cause more distal duodenal ulceration as seen in Zollinger-Ellison syndrome (see Chapters 35 and 109).

Nonulcer dyspepsia

The pathogenesis of NUD is not as well characterized as peptic ulcer disease and is likely to be multifactorial (Fig. 5.4). Initial attention focused on gastric pH but most studies have found that basal and peak gastric acid is similar between NUD patients and asymptomatic controls.[8] It is possible that NUD patients have an increased sensitivity to acid as direct instillation of acid into the duodenum can reproduce dyspepsia is some cases.[9]

Many NUD patients complain of early satiety, nausea, and abdominal bloating, which suggest a disorder of upper gastrointestinal motility. Indeed, studies indicate that 30–70% of NUD patients have abnormal gastrointestinal motility. This includes delayed gastric emptying, gastric dysrhythmias, impaired accommodation to a meal, antral hypomotility, and duodeno-jejunal dysmotility.[10] The mechanisms that cause these abnormalities are uncertain but may relate to disorders of gastrointestinal parasympathetic or sympathetic function. Although abnormal gastric emptying is common in NUD patients there is a poor correlation between dysmotility and dyspeptic symptoms. This suggests there are other mechanisms that produce symptoms in NUD patients.

Studies have reported that NUD patients have heightened upper gastrointestinal visceral sensation compared to healthy controls and patients with organic disease.[11] Balloon distention of the stomach induces abdominal pain at lower pressures in NUD patients compared to controls whereas there was no difference in the perception of painful somatic stimuli.[12] It is unclear whether abnormal visceral sensation is due to disordered mechanoreceptor function or abnormal processing of the sensory information either at the spinal or central nervous system level.

Psychological factors are also likely to have a role in NUD. Patients with NUD have higher anxiety, depression, and hypochondriasis scores than healthy controls or those with organic disease.[13] In addition, these factors will make subjects more likely to seek medical attention if they have dyspepsia symptoms.

CAUSES

Peptic ulcer disease (see Chapter 35)

Helicobacter pylori is still the cause of most duodenal and gastric ulcers in most countries. The majority of the remaining ulcers are caused by NSAIDs with more rare diagnoses such as Zollinger-Ellison syndrome and Crohn's disease (see Chapter 54) each accounting for approximately 1% of the total ulcer burden. In areas with a low prevalence of *H. pylori* (such as parts of the USA and Australia where only 5% of young adults harbor the infection), peptic ulcer disease has become an infrequent diagnosis. In these areas, the relative proportion of ulcers caused by NSAIDs and rarer diagnoses will increase although the absolute numbers of ulcers attributable to these factors will remain unchanged.

Physical stress is an important cause of peptic ulcers that develop in a hospital setting, particularly in those admitted to intensive care. There is evidence of mucosal injury in the majority of intensive care patients with significant gastrointestinal hemorrhage occurring in 1–4% of cases.[14]

Nonulcer dyspepsia

The etiological factors in NUD are unclear. Dyspepsia symptoms resolve more frequently with *H. pylori* eradication compared to placebo in randomized controlled trials although the effect size is small in NUD.[15] It is possible that patients responding to *H. pylori* eradication have an ulcer diathesis but did not have an ulcer at the time of their endoscopy. A subset

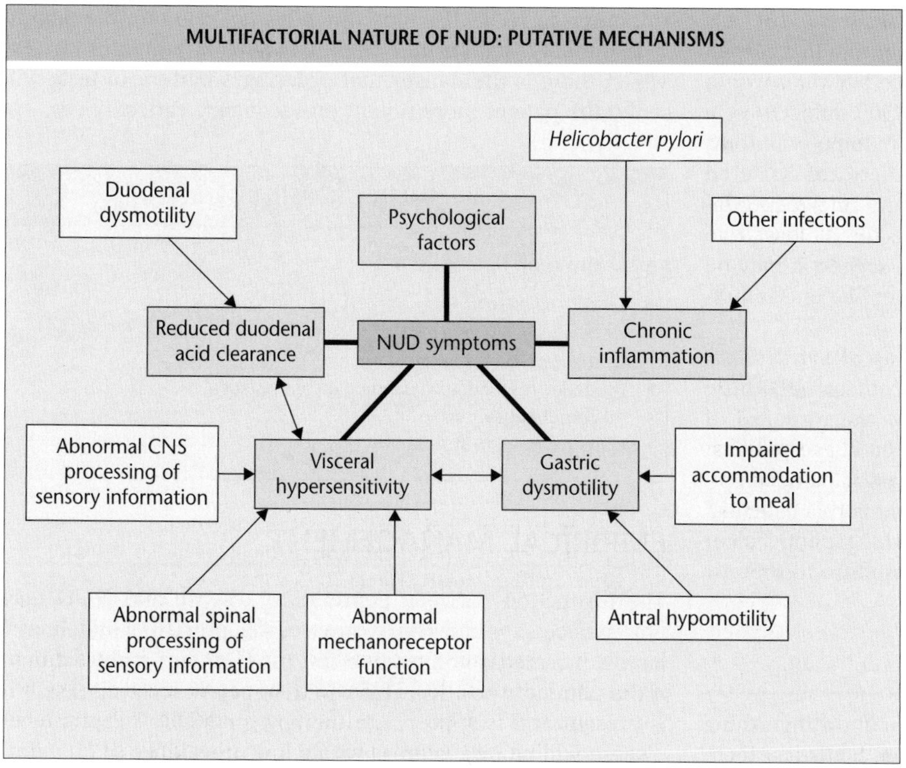

Fig. 5.4 Multifactorial nature of NUD. Multifactorial nature of NUD: putative mechanisms.

of NUD patients responds to proton pump inhibitor therapy,[16] although it is possible that these patients have atypical nonerosive gastroesophageal reflux disease.

NUD may be caused by an acute gastrointestinal infection in a subset of patients. One study suggested 17% of patients had clinical evidence of an acute infection followed by the abrupt onset of dyspepsia symptoms; however, there was no adequate control group in this study.[17] A significantly greater proportion of patients with presumed 'postinfectious' NUD had impaired gastric accommodation compared with other NUD patients.

CAUSES OF PEPTIC ULCER DISEASE

COMMON
- *Helicobacter pylori*
- Nonsteroidal anti-inflammatory drugs

UNCOMMON
- Stress ulceration*
- Crohn's disease
- Gastrinoma (isolated (Zollinger-Ellison syndrome), multiple endocrine neoplasia type 1)
- Mastocytosis
- Vascular insufficiency
- Herpes simplex type I
- Cytomegalovirus
- Chemotherapy induced
- Radiotherapy induced
- Idiopathic

* Uncommon in terms of overall population figures but common in intensive care units.

SYMPTOM COMPLEXES

Dyspepsia symptoms have been commonly divided into reflux-like, ulcer-like, and dysmotility-like. A cluster analysis of subjects in the general population would support the concept that certain symptoms cluster together more closely together than would be expected by chance. A re-analysis of 8505 subjects in a population-based dyspepsia study[18] suggests that the symptoms of nausea, vomiting, dysphagia, and early satiety are clustered together as are epigastric pain, heartburn, and acid regurgitation. There is therefore statistical evidence for at least two subgroups of symptoms although these data suggest it may be more difficult to differentiate those with ulcer-like and reflux-like dyspepsia.

Unfortunately, there is considerable overlap of symptoms[19] between the three subgroups and they appear to have little value in predicting endoscopic diagnosis or the response of symptoms to therapy.[20] It has therefore been suggested that the predominant symptom (heartburn, epigastric pain, or epigastric discomfort) should be used to classify dyspepsia patients.[3] The validity of this approach in distinguishing peptic ulcer disease from NUD patients or predicting response to therapy has yet to be prospectively tested.

DIAGNOSIS

Unaided clinical diagnosis is notoriously poor at distinguishing peptic ulcer disease from nonulcer dyspepsia. Statistical techniques such as logistic regression and discriminant analysis have been applied to a detailed history obtained by questionnaire. This approach initially showed promise in selected patients[21] but when prospectively applied to primary care patients the computer models did little better than chance.[22] Measuring the sensitivity and specificity at various cut-off points gives the area under a receiver operator curve (ROC). This was calculated at 61% (95% CI=56–66%) for the dyspepsia symptom computer model with an area under the ROC of 50% representing what would be achieved by chance alone.

In patients who require investigation, invasive tests are required to distinguish peptic ulcer disease from NUD reliably. Upper gastrointestinal endoscopy is the method of choice and has largely superseded barium meal examination. There is a paucity of literature on the accuracy of endoscopy in diagnosing peptic ulcer disease but it appears to have a sensitivity and specificity of greater than 95%. If a peptic ulcer is found it is important to test for *H. pylori* either by rapid urease test or histology and to reassess the history for any indication of NSAID intake. If the patient is *H. pylori* negative and is not taking NSAIDs it is likely that the initial assessment gave a false-negative result and the patients should again be tested for *H. pylori* with a urea breath test and/or serology. If this also confirms the patient is *H. pylori* negative, more rare causes of peptic ulcer disease should be evaluated.

Nonulcer dyspepsia is a diagnosis of exclusion, so by definition patients have had a normal endoscopy. In some cases, an abdominal ultrasound to exclude gallstones will be appropriate. Other tests such as an abdominal computed tomography (CT) scan and magnetic resonance cholangiopancreatography (MRCP) to exclude pancreatic pathology, small bowel meal to exclude Crohn's disease, or 24-h esophageal pH to exclude atypical reflux disease should only be carried out if there are other clinical features that suggest an organic disease is likely. Similarly, there is rarely a need for gastric emptying studies outside the research setting. In general, it is important to keep invasive tests to a minimum in NUD. If endoscopy does not reassure the patient it is unlikely that further tests will have any greater success whilst there is the danger that ordering a battery of tests will make the patient more reliant on secondary care services.

DIAGNOSTIC METHODS

- Gastroscopy

If clinically indicated:
- Ultrasound
- Computed tomography
- Magnetic resonance cholangiopancreatography
- 24-h esophageal pH
- Gastric emptying studies

EMPIRICAL MANAGEMENT

The distinction between peptic ulcer disease and NUD may not be necessary in primary care (see Chapter 26). Guidelines[23] have advocated a noninvasive test for *H. pylori* and treatment if the patient is positive. This will treat peptic ulcer disease if it is present and is appropriate therapy for NUD.[24] Peptic ulcer disease will be rare in areas with a low prevalence of *H. pylori* and empirical proton pump inhibitor (PPI) therapy may be the most cost-effective strategy for these populations (Fig. 5.5).

SOURCES OF INFORMATION FOR PATIENTS AND DOCTORS

http://patients.uptodate.com/topic.asp?file=digestiv/7283
http://www.patient.co.uk/showdoc.asp?doc=260

CURRENT CONTROVERSIES

- Relative cost benefit of 'test and treat' vs gastroscopy
- Definition of dyspepsia for patients, doctors and clinical trials
- Eradication of *H. pylori* in patients with no endoscopic abnormality
- Empiric treatment vs investigation

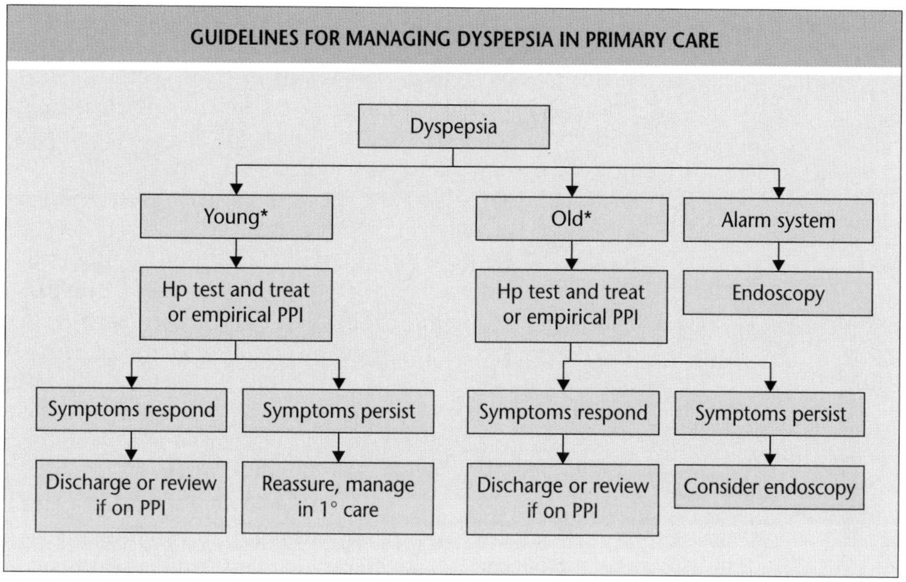

Fig. 5.5 Guidelines for managing dyspepsia in primary care. *Definitions of young and old depend on the local prevalence of upper GI malignancy. In England and Wales, young patients will usually be <55 years of age. PPI, proton pump inhibitor; Hp, *Helicobacter pylori*. (Adapted from Dyspepsia: managing adults in primary care. NICE guidelines, Department of Health, HMO London, UK, 2004. http://www.nice.org.uk, Copyright Scottish Intercollegiate Guidelines Network 2003.)

REFERENCES

1. Scottish Intercollegiate Guidelines Network: Dyspepsia, No 68, March 2003. http://www.sign.ac.uk
2. Management of dyspepsia: report of a working party. Lancet 1988; 1(8585):576–579.
3. Talley NJ, Stanghellini V, Heading RC et al. Functional gastroduodenal disorders. Gut 1999; 45 (Suppl 2):II37–II42.
4. Delaney B, Moayyedi P. Dyspepsia. In: Stevens A, Raftery J, Mant J, eds. Health Care Needs Assessment: The epidemiologically based needs assessment reviews, 3rd series. Oxford: Radcliffe Medical Press; 2004.
5. Endoscopic diagnoses after finished consulting episode. http://www.dh.gov.uk/PublicationsAndStatistics/Statistics/HospitalEpisodeStatistics/HESFreeData/fs/en; 2003.
6. Calam J, Baron JH. ABC of the upper gastrointestinal tract: Pathophysiology of duodenal and gastric ulcer and gastric cancer. BMJ 2001; 323:980–982.
7. Chan FK, Leung WK. Peptic-ulcer disease. Lancet 2002; 360(9337):933–941.
8. Jebbink HJA, Vanbergehenegouwen GP, Smout AJPM. Pathophysiology and treatment of functional dyspepsia. Scand J Gastroenterol 1993; 28:8–14.
9. Samsom M, Verhagen MAMT, vanBerge Henegouwen GP, Smout AJPM. Abnormal clearance of exogenous acid and increased acid sensitivity of the proximal duodenum in dyspeptic patients. Gastroenterology 1999; 116:515–520.
10. Thumshirn M. Pathophysiology of functional dyspepsia. Gut 2002; 51:I63–I66.
11. Camilleri M, Fried M, Thumshirn M. Visceral perception in gastroenterology. Gut 2002; 51:I1.
12. Thumshirn M, Camilleri M, Saslow SB et al. Gastric accommodation in non-ulcer dyspepsia and the roles of *Helicobacter pylori* infection and vagal function. Gut 1999; 44:55–64.
13. Whitehead WE. Psychosocial aspects of functional gastrointestinal disorders. Gastroenterol Clin North Am 1996; 25:21–34.
14. Fennerty MB. Pathophysiology of the upper gastrointestinal tract in the critically ill patient: Rationale for the therapeutic benefits of acid suppression. Crit Care Med 2002; 30:S351–S355.
15. Moayyedi P, Deeks J, Talley NJ, Delaney B, Forman D. An update of the Cochrane systematic review of *Helicobacter pylori* eradication therapy in nonulcer dyspepsia: Resolving the discrepancy between systematic reviews. Am J Gastroenterol 2003; 98:2621–2626.
16. Moayyedi P, Delaney B, Vakil N, et al. The effect of proton pump inhibitors in non-ulcer dyspepsia: a systematic review and economic analysis. Gastroenterology 2004; 127:1329–1337.
17. Tack J, Demedts I, Dehondt G et al. Clinical and pathophysiological characteristics of acute-onset function dyspepsia. Gastroenterology 2002; 122:1738–1747.
18. Moayyedi P, Forman D, Braunholtz D et al. The proportion of upper gastrointestinal symptoms in the community associated with *Helicobacter pylori*, lifestyle factors, and nonsteroidal anti-inflammatory drugs. Am J Gastroenterol 2000; 95:1448–1455.
19. Talley NJ, Zinsmeister AR, Schleck CD, Melton LJ. Dyspepsia and dyspepsia subgroups – a population-based study. Gastroenterology 1992; 102:1259–1268.
20. Bytzer P, Talley NJ. Dyspepsia. Ann Intern Med 2001; 134:815–822.
21. Horrocks JC, Lambert DE, Mcadam WAF et al. Transfer of computer-aided diagnosis of dyspepsia from one geographical area to another. Gut 1976; 17:640–644.
22. Bytzer P, Hansen JM, Schaffalitzky De Muckadell OB, Malchow-Moller A. Predicting endoscopic diagnosis in the dyspeptic patient. The value of predictive score models. Scand J Gastroenterol 1997; 32:118–125.
23. Dyspepsia: managing adults in primary care. NICE guidelines, Department of Health, HMO London, UK, 2004. http://www.nice.org.uk
24. Moayyedi P, Deeks J, Talley NJ, Delaney B, Forman D. An update of the Cochrane systematic review of *Helicobacter pylori* eradication therapy in nonulcer dyspepsia: resolving the discrepancy between systematic reviews. Am J Gastroenterol 2003; 98:2621–2626.

Chapter 6

Nausea and vomiting

Jan Tack

INTRODUCTION

Nausea and vomiting are frequently occurring symptoms, in the general population as well as in general practitioners' consultations and gastroenterological consultations.

- Nausea is the unpleasant sensation of the imminent need to vomit. The symptoms usually comprise epigastric discomfort as well as a generalized feeling of sickness.
- Vomiting is the forceful oral expulsion of gastric contents associated with contraction of the abdominal and chest wall muscles. Vomiting is usually preceded by and associated with retching.
- Retching is repetitive contractions of the abdominal wall without expulsion of gastric contents. Vomiting needs to be distinguished from regurgitation.
- Regurgitation is characterized by the effortless return of food back into the mouth, in the absence of contraction of the abdominal and chest wall muscles. Regurgitation is not preceded by nausea or retching and results from esophageal disorders like achalasia or severe reflux disease.
- Rumination is another entity that needs to be distinguished from vomiting. Rumination is characterized by the effortless regurgitation of undigested food after every meal. Although the mechanism is a transient voluntary increase in abdominal pressure, occurring during or soon after finishing the meal, the act is usually not conscious. Rumination is not preceded by nausea or retching and the food has no acid taste. The patient may spit out or re-swallow the food.

Two disorders frequently associated with nausea and vomiting are functional dyspepsia and gastroparesis:

- Dyspepsia is defined by persistent or recurrent pain or discomfort centered in the upper abdomen without evidence of organic disease likely to explain the symptoms.[1]
- Gastroparesis is characterized by delayed gastric emptying in the absence of mechanical obstruction.

DIFFERENTIAL DIAGNOSIS

Nausea and vomiting are controlled by the vomiting center in the medulla oblongata in the brainstem. A variety of stimuli can activate the vomiting center. Inputs to the vomiting center include vagal sensory pathways from chemo- or mechanoreceptors in the gastrointestinal tract, neural pathways from the labyrinth of higher centers of the cortex, intracranial baroreceptors, and the chemoreceptor trigger zone (CTZ), which is activated by a variety of drugs and toxins (Fig. 6.1).

Nausea and vomiting may occur as a result of several systemic and gastroenterological disorders. In spite of the long and varied list of potentially involved disorders, most causes of nausea and vomiting can be readily diagnosed on routine clinical grounds.

Gastrointestinal as well as extraintestinal infections may be associated with acute nausea and vomiting. Gastric or intestinal obstruction as well as a number of acute abdominal disorders may manifest themselves through or may be associated with nausea and vomiting. A number of substances, either given as drug therapy or accidentally ingested, may stimulate the chemoreceptor trigger zone. Extensive lists of drugs that may induce nausea and vomiting are available in the literature.[2] Several metabolic and endocrine disorders may also be associated with nausea and vomiting, which may sometimes be the presenting symptom.

Functional motor disorders are important causes of nausea and vomiting, and should be considered once organic disease has been ruled out. Gastroparesis and dyspepsia are the most important causes, but less frequent conditions like pseudo-obstruction syndrome, or the so-called cyclical nausea and vomiting, a rare idiopathic disorder characterized by acute episodes of nausea and vomiting, separated by intervening asymptomatic periods, may also occur. Postoperative nausea and vomiting may be in part related to the use of drugs in the perioperative setting, and in part to the associated derangement in gastrointestinal motor function. Finally, a number of central nervous system disorders and primary psychiatric syndromes may present with or be complicated by nausea and vomiting.

COMPLICATIONS

Loss of water and electrolytes, caused by severe and/or prolonged vomiting episodes, may lead to dehydration and hypokalemic metabolic alkalosis, mainly due to the loss of hydrochloric acid-containing gastric secretions. Profound hypokalemia may induce abnormalities of cardiac rhythm, and of skeletal muscle control.

CLINICAL APPROACH

As usual, history taking should identify the principal and associated symptoms, their course of onset, frequency, and duration. Careful history taking will allow the differentiation of vomiting from regurgitation and rumination, and will identify associated symptoms suggestive of reflux disease, peptic ulcer, obstruction, etc.

The timing and duration of the symptoms may help to indicate the most likely etiology. Nausea and vomiting of recent

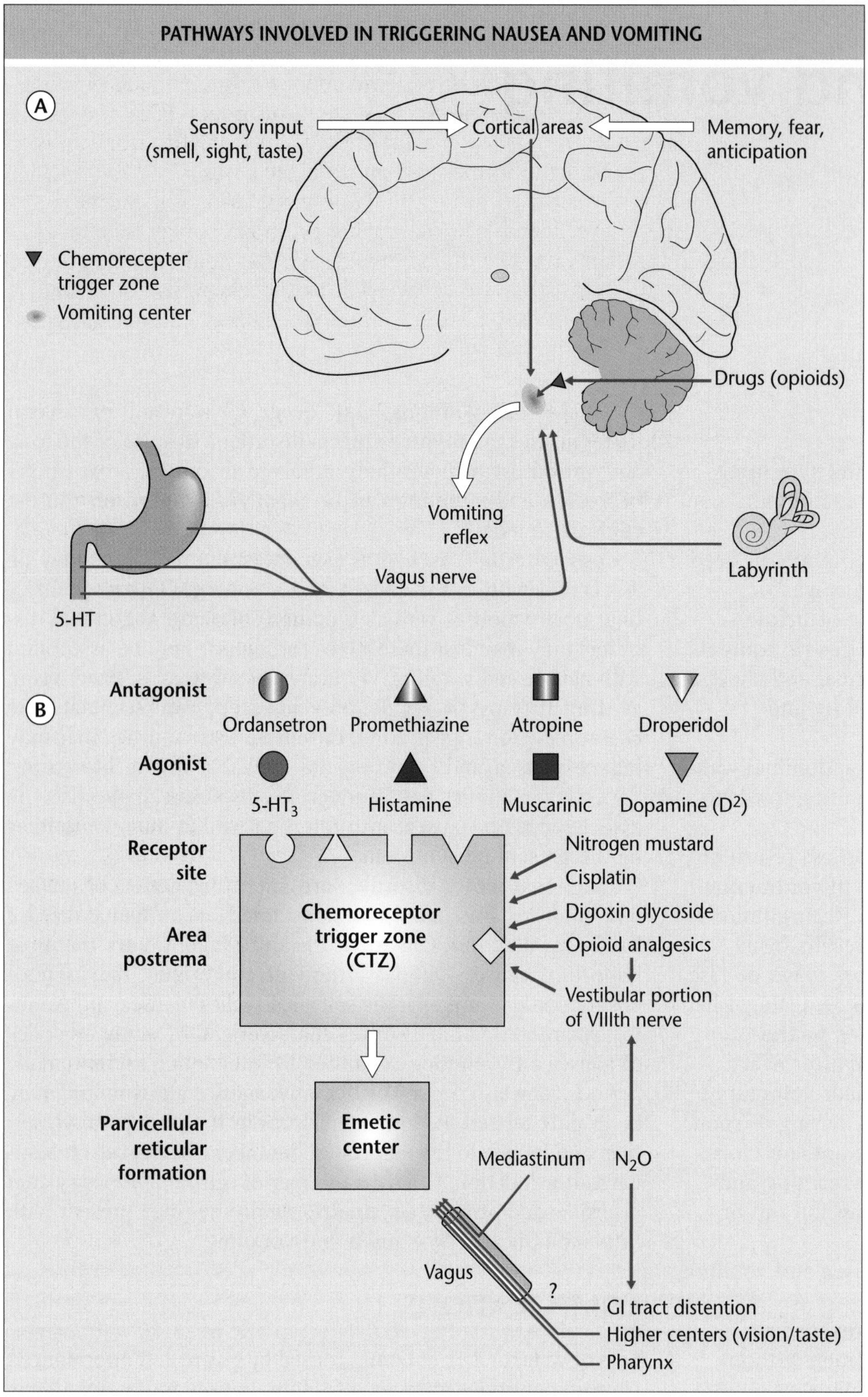

Fig. 6.1 Pathways. A, B. Pathways involved in triggering nausea and vomiting.

onset is most suggestive of an infectious cause (gastroenteritis), acute abdominal events (pancreatitis, obstruction), or drug-induced vomiting. The timing of vomiting may also provide clues to the underlying disorder. Early morning vomiting, before breakfast, is most suggestive of pregnancy, intracranial hypertension or uremia, or may be alcohol related. Late postprandial vomiting is most compatible with gastroparesis or obstruction, whereas vomiting that occurs during or immediately after food ingestion is more suggestive of a psychogenic cause. In adults, projectile vomiting, forceful and not preceded by nausea, is a sign of intracranial hypertension. Conditioned, 'learned' vomiting may lead to persisting symptoms once the acute cause has regressed, as shown in late chemotherapy-induced vomiting and after a transient organic disorder.[3]

The physical examination will look for signs that reveal the etiology of nausea and vomiting and will also assess signs suggestive of complications of nausea and vomiting. In addition, a neurological examination is indispensable as it may provide clues for a central nervous system cause for the symptoms.

Initial diagnostic evaluations will be aimed at identifying underlying causes suspected from the clinical evaluation, and ruling out peptic ulcer and obstruction. Routine laboratory testing will be done in all patients to assess the influence on blood electrolytes and in women of childbearing potential, a pregnancy

CAUSES
ORGANIC GASTROINTESTINAL DISEASES
• Peptic ulcer
• Mechanical obstruction
• Biliary colic
• Pancreatic tumors
• Secondary gastroparesis (diabetes, vagotomy, scleroderma, etc.)
• Peritonitis (cholecystitis, pancreatitis, appendicitis, etc.)
• Hepatitis
• Gastrointestinal ischemia
TOXIC OR DRUG INDUCED
• Ethanol
• Cancer chemotherapy
• Radiotherapy
• Miscellaneous drugs (analgesics, antibiotics, cardiovascular drugs, etc.)
• Miscellaneous intoxications
ENDOCRINE/METABOLIC DISORDERS
• Pregnancy
• Diabetic ketoacidosis
• Hyperthyroidism
• Uremia
• Addison's disease
• Parathyroid disorders
GASTROINTESTINAL MOTOR AND FUNCTIONAL DISORDERS
• Functional dyspepsia
• Idiopathic gastroparesis
• Chronic idiopathic intestinal pseudo-obstruction
• Idiopathic nausea and vomiting syndrome
• Roux-en-Y syndrome
• Cyclical nausea and vomiting disorder
POSTOPERATIVE NAUSEA AND VOMITING
CNS disorders
• Migraine
• Increased intracranial pressure (tumor, hemorrhage, infection, etc.)
• Seizure disorders
Labyrinthine disorders (motion sickness, labyrinthitis, Meniere's disease, etc.)
PSYCHIATRIC DISORDERS
• Psychogenic nausea and vomiting
• Bulimia nervosa

test is added. An electrocardiogram may provide additional information on the impact of electrolyte imbalance. The laboratory tests should include a screening thyroid-stimulating hormone measurement. The presence of hyponatremia may provide a clue to possible Addison's disease, especially if accompanied by hyperkalemia. Serum drug levels for patients on digoxin or theophylline may rule out or confirm drug toxicity-related symptoms.

In case of suspected severe underlying disease (e.g., obstruction), or in case of complications (e.g., dehydration, electrolyte imbalance), the patient will need to be hospitalized. In less urgent cases, additional investigations like endoscopy and barium X-rays may be performed on an outpatient basis. Where there is a readily identifiable or self-limited cause (e.g., drug adverse effect or viral gastroenteritis), removal of the cause and symptomatic treatment may be the only interventions necessary. In more complex cases, additional examinations are performed to rule out gastrointestinal obstruction (abdominal computed tomography scan (CT), small bowel X-ray, etc.), metabolic disorders (thyroid function, cortisol, pregnancy test, etc.) and central nervous system disorders (CT scan or magnetic resonance imaging (MRI)). A psychiatric work-up is required for refractory and unexplained cases.

In the absence of identifiable organic disorders and in the absence of identifiable underlying psychopathology, functional or motor disorders can be considered. The yield of performing motility studies is controversial, as the diagnostic yield and therapeutic impact of, for example, finding delayed gastric emptying, is limited.

ASSESSMENT OF GASTRIC MOTOR FUNCTION

Gastric motor disorders are often considered in refractory cases. The most popular test is the measurement of gastric emptying. Antro-duodeno-jejunal manometry can be considered in case of suspected generalized motor dysfunction, but the low yield makes this investigation debatable. Electrogastrography should be considered an experimental investigation.

Radionuclide gastric emptying is still considered the standard method to assess gastric emptying rate.[4] Solid and liquid emptying can be assessed separately or simultaneously. The solid and/or liquid meals are labeled with a (different) radioisotope, usually technetium 99m or indium 111 (^{111}In). The number of counts in a given region of interest (proximal, distal or total stomach, small intestine) is measured during a certain period of time after ingestion of a meal using a gamma camera. Correction factors for distance to the camera and decay of the isotope are taken into consideration. Mathematical processing with curve fitting allows calculating half emptying time, lag phase, and percentage of retention at different time points after the meal. Although not routinely used, the radioisotope technique also provides information on distribution within the stomach (proximal vs. distal). The disadvantage is the use of radioactive labels, its high costs and its poor level of standardization of meal composition and measuring times between different laboratories.

^{13}C breath tests are increasingly considered to be a valid and practical alternative to the scintigraphic emptying test. The solid or liquid phase of a meal is labeled with a ^{13}C-containing substrate (octanoic acid, acetic acid, glycin, or spirulina).[5–8] As soon as the labeled substrate leaves the stomach, it is rapidly absorbed and metabolized in the liver to generate $^{13}CO_2$, which is exhaled.[8] Breath sampling at regular intervals and mathematical processing of its $^{13}CO_2$ content over time allows a gastric emptying curve to be calculated. The advantages of this test are its nonradioactive nature and the ability to perform the test outside a hospital setting. Disadvantages are the absence of standardization of meal and substrate.

Antro-pyloro-duodenal manometry allows the investigation of mechanisms that are involved in the regulation of normal and abnormal gastric emptying. This is mainly a research tool, with clinical application in the investigation of generalized motility disorders including chronic idiopathic intestinal pseudo-obstruction (CIIP).

Cutaneous electrodes allow the electrical activity of the stomach to be measured. This so-called electrogastrography (EGG) provides information on frequency and regularity of gastric pacemaker activity, as well as changes in power of the signal after meal ingestion. EGG is largely an experimental tool.[9]

TREATMENT

Anti-emetic agents are often administered as a symptomatic treatment, regardless of the underlying cause. The principal anti-emetic drugs are dopamine receptor antagonists, antihistamines, and anticholinergic drugs.

Dopamine receptors in the area postrema are the target for anti-emetic drugs like:

- chlorpromazine;
- promethazine;
- haloperidol;
- metoclopramide; and
- domperidone.

The older dopamine antagonists of the phenothiazine (e.g., chlorpromazine, promethazine) and butyrophenone (e.g., haloperidol, droperidol) class have important central nervous system side effects such as sedation, drowsiness, orthostatic hypotension, and extrapyramidal symptoms.

Metoclopramide and domperidone are dopamine antagonists with gastroprokinetic properties and are therefore often used in gastroparesis- or dyspepsia-associated nausea and vomiting. They have less sedative side effects than the older dopamine antagonists. Metoclopramide often induces extrapyramidal symptoms, but domperidone, which crosses the blood–brain barrier poorly, is almost free from these adverse events. All dopamine receptor antagonists may induce hyperprolactinemia and galactorrhea.

Histamine1 receptor antagonists have central anti-emetic effects, but this is often associated with drowsiness. Drugs like dramamine or cinnarizine are mainly used in the treatment of motion sickness.

Anticholinergic drugs are not widely used in the treatment of nausea and vomiting because of lack of specificity and the occurrence of anticholinergic side effects. The only exception is the use of scopolamine in the treatment of motion sickness.

5-HT3 receptor antagonists, developed for the treatment of chemotherapy-induced nausea and vomiting, are more expensive and can be used as second-line drugs. They act on serotonin$_3$ receptors on the chemoreceptor-trigger zone and on vagal afferents. Examples of this class of drugs are:

- ondansetron;
- granisetron; and
- tropisetron.

The use of these drugs in nonchemotherapy-induced nausea and vomiting has been poorly studied.

Corticosteroids and benzodiazepines, both used in chemotherapy-induced vomiting, have no established application in other causes of nausea and vomiting. Cannabinoids have occasionally been used in refractory nausea and vomiting or chemotherapy-induced nausea and vomiting.[10] Tachykinin receptor antagonists are currently being evaluated for the treatment of chemotherapy-induced nausea and vomiting.[11]

Prokinetic agents are mainly used for the treatment of chronic nausea and vomiting resulting from gastroparesis or dyspepsia. Cholinomimetics like bethanechol have been abandoned for lack of specificity and cholinergic side effects. As described above, dopamine antagonists like domperidone and metoclopramide have gastroprokinetic properties and studies have established efficacy in gastroparesis and dyspepsia.[12–14]

Several studies have reported on the successful use of cisapride, a 5-HT4 receptor agonist, in gastroparesis and dyspepsia.[15,16] However, because of an enhanced risk of QT prolongation with cardiac arrhythmias, the availability of cisapride has been suspended.[17] Tegaserod, a new prokinetic 5-HT4 agonist, is currently under evaluation for the treatment of functional dyspepsia and gastroparesis.[18,19]

Short-term studies in diabetic and postsurgical gastroparesis have reported beneficial effects of treatment with the motilin receptor agonist erythromycin (3×250–500 mg).[20] This macrolide antibiotic acts as a motilin receptor agonist and has prokinetic properties. Attempts to develop macrolide prokinetics devoid of antibiotic properties have been disappointing.[21,22]

Gastric electric stimulation

Gastric electric stimulation (GES) with an implanted neurostimulator is an emerging therapy to treat patients with intractable nausea and vomiting and gastroparesis.[23, 24] However, the only controlled trial of this expensive treatment approach was of short duration and only partially convincing.[24] Until further data are available, GES should be reserved for refractory and incapacitating cases.

Nutritional intervention

Endoscopic placement of a percutaneous endoscopic feeding gastrostomy or jejunostomy may provide adequate calorie intake and some symptom relief but is not devoid of complications.[25]

Surgery

Although there are selected reports of favorable outcome, surgical treatment for refractory symptoms of gastroparesis and motility disorders has proven unpredictable and often disappointing.[23] Completion gastrectomy seems to provide benefit in refractory postoperative gastroparesis.

SOURCES OF INFORMATION FOR PATIENTS AND DOCTORS

http://www.nlm.nih.gov/medlineplus/nauseaandvomiting.html

Chemotherapy:

http://www.royalmarsden.org/patientinfo/booklets/coping/nausea.asp

REFERENCES

1. Talley NJ, Stanghellini V Heading RC et al. Functional gastroduodenal disorders. Gut 1999; 45(Suppl 2):37–42.
2. Quigley EEM, Hasler WL, Parkman HP. AGA technical review on nausea and vomiting. Gastroenterology 2001; 120:263–286.
3. Muraoka M, Mine K, Nakai Y, Nakagawa T. Psychogenic vomiting: the relation between patterns of vomiting and psychiatric diagnoses. Gut 1990; 31:526–528.
4. Harding K, Notghi A, Kumar DWD, eds. An illustrated guide to gastrointestinal motility, 2nd edn. London: Churchill Livingstone; 1993; 16 Radioscintigraphy: 228–241.
5. Ghoos YF, Maes BD, Geypens BJ et al. Measurement of gastric emptying rate of solids by means of a carbon-labeled octanoic

acid breath test. Gastroenterology 1993; 104:1640–1647.
6. Maes BD, Ghoos YF, Geypens BJ et al. Combined carbon-13-glycine/carbon-14-octanoic acid breath test to monitor gastric emptying rates of liquids and solids. J Nucl Med 1994; 35:824–831.
7. Braden B, Adams S, Duan LP et al. The [^{13}C]acetate breath test accurately reflects gastric emptying of liquids in both liquid and semisolid test meals. Gastroenterology 1995; 108:1048–1055.
8. Lee JS, Camilleri M, Zinsmeister AR et al. A valid, accurate, office based non-radioactive test for gastric emptying of solids. Gut 2000; 46:768–773.
9. Debinski HS, Ahmed S, Milla PJ, Kamm MA. Electrogastrography in chronic intestinal pseudoobstruction. Digestion 1996; 41:1292–1297.
10. Tramer MR, Carroll D, Campbell FA et al. Cannibinoids for control of chemotherapy induced nausea and vomiting: quantitative systemic review. BMJ 2001; 323:16–21.
11. Diemunsch P, Grelot L. Potential of substance P antagonists as antiemetics. Drugs 2000; 60:533–546.
12. Soo S, Moayyedi P, Deeks J et al. Pharmacological interventions for non-ulcer dyspepsia. Cochrane Database Syst Rev 2000; 2:CD001960.
13. Sturm A, Holtmann G, Goebell H, Gerken G. Prokinetics in patients with gastroparesis: a systematic analysis. Digestion 1999; 60:422–427.
14. Finney JS, Kinnersley N, Hughes M, O'Bryan-Tear CG, Lothian J. Meta-analysis of antisecretory and gastrokinetic compounds in functional dyspepsia. J Clin Gastroenterol 1998; 26:312–320.
15. Veldhuyzen van Zanten SJ, Jones MJ, Verlinden M, Talley NJ. Efficacy of cisapride and domperidone in functional dyspepsia: a meta-analysis. Am J Gastroenterol 2001; 96:689–696.
16. Corinaldesi R, Stanghellini V, Raiti C et al. Effect of chronic administration of cisapride on gastric emptying of a solid meal and on dyspeptic symptoms in patients with idiopathic gastroparesis. Gut 1987; 28:300–305.
17. Enger C, Cali C, Walker AM. Serious ventricular arrhythmias among users of cisapride and other QT-prolonging agents in the United States. Pharmacoepidemiol Drug Saf 2002; 11:477–486.
18. Tack J, Delia T, Ligozio G. A phase II placebo controlled randomized trial with tegaserod in functional dyspepsia patients with normal gastric emptying. Gastroenterology 2002; 122:A154.
19. Degen L, Matzinger D, Merz M et al. Tegaserod, a 5-HT4 receptor partial agonist, accelerates gastric emptying and gastrointestinal transit in healthy male subjects. Aliment Pharmacol Ther 2001; 15:1745–1751.
20. Janssens J, Peeters TL, Vantrappen G et al. Improvement of gastric emptying in diabetic gastroparesis by erythromycin. N Engl J Med 1990; 332:1028–1031.
21. Talley NJ, Verlinden M, Snape W et al. Failure of a motilin receptor agonist (ABT-229) to relieve the symptoms of functional dyspepsia in patients with and without delayed gastric emptying: a randomized double-blind placebo-controlled trial. Aliment Pharmacol Ther 2000; 14:1653–1661.
22. Talley NJ, Verlinden M, Geenen DJ et al. Effects of a motilin receptor agonist (ABT-229) on upper gastrointestinal symptoms in type 1 diabetes mellitus: a randomised, double blind, placebo controlled trial. Gut 2001; 49:395–401.
23. Abell TL, Van Cutsem E, Abrahamsson H et al. Gastric electrical stimulation in intractable symptomatic gastroparesis. Digestion 2002; 66:204–212.
24. Abell T, McCallum R, Hocking M et al. Gastric electrical stimulation for medically refractory gastroparesis. Gastroenterology 2003; 125:421–428.
25. Jones MP, Maganiti P. A systematic review of surgical therapy for gastroparesis. Am J Gastroenterol 2003; 98:2122–2129.

Chapter 7

Bloating and early satiety

Paul Moayyedi

INTRODUCTION

Bloating and early satiety are common symptoms that are often overlooked by clinicians. These symptoms can represent anything from benign functional disorders to severe organic disease.

WHAT IS IT?

The ROME-II working group (see Chapter 13)[1] have defined early satiety as 'a feeling that the stomach has overfilled soon after starting to eat, out of proportion to the size of the meal being eaten, so that the meal cannot be finished.' Abdominal bloating was described as 'a feeling of abdominal fullness; it should be distinguished from visible abdominal distention.' Thus, the definition of early satiety is closely related to meals whereas bloating is a sensation that may or may not relate to food. Furthermore, abdominal bloating can be subdivided into upper abdominal bloating and generalized bloating. The former can occur in isolation but is usually associated with early satiety whereas generalized abdominal bloating is a feature of irritable bowel syndrome and organic lower gastrointestinal disease. This chapter will focus on upper abdominal bloating and early satiety as a symptom complex.

HOW COMMON IS IT?

The prevalence of early satiety in the population has been reported to vary between 7.5% and 18% with bloating reported in the range between 11.5% and 31%.[2–4] There is a slight preponderance of women with early satiety (odds ratio (OR) = 1.6; 95% confidence interval (CI) 1.05–2.5) and a more marked female gender preference for abdominal bloating (OR = 3.5; 95% CI 2.5–4.8).[2] The ethnic and geographical differences in prevalence are poorly described.

PATHOPHYSIOLOGY

This is uncertain but is likely to be due to disturbed gastroduodenal motor and/or sensory function. Two-thirds of patients with early satiety have impaired relaxation of the proximal stomach.[5] The mechanism for generalized abdominal bloating may also relate to motor and sensory function rather than excess gas production but the precise mechanisms remain unclear.

CAUSES

Over 80% of the general population with predominant early satiety and bloating will have a functional disorder. The commonest organic cause of impaired gastric motor function is autonomic neuropathy secondary to diabetes mellitus. The commonest cause of mechanical obstruction is gastric malignancy. Early satiety as a secondary symptom to epigastric pain or heartburn may be due to peptic ulcer or gastroesophageal reflux disease. Generalized abdominal bloating is usually associated with irritable bowel syndrome or lactose intolerance but can be due to an obstructing lesion or an organic cause of intestinal motor impairment.

SYMPTOM COMPLEXES

Data on the overlap of early satiety, bloating, and other gastrointestinal symptoms are limited. We conducted an analysis of a large population survey[6] and found that in the 3234 subjects that had upper gastrointestinal symptoms, early satiety overlapped with heartburn and/or epigastric pain in 25% and was an isolated symptom in 12% of cases (Fig. 7.1).

CAUSES OF EARLY SATIETY AND UPPER ABDOMINAL BLOATING

- Functional
- Diabetes mellitus
- Pyloric stenosis
  - Gastric cancer
  - Peptic ulcer disease
  - Congenital
- Postsurgical
- Cachexia–anorexia syndrome
  - Tumor associated (e.g., carcinoma of lung, pancreas)
  - Anorexia nervosa
  - Human immunodeficiency virus
  - Parasitic diseases
  - Inflammatory bowel disease
  - Cardiovascular disease
  - Obstructive pulmonary disease
- Hypothyroidism
- Hypokalemia
- Drugs
  - Opioid analgesics
  - Anticholinergics
  - Levodopa
  - α-adrenergic agonists
- Amyloidosis
- Progressive systemic sclerosis
- Autonomic degeneration
- Brain stem tumor
- Spinal cord injury

OVERLAP BETWEEN HEARTBURN, EPIGASTRIC PAIN AND EARLY SATIETY

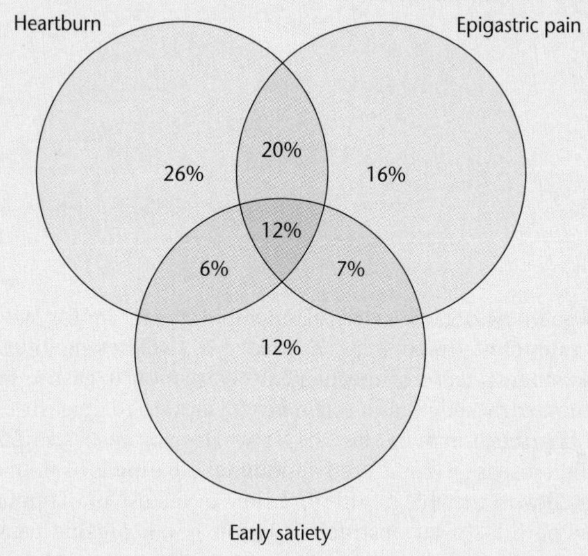

Fig. 7.1 Overlap of gastrointestinal symptoms. Overlap between heartburn, epigastric pain, and early satiety in 3234 subjects from the general population with upper gastrointestinal symptoms. Figures do not add up to 100% due to rounding errors.

DIAGNOSIS

Diagnostic tests, if needed to exclude serious underlying pathology, may include:

- blood tests to assess biochemical and endocrine abnormalities;
- endoscopy to exclude malignant or other mechanical obstruction; and
- gastric emptying studies to delineate the problem objectively in patients with severe symptoms.

DIAGNOSTIC METHODS
• Full blood count • Urea and electrolytes • Blood sugar • Thyroid function tests • Barium meal • Upper gastrointestinal endoscopy • Gastric emptying studies • Scintigraphy • Ultrasound • ^{13}C-Octanoic breath test

SOURCES OF INFORMATION FOR PATIENTS AND DOCTORS

http://www.patient.co.uk/showdoc/40000086/
http://patients.uptodate.com/frames.asp?page=topic.asp&file=digestiv/7452-33k
http://www.gastro.org/clinicalRes/brochures/gas.html
http://www.medicinenet.com/intestinal_gas_belching_bloating_flatulence/article.html

REFERENCES

1. Talley NJ, Stanghellini V, Heading RC et al. Functional gastroduodenal disorders. Gut 1999; 45 (Suppl 2):II37–II42.
2. Talley NJ, Boyce P, Jones M. Identification of distinct upper and lower gastrointestinal symptom groupings in an urban population. Gut 1998; 42:690–695.
3. Tougas G, Chen Y, Hwang P, Liu MM, Eggleston A. Prevalence and impact of upper gastrointestinal symptoms in the Canadian population: findings from the DIGEST study. Domestic/International Gastroenterology Surveillance Study. Am J Gastroenterol 1999; 94:2845–2854.
4. Stanghellini V. Three-month prevalence rates of gastrointestinal symptoms and the influence of demographic factors: results from the Domestic/International Gastroenterology Surveillance Study (DIGEST). Scand J Gastroenterol 1999; Supplement 231:20–28.
5. Tack J, Piessevaux H, Coulie B, Caenepeel P, Janssens J. Role of impaired gastric accommodation to a meal in functional dyspepsia. Gastroenterology 1998; 115:1346–1352.
6. Moayyedi P, Forman D, Braunholtz D et al. The proportion of upper gastrointestinal symptoms in the community associated with *Helicobacter pylori*, lifestyle factors and non-steroidal anti-inflammatory drugs. Am J Gastroenterol 2000; 95:1448–1455.

Chapter 8

Belching and rumination

Alexander C Ford and Paul Moayyedi

INTRODUCTION

Belching is a normal phenomenon in humans. Perceived disorders are usually benign in nature and arise from either an inability to belch or an excess of belching. Rumination is a disorder of gastroesophageal function and was first described in the seventeenth century by the Italian Fabricius ab Aquapendente.

WHAT IS IT?

Belching is the expulsion of gas from the stomach via the mouth whilst retaining semi-solid and fluid material. Individual differences in ease of eructation make the definition of abnormality difficult. Rumination also requires the regurgitation of stomach contents but, unlike belching, solids and gas are not distinguished. Recently ingested food is effortlessly regurgitated, with subsequent remastication and swallowing or ejection of the regurgitant, often depending on the social situation.

HOW COMMON IS IT?

Disorders of belching are commonly associated with non-organic gastrointestinal diseases, such as functional dyspepsia and aerophagia. In a community survey of 8351 subjects, excessive belching was reported in 17% with a similar frequency in males and females. Rumination is well described in infants and mentally impaired adults. More recently, it has been recognized to occur in adults of normal intelligence. Limited reporting by patients and lack of recognition by physicians make the true prevalence of this disorder difficult to estimate.

PATHOPHYSIOLOGY

The belch reflex is a normal physiological process. The sequence of events begins with transient relaxation of the lower esophageal sphincter in response to gaseous distention of the stomach. This allows a common cavity to be established between the stomach and the esophagus, causing pressure equalization and gastroesophageal reflux of gas. At this point the individual feels no impulse to belch, and gas that is confined to the distal esophagus tends to be returned to the stomach by secondary peristalsis. If, however, the proximal esophagus is distended with gas there is relaxation of the upper esophageal sphincter, and this is when the individual becomes aware of a need to belch. The result is esophago-pharyngeal gas reflux. The process is thought to be vagally mediated. The pathophysiology of rumination is poorly understood. There are two main theories to explain the phenomenon: the first suggests lower esophageal sphincter relaxation and increased intra-abdominal pressure cause retropulsion of the gastric contents; and the second suggests that it is a learned adaptation of the belch reflex.

CAUSES

The causes of disorders of belching can be divided into two categories. The gastric hypersensitivity described in some patients with functional dyspepsia is consistently associated with belching.[1] It is also described in gastroesophageal reflux disease, presumably because of the transient relaxations of the lower esophageal sphincter that occur in this condition. Aerophagia is an unusual, benign disorder in which there is a repetitive pattern of swallowing air and belching. Inability to belch is well recognized in achalasia, and can also occur as a result of anti-reflux surgery, when it is known as the 'gas-bloat' syndrome. Rumination occurs in several organic and psychiatric diseases, but can also occur in isolation when it is referred to as rumination syndrome. This is associated in some patients with abnormalities of gastroesophageal function including a low pressure and an ability to prolapse the valve back into the esophagus.[2–4]

SYMPTOM COMPLEXES

Frequent belching occurs as part of the symptom complex of dyspepsia, either organic or functional. From a large cross-sectional survey of gastrointestinal symptoms in the community of the 3234 individuals who described upper gastrointestinal symptoms[5] belching overlapped with heartburn and/or epigastric pain in 30% and occurred as an isolated symptom in 15% (Fig. 8.1).

DIAGNOSIS

The diagnosis of disordered belching may be difficult, largely because of the uncertainty in defining the threshold when a normal phenomenon becomes pathological. If there is any suspicion of an underlying organic cause for the symptom then upper gastrointestinal investigation is warranted in the form of endoscopy, and pH and manometric assessment. Aerophagia is usually a clinical diagnosis based on observation of air swallowing by the patient.[6] Similarly, the exclusion of structural causes in patients with rumination may be required. The diagnosis of rumination syndrome can be made on clinical grounds alone, but can be confirmed by manometric studies of esophagus, stomach, and small intestine. These often reveal the occurrence of 'pressure spikes' (R waves) at all levels below the esophagus due to increased intra-abdominal pressure, which are synchronous with episodes of rumination.[2]

OVERLAP BETWEEN HEARTBURN, EPIGASTRIC PAIN AND BELCHING

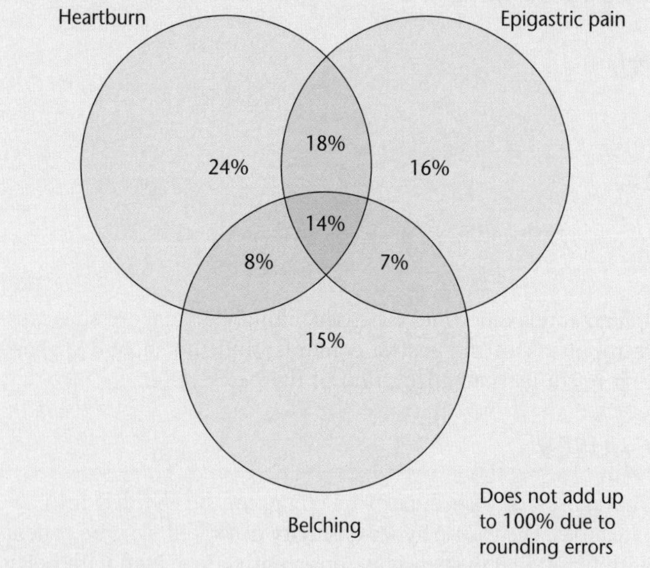

Fig. 8.1 Overlap of upper gastrointestinal symptoms. Overlap between heartburn, epigastric pain, and belching in 3234 subjects from the general population with upper gastrointestinal symptoms.

SOURCES OF INFORMATION FOR PATIENTS AND DOCTORS

http://patients.uptodate.com/topic.asp?file=digestiv/7452
Halitosis:
http://www.findarticles.com/p/articles/mi_m3225/is_n3_v53/ai_18134917

CAUSES

CAUSES OF DISORDERED BELCHING

- Increased belching:
  dyspepsia
  gastroesophageal reflux disease
  aerophagia
- Inability to belch:
  achalasia
  'gas-bloat' syndrome

CAUSES OF RUMINATION

- Pharyngeal:
  pharyngeal pouch
- Esophageal:
  abnormal gastroesophageal sphincter function
  esophageal stricture
  achalasia
- Gastric:
  hiatus hernia
  gastric outlet obstruction
  gastroparesis
- Neurological:
  hydrocephalus
  tumor
- Psychiatric:
  bulimia nervosa
  anorexia nervosa
- Functional:
  nonulcer dyspepsia
  psychogenic vomiting
- Drugs:
  neuroleptics

REFERENCES

1. Tack J, Caenepeel P, Fischler B, Piessevux H, Janssens J. Symptoms associated with hypersensitivity to gastric distension in functional dyspepsia. Gastroenterology 2001; 121:528–535.
2. Clouse RE, Richter JE, Heading RC, Janssens J, Wilson JA. Functional oesophageal disorders. Gut 1999; 45 (Suppl 2):II31–II36.
3. Thumshirn M, Camilleri M, Hanson RB et al. Gastric mechanosensory and lower esophageal sphincter function in rumination syndrome. Am J Physiol 1998; 275:G314–321.
4. Hasler WL. New insights into the pathogenesis of rumination: what's coming up next? Gastroenterology 1999; 116:1006–1008.
5. Moayyedi P, Forman D, Braunholtz D et al. The proportion of upper gastrointestinal symptoms in the community associated with *Helicobacter pylori*, lifestyle and non-steroidal anti-inflammatory drugs. Am J Gastroenterol 2000; 95:1448–1455.
6. Talley NJ, Stanghellini V, Heading RC et al. Functional gastroduodenal disorders. Gut 1999; 45 (Suppl 2):II37–II42.

Chapter 9

Diarrhea

Matthew R Banks and Michael J G Farthing

INTRODUCTION

Diarrhea is responsible for the deaths of several million people each year worldwide. Although acute infectious diarrhea is by far the most common clinical problem, chronic diarrhea presents the clinician with complex diagnostic and therapeutic challenges.

WHAT IS IT?

The formal definition of diarrhea requires that the daily stool output exceeds 200 g for adults in the developed world and up to 400 g in the developing world. However, there is great variability between individuals and an increase from the normal average stool weight or passage of two or more loose stools per day can be used most often to define diarrhea. The differentiation between acute and chronic diarrhea is often arbitrary: a cutoff of 14 days may be used. Bloody diarrhea, often termed 'dysentery,' suggests severe intestinal inflammation resulting in ulcer formation and subsequent bleeding.

Fecal urgency, a reflection of abnormal rectal physiology or sensation (see Chapter 66), is often wrongly described as 'diarrhea.'

HOW COMMON IS IT?

In the developing world diarrhea is one of the principal causes of morbidity and mortality among children. Although there has been a decline over the past 40 years, 2.5 million children still died from diarrheal disease annually in the 1990s.[1] The incidence of diarrhea is highest amongst children aged 6–11 months, who experience a median of 4.8 episodes of diarrhea per year, with the incidence falling progressively to 1.4 episodes per year in 4-year-olds. Although far less common in affluent countries, diarrhea still remains one of the two most common reasons for emergency attendance.

PATHOPHYSIOLOGY

The intestine functions as both a secretory and an absorptive organ; 10 litres of fluid enter the small intestine each day by mouth and from secretions from salivary glands, stomach, pancreas, and bile ducts, as well as the small intestine. Approximately 7.5 litres are absorbed in the small intestine and the remainder is absorbed by the colon, with less than 200 mL constituting normal stool volume. Broadly speaking, the majority of intestinal fluid secretion occurs in the crypts, whereas absorption occurs in the villi (Fig. 9.1).

Four processes can cause diarrhea: secretion, inhibition of absorption, osmotic agents, and increased intestinal motility. Most diarrhea is, however, multifactorial, with overlap of these four different pathophysiologic processes.

Active secretion

Stimulation of active intestinal secretion occurs as a result of secretagogues which bind to the enterocyte and activate three principal second messengers – cyclic AMP, cyclic GMP, and calcium – to cause the opening of apical (luminal) chloride channels and the induction of a phosphorylation cascade, resulting in active secretion of chloride ions. This is followed by the passive transport of sodium and water.

Pro-secretory agents include bacterial enterotoxins, hormones such as serotonin (5-hydroxytryptamine; 5-HT), many inflammatory mediators including histamine and prostaglandin E_2, and bile acids (Fig. 9.1).

Vibrio cholera produces an enterotoxin that causes diarrhea both by direct actions on enterocytes and also through activation of the enteric nervous system.[2] Once bound to the enterocytes, cholera toxin causes the release of serotonin to activate sensory neurons and initiate an excitatory neural cascade, culminating in the release of secretomotor neuropeptides such as vasoactive intestinal peptide and stimulating enterocyte secretion.

Inhibition of absorption

Many secretagogues also directly inhibit the enterocyte absorption, as does the activation of inhibitory neural secretory reflexes. Diarrhea can result from a reduced absorptive surface, with villus atrophy induced by celiac disease or infection with *Giardia lamblia* (Fig. 9.2) or following intestinal resection. Patients with less than 100 cm of small intestine experience persistent diarrhea (see Chapter 45).

Osmotic diarrhea

Nonabsorbed or poorly absorbed aqueous solutes increase the osmotic potential of the intestinal lumen (Fig. 9.3), attenuate the absorption and promote the passive inward movement of fluid and electrolytes. Osmotic solutes may be ingested (e.g., lactulose and sorbitol) or accumulate because of villus atrophy or lactase deficiency, with increased luminal carbohydrate.

Altered intestinal motility

Increasing intestinal transit with pro-motility agents such as erythromycin reduces the intestinal capacity to absorb, thus leading to diarrhea. Conversely, ineffective peristalsis due to autonomic neuropathy or systemic sclerosis promotes

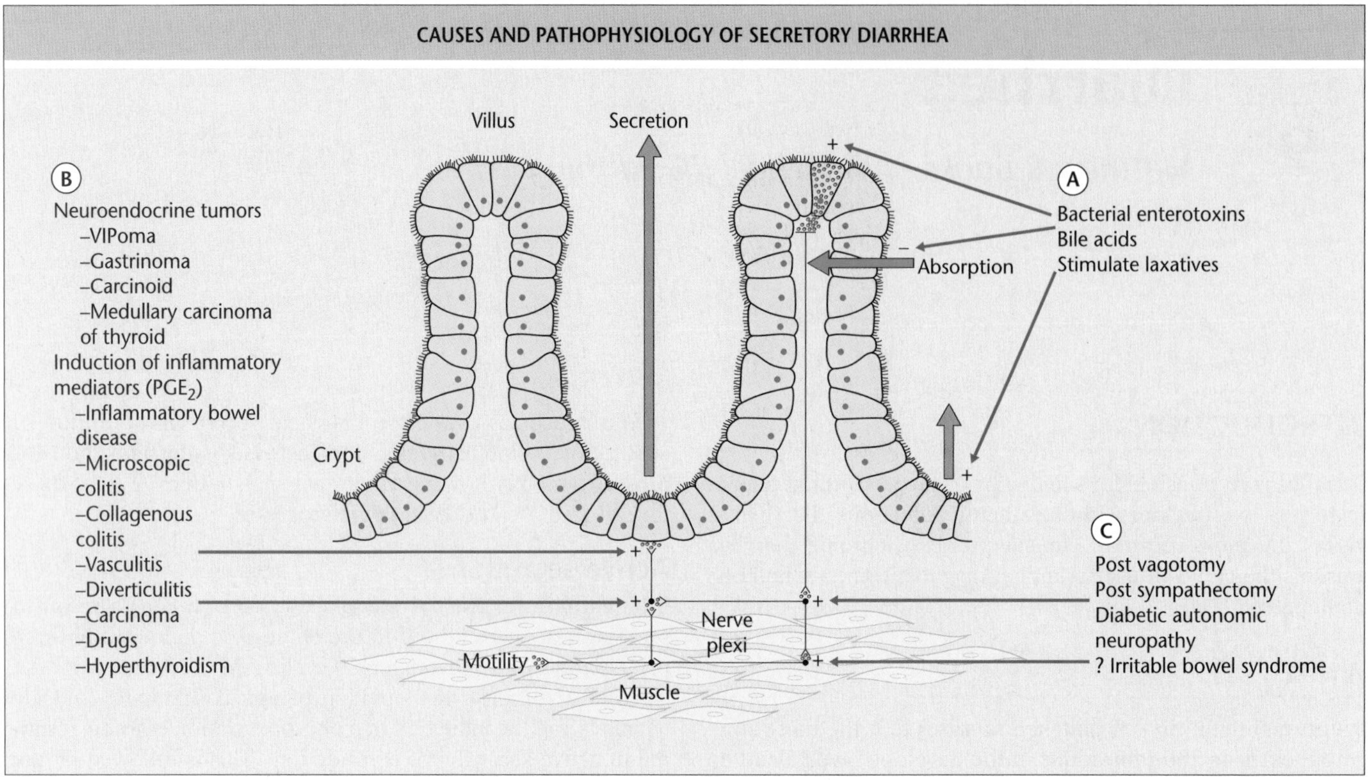

Fig. 9.1 Causes and pathophysiology of secretory diarrhea. A. Luminal secretagogs bind to the epithelium and induce secretion and inhibit absorption either directly or indirectly through the activation of nerve circuits. **B.** Mural secretagogues may induce secretion by binding to the serosal surface of the epithelium or activating the secretomotor nerves. These include intestinal hormones such as vasoactive intestinal peptide (VIP) and inflammatory mediators such as prostaglandin E_2 and histamine. **C.** Functioning of the enteric nervous system can be influenced by surgery, neuropathy, and possibly irritable bowel syndrome, such that secretion is augmented and motility altered.

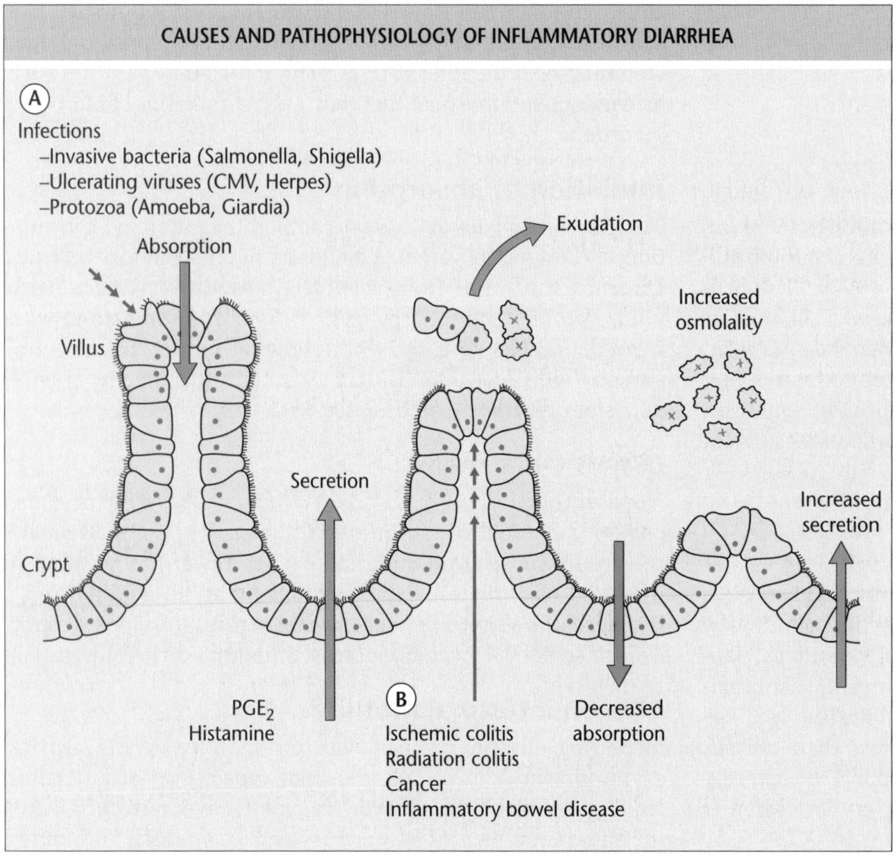

Fig. 9.2 Causes and pathophysiology of inflammatory diarrhea. Destruction of the intestinal mucosa with loss of villi. Luminal invasive infections **(A)** and intrinsic causes of intestinal inflammation **(B)** result in cell apoptosis. This process favors secretion through three mechanisms: (1) villus destruction reduces the absorptive capacity of the intestine and causes malabsorption and an increase in luminal osmolality; (2) cell exudation further increases the luminal osmolality; (3) immune recruitment of inflammatory mediators such as prostaglandin E_2 and histamine induces active secretion directly and through intermediate neural and cellular pathways.

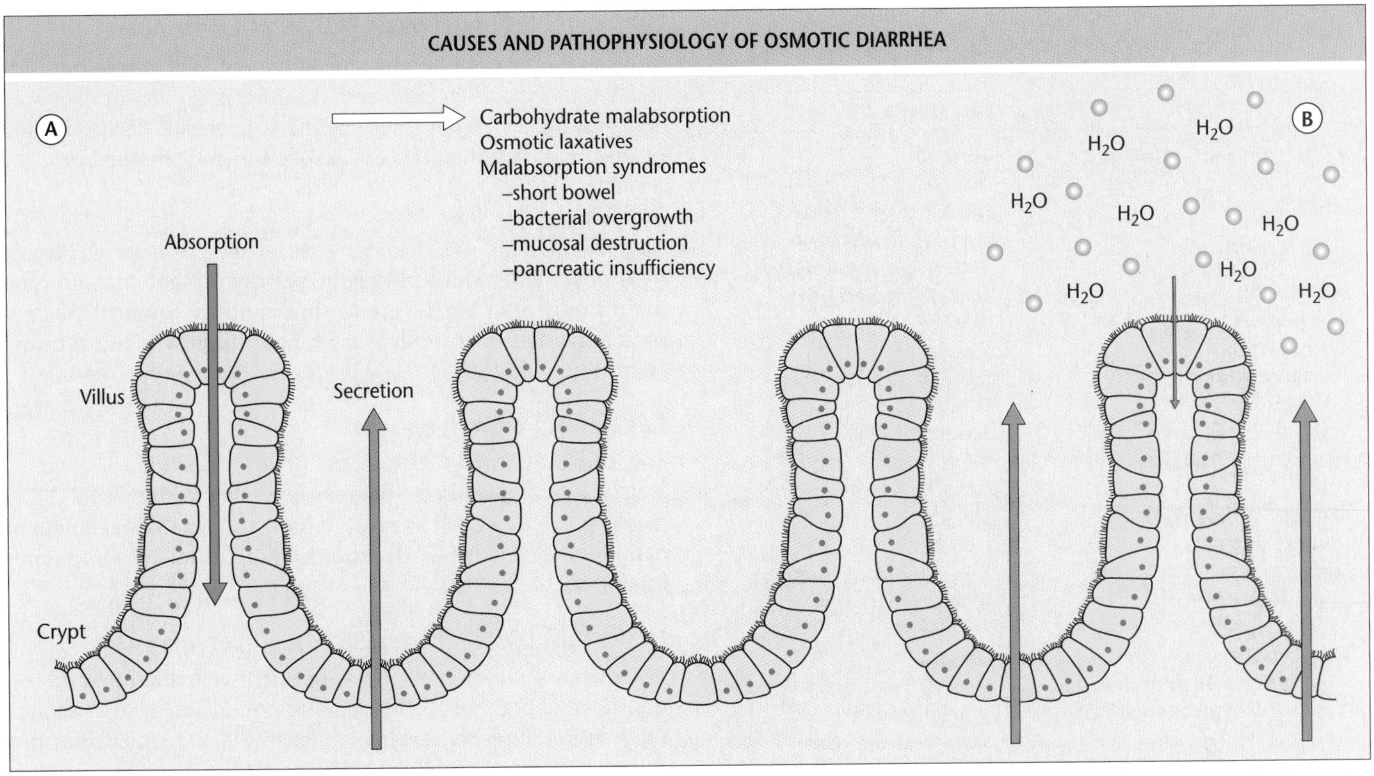

Fig. 9.3 Causes and pathophysiology of osmotic diarrhea. Pro-secretory effects of osmotic agents on intestinal fluid movement. **A.** Normal luminal environment. **B.** Effects of osmotic agents such as nonabsorbed carbohydrates. The intestine is thus capable of transporting very large volumes of fluid and electrolytes, and diarrhea is a consequence of disruption in the balance between absorption and secretion favoring a net increase in secretion. Some antibiotics, such as erythromycin, induce diarrhea through pro-motility effects, although most antibiotics that cause diarrhea do so as a result of undefined mechanisms. Laxatives induce diarrhea either by stimulating motility and secretion or by virtue of their osmotic potential.

bacterial overgrowth, leading to bile salt deconjugation and fat malabsorption.

CAUSES

Infection (see also Chapter 49)

Infections are responsible for the vast majority of acute diarrhea illnesses. Common *viral causes* of diarrhea include rotavirus, enteric adenovirus (types 40 and 41), caliciviruses and astroviruses, all of which induce a self-limiting, although occasionally severe, diarrheal illness, often associated with nausea and vomiting. Viruses induce diarrhea through epithelial invasion, causing inflammation and cell destruction, which impairs absorption (see Fig. 9.2).

Most *bacterial diarrhea* is acute, although some bacteria also cause chronic illness. Common enteropathogenic bacteria include *Escherichia coli, Campylobacter* spp., *Salmonella* spp., *Shigella* spp., and *Clostridium difficile*. Bacteria cause diarrhea by direct invasion, inducing an inflammatory response, and through the production of secretory toxins. Some bacteria, such as *Shigella dysenteriae*, produce cytolytic toxins (shiga toxin) which destroy epithelial cells causing inflammation and impairing absorption.

Protozoal causes of diarrhea are dealt with in Chapter 52.

Inflammation (see also Chapters 53 and 54)

Ulcerative colitis and Crohn's disease cause diarrhea by several mechanisms. Mucosal damage attenuates absorption (see Fig. 9.2). Inflammatory mediators induce active secretion and downregulate absorption (see Fig. 9.1). Intestinal resection reduces absorption. Bile salt malabsorption is common in patients with Crohn's disease, particularly after ileal resection.

Other inflammatory causes of diarrhea include vasculitis, such as systemic lupus erythematosus, and radiation-induced enteritis.

Drugs (see also Chapter 68)

Drugs can cause diarrhea directly (e.g., pro-motility effects of erythromycin) or indirectly (e.g., pseudomembranous colitis caused by *Clostridium difficile* (see Chapter 49) following treatment with broad-spectrum antibiotics).

Other drug causes of diarrhea are listed in Table 9.1.

Hormones (see also Chapter 109)

Hormone-secreting tumors are rare, but induce diarrhea by directly inducing active secretion (see Fig. 9.1). These tumors are typically found in the proximal intestine or the pancreas, and include vasoactive intestinal polypeptide-secreting tumors (VIPomas),[3] carcinoid tumors (see Chapter 110), gastrinomas, and medullary carcinoma of the thyroid, the latter secreting calcitonin, which stimulates secretion. The association between thyrotoxicosis and diarrhea is well known.

Inherited diarrhea

Nutrient malabsorption can result from a rare inherited impairment of brush border enzymes, such as glucose–galactose

TABLE 9.1 COMMON DRUG CAUSES OF DIARRHEA

Drug	Mechanism
5-Aminosalicylates, especially olsalazine	Secretion
Antibiotics	Change in bacteria flora, pseudomembranous colitis
Auranofin	Secretion, mucosal injury
Azathioprine	Toxic shock syndrome
Beta-blockers	Motility
Calcitonin	Secretion
Chemotherapeutic agents	Mucosal injury, secretion
Cisapride	Motility
Colchicine	Secretion/motility
Erythromycin (macrolides)	Motility
Iron	?Irritant
Laxatives, stimulant (abuse)	Secretion
Laxatives (osmotic)	Osmotic
Methyldopa	?Altered adrenergic activity
Metformin	Reported as the commonest cause of diabetic diarrhea
Magnesium (antacids and laxatives)	Osmotic
NSAIDs, especially mefenamic acid	Mucosal injury, direct secretion
Prostaglandins (misoprostol)	Secretion, motility
Proton pump inhibitors	Superinfection, ?other mechanisms
Statins	?Inflammation
Thyroxine	Motility
Ticlopidine	Lymphocytic colitis

malabsorption and sucrase–isomaltase, leading to carbohydrate malabsorption. Other rare disorders include defects in enterocyte membrane Na/H and Cl/HCO_3 exchange proteins.

Autonomic neuropathy (see also Chapter 41)

Idiopathic or secondary autonomic neuropathy due to conditions such as diabetes can be associated with both diarrhea and constipation (see Fig. 9.1). The pathogenesis is complex, but probably results from alterations in the regulation of fluid transport with destruction of either secretory or absorptive neural pathways. Changes in motility and transit may also result from neuropathy.

Intestinal neoplasms (see also Chapter 60)

Rectal villous adenomas typically cause an intermittent mucoid diarrhea resulting in marked fecal urgency due to the frequent accumulation of rectal fluid. Colorectal cancers occasionally present with a change in stool consistency and bloody mucous stools. The mechanisms of symptom production may include altered transit due to stricturing, mucous secretion, and local inflammatory mediators.

Bile salt malabsorption (see also Chapter 47)

Bile salts are normally recycled in the enterohepatic circulation after reabsorption in the terminal ileum. Malabsorption results in exposure of the colon to bile salts, which directly induce secretion (see Fig. 9.1). Bile salt malabsorption occurs idiopathically in some otherwise normal individuals, with disease or resection of the terminal ileum, and following vagotomy and cholecystectomy.[4]

Bacterial overgrowth (see also Chapter 46)

The small intestinal lumen is usually relatively sterile but bacterial numbers can increase with disordered motility or disrupted anatomy (e.g., jejunal diverticulosis). Bacterial deconjugation of bile acids results in fat malabsorption and steatorrhea.

Surgery

Surgery induces diarrhea by several mechanisms, including dysmotility and reduced absorptive capacity. Vagotomy and sympathectomy alter both secretion and motility. Surgical creation of 'blind loops' may result in bacterial overgrowth. Short bowel syndrome following surgery has been discussed previously.

Factitious diarrhea

The clinician should always be on the lookout for laxative abuse. In rare instances, patients have been known to dilute stools with fluids such as urine, water, and tea. Management of patients with 'factitious' diarrhea is complex and often requires inpatient assessment.[5]

HIV-associated diarrhea (see also Chapter 49)

Diarrhea associated with HIV is frequently attributed to opportunistic infections and is dependent upon the degree of immune suppression. Typical causative organisms include microsporidia, cytomegalovirus, cryptosporidia, and *Mycobacterium avium* complex. In addition, use of protease inhibitors in treatment has been found to induce diarrhea in 12–56% of patients.[6]

SYMPTOM COMPLEXES

Acute diarrhea (see also Chapter 49)

In the developed world, rapid-onset diarrhea lasting for several days to weeks is most commonly due to viruses and bacteria such as *Campylobacter jejuni* or *Salmonella* spp. Large outbreaks, notably on cruise ships or in residential homes or hospitals, imply a viral cause (e.g., Norwalk virus). Bacterial diarrhea often results from poor food handling or undercooking, and tends to affect limited numbers of people.

Travelers' diarrhea affects visitors to resource-poor regions and is usually due to enterotoxigenic *E. coli* (ETEC), which produces two secretory enterotoxins, heat-labile and heat-stable toxins (see Chapter 50). Cholera is classically related to poor sanitation, the source of infection typically being contaminated water supplies, and is endemic in many parts of the world including the Indian subcontinent, Africa, and Latin America.

Protozoa such as *Entamoeba histolytica* and *Giardia intestinalis* may present as acute diarrhea.

Inflammatory bowel disease (IBD) may present for the first time as acute diarrhea, although it invariably progresses to a persistent diarrhea.

Chronic diarrhea

Any diarrhea persisting for more than 2 weeks is termed chronic. The most common causes are infection and IBD.

Bacteria that typically cause chronic diarrhea include *Shigella* spp., *Mycobacterium tuberculosis*, *Salmonella* spp., *Yersinia enterocolitica*, and *Tropheryma whippelii* (the cause of Whipple's disease).

Protozoa such as *Giardia intestinalis*, *Entamoeba histolytica*, and *Cyclospora cayetanensis* give rise to diarrhea lasting for many months if untreated (see Chapter 49).

Rarer causes of persistent diarrhea include hormone-secreting tumors (see Chapter 109), pancreatic insufficiency (see Chapter 72), and autonomic neuropathies.

A useful diagnostic approach to chronic diarrhea is to consider the characteristics of the diarrhea in terms of three categories: watery (secretory or osmotic), inflammatory, and fatty diarrhea. However, as discussed in the section on pathophysiology, the etiologies with complex mechanisms may overlap different categories.

Watery diarrhea (see Figs 9.1 and 9.3)

Large-volume watery diarrhea is generally due to either the promotion of active intestinal secretion or an osmotic load. Secretory diarrhea persists on fasting, whereas osmotic diarrhea occurs only after ingestion of the causative food or drug. If the history is unclear, inpatient assessment with stool collection and food challenge may be useful.

Inflammatory diarrhea (see Fig. 9.2)

Characteristics of inflammatory diarrhea may include abdominal pain, pyrexia, and bloody diarrhea. Peripheral leukocytosis and raised inflammatory markers are useful indicators, and examination of the stool may reveal blood and leukocytes.

Fatty diarrhea

Fatty stools are typically described as pale stools with an oily texture that float in the toilet pan and are difficult to wash away. The most common cause is pancreatic insufficiency (see Chapter 72) with reduction of pancreatic lipases; however, loss of small intestinal absorptive capacity following *Giardia* infection or celiac disease may also lead to fat malabsorption.

DIAGNOSIS

History and examination

A careful history may be sufficient to suggest a likely diagnosis, and helps to direct and focus investigations. For example, a history of bloody diarrhea suggests colitis, whereas profuse large volume diarrhea suggests small intestinal etiology. History and examination should be used to assess the impact of the diarrhea on the patient's general state of health and quality of life, as well as systemic manifestations of diarrheal illnesses (e.g., erythema nodosum or arthritis).

Laboratory blood tests

A full blood count is helpful in starting to discriminate organic from functional disease. Depending on its characteristics, anemia may indicate iron deficiency due to intestinal blood loss (e.g., cancer or colitis), folate deficiency (e.g., malabsorption), B_{12} deficiency (ileal resection or disease), or chronic disease. Leukocytosis implies inflammation. A raised platelet count, often neglected, indicates bleeding, inflammation, or malignancy, and is often the first clue to Crohn's disease or cancer.

Biochemistry

Potassium levels may be reduced with secretion and urea raised with dehydration. A depressed level of thyroid-stimulating hormone indicates thyrotoxicosis. Clinicians should establish a common understanding on requests for stool and urine laxative screening ('anthroquines, etc.' is sufficiently cryptic) because writing 'laxatives' on the card usually prompts non-compliance.

Serology

For ongoing diarrhea, antiendomysial antibodies are very useful as screening tests for celiac disease. Other serological markers exist for amebiasis and strongyloidiasis. Antinuclear antibody can indicate vasculitis and depressed IgA deficiency. Rotavirus is the most common cause of acute severe diarrhea in young children and may contribute in adults. Other viruses include astroviruses, caliciviruses, enteric adenoviruses, and coronoviruses, and can be detected in stool using immunoassays or molecular biology techniques.[7]

Stool examination

Stool inspection, often neglected, is important to confirm the diagnosis and assess color, blood, and fatty appearance.

Stool microscopy and culture

In acute community-acquired diarrhea, stools should be cultured for *Salmonella* spp., *Shigella* spp., *Campylobacter* spp., and *E. coli* O157:H7 (see Chapter 49), and screened for *Clostridium difficile* if there has been antibiotic use.

Hospital-acquired diarrhea is commonly due to *C. difficile*,[8,9] acquired nosocomially or because of antibiotic use.

A wider range of infections, such as with *Giardia, Cryptosporidium, Cyclospora*, and *Isospora belli*, should be considered in patients with neutropenia or HIV infection (see Chapter 111) or with persistent diarrhea.

Quantitative stool evaluation

In difficult cases, quantitative stool collection over 48–72 h can be used to confirm the presence of a 'true' diarrhea (>200 g per 24 h), its magnitude, sodium content, and the presence of an osmotic gap. During the collection period, all drugs influencing stool output such as opiates should be stopped, and a normal diet should be adhered to, unless fasting is required to look for secretory diarrhea. If factitious diarrhea or laxative abuse is suspected, stool collection should ideally be supervised as an inpatient.

The stool osmotic gap can be measured using the expression: $290 - 2([Na^+] + [K^+])$. Osmotic diarrhea is characterized by an osmotic gap greater than 50 mOsm/kg, whereas secretory diarrhea typically has an osmotic gap of less than 50 mOsm/kg. Although most diarrhea is mixed, characterization of an osmotic or secretory diarrhea can greatly aid diagnosis. Directly measured stool osmolality is normally 290 mOsm/kg or above, and low values suggest dilution of stool with urine or water. When analyzing stools for evidence of carbohydrate malabsorption, $pH < 5$ is highly suggestive. Alternatively, Clinitest can be used to test for reducing sugars (glucose, galactose, fructose, maltose, and lactose).

Laxatives can be detected in both stool and urine, although available assays should be discussed with the laboratory.

Assessing stools for abnormal fat content is unpopular with laboratories and not very reliable as diarrhea of any cause attenuates normal fat absorption. Therefore, although fecal fat of up to 7 g per day (9% of dietary intake) is normal, it may exceed 13 g daily in diarrhea. More than 14 g/day is thus considered to be more specific for diseases primarily affecting fat digestion such as pancreatic insufficiency, bile salt disorders, and small intestinal enteropathies. Stool microscopy, with Sudan staining, is of some value.

Gut hormones (see Chapter 109)

VIP-secreting tumors are rare, but give rise to pancreatic cholera syndrome and can be diagnosed by a raised blood VIP level. Other tests for neuroendocrine tumors that cause diarrhea include urinary 5-hydroxyindole acetic acid (for carcinoid), serum gastrin (for gastrinoma), urinary vanillylmandelic acid (for pheochromocytoma), and serum calcitonin (for medullary thyroid carcinoma).

Endoscopy

Endoscopic inspection of the colon is indicated in acute diarrhea where a noninfectious etiology is suspected such as IBD, and in chronic diarrhea (see Chapter 120). Flexible sigmoidoscopy and biopsy is a safe and cost-effective primary investigation,[10] with colonoscopy where malignancy, right-sided colitis, or ileal pathology is suspected.

If signs and symptoms are suggestive of small intestinal disease, biopsy and aspiration of the distal duodenum or jejunum is indicated (see Chapter 119).

Breath testing

Breath tests are used to detect malabsorption of carbohydrates (lactose breath test) and small intestinal bacterial overgrowth (glucose and lactulose breath tests).

Lactose breath test

Principle: In lactase-deficient individuals, ingested lactose transits unabsorbed to the colon, where it is fermented by bacteria to produce metabolites including hydrogen (H_2), which in turn is absorbed and expired by the lungs where it can be measured by gas chromatography.

Protocol: Fasted patients are given 25 g oral lactose and H_2 levels are measured at baseline and every 30 min. A rise in H_2 of 20 parts per million at 4 h is considered positive. If the lactose breath test is not available, assessment of symptoms following a lactose load and dietary exclusion may be useful.

Value: Though generally reliable, lactose breath tests need to be interpreted with caution. Transient lactase deficiency may follow viral gastroenteritis. Some individuals do not possess bacteria that ferment lactose to produce H_2. Early rises in breath H_2 levels may be due to bacterial overgrowth.

Glucose breath test

Fasted patients are given 100 g oral glucose; H_2 levels are measured at baseline and every 30 min. In small intestinal bacterial overgrowth, the glucose is fermented by small bowel bacteria resulting in an early rise in breath H_2 concentration. A rise in breath H_2 of 20 parts per million at 30 min is abnormal.

Lactulose breath test

In normal individuals, lactulose reaches the colon after about 90 min, where it is fermented to give a rise in breath H_2 concentration that can be used to measure small bowel transit time. With small bowel bacterial overgrowth there is an additional early rise in breath hydrogen of 20 parts per million is abnormal.

Other tests of bacterial overgrowth

Although not commonly used, two other breath tests have been validated. The first uses the bile acid, [^{14}C]glycocholate, which is deconjugated by intestinal bacteria and metabolized to $^{14}CO_2$, which is then measured in expired air. The second uses [^{14}C]xylose, which is fermented by small intestinal bacteria to produce $^{14}CO_2$, which again is measured in expired air.

Bile salt malabsorption

See Chapters 43 and 47 for the use of xylose in the diagnosis of malabsorption.

Loss of bile salt retention from the enterohepatic circulation can be measured using the labeled bile salt ^{75}seleno homocholic acid–taurine (SeHCAT). Patients are given 0.4 MBq of SeHCAT. Whole-body radiation is scanned at baseline and after 7 days. Retention of less than 5% of SeHCAT is highly suggestive of bile salt malabsorption and correlates positively with response to therapy with bile salt sequestrants.[11]

Radiology

Barium studies of the small intestine may be useful in defining abnormal anatomy of the small intestine in chronic diarrhea, for example if Crohn's disease, lymphoma, jejunum diverticulosis, or systemic sclerosis is suspected. Barium is either drunk and followed through the small bowel or infused into the small intestine via a nasogastric tube[12] (see Chapter 125).

Computed tomography has a limited role but can detect abdominal lymph nodes associated with tuberculosis or lymphoma, and some structural intestinal abnormalities (see Chapter 126).

DIAGNOSTIC APPROACH TO DIARRHEA

Figure 9.4 is a suggested algorithm for a diagnostic approach for all presentations of diarrhea. Having characterized the diarrhea to a particular disease pattern, such as acute,[13] chronic,[14] or HIV associated,[6] the specific investigation pathways can be followed in Figures 9.5, 9.6, and 9.7.

DIAGNOSTIC METHODS

SPECIFIC INVESTIGATIONS FOR FATTY DIARRHEA

- **Small intestinal biopsy**
- **Breath tests**
  Hydrogen, glucose, or lactulose breath test for bacterial overgrowth
- **Pancreatic radiology**
  Pancreatic protocol computed tomography (CT) or magnetic resonance cholangiopancreatography (MRCP)
- **Pancreatic function testing**
  Fecal elastase, secretin test, pancreolauryl test, trial of pancreatic enzymes
- **Small intestinal barium study**

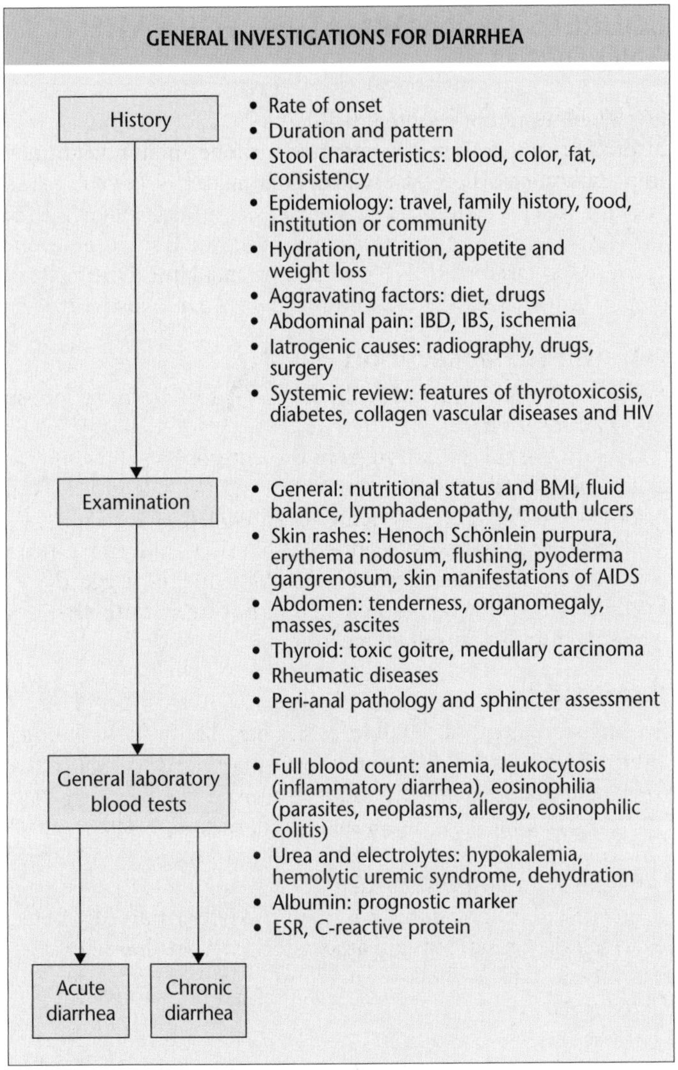
GENERAL INVESTIGATIONS FOR DIARRHEA
History
• Rate of onset
• Duration and pattern
• Stool characteristics: blood, color, fat, consistency
• Epidemiology: travel, family history, food, institution or community
• Hydration, nutrition, appetite and weight loss
• Aggravating factors: diet, drugs
• Abdominal pain: IBD, IBS, ischemia
• Iatrogenic causes: radiography, drugs, surgery
• Systemic review: features of thyrotoxicosis, diabetes, collagen vascular diseases and HIV
Examination
• General: nutritional status and BMI, fluid balance, lymphadenopathy, mouth ulcers
• Skin rashes: Henoch Schönlein purpura, erythema nodosum, flushing, pyoderma gangrenosum, skin manifestations of AIDS
• Abdomen: tenderness, organomegaly, masses, ascites
• Thyroid: toxic goitre, medullary carcinoma
• Rheumatic diseases
• Peri-anal pathology and sphincter assessment
General laboratory blood tests
• Full blood count: anemia, leukocytosis (inflammatory diarrhea), eosinophilia (parasites, neoplasms, allergy, eosinophilic colitis)
• Urea and electrolytes: hypokalemia, hemolytic uremic syndrome, dehydration
• Albumin: prognostic marker
• ESR, C-reactive protein
Acute diarrhea
Chronic diarrhea

Fig. 9.4 General investigations for diarrhea.

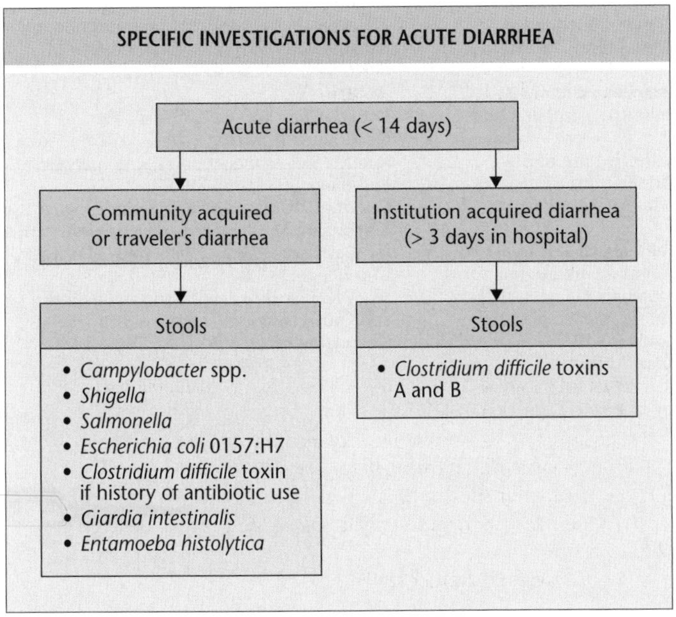
SPECIFIC INVESTIGATIONS FOR ACUTE DIARRHEA
Acute diarrhea (< 14 days)
Community acquired or traveler's diarrhea
Institution acquired diarrhea (> 3 days in hospital)
Stools
• Campylobacter spp.
• Shigella
• Salmonella
• Escherichia coli 0157:H7
• Clostridium difficile toxin if history of antibiotic use
• Giardia intestinalis
• Entamoeba histolytica
Stools
• Clostridium difficile toxins A and B

Fig. 9.5 Specific investigations for acute diarrhea.

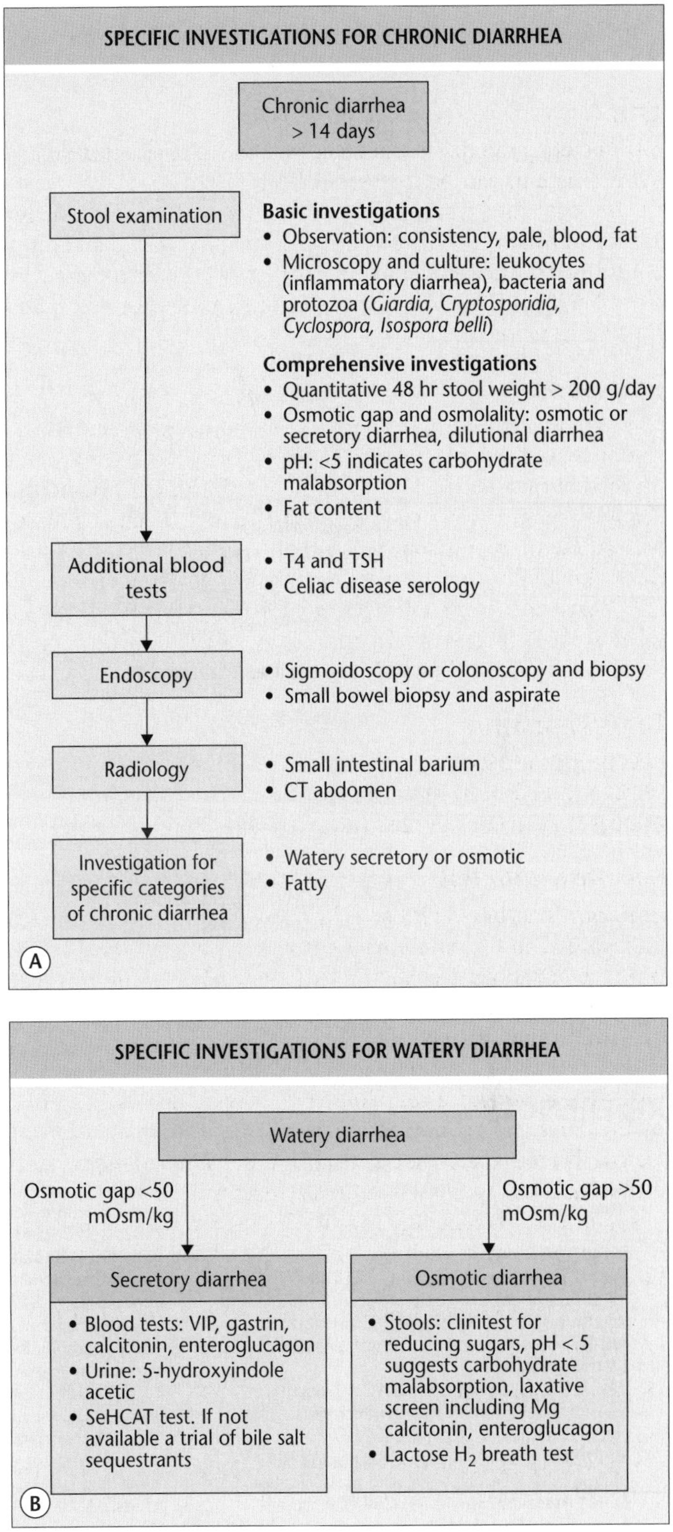
SPECIFIC INVESTIGATIONS FOR CHRONIC DIARRHEA
Chronic diarrhea > 14 days
Stool examination
Basic investigations
• Observation: consistency, pale, blood, fat
• Microscopy and culture: leukocytes (inflammatory diarrhea), bacteria and protozoa (Giardia, Cryptosporidia, Cyclospora, Isospora belli)
Comprehensive investigations
• Quantitative 48 hr stool weight > 200 g/day
• Osmotic gap and osmolality: osmotic or secretory diarrhea, dilutional diarrhea
• pH: <5 indicates carbohydrate malabsorption
• Fat content
Additional blood tests
• T4 and TSH
• Celiac disease serology
Endoscopy
• Sigmoidoscopy or colonoscopy and biopsy
• Small bowel biopsy and aspirate
Radiology
• Small intestinal barium
• CT abdomen
Investigation for specific categories of chronic diarrhea
• Watery secretory or osmotic
• Fatty
A
SPECIFIC INVESTIGATIONS FOR WATERY DIARRHEA
Watery diarrhea
Osmotic gap <50 mOsm/kg
Osmotic gap >50 mOsm/kg
Secretory diarrhea
• Blood tests: VIP, gastrin, calcitonin, enteroglucagon
• Urine: 5-hydroxyindole acetic
• SeHCAT test. If not available a trial of bile salt sequestrants
Osmotic diarrhea
• Stools: clinitest for reducing sugars, pH < 5 suggests carbohydrate malabsorption, laxative screen including Mg calcitonin, enteroglucagon
• Lactose H2 breath test
B

Fig. 9.6 Specific investigations for (A) chronic diarrhea and (B) watery diarrhea.

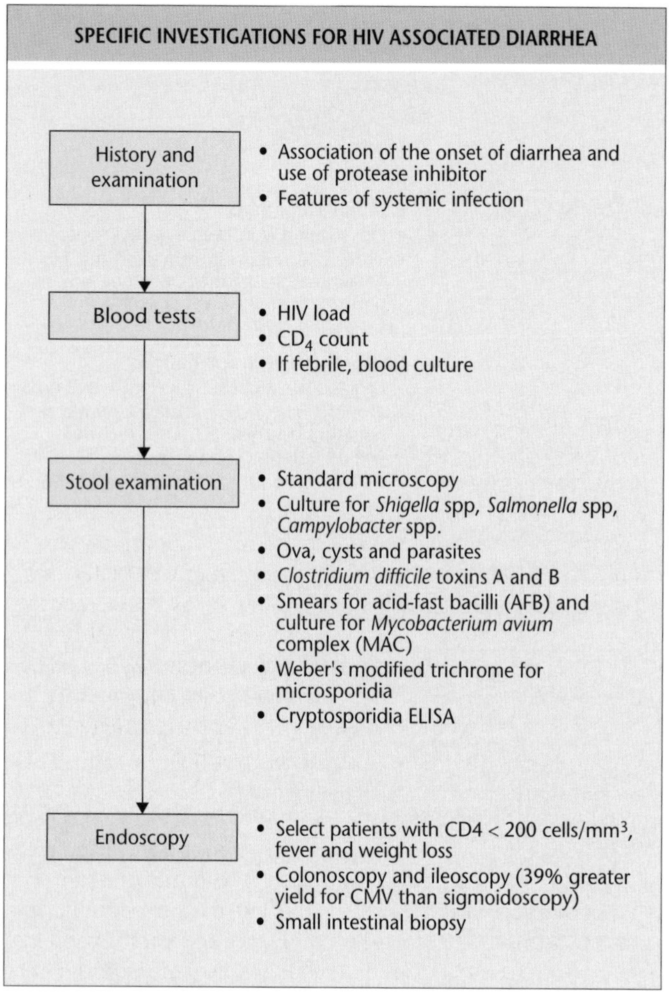
SPECIFIC INVESTIGATIONS FOR HIV ASSOCIATED DIARRHEA
History and examination
• Association of the onset of diarrhea and use of protease inhibitor
• Features of systemic infection
Blood tests
• HIV load
• CD_4 count
• If febrile, blood culture
Stool examination
• Standard microscopy
• Culture for *Shigella* spp, *Salmonella* spp, *Campylobacter* spp.
• Ova, cysts and parasites
• *Clostridium difficile* toxins A and B
• Smears for acid-fast bacilli (AFB) and culture for *Mycobacterium avium* complex (MAC)
• Weber's modified trichrome for microsporidia
• Cryptosporidia ELISA
Endoscopy
• Select patients with CD4 < 200 cells/mm^3, fever and weight loss
• Colonoscopy and ileoscopy (39% greater yield for CMV than sigmoidoscopy)
• Small intestinal biopsy

Fig. 9.7 Specific investigations for HIV-associated diarrhea.

SOURCES OF INFORMATION FOR PATIENTS AND DOCTORS

http://www.patient.co.uk/showdoc/249/
http://www.medic8.com/healthguide/articles/diarrhoea.html
http://www.gastro.org/generalPublic.html

REFERENCES

1. Kosek M, Bern C, Guerrant RL. The global burden of diarrhoeal disease, as estimated from studies published between 1992 and 2000. Bull World Health Organ 2003; 81:197–204.
2. Turvill JL, Connor P, Farthing MJ. The inhibition of cholera toxin-induced 5-HT release by the 5-HT(3) receptor antagonist, granisetron, in the rat. Br J Pharmacol 2000; 130:1031–1036.
3. Bloom SR, Polak JM, Pearse AG. Vasoactive intestinal peptide and watery-diarrhoea syndrome. Lancet 1973; ii:14–16.
4. Smith MJ, Cherian P, Raju GS, Dawson BF, Mahon S, Bardhan KD. Bile acid malabsorption in persistent diarrhoea. J R Coll Physicians Lond 2003; 34:448–451.
5. Pollok RC, Banks MR, Fairclough PD, Farthing MJ. Dilutional diarrhoea—underdiagnosed and over-investigated. Eur J Gastroenterol Hepatol 2000; 12:609–611.
6. Oldfield EC. Evaluation of chronic diarrhea in patients with human immunodeficiency virus infection. Rev Gastroenterol Disord 2002; 2:176–188.
7. Wilhelmi I, Roman E, Sanchez-Fauquier A. Viruses causing gastroenteritis. Clin Microbiol Infect 2003; 9:247–262.
8. Hines J, Nachamkin I. Effective use of the clinical microbiology laboratory for diagnosing diarrheal diseases. Clin Infect Dis 1996; 23:1292–1301.
9. Bauer TM, Lalvani A, Fahrenbach J. Derivation and validation of guidelines for stool cultures for enteropathogenic bacteria other than *Clostridium difficile* in hospitalized adults. JAMA 2001; 285:313–319.
10. Marshall JB, Singh R, Diaz-Arias AA. Chronic, unexplained diarrhoea: are biopsies necessary if colonoscopy is normal? Am J Gastroenterol 1995; 90:372–376.
11. Wildt S, Norby Rasmussen S, Lysgard Madsen J, Rumessen JJ. Bile acid malabsorption in patients with diarrhoea: clinical value of SeHCAT test. Scand J Gastroenterol 2003; 38:826–830.
12. Ott DJ, Chen YM, Gelfand DW, Van Swearingen F, Munitz HA. Detailed per-oral small bowel examination vs. enteroclysis. Radiology 1985; 155:29–31.
13. Guerrant RL, Van Gilder T, Steiner TS, Thielman NM, Slutsker L. Practice guidelines for the management of infectious diarrhoea. Clin Infect Dis 2001; 32:331–351.
14. AGA technical review on the evaluation and management of chronic diarrhoea. Gastroenterology 1999; 116:1464–1486.

Chapter 10

Fecal incontinence

Satish S C Rao

INTRODUCTION

The involuntary leakage of stool material or gas is a most distressing and disabling symptom that significantly impacts quality of life. Today, through rational diagnostic approaches and therapy, it is possible to improve fecal incontinence, thus restoring dignity and quality of life.

WHAT IS IT?

Fecal incontinence is defined as the recurrent uncontrolled passage of fecal material for a period of at least 1 month.[1] There are three clinical subtypes: (1) passive incontinence, i.e., the involuntary discharge of stool or gas without awareness; (2) urge incontinence, i.e., the discharge of fecal matter in spite of active attempts to retain bowel contents; and (3) fecal seepage, i.e., the leakage of small amount of stool without awareness or staining of undergarments following an otherwise normal evacuation.[2] The severity of incontinence can range from unintentional elimination of flatus via the seepage of liquid fecal matter to complete evacuation of bowel contents. It significantly impairs quality of life.

HOW COMMON IS IT?

The prevalence estimates vary from 2.2% to 18.4% depending on the definition of incontinence, the frequency of occurrence, and the clinical setting.[1,2,3] Although fecal incontinence affects people of all ages, its prevalence is disproportionately higher in women, in nursing home residents, and the elderly.[2]

PATHOPHYSIOLOGY AND CAUSES

Several structural and functional elements of the anorectal unit play a crucial role in maintaining continence (Fig. 10.1). Usually, incontinence is a consequence of multiple factors (Table 10.1). Disruption or weakness of the external anal sphincter muscle causes urge-related or diarrhea-associated fecal incontinence. In contrast, damage to the internal anal sphincter muscle or the anal endovascular cushions may lead to a poor seal and an impaired sampling reflex that causes incontinence under resting conditions. The most common cause for anal sphincter disruption is vaginal delivery. Both sphincters may be damaged. Up to a third of women may sustain an occult injury of the anal sphincter during vaginal delivery, particularly following forceps or breech delivery. Other causes include surgical trauma, neuropathy that is secondary to repeated and excessive straining, neurological disease or spinal cord injury, or drugs.

Intact sensation not only provides warning of imminent defecation but also helps to discriminate between formed stool, liquid feces, or flatus. Conversely, an impaired anorectal sensation predisposes to fecal incontinence. The elderly, physically and mentally challenged individuals, and children with functional fecal incontinence often exhibit blunted rectal sensation. The impaired sensation also leads to excessive accumulation of stool leading to fecal impaction, megarectum, and overflow. Impaired rectal sensation may occur as a result of neurological damage such as multiple sclerosis, diabetes mellitus, or spinal cord injury. Although less well known, analgesics and antidepressants may also lead to impaired rectal sensation and fecal incontinence.

The rectum is a compliant reservoir that stores stool until social conditions are conducive for its evacuation. If the rectal compliance is impaired, then a small volume of stool may generate high intrarectal pressures that may overwhelm anal resistance and cause incontinence. Rectal accommodation may be compromised due to inflammatory bowel disease, radiation enteritis, rectal surgery, and aging.

An intact innervation of the pelvic floor is essential for preserving continence. An injury to the terminal portion of the pudendal nerve, its nerve roots, the spinal cord, or the central nervous system may each predispose to incontinence. A neuropathy may not only cause weakness of the anal sphincter muscle, but also impair anorectal sensation and reflexes. Stools that are large in volume and are liquid in consistency or those that contain mucus or irritants such as bile salts may cause incontinence.

DIAGNOSIS

The first step in diagnosis of fecal incontinence is eliciting the history. Frequently, patients are reluctant to mention this

TABLE 10.1 PATHOPHYSIOLOGICAL MECHANISMS INVOLVED IN FECAL INCONTINENCE

- Weak or damaged external anal sphincter muscle
- Weak or damaged internal anal sphincter muscle
- Loss of endovascular cushions
- Weak pelvic floor or puborectalis muscle
- Impaired anorectal sensation
- Impaired compliance or loss of rectal accommodation
- Pudendal, sacral, spinal, or central nervous system neuropathy
- Incomplete evacuation of stool
- Large volume and/or liquid stools

CAUSES

TRAUMATIC
- Obstetric
- Postsurgical
- Sexual
- Accidental

NEUROLOGICAL
- Diabetes mellitus
- Pudendal neuropathy
- Cauda equina lesions
- Cerebrovascular injury
- Multiple sclerosis
- Polyneuropathies
- Dementia
- Developmental disability

INFLAMMATORY
- Ulcerative colitis/Crohn's disease
- Radiation proctitis

MISCELLANEOUS
- Idiopathic bile salt malabsorption
- Lactose intolerance
- Secretory diarrhea
- Laxative abuse
- Irritable bowel syndrome
- Fecal impaction with overflow

symptom and the physician should initiate the discussion. A detailed history should then be obtained with an assessment of its nature (i.e., incontinence of flatus, liquid or solid stool), the timing and duration, and its impact on the quality of life. The use of pads or other devices and the ability to discriminate between formed or unformed stool and gas should be documented. A detailed inquiry of obstetric history and coexisting problems such as diabetes mellitus, pelvic radiation, neurological problems, spinal cord injury, dietary history, and urinary incontinence is useful. A prospective stool diary may also be helpful.[2] Based on clinical features, several grading systems have been proposed.[4] These can provide an objective method of quantifying the degree of incontinence and it can also be useful for assessing the efficacy of therapy.

A detailed physical and neurological examination should be performed to rule out a systemic or neurological disorder. A digital rectal examination should assess the resting sphincter tone, length of anal canal, integrity of the puborectalis sling, acuteness of the anorectal angle, and the strength of the anal muscle during voluntary squeeze. The positive predictive value of digital rectal examination as an objective test of evaluating anal sphincter function is very low, but may be helpful in guiding further diagnostic strategies.[2]

Investigations of fecal incontinence

A flexible sigmoidoscopy or colonoscopy is usually desirable in most patients with diarrhea to exclude mucosal disease or colon cancer. However, in patients with long-standing fecal incontinence without diarrhea, these procedures may not be necessary if not required for other reasons, e.g., colon cancer screening. Several specific tests that are complementary are available for defining the underlying mechanisms of fecal incontinence.[2,5,6] The selection of diagnostic tests will depend on probable cause, symptom severity, and impact on quality of life.

Anorectal manometry

Anorectal manometry provides an assessment of sphincter pressures and reflexes. Currently, several types of probes and pressure recording devices are available.[5] Typically, a probe with

FUNCTIONAL ANATOMY OF THE ANORECTUM

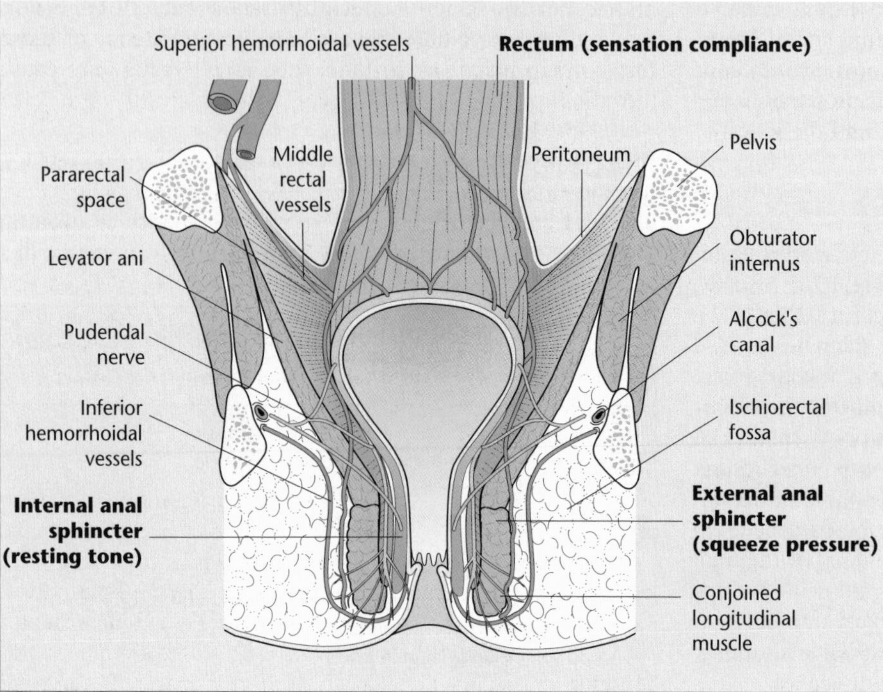

Fig. 10.1 Functional anatomy of the anorectum. Adapted from Keighley MRB, Williams NS. Surgery of the anus, rectum and colon, 2nd edn. London: W.B. Saunders; 2001.

multiple pressure sensors and a balloon is placed in the rectum and anal canal and the resting and squeeze sphincter pressures are assessed.[2,5,6]

A reduced resting pressure correlates with internal sphincter abnormality and reduced squeeze pressures with external sphincter defects.[2,5] Two large studies have reported that maximum squeeze pressure has the greatest sensitivity and specificity for discriminating incontinent patients.[2,5] The ability of the external anal sphincter to contract by reflex is assessed by having the subject cough.[2,5] This reflex response causes sphincter pressure to rise above the intra-abdominal pressure to preserve continence. This reflex response is absent in patients with lesions of the cauda equina or sacral plexus.[2] Anorectal manometry is also useful in evaluating the responses to biofeedback training or surgery.[2,7]

Rectal sensory testing and compliance

Rectal sensation and compliance are commonly measured by incremental balloon distention. A higher threshold for rectal sensory perception is associated with autonomic neuropathy, or congenital neurogenic anorectal malformation.[1,2,5] In some patients, rectal sensory thresholds may be altered because of changes in the compliance of the rectal wall.[1] Rectal compliance reflects both the distensibility and the ability of the rectum to accommodate. Patients with incontinence often have lower rectal compliance. Rectal compliance is also reduced in patients with colitis,[2] low spinal cord lesions, and diabetics.

Anal endosonography

Anal endosonography is performed using either a 7-mHz rotating transducer or 10–15-mHz transducer.[2,5,8] It provides an assessment of the thickness and structural integrity of the anal sphincter muscle and the presence of scarring. Anal endosonography is a simple and inexpensive method of imaging the anal sphincters.[2,5,8]

Defecography

In this radiographic test, approximately 150 mL of contrast material is placed into the rectum and the subject is asked to squeeze, cough, or expel the contrast.[2,5] It is used to assess anorectal angle, pelvic floor descent, length of anal canal, presence of rectocele, rectal prolapse, or mucosal intussusception. There is poor agreement between observers when measuring the anorectal angle.[5] Many have also questioned the rationale for performing defecography.[2,5]

Magnetic resonance imaging (MRI)

MRI (see Chapter 127) is the only imaging modality that can visualize the anal sphincters and the global pelvic floor motion in real time without radiation exposure.[9] Endoanal MRI has been shown to provide superior imaging with better spatial resolution of external anal sphincter. MRI and endosonography have been compared for the evaluation of anal sphincters. The internal anal sphincter is seen more clearly on anal endosonography, whereas the external anal sphincter is seen more clearly on MRI.[9] Disadvantages of MRI defecography include limited availability and lack of data comparing symptomatic with normal volunteers.

Pudendal nerve terminal latency (PNTML)

The pudendal nerve terminal motor latency measures the functional integrity of the terminal portion of the pudendal nerve and helps to distinguish whether a weak sphincter muscle is due to muscle or nerve injury.[2] A prolonged nerve latency time suggests pudendal neuropathy and this may occur following obstetric or surgical trauma, excessive perineal descent, or idiopathic fecal incontinence.[2] A normal PNTML does not exclude pudendal neuropathy.

Clinical utility of tests for fecal incontinence

History and physical examination alone detected an underlying cause in only 9 of 80 patients (11%), whereas anorectal physiologic tests revealed an abnormality in 66% of patients.[1,2] In another prospective study, physiological testing confirmed clinical impression and management was altered in 76% of patients.[1,2]

MANAGEMENT OF PATIENTS

The goal of treatment is to restore continence and to improve the quality of life. The following strategies may be useful.

Supportive measures

The underlying predisposing condition(s) such as fecal impaction, dementia, neurological problems, and inflammatory bowel disease should be treated. Hygienic measures such as changing undergarments, cleaning the perianal skin immediately following a soiling episode, and the use of moist tissue paper (baby wipes) rather than dry toilet paper and barrier creams such as zinc oxide and calamine lotion may be useful.[1,2]

Pharmacologic therapy

A placebo-controlled study showed that loperamide 4 mg t.i.d. (see Chapter 136) reduced stool frequency and urgency, increased colonic transit time, reduced stool weight, and increased anal resting sphincter pressure.[2] Clinical improvement was also reported with diphenoxylate/atropine (Lomotil), but objective improvement was lacking.[2]

Biofeedback therapy

The goals of biofeedback therapy are: (1) to improve the strength of the anal sphincter muscles; (2) to improve coordination during voluntary squeeze and following rectal perception; and (3) to enhance the anorectal sensory perception. Biofeedback training is often performed using either visual, auditory, or verbal feedback techniques.[1,2,7,10]

One prospective study showed that 1 year after starting therapy there was a significant increase in squeeze pressure, rectal sensation, and capacity.[7] Similar results were reported in other studies.[10] In a study of 100 patients, two-thirds showed improvement, and those with urge incontinence alone faired better than those with passive incontinence (55% vs 23%).[2,10] In a randomized controlled trial of biofeedback therapy with standard care, Kegel exercises, and home treatment, similar improvement was seen in all four groups.[10]

Surgery

In 80% of patients with obstetrical damage, anterior overlap repair of the external anal sphincter resolves symptoms, at least temporarily.[2] In patients with incontinence due to a weak but intact anal sphincter, post anal repair has been tried but success rates are low.[2] Over time, the success of sphincter repair seems to wear off and less than one-third of patients are still continent to liquid or solid stool after 5 years.[2] If the anal sphincter is irreparably damaged, reconstruction of the sphincter may be required. The technique of stimulated gracilis muscle transposition (dynamic gracioplasty) has been used but there are significant device-related adverse events and comorbidity.[11]

Sacral nerve stimulation

This new therapeutic approach is less invasive. Temporary electrodes are placed percutaneously through the sacral foramina. If the test period of 2–3 weeks shows satisfactory continence, the permanent electrode is placed and a neurostimulator is implanted. In the short term, continence was restored in 8 of 9 patients and similar results were obtained in the medium term.[2]

Other procedures

The Malone or ante-grade continent enema procedure consists of fashioning a caceostomy button or appendicostomy,[2] which allows ante-grade wash-out of the colon and may be suitable for children and patients with neurological lesions.[2] In the long term, fibrosis of the stoma site may lead to a loss of response but overall long-term success rate was 61%. If none of these techniques are suitable or have failed, a colostomy is a safe option, although esthetically less preferable.[2]

CURRENT CONTROVERSIES

Fecal incontinence is a symptom with complex etiology and pathogenesis and scant evidence-based data for management. A detailed history, digital rectal examination, and in some cases colonoscopy with biopsy may identify common disorders. Anorectal physiological tests may help in the evaluation of functional abnormalities and anal endosonography in the assessment of sphincter defects. While the results of these tests often guide further management, abnormal findings demonstrated by these procedures do not predict severity of incontinence or response to treatment. Biofeedback therapy is successful in 60–80% of patients and should be offered as first-line treatment, but whether a home-based or office-based treatment program is more effective and whether it should include muscle strengthening alone or a combination of coordination training and sensory training is unclear. If a well-defined sphincter defect with no pudendal neuropathy is identified, sphincteroplasty may be effective but long-term results are disappointing. If the sphincter is badly damaged, dynamic graciloplasty or artificial sphincter reconstructive surgery may be considered. However, these procedures are only performed in a few specialist centers; there are no randomized controlled trials or comparative treatments with medical or biofeedback therapy, and complications are frequent. Several experimental approaches, including bulking of the anal sphincter, sacral nerve stimulation, and the delivery of radiofrequency energy to the anal canal are currently being evaluated.

SOURCES OF INFORMATION FOR PATIENTS AND DOCTORS

http://www.google.co.uk/search?hl=en&as_qdr=all&q=incontinence+patient+information&btnG=Search&meta=

http://patients.uptodate.com/frames.asp?page=topic.asp&file=digestiv/6793

http://unthsc-dl.slis.ua.edu/patientinfo/urology/incontinence.htm

http://www.clevelandclinic.org/gastro/motility/patient/incontinence.htm

REFERENCES

1. Whitehead WE, Wald A, Diamant NE et al. Functional disorders of the anus and rectum. Gut 1999; 45:II55–II59.
2. Rao SS. Practice guidelines: Diagnosis and management of fecal incontinence. Am J Gastroenterol 2004; 99:1585–1604.
3. Perry S, Shaw C, McGrother C et al. Prevalence of faecal incontinence in adults aged 40 years or more living in the community. Gut 2002; 50:480–484.
4. Vaizey CJ, Carapeti E, Cahill JA, Kamm MA. Prospective comparison of faecal incontinence grading systems. Gut 1999; 44:77–80.
5. Diamant NE, Kamm MA, Wald A, Whitehead WE. AGA technical review on anorectal testing techniques. Gastroenterology 1999; 116: 735–760.
6. Rao SS, Azpiroz F, Diamant N et al. Minimum standards of anorectal manometry. Neurogastroenterol Motil 2002; 14: 553–559.
7. Rao SS, Welcher KD, Happel J. Can biofeedback therapy improve anorectal function in fecal incontinence? Am J Gastroenterol 1996; 91:2360–2366.
8. Sultan AH, Kamm MA, Talbot IC, Nicholls RJ, Bartram CI. Anal endosonography for identifying external sphincter defects confirmed histologically. Br J Surg 1994; 81:463–465.
9. Bertschinger KM, Hetzer FH, Roos JE et al. Dynamic MR imaging of the pelvic floor performed with patient sitting in an open-magnet unit versus with patient supine in a closed-magnet unit. Radiology 2002; 223:501–508.
10. Norton C, Chelvanayagam S, Wilson-Barnett J et al. Randomized controlled trial of biofeedback for fecal incontinence. Gastroenterology 2003; 125:1320–1329.
11. Vaizey CJ, Kamm MA, Nicholls RJ. Recent advances in the surgical treatment of faecal incontinence. Br J Surg 1998; 85:596–603.

Chapter 11

Rectal bleeding

John H Bond

INTRODUCTION

Rectal bleeding is usually mild and either intermittent or self-limiting. Although such mild bleeding may not by itself be life-threatening, it may be a sign of a common underlying potentially fatal disease – colorectal cancer. Evaluation of such patients may be carried out in a deliberate, stepwise, nonemergent manner in the outpatient setting. Rectal bleeding may be occult, detectable only by a fecal occult blood test (FOBT). Such bleeding may cause chronic iron-deficiency anemia and, again, may be the only sign of an underlying serious colorectal neoplasm. About 10–15% of patients with acute gross rectal bleeding (hematochezia) have more severe, ongoing, or recurrent bleeding. These patients usually require hospitalization, immediate resuscitation, careful monitoring, and relatively urgent evaluation and treatment. A large number of diverse conditions cause each type of rectal bleeding.

Evaluation and treatment should be tailored to the individual features of each case, including the type and rate of bleeding, patient characteristics, and diagnostic findings. As abnormalities in the large bowel are the most frequent cause of rectal bleeding, urgent or elective colonoscopy has become the preferred diagnostic approach for most of these patients. It is the most accurate method for diagnosing both the site and the cause of bleeding, and it offers an opportunity for nonsurgical treatment for many patients with severe rectal bleeding.

This chapter reviews the epidemiology, causes, and general management of each type of rectal bleeding.

WHAT IS IT?

Table 11.1 lists the different types of rectal bleeding. Occult rectal bleeding is defined as blood in the stool that is not visible and must be detected by a FOBT. Rectal outlet bleeding is defined as the intermittent passage of scant to modest amounts of bright red blood that is not mixed in with the stool and that usually follows a bowel movement. Often blood is noticed in these cases mainly on toilet tissue or in the toilet bowl following passage of stool, and is not usually accompanied by a clinically significant loss of blood volume or a drop in hemoglobin levels. The occasional passage of bright red blood mixed in with the stool or the passage of dark or maroon blood or stools, with or without the development of iron-deficiency anemia, usually comes from a source proximal to the anorectum. Acute severe rectal bleeding is a medical emergency requiring hospitalization, rapid resuscitation, and careful monitoring. Such bleeding is often self-limiting, although these patients are at high risk for recurrent bleeding and a complicated outcome. Lastly, the least common type of rectal bleeding is massive, continuous rectal bleeding. Patients with this type of rectal bleeding require emergent surgery and have a high mortality rate.

HOW COMMON IS IT?

Depending on the sensitivity for blood of the test used, 2–10% of asymptomatic people over the age of 50 years screened for colorectal cancer with a FOBT will have a positive result that requires the performance of colonoscopy.[1] In the USA approximately 2% and 5% of men and women, respectively, have iron-deficiency anemia. In women who are beyond their reproductive years, and in most men, chronic iron-deficiency anemia often is due to chronic occult rectal bleeding. Population-based surveys show that scant bright red rectal bleeding is very common in adults of all ages. Talley and Jones conducted a population-based survey in Olmsted County, Minnesota.[2] Scant bright red blood per rectum was reported by 13% and was more common among younger adults. Only 14% of people with any type of rectal bleeding had consulted their physician about the problem. Acute severe rectal bleeding requiring hospitalization and resuscitation has been estimated to occur about one-fifth, as commonly as serious bleeding from the upper GI tract.[3] The annual incidence rate is estimated to be 20.5–27 cases per 100 000 of the adult population. Severe rectal bleeding is significantly more common in men than in women, and the incidence increases dramatically with age, with a greater than 200-fold increase from the third to the ninth decades of life. In a large series from the Mayo Clinic the mean age of patients admitted for severe rectal bleeding was 71 years.[4] Patients with serious acute rectal bleeding not only tend to be older, they also are much more likely to have complicating co-morbidity (e.g., cardiovascular, pulmonary, renal, or hepatic disease) that must be managed concomitantly.

TABLE 11.1 DIFFERENT TYPES OF RECTAL BLEEDING
• Asymptomatic patient with a positive fecal occult blood test
• Occult rectal bleeding with chronic iron-deficiency anemia
• Intermittent scant outlet rectal bleeding
• Intermittent passage of dark or maroon stools, or blood mixed in with stool
• Acute severe rectal bleeding
• Massive, continuous rectal bleeding

Fortunately, the number of patients with massive, continuous rectal bleeding that requires immediate surgery constitutes only 1–2% of patients in most series.

CAUSES

Occult rectal bleeding in asymptomatic patients often results from colorectal cancer or advanced large adenomatous polyps, but may be due to a large number of other, benign, inflammatory conditions and mucosal lesions throughout the upper and lower GI tract. Scant outlet hematochezia most often results from anorectal disease, such as hemorrhoids, fissures, or proctitis. Intermittent passage of dark or maroon stools, or blood that is mixed in with the stool, usually originates from the more proximal colon, the small bowel, or sometimes the upper GI tract. Colorectal cancer or advanced adenomatous polyps in the proximal colon may be the cause of this type of bleeding. Such bleeding is also commonly the result of vascular anomalies, ulceration, or colitis (idiopathic, or infectious, ischemic, or radiation induced).

CAUSES AND DIFFERENTIAL DIAGNOSIS
COMMON CAUSES OF EACH TYPE OF RECTAL BLEEDING
OCCULT STOOL BLOOD
Cancer or advanced adenomatous polyps
Angiodysplasia
Other mucosal lesions or disease in colon, small bowel, or upper GI tract
SCANT OUTLET HEMATOCHEZIA
Hemorrhoids
Anal fissures
Proctitis
Distal cancer or polyps
DARK OR MAROON STOOLS, BLOOD MIXED WITH STOOL
Proximal colonic cancer or polyps
Angiodysplasia
Colitis (inflammatory bowel disease, infectious, ischemic)
Colonic ulceration
Small bowel or upper GI tract lesions or disease
ACUTE SEVERE RECTAL BLEEDING
Diverticulosis
Angiodysplasia
Colitis (inflammatory bowel disease, radiation, ischemic)
Cancer or advanced adenomatous polyps
Postpolypectomy bleeding
Ulceration (colonic, rectal)

In the large Mayo Clinic series, and most others, diverticulosis was the most common cause of acute severe rectal bleeding.[4] Other common causes included angiodysplasia, postpolypectomy bleeding, ischemic or radiation-induced colitis, colonic or rectal ulceration, inflammatory bowel disease, and cancer. Approximately 26% of Mayo Clinic patients with acute rectal bleeding remained undiagnosed following an in-hospital evaluation. Jensen and Machicado reported that the site of bleeding in 80 consecutive patients hospitalized for acute severe rectal bleeding was large bowel 74%, upper GI tract 11%, small bowel 9%, and no site found 6%.[5]

DIAGNOSIS

The adult patient with a positive screening FOBT, with or without iron-deficiency anemia, requires a prompt, elective evaluation with colonoscopy to rule out colorectal neoplasia. A more extensive evaluation, including the performance of upper GI and small bowel endoscopic and radiologic studies, is indicated in patients with chronic occult bleeding of obscure origin causing iron-deficiency anemia. New-onset outlet rectal bleeding may initially be evaluated with flexible sigmoidoscopy. Although such bleeding can come from a low-lying neoplasm, it usually arises from benign anorectal pathology (i.e., hemorrhoids, fissures, proctitis). If no cause of scant outlet rectal bleeding is found by flexible sigmoidoscopy, or if intermittent bleeding persists in spite of treatment of a benign lesion, colonoscopy usually should be performed regardless of the patient's age to rule out proximal colonic neoplasia. Intermittent passage of dark or maroon stools, or of blood that is mixed in with the stool, usually comes from a benign source in the more proximal bowel. Nevertheless colonoscopy is imperative to rule out advanced colorectal neoplasia in these individuals, regardless of age.

Acute major rectal bleeding requiring hospitalization tends to be a more difficult diagnostic and therapeutic challenge than serious upper GI bleeding. An effective management plan for these patients is quickly to assess the severity of bleeding (rate and volume), appropriately resuscitate and stabilize the patient if necessary, attempt to diagnose the site and cause of bleeding, apply therapy in some cases, and, perhaps most importantly, attempt to prevent recurrence. As in the upper GI tract, recurrent bleeding that occurs in hospital in these patients is a predictor of a poorer outcome and increased mortality. In the rare case of massive continuous bleeding there may not be an opportunity for complete resuscitation or any definitive diagnostic studies; the only chance to prevent death may be emergency surgery.

Acute severe rectal bleeding

In the majority of cases of acute severe rectal bleeding the bleeding is intermittent, so there usually is a window of opportunity within the first 24 h to evaluate the patient quickly and thoroughly. A careful history should be obtained of past upper or lower GI tract disease, as this information will often direct the clinician to the correct site and cause of bleeding. Features that predict a higher risk of complications and mortality include the presence of hemodynamic instability, serious active comorbid disease, advanced age, persistent or recurrent bleeding, the need for multiple blood transfusions, or evidence of an acute surgical abdomen. A gastroenterologist and a general surgeon should be involved early in the management of these high-risk patients. Increasing numbers of patients with serious lower GI bleeding are anticoagulated, or are taking antiplatelet agents for cardiovascular disease; their clotting studies often exceed the therapeutic range. The most crucial and effective management of these patients often is quickly to correct their coagulation status.

Diagnosing the cause of acute severe rectal bleeding

Diagnosis of the site and cause of serious lower tract bleeding can be made in four ways: flexible sigmoidoscopy with or without anoscopy, colonoscopy, radionuclide scanning and angiography, or barium enema. Of these, endoscopy has become the first and most important diagnostic approach, with radionuclide scans and angiography reserved for selected patients. Barium enema should rarely, if ever, be used because of its insensitivity; also the barium-filled colon reduces the chances of making a definitive diagnosis or treating the patient with either colonoscopy or angiography.

An initial flexible sigmoidoscopy might be done for selected patients in whom active bleeding appears to be coming from the perianal area or the rectum, or if it seems important because of the patient's history to rule out diffuse colitis. However, without a bowel preparation or in the presence of ongoing bleeding, it may be difficult to visualize the colon. Furthermore, if a potential bleeding site is identified but is not bleeding at the time, it may be impossible to be sure there is not another bleeding source higher up in the colon.

When a patient presents with acute, severe rectal bleeding there is a natural tendency to focus only on a possible colonic source. However, it is crucial to keep in mind that acute rectal bleeding may be coming from an upper GI lesion. The study by Jensen and Machicado showed that 11% of their patients with acute serious rectal bleeding were actually bleeding from a site in the upper tract.[5] An upper GI tract source should be considered particularly if the patient has had epigastric pain, is on nonsteroidal anti-inflammatory medication, or has an unexplained disproportionately raised blood urea nitrogen (BUN) level. A nasogastric tube can quickly be placed and the aspirate observed for blood and bile. If a significant amount of blood is found, or if a clear aspirate contains no bile, a quick upper GI endoscopy should be performed as soon as the patient is stable to rule out an upper GI source such as a bleeding duodenal ulcer. Used in this way, nasogastric aspiration has been shown to have an accuracy of 94–98%.[6] Depending on the clinical suspicion and stability of the patient, an alternative approach is to prepare the patient for colonoscopy as detailed below, and perform the colonoscopy first; if negative, do the upper endoscopy.

Bowel preparation needs to be vigorous and quick to clear the colon of blood. The best approach is to give 3–4 liters of a lavage prep through a small (less uncomfortable) nasogastric tube (12 Fr). Taking the lavage prep orally is often less efficacious in bedridden ill or frail patients. The timing of colonoscopy can be very important in these cases. Usually bleeding stops, at least for a time, and at some time in the first 12–24 h the patient can be adequately prepped and examined. As soon as the prep is completed, the examination should be started. Sometimes, the colonoscopy can be timed to coincide with rebleeding after the initial hemorrhage has stopped. There is little value in trying to colonoscope the patient without first doing a bowel-cleansing prep: blood and stool will greatly diminish the chances of diagnostic and therapeutic success.

If bleeding continues or recurs and colonoscopy is unsuccessful, a technetium-red cell scan can be performed to localize the bleeding site. If the scan is positive, subsequent angiography, sometimes with vasopressin or embolization therapy, may detect and control the bleeding.[7] Surgery may prove necessary, and is most successful in cases where the bleeding site has first been accurately located.

In one large series of 107 patients with severe lower GI bleeding at the Massachusetts General Hospital, this approach was successful in most patients.[8] Emergency colonoscopy after a lavage prep revealed the site and cause of bleeding in 90% and provided definitive endoscopic treatment in 19%. Nuclear scanning followed by angiography was successful in 48% of patients in whom this investigation was used, and allowed for treatment in 22% of the patients. Barium enema and flexible sigmoidoscopy rarely revealed the source when the bleeding was severe.

COLONOSCOPIC THERAPY

Depending on the cause of bleeding, there are several therapeutic options to control colonic bleeding using colonoscopy.[9] Injection in and around the bleeding site with an epinephrine solution is usually the first treatment given. Bipolar coagulation often is combined with injection therapy, especially for angiodysplastic lesions, a nonbleeding visible vessel, or active arterial bleeding, because the combination of injection and cautery is more effective in preventing rebleeding. The argon plasma coagulator is a very effective noncontact way to treat angiodysplastic lesions, radiation colitis, or similar, more diffuse, areas of bleeding. If the point of bleeding is small and discrete, the hemoclip device may be used in patients with an uncorrectable coagulopathy in whom coagulation could induce more bleeding.

Although colonoscopic treatment of bleeding can be very effective in selected patients, overall success is less than for endoscopic treatment of upper tract bleeding. In the large Mayo Clinic series, treatment was successful in 25%.[4] Endoscopic treatment was most likely to be possible when the bleeding was coming from a polypectomy site, angiodysplasia, exophytic lesions such as polyps and cancer, or benign cecal or rectal ulcers. In a small nonrandomized study of 27 patients, Jensen et al. demonstrated that colonoscopic treatment of bleeding diverticula prevented recurrent bleeding and the need for surgery, and substantially shortened hospital stay.[10]

CURRENT CONTROVERSIES

When a patient is screened for colorectal cancer and has a positive FOBT and a negative subsequent colonoscopy, some recommend that an upper GI evaluation must be done to rule out serious upper tract disease. However, most large studies of this issue indicate that, although upper GI abnormalities are commonly found in these asymptomatic patients, they rarely are clinically important or require treatment.[11] The prevalence of curable gastric cancer in these cases is negligible unless the patient also has upper GI tract symptoms or unexplained iron-deficiency anemia.

Many gastroenterologist experts in the USA advocate full colonoscopy for all patients with hematochezia, regardless of their age or the nature of the bleeding. Several studies that have carefully documented the nature of scant hematochezia, however, showed that patients with outlet-type rectal bleeding can effectively be evaluated initially with flexible sigmoidoscopy. Eckardt et al. performed structured preprocedure interviews in 4265 patients referred for colonoscopy for scant hematochezia.[12] Those with outlet-type bleeding (bright red blood on top of the stool and/or on toilet paper) had no increased prevalence of neoplasms located above 50 cm in the colon compared to an equivalent matched group of patients undergoing colonoscopy who did not have bleeding or other risk factors for colorectal cancer.

A number of reviews and studies have questioned the timing of colonoscopy in patients hospitalized with acute severe rectal bleeding. Traditionally, colonoscopic evaluation in such patients was delayed because of fear of increased procedural risks, the need for thorough bowel cleansing, and the lack of proven therapeutic interventions. Several recent studies, however, have shown that urgent colonoscopy (performed within 12h of admission) is safe and effective.[13] Early colonoscopy improves diagnostic yield, and endoscopic therapy can prevent recurrent bleeding and the need for surgical intervention.[13] In addition, studies now indicate that early colonoscopic evaluation may reduce the duration and cost of hospitalization.[14]

SUMMARY

There are several types of rectal bleeding: occult, scant outlet hematochezia, scant passage of changed blood or blood mixed in with stool, or acute severe rectal bleeding. Most causes of rectal bleeding are found in the colon and rectum. Evaluation and management should be tailored to the type of bleeding as well as the individual characteristics of each patient. Minor rectal bleeding rarely is clinically important in itself, although it may be a sign of an underlying colorectal cancer. Acute severe bleeding requiring hospitalization and urgent resuscitation has a higher risk of complications and mortality, especially when it occurs in patients with important co-morbidity or advanced age.

The cornerstone of evaluation and management of patients with acute severe bleeding now is urgent colonoscopy performed in the first 24–48h. In this setting, colonoscopy is safe and often accurately defines both the site and cause of bleeding. In an important minority of patients, endoscopic therapy is possible and obviates the need for other invasive studies or surgery, prevents recurrent bleeding, and frequently shortens hospital stay.

SOURCES OF INFORMATION FOR PATIENTS AND DOCTORS

http://www.patient.co.uk/showdoc/40000118/

REFERENCES

1. Bond JH. Fecal occult blood test screening for colorectal cancer. Gastrointest Endosc Clin N Am 2002; 12:11–22.
2. Talley NJ, Jones M. Self-reported rectal bleeding in a United States community: prevalence, risk factors and health care seeking. Gastroenterology 1998; 93:2179–2183.
3. Zuckerman GR, Prakash C. Acute lower intestinal bleeding: clinical presentation and diagnosis. Gastrointest Endosc 1998; 48:606–616.
4. Gostout CJ, Wang KK, Ahlquist DA et al. Acute gastrointestinal bleeding: experience of a specialized management team. J Clin Gastroenterol 1992; 14:260–267.
5. Jensen DM, Machicado GA. Diagnosis and treatment of severe hematochezia: the role of urgent colonoscopy after purge. Gastroenterology 1998; 95: 1569–1574.
6. Luk GD, Bynum TE, Hendrdix TR. Gastric aspiration in localization of gastrointestinal hemorrhage. JAMA 1979; 241:576–578.
7. Zuccaro G, Prakash C. Management of the adult patient with acute lower gastrointestinal bleeding. Am J Gastroenterol 1998; 93: 1202–1208.
8. Richter JM, Christensen MR, Kaplan LM, Nishoika NS. Effectiveness of current technology in the diagnosis and management of lower gastrointestinal hemorrhage. Gastrointest Endosc 1995; 41:93–98.
9. Jensen DA, Machicado GA. Colonoscopy and severe hematochezia. In Waye JD, Rex DK, Williams CB, eds. Colonoscopy: principles and practice. Malden, Massachusetts: Blackwell; 2003:561–572.
10. Jensen DM, Machicado DA, Jutabha R, Kovacs TO. Urgent colonoscopy for the diagnosis and treatment of severe diverticular hemorrhage. N Engl J Med 2000; 342:78–82.
11. Chen YK, Gladden DR, Kestenbaum DJ. Is there a role for upper gastrointestinal endoscopy in the evaluation of patients with occult blood-positive stool and negative colonoscopy? Am J Gastroenterol 1993; 88:2026–2029.
12. Eckardt VF, Schmitt T, Kanzier G et al. Does scant hematochezia necessitate the performance of total colonoscopy? Endoscopy 2002; 34: 599–603.
13. Zuccao G for the Practice Parameters Committee of the American College of Gastroenterology. Management of the adult patient with acute lower gastrointestinal bleeding. Am J Gastroenterol 1998; 93:1202–1208.
14. Strate LL, Syngal S. Timing of colonoscopy: impact on length of hospital stay in patients with acute lower intestinal bleeding. Am J Gastroenterol 2003; 98:317–322.

Chapter 12

Anorectal pain and pruritus ani

Steven D Wexner and Giovanna M da Silva

ANORECTAL PAIN

INTRODUCTION

Anorectal pain refers to pain localized in the anorectal area, the origin of which may be organic or functional. It is a very common complaint that is usually caused by benign conditions. Organic causes of anorectal pain are very common and are described in Chapter 70. Functional pain is estimated to occur in 6–19% of the population, with a slightly higher prevalence in women.[1] Although effective treatment options exist for many of the organic causes of anorectal pain, functional anorectal pain is often challenging, even for the most experienced specialists.

PATHOPHYSIOLOGY

The pain pathway uses three neurons to convey pain information from peripheral sensory receptors to the conscious level of the cerebral cortex. The anal region is richly supplied with free nerve endings of C fibers, which are activated by a cut, burn, tear, or bump. The afferent nerves of the viscera and pelvic floor musculature cannot localize noxious stimuli as precisely as nerves from the skin. As a result, patients with pain related to the pelvic floor muscles may not perceive it as originating in the pelvic musculature. Conversely, they may have symptoms from visceral structures surrounding and attached to the pelvic floor (urinary urgency, rectal pain, dyspareunia). In addition, because neural pathways lead to the limbic centers, they can also experience varying degrees of emotional distress.[2]

CAUSES/DIFFERENTIAL DIAGNOSIS

Common anorectal diseases are generally the cause of organic anorectal pain including anal fissure, anorectal abscess, hemorrhoidal pain related to thrombosed external hemorrhoids, rectal inflammation (proctitis, Crohn's disease, ulcerative colitis, radiation). Prior surgery may also produce anorectal pain due to adhesion formation, fibrosis, traumatic neuropathy (pelvic procedures), muscle spasm, or stenosis (anorectal procedures). Neoplastic lesions in or around the anal canal may initially present with insidious pain. Rectal cancer is seldom painful unless there is invasion of the sphincter muscle. Finally, benign or malignant organic diseases of any pelvic organ and/or structure can lead to anorectal pain. This pain is often associated with other symptoms related to the affected organ.

The most common causes of functional pain are levator ani syndrome and proctalgia fugax. Levator ani syndrome is a vague, dull ache or pressure sensation in the rectum that usually worsens when supine or sitting and may last for 20 min or longer. Levator ani syndrome should be differentiated from coccygodynia, which is often described as an aching or gnawing, sometimes sharp, pain, that may radiate into the buttocks. Although some authors have considered coccygodynia as a variant of the anorectal pain syndromes, it is a distinct condition and should be used only when there is a true orthopedic coccygeal disorder. Proctalgia fugax is a sudden onset of severe sharp, stabbing, or crampy rectal pain that lasts for seconds to minutes and then disappears, sometimes awakening the patient from sleep. It may occur in clusters as often as three to four times weekly, several times each year.

CAUSES AND DIFFERENTIAL DIAGNOSIS
CAUSES OF ANORECTAL PAIN
ORGANIC
Anorectal disorders – fissure, abscess, thrombosed hemorrhoids, and sexually transmitted diseases
Proctitis – ulcerative colitis, Crohn's disease, radiation, infectious
Previous surgery – low anterior resection, stenosis
Malignancy – of any pelvic organ, nerve, muscle, or bone
Gynecologic abnormalities – torsed ovarian cyst, endometriosis, ectopic pregnancy
Urinary abnormalities – prostatitis
Neurologic abnormalities – nerve compression (pudendal entrapment), multiple sclerosis
Orthopedic causes – coccygodynia, degenerative disease of the lumbosacral spine
FUNCTIONAL
Levator ani syndrome
Proctalgia fugax
Chronic idiopathic pain
Psychogenic

SYMPTOM COMPLEXES

Pain associated with bleeding is usually a sign of anorectal abnormality such as anal fissure and thrombosed hemorrhoids, which are often associated with constipation. The presence of fever associated with pain denotes an infectious process, most commonly an abscess. Pain, bleeding, and diarrhea may suggest inflammation of the bowel including radiation proctitis and inflammatory bowel disease. In males, pain associated with urinary symptoms may suggest prostatitis or any other urologic disorder. The presence of gynecologic symptoms in females warrants gynecologic examination. Patients with functional pain usually have associated functional gastrointestinal complaints. In a study conducted in 60 consecutive patients with chronic intractable rectal pain, 95% had one or more associated factors of constipation or dyschezia (57%), prior pelvic surgery (43%), prior anal surgery (32%), prior spinal surgery (8%), irritable bowel syndrome (10%), or psychiatric disorder (depression or anxiety, 25%).[3]

DIAGNOSIS

The evaluation of anorectal pain includes a detailed history and careful physical examination. The nature of the pain and its relationship to bowel movements frequently helps to distinguish the etiologic factor. Inspection, palpation, digital examination if tolerable, anoscopy, and sigmoidoscopy will reveal most common anorectal pathologies. Colonoscopy may be indicated in selected patients, especially in the presence of bleeding and change in bowel habits. If the rectal pain is not associated with an obvious benign condition and the patient cannot tolerate thorough office examination, an examination under anesthesia is warranted. Diagnostic imaging including computed tomography (CT), magnetic resonance imaging (MRI), and endorectal ultrasonography may be helpful to rule out a tumor or abscess.

A diagnosis of functional pain is made after all organic causes have been excluded. In patients with levator ani syndrome, the pain may be elicited by rectal massage, usually greater on the left than on the right side. Coccygodynia denotes pain with coccygeal manipulation. The diagnosis of proctalgia fugax is obtained from the patient's history as there are no physical findings or tests for diagnosing this condition. A complete work-up including anorectal physiology studies, CT, colonoscopy, and MRI may be employed in addition to gastroenterologic, gynecologic, pain management, neurologic, and psychologic evaluation. Multiple negative testing should be used to provide reassurance, not dismissal of patients' concerns.

DIAGNOSTIC METHODS
DIAGNOSIS OF ANORECTAL PAIN
• Detailed history • Inspection • Palpation (digital examination) • Anoscopy • Flexible sigmoidoscopy • Colonoscopy • Rectal ultrasonography • Computed tomography (CT) • Magnetic resonance imaging (MRI)

PRURITUS ANI (see also Chapter 17)

INTRODUCTION

Pruritus ani is an unpleasant cutaneous sensation around the perianal area that provokes the desire to scratch and has also been described as a burning sensation. Pruritus ani is a symptom with a wide spectrum of etiologies, which often makes the diagnosis and treatment difficult. Like pain, acute itch serves as a protective function; however, this may become a chronic cycle of itching and scratching, resulting in significant skin excoriation and soreness, with a great impact on the patient's quality of life. Pruritus ani is an extremely common symptom in the colorectal practice, affecting 1–5% of the general population, with a greater incidence in males than in females (4:1) in the fifth and sixth decades of life. This condition is rare in children and is usually associated with infection.

PATHOPHYSIOLOGY

Although pruritus ani and pain share a common neurologic pathway, it has been demonstrated that pruritus is mediated by a distinct subset of afferent C fibers that are insensitive to mechanical stimuli but responsive to histamine and other pruritogens. These are elicited by local irritation from excoriation, alkaline secretions, and various chemical irritants.[4] The complex interactions between pain and itch may explain the antipruritic effect of scratching.

CAUSES/DIFFERENTIAL DIAGNOSIS

Despite comprehensive evaluation to elucidate the etiologic factor of pruritus, 50–90% of cases are considered idiopathic in nature; the remainder are secondary to local or systemic diseases.

Most commonly, pruritus is secondary to inappropriate local hygiene. Both inadequate and excessive cleansing may lead to symptoms. Adequate hygiene may be particularly deficient in obese people or those with deep anal clefts, excessive hair, and who wear tightfitting clothing, especially in hot weather. In diarrheal conditions, such as with inflammatory bowel disease and laxative abuse, the skin may be directly affected by both stool contact and frequent cleaning.

Diet is another common reason for pruritus, changing stool consistency and leading to increased stool leakage and irritation as well as having a direct affect on the anus. It is known that caffeine, milk products, and alcohol, specifically beer and wine, may cause severe perianal irritation. Citrus foods, tomatoes, and spicy foods can also lead to intense pruritus.

Dermatologic conditions such as seborrhea, atopic eczema, lichen sclerosis, contact dermatitis, and psoriasis (Fig. 12.1) may be primarily responsible for anal pruritus. In a series of 40 consecutive patients with pruritus ani referred for a combined colorectal and dermatologic evaluation, Dasan et al. found recognizable dermatoses in 34 patients.[5]

Primary anorectal pathologies including fistula, fissure, anal tags, and mucosal prolapse may be a causative or contributory factor in approximately 25% of patients. Other causes include infectious diseases such as scabies (Fig. 12.2) and fungal infections (Fig. 12.3). In children, pinworm infection should be suspected.

Very importantly, pruritus ani may be the main complaint in patients with anal cancer or premalignant disease.[6] Rectal tumors or large polyps may result in excessive seepage secondary to a loss of rectal compliance or excessive secretions from the lesion.

Systemic diseases such as cholestatic jaundice, chronic renal failure, vitamin deficiency (specifically vitamins A, C, and D),

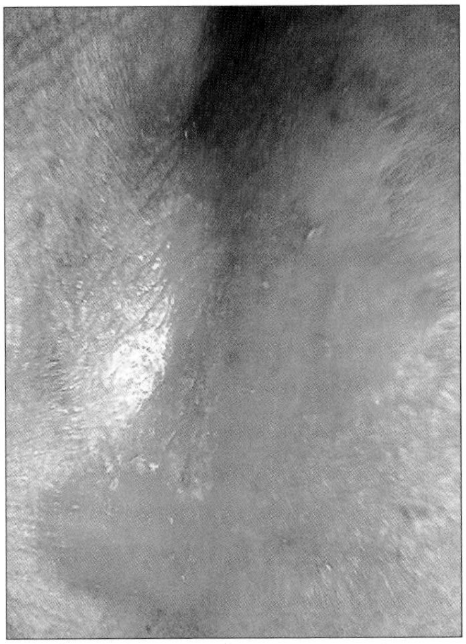

Fig. 12.1 Psoriasis. From Shahbaz A, Dermatlas; http://www.dermatlas.org

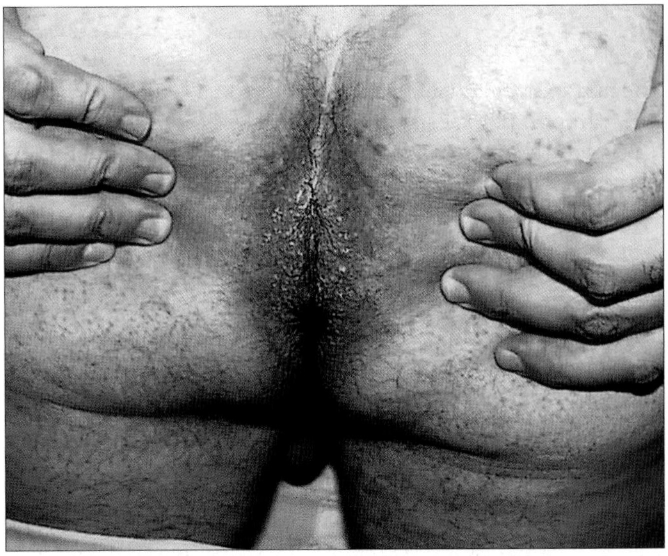

Fig. 12.3 Tinea circinata. From Shahbaz A, Dermatlas; http://www.dermatlas.org

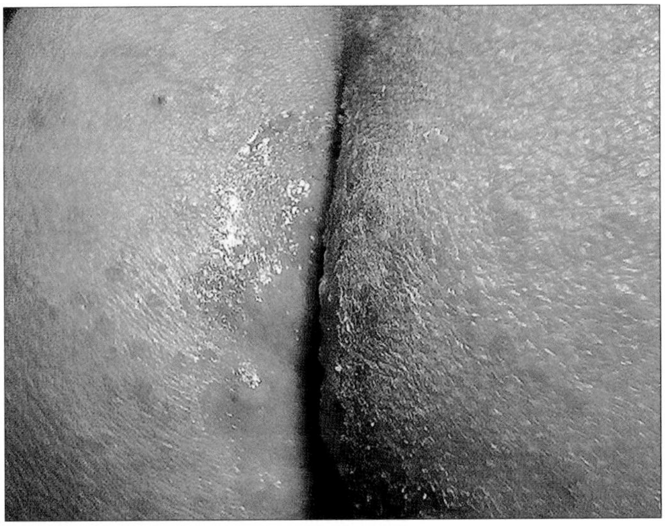

Fig. 12.2 Scabies. From Kosman Sadek Zikry, Dermatlas; http://www.dermatlas.org

CAUSES AND DIFFERENTIAL DIAGNOSIS
CAUSES OF PRURITUS ANI

- Idiopathic
- Hygiene habits – vigorous cleaning and poor hygiene
- Diet – tomatoes, caffeinated beverages, chocolate, citrus juice or fruit, spicy foods, beer, milk products, vitamin A and D deficiencies, fat substitutes
- Diarrheal states – irritable bowel syndromes, Crohn's disease, ulcerative colitis
- Dermatologic conditions – psoriasis, seborrheic dermatitis, intertrigo, atopic dermatitis, lichen planus, and lichen sclerosis; radiodermatitis
- Benign anorectal pathologies – fistula, fissure, skin tags, prolapsing papilla, mucosal prolapse, stool leakage
- Gynecologic conditions – pruritus vulvae, vaginal discharge
- Infections – parasites (pinworms, pediculosis, scabies), viruses (condyloma, herpes), bacteria (syphilis), fungi or yeasts, sexually transmitted diseases
- Neoplasms – Bowen's disease, extramammary Paget's disease, squamous cell carcinoma, malignancy, anorectal polypoid lesions
- Systemic disease – jaundice, diabetes mellitus, chronic renal failure, iron deficiency, thyrotoxicosis, myxedema, Hodgkin's lymphoma, polycythemia vera
- Exposures – systemic (quinidine, colchicine, tetracycline) and topical (soaps, perfumes, and ointments that may contain alcohol)

polycythemia vera (secondary to histamine release), thyrotoxicosis, myxedema, diabetes mellitus (candida infection), and Hodgkin's disease can cause isolated anal itching.

Finally, numerous drugs are known contributors to pruritus ani, including oral and intravenous systemic medications and topical substances. Systemic medications include quinidine, colchicines, oral mineral oil, tetracycline, and hydrocortisone. Any topical ointment applied to the perianal area may cause or exacerbate pruritus ani, usually secondary to a contact dermatitis. Other agents include alcohol, perfumes, and formaldehyde.

SYMPTOM COMPLEXES

Patients complaining of pruritus and anal pain, lump, or other local abnormality suggest the local condition as the causative factor of the pruritus. Pruritus secondary to systemic disease may be associated with features of a specific disease that help isolate the etiologic factor. For example, cholestatic jaundice may occur secondary to oral contraceptives, testosterone, and chlorpromazine use. Pruritus is common in patients undergoing hemodialysis for chronic renal failure. Evidence of concomitant anemia may suggest iron deficiency as a causative factor of the pruritus, although anemia may be absent. A history of pruritus exacerbated by alcohol may be indicative of Hodgkin's disease, whereas pruritus aggravated by bathing may suggest polycythemia vera. Patients with diet-induced pruritus often associate the onset of the symptom with ingestion of a specific food or drink.

DIAGNOSIS

The diagnosis of idiopathic pruritus should be made by exclusion only after all potential secondary causes have been excluded. The history should consider diet, clothing habits, medication use, diarrheal states, hygiene practices, sexual activity, anorectal pathologies, and previous surgery, as well as systemic illnesses such as diabetes, chronic renal failure, polycythemia vera, and others. Vaginal discharge and other gynecologic conditions should also be investigated in females. Psychologic factors such as stress and anxiety should be discussed as they may play an important role in this condition, but be dismissed by patients.

Physical examination begins with a careful skin evaluation of the entire body in order to identify psoriasis, seborrheic dermatitis, fungal or other infections. The perianal area is then examined for signs of moisture, soiling, excoriation, skin maceration, or perianal dermatoses. Patch testing, cultures, biopsies or scraping of lesions are acquired, as indicated. The anal tonus is then assessed by digital examination. Proctoscopy, sigmoidoscopy, or colonoscopy may be useful to rule out proctitis, inflammatory bowel disease, rectal lesions, or active infections causing pruritus. Laboratory tests should include blood count and stool examination for ova and parasites. Anorectal physiology studies may indicate minor leakage secondary to abnormal transient internal sphincter relaxation as a cause of idiopathic pruritus ani.[7] Finally, a combined evaluation with a dermatologist may be greatly beneficial in the diagnosis and treatment of patients with pruritus ani.

DIAGNOSTIC METHODS
DIAGNOSIS OF PRURITUS ANI
• Detailed history • Physical examination • Inspection • Digital examination • Anoscopy • Flexible sigmoidoscopy or colonoscopy • Patch testing, cultures, biopsies, scraping • Laboratory testing (blood, stool) • Anorectal physiology

SOURCES OF INFORMATION FOR PATIENTS AND DOCTORS

http://www.patient.co.uk/showdoc/942/
http://www.patient.co.uk/showdoc/40000238/
http://cchs-dl.slis.ua.edu/patientinfo/gastroenterology/lower/anorectal/pruritus-ani.htm
http://www.betterhealth.vic.gov.au/bhcv2/bhcarticles.nsf/pages/Anal_fissure?Open

REFERENCES

1. Wald A. Functional anorectal and rectal pain. Gastroenterol Clin N Am 2001; 30:243–251.
2. Weiss J. Chronic pelvic pain and myofascial trigger points. Pain Clinic 2000; 2:13–18.
3. Ger GC, Wexner SD, Jorge JM et al. Evaluation and treatment of chronic intractable rectal pain—a frustrating endeavor. Dis Colon Rectum 1993; 36:247–248.
4. Ikoma A, Rukwied R, Stander S et al. Neurophysiology of pruritus. Interaction of itch and pain. Arch Dermatol 2003; 139:1475–1478.
5. Dasan S, Neill SM, Donaldson DR, Scott HJ. Treatment of persistent pruritus ani in a combined colorectal and dermatological clinic. Br J Surg 1999; 86:1337–1340.
6. Handa Y, Watanabe O, Adachi A, Yamanaka N. Squamous cell carcinoma of the anal margin with pruritus ani of long duration. Dermatol Surg 2003; 29:108–110.
7. Farouk R, Duthie GS, Pryde A, Bartolo DC. Abnormal transient internal sphincter relaxation in idiopathic pruritus ani: physiological evidence from ambulatory monitoring. Br J Surg 1994; 81:603–606.

Chapter 13

Functional gastrointestinal disease

The editors

A high proportion of gastrointestinal disorders are functional. Functional disorders are those in which significant gastrointestinal symptoms are not associated with organic disease but to metabolic, infectious, neoplastic, or other structural abnormalities. A number of functional symptoms have been recognized, based on clusters of symptoms. There have been a number of attempts to define these as precisely as possible, of which the Rome II[1] criteria are the most recent and best developed.

These criteria have been found to be useful in clinical trials. In clinical practice there is a dilemma in that the more precise the definition, the lower the proportion of patients that are encompassed by it,[2] so that many of the Rome II criteria exclude patients who might attract a particular 'label' in more informal clinical practice. Whether the current criteria are too narrow, whether informal approaches adopted in practice are too lax, and whether a symptom rather than a syndrome based approach to functional gastrointestinal disorders would be more productive are all unanswered questions. To assist readers in considering these issues, the overall classification of functional gastrointestinal disorders (Table 13.1) and the formal diagnostic criteria for establishing them (Tables 13.2–13.8) are reproduced here.[3]

TABLE 13.1 FUNCTIONAL GASTROINTESTINAL DISORDERS

A. ESOPHAGEAL DISORDERS
- A1. Globus
- A2. Rumination syndrome
- A3. Functional chest pain of presumed esophageal origin
- A4. Functional heartburn
- A5. Functional dysphagia
- A6. Unspecified functional esophageal disorder

B. GASTRODUODENAL DISORDERS
- B1. Functional dyspepsia
  - B1a. Ulcer-like dyspepsia
  - B1b. Dysmotility-like dyspepsia
  - B1c. Unspecified (nonspecific) dyspepsia
- B2. Aerophagia
- B3. Functional vomiting

C. BOWEL DISORDERS
- C1. Irritable bowel syndrome
- C2. Functional abdominal bloating
- C3. Functional constipation
- C4. Functional diarrhea
- C5. Unspecified functional bowel disorder

D. FUNCTIONAL ABDOMINAL PAIN
- D1. Functional abdominal pain syndrome
- D2. Unspecified functional abdominal pain

E. FUNCTIONAL DISORDERS OF THE BILIARY TRACT AND THE PANCREAS
- E1. Gallbladder dysfunction
- E2. Sphincter of Oddi dysfunction

F. ANORECTAL DISORDERS
- F1. Functional fecal incontinence
- F2. Functional anorectal pain
  - F2a. Levator ani syndrome
  - F2b. Proctalgia fugax
- F3. Pelvic floor dyssynergia

G. FUNCTIONAL PEDIATRIC DISORDERS
- G1. Infant regurgitation
  - G1a. Infant rumination syndrome
  - G1b. Cyclic vomiting syndrome
- G2. Abdominal pain
  - G2a. Functional dyspepsia
    - G2a1. Ulcer-like dyspepsia
    - G2a2. Dysmotility-like dyspepsia
    - G2a3. Unspecified (nonspecific) dyspepsia
  - G2b. Irritable bowel syndrome
  - G2c. Functional abdominal pain
  - G2d. Abdominal migraine
  - G2e. Aerophagia
- G3. Functional diarrhea
- G4. Disorders of defecation
  - G4a. Infant dyschezia
  - G4b. Functional constipation
  - G4c. Functional fecal retention
  - G4d. Functional nonretentive fecal soiling

TABLE 13.2 FUNCTIONAL ESOPHAGEAL DISORDERS

A1. GLOBUS
At least 12 weeks, which need not be consecutive, in the preceding 12 months of:
1. The persistent or intermittent sensation of a lump or foreign body in the throat;
2. Occurrence of the sensation between meals;
3. Absence of dysphagia and odynophagia; *and*
4. Absence of pathologic gastroesophageal reflux, achalasia, or other motility disorder with a recognized pathologic basis (e.g., scleroderma of the esophagus).

A2. RUMINATION SYNDROME
At least 12 weeks, which need not be consecutive, in the preceding 12 months of:
1. Persistent or recurrent regurgitation of recently ingested food into the mouth with subsequent remastication and swallowing or spitting it out;
2. Absence of nausea and vomiting;
3. Cessation of the process when the regurgitated material becomes acidic; *and*
4. Absence of pathologic gastroesophageal refluex, achalasia, or other motility disorder with a recognized pathologic basis as the primary disorder.

A3. FUNCTIONAL CHEST PAIN OF PRESUMED ESOPHAGEAL ORIGIN
At least 12 weeks, which need not be consecutive, within the preceding 12 months of:
1. Midline chest pain or discomfort that is not of burning quality; *and*
2. Absence of pathologic gastroesophageal efflux, achalasia, or other motility disorder with a recognized pathologic basis.

A4. FUNCTIONAL HEARTBURN
At least 12 weeks, which need not be consecutive, in the preceding 12 months of:
1. Burning retrosternal discomfort or pain; *and*
2. Absence of pathologic gastroesophageal reflux, achalasia, or other motility disorder with a recognized pathologic basis.

A5. FUNCTIONAL DYSPHAGIA
At least 12 weeks, which need not be consecutive, in the preceding 12 months of:
1. Sense of solid and/or liquid foods sticking, lodging, or passing abnormally through the esophagus; *and*
2. Absence of pathologic gastroesophageal reflux, achalasia, or other motility disorder with a recognized pathologic basis.

A6. UNSPECIFIED FUNCTIONAL ESOPHAGEAL DISORDER
At least 12 weeks, which need not be consecutive, in the preceding 12 months of:
1. Unexplained symptoms attributed to the esophagus that do not fit into the previously described categories; *and*
2. Absence of pathologic gastroesophageal reflux, achalasia, or other motility disorder with a recognized pathologic basis.

The diagnosis of a functional esophageal disorder always presumes the absence of a structural or biochemical explanation for the symptoms.

TABLE 13.3 FUNCTIONAL GASTRODUODENAL DISORDERS

B1. FUNCTIONAL DYSPEPSIA
At least 12 weeks, which need not be consecutive, in the preceding 12 months of:
1. Persistent or recurrent symptoms (pain or discomfort centered in the upper abdomen);
2. No evidence of organic disease (including at upper endoscopy) that is likely to explain the symptoms; *and*
3. No evidence that dyspepsia is exclusively relieved by defecation or associated with the onset of a change in stool frequency or stool form (i.e., not irritable bowel).

B1a. Ulcer-like dyspepsia
Pain centered in the upper abdomen is the predominant (most bothersome) symptom.

B1b. Dysmotility-like dyspepsia
An unpleasant or troublesome nonpainful sensation (discomfort) centered in the upper abdomen is the predominant symptom; this sensation may be characterized by or associated with upper abdominal fullness, early satiety, bloating, or nausea.

B1c. Unspecified (nonspecific) dyspepsia
Symptomatic patients whose symptoms do not fulfil the criteria for ulcer-like or dysmotility-like dyspepsia.

B2. AEROPHAGIA
At least 12 weeks, which need not be consecutive, in the preceding 12 months of:
1. Air swallowing that is observed objectively; *and*
2. Troublesome repetitive belching.

B3. FUNCTIONAL VOMITING
At least 12 weeks, which need not be consecutive, in the preceding 12 months of:
1. Frequent episodes of vomiting, occurring on at least three separate days in a week over 3 days;
2. Absence of criteria for an eating disorder, rumination, or major psychiatric disease according to DSM-IV;
3. Absence of self-induced and medication-induced vomiting; *and*
4. Absence of abnormalities in the gut or central nervous system, and metabolic diseases to explain the recurrent vomiting.

The diagnosis of a functional gastroduodenal disorder always presumes the absence of a structural or biochemical explanation for the symptoms.

TABLE 13.4 FUNCTIONAL BOWEL DISORDERS

C1. IRRITABLE BOWEL SYNDROME
At least 12 weeks, which need not be consecutive, in the preceding 12 months of:
1. Relieved with defecation; *and/or*
2. Onset associated with a change in frequency of stool; *and/or*
3. Onset associated with a change in form (appearance) of stool.

Symptoms that cumulatively support the diagnosis of irritable bowel syndrome:
- Abnormal stool frequency (for research purposes 'abnormal' may be defined as more than three bowel movements per day and fewer than three bowel movements per week);
- Abnormal stool form (lumpy/hard or loose/watery stool);
- Abnormal stool passage (straining, urgency, or feeling of incomplete evacuation);
- Passage of mucus;
- Bloating or feeling of abdominal distention.

C2. FUNCTIONAL ABDOMINAL BLOATING
At least 12 weeks, which need not be consecutive, in the preceding 12 months of:
1. Feeling of abdominal fullness, bloating, or visible distention; *and*
2. Insufficient criteria for a diagnosis of functional dyspepsia, irritable bowel syndrome, or other functional disorder.

C3. FUNCTIONAL CONSTIPATION
At least 12 weeks, which need not be consecutive, in the preceding 12 months of:
1. Straining in more than a quarter of defecations;
2. Lumpy or hard stools in more than a quarter of defecations;
3. Sensation of incomplete evacuation in more than a quarter of defecations;
4. Sensation of anorectal obstruction/blockage in more than a quarter of defecations;
5. Manual maneuvers to facilitate more than a quarter of defecations (e.g., digitial evacuation, support of the pelvic floor); *and/or*
6. Less than three defecations per week.

Loose stools are not present, and there are insufficient criteria for irritable bowel syndrome.

C4. FUNCTIONAL DIARRHEA
At least 12 weeks, which need not be consecutive, in the preceding 12 months of:
1. Loose (mushy) or watery stools
2. Present more than three-quarters of the time; *and*
3. No abdominal pain.

C5. UNSPECIFIED FUNCTIONAL BOWEL DISORDER
Bowel symptoms in the absence of organic disease that do not fit into the previously defined categories of functional bowel disorder.

The diagnosis of a functional bowel disorder always presumes the absence of a structural or biochemical explanation for the symptoms.

TABLE 13.5 FUNCTIONAL ABDOMINAL PAIN

D1. FUNCTIONAL ABDOMINAL PAIN SYNDROME
At lease 6 months of:
1. Continuous or nearly continuous abdominal pain; *and*
2. No or only occasional relationship of pain with physiologic events (e.g., eating, defecation, or menses); *and*
3. Some loss of daily functioning; *and*
4. The pain is not feigned (e.g., malingering), *and*
5. Insufficient criteria for other functional gastrointestinal disorders that would explain the abdominal pain.

D2. UNSPECIFIED FUNCTIONAL ABDOMINAL PAIN
This is functional abdominal pain that fails to reach criteria for functional abdominal pain syndrome.

The diagnosis of functional abdominal pain always presumes the absence of a structural or biochemical explanation for the symptoms.

TABLE 13.6 FUNCTIONAL DISORDERS OF THE BILIARY TRACT AND THE PANCREAS

E1. GALLBLADDER DYSFUNCTION
Episodes of severe steady pain located in the epigastrium and right upper quadrant, and all of the following:
1. Symptom episodes last 30 min or more, with pain-free intervals;
2. Symptoms have occurred on one or more occasions in the previous 12 months;
3. The pain is steady and interrupts daily activities or requires consultation with a physician;
4. There is no evidence of structural abnormalities to explain the symptoms; *and*
5. There is abnormal gallbladder functioning with regard to emptying.

E2. SPHINCTER OF ODDI DYSFUNCTION
Episodes of severe steady pain located in the epigastrium and right upper quadrant, and all of the following:
1. Symptom episodes last 30 min or more, with pain-free intervals;
2. Symptoms have occurred on one or more occasions in the previous 12 months;
3. The pain is steady and interrupts daily activities or requires consultation with a physician; *and*
4. There is no evidence of structural abnormalities to explain the symptoms.

The diagnosis of a functional disorder of the biliary tract and pancreas always presumes the absence of a structural or biochemical explanation for the symptoms.

TABLE 13.7 FUNCTIONAL DISORDERS OF THE ANUS AND RECTUM

F1. FUNCTIONAL FECAL INCONTINENCE
Recurrent uncontrolled passage of fecal material for at least 1 month, in an individual with a developmental age of at least 4 years, associated with:
1. Fecal impaction; *or*
2. Diarrhea; *or*
3. Nonstructural anal sphincter dysfunction.

F2. FUNCTIONAL ANORECTAL PAIN
F2a. Levator ani ayndrome
At least 12 weeks, which need not be consecutive, in the preceding 12 months of:
1. Chronic or recurrent rectal pain or aching;
2. Episodes last 20 min or longer; *and*
3. Other causes of rectal pain such as ischemia, inflammatory bowel disease, cryptitis, intramuscular abscess, fissure, hemorrhoids, prostatitis, and solitary rectal ulcer have been excluded.

F2b. Proctalgia fugax
1. Recurrent episodes of pain localized to the anus or lower rectum;
2. Episodes last from seconds to minutes; *and*
3. There is no anorectal pain between episodes.

F3. PELVIC FLOOR DYSSYNERGIA
1. The patient must satisfy diagnostic criteria for functional constipation in Diagnostic Criterion C3;
2. There must be manometric, electromyogenic, or radiologic evidence for inappropriate contraction or failure to relax the pelvic floor muscles during repeated attempts to defecate;
3. There must be evidence of adequate propulsive forces during attempts to defecate, *and*
4. There must be evidence of incomplete evacuation.

The diagnosis of a functional disorder of the anus and rectum always presumes the absence of a structural or biochemical explanation for the symptoms.

TABLE 13.8 CHILDHOOD FUNCTIONAL GASTROINTESTINAL DISORDERS

G1. VOMITING
G1a. Infant regurgitation
1. Regurgitation two or more times for 3 weeks or more;
2. There is no retching, hematemesis, aspiration, apnea, failure to thrive, or abnormal posturing;
3. The infant must be 1–12 months of age and otherwise healthy; *and*
4. There is no evidence of metabolic, gastrointestinal, or central nervous system disease to explain the symptom.

G1b. Infant rumination syndrome
At least 2 months of stereotypical behavior beginning with repetitive contractions of the abdominal muscles, diaphragm, and tongue, and culminating in regurgitation of gastric contents into the mouth, which is either expectorated or rechewed and reswallowed, and three or more of the following:
a. Onset between 3 and 8 months of age;
b. Does not respond to management for gastroesophageal efflux disease, anticholinergic drugs, hand restraints, formula changes, and gavage or gastrostomy feedings;
c. Unaccompanied by signs of nausea or distress; *and/or*
d. Does not occur during sleep and when the infant is interacting with individuals in the environment.

G1c. Cyclic vomiting syndrome
1. A history of three or more periods of intense, acute nausea, and unremitting vomiting lasting from hours to days, with intervening symptom-free intervals lasting from weeks to months;
2. There is no metabolic, gastrointestinal, or central nervous system structural or biochemical disease.

G2. ABDOMINAL PAIN
G2a. Functional dyspepsia
In children mature enough to provide an accurate pain history, at least 12 weeks, which need not be consecutive, in the preceding 12 months of:
1. Persistent or recurrent pain or discomfort centered in the upper abdomen (above the umbilicus);
2. No evidence of organic disease (including at upper endoscopy) that is likely to explain the symptoms; *and*
3. No evidence that dyspepsia is exclusively relieved by defecation or associated with onset of a change in stool frequency or stool form (i.e., not irritable bowel).

TABLE 13.8 CHILDHOOD FUNCTIONAL GASTROINTESTINAL DISORDERS—cont'd

G2a1. Ulcer-like dyspepsia
Pain centered in the upper abdomen is the predominant (most bothersome) symptom.

G2a2. Dysmotility-like dyspepsia
An unpleasant or troublesome nonpainful sensation (discomfort) centered in the upper abdomen is the predominant symptom; this sensation may be characterized by early satiety, upper abdominal fullness, bloating, or nausea.

G2a3. Unspecified (nonspecific) dyspepsia
Symptomatic patients whose symptoms do not fulfil the criteria for either ulcer-like or dysmotility-like dyspepsia.

G2b. Irritable bowel syndrome
In children old enough to provide an accurate pain history, at least 12 weeks, which need not be consecutive, of continuous or recurrent symptoms during the preceding 12 months of:

1. Abdominal discomfort or pain that has two out of three features:
   a. Relieved with defecation; *and/or*
   b. Onset associated with a change in frequency of stool; *and/or*
   c. Onset associated with a change in form (appearance) of stool.
2. There are no structural or metabolic abnormalities to explain the symptom.

Symptoms that cumulatively support the diagnosis of irritable bowel syndrome:

- Abnormal stool frequency (for research purposes 'abnormal' may be defined as more than three bowel movements per day and fewer than three bowel movements per week);
- Abnormal stool form (lumpy/hard or loose/watery stool);
- Abnormal stool passage (straining, urgency, or feeling of incomplete evacuation);
- Passage of mucus;
- Bloating or feeling of abdominal distention.

G2c. Functional abdominal pain
At least 12 weeks of:

1. Continuous or nearly continuous abdominal pain in the school-aged child or adolescent; *and*
2. No or only occasional relationship of pain with physiologic events (e.g., eating, menses, defecation); *and*
3. Some loss of daily functioning; *and*
4. The pain is not feigned (e.g., malingering); *and*
5. Insufficient criteria for other functional gastrointestinal disorders that would explain the abdominal pain.

G2d. Abdominal migraine

1. In the preceding 12 months, three or more paroxysmal episodes of intense, acute, midline abdominal pain lasting from 2 h to several days, with intervening symptom-free intervals of weeks to months; *and*
2. Evidence of metabolic, gastrointestinal, and central nervous system structural or biochemical diseases is absent; *and*
3. Two of the following features:
   a. Headache during episodes;
   b. Photophobia during episodes;
   c. Family history of migraine;
   d. Headache confirmed to one side only; *and*
   e. An aura or warning period consisting of either visual symptoms (e.g., blurred or restricted vision) or sensory symptoms (e.g., numbness or tingling), or motor symptoms (e.g., slurred speech, inability to speak, paralysis).

G2e. Aerophagia
At least 12 weeks, which need not be consecutive, in the preceding 12 months, or two or more of the following signs and symptoms:

1. Air swallowing;
2. Abdominal distention due to intraluminal air; *and*
3. Repetitive belching and/or increased flatus.

G3. FUNCTIONAL DIARRHEA (ALSO CALLED TODDLER'S DIARRHEA, CHRONIC NONSPECIFIC DIARRHEA, IRRITABLE COLON OF CHILDHOOD)
For more than 4 weeks, daily painless, recurrent passage or three or more large, unformed stools, in addition to all these characteristics:

1. Onset of symptoms begins between 6 and 36 months of age;
2. Passage of stools occurs during waking hours; *and*
3. There is no failure-to-thrive if caloric intake is adequate.

G4. DISORDERS OF DEFECATION
G4a. Infant dyschezia
At least 10 min of straining and crying before successful passage of soft stools in an otherwise healthy infant less than 6 months of age.

G4b. Functional constipation
In infants and children, at least 2 weeks of:

1. Scybalous, pebble-like, hard stools for a majority of stools; *or*
2. Firm stools two or fewer times/week; *or*
3. There is no evidence of structural, endocrine, or metabolic disease.

TABLE 13.8 CHILDHOOD FUNCTIONAL GASTROINTESTINAL DISORDERS—cont'd

G4c. Functional fecal retention

From infancy to 16years of age, a history of at least 12weeks of:

1. Passage of large-diameter stools at intervals of less than twice per week; *and*
2. Retentive posturing, avoiding defecation by purposefully contracting the pelvic floor. As pelvic floor muscles fatigue, the child uses gluteal muscles, squeezing buttocks together.

Accompanying symptoms may include fecal soiling, irritability, abdominal cramps, decreased appetite, and/or early satiety. The accompanying symptoms disappear immediately following passage of a large stool.

G4d. Functional nonretentive fecal soiling

Once a week or more for the preceding 12weeks, in a child older than 4years, a history of:

1. Defecation in places and at times inappropriate to the social context;
2. In the absence of structural or inflammatory disease; *and*
3. In the absence of signs of fecal retention (listed in G4c above).

The diagnosis of a childhood functional gastrointestinal disorder always presumes the absence of a structural or biochemical explanation for the symptoms.

REFERENCES

1. Drossman DA.The functional gastrointestinal disorders. In: Corazziarie E, Talley NJ, Thompson WG, Whitehead WE, eds. Rome II, 2nd edn. McLean, VA: Degnon Associates, 2000:1–31.
2. Hungin AF, Whorwell PJ, Tack J, Mearin F. The prevalence, patterns and impact of irritable bowel syndrome: an international survey of 40000 subjects. Aliment Pharmacol Ther 2003; 17:643–650.
3. Drossman DA. The functional gastrointestinal disorders and the Rome II process. Gut 1999; 45:111–115. Tables reproduced with permission from the BMJ Publishing Group.

Chapter 14

Anorexia and eating disorders

Tomas J Silber

INTRODUCTION

Eating disorders are usually considered as belonging to the field of mental health. However, the reality is that there are serious medical complications, including death, that require patients to be monitored and treated by physicians. This chapter has been written to facilitate a clinician's ability to:

- diagnose anorexia nervosa, bulimia nervosa, and eating disorders, not otherwise specified
- consider a differential diagnosis
- select the appropriate laboratory assessments
- understand the physiopathology of starvation and electrolyte imbalance
- anticipate and detect potential medical complications
- recognize water loading
- identify and prevent the refeeding syndrome
- make judicious use of medication.

WHAT IS IT?

Anorexia nervosa is a condition that is usually suspected whenever a young person, who is otherwise healthy, is brought to medical attention because of marked weight loss, or, consulting for another reason, is found to be malnourished. These patients often consider themselves fit and resist the idea that they have a medical problem. 'There is nothing wrong with me' is the typical comment. The distinguishing features are: fanatical pursuit of thinness, loss of 15% or more of bodyweight, amenorrhea, phobic fear of weight gain or fatness, body image distortion, and denial of the seriousness of the condition. Patients may or may not purge.

Bulimia nervosa is a condition characterized by binge eating followed by purging. This usually consists of self-induced vomiting (manually, with instruments or with ipecac), but may also be done by laxatives, diuretics, and/or compulsive exercising. Purging is a solitary and secretive activity practiced by patients who may be of normal weight. Therefore it may be difficult to detect unless the patient self-reports, is 'caught in the act,' or medical complications ensue.

Finally, there is an even greater number of people who have subthreshold presentations, whose eating habits are clearly disordered, who may engage in frequent fasting, binging, and purging, but who do not fit the criteria for either anorexia nervosa or bulimia. They are often malnourished and in need of treatment, and are all subsumed under the diagnosis of Eating Disorders, NOS (not otherwise specified).

The psychiatric diagnosis of an eating disorder is established following Diagnostic and Statistical Manual of Medical Disorders (DSM-IV TR) criteria[1] (Table 14.1).

TABLE 14.1 DIAGNOSTIC CRITERIA

ANOREXIA NERVOSA

1. Refusal to maintain bodyweight at or above a minimally normal weight for age and height (85% of expected), via:
   a) weight loss
   b) failure to make expected weight gain during period of growth.
2. Intense fear of gaining weight or becoming fat, even though underweight.
3. Disturbance in the way in which bodyweight or shape is experienced, undue influence of body weight or shape on self-evaluation, or denial of the seriousness of the current low bodyweight.
4. In postmenarchal females, amenorrhea (i.e., the absence of at least three consecutive menstrual cycles). (A woman is considered to have amenorrhea if her periods occur only following hormone [e.g., estrogen] administration.)

BULIMIA NERVOSA

1. Recurrent episodes of binge eating, characterized by both of the following:
   a) Eating, in a discrete period of time (e.g., within any 2-h period), an amount of food that is definitely larger than most people would eat during a similar period of time and under similar circumstances
   b) A sense of lack of control over eating during the episode (e.g., a feeling that one cannot stop eating or control what or how much one is eating).
2. Recurrent inappropriate compensatory behavior in order to prevent weight gain, such as:
   a) self-induced vomiting
   b) misuse of laxatives, diuretics, enemas, or other medications
   c) fasting
   d) excessive exercise.
3. Binge eating and inappropriate compensatory behaviors both occur, on average, at least twice a week for 3 months.
4. Self-evaluation is unduly influenced by body shape and weight.
5. The disturbance does not occur exclusively during episodes of anorexia nervosa.

Adapted and reprinted with permission from the *Diagnostic and Statistical Manual of Mental Disorders*, Text Revision, © 2000, American Psychiatric Association.

HOW COMMON IS IT?

The lifetime prevalence of anorexia nervosa is approximately 0.5%; close to half of individuals with anorexia nervosa will eventually develop bulimia nervosa. Moreover, the lifetime prevalence for the latter is estimated to be between 1% and 3%. The incidence of Eating Disorders, NOS is unknown, but certainly much higher. The ratio of female to male patients with eating disorders ranges from 10:1 to 20:1. These conditions can begin in childhood, almost always arise during adolescence and young adulthood, and seldom develop after the age of 40 years. There is an increased risk of anorexia nervosa among first-degree biologic relatives. The concordance rate for monozygotic twins is significantly higher than for dizygotic twins. The long-term mortality rate is close to 20% for anorexia nervosa and unknown for bulimia nervosa.[2]

PATHOPHYSIOLOGY

Patients with anorexia nervosa who are pure food restrictors develop severe malnutrition, whereas anorexic patients who purge, patients with bulimia nervosa, and in general all those who self-induce vomiting or abuse laxatives, tend to have complications relating to electrolyte imbalances. Dramatic and dangerous physiologic changes may take place during refeeding attempts[3–7] (Table 14.2).

Malnutrition eventually results in emaciation, amenorrhea, hypothermia, bradycardia, hypotension, orthostasis, and chronic depression. It is useful to understand the physiology of starvation. The organism's attempts at adaptation to lack of food take place at a metabolic and neuroendocrine level. These metabolic changes can be understood as an attempt to maintain glucose homeostasis (initial phase) and to conserve protein (final phase). Initially there is an acceleration of hepatic gluconeogenesis (alanine produced by the muscles is its main substrate). When starvation is prolonged, the organism responds to the depletion of protein with a metabolic shift to the burning of fat and production of ketone bodies, thus giving priority to protein conservation.

Ketonemia has a special role. Acetone gradually replaces glucose as fuel for the brain. In addition, the ketones send signals to the muscles to reduce their catabolic rate. If malnutrition is allowed to progress, a persistent hypometabolic state follows with amenorrhea, hypothermia, marked bradycardia, hypotension, and orthostasis. As starvation continues unabated, the patient develops an organic brain syndrome that progresses to obtundation, lethargy, coma, and death.

Hypophosphatemia, in its protean manifestations, more commonly occurs when hospitalized patients receive an excessive nutritional treatment. This is known as the 'refeeding syndrome'.[4–7] Hypophosphatemia is exceptional in the untreated anorexic because phosphorus is found in nearly all foods. During the phase of starvation, phosphorus is not needed for fat metabolism. By contrast, metabolism of glucose requires the presence of phosphate. With the arrival of food, the extracellular phosphorus enters the cells and hypophosphatemia ensues. Hypophosphatemia will manifest with nausea, vomiting, weakness, and anorexia. In severe cases there may be hemolytic anemia, rhabdomyolysis, cardiomyopathy, and respiratory insufficiency. The central nervous system is sensitive to hypophosphatemia, responding with confusion, delirium, psychosis, convulsions, and even death. Therefore, patients with anorexia and severe malnutrition should avoid parenteral glucose or brisk realimentation. Whenever increased nourishment is to be given, it is necessary also to provide phosphorus.

Occasionally, anorectic patients fearful of being 'punished' or hospitalized due to weight loss discover that they can 'fake weight gain' through the process of 'waterloading' – drinking large amounts of water shortly before their 'weigh in.' This can cause dilutional hyponatremia, with weakness, irritability, and confusion. When sodium concentration falls below 120 mEq/L, water intoxication can lead to brain edema, induce seizures, and be a cause of death.[4,5]

Patients who purge by self-induced vomiting develop metabolic abnormalities. This is due to the fact that they lose chlorhydric acid. Sodium chloride has osmotic properties, so that the loss of chloride interferes with maintenance of an effective arterial blood volume. This results in a compensatory hyperaldosteronism with reabsorption of renal tubular sodium (as bicarbonate) and excretion of potassium; hence the bulimic's hypokalemic, hypochloremic alkalosis. Patients who abuse laxatives tend to become acidotic.[4–6]

TABLE 14.2 PHYSIOPATHOLOGY OF HUMAN STARVATION, PURGING, WATER INTOXICATION, AND REFEEDING

STARVATION
- Initial phase – accelerated hepatic gluconeogenesis
- Final phase – ketosis, reduction of protein catabolism
- Glycogen depletion, hypoglycemia, low T_3 levels, hypercholesterolemia, hypercarotenemia
- Hypometabolic state – amenorrhea, bradycardia, hypotension, orthostasis, hypothermia, lanugo, organic brain syndrome, confusion, lethargy, coma, death

PURGING, WATER INTOXICATION, AND REFEEDING
- Hypokalemic alkalosis, hypochloremia, hyponatremia (secondary hyperaldosteronism)
- Acidosis (laxative abuse)
- Hyponatremia, dilutional ("water loading")
- Hypomagnesemia, hypocalcemia, zinc deficiency (starvation)
- Hypophosphatemia, hypomagnesemia ("refeeding syndrome," extracellular phosphorus level falls abruptly as it becomes intracellular, intravenous glucose)
- Seizures, delirium, arrhythmias, sudden death

CAUSES/DIFFERENTIAL DIAGNOSIS

The eating disorders have been described for centuries, ranging from behaviors manifested in the Roman 'vomitoriums' to the feats of the starving saints. The causes are multifactorial in that there is a strong genetic component (probably relating to traits such as perfectionism and obsessiveness), an important sociocultural component (influencing the role of body image), and a significant psychologic component (sense of ineffectiveness and loss of control in anorexia nervosa, impulse disorder and addictive tendencies in bulimia nervosa). Triggering factors have been described often, such as losses (a move, a sibling going to college, a death in the family) or critical remarks about the young person's body. Past episodes of sexual abuse are being increasingly detected. Biologic factors such as hypothalamic malfunction and abnormalities involving leptin and ghrelin, among others, have also been implicated.[8]

Not every young person with weight loss and amenorrhea has anorexia nervosa, nor does everybody with weight concerns and recurrent vomiting have bulimia nervosa (see Chapter 15).[1] The reason for this is that dissatisfaction with body image and dieting are almost universal preoccupations, and therefore may simply coincide with another illness. There is a long list of differential diagnoses to consider. The most common error is overdiagnosis relating to *gastrointestinal pathologies*. Crohn's disease can be overlooked, especially when it follows an indolent course, with scant symptoms such as a very slow progression of puberty, weight loss, and growth deceleration (see Chapter 54).

CAUSES AND DIFFERENTIAL DIAGNOSIS
DIFFERENTIAL DIAGNOSIS OF THE EATING DISORDERS
GASTROINTESTINAL PATHOLOGY
Inflammatory bowel disease
Celiac and other malabsorption syndromes
Achalasia
Superior mesenteric artery syndrome
ENDOCRINE PATHOLOGY
Hyperthyroidism
Diabetes mellitus type 1
Addison's disease
Hypothalamic tumors
Sheehan's syndrome
BEHAVIORAL OR PSYCHIATRIC PATHOLOGY
Major depression, psychosis, or schizophrenia
Substance abuse (cocaine, amphetamines)
Social phobia
Obsessive compulsive disorder
Dysmorphophobia
MISCELLANEOUS
Hyperemesis gravidarum
Emaciating diseases (AIDS, tuberculosis, metastatic cancer)

Celiac disease and other malabsorption syndromes may also mimic anorexia nervosa. Weight loss may occur years after the initial diagnosis has been forgotten; typically, with the beginning of adolescence and the desire to be 'like everybody else,' the gluten-free diet is abandoned and the malnutrition ensues (see Chapters 43 and 44).

Achalasia can lead to severe weight loss and amenorrhea as a result of dysphagia, which may be ignored as 'typical manipulation of patients with eating disorders,' unless a barium swallow demonstrates the condition.

The **superior mesenteric artery syndrome** may induce remarkable weight loss secondary to recurrent vomiting. It is caused by intermittent compression of the second portion of the duodenum, clamped between the superior mesenteric artery and the aorta, in patients who have experienced rapid weight loss (e.g., following bariatric surgery). The patients assume a typical position when eating: they bend forward. This syndrome can be a complication of anorexia nervosa.

Endocrine disorders can also result in marked weight loss and amenorrhea. Hyperthyroidism can present with rapid and progressive malnutrition, but is easily differentiated from anorexia nervosa because of tachycardia, hypertension, and a hypermetabolic state. The simple observation of the hyperphagic hyperthyroid adolescent is sufficient to rule out anorexia nervosa.

Diabetes type 1 can also present with rapid weight loss. However, these patients are polydipsic, polyphagic, and polyuric, and deteriorate rapidly into ketoacidosis.

Addison's disease manifests with fatigue, anorexia, recurrent vomiting, and hypotension. The patient is very weak and develops brownish skin pigmentation. The diagnosis is suspected by electrolyte abnormalities and confirmed by endocrine testing. Sheehan's syndrome occurs in young women following a hypothalamic injury as the result of a massive postpartum hemorrhage, resulting in weight loss, weakness, and amenorrhea due to panhypopituitarism.

A variety of tumors and hypothalamic lesions can induce abnormal eating behaviors and weight loss, which is not surprising because the hypothalamus regulates appetite. However, these lesions are associated with findings suggestive of a central nervous system disorder, such as headaches, abnormal thirst, diplopia, papilledema, and spontaneous projectile vomiting.

Systemic conditions such as severe infections (tuberculosis), immunologic disorders (AIDS), chronic conditions (cystic fibrosis), and malignancies may lead to emaciation and amenorrhea, but these patients appear much sicker than those with eating disorders.

Pregnancy may be confused with bulimia nervosa in secretive adolescents developing hyperemesis gravidarum. A complete sexual history and pregnancy testing should always be part of the evaluation.

Psychiatric conditions may lead to emaciation. Patients with major depression may suffer psychomotor retardation, neurovegetative signs, and profound lack of appetite. On the other hand, severe malnutrition can result in marked depression. Schizophrenia or other psychotic conditions may manifest with bizarre ideas, such as the fear of being poisoned, with the resulting food refusal. Social phobias may incline to the avoidance of being seen eating. Obsessive compulsive disorder may involve unusual eating rituals.

Substance abuse can cause malnutrition, especially if it involves powerful appetite suppressors (cocaine or amphetamines). Patients with bulimia nervosa, who often have an impulse disorder, may harbor drug addictions and alcoholism.

SYMPTOM COMPLEXES

Symptoms vary depending on whether starving or purging predominates[4–7] (Fig. 14.1). In anorexia nervosa, semistarvation leads to constipation, abdominal pain, and postprandial discomfort. Most patients develop delayed gastric emptying and impaired intestinal motility. They suffer from cold intolerance, become hypothermic, and develop acrocyanosis and lanugo. Dehydration and orthostasis are common. Peripheral edema on refeeding or cessation of the use of laxatives and diuretics can be dramatic. Yellow skin color can be distinguished from jaundice because the mucosa is not affected; it is due to raised levels of carotene. Petechiae may indicate a bleeding diathesis. Many develop normochromic normocytic anemia, impaired renal function, and cardiovascular symptoms due to impaired myocardial contractility, mitral valve prolapse, and arrhythmias. Prolonged amenorrhea and reduced estrogen secretion may result in osteopenia, osteoporosis, and fractures.

SYMPTOM COMPLEXES

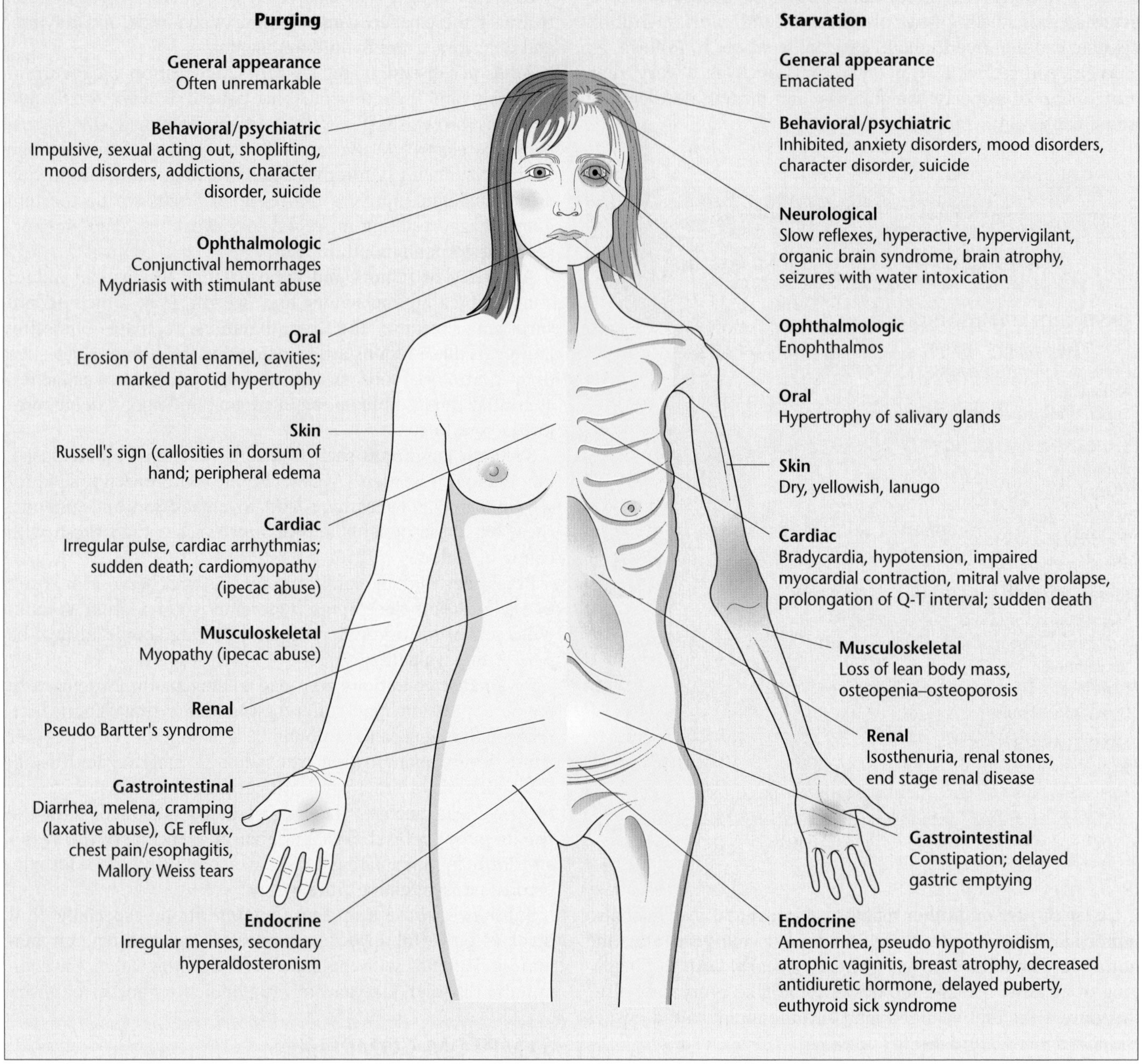

Fig. 14.1 Symptom complexes in patients with eating disorders. The right side shows the general appearances in patients who starve themselves, and the left side shows appearances in those who purge. Symptoms may overlap as patients with anorexia nervosa who purge will develop complications associated with purging, and patients with bulimia nervosa may also fast or diet, becoming malnourished.

Patients with bulimia nervosa are at risk for loss of dental enamel. Their teeth become chipped and appear 'moth-eaten,' with increased dental cavities. They also develop marked parotid hypertrophy and conjunctival hemorrhages. Those that stimulate the gag reflex manually develop calluses on the dorsal surface of their hand (Russell's sign). Deadly cardiomyopathies and muscle injury may result from the use of ipecac to induce emesis. Recurrent vomiting can induce chest pain (see Chapter 2), esophagitis, and Barrett's esophagus (see Chapter 31). Many become laxative dependent and develop melanosis coli, cathartic colon, and rectal prolapse, sometimes with bleeding. Electrolyte changes stemming from purging can result in fatal arrhythmias. Other potentially fatal complications include esophageal tears, gastric rupture, and acute dilatation of the stomach (see Chapters 22 and 23).

It always needs to be remembered that psychiatric co-morbidity is common in patients with eating disorders, including mood disorders, anxiety disorders, obsessive compulsive disorder, personality disorders, and addictive disorders. Suicide is a leading cause of death in patients with eating disorders.

DIAGNOSIS

The term anorexia is a misnomer because these patients do not suffer from loss of appetite. After recovery from the illness, many confess to have suffered from chronic hunger. Most patients will insist that they 'eat healthily.' Patients who binge–purge keep this shrouded in an area of secrecy and usually admit to it only when 'caught in the act.'

The **diagnosis** needs to be based on more than malnutrition and amenorrhea, requiring the presence of positive data, such as distorted body image, fanatic pursuit of thinness, binge eating followed by purging, etc. A series of screening questions may help to elicit the data necessary to fulfill DSM-IV criteria.[1–7] They include inquiry about eating patterns, bingeing, purging, exercise, degree of satisfaction with the body, undue influence of shape and weight on self-evaluation, fear of being or becoming fat (in an underweight individual), refusal to reach or maintain a medically recommended bodyweight, and denial of the seriousness of the condition.

The **physical examination** may detect elements of the hypometabolic states or evidence of purging as outlined under the symptom complexes (Fig. 14.1). Anthropometric measurements should include a careful assessment of height and weight for calculation of the body mass index (BMI). This is obtained by dividing weight in kilograms by height in meters squared. A BMI of 16 kg/m^2 or less is characteristic of anorexia nervosa.

Laboratory assessment

Laboratory findings can be falsely reassuring, as many patients have been known to die with 'normal lab values'.[4] A complete blood count may show hemoconcentration, leukopenia with low total lymphocyte count. Prealbumin and transferrin may be useful markers for fasting, as their half-life is much shorter than that of albumin.

Malnutrition can cause fatty liver infiltrate and raised liver enzyme levels (see Chapter 21). Persistent hypoglycemia is an ominous sign. Hormonal profile in amenorrheic patients shows prepubertal gonadotropins and low estradiol levels. Triiodothyronine (T_3), the bioactive form of thyroid hormone, is low in starvation states. The presence of a normal thyroid stimulating hormone concentration rules out hypothyroidism. Urinalysis may show proteinuria (increased exercise), ketonuria (fasting), isostenuria, or abnormal microscopy findings (dehydration).

Bone density by dexa-scanning may reveal osteopenia or osteoporosis. Neuroradiology can demonstrate brain atrophy, mostly of white matter but also of some gray matter, which may be only partially reversible. Patients who vomit frequently may demonstrate hypochloremic, hypokalemic, hyponatremic metabolic alkalosis as well as increased levels of amylase (salivary). Electrocardiography can rapidly detect hypokalemia, prolongation of the QT interval, and arrhythmia. Hospitalized patients may require cardiac monitors.

DIAGNOSTIC METHODS

DIAGNOSTIC ASSESSMENT AND LABORATORY EVALUATION

Test	Significance
Full blood count	Hemoglobin concentration, leukopenia, thrombocytopenia
Erythrocyte sedimentation rate	Increase suggests another illness
Clinical chemistry	Reduced blood sugar, calcium, magnesium, phosphate Reduced urea, electrolyte abnormalities. Abnormal liver function test results
Nutritional parameters	Transferrin low with fasting. Total protein, prealbumin, cholesterol (low or high), T_3 Low albumin may imply other disease
Urine analysis Pregnancy test	Confirm or question report of menstruation
ECG	Bradycardia, hypokalemia, arrhythmia
Sex hormones	
Serum osmolality	
Decrease in water loading	
Investigation for celiac or inflammatory bowel disease	Gastrointestinal disease, differential diagnosis
Vitamin levels	Anemia type, scurvy, pellagra
Zinc	Acrodermatitis
Urine tests for substance abuse	
Neuroimaging	If headaches, organic brain syndrome, ?tumor or brain atrophy
Bone density by dexa scan	Osteopenia or osteoporosis with more than 6 months of arrhythmia
Genetic markers Bone metabolites Functional MRI, etc.	Research tests

CURRENT CONTROVERSIES/TREATMENT

The eating disorders are considered psychiatric illnesses and there is still ongoing debate as to the best treatment. Currently there is consensus that specialized multidisciplinary treatment teams might offer the best possibility for recovery.[1–7] Nutritional rehabilitation is at the heart of recovery (see Chapters 138 and 139). Family therapy is the most helpful treatment for children and adolescents, with individual therapy for young adults. The 'Maudsley' approach trains parents on how to best help their child by taking care of the nutritional rehabilitation first, and, once this is achieved, there is follow-up with adolescent and family issues.[9] Cognitive behavioral therapy seems to be of great help to patients with bulimia.[7]

Treatments based on standard protocols are gaining ascendance.[7,8] Hospitalization is recommended when there is severe malnutrition or out-of-control purging, not only because these situations are dangerous, but also because therapy is not possible under these circumstances.[1–7] Various behavioral therapeutic inpatient programs have been successful in the acute-care phase, including nocturnal nasogastric pump refeeding as the initial approach to nutritional rehabilitation rather than as a treatment of last resort.[10] Degree of nutritional rehabilitation is a crucial variable: patients discharged before reaching 90% of ideal bodyweight have a much higher incidence of rehospitalization.[11]

Medications are somewhat helpful in the treatment of anorexia nervosa. Chlorpropamide given 20 min before meals can alleviate delayed gastric emptying. Phosphorus is essential during refeeding. The treatment of osteopenia is controversial; birth control pills seem to be helpful only when there is also weight recovery. Nasal calcitonin, oral alendronate, and dehydroepiandrosterone (DHEA) have also been proposed. Multivitamins and calcium need to be supplemented. Psychopharmacologic treatment is indicated for psychiatric co-morbidity. Fluoxetine has been used to stabilize the weight of chronically ill anorexics. Patients with bulimia nervosa often respond to treatment with selective serotonin reuptake inhibitors (SSRIs). Ondansetron and topotecan are being investigated.[12]

Practice guidelines have been proposed by the American Psychiatric Association,[3] the American Academy of Pediatrics,[4] the Society for Adolescent Medicine,[5] the American Dietetic Association,[6] and most recently by the UK National Institute for Clinical Excellence.[13]

Prognosis

Contrary to general belief, most patients receiving relatively long treatments will recover. Patients diagnosed early may respond to brief interventions. A minority of seriously ill or chronically ill patients will require care in specialized programs and residential centers. Anorexia nervosa, however, has a disturbingly high long-term mortality rate of 20%. Death is mostly due to starvation and suicide, but many die from arrhythmias, renal failure, and ipecac abuse. However, even among those who have been seriously ill for many years, recovery is still possible.[1–7]

SOURCES OF INFORMATION FOR PATIENTS AND DOCTORS

http://www.patient.co.uk/showdoc/733/
http://www.patient.co.uk/showdoc/23069106/
http://www.aafp.org/afp/20040401/1729ph.html
http://www.mentalhealth.com/dis/p20-et02.html
Eating disorders – general:
http://www.edauk.com
http://www.healthcyclopedia.com/mental-health/disorders/eating.html

REFERENCES

1. American Psychiatric Association. Diagnostic and statistical manual of mental disorders, 4th edn, text revision. Washington, DC: American Psychiatric Association; 2000.
2. Robb AS, ed. Eating disorders. Child Adolesc Psychiatric Clin N Am 2002; 11:163–441.
3. American Psychiatric Association. Practice guideline for the treatment of patients with eating disorders. Am J Psychiatry Suppl 2000; 157:1–39.
4. American Academy of Pediatrics. Committee on Adolescence. Policy statement. Identifying and treating eating disorders. Pediatrics 2003; 111:204–211.
5. Society for Adolescent Medicine. Eating disorders in adolescents. Position paper of the Society for Adolescent Medicine. J Adol Health 2003; 33:496–503.
6. American Dietetic Association. Nutrition intervention in the treatment of anorexia nervosa, bulimia nervosa, and eating disorder not otherwise specified (EDNOS). Position paper. J Am Diet Assoc 2001; 101:810–819.
7. Kleinman RE, ed. Pediatric nutrition handbook, 5th edn. Washington, DC: American Academy of Pediatrics; 2004.
8. Garner DM, Garfinkel PE, eds. Handbook of treatment for eating disorders, 2nd ed. New York: Guilford Press; 1997.
9. Lock J, Le Grange D, Agras WS et al. Treatment manual for anorexia nervosa. A family based approach. New York: Guilford Press; 2001.
10. Robb AS, Silber TJ, Orrell-Valente JK et al. Supplemental nocturnal nasogastric refeeding for better short-term outcome in hospitalized adolescent girls with anorexia nervosa. Am J Psychiatry 2002; 159:1347–1353.
11. Baran SA, Weltsin TE, Kaye WH. Low discharge weight and outcome in anorexia nervosa. Am J Psychiatry 1995; 152: 1070–1072.
12. Casper RC. How useful are pharmacological treatments in eating disorders? Psychopharmacol Bull 2002; 36:88–104.
13. National Institute for Clinical Excellence website (www.nice.org.uk). Quick reference guide (16 pp); NICE guidelines (35 pp); full guidelines (260 pp, Plus CD-ROM), 2004.

Chapter 15

Weight loss

Carol M Reife

INTRODUCTION

Unintentional weight loss is a common finding in clinical practice and one that raises concern for both physician and patient. Involuntary weight loss has been associated with both increased morbidity and mortality especially in the elderly population.[1–6] Although cancer is an often feared cause of weight loss, especially in older patients, other etiologies including depression and benign gastrointestinal illnesses are common as well. The etiology of weight loss in a specific patient may be elusive at first. However, careful history, physical examination, and directed testing will lead to a diagnosis in most cases.

WHAT IS IT?

Weight loss may occur in patients on special diets and in those modifying food intake in order to lose weight. This weight loss is considered intentional or voluntary and is most often not a cause for concern. Periods of slight positive or negative energy balance and bodyweight fluctuation occur as a normal part of life. However, when significant unintentional weight loss is found, evaluation should be sought, as this may be associated with increased morbidity and mortality.[2,6,7] Beginning at approximately the third decade of life, adipose tissue increases and lean muscle mass decreases by about 0.3 kg per year. At 70–75 years of age, weight begins to decline at a rate of about 0.1–0.2 kg/year.[8] Weight loss beyond this amount should not be considered a normal part of the aging process.

It is important to record a patient's weight at each visit and to compare readings with previous examinations. Height should be recorded as well. Body mass index (BMI), calculated as weight in kilograms divided by height in meters squared (wt/ht^2), allows comparison of the patient's data with published norms. In patients for whom no prior weight measurement is available, assessment of clothing fit or belt-notch use may give information regarding prior weight. Patients are often incorrect when asked about the amount of weight lost or gained. Confirmation by a family member is often helpful. In up to half of patients reporting weight loss, charted weights do not confirm that weight was actually lost.[7]

The range of weight loss cited in the literature as clinically important is variable and has been defined in different ways by different authors. Most often, a weight loss of 5% over 6–12 months is considered significant. Weight loss in excess of 20% implies severe protein energy malnutrition and is associated with impaired physiologic function, including impaired cell-mediated and humoral immunity.[9] Weight loss has been correlated with poorer wound healing, infectious complications, decreased performance status and response to medical therapy, and increased mortality.[1]

HOW COMMON IS IT?

There are limited data regarding the incidence of unintentional weight loss, but in available studies it appears to be common. Absolute numbers are difficult to determine as populations cited are variable. Unintentional weight loss has been found to have an incidence as high as 13.1% annually in a population of older veteran outpatients.[1] Significant weight loss was found in more than 25% of older dependent persons receiving home care services.[8] A study of 4714 community dwelling individuals aged 65 years or greater showed a greater than 5% weight loss in 19% of men and 16% of women.[9] Involuntary weight loss in a group of nursing home residents was found to be 36%.[10,11]

PATHOPHYSIOLOGY

Bodyweight is maintained at a fixed 'set point,' regulated by complex interactions between multiple neural and hormonal factors. In most instances, it is difficult to lose weight, even with voluntary changes in exercise and food intake. Fluid shifts and fluid losses may account for the initial decreases in weight over a period of several days. Decreases in weight that persist over weeks to months are almost invariably due to loss of tissue mass. Weight loss occurs when energy expenditure exceeds calories available for energy utilization. Weight loss is a consequence of decreased caloric intake or absorption, alterations in energy metabolism or expenditure, or loss of calories from the skin or in urine or stool (Fig. 15.1).

Neuropeptides induce anorexia by acting centrally on satiety centers of the hypothalamus. Gastrointestinal peptides, released secondary to gut distention and other factors, may induce satiety through vagal or other mechanisms. Leptin, produced by adipose tissue, acts to decrease food intake and increase energy expenditure. Cytokines, such as tumor necrosis factor, which may be increased in cancer, severe infection, and chronic inflammatory conditions, can cause anorexia and contribute to weight loss. Alterations in taste or smell, various social, psychological, and cultural factors, and food availability and accessibility may alter caloric intake as well[12] (Fig. 15.2).

Absorption of nutrients may be impaired due a variety of factors including surgery (postgastrectomy, ileal resection), pancreatic insufficiency, tumor, liver disease (parenchymal or cholestatic), bacterial overgrowth (from anatomic or functional stasis), inflammatory bowel disease, radiation changes, sprue,

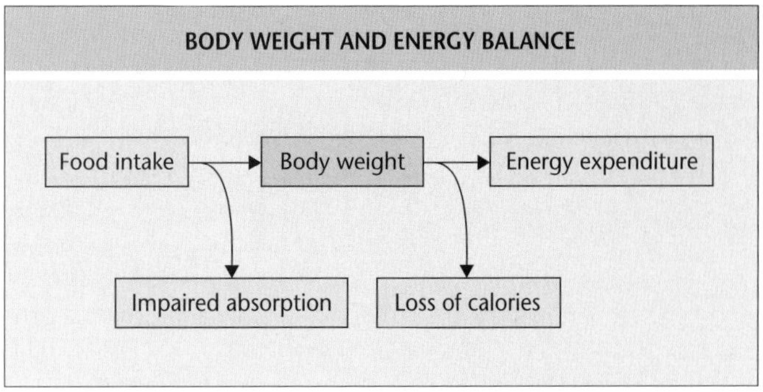

Fig. 15.1 Bodyweight and energy balance. Bodyweight is a result of the balance between energy available and energy expenditure.

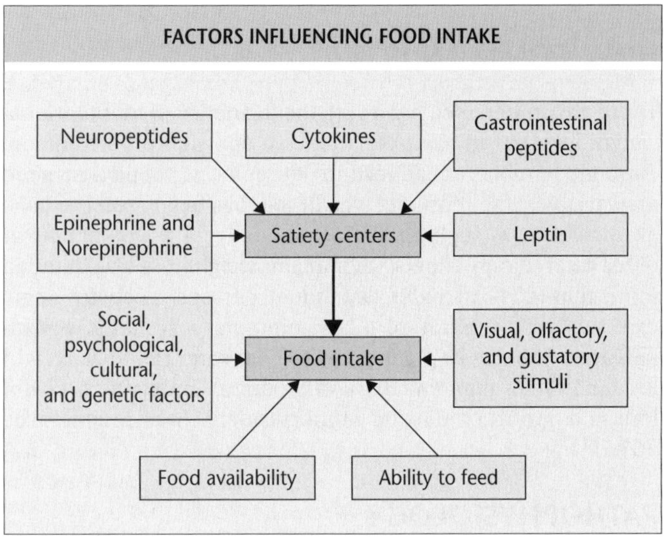

Fig. 15.2 Factors influencing food intake. Input from a variety of sources plays a role in determining food intake.

CAUSES AND DIFFERENTIAL DIAGNOSIS

FACTORS AFFECTING ABSORPTION OF NUTRIENTS AND LOSS OF CALORIES

FACTORS THAT MAY DECREASE ABSORPTION OF NUTRIENTS

Surgery
Pancreatic insufficiency
Tumor
Liver disease
Bacterial overgrowth
Inflammatory bowel disease
Radiation enteritis
Infiltrative diseases
Sprue
Endocrine disorders
Genetic disorders
Lymphatic disorders
Circulatory disorders
Medication

FACTORS THAT MAY CAUSE LOSS OF CALORIES

Vomiting
Diarrhea
Glycosuria
Proteinuria
Fistulous drainage

infiltrative diseases, genetic disorders, lymphatic or circulatory disorders, endocrine disorders (diabetes, hyperthyroidism), or medication effect. Total energy expenditure encompasses basal or resting energy expenditure (50–75% of total), thermic expenditures of digestion, absorption and food metabolism (10%), and physical exercise (15–40%). Excessive loss of calories can result from vomiting, diarrhea, glycosuria, fistulous drainage, and diseases of the skin and kidneys.

Unintentional weight loss is a nonspecific finding with an extensive differential diagnosis. One or more factors may play a key role, but a specific cause may not be identified in up to one-fourth of cases. Data suggest that, when a cause of weight loss is determined, cancer, benign gastrointestinal disease, and depression are the most common etiologies (Table 15.1). When cancer is the cause of weight loss, the diagnosis is rarely obscure. Almost any illness can cause weight loss either through direct

TABLE 15.1 CAUSES OF INVOLUNTARY WEIGHT LOSS IN PUBLISHED STUDIES

	Marton et al.[7]	Rabinovitz et al.[6]	Thompson & Morris[8]	Morley & Kraenzle[10]	Lankisch et al.[9]
No. of patients	91	154	45	185	158
Male : female (%)	99 : 1	45 : 55	33 : 67	11 : 89	44 : 56
Mean age (years)	59	64	72	80	68
Outpatient : inpatient : nursing home (%)	70 : 30 : 0	0 : 100 : 0	100 : 0 : 0	0 : 0 : 100	0 : 100 : 0
Cause (%)					
Cancer	19	36	16	7	24
Benign GI disorder	14	17	11	10	19
Psychiatric diagnosis	9	10	18	42	11
Endocrine disorder	4	4	9	N/A	11
Medication	2	N/A	9	7	N/A
Neurologic diagnosis	2	2	7	3	N/A
Other	24	8	6	28	25
Unknown	26	23	24	3	16

CAUSES AND DIFFERENTIAL DIAGNOSIS
COMMON CAUSES OF UNINTENTIONAL WEIGHT LOSS
• **Cancer** Gastrointestinal Lung Hematologic Breast Ovary Prostate • **Gastroenterologic disorders** Inflammatory bowel disease Peptic ulcer disease Gastroesophageal reflux Dysmotility syndromes Chronic pancreatitis Celiac disease Atrophic gastritis Constipation • **Depression** • **Infection** Tuberculosis AIDS Subacute bacterial endocarditis Occult abscess • **Oral problems** Poor dentition Periodontal disease Dentures Xerostomia • **Medications** • **Endocrine diseases** Diabetes mellitus Hyperthyroidism and hypothyroidism Hyperparathyroidism • **Neurologic disease** Stroke Dementia Parkinson's disease • **Chronic cardiovascular disease** • **Chronic pulmonary disease** • **Chronic renal disease** • **Rheumatologic diseases** • **Psychologic and social factors**

effects or by inducing anorexia, nausea, or emotional or psychological stresses.

Cancer is common among organic etiologies, accounting for about one-third of cases. Cancer of any kind may present with weight loss, although cancers of the gastrointestinal tract and lung commonly do so. Lymphoma and cancers of the breast, ovaries, or prostate should be excluded as well.

Benign gastrointestinal disorders are the most common non-malignant causes of unintentional weight loss, accounting for about 6–19% of cases. Nonulcer dyspepsia, peptic ulcer disease, inflammatory bowel disease, and dysmotility syndromes are common causes. Chronic pancreatitis, celiac disease, and atrophic gastritis are more remote possibilities. Diarrhea and constipation may cause anorexia and lead to weight loss as well. Oral problems such as poor dentition, periodontal disease, and poorly fitting dentures are common in the elderly and may lead to decreased oral intake. Mucositis and xerostomia, either from primary disease or as a side effect of medication, may make food less palatable.

Hypothyroidism and hyperthyroidism may both present with weight loss. Energy expenditure in hyperthyroidism may be greatly increased leading to excess consumption of calories. 'Apathetic hyperthyroidism' may occur, especially in the elderly, with weight loss being the only apparent symptom. Hypothyroidism may lead to apathy and anorexia with subsequent decreased oral intake and loss of weight. Diabetes, especially when poorly controlled, may be associated with loss of calories in the urine. Less common endocrine causes of weight loss include hyperparathyroidism, pheochromocytoma, hypopituitarism, and adrenal insufficiency.

Infection should be excluded. Based on risk factors, HIV, tuberculosis, bacterial endocarditis, and occult abscess are possible causes of weight loss.

Medications, especially when multiple, may result in anorexia, nausea, dysgeusia, abdominal discomfort, delayed gastric emptying and diarrhea, and subsequent loss of weight. Centrally acting medications may cause fatigue, sedation, and decreased desire to eat. Adverse effects of medications may be more pronounced in the elderly.

Chronic pulmonary and cardiac disease may increase metabolic demands and contribute to weight loss. Cardiac cachexia is a known complication of severe congestive heart failure. Dyspnea or chest discomfort with eating may lead to decreased food intake. Low fat and low salt diets may make food less palatable and decrease food intake as well. Chronic renal disease may result in anorexia and nausea. Proteinuria may result in loss of calories. Chronic rheumatologic diseases may lead to swallowing difficulties, impaired gastrointestinal motility, bacterial overgrowth, and impaired absorption.

Depression is common in the elderly, especially in residents of long-term care facilities. As many as 15% of elderly people have depressive symptoms, with approximately 4% meeting criteria for major depression.[13] Depression may lead to apathy and decreased enjoyment of food, as well as decreased ability to obtain and prepare food. Anxiety can be associated with functional gastrointestinal disorders including nonulcer dyspepsia. Anxiety-related increase in activity, including pacing, may cause increased consumption of calories. Functional or social problems such as alcoholism, social isolation, and poverty may interfere with ability to obtain food, and contribute to weight loss.

Neurologic disease such as stroke and dementia may cause decreased mobility and decreased ability to obtain food, bring it to the mouth, and chew. Parkinson's disease may cause decreased ability to feed, as well as intestinal dysmotility. In a study of patients with Alzheimer's disease, twice as many patients experienced a weight loss of 5% or more compared with controls.[14]

SYMPTOMS

Unintentional weight loss may encompass a wide range of presentations. Patients may feel well and exhibit no other signs or symptoms. On the other hand, patients with malignancy or AIDS may present with progressive inanition and wasting as a manifestation of the anorexia–cachexia syndrome. Unintentional weight loss as well as low bodyweight have

CAUSES AND DIFFERENTIAL DIAGNOSIS

MEDICATIONS ASSOCIATED WITH UNINTENTIONAL WEIGHT LOSS

- Analgesics (aspirin, NSAIDs, opioids)
- Supplements (iron, calcium, vitamins)
- Antibiotics (erythromycins, tetracyclines, sulfonamides)
- Cardiovascular medications (digoxin, antiarrythmics, antihypertensives, ACE inhibitors, beta-blockers, calcium channel blockers, diuretics)
- Oral hypoglycemic medications (metformin)
- Antidepressant medications (SSRIs)
- Bisphosphonates
- Oral contraceptives
- Anti-parkinsonian agents (levodopa, bromocriptine)
- Anticonvulsants (topiramate, phenytoin)
- Medications for gout (allopurinol, colchicine)
- Theophyllines
- Nicotine

been associated with increased rates of infection and poor wound healing.[1] Weight loss has been linked to both poor performance status and decreased response to therapy in patients with cancer. Quality of life is lower and median survival is shorter in patients with cancer and weight loss than those without weight loss. The increase in mortality rate with weight loss occurs irrespective of underlying diagnosis or cause of death.[1–5]

DIAGNOSIS (Fig. 15.3)

In most cases a careful history and physical examination will yield clues that can help target a diagnostic approach. Even profound weight loss may result from benign disorders. Signs and symptoms are often subtle. The history should begin with the amount of weight lost and the period of time over which it was lost. Information about changes in diet or dietary restrictions may be helpful. Symptoms of anorexia, nausea, and dysgeusia are nonspecific but may point to decreased food intake as the cause of weight loss. Oral difficulties, pain with eating, bloating, early satiety, diarrhea, and flatulence may cause a patient to decrease food intake and should prompt early evaluation of the mouth and gastrointestinal systems. A complete review of systems, including questions regarding fever or sweats, pain in any body area, chest discomfort, palpitations, shortness of breath, polyuria, hematuria, and change in color or consistency of the stool, should be ascertained. Information regarding prior weight loss, prior illnesses, surgery, history of infection, travel, lifestyle risk factors, medications, and cigarette or alcohol use should also be obtained. Search should be made for relevant psychosocial issues, particularly unrecognized depression, isolation, and financial difficulties. In selected patients, a standard tool for detecting depression may be useful. A dietary history including type and amount of foods consumed should be obtained.

Physical examination should confirm any diagnostic possibilities arising from the history. Search for abnormalities of the skin, mouth, lymph glands, breasts, chest, abdomen and pelvis, rectum, and prostate may yield other areas of concern. Stool should be tested for occult blood. Neurologic examination with assessment of cognitive function and screening for depression may provide additional information in certain patients.

EVALUATION OF UNINTENTIONAL WEIGHT LOSS

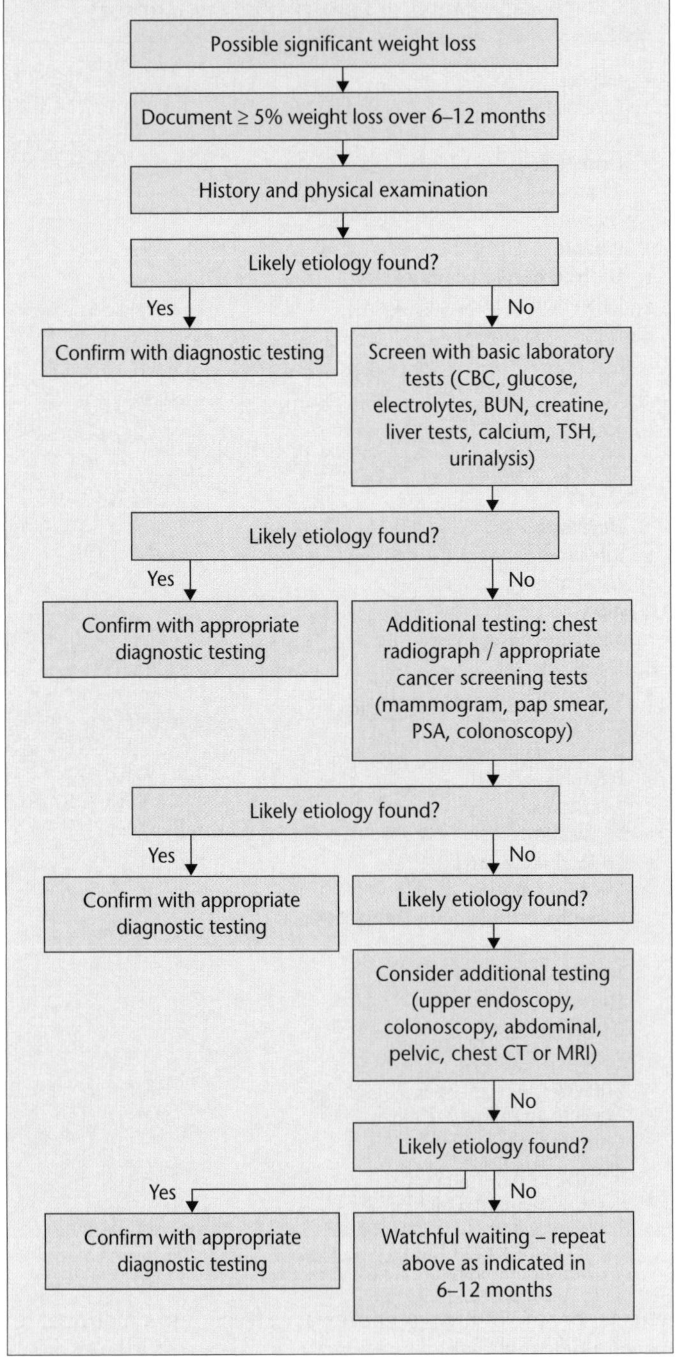

Fig. 15.3 Algorithm for the evaluation of unintentional weight loss.

Basic laboratory tests should be performed, including:

- complete blood count with differential
- biochemical profile with renal and liver function, calcium, thyroid function testing
- urinalysis.

Chest radiography should be obtained if evaluation remains unrevealing or there is reason to suspect chest pathology. Recommended periodic cancer screening tests such as mammography, Pap smear, and colonoscopy should be updated based on the patient's age and risk factors. More targeted diagnostic procedures such as abdominal ultrasonography, magnetic resonance imaging, or computed tomography of the chest, abdomen, or pelvis, and upper or lower endoscopy should be performed based on specific concerns or to follow-up abnormalities identified on initial testing. Patients with negative evaluations are unlikely to have serious organic causes of weight loss. A period of watchful waiting with early follow-up is generally preferable to blind pursuit of additional diagnostic testing that may yield few useful data.

TREATMENT

Although nutritional supplements can improve certain parameters and result in weight gain, their ability to improve clinical outcomes has not been well established.[15] Management should be directed at treating the underlying cause of weight loss when possible, and providing nutritional support. Medications should be reviewed; those that are unnecessary should be discontinued. Patients with depression may regain weight when treated with counseling or antidepressant medications. Social intervention may decrease isolation and provide better access to nutritious foods. Lifting of dietary fat and salt restrictions, and attempting to meet food preferences, may make food more palatable.

In some cases, lost weight is not regained even after treatment of underlying conditions. In other cases, no cause of weight loss is found. Consultation with a dietitian for nutritional assessment and patient education should be considered in these cases. Use of high-calorie snacks or dietary supplements between meals should be a first step in attempting weight gain. Exercise, with even small increases in daily physical activity, may be beneficial by increasing appetite and sense of wellbeing, increasing metabolism, and increasing lean body mass. Parenteral nutrition should be reserved for selected patients.

Treatment of specific processes or symptoms with medication to relieve symptoms may increase food intake. Medication to decrease acid secretion, fiber or laxatives for constipation, antidiarrheals, antispasmodics, or antiemetics may prevent or reverse weight loss. Prokinetic agents such as metoclopramide may decrease bloating, nausea, or anorexia in patients with gastroparesis or postoperative slowing of the bowel. However, adverse effects of treatment may include depression, dystonia, and parkinsonism, especially in elderly patients.

Certain orexigenic agents have been used to stimulate appetite and promote weight gain in patients with AIDS and those with cancer, but have not been well studied in other populations. The US Food and Drug Administration has not labeled these drugs for treatment of weight loss in the elderly. Corticosteroids have been used for appetite stimulation in patients with cancer cachexia, but weight gain tends to be short lived. Adverse effects such as muscle wasting and weakness, immunosuppression, diabetes, and mental status changes may limit their use.[16] The serotonin antagonist cycloheptadine may produce a mild increase in appetite without substantial weight gain, but may also cause dizziness and drowsiness as side effects. The use of dronabinol (Marinol), a cannabinoid indicated for the treatment of anorexia and weight loss in patients with AIDS, has been associated with improvement in appetite, decrease in nausea, and improvement in bodyweight.[8] However, dizziness, confusion, and somnolence may occur with its use. Megestrol acetate (Megace), a progestational agent indicated for palliative treatment of breast and endometrial cancers, has been used successfully to treat cachexia in patients with AIDS and cancer. Studies using doses ranging from 160 to 240 mg daily have shown improved appetite, weight, and energy level.[15] Adverse effects such as edema and thromboembolism may be troublesome.

REFERENCES

1. Wallace JI, Schwartz RS, LaCroix AZ et al. Involuntary weight loss in older outpatients: incidence and clinical significance. J Am Geriatr Soc 1995; 43:329–337.
2. Murden RA, Ainslie NK. Recent weight loss is related to short-term mortality in nursing homes. J Gen Intern Med 1994; 9:648–650.
3. Ryan C, Bryant E, Eleazer P et al. Unintentional weight loss in long term care: predictor of mortality in the elderly. South Med J 1995; 88:721–724.
4. Fabiny AR, Kiel DP. Assessing and treating weight loss in nursing home patients. Clin Geriatr Med 1997; 13:737–751.
5. Fischer J, Johnson MA. Low body weight and weight loss in the aged. J Am Diet Assoc 1990; 90:1697–1706.
6. Rabinovitz M, Pitlik SD, Leifer M et al. Unintentional weight loss. A retrospective analysis of 154 cases. Arch Intern Med 1986; 146: 186–187.
7. Marton KI, Sox HC, Krupp JR. Involuntary weight loss: diagnostic and prognostic significance. Ann Intern Med 1981; 95:568–574.
8. Thompson MP, Morris LK. Unexplained weight loss in the ambulatory elderly. J Am Geriatr Soc 1991; 39:497–500.
9. Lankisch PG, Gerzmann M, Gerzmann JF et al. Unintentional weight loss: diagnosis and prognosis. The first prospective follow up study from a secondary referral centre. J Intern Med 2001; 249:41–46.
10. Morley JE, Kraenzle D. Causes of weight loss in a community nursing home. J Am Geriatr Soc 1994; 42:583–585.
11. Wallace JI, Schwartz RS. Epidemiology of weight loss in humans with special reference to wasting in the elderly. Int J Cardiol 2002; 85:15–21.
12. Reife C. Weight loss. In: Braunwald E, Fauci AS, Kasper DL et al., eds. Harrison's principles of internal medicine. New York: McGraw Hill, 2000:250–251.
13. Morley JE, Silver AJ. Anorexia in the elderly. Neurobiol Aging 1988; 9:9–16.
14. White H, Pieper C, Schmader K et al. Weight change in Alzheimer's disease. J Am Geriatr Soc 1996; 44:265–272.
15. Wallace JI, Schwartz RS. Involuntary weight loss in elderly outpatients: recognition, etiologies, and treatment. Clin Geriatr Med 1997; 13:717–735.
16. Ottery FD, Walsh D, Strawford A. Pharmacologic management of anorexia/cachexia. Semin Oncol 1998; 25(Suppl 6):35–44.

Chapter 16

Gastrointestinal causes of anemia and occult bleeding

Gareth S Dulai and Vincent P De Rosa

INTRODUCTION

Iron deficiency anemia and occult gastrointestinal (GI) bleeding are common sources of referral to gastroenterologists. Good evidence exists to support a standardized approach to evaluation of these clinical syndromes. The majority of these patients will improve with empiric or targeted therapy based on the results of a limited initial evaluation. A small subset of patients presenting with occult GI bleeding, and a fraction of those presenting with overt GI bleeding (see Chapters 11, 23, and 24), without a source of hemorrhage identified on initial evaluation will have recurrent bleeding and warrant further diagnostic evaluation. These patients fall into the category of GI bleeding of obscure origin.

In this chapter we present a rational approach to the evaluation of patients with iron deficiency anemia, occult GI bleeding, and obscure GI bleeding.

WHAT IS IT?

Iron deficiency anemia, occult GI bleeding, and obscure GI bleeding may have significant overlap and are often confused. These interrelated syndromes have distinct diagnostic and therapeutic implications. Thus, it is essential to offer a clear definition of terms.

The suggested World Health Organization cutoff points for abnormally low blood hemoglobin levels are 14 g/dL for adult men, 12 g/dL for adult nonpregnant women, and 11 g/dL for pregnant women. Iron deficiency is most readily diagnosed by measurement of the serum ferritin level, and is best defined as the depletion of iron stores in the bone marrow, liver, and spleen as a result of chronic negative iron balance from bleeding, inadequate dietary intake, increased requirements, or malabsorption.

Occult bleeding refers to the detection of fecal occult blood test (FOBT)-positive stool, with or without iron deficiency anemia or GI symptoms, in a patient without a history of overt GI bleeding (i.e., passage of visible blood per os or per rectum). The amount of luminal GI blood loss required for visual detection of blood in the stool may depend on the location of the lesion, the rate of bleeding, the degree of heme degradation, the transit time, and the eye of the beholder. Patients with as much as 100 mL gastroduodenal blood loss per day may have normal-appearing stools, whereas those with much smaller volumes lost distally may have visible blood.

Gastrointestinal bleeding of obscure origin is defined as persistent or recurrent bleeding, despite negative initial GI evaluation (i.e., colonoscopy and upper panendoscopy).[1] Obscure GI bleeding should be further characterized as overt (passage of visible blood) or occult (FOBT-positive only).

HOW COMMON IS IT?

Iron deficiency anemia is the most common cause of anemia, leading to 4% of all referrals to gastroenterologists.[2] The prevalence is approximately 1–2% among adults in the USA,[3] but patients older than 65 years have shown levels as high as 5%, with the most common etiology being chronic GI bleeding.

The majority of cases of occult bleeding are found in the course of colorectal cancer screening or during the evaluation of iron deficiency anemia. Colorectal cancer screening studies have demonstrated that 2–16% of average-risk patients older than 50 years of age test positive with FOBT.[4] However, false-positive results (associated with red meat consumption, dietary peroxidases, and sample rehydration) and false-negative results (associated with hemoglobin degradation, storage, and vitamin C consumption) are not uncommon.[4]

The prevalence of recurrent, obscure GI bleeding is rare.[5] Although the source of bleeding will not be found on initial endoscopic evaluation in up to half of all patients with fecal occult bleeding, a very small number of these patients will develop clinically significant bleeding. Similarly, the proportion of patients with recurrent GI bleeding after a negative initial evaluation is very small.

PATHOPHYSIOLOGY

The amount of blood normally lost from the gastrointestinal tract (approximately 0.5–1.5 mL per day) is not typically detected by FOBT, nor substantial enough to cause iron deficiency anemia. It is generally believed that a steady blood loss of 3–4 mL/day (equivalent to 1.5–2 mg iron) is sufficient to cause a negative iron balance. This degree of blood loss is usually assumed to originate from the bowel[6] unless the history dictates otherwise. Two uncommon exceptions are pulmonary hemosiderosis (iron deposition in the lung) and paroxysmal nocturnal hemoglobinuria (occult urinary loss of iron).

There are several sources of impaired absorption leading to iron deficiency anemia. Celiac disease is the most common cause of iron malabsorption. Gastrectomy (total or partial) and vagotomy with gastroenterostomy may lead to impaired iron absorption as well, via reduction in gastric acidity and rapid transit.

CAUSES

Occult GI bleeding is by far the most common source of iron deficiency anemia. A broad range of lesions can lead to occult

CAUSES AND DIFFERENTIAL DIAGNOSIS	
ETIOLOGY OF IRON DEFICIENCY ANEMIA	
	Frequency (%)[a]
GASTROINTESTINAL BLEEDING	56
Site unknown	16
Hemorrhoids	10
Salicylate ingestion	8
Peptic ulcer disease	7
Hiatal hernia	7
Diverticulosis	4
Neoplasm	2
Ulcerative colitis	1
Hookworm	–[b]
Milk allergy in infants	–
Meckel's diverticulum	–
Schistosomiasis	–
Trichuriasis	–
IMPAIRED ABSORPTION	
Chlorhydria	41
Gastric surgery	10
Celiac disease	6
Pica	–
Excessive menstrual flow	29
Dietary deficiency	19
Idiopathic hypochromic anemia	17
Pregnancy	6

[a] Based on 371 adult patients with iron deficiency anemia;[13] frequencies total more than 100% because the cause of anemia in the cohort was multifactorial.
[b] Up to 33% in endemic areas.

CAUSES AND DIFFERENTIAL DIAGNOSIS	
ETIOLOGY OF OCCULT BLEEDING	
	Frequency (%)[a]
UPPER GI LESIONS	29–36
Peptic ulcer disease	7–10
Esophagitis	6–9
Angiodysplasia	3–13
Gastritis or erosions	
Duodenitis or erosions	
Gastric or duodenal polyps	
Gastric cancer	
Esophageal or gastric varices	
Watermelon stomach	
Crohn's disease	
Dieulafoy's lesion	
Hemosuccus pancreaticus	
Hemobilia	
Long-distance running	
Parasitic infection (hookworm)	
Hemoptysis	
Epistaxis	
LOWER GI LESIONS	22–26
Colonic adenoma >1 cm	12–14
Colorectal cancer	5–6
Angiodysplasia	3–13
Colonic ulcers	
Ulcerative colitis	
Infectious colitis	
Colitis (nonspecific)	

[a] Percentage ranges given for the three most common causes of occult bleeding.[6,7]

GI bleeding, with or without iron deficiency anemia. The upper GI tract is the more common source than the lower GI tract, for both occult bleeding and iron deficiency anemia.[7,8]

Obscure bleeding can be organized into three main categories and sources: (1) upper GI lesions within reach of an endoscope; (2) small bowel lesions beyond the reach of an endoscope; and (3) lower GI lesions within reach of an endoscope. In the evaluation of obscure bleeding, common causes that have been missed on a previous endoscopy may be found on re-examination. Upper GI lesions that are not uncommonly missed include erosions within large hiatal hernias (Cameron's lesions) and gastric antral vascular ectasia (Watermelon stomach); the latter may be originally mistaken as 'gastritis.'

Angiodysplasia is by far the most common source of small bowel bleeding. With the introduction of wireless capsule endoscopy, a substantial number of small bowel erosions have been detected in healthy subjects not taking nonsteroidal anti-inflammatory drugs (NSAIDs). However, patients on NSAIDs have an increased prevalence of small bowel erosions, perhaps suggesting NSAID enteropathy as a potential source of small bowel blood loss and iron deficiency anemia.[9]

Missed colonic lesions apart from more commonly recognized causes include angiodysplasia or internal hemorrhoids. In the latter instance the hemorrhoids may have been noted previously but their potential as a cause of obscure bleeding may not have been considered.

DIAGNOSIS

Patient history

A focused history is essential to help guide the diagnostic approach to anemia from occult and obscure bleeding. Age may be the most important and readily defined variable, especially in the evaluation of obscure GI bleeding. Inquiring about NSAID, steroid, bisphosphate, or tetracycline (pill-induced esophagitis) use, as well as over-the-counter supplements and herbal preparations, is also imperative as these common medications theoretically may predispose patients to mucosal erosion and ulceration. Chronic anticoagulation with warfarin, within the appropriate therapeutic range, has not been shown to increase the risk of bleeding secondary to insignificant lesions.[10] Rather, these medications serve as 'stress tests,' inducing bleeding from pre-existing lesions before they would have bled if anticoagulants had not been given.

The past medical history may provide key clues. For instance, patients with aortic valve replacements as well as those with chronic renal failure have a predilection to develop intestinal angiodysplasias. Other previous surgical procedures that may lead to GI bleeding are repair of an aortic aneurysm (aortoenteric fistulae), bowel resection (anastomotic ulcers), and liver biopsy (hemobilia). In HIV infection, neoplastic lesions such as lymphoma and Kaposi's sarcoma need to be considered. A family history of an inherited polyposis syndrome, hereditary

CAUSES AND DIFFERENTIAL DIAGNOSIS

CAUSES OF OBSCURE GI BLEEDING

Within reach on upper endoscopy	Beyond the reach of endoscope	Within reach on colonoscopy[a]
Cameron's erosions	Angiodysplasia	Angiodysplasia
Esophagitis	Small bowel tumors[b]	Colonic polyps
Angiodysplasia	Small bowel ulcers	Colorectal cancer
Esophageal varices	Crohn's disease	Colonic diverticulosis
Peptic ulcer disease	Celiac sprue	Ulcerative colitis
Gastritis	Small bowel varices	Colonic ulcers
Gastric polyps	Lymphangioma	Hemorrhoids
Gastric antral vascular ectasia	Radiation enteritis	Parasitic infestation
Blue rubber bleb nevus syndrome	Blue rubber bleb nevus syndrome	
Osler-Weber-Rendu syndrome	Osler-Weber-Rendu syndrome	
Dieulafoy's lesion	Von Willebrand's disease	
Celiac sprue	Small bowel polyposis syndromes	
	Gardner's syndrome	
	Aortoenteric fistula	
	Amyloidosis	
	Meckel's diverticulum	

[a] Up to 25% of cases of lower intestinal bleeding remain undiagnosed after initial and sometimes exhaustive investigation.[1]

[b] Includes small bowel adenocarcinoma, metastatic lesions, lymphoma, leiomyoma, leiomyosarcoma, melanoma, carcinoid, and lipoma.

bleeding disorder (i.e., von Willebrand's disease), hereditary telangiectasia, or neurofibromatosis may be relevant. In addition to these unique associations, questioning about prior gastrointestinal malignancy (recurrence), extraintestinal malignancy (metastatic lesions), inflammatory bowel disease (erosions, ulcers, or tumors), alcohol abuse (erosive gastritis), gastroesophageal reflux disease (esophagitis), and liver disease (varices or portal hypertensive gastropathy) is essential.

The majority of patients presenting with anemia secondary to occult and obscure bleeding are asymptomatic. When present, symptoms such as reflux, epigastric pain, change in bowel habits or stool caliber are surprisingly unreliable in localizing the site of bleeding, and should not in and of themselves restrict evaluation to the upper or lower GI tract.

Diagnostic evaluation of iron deficiency anemia and occult bleeding

A FOBT should be among the first tests ordered in the evaluation of iron deficiency anemia. As false-negative FOBT results are not uncommon, GI evaluation is still indicated. Other serologic tests – such as a peripheral smear, bilirubin, lactate dehydrogenase, and haptoglobin to evaluate for hemolysis; antiendomysial and antitissue transglutaminase antibody assays to test for celiac disease; and blood eosinophil percentage with stool ova/parasite exams for possible parasitic infections – may be useful in detecting non-GI bleeding sources of anemia.

Endoscopy is the cornerstone of initial investigation for occult GI blood loss (Fig. 16.1). Deciding on which endoscopic procedure to pursue first depends mainly on the medical history variables already discussed. If a significant lesion consistent with bleeding is found, treatment should be performed without further investigations as multiple lesions are rare. One exception to this rule is patients over the age of 50 years who first receive upper endoscopy and treatment for an upper GI tract lesion. Because this age group is at considerable risk of colorectal cancer, these patients should also receive a colonoscopy for screening purposes. In this scenario, back-to-back upper and lower exams are an efficient alternative to exams on separate days, so patients should be prepped and consented for both.

If the initial endoscopic procedure is negative, a second endoscopic procedure in the opposite direction is recommended. Small bowel biopsy for celiac disease should be considered in appropriate patients who have not undergone serologic testing, as well as those with positive tests. Patients with negative bidirectional endoscopic findings, assuming adequate bowel preparation with good mucosal visualization, should be started on a 3-month trial of empiric iron supplementation. Up to 83% of patients with iron deficiency anemia and a negative bidirectional evaluation will respond, with no recurrence of anemia for at least 20 months.[11] Patients with continued evidence of occult bleeding or iron deficiency anemia despite iron supplementation meet the criteria for obscure-occult bleeding and need to undergo further evaluation to determine the location of blood loss.

Diagnostic evaluation of obscure bleeding

Although obscure bleeding accounts for only a small proportion of patients with GI blood loss, it is a significant source of morbidity (and even mortality) for affected patients, and a diagnostic challenge to clinicians. The first step in evaluation of these patients is to determine whether the blood loss is best characterized as obscure-occult or obscure-overt (Fig. 16.2).

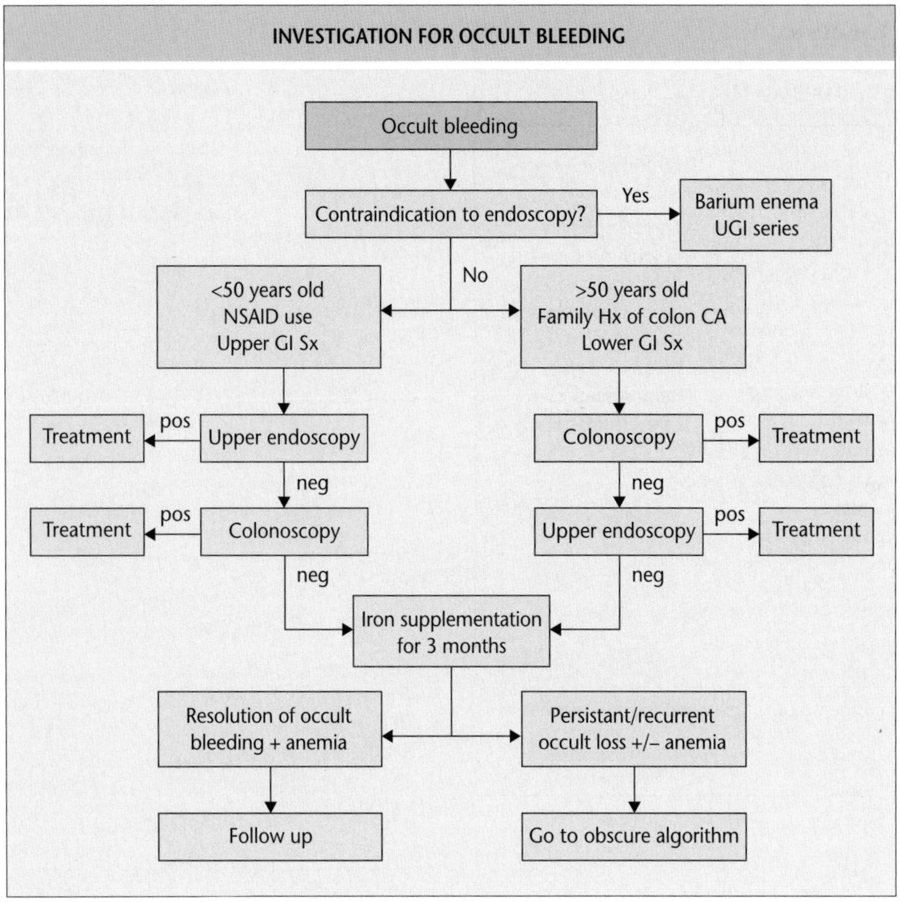

Fig. 16.1 Investigation of occult bleeding. Occult bleeding algorithm.

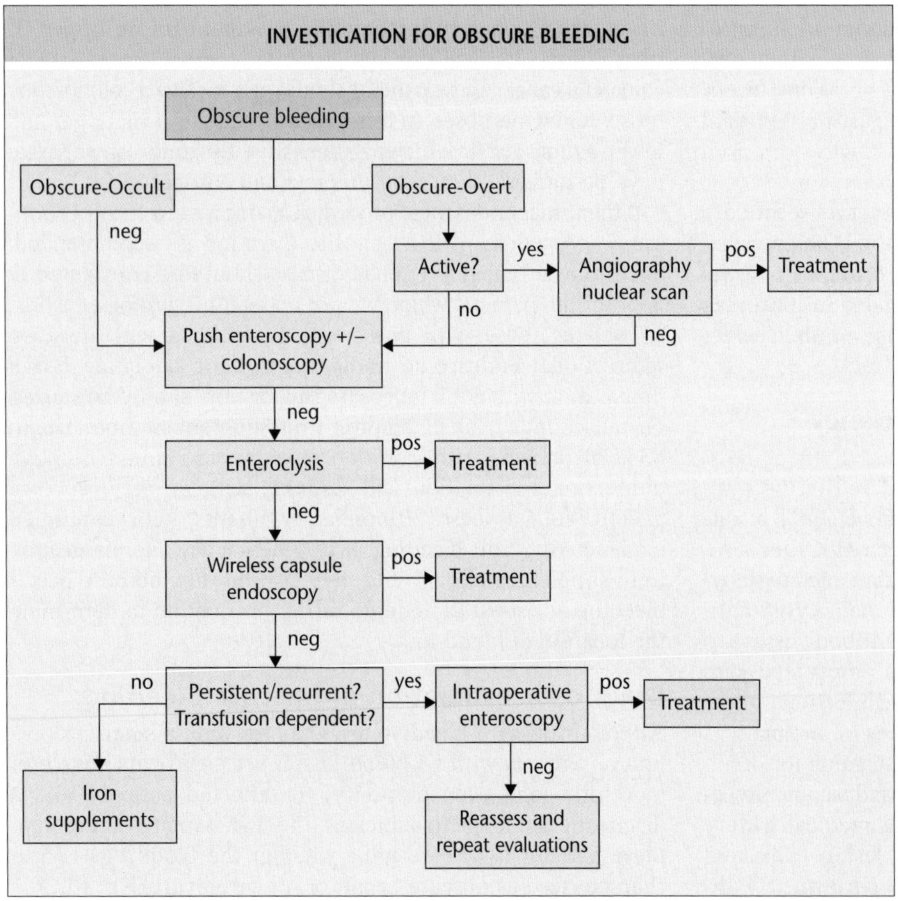

Fig. 16.2 Investigation of obscure bleeding. Obscure bleeding algorithm.

Technetium-99m-labeled red blood cell scans may be useful in the setting of overt bleeding, but require an active bleeding rate of more than 0.1–0.4 mL/min for a positive result. Moreover, the sensitivity of localizing the bleeding site varies considerably depending on when the scan becomes positive during the procedure. Late positive scans may indicate areas of pooled blood rather than the actual site of bleeding. Angiography is usually required to confirm the location of hemorrhage. Rarely, angiography can identify angiodysplasia or neoplastic lesions strictly by typical vascular patterns. Localization of an active bleeding site requires more than 0.5 mL/min for a positive result. Provocative angiography using selective arterial injection of vasodilators, thrombolytics, or anticoagulants has a greater risk of complications, but may be warranted in difficult cases to increase the diagnostic yield.[12]

Repeat bidirectional endoscopy is indicated because the cause of bleeding can frequently be missed on the initial evaluation. However, repeat upper endoscopy should be performed using a small bowel enteroscope with the thought of continuing to push enteroscopy if no proximal lesions are found. Push enteroscopy can be very useful, as it allows a broad range of diagnostic (e.g., biopsy, irrigation, insufflation, suction) and therapeutic options. Patients with normal repeat evaluations will require further investigation of the small bowel further downstream.

Intraoperative enteroscopy has been the gold standard for determining the site of a small bowel lesion out of reach of the push enteroscope. However, the development of wireless capsule endoscopy (WCE) has added a new noninvasive diagnostic alternative. At present, the only commercially available WCE device (Given Imaging, Yoqneam, Israel) can easily be swallowed by most subjects. Two images per second are transmitted to a data-recording device worn on the patient's waist for the 6–8-h battery life of the capsule. The images are then downloaded to a computer workstation for viewing. The capsule is normally passed in the stool. Unexpected impaction in a small bowel stricture or mass occurs in less than 1% of cases, but requires surgical excision.

Several case series suggest that WCE has better diagnostic yield than push enteroscopy, but these comparisons are limited by the definition and location of positive findings. No studies have convincingly demonstrated an improvement in clinically relevant outcomes with WCE over push enteroscopy. Given available data, we recommend that push enteroscopy be performed before the use of WCE in the evaluation of obscure bleeding. Because of the risk, albeit small, of bowel impaction and obstruction with WCE, enteroclysis should be considered after push enteroscopy to screen for distal strictures or masses prior to the capsule examination. A dissolvable capsule-like device for detecting small bowel strictures before WCE is being developed, and may obviate the need for GI contrast studies. If push enteroscopy, enteroclysis, and WCE are not revealing, then exploratory laparotomy with intraoperative endoscopy is recommended for diagnosis and treatment.

CURRENT CONTROVERSIES AND THEIR FUTURE RESOLUTION

Future studies need to answer the following questions, which have yet to be resolved:

- *What is the optimal sequence of diagnostic tests for evaluation of obscure GI bleeding?* The approach recommended in this chapter is based on the current literature and expert opinion: both can be improved significantly by further studies.
- *How valid are findings on wireless capsule endoscopy?* The diagnostic lexicon ('red spots,' 'bleeding without focal lesion,' 'probable angiodysplasia') emerging from initial studies of the capsule needs to be validated by studies that include either surgical pathology or long-term outcome evaluation in at least a subset of cases. The reliability of these findings and the amount of training required also need to be established.
- *What are the consequences of false-positive capsule exams?* Overevaluation and treatment of incidental lesions may subject patients to unnecessary morbidity and even mortality, but current outcome data are limited.
- *What is the prevalence, importance, and best management strategy for small-bowel NSAID enteropathy?* The risk of gastric erosion and ulceration secondary to NSAID use has been established with corresponding effective treatment strategies. WCE has provided preliminary data on the prevalence of NSAID enteropathy. Ongoing trials are evaluating the mechanism, consequences, and treatment of this relatively novel entity.

SOURCES OF INFORMATION FOR PATIENTS AND DOCTORS

http://www.patient.co.uk/showdoc/27000442/

REFERENCES

1. Zuckerman GR, Prakash C, Askin MP, Lewis BS. AGA technical review on the evaluation and management of occult and obscure gastrointestinal bleeding. Gastroenterology 1999; 118:201–221.
2. Moses PL, Smith RE. Endoscopic evaluation of iron deficiency anemia. Postgrad Med 1995; 98:213–224.
3. Looker AC, Dallman PR, Carroll MD et al. Prevalance of iron deficiency in the United States. JAMA 1997; 277:973–996.
4. Mandel JS, Bond JH, Church TR et al. Reducing mortality from colorectal cancer by screening for fecal occult blood. N Engl J Med 1993; 328:1365–1371.
5. Dulai GS, Jensen DM. Severe gastrointestinal bleeding of obscure origin. Gastrointest Endosc Clin N Am 2004; 14:101–113.
6. Kandel GP, Rasul I. An approach to iron deficiency anemia. Can J Gastroenterol 2001; 15:739–747.
7. Zuckerman G, Benitez J. A prospective study of bi-directional endoscopy (colonoscopy and upper endoscopy) in the evaluation of patients with occult gastrointestinal bleeding. Am J Gastroenterol 1992; 87:62–66.
8. Rockey DC, Koch J, Cello JP, Sanders LL, McQuaid K. Relative frequency of upper gastrointestinal and colonic lesions in patients with positive fecal occult blood tests. N Engl J Med 1998; 339:153–159.
9. Goldstein J, Eisen G, Lewis B et al. Abnormal small bowel findings are common in healthy subjects screened for a multi-center, doubleblind, randomized, placebo-controlled trial using capsule endoscopy. Gastroenterology 2003; 124(Suppl 1):A37.
10. Greenberg PD, Cello JP, Rockey DC. Asymptomatic chronic gastrointestinal blood loss in patients taking aspirin or warfarin for cardiovascular disease. Am J Med 1996; 100:598–604.
11. Rockey DC, Cello JP. Evaluation of the gastrointestinal tract in patients with iron deficiency anemia. N Engl J Med 1993; 329: 1691–1695.
12. Bloomfeld RS, Smith TP, Schneider AM, Rockey DC. Provocative angiography in patients with gastrointestinal hemorrhage of obscure origin. Am J Gastroenterol 2000; 95:2807–2812.
13. Beveridge BR, Bannerman RM, Evanson JM et al. Hypochromic anemia. A retrospective study and follow-up of 378 in-patients. Q J Med 1965; 34:145–161.

Chapter 17

Pruritus

Nora V Bergasa

INTRODUCTION

Pruritus or itch is one of the symptoms associated with cholestasis. It can have a marked negative impact on the quality of life of patients and it may lead to suicidal ideations. Severe pruritus may be an indication for liver transplantation.

WHAT IS IT?

Hafenreffer, in 1660, defined pruritus as an unpleasant sensation that elicits the need to scratch. Scratching is the behavior that universally results from pruritus; it appears to have evolved as a protective reflex.

HOW COMMON IS IT?

The reported range of patients with primary biliary cirrhosis (PBC) that present with pruritus is 25–70%.[1] A recent survey conducted via the Internet through the website of the PBCers' organization revealed that 68% of the 242 patients who responded to the survey experienced pruritus. In 75% of the patients with pruritus, the symptom had been present for 2–5 years prior to the diagnosis of PBC (Rishe and Bergasa, 2002, unpublished data). The range of pruritus prevalence in primary sclerosing cholangitis (PSC) has been reported to range from 5% to 23%. Retrospective studies report the prevalence of pruritus in liver disease secondary to chronic hepatitis C to be around 5%.

PATHOPHYSIOLOGY

The pathogenesis of the pruritus of cholestasis is unknown. It has been assumed that it results from the stimulation of peripheral nerve fibers by substances that accumulate in the body as a result of cholestasis; the nature of those substances is unknown. Bile acids accumulate in tissues in cholestasis and they have been considered the pruritogens. Arguments proposed in support of this idea include: (1) the reported pruritogenic effect of bile acids when injected into the skin of normal volunteers (however, this experiment is not a model of the pruritus of cholestasis), and (2) the reported amelioration of the pruritus associated with interventions aimed at a decrease in the enterohepatic circulation of bile acids, including the intake of cholestyramine (a nonabsorbable resin that binds anions in the small intestine), and partial external diversion of bile, and ileal diversion.[1] However, cholestyramine may exert other effects that may result in a decrease in the perception of pruritus, and the surgical interventions stated above may remove, in addition to bile acids, substances that may be involved in the pruritus. In the context of bile acids, not all patients with cholestasis and elevated serum concentrations of these compounds report pruritus. The pruritus of cholestasis may spontaneously remit independently from changes in serum bile acids, and some patients with liver disease and pruritus do not have increased bile acid concentrations in serum. It is possible that a certain profile of bile acids is necessary for these substances to mediate pruritus but a role of bile acids in the mediation of the pruritus of cholestasis has not been proven.

Central effects: Pruritus can also be of central origin, from increased central opioidergic tone.[2] A link between opioid receptors and pruritus and scratching of central origin is well established[3]: (1) the pharmacological increase in opioidergic tone (e.g., central administration of morphine) is associated with pruritus and scratching in human beings and in laboratory animals; and (2) this type of pruritus and scratching is ameliorated and/or prevented by opiate antagonists, suggesting that it is opioid-receptor mediated.[3] That cholestasis is associated with increased central opioidergic tone in human beings is suggested by the opiate withdrawal-like syndrome that patients with cholestasis can experience at the administration of opiate antagonists.[4] Thus, if increased opioidergic tone results in pruritus, the increased opioidergic tone of cholestasis may mediate this type of pruritus. The reason for increased opioidergic tone in cholestasis is unknown; however, increased availability of opioid ligands from peripheral sources may be an explanation, as suggested by the increased serum concentration of some of the opioid peptides in patients with cholestasis.[4] The source of opioid peptides in cholestasis is unknown but the cholestatic liver is a possibility.[3] In this context, periphery-derived endogenous opioids may reach itch-mediating centers including the medullary dorsal horn in the central nervous system.[3]

Objective measurement: The subjective nature of pruritus has been recognized as a research challenge. Instruments that recorded limb movements as an index of 'scratching' were developed in the 1970s.[2] A ground breaking piece of work was the development of a scratching activity monitoring system (SAMS),[2,5] which used a piezo film sensor attached to a finger. Signals are derived from vibrations of the fingernail as they traverse the skin in the act of scratching and are independent from gross body movements. The SAMS has been used in clinical trials of therapeutic interventions for pruritus of cholestasis with a well-defined end-point, i.e., change in scratching activity. The SAMS has been adapted for ambulatory use; thus, clinical trials that record scratching behavior from participating subjects in their living environment are now possible.

Complete resolution of biliary obstruction results in relief of pruritus; this observation tends to suggest that the pruritogen(s) is excreted in bile. Liver transplantation also results in the relief of the pruritus of cholestasis; this observation supports the idea that the pruritogen or cofactors required for the pruritus to be perceived are synthesized in the liver. The pruritus of cholestasis, however, does not consistently respond to treatments directed at the liver disease. Accordingly, it requires treatment that is directed at the symptom, some of which are listed in Table 17.1. The treatment of the pruritus of cholestasis had tended to be empirical and sometimes lacking a clear rationale. In Table 17.1 the proposed aim behind each listed treatment is given. Recently, however, progress has been made. The hypothesis that the endogenous opioid system contributes to the pruritus of cholestasis was tested in controlled clinical trials in which the SAMS was used to collect behavioral data. In these studies, the administration of the opiate antagonists naloxone and nalmefene was associated with a decrease in scratching activity.[5] The use of opiate antagonists can be accompanied by an opiate withdrawal-like syndrome.[4] Starting treatment with opiate antagonists at low doses tends to decrease or avoid this reaction.[1]

The use of objective methodology revealed a 24-h rhythm in the scratching behavior of some patients[5] (Fig. 17.1). This led to the idea of exploring the use of light, which regulates biological rhythms via retinothalamic pathways, to decrease pruritus and scratching. A pilot study using bright light therapy (10 000 lux, ultraviolet filtered) that applied quantitative methodology revealed that seven of the eight patients studied scratched less after 8 weeks of therapy than at baseline and that the outbursts of scratching behavior were significantly decreased in all cases[6] (Fig. 17.2). These results tend to support the idea that pruritus and scratching are centrally regulated, but randomized controlled trials should be carried out to confirm this result.

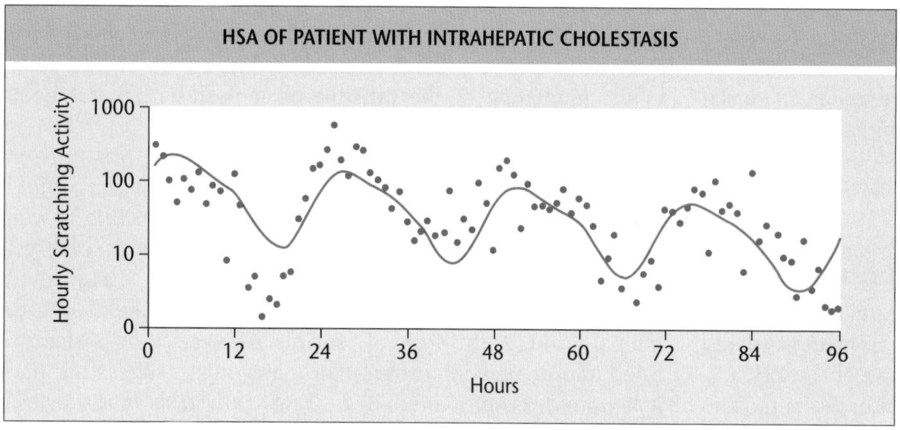

Fig. 17.1 Mean hourly scratching activity (HSA) of a patient with intrahepatic cholestasis. HAS during the 96-h study period of a patient with benign recurrent intrahepatic cholestasis who participated in a study of naloxone infusions for the pruritus of cholestasis. The continuous line indicates the 24-h rhythm that best fits the observation. The line has a significant downward trend, which is consistent with the sequence of infusion (placebo, placebo, naloxone, naloxone) indicating that the patient scratched less on the study drug. Reproduced with permission from Bergasa NV et al. Effects of naloxone infusions in patients with the pruritus of cholestasis. A double-blind, randomized, controlled trial. Ann Intern Med 1995; 123:161–167.

TABLE 17.1 SELECTED TREATMENTS OF THE PRURITUS OF CHOLESTASIS

Medication/postulated antipruritic mechanism/ reference	Dose/mode of administration/ frequency	Type of study/ duration	*n*	End-points	Results	Possible side effects
Cholestyramine/ increased excretion of pruritogen(s)/ Datta and Sherlock[9]	3.3–12 g PO/day	Single blind, open label/placebo controlled crossover/ 6–32 months	27	Not reported	23 patients experienced relief of pruritus[a]	Bloating, constipation, malabsorption of nutrients
Rifampicin/unknown/ Ghent and Carruthers[10]	150 mg PO/BID if serum bilirubin >3 mg/dl; 150 mg PO/TID if serum bilirubin <3 mg/dl	Double blind, randomized, placebo controlled crossover/4 weeks	9	Change in VAS	Highly significant decrease in the 7-day summed VAS[b]	Hepatotoxicity
Naloxone/decrease in opioidergic tone	0.2 μg/kg/min/IV continuous infusions preceded by 0.4 mg IV bolus	Double blind, placebo controlled, randomized crossover/4 consecutive days	29	Change in HSA	Geometric mean HSA 34% lower on naloxone than on placebo	Opiate withdrawal-like syndrome

[a]Compared to an observational control group that did not receive cholestyramine but that received norethandrolone or no treatment.
[b]Patients were allowed to continue taking cholestyramine; during the study, the number of cholestyramine packs per day was counted. Mean change in VAS not reported; VAS graphed per patient.

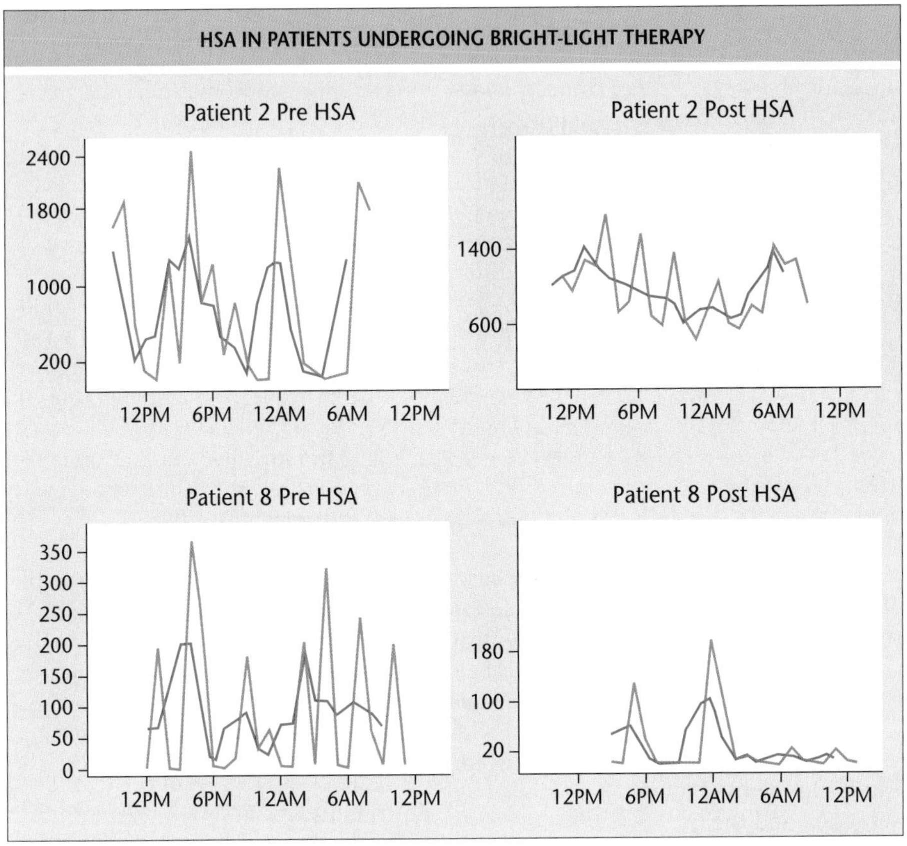

Fig. 17.2 Hourly scratching activity (HSA) in patients undergoing bright-light therapy. HSA in two patients with chronic liver disease who participated in a study of bright-light therapy for the pruritus of cholestasis. y-axis, HAS; x-axis, time of day. Pre HSA indicates data at baseline and post HSA indicates data after 8 weeks of therapy. The solid line represents raw data and the interrupted line represents the same data after having been smoothed out with a moving average smoother. In both patients, HSA was less after bright-light therapy. The data represented by the solid line were highly volatile, as indicated by the peaks and valleys of HSA, which represent outbursts of scratching behavior. The volatility was less after bright-light therapy, as suggested by the smoother curves. Reprinted from American Journal of Gastroenterology, vol 96, Bergasa NV et al. Pilot study of bright-light therapy reflected toward the eyes for the pruritus of chronic liver disease, 1563–1570, 2001, with permission from American College of Gastroenterology.

Other mediators: Attention is being paid to other systems of neurotransmission. Controlled trials of ondansetron, a serotonin antagonist, have yielded inconsistent results, although initial case reports were encouraging.[1] Review of data collected prospectively from symptom diaries from patients with PBC reported that the use of sertraline, a serotonin re-uptake inhibitor, was associated with a decrease in pruritus.[7] Three patients were reported to experience relief of their intractable pruritus after taking dronabinol, an agonist at the central cannabinoid receptor.[8] These observations are anecdotal; however, they merit follow-up with properly controlled quantitative studies. A clinical trial on the drug gabapentin (reported to change nociceptive threshold) to treat the pruritus of cholestasis has recently been completed (Bergasa, unpublished data).

CAUSES AND DIFFERENTIAL DIAGNOSIS

Table 17.2 includes some of the hepatic conditions that have been associated with pruritus. It appears that most types of liver disease can be associated with pruritus, irrespective of the serum liver profile. Why some patients with cholestasis experience this symptom and others do not still remains a mystery.

Pruritus is the most common symptom of skin disorders. The skin of patients with the pruritus of cholestasis may display excoriations and prurigo nodularis (Fig. 17.3), when scratching has been chronic. Hyperpigmentation may be a clue to the presence of some cholestatic conditions such as PBC and PSC, but this finding is independent from pruritus.

When the cause of pruritus is not apparent (e.g., in the absence of a diagnostic rash) diagnostic investigations must include a thorough review of systems and appropriate radiographic and laboratory tests, including those designed to diagnose liver disease.

TABLE 17.2 HEPATIC CONDITIONS ASSOCIATED WITH PRURITUS

CHILDHOOD	ADULTHOOD
Progressive familial intrahepatic cholestasis	Primary biliary cirrhosis
Allagille's syndrome	Primary sclerosing cholangitis
Biliary atresia	Chronic viral hepatitis
Primary sclerosing cholangitis	Drug-induced cholestasis with and without ductopenia
Drug-induced cholestasis with and without ductopenia	Biliary obstruction
Cystic fibrosis[a]	Pregnancy
Biliary obstruction	Hepatic sarcoidosis[b]
Alpha-1-antitrypsin deficiency	Cirrhosis secondary to alcohol
	Alpha-1-antitrypsin deficiency

[a]Pruritus was reported in one publication on patients with cholestasis and cystic fibrosis.
[b]Ductopenia may be associated with hepatic sarcoidosis. Pruritus secondary to cholestasis in sarcoidosis is well documented in adults but not in children.

SYMPTOM COMPLEXES

In general, patients with liver disease and pruritus describe their symptom as 'irritation,' 'pins and needles,' 'crawling' sensation. Twenty-five per cent of the patients with PBC who participated in the Internet survey reported that the degree of pruritus increased prior to menstruation (Rishe and Bergasa, 2002, unpublished data). The majority of patients with liver disease and pruritus report that it is worse at night, when they return home from their daily activities.

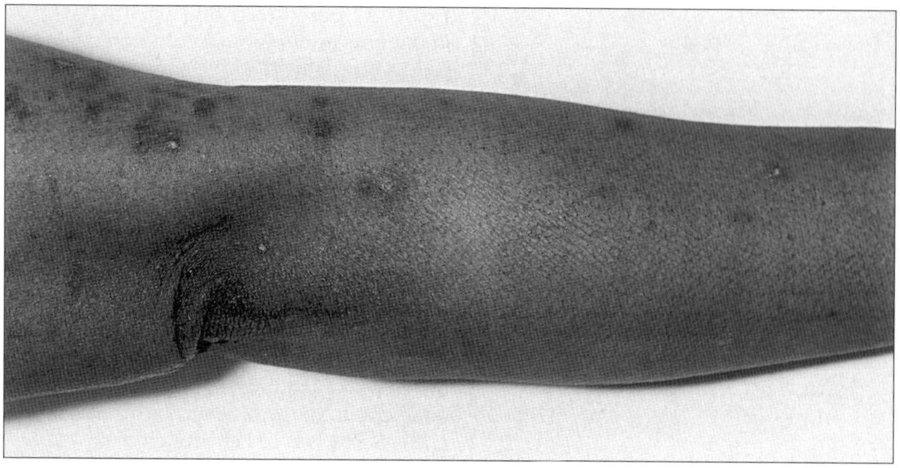

Fig. 17. 3 Skin of a patient with cholestasis and pruritus exhibiting prurigo nodularis secondary to chronic scratching.

DIAGNOSIS

Pruritus can precede the diagnosis of liver disease by years. The diagnosis of pruritus is made by taking a thorough history.

CURRENT CONTROVERSIES AND THEIR FUTURE RESOLUTION

It is necessary to develop methodology to study the neurophysiology and pathophysiology of the itch sensation and the resulting protective scratching reflex in human beings.

Anecdotal observations on the ameliorating effect of the pruritus of cholestasis by reasonable interventions should be followed by controlled clinical trials that include objective methodology to be used in the ambulatory setting. Objective data obtained via quantitative methodology can be standardized and generalized with the final aim of developing effective and specific therapies for pruritus in cholestasis.

REFERENCES

1. Bergasa NV. Pruritus and fatigue in primary biliary cirrhosis. Clin Liver Dis 2003;7:879–900.
2. Jones EA, Bergasa NV. The pruritus of cholestasis: from bile acids to opiate agonists. Hepatology 1990;11:884–887.
3. Bergasa NV, Jones EA. The pruritus of cholestasis: potential pathogenic and therapeutic implications of opioids. Gastroenterology 1995; 108:1582–1588.
4. Thornton JR, Losowsky MS. Opioid peptides and primary biliary cirrhosis. Br Med J 1988; 297:1501–1504.
5. Bergasa NV, Alling DW, Talbot TL et al. Naloxone ameliorates the pruritus of cholestasis: results of a double-blind randomized placebo-controlled trial. Ann Intern Med 1995; 123:161–167.
6. Bergasa NV, Link MJ, Keogh M et al. Pilot study of bright-light therapy reflected toward the eyes for the pruritus of chronic liver disease. Am J Gastroenterol 2001; 96:1563–1570.
7. Browning J, Combes B, Mayo MJ. Long-term efficacy of sertraline as a treatment for cholestatic pruritus in patients with primary biliary cirrhosis. Am J Gastroenterol 2003; 98:2736–2741.
8. Neff GW, O'Brien CB, Reddy KR et al. Preliminary observation with dronabinol in patients with intractable pruritus secondary to cholestatic liver disease. Am J Gastroenterol 2002; 97:2117–2119.
9. Datta DV, Sherlock S. Cholestyramine for long term relief of the pruritus complicating intrahepatic cholestasis. Gastroenterology 1966; 50:323–332.
10. Ghent CN, Carruthers SG. Treatment of pruritus in primary biliary cirrhosis with rifampin. Results of a double-blind, crossover, randomized trial. Gastroenterology 1988; 94:488–493.

Chapter 18

Jaundice

Adrian Reuben

INTRODUCTION

The term jaundice denotes yellowness that is seen in the sclerae, skin, and mucous membranes when circulating bilirubin levels rise approximately 3-fold or more above normal, i.e., when serum bilirubin levels exceed about 3 mg/dL (51 µmol/L). Such hyperbilirubinemia can occur either when too great a load of bilirubin is presented to the normal liver or, more commonly, when any hepatobiliary condition causes defective hepatic uptake, processing, or biliary excretion of bilirubin.

The word jaundice comes from the Middle English *jaunice* (*jaunisse*) that was adopted from *jaune* (*jalne*), the French word for yellow, as far back as the 12th century CE; the 'd' in the form *jaundice* was acquired a couple of hundred years later, by so-called phonetic accretion. The term *icterus* means exactly the same as jaundice, namely yellowness, even though some physicians mistakenly insist on reserving the adjective *icteric* to describe yellow eyes and use *jaundice* to describe yellowness elsewhere in the body. The word icterus is derived from the Greek *ikteros* for oriole, the yellow-breasted bird that many Greeks kept as pets, the mere sight of which was thought to cure jaundice.[1]

WHAT IS IT?

Jaundice or icterus is defined as an abnormally yellow hue to tissues that are ordinarily white (or relatively white) but become visibly stained with bilirubin (and possibly biliverdin too), which binds to them after diffusing from the blood. Jaundice does not cause any unusual sensation in the skin or the eyes apart from the extremely rare experience of *xanopsia* (seeing yellow). Jaundice is first detected in the sclerae of the eyes, where there is abundant elastic tissue to which bilirubin readily binds. This is followed by yellowing of the skin and mucous membranes, being particularly noticeable in the frenulum of the tongue. Scars, edematous areas, and parts that are paralyzed or immobilized are usually spared. Jaundice also affects bodily secretions and fluids (especially those that are protein-rich), such as tears, sweat, semen, milk, sputum, and ascites; even cerebrospinal fluid may be yellow in jaundiced patients, so that xanthochromia may be misdiagnosed. Jaundice itself may be misdiagnosed too when yellow discoloration of the skin is not caused by bilirubin staining but by xenobiotics, such as quinacrine (mepacrine), an acridine derivative that was once used to treat malaria, or carotenes in individuals who consume large amounts of yellow vegetables and fruits, such as tomatoes, carrots, squashes, pumpkins, and papaya; in neither case are the sclerae yellow. In Victorian times, jaundice was often spuriously diagnosed by being mistaken for many other conditions that were recognized because of an abnormal skin color,[2] such as the yellow-green countenance of the severe anemic state known then as chlorosis, the grayish-yellow of the cancer patient, the dusky yellow of the chronic malaria sufferer, a weather-beaten outdoors complexion, the bronzing of Addison's hypoadrenalism, and hemochromatosis. Also, factitious jaundice may be produced by malingerers who paint their skin with tinctures of yellow pigment, such as turmeric or saffron, and water-fast dyes. Finally, it may be difficult to tell whether jaundice is present in the eyes of non-Caucasians, whose natural pigmentation may give an appearance to the sclerae that is usually described as being 'muddy,' making any yellowness there difficult to discern.

HOW COMMON IS IT?

Jaundice is obviously a defining feature of any disorder that interferes with the metabolism of bilirubin sufficiently to raise its serum level above 3 mg/dL. It follows that jaundice is common in hepatobiliary disorders that impair bilirubin handling and excretion, as well as in hematologic and other disorders in which heightened degradation of heme and/or other hemoproteins yields an increased bilirubin load for excretion by the liver. Jaundice can also complicate extrahepatic conditions that impede hepatic bilirubin metabolism and/or clearance without causing structural liver injury per se, such as sepsis, pregnancy, or the use of drugs that inhibit some aspect of hepatic bilirubin transport. Drugs can displace bilirubin from binding at extrahepatic sites, which can increase the load for the liver to process, as well as cause cerebral toxicity in infants (kernicterus) by displacing unconjugated bilirubin into the brain, e.g., with aspirin and sulfonamides.

Parenchymal liver injury that causes moderate to severe hepatocyte necrosis is often characterized by jaundice; this is seen especially in alcoholic hepatitis and also in viral or drug-related hepatitis. The prevalence of jaundice in viral hepatitis is greater in older patients, who also fare less well than younger patients. Similarly, the development of jaundice in patients with drug-induced hepatitis is a harbinger of a poor outcome,[3] which may amount to an approximately 10% fatality rate. Hepatobiliary diseases that are characterized by a reduction in bile formation, the so-called cholestatic disorders,[4,5] are more likely to show jaundice early in the course of the disease than later, whether the lesion is (1) at the level of the canalicular membrane transport system, (2) in injured bile ductules and intrahepatic bile ducts, for example in immunologically determined diseases such as primary biliary cirrhosis and chronic liver allograft rejection, etc., and with drug-induced bile ductular and ductal inflammation (caused by chlorpromazine, amoxicillin–clavulanic acid, or other drugs[6]), or (3) due to mechanical obstruction of the extrahepatic biliary tree by gallstones, pancreatic cancer, major bile duct injury, sclerosing cholangitis, bile duct parasitic infestation, and the like. Paradoxically, some patients with cholestatic disorders do not present with jaundice initially but complain of pruritus well before jaundice supervenes, whereas a third of patients who develop cholestasis due to sepsis become jaundiced before the infection is apparent to the patient or physician.[7] With so many different etiologies of jaundice, the distribution of causes varies between populations, depending on the age of the patient, lifestyle, geography. and socioeconomics.[8]

METABOLISM AND TRANSPORT OF BILIRUBIN: NORMAL PHYSIOLOGY

The best way to understand the pathophysiology of jaundice is to start by appreciating the normal physiology of bilirubin metabolism and transport, from formation to entry into canalicular fluid (primary bile) (Fig. 18.1).

(a) Bilirubin is the end-product of the degradation of heme, of which 80% comes from senescent red cell hemoglobin that is released in the spleen, bone marrow, and other tissues; the rest is derived from the turnover of other hemoproteins, such as myoglobin, tissue mitochondrial and microsomal cytochromes, catalase, peroxidase, and tryptophan pyrrolase. There is a small pool of free heme in hepatocytes and some newly synthesized heme is degraded in the bone marrow as a result of so-called 'ineffective erythropoiesis.' Heme, the iron atom-containing heterocyclic tetrapyrrole ring, ferroprotoporphyrin IX, is catalytically cleaved to the water-soluble linear tetrapyrrole biliverdin, by microsomal heme oxygenase that oxidizes and opens the alpha-carbon bridge with the loss of iron and carbon monoxide (Fig. 18.2). The green pigment biliverdin is reduced by cytosolic biliverdin reductase to generate 250–400 mg of water-insoluble orange-yellow bilirubin each day in healthy adult humans. The benefits to humans and other mammals of reducing biliverdin to bilirubin, a lipophilic product that requires conjugation for excretion, are unknown. It has been reasoned that generation of lipophilic bilirubin permits removal from the fetus, by the placenta, of products of heme catabolism, and it also provides both an antioxidant of possible physiologic importance and a major physiologic cytoprotectant.[9]

(b) The problem of transporting a water-insoluble waste product in the circulation is solved for bilirubin, as it is for many drugs and other hydrophobic compounds, by reversible binding to albumin that carries it in the plasma to the liver for processing.

(c) The obstacle to bilirubin elimination from the body via aqueous secretions, such as bile and urine, is overcome by conjugation in the liver with glucuronic acid, which converts bilirubin to its water-soluble glucuronides. The rate-determining step in the conjugation of bilirubin is the uptake of unconjugated bilirubin into the hepatocytes from sinusoidal blood. In the liver sinusoids, bilirubin dissociates from albumin, to be taken up

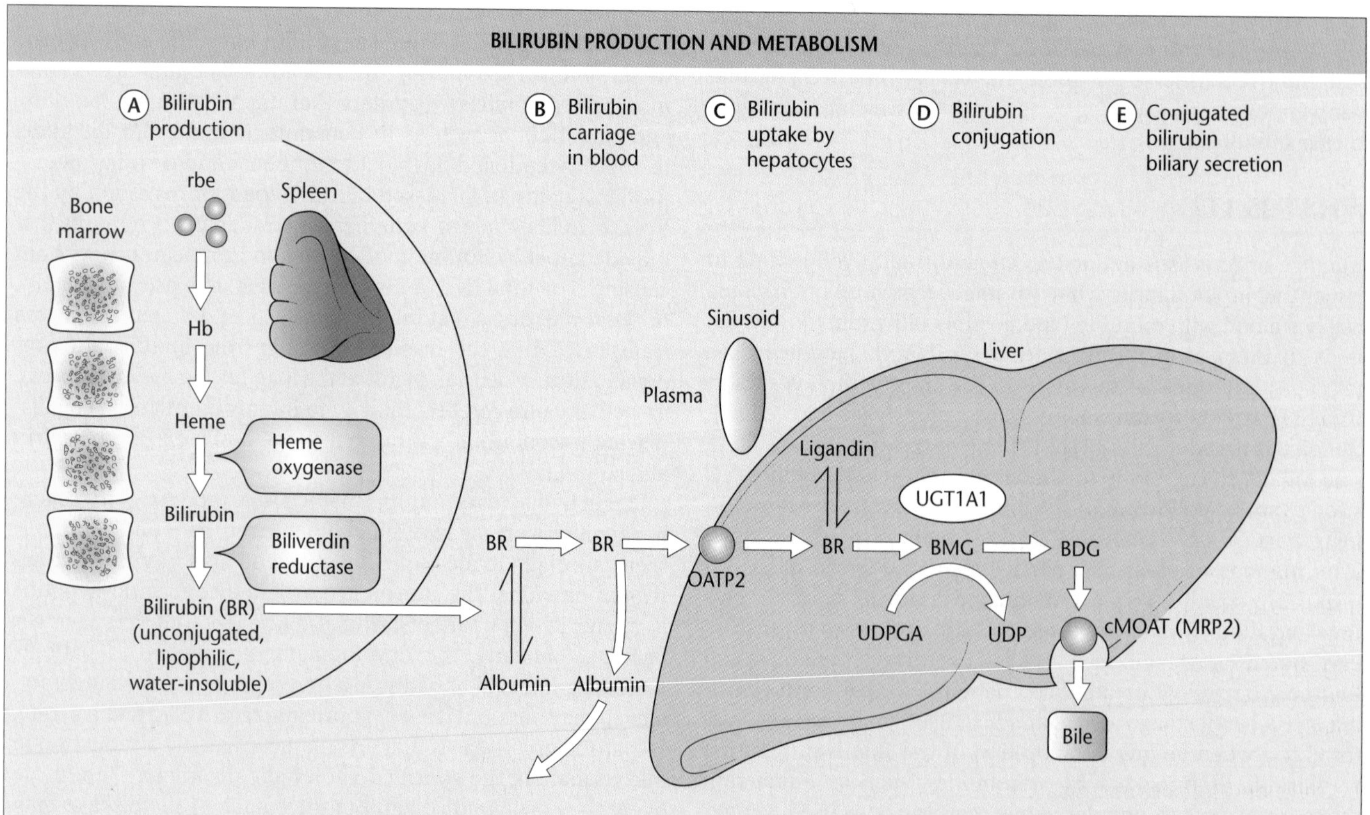

Fig. 18.1 Bilirubin production and metabolism. Overview of bilirubin production, transport in blood, hepatocyte uptake, conjugation, and biliary secretion. BDG, bilirubin diglucuronide; BMG, bilirubin monoglucuronide; BR, bilirubin; cMOAT, canalicular multispecific organic anion transporter; Hb, hemoglobin; MRP2, multidrug resistance-associated protein 2; OATP2, organic anion-transporting polypeptide 2; rbc, red blood cells; UDPGA, uridine disphosphoglucuronic acid; UGT1A1, bilirubin-specific isoform of uridine diphosphoglucuronosyltransferase.

BILIRUBIN SYNTHESIS

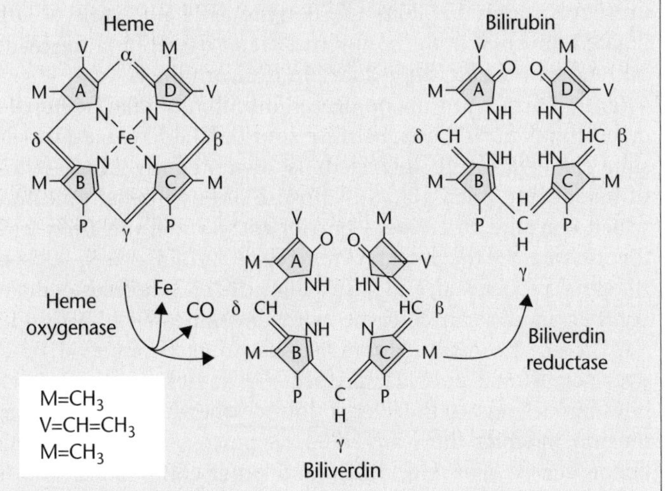

Fig. 18.2 Bilirubin synthesis. Conversion of heme to biliverdin and then to bilirubin. Heme ring-opening at the alpha-carbon bridge of heme is catalyzed by heme oxygenase, resulting in the formation of bilirubin and release of the iron atom and carbon monoxide. This is followed by reduction of biliverdin to bilirubin in a reaction catalyzed by biliverdin reductase. Adapted from Chowdhury NR, Chowdhury JR. Bilirubin metabolism. UpToDate Online 12.1, October 22, 1999. http://www.uptodate.com

(without the albumin) at the hepatocyte sinusoidal (basolateral) plasma membrane, probably by carrier-mediated facilitated diffusion, although the role of the organic anion-transporting polypeptide 2 (OATP2), the proposed membrane carrier protein, is controversial.[10,11] Bilirubin is then trapped in the hepatocyte cytosol by binding to glutathione-*S*-transferases (originally identified as the aminoazodye-binding protein, ligandin) and probably to some extent to fatty acid-binding protein too, so that bilirubin reflux back into the blood is retarded.

(d) Conjugation of bilirubin is a two-stage sequential reaction that takes place in the endoplasmic reticulum and is mediated by the bilirubin-specific isoform of the uridine diphosphoglucuronosyltransferase (UGT) family of enzymes that uses uridine diphosphoglucuronic acid (UDPGA) to form bilirubin monoglucuronide first, and then the major conjugate, bilirubin diglucuronide. Human UGTs are divided into two families; UGT1 family members, which include the bilirubin-specific isoform UGT1A1, are encoded by the UGT1A locus on chromosome 2q37.

(e) Conjugated bilirubin is secreted into bile by an ATP-dependent active transport mechanism, which is mediated by the canalicular isoform of the multidrug resistance-associated protein 2 (MRP2), which is also known as the canalicular multispecific organic anion transporter (cMOAT).[4]

(f) Finally, bile flows from the canaliculi into the ducts of Hering, and thence, successively, to the bile ductules (cholangioles), intralobular (terminal) bile ducts, and conducting area and segmental bile ducts. Eventually, bile leaves the liver via the right and left hepatic ducts, which converge and form the common hepatic duct. Bile then enters the gallbladder for temporary storage and/or traverses the common bile duct to enter the second part of the duodenum through the papilla of Vater. The water and electrolyte content of bile is modified during passage and storage, by the epithelium of the biliary tree.

ABNORMAL METABOLISM AND TRANSPORT OF BILIRUBIN: PATHOPHYSIOLOGY AND CAUSES

The pathophysiology of many causes of jaundice is now explicable in terms of primary specific molecular defects in one or more of the steps in the physiology of bilirubin reviewed above. Of equal interest is the continuing discovery of molecular defects in physiology in hepatobiliary diseases associated with jaundice. Such molecular defects are secondary to the main pathologic process of injury, inflammation, and/or obstruction,[12] but nonetheless can enhance the explanation of how these conditions cause jaundice, and may suggest new and creative remedies. The different mechanisms that lead to jaundice are classified below, corresponding to the physiologic steps enumerated above.

CAUSES AND DIFFERENTIAL DIAGNOSIS

CAUSES OF JAUNDICE

- **Bilirubin overproduction**
  Excessive red cell breakdown (hemolysis, hematomas, etc.)
  Ineffective erythropoiesis
  Nonhemoglobin hemoprotein degradation (myoglobin)
- **Disordered plasma transport of bilirubin**
  Intravenous albumin infusion
  Conjugated bilirubin–albumin, irreversibly bound
- **Impaired uptake of bilirubin by hepatocytes**
  Disruption of sinusoid–hepatocyte interface (cirrhosis)
  Reduced or bypassed hepatic blood flow
  Xenobiotic competition for bilirubin uptake (rifampin, probenecid, flavaspidic acid)
- **Reduced intrahepatic bilirubin conjugation**
  Immature UGT1A1 enzyme (physiologic jaundice of the newborn)
  Defective UGT1A1 enzyme biosynthesis (Gilbert and Crigler-Najjar syndromes)
  Xenobiotic competition for UGT1A1 activity (indinavir)
- **Obstructive and nonobstructive cholestatic syndromes and other disorders**

(a) Bilirubin overproduction from hemoglobin is caused by an excessive breakdown of red cells that is not accounted for by normal senescence. Consequently, hepatic uptake of unconjugated bilirubin becomes saturated and leads to a rise in serum bilirubin concentration that rarely exceeds 4 mg/dL, unless there is coexisting hepatobiliary disease. Although only 4% of bilirubin in normal plasma is conjugated, the diazo assay used in clinical laboratories overestimates this component to be 10–15%, which is therefore the maximum so-called 'direct' bilirubin fraction that is seen in conditions of isolated bilirubin overproduction, or impairment of hepatic uptake and/or conjugation. Bilirubin overproduction results from: (1) hemolysis due to abnormal red cell morphology, as occurs in sickle cell disease and hereditary spherocytosis; (2) mechanical hemolysis due to prosthetic heart valves, disseminated intravascular coagulation, hemolytic-uremic syndrome, etc.; and (3) immune and drug-induced hemolytic anemia. When there is ineffective erythropoiesis, as occurs in thalassemia, pernicious anemia, sideroblastic anemias, severe iron deficiency, lead poisoning, and the rare congenital dyserythropoietic anemias, hemoglobin incorporation into red cells is impaired and its heme is degraded. Increased breakdown of other tissue hemoproteins, especially myoglobin that is released when there is an extensive muscle damage (rhabdomyolysis), can add to the bilirubin load. The jaundice in hemolytic anemias is said to be lemon-yellow, in contrast to the orange-yellow of hepatocellular jaundice that occurs in hepatitis and the green-yellow pigmentation seen in obstructive or cholestatic jaundice (Fig. 18.3). Although these color differences are subtle when jaundice is mild and may be difficult to distinguish in artificial light, the absence of bilirubin from the urine, *acholuria*, is a hallmark of hemolytic jaundice and other unconjugated hyperbilirubinemias. When cholestatic jaundice is prolonged, the skin becomes hyperpigmented (darkened) with melanin, and lipid deposits may appear around the eyes (*xanthelasmas*) and at pressure points in the skin (*xanthomas*).

(b) Theoretically, compounds that displace unconjugated bilirubin from albumin could interfere with hepatic uptake of bilirubin, but this is not discernible in clinical practice. However, if the serum albumin level is increased by an intravenous albumin infusion, this may lead to a rise in serum bilirubin due to further binding to albumin of unconjugated bilirubin that diffuses into the blood from tissue sites. In contrast to the indirectly reacting unconjugated bilirubin that is carried noncovalently bound to albumin, a conjugated bilirubin fraction can become nonenzymatically and irreversibly covalently bound to albumin during periods of prolonged conjugated hyperbilirubinemia. This directly reacting bilirubin–albumin species has a half-life determined by the albumin in the complex, and its presence readily explains the persistently high levels of conjugated bilirubin in the serum that is not excreted in the urine, but endures during the resolution of liver injury.

(c) Impairment of unconjugated bilirubin uptake by hepatocytes occurs in cirrhosis, because sinusoidal microanatomy (the sinusoid–hepatocyte interface) is disrupted by fibrosis, loss of hepatocyte microvilli, and closure of endothelial fenestrae, which conspire to create a barrier to bilirubin diffusion from the plasma to the hepatocytes. Also, certain drugs, such as rifampin, probenecid, and flavaspidic acid, and cholecystographic contrast media can compete with unconjugated bilirubin for hepatic uptake, leading to an increase in its serum level. When liver perfusion is poor, as may occur in heart failure and shock, bilirubin delivery to the liver is slowed, whereas in portal hypertension, in which there are extensive portosystemic collaterals, unconjugated bilirubin, drugs, and other compounds may be diverted away from the liver at the 'first pass,' into the systemic circulation. In both cases, reduced or delayed hepatic uptake contributes further to unconjugated hyperbilirubinemia. In parenchymal liver injury, any reduction in availability of cytosolic binding sites due to reduced cytosolic protein concentrations or increased binding by other compounds could theoretically increase reflux of unconjugated bilirubin into plasma following hepatocyte uptake, but this has not been defined clinically.

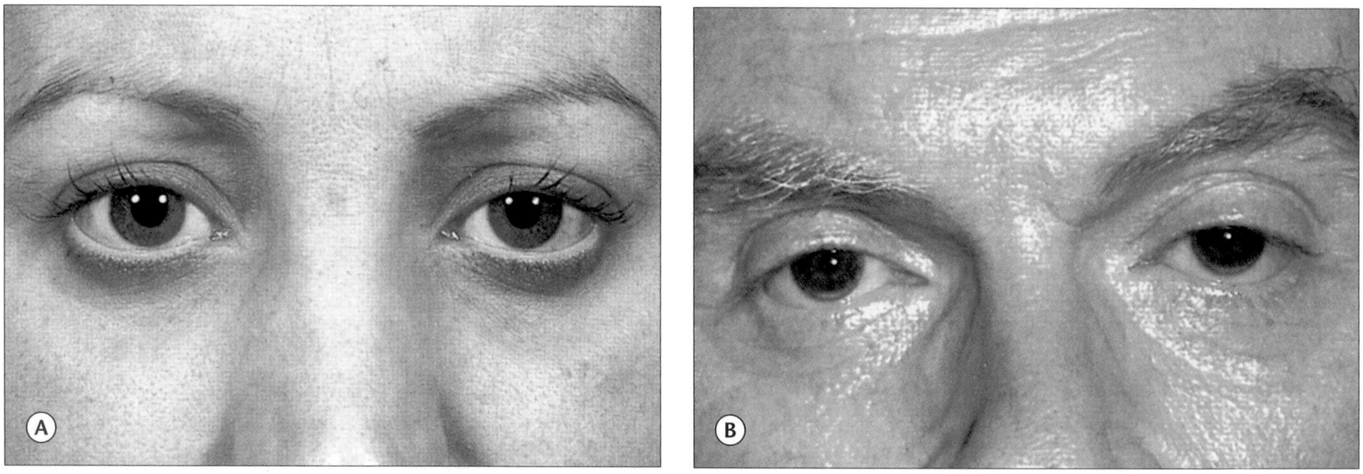

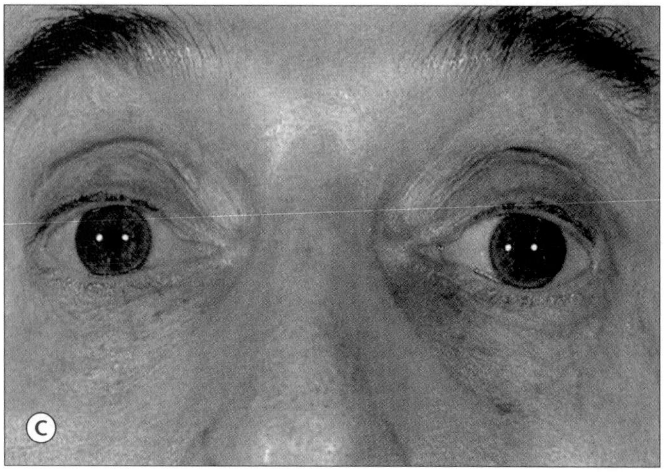

Fig. 18.3 Three faces of jaundice. (A) Lemon-yellow jaundice of hemolytic anemia. (B) Orange-yellow jaundice of hepatitis. (C) Green-yellow jaundice of cholestasis, showing skin hyperpigmentation. Reproduced with permission from Sherlock S, Summerfield JA. A colour atlas of liver disease. London: Wolfe Medical Publications; 1979.

(d) The discovery of defective bilirubin conjugation due to a variety of hereditary and acquired anomalies of the unique UGT catalyst of bilirubin conjugation, UGT1A1, demonstrates the value of elucidating the molecular basis of bilirubin physiology.[13] The commonest hereditary anomaly of UGT1A1, the variant allele UGT1A1*28, underlies a benign autosomal recessive partial defect of bilirubin conjugation known as Gilbert's syndrome, which affects up to 10% of Western populations and, in a subset of individuals, may be associated with reduced red cell survival and/or impaired hepatocyte uptake of bilirubin. In Gilbert's syndrome, the only clinical manifestation is mild unconjugated hyperbilirubinemia (serum bilirubin level 5mg/dL), which can be exacerbated by calorie restriction or an intercurrent illness that often prompts recognition of the syndrome. Some individuals with Gilbert's syndrome may be susceptible to the adverse effects of medications that are metabolized by bilirubin UGT, such as the semisynthetic cytotoxic alkaloid irinotecan, the active metabolite of which (SN-38) can cause severe diarrhea and neutropenia if it is not glucuronidated.[14]

In Gilbert's syndrome, the genetic defect that results in 80% loss of bilirubin UGT activity is the addition of a seventh TA dinucleotide to the TATA box of the gene promoter, which lies just upstream of the first exon. In contrast, in the severe familial unconjugated hyperbilirubinemia known as the Crigler-Najjar syndrome, bilirubin UGT activity is completely abolished in the lethal type I variant, or reduced to less than 10% (albeit, still phenobarbitone-inducible) in the type II variant, which are both due to a variety of defects in UGT1A1 exons. These exon errors result in premature stop codons or single amino acid substitutions (type 1), or are due to point mutations that substitute single amino acids (type II). Immaturity of genetically normal bilirubin UGT is common in neonates, causing so-called physiologic jaundice that may be exacerbated by hemolysis due to ABO and Rhesus incompatibility. In premature infants especially, serum unconjugated bilirubin levels can rise sufficiently high (above 20mg/dL) to cause kernicterus in some cases. Exposure of the affected infant to ultraviolet light produces unstable water-soluble photoisomerization of unconjugated bilirubin, which lasts long enough to permit biliary excretion and lower serum bilirubin to safe levels. Finally, although bilirubin UGT activity is not commonly impaired in parenchymal liver disease sufficiently to aggravate jaundice, the enzyme can be inhibited by a factor present in maternal milk, which causes so-called breast milk jaundice, and by drugs. Indinavir, a viral protease inhibitor that is used to treat HIV-infected patients, often causes unconjugated hyperbilirubinemia that results in part from bilirubin UGT inhibition and partly from hemolysis.

(e) Cholestatic liver disease represents a very large group of overlapping disorders in adults and children in which the common theme is failure or impairment of bile secretion. For many of these disorders, particularly those that are hereditary diseases of childhood, precise molecular abnormalities of the bile secretory transport apparatus (Fig. 18.4) have been identified,[4] some of which are represented in adults too. In adults, however, most cases of cholestasis are acquired, of which some may be due to inhibition of bile secretion without overt liver injury. Even in the more common acquired forms of cholestasis, in which microscopic or macroscopic lesions of the biliary tree are found, secondary changes can be identified in the molecular biliary secretory apparatus that contribute to the cholestatic syndrome.[12] Of course, cholestasis can occur in any kind of liver disease, for which the secondary molecular defects have yet to be identified. These discoveries provide ample justification, if any were needed, for research that defines canalicular transport at the molecular level, as summarized in Figure 18.4. The rest of this section will therefore focus on cholestatic disorders in which the pathophysiology has been addressed at the molecular level.

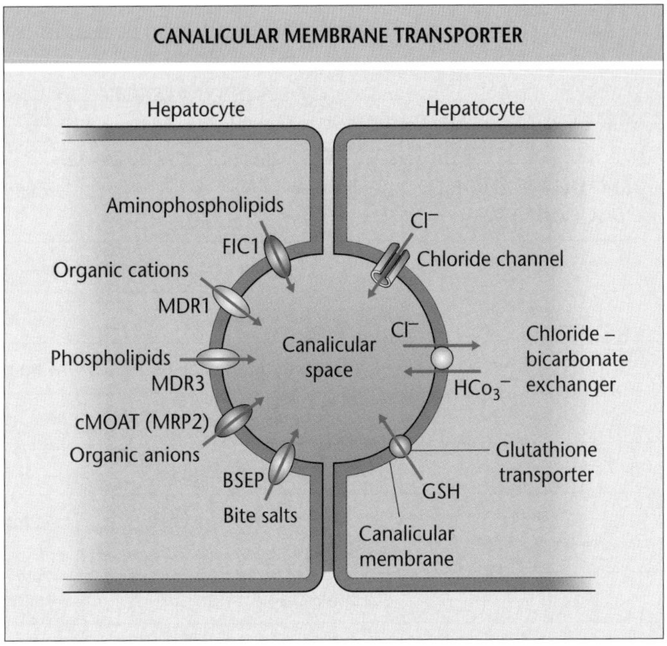

Fig. 18.4 Canalicular membrane transporters. A canaliculus between two neighboring hepatocytes is represented. The canalicular membranes contain several ATP-dependent export pumps: the multidrug resistance-1 P-glycoprotein (MDR1) that transports organic cations into bile; the phospholipid transporter multidrug resistance-3 P-glycoprotein (MDR3); the canalicular multispecific organic anion transporter (cMOAT), which is also termed the multidrug resistance-associated protein 2 (MRP2); and the canalicular bile salt export pump (BSEP), which is also known as the 'sister of P-glycoprotein' (SPGP). The canalicular membrane also contains ATP-dependent transport systems for chloride extrusion into bile, chloride–bicarbonate exchange, glutathione (GSH) transport, and the product of the *FIC1* (familial intrahepatic cholestasis type 1) gene, which has been redesignated *ATP8B1*, a P-type ATPase that probably transports aminophospholipids.

Hereditary, familial, and related cholestatic syndromes

Bile formation and the transport of solutes into bile are mediated by an array of channels, exchangers, and transporters that are embedded in the canalicular membrane (Fig. 18.4). Genetic defects have been reported that are responsible for several rare homozygous recessive disorders of infancy, originally collected under the rubric of progressive familial intrahepatic cholestasis (PFIC). PFIC can now be subdivided according to the mutation of genes that encode for specific canalicular transporters and their corresponding phenotypic expression. These syndromes are described in greater detail in Chapter 99. PFIC-1 was previously recognized as Byler's disease and is due to a mutation in an aminophospholipid transporter that results in progressive cholestasis, malabsorption, and pancreatitis. This genetic

CAUSES AND DIFFERENTIAL DIAGNOSIS		
CAUSES OF CHOLESTASIS		
	Adults	**Children**
OBSTRUCTIVE AND BILE DUCT DISEASES	Gallstones	Biliary atresia
	Cancer of pancreas or bile ducts	Inspissated bile or mucous plug
	Primary biliary cirrhosis	Gallstones or sludge
	Primary sclerosing cholangitis	Choledochal cysts
	Biliary stricture	Bile duct paucity syndromes
	Ischemic bile duct injury	Cystic fibrosis
	Acute or chronic transplant rejection	As for adults
	Graft-versus-host disease	As for adults
	Vanishing bile duct syndromes	Alagille syndrome
NONOBSTRUCTIVE		
Infections	Viral hepatitides, herpes family and other viral infections, sepsis, bacteremia, AIDS, etc.	As for adults
Toxic	Drugs, total parenteral nutrition	As for adults
Metabolic	Wilson disease	Alpha$_1$-antitrypsin deficiency
		Galactosemia, tyrosinemia, fatty acid oxidation defects
Infiltration and storage	Amyloidosis	Glycogen, lipids, peroxisomal disorders, histiocytosis X
	Metastatic cancer	
Canalicular transport	Cholestasis of pregnancy	
	Dubin-Johnson syndrome	As for adults
	Benign recurrent intrahepatic cholestasis (BRIC)	Progressive familial intrahepatic cholestasis (PFIC)
		Bile acid biosynthesis defects
		North American Indian cholestasis
		Norwegian cholestasis (Aagenaes syndrome)
Miscellaneous	Rotor syndrome, shock, hypoperfusion, hypoxemia, hepatic sickle cell crisis	As for adults
	Hodgkin disease	
	Paraneoplastic syndromes	

Modified from Li MK, Crawford JM. The pathology of cholestasis. Semin Liver Dis 2004; 24:1–39.

defect is thought to be related to the rare syndrome in adults of benign recurrent intrahepatic cholestasis. A defect in the bile salt export pump, BSEP (also known as the 'sister of P-glycoprotein;' SPGP), is responsible for PFIC-2 (Byler's syndrome), which causes jaundice in infancy associated with a nonspecific giant cell hepatitis. Mutations of the *MDR3* gene abolish phospholipid secretion into bile and this leads to liver damage with extensive bile ductular proliferation, pruritus, and cirrhosis (PFIC-3) in childhood. The same defect may be related to intrahepatic cholestasis of pregnancy. Mutation of the canalicular organic anion transporter, cMOAT (also known as the multidrug resistance-associated protein 2; MRP-2) is responsible for the benign conjugated hyperbilirubinemia known as Dubin-Johnson syndrome. The defect responsible for Rotor syndrome, a conjugated hyperbilirubinemia that is benign and clinically somewhat similar to Dubin-Johnson syndrome, appears not to be a biliary transport anomaly but a fault in intrahepatic storage of conjugated organic anions that reflux into plasma. Finally, the syndromic form of familial paucity of intrahepatic bile ducts, known as Alagille syndrome or arteriohepatic dysplasia, is not due to a primary canalicular transport abnormality but rather is related to an autosomal dominant mutation of the *Jagged 1* gene, which encodes a ligand of Notch 1, one of four members of a family of transmembrane receptor proteins.

Extrahepatic causes of cholestasis

Factors originating outside the hepatobiliary system can cause cholestasis, sometimes without causing inflammation, injury, or infiltration in the liver and biliary system. However, hepatic changes that are secondary to cholestasis itself may be visible histologically. Bile retention is seen in hepatocytes, bile canaliculi, and other parenchymal elements that represent the pathologist's view of cholestasis. In addition, a feathery rarified appearance is imparted to the hepatocyte cytoplasm that is termed pseudoxanthomatous change because it simulates lipid droplets, or is referred to as *cholestasis*, which implies that liver cell injury is due to the toxic effect of retained bile salts. Pure or bland cholestasis is also the histologic picture seen in heart failure, sickle cell disease, functional bile flow impairment after liver transplantation, and in the early stage of some of the hereditary canalicular transport defects. Several drugs can inhibit canalicular transporters to cause jaundice.[15] Estrogens and androgens cause cholestasis, the former via a combination of a dose-related effect and genetic susceptibility. C_{17}-alkylated anabolic steroids, ciclosporin, and synthetic progestogens cause dose-related cholestasis. Rarer associations occur with some antimicrobials and nonsteroidal anti-inflammatory drugs. Cholestasis of pregnancy, which has some connection with aberrant canalicular *MDR3* expression, appears to be related to circulating estrogen levels in genetically susceptible individuals, a few of whom also experience cholestasis when treated with oral contraceptive steroids. These conditions contrast with most drug-induced cholestatic jaundice, which is due to cholestatic hepatitis or cholangiolitis.

Sepsis, septic shock, and the hemodynamic, metabolic, and immune alterations that occur during recovery from major trauma have been characterized as the 'systemic inflammatory response syndrome' (SIRS), which is a potent cause of cholestasis. The mechanism of cholestasis of sepsis is complex,[16] involving many inflammatory cell types in the sinusoids and portal tracts, and the hepatocytes, with impairment of bile formation by endotoxin-mediated tumor necrosis factor alpha (TNFα) and proinflammatory cytokines. In sepsis, there is downregulation of transporters in both the sinusoidal and canalicular plasma membranes that is mediated in part via corresponding changes in gene expression. Cholestasis of sepsis is seen with a variety of microorganisms, not only *Escherichia coli* but also *Staphylococcus* and other Gram-positive organisms. The primary site of infection may be intra-abdominal, but the infection can also be pneumonia, endocarditis, pyelonephritis, and abscesses. In the preantibiotic era, right lower lobe pneumonia associated with cholestasis of sepsis could mimic acute cholangitis because of the triad of right upper abdominal pain (that was actually pleurisy), fever, and jaundice.

Secondary changes in hepatocyte transport in acquired cholestatic liver disease

The tools of cellular and molecular biology that have been used to elucidate the mechanism of hepatic transport and bile formation over the past 20 years have recently been applied to determine changes that take place in the activity and cellular distribution of transporters in acquired cholestatic disorders.[4,12] For the most part, animal models of cholestasis have been used for these studies. Animal models of cholestasis have included bile duct ligation and estrogen/ethinylestradiol and endotoxin administration.[4,12,17] In general, the pattern of response to cholestasis from any cause is a tendency to protect hepatocytes from the accumulation of toxic compounds, notably bile salts. Thus, there is downregulation of the normal sinusoidal membrane transporters by which bile salts and other organic anions enter hepatocytes from sinusoidal blood. At the same time, bile salt export pumps continue to be expressed and, in some cases, upregulated at the canalicular pole. A few transporters are downregulated. Upregulation of the expression of exporters on the sinusoidal membrane may provide a compensatory efflux pump for hepatocytes that cannot export into the canalicular space. It remains to be seen whether adaptive responses of bile salt transport on cholangiocytes, in the kidney and the intestine, may help rid the body of potentially toxic compounds that the liver can no longer expel.

DIAGNOSIS OF THE CAUSE OF JAUNDICE

All the usual modalities of clinical investigation are used to diagnose the cause of jaundice, including standard and special laboratory blood tests, some form of hepatobiliary imaging, and, frequently, liver biopsy. Nonetheless, the importance of acquiring an exhaustive clinical history and of performing a careful and thorough physical examination, cannot be overemphasized.

History

The age and sex of the patient should be taken into account because of the relationship between these variables and different causes of jaundice, especially cholestasis. The duration of jaundice, the patient's age at onset (especially in childhood), and a persistent or relapsing nature all relate to different causes. If jaundice is episodic or intermittent, its periodicity should be noted and contemporary events should be ascertained, such as pain (and all the usual associated features), intercurrent illness, all medication use (both current and over the past 6 months), fever, and other co-morbid events, such as pregnancy, heart failure, anemia, episodes of hypotension or hypoxemia, recent or distant surgery (especially abdominal), abdominal injury, blood transfusions, intentional or unintentional weight loss, and injury with hematoma formation. Alcohol use should be quantified and psychosocial evidence sought for alcohol and/or other substance dependency. The family history should seek liver disease and jaundice in close relatives, with questions about connective tissue disorders and other autoimmune processes, as well as any history of unusual anemia.

Physical examination

A detailed discussion of the physical signs of liver disease can be found in Chapter 19. In brief, jaundice should be confirmed in good light by careful examination of the whole sclera of the eyes, the mucous membranes (especially the frenulum), and the skin, including the palms of the hands and soles of the feet. Dermovascular signs of chronic liver disease, namely spider nevi, palmar erythema, 'paper money' skin, petechiae or ecchymoses, finger clubbing, and abdominal wall veins, should be sought. Signs of heart failure and other evidence and causes of raised systemic venous pressure and hypoxemia must be checked. The characteristic facies of Alagille syndrome and its other signs should be looked for in children and young adults. Obviously, the size of the liver, presence of splenomegaly, ascites, other abdominal masses, lymphadenopathy, and peripheral edema should be noted, in addition to the patient's level of consciousness, cognitive function, and asterixis, or other neuromuscular and neurologic abnormalities.

Laboratory tests

These should include a full hemogram including red cell indices, red cell morphology (especially to look for causes of hemolytic anemia, such as spherocytosis, sickling, and spur cells), white cell count and differential (including eosinophils), and platelet count. The hepatic panel should include both aspartate (AST) and alanine (ALT) aminotransferases, alkaline phosphatase, both total and direct bilirubin, total protein, and albumin. Gamma-glutamyltransferase is occasionally useful in identifying a liver origin for raised alkaline phosphatase levels, and also helps to distinguish between the different forms of PFIC. In addition to blood urea nitrogen, creatinine, and electrolytes, serum urate measurement may be helpful. Serum protein electrophoresis can give clues to a generalized hepatic inflammatory state, autoimmune disease, paraproteinemia, alpha$_1$-antitrypsin deficiency, and immunoglobulin deficiency. Viral hepatitis serology should include testing for both infection and immunity. More specialized hematologic testing may be needed to look for specific hemolytic syndromes, as well as causes of ineffective erythropoiesis. Testing for specific causes of liver disease is guided by the history and physical examination, and the results of standard liver tests.

Hepatobiliary imaging

This usually includes some form of cross-sectional scan to look for evidence of biliary dilatation and its cause, evidence of other biliary diseases, liver size, contour, liver substance, and signs of portal hypertension. The choice between ultrasonography, computed tomography, magnetic resonance imaging, and positron emission tomography is considered elsewhere in this book. Similarly, direct biliary imaging by endoscopic retrograde cholangiopancreatography or percutaneous transhepatic cholangiography is covered elsewhere.

Liver biopsy

Liver biopsy is not usually necessary in acute jaundice but is used to make the diagnosis of chronic hepatitis or cirrhosis, to find evidence for and possible causes of prolonged drug reactions, and to distinguish among various cholestatic syndromes, especially those of bile duct loss, infiltration and storage disorders.

SOURCES OF INFORMATION FOR PATIENTS AND DOCTORS

http://www.patient.co.uk/showdoc/900/

REFERENCES

1. Reuben A. By indirections find directions out. Hepatology 2002; 35:1287–1290.
2. Murchison C. Spurious jaundice. Lecture IX. Jaundice. In: Clinical lectures and disease of the liver. Jaundice and abdominal dropsy, including the Croonian Lectures on functional derangements of the liver delivered at the Royal College of Physicians in 1874. 2nd edn. London: Longmans, Green; 1877:310–313.
3. Reuben A. Hy's law. Hepatology 2004; 39: 574–578.
4. Trauner M, Meier PJ, Boyer JL. Molecular pathogenesis of cholestasis. N Engl J Med 1998; 339:1217–1227.
5. Hutchins GF, Gollan JL. Recent developments in the pathophysiology of cholestasis. Clin Liver Dis 2004; 8:1–26.
6. Desmet VJ. Vanishing bile duct syndromes in drug-induced liver disease. J Hepatol 1997; 20(Suppl 1):31–35.
7. Franson TR, Hierholzer WJ Jr, LaBrecque DR. Frequency and characteristics of hyperbilirubinemia associated with bacteremia. Rev Infect Dis 1985; 7:1–9.
8. Reisman Y, Gips CH, Lavelle SM, Wilson JH. Clinical presentation of (subclinical) jaundice—the Euricterus product in the Netherlands. United Dutch Hospitals and Euricterus Project Management Group. Hepatogastroenterology 1996; 43:1190–1195.
9. Baranano DE, Rao M, Ferris CD, Snyder SH. Bilirubin reductase: a major physiologic cytoprotectant. Proc Natl Acad Sci USA 2002; 99:16093–16098.
10. Cui Y, König J, Leier I, Buchholz U, Keppler D. Hepatic uptake of bilirubin and its conjugates by the human organic anion transporter SLC21A6. J Biol Chem 2001; 276:9626–9630.
11. Wang P, Kim RB, Chowdhury JR, Wolkoff AW. The human organic anion transporter protein SLC21A6 is not sufficient for bilirubin transport. J Biol Chem 2003; 278:20695–20699.
12. Jansen PLM, Roskams T. Why are patients with liver disease jaundiced? ATP-binding cassette transporter expression in human liver disease. J Hepatol 2001; 35:811–813.
13. Bogma PJ. Inherited disorders of bilirubin metabolism. J Hepatol 2003; 38:107–117.
14. Innocenti F, Undevia SD, Tyer L et al. Genetic variants in the *UDP-glucuronosyltransferase1A1* gene predict the risk of severe neutropenia of irinotecan. J Clin Oncol 2004; 22:1382–1388.
15. Bohan A, Boyer JL. Mechanism of hepatic transport of drugs; implications of cholestatic drug reactions. Semin Liver Dis 2002; 22: 123–136.
16. Moseley RH. Sepsis and cholestasis. Clin Liver Dis 2004; 8:83–94.
17. Trauner M, Boyer JL. Bile salt transporters: molecular characterization, function and regulation. Physiol Rev 2003; 83:633–671.

Chapter 19

Spotting and dealing with signs of chronic liver disease: a guided tour

Adrian Reuben

INTRODUCTION

Clinical hepatology is a treasure trove of physical signs, which, though not necessarily pathognomonic, can indicate the presence of liver disease, gauge its severity and, together with the history, give insight into its cause. The classical armamentarium of inspection, percussion, palpation, auscultation and, even olfaction, is put to good use in the evaluation of the liver patient and, together with the findings of a comprehensive history and results of preliminary blood tests, can provide a rational basis for choosing laboratory, imaging, and invasive tests for patient investigation.

A reasonable scheme for classifying physical signs would be to catalog them by organ system, however, a more practical approach is to categorize signs by their bodily location during the conduct of the physical examination, starting with an overall assessment of the patient, followed by specific examinations of the face, head and neck, chest, and so forth.

GENERAL APPEARANCE

For the patient who is lethargic, jaundiced, gaunt and edematous, with prominent spider nevi and an abdomen grossly distended with ascites, a single glance confirms the presence of liver disease and judges its severity. In general, however, one begins by noting if the patient looks well or ill, is alert or drowsy, and well nurtured or not. Fever may occur in chronic hepatitis and/or cirrhosis (especially alcoholic), but its presence should always prompt a search for infection. **The nutritional state**, which can give clues to the nature and severity of liver disease and its outcome,[1] is as well appraised using clinical judgment as it is using sophisticated anthropometric and laboratory measurements. Most useful is the so-called Global Subjective Assessment[1] that includes components of history – weight change, appetite, satiety, taste, dietary intake, gastrointestinal symptoms, energy and activity levels; physical appearance – muscle wasting, fat stores, ascites, and edema; and a rating of the degree of nurture that ranges from severely malnourished to well nourished. **Obesity**, which is quantified by calculating the body mass index from the dry weight and height (weight/height^2 in kg/m^2), may be associated with nonalcoholic fatty liver disease. Protein-calorie malnutrition can be masked by obesity, and both adversely impact survival from liver disease and liver transplantation.[1,2]

REGIONAL PHYSICAL SIGNS

Face, head, and neck

Face: The patient's face is a rich site for physical signs. Muscle loss in advanced cirrhosis or cancer is evident as temporal wasting and sunken cheeks; occasionally, the characteristic facies of a **childhood storage disorder**, or the widely set eyes, flat forehead, and small pointed chin of **Alagille syndrome** give a clue to the diagnosis. **Jaundice** is seen first in the sclerae (see Fig. 18.3) and later in the skin and mucous membranes, especially beneath the tongue; hyperpigmentation of the skin due to melanin deposition complicates longstanding cholestasis (see Fig. 18.3). In prolonged cholestasis, lipids are deposited in the skin as creamy-yellow excrescences called **xanthelasmas** when they occur around the eyes and xanthomas when they are elsewhere (Fig. 19.1), usually in areas that are exposed or subject to trauma, such as the ears, elbows, knees, in creases on the palms of the hands, and over tendons. **Petechiae** and **ecchymoses** localize to sites of trauma and where subcutaneous tissues are sparse in patients with thrombocytopenia, but periorbital bruising suggests amyloidosis.

Telangiectasias are common in liver cell failure, particularly spider angiomas or spider nevi[3] (Fig. 19.2); infrequently there are mat-shaped telangiectasias, white spots, and fine thread-like vessels in the skin that are reminiscent of the silk threads in paper US dollar bills (**paper money skin**)(Fig. 19.3A). Spider nevi, which are the surface manifestation of enlarged coiled skin arterioles, occur predominantly on the face, neck, shoulders, and chest, with fewer on the arms, hands and abdomen, rarely on the legs, but sometimes even on mucous membranes. As the arteriole reaches the surface and numerous branches radiate to form the spider's 'legs,' its terminus is seen as a central red spot that pulsates under light pressure; heavy pressure blanches the whole spider. Spider nevi occur in pregnancy, estrogen treatment, and in some normal individuals, and must be distinguished from telangiectasias seen in sun-exposed areas and in hereditary hemorrhagic telangiectasia (Osler-Weber-Rendu syndrome). Spider nevi are especially common in alcoholic liver disease and are associated with palmar erythema, digital clubbing, esophageal varices, and a poor outcome of cirrhosis.[3] Spider number greater than 20, size greater than 15 mm and an atypical location, correlate with an increased risk of esophageal variceal rupture.[3]

Parotid gland enlargement is typical of alcoholism (Fig. 19.3B), but though flushing in rosacea (Fig. 19.4) is exacerbated by alcohol, it is unclear if this skin disease per se or its rhinophyma complication are alcohol induced. The skin of the face may be **bronzed** in patients with hemochromatosis, tight and thickened in scleroderma (an association of primary biliary cirrhosis), or marked with acne in alcohol abuse, autoimmune hepatitis and steroid treatment.

Feminization: The **soft skin, fine hair** and **sparse beard** of feminization, predominantly in men with alcoholic cirrhosis, results from low androgen relative to estrogen activity. Exacerbation of acne and psoriasis, the presence of various dermati-

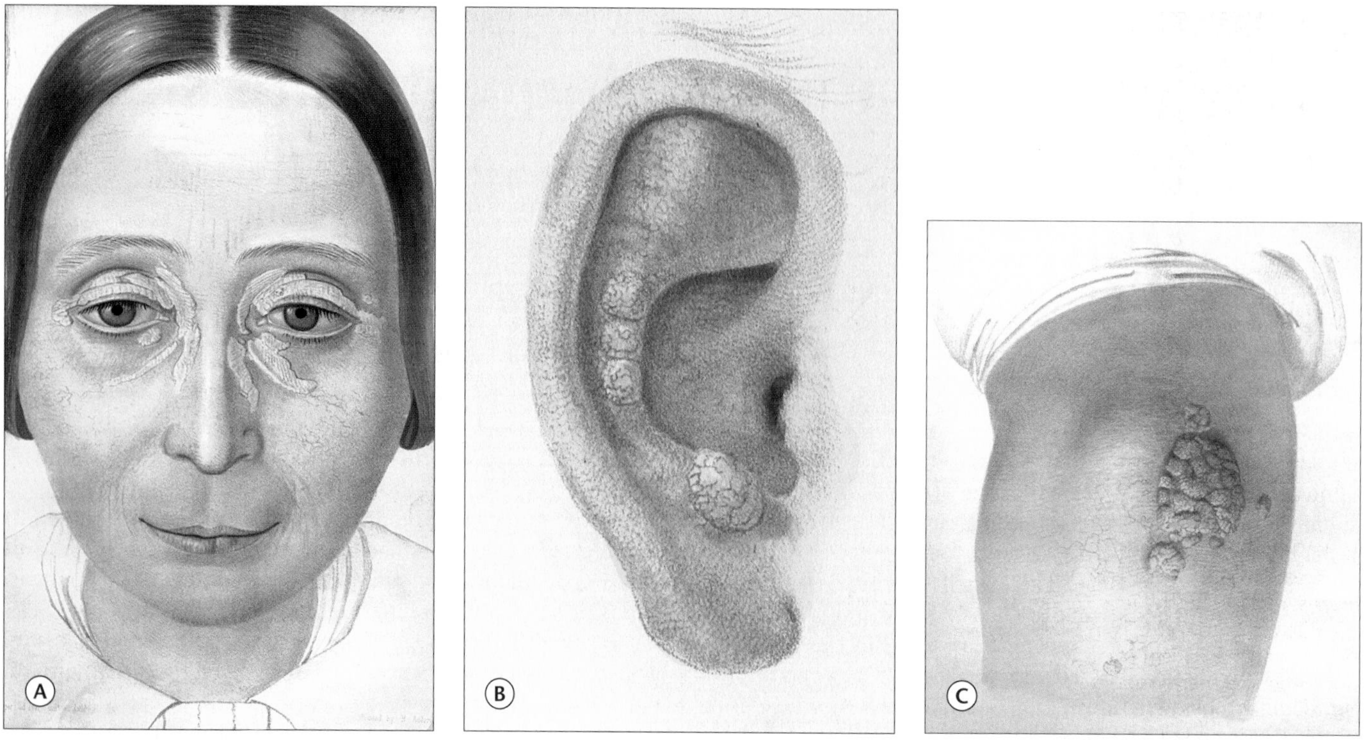

Fig. 19.1 Xanthelasmas and xanthomas. Xanthelasmas around the eyes (A), and xanthomas on the ear (B) and knee (C) in chronic cholestasis. (Reproduced from the color plates of J. L. Tupper, in: Addison T, Gull W. On a certain affection of the skin, Vitiligoidea – α plana, β tuberosa. With remarks and plates. Guys Hosp Rep 1851; 7:265–276. Images courtesy of Information Services and Systems Department of GKT, Kings College London.

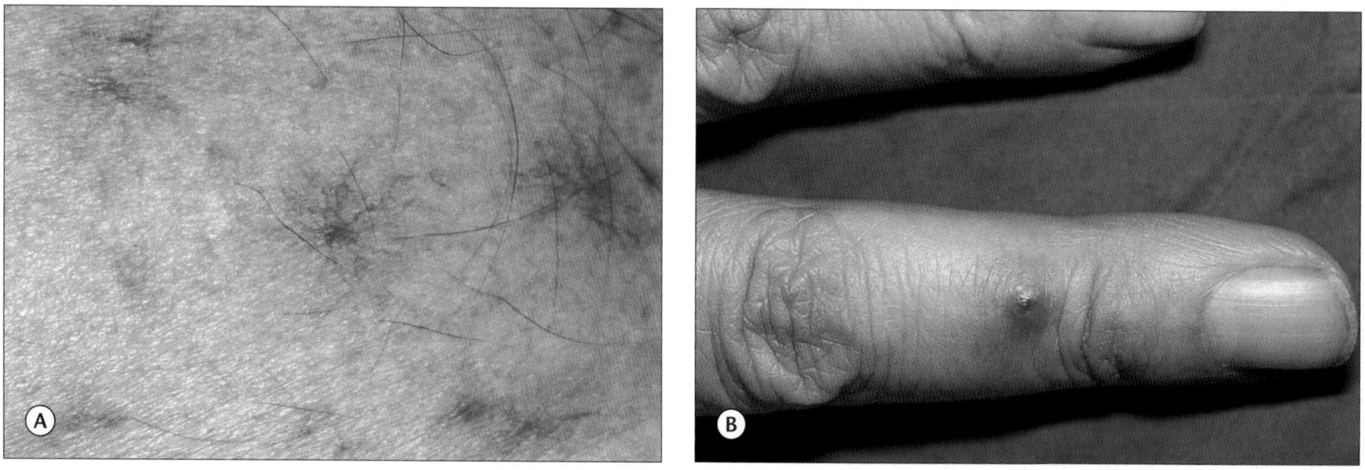

Fig. 19.2 Spider nevi. A. Truncal. **B.** On finger. Note the larger than average central feeding arteriole.

tides, or the characteristic skin fragility and blistering of porphyria cutanea tarda, should prompt an inquiry for alcohol misuse.[4]

Eyes: Aside from jaundice, the eyes may show other lesions in liver disease, such as the characteristic **Kayser-Fleischer rings** of Wilson's disease (see Chapter 91) that are seen as golden-brown or greenish pigment at the margin of the cornea near the limbus, from copper deposition on the inner surface of the cornea in Descemet's membrane. These rings, which are often complete, nearly always bilateral, and most intense and wide at the superior and inferior aspects of the cornea, constitute the single most important diagnostic sign of Wilson's disease and should be confirmed by slit-lamp examination. Kayser-Fleischer rings are seen occasionally in non-Wilsonian liver disease and sometimes in patients with prolonged cholestasis that leads to corneal pigmentation from bilirubin deposition. The eyes in Wilson's disease may show characteristic sunflower cataracts, whereas common cataracts may be seen in liver patients treated with steroids. The deformity of the anterior chamber of the eye known as posterior embryotoxon is characteristic of Alagille's syndrome, but this and other intraocular abnormalities in liver patients are generally signs for the ophthalmologist.

The **mouth** should be inspected for lesions that occur in systemic disorders, e.g., the **glossitis** and **angular stomatitis** that

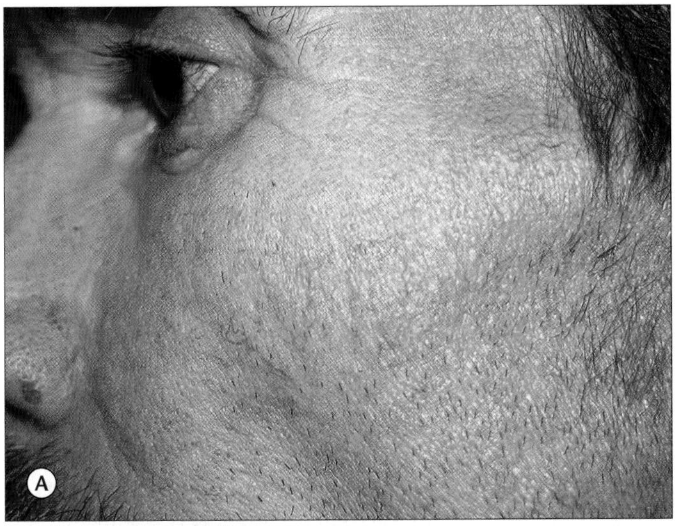

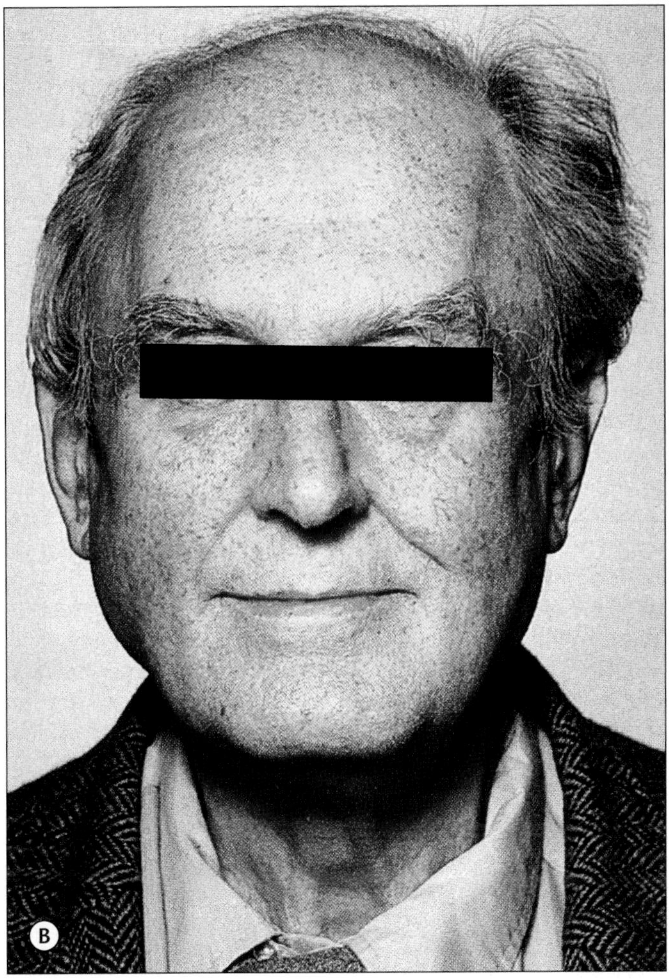

Fig. 19.3 Signs – face, head, and neck. A. Paper money skin. Fine thread-like superficial veins on the face of a patient with alcoholic cirrhosis, resembling the finely chopped red and blue silk threads embedded in US dollar bills. **B.** Parotid gland enlargement in an alcoholic patient. Patient also has paper money skin. Figure 19.2B reproduced with permission from Misiewicz JJ et al. A slide atlas of gastroenterology: Unit 18. Produced and published by Gower Medical Publishing Ltd, London UK for Glaxo, Research Triangle Park, Durham, North Carolina 27709. 1987.

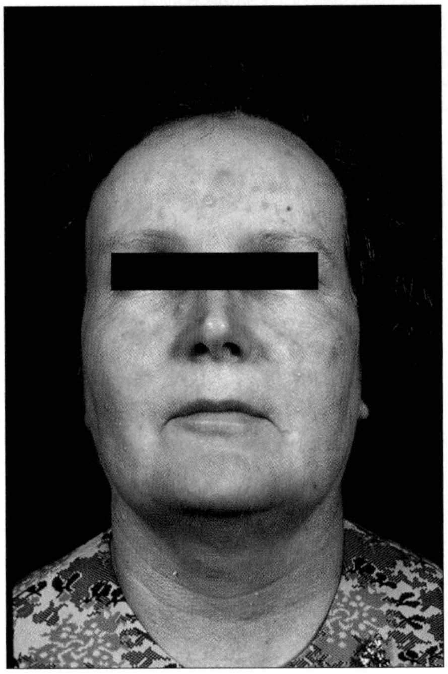

Fig. 19.4 Rosacea in a patient with alcoholic liver disease.

are common in vitamin B deficient alcoholics, telangiectasias that decorate the lips in Osler-Weber-Rendu syndrome, and lichen planus that may be associated with chronic hepatitis C infection and primary biliary cirrhosis. Also, the dental hygiene of the liver transplant candidate must be checked when screening for risks of perioperative infection. In children, prolonged cholestasis discolors the growing teeth (**chlorodontia**). Central **cyanosis**, recognized as a blue discoloration of the lips, tongue, and other mucous membranes, points to hypoxemia that may be due to hepatopulmonary syndrome or other lung disorders, some of which are causally associated with liver disease, e.g., cystic fibrosis and alpha$_1$-antitrypsin deficiency. Cyanosis may be inapparent, however, if the patient is anemic. Finally, once whiffed, the characteristic 'mousey' odor of the breath of patients with liver failure, the fetor hepaticus, is hard to forget.

Jugular veins: One cannot overstate the importance of looking for jugular venous pressure elevation, especially if it is exacerbated by deep inspiration, as its presence should make the examiner suspicious that a patient's ascites is due to constrictive pericarditis and not cirrhosis. Jugular venous pressure elevation may also be caused by fluid overload, tricuspid regurgitation, systolic or diastolic dysfunction, and pulmonary hypertension that is often a consequence of portal hypertension. These cardiac abnormalities can explain or aggravate hepatomegaly and adversely affect patient outcome and transplant candidacy. When eliciting the '**hepatojugular reflux**' **sign**, which relies on increasing venous return through the inferior vena cava, abdominal pressure should be applied anywhere but over a liver that is enlarged, congested, and tender in the patient who is likely to show a positive response.

Arms and hands

Characteristic albeit nonspecific signs of liver disease are seen in the hands, but examining the rest of the upper limbs is rewarding too. The arms should be inspected for the loss of **muscle bulk** of advanced cirrhosis, for excoriations and prurigo nodularis that indirectly measure the severity of a patient's pruritus, and for axillary hair loss in men that is further evidence of **feminization**. **Tattoos** and **needle marks** may indicate a lifestyle that is conducive to viral hepatitis acquisition. Hypotension, which is not usually thought of as a physical sign, is a predictor of reduced survival in cirrhosis,[5] and is common in patients with advanced liver disease because systemic arterial vasodilatation is a consequence of portal hypertension. Common too are warm hands and a bounding pulse, which are peripheral signs of the hyperdynamic circulation of advanced cirrhosis. Measurement of postural changes in pulse and blood pressure are important when evaluating a patient for reduced blood volume due to bleeding or fluid loss, since supine blood pressure may be normal in this setting. Reduced skin turgor may help in the diagnosis of fluid depletion too. **Petechiae** may appear on the arm following blood pressure measurement in patients with thrombocytopenia, platelet dysfunction, or capillary fragility if the cuff is held inflated between venous and arterial pressure for more than a few moments.

The arms and hands of chronic liver disease patients may show the same skin changes that affect the face and neck, especially lesions that are exacerbated by sunlight exposure. **Vitiligo** may accompany autoimmune liver diseases, e.g., primary biliary cirrhosis. The particular form of palmar erythema that localizes to the thenar and hypothenar eminences (Fig. 19.5A), which can also involve both palmar and dorsal surfaces of the distal phalanges, is typical of cirrhosis but it can also occur in rheumatoid arthritis, thyrotoxicosis, pregnancy, bronchogenic carcinoma, and some normal individuals. Similarly, the Hippocratic sign of **finger clubbing** (Fig. 19.5A and B) occurs not only in cirrhosis but also in heart disease (cyanotic congenital deformities, spontaneous bacterial endocarditis, and atrial myxoma), lung disease (pyogenic abscess, bronchiectasis, carcinoma, interstitial fibrosis, and mesothelioma), and inflammatory bowel disease (especially Crohn's disease). If hypoxemia complicates cirrhosis, clubbing may be noticeable but disappears with

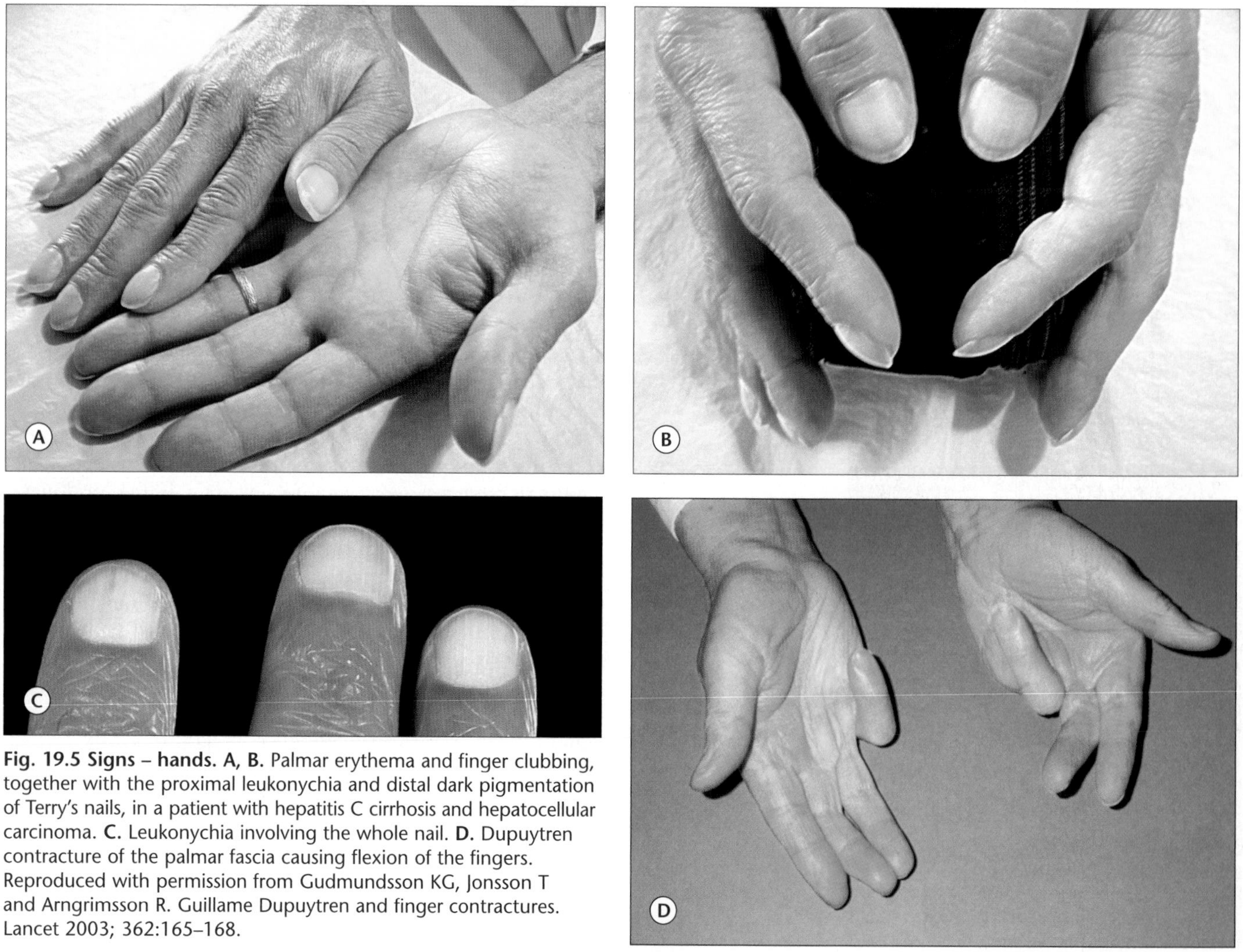

Fig. 19.5 Signs – hands. A, B. Palmar erythema and finger clubbing, together with the proximal leukonychia and distal dark pigmentation of Terry's nails, in a patient with hepatitis C cirrhosis and hepatocellular carcinoma. **C.** Leukonychia involving the whole nail. **D.** Dupuytren contracture of the palmar fascia causing flexion of the fingers. Reproduced with permission from Gudmundsson KG, Jonsson T and Arngrimsson R. Guillame Dupuytren and finger contractures. Lancet 2003; 362:165–168.

successful liver transplantation. When finger clubbing coincides with **palmar erythema** and **spider nevi** cirrhosis is virtually assured, yet it must be admitted that there is considerable interobserver variation and a lack of objective diagnostic criteria in the diagnosis of clubbing. Besides clubbing and hypertrophic osteoarthropathy, the hands may show other disfigurements.

The **nails** in cirrhosis may be thickened, ridged, brittle, flat, or even concave. Nail discoloration includes reddened lunulae in alcoholism (without cirrhosis), blue lunulae in Wilson's disease, and streaks of green that bear witness to prior cholestasis. Whitening (**leukonychia**), which occurs in hypoalbuminemia, cirrhosis, heart failure, renal failure, and diabetes, may involve the whole nail (Fig. 19.5C) or occur in bands only (**Muehrcke's lines**), or may be associated with distal reddening (**Terry's nails**) that is probably due to telangiectasias (Fig. 19.5A). A curious deformity of the hand and fingers described by Felix Platter in seventeenth century Basel was popularized by French surgeon Baron Guillaume Dupuytren in the nineteenth century, and was recognized by him as a fibrotic contracture of the palmar fascia that involves the digits, usually beginning with flexion of the ring and/or little finger (Fig. 19.5D). **Dupuytren contracture** occurs in both genders and all ethnic groups, but it is predominantly a disease of older men of northern European ancestry and, by repute, it originated with the Vikings.[6] Dupuytren contracture, which is a feature of alcoholism rather than liver disease as such, also complicates diabetes, seizure disorders, cigarette smoking, and probably vibration-induced hand injury, especially in genetically susceptible individuals. Finally, testing for the flapping irregular tremor of asterixis is usually done during examination of the hands.

Chest

Telangiectasias that occur in sunlight-exposed skin must be distinguished from spider nevi. **Extensive scratching** because of pruritus causes hyperpigmentation of the skin, whereas there is sparing of the unreachable central area of the back that remains pale in a characteristic 'butterfly' configuration (Fig. 19.6A). **Loss of muscle** may be conspicuous in the pectoral girdle and especially the back, where the vertebrae and bony outlines of the scapulae may be prominent (Fig. 19.6B).

Gynecomastia (Fig. 19.7), i.e., breast tissue enlargement, either bilateral or unilateral, is another feature of feminization, but it may also be caused by spironolactone therapy (in which the breasts are often tender) and can be a presenting sign of fibrolamellar carcinoma, possibly related to aromatase expression by the tumor. Gynecomastia can be mistaken for a variety of primary and metastatic breast lesions and should be investigated further by imaging or biopsy, if there is doubt.

The **heart** should be examined for signs of a hyperdynamic circulation and for pulmonary hypertension, both of which are complications of cirrhosis and portal hypertension. The **respiratory examination** may show a right-sided pleural effusion, usually but not invariably associated with ascites, i.e., a hepatic hydrothorax, but a left-sided effusion should arouse suspicion of infection, malignancy, trapped lung, or heart failure. Finally, the degree of inflation of the lungs and the positions and

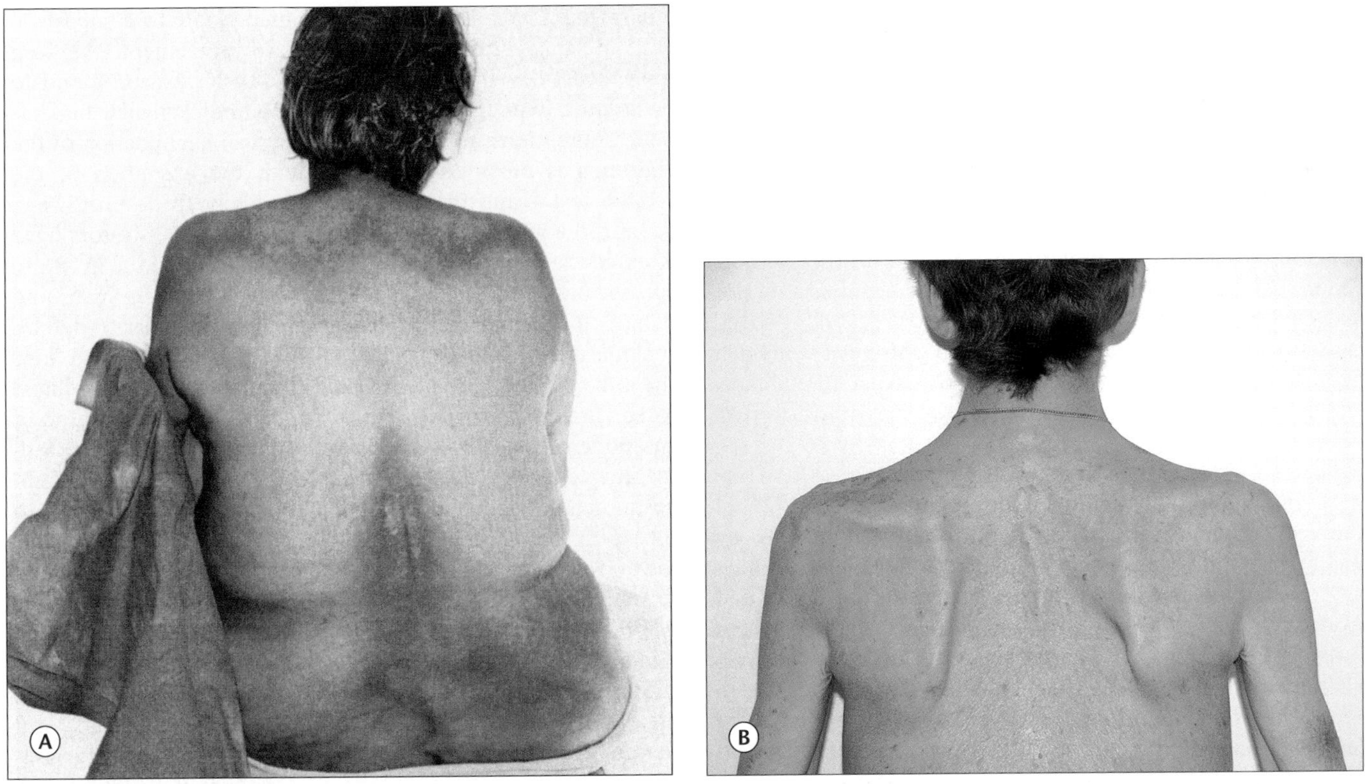

Fig. 19.6 Signs – back. A. The back of a patient with severe pruritus showing a pigmented peripheral region that has been repeatedly scratched, and a pale 'butterfly' area of skin that the patient could not reach with the fingernails. (Reproduced with permission from Reynolds TB. The 'butterfly' sign in patients with chronic jaundice and pruritus. Ann Int Med 1973; 78:595–596.) **B.** Prominent muscle wasting of the back in a patient with alcoholic cirrhosis, revealing the spines of vertebrae and the bony outlines of the scapulae. A very large spider nevus is also visible on the patient's right upper arm.

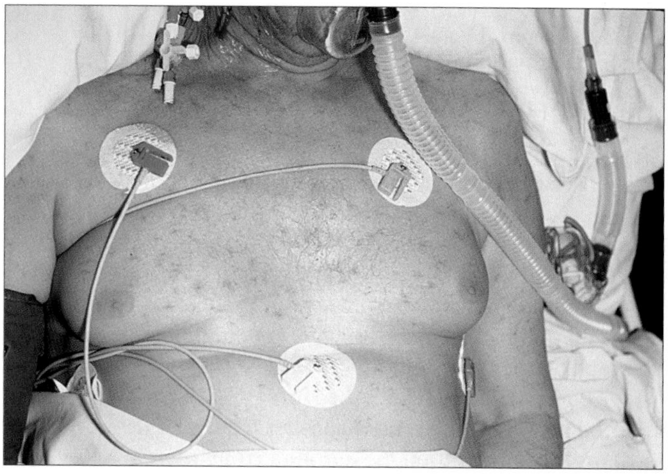

Fig. 19.7 Gynecomastia (with spider nevi restricted to upper trunk) in a male patient with alcoholic cirrhosis.

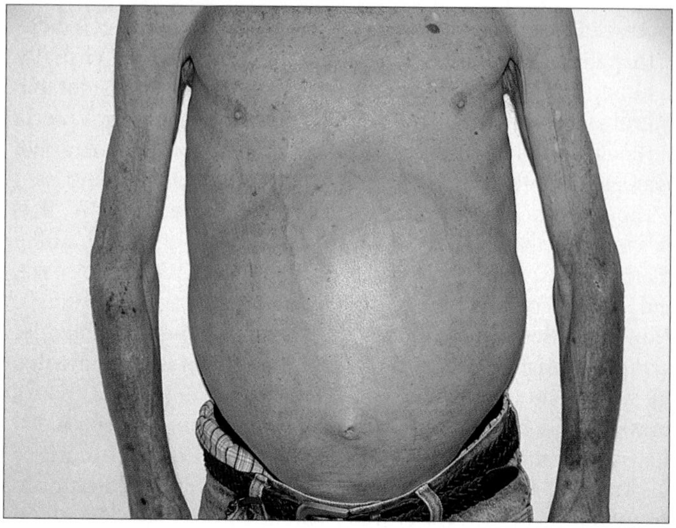

Fig. 19.8 Signs – abdomen. Distended abdomen with ascites and dilated superficial veins.

mobility of the hemidiaphragms, ascertained easily by percussion, help in the interpretation of abdominal findings, particularly distention and palpability of the liver.

Abdomen

Abdominal wall striae document new or prior distention, from obesity, ascites, pregnancy, or immense organomegaly, as may occur in polycystic disease. Spider nevi are infrequent on the abdomen, especially below the umbilicus, and are sometimes mistaken for cherry angiomas (Campbell de Morgan spots), those benign flat or slightly raised, bright red or purple circular angiokeratoses that appear with advancing years and do not blanch with pressure. **Dilated superficial abdominal wall veins** with cephalad blood flow are often seen in the upper abdomen in cirrhosis. These cutaneous veins carry blood from a recanalized umbilical vein or paraumbilical veins in portal hypertension, or bypass an obstructed inferior vena cava that is either compressed by an enlarged liver (usually the caudate lobe) or is constricted intrinsically or extrinsically by other causes, including thrombosis in association with the Budd-Chiari syndrome. Caudal flow in cutaneous abdominal veins signifies superior vena cava obstruction. However, it is rare to see a fully-fledged caput medusae, the radiating system of hepatofugal veins that emanate from the umbilicus, even if there is a patent umbilical vein in patients with cirrhosis and portal hypertension (Fig. 19.8).

Ascites is a hallmark of decompensation in cirrhosis, and one that is likely to progress with a poor prognosis.[5] Until 1–2 L of fluid collect, however, ascites is only detected reliably by imaging, i.e., ultrasonography, computed tomography, or magnetic resonance imaging. As ascites increases, the flanks and abdomen bulge (see Fig. 19.8) and fluid collects in the pelvis to form a U-shaped region of dullness to percussion in the abdomen when the patient is supine. That abdominal distention is due to free fluid in the peritoneal cavity is best corroborated by demonstrating 'shifting' of the dullness when the patient turns from one side to the other. Shifting dullness may also be found in the occasional patient with diarrhea or a large fat pannus. With gross ascites it is possible but scarcely necessary to elicit a 'fluid wave' in the supine patient, by tapping one flank and feeling the percussion ripple at the other, provided that vibration through the anterior abdominal wall is dampened by gentle hand pressure. Massive ascites causes umbilical herniation that can lead to bowel or omental incarceration, or rupture that occurs when the hernia sac is thin and the overlying skin is eroded, with its attendant morbidity and high mortality.[7]

Abdominal examination for the diagnosis of chronic liver disease, specifically for cirrhosis, has been scrutinized repeatedly and found wanting,[8] although the methodology to assess it was often insufficient. Clinical estimates of liver size, splenic enlargement, and ascites have been inadequate by comparison with imaging results. Between-observer agreement and, to a lesser extent, within-observer variability have been found to be at fault. Even the localization of the mid-clavicular line has been contentious. Yet, for all that, physical examination of the abdomen is of value – perhaps with the exception of the scratch test – and findings are more likely to be positive in advanced compared to early disease. Some investigators have stressed the value of percussion over palpation of the liver and spleen, but both are used together to assess liver span, and palpation best assesses liver consistency and nodularity, detects the pulsatile hepatomegaly of tricuspid regurgitation, and finds the enlarged left lobe of cirrhosis in the epigastrium. Dullness to percussion of Traube's space,[9] the crescent-shaped region of gastric resonance above the left costal margin, is an early finding in splenomegaly before the spleen is palpable. A right subcostal mass may be a distended gallbladder in malignant jaundice with distal biliary obstruction, a Reidel's lobe, or even the lower pole of an anteriorly placed right kidney. The abdominal examination includes the inguinal regions and the genitalia, where edema and ascites may collect, and where fluid and dilated veins in the inguinal canal in patients with portal hypertension can mimic an inguinal hernia. Auscultation of the abdomen may disclose the arterial bruit of a liver tumor or a venous hum from dilated veins in portal hypertension (Cruveilhier-Baumgarten syndrome). Finally, in patients with atypical abdominal pain, the examination is not complete unless the abdominal muscles are flexed to distinguish superficial from deep intra-abdominal tenderness, and the spine is interrogated for a cause of referred pain.

KEY PHYSICAL SIGNS IN CHRONIC LIVER DISEASE	
Signs	**Comments**
FACE, HEAD AND NECK	
Jaundice (icterus)	• First seen in sclerae, then in mucous membranes and skin • Distinguish from exogenous yellow pigment that does not color sclerae, e.g., carotene
Spider nevi (spider angiomas)	• Also seen on chest, back, and arms; very uncommon on abdomen and legs • Distinguish from other telangiectasias (e.g., solar telangiectasias and Osler-Weber-Rendu syndrome) and cherry angiomas • Also seen in pregnancy and estrogen therapy • Due to relative estrogen to androgen excess, caused by liver cell failure
Temporal wasting	• Part of generalized muscle loss in cirrhosis, due to impaired protein metabolism • Also affects the muscles of the back, arms, shoulders, and legs
Xanthelasmas	• Lipid deposits in periocular skin, secondary to hyperlipidemia of cholestasis • Associated with cutaneous lipid deposits (xanthomas) on areas exposed or subject to trauma • Also occurs in disorders of severe hyperlipidemia or dyslipidemia
Paper money skin	• Fine thread-like telangiectasias on face due to relative estrogen to androgen excess, caused by liver cell failure • Also occurs on chest
Feminization	• Soft skin and sparse beard • Associated with sparse hair in axillae and elsewhere, and with gynecomastia
Kayser-Fleischer rings	• Typical brown-green pigmentation of cornea in Wilson's disease; due to copper deposition in Descemet's membrane • Also occurs in cholestatic and occasionally non-cholestatic chronic liver disease
Sunflower cataracts	• Typical of Wilson's disease
Central cyanosis	• Indicates hypoxemia that may be due to hepatopulmonary syndrome or other cardiopulmonary disease
Elevated jugular venous pressure	• May indicate pulmonary hypertension due to cirrhosis, but can result from other cardiac dysfunction
HANDS AND ARMS	
Finger clubbing	• Especially likely in cirrhosis if patient is hypoxemic • Also seen in certain cardiac, respiratory, and bowel disorders • May be accompanied by hypertrophic osteoarthropathy
Nail discoloration	• White nails (leukonychia), also seen in diabetes, hypoalbuminemia, heart failure, and renal failure • White nail color may be uniform or show lines (Muehrcke's) or bands (Beau's), or distal dusky redness (Terry's nails) • Green streaks from previous cholestasis
Nail disfigurement	• Brittle, ridged, concave, or convex nails
Dupuytren contracture	• Thickening and nodularity of palmar fascia • Causes flexion deformities of digits, especially ring and little fingers • Occurs infrequently in feet • A feature of alcoholism rather than liver disease per se, also seen in diabetes, epilepsy, cigarette smoking, and vibration injury; genetic predisposition
CHEST AND BACK	
Muscle wasting	• Especially of shoulders, back, and upper arms
Gynecomastia	• May be bilateral or unilateral • Breasts tender with spironolactone use • Due to relative estrogen to androgen excess, caused by liver cell failure • Can occur with fibrolamellar carcinoma
Pleural effusion (hepatic hydrothorax)	• Derived from ascites that may or may not be apparent • Almost always right-sided
Cardiac signs of pulmonary hypertension	• Tricuspid regurgitation may follow
ABDOMEN	
Ascites	• Detectable clinically when more than 1–2 L fluid present • Confirmed by demonstrating shifting dullness • Diarrhea and fat pannus can give shifting dullness too
Dilated superficial abdominal wall veins	• Flow is cephalad or caudal in obstruction of inferior or superior vena cava, respectively • Caput medusae rarely seen • Associated with recanalization of umbilical vein or IVC compression
Abdominal wall striae	• Secondary to prior or current abdominal distention of any cause
Umbilical hernia	• Secondary to increased intra-abdominal pressure • Erosion and leakage creates medical emergency with high mortality
LEGS AND FEET	
Clubbing of toes, plantar erythema, plantar Dupuytren contracture	• All uncommon compared to finger clubbing, but carry same implications
Edema	• Check near Achilles tendon and sacrum for gravity-dependent edema during recumbency

Legs and feet

Plantar erythema, **clubbing of the toes**, and **plantar fascia contractures** (i.e., palmar fibromatosis or the lederhosen syndrome) are the infrequent pedal counterparts of respective signs in the hands, and have the same clinical significance. **Loss of muscle bulk** in the thighs may be less noticeable than in the arms and shoulders but, in contrast, **edema** is obviously much more common in the legs and feet than in the upper limbs because extravascular fluid accumulation is gravity dependent. There is no generally agreed grading scheme or scale for edema but, for purposes of description and comparison, it is suggested that the terms trace, mild, moderate, and severe be applied that take account of the depth, compressibility, and distribution of the edema in feet, legs, sacral region, and abdominal wall. When patients have been recumbent for more than 12h, it is important to press near the Achilles tendons and in the sacral region, otherwise edema that has gravitated there might be neglected. Other physical signs that are common in the legs and feet of patients with liver disease are **petechiae** due to thrombocytopenia, and the petechial rash, palpable purpura, and ulceration associated with **cryoglobulinemic vasculitis**, which afflicts those with chronic hepatitis C.

SOURCES OF INFORMATION FOR PATIENTS AND DOCTORS

http://www.patient.co.uk/showdoc/23068925/
http://patients.uptodate.com/topic.asp?file=livr_dis/4490

REFERENCES

1. Stephenson GR, Moretti EW, El-Moalem H, Clavien PA, Tuttle-Newhall JE. Malnutrition in liver transplant patients: preoperative subjective global assessment is predictive of outcome after liver transplantation. Transplantation 2001; 72:666–670.
2. Nair S, Verma S, Tuluvath PH. Obesity and its effect on survival in patients undergoing orthotopic liver transplantation in the United States. Hepatology 2002; 35:105–109.
3. Reuben A. Along came a spider. Hepatology 2002; 35:735–756.
4. Higgins EM, du Vivier AWP. Cutaneous disease and alcohol misuse. Br Med Bull 1994; 50:85–98.
5. Fernandez-Esparrach G, Sanchez-Fueyo A, Gines P et al. A prognostic model for predicting survival in cirrhosis with ascites. J Hepatol 2001; 34:46–52.
6. Flatt AE. The Vikings and Baron Dupuytren's disease. Baylor Uni Med Center Proc 2001; 14:378–384.
7. Maniatis AG, Hunt CM. Therapy for spontaneous umbilical hernia rupture. Am J Gastroenterol 1995; 90:310–312.
8. de Bruyn G, Graviss EA. A systematic review of the diagnostic accuracy of physical examination for the detection of cirrhosis. BMC Med Inform Decis Mak 2001; 1:6.
9. Castell DO, Frank BB. Abdominal examination: role of percussion and auscultation. Postgrad Med 1977; 62:131–134.

Chapter 20

Ascites

Andrés Cárdenas, Pere Ginès, and Vicente Arroyo

INTRODUCTION AND SYMPTOM DEFINITION

Ascites is the pathological accumulation of free fluid in the peritoneal cavity. The most common cause of ascites is portal hypertension secondary to cirrhosis, which accounts for over 80% of patients with ascites.[1] Malignancy, congestive heart failure, tuberculosis, and other causes are the etiology of ascites in approximately 20% of cases.[1] The development of ascites is a major complication of cirrhosis associated with a decreased quality of life, increased risk for infections, renal failure, and decreased survival. The development of ascites in cirrhosis is an important prognostic feature, as 50% of these patients will die in approximately 3–4 years.[2]

HOW COMMON IS IT?

The epidemiology of ascites is difficult to assess given its multiple causes. However, among patients with compensated cirrhosis nearly 50-60% of patients will develop ascites in the natural history of their disease.[3] Regarding chylous ascites, one large study reported an incidence of one in 20 000 admissions to a large university-based hospital over a 20-year period.[4] For other causes of ascites estimated figures of incidence and prevalence are lacking.

PATHOPHYSIOLOGY

The pathogenesis of ascites depends on the underlying cause. In cirrhosis, increased intrahepatic resistance leads to sinusoidal and portal hypertension that in turn leads to collateral vein formation with shunting of blood to the systemic circulation. As portal hypertension develops, splanchnic arterial vasodilation occurs due to the enhanced local production of vasodilators. Splanchnic vasodilation decreases effective arterial blood volume and causes a homeostatic activation of vasoconstrictor and anti-natriuretic factors as a compensatory response. This event leads to sodium retention, renal function abnormalities, and local splanchnic capillary pressure changes that are responsible for the accumulation of fluid in the abdominal cavity (Fig. 20.1).[5]

In **malignancy-associated ascites**, direct or metastatic involvement of the peritoneum by cancer leads to significant alterations in the permeability of the peritoneum or to obstruction of peritoneal lymphatics. Other patients develop ascites due to massive liver metastases or hepatocellular carcinoma causing portal hypertension or lymphatic obstruction.

Chylous ascites is a milky appearing peritoneal fluid that is rich in triglycerides and is due to the presence of thoracic or intestinal lymph in the abdominal cavity.[4] It develops when there is disruption of the lymphatic system, which occurs as a result of traumatic injury or obstruction (from benign or malignant causes).

Other forms: In tuberculous peritonitis, the formation of ascites is related to direct involvement of the peritoneum by mycobacteria causing a chronic inflammation with exudates.[6] The underlying pathogenesis of pancreatic ascites is related to the disruption of the pancreatic duct or leakage from a pseudocyst, which may occur in the setting of either acute or chronic pancreatitis.[7] Bile ascites typically occurs after biliary tract surgery and trauma to the abdomen; other rare causes include percutaneous liver biopsy, transhepatic cholangiography, and rupture of the gallbladder. Finally, in myxedema ascites, the pathogenesis of ascites formation seems to be related to an increased capillary permeability, impaired lymphatic drainage, and congestive heart failure due to low levels of circulating thyroid hormones.[8]

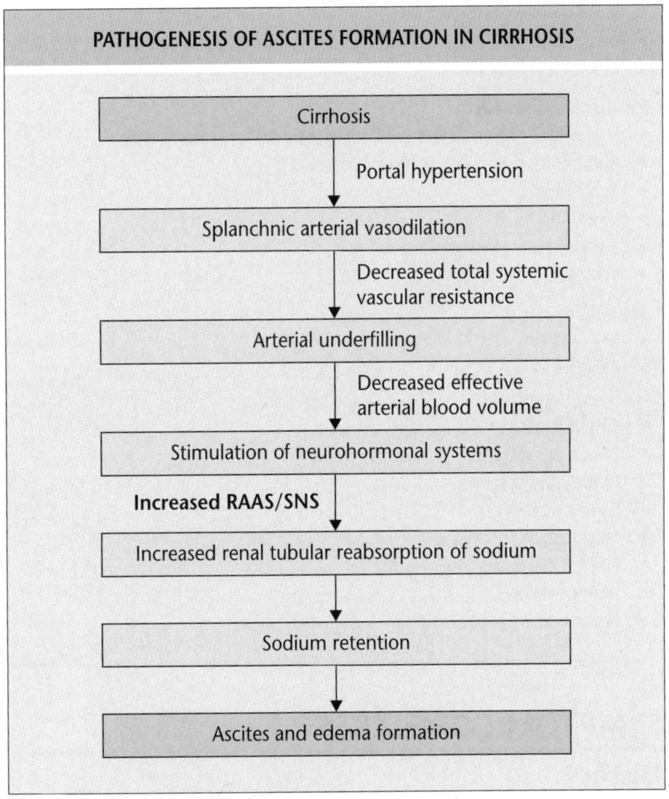

Fig. 20.1 Pathogenesis of ascites formation in cirrhosis. RAAS, renin angiotensin aldosterone system; SNS, sympathetic nervous system.

CAUSES

The etiology of ascites can be divided into three categories: related to portal hypertension, related to peritoneal diseases, and related to other miscellaneous diseases.

Liver disease: Nearly 90% of cases are due to portal hypertension, and in this category cirrhosis is responsible for the majority. Other less common causes of portal hypertension-related ascites include congestive heart failure, constrictive pericarditis, Budd-Chiari syndrome, and liver metastases. Among peritoneal diseases, carcinomatosis and mesothelioma are the most common malignancies associated with ascites. Tuberculous peritonitis is still a common cause, particularly in developing countries. Other miscellaneous causes such as chylous ascites are also commonly seen in association with cirrhosis and malignancy such as lymphoma. Pancreatic ascites and bile ascites can occur when there is disruption of the pancreatic duct and biliary tree. Myxedema is a rare cause of ascites, but can occur in patients with clinically significant hypothyroidism. Patients with severe hypoalbuminemia secondary to protein-losing enteropathy or nephrotic syndrome can occasionally present with ascites. Ovarian causes include Meig's syndrome (benign ovarian tumor, usually a fibroma with reactive ascites, usually a transudate, and right plural effusion).

CAUSES OF ASCITES

PORTAL HYPERTENSION RELATED
- Cirrhosis
- Alcoholic hepatitis
- Fulminant hepatic failure
- Heart failure
- Constrictive pericarditis
- Budd-Chiari syndrome and hepatic veno-occlusive disease
- Liver metastases

Peritoneal diseases
- Malignancy (peritoneal carcinomatosis and mesothelioma)
- Tuberculosis and other fungal infections
- Sarcoidosis
- Vasculitis
- Eosinophilic gastroenteritis
- Whipple disease

Miscellaneous
- Myxedema
- Ovarian disease (tumor, ovarian hyperstimulation syndrome and Meig's syndrome)
- Chylous ascites
- Pancreatic ascites
- Bloody ascites
- Biliary ascites
- Nephrogenous ascites
- Nephrotic syndrome
- Malnutrition
- Protein-losing enteropathy

SYMPTOM COMPLEXES

History

Ascites commonly presents as the first manifestation of decompensated liver disease. Patients usually complain of a progressive increase in abdominal girth, occasionally with abdominal pain depending on the cause.

In patients with known cirrhosis, the presence of precipitating events leading to ascites such as excessive salt intake, alcohol consumption, infections, medications such as nonsteroidal anti-inflammatory drugs, and diuretic noncompliance should be investigated. Worsening liver disease, portal vein thrombosis, renal failure (i.e., glomerular diseases), and development of hepatocellular carcinoma may also precipitate the development of ascites in patients with cirrhosis. In the setting of acute alcoholic hepatitis, ascites forms rapidly but it usually resolves following alcohol abstinence. More commonly, ascites develops insidiously over the course of weeks to months. The main symptoms associated with ascites in cirrhosis are increased abdominal girth along with lower extremity edema. In patients with large and tense ascites, respiratory function and physical activity may be impaired. Dyspnea occurs as a consequence of increasing abdominal distention and/or the presence of pleural effusions. Patients with ascites and spontaneous bacterial peritonitis can present with fever, chills, abdominal pain, encephalopathy, and rebound abdominal tenderness. However, often they are asymptomatic and the diagnosis relies on examination of the peritoneal fluid. Other common manifestations of patients with ascites include dull abdominal pain, anorexia, malaise, weakness, difficulty in sleeping, and muscle cramps.

Other patients: In patients without liver disease, the presence of ascites usually is a manifestation of the underlying disease but occasionally may manifest as an initial symptom. Therefore, the evaluation of ascites should include a detailed history of previous cardiac disease, history of any malignancy, or ongoing symptoms of cancer (such as lymphadenopathy, weight loss, night sweats, and fever), history of travel, nutritional status, medications, and other concomitant diseases such as kidney, thyroid, infectious, ovarian, or autoimmune diseases. Finally, a detailed history of any previous abdominal trauma or surgery should always be obtained.

Physical examination

Physical examination is not completely reliable for detecting fluid in the abdominal cavity. Patients must have approximately 1500 mL of fluid to be detected reliably by examination.[9] A common pitfall is the obese patient in which it may be very difficult to distinguish between significant adipose tissue of the abdominal wall and ascites. In these cases, an abdominal ultrasound establishes the presence of fluid as this diagnostic test can detect as little as 100 mL of fluid in the abdomen. A distended abdomen with bulging flanks and dullness to percussion in these areas indicates the presence of ascites. When free fluid is present in the abdominal cavity, it moves to the flanks and the intestines float upward when the patient is supine. The air–fluid level is higher than that normally found on the lateral aspect of the abdomen, if the patient is turned on his/her side the dullness will shift and percussion over the uppermost part becomes tympanic, because that area is occupied by intestines as fluid shifts to the other side. This maneuver is called shifting dullness and is very sensitive for detecting ascites.[10] Other maneuvers to detect ascites such as the fluid wave and puddle sign are less reliable. Mild or moderate pleural effusions are common in patients with ascites. Large pleural effusions (usually greater than 500 mL) in cirrhotic patients without cardiopulmonary disease are known as hepatic hydrothorax and are uncommon.

Determining the cause: The cause of ascites can usually be determined on the basis of clinical history and physical examination. Since the most common cause of ascites is cirrhosis, the examiner should look for signs indicative of the presence of portal hypertension and cirrhosis. Nonetheless, a thorough physical exam must be performed in order to help rule out noncirrhotic causes of ascites. The neck veins of patients with ascites should always be examined as constrictive pericarditis is a curable cause of ascites. The majority of patients with cardiac ascites have a dramatic jugular venous distention and a positive hepatojugular reflex. Tender hepatomegaly in the presence of ascites is characteristic of acute alcoholic hepatitis or Budd-Chiari syndrome. The presence of large abdominal wall veins with centrifugal flow is characteristic of portal hypertension, whereas cephalad flow suggests inferior vena cava obstruction. Patients with anasarca and ascites usually have advanced congestive heart failure or nephrotic syndrome with severe hypoalbuminemia, although some patients may have advanced cirrhosis.

Firm lymph nodes in the left supraclavicular region or umbilicus may suggest intra-abdominal malignancy. An immobile mass in the umbilicus (Sister Mary Joseph nodule) is suggestive of peritoneal carcinomatosis. Umbilical hernias may appear in patients with cirrhosis and long-standing ascites, and their size increases progressively if ascites is not treated. Unfortunately, they can sometimes cause significant complications such as strangulation and rupture due to the formation of an ulcer on the overlying skin. Rupture is associated with infection of the ascitic fluid and delayed wound healing. In patients with incisional hernias and ascites, the use of prosthetic meshes should be avoided due to the risk of bacterial infection. In cases of advanced cirrhosis, a hyperdynamic state characterized by resting tachycardia, low arterial blood pressure, and bounding peripheral pulses is present. Most patients are malnourished and have signs of muscle wasting, palmar erythema, spider angiomata, and lower extremity edema.

DIAGNOSIS

In all patients presenting with ascites, standard electrolytes, liver, renal, hematology, and coagulation tests should be performed. Liver tests required include aminotransferases, bilirubin, albumin, total protein, alkaline phosphatase, prothrombin time, and alpha fetoprotein. The majority of patients presenting with ascites of any origin will require some form of imaging of the abdomen to evaluate the liver, pancreas, biliary system, kidneys, adrenal glands, and pelvic organs. In patients with cirrhosis and ascites an abdominal ultrasound or CT scan are required to rule out hepatocellular carcinoma, evaluate the patency of portal and hepatic flow and, in some cases, confirm the presence of ascites. In patients with previously unknown liver disease, the diagnosis of cirrhosis can be confirmed either histologically or by a combination of exploratory, ultrasonographical, and endoscopic findings. A percutaneous liver biopsy should only be performed after resolution of ascites, because its presence increases the risk of complications. In patients with coagulopathy and ascites, the liver biopsy, if required, may be performed through a transjugular approach. Finally, a 24-h urine collection on a low-salt diet and off diuretics for at least 4 days for determination of volume and urinary sodium excretion is helpful in determining prognosis and response to therapy.

Diagnostic paracentesis is required in all patients presenting with ascites *de novo*. The ascitic fluid must always be visually inspected. The ascitic fluid in cirrhotics is transparent and yellow/amber in color. An opalescent and/or turbid ascitic fluid suggests the presence of a high amount (>1000/mm^3) of white blood cells. Milky appearing fluid suggests increased triglycerides (i.e., chylous ascites). Bloody ascites may be caused by a traumatic tap, malignancy, cirrhosis, or tuberculosis.

Basic parameters to be determined in ascitic fluid are cell count, culture in blood culture bottles, albumin, and total protein. Glucose, lactate dehydrogenase, amylase, triglycerides, tuberculosis smear, and cytological analysis should be measured depending on the suspected cause of ascites. The cell count is the most helpful test in determining bacterial infection in cirrhotic patients. In uninfected ascites, the white blood cell count is less than 500 per mm^3 in most cases, with predominance of mononuclear cells (>75%) and a very low number of polymorphonuclear (PMN) cells. The diagnosis of spontaneous bacterial peritonitis (SBP) is made when the fluid sample has a PMN count greater than 250/mm^3 (see Chapter 98).[11] Bloody ascites may lead to a higher PMN count in the absence of infection. Chylous ascites is defined when the triglyceride values are above 200 mg/dL, although some authors use a cutoff value of 110 mg/dL.[5] The red blood cell (RBC) count in ascitic fluid is usually low in patients with cirrhosis (below 1000 cells/mm^3). Bloody ascites (more than 50 000 RBC/mm^3) may be observed in patients with a traumatic tap or hepatocellular carcinoma.

Tuberculous peritonitis: The ascitic fluid protein exceeds 3.0 g/dL in more than 95% of cases.[12] The white blood cell count ranges from 150 to 4000/mm^3 with a predominance of lymphocytes.[6] Acid-fast smears have a very low yield and cultures of the ascitic fluid may require up to 6 weeks to grow mycobacteria. Polymerase chain reaction analysis for rapid detection of the mycobacteria is promising, but its utility has not been well established in clinical practice. Adenosine deaminase (ADA) is an enzyme involved in the conversion of adenosine to inosine, which is released by macrophages and lymphocytes during the cellular immune response. ADA values in peritoneal fluid are used as an indirect guide for the diagnosis of tuberculous effusions. Studies outside the US have reported high sensitivity (100%) and specificity (97%) in the diagnosis of tuberculous peritonitis in areas of high prevalence for tuberculosis without cirrhosis.[13] In the setting of cirrhosis, the sensitivity is lower and its utility is very limited. Laparoscopy with peritoneal biopsy is the gold standard for the diagnosis of peritoneal tuberculosis.

In pancreatic ascites, there is a high amylase content, usually above 1000 IU/L and the ascitic fluid to serum ratio is approximately 6.0.[14] In patients with bile ascites, the ascitic fluid is dark yellow with a bilirubin level greater than 6 mg/dL and usually exceeding the serum bilirubin.

The difference between serum albumin concentration and ascites albumin concentration (serum–ascites albumin gradient) in patients with cirrhosis is usually greater than 1.1 g/dL. Values lower than 1.1 g/dL suggest a cause of ascites other than portal hypertension.[15] Most patients with cirrhosis have a total ascitic fluid protein concentration of less than 1.0 g/dL. However, values greater than 1.0 g/dL are not uncommon. Patients with a protein concentration in ascitic fluid lower than 1.0 g/L have a greater risk of developing SBP. The mobilization of ascites with diuretics may lead to a slight increase in the concentration of proteins in the ascitic fluid.

SOURCES OF INFORMATION FOR PATIENTS AND DOCTORS

http://patients.uptodate.com/topic.asp?file=livr_dis/4490
http://www.patient.co.uk/showdoc/40002410/

DIFFERENTIAL DIAGNOSIS

DIFFERENTIAL DIAGNOSIS OF ASCITES BY THE SERUM–ASCITES ALBUMIN GRADIENT[a]

High gradient (≥ 1.1) g/dL)	Low gradient (< 1.1) g/dL)
Cirrhosis	Peritoneal carcinomatosis
Congestive heart failure	Tuberculosis (without cirrhosis)
Fulminant hepatic failure	Pancreatitis (without cirrhosis)
Portal vein thrombosis	Biliary (without cirrhosis)
Liver metastases	Nephrotic syndrome
Alcoholic hepatitis	Connective tissue diseases
Budd-Chiari syndrome	Chlamydia/gonococccal infection
Veno-occlusive disease	
Myxedema	

[a]Serum ascites–albumin gradient = serum albumin concentration minus ascites albumin concentration.

REFERENCES

1. Runyon BA. Care of patients with ascites. N Engl J Med 1994; 330:337–342.
2. Salerno F, Borroni G, Moser P et al. Survival and prognostic factors of cirrhotic patients with ascites: a study of 134 outpatients. Am J Gastroenterol 1993; 88:514–519.
3. Ginès P, Quintero E, Arroyo V et al. Compensated cirrhosis: natural history and prognostic factors. Hepatology 1987; 7:122–128.
4. Cardenas A, Chopra S. Chylous ascites. Am J Gastroenterol 2002; 97:1896–1900.
5. Cardenas A, Bataller R, Arroyo V. Mechanisms of ascites formation. Clin Liver Dis 2000; 4:447–465.
6. Marshall JB. Tuberculosis of the gastrointestinal tract and peritoneum. Am J Gastroenterol 1993; 88:989–999.
7. Gomez-Cerezo J, Barbado Cano A, Suarez I, Soto A, Rios JJ, Vazquez JJ. Pancreatic ascites: study of therapeutic options by analysis of case reports and case series between the years 1975 and 2000. Am J Gastroenterol 2003; 98:568–577.
8. de Castro F, Bonacini M, Walden JM, Schubert TT. Myxedema ascites. Report of two cases and review of the literature. J Clin Gastroenterol 1991; 13:411–414.
9. Runyon B. Approach to the patient with ascites. In: Yamada T, ed. Textbook of gastroenterology, 3rd edn. Philadelphia: Lippincott Williams & Wilkins; 1999:966.
10. Williams JW Jr, Simel DL. Does this patient have ascites? How to divine fluid in the abdomen. JAMA 1992; 267:2645–2648.
11. Such J, Runyon BA. Spontaneous bacterial peritonitis. Clin Infect Dis 1998; 27:669–674.
12. Manohar A, Simjee AE, Haffejee AA, Pettengell KE. Symptoms and investigative findings in 145 patients with tuberculous peritonitis diagnosed by peritoneoscopy and biopsy over a five year period. Gut 1990; 31:1130–1132.
13. Hillebrand DJ, Runyon BA, Yasmineh WG, Rynders GP. Ascitic fluid adenosine deaminase insensitivity in detecting tuberculous peritonitis in the United States. Hepatology 1996; 24: 1408–1412.
14. Runyon BA. Amylase levels in ascitic fluid. J Clin Gastroenterol 1987; 9:172–174.
15. Runyon BA, Montano AA, Akriviadis EA et al. The serum-ascites albumin gradient is superior to the exudate-transudate concept in the differential diagnosis of ascites. Ann Intern Med 1992; 117:215–220.

Chapter 21

Abnormal liver function tests

Kevin M Comar and Arun J Sanyal

INTRODUCTION

Liver function tests (LFTs) are commonly ordered when evaluating the liver. Broadly, these are classified as (1) markers of liver injury or (2) tests of liver function. Due to the potential limitations of these tests, one must consider them in the context of the clinical picture in order to evaluate a person with liver disease.

EPIDEMIOLOGY AND CLINICAL FEATURES

Typically, laboratories define the upper limit of normal values as two standard deviations from the mean of a group of apparently normal individuals. Thus, approximately 5% of normal individuals have elevated LFTs. It is estimated that 7.9% of the US population have elevated LFTs. The most common conditions associated with persistently elevated LFTs are hepatitis C and nonalcoholic fatty liver disease (NAFLD). The clinical features associated with abnormal LFTs depend on its cause, mode of presentation (acute vs. chronic), and the severity of injury. The clinical features can vary from non-specific symptoms, e.g., nausea and fatigue, to the stigmata of chronic liver disease, e.g., spider, palmar erythema, gynecomastia, caput medusae.

PATHOGENESIS

Markers of liver injury

Markers of parenchymal liver injury

Aspartate aminotransferase (AST), also known as serum glutamic-oxaloacetic transaminase (SGOT), and alanine aminotransferase (ALT), also known as serum glutamate-pyruvate transaminase (SGPT), are common markers of hepatocellular injury. These two enzymes catalyze the transfer of amino groups between amino acids and carboxylic acids. While both are found in the cytoplasm of hepatocytes, AST is also found in the mitochondria.[1] Neither enzyme is liver specific; however, both are present at the highest concentration in the liver. AST is also found in significant amounts in several other tissues, e.g., myocardium, striated muscle, etc. Thus, isolated or disproportionate elevation of AST should prompt an investigation for pathology outside the liver (see Table 21.1).

Like many other laboratory standards, the normal range of AST and ALT were based on the values obtained in self-reported normal individuals. Many of these individuals may have had underlying nonalcoholic fatty liver disease (NAFLD) or hepatitis C. Also, normal males, nonwhites, and individuals with larger body mass have a tendency to have higher levels of aminotransferases.[2] Finally, the upper limit of normal for these enzymes may vary from one laboratory to another due to differences in the methods used. Despite these limitations, most laboratories consider a value of about 40 IU/L to be the upper limit of normal.

Markers of cholestasis

Alkaline phosphatase (AP)

This enzyme catalyzes the hydrolysis of phosphate esters and is present in many organs including the liver, biliary tree, intestine, placenta, kidney, and bone (Table 21.2).[3] The serum levels normally reflect the activities of the enzyme in these organs. AP is increased in cholestatic disorders. The plasma concentration of AP ranges from 25 to 85 IU/L; however, during adolescence, pregnancy, and periods of bone growth, the physiologic levels of AP are elevated.

Gamma glutamyl transferase (GGT)

This is a microsomal enzyme and is found in many tissues including the liver. GGT levels are very sensitive to minor degrees of liver injury, which greatly reduces its diagnostic

TABLE 21.1 NONHEPATIC SOURCES OF ELEVATED AST LEVELS
HEART
Acute myocardial infarct
Pericarditis
SKELETAL MUSCLE
Acute skeletal muscle injury
Muscle inflammation
Muscular dystrophy
Recent surgery
Delirium tremens
KIDNEY
Acute injury or damage
Renal infarct
OTHER
Intestinal infarction
Shock
Cholecystitis
Acute pancreatitis
Pancreatic carcinoma
Lymphoma
Hypothyroidism
Heparin therapy (60–80% of cases)

TABLE 21.2 NONHEPATIC SOURCES OF ELEVATED AP LEVELS

BONE ORIGIN
Physiologic adolescent bone growth
Metastatic tumor with osteoblastic reaction
Fracture healing
Paget's disease of bone
CAPILLARY ENDOTHELIAL ORIGIN
Granulation tissue formation
PLACENTAL ORIGIN
Pregnancy
Parenteral albumin preparations
OTHER
Thyrotoxicosis
Benign transient hyperphosphatasemia
Primary hyperparathyroidism
Sepsis
Chronic renal failure
Drugs

utility. In addition to serving as a marker of liver injury in cases of isolated AP elevation, an isolated persistent elevation of GGT may be seen with alcohol abuse.[4]

Tests of liver function

Serum bilirubin

Bilirubin is a breakdown product of hemoglobin and is derived from destroyed red blood cells. It is very hydrophobic and is carried to the liver by binding to albumin. It is taken up from sinusoidal circulation via uptake by the hepatocyte basolateral membrane transporters, which have not been fully characterized. Within hepatocytes, it is conjugated to bilirubin mono- and diglucuronide, which are water-soluble and excreted into bile by the canalicular multiple organic anion transporter (cMOAT). This is the rate-limiting step in bilirubin excretion. In the intestinal lumen, bilirubin is degraded mainly to urobilinogen, which is reabsorbed and excreted by the kidneys.

Serum bilirubin is measured by a colorimetric assay where a purple color is produced by the reaction of a diazo reagent with bilirubin in the presence (total bilirubin) or absence (conjugated or direct bilirubin) of an accelerator, e.g., alcohol. Indirect bilirubin is the difference between total and direct bilirubin levels and reflects unconjugated bilirubin. The normal range of serum bilirubin is between 3 and 15 μmol/L (0.3–0.8 mg/dL). Hyperbilirubinemia and jaundice results from increased production or decreased clearance of bilirubin. Unconjugated hyperbilirubinemia (>85% of total bilirubin) results from increased production, i.e., hemolysis or decreased hepatic uptake and conjugation (Gilbert syndrome, Crigler-Najjar syndrome), while conjugated hyperbilirubinemia (>50% of total bilirubin is conjugated) results from either parenchymal liver injury or cholestasis (Table 21.3).

Albumin

Albumin is a plasma protein that is produced by the liver. The normal plasma concentration range of albumin is 3.5–5.0 g/dL. While hepatocellular dysfunction and liver failure cause low albumin levels, the levels may also be lowered by increased clearance, e.g., renal losses in nephrotic syndrome, burns, protein-losing enteropathy, or decreased delivery of amino acids to the liver due to malnutrition (Table 21.4). Differentiation between the latter and liver failure may be difficult because they frequently coexist. The degree of hypoalbuminemia correlates with outcomes and is part of the Child-Pugh scoring system to assess prognosis of advanced liver disease.[5]

Prothrombin time

The prothrombin time (PT) is a direct measurement of the conversion rate of prothrombin to thrombin and the activity of

TABLE 21.3 DIFFERENTIAL DIAGNOSIS OF HYPERBILIRUBINEMIA

UNCONJUGATED HYPERBILIRUBINEMIA
1. Increased bilirubin production
Hemolysis
Dyserythropoiesis
Blood transfusion
Extravasation
2. Decreased hepatocellular uptake
Drugs (e.g., rifampicin)
Gilbert's syndrome
3. Decreased conjugation
Gilbert's syndrome
Crigler-Najjar syndrome
Physiologic jaundice of the newborn
CONJUGATED HYPERBILIRUBINEMIA
1. Parenchymal
Hepatocellular injury
Viral hepatitis
Hepatotoxins (e.g., acetaminophen)
Drugs (e.g., isoniazid)
Alcoholic hepatitis
Sepsis or ischemia (e.g., hypotension)
Metabolic disorders (e.g., Wilson's disease, Reye's syndrome)
Pregnancy-related (e.g., acute fatty liver of pregnancy, preeclampsia)
Autoimmune hepatitis
Metabolic (hemochromatosis, nonalcoholic steatohepatitis, α1-antitrypsin deficiency)
2. Cholestasis
Infiltrative disorders
Granulomatous diseases (e.g., mycobacterial infections, sarcoidosis, lymphoma)
Amyloidosis
Malignancy
Obstruction or inflammation of the bile ducts
Gallstones
Primary sclerosing cholangitis
AIDS cholangiopathy
Postsurgical strictures
Neoplasms
Extrinsic compression of the biliary tree
Neoplasms
Pancreatitis
Vascular enlargement (e.g., aneurysm)

TABLE 21.4 DISEASES ASSOCIATED WITH HYPOALBUMINEMIA
DECREASED SYNTHESIS
Liver dysfunction
Malnutrition
INCREASED CATABOLISM
Stress
Sepsis
Trauma
Surgery
INCREASED LOSS
Renal disease
Protein-losing enteropathy
Burns
Lymphatic blockage or mucosal disease (e.g., inflammatory bowel disease, sprue, and bacterial overgrowth)
Gastrointestinal bleeding
REDISTRIBUTION
Hemodilution (e.g., congestive heart failure, ascites)

coagulation factors II, V, VII, and X. The normal prothrombin time is 11–15 s, depending on the source of the thromboplastin used in the test. Coagulation factors II, V, VII, and X are vitamin K dependent; thus, when vitamin K deficiency occurs, e.g., as in malnutrition, altered gut flora or cholestasis, the prothrombin time is prolonged (Table 21.5). In such cases, vitamin K administration should correct the PT within 24 h. In the absence of vitamin K deficiency, prolonged PT is a reliable marker of liver dysfunction. However, it is not a sensitive measure of liver function and over 80% of the hepatic functional reserve has to be compromised before the PT becomes abnormal.[6] Acute liver failure is associated with the highest PT levels and correlates with mortality.

DIAGNOSIS

An integrated approach to evaluation of abnormal LFTs

There are three fundamental steps in the assessment of a patient with liver disease: (1) to determine the nature of the liver disease, i.e., parenchymal vs cholestatic vs mixed pattern; (2) to determine the etiology of liver disease; and (3) to assess the prognosis of the patient.

TABLE 21.5 DISEASES ASSOCIATED WITH ELEVATED PROTHROMBIN TIME
Afibrinogenemia
Anticoagulants
Disseminated intravascular coagulation
Drugs
Dysfibrinogenemia
Liver disease
Vitamin K deficiency

Identification of the nature of liver disease

Parenchymal liver diseases are those where the hepatocytes are the primary target of injury. They are associated with elevated AST and ALT levels. Diseases characterized by cholestasis are associated with elevated AP levels. The ALT/AP (both expressed as the fold elevation above upper limit of normal) ratio is typically >5 in parenchymal diseases while it is <2 in cholestatic disorders (Fig. 21.1).[7] Parenchymal diseases with a cholestatic component, e.g., drug toxicity or cholestatic diseases with ongoing hepatocellular necrosis may present with a mixed pattern of LFT abnormality and an ALT/AP ratio between 2 and 5.

Identification of the etiology of liver disease

Parenchymal liver disease

A 10-fold or greater elevation of AST and ALT are specific findings of active hepatocellular necrosis. Lower degrees of ALT elevation do not correlate well with histologic findings. A >10-fold increase in AST and ALT is associated with viral hepatitis, drug or toxin-mediated injury, ischemia, autoimmune hepatitis, and Wilson's disease. Hepatitis A, B, C, D, and E can all cause acute hepatitis and active hepatocellular necrosis. Ischemic and toxic liver injury cause the highest ALT values (>1000). The passage of a gallstone may also cause a marked elevation of AST, which rapidly returns to baseline values once the stone has passed.

AST and ALT values that are <10-fold the upper limit of normal can be seen in those with lesser degrees of hepatocellular necrosis, e.g., chronic liver diseases or milder forms of acute liver injury. Acute microvesicular steatosis, e.g., Reye's syndrome, is usually associated with modest ALT elevation. Hepatitis B, C, and D are common causes of chronic viral hepatitis. Alcoholic liver injury is usually associated with AST and ALT values below 300–400 IU/L. The AST/ALT ratio is often greater than 2 in alcoholic liver disease[8] whereas values between 1 and 2 can often be seen in cirrhosis and Wilson's disease. Other common causes of AST and ALT values that are elevated <10-fold and should be assessed by appropriate laboratory tests are listed in Fig. 21.2. When common causes of AST and ALT have been excluded, the presence of underlying NAFLD must be considered, especially in those with obesity, diabetes, and other features of the metabolic syndrome.[9] A liver biopsy is needed for the definitive diagnosis of steatohepatitis. Fatty liver can usually be detected by ultrasonography.

ETIOLOGY OF ABNORMAL LIVER FUNCTION TESTS

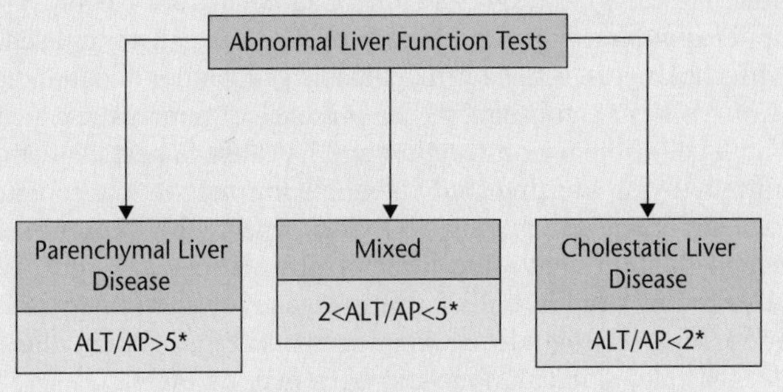

Fig. 21.1 Etiology of abnormal liver function tests. *ALT/AP is expressed as the fold elevation above the upper limit of normal.

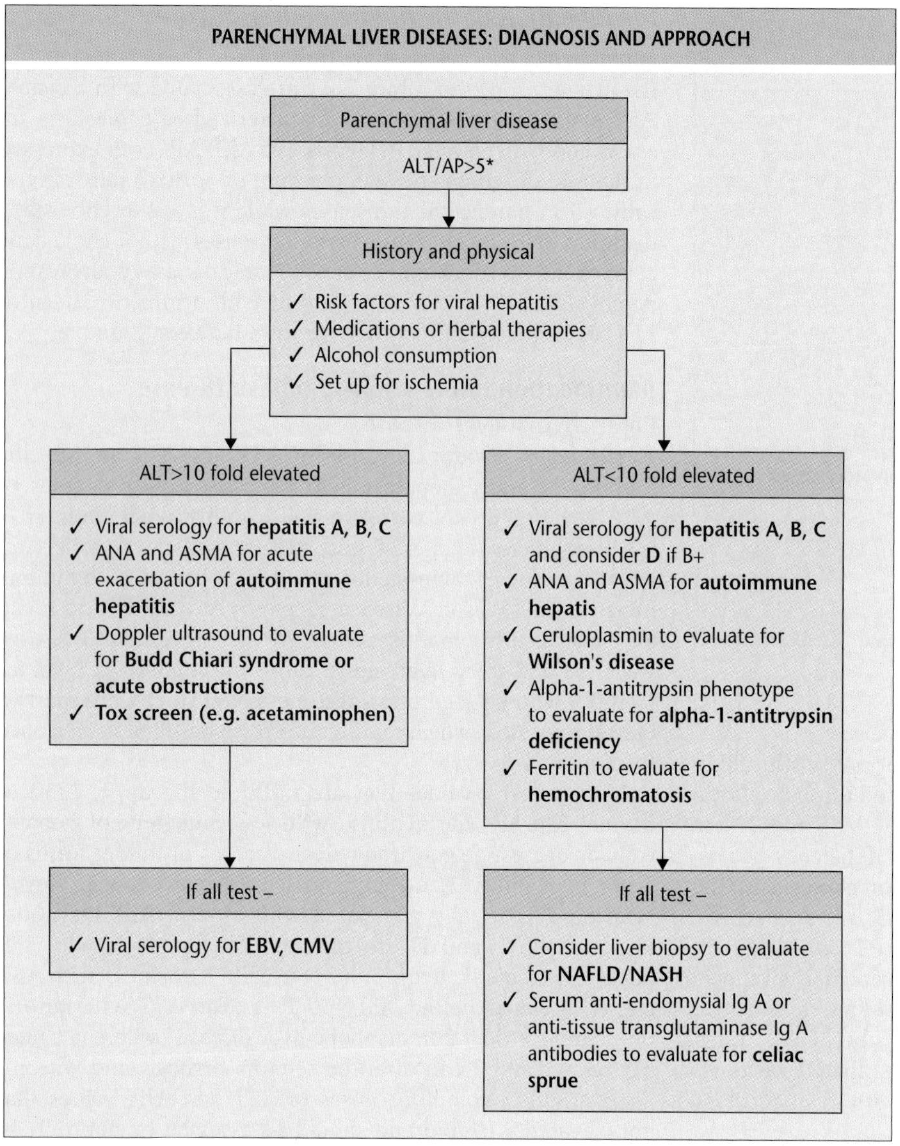

Fig. 21.2 Diagnosis and approach to parenchymal liver diseases. *ALT/AP is expressed as the fold elevation above the upper limit of normal.

Cholestatic liver diseases

In asymptomatic persons with an isolated elevation of AP, the presence of a cholestatic disorder can be verified by checking for an elevated GGT value or the AP isoforms. Cholestatic disorders can be broadly categorized as those due to mechanical biliary obstruction versus those due to medical cholestasis. A large number of conditions can cause mechanical biliary obstruction (Fig. 21.3). The presence of Charcot's triad (fever, right upper quadrant pain, and jaundice) suggests gallstone disease with cholangitis, while a firm, palpable gallbladder and jaundice (Courvoisier's sign) suggests the presence of pancreatic cancer. The level of biliary obstruction and its cause is best evaluated initially by an imaging study (sonography, magnetic resonance cholangiopancreatography (MRCP)) where the presence of ductal dilation above the level of obstruction is sought. The obstruction can be both confirmed and often treated using endoscopic retrograde cholangiography (ERC). When this is not feasible, a percutanous approach may be taken.

Medical cholestasis refers to conditions where cholestasis is due to diseases of intrahepatic microscopic bile ducts (e.g., primary biliary cirrhosis), infiltrative conditions (e.g., lymphoma), or hepatocellular diseases (e.g., estrogen toxicity). Once the presence of biliary obstruction and a hepatic space-occupying lesion are excluded by an imaging test (sonography, CT scan, or MRI), the diagnosis is established by the appropriate laboratory tests (Fig. 21.3) (e.g., antimitochondrial antibody for primary biliary cirrhosis) and liver biopsy. A thorough clinical assessment may obviate the need for liver biopsy, e.g., in disseminated cancer.

Mixed pattern (ALT/AP ratio 2<R<5)

The most important cause of this pattern of injury is drug-induced liver injury. Iatrogenic liver disease is now considered to be a major cause of liver failure in North America. Diagnosis of iatrogenic liver disease can be made from the enzyme pattern along with the clinical history, after excluding other common causes of parenchymal liver injury. When more than one pathologic process is suspected, the appropriate laboratory tests along with liver biopsy are required to make the diagnosis, e.g., acute rejection of liver allograft along with CMV infection.

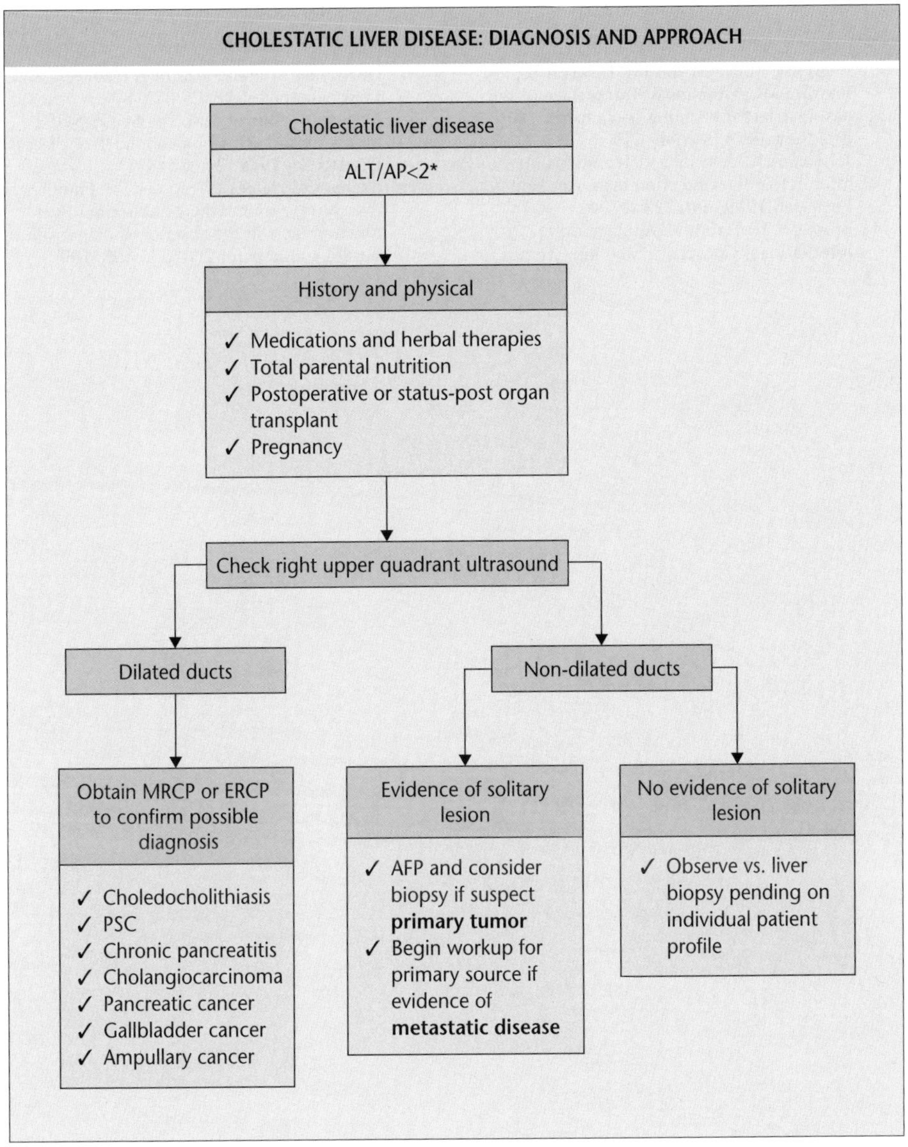

Fig. 21.3 Diagnosis and approach to cholestatic liver diseases. *ALT/AP is expressed as the fold elevation above the upper limit of normal.

PROGNOSIS

Prognosis of patients with liver disease depends on: (1) the degree of liver failure; and (2) the presence of complications of liver disease. Liver function is assessed using serum bilirubin and albumin levels, and PT. The presence of complications, e.g., ascites, spontaneous bacterial peritonitis, variceal hemorrhage, and encephalopathy, further contribute to mortality and thus are important determinants of prognosis. The presence of renal failure is an ominous sign in those with advanced liver disease. Several algorithms have been developed to assess the prognosis of those with acute and chronic liver disease. These include the Child-Pugh score and the model for end-stage liver disease (MELD) score, which includes bilirubin, international normalized ratio (INR), and creatinine.

SUMMARY

A medical misnomer, LFTs not only provide information on the liver biosynthetic function but are also markers of liver injury. They can be used to direct the diagnostic evaluation of patients with liver disease and assess their prognosis. It is critically important to remember the factors that limit the diagnostic utility of individual tests. Ideally, the use of these tests should be combined with a comprehensive clinical evaluation. The clinical picture and the nature of liver enzyme abnormalities dictate the optimal sequence of tests.

SOURCES OF INFORMATION FOR PATIENTS AND DOCTORS

http://www.patient.co.uk/showdoc/27000446/

REFERENCES

1. Rej R. Aspartate aminotransferase activity and isoenzyme proportions in human liver tissues. Clin Chem 1978; 24:1971–1979.
2. Manolio TA, Burke GL, Savage PJ et al. Sex- and race-related differences in liver-associated serum chemistry tests in young adults in the CARDIA study. Clin Chem 1992; 38:1853–1859.
3. Kaplan MM. Alkaline phosphatase. Gastroenterology 1972; 62:452–468.
4. Whitehead TP, Clarke CA, Whitfield AG. Biochemical and haematological markers of alcohol intake. Lancet 1978; 1:978–981.
5. Pugh RN, Murray-Lyon IM, Dawson JL, Pietroni MC, Williams R. Transection of the oesophagus for bleeding oesophageal varices. Br J Surg 1973; 60:646–649.
6. Johnston DE. Special considerations in interpreting liver function tests. Am Fam Physician 1999; 59:2223–2230.
7. Bussieres JF, Habra M. Application of International Consensus Meeting Criteria for classifying drug-induced liver disorders. Ann Pharmacother 1995; 29:875–878.
8. Cohen JA, Kaplan MM. The SGOT/SGPT ratio – an indicator of alcoholic liver disease. Dig Dis Sci 1979; 24:835–838.
9. Skelly MM, James PD, Ryder SD. Findings on liver biopsy to investigate abnormal liver function tests in the absence of diagnostic serology. J Hepatol 2001; 35:195–199.

Chapter 22

Acute abdominal pain

Dileep N Lobo

INTRODUCTION

Sir William Osler once wrote 'Medicine is a science of uncertainty and an art of probability.' Acute abdominal pain, which accounts for a large proportion of gastrointestinal emergency work, poses problems of uncertainty where probability is an important component of management. Acute abdominal pain usually results from gastrointestinal disorders but other causes must not be forgotten.

WHAT IS IT?

Acute pain

Acute pain arises from nociceptor activation at sites of damage.[1] The local injury alters the response characteristics of the nociceptors, their central connections, and the autonomic nervous system in the region. Therefore, acute pain can be considered to be the initial phase of an extensive, persistent nociceptive and behavioral cascade triggered by tissue injury.[2] However, in malignant diseases, the invasion of body tissues can produce continuous acute pain.

Acute abdominal pain has loosely been described as pain occurring in the abdomen with an onset of less than 6–8 h. However, a more pragmatic definition is that of previously undiagnosed abdominal pain that arises suddenly and is of less than 7 days and usually less than 48 h duration. The likelihood of surgical intervention is greater if acute abdominal pain lasts for more than 6 h. The dichotomy between acute and chronic pain is now untenable[3] with a continuum between causes.

Visceral pain

Visceral pain, in contrast to somatic pain, is diffuse, difficult to localize, and is referred to cutaneous dermatomes. Patterns of referred sensations overlap considerably and can cause problems with differential diagnosis. Visceral pain does not arise from all viscera, and organs such as liver, kidney, most solid viscera, and lung parenchyma are not sensitive to pain. Distention of hollow viscera such as the bowel and bladder can produce pain in the absence of injury. Visceral pain can also be associated with motor and autonomic reflexes, such as nausea and vomiting.[4]

Referred pain

Pain as a result of irritation of an abdominal organ is usually not felt in the viscus, but in a somatic structure that may be at a considerable distance from it. This is known as referred pain and when visceral pain is both local and referred, it may seem to radiate from the local to the distant site. When pain is referred, it is usually to a structure that developed from the same embryonic segment or dermatome as the organ the pain originates from. Thus, pain that originates from the foregut is referred to the epigastrium (T8), that from the mid gut to the umbilical region (T10), and that from the hindgut to the hypogastrium (T12). A more dramatic form of referred pain is that from the diaphragm (innervated by the phrenic nerve C3–5) to the shoulder tip, which receives its cutaneous innervation from the same spinal segments.

HOW COMMON IS IT?

Acute abdominal pain is relatively common and accounts for 5% of visits to the emergency department.[5] Although most patients presenting with acute abdominal pain have minor problems, about 18–25% of patients have a serious enough condition to warrant hospital admission for investigation and treatment[5,6] and about 10% of patients need emergency or urgent surgery.[5] A large audit from the UK has shown that up to 50% of all general surgical admissions are emergencies, half of which are due to acute abdominal pain.[7] Missing the diagnosis in patients with acute abdominal pain can lead to major morbidity, mortality, and ensuing litigation.

PATHOPHYSIOLOGY

The abdominal viscera are connected to the cerebral cortex by three levels of sensory neurons (Figs 22.1 and 22.2). Nociceptive stimuli are detected by specialized transducers attached to A and C fibers and are transmitted almost exclusively by the sympathetic nervous system. The first-order neurons link the viscera to the spinal cord and pass through autonomic plexuses usually associated with a major artery supplying the organs such as the celiac, superior mesenteric, and inferior mesenteric arteries. Pain can be elicited by a wide variety of insults, which include mechanical, chemical, and thermal stimuli. Damaged tissue can release neurotransmitter-like substances such as substance P, potassium, histamine, prostaglandins, serotonin, bradykinin, γ-aminobutyric acid, neuropeptide Y, adenosine, noradrenaline, capsaicin, and a host of others.[3,4,8] Nociceptive nerve endings themselves may release substance P and other mediators, via axon reflexes originating in other branches, causing additional inflammation and edema. Signaling via second- and third-order neurons activates the limbic system thalamus and cingulate gyrus, giving pain its unpleasant nature.

Second-order or postsynaptic neurons begin in the dorsal horn and cross at the midline to the contralateral side and then travel within the ventrolateral quadrant of the spinal cord upward

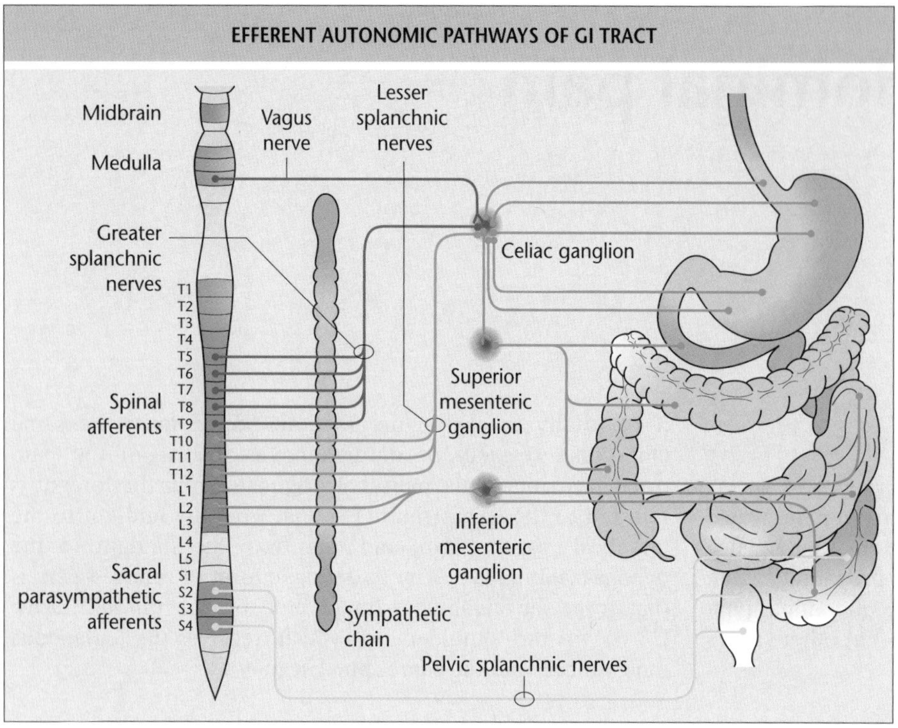

Fig. 22.1 Efferent autonomic pathways of the gastrointestinal tract. The parasympathetic pathways are shown in purple and the sympathetic pathways in red. (Redrawn from Mertz HR, Mayer EA. Functional gastrointestinal syndromes. In: Zinner MJ, Schwartz SI, Ellis H, eds. Maingot's abdominal operations. vol. 1, 10th ed. Stamford: Appleton & Lange; 1997: 361–378, with permission from McGraw Hill.)

toward the brainstem via pathways such as the spinothalamic tracts. Third-order neurons travel from the spinoreticular tracts to the frontal cortex and limbic system. Third-order neurons that ascend from the thalamus to the post central gyrus of the cerebral cortex form the pathway for the localization of pain and those that ascend from the intralaminar nuclei to cingulate gyrus (association cortex-limb system) form the pathway related to the unpleasantness of pain.

Nausea and diaphoresis are examples of autonomic responses provoked by visceral pain.

Referred visceral pain is thought to be the result of convergence of somatic and visceral afferents on the same spinal cord neurons. There is also evidence that single distal processes of dorsal root ganglia branch, with one branch going to body surface and one to viscera. This convergence-projection theory explains the features of referred pain.

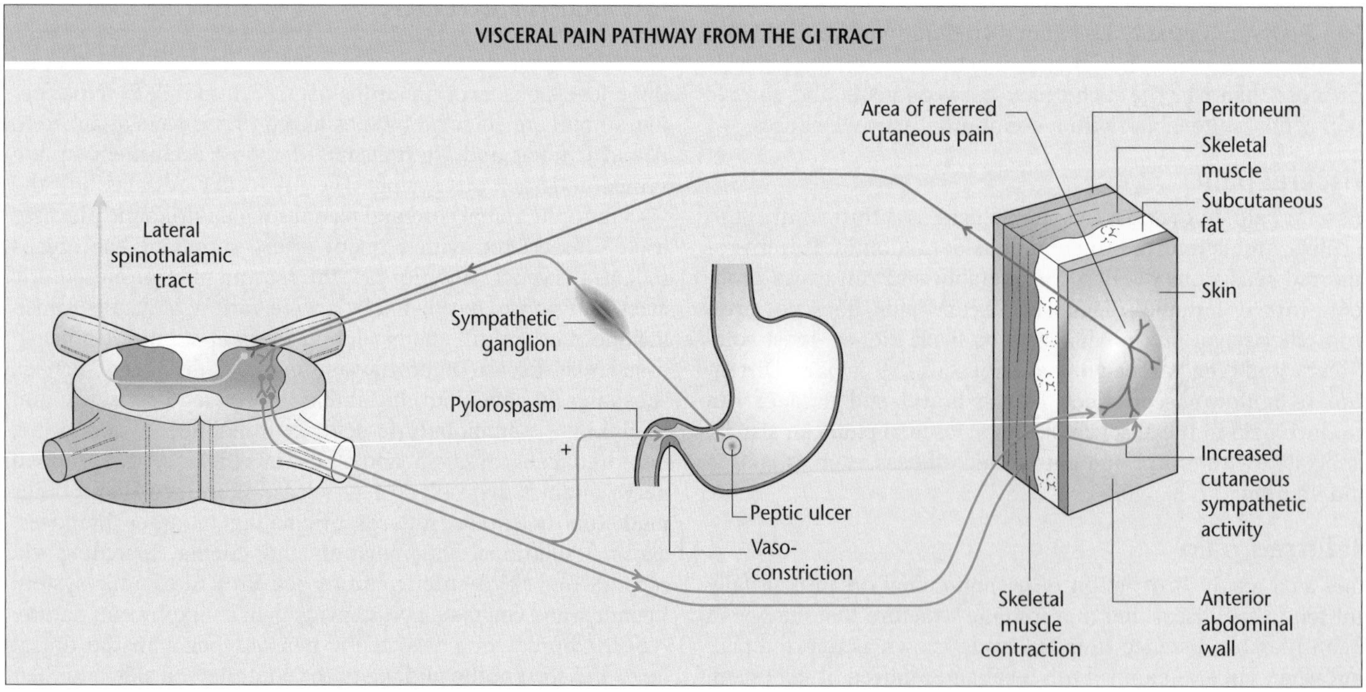

Fig. 22.2 Visceral pain pathway from the gastrointestinal tract.

CAUSES

Acute pain in the abdomen is usually due to luminal obstruction, inflammation, perforation, volvulus or torsion, and intestinal ischemia. The common causes of acute abdominal pain are listed in Tables 22.1 and 22.2 and depicted in Fig. 22.3.

SYMPTOM COMPLEXES

Luminal obstruction

Luminal obstruction usually starts with abdominal colic that is referred to the dermatomes supplying the part of the gut proximal to the obstruction. Vomiting is a prominent feature of gastric outlet obstruction and small bowel obstruction. If the ileocecal valve is competent, patients with large bowel obstruction may not vomit. Abdominal distention is more pronounced in patients with large bowel obstruction and this condition is usually associated with absolute constipation. Patients with small bowel obstruction may continue to pass small amounts of flatus and feces. Visible peristalsis may be observed and bowel sounds are usually hyperdynamic. Hernial orifices must be examined meticulously. If untreated, luminal obstruction may lead to adynamic ileus, strangulation, and perforation. Intestinal obstruction in patients who have had previous surgery is usually due to

TABLE 22.1 CAUSES OF ACUTE ABDOMINAL PAIN

Main pain location	Organ	Additional localization	Pathology
RUQ	Liver	Epigastrium Also referred to tip of shoulder	Hepatitis, abscess, infarction, bleed into tumor, expanding hematoma, congestive cardiac failure
	Biliary tract	May radiate to back along rib cage	Stones in gall bladder/cystic duct: colic, cholecystitis Stones in common bile duct: colic, ascending cholangitis Mucocele, empyema, gallbladder perforation
Epigastric	Pancreas	R & L hypochondria Radiates to back May be relieved by leaning forward	Acute pancreatitis or exacerbation of chronic pancreatitis Complications of pancreatitis, pancreatic cancer, obstruction (pancreas divisum and sphincter of Oddi dysfunction)
	Stomach	R and L upper quadrants[a]	Ulcer, volvulus, perforation, cancer, acute dilatation Gastric outlet obstruction, hiatus hernia
	Duodenum	R and L upper quadrants[a]	Ulcer, perforation, obstruction
	Esophagus	Retrosternal	Esophagitis, spasm, rupture, hiatus hernia
LUQ	Spleen	May radiate to flank	Splenomegaly, infarction, rupture, expanding splenic hematoma Sickle cell crisis
Central	Aorta	Epigastrium/periumbilical/ flank/ back/may become generalized	Ruptured/dissecting aneurysm
	Small bowel	May later localize to area of inflammation of parietal peritoneum[a]	Obstruction (adhesions, herniae, volvulus, tumor, stricture, gallstone ileus, bezoars, intussusception, tuberculosis) Perforation, ischemia, Crohn's disease, Meckel's diverticulum, mesenteric adenitis, gastroenteritis, motility disorders/IBS
	Appendix	Later localizes to R lower quadrant[a]	Acute appendicitis, appendicular abscess
	R colon	May later localize to area of inflammation of parietal peritoneum[a]	Obstruction (malignant/benign strictures, volvulus) Perforation, ischemia, acute diverticulitis and its complications Inflammatory bowel disease
Hypogastrium	L colon	May then localize to area of inflammation of parietal peritoneum or become generalized	Obstruction (malignant/benign strictures, volvulus) Perforation, ischemia, acute diverticulitis and its complications Constipation/fecal impaction Inflammatory bowel disease, amoebic colitis
	Urinary bladder	May radiate to base of penis	Cystitis, bladder calculus, acute urinary retention, obstructing bladder tumors
	Uterus, ovaries	R and L lower quadrants	Ectopic pregnancy, ovarian torsion, uterine perforation
	Fallopian tubes	May be referred to the inner thighs May be generalized	Pelvic inflammatory disease, acute salpingitis, ovarian cysts Endometriosis, mittelschmerz, dysmenorrhea
Loin to groin	Kidneys/ureters	May radiate to testes or labia	Calculi, infection, pyelonephritis, obstruction (e.g., tumor)
Scrotum	Testes	Hypogastrium, R and L lower quadrant	Torsion, trauma, epididymoorchitis
Other	Abdominal wall		Herniae, muscular contusions/hematoma, abdominal wall abscess, herpes zoster, entrapment neuropathy
	Abdominal trauma		Trauma to abdominal wall, hemoperitoneum, rupture of solid or hollow viscus Retroperitoneal hematoma
	Postoperative		Intra-abdominal bleeding, anastomotic dehiscence, intra-abdominal abscess Abdominal compartment syndrome

[a] Generalized in perforation.

TABLE 22.2 EXTRA-ABDOMINAL/SYSTEMIC CAUSES OF ACUTE ABDOMINAL PAIN

Lungs	Lobar pneumonia
	Pleurisy
	Pulmonary embolism
Heart	Acute myocardial infarction
	Congestive cardiac failure
	Myocarditis
Metabolic/endocrine	Porphyrias
	Diabetic ketoacidosis
	Lead poisoning
	Hypercalcemia
	Adrenal insufficiency
Vasculitis	Henoch-Schonlein purpura
	Systemic lupus
	Polyarteritis nodosa
	Familial Mediterranean fever

adhesions and it is worthwhile instituting a trial of nasogastric aspiration and intravenous fluids for 24–48 h. Surgery is indicated if the patient's condition fails to resolve, or at the first sign of deterioration (e.g., tachycardia, increasing white cell count, increasing pain and distention, feculent aspiration). Patients with large bowel obstruction should ideally undergo an unprepared lower gastrointestinal contrast study to rule out pseudo-obstruction.

Inflammation

Intraperitoneal inflammation usually arises from intra-abdominal organs such as the appendix, gallbladder, pancreas, small and large bowel (inflammatory bowel disease, diverticulitis), and pelvic organs. Primary peritonitis occurs rarely, in young girls and in patients with ascites (cirrhosis, nephrotic syndrome). Vomiting may be a vagal response to the pain. In most instances, the inflammation is secondary to infection or ischemia. Initially, the inflammation is confined to the organ of origin and the physical signs will be localized to the area of peritoneal inflammation, characterized by local tenderness with exacerbation on rebound. A large proportion of patients with inflammatory conditions respond to nonoperative management, but untreated and progressive inflammation will eventually lead to gangrene and necrosis, with consequent perforation of the viscus and resultant generalized peritonitis.

Peritonitis

Generalized peritonitis usually manifests with the classic signs of tenderness, guarding, rigidity, and rebound tenderness (see Table 22.4). The abdomen may be distended and bowel sounds may be absent if the condition is established. Bowel contents, bile, urine, and blood are irritant to the peritoneum and generalized peritonitis can be due to a perforated viscus, mesenteric ischemia, strangulation of the bowel secondary to an internal or external hernia, or a volvulus, an intraperitoneal bleed, and due to rupture of a localized abscess into the general peritoneal cavity. Free intraperitoneal gas is not always present on chest X-ray and this is particularly true of appendicular and gallbladder perforations. A laparotomy is usually necessary after adequate resuscitation and although a preoperative diagnosis of the etiology is desirable, time must not be wasted in over-investigating a critically ill patient.

Nonspecific abdominal pain

It has been estimated that a cause for acute abdominal pain is not discovered in up to 40% of patients who are admitted to hospital.[9,10] Although no cause for the pain is found, these patients may have very real and distressing symptoms and it is important to reassure the patients that the diagnosis of nonspecific abdominal pain does not necessarily mean that there is no pain or no cause for it. Some of these patients may have tenderness in addition to the pain, but the signs are usually not enough to make a diagnosis of peritonitis. Most patients are young and almost two-thirds are female. The diagnosis is one of exclusion and patients must be observed for 24–48 h in order to ensure that there is no progression of the symptoms and signs. The pain usually subsides spontaneously. Undiagnosed causes of nonspecific abdominal pain include viral infections, parasitic infestations, gastroenteritis, mesenteric adenitis, ovulatory pain, and torsion of the appendices epiploicae of the colon. Some patients may have irritable bowel syndrome (see Chapter 64).

Munchausen's syndrome (spurious abdominal pain)

Globally there are a few patients who seek admission to hospital in the absence of genuine symptoms prompted by the need for a bed, drugs, attention, or help. Such patients usually present to the accident and emergency department with a dramatic history of an acute abdominal event. They can usually simulate appropriate physical signs and often appear to be in a great deal of distress. Many of these patients may be admitted for observation for several days before the true diagnosis is revealed. Patients may visit hospitals some distance from their area of domicile and other clues include a very meticulous history, early and repeated demands for opiate analgesia, and many previous admissions to hospital. In the classical case of Munchausen's syndrome, there are also multiple abdominal scars.[11]

Even when the diagnosis is suspected it is difficult to confront the patient and it is prudent to investigate the background by contacting doctors who have treated the patient in the past. Demands for pain relief should be met by the offer of nonopiate analgesics. Most patients leave the hospital, often without informing the staff, once this process of enquiry starts or when they fail to obtain the treatment sought.

DIAGNOSIS

History and examination

The two immediate goals in the diagnosis of acute abdominal pain are to decide if the patient needs admission to hospital and to ascertain whether the patient needs urgent or emergency surgery. Resuscitation may be needed prior to investigation or sometimes simultaneously, e.g., in patients who have pain secondary to trauma or an intra-abdominal hemorrhage.

A careful clinical history and examination then helps narrow down the diagnosis. The clinician should have a mental picture of the topography of the abdomen and correlate the symptoms and signs with the underlying anatomical structures and possible pathological diagnoses. Questions that should be asked whilst taking the history are outlined in Table 22.3. The age of the patient must also be considered when making a differential diagnosis. However, it must be remembered, for example, that even the elderly can get acute appendicitis, albeit rarely.

CAUSES OF ACUTE ABDOMINAL PAIN

RIGHT UPPER QUADRANT

Organ	Additional localization
Liver	Epigastrium Also referred to tip of shoulder
Biliary tract	May radiate to back along rib cage

EPIGASTRIC

Organ	Additional localization
Pancreas	R & L upper quadrants Radiates to back May be relieved by leaning forward
Stomach	Right & left upper quadrants
Duodenum	Right & left upper quadrants
Esophagus	Retrosternal

RIGHT OR LEFT LOWER QUADRANTS

Organ	Additional localization
L Colon	May then localize to area of inflammation of parietal peritoneum or become generalized
Urinary bladder	May radiate to base of penis
Uterus, ovaries Fallopian tubes	Right and left lower quadrants May be referred to the inner thighs May be generalized

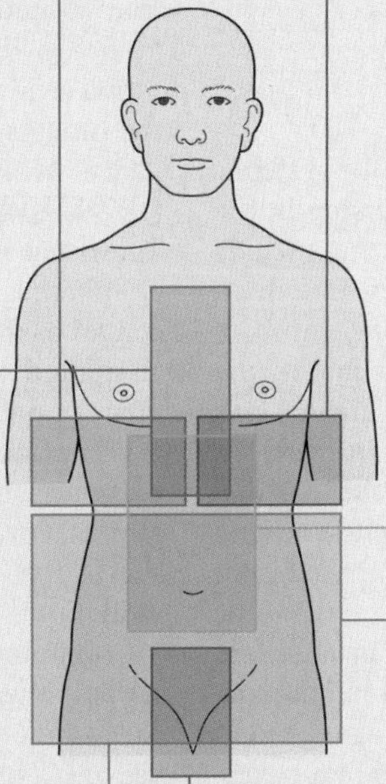

LEFT UPPER QUADRANT

Organ	Additional localization
Spleen	May radiate to flank

CENTRAL

Organ	Additional localization
Aorta	Epigastrium Periumbilical Flank Back May become generalized
Small bowel	May later localize to area of inflammation of parietal peritoneum
Appendix	Later localized to area of inflammation of parietal peritoneum or become generalized
R Colon	May then localize to area of inflammation of parietal peritoneum

LOIN TO GROIN

Organ	Additional localization
Kidneys/Ureters	May radiate to testes or labia

SCROTUM

Organ	Additional localization
Testes	Hypogastrium Right & left lower quadrant

OTHER

Abdominal wall	Abdominal trauma	Postoperative

Fig 22.3 Sites of acute abdominal pain.

TABLE 22.3 QUESTIONS TO ASK WHEN TAKING THE PATIENT HISTORY
When and where did the pain start?
Was the onset sudden and what brought the pain on?
Where is it now?
What is the character of the pain?
How severe is it?
Does the pain radiate elsewhere?
Are there any aggravating or relieving factors?
Has this happened before?
Are there any associated symptoms? (e.g., distention, nausea, vomiting, fever, diarrhea, absolute constipation, anorexia, jaundice, prutitus, gastrointestinal bleeding, dysuria, oliguria, chest pain)
When was your last period and is there any chance of you being pregnant?
History of alcohol intake
Drug (medicinal and recreational) history
History of previous surgery
History of pre-existing disease
History of travel, especially foreign travel
Family history

Patients with acute abdominal pain may manifest the systemic inflammatory response syndrome[12] and the initial step in the clinical examination is to document the vital signs that include pulse rate and rhythm, blood pressure, respiratory rate, temperature, and the Glasgow Coma Score.

The general physical examination must document the presence or absence of pallor, cyanosis, jaundice, edema, and lymphadenopathy. The abdomen should be examined with the patient lying supine with the arms at the side and the legs flat. The usual sequence of inspection, palpation, percussion, and auscultation must be followed with the abdomen exposed from nipples to mid thigh and the genitals covered.

Common clinical signs and their possible significance are listed in Table 22.4. The signs must be interpreted in conjunction with the history and the general condition, age, gender, and potential risk factors of the patient. The individual conditions listed in Tables 22.1 and 22.4 are described in more detail elsewhere in this textbook.

Initial management

The patient with acute abdominal pain may need resuscitation or emergency surgery and it is sensible to keep the patient nil by mouth and insert two large-bore venous cannulae at first contact. Intravenous fluids should be administered at an appropriate rate. Blood should be sampled at the time of insertion of the cannulae and sent to the laboratory for the investigations listed in Table 22.5. Arterial blood gas analysis should be performed if indicated. Laboratory tests may also help with the diagnosis of medical conditions such as diabetic ketoacidosis and adrenal crisis.

Patients who are hemodynamically unstable and those with copious vomiting or peritonitis will benefit from the insertion of a nasogastric tube and urinary catheter.

Pain relief

Many patients require substantial analgesia. A recent controlled trial[13] found no evidence that use of morphine affects diagnostic accuracy. Thus, establishing effective analgesia does not compromise investigation and treatment and probably facilitates the process.

Investigations and definitive management

The usual initial investigation is an erect chest and a supine abdominal X-ray (Table 22.5 and Figs 22.4–22.6). The widespread availability of high-quality ultrasonography and helical computed tomography (CT) has revolutionized the management of patients with acute abdominal pain.

Ultrasonography should be part of the routine work-up of these patients and in one study has been shown to increase the rate of correct diagnosis from 70% to 83%, leading to the suggestion that surgeons should develop expertise with this modality.[14]

Computed tomography (CT) scanning is very helpful in the stable patient (Figs 22.4, 22.6–22.8) and two recent prospective, randomized trials have demonstrated that routine early use of CT in the evaluation of acute abdominal pain can identify

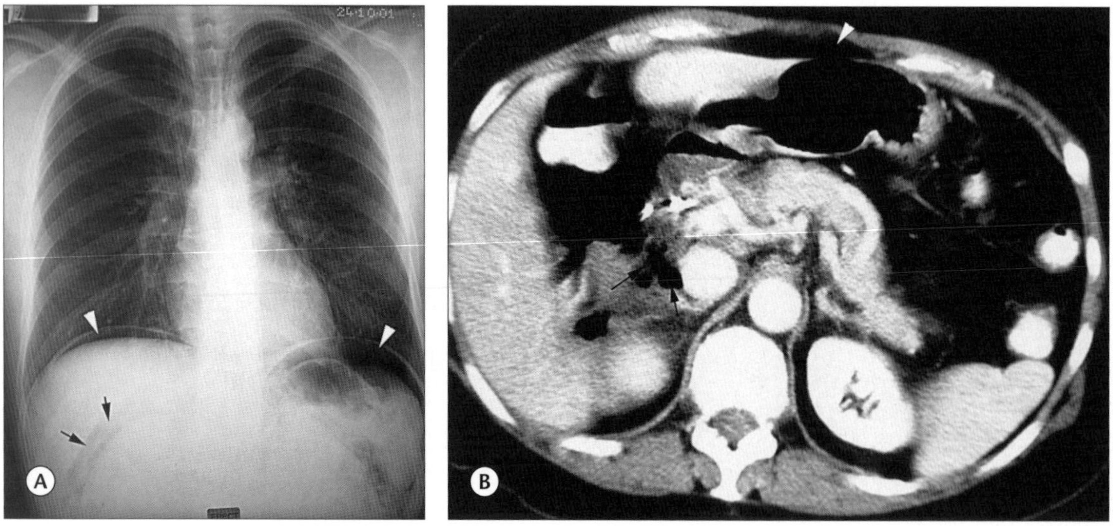

Fig. 22.4 Intraperitoneal and retroperitoneal gas. Chest X-ray **(A)** and abdominal CT scan **(B)** demonstrating both intraperitoneal (white arrowheads) and retroperitoneal (black arrows) gas. The patient had a duodenal perforation secondary to an endoscopic sphincterotomy.

TABLE 22.4 CLINICAL EXAMINATION OF THE ACUTE ABDOMEN

Sign	Definition/cautions	Implication
INSPECTION		
Distention		Ascites, obstruction, pseudo-obstruction, ileus, toxic dilatation, trauma, peritonitis, ovarian cyst
Bruising	Around umbilicus: Cullen's sign	Either can indicate: ruptured aortic aneurysm, acute pancreatitis
	In flank: Grey-Turner's sign	Grey-Turner also: retroperitoneal hemorrhage/inflammation
Visible peristalsis	May not be visible in the obese	Bowel obstruction
Regional fullness/ asymmetry		Organomegaly/mass
Hernia		Obstructed/strangulated hernia
Skin lesions	Scratch marks	Obstructive jaundice
	Pyoderma gangrenosum	Inflammatory bowel disease
	Sr. Joseph's nodule	Advanced cancer
	Acanthosis nigricans	Advanced cancer
Superficial veins	Caput medusae	Cirrhosis
	Caudal-cephalad flow	IVC obstruction
Surgical scars		Adhesions, recurrence of malignancy, incisional herniae
PALPATION		
Tenderness	Usually from parietal peritoneum	Patients can often accurately localize the site of most intense pain
Guarding	Voluntary	Peritoneal irritation
Rigidity	Involuntary, varies from minor to board-like	Established peritonitis
Rebound tenderness	Pain on rapid removal of hand, abdominal pain with coughing, Rovsing's sign (see Chapter 69)	Peritoneal irritation or peritonitis
Loin or costovertebral angle tenderness	Make the patient sit forward	Renal pathology, e.g., pyelonephritis
PERCUSSION		
Tympanic	Gaseous distention	Gas-filled bowel loops in obstruction Pneumoperitoneum
Dull	Usually fluid	Ascites, ovarian cyst, fluid-filled bowel loops
Shifting dullness, fluid thrill	Free fluid	Ascites, intraperitoneal bleed
AUSCULTATION		
Bowel sounds	Listen for at least a minute	
	Increased	Intestinal obstruction
	Tinkling	Paralytic ileus
	Absent	Paralytic ileus/peritonitis
Succussion splash	Shake patient with stethoscope on abdomen to elicit sloshing sound	Gas and fluid in an obstructed hollow organ (stomach or colon)
Bruit	Listen over aorta and renal vessels	Aneurysm or renal artery stenosis
Peritoneal rub	Similar to a pleural rub	Peritoneal irritation
OTHER TESTS		
Male genitalia		Hernias, hydroceles, torsions, and epididymoorchitis
Rectal examination	Feel the rectum, rectovesical (uterine) pouch and prostate. Inspect the stool on the glove	Rectal tumors, constipation, pelvic abscesses, rectal bleeding, and prostatic enlargement
Vaginal examination	In women with pelvic pain	Cervix, uterine and adnexal (ovarian, tubal) pathology
Psoas spasm	Inability to extend the hip completely	Psoas abscess, acute appendicitis (retrocecal)

unforeseen conditions and reduce length of hospital stay and overall mortality in patients with acute abdominal pain of unknown etiology.[15,16] However, the desire to obtain an accurate preoperative diagnosis should not be allowed to delay therapeutic intervention in the critically ill or unstable patient. Gastrointestinal contrast studies and endoscopy can be helpful in selected cases (Table 22.5) and early laparoscopy can provide a higher diagnostic accuracy and improved quality of life in patients with acute abdominal pain of uncertain etiology.[17] Finally, a laparotomy can be the ultimate diagnostic investigation in difficult cases, in addition to it being of therapeutic benefit.

TABLE 22.5 INVESTIGATIONS FOR ACUTE ABDOMINAL PAIN

Investigations	Subcategory/comment	Interpretation/usefulness
Full blood count	Hemoglobin ↓	Blood loss
	Hemoglobin ↑	Dehydration/hemoconcentration/polycythemia
	Leukocytes ↑	Inflammation or infection
	Leukocytes ↓	Overwhelming inflammation
	Platelets ↑	Active inflammatory bowel disease
	Platelets ↓	Overwhelming sepsis
Clinical chemistry	Creatinine ↑	Renal failure
	Urea ↑	Dehydration/hemoconcentration
	Electrolytes	
Serum amylase	Fourfold increase	Acute pancreatitis (but may be normal)
	Lesser increases	Almost any acute abdominal condition
Liver function tests	Biliary enzymes	Obstructive jaundice (but alkaline phosphatase slow to rise with acute obstruction)
	Transaminases/mixed	Acute liver injury, sepsis, cholangitis
Calcium	Calcium ↑	Medical cause of abdominal pain
Blood glucose	Glucose ↑	Ketoacidosis can cause abdominal pain
Culture	Urine/blood	Prelude to antibiotics
Group/cross match		Prelude to surgery, transfusion
Arterial blood gases	Acidosis and elevated lactate	?Mesenteric ischemia, illnesses severity, e.g., in acute pancreatitis
	PO_2	Latent hypoxia
Urinalysis	Stick tests	Blood and proteinuria (? infection) Ketones (starvation or ketoacidosis)
	Microscopy	Red cells, casts (? tubular necrosis), white cells (? infection)
	Culture	Infection
Pregnancy test		? Ruptured ectopic
Electrocardiogram		Myocardial infarction as cause of abdominal pain Preoperative investigation for patients over the age of 50 years
Supine abdominal X-ray	Intestinal lumen and wall pattern	Obstruction, ileus, IBD
	Calcification	Gallstones (10%), renal stones, pancreatic calcification, aortic rim
	Pneumobilia	Ascending cholangitis
	Foreign bodies	
	Skeletal abnormalities	
	Soft tissue masses	
Erect chest X-ray	Detection of free subdiaphragmatic air	Perforation. Also look at lung fields and cardiac contour
Lateral decubitus film	≥1 mL of free peritoneal gas can be visualized	Perforation
Abdominal ultrasound	Percutaneous ultrasound	Bile duct dilatation, gallstones, fluid collections, aortic aneurysms
	Transvaginal ultrasound	Gynecological causes
Abdominal CT scan	Value high especially with intravenous and intraluminal contrast enhancement	Multiple diagnoses Provides both anatomical and etiological diagnosis
Intravenous urography	Important if blood in the urine	Urological causes Useful in urological trauma
Magnetic resonance imaging	Not as popular as CT for the acute abdomen. MRCP	Excellent images of biliary tract pathology
Gastrointestinal contrast studies	Lower GI	Large bowel obstruction vs. pseudo-obstruction (may be therapeutic)
	Upper GI	Cryptic perforation or obstruction
Visceral angiography	Diagnostic	Intestinal ischemia, obscure bleeding
	Therapeutic	Embolization in gastrointestinal bleeding
Endoscopy	Upper and lower GI endoscopy	Helpful in selected cases
	Sigmoidoscopy	May be therapeutic for sigmoid volvulus
	ERCP	Therapeutic in biliary obstruction, especially ascending cholangitis
Laparoscopy	Increasingly popular, especially for the diagnosis of obscure acute abdominal pain	Therapeutic in duodenal ulcer perforations, acute cholecystitis, acute appendicitis, and gynecological conditions
Laparotomy	Ultimate arbiter in difficult cases	Also therapeutic

CONCLUSIONS

Over the past few decades there have been major advances in imaging modalities and laparoscopic techniques to facilitate the diagnosis of acute abdominal pain. Computer programs based on Bayesian reasoning and neural networks have been developed to help increase the diagnostic accuracy in this condition. However, despite the giant strides forward, only an astute clinician can obtain the information that is needed from a patient with acute abdominal pain, choose the best investigations, and plan appropriate treatment. The doctor who first

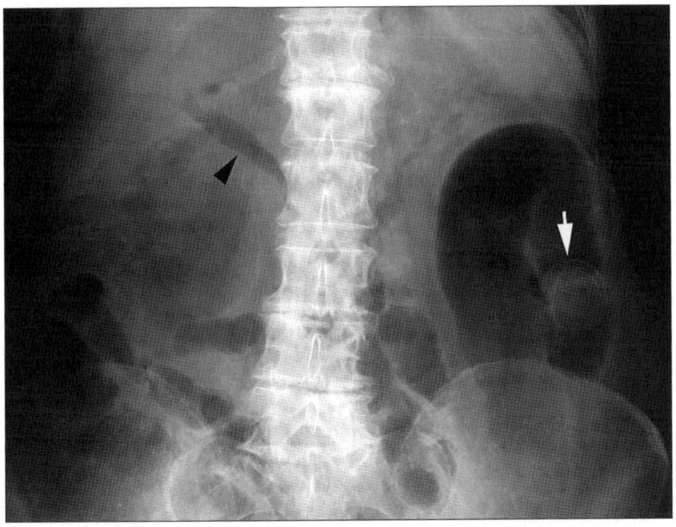

Fig. 22.5 **Gallstone ileus.** Supine abdominal X-ray demonstrating pneumobilia (black arrowhead) and a radiopaque gallstone obstructing the small bowel (white arrow).

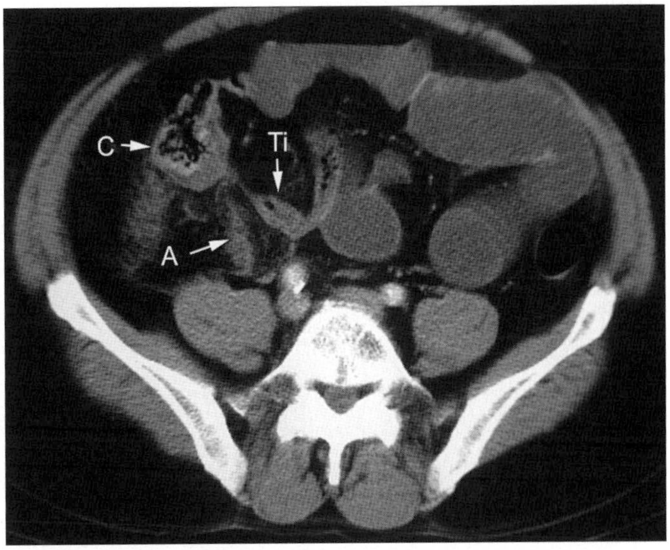

Fig. 22.7 Acute appendicitis. Pelvic CT scan of a patient with acute appendicitis. Ti, terminal ileum; C, cecum; A, inflamed appendix.

sees a patient with acute abdominal pain in hospital makes a correct diagnosis in 45% of cases. A combination of review of the patient by a senior clinician, analysis of the results of the investigations, and regular reassessment of the patient can improve the diagnostic accuracy to 75–80%. This leads to optimum treatment of the patient, with interventions planned at the appropriate time and a lower rate of negative surgical explorations.

If the patient deteriorates or fails to make progress after institution of treatment, the working diagnosis must be reassessed and the possibility of another coexisting condition must be entertained. Further investigations, and even the possibility of a diagnostic laparotomy must be considered in this situation. The acute abdomen has been likened to Pandora's box, containing all the evils of the world. Sometimes, it is necessary to open this box and let the evils out!

SOURCES OF INFORMATION FOR PATIENTS AND DOCTORS

http://www.patient.co.uk/showdoc/40000215/

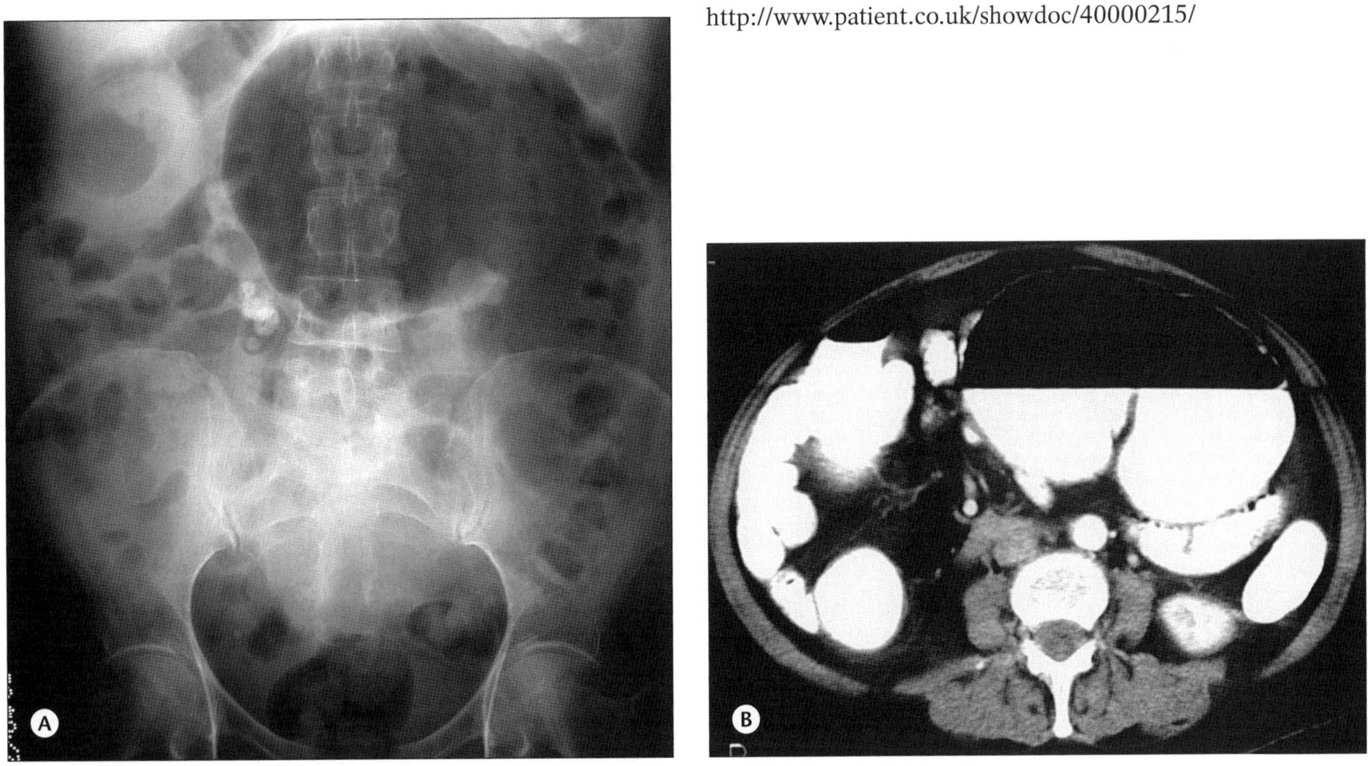

Fig. 22.6 Cecal volvulus. Supine abdominal X-ray **(A)** and contrast-enhanced CT scan **(B)** of a patient with a cecal volvulus.

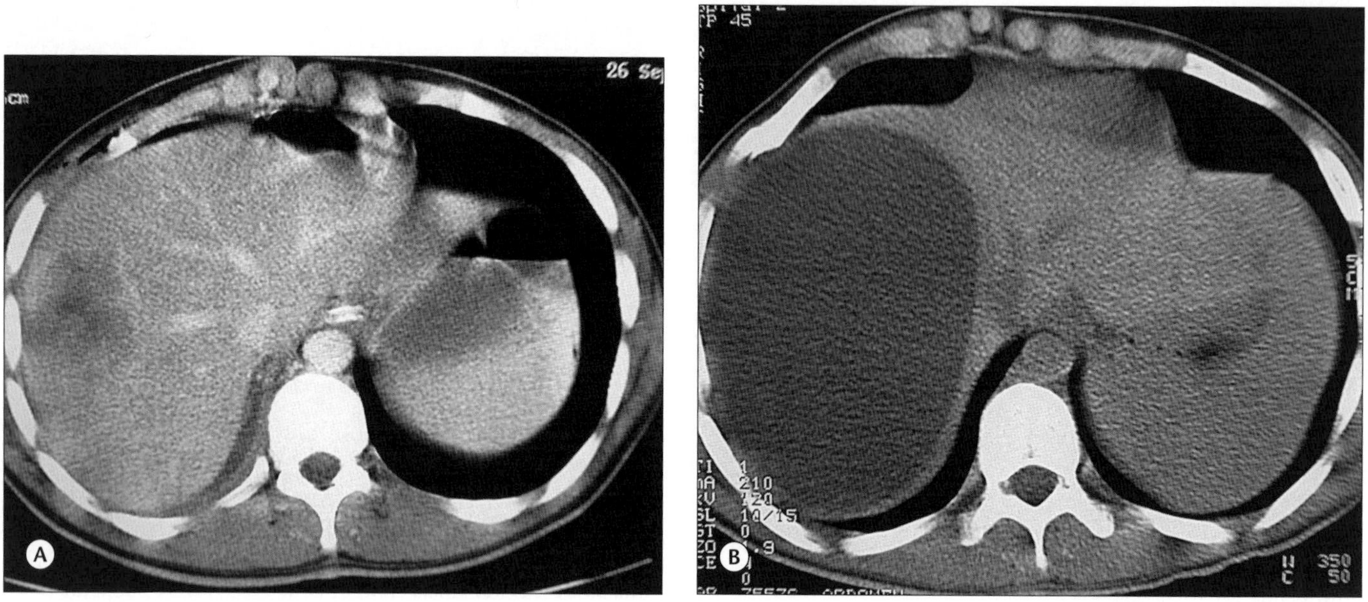

Fig. 22.8 Liver hematoma expansion. Abdominal CT scans done at admission **(A)** and 3 days later **(B)** showing expansion of a liver hematoma in a patient who sustained blunt abdominal trauma.

REFERENCES

1. Merskey H, Bogduk N. Classification of chronic pain: descriptions of chronic pain syndromes and definition of pain terms. Report by the International Association for the Study of Pain Task Force on Taxonomy, 2nd edn. Seattle: IASP Press; 1994.
2. Carr DB, Cousins MJ. Spinal route of analgesics: opioids and future options. In: Cousins MJ, Bridenbaugh PO, eds. Neural blockade in clinical anaesthesia and management of pain, 3rd edn. Philadelphia: Lippincott-Raven; 1998.
3. Carr DB, Goudas LC. Acute pain. Lancet 1999; 353:2051–2058.
4. Cervero F, Laird JM. Visceral pain. Lancet 1999; 353:2145–2148.
5. Kamin RA, Nowicki TA, Courtney DS, Powers RD. Pearls and pitfalls in the emergency department evaluation of abdominal pain. Emerg Med Clin North Am 2003; 21:61–72.
6. Graff IV LG, Robinson D. Abdominal pain and emergency department evaluation. Emerg Med Clin North Am 2001; 19:123–136.
7. Ellis BW, Rivett RC, Dudley HA. Extending the use of clinical audit data: a resource planning model. BMJ 1990; 301:159–162.
8. Besson JM. The neurobiology of pain. Lancet 1999; 353:1610–1615.
9. Gray DW, Collin J. Non-specific abdominal pain as a cause of acute admission to hospital. Br J Surg 1987;74:239–242.
10. Irvin TT. Abdominal pain: a surgical audit of 1190 emergency admissions. Br J Surg 1989; 76:1121–1125.
11. Huffman JC, Stern TA. The diagnosis and treatment of Munchausen's syndrome. Gen Hosp Psychiatry 2003; 25:358–363.
12. Bone RC. Sir Isaac Newton, sepsis, SIRS and CARS. Crit Care Med 1996; 24:1125–1128.
13. Thomas SH, Silen W, Cheema F et al. Effects of morphine analgesia on diagnostic accuracy in Emergency Department patients with abdominal pain: a prospective, randomized trial. J Am Coll Surg 2003; 196:18–31.
14. Allemann F, Cassina P, Rothlin M, Largiader F. Ultrasound scans done by surgeons for patients with acute abdominal pain: a prospective study. Eur J Surg 1999; 165:966–970.
15. Ng CS, Watson CJ, Palmer CR et al. Evaluation of early abdominopelvic computed tomography in patients with acute abdominal pain of unknown cause: prospective randomised study. BMJ 2002; 325:1387.
16. Tsushima Y, Yamada S, Aoki J, Motojima T, Endo K. Effect of contrast-enhanced computed tomography on diagnosis and management of acute abdomen in adults. Clin Radiol 2002; 57:507–513.
17. Decadt B, Sussman L, Lewis MP et al. Randomized clinical trial of early laparoscopy in the management of acute non-specific abdominal pain. Br J Surg 1999; 86:1383–1386.

Chapter 23

Hematemesis and melena

James Y W Lau and S C Sydney Chung

INTRODUCTION

Hematemesis is defined as vomiting of blood or blood clots whereas melena is defined as passage of dark, tarry stool with a characteristic foul smell (Fig. 23.1). Both are signs that suggest an upper gastrointestinal (GI) source of bleeding. Fresh hematemesis is often a reliable sign signifying ongoing or active bleeding. Occasionally, vomiting of swallowed blood from hemoptysis or bleeding from upper aerodigestive tract, e.g., nasopharynx, can confuse the diagnosis. Melena occurs when hemoglobin is converted to hematin or other hemochromes by bacterial degradation. This can be produced experimentally by the ingestion of as little as 100–200 mL of blood. An increased blood urea (BUN): creatinine ratio assuming a normal baseline level can aid the diagnosis of upper GI bleeding. Blood is absorbed by the small intestine causing raised blood urea. Some of this azotemia is probably secondary to hypovolemia as experimental ingestion of blood results in lower elevation in BUN of shorter duration.

If the volume of an upper GI hemorrhage is large, the patient may present with hematochezia (passage of fresh blood per rectum). An endoscopic examination should be considered if there is any question about the location of bleeding in a patient with hematochezia. Conversely, if the volume of bleeding is small but sufficient to supply enough hemoglobin for degradation, and if colonic motility is sufficiently slow, bleeding from the small bowel or proximal colon may cause melena. Small bowel bleeding is however uncommon. Bleeding from colonic sources, e.g., tumors, is either slow, leading to anemia or hemoccult positive stool, or rapid, such as in diverticular disease leading to hematochezia. A high BUN-to-creatinine ratio may indicate bleeding from an upper rather than a lower GI source.

Coffee ground vomiting is a good sign when it is witnessed. However, it can be confused with vomiting from bowel obstruction.

HOW COMMON IS IT?

Upper GI bleeding is a common medical emergency that carries a substantial mortality. In a recent UK population-based audit involving four health regions over a period of 4 months, a total of 4185 admissions with upper GI bleeding were identified.[1] The overall incidence was 103 cases per 100 000 adults/year. The median age of the sample population was 71 and only 44% were aged <60 years. Compared to historical series over the past few decades, this study found an aging population of patients with upper GI bleeding. Overall mortality for this cohort of patients was 14%. Mortality was 11% for those admitted because of upper GI bleeding and this increased to 33% when including those patients who developed bleeding, having already been admitted for another reason. Mortality among those admitted with bleeding increases with age: 3% in those <60 years to 20% in those >80 years. One or more co-morbidities were present in 83% of those who died from the condition.

CAUSES

In about 20% of patients, a diagnosis is not made. Among the remaining patients, peptic ulcers are the commonest cause, constituting 43% of cases.

For practical management, upper GI bleeding can also be categorized into variceal and nonvariceal bleeding because of their different prognosis.

DIAGNOSIS AND MORTALITY BY CAUSE OF BLEEDING[a]

Diagnosis	No. (%)	Mortality (%)
None made	1014 (25)	20
Peptic ulcer	1448 (35)	12
Malignancy	155 (4)	37
Varices	180 (4)	23
Mallory-Weiss syndrome	214 (5)	3
Erosive disease	444 (11)	7
Esophagitis	429 (10)	8
Other diagnosis	253 (6)	18
Total	4137	14

[a]Adapted from Rockall et al. BMJ 1995; 311:222–226.[1] With permission from the BMJ Publishing Group.

PATIENT ASSESSMENT

Figure 23.2 outlines an algorithm on the management of patients presenting with upper GI bleeding.[2,3]

Bleeding has already stopped spontaneously in about 80% of patients presenting with upper GI bleeding. In the management of patients with upper GI bleeding, it is essential to categorize patients into those with low or high risk of continued bleeding and death. Those judged to be of high risk should be admitted to high dependency areas and considered for urgent endoscopy.

Resuscitation is the first priority in the management of patients with upper GI bleeding. Table 23.1 provides a schema

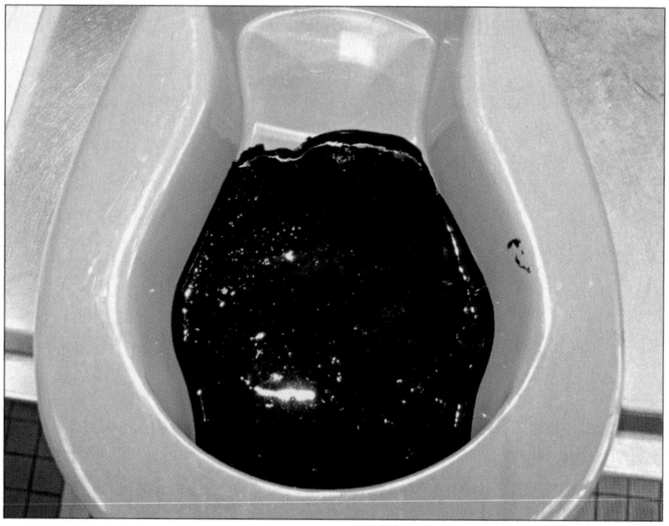

Fig. 23.1 Melena stool.

on the assessment of volume deficit. This should be corrected by fluid and blood in those judged to have had severe bleeding. In those with impaired mental status, their airways should be protected and often orotracheal intubation is required prior to endoscopy. Large-bore intravenous cannulae should be sited for rapid fluid administration. A urinary catheter is useful, especially with hemodynamic compromise, to detect dysuria. A central venous catheter is useful for monitoring volume replacement, particularly in those with incipient heart failure.

Physical examination may reveal stigmata of chronic liver disease that may call for specific treatments such as vasoactive drugs, antibiotics, and drugs to prevent encephalopathy. The findings of buccal pigmentation may alert to the diagnosis of Peutz-Jegher syndrome. A history of aortic surgery raises the possibility of an aorto-enteric fistula. Hemoglobin is a poor estimation of blood loss as even at an acute stage, hemoglobin drop may not be significant. Hematocrit is of value in assessing degree of dilution.

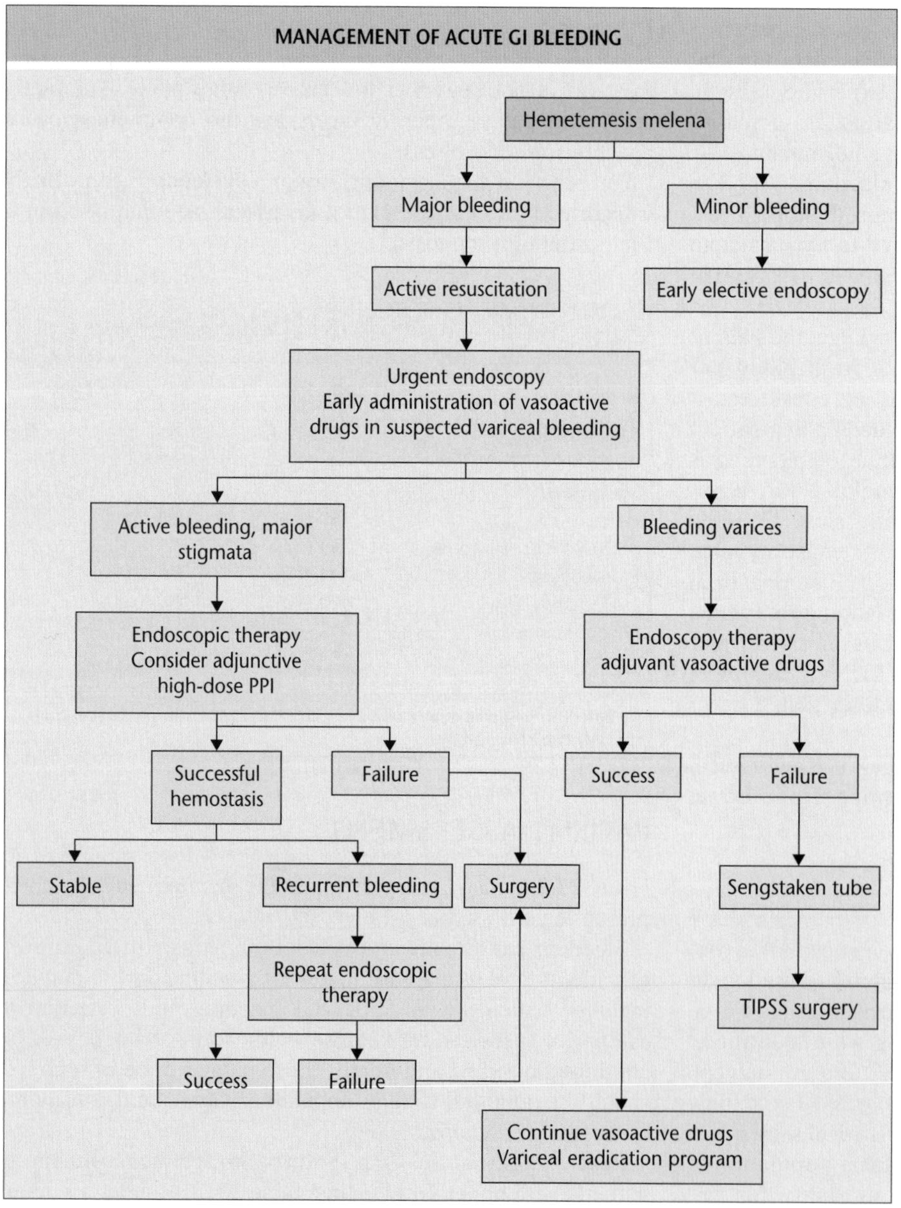

Fig. 23.2 Algorithm for the management of acute GI bleeding.

TABLE 23.1 HYPOVOLEMIC SHOCK: SYMPTOMS, SIGNS, AND FLUID REPLACEMENT

Blood loss (ml)	<750	750–1500	1500–2000	>2000
Blood loss (%)	<15	15–30	30–40	>40
Pulse rate	<100	>100	>120	>140
Blood pressure	Normal	Normal	Decreased	Decreased
Pulse pressure	Normal or increased	Decreased	Decreased	Decreased
Respiratory rate	14–20	20–30	30–40	>35
Urine output (ml)	>30	20–30	30–40	>35
Mental status	Slightly anxious	Mildly anxious	Anxious and confused	Confused and lethargic
Fluid replacement	Crystalloid	Crystalloid	Crystalloid and blood	Crystalloid and blood

Based on data derived from the National United Kingdom Audit, Rockall et al. defined independent risk factors predictive of death. These included age, co-morbidity, shock, and endoscopic findings (Table 23.2).[4] A score of 3 or less is associated with favorable prognosis whereas a score greater than 8 carries grave prognosis (Table 23.3). The decision for the need for urgent endoscopy and possible therapy is often a matter of clinical judgment based on the patient's age, the severity of bleeding episode, and co-morbidities. An elderly patient with end organ failure is unlikely to tolerate a large blood loss and therefore will benefit from earlier intervention. Fresh hematemesis and shock are signs of rapid exsanguination. Urgent endoscopy becomes mandatory after initial resuscitation with a view to stop bleeding.

ENDOSCOPY

Whether carrying out endoscopy early on improves a patient's outcome is controversial. The majority of endoscopic procedures can be scheduled for the next available session, ideally on the following morning. In a few selected patients with signs of ongoing bleeding, urgent endoscopy with therapy may however be lifesaving. Endoscopic procedures should be performed by medical or surgical gastroenterologists with expertise in therapeutic endoscopy in a unit supported by appropriate staff, and monitoring and resuscitation equipment. Endoscopy localizes the source of bleeding. The endoscopic appearance or stigmata of bleeding have prognostic implications. Therapy may be offered at the time of endoscopy to either stop active bleeding or prevent recurrent bleeding.

TABLE 23.2 ROCKALL SCORING SYSTEM FOR RISK OF REBLEEDING AND DEATH AFTER ADMISSION TO HOSPITAL FOR ACUTE GI BLEEDING

SCORE	0	1	2	3
Age (years)	<60	60–79	≥80	
Shock	No shock (systolic BP >100, pulse <100)	Tachycardia (systolic BP >100, pulse >100)	Hypotension (systolic BP <100, pulse >100)	
Co-morbidity	Nil major		Cardiac failure, ischemic heart disease, any major co-morbidity	Renal failure, liver failure, disseminated malignancy
Diagnosis	Mallory-Weiss tear, no lesion, and no SRH	All other diagnoses	Malignancy of upper GI tract	
Major SRH	None or dark spot		Blood in upper GI tract, adherent clot, visible or spurting vessel	

Each variable is scored and the total score calculated by simple addition.
SRH, stigmata of recent hemorrhage.

TABLE 23.3 OBSERVED REBLEED AND MORTALITY BY PRE-ENDOSCOPY SCORE AND COMPLETE RISK SCORE

Score	0	1	2	3	4	5	6	7	8+
OBSERVED MORTALITY BY PRE-ENDOSCOPY SCORE									
Deaths (%)	0.2	2.4	5.6	11.0	24.6	39.6	48.9	50.0	
OBSERVED REBLEEDING AND MORTALITY BY COMPLETE RISK SCORE									
Rebleed	4.9	3.4	5.3	11.2	14.1	24.1	32.9	43.8	41.8
Deaths (%)	0	0	0.2	2.9	5.3	10.8	17.3	27.0	41.1

BLEEDING PEPTIC ULCERS

Bleeding peptic ulcers are categorized into those that are actively bleeding (Forrest I; Fig. 23.3), ulcers that exhibit stigmata of recent bleeding (nonbleeding visible vessel defined as protuberant discoloration (II a; Fig. 23.4), an adherent clot (II b; Fig. 23.5), and flat pigmentations (II c; Fig. 23.6)), and a clean base ulcer (Forrest III; Fig. 23.7). Their prevalence, risks of further bleeding, and need for surgery is summarized in Table 23.4.

Endoscopic therapy is clearly indicated in ulcers that are actively bleeding. Therapy in ulcers with nonbleeding visible vessels reduces the risk of recurrent bleeding. It is controversial whether clots overlying ulcer craters should be removed. Findings from a small, randomized study suggested that removal of clots and treatment of underlying vessels reduced risk of recurrent bleeding.[6] A diligent search of ulcer craters should be made to look for a vessel. Most would use a combination of injection and thermocoagulation. Ulcers are preinjected with diluted epinephrine followed by coagulation of the bleeding vessel using a contact thermal device. Ulcers with flat pigmentations or a clean base are associated with small or negligible risk of recurrent bleeding. No endoscopic therapy

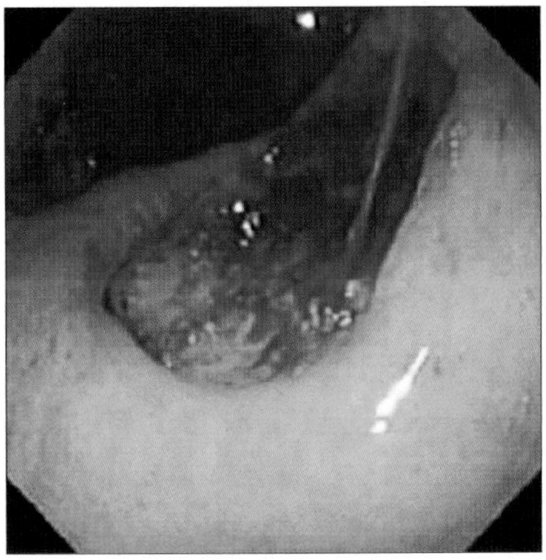

Fig. 23.3 Ulcer with spurting hemorrhage.

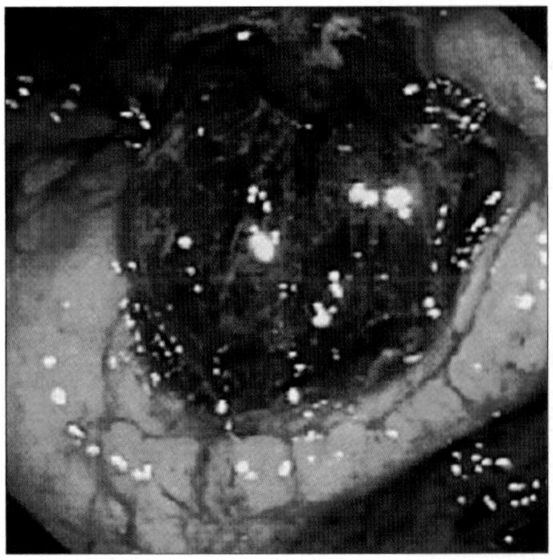

Fig. 23.5 Ulcer with an adherent clot.

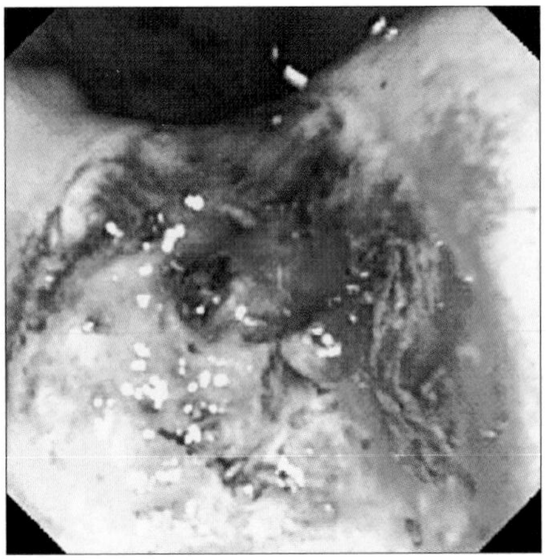

Fig. 23.4 Nonbleeding visible vessel ulcer.

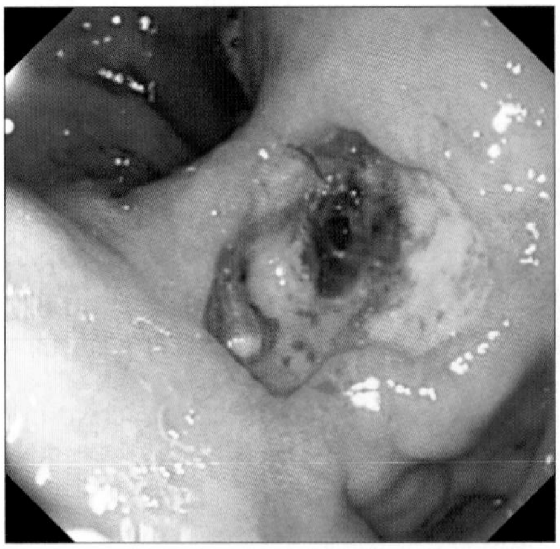

Fig. 23.6 Ulcer with a flat pigmentation.

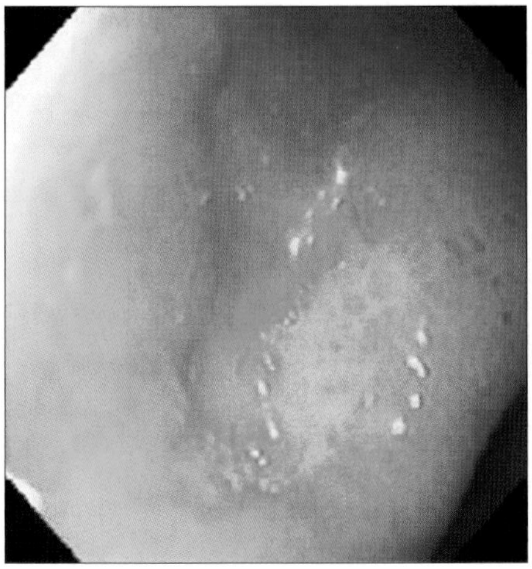

Fig. 23.7 Ulcer with a clean base.

is indicated. Patients can resume a normal diet soon after endoscopy and can be discharged early.

After securing hemostasis in actively bleeding ulcers and ulcers with high-risk stigmata, an adjuvant high-dose proton pump inhibitor (PPI) has been shown to reduce recurrent bleeding. Only a high-dose PPI can render intragastric pH neutral. This in theory promotes platelet aggregation and stabilizes clots overlying arteries. Peterson and Cook summarized the literature on published randomized studies that compared high-dose PPI to either placebo or histamine antagonist infusion and concluded that a high-dose PPI regimen would reduce further bleeding after endoscopic control of bleeding.[7] A subsequent large-scale single center placebo controlled trial confirmed that an adjuvant use of high-dose PPI was beneficial.[8]

Recurrent bleeding after initial endoscopic control carries substantial mortality. It is reasonable to repeat endoscopic therapy. Early recourse to surgery is however advisable in larger ulcers and in those with episodes of hypotension.[9] Surgery is considered the most definitive method of controlling bleeding. Postoperative mortality however occurs in around 20–25% of patients.

TABLE 23.4 BLEEDING ULCERS: PREVALENCE, RISK AND NEED FOR SURGERY

Endoscopic characteristics	Prevalence (%)	Further bleeding (%)	Surgery (%)	Mortality (%)
Clean base	42	5	0.5	2
Flat spot	20	10	6	3
Adherent clot	17	22	10	7
Nonbleeding visible vessel	17	43	34	11
Active bleeding	18	55	35	11

Data are from patients in prospective trials that did not receive endoscopic therapy. Modified from Laine L and Peterson WL. N Engl J Med 1994; 331:717–727.[5]

BLEEDING ESOPHAGOGASTRIC VARICES

The average mortality of the first episode of variceal bleeding approaches 50%. Mortality from subsequent bleeds decreases to around 5–50% depending on the severity of liver disease as indicated by the Child-Pugh grading system (Fig. 23.8).

The best treatment option for acute variceal bleeding includes vasoactive drugs and endoscopic therapy. Early administration of vasoactive drugs either in the form of vasopressin or its analog or somatostatin or its analogs reduces portal venous blood flow and variceal pressure.[10] This makes subsequent endoscopic treatment easier by stopping or slowing bleeding. Vasoactive drugs should be continued after endoscopic control to prevent recurrent bleeding. Ocasionally, with massive bleeding, temporary passage of a Sengstaken tube (with orotracheal protection of the airway) is a necessary prelude to endoscopy.

In up to 50% of cirrhotic patients presenting with upper GI bleeding, the bleeding source is nonvariceal. An urgent endoscopy enables the determination of the site and cause of bleeding. This has therapeutic and prognostic implications. Orotracheal intubation is often required in patients with variceal bleeding in order to protect their airways against aspiration, especially in those obtunded with encephalopathy.

Emergency endoscopic treatment is often associated with transient bacteremia. The administration of prophylactic antibiotics decreases the incidence of clinical infections such as bacterial peritonitis. Antibiotic prophylaxis is recommended for all patients with cirrhosis.

Band ligation is the preferred method in the treatment of esophagogastric varices as it is associated with less local complications when compared to endoscopic sclerotherapy. Gastric varices can be divided into those in continuity with esophageal varices and those that occur in isolation. Isolated fundal varices are associated with high risk of recurrent bleeding and death. In the control of acute bleeding, histoacryl glue injection appears to be the only effective method (Fig. 23.9). Many would consider a transjugular intrahepatic portosystemic shunt (TIPS) or early shunt surgery as an alternative.

In those patients where endoscopic therapy fails, a Sengstaken tube can tamponade bleeding in about 90% of cases; however, following deflation of the balloons, recurrent bleeding occurs in about 50%. A definitive plan is required including a repeat trial of endoscopic therapy, TIPSS, or surgery.

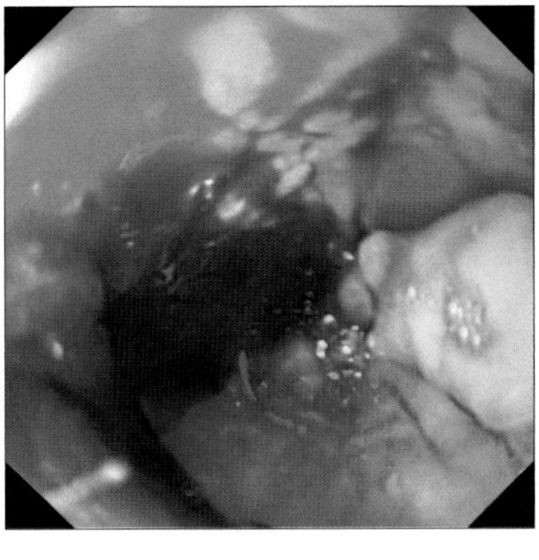

Fig. 23.8 A bleeding varix with a fibrin clot.

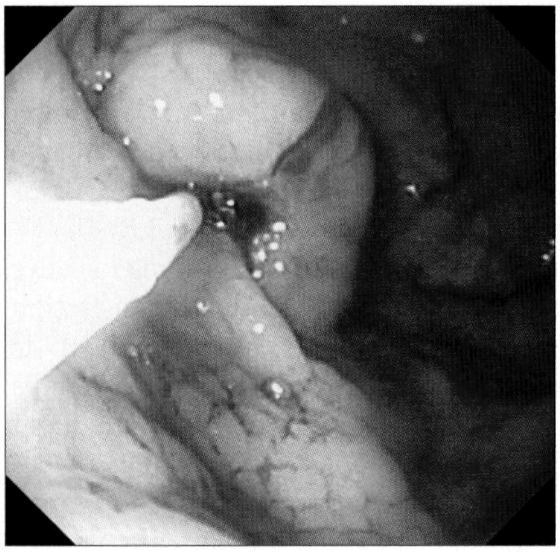

Fig. 23.9 Histoacryl glue injection of a gastric varix with a fresh clot.

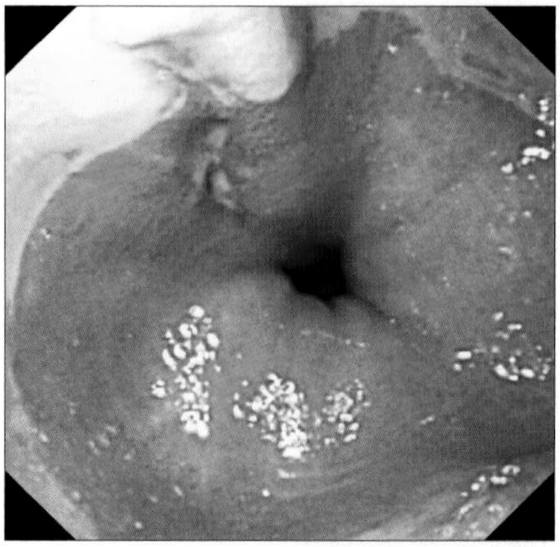

Fig. 23.10 Mallory-Weiss tear.

MISCELLANEOUS CAUSES OF UPPER GI BLEEDING

Other causes of upper GI bleeding are uncommon. Fresh hematemesis that occurs after emesis is typical of a Mallory-Weiss tear (Fig. 23.10). The condition is often self-limiting and carries an excellent prognosis. Other causes include neoplasms, vascular ectasia, and vascular malformations (Fig. 23.11).

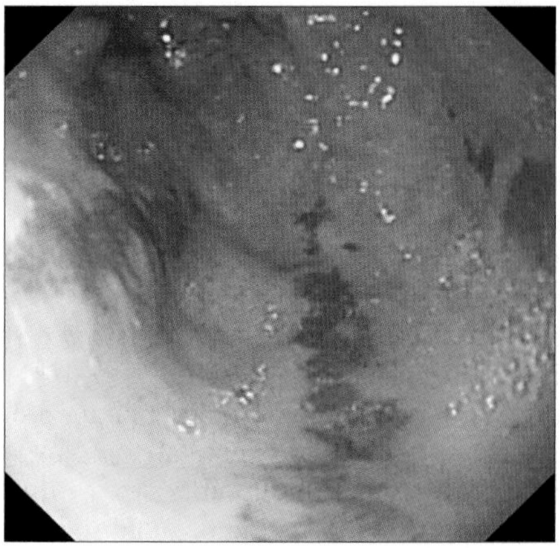

Fig. 23.11 Vascular malformation of gastric antrum.

SOURCES OF INFORMATION FOR PATIENTS AND DOCTORS

http://www.clevelandclinic.org/gastro/endoscopy/patient/bleeding.htm

REFERENCES

1. Rockall TA, Logan RFA, Devlin HB et al. Incidence of and mortality from acute upper gastrointestinal haemorrhage in the United Kingdom. BMJ 1995; 311:222–226.
2. British Society of Gastroenterology Endoscopy Committee. Non-variceal upper gastrointestinal haemorrhage: guidelines. Gut 2002; 51(Suppl 4):iv1–iv6.
3. Jalan R, Hayes PC. UK guidelines on the management of variceal haemorrhage in cirrhotic patients. Gut 2000; 46(Suppl 3):iii1–iii15.
4. Rockall TA, Logan RFA, Devlin HB et al. Risk assessment following acute gastrointestinal haemorrhage. Gut 1996; 38:316–321.
5. Laine L, Peterson WL. Bleeding peptic ulcer. N Engl J Med 1994; 331:717–727.
6. Jensen DM, Kovacs TO, Jutabha R et al. Randomized trial of medical or endoscopic therapy to prevent recurrent ulcer hemorrhage in patients with adherent clots. Gastroenterology 2002; 123:407–413.
7. Peterson WL, Cook DJ. Antisecretory therapy for bleeding peptic ulcer. JAMA 1998; 280: 363–365.
8. Lau JY, Sung JJ, Lee KK et al. Effect of intravenous omeprazole on recurrent bleeding after endoscopic treatment of bleeding peptic ulcers. N Engl J Med 2000; 343:310–316.
9. Lau JY, Sung JJ, Lam YH et al. Endoscopic retreatment compared with surgery in patients with recurrent bleeding after initial endoscopic control of bleeding ulcers. N Engl J Med 1999; 340:751–756.
10. Cales P, Masliah C, Bernard B et al. Early administration of vapreotide for variceal bleeding in patients with cirrhosis. French Club for the study of portal hypertension. N Engl J Med 2001; 344:23–28.

Chapter
24

Acute lower gastrointestinal bleeding

Thomas O G Kovacs and Dennis M Jensen

INTRODUCTION

Acute lower gastrointestinal (LGI) bleeding, defined as bleeding from a site distal to the duodenum (most commonly the colon), has an annual hospitalization rate of about 20 per 100 000 adults.[1,2] If the patient presents with severe hematochezia, clinicians cannot determine the site of the lesion clinically as foregut, midgut, or colon. Even without a history or signs of upper gastrointestinal (UGI) lesions, approximately 15–20% of patients hospitalized with severe hematochezia have a foregut (UGI or proximal jejunum) source of the severe hematochezia. In most ambulatory patients with hematochezia, the bleeding stops spontaneously, permitting elective diagnostic evaluation. However, some patients with severe hematochezia require urgent attention to minimize further bleeding and complications. Mortality rates still range between 3% and 5% because the incidence of LGI bleeding increases markedly in the elderly, and these patients frequently have significant co-morbidity.[1,3]

WHAT IS IT?

The primary criterion for identifying a definitive source of bleeding is visualized stigmata of recent hemorrhage (active bleeding, nonbleeding visible vessel, an adherent clot for colonic lesions, or flat spots for ulcers) on the lesion. A lesion is classified as the 'presumptive cause' of the bleeding when fresh blood is in that location (such as the colon) or a lesion is found there without stigmata and no other likely bleeding sites are identified on colonoscopy, anoscopy, and enteroscopy. The term angioma as used here is synonymous with others' usage of angiodysplasia, arteriovenous malformations, and vascular ectasia.

In a large series of patients with severe hematochezia of presumed LGI origin, 15.3% had an UGI source (such as an ulcer, varices, or angioma), 1.3% had a small bowel source, and 2.4% had no identified source.[4] The most common colonic cause was diverticulosis (either presumed or definitive), followed by internal hemorrhoids, ischemic colitis, rectal ulcers, delayed bleeding from postpolypectomy ulcers, colonic polyps or cancer, and colonic angiomas or radiation telangiectasia[4] (Table 24.1). The findings at urgent colonoscopy permit triage of low-risk patients (without stigmata of hemorrhage and/or severe comorbidity) to less intensive and less expensive care, which often facilitates early discharge.

CAUSES

Diverticulosis

Diverticular bleeding is the most common cause for patients hospitalized with severe hematochezia. Although diverticulosis most often involves the sigmoid and descending colon, about 50% of diverticular bleeding originates proximal to the splenic flexure. Definitive diverticular hemorrhage[5,6] is treated with epinephrine injection, multipolar probe coagulation, and metallic clips at sites of active bleeding (Fig. 24.1), visible vessel (Fig. 24.2), or adherent clot (Fig. 24.3) associated with a specific diverticulum. Approximately 20% of patients with diverticular bleeding have stigmata of definitive hemorrhage, 30% have presumed diverticular bleeding, and 50% have incidental diverticulosis with another definitive site.[5] Rebleeding and complications are rare from endoscopic therapy. Medical therapy should consist of fiber and stool softeners to control constipation; risk factors for rebleeding include aspirin, nonsteroidal antiinflammatory drugs (NSAIDs), anticoagulants, and ginkgo. Clearly the use of NSAIDs may be essential in some patients with debilitating arthritis, and some patients require anticoagulation for potentially life-threatening cardiac events. In those settings the physician must make a risk–benefit assessment. Some advocate the longstanding admonition to avoid small hard seeds, popcorn, and nut shells. Approximately 3% will rebleed during the next 3 years.

Management: Active bleeding (see Fig. 24.1) or adherent clots (see Fig. 24.3) should be treated with a 1:10 000 epinephrine:saline injection in 1–2-mL aliquots for shallow broad-based diverticula.[5,6] After epinephrine injection, adherent clots can be safely guillotined off with a snare, similar to peptic ulcers with adherent clots. After the bleeding stops and for nonbleeding visible vessels (see Fig. 24.2), multipolar coagulation with 10–14 watts of power can then be applied using moderate pressure and a 1-s pulse duration until the vessel is flattened and

TABLE 24.1 SOURCE OF COLONIC BLEEDING IN 300 PATIENTS HOSPITALIZED WITH SEVERE HEMATOCHEZIA[4]

Diagnosed lesion	Frequency (%)[a]
COLONIC SOURCE	81.0
Diverticulosis	29.6
Internal hemorrhoids	14.0
Ischemic colitis	12.3
Rectal ulcers	9.1
Ulcerative colitis, Crohn's disease, other colitis	8.2
Postpolypectomy ulcer	7.4
Colonic polyp or colonic cancer	6.2
Colon angiomas or radiation telangiectasia	5.7
Other LGI diagnosis	7.5

[a] Expressed as a percentage of total colorectal sources.

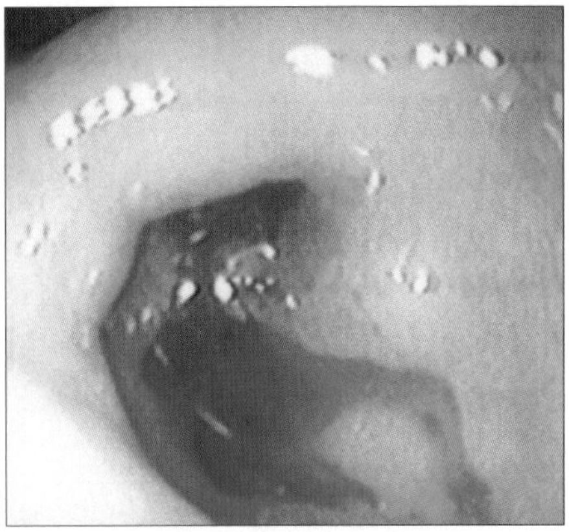

Fig. 24.1 Bleeding diverticulum.

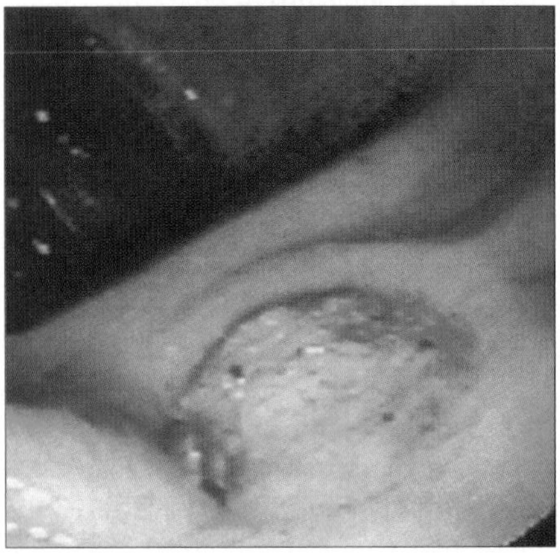

Fig. 24.2 Diverticulum with nonbleeding visible vessel.

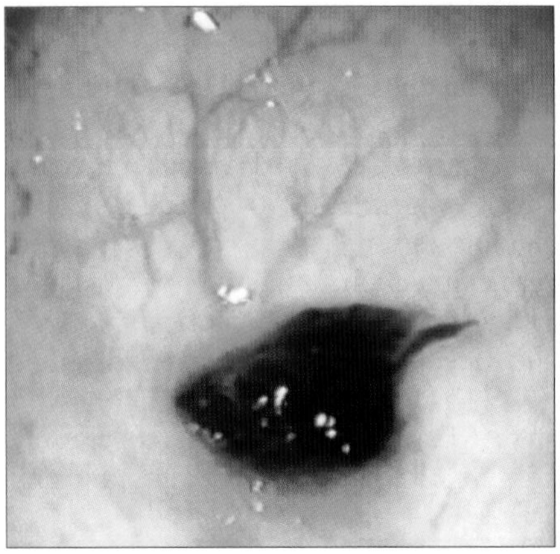

Fig. 24.3 Clot on diverticulum.

adequate coagulation has been achieved. India ink labeling of the diverticulum with the major stigmata (active bleed, visible vessel, or clot) after successful endoscopic hemostasis will facilitate localization, endoscopic retreatment (if necessary), surgery in case of early rebleeding, and histopathologic correlation.

Internal hemorrhoids

Internal hemorrhoids are the most common cause of LGI bleeding in outpatient ambulatory adults, and the second most common cause of severe hematochezia in patients hospitalized with presumed LGI hemorrhage.[7] Most patients with internal hemorrhoids have self-limiting, mild bleeding manifested by bright red blood on the toilet tissue. Medical therapy consists of fiber supplementation, stool softeners, low-dose hydrocortisone containing suppositories designed for treatment of hemorrhoids, and Sitz baths. Despite medical treatment, bleeding may be recurrent and frequent, resulting in iron deficiency and anemia. Occasionally, internal hemorrhoids may bleed profusely and require emergency hemostasis[8] (Fig. 24.4).

Management: The anal canal should be examined by anoscopy and, if not diagnostic, by retroflexion in the rectum with a flexible sigmoidoscope. With a slotted anoscope, active bleeding from internal hemorrhoids or stigmata of hemorrhage (such as an adherent clot) will confirm the diagnosis and facilitate bedside treatment. For inpatients, rubber-band ligation can be used for emergency hemostasis of bleeding internal hemorrhoids[8] (Fig. 24.4). Emergency colonoscopy can be obviated in such cases. Surgery is required for patients with continued severe bleeding not responding to anoscopic treatment.

Focal ulcers or colitis

Focal ulcers proximal to the sigmoid colon are an uncommon cause of severe LGI hemorrhage. In one large series these accounted for the bleeding site in 8% of patients[4] (Table 24.1). Bleeding colonic ulcers were caused by: recent polypectomy with ulceration (Fig. 24.5), inflammatory bowel disease (IBD), ischemic ulcers (Fig. 24.6), or infectious colitis (e.g., pseudomembranous colitis, cytomegalovirus ulcers). The most common cause was delayed bleeding from an induced ulcer, 3–10 days after piecemeal polypectomy of a large sessile polyp (see Fig. 24.5). This is more common in patients who resume aspirin, NSAIDs, anticoagulants, or ginkgo after polypectomy. Patients with severe hematochezia after recent polypectomy should have an oral

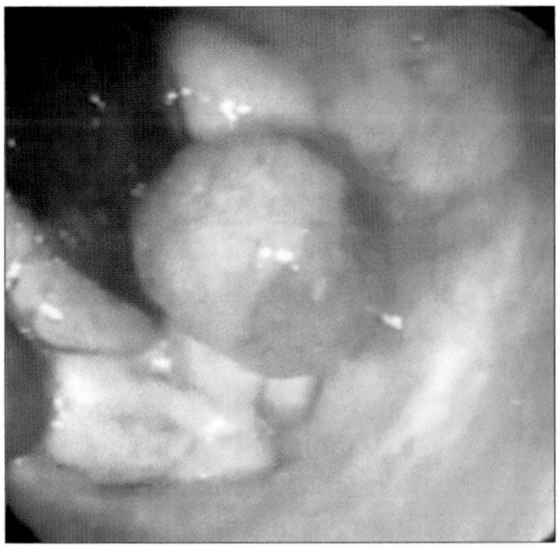

Fig. 24.4 Internal hemorrhoids – postbanding.

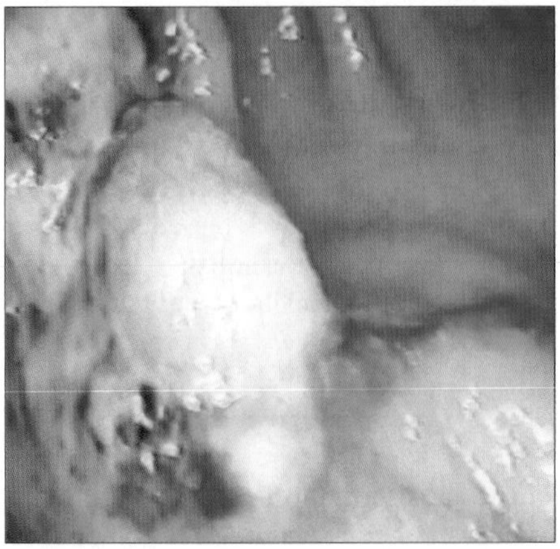

Fig. 24.5 Clot on postpolypectomy ulcer.

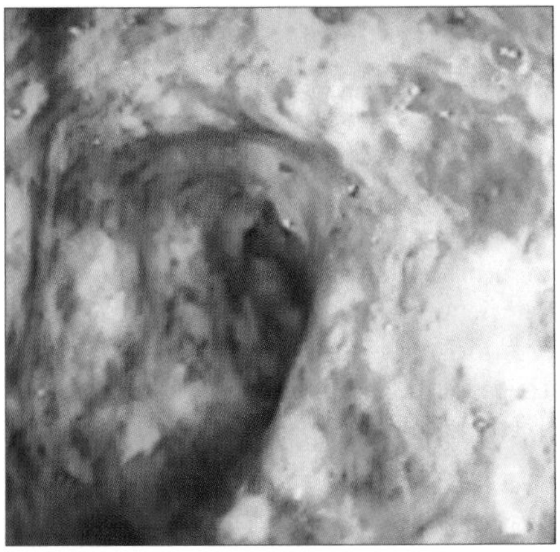

Fig. 24.6 Ischemic colitis.

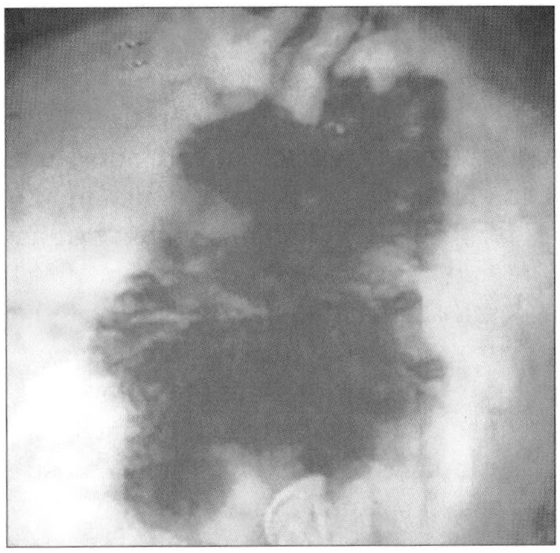

Fig. 24.7 Large angioma in the ascending colon.

purge prior to colonoscopy. Colonoscopy usually reveals an ulceration at the site of a recent polypectomy with either active bleeding, adherent clot, or a nonbleeding visible vessel. Such stigmata should be treated with endoscopic hemostasis, similar to peptic ulcer hemostasis treatment.[9]

Focal, discrete colonic ulcers secondary to infection, ischemia, or IBD are much less common causes of severe LGI hemorrhage (Fig. 24.6).

Rectal ulcers

Solitary or multiple rectal ulcers may be a cause of severe LGI hemorrhage, especially in elderly or debilitated patients, associated with fecal impaction, rectal prolapse, ischemia, or trauma. In one series of patients with severe hematochezia, 8% of patients had rectal ulcers found during colonoscopy.[10]

Management: Half will have major stigmata of recent hemorrhage (active bleeding, visible vessel, or adherent clot) and should be treated endoscopically with epinephrine injection and bipolar coagulation.[10] Although initial hemostasis is usually successful, recurrent bleeding is frequent, suggesting that this group of patients is at especially high risk for rebleeding.

Colonic tumors

Colonic tumors, either cancer or gastrointestinal stromal tumors, occasionally present with hematochezia and may occur anywhere in the rectum or colon. Overt bleeding suggests that the lesion has ulcerated. Although endoscopic therapy with thermal devices, injection, or a combination of both usually produces temporary hemostasis, surgical resection is the best long-term treatment.[7,9]

Colonic angiomas

Bleeding colonic angiomas most often occur in the right colon and are usually multiple (Fig. 24.7). They may be associated with advanced age and medical conditions such as chronic renal insufficiency, cirrhosis, valvular heart disease, and connective tissue disorders. Bleeding from angiomas is usually mild to moderate, intermittent, and self-limiting, and presents with chronic iron deficiency anemia.

Treatment with multipolar coagulation has lower complication rates than heater probe.[7,11] Patients usually require more than one session of endoscopic hemostasis to obliterate multiple colonic angiomas. The main risk of endoscopic coagulation of angiomas is severe delayed bleeding and postcoagulation syndrome (in 3% and 1.7% of patients respectively).[11] Perforation is rare but has been reported.

Radiation proctitis

Radiation proctitis can occasionally cause severe hematochezia, although it is most often associated with mild, chronic rectal bleeding. Chronic injury develops 6–18 months after radiation therapy for prostatic, gynecologic, rectal, or bladder tumors, and damage is caused by altered vascularity and ensuing mucosal ischemia. Rectal telangiectasia and friability are the endoscopic features of radiation proctitis. Endoscopic hemostasis with thermal treatment has been effective for patients with recurrent bleeding when medical therapy has failed.[11]

GENERAL MEASURES AND DIAGNOSIS

An initial hematocrit of less than 35%, the presence of abnormal vital signs 1 h after initial medical evaluation, and gross blood on initial rectal examination are independent predictors of severe LGI bleeding and adverse outcome.[12] For patients who present with severe hematochezia, the diagnostic and therapeutic approach is not standardized in most medical centers.[2,3] The following standardized approach has been evaluated and found to be effective, safe, and cost-effective.

Resuscitation: Patients with persistent, severe hematochezia should initially have aggressive resuscitative measures in a monitored care setting.[9] A consultation with a general or gastrointestinal surgeon should be obtained at an early stage. Orogastric or nasogastric lavage will determine whether UGI bleeding (coffee grounds, blood clots) is present. Patients with hematochezia from an upper source will usually have significant anemia and hypotension, along with nasogastric tube evidence of bleeding. If there is bile without blood in the nasogastric aspirate, a lesion proximal to the ligament of Treitz is unlikely with ongoing hematochezia. In patients with hematochezia, return of clear fluid without bile should not be considered a negative nasogastric tube aspirate as the patient may have a duodenal ulcer or other duodenal lesions. Some 1–3% of patients who present with severe hematochezia have a small bowel source of hemorrhage.[9]

Endoscopy: If there is no evidence of an UGI source, rapid oral lavage should be given to cleanse the colon, followed by urgent anoscopy and colonoscopy. Urgent colonoscopy provides an accurate diagnosis and, if required, an opportunity for hemostasis during the same examination. If urgent colonoscopy and anoscopy are not diagnostic for a bleeding site, push enteroscopy is recommended. This approach improves the diagnostic and therapeutic efficacy while reducing direct costs of patient care.[7,13]

Colonoscopy

Prior to preparation for emergency colonoscopy, tapwater enemas are recommended to clear the distal colon and permit examination of the rectosigmoid colon and anal canal with anoscopy, followed by flexible sigmoidoscopy with retroflexion in the rectum. This is indicated particularly in patients with a history of bleeding, internal hemorrhoids, anorectal disease, or distal colitis. Rigid sigmoidoscopy is not adequate because of the blind area of the rectum not visualized with a rigid instrument.

If the above tests are unrevealing, cleansing the colon with an oral purge is recommended, followed by urgent colonoscopy in the intensive care unit or monitored bed area. The diagnostic yield of colonoscopy in severe hematochezia ranges from 48% to 90%. Several factors determine the 'yield,' including timing of colonoscopy, thoroughness of colonic preparation, and definition of what is the source of bleeding.

Should the push enteroscopy and colonoscopy not be diagnostic, then scintigraphy and angiography are warranted. For those patients who stop bleeding or present with less severe bleeding, colonoscopy within 24h of presentation should still be considered the initial diagnostic and therapeutic procedure of choice.

Scintigraphy

The threshold rate of GI bleeding for localization with radioisotope scanning is about 0.1mL/min or more. Scintigraphy may be particularly useful for identification of small bowel or colonic sites with moderate to severe active bleeding.[3] Two different types of scintigraphy are available: (1) sulfur colloid with technetium, and (2) autologous red blood cells (RBCs) tagged with technetium. Sulfur colloid is used less commonly now owing to more rapid clearance of the labeled material. In many institutions, scintigraphy has replaced emergency visceral angiography as an adjunct to colonoscopy, because scintigraphy is more sensitive, less expensive, and has significantly lower morbidity than angiography. Injection of labeled RBCs and early scanning (at least 30min, 60min, and 4h) is recommended to identify potential bleeding sites. As specific localization and etiologic diagnosis are not possible with RBC scanning, confirmatory examinations such as angiography and/or endoscopy are recommended prior to surgical exploration. Delayed scans (12–24h) are not reliable for localization in the gut.

Angiography, magnetic resonance imaging, computed tomography, and barium radiography

If the rate of ongoing arterial bleeding is at least 0.5mL/min, selective visceral angiography may show extravasation of contrast into the lumen to identify a bleeding site.[3] Emergency visceral angiography can be useful for diagnosis and treatment of colonic, small bowel, or UGI lesions.

Abdominal computed tomography (CT) or magnetic resonance imaging (MRI) may be helpful for diagnosis of an aortoenteric fistula in selected patients with a previous diagnosis of severe peripheral vascular disease or abdominal aneurysm with or without surgery. The physician should consider performing one of these investigations if colonoscopy and enteroscopy do not identify a bleeding site. Most patients with severe hematochezia do not require such diagnostic testing because they do not have large abdominal aneurysms or a past surgery for this diagnosis.

Barium studies (barium enema or small bowel follow-through) have no role in the assessment of severe hematochezia as they cannot show active bleeding. Barium also interferes with subsequent evaluation by colonoscopy or angiography.

Small bowel evaluation

As an emergency examination, a small bowel evaluation with push enteroscopy is indicated for patients with negative colonoscopy and upper endoscopy findings. Enteroscopy provides examination of the proximal 60–80cm of the jejunum.[4] Video capsule endoscopy may have a role in selected patients with recurrent hematochezia and when no diagnosis or localization has been made by urgent colonoscopy, push enteroscopy, and RBC scanning.

Emergency surgery

Emergency surgery should be considered for persistent or recurrent severe hematochezia with: (1) hypotension or shock, despite resuscitative efforts; (2) continued bleeding with transfusion of 6units blood or more, and no diagnosis by emergency endoscopy; and (3) when severe active bleeding can not be controlled by colonoscopy or angiography.

CURRENT CONTROVERSIES AND FUTURE DIRECTIONS

The availability of clinical prognostic criteria to identify patients with a high and low risk of recurrent bleeding is essential for improvement of the management and outcomes of patients with severe hematochezia. Further, clinical factors that may be predictive of the location of the source of severe hematochezia (UGI versus LGI) need to be evaluated more fully in prospective studies. In a preliminary study, positive nasogastric lavage results, severe liver disease, chronic NSAID use, and hematocrit level (<28%) were predictive of the UGI site of hemorrhage. Early colonoscopy (within 24h of presentation) has been associated with both decreased duration of hospitalization and reduced cost of patient care,[13] so should be used more widely as the initial diagnostic and therapeutic procedure of choice.

Stigmata of recent hemorrhage in patients with severe hematochezia and diverticulosis, such as active bleeding, nonbleeding visible vessel, or adherent clot, need to be better appreciated. Appropriate therapeutic intervention targeting these lesions may then improve improve patient outcomes. Finally, improved devices for even more effective and safe colonoscopic hemostasis (e.g., improved hemoclips) need to be developed and tested.

SUMMARY

Severe hematochezia remains a challenging medical problem. For patients whose bleeding persists, identification of the cause is essential for management. Urgent colonoscopy should be performed by experienced endoscopists skilled in the recognition of the stigmata of hemorrhage and use of hemostasis techniques. With this approach, patients will be managed effectively, with decreased rebleeding, morbidity, and mortality rates.

SOURCES OF INFORMATION FOR PATIENTS AND DOCTORS

http://www.patient.co.uk/showdoc/40000118/

REFERENCES

1. Longstreth GF. Epidemiology and outcome of patients hospitalized with acute lower gastrointestinal hemorrhage. A population-based study. Am J Gastroenterol 1997; 92:419–424.
2. Zuccaro G Jr. Management of the adult with acute lower gastrointestinal bleeding. Am J Gastroenterol 1998; 93:1202–1208.
3. Bounds BCS, Friedman L. Lower gastrointestinal bleeding. Gastroenterol Clin North Am 2003; 32:1107–1125.
4. Kovacs TOG, Jensen DM. Upper or small bowel hemorrhage that presents as hematochezia. Tech Gastrointest Endosc 2001; 3:206–215.
5. Jensen DM, Machicado GA, Jutabha R, Kovacs TO. Urgent colonoscopy for the diagnosis and treatment of severe diverticular hemorrhage. N Engl J Med 2000; 342:38–82.
6. Jensen DM. Diverticular bleeding. An appraisal based on stigmata of recent hemorrhage. Tech Gastrointest Endosc 2001; 3:192–198.
7. Savides TJ, Jensen DM. Evaluation and endoscopic treatment of severe lower gastrointestinal bleeding. Tech Gastrointest Endosc 2003; 5:148–154.
8. Jutabha R, Miura-Jutabha C, Jensen DM. Current medical, anoscopic, endoscopic and surgical treatment for bleeding internal hemorrhoids. Tech Gastrointest Endosc 2001; 3:199–120.
9. Kovacs TOG, Jensen DM. Recent advances in the endoscopic diagnosis and therapy of upper gastrointestinal, small intestinal and colonic bleeding. Med Clin N Am 2002; 86:1319–1356.
10. Kanwal F, Dulai G, Jensen DM et al. Major stigmata of recent hemorrhage on rectal ulcers in patients with severe hematochezia: endoscopic diagnosis, treatment and outcomes. Gastrointest Endosc 2003; 57:462–468.
11. Machicado GA, Jensen DM. Bleeding colonic angiomas and radiation telangiectasias: endoscopic diagnosis and treatment. Tech Gastrointest Endosc 2001; 3:185–191.
12. Velayos FS, Williamson A, Sousa KH et al. Early predictors of severe lower gastrointestinal bleeding and adverse outcomes: a prospective study. Clin Gastroenterol Hepatol 2004; 2:485–490.
13. Jensen DM, Machicado GA. Colonoscopy for diagnosis and treatment of severe lower gastrointestinal bleeding. Routine outcomes and cost analysis. Gastroenterol Clin North Am 1997; 7:477–498.

Chapter 25

Being on nonsteroidal anti-inflammatory drugs

Neville D Yeomans and Francis K L Chan

INTRODUCTION

Humans have used nonsteroidal anti-inflammatory drugs (NSAIDs) for several thousand years, ever since the analgesic and 'antiphlogistic' (anti-inflammatory) properties of the salicylate-containing willow bark were recognized. Recently, their use has reached unprecedented levels, as the increasing longevity of populations increases the burden of painful degenerative joint disease, and as the recognition of the antiplatelet and anticancer properties of aspirin creates new uses for this old drug.

This chapter deals with the features, causation, and epidemiology of the adverse effects of NSAIDs on the gastrointestinal (GI) tract. It does not discuss their treatment, which is dealt with elsewhere in this book under each individual disorder.

WHAT SYMPTOMS AND DISORDERS DO NSAIDS CAUSE?

The problems that NSAIDs cause, or have been postulated to cause, in the GI tract are listed in Table 25.1.

Dyspepsia (epigastric discomfort or pain) is a common consequence of NSAID treatment and is also experienced (although less frequently) when patients take cyclo-oxygenase 2 (COX-2)-selective NSAIDs. There is some evidence that NSAIDs also can provoke GI reflux, based on a crossover study measuring 24-h esophageal pH before and during NSAID treatment, and one case–control study of patients with heartburn.[1]

Erosions are shallow abrasions that, by definition, do not extend deeper in the wall than the mucosa. Some are visible only with microscopy, but many are seen at endoscopy as areas of denuded surface 1mm or so in size (Fig. 25.1A). They normally do not cause symptoms, and heal in a matter of days without ever coming to clinical attention.

Ulcers (Fig. 25.1B) are deeper and larger lesions that arise when one or more erosions enlarges instead of healing as usual, and extends down to the submucosa or muscularis of the gastric or duodenal wall (see Chapter 35). The more common site for NSAID-induced ulcers is the stomach, although they also occur in the duodenum – even in the absence of *Helicobacter pylori* infection.

Small intestine imaging with either capsule endoscopy (see Chapter 123) or enteroscopy shows that erosions and ulceration are also common in the small bowel mucosa.[2] An example of an intestinal ulcer is shown in Figure 25.2.

There is also reasonable agreement that NSAIDs can exacerbate colitis, based on case–control data as well as quite a large number of anecdotal case reports (see also Chapter 53). Worsening of colitis has been reported during treatment with selective COX-2 inhibitors as well, but whether the relationship is causal is currently less clear than with nonselective NSAIDs.

Abnormalities of liver function occur in about 1% of patients on NSAIDs, including COX-2 inhibitors, and appear to be more common with diclofenac than with other NSAIDs. Clinical hepatitis occurs uncommonly and is reversible on drug withdrawal, so monitoring is wise, especially in the first 6 months of use.

HOW COMMON ARE THESE PROBLEMS?

Table 25.2 sets out prevalence and incidence for the problems of ulcers, erosions, and their complications, together with estimates of relative risk for some of the other GI adverse consequences of NSAIDs. The information on small intestinal damage is very recent, taking advantage of the development of capsule endoscopy. The prevalence of small intestinal lesions given here represents a composite prevalence for large erosions plus frank ulcers, because these cannot be reliably distinguished from one another at present by capsule endoscopy.

PATHOPHYSIOLOGY

The mechanism of NSAID injury is probably multifactorial, but inhibition of prostaglandin synthesis via blockade of cyclo-oxygenase is a major contributor. Constitutive production of prostaglandins in the gastric mucosa is due mainly to the COX-1 isoenzyme, and this was the rationale for developing highly selective COX-2 inhibitors in order to spare the COX-1 generation of gastric prostaglandins. The story is a little more complicated, though, as animal studies indicated a need to block both COX-1 and COX-2 before substantial gastric damage resulted.[3]

There is also some evidence for direct damage to gastric cells by some NSAIDs, especially aspirin, as they traverse the lumen.

TABLE 25.1 ADVERSE EFFECTS OF NSAID THERAPY ON THE GASTROINTESTINAL SYSTEM

- NSAID dyspepsia
- Exacerbation or induction of gastroesophageal reflux disease (GERD)
- Gastric and duodenal erosions
- Gastric and duodenal ulcers
- Small bowel erosions and ulcers
- Exacerbation of colitis
- Drug-induced hepatitis

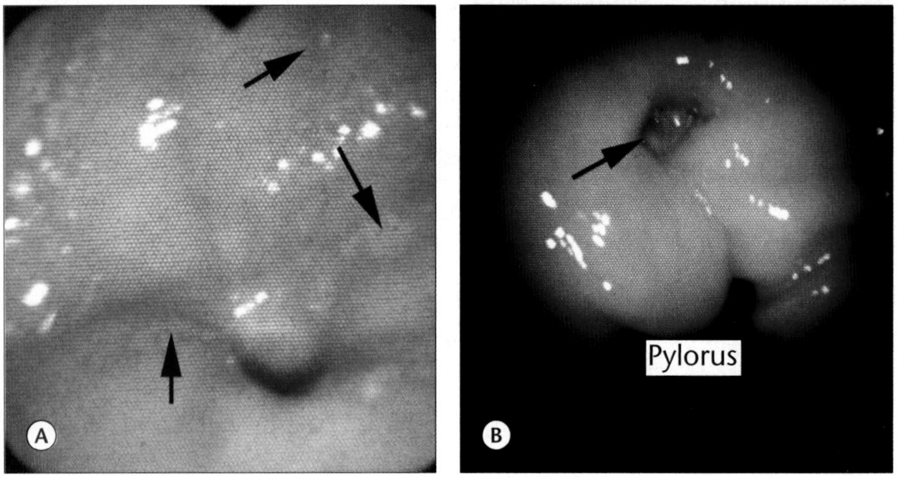

Fig. 25.1 Endoscopic appearance of lesions causes by NSAIDs. A. Antral erosions in vicinity of pylorus in a patient taking aspirin for several days (arrows). **B.** Prepyloric ulcer (arrow) in a patient who had been taking a nonselective NSAID for several months.

For most NSAIDs this is a minor component of damage, as rectal and even transcutaneous administration still produce gastroduodenal erosions and ulcers.

The pH of the gastric lumen appears to play an important part in gastric and probably duodenal injury, however. Figure 25.3 illustrates that indometacin damage in rats is much less when the luminal pH is above 4.0.[4] The success of proton pump inhibitors in reducing NSAID gastric and duodenal ulcers in humans is presumably a manifestation of this.[5]

Damage to the small intestine and colon is unlikely to be mediated by acid. One study with capsule endoscopy after administration of a dual COX inhibitor plus an acid suppressant appears to bear this out. COX-2 inhibitors have been shown to cause less intestinal damage than dual COX inhibitors, indicating that, as in the stomach, inhibition of COX-2 alone is probably not the major contributor to injury.[6]

The life-threatening complication of ulcer hemorrhage may be aggravated by impaired platelet aggregation when dual COX inhibitors are used. This is likely to be most important with aspirin, because of its long-lasting antiplatelet effect.

The mechanism of NSAID dyspepsia is poorly understood. There is only a weak correlation with the macroscopic damage, although it has been suggested that acid diffusing back into the mucosa as a result of widespread microscopic damage activates nociceptive nerves in some people.[7]

CONTRIBUTING CAUSES (RISK FACTORS) FOR NSAID ULCERS AND EROSIONS

A number of factors are now known to contribute to the risk of NSAID gastric and duodenal ulcers and their complications. Much less is known about risk factors for the other GI adverse

TABLE 25.2 FREQUENCY OF GI EVENTS IN PATIENTS TAKING NSAIDS

	Prevalence, incidence, or relative risk	Comments
Gastric erosions	50–100% point prevalence	Much less common with COX-2 inhibitors
Gastric or duodenal ulcers	15–30% point prevalence and 3-month incidence	Reduced by >70% with COX-2 inhibitors
Ulcer complications (hemorrhage, perforation)	1–2 per 100 patient-years	Much higher if prior ulcer complication. Reduced by median of about 65% with COX-2 inhibitors
Small intestinal erosions or ulcers	Approx. 25%	Based on recent capsule endoscopy data.[1] Substantially less frequent with COX-2 inhibitors
Dyspepsia	10–20%	
Gastroesophageal reflux disease (GERD)	Relative risk approx. 2	Based on one case–control study[2]
Exacerbation of colitis	Relative risk approx. 2–6	From case–control studies
Hepatic reactions	<1% clinically significant liver function test increases for most NSAIDs; severe liver injury in <1 per 10000	

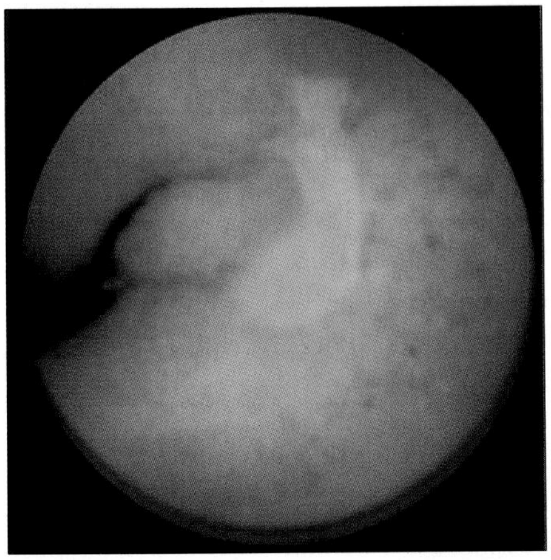

Fig. 25.2 Endoscopic appearance of ulcer in small intestine. Ulcer in small intestine, visualized by M2A™ capsule endoscopy, in a patient taking nonselective NSAIDs. Photo by courtesy of Given Imaging Ltd.

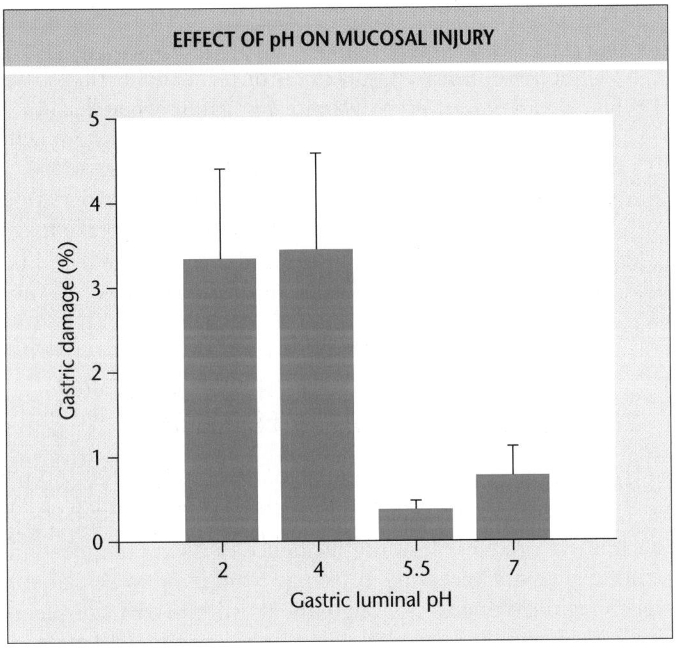

Fig. 25.3 Effect of pH on mucosal injury. Acute mucosal injury by a NSAID (indometacin) depends on luminal pH. After Elliott et al.,[4] with permission.

events of NSAIDs. It is useful to divide these risk factors into those that relate to the NSAID itself and those that are intrinsic to the particular patient.

NSAID-related risk factors

The class of NSAID is one important determinant. Although there is still a little controversy about how much safer are the COX-2 inhibitors (see Current controversies below), there is little doubt that overall there are fewer ulcers and fewer complications produced by the coxibs than by classical NSAIDs, so long as low-dose aspirin is not added in as well (essentially to reconstitute a dual COX inhibitor).

The dose of NSAID is the second important determinant of risk. This has been particularly well shown for ibuprofen, where the very low end of the marketed dosage scale carries little more risk than placebo. Aspirin damage is also broadly dose related, but doses even as low as 75 mg daily still carry a significant ulcer and ulcer-bleeding risk.[8]

Finally, within the classical NSAID group, the longer-acting NSAIDs seem to be generally more damaging than the short- to medium-duration drugs. This might be due to members of this group being marketed at relatively higher doses, although there is a theoretic basis to believe that there might be a real difference in gastric toxicity.

Risk factors in the individual patient

Age

Older patients are at increased risk of NSAID ulcers, and also at increased risk of succumbing to an ulcer bleed (see Chapter 27). The increase with age is curvilinear upwards, but there is no particular age at which a sudden step-up in risk occurs, so it is not practicable to define one particular age as the dividing point between low and high risk.

Past ulcer history

A history of previous peptic ulcer increases the risk of a NSAID ulcer and ulcer hemorrhage several-fold. The risk is particularly high if the patient recently had a *bleeding* ulcer whilst on NSAIDs – amounting to almost 20% recurrent bleeding in 6 months in one recent study.[9]

Helicobacter pylori

There has been controversy about whether coexistent *H. pylori* infection is a risk factor for NSAID gastric ulcers (see Current controversies below; see also Chapter 34), but the evidence does support an interaction between *H. pylori* and NSAIDs in causing duodenal ulcers.

Other co-administered drugs

Corticosteroids modestly increase the risk of NSAID ulcer complications. Aspirin can be thought of as effectively increasing the total NSAID dose (and hence ulcer risk), whereas other anticoagulants and antiplatelet agents increase the risk of bleeding from NSAID ulcers without increasing the underlying rate of ulceration. In the case of warfarin-like anticoagulants, the relative risk for bleeding in patients taking these in combination with an NSAID can be as high as 20-fold compared with that in patients taking neither of these medications. (See also Chapter 68, Drug-induced diseases of the small and large bowel.)

SYMPTOM COMPLEXES

Dyspepsia, described as burning, discomfort, or pain in the upper abdomen, is common during NSAID therapy, with reported prevalences ranging from about 10% to as high as 40%. Several studies have shown that it is less common during treatment with COX-2 inhibitors. There is nothing very specific about these symptoms, which are similar to those described by some patients with peptic ulcer and by patients not taking NSAIDs who are labeled as having nonulcer dyspepsia.

These symptoms are a poor predictor of whether the patient has macroscopic injury in the stomach or duodenum. Erosions are usually asymptomatic, as indeed are many frank ulcers in NSAID users. In one recent study of ulcer prevalence and incidence in patients taking low-dose aspirin, those with an ulcer complained of dyspeptic symptoms no more often than patients who turned out to be ulcer free. Other studies have shown that new dyspepsia, arising after patients have been taking NSAIDs for some time, does give some indication (albeit with a sensitivity and specificity of only about 50%) that an ulcer may have developed.

The important symptoms of hematemesis or melena in patients taking NSAIDs will be readily recognized, and point to the likelihood of a gastric, duodenal, or small intestinal ulcer in roughly that order of frequency. Similarly, the development of sudden, severe epigastric pain, with features of shock and signs of peritonismus, will immediately raise the suspicion of peptic ulcer perforation.

Symptoms of anemia developing in patients taking NSAIDs should raise the possibility of chronic blood loss, which can occur from erosions as well as ulcers, and again may originate from the upper gut or mid gut, or both. Of course, more sinister causes such as bleeding from a colonic neoplasm normally need to be ruled out. As mentioned above, exacerbation of colitis in inflammatory bowel disease is probably also a consequence of NSAID treatment in some patients.

DIAGNOSIS

The investigation of NSAID dyspepsia rationally depends on when the dyspepsia develops and whether there are any associated features, such as overt bleeding or anemia, to point to ulcer development. Dyspepsia that begins *immediately* with the commencement of a NSAID is highly unlikely to be due to the development of a new ulcer. Investigation of such patients is therefore usually not needed. In practice, clinicians often stop or switch NSAIDs in such patients, and recent data show that treatment with a proton pump inhibitor can also be effective in reducing dyspepsia (see Chapter 5).

On the other hand, it is important to remember that ulcers can develop quickly – even a week is sufficient – so dyspepsia that develops a little after the onset of NSAID treatment may warrant gastroscopy, and the onset of bleeding *certainly* warrants upper GI endoscopy. Barium studies have low sensitivity for diagnosing small lesions and have little place for diagnosis in most patients. Figure 25.4 illustrates the endoscopic appearance of an ulcer with active bleeding. The management of such bleeding ulcers is considered in Chapter 35.

Gastroscopy may also be useful for gauging the severity of esophagitis (and hence to some extent the need for or choice of acid suppressant therapy) in patients who develop heartburn while taking NSAIDs.

The recently introduced tool of capsule endoscopy (see Chapter 129) can be useful for investigating the patient with NSAID-associated anemia who has negative upper and lower gastrointestinal endoscopy findings.

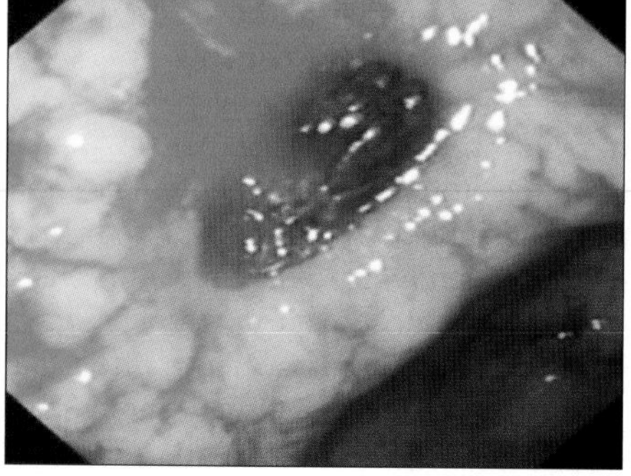

Fig. 25.4 Endoscopic appearance of a bleeding ulcer. Bleeding ulcer in a patient taking NSAIDs.

CURRENT CONTROVERSIES AND THEIR FUTURE RESOLUTION

The role of *H. pylori* as a risk factor for NSAID-associated ulcer is highly controversial. Current evidence indicates that *H. pylori* increases the risk of NSAIDs causing duodenal ulcers. *H. pylori* also contributes to ulcer bleeding associated with low-dose aspirin. However, several important questions remain unresolved. Their resolution will await future clinical trials and epidemiologic studies.

CURRENT CONTROVERSIES
SOME CONTROVERSIES AND UNRESOLVED ISSUES
• Is it cost-effective to test for *H. pylori* and eradicate the infection if present before starting NSAIDs? • How does *H. pylori* infection influence the risk of developing gastric ulcers associated with NSAIDs? • What is the long-term risk of ulcer bleeding with low-dose aspirin after the eradication of *H. pylori*? • What is the optimal management strategy for patients with prior ulcer complications who require NSAIDs? • Do COX-2 inhibitors increase the risk of coronary events?

Recently, the enthusiasm for COX-2 inhibitors as gastric-sparing NSAIDs has been challenged. The Celecoxib Long-term Arthritis Safety Study (CLASS) (a randomized comparison of celecoxib with diclofenac and ibuprofen) failed to show a significant reduction in the incidence of ulcer complications among patients receiving celecoxib compared with patients receiving diclofenac.[10] Among patients with prior ulcer bleeding, a recent study showed that neither celecoxib nor diclofenac and omeprazole could adequately prevent recurrent bleeding.[11] Post hoc subgroup analysis of the VIGOR study failed to demonstrate superiority of rofecoxib over naproxen in patients with prior upper GI events.[12] An excess of acute coronary events associated with rofecoxib has raised concern about the cardiovascular safety of COX-2 inhibitors.[13]

SOURCES OF INFORMATION FOR PATIENTS AND DOCTORS

http://www.patient.co.uk/showdoc/27000440/
http://www.2reduce.org/
http://uconnsportsmed.uchc.edu/patientinfo/whathurts/treatment/nsaids.html
http://www.arthritis.about.com/od/vioxxgeninfo/

REFERENCES

1. Kotzan J, Wade W, Yu HH. Assessing NSAID prescription use as a predisposing factor for gastroesophageal reflux disease in a Medicaid population. Pharm Res 2001; 18:1367–1372.
2. Graham D, Qureshi WA, Willingham K et al. A controlled study of NSAID-induced small bowel injury using video capsule endoscopy. Gastroenterology 2003; 124(Suppl 1):A19.
3. Wallace JL, McKnight W, Reuter BK et al. NSAID-induced gastric damage in rats: requirement for inhibition of both cyclooxygenase 1 and 2. Gastroenterology 2000; 119:706–714.
4. Elliott SL, Ferris RJ, Giraud AS et al. Indomethacin damage to rat gastric mucosa is markedly dependent on luminal pH. Clin Exp Pharmacol Physiol 1996; 23:432–434.
5. Yeomans ND, Tulassay Z, Juhász L et al. A comparison of omeprazole with ranitidine for ulcers associated with nonsteroidal antiinflammatory drugs. N Engl J Med 1998; 338:719–726.
6. Goldstein JL, Eisen G, Lewis B et al. Celecoxib is associated with fewer small bowel lesions than naproxen plus omeprazole in healthy subjects as determined by capsule endoscopy. Am J Gastroenterol 2003; 98:S298.
7. Holtmann G, Gschossmann J, Buenger L et al. Do changes in visceral sensory function determine the development of dyspepsia during treatment with aspirin? Gastroenterology 2002; 123:1451–1458.
8. Weil J, Colin-Jones D, Langman M et al. Prophylactic aspirin and risk of peptic ulcer bleeding. BMJ 1995; 310:827–830.
9. Chan FKL, Chung SCS, Suen BY et al. Preventing recurrent upper gastrointestinal bleeding in patients with *Helicobacter pylori* infection who are taking low-dose aspirin or naproxen. N Engl J Med 2001; 344:967–973.
10. Silverstein FE, Faich G, Goldstein JL et al. Gastrointestinal toxicity with celecoxib vs nonsteroidal anti-inflammatory drugs for osteoarthritis and rheumatoid arthritis: the CLASS study: a randomized controlled trial. Celecoxib Long-term Arthritis Safety Study. JAMA 2000; 284:1247–1255.
11. Chan FKL, Hung LCT, Suen BY et al. Celecoxib versus diclofenac and omeprazole in reducing the risk of recurrent ulcer bleeding in patients with arthritis. N Engl J Med 2002; 347:2104–2110.
12. Laine L, Bombardier C, Hawkey CJ et al. Stratifying the risk of NSAID-related upper gastrointestinal clinical events: results of a double-blind outcomes study in patients with rheumatoid arthritis. Gastroenterology 2002; 123:1006–1012.
13. Bombardier C, Laine L, Reicin A et al. Comparison of upper gastrointestinal toxicity of rofecoxib and naproxen in patients with rheumatoid arthritis. N Engl J Med 2000; 343:1520–1528.

Chapter 26

Gastrointestinal problems in primary care

Julia L Newton

INTRODUCTION

Across most of Europe and North America, primary care is a specific specialty that exists within a range of healthcare systems and cultures. It is at the forefront of care for most patients, and a primary care physician is generally the first point of medical input when a person chooses to consult.

In primary care gastrointestinal (GI) problems tend to be undifferentiated, and in those under the age of 55 years who do not have alarm symptoms the probability of serious pathology is low. Management is largely symptom driven and an empiric approach in primary care is often more appropriate than the diagnostic model generally used in secondary care, where investigation rates tend to be higher. In primary care the predictive value of symptoms for a specific diagnosis is small where there is a low prevalence of pathology.

The many roles of the primary care physician in the management of GI problems are outlined in Table 26.1. It is important to recognize that much of the evidence for the management of GI disease in primary care is derived from populations based in secondary care and that results obtained in highly selected clinical trials do not necessarily reflect practice in the real world.

In this chapter several areas in the field of gastroenterology that are frequently encountered in primary care will be discussed. Reference should be made to the relevant clinical chapters when considering management of specific conditions.

TABLE 26.1 ROLE OF THE PRIMARY CARE PHYSICIAN IN MANAGING GASTROINTESTINAL PROBLEMS

- Diagnose and refer to secondary care acute medical and surgical GI problems.
- Identify subacute and chronic GI problems and refer as appropriate.
- Use well validated screening tools that identify those at risk of malignant versus nonmalignant diseases.
- Determine according to local and national policies and expertise whether referral would be more appropriate to open-access clinics or gastroenterology services.
- Maintenance of relapse of GI diseases.
- Manage chronic relapsing or recurring GI diseases.
- Identifying in family practice those people who would benefit from eradication of *H. pylori* infection.
- Screening of asymptomatic people at risk of GI malignancy.

HOW COMMON IS IT?

The true prevalence of GI symptoms in the community is unclear and depends upon the population studied, the setting, and the definition of symptoms. In one systematic review, the prevalence of upper GI symptoms ranged between 5% and 54%, whereas the prevalence of heartburn and regurgitation ranged between 21% and 59%.[1]

In the majority of people presenting with abdominal symptoms in primary care the problem is self-limiting, frequently relapsing; often no definitive cause is found and the symptoms are managed entirely in primary care. The prognosis for all symptoms is generally good. The decision by a patient to consult a clinician can be driven by psychologic factors, symptom-related anxiety, the frequency of symptoms, and the fear of serious disease, particularly cancer.

SCREENING FOR *HELICOBACTER PYLORI* INFECTION IN PRIMARY CARE

(see also Chapters 26 and 38)

Guidelines have been developed for the primary care management of *H. pylori*, and the European *H. pylori* Study Group has set goals for optimal therapy in primary care.[2–4]

The recommendations for eradication of *H. pylori* do not differ in primary or secondary care. *H. pylori* eradication should be considered in patients with a current or previous diagnosis of peptic ulcer disease and in those with a personal or family history of gastric cancer and gastric MALToma (mucosa-associated lymphoid tumor). In addition, a test and treat strategy (see Chapters 5 and 34) is considered appropriate for those with dyspepsia and for asymptomatic subjects infected with *H. pylori* in whom the natural history of the ulcer diathesis could be altered.

The mainstay of testing for *H. pylori* in primary care involves noninvasive tests such as serology and breath tests; ensuring that these forms of testing are used in appropriate groups of patients is critical. Near-patient testing kits are not recommended because of their high sensitivity and low specificity. In primary care, testing to confirm successful eradication is regarded as a counsel of perfection. Pragmatically, it can be reserved for patients whose symptoms recur or for those with a history of ulcer complications such as hematemesis (see Chapters 34 and 35).

SCREENING FOR LOWER GI DISEASES IN PRIMARY CARE (see Chapter 60B)

Each primary care physician in the UK will see at least one new case of colorectal cancer (CRC) each year. CRC screening reduces morbidity and mortality, is cost effective, and is often carried out by primary care physicians. Early and accurate diagnosis of CRC improves the 5-year survival rate and also leads to less complicated surgery. In primary care CRC screening practices can vary considerably. Ensuring the appropriate use of screening tools and offering screening to appropriate groups will optimize early detection of CRC.[5]

For effective implementation of CRC screening strategies, risk stratification is essential. Genetic factors are important in CRC. Once a diagnosis of CRC has been made in an index case, it is important that primary care physicians recognize that eliciting a family history and implementation of appropriate screening strategies from recommended guidelines with notification of at-risk relatives is essential. Referral criteria for further investigation and genetic testing in those with a family history of colonic cancer, as recommended by the British Society of Gastroenterology, are outlined in Figure 26.1.[6]

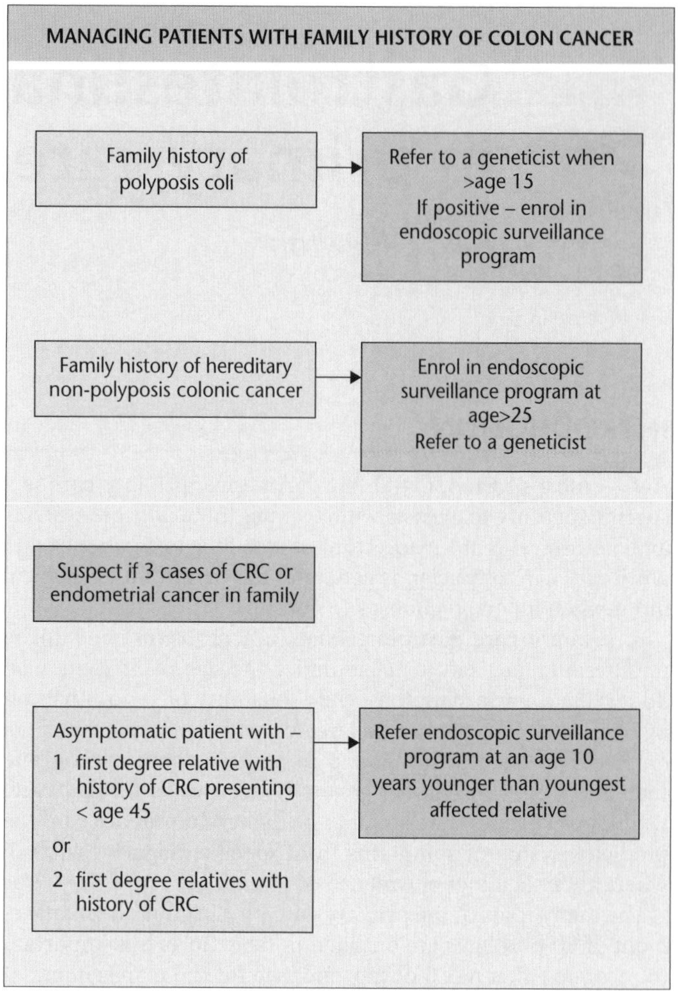

Fig. 26.1 Managing patients with family history of colonic cancer.

WHO AND WHEN TO REFER?

Identifying people who cannot be entirely managed in primary care and need referral to secondary care may be difficult; the differentiation of organic from nonorganic disease is critical. Sometimes there may be a gray area between 'sinister' and 'nonsinister' symptoms, or presentation with acute, subacute, and chronic symptoms. How clinicians in primary care interpret these gray areas may vary, and studies are needed to standardize ambiguities. Furthermore, the availability of over-the-counter (OTC) medications provides ample opportunity for patients to self-medicate before consulting; therefore clinicians frequently see patients who have persistent symptoms after a trial of OTC remedies.

Primary care referral patterns vary hugely, and adherence to guidelines is critical. It is, however, important that guidelines are adaptable and applicable to primary care physicians in a variety of health delivery systems.

Many guidelines are dependent upon the presence or absence of 'sinister' symptoms which, if present, should initiate referral for investigation. In the upper GI tract, guidelines recommend a 'test and treat' strategy which pivots upon whether the patient is infected with *H. pylori*. In these strategies, eradication of *H. pylori* or empiric treatment is recommended in younger patients, whereas in older patients (until recently above the age of 45 years, and more recently above 55 years of age) referral is advocated because of the increased prevalence of pathology in older age groups.

It is important to recognize that this approach rations the use of diagnostic endoscopy and begs the question of whether we are underusing this diagnostic investigation.

There are differences in how primary care physicians, gastroenterologists, and surgeons interpret referral criteria for open-access gastroscopy and colonoscopy; inappropriate referrals for colonoscopy tend to be higher than for gastroscopy. The reason why different specialties request investigations differently requires clarification.

MANAGING UPPER GI SYMPTOMS IN PRIMARY CARE (see Chapters 4 and 5)

In primary care, dyspepsia accounts for up to 5% of all consultations[7] and for 10% of drug expenditure. Together, prescriptions for ulcer-healing drugs and endoscopy costs represent major expenditures for dyspepsia in primary care. However, the proportion of patients who actually consult a doctor comprises a minority of the total population with dyspepsia. In general practices in the UK, 0.82% of the population were taking acid-suppressive medication and in 19% no diagnosis had ever been reached.[8] In younger patients, the 'test and treat' *H. pylori* management strategy appears to be as effective and safe as prompt endoscopy in primary care[9] in those presenting with more than 2 weeks of epigastric pain but no alarm symptoms. Patients, however, are less happy with their treatment (Fig. 26.2).

Guidelines for dyspepsia management have been developed[10,11] which, if adhered to, would have a major impact upon primary care in terms of workload and financial implications should all currently undiagnosed dyspeptics be investigated.

The treatment of upper abdominal pain in primary care hinges greatly upon the use of medications that suppress gastric acid. Treating younger patients with high doses of medication that

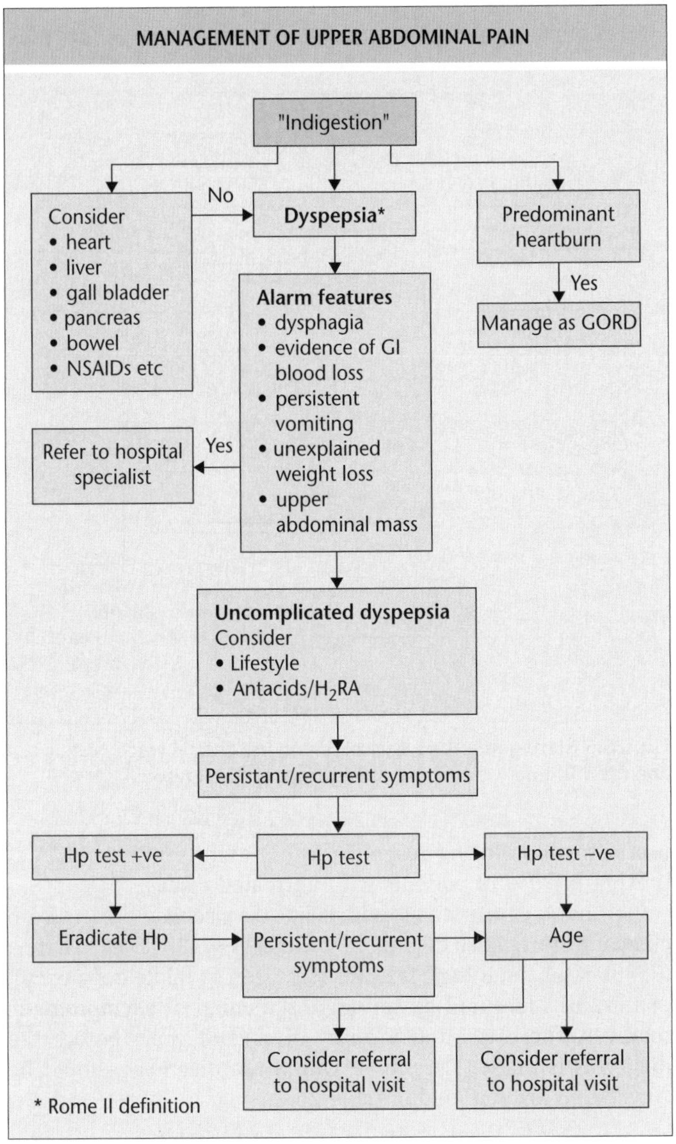

Fig. 26.2 Management of upper abdominal pain. Algorithm for the management of upper abdominal pain in primary care, as recommended by the Scottish Intercollegiate Guideline Network (SIGN; www.sign.ac.uk).

are reduced as symptoms resolve (step-down), rather than starting at a low dose and increasing if symptoms persist (step-up), has been shown in primary care to offer improved symptom relief and quality of life.[11] However, it may be that empiric treatment with prokinetic therapies and antisecretory medication in undiagnosed dyspepsia is equally effective.

MANAGING LOWER GI SYMPTOMS IN PRIMARY CARE

Colorectal cancer (see Chapter 60)

The prevalence of cancer increases with advancing age. However, signs and symptoms of colonic cancer in a primary care setting are poorly predictive of pathology.[4] The patients that primary care physicians are likely to encounter who have CRC are patients presenting with large bowel symptoms, such as rectal bleeding or altered bowel habit, those with clinical signs or results of investigations suggestive of CRC, principally iron deficiency anemia (Fig. 26.3), or asymptomatic patients with a positive family history of CRC or endometrial cancer. In those presenting with new large bowel symptoms and over 45 years of age, and patients of any age with alarm features or a strong family history of GI cancer, referral for investigation is mandatory (Figs 26.1, 26.3 and 26.4). Total colonoscopy and flexible sigmoidoscopy with barium enema are the investigations of choice and should be chosen with regard to local services and expertise.[5,6]

Irritable bowel syndrome (see Chapters 11 and 64)

Many patients have functional lower GI symptoms without pathology to explain these symptoms. Irritable bowel syndrome (IBS) is a common, chronic, fluctuating, nonlife-threatening condition that predominantly affects women. IBS has a significant impact on quality of life and affects 17% of the UK population, three-quarters of whom rely on self-care. IBS is characterized by the presence of abdominal pain that is associated with altered bowel habit in the absence of an identifiable structural or biochemical disorder. There are four key symptoms: pain, constipation, diarrhea, and abdominal bloating. The diagnosis is often presumptive, but alternative diagnoses such as celiac disease or, where symptoms develop in older patients, colonic cancer may need to be ruled out.

The treatment of IBS remains controversial. Drug therapy should target the patient's most troublesome symptoms. Lifestyle advice such as a high-fibre diet and supplementation with bran are of conflicting benefit. The role of diet remains controversial, but some patients report that their symptoms are related to specific foodstuffs. Nonpharmacologic therapies such as hypnosis, cognitive behavioral therapy, biofeedback, and psychotherapy have been shown to be effective.[13]

MANAGING ANEMIA IN PRIMARY CARE

Anemia is a common hematologic abnormality encountered in primary care. Abnormalities of the GI tract can be involved in a number of types of anemia that frequently present for the first time in primary care. In the first instance, defining the type

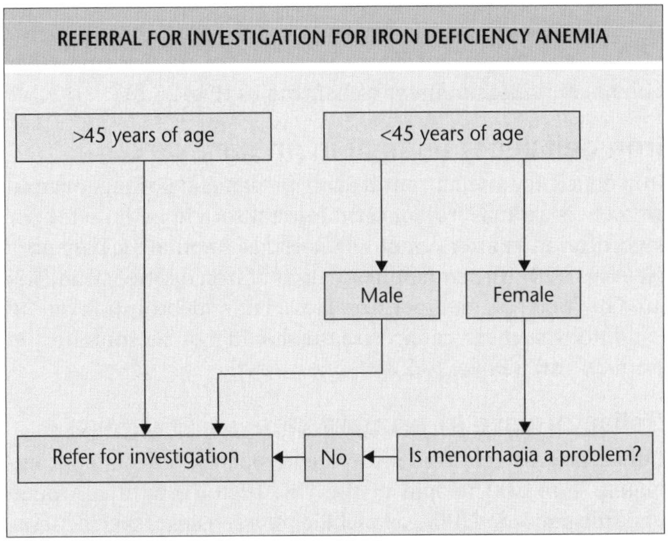

Fig. 26.3 Referral for investigation for iron deficiency anemia. Who should be referred for investigation for iron deficiency anemia in primary care?

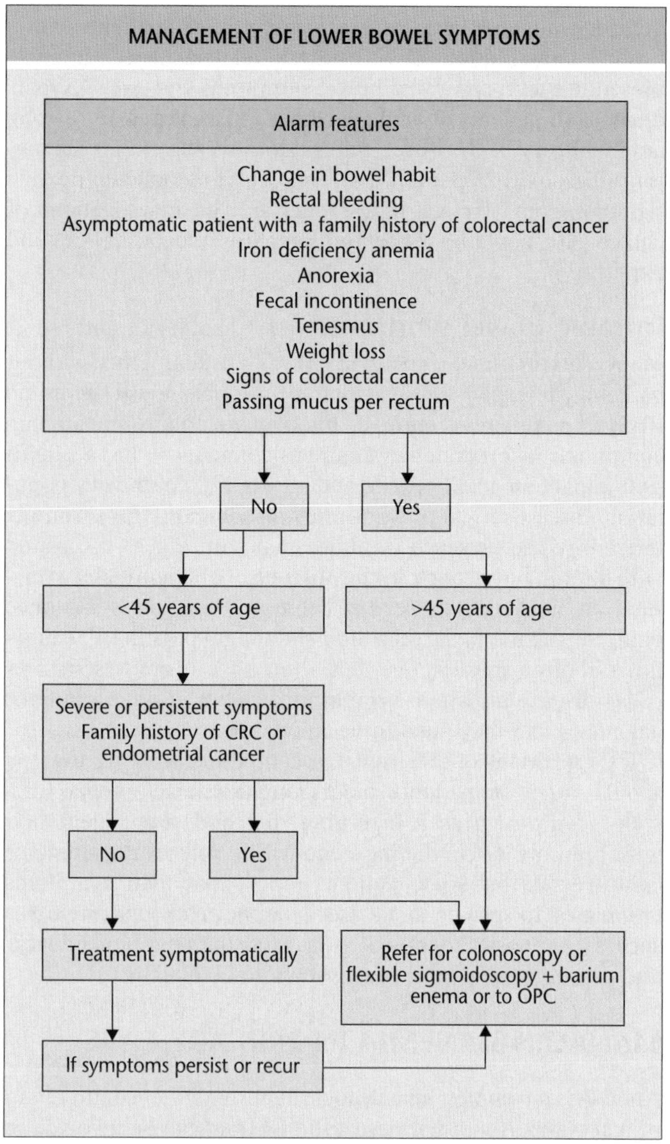

Fig. 26.4 Management of lower bowel symptoms. Algorithm for the management of lower bowel symptoms in primary care.

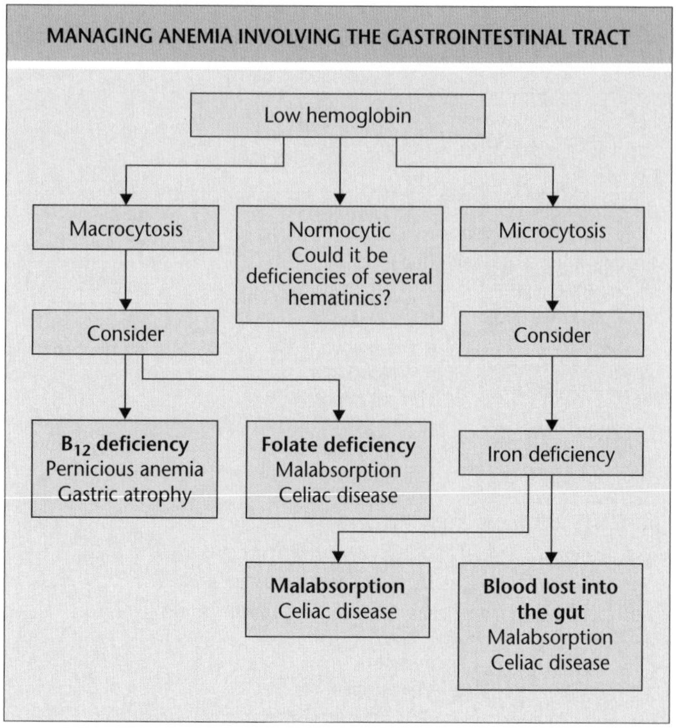

Fig. 26.5 Management of anemia involving the GI tract. Managing anemia in primary care: how the GI tract can be involved.

of anemia is important by measurement of mean corpuscular volume and measurement of hematinics (Fig. 26.5).

Iron deficiency anemia in primary care

Iron deficiency anemia, particularly in men and postmenopausal women, is a cause for concern; referral should be initiated for investigation in both symptomatic and asymptomatic patients[14] (see Fig. 26.3). The commonest causes of iron deficiency anemia are GI blood loss and menstrual loss, but malabsorption due to conditions such as celiac disease should not be forgotten in primary care (Table 26.2).

Celiac disease in primary care (see Chapter 44)

Celiac disease (gluten-sensitive enteropathy) affects approximately 1 in 300 people in the UK. Historically it has been underdiagnosed, but the availability of a sensitive, specific serological screening test has improved diagnosis and is particularly applicable to primary care physicians. Endomysial antibody (EMA) testing is the initial screening test of choice and is also useful for monitoring response to a gluten-free diet. EMA is present in 90% of patients with untreated disease.[15]

In primary care, patients with celiac disease may present with clinical features such as general tiredness (80–90%) or diarrhea (75–80%), hematologic features (e.g., iron or folate deficiency), or may be identified by serologic screening of asymptomatic relatives. There is often a delay of several years before the diagnosis is made. Patients in whom the diagnosis should be considered are outlined in Table 26.2.

MANAGING PATIENTS WITH ABNORMAL LIVER FUNCTION TEST RESULTS IN PRIMARY CARE (see Chapter 21)

Standard laboratory tests for liver function are often requested by primary care physicians in patients with nonspecific symptoms such as tiredness, abdominal pain, dyspepsia, and weight loss. It is unclear what are the implications of mildly abnormal results in patients with no signs suggestive of liver disease, and what is appropriate follow-up. Importantly, early diagnosis of chronic liver diseases such as viral and autoimmune liver diseases can improve prognosis.

Liver function test results can be transiently abnormal after acute alcohol excess, minor viral illness, or a drug reaction. After discovery of an abnormal test result, repeating liver function tests after several weeks of alcohol abstention if no other clinical diagnostic clues are apparent would be the first step. The pattern of changes in liver function test results can suggest a diagnosis, but even large increases are nonspecific. However, it is important to recognize that normal liver blood test findings do not exclude major chronic liver disease.

Persistently abnormal test results for liver function require investigation as they may indicate potentially communicable and/or treatable diseases. A battery of serologic tests, including

TABLE 26.2 MANAGING CELIAC DISEASE IN PRIMARY CARE

- **Consider celiac disease in patients with:**
  Iron or folate deficiency anemia
  Tired all the time or chronic fatigue
  Unexplained diarrhea.
- **Particularly if the patient also has:**
  A family history of celiac disease
  Insulin-dependent diabetes mellitus
  Autoimmune thyroid disease
  Osteoporosis
  Infertility
  An undefined neurologic disorder.

hepatitis B surface antigen, hepatitis C antibody, an autoantibody screen, and concentrations of immunoglobulins and ferritin, can identify some of the more important diagnoses. Patients with persistently abnormal test results in primary care should be referred to a hepatologist or gastroenterologist.[16]

Mild abnormalities often turn out to be associated with one of the fatty liver syndromes.

OPEN ACCESS OR GASTROENTEROLOGIST?

There are wide variations in the referral behavior of primary care physicians. Local policies need to be established with close links between primary care, gastroenterology, and surgical services to ensure that people are referred and seen quickly, particularly those with signs or symptoms suggestive of cancer.

Referral to open-access or hospital outpatient clinics will be determined by local waiting lists, funding priorities, and policies. In a UK survey, 90% of primary care physicians chose direct-access endoscopy referral for all patients with dyspepsia; however, these are predominantly younger patients and as a result diagnostic rates appear low.[17]

Many primary care physicians have responsibility for their own budget. As a result, units providing endoscopy in primary care have been developed, often with primary care physicians as endoscopist. These units have proved popular, being local and convenient.

Before working in primary care units, endoscopists must be suitably trained in an approved unit, and have at least 5 years' experience in hospital endoscopy. In order to maintain skills, it is recommended that every endoscopist should be performing 200 procedures per year.[18]

CURRENT CONTROVERSIES

In general, there are few prospective studies to guide primary care physicians; as a result, primary care physicians are largely required to extrapolate evidence from secondary care. This lack of evidence-based practice needs to be addressed with pragmatic randomized controlled trials.

It is essential that 'regional platforms' are developed where primary care physicians and specialists develop guidelines, priorities, and patient pathways (e.g., Scottish Intercollegiate Guideline Network; SIGN).

Consistent GI symptom definitions are a priority to enable valid population prevalence studies to be performed and to allow comparisons to be drawn between them.

Primary care physicians are eager for shared care, continuing education, and closer links with gastroenterologic colleagues. Moving towards integrated care pathways based on evidence-based guidelines is critical.

Protocols for managing GI problems must be validated in primary care.

SOURCES OF INFORMATION FOR PATIENTS AND DOCTORS

http://www.patient.co.uk/showdoc/108/
http://www.patient.co.uk/showdoc/23068673/

REFERENCES

1. Heading RC. Prevalence of upper gastrointestinal symptoms in the general population: a systematic review. Scand J Gastroenterol Suppl 1999; 231:3–8.
2. Malfertheiner P, Mégraud F, O'Morain C et al. Current concepts in the management of *Helicobacter pylori* infection – the Maastricht 2-2000 Consensus Report. Aliment Pharmacol Ther 2002; 16:167–180.
3. Childs S, Roberts A, Meineche-Schmidt V, de Wit N, Rubin G. The management of *Helicobacter pylori* infection in primary care: a systematic review of the literature. Fam Pract 2000; 17:S6–11.
4. Verma S, Giaffer MH. *Helicobacter pylori* eradication ameliorates symptoms and improves quality of life in patients on long-term acid suppression. A large prospective study in primary care. Dig Dis Sci 2002; 47: 1567–1574.
5. British Society of Gastroenterology. Guidelines for colorectal cancer screening in high risk groups. Online. Available: http://www.bsg.org.uk/clinical_prac/guidelines/colorectal.htm
6. Primary Care Society for Gastroenterology. Guidelines for the early detection of colorectal cancer in primary care. Online. Available: www.pcsg.org.uk
7. British Society of Gastroenterology. Dyspepsia management guidelines. Online. Available: http://www.bsg.org.uk/clinical_prac/guidelines/dyspepsia.htm
8. Morbidity statistics from general practice, 4th national study 1991–2. London: Office of Population Censuses and Surveys; 1995.
9. Lassen AT, Pedersen FM, Bytzer P, Schaffalitzky de Muckadell OB. *Helicobacter pylori* test-and-eradicate versus prompt endoscopy for management of dyspeptic patients: a randomised trial. Lancet 2000; 356:455–460.
10. Bodger K, Eastwood PG, Manning SI, Daly MJ, Heatley RV. Dyspepsia workload in urban general practice and implications of the British Society of Gastroenterology Dyspepsia guidelines (1996). Aliment Pharmacol Ther 2000; 14:413–420.
11. Scottish Intercollegiate Guidelines Network. Dyspepsia. Guideline no. 68, March 2003. Online Available: http://www.sign.ac.uk
12. Ofman JJ, Dorn GH, Fennerty MB, Fass R. The clinical and economic impact of competing management strategies for gastrooesophageal reflux disease. Aliment Pharmacol Ther 2002; 16:261–273.
13. British Society of Gastroenterology. Guidelines for the management of the irritable bowel syndrome. Online. Available: http://www.bsg.org.uk/clinical_prac/guidelines/man_ibs.htm
14. British Society of Gastroenterology. Guidelines for the management of iron deficiency anaemia. Online. Available: http://www.bsg.org.uk/clinical_prac/guidelines/iron_def.htm
15. British Society of Gastroenterology. Interim guidelines for the management of patients with coeliac disease: http://www.bsg.org.uk/clinical_prac/guidelines/coeliac.htm
16. Sherwood P, Lyburn I, Brown S, Ryder S. How are abnormal results for liver function tests dealt with in primary care? Audit of yield and impact. BMJ 2001; 322:276–278.
17. Asante MA, Patel P, Mendall M, Jazrawi R, Northfield TC. The impact of direct access endoscopy, *Helicobacter pylori* near patient testing and acid suppressants on the management of dyspepsia in general practice. Int J Clin Pract 1997; 51:497–499.
18. British Society of Gastroenterology. Gastrointestinal endoscopy in general practice. Online. Available: http://www.bsg.org.uk/clinical_prac/guidelines/gi_endo.htm

Chapter 27

Gastrointestinal problems in the elderly

Julia L Newton

KEY POINTS
• *Helicobacter pylori* is more prevalent in the elderly • The elderly have impaired mucosal defences (prostaglandin, mucus, and bicarbonate production) and repair mechanisms • Admission rates for bleeding peptic ulcer are increasing in the elderly, in whom the mortality rate is highest • The elderly have an increased incidence of small bowel bacterial overgrowth due to dysmotility • Irritable bowel rarely presents in old age – exclude colorectal cancer

INTRODUCTION

Older people are an increasing proportion of the population and, although there are no gastrointestinal diseases specific to older people, many symptoms and diseases such as gastrointestinal cancers, peptic ulcer disease, and diverticulosis become more common in older age groups. As the population ages, the number of older people consulting with gastrointestinal symptoms will increase. The challenges of managing gastrointestinal disease in older people are outlined in Table 27.1.

Evidence-based studies examining the management of gastrointestinal problems in older people are rare, and in most of the current literature older people are specifically excluded from studies. As a result, a great deal of clinical practice in the elderly is extrapolated from studies in the young. It is often difficult to be sure how the results of what might be regarded as landmark trials translate into the clinic when faced with a frail 80-year-old with dyspepsia.

TABLE 27.1 WHY GASTROENTEROLOGY IN AN AGING POPULATION IS MORE DIFFICULT
• Young people with gastrointestinal diseases become old. • Gastrointestinal diseases can present for the first time in older people. • Many gastrointestinal diseases increase in prevalence in the elderly. • Polypharmacy is common in older people. • Older people are more sensitive to the effect of drugs. • Older people can present nonspecifically. • The elderly may not be suitable for investigations that are routine in younger patients. • They may not be considered suitable for surgery. • Older people have a high prevalence of co-morbidity. • Diseases in older people frequently have a different clinical course.

For those interested in the science of aging, the gastrointestinal tract is an ideal organ in which to study the aging process, as the mucosa is constantly exposed to damaging agents, has an increased cell turnover, and is readily accessible for repeated in vivo sampling.

In this chapter changes in gastrointestinal physiology in the elderly are reviewed and details specific to the diagnosis, investigation, and management of gastrointestinal symptoms and diseases in older people are discussed. Further details of individual conditions should be sought in relevant chapters.

CAUSES AND DIFFERENTIAL DIAGNOSIS
COMMON SYMPTOMS AND PATHOLOGY IN OLDER PEOPLE
• Dysphagia • Gastroesophageal reflux disease (GERD) • Esophageal dysmotility • Esophageal cancer • Gastric cancer • Peptic ulcer disease • Gastric atrophy • Bacterial overgrowth • Colonic cancer • Constipation • Diarrhea • Diverticular disease • *Clostridium difficile* diarrhea

HOW COMMON IS IT?

Nearly 50% of older people suffer from gastrointestinal symptoms. The elderly are more likely to consult a doctor about their symptoms, which has implications as those with gastrointestinal symptoms have significant healthcare utilization and poorer quality of life. Abdominal symptoms in the majority of older people are self-limiting and frequently relapsing. Despite this, the prognosis of all symptoms appears good.[1,2]

INVESTIGATING GASTROINTESTINAL SYMPTOMS IN OLDER PEOPLE

Taking a history from an elderly patient can be challenging and examination requires an open mind.[3] In terms of investigation, older people tolerate upper gastrointestinal endoscopy and colonoscopy well (see Chapter 119) and should not be denied the benefits of diagnostic investigation. It might sometimes be felt that seeking a diagnosis is not appropriate if ultimately little can be offered in the way of treatment. However, older people also tolerate surgery well; even when extensive curative surgery is not appropriate, palliation of symptoms might be possible.

Many national and international guidelines recommend an age threshold for investigations such as endoscopy.[4] Although this is in part to increase the specificity and sensitivity of the test, it should also be acknowledged that an age threshold is a means of limiting endoscopy based upon the fact that the incidence of malignancy increases with age.

EFFECT OF AGING ON NUTRITION AND APPETITE (see also Chapters 1, 15, and 138)

Older people are at increased risk of impaired nutrition and nutritional deficiency, although the absolute prevalence depends on the population studied and definitions used. It is unclear whether aging alone results in dysfunction of the gastrointestinal tract leading to undernutrition, or whether undernutrition in older people points to another disease or simply reflects social or physical conditions such as inability to chew, poverty, and social isolation. Poor oral health (Fig. 27.1) has been consistently correlated with malnutrition and, although the prevalence of edentulousness among older independent adults is projected to decrease, because of demographic changes the absolute number of edentulous elderly will remain high.[5]

CAUSES AND DIFFERENTIAL DIAGNOSIS
CAUSES OF UNDERNUTRITION IN OLDER PEOPLE
• Decreased food intake • Gastrointestinal diseases • Maldigestion • Malabsorption • Hypermetabolism

AGE-RELATED CHANGES IN HISTOLOGY AND STRUCTURE IN THE GASTROINTESTINAL TRACT (see also Chapter 138)

Changes in gastrointestinal physiology with age are summarized in Figure 27.2. Inflammation in the upper gastrointestinal tract increases with age, and the prevalence of gastric atrophy is commoner in older people partly, but not entirely, related to the increased prevalence of *Helicobacter pylori* in older people.

Gastrointestinal transit time is slower in older people owing to age-related changes in the innervation and composition of neuronal tissue in the gut wall. This reduced transit can lead to conditions that include esophageal dysmotility, decreased gastric emptying, diverticular disease, and constipation.

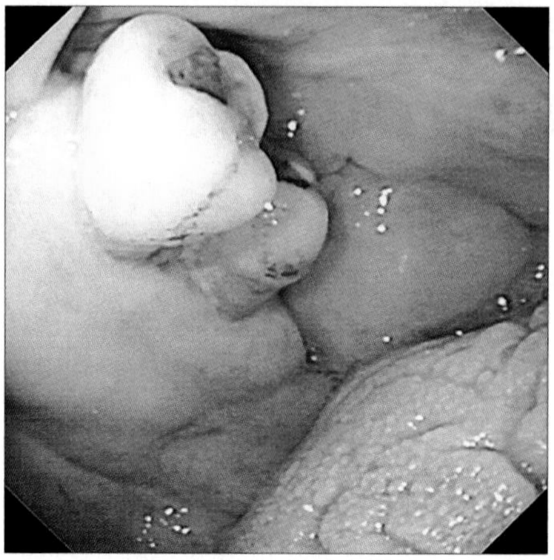

Fig. 27.1 Poor oral health. Inside the mouth of an 89-year-old man with some of his own teeth remaining.

CHANGES IN GASTROINTESTINAL MUCOSAL PROTECTION WITH AGE

In the human gastrointestinal tract there is a balance between aggressive factors and mucosal protective mechanisms; when this equilibrium is disrupted pathology results (Fig. 27.3). There are no age-related increases in the endogenous aggressors: acid and pepsin. Therefore, the imbalance that leads to diseases seen more commonly in older people, such as cancer or ulceration, is due to an age-associated impairment of mucosal protective mechanisms (see Fig. 27.2).

Prostaglandins

Prostaglandins are molecules involved in mucosal protection, via mucus, bicarbonate secretion, and blood flow. One study has suggested that their concentration may be reduced with advancing age.[6] Medications such as nonsteroidal anti-inflammatory drugs (NSAIDs), which also inhibit the production of prostaglandins, are used widely by older people, making them particularly vulnerable (see Chapters 27 and 35).

Mucus

Mucus covers the gastrointestinal tract with an adherent gel, with some barrier properties and a 'sloppy' luminal layer, which acts as a lubricant (Fig. 27.3). The amount of mucus, its quality, and the number of mucus-producing cells in the stomach are reduced with age and *H. pylori* infection,[7] and may contribute to the risk of ulcer development in older people.

Bicarbonate

Bicarbonate neutralizes gastric acid and inactivates pepsin by increasing pH. Bicarbonate secretion may be lower in the elderly, and the ability of the gastric mucosa to produce bicarbonate in response to prostaglandins is impaired.[8]

Repair mechanisms

In animals aging is associated with decreased reparative ability in the gastric mucosa, and with delays in both resolution of mucosal injury and regeneration of injured gastric mucosa. It is unclear whether this also occurs in the human stomach.

Blood flow to an injured area is important during repair, to bring nutrients and remove waste. Reduction in blood flow alone is sufficient to cause ulceration in the mucosa and likely to contribute to human disease. In aged rats, basal gastric blood flow and flow in response to injury is reduced.

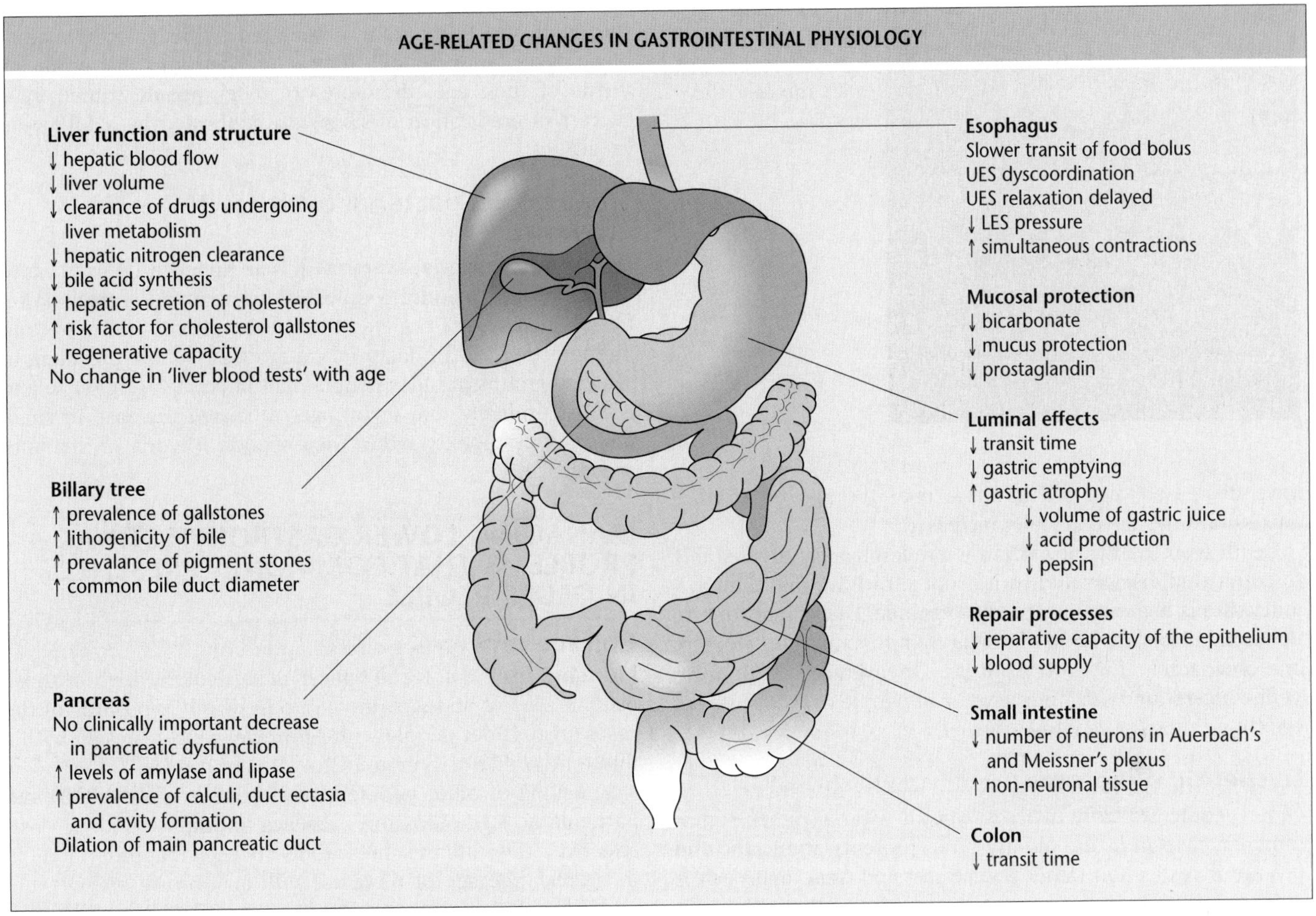

Fig. 27.2 Age-related changes in gastrointestinal physiology.

MANAGING UPPER GASTROINTESTINAL PROBLEMS COMMONLY PRESENTING IN OLDER PEOPLE

Gastroesophageal reflux disease/heartburn (see also Chapter 29)

Gastroesophageal reflux disease (GERD) becomes more prevalent with age. The prevalence in older people may be as high as 20%, although many do not report heartburn and self-medicate in the community without presenting to clinicians. Older people may present for the first time with the complications of longstanding reflux, such as benign esophageal stricture. Despite the management of GERD being established,[9] studies specific to older people are rare. In one small study patients over the age of 60 years were less likely to receive advice regarding lifestyle modification compared to those aged less than 60 years.[10]

Reflux symptoms are treated using a symptom-driven approach with a proton pump inhibitor.[9] There is no evidence to recommend whether stepping up treatment according to symptoms or stepping down when symptoms have resolved, or the use of empiric treatment without endoscopy, is most appropriate in older people. In view of the tendency for atypical presentation in older people, caution suggests referral for endoscopy to exclude malignancy.

Peptic ulceration (see also Chapter 35)

Peptic ulceration is more common in the elderly (Fig. 27.4). Increased NSAID use in older age groups is in part responsible for this. Older people are more likely to suffer the ulcer complications of perforation and bleeding, and, although admissions

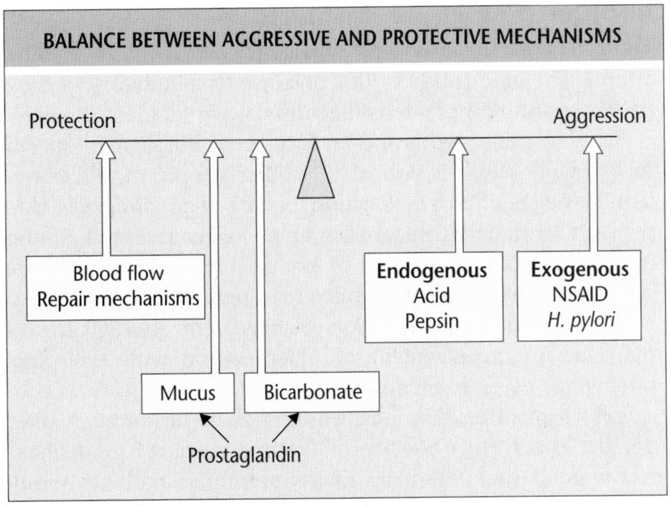

Fig. 27.3 Balance between aggressive and protective mechanisms. Disruption of the balance between aggressive and protective mechanisms in the human stomach leads to pathology.

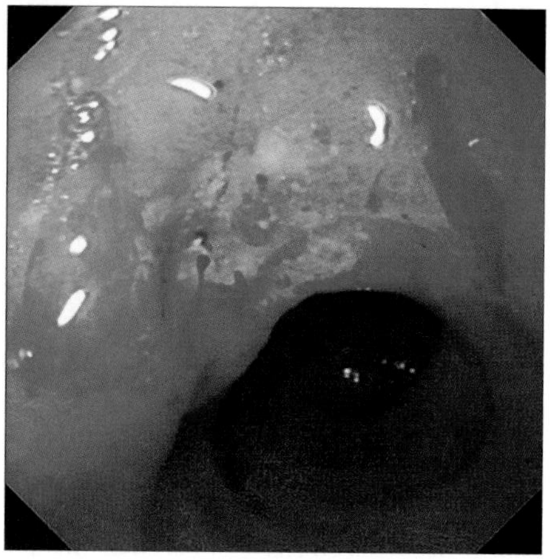

Fig. 27. Peptic ulcer. Peptic ulcer in a 67-year-old presenting with iron deficiency anemia.

have decreased over all, in those over the age of 75 years admission rates have actually increased.

Death from peptic ulceration is predominantly attributable to co-morbid disease, and so it is not surprising that the mortality rate is highest amongst older people. Death rates due to duodenal ulcers are higher in older men than in older women, but comparable for gastric ulcers. On average, death from peptic ulceration is 20 times greater in people over 75 years of age than in those aged 45–64 years.[11]

Dyspeptic symptoms (see also Chapters 4 and 5)

Older people are more likely to consult with dyspeptic symptoms. Dyspepsia in the elderly often presents atypically, and prompt investigation rather than a 'test and treat' approach is more appropriate in this age group, considering the high likelihood of organic disease, particularly malignancy.[4] This advice may be changing, and a number of guidelines now discourage referral for investigation solely on grounds of age. Moreover, in the frail elderly considered unfit for investigation, the adoption of an empiric treatment approach may be appropriate.

Generally there is poor agreement between the presence of gastritis or duodenitis and symptoms of dyspepsia, and older people report fewer symptoms despite having higher rates of pathology.

Management of *Helicobacter pylori* infection in older people (see also Chapter 34)

There is a particularly high prevalence of *H. pylori* in older people. The eradication of this organism is mandatory in those with a recent and previous diagnosis of peptic ulcer disease.

H. pylori guidelines have been developed; although not specific to older people, it is critical that older people should not be denied the benefits of eradication therapy. Suggestions that older people remain on H_2 antagonists are no longer accepted. Studies in older people are needed to evaluate eradication rates and side effects in the group in which the prevalence is the highest.

A 'test and treat' *H. pylori* management strategy has no place in the management of older people with their high prevalence of sinister pathology.[12]

Follow-up after *H. pylori* eradication is different in older people. The British Society of Gastroenterology guidelines[12] recommend that follow-up in asymptomatic patients should ideally be by breath test, but only when symptoms persist or recur, and in all subjects who would otherwise be given long-term antisecretory treatment to prevent recurrence. In view of the high mortality rate associated with gastrointestinal bleeding in older people, they would fall into this group by virtue of their age; therefore, all older people should have successful eradication of *H. pylori* confirmed by a follow-up breath test.

Small bowel bacterial overgrowth (see also Chapter 46)

Small bowel bacterial overgrowth is an under-recognized cause of malnutrition in older people. Colonization of the small bowel by colonic bacteria can lead to malabsorption of nutrients and vitamins (Fig. 27.5). Bacterial overgrowth is more prevalent in selected groups of older people than in young age groups, and is most probably due to an age-associated increase in small intestinal dysmotility rather than hypochlorhydria or immunosenescence.[13]

MANAGING LOWER GASTROINTESTINAL PROBLEMS THAT COMMONLY PRESENT IN OLDER PEOPLE

Colonic cancer (see also Chapter 60)

Mortality from colorectal cancer is particularly high in those over the age of 65 years, the group in whom two-thirds of the cases arise. Older people with colorectal cancer present with a different profile of symptoms to younger groups.[14]

Screening of older people by fecal occult blood (FOB) and particularly sigmoidoscopy reduces mortality and is cost-effective.[15] Despite this, these tools are used inappropriately in those over the age of 65 years, with an overuse of FOB and underuse of sigmoidscopy. Furthermore, older people do not appear to recognize the significance of 'sinister' lower gastrointestinal symptoms such as rectal bleeding.

A change in bowel habit in those over 45 years of age is an immediate cause for concern, requiring prompt referral for secondary investigations. Irritable bowel rarely presents for the first time in the elderly and should be a diagnosis of exclusion. Although treatment is generally surgical, older people are more often referred to medical or geriatric units.

Functional constipation (see also Chapters 9, 68, 70 and 71)

Constipation impacts hugely upon the quality of life of older people and is a common cause of consultations in the elderly. Once serious pathology has been ruled out, management

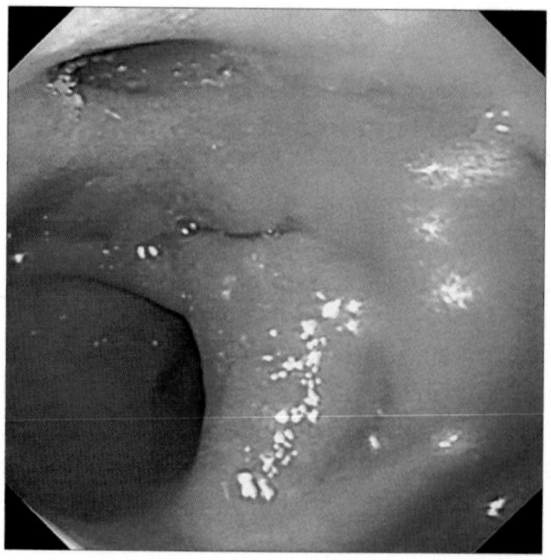

Fig. 27.5 Small bowel bacterial overgrowth. View taken during gastroscopy in a 93-year-old woman with malnutrition showing a duodenal diverticulum that is causing small bowel overgrowth.

generally involves the use of eperients; laxative use is common in older patients. Laxatives improve bowel movement frequency, stool consistency, and symptoms, but there is currently little evidence for marked differences in effectiveness between laxatives. Further good-quality trial evidence is required in the management of constipation in older people.

Clostridium difficile (see also Chapters 49 and 59)

Clostridium difficile causes gastrointestinal infections ranging from asymptomatic colonization to severe diarrhea, pseudomembranous colitis, and toxic megacolon.[16] It is the most frequent cause of nosocomial diarrhea. A history of antibiotic treatment is identifiable in virtually all patients. Infection with *C. difficile* increased 4-fold in all age groups between 1994 and 1997; however, reports in over 65-year-olds increased 6-fold over the same period, with more than 80% of cases in those aged over 65 years. Once acquired, the infection may be more severe in the elderly. Older age and frailty are predictors for recurrent disease.

Chronic diarrhea (see also Chapter 9)

Chronic diarrhea is one of the most common reasons for referral to gastroenterologists. It is commoner in older people, with prevalence rates of 7–14% in an elderly population.[17] Causes of chronic diarrhea to consider in older people, and signs and symptoms that should initiate prompt further investigation, are shown in Table 27.2.

AGE-RELATED CHANGES IN THE PANCREAS, LIVER, AND BILIARY TREE (see also Chapter 27)

Liver disease is increasing in older people, in part because of the increase in systemic diseases that affect the liver and also due to improved management of liver diseases, which enables those with liver disease to live into older age. There appear to be no liver diseases specific to older age; however, presentation, clinical course, and management of liver disease may be different in older people than in younger age groups. Age-related changes in the pancreas, liver, and biliary tree are summarized in Figure 27.2.

TABLE 27.2 REASONS FOR FURTHER INVESTIGATION OF DIARRHEA IN THE ELDERLY

- History of diarrhea of > 3 months
- Predominantly nocturnal diarrhea
- Continuous rather than intermittent diarrhea
- Weight loss
- Steatorrhea
- Passage of malodorous pale stools
- Mucus
- Blood
- Family history – neoplastic, inflammatory bowel or celiac disease

CAUSES AND DIFFERENTIAL DIAGNOSIS

DIFFERENTIAL DIAGNOSIS OF DIARRHEA IN OLDER PEOPLE

- Previous gastrointestinal surgery, particularly of the ileum and right colon
- Lack of absorptive surface – fat and carbohydrate malabsorption
- Decreased transit time
- Malabsorption of bile acids
- Bacterial overgrowth
- Previous pancreatic disease
- Systemic disease
- Thyrotoxicosis
- Parathyroid disease
- Diabetes mellitus
- Alcohol
- Drugs
- Recent overseas travel or other potential sources of infectious gastrointestinal pathogens
- Recent antibiotic use and *C. difficile* infection
- Lactase deficiency

SUMMARY

- The demographics of the population is changing as the proportion of older people increases.
- Gastrointestinal symptoms and diseases are a major cause of morbidity and mortality in older people and impact hugely upon quality of life.
- Research needs to be directed towards a better understanding of the underlying changes that occur in the gastrointestinal tract with aging, to help explain why older people are more susceptible to diseases such as peptic ulcer.
- Clinical studies carried out specifically in older people are required to confirm that management of common gastrointestinal syndromes is effective and efficient in older people.
- An examination of why older people are more likely to suffer from malnutrition is high on the research agenda.

SOURCES OF INFORMATION FOR PATIENTS AND DOCTORS

http://www.patient.co.uk/showdoc/214/
http://www.patient.co.uk/showdoc/23068673/

REFERENCES

1. Stanghellini V. Three month prevalence rates of gastrointestinal symptoms and the influence of demographic factors: results from the Domestic/International Gastroenterology Surveillance Study (DIGEST). Scand J Gastroenterol Suppl 1999; 231:20–28.
2. Chaplin A, Curless R, Thomson R, Barton R. Prevalence of lower gastrointestinal symptoms and associated consultation behaviour in a British elderly population determined by face to face interview. Br J Gen Pract 2000; 50:798–802.
3. Barry PP. An overview of special considerations in the evaluation and management of the geriatric patient. Am J Gastroenterol 2000; 95:8–10.
4. British Society of Gastroenterology. Dyspepsia management guidelines. Online. Available: http://www.bsg.org.uk/clinical_prac/guidelines/dyspepsia.htm
5. Budtz-Jorgenson E, Chung JP, Rapin CH. Nutrition and oral health. Best practice and research. Clin Gastroenterol 2001; 15: 885–896.
6. Lee M, Feldman M. The ageing stomach: implications for NSAID gastropathy. Gut 1997; 41:575–576.
7. Allen A, Newton J, Oliver L et al. Mucus and *H. pylori*. J Physiol Pharmacol 1997; 48: 297–305.
8. Guslandi M, Pellegrini A, Sorghi M. Gastric mucosal defences in the elderly. Gerontology 1999; 45:206–208.
9. Ferriman A. NICE issues guidance for heartburn and indigestion. BMJ 2000; 321:197.
10. Blair DI, Kaplan B, Speigler J. Patient characteristics and lifestyle recommendations in the treatment of gastroesophageal reflux disease. J Fam Pract 1997; 44:266–272.
11. Rockall TA, Logan RF, Devlin HB, Northfield TC. Incidence of and mortality from acute upper gastrointestinal haemorrhage in the United Kingdom. Steering committee and members of the National Audit of Acute Upper Gastrointestinal Haemorrhage. BMJ 1995; 311:222–226.
12. European Society for Primary Care Gastroenterology. The management of *H. pylori* infection. Online. Available: http://www.espcg.org/ guidelines/hpguide.html
13. Lewis SJ, Potts LF, Malhotra R, Mountford R. Small bowel bacterial overgrowth in subjects living in residential care homes. Age Ageing 1999; 28:181–185.
14. Curless R, French J, Williams G, James O. Comparison of gastrointestinal symptoms in colorectal carcinoma patients and community controls with respect to age. Gut 1994; 35:1267–1270.
15. British Society of Gastroenterology. Guidelines for colorectal cancer screening in high risk groups. Online. Available: http://www.bsg.org.uk/clinical_prac/guidelines/colorectal.htm
16. Kyne L, Farrell RJ, Kelly CP. *Clostridium difficile*. Gastroenterol Clin North Am 2001; 30:753–777.
17. British Society of Gastroenterology. Guidelines for the investigation of chronic diarrhoea. Online. Available: http://www.bsg.org.uk/ clinical_prac/guidelines/chronic_diarr.htm

Chapter 28

Problems in pediatrics

Simon Murch

KEY POINTS

- GI problems in childhood assume greater significance due to the impact on growth and development
- Autoimmune enteropathy is a rare but important cause of severe persistent diarrhea in infancy
- GOR is common in infancy but tends to improve with growth
- Allergic dysmotility is an increasingly recognized cause of reflux
- Some food allergies (e.g., peanuts) are becoming more common
- Two major groups of constipation are slow transient and outflow obstruction
- Classic presentation of celiac disease in childhood represents only the minority of cases
- IBD is rare under 2 years of age – inherited immunological conditions should be looked for
- Current trends in IBD include early aggressive treatment (e.g., azathioprine) and nutritional intervention rather than corticosteroid use

INTRODUCTION

The nutritional requirements of infants and young children are relatively higher than for adults, because of the requirements for growth. There is also relative functional immaturity of the immune system in early life, and thus an increased tendency for sensitization to dietary components. The spectrum of gastrointestinal problems in children is therefore different from that in adults, and conditions that may have relatively minor significance in adults may compromise growth and weight gain in children. Inherited abnormalities play a greater role in young infants presenting with gastrointestinal disease, whilst immunodeficiency may be unmasked by postnatal infections or antigen challenge, resulting in chronic diarrhea or apparent food allergy.

There is now an increasing incidence of inflammatory bowel disease (IBD), notably Crohn's disease, in children, including apparently those in the 3–7 years age range where it was previously extremely rare. Basic principles of management are shared with adults, with special considerations related to growth and development.

GASTROENTEROLOGICAL PROBLEMS IN INFANCY

Congenital abnormalities of intestinal structure may present in the first hours or days of life with symptoms of obstruction. The initial features may be nonspecific, and there may be similar symptoms in infants with sepsis. Sepsis may also mimic congenital metabolic disorders and cause neonatal jaundice.

Hirschsprung's disease

This condition is due to defective innervation of the rectum, with loss of nitric oxide (NO) mediation of nonadrenergic noncholinergic (NANC) inhibitory nerves. Molecular genetic analyses suggest that Hirschsprung's disease is a complex oligo/polygenic disorder with several genes (e.g., RET, GDNF, EDNRB, EDN3, and SOX10) implicated.[1]

Hirschsprung's disease may present initially with delayed passage of meconium, but this may be missed and the diagnosis delayed until later infancy, or even childhood. In addition to constipation, Hirschsprung's disease may be complicated by the development of severe enterocolitis.

Diagnosis requires full thickness rectal biopsy, best performed as a formal surgical procedure. Long-term management is required, and many children have significant problems despite surgical resection of the aganglionic segment. There have been important recent advances in the understanding of Hirschsprung's disease.

Necrotizing enterocolitis (NEC)

This is a severe and frequently life-threatening intestinal disease, which may result in fatal intestinal perforation. NEC is characterized by diffuse or patchy ischemic lesions of the mucosa or submucosa of the small and/or large intestine (Fig. 28.1), causing ulceration of the distal small intestine and colon, frequently progressing to necrosis and perforation.[2]

NEC is associated with birth asphyxia, umbilical catheterization, polycythemia or sepsis, and extreme prematurity without other predisposing factors (Table 28.1). NEC frequently affects the terminal ileum, a vascular 'watershed' area, suggesting that mesenteric blood flow is an important determinant. Other risk factors may include dysmotility, hypoxia, ischemia with reperfusion, luminal bacteria, and high osmolality enteral feeds, particularly containing casein and lactose. Certain bacteria, particularly *Clostridia*, have been implicated in localized outbreaks, but most cases are sporadic.

Infants often present with gastric stasis, abdominal distention, or acidosis and thrombocytopenia. Management is then based on stopping enteric feeds and commencing antibiotics, and many cases are self-limiting. The disease may progress, with increasing distention and signs of perforation or sepsis. Characteristic X-ray findings include distended bowel loops with wall thickening, and free gas in the peritoneum or biliary tree (Fig. 28.1). Laparotomy is often required and affected bowel may appear ischemic or frankly gangrenous. Late consequences of NEC include stricturing and short bowel syndrome.

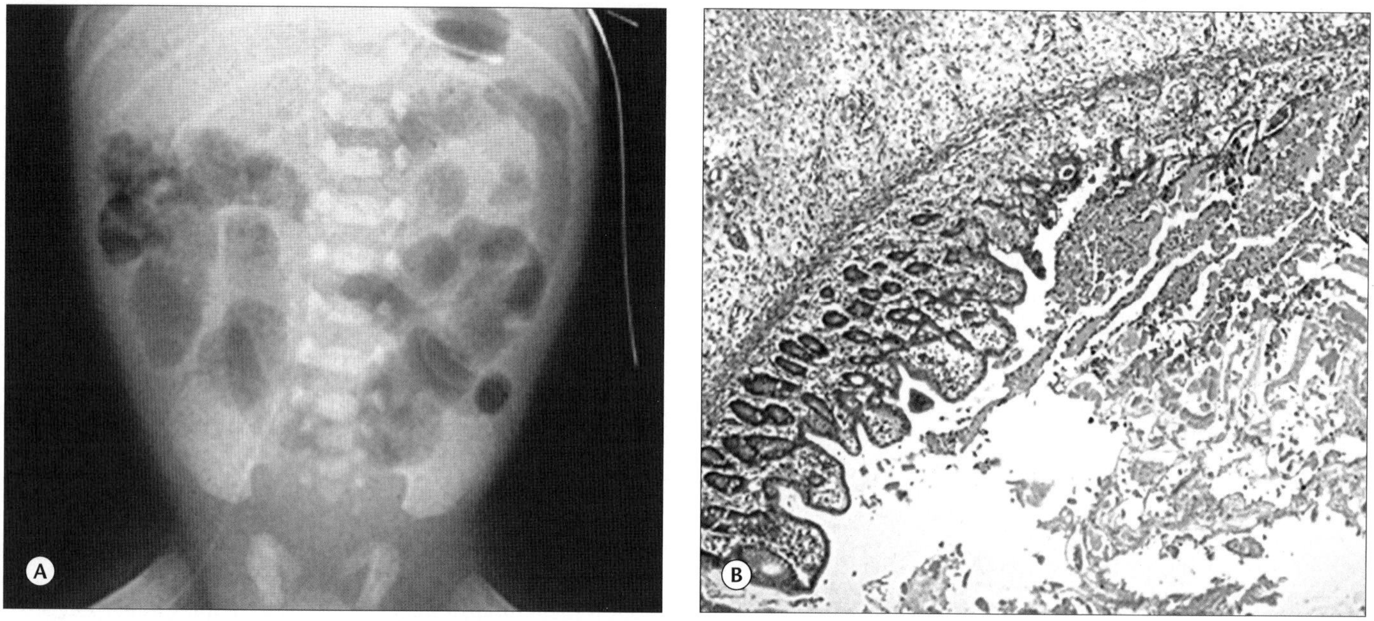

Fig. 28.1 Findings on investigation of necrotizing enterocolitis. A. Plain abdominal X-ray of an infant with acute NEC, showing loops of distended small bowel and colon, with bowel wall thickening. **B.** Full thickness resection specimen shows focal mucosal ulceration, with relatively minor inflammatory infiltrate.

Neonatal diarrhoea

It is uncommon for neonates to present with diarrhea, and this may point to an underlying inherited abnormality (Table 28.2). It is important to differentiate between osmotic and secretory diarrhea. Two rare conditions, **chloridorrhea** and **sodium diarrhea,** present with secretory diarrhea so watery it can be mistaken for urine. Antenatal ultrasound examination can show dilated echogenic loops of bowel. Early recognition is important to prevent CNS and renal complications, but subsequent treatment is straightforward and dependent on electrolyte replacement.

By contrast, in **glucose-galactose malabsorption,** due to mutations in the sodium-glucose cotransporter (SGLT-1), the diarrhea is entirely osmotic. An important clinical clue is perianal burning due to carbohydrate malabsorption. Treatment is based on fructose-based milk formulae, as fructose is absorbed by a separate transporter (Glut 5).

Much less frequently, the onset of persistent diarrhea in infancy is a manifestation of one of the intractable diarrhea syndromes.[3] Primary epithelial abnormalities, including microvillous inclusion disease and tufting enteropathy, usually present in the first few days of life. These cause intestinal failure, requiring long-term TPN therapy. Microvillous inclusion disease is characterized by abnormal development of the microvilli and glycocalyx, with characteristic ultrastructural findings of vesicles containing microvilli (Fig. 28.2). In tufting enteropathy cell adhesion is disturbed, causing characteristic tufts of extruding epithelium. Both disorders are lethal unless long TPN is maintained, and small bowel transplantation is increasingly attempted. Hopes for the future include gene transfer, when the molecular basis is established.

Infant protein-losing enteropathy is most frequently due to lymphangiectasia, but rare causes include enterocyte heparan sulfate deficiency. Similar presentations may occur as a rare

TABLE 28.1 RISK FACTORS FOR THE DEVELOPMENT OF NECROTIZING ENTEROCOLITIS
FACTORS AFFECTING EPITHELIAL INTEGRITY
Prematurity (particularly extreme prematurity below 26 weeks' gestation)
Systemic infection (neonates are relatively immune compromised)
Hypoxia (e.g., severe respiratory distress syndrome, meconium aspiration)
FACTORS AFFECTING MESENTERIC BLOOD SUPPLY
Placental insufficiency
Reversed umbilical arterial diastolic flow
Polycythemia
Cyanotic congenital heart disease
Indomethacin treatment (patent ductus arteriosus)
Maternal cocaine abuse
LUMINAL FACTORS (GUT FLORA, DIETARY ANTIGENS)
Formula feeds (breast feeding is protective)
Intestinal obstruction (e.g., congenital malformation, meconium ileus, Hirschsprung's disease)
Intestinal bacteria (individual pathogens only rarely found)

TABLE 28.2 POTENTIAL CAUSES OF PERSISTENT DIARRHEA IN INFANTS AND YOUNG CHILDREN
Misdiagnosis or poor treatment of recognized food-sensitive enteropathy
Unrecognized immunodeficiency and/or infection
Inflammatory enteropathy or colitis
Anatomical abnormalities or dysmotility syndromes (pseudo-obstruction)
Primary specific absorption failures (e.g., chloridorrhea)
Enteropathy associated with primary metabolic diseases (e.g., mitochondrial cytopathy, abetalipoproteinemia, congenital disorders of glycosylation)
True intractable diarrhea syndromes:
Epithelial – microvillous inclusion disease, tufting enteropathy, heparan sulfate deficiency
Autoimmune enteropathy syndromes, e.g., IPEX syndrome

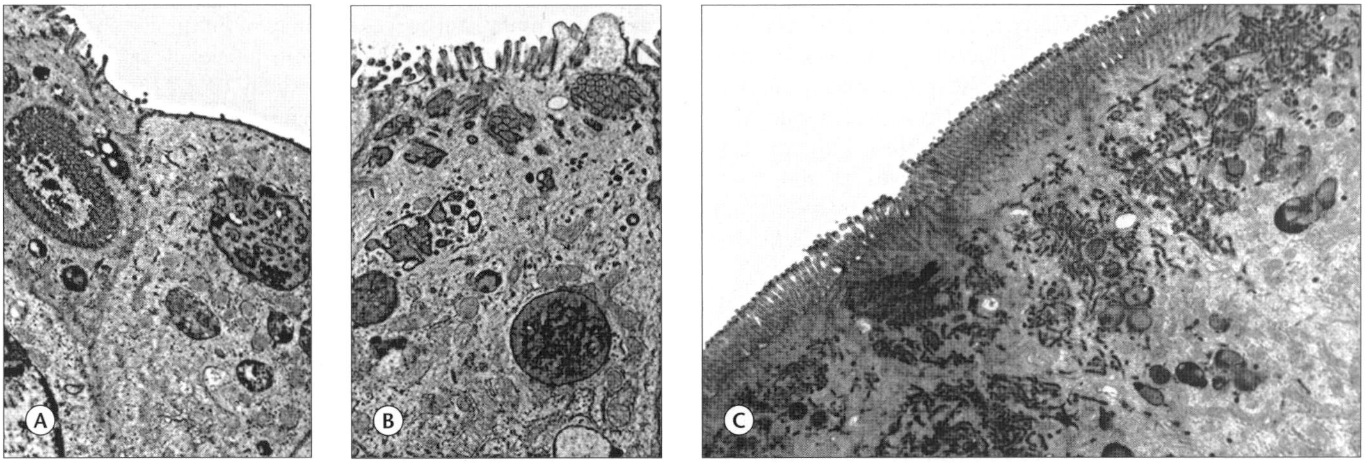

Fig. 28.2 Electron microscopic features of microvillous inclusion disease/microvillous atrophy. A,B. Characteristic findings of disrupted surface microvilli on villous epithelium, with intracellular vesicles containing microvillous components. **C.** Note crypt epithelium, with intact surface microvilli, but the presence of intracellular secretory granules. The molecular basis has yet to be determined. (Courtesy of Dr Alan Phillips.)

manifestation of other primary disorders, including mitochondrial cytopathies, immunodeficiencies and congenital disorders of glycosylation.

Autoimmune enteropathy

This is an uncommon, but important cause of severe persistent diarrhea in infancy, due to an autoimmune response to the gut epithelium (Fig. 28.3). Inflammation may be confined to the intestine or be part of a multisystem process, often in association with endocrinopathy. There have been important recent advances in the molecular basis of autoimmune enteropathy syndromes. The immune polyendocrinopathy X-linked (IPEX) syndrome is due to mutation in the transcription factor FOXP3, a master regulator of regulatory lymphocyte generation.[4] Affected infants cannot generate normal regulatory lymphocytes, and thus present with a multifocal autoimmune disease, characterized by hyper-IgE, intractable diarrhea, eczema, and a variety of endocrinopathies. The disease is of major conceptual interest, despite its rarity, and bone marrow transplantation may potentially be curative.

The autoimmune polyendocrinopathy-candidosis-ectodermal dystrophy (APECED) syndrome presents in later childhood and is due to mutations in the autoimmune regulator gene *Aire*, which is expressed in the thymus.[3] Other cases have been associated with T cell activation deficiencies, and it is likely that bone marrow transplantation may become a more widely used form of treatment. Medical therapy is based otherwise upon a combination of TPN and immunosuppression.

Gastroesophageal reflux

Gastroesophageal reflux (GOR) is common in infancy. It is mainly caused by mechanical factors, and is in part due to the relatively straight gastroesophageal alignment in early infancy. Additional neural immaturity makes reflux almost universal in very preterm infants, while neurological abnormalities of any kind predispose to later reflux. Impedance monitoring has shown that the great majority of reflux episodes are nonacid, and thus go undetected on standard 24-h pH testing. Symptoms are variable, with some infants showing clear evidence of vomiting or pain, while others present more insidiously with

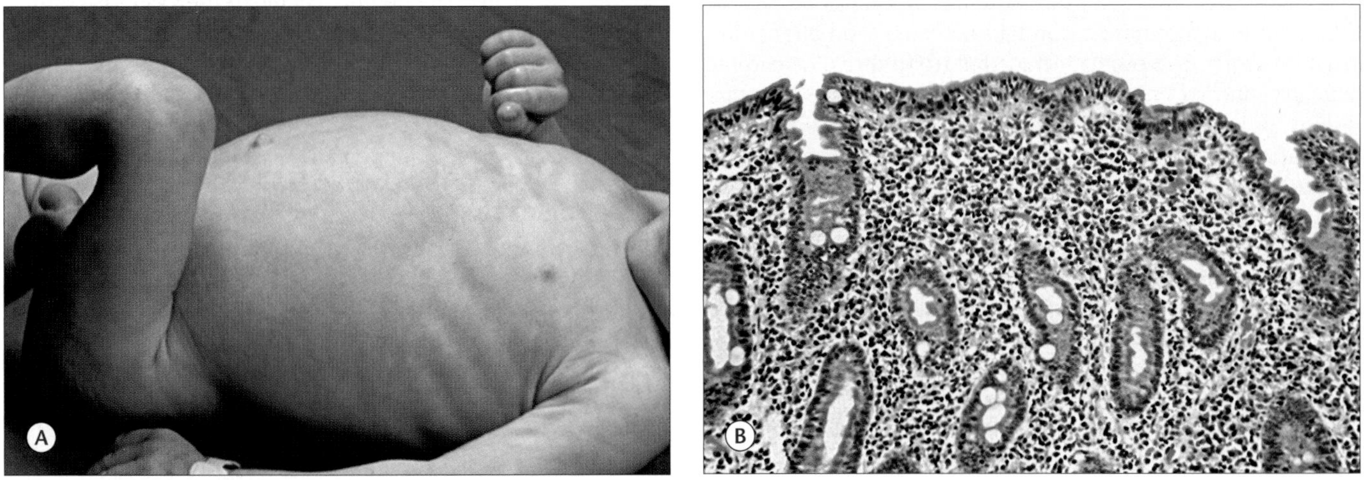

Fig. 28.3 A case of autoimmune enteropathy, due to IPEX syndrome. A. Note the characteristic abdominal distention and buttock wasting. **B.** Histological features in the duodenum, with crypt hyperplastic villous atrophy. Unlike celiac disease, the intraepithelial lymphocyte density is often normal.

signs of aspiration or of feeding refusal. Treatment has been based on posture control, feed thickening, acid-suppressing agents (ranitidine or omeprazole), and prokinetics (domperidone). Nissen's fundoplication is a last resort in infants with intractable reflux (usually due to neurological impairment).[5] Gastroesophageal reflux classically improves as the infant grows, and may become less evident as the infant weans onto solids, but inadequate treatment predisposes to later feeding difficulty.

Recently, a second important cause of GOR has been recognized. In allergic dysmotility, GOR is precipitated by ingested dietary antigen, most commonly milk. Multiple food antigens have now been implicated, and induced mast cell and eosinophil degranulation is thought to be the likely mechanism of the induced dysmotility.[6] Thus, antigen exclusion may need to be combined with conventional therapy in the management of infants with reflux, and empirical antigen restriction is attempted in most cases resistant to classic therapy (see Chapter 57).

Food allergies

Food allergies now affect 5% or more of children in most developed countries.[7] Previously uncommon allergies such as to peanut have become much more prevalent.[8] Current theories include changing antigen intake in infancy, and reduced infectious exposures.[9] IgE-mediated allergies generally present soon after ingestion, and the diagnosis is usually supported by positive skin prick and specific-IgE tests. Non-IgE-mediated allergies usually present later after ingestion, and the causative antigen may be more difficult to detect, particularly as tests for immediate allergies are often negative.

In IgE-mediated reactions, children may complain of tingling of the tongue or lips, or simply appear apprehensive. This may be followed rapidly by skin rash, urticari, or wheezing. Angioneurotic edema can follow, and in more severe cases, the airway may become compromised or anaphylactic shock may develop. Specific therapy includes antihistamines such as chlorphenamine (chlorpheniramine), together with inhaled bronchodilators as appropriate. Some children manifest a biphasic response, with a relatively modest initial reaction followed several hours later by a potentially life-threatening response. Severe food allergic reactions require urgent assessment, and adrenaline therapy is required if there is any evidence of airway obstruction or systemic hypotension.[10]

Late-onset symptoms of non-IgE-mediated food allergy are often insidious. Symptoms include failure to thrive or chronic diarrhea, due to enteropathy or colitis, as well as eczema, rhinitis, or rectal bleeding. These symptoms are mediated by T cells or eosinophils in a delayed hypersensitive reaction, and may not be recognized as due to food ingestion. They may also occur in exclusively breast-fed infants in response to maternally ingested antigen. Although intestinal biopsy may show evidence of enteropathy or mucosal eosinophilia, both skin prick tests and specific IgE tests may be negative. Effective food elimination relieves all the symptoms and challenge causes return of symptoms.

Food-sensitive enteropathy

The major mucosal manifestation of food allergy is food sensitive enteropathy, in which an immunologically mediated lesion disturbs small intestinal function. Features of enteropathy include excess lymphocyte infiltration, epithelial abnormality, or architectural disturbance. This may often impair absorption, causing either covert micronutrient deficiency or frank malabsorption. Modern diagnosis is usually based on histological features at initial biopsy and clinical response to antigen exclusion and challenge, without the sequential biopsies previously performed. By contrast to celiac disease, such enteropathies are usually restricted to early life, and later challenge with the protein is usually tolerated. The mucosal lesion is classically patchy, and less severe than seen in celiac disease.

The food protein-induced enterocolitis syndrome (FPIES) is a severe and sometimes life-threatening form of mucosal food hypersensitivity. It is classically associated with cows' milk or soya ingestion in infants, but has recently been reported in older children in response to several foods of usually low antigenicity, including rice, oat, barley, vegetables, and poultry.[11] It is also common for allergic colitis to occur in exclusively breast-fed infants, triggered by milk protein in the mother's diet. Negative skin prick tests do not exclude this diagnosis, and the majority of cases are in fact negative. Mild cases present with loose stools containing mucus or blood, with evidence of thrombocytosis and mucosal eosinophilia, and respond rapidly to exclusion of cows' milk from the diet (cows' milk colitis). More severe cases present with vomiting and diarrhea or melena, and may result in dehydration and shock.

If colonoscopy is performed, changes are usually milder than with classic IBD, and the macroscopic findings are dominated by loss of vascular pattern, prominent lymphoid follicles with a rim of perifollicular erythema (red halo sign), and an easily traumatized mucosa. Histological features include infiltration of lymphocytes, plasma cells and eosinophils, and focal crypt abscesses. Lymphoid follicles are seen in the majority of colonic biopsies, and ileal lymphoid hyperplasia is also characteristic.

Constipation

Constipation is a relatively common problem in children, with prevalence in otherwise normal children up to 8%. Development of severe constipation in infancy raises the possibility of structural or neurological abnormality, and makes neurological assessment and rectal examination important. Most cases do not have a clear structural basis, and are labeled functional constipation. Two major groups can be differentiated by transit studies: either due to slow transit throughout the colon, or outflow obstruction (rectal impaction) due to local dysmotility of the sphincter mechanisms. General pediatricians manage the majority of cases, and referral to pediatric gastroenterologists is usually reserved for severe or treatment-resistant cases. Some cases of apparently intractable constipation may be relieved by exclusion diets,[12] but many remain resistant to medical therapy.

Celiac disease

The incidence of celiac disease in childhood is much higher than previously thought. It is important to recognize that the classical presentation of a child with steatorrhea, abdominal distention, poor growth, and anemia is actually quite uncommon in childhood celiac disease (Fig. 28.4). These children represent the 'tip of the iceberg' of total celiac disease cases.

Estimates of incidence have increased from 1 in 2000 in UK children and 1 in 600 in Irish children during the 1970s to more than 1 in 100 of Finnish children in 2000.[13] This is because of better detection by specific serology. Population-based serological studies have demonstrated that silent or

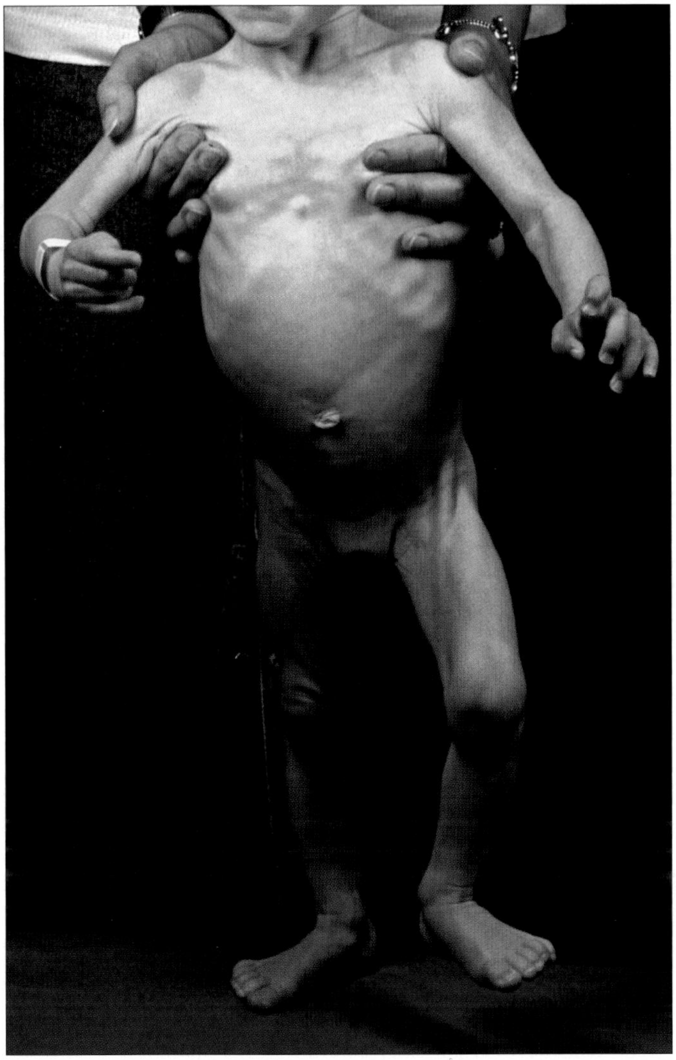

Fig. 28.4 Celiac disease. Classical appearance of celiac disease, with abdominal distention and wasting of the buttocks and thighs. Many current cases show less florid features, and celiac serology is being performed increasingly readily in pediatric practice (e.g., in Down's syndrome, unexplained epilepsy, diabetes).

atypical celiac disease is far more common than usually appreciated.[13]

Early weaning of infants has an important influence on presentation of celiac disease. In the UK, its incidence apparently rose from the 1950s to the 1970s, due to earlier introduction of solids, and then fell sharply as weaning recommendations changed. An even more striking demonstration was seen in Sweden, in which there was a major increase in infant presentation when a high wheat-containing weaning diet was recommended, and a dramatic fall when recommendations changed.[14] However, it is not known whether this will lead to a true reduction in incidence or an increase in the numbers of children presenting late and atypically.

The pathogenesis of celiac disease in childhood is similar to adult celiac disease (see Chapter 44). The lesion is driven by pathogenic T cell clones, which recognize gliadin peptide sequences that have been deamidated by tissue transglutaminase, a tissue repair molecule that is itself the subject of an autoimmune response. In contrast to adult celiac disease, in which there are clearly a very few immunodominant peptide sequences in the gliadin molecule, responses in children may be directed to a large number of peptide sequences in both gliadin and gluten.[15]

As in adult celiac disease, the only current treatment is a lifelong strict gluten-free diet. There are a very small number of children who develop apparent celiac disease in the first 2 years of life, but then recover on a gluten-free diet and do not relapse subsequently (transient gluten intolerance of infancy). Such early onset makes advisable a later formal gluten challenge, including serial biopsies on and off gluten. However, for all children diagnosed after 2 years of age, current ESPGHAN recommendations suggest that a single abnormal biopsy is diagnostic if specific serology is positive.

Inflammatory bowel disease

True IBD is extremely uncommon in young infants, and many such cases represent inherited immunological conditions. Thus, any case of apparent IBD in a child below 2 years of age warrants in-depth immunological assessment. Histological findings of granulomata in such cases make exclusion of chronic granulomatous disease important. Other conditions to exclude in the very young child with apparent IBD include Behçet's disease and autoimmune enteropathy.

In older children, however, classic IBD occurs, and the manifestations are broadly similar to adult disease, with the additional effects of growth impairment and pubertal delay. There has been recent evidence of substantial increase in the incidence of Crohn's disease and ulcerative colitis in children and adolescents.[16] Many cases present without the classic features of diarrhea, weight loss, and pain, but with unexplained short stature.[17] Thus, diagnostic delay is unfortunately common. A simple check of inflammatory markers will identify most cases.[18]

The essential lesion of IBD is similar in children to that seen in adults (Fig. 28.5). For initial diagnosis, it is important to perform full ileocolonoscopy, with upper endoscopy.[16] The use of sigmoidoscopy alone is suboptimal, particularly in view of the increasing incidence of indeterminate colitis in pediatric patients.

Because the disease is often of relatively recent onset in young people, there are increased potential opportunities for treatment. In general, there is now a trend towards early aggressive therapy, with earlier use of azathioprine, either at first relapse, or even at diagnosis.[19] The ideal aim of therapy is to induce and maintain clinical and histological remission, rather than just symptomatic improvement. Successful treatment should allow children to achieve their full potential for growth and educational attainment, without deprivation of normal social interaction. Treatment modalities are similar to those used in adult patients, although therapies for children should not interfere with growth and pubertal development. Thus, there is an increased use of nutritional intervention, and reduced use of corticosteroids in children.

Although active IBD, particularly Crohn's disease, impairs linear growth and retards puberty, growth failure may be compounded by use of corticosteroids. Thus, enteral nutrition therapy is often used as first line treatment for Crohn's disease, and meta-analysis shows equal efficacy to steroids in pediatric practice.[20]

There has been significant advance in the understanding of basic pathogenesis, and the important finding of a specific

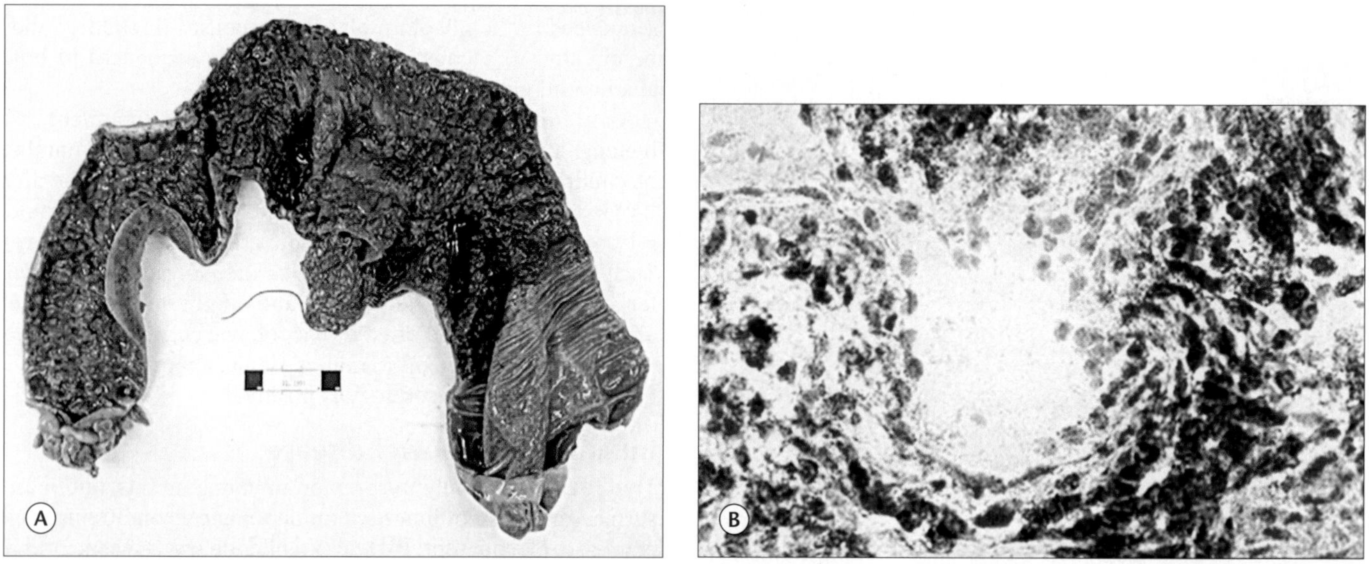

Fig. 28.5 Pediatric IBD may be severe. A. Colon resected from a 12-year-old child as an emergency because of fulminant ulcerative colitis. There is a sharp demarcation between severely affected and relatively normal colon. (Photograph courtesy of Dr Alan Bates). **B.** Submucosal vessel from the ileum of a 14-year-old child with Crohn's disease, which was resected because of intractable disease causing growth failure and pubertal delay. The vessel is surrounded by multiple TNF-α immunoreactive cells (stained red).

disease-associated gene, Nod-2 (CARD 15), which is associated with increased growth suppression in pediatric patients. Such genetic stratification may allow insight into optimal treatment strategies on an individual basis. However, the inflammatory bowel diseases remain difficult to treat, and fundamental uncertainties remain about optimal management approaches. While new biological agents offer great promise, they are likely to be extremely expensive, and thus not available to all.

An important consequence of uncontrolled IBD in childhood is the retardation of growth and pubertal development. Although candidate cytokines have been proposed, notably IL-6 and TNF-α,[16] the immunological basis of growth failure has not been determined (Fig. 28.5). Further study of the systemic response to gut inflammation is important, as growth failure is an important cause of impaired quality of life.

SOURCES OF INFORMATION FOR PATIENTS AND DOCTORS

http://www.cdhnf.org/pdf/GERDInfants.pdf
http://www.cdhnf.org/
http://pcca.hypermart.net/

REFERENCES

1. Pusch CM, Sasiadek MM, Blin N. Hirschsprung, RET-SOX and beyond: the challenge of examining non-mendelian traits. Int J Mol Med 2002; 10:367-370.
2. Walker-Smith JA, Murch SH. Necrotizing enterocolitis. In: Diseases of the small intestine in childhood, 4th edn. Oxford: Isis Medical Media; 1999:343-352.
3. Murch SH. Towards a molecular understanding of complex childhood enteropathies. J Pediatr Gastroenterol Nutr 2002; 34:S4-S10.
4. Gambineri E, Torgerson TR, Ochs HD. Immune dysregulation, polyendocrinopathy, enteropathy, and X-linked inheritance (IPEX), a syndrome of systemic autoimmunity caused by mutations of FOXP3, a critical regulator of T-cell homeostasis. Curr Opin Rheumatol 2003; 15:430-435.
5. Salvatore S, Vandenplas Y. Gastro-oesophageal reflux disease and motility disorders. Best Pract Res Clin Gastroenterol 2003; 17:163-179.
6. Heine RG, Elsayed S, Hosking CS, Hill DJ. Cow's milk allergy in infancy. Curr Opin Allergy Clin Immunol 2002; 2:217-225.
7. Wood RA. The natural history of food allergy. Pediatrics 2003; 111:1631-1637.
8. Hourihane JO. Peanut allergy – current status and future challenges. Clin Exp Allergy 1997; 27:1240-1246.
9. Murch SH. The immunologic basis for intestinal food allergy. Curr Opin Gastroenterol 2000; 16:552-557.
10. Sampson HA. Anaphylaxis and emergency treatment. Pediatrics 2003; 111:1601-1608.
11. Nowak-Wegrzyn A, Sampson HA, Wood RA, Sicherer SH. Food protein-induced enterocolitis syndrome caused by solid food proteins. Pediatrics 2003; 111: 829-835.
12. Iacono G, Cavataio F, Montalto G et al. Intolerance of cow's milk and chronic constipation in children. New Engl J Med 1998; 339:1100-1104.
13. Maki M, Mustalahti K, Kokkonen J et al. Prevalence of celiac disease among children in Finland. N Engl J Med 2003; 348: 2517-2524.
14. Hernell O, Ivarsson A, Persson LA. Coeliac disease: effect of early feeding on the incidence of the disease. Early Hum Devel 2001; 65:S153-S160.
15. Vader W, Kooy Y, van Veelen P et al. The gluten response in children with celiac disease is directed toward multiple gliadin and glutenin peptides. Gastroenterology 2002; 122:1729-1737.
16. Buller H, Chin S, Kirschner B et al. Inflammatory bowel disease in children and adolescents: working group report of the first world congress of pediatric gastroenterology, hepatology, and nutrition. J Pediatr Gastroenterol Nutr 2002; 35:S151-S158.
17. Sawczenko A, Sandhu BK. Presenting features of inflammatory bowel disease in Great Britain and Ireland. Arch Dis Child 2003; 88:995-1000.
18. Beattie RM, Walker-Smith JA, Murch SH. Indications for investigation of chronic gastrointestinal symptoms. Arch Dis Child 1995; 73:354-355.
19. Markowitz J, Grancher K, Kohn N, Lesser M, Daum F. A multicenter trial of 6-mercaptopurine and prednisone in children with newly diagnosed Crohn's disease. Gastroenterology 2000; 119:895-902.
20. Heuschkel RB, Menache CC, Megerian JT, Baird AE. Enteral nutrition and corticosteroids in the treatment of acute Crohn's disease in children. J Pediatr Gastroenterol Nutr 2000; 31:8-15.

Chapter 29

Gastroesophageal reflux disease

Ronnie Fass and Wai-Man Wong

KEY POINTS

- There are three phenotypic presentations of gastroesophageal reflux disease (GERD): nonerosive reflux disease (NERD), erosive esophagitis, and Barrett's esophagus.
- NERD is defined as present in an individual who experiences typical symptoms of GERD, due to reflux of gastric contents into the esophagus, and who lacks endoscopic evidence of esophageal mucosal injury.
- The current definition of erosive esophagitis requires the presence of esophageal mucosal breaks for diagnosis.
- The Los Angeles classification of endoscopic esophagitis is a highly reproducible and well validated reporting system that classifies esophageal mucosal injury into grades A through D, according to severity of esophageal inflammation.

INTRODUCTION AND DEFINITION

Gastroesophageal reflux disease (GERD) is a very common disorder affecting between 10% and 30% of the Western population (Fig. 29.1). According to the Genval Workshop Report (an evidence-based appraisal of GERD management), 'the term GERD should be used to include all individuals who are exposed to the risk of physical complications from gastroesophageal reflux disease, or who experience clinically significant impairment of health-related well-being (quality of life) due to reflux-related symptoms, after adequate reassurance of the benign nature of their symptoms'.[1] GERD is the digestive disease with the highest annual direct cost in the United States (US$ 9.3 billion).[2]

Traditionally, GERD has been regarded as a continuum with potential progression from nonerosive reflux disease to erosive esophagitis, and, possibly, in subset of patients, to Barrett's esophagus. An alternative conceptual framework is that there are three unique phenotypic presentations of GERD: nonerosive reflux disease (NERD), erosive esophagitis, and Barrett's esophagus.[3] This framework proposes that patients usually remain within one of these three phenotypic presentations, with very little transition over time into another GERD group. The complications of GERD such as esophageal stricture and Barrett's esophagus are discussed in Chapters 30 and 31.

Nonerosive reflux disease or *endoscopy-negative reflux disease* is characterized by the presence of GERD symptoms but without endoscopically visible breaks (erosions or ulcers) in the esophageal mucosa. As acid may not be the only stimulus that leads to heartburn (see Chapter 2), NERD could also be defined as 'the presence of typical symptoms of GERD caused by intra-esophageal gastric content, in the absence of visible esophageal mucosal injury at endoscopic examination'.[3]

The Los Angeles classification is a validated and reproducible standardized classification to describe the extent of esophageal mucosal injury (Fig. 29.2). It has a good correlation with the degree of esophageal acid exposure as measured by 24-h esophageal pH monitoring, severity of heartburn symptoms, response to proton pump inhibitor (PPI) therapy as well as the risk of symptomatic relapse after 6 months of therapy.[4]

EPIDEMIOLOGY

Some 50–70% of patients with heartburn have a normal-appearing mucosa at endoscopy. The prevalence of erosive esophagitis in Europe and Asia has been estimated as 1.2–2.4%, and esophageal stricture as 0.1% (Table 29.1).[5] Most patients with GERD-related symptoms never seek medical attention. Therefore, those who do seek medical attention represent just the tip of the GERD 'iceberg.'

Patients with NERD are more commonly females, usually leaner, report a shorter symptom duration and have a lower incidence of hiatus hernia compared with patients with erosive esophagitis. Furthermore, complicated GERD is more commonly seen in caucasian men, and is associated with increased age. There appears to be an association between aspirin and nonsteroidal anti-inflammatory drug (NSAID) use and the presence of erosive esophagitis or esophageal stricture.

Of all ethnic groups, caucasians demonstrate the highest rates of GERD and esophageal adenocarcinoma. GERD is less commonly seen in the Asia-Pacific region.[6] Furthermore, erosive

PREVALENCE OF GERD IN THE WORLD

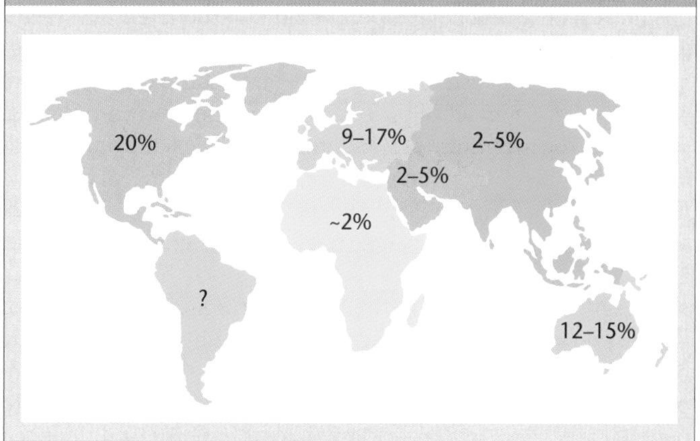

Fig. 29.1 Prevalence of GERD in the world.

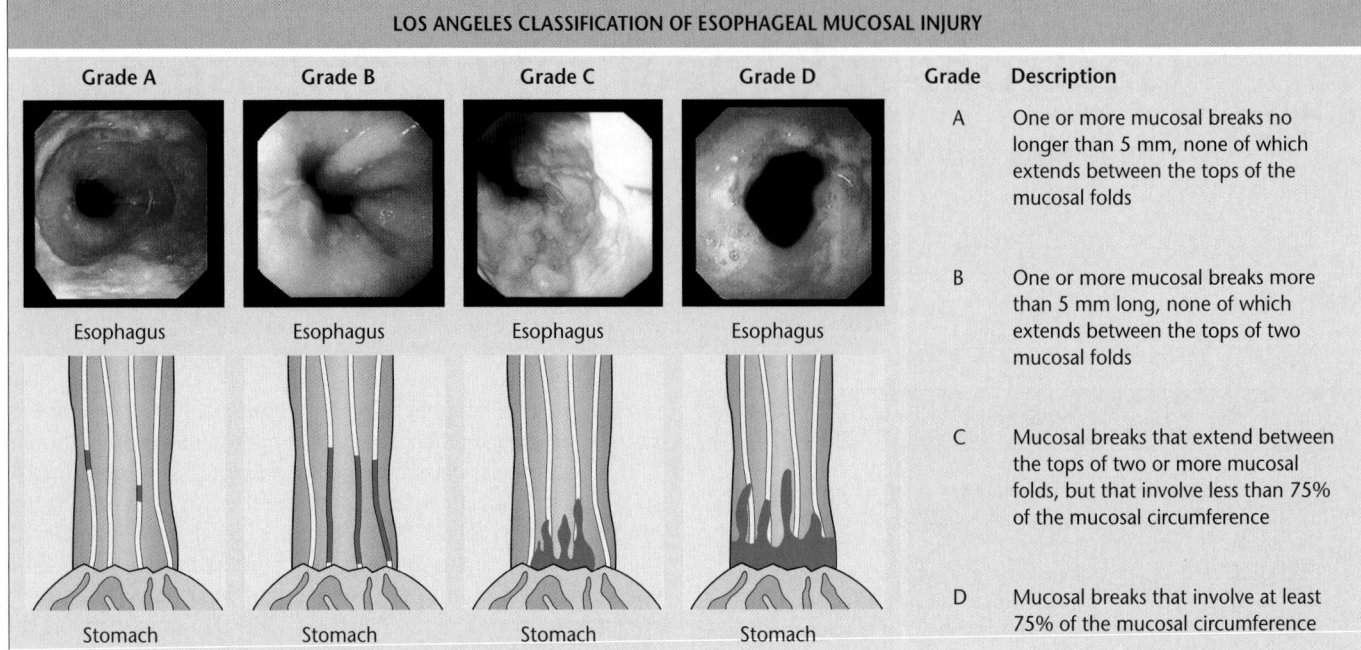

LOS ANGELES CLASSIFICATION OF ESOPHAGEAL MUCOSAL INJURY

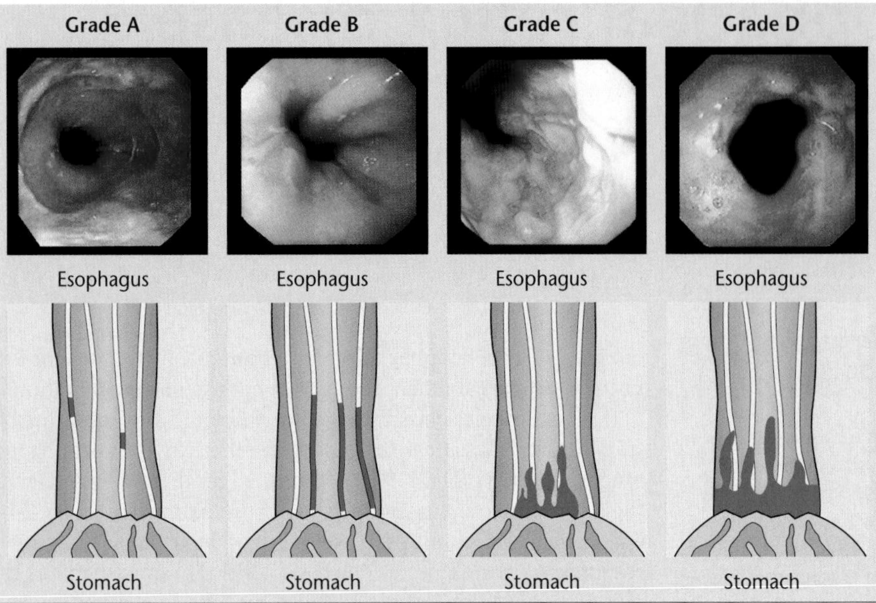

Grade	Description
A	One or more mucosal breaks no longer than 5 mm, none of which extends between the tops of the mucosal folds
B	One or more mucosal breaks more than 5 mm long, none of which extends between the tops of two mucosal folds
C	Mucosal breaks that extend between the tops of two or more mucosal folds, but that involve less than 75% of the mucosal circumference
D	Mucosal breaks that involve at least 75% of the mucosal circumference

Fig. 29.2 The Los Angeles classification of esophageal mucosal injury.

esophagitis is usually milder in Asia (predominantly Los Angeles grade A and B) and complications such as esophageal stricture, Barrett's esophagus, and esophageal adenocarcinoma are exceedingly rare.[7] The prevalence of GERD in other parts of the world, such as Africa or South America, is largely unknown. An estimated prevalence of weekly reports of heartburn in different parts of the world is presented in Figure 29.1.

The prevalence of hiatus hernia varies between 29% and 96% in patients with GERD,[8] and the prevalence is much lower in patients with no reflux symptoms, indicating the importance of hiatus hernia in the pathophysiology of GERD. It has been demonstrated that 96% of patients with long-segment (≥3 cm) Barrett's esophagus, 72% with short-segment (<3 cm) Barrett's esophagus, 71% with erosive esophagitis, and 29% with NERD have hiatus hernia.[8]

CAUSES, RISKS FACTORS, DISEASE ASSOCIATIONS

Risk factors purported to be associated with GERD include cigarette smoking; alcohol; coffee; obesity; high fat diet; food products such as chocolate, peppermint, carbonated beverages, and citrus juices; and drugs.[5] GERD is more common in pregnant women because of increased intra-abdominal pressure and the relaxing effect of progesterone on the lower esophageal sphincter. Furthermore, scleroderma–CREST syndrome (cutaneous calcinosis, Raynaud's phenomenon, esophageal dysfunction, sclerodactyly, and telangiectasia) Sjögren's syndrome, and diabetes mellitus are associated with a higher incidence of GERD. Table 29.2 lists the conditions associated with erosive esophagitis. Depending on the clinical presentation, various of these clinical entities should be considered before labeling the patient as having GERD. For example, in the immunocompromised patient, infectious causes should be considered. In patients of all ages with new-onset apparent GERD, pill-induced esophagitis should be excluded.

The relationship between *Helicobacter pylori* and GERD has been controversial. Some studies suggested that *H. pylori* conferred protection from GERD and that its eradication, as in the treatment of duodenal ulcer, was associated with an increased risk of erosive esophagitis. A post hoc analysis of eight double-blind prospective trials revealed that eradication of *H. pylori* in patients with duodenal ulcer was not associated with the development of erosive esophagitis, new symptomatic GERD, or worsening of symptoms in patients with pre-existing GERD.[9]

PATHOGENESIS

The pathogenesis of heartburn was discussed in Chapter 2; several factors have been proposed to be important in the pathophysiology of GERD. They include the antireflux barrier, hiatus hernia, esophageal dysmotility, gastric acid hypersecretion, duodenogastroesophageal reflux, gastric dysmotility, impaired esophageal mucosal defense mechanisms, and genetic factors (Fig. 29.3).

TABLE 29.1 POPULATION PREVALENCE OF GASTROESOPHAGEAL REFLUX DISEASE

	Prevalence (%)
GERD symptoms at least once in past year	59
Monthly symptoms of GERD	44
Weekly symptoms of GERD	20
Erosive esophagitis	1.2–2.4
Esophageal stricture	0.1
Barrett's esophagus	0.4
Esophageal adenocarcinoma	0.0025

Adapted from Sonnenberg A. Epidemiologic aspects in the occurrence and natural history of gastroesophageal reflux disease. In: Fass R, ed. GERD/dyspepsia. Philadelphia: Hanley & Belfus; 2004:1–22.

TABLE 29.2 CAUSES OF EROSIVE ESOPHAGITIS
• **Gastroesophageal reflux disease**
• **Infections**
Candida
Viral (cytomegalovirus, herpes virus, human immunodeficiency virus)
Bacterial (*Nocardia*, syphilis)
Mycobacterium (tuberculosis, atypical mycobacteria)
Parasitic (Chagas' disease)
• **Systemic disease**
Skin pathology (epidermolysis bullosa, pemphigus, drug induced)
Behçet's disease
Graft versus host disease
Inflammatory bowel disease
Sarcoidosis
Metastatic cancer
Collagen vascular disease (scleroderma, CREST syndrome, Sjögren's syndrome)
• **Iatrogenic**
Pill-induced esophagitis (tetracycline, potassium chloride, alendronate, NSAIDs)
Radiation-induced esophagitis
Chemotherapy-induced esophagitis
Sclerotherapy-induced erosions/ulcerations
• **Nasogastric tube (Ryle's tube) induced trauma**
• **Zollinger-Ellison syndrome**

Adapted from Oviedo J et al. Erosive esophagitis. In: Fass R, ed. GERD/dyspepsia. Philadelphia: Hanley & Belfus; 2004:83–99.

Antireflux barrier

It is presently accepted that the major elements that compose the antireflux barrier are the lower esophageal sphincter (LES) and the crural diaphragm. The LES is a thickened ring of circular smooth muscle located at the distal 2–3 cm of the esophagus and serves as a mechanical barrier between the stomach and the esophagus. The right crus of the diaphragm encircles the LES and thus provides additional mechanical support. The variations in LES pressure are usually coupled with esophageal and gastric contractions, whereas the pressure contributed by the crural diaphragm is in response to physical activity such as inspiration, coughing, Valsalva maneuver, abdominal compression, and others. Traditionally, gastroesophageal reflux is thought to occur across a hypotensive LES in the presence of hiatal hernia. However, the LES basal pressure in most cases is within normal limits. In fact, for most patients with GERD, the predominant mechanism of gastroesophageal reflux is transient lower esophageal sphincter relaxation (TLESR), in which spontaneous (not preceded by a swallow), prolonged relaxations of the LES are triggered primarily by fundic relaxation (mostly postprandial) and mediated by a vagovagal reflex. TLESRs have been established as the primary mechanism for gastroesophageal reflux in normal subjects and patients with GERD, as well as the underlying mechanism for belching.[5,8,10] Although recent trials found no increased rate of TLESR in patients with GERD, a TLESR was more likely to be associated with acid reflux in patients with GERD when compared to healthy controls.[5,11]

The presence of a hiatal hernia is associated with increased severity of GERD, particularly if the hiatal hernia is large (Fig. 29.4). The presence of a nonreducible hiatal hernia disrupts the integrity of the sphincter mechanism and prolongs esophageal clearance, leading to increased esophageal acid exposure. Patients with GERD and hiatus hernia have a substantial additional number of reflux episodes during swallow-induced LES relaxations, compared with those without hiatus hernia.[12]

Esophageal dysmotility

The most common physiologic aberration causing increased acid contact time is ineffective refluxate clearance. Impairment of acid clearance can be secondary to either peristaltic dysfunction and/or re-reflux (the to-and-fro movement of reflux fluid), which is seen in association with hiatus hernia.

Peristaltic dysfunction in GERD is well documented[13,14] and is increasingly observed with more severe grades of esophagitis. There has been a longstanding argument as to whether the dysmotility precedes or is caused by GERD.[13] Elimination of reflux does not result in normalization of motility, but it may be that severe reflux has permanently damaged the distal esophageal 'pump.'

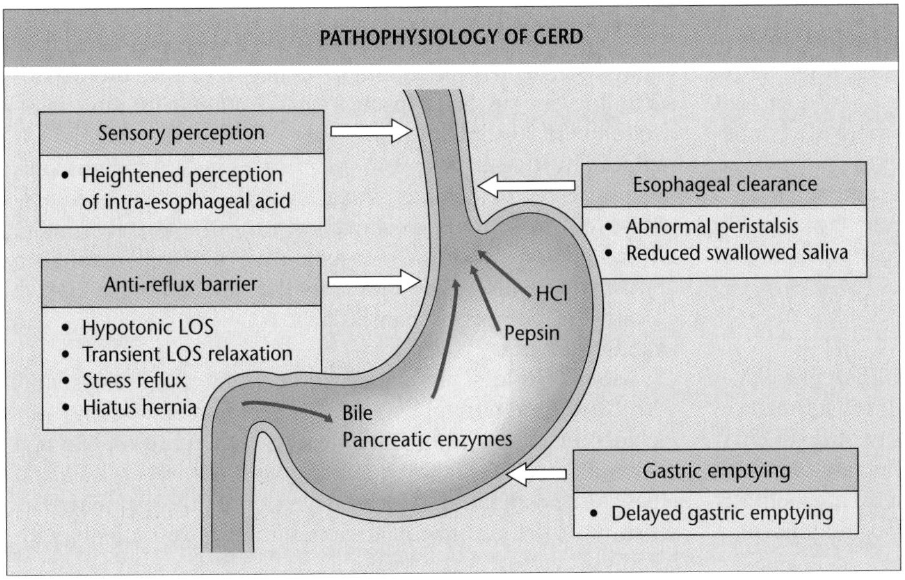

Fig. 29.3 Pathophysiology of GERD.

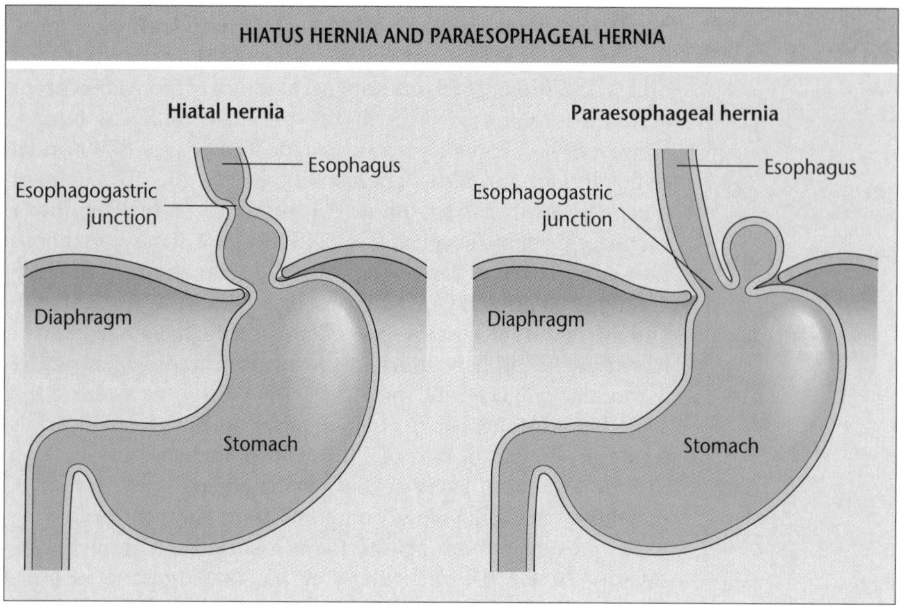

Fig. 29.4 Schematic representation of hiatus hernia and paraesophageal hernia. Note the proximal displacement of the esophagogastric junction in hiatus hernia, whereas in paraesophageal hernia the anatomic location of the esophagogastric junction is preserved.

Nontransmitted peristalsis or simultaneous esophageal contractions are ineffective in clearing the volume of the refluxate. Ineffective esophageal motility, defined by the presence of abnormally low amplitude (<30 mmHg) contractions in the distal esophagus (30% or more of wet swallows), was also found to be associated with prolonged esophageal acid clearance in both the upright and recumbent positions.

Gastric acid secretion

There is no strong evidence to suggest that hypersecretion of gastric acid plays an important role in the pathogenesis of GERD.[5,8,11] However, in patients with moderate to severe oxyntic gland (fundus and body) gastritis, eradication of *H. pylori* may improve gastric hyposecretion and lead to more acid gastroesophageal reflux in subjects with a pre-existing, subclinical incompetent gastroesophageal barrier.

Duodenogastroesophageal reflux

It has been suggested that duodenogastroesophageal reflux itself does not cause significant damage to the esophageal mucosa but may act synergistically with acid reflux to produce erosive esophagitis. By using 24-h esophageal pH monitoring and Bilitec 2000 (a spectrophotometric system that measures bilirubin concentration within the esophagus, independent of pH) in patients with GERD, investigators demonstrated that 28% of heartburn episodes were associated with acid reflux alone, 60% with duodenogastroesophageal reflux alone, and 12% with mixed acid and duodenogastroesophageal reflux.[5,11]

Gastric dysmotility

Approximately 20% of the patients with GERD may have delayed gastric emptying, but there is no direct correlation between the degree of the delay and the severity of GERD.[5,8,15] However, slow proximal gastric emptying in patients with GERD correlated with increased 24-h esophageal pH monitoring, number of reflux episodes per hour, and postprandial acid exposure.

Esophageal mucosal defense mechanisms

Esophageal mucous and bicarbonate layer, cell membranes, intercellular junctional complexes, and an adequate mucosal blood flow are important defense mechanisms against injury by gastroesophageal reflux. Increased esophageal permeability and reduced mucin production improve after antisecretory therapy, suggesting that these abnormalities are caused by gastroesophageal reflux.

Genetic factors

A large twin study has shown an increased concordance for GERD in monozygotic pairs, compared with dizygotic pairs, suggesting that genetic factors accounted for 31% of the liability to GERD in a US population.[5] Furthermore, a genetic linkage study in a pediatric GERD population mapped a locus in chromosome 13q14. Although the importance of this locus was refuted by a subsequent study, it did not completely exclude the possibility of genetic factors in GERD.

PATHOLOGY

Figure 29.2 depicts the different grading of erosive esophagitis according to the Los Angeles classification.[4] In this classification, the histopathologic term – erosive esophagitis – is replaced by a descriptive term – mucosal break. An endoscopic mucosal break is defined as 'an area of slough or erythema with a discrete line of demarcation from the adjacent, more normal looking mucosa.' Documenting mucosal breaks on endoscopy is an indication for the presence of erosive esophagitis, but minor changes such as erythema, edema, and friability are not.

Various histologic findings have been described in patients with GERD and normal-appearing mucosa on endoscopy. They include the presence of inflammatory cells (neutrophils and eosinophils), epithelial hyperplasia (basal cell hyperplasia and elongated papillae), and dilated vessels in the papillae. The sensitivity of these histopathologic findings in patients with NERD is unclear.

CLINICAL PRESENTATION

Heartburn is the hallmark symptom of reflux disease (see Chapter 2). According to the Genval Workshop: 'When heartburn is a major or sole symptom, GERD is the cause in at least 75% of the individuals.' Heartburn is thus a reliable pointer to the diagnosis but other symptoms are related to GERD. These include acid regurgitation, belching, and water brash (see Chapter 2). Angina-like chest pain, globus sensation, chronic cough, hoarseness, and asthma are considered atypical manifestations of GERD (see Chapter 2). Dysphagia and odynophagia usually suggest the presence of esophageal mucosal injury. GERD symptom frequency or severity is not correlated with the extent of esophageal mucosal involvement in patients with erosive esophagitis.

Natural history of GERD

The few retrospective studies that evaluated the natural course of NERD revealed limited progression to erosive esophagitis, and no evidence to support progression to Barrett's esophagus. Similarly, there are no data in the literature to support the view that patients with erosive esophagitis, without underlying Barrett's mucosa, will progress over time to develop overt Barrett's esophagus. Furthermore, as with the NERD group, patients with erosive esophagitis almost always relapse when antireflux medications are discontinued. Patients with Barrett's esophagus, on the other hand, demonstrate very little, if any, evidence of regression or progression of the metaplastic epithelium over the years. Patients with Barrett's esophagus are almost always diagnosed on first endoscopy, and the length of patients' Barrett's mucosa remains unchanged during their lifetime. Overall, there appears to be very limited movement between the different GERD groups (NERD, erosive esophagitis, and Barrett's esophagus)[3]

DIFFERENTIAL DIAGNOSIS

Although heartburn is strongly associated with the diagnosis of GERD, it should be borne in mind that patients with peptic ulcer disease, gastric cancer, and delayed gastric emptying may present with heartburn. Furthermore, sudden and isolated attacks of heartburn may be caused by pill-induced esophagitis or corrosive injury, emphasizing the importance of a careful drug history. In patients who present with alarm symptoms such as anorexia, weight loss, anemia, dysphagia, and hematemesis, early upper endoscopy is indicated. The presence of erosive esophagitis in patients undergoing upper endoscopy is usually indicative of GERD, but other etiologies have been identified and should be considered (see Table 29.2).

DIAGNOSTIC METHODS

The diagnostic methods available for GERD include clinical evaluation, barium esophagography, upper endoscopy, ambulatory 24-h esophageal pH monitoring, esophageal manometry, multichannel intraluminal impedance, and use of the empiric PPI test.[5]

Clinical evaluation

The clustering of symptoms in the postprandial period and rapid relief by antacids are useful positive diagnostic criteria. Several validated GERD symptom questionnaires have been developed, but their usage has been limited to clinical trials.[16]

Empiric proton pump inhibitor (PPI) test

The empiric PPI test is a simple noninvasive diagnostic as well as a therapeutic tool for GERD that is widely available to community-based physicians (see Chapter 131).[17] The PPI test is the usage of a short course (1–4 weeks) of high-dose PPI given twice daily for the diagnosis of GERD in patients with typical, atypical, or extraesophageal manifestations of GERD. Several trials in patients with typical symptoms of GERD have demonstrated that the sensitivity of the PPI test ranges from 66% to 89%, and the specificity from 35% to 73%. However, there is still no consensus about the desired level of symptom response (cutoff level), optimal dose, frequency, or duration of the empiric treatment for GERD.

Barium esophagography

Barium esophagography has shown a low sensitivity (20%) in the diagnosis of GERD.[5,16] The sensitivity of these tests improves in patients with more severe erosive esophagitis and complicated GERD (stricture and ulceration). The tests are not sensitive for Barrett's esophagus but may help in determining the presence and size of hiatus hernia as well as the length of the esophagus.

Upper endoscopy

Endoscopy only has a sensitivity of about 30–50% in patients with typical symptoms of GERD, as most patients with GERD have NERD. However, the test is the gold standard for diagnosing erosive esophagitis, GERD complications, and Barrett's esophagus. Additionally, endoscopy allows an assessment of the degree of esophageal mucosal injury. The value of histopathologic examination of normal-appearing esophageal mucosa to confirm or exclude pathologic acid reflux remains controversial. Ultra-thin transnasal endoscopy has been introduced as a rapid, ambulatory, and well tolerated method of examining the esophageal mucosa. However, patient preferences for being 'sedated' during endoscopic procedures may limit the utilization of this technique.

Ambulatory 24-h esophageal pH monitoring

This test involves the transnasal placement of a flexible pH-recording probe into the distal esophagus.[18] The tip of the probe is positioned 5 cm above the proximal margin of the LES. The test allows assessment of 24-h esophageal acid exposure and the relationship between patient symptoms and acid reflux events.

Esophageal pH monitoring is normal in 25% of patients with erosive esophagitis and in up to 50% of those with NERD.[16] Because of nasal and pharyngeal discomfort, patients often limit their daily activity during pH monitoring, which may decrease the accuracy of the test. Migration of the pH probe into the stomach during the test may lead to erroneous results. Despite these drawbacks, ambulatory 24-h esophageal pH monitoring should be considered in the following circumstances:

- patients with NERD being considered for antireflux surgery
- patients after antireflux surgery who continue to be symptomatic

- patients with GERD-related symptoms despite PPI treatment (including symptoms of noncardiac chest pain, suspected otolaryngologic manifestations of GERD, adult-onset refractory asthma)

Patients who fail a PPI test (see above) should undergo 24-h pH monitoring whilst continuing to take the treatment.

The wireless pH capsule (Bravo; Medtronics, Minneapolis, Minnesota, USA) (Fig. 29.5), a radiotransmitter pH system, was introduced as a more patient-friendly pH system. The capsule is attached to the distal esophageal mucosa using a delivery system either after endoscopy or esophageal manometry.[5] The capsule transmits pH changes via radio signals to a receiver worn by the patient around the waist. The capsule appears to have less effect on the patient's daily activities, potentially can be placed at any level of the esophagus, and can provide 48h of pH recording.

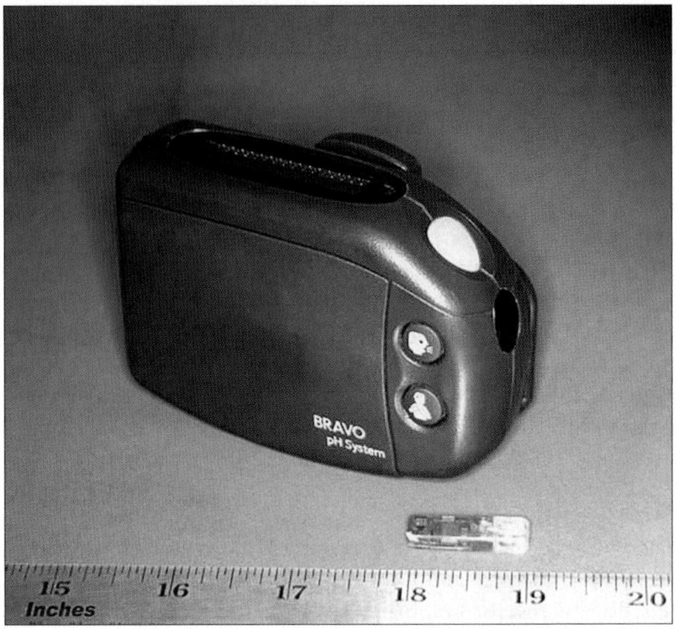

Fig. 29.5 The wireless pH capsule and the recorder device (pH data logger).

Esophageal manometry

While esophageal manometry has no role in the diagnosis of GERD, it is routinely performed to determine the proper location of the LES prior to placement of a pH probe. Additionally, esophageal manometry is commonly used to evaluate patients with GERD who are candidates for antireflux surgery, in order to exclude esophageal motility abnormalities.

Multichannel intraluminal impedance

Improved impedance probes with integrated pH sensors allow further assessment of refluxate composition and its relationship to symptoms.[19] Because the electrical conductivity of the esophageal muscular wall, air, and any given bolus is different, the presence of different substances in the esophageal lumen provides different impedance patterns.[19] With a highly conductive bolus (e.g., saliva), the impedance decreases; with poorly conductive material (e.g., air), the impedance increases.

The combination of an impedance catheter and a pH probe provides a unique opportunity to study physiologic and pathologic events within the esophagus and their relationship to symptoms. In addition, the recording assembly can disclose the characteristics of the gastric refluxate (acid, nonacid, gas, and mixed gas and liquid). The value of this technique has been demonstrated by showing that nonacidic reflux is not uncommon in patients with PPI failure and may lead to classic heartburn symptoms as well.[19]

DIAGNOSTIC METHODS

COMMONLY USED METHODS FOR THE DIAGNOSIS OF GERD

Test	Advantages	Disadvantages	Recommended use
Barium swallow	Noninvasive Widely available	Poor sensitivity and specificity	For patients with GERD who present with dysphagia
Upper endoscopy	Highly sensitive for the diagnosis of erosive GERD and GERD complications Obtain tissue biopsies Treat peptic strictures	Limited sensitivity for general GERD Invasive Expensive Not always readily available	GERD with alarm symptoms Detection of Barrett's esophagus
24-h esophageal pH monitoring Conventional catheter	Assesses esophageal acid exposure Correlation of symptoms with acid reflux events	Transnasal intubation is not well tolerated by patients Limitation in everyday activities during the study may affect accuracy	Failure of PPI therapy (twice daily) Before antireflux surgery (NERD) Following antireflux surgery after symptom recurrence
Bravo capsule	Avoids the need for nasal intubation	Endoscopy may be required for placement of capsule	
PPI test	Widely available Noninvasive Cost effective	Subjective outcome Limited specificity in GERD	Atypical symptoms of GERD

Modified from Sunil J et al. Gastroesophageal reflux disease: diagnosis of GERD. In: Fass R, ed. GERD/dyspepsia. Philadelphia: Hanley & Belfus; 2004:41–54.

Esophageal impedance techniques need to be standardized and further studies are required to determine their proper clinical utility in GERD. However, future usage may further expand our understanding of symptom generation in patients with different presentations of GERD.

TREATMENT

The aims of GERD management include: (1) confirmation of the diagnosis of GERD; (2) adequate relief of GERD symptoms; (3) healing of erosive esophagitis, if present; and (4) improvement of patient-reported quality of life.

For patients with mild and infrequent reflux symptoms, antacids and lifestyle modifications (weight loss, cessation of smoking, elevation of head of the bed, and avoidance of aggravating foods) may provide adequate treatment. Most gastroenterologists no longer prescribe antacids for more than just occasional symptoms, and may start with a H_2-receptor antagonist or PPI. In parallel, these physicians often consider that the availability of drugs to supersede indefinite antacids may also obviate the need for routine elevation of the head of the bed. However, many patients with typical GERD symptoms will require a more definitive treatment.[16]

PPIs (see Chapter 136) allow an effective control of symptoms that is unsurpassed by any other medical therapy for GERD, high rate of healing of erosive esophagitis, and diagnosis of GERD by relieving symptoms. In a meta-analysis of 7635 patients with erosive esophagitis, PPIs provided the highest healing rate (84%), when compared with H_2-receptor antagonists (52%), sucralfate (39%), or placebo (28%).[20] Furthermore, complete relief of heartburn was the highest with PPIs (77%), versus 48% with H_2-receptor antagonists. Failure of a 4-week course of initial therapy with a PPI should prompt a review of the diagnosis.

A once-daily morning dosing of PPI, half an hour before a meal, is generally the most appropriate initial therapy, but may fail in up to 30% of patients. For those who do not respond adequately to once-daily PPI, the addition of a second daily dose before the evening meal is commonly practised.[16] A suggested algorithm for the management of patients with GERD is provided in Figure 29.6. Patients with NERD have demonstrated a lower symptom response rate to PPIs than patients with erosive esophagitis.[3,5,21] GERD is primarily a chronic relapsing disorder. Long-term maintenance treatment with a PPI may be delivered daily, intermittently, or on demand.

Treatment for GERD may follow three different clinical strategies: step-up, step-down or step-in. The step-up approach initiates patients on the least effective antireflux modality and upgrades treatment if satisfactory control of symptoms is not achieved. The step-down approach initiates patients on the most potent antireflux modality and downgrades patients to a therapeutic modality that still controls their symptoms effectively. The step-in approach initiates and maintains patients on the most potent antireflux modality.[22,23]

It is inappropriate to withdraw therapy in patients with severe erosive esophagitis (Los Angeles grade C or D) as all patients will invariably relapse upon cessation of therapy.[16] However, for patients with mild to moderate erosive disease (Los Angeles grade A or B), or those with NERD, there is increasing support for the usage of an on-demand or intermittent approach as maintenance therapy. Both on-demand and intermittent therapy have demonstrated an efficacy in reducing symptoms and improving quality of life, patient satisfaction, and cost effectiveness.

Antacids and alginates (see Chapter 136)

Antacids are basic compounds composed of different combinations of acid-neutralizing agents such as aluminum and magnesium hydroxide, calcium carbonate, sodium citrate, and sodium bicarbonate. They provide transient symptom relief but do not contribute to the healing or prevention of GERD complications.[24,25] Nevertheless, antacids are a very popular on-demand treatment for patients seeking rapid symptom relief. Alginates create a foamy raft above the gastric content; they provide rapid, transient relief of symptoms but play no proven role in healing erosive esophagitis or preventing symptom relapse or GERD complications.

Sucralfate (see Chapter 136)

Sucralfate provides mucosal protection by creating an adherent complex with the proteinaceous exudates of denuded esophageal mucosa. It also has pepsin binding and bile acid-binding capacities that enhance tissue resistance. Sucralfate has lost favor as an antireflux treatment because of limited efficacy and the need for multiple (four times daily) dosing.

Promotility/prokinetic drugs (see Chapter 136)

Motility-modifying drugs may affect gastroesophageal reflux by increasing LES pressure, improving esophageal peristalsis and thus acid clearance, and facilitating gastric emptying.

Metoclopramide is a dopamine antagonist and cholinomimetic that crosses the blood–brain barrier and neutralizes the inhibitory effect of dopamine in the central nervous system and on the gastrointestinal smooth muscle. Its therapeutic efficacy in GERD is limited because of multiple adverse effects of a neurologic or psychotropic nature, including lethargy, mental status changes, and extrapyramidal abnormalities, which are not reversible after discontinuation of the drug.

Domperidone is a potent peripheral dopamine antagonist whose properties are similar to those of metoclopramide. Unlike metoclopramide, however, it does not readily cross the blood–brain barrier. Domperidone is commonly used to treat GERD in patients who have delayed gastric emptying.

Tegaserod, a partial 5-hyydroxytryptamine type 4 ($5\text{-}HT_4$) receptor agonist, has been prescribed primarily for women with constipation-predominant irritable bowel syndrome. A potent promotility agent throughout the gastrointestinal tract, tegaserod may improve delayed gastric emptying in patients with GERD but its specific role has not been clearly established.

Histamine type 2 receptor antagonists (see Chapter 136)

Histamine type 2 receptor antagonists (H_2RAs) are still widely used for the treatment of GERD. This class of drugs reduces gastric acid output by competitive inhibition of histamine at H_2 receptors on the parietal cells.[26] Standard doses have been proven to be effective in controlling symptoms and in healing mild to moderate erosive esophagitis.

The potential effect of H_2RAs on night-time histamine-driven surge of gastric acid secretion led to the popular use of these drugs at bedtime by patients who continued to be symptomatic on a standard or double-dose PPI therapy.[27] However,

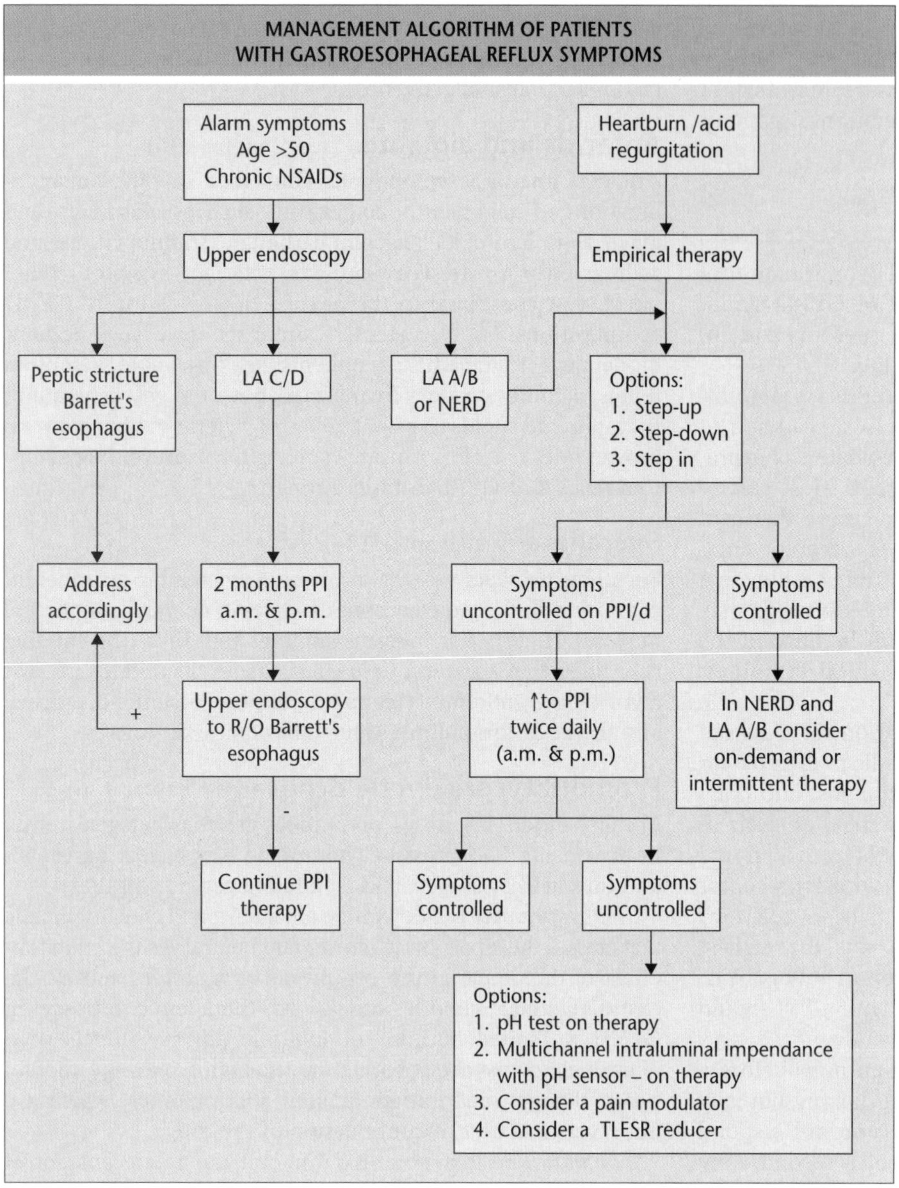

Fig. 29.6 Management algorithm for patients with symptoms of gastroesophageal reflux. LA, Los Angeles classification; NERD, nonerosive reflux disease; PPI, proton pump inhibitor; TLSER, transient lower esophageal sphincter relaxation.

tachyphylaxis develops quickly with H_2RAs, limiting their regular use in clinical practice.[28] The main appeal of H_2RAs is their rapid effect on GERD symptoms, unsurpassed by any of the currently available PPIs.

Antireflux surgery and new endoscopic therapies (see Chapters 151 and 152)

Antireflux surgery is offered to patients in the hope of obviating the need for continuous medical therapy, which may result in patient inconvenience, increased costs, and concerns about safety.[29] Nissen fundoplication remains the most commonly performed operation and consists of a 360° wrap of the gastric fundus around the distal esophagus, which results in augmentation of LES basal pressure and a decrease in the rate of TLESR. At this time fundoplication is commonly done laparoscopically (see Chapter 152). Complications due to antireflux surgery are determined by the expertise of the surgeon, which has been shown to correlate closely with the number of procedures performed.

Offering surgery to young patients because of the prospect of long-term medical therapy should be individualized and discussed in an unbiased way. Ultimately, the success of antireflux surgery depends on selecting the appropriate patients and surgeon. Presurgical evaluation includes esophageal manometry, primarily to exclude achalasia and ineffective peristalsis (amplitudes of esophageal body contractions <30 mmHg), upper endoscopy, and 24-h esophageal pH monitoring in those patients without erosive esophagitis.

As discussed in Chapter 152, a positive response to medical therapy is the best predictor of successful surgical outcome. However, approximately half of the patients are referred for antireflux surgery because medical therapy has failed.[30] When clinical outcome of antireflux surgery was compared with treatment with omeprazole, as long as patients were allowed to adjust the needed dose no greater difference in treatment failure was observed between the two therapeutic strategies.[31] However, 10 years after antireflux surgery, more than half of the patients require medical therapy (many on PPIs) to control their GERD symptoms.[32]

Several endoscopic techniques have been introduced for the treatment of GERD. They include endoscopic suturing, radiofrequency energy procedure, and submucosal bulking. The primary aim of the various endoscopic techniques is to augment LES basal pressure and possibly reduce the rate of TLESR. Thus far, most of the studies published have shown a good safety profile, patient satisfaction with the clinical outcome, and good feasibility in performing these procedures, but long-term data are required with the same scrutiny as has been asked of surgeons who perform fundoplications.

COMPLICATIONS AND THEIR MANAGEMENT

Complications of GERD include upper gastrointestinal bleeding due to erosive esophagitis or bleeding esophageal ulcers, esophageal stricture, which commonly presents as dysphagia (see Chapter 30), and Barrett's esophagus (see Chapter 31), which increases the risk of developing adenocarcinoma of the esophagus. Other complications include involvement of the oropharynx, larynx, and respiratory system, resulting in symptoms and signs termed extraesophageal manifestations of GERD (hoarseness, chronic cough, asthma, etc.). Other complications may include sleep disturbances, obstructive sleep apnea and linked cardiac angina.

PROGNOSIS WITH AND WITHOUT TREATMENT

In patients with erosive esophagitis, the disease will invariably relapse after cessation of therapy. Similarly, for patients with NERD, only 25% of those who initially achieved complete symptom resolution while taking PPIs remain asymptomatic after 6 months of not receiving any antireflux treatment. Interestingly, the superiority of PPIs over H_2-receptor antagonists is preserved in patients with NERD.[3,5,21] For patients with complicated GERD, such as esophageal stricture and potential Barrett's esophagus, long-term lifelong maintenance treatment with PPIs is needed.

Harmful consequences of medical treatment

The safety of long-term use of PPIs has been of potential concern for many physicians and patients alike. Initial reports suggested that long-term acid suppression with a PPI may potentially lead to metaplastic changes in the gastric mucosa and subsequently to the development of gastric cancer. However, with almost 20 years of extensive global experience with PPIs, studies thus far have failed to document malignant transformation in long-term users. Studies of patients who are infected with *H. pylori* and require long-term PPI therapy have suggested that gastric atrophy and potential intestinal metaplasia (the precursor for adenocarcinoma of the stomach) may develop. Consequently, some authorities have recommended testing for the presence of *H. pylori* infection prior to commencement of long-term PPI therapy in patients with GERD.[33] Vitamin B_{12} may be reduced with long-term PPI treatment, but this phenomenon is clinically significant only in patients with pre-existing atrophic gastritis.

The safety of PPIs has not been fully established in pregnant women. The drug has been assigned category B (omeprazole – C), suggesting that proper human studies substantiating the safety of the compound in pregnant women are still lacking.

Patients should be advised not to stop PPIs abruptly if they have been taking a PPI for several months or more. *Never leave home without them* is a good motto. The reason is that rebound hypersecretion may provoke symptoms that are worse even than those that led to the prescription of a PPI in the first place. There is no defined regimen for PPI withdrawal, for example after antireflux surgery or prior to performing 24-hour pH monitoring. One approach is to taper by reducing to q.d. dosage if they were on bid for 2 weeks, and then every other day q.d. dosage for 2–3 weeks before stopping. During the withdrawal, H_2 antagonists can be used on a p.r.n. basis for breakthrough symptoms.

Complications and side effects of antireflux surgery

With the advancement and the availability of minimally invasive antireflux procedures, the overall perioperative complication rate of antireflux surgery is around 5%, with a mortality rate of only 0.08%.[5] The most common complications are pneumothorax (1%), esophageal perforation (0.78%), gastrointestinal bleeding (0.75%), pneumonia (0.57%), wound infection (0.26%), and splenic injury (0.24%). Postoperative side effects of antireflux surgery may include dysphagia, bloating, flatulence, diarrhea, and others.

As is also stressed in Chapter 152, patients who are 'refractory to medical therapy' are unlikely to benefit from antireflux surgery.

SOURCES OF INFORMATION FOR PATIENTS AND DOCTORS

Reassurance of patients about the benign nature of the disease is important and relieves anxiety associated with the fear of cancer. Patients should be instructed to report any change in their symptoms over time, primarily the development of alarm symptoms such as dysphagia, odynophagia, anorexia, and weight loss. Some websites helpful for patient education are listed below.

- American College of Gastroenterology: http://www.acg.gi.org
- American Gastroenterological Association: http://www.gastro.org
- National Library of Medicine: http://www.nlm.nih.gov/medlineplus
- National Institute of Diabetes & Digestive & Kidney Diseases: http://www.niddk.nih.gov
- Heartburn-help: http://heartburn-help.com
- National Digestive Diseases Information Clearinghouse (NDDIC): http://digestive.niddk.nih.gov

CURRENT CONTROVERSIES AND THEIR FUTURE RESOLUTION

Controversies that have emerged in the past decade include: the natural course of GERD, the role of genetic factors, mechanisms for symptoms in patients GERD who fail PPI treatment, the role of pH and impedance monitoring, antireflux surgery versus endoscopic therapy versus medical therapy, and the extent of causality between GERD and putative extraesophageal symptoms.

Achieving solutions for most of these controversies will require well designed, long-term studies, development of better tools to assess pain perception, and the inclusion of brain imaging in future studies. However, to date, research in GERD has been driven largely by interest groups such as drug and equipment companies assessing new therapeutic and diagnostic techniques. Although these initiatives have had some success in advancing the field, there is still a major need for research into the mechanisms of GERD and the pathophysiology of treatment responses and failures.

REFERENCES

1. Dent J, Brun J, Fendrick AM et al. An evidence-based appraisal of reflux disease management – The Genval Workshop Report. Gut 1999; 44(Suppl 2):S1–S16.
   A document of the first international GERD consensus meeting that involved experts in the field from around the world.
2. Sandler RS, Everhart JE, Donowitz M et al. The burden of selected digestive diseases in the United States. Gastroenterology 2002; 122:1500–1511.
3. Fass R. Gastroesophageal reflux disease revisited. Gastroenterol Clin N Am 2002; 31(Suppl):S1–S10.
4. Lundell LR, Dent J, Bennett JR et al. Endoscopic assessment of oesophagitis: clinical and functional correlates and further validation of the Los Angeles classification. Gut 1999; 45:172–180.
5. Sonnenberg A. Epidemiologic aspects in the occurrence and natural history of gastroesophageal reflux disease. In: Fass R, ed. Hot topics: GERD/dyspepsia. Philadelphia: Hanley & Belfus; 2004:1–22.
6. Fock KM, Talley NJ, Hunt R et al. Report of the Asia-Pacific consensus on the management of gastroesophageal reflux disease. J Gastroenterol Hepatol 2004; 19:357–367.
7. Wong WM, Lam SK, Hui WM et al. Long-term prospective follow-up of endoscopic oesophagitis in Southern Chinese – prevalence and spectrum of the disease. Aliment Pharmacol Ther 2002; 16:2037–2042.
8. Cameron AJ. Barrett's esophagus: prevalence and size of hiatal hernia. Am J Gastroenterol 1999; 94:2054–2059.
9. Laine L, Sugg J. Effect of *Helicobacter pylori* eradication on development of erosive esophagitis and gastroesophageal reflux disease symptoms: a post hoc analysis of eight double blind prospective studies. Am J Gastroenterol 2002; 97:2992–2997.
10. Dodds WJ, Dent J, Hogan WJ et al. Mechanisms of gastroesophageal reflux in patients with reflux esophagitis. N Engl J Med 1982; 307:1547–1552.
11. Penagini R, Carmagnola S. Cantu P. Gastro-esophageal reflux disease – pathophysiological issues of clinical relevance. Aliment Pharmacol Ther. 20002; 16(Suppl 4):65–71.
12. van Herwaarden MA, Samsom M, Smout AJ. Excess gastroesophageal reflux in patients with hiatus hernia is caused by mechanisms other than transient LES relaxations. Gastroenterology 2000; 119:1439–1446.
13. Singh P, Adamopoulos A, Taylor RH, Colin-Jones DG. Oesopahgeal motor function before and after healing of oesophagitis. Gut 1992; 33:1590–1596.
14. Lin S, Ke M, Xu J, Kahrilas PJ. Impaired esophageal emptying in reflux disease. Am J Gastroenterol 1994; 89:1003–1006.
15. Helm JF, Dodds WJ, Pelc LR et al. Effect of esophageal emptying and saliva on clearance of acid from the esophagus. N Engl J Med 1984; 310:284–288.
16. Dent J. Management of reflux disease. Gut 2002; 50(Suppl 4):iv67–71.
17. Fass R. Empirical trials in treatment of gastroesophageal reflux disease. Dig Dis 2000; 18:20–26.
18. Locke GR III, Talley NJ, Fett SL et al. Prevalence and clinical spectrum of gastroesophageal reflux: a population-based study in Olmsted County, Minnesota. Gastroenterology 1997; 112:1448–1456.
   An important community-based epidemiologic study that evaluated the prevalence and demographics of GERD and its associated symptoms.
19. Vela MF, Camacho-Lobato L, Srinivasan R et al. Simultaneous intraesophageal impedance and pH measurement of acid and nonacid gastroesophageal reflux: effect of omeprazole. Gastroenterology 2001; 120:1599–1606.
   One of the first studies to evaluate the role of intraesophageal multichannel impedance with pH measurement in patients on PPI therapy.
20. Chiba N, De Gara CJ, Wilkinson JM, Hunt RH. Speed of healing and symptom relief in grade II to IV gastroesophageal reflux disease: a meta-analysis. Gastroenterology. 1997; 112:1798–1810.
21. Fass R. Epidemiology and pathophysiology of symptomatic gastroesophageal reflux disease. Am J Gastroenterol 2003; 98(Suppl):S2–S7.
   A comprehensive review of what is currently known about the epidemiology and pathophysiology of NERD.
22. Howden CW, Henning JM, Huang B, Lukasik N, Freston JW. Management of heartburn in a large, randomized, community-based study: comparison of four therapeutic strategies. Am J Gastroenterol 2001; 96:1704–1710.
23. Inadomi JM, Jamal R, Murata GH et al. Step-down management of gastroesophageal reflux disease. Gastroenterology 2001; 121:1095–1100.
24. Weberg R, Berstad A. Symptomatic effect of a low-dose antacid regimen in reflux oesophagitis. Scand J Gastroenterol 1989; 24:401–406.
25. Grove O, Bekker C, Jeppe-Hansen MG et al. Ranitidine and high-dose antacid in reflux oesophagitis. A randomized, placebo-controlled trial. Scand J Gastroenterol 1985; 20:457–461.
26. Fass R, Hixson LJ, Ciccolo ML et al. Contemporary medical therapy for gastroesophageal reflux disease. Am Fam Physician 1997; 55:205–212.
27. Peghini PL, Katz PO, Castell DO. Ranitidine controls nocturnal gastric acid breakthrough on omeprazole: a controlled study in normal subjects. Gastroenterology 1998; 115:1335–1339.
28. Fackler WK, Ours TM, Vaezi MF et al. Long-term effect of HSRA therapy on nocturnal gastric acid breakthrough. Gastroenterology 2002; 122:625–632.
29. Fass R, Sampliner RE. Gastroesophageal reflux disease and Barrett's esophagus. In: DiMarino AJ Jr, Benjamin SB, eds. Gastrointestinal disease approach. Thorofare, NJ: Slack; 2002:191–214.
30. Vakil N, Shaw M. Kirby R. Clinical effectiveness of laparoscopic fundoplication in a US community. Am J Med 2003; 114:1–5.
   Community-based assessment of the role of laparoscopic fundoplication in patients with GERD.
31. Lundell LR, Miettinen P, Myrvold HE et al. Continued (5-year) followup of a randomized clinical study comparing antireflux surgery and omeprazole in gastroesophageal reflux disease. J Am Coll Surg 2001; 192:172–179.
   A large long-term multicenter comparative trial of antireflux surgery versus medical therapy (omeprazole) in patients with GERD.
32. Spechler SJ, Lee E. Ahnen D et al. Long-term outcome of medical and surgical therapies for gastroesophageal reflux disease: follow-up of a randomized controlled trial. JAMA 2001; 285:2331–2338.
   A follow-up study (11–13 years) of patients with severe GERD who were originally enrolled in a comparative trial of medical versus surgical therapy. This was the first study to report that about 10 years after antireflux surgery most patients with GERD are back on antisecretory medication.
33. Malfertheiner P, Megraud F, O'Morain C et al. Current concepts in the management of *Helicobacter pylori* infection – the Maastricht 2-2000 Consensus Report. Aliment Pharmacol Ther 20002; 16:167–180.

Chapter 30

Benign esophageal strictures and caustic esophageal injury

H Worth Boyce

KEY POINTS

- Most caustic injuries are due to accidental ingestion by children, or deliberate self harm in adults
- Esophageal dilatation should be commenced within 3 weeks of caustic injury
- Benign mid-esophageal strictures may be due to eosinophilic esophagitis, GERD or Barrett's
- Solid food dysphagia occurs when the lumen is reduced by 50%
- Peptic strictures are often preceded by a history of heartburn and intermittent dysphagia, unlike those with Schatzki rings
- Achalasia is characterized by dysphagia for both liquids and solids
- A series of gentle therapeutic dilatations is safer than a single session
- Esophageal stents are not recommended for benign strictures

INTRODUCTION, INCLUDING DEFINITION

There are many etiologies of esophageal strictures with considerable variation in both pathologic features and symptom severity. The type of esophageal narrowing, either stenosis or stricture, requires definition as appropriate treatment varies with different pathologic states.[1] The generic term stenosis is defined here as 'any narrowing or contraction of the esophagus' without reference to specific etiology or pathogenesis. Stenosis may be due to spasm, inflammation, compression, or deposition of fibrotic or neoplastic tissue (Fig. 30.1). The definition of benign stricture used here is 'an abnormal narrowing of the esophagus due to deposition of fibrous tissue.'

EPIDEMIOLOGY

More than 80% of benign esophageal strictures in the United States are due to acid reflux. These strictures are present in 10% of patients with acid reflux symptoms, are more common in men, and far more common in Caucasians than in African Americans.[2] Another major cause of benign strictures is caustic injury, with 25 000 episodes annually in the USA. Of these, 17 000 involve accidental ingestion by children, over half of whom are under the age of 4 years. The majority of adult cases occur as suicidal attempts.[3]

CAUSES, RISK FACTORS, DISEASE ASSOCIATIONS

Peptic strictures develop in patients with severe reflux esophagitis. Strictures in the mid-esophagus are usually associated with Barrett's esophagus.

Prolonged nasogastric intubation is another contributing mechanism for reflux esophagitis and stricture. These strictures involve a longer segment and are related to increased acid exposure as well as possible direct mucosal injury from tube compression.

Rings: The mid-esophageal stricture of the ringed esophagus is associated with eosinophilic esophagitis and/or gastroesophageal acid reflux. There is no good evidence that true lower esophageal (Schatzki) rings evolve into strictures.

Caustic ingestion in children is primarily due to lack of close supervision and inadequate storage of common household caustic agents. Adults and adolescents use caustic agents with suicidal intent. About 30% of persons who ingest corrosive agents develop esophageal strictures.

Radiation therapy (see Chapter 113): Esophageal strictures develop after irradiation for esophageal cancer (in 25–67% of patients), head and neck cancer, and after mediastinal radiation for other malignancies.[4]

Anastomotic stricture: The incidence is dependent upon the type of surgical procedure: retrosternal surgical approach (50%), antiperistaltic interposition (30%), two-layer anastomosis (10%), lack of gastric drainage procedure (58%), and the occurrence of anastomotic leaks.[5]

DEFINITION OF STENOSIS

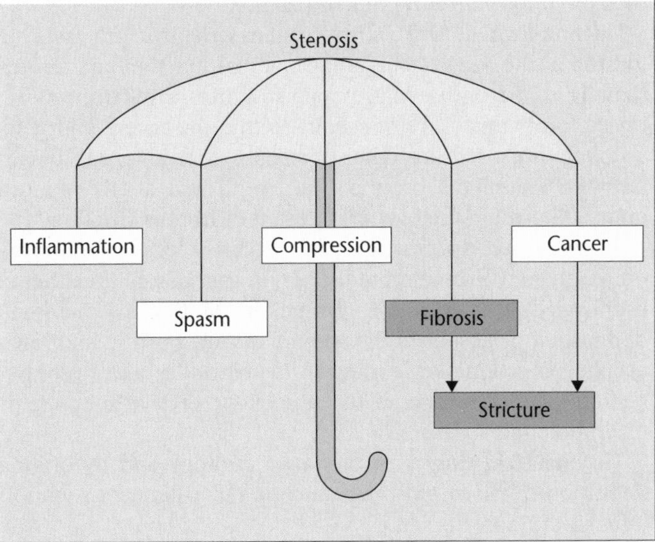

Fig. 30.1 Definitions of stenosis. The term stenosis should be considered a generic esophageal narrowing covering five different processes, i.e., an umbrella. Stricture confirmation requires evidence of deposition of abnormal tissue, either fibrosis or cancer.

CAUSES, RISK FACTORS, ASSOCIATIONS
• Acid reflux esophagitis Nasogastric intubation Scleroderma Zollinger-Ellison syndrome (gastrin-hypersecreting tumor) Gastroparesis Esophagogastrostomy Hyperemesis syndromes • Schatzki ring • Radiation injury • Caustic injury • Webs • Esophagitis Eosinophilic ("ringed" esophagus) *Candida* Drug/pill-induced – NSAIDs, potassium chloride, quinidine, alendronate • Photodynamic therapy (PDT) • Thermal laser therapy (NdYAG) • Sclerotherapy (variceal) • Epidermolysis bullosa • Congenital atresia • Ischemia • Lichen planus

Photodynamic laser therapy with Photofrin (QLT Phototherapeutics, Vancouver, B.C., Canada) for high-grade dysplasia in Barrett's esophagus causes stricture in 29% of patients.[6]

PATHOGENESIS AND PATHOLOGY

Benign strictures result from intramural esophageal injury. The volume, dwell time, concentration, and depth of injury produced by the causative agent, or the severity of the associated systemic disorder, determine the severity of the stricture. If there is continuing or repeated injury of a pre-existing stricture from a noxious agent (e.g., acid, pill injury, or radiation), the resulting acute inflammation, edema, and enhanced fibrosis further compromise the lumen patency.

Uncomplicated acid reflux-related strictures are typically located at the squamocolumnar mucosal junction and are less than 1 cm in length.[7] Mild peptic strictures result from reflux injury to the mucosal layer alone. With more severe injury, the esophagitis extends into the submucosa, and, in rare instances, into the muscularis propria. The length and depth of mural injury determine the eventual degree of fibrous stricture.

Scleroderma: In 50–80% of patients with scleroderma, esophageal involvement predisposes to gastroesophageal reflux, esophagitis, and stricture formation. Motility is markedly diminished or absent in the smooth muscle portion and lower esophageal sphincter, leading to hypomotility and decreased resting sphincter tone, with subsequent erosive esophagitis, ulceration and stricture.[8]

The Schatzki ring is of unknown etiology and by original definition involves only the mucosa and submucosa without inflammation or fibrosis.

Chemical injury (caustics, quinidine, potassium chloride, and sclerosants), ischemia, photodynamic and Nd:YAG laser therapy, and surgical anastomosis are likely to result in deep to full-thickness esophageal wall injury with severe fibrosis. After caustic injury, an inflammatory response and vascular thrombosis with ischemia is followed by bacterial invasion. Initially, there is sloughing of tissue and proliferation of granulation tissue, followed by fibrosis and retraction of the fibrous tissue, producing a stricture. In patients with third-degree burns with loss of epithelium, ulceration, and evidence of granulation there is an 80–100% chance of stricture.[3] For most other etiologies, the pathologic process may be similar but more gradual and less severe. Strictures with this pathogenesis are tighter, longer, of higher risk, and less responsive to dilatation.

Anastomotic strictures most often develop after anastomotic leaks but also are related to the type of surgical procedure, technical expertise, and gastric stasis with acid reflux.[5] The degree of fibrosis also is influenced by individual tissue reaction to suture material or staples at the anastomosis.

CLINICAL PRESENTATION

Dysphagia is the primary symptom of any type of esophageal obstruction (see Chapter 3). Dysphagia associated with esophageal stricture is a relatively late symptom. Solid food dysphagia is predictable and permanent when the lumen diameter is reduced to about 13 mm (50% of normal), but may be provoked earlier by larger, solid food bolus challenges.

Patients may ignore warning symptoms for months or years, and may even deny that food ever 'got stuck' before. Patients compensate by eating softer or blenderized food, eating slowly, and using large amounts of fluid to 'wash the food down.' When complete obstruction occurs acutely – not uncommonly during a restaurant meal – the physician is challenged with difficult, emergency management of a far advanced lesion.

A long history of heartburn with intermittent dysphagia for solids over a period of months to years without weight loss is typical for a benign peptic stricture. Lower esophageal rings (Schatzki) have a distinct anatomic appearance and a similar presentation, but with minimal or no heartburn.

Impact pain occurs within seconds after swallowing a solid bolus and results from the increased intraesophageal pressure and distention.

Regurgitation, the spontaneous projection of gastric or esophageal content into the pharynx and mouth, is easily separated from vomiting because it is not associated with nausea. A sour taste indicates free reflux from the stomach to the pharynx, whereas an unaltered taste of recently swallowed food indicates that the food never reached the stomach.

CLINICAL PRESENTATION
• Dysphagia – intermittent with solid food, rarely a problem with liquids • Odynophagia – bolus impact pain, disappears with transition to softer diet • Associated symptoms – heartburn; symptoms and signs of systemic disease • History of esophageal injury – caustic, radiation, pills • Regurgitation – usually in advanced cases only • Sialorrhea – excess salivation or "water brash;" related to severity of obstruction or acid reflux • Upper aerodigestive symptoms – cough, sore throat, hoarseness, bronchitis, or asthma; suggest regurgitation with aspiration • Weight loss – uncommon with benign strictures

Caustic ingestion: During acute and subacute phases, odynophagia and variable degrees of dysphagia occur. Signs and symptoms do not accurately predict esophageal injury acutely, but patients with sialorrhea, drooling, stridor, and vomiting are the most likely to have had esophageal injury.

DIFFERENTIAL DIAGNOSIS

Once obstructive dysphagia is identified, the physician has to decide whether it is the result of dysmotility or mechanical obstruction. Early cases of reflux esophagitis with dysphagia may be due to inflammation and spasm, rather than cicatricial narrowing.[1] Barium radiography is helpful in evaluating a narrow segment, which may be shown to open up intermittently, suggesting inflammatory stenosis or spasm as the cause.[9]

Once a true stricture has been confirmed, the challenge is to determine the etiology as benign or malignant by endoscopy, biopsy, and cytologic examination.[10] There are numerous potential etiologies that may be determined primarily by a proper medical history and objectively by radiography, endoscopy, and biopsy.

The tight lower esophageal sphincter of achalasia may be confused with a distal stricture, but the correct diagnosis is confirmed by symptoms of both liquid and solid food dysphagia, proper barium esophagraphy, endoscopy, and manometry.

DIAGNOSTIC METHODS

The following are essentials for the medical history: duration of dysphagia, location of the sensation, associated events such as cough or choking, nasal regurgitation, neck or chest pain, provocative food consistencies, most bothersome food at onset of dysphagia, weight loss, problems with sialorrhea (recognized as foamy mucus), regurgitation, and evidence of other medical illness or family history of dysphagia.

Barium contrast studies are the next logical diagnostic step. Liquid barium is usually diagnostic for oropharyngeal dysphagia and stricture. The location and anatomic features of the stricture provide clues to etiology (Fig. 30.2A). If the standard column barium study is negative, a bolus challenge, such as a pill or marshmallow, will identify the level of obstruction without risk of prolonged impaction of the esophagus (see Chapter 3).

Video endoscopy is indicated in every patient with an esophageal stricture.[7] The endoscopic features and biopsy can settle the important differential diagnosis between benign and malignant etiology (Fig. 30.2B). Biopsies beyond the stricture may be impossible during the initial endoscopy unless dilatation is performed. Endoscopy showing neither mucosal abnormality nor resistance does not rule out significant narrowing. In such instances, barium esophagraphy with bolus challenge can confirm the location of a significant narrowing (see Chapter 3).

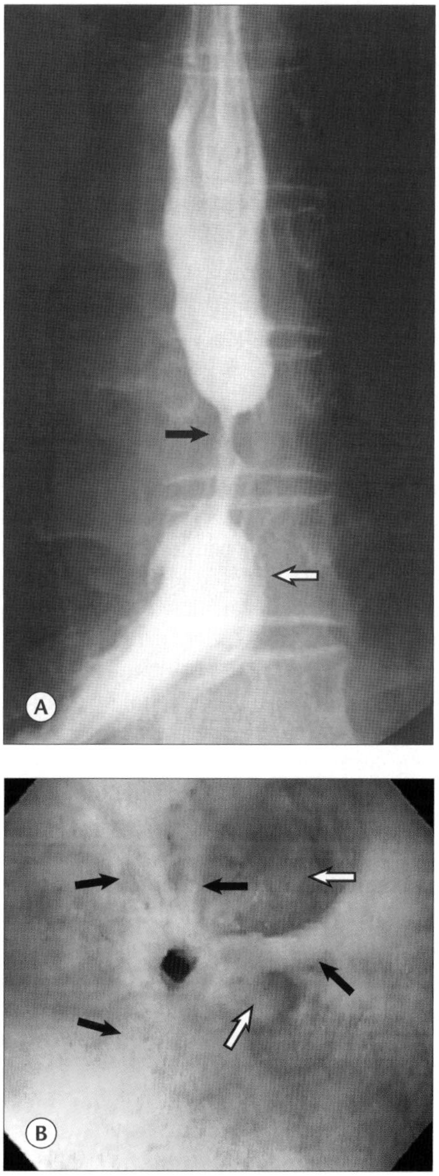

Fig. 30.2 Benign distal esophageal peptic stricture. **A.** Barium esophagraphy reveals a benign distal esophageal peptic stricture (closed arrow) complicated by pill injury at the esophagogastric junction proximal to a hiatal hernia (open arrow). **B.** The endoscopic appearance of this stricture is shown. A pre-existing peptic stricture was complicated by daily impactions of three NSAID tablets producing a marked increase in dysphagia. Note the fibrous subepithelial bands radiating from the stricture (closed arrows) and the pseudodiverticula at the one and four o'clock positions (open arrows).

DIAGNOSTIC METHODS
• **Radiography** Standard column esophagraphy – best initial study Bolus challenge – barium pill, marshmallow when standard esophagram negative Double contrast for esophagitis and mucosal detail • **Endoscopy** Standard videoendoscope Thin-caliber videoendoscope – for severe strictures Endoscopic biopsy/cytology • **Studies as indicated for systemic and infectious disease etiologies**

TREATMENT AND PREVENTION

Every stricture has its distinctive 'personality' and deserves careful evaluation before therapy begins. Potential difficulties with future stricture therapy can be predicted by determining several factors: etiology, pathogenesis, lumen diameter, angulations and associated inflammation, ulceration, or diverticula. Strictures due to transmural injury initially require a Savary-type dilator over a guide wire for optimal dysphagia relief and safety.[7]

The first principle of stricture therapy is to avoid attempting full dilatation of a severe stricture at one sitting. Most strictures have been present for months to many years, and the treatment program should not be limited to one session. A good practice is to pass no more than three dilators per sitting (the 'Rule of 3'), after more than moderate resistance is encountered.[7]

The second principle is to be aware of the position or location of the dilator and/or guidewire at all times to ensure safety and optimal dilatation. An experienced operator can safely dilate many simple benign strictures without fluoroscopy, but for tight or tortuous strictures there is general agreement that using a guidewire with fluoroscopic control is a wise practice. Fluoroscopic control is the safest method for proper positioning and utilization of all peroral dilators.

Dilators passed under fluoroscopy over a wireguide (Savary) or tantalum-filled bougies (Maloney) are best suited for severe strictures. Most benign, simple strictures (reflux-related and rings) are safely and effectively treated with the above dilators or through-the-scope hydrostatic dilators. The frequency of dilatation is determined by the type of stricture and associated inflammation.

For caustic strictures, esophageal dilatation should be started at the latest by the end of the third week after injury.[11] Dilatation over a guidewire under fluoroscopic control at least weekly to maintain patency and reduce the degree of stricture occlusion should be continued indefinitely at increasing intervals, depending on patient need.

Refractory strictures: Where refractoriness to standard peroral dilatation techniques is expected during the initial evaluation, it is important to determine an accurate prognosis and develop an effective realistic long-term treatment plan.

Severe strictures significantly alter quality of life and social activities. Nutrition and hydration are impaired, meals represent agony not pleasure, oral secretions cannot be handled adequately, and bronchopulmonary aspiration is a constant threat. These problems are enhanced by the fact that most patients with advanced esophageal obstruction produce large amounts of saliva (sialorrhea). Restoration of an adequate lumen will reduce dysphagia and sialorrhea. The goal of therapy is to establish and maintain a patent esophagus with relief of dysphagia suitable for the patient's need at the lowest risk and cost.

Prevention is easier than treating a far advanced stricture; therefore, avoidance of injury and/or early treatment cannot be overemphasized. Adequate therapy for acid reflux with proton pump inhibitors (PPIs) will prevent stricture occurrence or progression. Acid suppression plus antireflux measures should be used in all patients who must undergo prolonged nasogastric intubation. Patients should be instructed on the proper method for taking medications to prevent either primary or secondary drug-induced injury.[12] Early postoperative dilatation and use of proper doses of PPI therapy will reduce or eliminate the need for dilatation of anastomotic strictures.[5] After the ingestion of corrosives and irradiation therapy, early, properly performed, peroral dilatation is safe and will reduce the severity of stricture formation.

COMPLICATIONS AND THEIR MANAGEMENT

Pulmonary: Aspiration pneumonia is a serious complication of esophageal stricture with obstruction. The patient may be treated for nocturnal cough, wheezing from 'asthma,' or recurrent bouts of pneumonia without the primary problem of dysphagia and aspiration being recognized. All patients with recurrent pulmonary infections or unexplained persistent (particularly nocturnal) cough require evaluation for dysfunction of the oropharynx and esophagus.

TREATMENT AND PREVENTION

TREATMENT

- Dilatation plan based on stricture classification (etiology, pathology, diameter, length):
  Simple strictures (reflux, rings, webs)
  Complex transmural strictures (radiation, caustic, pill-induced, etc.)
- Dilator selection:
  Simple strictures – Maloney, Savary (wire-guided) or hydrostatic balloon (through-the-scope)
  Complex strictures – Savary (wire-guided), Maloney
- Fluoroscopy for dilatation:
  Simple strictures – optional, based on anatomic features by radiography
  Complex strictures – recommended as the safest procedure
- Stents – not recommended for benign strictures
- Pharmacotherapy – proton pump inhibitors (PPIs) for active reflux esophagitis, antifungal drugs for *Candida*

PREVENTION

- Adequate acid suppression (PPI) for gastroesophageal reflux disease to prevent strictures
- Prophylactic PPIs during nasogastric intubation and after esophagogastrostomy
- Proper labeling and storage of caustic chemicals
- Early dilatation after caustic and radiation injury

Carcinoma complicates caustic strictures of the esophagus in 3–5% of patients, usually after 10–30 years, and is usually not detected early. Patients with radiation stricture and a history of head/neck cancer also are at higher risk for developing esophageal squamous cancer and may benefit from periodic endoscopic surveillance. Surveillance using staining by iodine chromoendoscopy can detect dysplasia or early squamous carcinoma, and permit curative therapy.

Esophageal perforation due to dilatation is a life-threatening complication and should occur in less than 0.2% of cases when the correct technique is used.[13] Early diagnosis and therapy are essential. Postdilatation chest pain, tachycardia, mediastinal and subcutaneous emphysema, pleural effusion, and odynophagia suggest the diagnosis. Suspicion of perforation should be followed by prompt examination of the neck and chest, posteroanterior/lateral chest radiography, and water-soluble contrast esophagraphy. If the initial esophagram is negative, a barium contrast and possibly CT should be done. Early surgical consultation is essential.

PROGNOSIS WITH AND WITHOUT TREATMENT

The patient should be counseled properly regarding the predicted long-term dilatation treatment plan and prognosis. Misunderstanding and disappointment can be minimized if the patient is properly informed about strictures, usually the complex type, most likely to require either a prolonged initial series of dilatation sessions or periodic dilatations in the future. Transmural strictures always require periodic dilatation indefinitely to maintain lumen patency, whereas simple reflux strictures and rings respond well to only several initial dilatations. Esophagectomy has a high risk of morbidity and mortality, and is rarely needed for benign strictures.

SOURCES OF INFORMATION FOR PATIENTS AND DOCTORS

Concise, accurate pamphlets on esophageal strictures and dilatation are available from the American Society for Gastrointestinal Endoscopy. Patient-oriented books on gastroesophageal reflux disease and peptic strictures provide good information: *Coping with Chronic Heartburn* by Elaine Fantle Shimberg, St Martin's Press, 175 Fifth Avenue, New York, NY 10010, is recommended.

Reliable information for patients on strictures is available via the following internet sites:

http://www.gastromd.com/education/print_esophagealstrictures.html
http://www.gicare.com/pated/ecdgs05.htm
http://www.health.discovery.com/encyclopedias/220.html
http://www.patient.co.uk/showdoc/40024630/
http://www.patient.co.uk/showdoc/40002339/

REFERENCES

1. Boyce HW. Definitions, diagnoses and documentation. Editorial. Gastrointest Endosc 1995; 41:264–265.
2. Johnston MH, Wong R. Esophageal strictures. In: Castell DC, Richter JE, eds. The esophagus, 4th edn. Philadelphia: Lippincott Williams & Wilkins; 2004:507–517.
3. Spiegel JR, Sataloff RT. Caustic injuries of the esophagus. In: Castell DO, Richter JE, eds. The esophagus, 4th edn. Philadelphia: Lippincott Williams & Wilkins; 2004:602–610.
4. Vanagunas A, Jacob P, Olinger E. Radiation-induced esophageal injury: a spectrum from esophagitis to cancer. Am J Gastroenterol 1990; 85:808–812.
5. Lerut T, Coosemans W, Decker G et al. Anastomotic complications after esophagectomy. Dig Surg 2002; 19:92–98.
6. Panjehpour M, Overholt BF, Haydek JM et al. Results of photodynamic therapy for ablation of dysplasia and early cancer in Barrett's esophagus and effect of oral steroids on stricture formation. Am J Gastronterol 2000; 95:2177–2184.
7. Boyce HW. Hiatal hernia and peptic diseases of the esophagus. In: Sivak MV, ed. Gastroenterologic endoscopy, 2nd edn. Philadelphia: WB Saunders; 2000:580–597.
8. Richter JE. Peptic strictures of the esophagus. Gastroenterol Clin North Am 1999; 28:875–891.
9. Luedtke P, Levine MS, Rubesin SE et al. Radiologic diagnosis of benign esophageal strictures: a pattern approach. Radiographics 2003; 23:897–909.
10. Miller LS, Jackson W, McCray W et al. Benign nonpeptic esophageal strictures: diagnosis and treatment. Gastroenterol Clin North Am 1998; 8:329–355.
11. Choudhry U, Boyce HW. Treatment of esophageal disorders caused by modifications, caustic ingestion, foreign bodies and trauma. In: Wolfe E, ed. Therapy of digestive disorders. Philadelphia: WB Saunders; 2000:37–53.
12. Kikendall JW. Pill-induced esophageal injury. In: Castell DO, Richter JE, eds. The esophagus, 4th edn. Philadelphia: Lippincott Williams & Wilkins; 2004:572–584.
13. Tulman AB, Boyce HW. Complications of esophageal dilation and guidelines for their prevention. Gastrointest Endosc 1981; 27:229–234.

Chapter 31

Barrett's esophagus

John A Bonino and Prateek Sharma

KEY POINTS

- Barrett's esophagus is the precursor lesion in most cases of esophageal adenocarcinoma, with an annual cancer risk of 0.5% per year
- 10–12% of patients with gastroesophageal reflux disease have Barrett's esophagus at endoscopy
- Barrett's esophagus is primarily a disease of white middle-aged men
- Loss of heterozygosity is a key genetic mechanism in the etiology of esophageal adenocarcinoma
- COX-2 inhibitors have a potential chemopreventive role by promoting apoptosis
- Patients over 50 years old with longstanding reflux symptoms should be screened for Barrett's esophagus
- The diagnosis requires consensus between endoscopic recognition of a displaced squamocolumnar junction and confirmation of intestinal metaplasia
- It is unclear whether surveillance programs result in a true survival advantage – identifying high-risk individuals by the presence of biomarkers may offer better prediction of risk in the future
- It is not known whether acid suppression reduces cancer risk

INTRODUCTION

Barrett's esophagus is a metaplastic change in the esophagus that results in replacement of the normal squamous lined epithelium with a columnar type. This metaplastic lesion carries an increased risk for the development of esophageal adenocarcinoma. The incidence of esophageal adenocarcinoma has increased substantially around the world[1–2] but the explanation for this trend is unknown. Barrett's esophagus is found as a precursor lesion in most cases of esophageal adenocarcinoma. Patients with Barrett's esophagus are thought to have an annual risk of developing esophageal cancer of 0.5% per year, substantially higher than the general population.[2] Although the relative risk of individuals in the US with Barrett's esophagus developing esophageal adenocarcinoma is high, the absolute risk is extremely low due to the small number of cases.

The metaplastic change of Barrett's esophagus is thought to develop as a consequence of chronic gastroesophageal reflux disease. Currently, it is estimated that as much as 10% of the adult US population experiences daily heartburn.[3] Furthermore, of those who undergo upper endoscopy for symptomatic gastroesophageal reflux disease, as many as 10–12% have Barrett's esophagus.[4]

Investigators have suggested that although reflux disease probably plays a role in Barrett's esophagus and cancer development, many genetic determinants potentially influence the epithelial response to such stimulus and affect malignant transformation. Since most cases of esophageal adenocarcinoma present clinically at incurable stages, questions have arisen regarding the appropriate methods and frequency of screening and surveillance, as well as those who would benefit from intervention. Much interest and research also surrounds the development of both chemotherapeutic and endoscopic interventions that could be used to halt or reverse the progression of Barrett's esophagus and prevent adenocarcinoma.

EPIDEMIOLOGY

Although gastroesophageal reflux disease is a common problem, many previous studies of Barrett's esophagus may have actually underestimated prevalence rates by focusing on patients who had symptomatic reflux. The diagnosis of Barrett's esophagus is frequently made in the elderly with a mean age at diagnosis of approximately 60 years. Barrett's esophagus is twice as common in men as in women.[3] Barrett's esophagus is primarily a disease of white men. Although Barrett's esophagus is considered an acquired phenomenon, there is probably some genetic predilection to the metaplastic change.[4]

Adenocarcinoma is now the dominant form of esophageal carcinoma in white males in the US and Western Europe.[5, 6] The incidence of adenocarcinoma of the esophagus in American white males is approximately 4–6 per 100 000, an increase of over 300% when compared to previously documented annual rates from the mid 1970s.[4]

CAUSES, RISK FACTORS, DISEASE ASSOCIATIONS

Chronic reflux disease is generally considered the most recognizable trigger for the development of Barrett's esophagus. Otherwise, very few risk factors have been elucidated. Advanced age, history of reflux symptoms at an early age, increased duration of symptoms, increased severity of nocturnal reflux symptoms, and increased complications commonly associated with gastroesophageal reflux disease (ulcers, bleeding, etc.) are also cited as increasing the risk.[2–4] Conversely, the risk factors for the development of esophageal adenocarcinoma are better established. The presence of Barrett's esophagus, increasing age, and obesity are all important risk factors for esophageal adenocarcinoma.[7] The predilection for white males is a great mystery.

CAUSES AND RISK FACTORS
RISK FACTORS FOR ESOPHAGEAL ADENOCARCINOMA
1) Male gender 2) Elevated body mass index 3) Tobacco use 4) Advanced age 5) Gastroesophageal reflux symptoms 6) Lower esophageal sphincter-relaxing drugs 7) Barrett's esophagus with: – increasing length of Barrett's esophagus – high-grade dysplasia – biomarkers[a]

[a] Biomarkers as predictors of esophageal adenocarcinoma remains controversial.

PATHOGENESIS

Barrett's esophagus, stimulated by gastroesophageal reflux, is a direct result of esophageal mucosal injury. This injury probably begins with both genetic and environmental triggers that initiate pluripotent stem cells to undergo differentiation resulting in the proliferation of an altered phenotype, in this case intestinal metaplasia.[8] It is likely, given the small percentage of patients with reflux disease who develop Barrett's esophagus, that other important factors such as the composition of the refluxed matter itself and the duration of reflux exposure, amongst others, also contribute to this change. Accordingly, risk factors such as decreased lower esophageal sphincter tone, increased severity of reflux symptoms, and night-time reflux symptoms all appear to increase an individual's risk of development of Barrett's esophagus.[7]

The **evolution of Barrett's esophagus to neoplasia** is proposed to arise from a combination of both mutation and natural selection. Genomic instability is believed to initiate a clonal evolution early in Barrett's metaplasia following mutations that give a selective advantage to a line of 'abnormal' cells over genetically 'normal' ones. At least three abnormalities have been described in Barrett's epithelial cells during this clonal evolution: chromosomal aberrations, genetic mutations, and DNA methylation (of the promoter), which can silence a tumor suppression gene.[8] Loss of heterozygosity is believed to be the single most common mechanism by which genetic lesions occur in esophageal adenocarcinoma. Loss of heterozygosity is described as a loss of genetic regions from various chromosomes, which in this case may result in loss of regulation in the transition from the G1 phase to the S phase in the cell cycle (e.g., loss of p53 and p16). This loss of suppressor genes allows genetically abnormal cells to divide and proliferate, setting the stage for dysplastic evolution.[8–9]

Experimental studies have demonstrated that exposing cultured intestinal metaplasia to acid for an extended period of time results in an increase in proliferation and expression of proteins inhibiting cell death. One of the antiapoptotic proteins under investigation has been cyclooxygenase-2 (COX-2). COX-2 is induced by cell injury and leads to increased production of prostaglandin E2.[8] This prostaglandin is known to affect apoptosis and has generated interest in evaluating COX-2 inhibitors as potential chemopreventive agents. This interest has been further nurtured by clinical studies showing the possible chemoprotective effects of cyclooxygenase inhibitors in other gastrointestinal malignancies.

CLINICAL PRESENTATION

There are no symptoms proven to be specific for patients with Barrett's esophagus. In fact, the symptoms in patients with Barrett's esophagus are usually the same as those in patients with gastroesophageal reflux without Barrett's esophagus. Attempts have been made to assess the probability of Barrett's esophagus based on symptoms, e.g., heartburn, nocturnal chest pain, or odynophagia.[10] However, a considerable number of patients with Barrett's esophagus or Barrett's-associated adenocarcinoma may be asymptomatic with respect to gastroesophageal reflux.[10–11] The American College of Gastroenterology guidelines for the diagnosis and treatment of Barrett's esophagus suggest that any patient greater than 50 years of age with longstanding reflux symptoms should have an upper endoscopy to assess for possible Barrett's esophagus (i.e., screening).[12] However, the cost effectiveness in identifying individuals at increased risk for development of Barrett's esophagus and its impact on mortality rates from esophageal adenocarcinoma have not been established.

DIAGNOSIS

The definition of Barrett's esophagus has evolved over time. Barrett's esophagus was recently defined during a workshop sponsored by the American Gastroenterological Association in February 2003 (Barrett's Esophagus Chicago Workshop) as 'a displacement of the squamocolumnar junction proximal to the gastroesophageal junction with the presence of intestinal metaplasia' (Fig. 31.1A,B).[12] Given that intestinal metaplasia is the precursor lesion associated with adenocarcinoma, the goal of this definition is to adequately identify individuals at risk for adenocarcinoma in whom a program of surveillance or intervention would probably be beneficial.

Endoscopic recognition of columnar mucosa in the distal esophagus is at times complicated by the clinician's ability to clearly identify both the gastroesophageal and the squamocolumnar junctions. The squamocolumnar junction is identified by the endoscopically appreciated 'Z-line,' which represents the junction of the squamous epithelium with the columnar epithelium.[2] Frequently, however, the endoscopist may have difficulty identifying the gastroesophageal junction due to a large hiatal hernia, inflammation, a patulous lower esophageal sphincter, or other entities that may distort the anatomical landmarks. Proximal displacement of the squamocolumnar junction, relative to the gastroesophageal junction, recognized during endoscopy suggests the diagnosis of Barrett's esophagus.

In vivo staining: Today, a variety of endoscopically applied staining techniques are helpful in highlighting the squamocolumnar junction as well as accentuating patterns of intestinal metaplasia in the distal esophagus. Lugol's iodine, toluidine blue, indigo carmine, and methylene blue are all different type of stains used for this purpose (Fig. 31.2).[13] Although not routinely required, their application in specific circumstances can be useful to diagnose Barrett's esophagus. It has also been noted that recognition of intestinal metaplasia on biopsy specimens is enhanced with use of alcian blue stain at a pH of 2.5, allowing the pathologist to appreciate the presence or absence

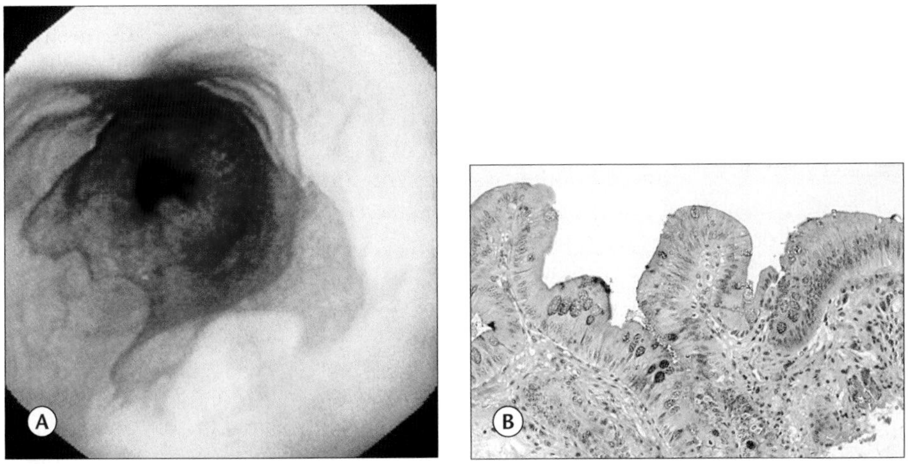

Fig. 31.1 Columnar lined distal esophagus and intestinal metaplasia. A. Endoscopic view of the columnar lined distal esophagus. **B.** Intestinal metaplasia. Reproduced from Sharma P. Recent advances in Barrett's esophagus: short-segment Barrett's esophagus and cardia intestinal metaplasia. Sem Gastrointest Dis 1999; 10:93–101 with permission from Elsevier.

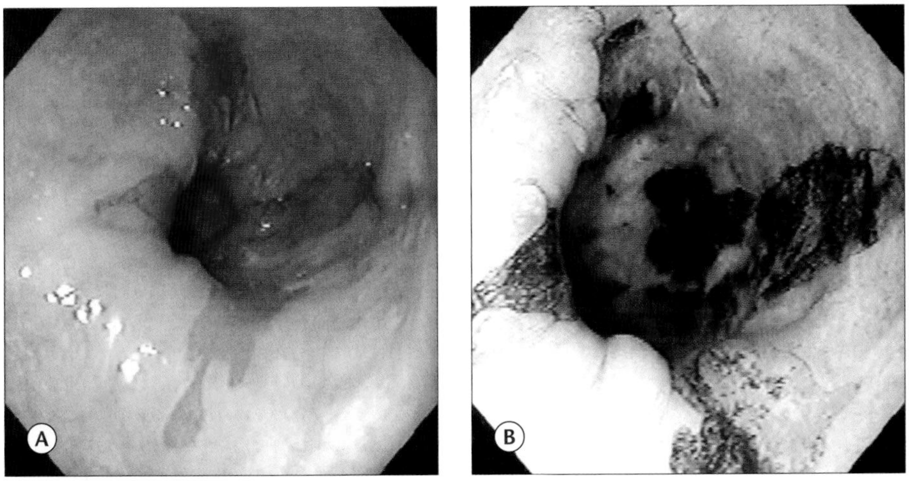

Fig. 31.2 Chromoendoscopy. An example of chromoendoscopy using methylene blue showing areas of staining within the columnar mucosa. Reproduced from Sharma P et al. Methylene blue chromoendoscopy for detection of short-segment Barrett's esophagus. Gastrointest Endosc 2001; 54:2889–2893 with permission from Elsevier.

of goblet cells, which are pathognomonic of the metaplastic changes, and to avoid overdiagnosis of the presence of goblet cells.[14]

For the purposes of research studies and transmitting information at the clinical practice level patients with <3 cm of Barrett's esophagus are considered to have short-segment Barrett's, while those with longer areas of affected esophagus have long-segment disease.[15] The clinical significance with regards to prognosis and treatment between the two types has not been firmly demonstrated to date, though preliminary data suggests that increasing lengths of Barrett's esophagus correspond to increased risk of development of adenocarcinoma.[2]

SURVEILLANCE AND TREATMENT

No prospective trials have been conducted in patients with Barrett's esophagus to attempt to show a survival advantage in those who have undergone endoscopic surveillance compared with nonsurveyed patients. Several retrospective trials, however, have suggested mortality rate improvement with the use of endoscopic surveillance programs in individuals identified with Barrett's esophagus.[16–18] These reports have shown that individuals undergoing surveillance are more likely to be recognized with adenocarcinoma at an earlier stage, resulting in improved survival rates compared to those not under surveillance. These studies are obviously limited by small numbers of patients, and lead and length time biases.

Economics: In one model, the cost of endoscopic surveillance of Barrett's esophagus was more economical than mammography for breast cancer screening: the cost per life year saved for the Barrett's adenocarcinoma patient was US$4151 while that for the breast cancer patient was US$57 926.[19] Another study employed a cost-utility analysis of surveillance for Barrett's esophagus and concluded that screening 'high-risk' individuals with gastroesophageal reflux, followed by surveillance of only those with dysplasia, would probably be cost effective.[20]

Clearly, a high-risk group needs to be identified so that resources may be focused on those with a higher likelihood of developing carcinoma compared with the vast majority of Barrett's esophagus patients who will never get carcinoma.

Current practices and guidelines hold that patients with Barrett's esophagus should undergo surveillance endoscopy with an interval based on the degree of dysplasia detected on biopsy. These recommendations (not evidence based) are summarized in a report by the American College of Gastroenterology (see Table 31.1).[12]

Biopsy: For the detection of dysplasia in patients with Barrett's esophagus, it is generally recommended that four quadrant biopsies be taken every 2 cm in routine circumstances and every 1 cm in high-grade dysplasia or in extensive low-grade

TABLE 31.1 ENDOSCOPIC SURVEILLANCE OF BARRETT'S ESOPHAGUS

SUMMARY OF RECOMMENDATIONS BY AMERICAN COLLEGE OF GASTROENTEROLOGY ON ENDOSCOPIC SURVEILLANCE OF INDIVIDUALS WITH BARRETT'S ESOPHAGUS	
Dysplasia	**Surveillance**
No dysplasia	Yearly until two negative exams, then every 3 years
Low-grade dysplasia	Repeat every year until **no** dysplasia
High-grade dysplasia	Repeat every 3 months or remove

dysplasia. In addition, biopsies should be taken of any mucosal abnormalities such as bumps, erosions, or ulcers. Given that these biopsies are random in nature and sample only a small surface area of the Barrett's segment, a number of new techniques (i.e., magnification endoscopy, spectroscopy, optical coherence tomography, etc.) are being evaluated to increase the yield of detecting dysplastic and cancerous tissue (Fig. 31.3).[21] These technologies are not yet ready for routine clinical use but, if validated, would dramatically change how patients with Barrett's esophagus are surveyed in the future.

Identifying 'high-risk' individuals through the use of biological markers would increase the cost-effectiveness of screening and surveillance techniques. The intent of using 'biomarkers' would be to help predict those individuals with Barrett's esophagus that may eventually develop esophageal adenocarcinoma. In total, more than 60 putative biomarkers have been proposed in Barrett's esophagus. The focus has been on p53 tumor suppressor marker mutations and aneuploidy with flow cytometry.[9,22] Any marker studies for prediction of heightened cancer risk will require large-scale multicenter studies. If markers are found to be predictive they might actually be in the form of a 'basket of markers,' analogous to the marker basket used commonly in lymphoma diagnosis and differential diagnosis.

Management: A reasonable initial step in treatment of Barrett's esophagus is the elimination of symptoms of reflux and healing esophagitis. Gastroesophageal reflux symptoms may be controlled by initiating and titrating proton pump inhibitor therapy. However, even symptomatic eradication with proton pump inhibitor therapy did not ensure normalization of esophageal pH in up to 38% of patients, a fact that has been reproduced in other studies.[23] The importance of reflux control has been proposed by further studies that concluded that acid reflux predisposed to progression of cell proliferation, and some studies have even cited gastroesophageal reflux in the activation of protein kinase-regulated pathways resulting in decreased apoptosis in cell lines exposed to acid.[24] Acid suppression therapy, however, has not yet clearly demonstrated a reduction in cancer risk.

Surgery: This option can be considered in some individuals with Barrett's esophagus for the treatment of their underlying gastroesophageal reflux disease. Although studies in the surgical literature argue for histological regression in individuals after antireflux surgery, cases of high-grade dysplasia and cancer have been reported even after these procedures. From a meta-analysis it was concluded that the risk of adenocarcinoma in individual's with Barrett's esophagus was not significantly decreased by antireflux surgical procedures.[25] Many questions still remain on the ability of both medical and surgical treatments to reverse Barrett's metaplasia and reduce cancer risk.

Endoscopic therapies for the treatment of Barrett's esophagus are still largely an investigational mode of therapy. A variety of endoscopic ablative therapies including thermal, chemical, and mechanical methods have been applied in patients with both dysplastic and nondysplastic Barrett's esophagus. Although the majority of the area of Barrett's esophagus can be replaced by neo-squamous mucosa, persistent metaplastic tissue may be found beneath the squamous tissue and cases of adenocarcinoma have been reported after such 'successful' ablation therapy.[26] Other side effects include stricture formation and perforation. Given the low risk of cancer in patients with nondysplastic Barrett's esophagus or even in those with low-grade dysplasia, endoscopic ablation treatments cannot be recommended outside of protocols in these patients. In patients

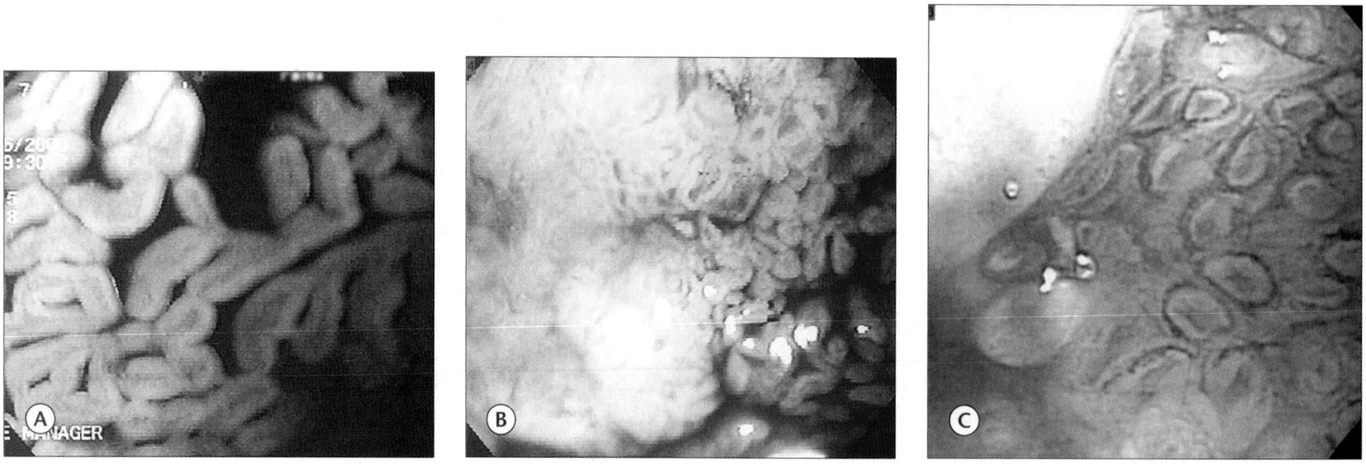

Fig. 31.3 Magnification endoscopy. Use of magnification endoscopy in patient's with Barrett's esophagus showing three distinct patterns observed under magnification (115×) after spraying with indigo carmine: ridge villous **(A)**; irregular/distorted **(B)**; and circular **(C)**. Reproduced from Sharma P et al. Magnification chromoendoscopy for the detection of intestinal metaplasia and dysplasia in Barrett's esophagus. Gut 2003; 52:24–27 with permission from the BMJ Publishing Group.

with high-grade dysplasia, however, the risk of progression to cancer can be as high as 25–37%.[12,26] In these patients, aggressive surveillance, early surgical resection, endoscopic mucosal resection for localized lesions, or endoscopic ablation should be considered. Esophagectomy – although a procedure with considerable morbidity – for cure of high-grade dysplasia and early adenocarcinoma is the gold standard against which other therapies must be measured in terms of durability and lack of recurrence.

Chemoprevention is an increasingly intense area of research interest in Barrett's esophagus and in other conditions associated with an increased risk of cancer. Some epidemiological studies have also shown a risk reduction in esophageal cancer in aspirin users compared to nonusers.[27] A rat model of esophageal cancer has also shown a reduction of esophageal cancer with the use of cyclooxygenase inhibitors. [27]

WHAT TO TELL PATIENTS

Gastroesophageal reflux disease is a very common digestive problem, while esophageal adenocarcinoma is uncommon. Barrett's esophagus occurs as a result of chronic reflux and is probably an intermediate step in the development of adenocarcinoma of the esophagus. Owing to a variety of factors, reflux of contents from the stomach causes damage to the lining of the esophagus and results in a change of cell types lining the esophagus. This process is called metaplasia and this condition in the esophagus is termed Barrett's esophagus. These newly 'displaced' cells can potentially undergo malignant transformation, but this process occurs only in a minority of patient's with Barrett's esophagus.

The symptoms of Barrett's esophagus are the same as those of uncomplicated gastroesophageal reflux without Barrett's esophagus. Controlling reflux symptoms is extremely important and various acid suppression medications (i.e., proton pump inhibitors) are used for this purpose. Though not all patients with gastroesophageal reflux will benefit from endoscopy, individuals over 50 years of age with chronic symptoms of reflux should discuss with their physician whether a screening endoscopy would be appropriate for them. Individuals found to have Barrett's esophagus should then be considered for enrollment in an endoscopic surveillance program, although there are scant data suggesting that this changes outcomes. Informing one's physician of uncontrolled reflux symptoms is of importance in identifying and treating this disorder and its possible complications. Special attention should be paid to problems such as dysphagia, anemia, or weight loss, which should lead to early endoscopy for further evaluation.

CURRENT CONTROVERSIES AND THEIR FUTURE RESOLUTION

Several controversies surround the area of Barrett's esophagus. Current strategies for identifying all those with Barrett's esophagus are unlikely to have a significant impact on mortality from esophageal adenocarcinoma. The premise of, 'Whom to screen?' is still a question unanswered. Although some risk factors for Barrett's esophagus have been suggested, a category of high-risk individuals who would substantially benefit from a screening protocol have not yet been identified. Similarly, surveillance of Barrett's esophagus is of unproven value. High-risk individuals clearly need to be identified. To this end, the clinical utility of biomarkers needs to be evaluated in controlled studies.

A second area of controversy involves acid suppression and chemoprevention. Even controlling reflux symptoms, however, does not equate into achieving successful acid suppression. Some would suggest performing 24-h ambulatory esophageal monitoring to titrate such treatment. Unfortunately, this is not practical. Instead, most practitioners seek symptom control as an end-point of therapy. Evidence is lacking to support the idea that the control of esophageal acid exposure in Barrett's esophagus results in lower rates of adenocarcinoma. The best guide for clinicians, at this point, is to titrate acid suppression therapies for reflux symptom control. Aspirin and cyclooxygenase-2 inhibitor therapy also appears to be a promising area of potential chemoprevention, but further studies are needed.

Endoscopic ablation remains yet another subject of controversy. To date, no prospective randomized trials have demonstrated the long-term benefit of this therapy in nondysplastic Barrett's esophagus patients. Subsquamous areas of Barrett's mucosa can remain after various ablative therapies. Although much of the high-grade dysplasia may resolve as a result of the therapy, do the genetic abnormalities persist? What is the clinical significance if they do? The clinical role of such ablative therapies has yet to be clearly defined, but may be beneficial in a special subset of patient's with high-grade dysplasia or early adenocarcinoma who for other medical reasons would not be candidates for esophagectomy. Endoscopic mucosal resection (EMR) of localized defined areas of high-grade dysplasia can be accomplished but more and longer follow-up studies are needed to determine the durability of the therapy in regards to the remaining Barrett's mucosa.

SOURCES OF INFORMATION FOR PATIENTS AND DOCTORS

http://www.clevelandclinic.org/gastro/barretts/patient/
http://www.patient.co.uk/showdoc/27000642/

REFERENCES

1. Shaheen NJ, Crosby MA, Bozymski EM, Sandler RS. Is there publication bias in the reporting of cancer risk in Barrett's esophagus? Gastroenterology 2000; 119:333–338.
2. Spechler SJ. Barrett's esophagus. N Engl J Med 2002; 346:836–842.
3. Castell DO, Tutuian R. Barrett's esophagus: prevalence and epidemiology. Gastrointest Endosc Clin North Am 2003; 13:227–232.
4. Falk GW. Barrett's esophagus. Gastroenterology 2002; 122:1569–1591.
5. Devesa SS, Blot WJ, Fraumeni JF. Changing patterns in the incidence of esophageal and gastric carcinoma in the United States. Cancer 1998; 83:2049–2053.
6. Reed PI. Changing pattern of oesophageal cancer. Lancet 1991; 338:178.
7. Lagergren J, Bergstrom R, Lindgren A, Nyren O. Symptomatic gastroesophageal reflux as a risk factor for esophageal adenocarcinoma. New Engl J Med 1999; 340:825–831.
8. Fitzgerald RC, Cantab MA, Farthing MJ. The pathogenesis of Barrett's esophagus. Gastrointest Endosc Clin North Am 2003; 13:2233–2255.
9. Reid BJ, Blount PL, Rabinovitch PS. Biomarkers in Barrett's esophagus. Gastrointest Endosc Clin North Am 2003; 13:369–397.
10. Gerson LB, Edson R, Lavori PW, Triadafilopoulos G. Use of a simple symptom questionnaire to predict Barrett's esophagus in patients with symptoms of gastroesophageal

reflux. Am J Gastroenterol 2001; 96: 2005–2011.
11. Winters C, Spurling TJ, Chobanian SJ et al. Barrett's esophagus: a prevalent, occult complication of gastroesophageal reflux disease. Gastroenterology 1987; 92:118–124.
12. Sampliner RE and The Practice Parameters Committee of the American College of Gastroenterology. Updated Guidelines on the Diagnosis, Surveillance, and Therapy of Barrett's Esophagus. Am J Gastroenterol 2002: 97:1888–1895.
13. Connor M, Sharma P. Chromoendoscopy and magnification endoscopy in Barrett's esophagus. Gastrointest Clin North Am 2003; 13:269–277.
14. Weinstein WM, Ippoliti AF. The diagnosis of Barrett's esophagus: Goblets, goblets, goblets. Gastrointest Endosc 1996; 44:91–95.
15. Sharma P, Morales TG, Sampliner RE. Short segment Barrett's esophagus: The need for standardization of the definition and of endoscopic criteria. Am J Gastroenterol 1998; 93:1033–1036.
16. Streitz JM et al. Endoscopic surveillance of Barrett's esophagus. Does it help? J Thorac Cardiovasc Surg 1993; 105:383–388.
17. Peters JH, Clark GWB, Ireland AP et al. Outcome of adenocarcinoma arising in Barrett's esophagus in endoscopically surveyed and nonsurveyed patients. J Gen Thoracic Surg 1994; 108:813–821.
18. Van Sandick JW, vanLanschot JB, Kuiken BW et al. Impact of endoscopic biopsy surveillance of Barrett's oesophagus on pathological stage and clinical outcome of Barrett's carcinoma. Gut 1998; 43:216–222.
19. Streitz JM, Ellis FH, Tilden RL, Erickson RV. Endoscopic surveillance of Barrett's esophagus: a cost-effectiveness comparison with mammographic surveillance for breast cancer. Am J Gastroenterol 1998; 93:911–915.
20. Inadomi JM, Sampliner R, Lagergren J et al. Screening and surveillance for Barrett's esophagus in high-risk groups: A cost utility analysis. Ann Int Med 2003; 138:176–186.
21. Sharma P, Weston AP, Topalovski M, Sampliner RE et al. Magnification chromoendoscopy for the detection of intestinal metaplasia and dysplasia in Barrett's oesophagus. Gut 2003; 52:24–27.
22. Weston AP, Banerjee SK, Sharma P et al. P53 protein overexpression in low grade dysplasia (LGD) in Barrett's esophagus: Immunohistochemical marker predictive of progression. Am J Gastroenterol 2001; 96:1355–1361.
23. Ouatu-Lascar R, Triadafilopoulos G. Complete elimination of reflux symptoms does not guarantee normalization of intraesophageal acid reflux in patient's with Barrett's esophagus. Am J Gastroenterol 1998; 93:711–716.
24. Souza RF, Shewmake K, Terada LS, Spechler SJ. Acid exposure activates the mitogen-activated protein kinase pathways in Barrett's esophagus. Gastroenterology 2002; 122:299–307.
25. Corey KE, Schmitz SM, Shaheen NJ. Does a surgical antireflux procedure decrease the incidence of esophageal adenocarcinoma in Barrett's esophagus: A meta-analysis. Am J Gastroenterol 2003 98:2310–2314.
26. Booger JV, Hillegersberg RV, Siersema PD, de Bruin RWF, Tilanus HW. Endoscopic ablation therapy for Barrett's esophagus with high-grade dysplasia: A review. Am J Gastroenterol 1999; 94:1153–1158.
27. Souza RF, Spechler SJ. Barrett's esophagus: Chemoprevention. Gastrointest Endosc Clin North Am 2003; 13:419–432.

Chapter 32

Esophageal cancer

Elizabeth J Carey and David E Fleischer

KEY POINTS

- The majority of esophageal cancers are squamous cell carcinomas and adenocarcinomas
- Esophageal cancer remains a highly fatal disease; the overall 5-year survival rate is 13%
- The incidence of squamous cell carcinoma varies widely by geographic region and the incidence is steady or decreasing
- Adenocarcinoma is more common in developed countries, where the incidence has doubled over the past 30 years
- The treatment and prognosis of patients with esophageal cancer is strongly related to the stage at presentation
- Stent placement is the preferred endoscopic therapy for advanced disease

INTRODUCTION

Approximately 400 000 new cases of esophageal cancer occur each year, and esophageal cancer is the sixth leading cause of cancer death worldwide.[1] More than 90% of esophageal cancer is squamous cell carcinoma (SCC) or adenocarcinoma (ACA); this chapter focuses on these important epithelial tumors. Despite their histologic differences, the clinical presentation, testing leading to diagnosis, and treatment of esophageal SCC and ACA are similar.

EPIDEMIOLOGY

Squamous cell carcinoma

The incidence of esophageal SCC varies widely by geography, sex, and race. In the United States, the overall incidence is approximately 3–4 per 100 000, with a steady decline over the past 25 years.[2] SCC occurs most commonly in African American men, with an incidence of approximately 12.9 per 100 000, compared with 2.2, 3.6, and 0.9 per 100 000 for caucasian men, African American women, and caucasian women, respectively.[3]

Worldwide, the incidence of SCC shows dramatic variation. In Europe, the incidence of SCC in men ranges from 1.8 per 100 000 in Finland to 13.6 per 100 000 in France, with most countries falling in the range of 2–3 per 100 000. Foci of high-incidence esophageal SCC exist in the 'esophageal cancer belt,' encompassing an area stretching from Iran eastward through Turkmenistan, northern Afghanistan, Uzbekistan, Kazakhstan, and into northern China. The incidence of SCC in these regions reaches as high as 144 per 100 000. Although SCC occurs more commonly in men than in women in areas of low incidence, high-incidence areas do not show a strong sex difference.

Adenocarcinoma

Esophageal ACA is largely a disease of developed nations. The United States, Europe, and Canada have higher rates than developing countries in Asia or Africa. Although the rate of SCC in developed countries has steadily declined over the past three decades, the incidence of ACA of the esophagus has risen dramatically.[4] Since the 1970s the incidence of ACA has doubled in the USA and similar trends have been reported in Australia, western Europe, and New Zealand.[5]

The incidence of ACA in the USA has shown an annual increase of 4–10% since the 1970s, and is the fastest rising malignancy among caucasian men. In 1998, the incidence for caucasian men in the United States was 3.3 per 100 000, up from 0.5 per 100 000 in 1973. Men are 6–8-fold more likely than women to suffer from esophageal ACA, and caucasians are 3–4-fold more likely than African Americans.

CAUSES, RISK FACTORS, DISEASE ASSOCIATIONS

Squamous cell carcinoma

There are a number of well characterized risk factors for SCC of the esophagus. Alcohol, tobacco, dietary factors, underlying esophageal disease, and congenital conditions all confer an increased risk for developing this malignancy.

Tobacco

Tobacco use (in any form) constitutes the largest modifiable risk factor for SCC. Tobacco tars and cigarette smoke contain multiple carcinogens that, over time, cause epithelial hyperproliferation and eventual malignant transformation. The relative risk (RR) increases from 2.0 in people who smoke 15 cigarettes per day to 6.2 for those smoking more cigarettes daily. Alcohol enhances the carcinogenicity of tobacco. Similar to the relationship between tobacco and lung cancer, quitting smoking is associated with a decreased risk of SCC after 10 years of abstinence.

Alcohol

The quantity and type of alcohol consumed are related to SCC, with distilled spirits conferring the greatest risk. Although the relationship between alcohol and SCC is well described, causality is difficult to prove. In the USA, the population attributable risk of alcohol is 45% for those consuming more than 30 drinks per week.[6]

Dietary factors

A number of dietary factors have been implicated in esophageal SCC. This is due to the high incidence of SCC in areas where diets have nutritional deficits, but no single causative deficiency has been identified.

N-nitroso compounds are concentrated in foods in Linxian Province of China, where the incidence of SCC is one of the highest in the world. Nitrosamines, found in pickled vegetables and produced by local fungi, are known to be carcinogenic in animals, and have been implicated in the pathogenesis of esophageal SCC. Betel nut chewing, a common activity in more than 10% of the world's population, is associated with a 5–13-fold relative risk increase for SCC.[7]

Underlying esophageal disease

Longstanding achalasia leads to an increased risk of 33–197 times that of the baseline population, with a prevalence of SCC of approximately 3%.[8] The interval between the onset of symptoms of achalasia and the development of cancer is approximately 15–20 years. SCC is presumably the result of chronic irritation from retained food, which also allows for increased local absorption of toxins.

A history of caustic strictures from lye ingestion is also a risk factor for SCC. Cancer in these patients usually appears 40–50 years after the initial injury. Chronic inflammation, epithelial hyperplasia, and stasis of food may contribute to malignant transformation.

Other factors

Plummer-Vinson syndrome (also known as the Patterson-Kelly syndrome) is a rare syndrome of esophageal webs, iron deficiency anemia, and epithelial lesions, and patients with this disorder have a 3–15% risk of developing esophageal cancer. The pathophysiologic mechanism is not understood.

Human papilloma virus (HPV), especially HPV-16 and HPV-18, is associated with SCC. The DNA HPV virus infects squamous epithelial cells with subsequent replication and production of oncogenic proteins that contribute to malignant transformation. A similar process exists to a lesser degree with Epstein-Barr virus.

Patients with head and neck squamous cell carcinoma have an increased risk of esophageal SCC. Incidental esophageal cancer is found at presentation in 1–2% of patients with head and neck cancer, and develops at an annual rate of 3–7%. Screening endoscopy is recommended for these patients.

Tylosis, an autosomal dominant disorder resulting in hyperkeratosis of the palms and the soles, is associated with SCC of the esophagus and oropharyngeal leukoplakia. Some 50% of patients with tylosis develop SCC of the esophagus by the age of 45 years, and up to 95% by age 55. Screening endoscopy is recommended both for patients and for their families.

Drinking exceptionally hot liquids (>70° C) is a common habit in certain populations of Iran and Turkey, where SCC rates are high; thermal injury has been suggested as a contributing factor in these regions. Ionizing radiation, celiac sprue, esophageal diverticula, and a history of partial gastrectomy have also been linked to SCC.

Protective factors

Green and yellow vegetables, β-carotene, folic acid, riboflavin, and vitamins A, C, E, and B_{12} have all been associated with a decreased rate of esophageal cancer. In the General Population Trial in Linxian, China, people who received supplemental selenium, β-carotene, and vitamin E were found to have a 9% reduction in the overall mortality and esophageal cancer rates.[9] High serum levels of α-tocopherol and selenium were also associated with a decreased risk in this population.

CAUSES AND RISK FACTORS

RISK FACTORS FOR SCC
- Geographic location
- Tobacco and alcohol
- Untreated achalasia
- History of caustic injury
- Dietary factors

RISK FACTORS FOR ACA
- Barrett's esophagus (associated with a 0.5% annual rate of ACA)
- Gastroesophageal reflux and obesity
- Medications that relax the lower esophageal sphincter
- *Helicobacter pylori* colonization may decrease risk

Adenocarcinoma

Unlike SCC, tobacco and alcohol use are associated with minimal, if any, increased incidence of ACA. In contrast, gastroesophageal reflux and obesity are the best characterized risk factors.

Gastroesophageal reflux and Barrett's esophagus

The majority of esophageal ACA arises in the setting of Barrett's esophagus, a complication in 5–8% of patients with longstanding gastroesophageal reflux.[10] Barrett's esophagus is a transformation of the epithelial lining from the normal squamous epithelium to columnar epithelium of the specialized intestinal type. The natural history of Barrett's esophagus is not fully understood, but the incidence of ACA in this group is clearly increased. The annual incidence of ACA in patients with Barrett's esophagus is 0.5–0.8%, a 30–60-fold increase over that in the general population. The risk of ACA in short-segment Barrett's (<3 cm) is no different to that in long-segment Barrett's (>3 cm). Although most Barrett's esophagus is thought to occur sporadically, familial clustering has been noted in up to 20% of cases.

Gastroesophageal reflux is the strongest risk factor for ACA, and some authors postulate that the strength of the relationship implies causality.[11] Although over half of patients with ACA of the esophagus do not have a history of symptomatic gastroesophageal reflux, studies have found a strong association between symptoms of reflux and ACA. Antireflux surgery does not reduce the risk of ACA.[12]

Medications that relax the lower esophageal sphincter have been linked with an increased risk of ACA.[13] Daily, long-term (>5 years) use of nitroglycerines, aminophylline, beta-blockers, anticholinergics, and benzodiazepines is associated with an adjusted incidence risk ratio of 3.8 for ACA, but not for SCC. The relationship disappears after adjusting for symptoms of reflux, suggesting a causative role of gastroesophageal reflux.

Obesity

Obesity is the second greatest risk factor for esophageal ACA.[14] Obese persons (those with a body mass index (BMI) of greater than 30 kg/m^2) have an odds ratio of 16.2 compared with that in lean persons.

Protective factors

At least one population-based study has indicated a lower prevalence of ACA in wine drinkers. Colonization with *Helicobacter pylori*, particularly strains with cag pathogenicity, is associated with a decreased risk of gastroesophageal reflux and may be protective against ACA. Use of aspirin or other nonsteroidal anti-inflammatory agents (NSAIDs) may also reduce the risk of ACA. A meta-analysis of observational studies found an inverse relationship between the use of aspirin or NSAIDs and the risk of ACA or SCC.

PATHOGENESIS

Squamous cell carcinoma

The progression of a normal cell to a cancerous one is the result of a series of mutations that culminates in unregulated growth and reproduction. Activation of oncogenes, inactivation of tumor suppressor genes, and dysregulation of cell cycle growth factors are some of the key changes in the process.[15] Overexpression of the oncogene *Cyclin D1* is thought to be an early event in the pathogenesis of squamous cell carcinoma. It is overexpressed in up to half of esophageal SCCs and is associated with a poor prognosis. Overexpression of epidermal growth factor (EGF) receptor correlates with the degree of dysplasia in SCC. The *p53* tumor suppressor gene is mutated in up to 70% of esophageal SCCs. Normal functions of the *p53* protein product include cell cycle regulation, induction of apoptosis, transcriptional regulation, and DNA replication.

Adenocarcinoma

Esophageal ACA usually, if not always, develops within a focus of Barrett's intestinal metaplasia. Similar to the adenoma–carcinoma sequence in colorectal cancer, esophageal ACA follows a predictable sequence of metaplasia–dysplasia–adenocarcinoma. Aneuploidy is one of the earliest genetic changes seen in Barrett's esophagus. Oncogene activation occurs, with overexpression of *Cyclin D1*. Growth factor alterations can also lead to increased expression of *Cyclin D1*, promoting cell proliferation.[16] EGF and transforming growth factor-α (TGF-α) have been implicated in the development of esophageal carcinoma. Alterations in tumor suppressor genes further increase the risk of progression to cancer. Overexpression of cyclooxygenase-2 (COX-2) may enhance the ability of cancerous cells to resist apoptosis.

PATHOLOGY

ACA and SCC comprise more than 90% of esophageal cancers. ACA usually develops in the distal esophagus, whereas SCC may arise at any location in the esophagus (Figs 32.1 and 32.2). Invasion of the submucosa occurs early in SCC, with proximal extension of tumor along the mucosal surface. Invasion of the lymphatic system is another early event in SCC due to the superficial location of lymph nodes in the mid-esophagus. After involvement of the regional nodes, spread to the celiac and periaortic lymph nodes occurs. Local invasion may result in esophagorespiratory fistulas or erosion into the aorta. Distant metastases occur in 30% of patients, most commonly to the liver, bone, and lung. Because of the more distal location of most ACAs, involvement of the celiac and perihepatic nodes is more common than in SCC.

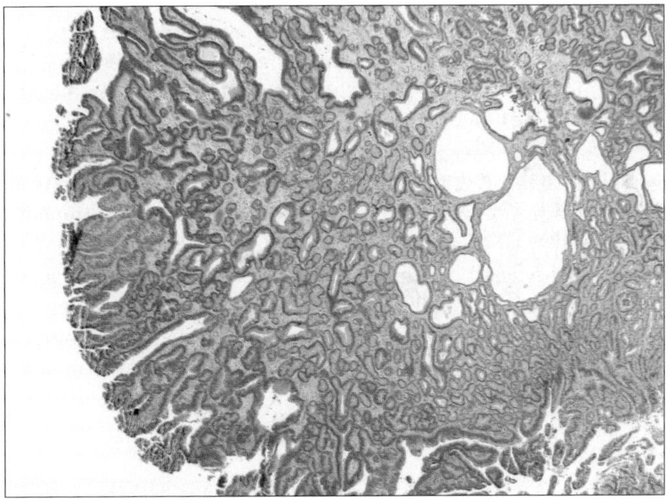

Fig. 32.1 Adenocarcinoma. Low-power (×40) view of invasive adenocarcinoma showing neoplastic glands throughout the field extending deep in the wall of the esophagus.

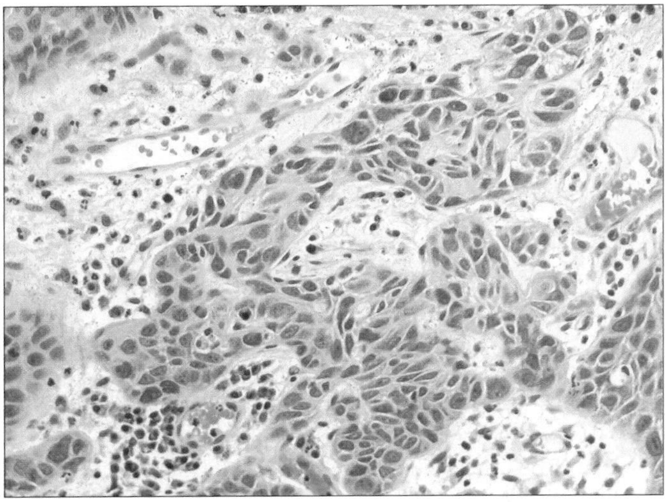

Fig. 32.2 Squamous cell carcinoma. High-power view (×400) of invasive squamous cell carcinoma with infiltrating sheets of neoplastic cells.

CLINICAL PRESENTATION

Most patients with esophageal cancer do not develop symptoms until the tumor is large enough to cause mechanical obstruction, usually when the esophageal lumen is narrowed to approximately 13 mm. At presentation, the most common symptoms are dysphagia, odynophagia, and weight loss or anorexia. Other common symptoms include heartburn, gastroesophageal reflux, nausea, and vomiting. Chest pain may indicate invasion into the mediastinum. Cough and recurrent pneumonia may indicate an esophagorespiratory fistula, compression of the trachea, or aspiration. Hoarseness may occur if there is involvement of the recurrent laryngeal nerve. Bone pain may herald the onset of bony metastases. Esophageal cancer may rarely present with gastrointestinal bleeding in the form of melena or heme-positive stools.

Esophageal cancer tends to present at an advanced stage. The esophagus has a rich lymphovascular supply and lacks a serosal lining. This frequently permits invasion of cancer into the surrounding tissue before luminal compromise occurs and also permits early invasion of regional lymph nodes. Many esophageal cancers may be more advanced than staging suggests; when rib biopsy is performed at the time of surgery, up to 90% of patients undergoing esophagectomy for curative intent have micrometastases to the bone marrow.

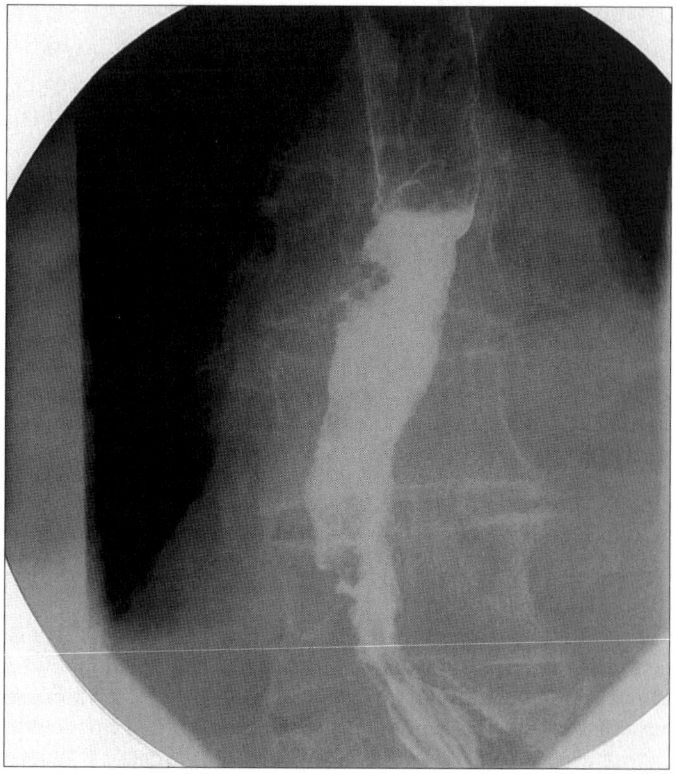

Fig. 32.3 Barium esophagogram of a patient with adenocarcinoma. There is a markedly irregular area of ulceration and mucosal irregularity in the distal esophagus extending for a distance of approximately 6 cm, almost to the gastroesophageal junction.

CLINICAL PRESENTATION

- Dysphagia is the most common presenting symptom
- Over 50% of patients present at an incurable stage
- Endoscopic surveillance programs in high-risk individuals may identify cancers at an early stage
- ACA usually occurs in the distal esophagus; SCC may occur throughout the esophagus
- Weight loss at the time of presentation is an indicator of poor prognosis

DIFFERENTIAL DIAGNOSIS

The differential diagnosis for a patient presenting with dysphagia and an esophageal mass is small: it is usually SCC or ACA. Rare causes of esophageal cancer include verrucous carcinoma, spindle cell carcinoma, small cell carcinoma, leiomyosarcoma, Kaposi's sarcoma, lymphoma, and malignant melanoma. Cancers that may metastasize to the esophagus include melanoma, breast, lung, germ cell tumor, and renal cell carcinomas. Benign lesions in the esophagus include squamous papilloma, leiomyomas, fibrovascular polyps, lymphangiomas, and lipomas, although these lesions rarely cause dysphagia. Pseudoachalasia can occur when there is submucosal cancer infiltration at the gastroesophageal junction; this should be considered in patients with normal imaging.

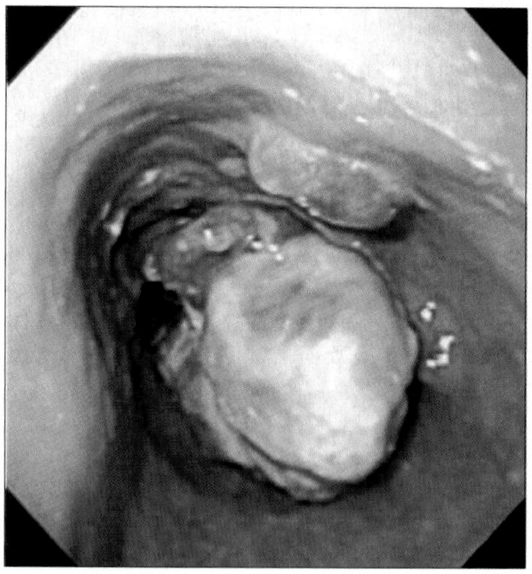

Fig. 32.4 Endoscopic image of invasive adenocarcinoma in the distal esophagus. A friable exophytic mass partially obstructs the lumen.

DIAGNOSTIC METHODS

Upon presentation, a thorough history of gastroesophageal reflux symptoms (including duration and severity), tobacco and alcohol use, and residence in an endemic area is of importance. On physical examination, lymphadenopathy, cachexia, presence of fecal occult blood, or hepatomegaly should be noted. Laboratory studies may reveal iron deficiency anemia or signs of malnutrition such as hypoalbuminemia or prolonged prothrombin time.

Although patients presenting with dysphagia may undergo barium esophagography (Fig. 32.3), it is now more common to perform endoscopy, with tissue biopsy and, if appropriate, treatment (Fig. 32.4).[17] Early cancers may appear as a superficial plaque or ulcer. Advanced cancerous lesions appear as polypoid, friable, often ulcerated, eccentric, or circumferential masses. Biopsies are essential and the diagnostic accuracy increases with the number of biopsies taken. On rare occasion, tumor infiltration may involve only the submucosa, resulting in a normal-appearing esophagus on endoscopy. In such cases, superficial endoscopic biopsies may be nondiagnostic.

Chromoendoscopy, the endoscopic evaluation of mucosa after application of a dye, can be used to highlight neoplastic tissue that is not visible to the naked eye.[18] Lugol's iodine solution and toluidine blue are typically used for the early detection of SCC, whereas methylene blue is preferred for Barrett's esophagus and ACA. Iodine stains are picked up by normal glycogen-containing squamous epithelial cells but are not absorbed by glycogen-depleted malignant cells (Fig. 32.5).

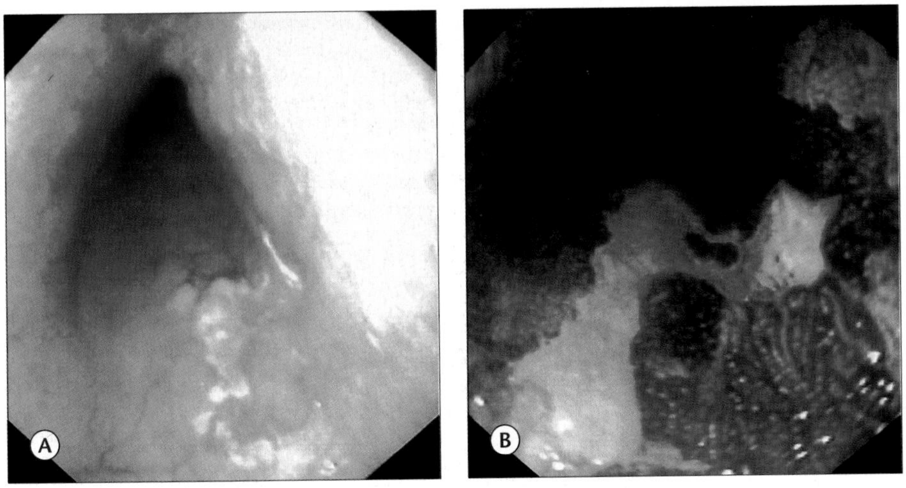

Fig. 32.5 Chromoendoscopy images. **A.** White plaque represents biopsy-proven squamous cell carcinoma. **B.** After staining with Lugol's iodine, the lesion is more precisely defined.

Computed tomography (CT) of the chest and abdomen with intravenous contrast is recommended to detect metastatic disease (Fig. 32.6), as well as endoscopic ultrasonography (EUS) for local invasion and regional lymph nodes.[19] EUS is recommended as the most accurate method of assessing disease stage if no distant metastasis are present (Fig. 32.7).[20] Fine-needle aspiration of regional lymph nodes can be performed, which increases the accuracy to over 90%. EUS is also useful after neoadjuvant therapy to assess response and resectability.[21] Positron emission tomography (PET) with [^{18}F]fluorodeoxyglucose is emerging as a more sensitive method than CT to detect metastatic disease (Fig. 32.8).[22]

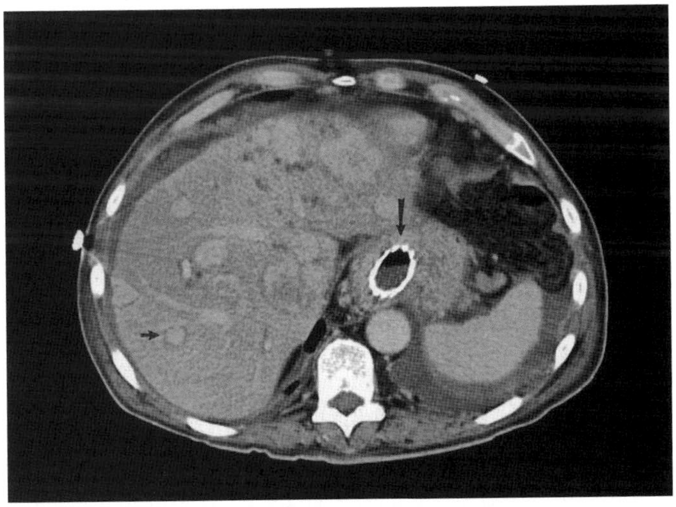

Fig. 32.6 Computed tomogram showing metastatic adenocarcinoma of the distal esophagus. A metal stent is located in the distal esophagus and there is diffuse and irregular mucosal thickening of this area (long arrow). Multiple metastatic lesions are seen in the liver (short arrow).

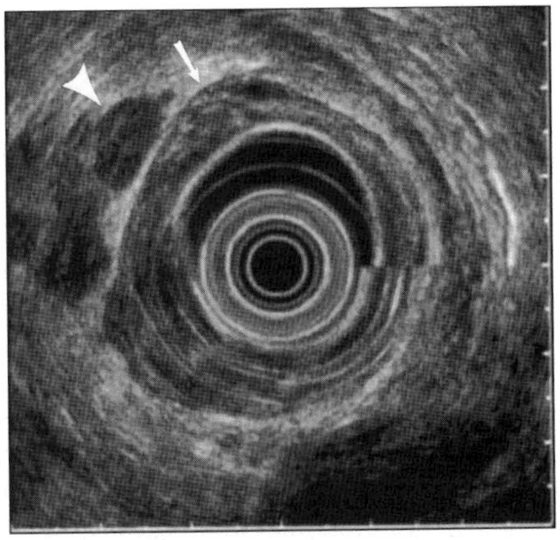

Fig. 32.7 T3 squamous cell carcinoma. Endoscopic ultrasonography image of a T3 squamous cell carcinoma (arrow) with an enlarged lymph node (arrowhead).

Staging of esophageal cancer is performed using the 2002 American Joint Committee on Cancer tumor node metastasis (TNM) system (Table 32.1). The 5-year survival rate ranges from 95% for stage 0 disease to 4% for stage IV disease (Table 32.2).[23]

CLINICAL TIPS

- Ask patients what they can and can't eat. Patients will often unconsciously modify their diet and deny dysphagia
- Endoscopic biopsy usually leads to the diagnosis. In some cases, malignant cells may be submucosal, and repeated deep biopsies or EUS/fine-needle aspiration cytology may be necessary
- Respiratory problems with esophageal cancer may be related to esophagorespiratory fistulae, aspiration, or tracheal invasion
- Staging is the key to management of esophageal cancer. It is the key to treatment and the key to prognosis
- Differences in management of SCC and ACA are a result of different locations. With distal tumors (usually ACA), stent placement violates the gastroesophageal junction and may exacerbate gastroesophageal reflux. High cervical tumors (usually SCC) pose a technical challenge for stenting
- Esophageal cancer usually recurs after initial therapy
- Palliative measures (stenting, percutaneous endoscopic gastrostomy, analgesia, hospice care) are extremely important in minimizing suffering in the late stages of the disease

TREATMENT AND PREVENTION

Treatment

The treatment of esophageal cancer is dependent on the stage of disease (Table 32.3). Unfortunately, esophageal cancer is rarely detected in the early stages and over half of patients have irresectable disease at the time of diagnosis. The overall 5-year survival rate is 13% (see Table 32.2).

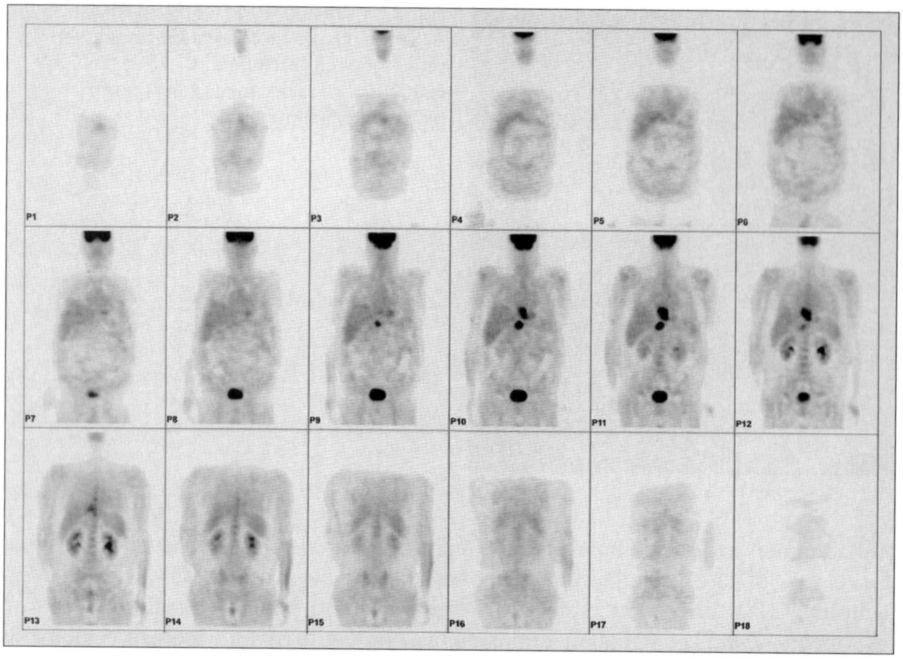

Fig. 32.8 Metastatic adenocarcinoma of the esophagus. Positron emission tomogram from a patient with metastatic adenocarcinoma of the esophagus. Abnormal [^{18}F]fluorodeoxyglucose accumulation is seen at the site of the distal esophageal carcinoma. There is also intense abnormal accumulation at an enlarged supraceliac lymph node, the smaller adjacent gastrohepatic ligament, and distal paraesophageal lymph nodes.

Stage 0–I disease

The goal of therapy for stage 0–1 disease (Barrett's esophagus with high-grade dysplasia (carcinoma in situ) and stage I esophageal cancer) is surgical resection with intent to cure.[24] In Barrett's esophagus, high-grade dysplasia and carcinoma in situ are synonymous. The convention is to use high-grade dysplasia as the preferred term. High-grade dysplasia (carcinoma in situ) is rarely detected outside of surveillance programs, but outcomes are excellent when cancer is detected at an early stage. Conventional teaching is that esophageal cancer requires a complete esophagectomy. The perioperative mortality rate for esophagectomy is approximately 4%; common complications include anastomotic leaks, anastomotic strictures, respiratory or cardiovascular problems, and recurrent laryngeal nerve injury.

Concern about the morbidity and mortality of esophagectomy has led to the investigation of endoscopic mucosal resection (EMR) for the excision of lesions limited to the mucosa (Fig. 32.9).[25] Lesions confined to the lamina propria have a minimal risk of lymph node or distant metastasis, so an effective means of local resection could obviate the risks of surgery for patients with mucosal disease. Small trials using EMR to resect early esophageal cancer or foci of high-grade dysplasia have demonstrated 5-year survival rates of up to 95%. Therefore, EMR is an option for patients with limited disease and particularly those who are not surgical candidates.

Stage II–III disease

Surgical resection with intent to cure or long-term remission is recommended for operative candidates with stage II and T3 stage III lesions. Although survival decreases with increasing tumor stage, some patients with stage II–III disease have good long-term outcomes.

Radiation alone

Radiation alone has provided up to 20% 5-year survival rates in some patients with localized esophageal cancer. The superior results of combined therapy, however, have minimized the role of radiotherapy alone, except for patients who are unwilling or unable to receive chemotherapy.

Chemoradiation without surgery

Unlike surgery, chemoradiation has the advantage of treating both local disease and distant micrometastases. Chemoradiation alone may result in similar outcomes without subjecting patients to the morbidity and mortality of esophagectomy. Chemoradiation is superior to radiation alone and is the standard of care for patients who are not surgical candidates.[26] A combination of cisplatin and 5-fluorouracil (5-FU) is the mainstay for treatment of esophageal cancer, although paclitaxel, carboplatin, and irinotecan may also be used.

Neoadjuvant chemoradiation

The frequent occurrence of distant metastases after surgical resection has prompted the investigation of multimodality therapy for localized esophageal cancer. Neoadjuvant chemoradiation compared to surgery alone has been the subject of a number of trials showing a trend towards better survival with neoadjuvant chemoradiation that did not reach statistical significance.[27] Preoperative chemoradiation was associated with a higher likelihood of achieving complete resection at the time of surgery. National guidelines currently support either surgery alone or surgery with neoadjuvant chemoradiation for patients with operable T1–T3 tumors.

Stage III–IV disease

The goal of T4 stage III and stage IV disease is nonsurgical palliation. Patients may benefit from radiation, chemotherapy, or endoscopic therapy. Surgical resection for palliation is not usually considered because of the morbidity of the operation, but may be an appropriate option in selected patients.

Radiation

Radiation is well tolerated and very effective for maintenance of local disease control and for palliation of dysphagia. Radiation improves dysphagia in 71% of patients and provides adequate

TABLE 32.1 CANCER STAGING FOR ESOPHAGEAL CANCER

PRIMARY TUMOR (T)			
TX	Primary tumor cannot be assessed		
T0	No evidence of primary tumor		
Tis	Carcinoma in situ		
T1	Tumor invades lamina propria or submucosa		
T1a	Tumor invades mucosa or lamina propria		
T1b	Tumor invades submucosa		
T2	Tumor invades muscularis propria		
T3	Tumor invades adventitia		
T4	Tumor invades adjacent structures		
REGIONAL LYMPH NODES (N)			
NX	Regional lymph nodes cannot be assessed		
N0	No regional lymph node metastasis		
N1	Regional lymph node metastasis		
N1a	1 to 3 nodes involved		
N1b	4 to 7 nodes involved		
N1c	>7 nodes involved		
DISTANT METASTASIS			
MX	Distant metastasis cannot be assessed		
M0	No distant metastasis		
M1	Distant metastasis		
Tumors of the lower thoracic esophagus			
M1a	Metastasis in celiac lymph nodes		
M1b	Other distant metastasis		
Tumors of the mid-thoracic esophagus			
M1a	Not applicable		
M1b	Nonregional lymph nodes and/or other distant metastasis		
Tumors of the upper thoracic esophagus			
M1a	Metastasis in cervical nodes		
M1b	Other distant metastasis		
STAGE GROUPING			
Stage 0	Tis	N0	M0
Stage I	T1	N0	M0
Stage IIA	T2	N0	M0
	T3	N0	M0
Stage IIB	T1	N1	M0
	T2	N1	M0
Stage III	T3	N1	M0
	T4	Any N	M0
Stage IV	Any T	Any N	M1
Stage IVA	Any T	Any N	M1a
Stage IVB	Any T	Any N	M1b

Used with the permission of the American Joint Committee on Cancer (AJCC), Chicago, Illinois. The original source for this material is the AJCC Cancer Staging Manual, Sixth Edition (2002) published by Springer-Verlag New York, www.springeronline.com[29]

TABLE 32.2 FIVE-YEAR SURVIVAL BY STAGE AT DIAGNOSIS

Stage	5-year survival (%)
0	>95
I	60
II	31
III	20
IV	4

TABLE 32.3 OPTIONS FOR TREATING ESOPHAGEAL CANCER

AJCC stage group	Primary treatment
Stage 0–I	Surgery Endoscopic mucosal resection Photodynamic therapy
Stage II	Surgery Chemoradiation ± surgery
Stage III	Surgery Chemoradiation ± surgery Palliation
Stage IV	Endoscopic therapy Palliation Chemoradiation

AJCC, American Joint Commission on Cancer.
Adapted from the National Comprehensive Cancer Network Clinical Practice Guidelines.[24]

control of symptoms until death in 54%. Unfortunately, radiation rarely results in sustained remission and the 5-year survival rate ranges from 0% to 10%.

Brachytherapy

Brachytherapy delivers a constant dose of localized radiation via an intraluminally implanted radioactive source. Early studies have suggested that brachytherapy is effective for relief of dysphagia but is associated with a 10% complication rate. The role of brachytherapy in the management of esophageal cancer remains to be defined, but current recommendations discourage use of concurrent brachytherapy and chemotherapy.

Chemotherapy

In general, multiagent chemotherapy is associated with a better response rate, although a survival benefit has not been demonstrated. The most common agents used are cisplatin, 5-FU, paclitaxel, and irinotecan. Regimens are chosen based on side-effect profile, provider preference, and patient performance status.

Endoscopic therapy

A number of endoscopically performed therapies are effective for palliation of symptoms. These include dilatation, neodynium: yttrium–aluminum–garnet (Nd:YAG) laser therapy, injection therapy, photodynamic therapy (PDT), electrocautery, and stent placement. The choice of modality is tailored to specific patient clinical characteristics. Endoscopic dilatation can temporarily relieve dysphagia, but symptom recurrence is universal unless repeated procedures are performed. Tumor ablation with Nd:YAG laser is associated with a high success rate; over 75% of patients with inoperable cancer have functional swallowing after laser therapy. Disadvantages of laser therapy include the expense, the need for prolonged endoscopic procedures, and a perforation rate of nearly 5%. Intratumoral injection of a chemotherapy-containing gel appears promising in pilot studies.

PDT uses the combination of a photosensitizing agent with a low-power laser. After intravenous administration, the agent accumulates in malignant tissue. Endoscopic laser treatment is applied to the affected area, producing ischemic damage to the

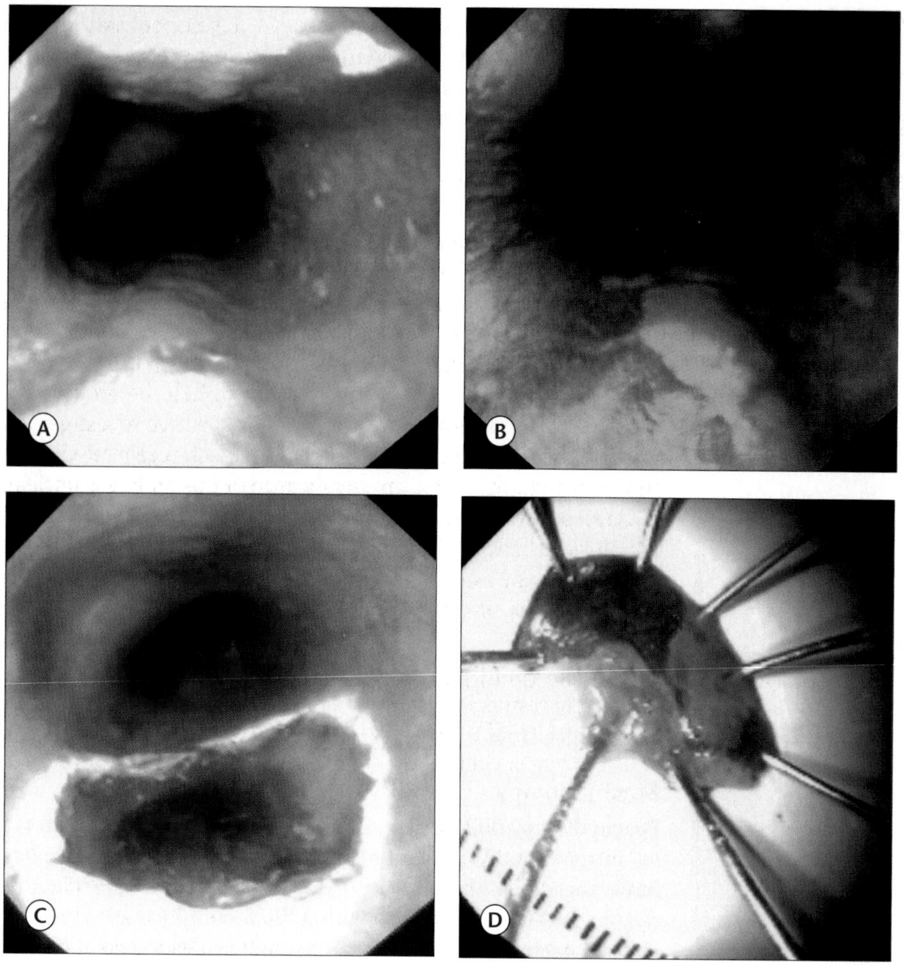

Fig. 32.9 Stage I esophageal cancer treated by endoscopic mucosal resection.
A. Endoscopic view. **B.** After iodine staining. **C.** Resection site after EMR. **D.** Pathologic specimen.

tissue. In comparative trials, PDT was found to be of comparable or superior efficacy to laser therapy.

Endoscopic stenting has become the standard of care for palliation of malignant dysphagia and for management of esophagorespiratory fistulae. Self-expanding metal stents (SEMSs) are effective, easy to insert, associated with few complications, and well tolerated by patients.[28] A SEMS is typically placed with the patient under conscious sedation using either endoscopic guidance, fluoroscopic guidance, or both. Stent characteristics should be individualized to the location and length of the tumor (Fig. 32.10). Some stents include features that are helpful in specific situations, such as proximal or distal release systems when precise deployment is essential, or a distal valve to prevent reflux when the stent crosses the gastroesophageal junction. After deployment, the SEMS slowly expands, with the final diameter dependent upon the radial force of the stent and characteristics of the tumor (Fig. 32.11). SEMSs with coated walls are recommended owing to the reduction of tumor ingrowth. Late complications are not uncommon, occurring in 20–40% of patients. Complications include stent migration, tumor ingrowth, tissue hyperplasia, chest pain, hemorrhage, and fistulization.

Supportive care

Percutaneous endoscopic gastrostomy (PEG) and hospice care play important roles in the management of patients with end-stage esophageal cancer. Not all patients will be interested in PEG feeding, but the option should be presented to patients with severe anorexia or dysphagia resistant to therapy. Hospice care is an invaluable aid to comfort patients and their families at the end of life.

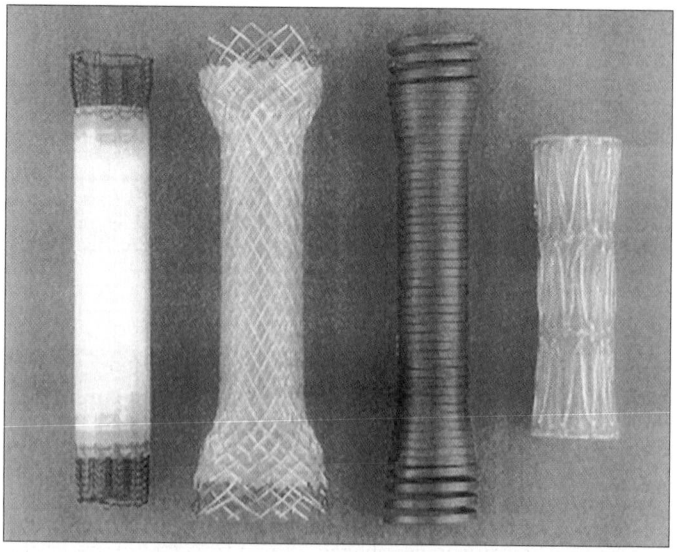

Fig. 32.10 Esophageal stents. Four types of esophageal stents. From left to right, Ultraflex (Microvasive, Boston Scientific, Natick, Massachusetts, USA), Wallstent (Microvasive, Boston Scientific), EsophaCoil (Instent, Minneapolis, Minnosota, USA), Z-stent (Wilson Cook, Winston Salem, North Carolina, USA).

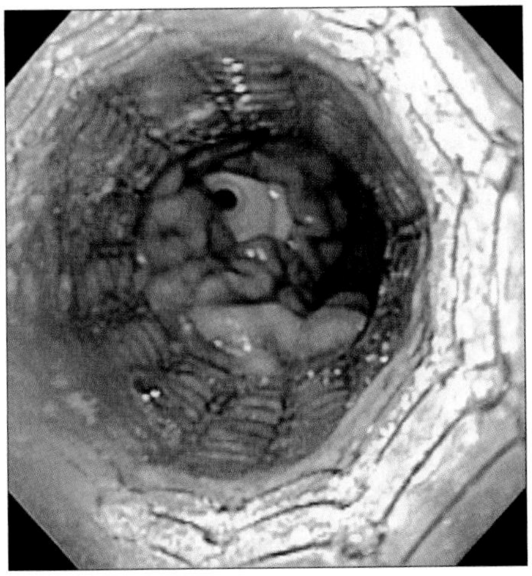

Fig. 32.11 Esophageal stent. Endoscopic image of a deployed (Ultraflex) stent in a patient with adenocarcinoma of the distal esophagus. The gastrostomy site is seen on the greater curvature of the stomach.

TREATMENT AND PREVENTION

- Surgical resection is recommended for patients with localized disease
- Endoscopic therapy may have a role in patients with disease limited to mucosa
- Advanced disease is treated with chemotherapy and radiation; long-term cure is rare
- Chemotherapy and radiation may provide effective palliation
- Multiple methods for endoscopic palliation exist
- Smoking cessation reduces the risk of SCC
- Diets high in fruits and vegetables may reduce risk
- Endoscopic screening of high-risk individuals may detect cancer at an early stage
- Endoscopic surveillance in patients with Barrett's esophagus may improve outcomes

COMPLICATIONS AND THEIR MANAGEMENT

- Esophagorespiratory fistulae occur in 5–10% of patients
- Fistulae may be a direct result of tumor invasion or a complication of therapy
- Approximately 50% of esophagorespiratory fistulae are related to chemoradiation; these may heal spontaneously when therapy is concluded
- Covered metal stents are effective for the palliation of esophagorespiratory fistulae

Prevention

Lifestyle modifications, primarily the minimization of tobacco and alcohol use, are the first line of prevention against SCC. Dietary changes may modify the risk for SCC in high-incidence areas. Diets rich in fresh fruits and vegetables may help to prevent SCC.

The late stage at which most patients present and the poor prognosis of advanced esophageal cancer underscore the importance of screening for this disease. In developed nations, the incidence of SCC is low enough that routine screening is not cost-effective, except in the highest risk groups, such as those with head and neck cancer, achalasia, or tylosis. In high-incidence regions, an effective screening method could have a dramatic impact on public health.

The primary risk factor for ACA is longstanding gastroesophageal reflux and Barrett's esophagus, so routine endoscopic screening is recommended for these patients. Medical therapy with proton pump inhibitors heals esophagitis but rarely reverses Barrett's esophagus. The frequency of screening depends on the presence of Barrett's esophagus and/or dysplasia.

The use of endoscopic ablative therapy to halt the progression of Barrett's esophagus to ACA is an area of active investigation. Foci of Barrett's metaplasia may persist beneath regenerated squamous mucosa; the long-term significance of this finding is unclear.

Chemoprevention may also play a role in the prevention of esophageal cancer. Observational and animal studies suggest that the use of aspirin and other NSAIDs is associated with a decreased risk of esophageal cancer.

WHAT TO TELL PATIENTS

The National Cancer Institute (NCI) maintains a website that is an excellent resource for patients and physicians (http://www.cancer.gov/cancerinfo/types/esophageal/). This site contains comprehensive and easily understandable information on everything from symptoms and risk factors to clinical trials. Sections are tailored to health professionals or patients to best serve the needs of each group, and a Spanish language version is available. Links to resources for social support, coping, and complmentary medicine are provided. The American Cancer Society website has general information about cancer and cancer therapies (http://www.cancer.org).

CURRENT CONTROVERSIES AND THEIR FUTURE RESOLUTION

Despite recent advances, esophageal cancer remains a highly fatal disease. Because prognosis is so closely related to stage at the time of diagnosis, an emphasis on early detection of esophageal cancer is required. High-risk populations need to be identified and reliable, cost-effective methods of screening and early detection are essential. An early marker of esophageal cancer could be useful for low-risk groups. More trials are needed to determine the optimal treatment approach for patients with stage II–III disease and to minimize the treatment-related side effects. Targeted therapy, such as with an epidermal growth factor receptor antagonist, may add to current chemotherapeutic regimens. Finally, prevention trials should be pursued as dietary changes and NSAIDs have shown promise in some populations.

SOURCES OF INFORMATION FOR PATIENTS AND DOCTORS

http://www.patient.co.uk/showdoc/929/
http://www.cancerhelp.org.uk/help/default.asp?page=4478

REFERENCES

1. Pisani P, Parkin DM, Bray F et al. Estimates of the worldwide mortality from 25 cancers in 1990. Int J Cancer 1999; 83:18–29.
2. Vizcaino AP, Moreno V, Lambert R et al. Time trends incidence of both major histologic types of esophageal carcinomas in selected countries, 1973–1995. Int J Cancer 2002; 99:860–868.
3. National Cancer Institute, DCCPS, Surveillance Research Program, Cancer Statistics Branch. SEER Program Public Use Data, 1973–1999 November 2001 Submission; issued April 2002.
4. El-Serag HB. The epidemic of esophageal adenocarcinoma. Hematol Oncol Clin North Am 2003; 17:421–440.
5. Bollschweiler E, Wolfgarten E, Gutschow C et al. Demographic variations in the rising incidence of esophageal adenocarcinoma in white males. Cancer 2001; 92:549–555.
6. Engel LS, Chow WH, Vaughan TL et al. Population attributable risks of esophageal and gastric cancers. J Natl Cancer Inst 2003; 95:1404–1413.
7. Phukan RK, Ali MS, Chetia CK et al. Betel nut and tobacco chewing; potential risk factors of cancer of oesophagus in Assam, India. Br J Cancer 2001; 85:661–667.
8. Dunaway PM, Wong RKH. Risk and surveillance intervals for squamous cell carcinoma in achalasia. Gastrointest Endosc Clin N Am 2001; 11:425–433.
9. Mark SD, Qiao YL, Dawsey SM et al. Prospective study of serum selenium levels and incident esophageal and gastric cancers. J Natl Cancer Inst 2000; 92:1753–1763.
10. Shaheen N, Ransohoff DF. Gastroesophageal reflux, Barrett esophagus, and esophageal cancer. JAMA 2002; 287:1972–1981.
11. Lagergren J, Bergstrom R, Lindgren A et al. Symptomatic gastroesophageal reflux as a risk factor for esophageal adenocarcinoma. N Engl J Med 1999; 340:825–831.
12. Ye W, Chow HW, Lagergren J et al. Risk of adenocarcinomas of the esophagus and gastric cardia in patients with gastroesophageal reflux diseases and after antireflux surgery. Gastroenterology 2001; 121:1286.
13. Lagergren J, Bergstrom R, Adami HO et al. Association between medications that relax the lower esophageal sphincter and risk for esophageal adenocarcinoma. Ann Intern Med 2000; 133:165–175.
14. Lagergren J, Bergstrom R, Nyren O. Association between body mass and adenocarcinoma of the esophagus and gastric cardia. Ann Intern Med 1999; 130:883.
15. Okano J, Snyder L, Rustgi AK. Genetic alterations in esophageal cancer. Methods Mol Biol 2003; 222:131–145.
16. Souza RF. Molecular and biologic basis of upper gastrointestinal malignancy – esophageal carcinoma. Surg Oncol Clin N Am 2002; 11:257–272.
17. Jacobson BC, Hirota W, Baron TH et al. The role of endoscopy in the assessment and treatment of esophageal cancer. Gastrointest Endosc 2003; 57:817–822.
18. Dawsey SM, Wang GQ, Weinstein WM et al. Squamous dysplasia and early esophageal cancer in Linxian region of China: distinctive endoscopic lesions. Gastroenterology 1993; 105:1333–1340.
19. Romagnuolo J, Scott J, Hawes RH et al. Helical CT versus EUS with fine needle aspiration for celiac nodal assessment in patients with esophageal cancer. Gastrointest Endosc 2002; 55:648–654.
20. Vazquez-Sequeiros E, Wiersema MJ, Clain JE et al. Impact of lymph node staging on therapy of esophageal carcinoma. Gastroenterology 2003; 125:1626–1635.
21. Willis J, Cooper GS, Isenberg G et al. Correlation of EUS measurement with pathologic assessment of neoadjuvant therapy response in esophageal carcinoma. Gastrointest Endosc 2002; 55:655–661.
22. Flamen P, Lerut A, Van Cutsem E et al. Utility of positron emission tomography for the staging of patients with potentially operable esophageal carcinoma. J Clin Oncol 2000; 18:3202–3210.
23. Younes M, Henson DE, Ertan A et al. Incidence and survival trends of esophageal carcinoma in the United States: racial and gender differences by histologic type. Scand J Gastroenterol 2002; 37:1359–1365.
24. Ajani J, D'Amico TA, Hayman JA et al. Esophageal cancer. Clinical Practice Guidelines in Oncology, Version 1, 2003, National Comprehensive Cancer Network. Online. Available: http://www.nccn.org/physician_gls/f_guidelines.html [29 September 2004].
25. Narahara H, Hiroyasu I, Tatsuta M et al. Effectiveness of endoscopic mucosal resection with submucosal saline injection technique for superficial squamous carcinomas of the esophagus. Gastrointest Endosc 2000; 52:730–734.
26. al-Sarraf M, Martz K, Herskovic A et al. Progress report of combined chemoradiotherapy versus radiotherapy alone in patients with esophageal cancer: an intergroup study. J Clin Oncol 1997; 15:277–284.
27. Urschel JD, Vasan H. A meta-analysis of randomized controlled trials that compared neoadjuvant chemoradiation and surgery to surgery alone for resectable esophageal cancer. Am J Surg 2003; 185:538–543.
28. Siersema PD, Schrauwen LS, van Blankenstein M et al. Self-expanding metal stents for complicated and recurrent esophagogastric cancer. Gastrointest Endosc 2001; 54:579–586.
29. Greene FL, Page DL, Fleming ID, et al. AJCC Cancer Staging Manual, Sixth Edition. New York: Springer-Verlag, 2002.

Chapter 33

Infections of the esophagus and stomach

David J Kearney and George B McDonald

KEY POINTS

- Esophageal and stomach infections usually occur in the context of immune impairment or gastric acid suppression
- Fungal causes include *Candida, Aspergillus* and *Histoplasma*
- Viral causes include herpes simplex virus, varicella zoster virus, Epstein-Barr virus, HIV, and human papilloma virus
- Diagnosis of Candida esophagitis should include esophageal brushings
- Fluconazole can be given empirically to patients with HIV, oral thrush and esophageal symptoms
- Apart from *Helicobacter pylori*, gastric infections are rare in healthy people
- Achlorhydria or proton pump inhibitor (PPI) treatment usually result in asymptomatic colonization
- Phlegmonous gastritis is caused by oral flora in immune deficient states (alcoholism, granulocytopenia)

INTRODUCTION

The esophagus and stomach may become infected with bacteria, fungi and viruses in the setting of immunologic impairment or gastric acid suppression. Infection is defined as the presence of organisms that invade or elicit an inflammatory response in the mucosa, in contrast to colonization. Nonspecific complaints may be the only clinical manifestations of infection in immunosuppressed patients. Effective treatment is available for most esophageal and gastric infections.

EPIDEMIOLOGY

The only common organisms that infect reasonably healthy people are *Candida albicans* (in elderly or diabetic patients) and, rarely, viruses (herpes simplex virus (HSV), varicella zoster virus (VZV), Epstein-Barr virus (EBV)).[1] In immunosuppressed patients, a wider range of organisms cause infection.[2] *Candida* infection is common. Cytomegalovirus (CMV) and HSV occur from reactivation of latent virus. Disseminated VZV may involve the esophagus. HIV infection is associated with idiopathic esophageal ulcers. Human papilloma virus (HPV) may cause esophageal condylomata and possibly contribute to carcinoma.

CAUSES, RISK FACTORS, DISEASE ASSOCIATIONS

Antibiotics disrupt the balance among bacteria and fungi; this permits *Candida* overgrowth. Immune deficiency involving T cells or granulocytes, whether genetic or acquired, increases the risk of infection. Fungal infections are common in AIDS patients not on highly active antiretroviral therapy (HAART), and in hematologic malignancies. Predisposing illnesses include diabetes mellitus, esophageal motility disorders, alcoholism, and advanced age. Corticosteroids, including corticosteroid inhalers, predispose to fungal esophagitis.

ESOPHAGEAL INFECTIONS (Table 33.1)

Fungal esophagitis

Pathology

Candida species colonize by superficial adherence. Invasion into epithelia requires a defect in cellular immunity. Infection is distinguished from colonization by the endoscopic and microscopic appearance, i.e., adherent plaques and masses of budding yeast. Other fungi such as *Aspergillus, Histoplasma, Cryptococcus*, and *Blastomyces* are rare causes of esophagitis.

Clinical presentation

Most patients have dysphagia or odynophagia. Associated symptoms often include retrosternal discomfort, heartburn, and nausea. In granulocytopenic patients, fever, sepsis, and abdominal pain suggest disseminated disease.

Differential diagnosis

The differential diagnosis includes benign or malignant strictures and esophagitis caused by viruses, pills, and acid-peptic reflux.

Diagnostic methods

Endoscopic brushing and biopsy should be performed.[3] Candida plaques are white/yellow and if dislodged show a raw surface

TABLE 33.1 ORGANISMS CAUSING ESOPHAGEAL INFECTIONS

Reasonably healthy population	Immunocompromised patients
COMMON	COMMON
Candida species	*Candida* species
UNCOMMON	CMV
HSV	HSV
EBV (mononucleosis)	HIV (HIV-associated ulcer)
RARE	UNCOMMON
VZV (disseminated)	Bacteria from the oral flora
Mycobacterium tuberculosis	*Aspergillus* species
Histoplasma	VZV
Other fungal organisms	

(Fig. 33.1). Brushings should be spread onto slides, air dried, and stained. Cultures are rarely helpful unless an unusual fungus or resistant *Candida* species are suspected. Radiographs are of limited value.

Treatment and prevention

Most patients with *Candida albicans* infection should receive oral fluconazole or a topical agent. Fluconazole (100–200 mg p.o. daily) is convenient and the choice for immunodeficient patients, but clotrimazole or nystatin troches (pastilles retained in the mouth for local delivery) are effective and lack side effects and drug–drug interactions.

In HIV infection, oral thrush with esophageal symptoms predicts *Candida* esophagitis, and empiric treatment with fluconazole is recommended, with endoscopy reserved for patients without a clinical response within 3–5 days (to exclude resistant *Candida* and viral infection). Itraconazole 200 mg daily is an effective alternative.

For febrile, granulocytopenic patients with disseminated infection, a liposomal amphotericin formulation is the treatment of choice (3–5 mg/kg/day). Fluconazole and itraconazole are effective in granulocytopenic patients with only mucosal infection.

Risk factors should be sought and eliminated. For HIV-infected patients, prophylaxis with fluconazole is effective, but a better strategy is HAART. For hematologic disorders, fluconazole or oral amphotericin B reduces recurrences.

Complications and their management

Yeast forms of *Candida* pass through the normal intestinal mucosa and disseminate. Rarely, esophageal ulcers penetrate into the mediastinum.

Viral esophagitis

Pathology

HSV esophagitis usually occurs after reactivation of virus within neurons. Histology reveals multinucleated giant cells, ballooning degeneration, and 'ground glass' intranuclear inclusions (Fig. 33.1). CMV infection is identified by large cells with intranuclear and cytoplasmic inclusions and a halo surrounding the nuclear inclusions. VZV shows ballooning degeneration and multinucleated giant cells with intranuclear eosinophilic inclusions (Fig. 33.1).

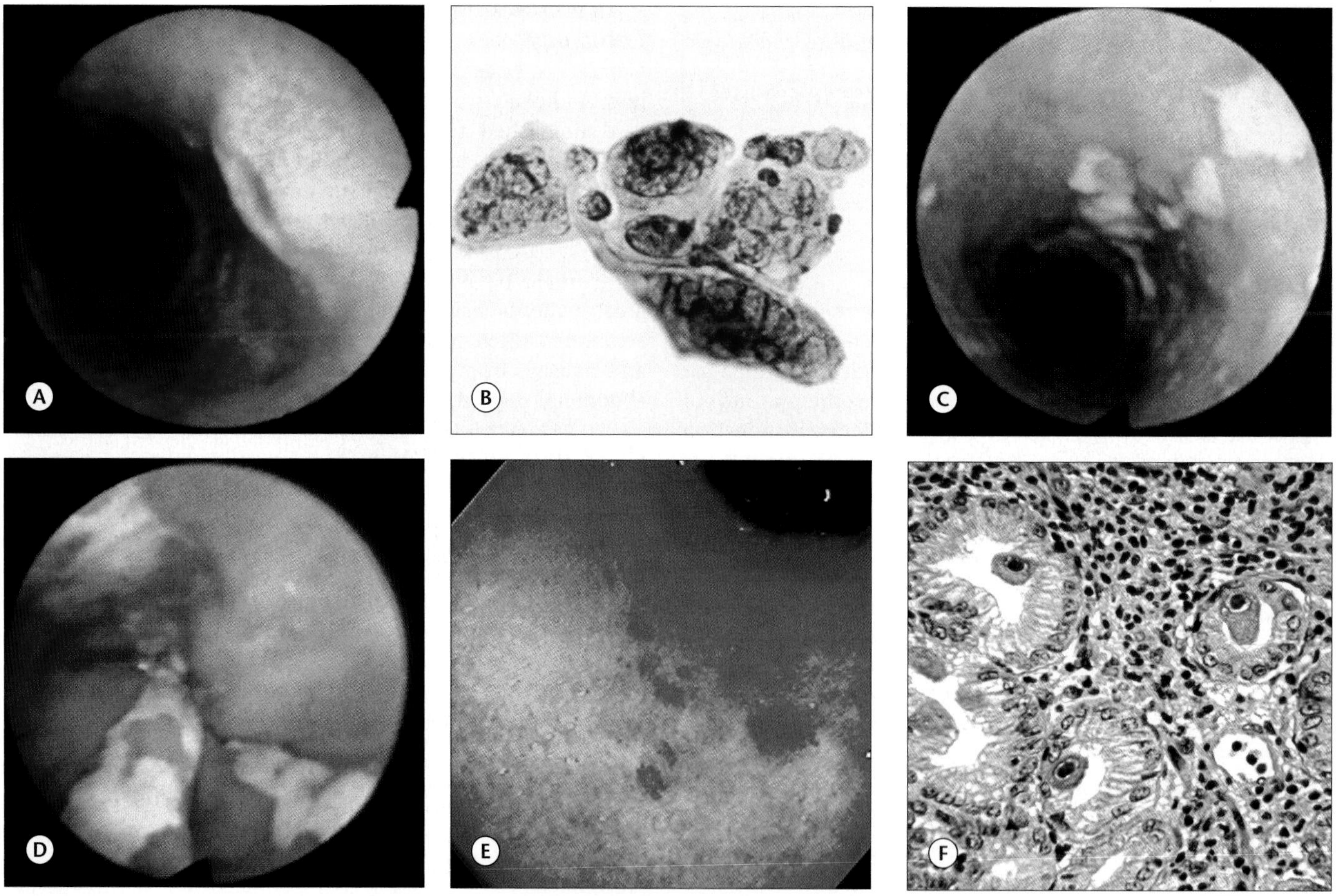

Fig. 33.1 Endoscopic and histologic features of esophageal and gastric infections. A. Endoscopy photograph of a volcano-like lesion caused by HSV in the esophagus. The crater of the volcano represents sloughed squamous epithelium, forming an ulcer. A diagnosis can be made by biopsy or brushing an edge of the ulcer. **B.** Photomicrograph of a cluster of multinucleate giant cells, typical of HSV infection of squamous epithelium. The specimen was obtained at endoscopy using a brush. **C.** Endoscopy photograph of adherent white plaques with reddened edges, typical of *Candida* esophagitis. **D.** Endoscopy photograph of linear ulcerations in the esophagus caused by CMV. This endoscopic appearance can be confused with *Candida* esophagitis. **E.** Endoscopy photograph of gastric mucosa, showing small punctate bleeding sites (overlying erosions), caused by CMV infection. **F.** Photomicrograph of a gastric biopsy, showing typical findings of CMV infection – three megaloid cells within crypt epithelium, each containing an inclusion surrounded by a light-colored rim. Lymphoid cells are increased in the lamina propria.

Clinical presentation

For CMV, fever, nausea, and vomiting often dominate the clinical picture. HSV causes odynophagia and nausea. Esophageal VZV infection is often of minor significance compared to encephalitis, pneumonia, and hepatitis. HIV-associated idiopathic ulcerations range from small aphthoid lesions to giant, deep ulcers. HPV lesions present as erythematous plaques or nodules and are usually asymptomatic.

Differential diagnosis

The differential diagnosis includes fungal esophagitis, reflux esophagitis, pill esophagitis, and, less likely, malignancy.

Diagnostic methods

Viral esophagitis is diagnosed by endoscopy.[4] Radiographs are not accurate. Specimens from ulcer bases lack epithelial cells and are inadequate to exclude HSV, whereas CMV-infected fibroblasts and endothelial cells reside in the ulcer base (Fig. 33.2). Immunohistology, PCR, and viral culture are more accurate than histology alone.

Therefore, biopsies for viral culture and histology should be obtained from ulcer margins, ulcer base, and surrounding mucosa. On endoscopy, HSV causes vesicles, erosions, or large superficial ulcers (Fig. 33.1). CMV appears as erosions or ulcers (Fig. 33.1). VZV esophagitis occurs with dermatologic VZV and results in vesicles and ulcers. Immunohistochemical staining is less sensitive than viral culture or PCR. HIV-associated idiopathic ulceration is a diagnosis of exclusion.

Treatment and prevention

HSV esophagitis is treated with intravenous acyclovir, 250 mg/m^2 every 8 h, then oral valacyclovir (1000 mg t.i.d.) for 7–10 days. Foscarnet (40 mg/kg t.i.d.) is effective for acyclovir-resistant HSV. Prophylaxis with oral acyclovir or valacyclovir prevents recurrences.

CMV esophagitis is treated with ganciclovir (5 mg/kg every 12 h for 2 weeks) or foscarnet (90 mg/kg intravenously every 12 h for 2–3 weeks). Recurrence is common if immunodeficiency persists (as in HIV). Maintenance therapy with ganciclovir or foscarnet is indicated. Screening of blood products prevents CMV disease among CMV-naïve transplant recipients.

VZV infection is treated with intravenous acyclovir. Foscarnet is effective for acyclovir-resistant VZV.

Idiopathic HIV-associated ulcers respond to prednisone (40 mg/day for 2 weeks, then a 1-month taper).[5] Another option is thalidomide (200 mg/day for 4 weeks).

Complications

Complications can include extensive mucosal necrosis, superinfection, Boerhaave syndrome, hemorrhage, strictures, HSV or VZV pneumonia, tracheoesophageal fistula formation, and disseminated infection.

Bacterial infections of the esophagus

Tuberculosis of the esophagus may occur via mediastinal extension. In granulocytopenic patients, bacteria from the oral flora may infiltrate esophageal tissues.

INFECTIONS OF THE STOMACH (Table 33.2)

In reasonably healthy people, gastric infections are rare (except *Helicobacter pylori* infection, see Chapters 26 and 38). Rotavirus involvement of gastric mucosa has been described as part of a generalized gut infection. Ingestion of raw fish can lead to acute gastric infection with Anisakis worms.

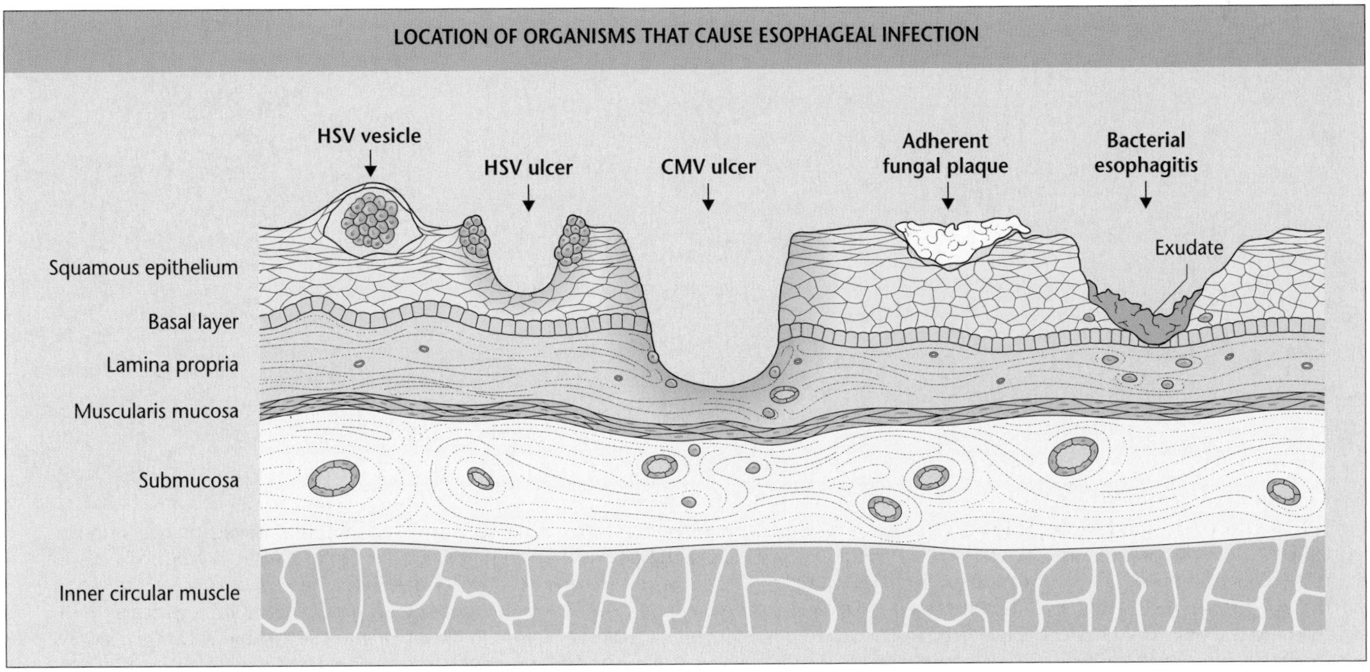

Fig. 33.2 Location of organisms causing esophageal infection. Schematic diagram of the esophageal mucosa showing the location of organisms that cause infection. HSV infects squamous epithelium whereas CMV infects only subepithelial cells (endothelial cells, fibroblasts). Fungal and bacterial esophagitis infect superficial layers of the mucosa but may extend more deeply.

TABLE 33.2 ORGANISMS CAUSING GASTRIC INFECTIONS

Reasonably healthy population	Immunocompromised patients
COMMON	**COMMON**
H. pylori (see Chapters 26, 38)	CMV
UNCOMMON	**UNCOMMON**
Rotavirus	VZV
Anisakis worms	Fungal infection (especially molds)
RARE	Phlegmonous gastritis
Spiral organisms	
Mycobacterium tuberculosis	
Treponema pallidum (syphilis)	
CMV	

In immunodeficient patients, gastric infections occur more commonly. For CMV and VZV, the spectrum of findings found in the esophagus may also be found in the stomach (Fig. 33.2). Bacterial overgrowth also occurs with achlorhydria or treatment with proton pump inhibitors, but manifests only as asymptomatic colonization. Phlegmonous (suppurative) gastritis, a rare infection of the submucosa of the stomach caused by bacteria from the oral flora, has been described in the setting of alcoholism, trauma, and granulocytopenia. It presents as an acute abdomen, usually with peritoneal signs, and endoscopy reveals erythematous or purple mucosa, submucosal narrowing of the gastric lumen, or cobblestoning.[6] Treatment consists of broad-spectrum antibiotics and, often, surgical intervention.

Gastritis can also rarely be caused by spiral-shaped bacteria (*Helicobacter heilmanni, H. felis*) other than *H. pylori*.[7] Gastric syphilis has been reported in the setting of HIV infection, and is characterized by an inflammatory infiltrate, erosions, ulcerations, and thickened folds. It responds to treatment for secondary syphilis. Gastric tuberculosis is rare. Cytomegalovirus has also been associated with marked gastric rugal hypertrophy and transient protein-losing enteropathy, similar to Menetrier's disease. Fungal gastric infections, including *Candida*, *Histoplasma* and *Zygomycetes*, can occur in granulocytopenic patients.

REFERENCES

1. Ramanathan, J, Rammouni M, Baran J, Khatib R. Herpes simplex virus esophagitis in the immunocompetent host: an overview. Am J Gastroenterol 2000; 95:2171–2176.
2. Greenson JK. Infections of the esophagus. Pathol Case Rev 2002; 7:19–26.
3. Baehr PH, McDonald GB. Esophageal infections: risk factors, presentation, diagnosis and treatment. Gastroenterology 1994; 106:509–532.
4. McDonald GB, Owens MM. Gastrointestinal infections after hematopoietic or solid organ transplantation. In: Bowden RA, Ljungman P, Paya CV, eds. Transplant infections, 2nd edn. Lippincott Williams Wilkins: Philadelphia; 2003:198–221.
5. Wilcox CM, Schwartz DA. Comparison of two corticosteroid regimens for the treatment of HIV-associated idiopathic esophageal ulcer. Am J Gastroenterol 1994; 89:2163.
6. Cohen M, Taylor MB. Phlegmonous gastritis. In: Taylor MD, ed. Gastrointestinal emergencies, 2nd edn. Williams & Wilkins: Philadelphia; 1997:219–223.
7. Fox JG. The non-*H. pylori* helicobacters: their role in gastrointestinal and systemic diseases. Gut 2002; 50:273–283.

Chapter 34

H. pylori: its diseases and management

Peter Malfertheiner

KEY POINTS
• *H. pylori* colonization of the gastric antrum is associated with hypergastrinemia, increased gastric acid, and duodenal ulcer • *H. pylori* colonization of the corpus or pangastritis is associated with impaired gastric acid secretion, gastric ulcer, and gastric cancer • *H. pylori* adapts to changing conditions, including modification of host signalling pathways • *H. pylori* is responsible for 90% of duodenal ulcers and 70% of gastric ulcers • *H. pylori* gives a lifetime risk of peptic ulcer of 5–10%, and a 3–6 fold increased risk of gastric cancer • Genotypes such as *vacA* and *cagA* are more ulcerogenic and carcinogenic • *H. pylori* is a type 1 carcinogen • Early stage mucosa-associated lymphoid tissue (MALT) lymphoma can be cured by *H. pylori* eradication • A test and treat strategy requires a background prevalence of 20%

INTRODUCTION

Helicobacter pylori affects approximately half of the world's population. Its colonization is limited strictly to gastric epithelium (Figs 34.1 and 34.2). Outside the stomach, *H. pylori* can be detected in areas of gastric metaplasia, and is encountered most frequently in the duodenum but also in Meckel's diverticulum (see Chapter 35). *H. pylori* colonization of the gastric mucosa always results in inflammation of the gastric mucosa (i.e., gastritis).

There are two main routes of disease development, based on distinct gastritis phenotypes:

- Antral predominant – associated with increased acid production and duodenal ulceration
- Corpus predominant or pangastritis – associated with impaired acid secretion, gastric ulcer, and gastric cancer (see Chapters 35 and 37).

Approximately 80% of patients, however, remain asymptomatic and free of clinical disease. The challenge at present is to identify individuals in whom *H. pylori* infection will progress to overt disease for early intervention and disease prevention.

MICROBIOLOGY AND PATHOGENESIS
(Figs 34.1–34.5)

H. pylori is a flagellated Gram-negative bacillus. It is microaerophilic, growing best in the presence of carbon dioxide, and is capable of producing large quantities of ammonia from urea because it contains high levels of the enzyme urease. It seems likely that this property enables it to evade initial acid killing and also provides the basis of several diagnostic tests. *H. pylori* is also specifically adapted to colonize only areas of gastric epithelium in the stomach of humans, its natural host.[1] The entire *H. pylori* genome has been fully sequenced.[2] It is, however, a remarkably diverse organism and there is evidence that diversity occurs rapidly in response to any change in the milieu by recombination and point mutation, so that subpopulations adapted to specific micro-niches can be detected within an individual stomach. Other important interactions that may facilitate survival include possession of an active type 4 secretion system that enables bacterial products to influence host signaling.[3,4] The vacuolating cytotoxin (Fig. 34.4) may contribute to survival by facilitating urea availability by increasing transmembrane and transcellular permeability (Fig. 34.5), immune evasion and subversion, and possibly effects on food intake and energy expenditure via influences on gastric leptin and ghrelin[1,4]

EPIDEMIOLOGY

The prevalence of *H. pylori* infection is still high in patients above the age of 50 years in many areas of the Western world (around 40%), whereas it is generally decreasing in the younger population (less than 10% in children).[5–8] In the developing world the infection still shows a high prevalence across all age groups (above 70%). The route of transmission is either oral–oral or fecal–oral. Recent studies have confirmed that the infection occurs usually in childhood after the second year of

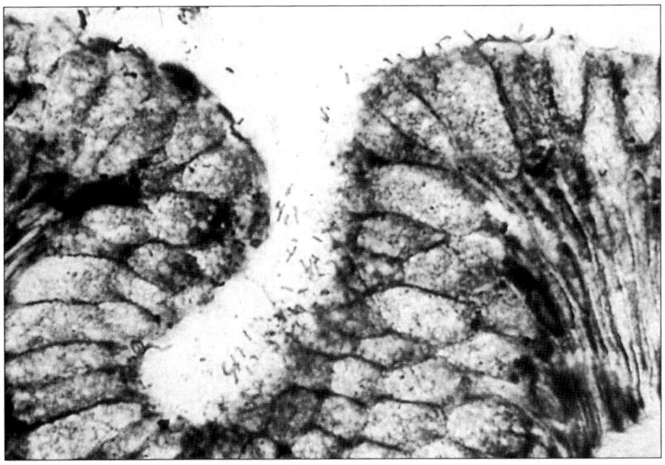

Fig. 34.1 Heavy *H. pylori* infection. Hematoxylin and eosin-stained section.

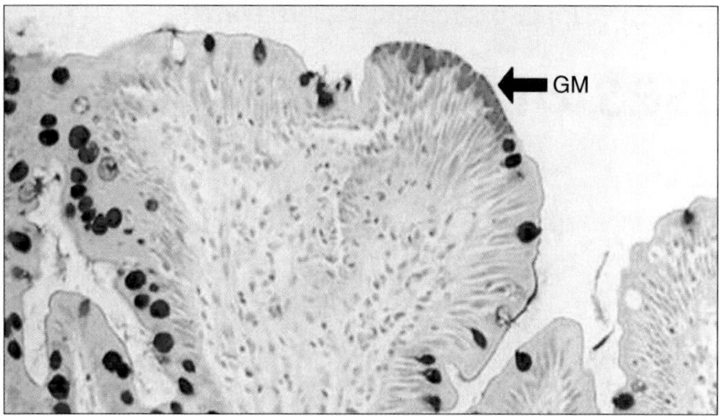

Fig. 34.2 Duodenal area of gastric metaplasia identified by staining for gastric mucins.

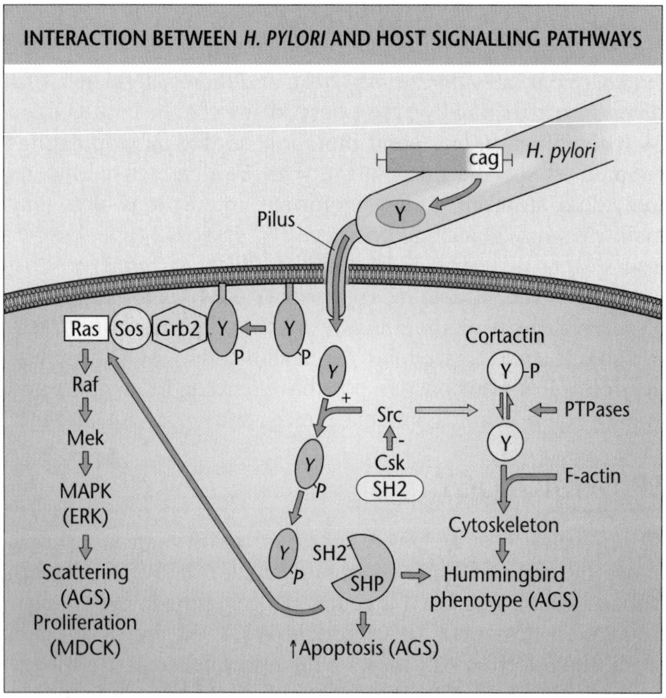

Fig. 34.3 Effect of *H. pylori* type 4 active secretory apparatus and CagA protein on host signalling pathways.

life, with a peak in infection transmission between the age of 2 and 3 years.

Intrafamilial transmission is the most frequent route, with mother to child transmission the commonest. A low socio-economic level and poor hygiene are major risks for the acquisition of *H. pylori* infection in childhood. Transmission of the infection among adults is not common. Reinfection after successful cure (apart from exceptions in certain areas) is rare (around 1%). *H. pylori* has been shown to have a causal relationship with upper gastrointestinal diseases, shown in Table 34.1.[9–14] There has been speculation regarding association with many other diseases (Table 34.2), but the evidence is sufficiently weak to discount a relationship as likely in such diseases.[15]

PATHOPHYSIOLOGY

H. pylori gastritis

Chronic active gastritis is the unequivocal result in all subjects infected with *H. pylori*[16] (Fig. 34.6). Gastritis may be suspected endoscopically, but it is a histologic not an endoscopic diagnosis. The currently accepted histologic diagnosis of gastritis is based on the revised Sydney classification (see Chapters 36 and 135), which includes assessment of mucosal morphology, and the topographic distribution of the inflammatory involvement. The validity and meaning of endoscopic gastritis is questioned by some. The histologic assessment includes:

- A description of the degree of inflammatory activity
- Grade of atrophy
- Presence of intestinal metaplasia
- Density of *H. pylori*.

Other possible etiologic factors are also considered in this classification. In the initial phase of infection the whole gastric mucosa from pylorus to cardia is homogeneously involved.[16] Although *H. pylori* usually persists in all areas, over time the distribution of inflammatory changes within the stomach becomes more distinctly defined (Fig. 34.7) as:

- Antrum predominant
- Corpus predominant
- Pangastritis.

These phenotypes may represent a spectrum rather than clear-cut, distinct entities.

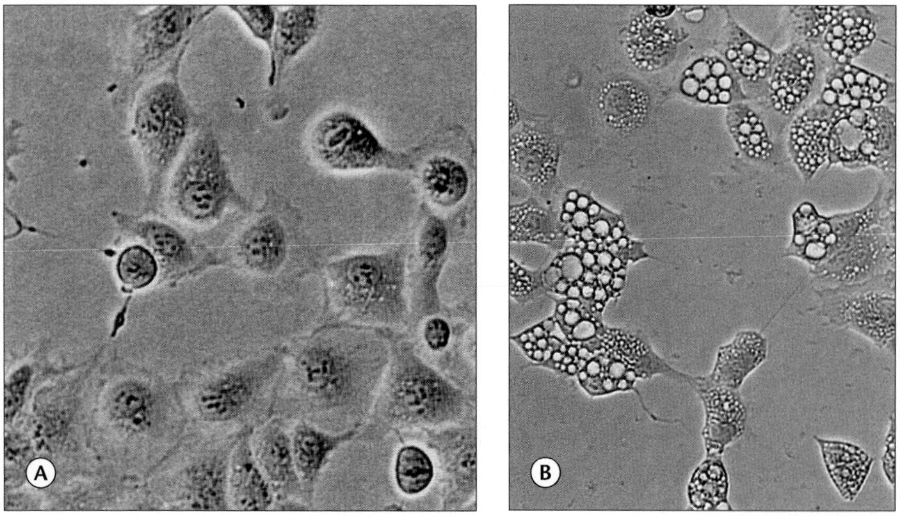

Fig. 34.4 Epithelial cell vacuolation with *H. pylori* toxin VacA. A. Untreated. **B.** VacA treated.

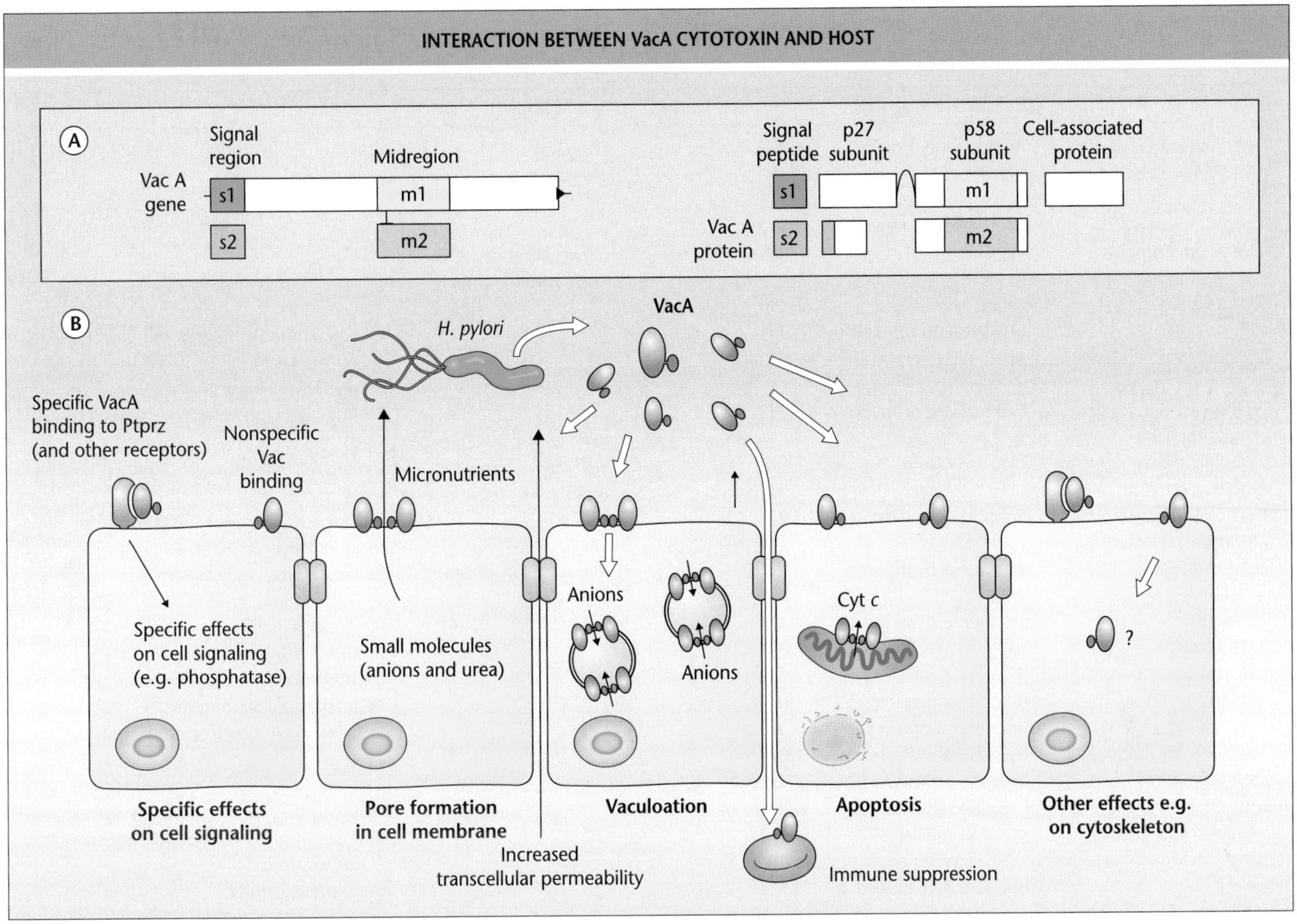

Fig. 34.5 Vacuolating cytotoxin, VacA. A. Pathogenic regions of VacA. **B.** Effects of VacA on the host.

The macroscopic appearance is often completely normal, or the patient may present with spotty or streaky reddening of the mucosal folds in the antrum with or without chronic erosions. Florid exudative erosions are uncommon in *H. pylori* infection. The histologic picture is characterized by *H. pylori* colonization of the superficial gastric epithelium and infiltration of neutrophils, lymphocytes, and plasma cells in the mucosa (see Fig. 34.6). The persistent inflammation leads to:

TABLE 34.1 DISEASES CAUSED BY *H. PYLORI*

Disease	Comment
Active gastritis	Causal
Atrophic gastritis	Develops from chronic active gastritis
Pernicious anemia	Develops via chronic atrophic gastritis in some cases
Lymphocytic gastritis	Likely cause
Ménétrièr's syndrome	Likely cause
Gastric ulcer	Most cases occur in absence of NSAID use
Duodenal ulcer	Most cases occur in absence of NSAID use
Gastric cancer	In most cases (classified as class 1 carcinogen)
MALT lymphoma	Most cases
Functional dyspepsia	Subset of cases

- Mucosal damage with mucus depletion
- Epithelial regeneration
- Development of focal intestinal metaplasia.

The expression of different patterns of gastritis is dependent on both the virulence of the infecting strain and the genetic predisposition of the host[17,18] (see Chapter 37). The topographic distribution of gastritis and the degree of gastritis activity/chronicity predispose to the development of different disease entities (Fig. 34.7). The most consistent significant outcomes of *H. pylori*-induced chronic gastritis are peptic ulcer (see Chapter 35) and gastric adenocarcinoma (see Chapter 37), and mucosa-associated lymphoid tissue (MALT) (see Chapter 38). Reasonable evidence exists favoring a role for *H. pylori* in at least some cases of lymphocytic colitis,[9,10] as a precursor to pernicious anemia,[11,12] and possibly in some cases of nonulcer dyspepsia.[13,14]

Interaction of H. pylori with the mucosal barrier

Colonization of the gastric mucosa by *H. pylori* evokes a local inflammatory response, which results in mucosal injury of varying degrees.[19] The acute inflammatory response starts with the release of epithelium-derived cytokines, predominantly interleukin (IL)-8. Bacterial products and cytokines orchestrate the acute inflammatory response, promoting an influx of neutrophils and macrophages into the gastric mucosa that subsequently release lysosomal enzymes, leukotrienes, and oxygen free radicals. The next step in the inflammatory cascade is the

TABLE 34.2 EXTRAINTESTINAL DISEASES IN WHICH A CAUSAL ROLE FOR *H. PYLORI* HAS BEEN POSTULATED (IN MOST CASES THE EVIDENCE IS WEAK)

Endpoint	Possible mechanism	Positive studies	Meta-analysis	Comment
Raised fibrinogen	Acute-phase protein	3/8	Negative	
White blood cell count	Inflammation	2/5	Negative	
CRP	Acute-phase protein	1/1		
TNF-α	Acute-phase protein	2/2		
Adverse lipid profile	Via CRP	3/14	Cholesterol negative HDL positive (small)	
Homocysteine	Folate deficiency	0/4		
HSP	Cross-reacting proteins	1/1		HSP65 antibodies higher with infection
Coronary heart disease	Acute-phase proteins	9/21		Many studies did not match controls for age, sex, or class
Cerebrovascular accident and peripheral vascular disease	Acute-phase proteins	2/3		Similar matching issues
Hypertension		3/10	Positive (small)	
Raynaud's disease	Immune activation	2/2		Includes uncontrolled treatment trial
Migraine		2/2		Includes uncontrolled treatment trial
Diabetes mellitus	Immune activation	3/5	Blood sugar: positive (small)	Some studies poorly controlled
Thyroiditis	Immune activation	1/2		No biologic basis
Acromegaly		1/3		Chance finding
Acne rosacea		3/5		Controlled studies negative
Psoriasis	Immune activation	0/2		Anecdotes not supported
Chronic urticaria	Immune complexes	3/6		Includes unblinded treatment trials
Rheumatoid arthritis	Immune activation	0/2		
Scleroderma	Immune activation	0/2		
Sjögren's syndrome	Immune activation	2/3		Small studies. No compelling evidence
Iron-deficiency anemia	Iron scavenging	1/2		Also case reports. Confounding by poverty not excluded
ITP	Autoantibody induction	1/1		Uncontrolled study
Hepatic encephalopathy	Ammonia	5/10		Recent abstract questions causal association
SIDS	IL-1-induced fever *H. pylori* aspiration	4/5		Uncontrolled data. Confounding by poverty not excluded
Childhood growth retardation	Chronic infection	5/7		May be true even after adjustment for poverty, but not all studies consistent

CRP, C-reactive protein; HDL, high density lipoprotein; HSP, heat shock protein; ITP, idiopathic thrombocytopenic purpura; SIDS, sudden infant death syndrome.

activation of T and B lymphocytes by bacterial antigens, with the release of further proinflammatory cytokines, including IL-1, IL-2, IL-6, and tumor necrosis factor (TNF)-α, as well as the generation of specific antibodies (IgA and IgG) directed against *H. pylori*. All of these factors concur in damaging the gastric mucosa (Fig. 34.8). Response is predominantly a T helper cell type 1 (Th1) response, and interventions such as infestation with enteric helminths can drive a Th2 response and reduce inflammation and gastric atrophy.[20]

H. pylori gastritis – clinical manifestations and symptoms

The majority of individuals (approximately 80%) with *H. pylori* infection and gastritis remain asymptomatic in the long term. Only in a small subset of patients is the presence of gastritis alone the true cause of dyspeptic symptoms (see Chapter 5). Dyspepsia is a symptom complex referable to the upper gastrointestinal tract, and most frequently includes epigastric pain, fullness, early satiety, and nausea. Despite several attempts at classifying dyspepsia, there is still no clear way of predicting underlying endoscopic or histologic findings based on any predominant symptom complex, or vice versa. It is important to note that gastritis is the histological entity. The term is often used inaccurately to refer to dyspeptic symptoms by many patients and even physicians.

H. pylori and functional dyspepsia

In the absence of notable macroscopic structural lesions in the stomach and duodenum, *H. pylori*-positive gastritis is a possible cause of functional dyspepsia. Treatment trials have shown only a subset of patients responding with symptom relief to *H. pylori* eradication.[18]

H. pylori and peptic ulcer

H. pylori is the most frequent cause of peptic ulcer disease. Successful eradication results in both ulcer healing and prevention of disease relapse. Epidemiologic studies have attributed a 4-fold increased risk of developing an ulcer in *H. pylori*-infected versus noninfected persons; this risk is estimated to be 25 times greater if the degree of inflammatory activity is high and antrum predominant.[5] Approximately 90% of patients with duodenal ulcer and 70% of those with gastric ulcers are infected with *H. pylori*[6] (see Chapter 35).

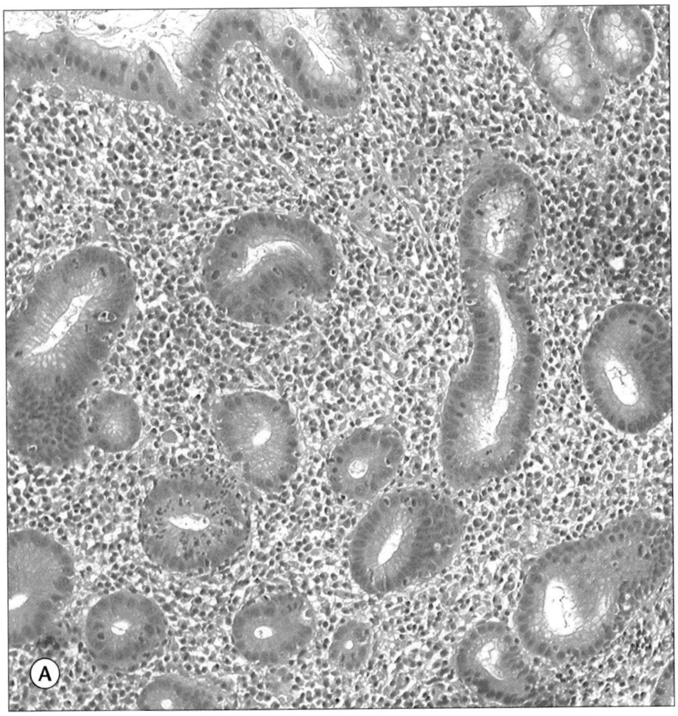

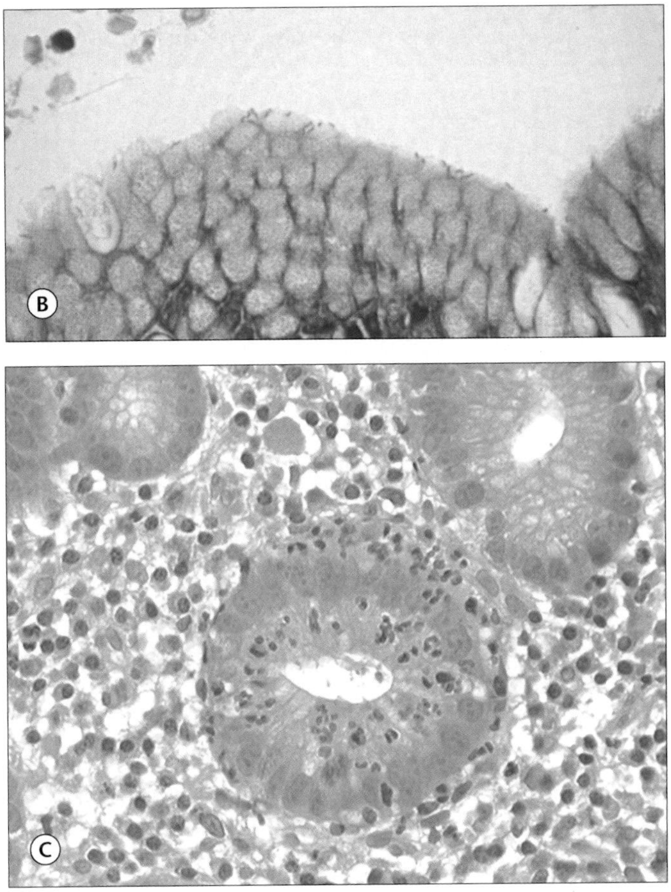

Fig. 34.6 Persistent active gastritis associated with *H. pylori* infection. A. Heavy mixed infiltrate throughout the mucosa. **B.** Surface *H. pylori.* **C.** Neutrophil invasion of a gastric gland. (Courtesy of Dr Philip Kaye, University Hospital, Nottingham.)

The difference in prevalence of *H. pylori* among patients with duodenal and gastric ulcers is due to the greater contribution of nonsteroidal anti-inflammatory drugs (NSAIDs) to gastric ulceration, although these drugs also contribute to development of duodenal ulcers. An estimate of the lifetime risk of peptic ulcer disease in *H. pylori*-infected subjects in Western industrialized countries is at least 5–10%. Approximately 80% of *H. pylori*-infected persons, however, will live with a persistent chronic gastric inflammation with no symptoms and without any further progression to relevant clinical disease.

Several factors influence whether peptic ulceration develops:

- Bacterial genotype and phenotype
- Host genotype and phenotype
- Pattern of gastritis
- Alterations in the homeostasis of gastric hormones and acid secretion
- Gastric metaplasia in the duodenum as a prerequisite for *H. pylori* colonization.

Ulcerogenic strains of H. pylori (see Chapter 35)

Pathogenetic properties (virulence factors) vary among strains. *H. pylori* isolated from patients with peptic ulcer disease

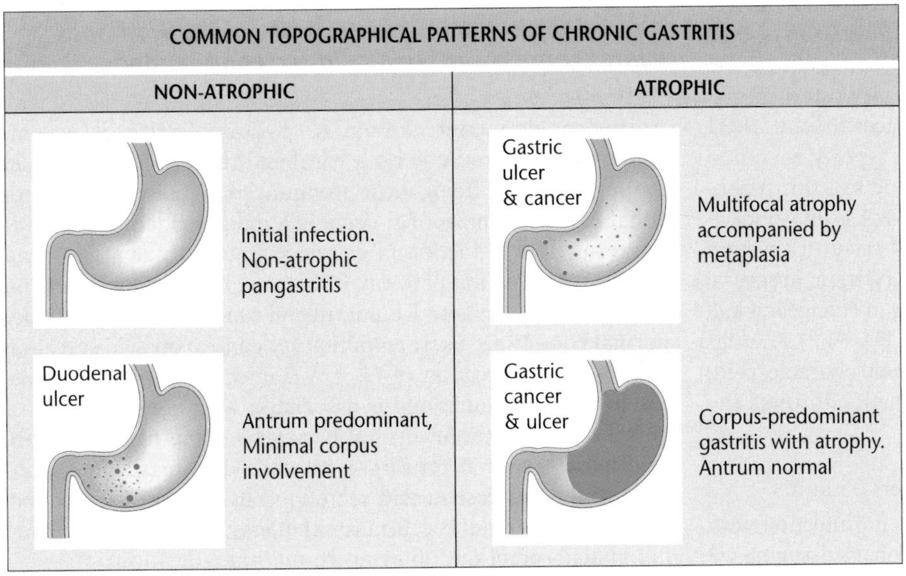

Fig. 34.7 Common topographic patterns of chronic active gastritis.

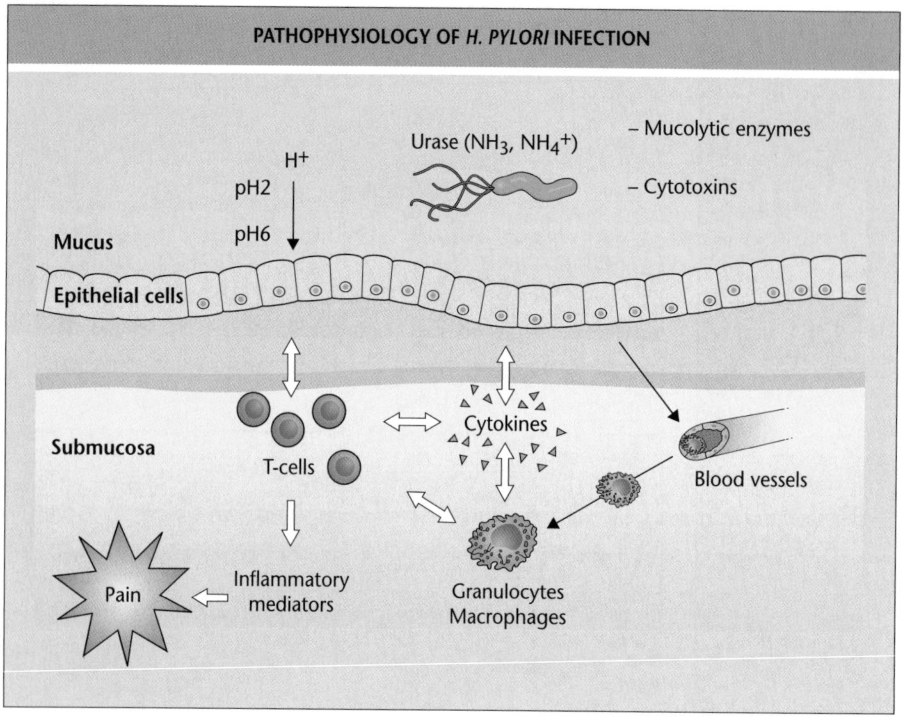

Fig. 34.8 Functional consequences of *H. pylori* infection.

appear to be more virulent. The most important genotypes are *vacA*$^+$ and *cagA*$^+$, present in almost all patients with peptic ulceration.[17,21,22] The *H. pylori*-derived vacuolating cytotoxin (VacA), an 87-kDa protein, causes vacuolar degeneration in cultured gastric cell preparations and gastric ulceration in experimental animals. Although present in all *H. pylori* strains, the *vacA* gene, depending on its allelic form, is expressed in only 60%, lending strong support to the hypothesis of strain-dependent virulence. Effects attributed to *vacA* include induction of apoptosis via pore formation in mitochondrial membranes, increased transcellular permeability, enhanced release of anions and urea into the lumen, and immune suppression (see Figs 34.4 and 34.5). The cytotoxin-associated gene A (*cagA*), part of a complex pathogenicity island that is restricted to cytotoxin-producing strains of *H. pylori*, encodes for a 120–160-kDa immunodominant protein that is now recognized as a marker of greater virulence, leading to an enhanced local inflammatory response. Among *H. pylori*-infected individuals, bacterial strains expressing CagA protein are closely associated with peptic ulcer (present in 92% of cases) and, to a lesser extent, with chronic gastritis (approximately 60% in Western populations). The *cag* pathogenicity island embraces a total of 31 genes that allow the formation of a complex type IV secretion system for introducing cagA and other products of this pathogenicity in the epithelial target cell. Injected CagA is phosphorylated, and this and other aspects of the type 4 secretory system lead to interaction, mostly by further phosphorylation, in several major signal transduction pathways, resulting in changes of cell morphology, proliferation, and apoptosis (see Fig. 34.3). A series of other genes (*NAP*, *oiPA*, *iceA*) have been characterized; their function is to enhance mucosal inflammation through the induction of proinflammatory cytokines.[23]

Genetic factors and H. pylori (see Chapters 35 and 37)

Twin studies confirm a genetic predisposition for infection with increased susceptibility in monozygotes versus dizygotes.[24] Lewis antigen association studies also support a genetic predisposition for peptic ulcer disease.[25] Other studies suggest a higher prevalence of the human lymphocyte antigen (HLA) type DQA1301 in patients with ulcer disease.

Pattern of gastritis in association with H. pylori (see Chapter 35)

The characteristic pattern of gastritis in patients with duodenal ulcer is the antrum-predominant distribution of *H. pylori* with a high density of the bacteria and a high degree of inflammatory activity in this location (see Figs 34.6 and 34.7). Following eradication therapy, gastric mucosal alterations are usually fully reversible in duodenal ulcer. In gastric ulcer, the topographic expression of gastritis is such that the body mucosa and antral mucosa are equally affected (see Fig. 34.6). Unlike duodenal ulcer, acid secretion is frequently impaired in patients with gastric ulceration, because of the more severe involvement of the body mucosa.

Alterations in the homeostasis of gastric hormones, neural connections, and acid secretion related to H. pylori

Antrum-predominant chronic *H. pylori* infection is accompanied by an increase in both basal and stimulated gastric acid output, the effect being most pronounced in patients with duodenal ulcer. The hormonal drive is hypergastrinemia, which is the result of a reduction in gastric somatostatin synthesis and release.[26] The neural pathway influenced by *H. pylori* infection is the disruption of antral–fundic neural connections which, under normal conditions, exert an inhibitory control on acid secretion (Fig. 34.9). Eradication of *H. pylori* infection rapidly resolves the hypergastrinemia and is associated with normalization of antral somatostatin levels, but it may be many months before acid hypersecretion returns to normal. Hypergastrinemia not only stimulates gastric acid secretion but also exerts a trophic effect on the parietal cell mass; this may explain the delayed fall in acid secretion following *H. pylori* eradication.

Gastric metaplasia in the duodenum is essential for H. pylori colonization (see Chapter 35)

Gastric acid hypersecretion and, more specifically, the acid overload in the duodenum leads to the development of gastric metaplasia in the duodenal bulb. This adaptive change permits *H. pylori* (which is adapted to colonize gastric epithelial cells) to infect areas of gastric metaplasia in the duodenum (see Fig. 34.9). The risk of developing a duodenal ulcer in the presence of gastric metaplasia and *H. pylori* appears to be 50 times that of controls.[5,6]

Therapeutic proof of causality: H. pylori and ulcers

All studies report that *H. pylori* eradication leads to ulcer healing and very low relapse rates for both duodenal and gastric ulcer. This led to the National Institutes of Health consensus statement[27] that antibiotic treatment in addition to antisecretory therapy is required for all patients with *H. pylori*-positive peptic ulcers, although some have questioned this approach for NSAID users.

H. pylori infection and NSAIDs combined

The relationship between *H. pylori* infection and NSAID-induced gastric toxicity is complex, with results that range in different studies from significantly increased to significantly reduced risks for NSAID users if they are infected with *H. pylori* (see Chapter 35). It seems that patients with *H. pylori* infection have a significantly reduced risk of ulceration if the infection is cured before the first exposure to NSAIDs,[28] whereas there appears to be no benefit of *H. pylori* eradication in patients who have already developed ulceration during NSAID intake.[29] Possible explanations include *H. pylori* induction of cyclo-oxygenase (COX) 2 synthesis, which may facilitate healing of NSAID-related ulcers, whilst for those taking proton pump inhibitors (PPIs) the benefit may come from the enhanced efficacy of PPIs in the presence of *H. pylori* (see Chapter 136).

A consequence of *H. pylori* infection is lifelong inflammation, including an active granulocyte component (Fig. 34.8). Pathology develops when the symbiotic relationship is lost and inflammation leads to mucosal ulceration, atrophy, or malignant change.

Gastric cancer (see Chapter 37)

Since 1994, *H. pylori* has been recognized as an established carcinogen type 1, according to World Health Organization criteria.[30] Further preclinical and clinical evidence has since strengthened the role of *H. pylori* as a key factor in gastric carcinogenesis.[31–35] Most epidemiologic studies report a 3–6-fold increase in risk of gastric cancer in *H. pylori*-infected individuals. The magnitude obviously depends upon the interval between testing and emergence of the disease. Based on the latest epidemiology findings, at least 70% of distal gastric adenocarcinomas are attributable to *H. pylori*. Several other disciplines have helped establish the scientific evidence for the role of *H. pylori* in gastric cancer (see Chapter 37). As with many cancers, it is the process of longstanding inflammation that results in malignant change (Fig. 34.9), with a fairly stereotyped evolution through premalignant changes, originally hypothesized by Correa[31] (Fig. 34.10).

Bacterial virulence

It has been shown in several studies that gastric cancer development is influenced by particular virulence characteristics of the bacterium, such as *cagA*. In addition, infection with *H. pylori* carrying *vacA* s1, *vacA* m1 has much stronger influence on neoplasia development.[17,21,22]

Host genetic factors

Host genetic factors contribute significantly to the clinical outcome of *H. pylori* infection.[12] There is good evidence for important host genetic factors that control both the host's innate immune response and its inflammatory response against *H. pylori* infection. Functional polymorphisms in the IL-1 receptor antagonist and TNF-α (TNF-A-308) genes increase the risk of noncardia gastric cancer (but not other upper gastrointestinal malignancies), and the risk seems to be significantly increased in the presence of proinflammatory genotypes of IL-1β and virulent *H. pylori* strains (see Fig. 34.8).[12] The risk applies to both intestinal and diffuse types of gastric adenocarcinoma. The sequence of biologic and gastric physiologic events in the pathway of gastric cancer is depicted in Figure 34.11 (see also Chapter 37).

Animal models and cell biologic aspects

A number of animal models have now been developed to examine gastric carcinogenesis in animals, the most widely used being ferrets, mice, and Mongolian gerbils.[36–38] A few studies in the Mongolian gerbil have proved for the first time that *H. pylori* can be a complete carcinogen, although more commonly it has been shown to act as a co-stimulant of cancer in the presence of a chemical carcinogen.[36–38] Another model of gastric carcinogenesis is the mouse infected by another *Helicobacter*, *H. felis*. Mice that mount a vigorous Th1 response develop atrophy, metaplasia, and gastric cancer.[39] In some *H. felis* models, male mice are more likely to develop gastric cancer than female mice. In general, animal studies have suggested that progression to gastric cancer is determined strongly by the host immune response, with ancillary influences such as a high-salt diet, and both atrophy and metaplasia can be reversed in whole or part.

H-PYLORI AND DUODENAL ULCERS

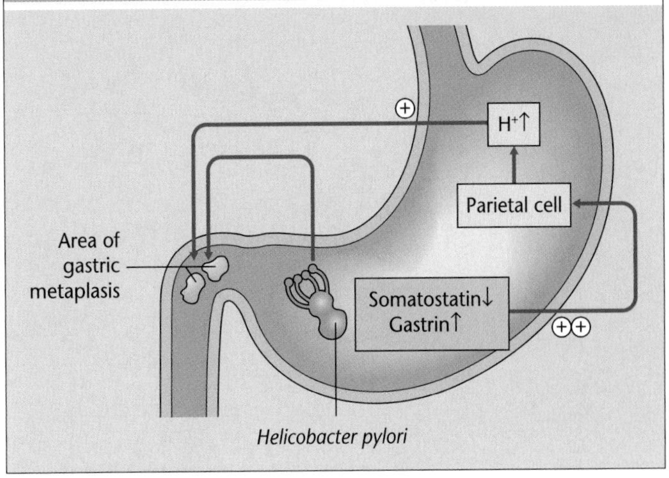

Fig. 34.9 How antral *H. pylori* causes duodenal ulcers. *H. pylori* colonizes duodenal gastric metaplasia and reduces antral somatostatin activity, resulting in increased gastrin and enhanced acid secretion by parietal cells.

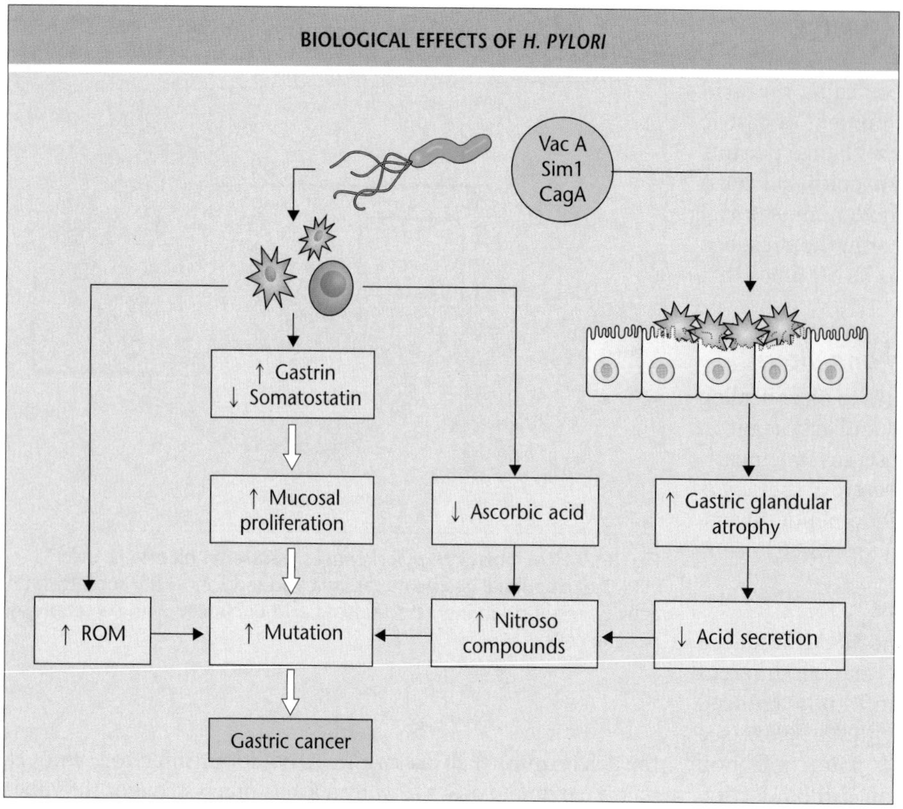

Fig. 34.10 Possible mechanisms linking *H. pylori* and cancer.

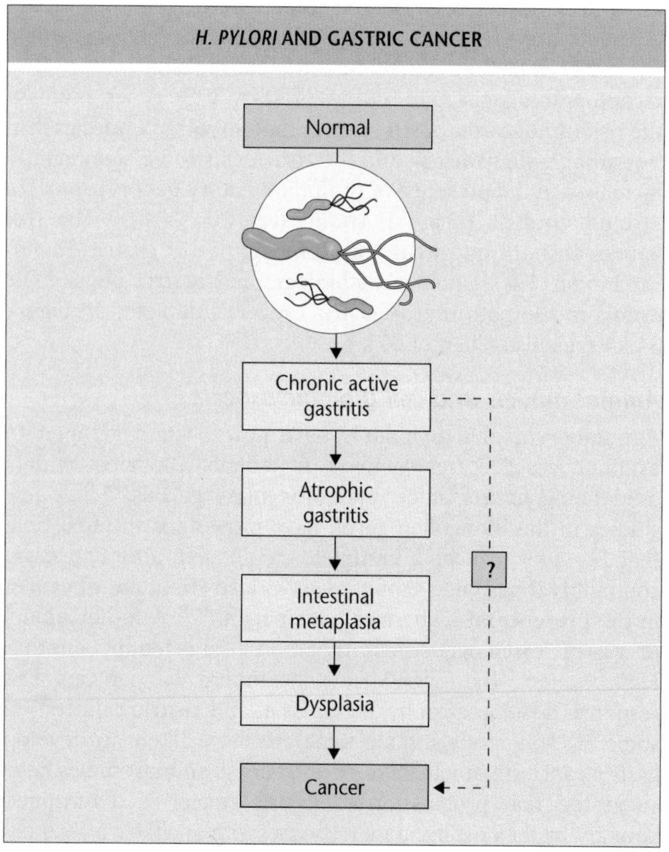

Fig. 34.11 Evolution of premalignant changes into cancer in patients with *H. pylori* infection.

Reversibility of molecular and histologic changes of preneoplastic lesions

Several molecular and genetic changes have been identified in gastric cancer cells,[33] including:

- A reduction in cellular adhesion due to mutations in E-cadherin (50% of diffuse cancers)
- α-Catenin (60%) and β-catenin (25%)
- Microsatellite instability (25–40%)
- Increased telomerase activity (in nearly all gastric cancers)
- Inactivation of tumor suppressor genes such as *p53* (60–70%) – this occurs in *H. pylori*-associated gastritis even before metaplasia
- Overexpression of cyclins D1 and D2
- Overexpression of COX-2 and ornithine decarboxylase.

Review of the literature indicates that, in studies with a control group that remains *H. pylori* positive, there is either no change or progression of atrophy and metaplasia. In contrast, atrophy and metaplasia do not progress in most patients who have had *H. pylori* eradicated.[35] In a subset of patients, regression of atrophic gastritis may occur, although many of the available studies have significant limitations in their design and the problem of bias in biopsy sampling. A recent randomized prospective study performed in China,[40] however, suggests that *H. pylori* eradication reduces the incidence of gastric cancer only in patients with gastritis that has not yet advanced and associated with atrophy or intestinal metaplasia. Even though regression of lesions may occur in some patients, at present there are no markers to indicate whether this may happen or not in individual patients. Therefore, eradication as early as possible seems appropriate, as the probability of progression to neoplasia is then lowest.

Gastric MALT lymphoma (see Chapter 38)

In its early stage MALT neoplasia is curable by *H. pylori* eradication. The chain of events in the pathogenesis of gastric MALT lymphoma starts with the acquisition of lymphatic tissue in the stomach following colonization with *H. pylori.*

Molecular studies show a stepwise transition from gastritis to lymphoma, with neoplastic B-cell clones as the starting point.[41] From a histologic perspective, the morphology of lymphoid cells is critical in the distinction between reactive and neoplastic infiltrate. The neoplastic lymphoid cells most frequently resemble centrocytes. For malignant transformation of B cells, *H. pylori* factors and activated T cells act synergistically.

A recent discovery indicates a role of a specific bacterial *H. pylori* virulence factor (HopZ) in the development of gastric B-cell lymphoma.[42] More than 90% of all MALT lymphomas appear to be associated with *H. pylori.* Latest results indicate that a lasting remission is obtained in around 70% of patients by eradication alone. Treatment response is dependent upon:

- Number of blasts in the infiltrate
- Depth of infiltration of the tumor
- Molecular genetic abnormality related to the presence of the translocation (t11,13).

The risk of relapse appears to be related to the persistence of a monoclonal B-cell population.

Extragastric disease associations

H. pylori has been reported to have a significant association with a variety of extragastric diseases.[15] The list of these associations (Table 34.2) has become long over the years, and includes main categories such as:

- Cardiovascular and cerebrovascular diseases
- Hepatologic diseases
- Skin and joint diseases.

However, definite proof with sound scientific evidence has not been provided for most associations, which therefore remain of anecdotal relevance. There are some proposed mechanisms, including the activation of focal gastric inflammatory mechanisms by *H. pylori* with systemic release of cytokines and other inflammatory mediators. In addition, mimicry between bacterial and host antigens has been proposed for the induction of systemic pathologies. Thus, there is no evidence base to recommend the treatment of *H. pylori* infection in patients with extra-alimentary conditions.

New *Helicobacter* species have been described in association with hepatobiliary and inflammatory bowel disease, but research in this field is still at an early phase.

DIAGNOSTIC METHODS

Tests for the detection of *H. pylori* infection embrace a large battery of methods based on several different principles.[43–49] Several different biologic samples, including gastric mucosal specimens, gastric juice, breath, blood, stool, and urine, can be used for the assessment of *H. pylori* infection. Tests can be divided into invasive (endoscopy-based tests) and noninvasive tests, based on bacterial degradation products measurable in breath, immune reactions by antibodies, or even direct bacterial products such as antigens or DNA in stool.[45,46]

DIAGNOSTIC METHODS

DIAGNOSTIC TESTS IN *H. PYLORI* INFECTION

	Sensitivity (%)	Specificity (%)
INVASIVE TESTS		
Urease test	85–95	95–100
Histology	90–95	95–98
Culture	80–95	100
NONINVASIVE TESTS		
C13 urea breath test	85–95	95–97
H. pylori antigen – stool test	85–95	90–95
Serum IgG ELISA	70–90	65–90

Invasive techniques

Urease test

In this test a mucosal biopsy from antrum and/or body (if on PPIs) is inoculated into a small well filled with agar containing urea and a pH indicator. The substantial urease activity associated with *H. pylori* converts the urea to ammonia, leading to a pH change detected as a red color in the test gelatin, usually within 1h (Fig. 34.12). The test is sensitive and specific. The best known urease test is the CLO™ Test. Optimal incubation is at body temperature (e.g., in the pocket). Urease activity diminishes markedly (particularly in the antrum) with PPI use because of suppression and redistribution of *H. pylori.* Ideally, patients should avoid PPIs prior to urease testing, but where this is not possible (for instance with biopsies that are not preplanned) there is evidence that doing an additional body urease test enhances sensitivity.

Histology

H. pylori can usually be easily detected on the epithelial surface in hematoxylin and eosin-stained sections (see Fig. 34.1). Special stains, such as silver stain and Genta stain (see Chapter 36), aid detection. In patients on PPIs or following recent antibiotic treatment, persistence of chronic gastritis (see Fig. 34.6) is a surrogate that indicates probable recent infection.

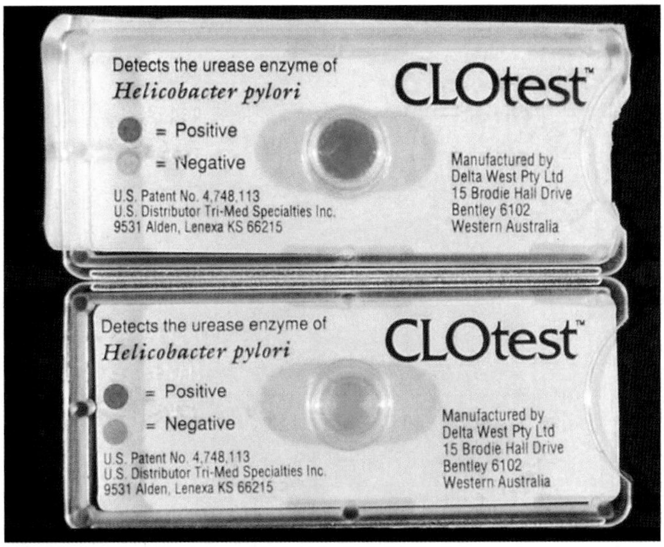

Fig. 34.12 Urease test. Top: positive; bottom: negative.

Culture

H. pylori's culture requirements are fastidious (37°C, microaerobic, 5% carbon dioxide), but culture is reliable if the organism is transported in suitable medium (e.g., Portagerm) and cultured as above.

Polymerase chain reaction (PCR)[46]

This can be used to detect *H. pylori* and to characterize whether there is expression of virulence factors such as CagA or VacA. PCR is seldom used outside research settings.

Noninvasive techniques

C13 urea breath test (Fig. 34.13)

As indicated by European *Helicobacter pylori* Study Group,[50] the C13 urea breath test should be regarded as the gold standard for noninvasive testing because of its specificity and sensitivity. As for urease testing, spurious negative results are obtained in patients taking PPIs or antibiotics currently or recently. The test is performed in a fasting state. The patient is given 75 mg [^{13}C]urea, a 2.5-g citric acid test meal (UBT-Lite), and a final breath sample is taken by direct exhalation into tubes 15 min after urea ingestion.[44] Citric acid has been shown to increase the sensitivity of the test by accelerating the appearance of isotope in the breath.

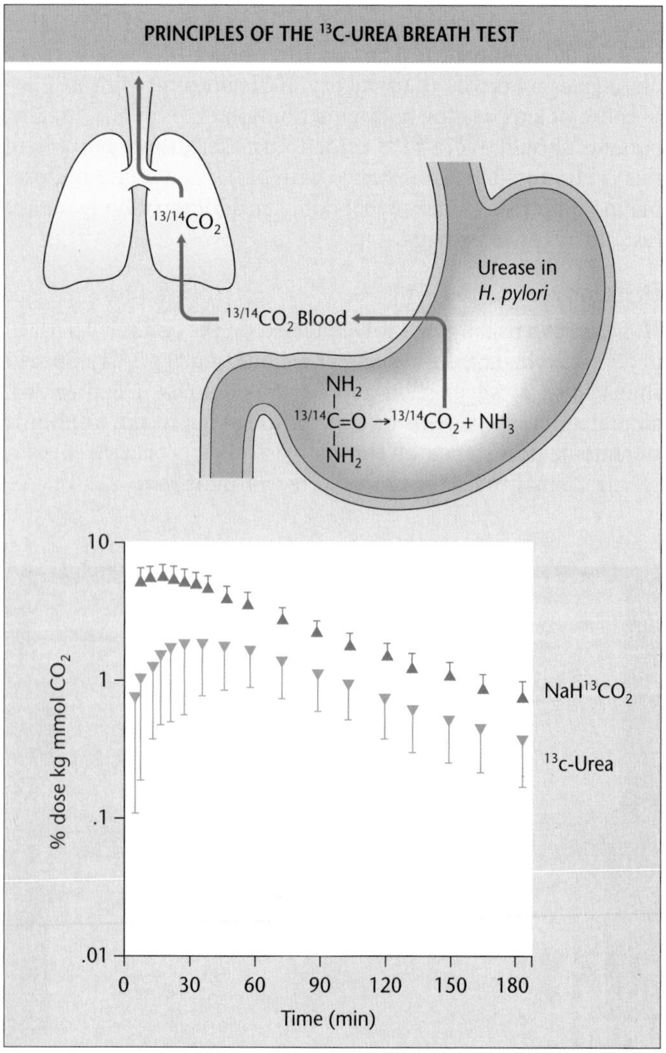

Fig. 34.13 Principles and results of C13 urea breath testing. Note the rapid rise in [^{13}C]carbon dioxide following administration of [^{13}C]urea.

H. pylori antigen stool test

A disadvantage of the C13 urea breath test is the need for specialist equipment for analysis; this means that the patient or breath sample has to be sent to a specialist center. The first generation of 'near patient' stick tests are too insensitive and nonspecific for practical use. An enzyme-linked immunosorbent assay (ELISA) or PCR-based test that detects *H. pylori* antigens or DNA in the stool[46,48] may overcome this problem. However, this test is not yet generally available and more data may be needed before its exact value is confirmed.

Serum IgG ELISA

This is a reliable test for demonstrating that a person has been infected with *H. pylori* at some time,[49] but its specificity is limited by variable antibody persistence after deliberate or incidental eradication. In general, antibodies fall during the year after eradication, but there is too much variability in the test for it to be used either to diagnose current infection or to demonstrate the success of eradication.

TREATMENT

Currently, standard treatment for *H. pylori* infection is by 'triple therapy'.[51] This consists of:

- A standard dose of a PPI given orally twice daily (see Chapter 136)
- Clarithromycin given orally twice daily
- Amoxicillin or metronidazole given orally twice daily.

Most use clarithromycin at a dose of 500 mg twice daily, as this is probably slightly more effective than a twice-daily dose of 250 mg. Amoxicillin is normally given as 1 g twice daily. Metronidazole is commonly given at a dose of 400 mg three times daily, although some argue that a higher dose is more effective and results in less drug resistance. In most parts of the world, triple therapy is given for 7 days. In the USA, where lower eradication rates have been seen with this regimen, it is more common to treat for 10 days or 2 weeks (see Chapter 136).

Modern triple therapy achieves eradication in approximately 90% of those treated[51] (Fig. 34.14) and results in permanent ulcer healing in most cases where deployed for this purpose (Fig. 34.15). Use of amoxicillin in first-line regimens should reduce development of metronidazole resistance, but gastrointestinal side effects, particularly diarrhea, are more common.

Treatment failure is frequently a result of either poor patient compliance or antibiotic resistance.[52–54] There is some evidence that compliance is improved with treatments of shorter duration, but these may be of reduced intrinsic effectiveness in some populations. The issue of antimicrobial primary resistance has become increasingly important. It has been estimated that the worldwide prevalence of primary resistance to metronidazole and clarithromycin is 20–70% and 1–12% respectively[54–56] (Table 34.3). These figures vary dramatically by region. Amoxicillin resistance appears to be extremely uncommon. Secondary resistance to metronidazole has been demonstrated in 60–70% of individuals[54] and that to clarithromycin in 30–50%.[55]

Consequently, second-line treatments have been developed. Many would use a second course of PPI–clarithromycin-based triple therapy, using a different third antibiotic (e.g.,

TREATMENT AND PREVENTION

TREATMENT FOR *H. PYLORI*

INITIAL TREATMENT

Standard triple therapy
- PPI[a] standard dose bd
- Clarithromycin 500 mg bd
- Amoxicillin 1 g bd or metronidazole 400 mg bd

Modern bismuth-based regimens
- Ranitidine bismuth citrate 400 mg bd
- Clarithromycin 500 mg bd
- Amoxicillin 1 g bd or metronidazole 400 mg bd

RETREATMENT

Standard triple therapy
- As above using a regimen different from that first employed (see text)

Quadruple therapy
- PPI[a] standard dose bd
- Tetracycline 4× 500 mg
- Metronidazole 3× 400 mg or 500 mg
- Ranitidine bismuth citrate 400 mg bd or bismuth subcitrate 4× 100 mg or bismuth subsalicylate 4× 600 mg

OPTIONS IF MULTIPLE FAILURES OCCUR

Resistance testing
- Portagerm transport medium – treatment based on susceptibility

Other regimens

Rifabutin-based (1–2 weeks)
- PPI double standard dose bd
- Rifabutin 150 mg bd
- Amoxicillin 1 g bd

Furazolidone-based (1 week)
- PPI double standard dose bd
- Bismuth chelate 240 mg bd
- Tetracycline 1 g bd
- Furazolidone 200 mg bd

[a]20 mg bd for omeprazole, esomeprazole, rabeprazole; 30 mg bd for lansoprazole; 40 mg bd for pantoprazole.

metronidazole the second time if amoxicillin was used initially). Alternatively, there are a number of regimens that are usually reserved exclusively for second-line therapy. These offer eradication rates of 70–80% and may be employed without the need for culture and antibiotic sensitivity testing. In principle, antibiotics other than those initially used should be employed. If second-line therapy fails, it is advisable to repeat a gastroscopy and obtain mucosal samples for culture and sensitivity analysis, as retreatment is unlikely to be successful with empiric (blind) therapy. Among the new emerging therapies in developed countries, the combinations of PPI plus amoxicillin and rifabutin, and PPI plus amoxicillin and levofloxacin, have been used successfully.

Indications for treatment

The current indications for therapy according to the European conference in Maastricht[50] are summarized in Table 34.4 along with supporting evidence. There are good data that *H. pylori* eradication reduces ulcer recurrence and ulcer complications, and is cost-effective where disease is due to *H. pylori*.[57–60]

TRIPLE THERAPY ERADICATION RATES

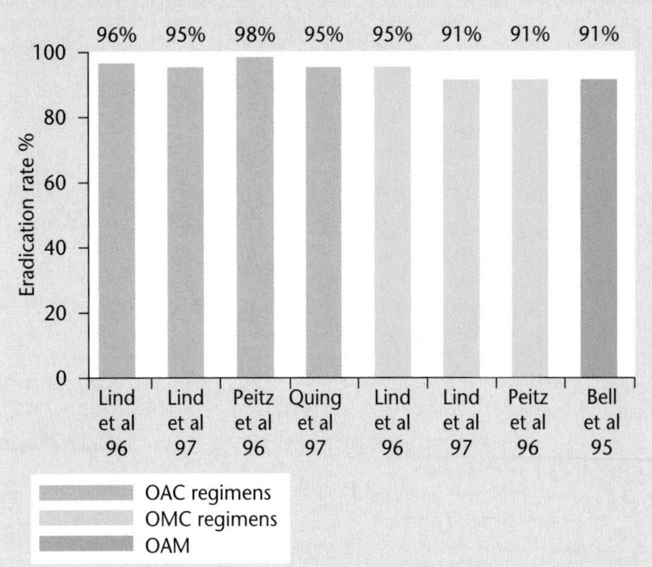

Fig. 34.14 Eradication rates with different triple therapy regimens.

Therapy without diagnosis

Because *H. pylori* is so prevalent and the cause of so much pathology, it has been suggested that it may be appropriate to treat the bacterium without diagnosing any underlying condition for which it is responsible.

Test and treat strategy

This is the most accepted noninvasive management strategy.[14,61,62] In this strategy, noninvasive *H. pylori* testing (C13 urea breath test, stool antigen assay) is undertaken as the first-line investigation in young people (age less than 45 years) who present with dyspepsia without alarm symptoms. Those who are *H. pylori* positive subsequently receive an accepted eradication therapy, whereas those who are not infected receive empiric symptomatic treatment. Such a strategy has advantages in reducing the endoscopy workload and is cost-effective in populations

TABLE 34.3 GLOBAL *H. PYLORI* RESISTANCE TO CURRENTLY USED ANTIBIOTICS

	H. pylori-resistant strains (%)	
	Clarithromycin	**Metronidazole**
USA	8	37
Germany	2–3	26
Netherlands	2	21
Spain	15	37
France	14	25
Bulgaria	12	29
China	8	50
Japan	12	13

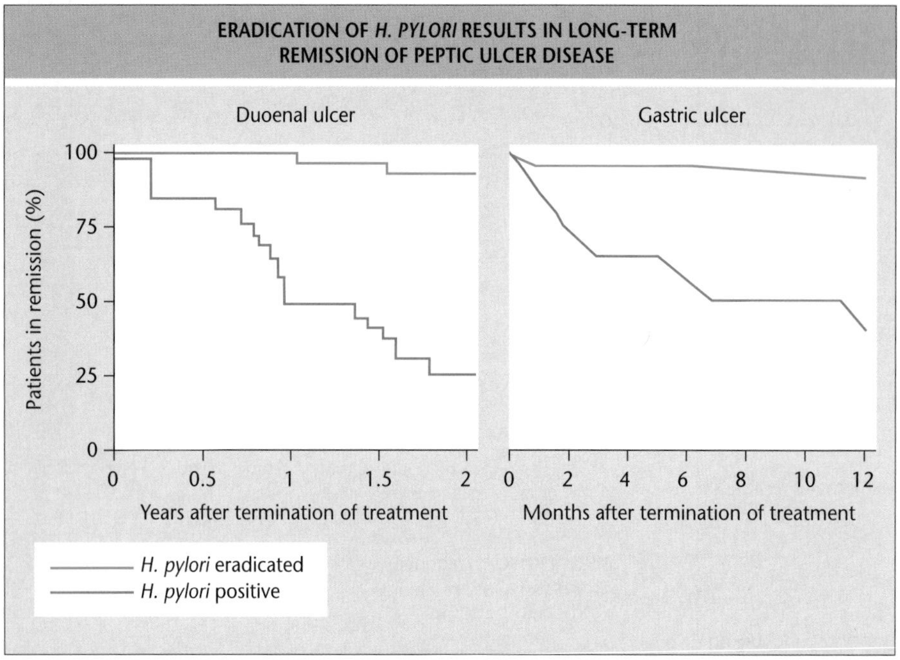

Fig. 34.15 Low relapse rate following *H. pylori* eradication in duodenal ulcer and gastric ulcer.

TABLE 34.4 *H. PYLORI* MANAGEMENT: MAASTRICHT 2 RECOMMENDATIONS

Indication	Scientific evidence
STRONGLY RECOMMENDED INDICATIONS	
Duodenal or gastric ulcer (active or not, including complicated peptic ulcer disease)	1
MALToma	2
Atrophic gastritis	2
Postgastritis cancer resection	3
Patients who are first-degree relatives of a patient with gastric cancer	3
Patient wishes (after full consultation with their physician)	4
DISCRETIONARY INDICATIONS AND RELEVANT STATEMENTS	
Functional dyspepsia	
• *H. pylori* eradication is an appropriate option	2
• This leads to long-term symptom improvement in a subset of patients	2
Gastroesophageal reflux disease (GERD)	
H. pylori eradication:	
• Is not associated with GERD development in most cases	3
• Does not exacerbate existing GERD	3
H. pylori should be eradicated, however, in patients requiring long-term profound acid suppression	3
NSAIDs	
H. pylori eradication:	
• Reduces the incidence of ulcer, given before NSAID use	2
• Alone, is insufficient to prevent recurrent ulcer bleeding in high-risk NSAID users	2
• Does not enhance healing of gastric or duodenal ulcers in patients receiving antisecretory therapy who continue to take NSAIDs	1
H. pylori and NSAIDs/aspirin are independent risk factors for peptic ulcer disease	2

with a background prevalence of infection greater than 20%. A strategy of empiric drug treatment for patients with dyspepsia may be more cost-effective where background prevalence is low (see Chapter 5).

'Search and treat'[63] serves two purposes:

- To identify patients taking chronic antisecretory therapy (PPI, H_2 receptor antagonists) for dyspeptic symptoms who may be naive *H. pylori*-positive ulcer patients – eradication will resolve their problems
- To identify *H. pylori* infection in first-degree relations of patients with gastric cancer – the aim is to eliminate the risk factor.

'Screen and treat' is, for many gastroenterologists, the ultimate way of resolving all *H. pylori*-related pathologies. However, the financial cost of current therapies and their side effects (including development of antibiotic resistance), as well as the falling prevalence of *H. pylori* in many parts of the world, preclude widespread adoption of this strategy.

PROGNOSIS AND WHAT TO TELL PATIENTS

Untreated peptic ulcer disease influences life expectancy.[64] Following successful *H. pylori* eradication, prognosis can be excellent, depending on the condition treated. Reinfection is rare in adult life and relapse of (non-NSAID) ulcers even rarer with true successful eradication and no reinfection. For most patients with gastric cancer, *H. pylori* eradication is of limited value, although there have been claims that early gastric cancers regress with treatment. Limited evidence also suggests that *H. pylori* eradication in advanced gastritis may reduce the risk of developing gastric cancer compared with noneradication, although more data are needed (see Chapter 37). Remarkably, *H. pylori* eradication alone results in regression of many cases of lymphoma (see Chapter 38). There is more controversy about the long-term impact of *H. pylori* eradication in healthy individuals. At present, there are no clear data to support the fear that diseases such as Barrett's esophagus (see Chapter 31), esophageal cancer (see Chapter 32), or proximal gastric cancer (see Chapter 37) will become more common.

SOURCES OF INFORMATION FOR PATIENTS AND DOCTORS

http://www.patient.co.uk/showdoc/349/
http://www.medhelp.org/HealthTopics/Helicobacter.html
http://digestive.niddk.nih.gov/ddiseases/pubs/hpylori/index.htm
http://www.gastro.org/generalPublic.html

CURRENT RESEARCH AND FUTURE TRENDS

Current research is dedicated to the identification of new molecules with selective anti *H. pylori* activity to be used as monotherapy. Various approaches to treat *H. pylori*-infected volunteers with vaccines have failed, but the use of vaccines as strategy of primary prevention still holds promise. Prevention or global screening and therapy of those infected holds the potential not only to close the chapter on 'peptic ulcer disease' (in the absence of NSAIDs) but probably also on gastric cancer in the distal stomach.

REFERENCES

1. Blaser MJ, Berg DE. *Helicobacter pylori* genetic diversity and risk of human disease. J Clin Invest 2001; 107:767–773.
2. Odenbreit S, Puls J, Sedlmaier B, Gerland E, Fischer W, Haas R. Translocation of *Helicobacter pylori* CagA into gastric epithelial cells by type IV secretion. Science 2000; 287:1497–1500.
3. Naumann M, Crabtree JE. *Helicobacter pylori*-induced epithelial cell signalling in gastric carcinogenesis. Trends Microbiol 2004; 12:29–36.
4. Blaser MJ, Atherton JC. *Helicobacter pylori* persistence: biology and disease. J Clin Invest 2004; 113:321–333.
5. Malfertheiner P. *H. pylori* infection and peptic ulcer disease. In: Olbe L (ed). Proton pump inhibitors. Basel: Birkhäuser; 1999: 173–191.
6. Mitchell H, Megraud F. Epidemiology and diagnosis of *Helicobacter pylori* infection. Helicobacter 2002; 7(Suppl 1):8–16.
7. Pilotto A, Malfertheiner P. An approach to *Helicobacter pylori* infection in the elderly. Aliment Pharmacol Ther 2002; 16:683–691.
8. Sherman PM. Appropriate strategies for testing and treating *Helicobacter pylori* in children: when and how? Am J Med 2004; 117(Suppl 5A):30S–35S.
9. Leontiadis GI, Sharma VK, Howden CW. Non-gastrointestinal tract associations of *Helicobacter pylori* infection. Arch Intern Med 1999; 159:925–940.
10. Marshall BJ, Armstrong JA, McGechie DB, Glancy RJ. Attempt to fulfil Koch's postulates for pyloric *Campylobacter*. Med J Aust 1985; 142:436–439.
11. Hocker M, Hohenberger P. *Helicobacter pylori* virulence factors – one part of a big picture. Lancet 2003; 362:1231–1233.
12. Macarthur M, Hold GL, El-Omar EM. Inflammation and cancer II. Role of chronic inflammation and cytokine gene polymorphisms in the pathogenesis of gastrointestinal malignancy. Am J Physiol Gastrointest Liver Physiol 2004; 286:G515–G520.
13. Hayat M, Arora DS, Dixon MF, Clark B, O'Mahony S. Effects of *Helicobacter pylori* eradication on the natural history of lymphocytic gastritis. Gut 1999; 45:495–498.
14. Madsen LG, Taskiran M, Bytzer P. Menetrier's disease. Another *Helicobacter pylori* associated disease? Ugeskr Laeger 2000; 162:4250–4253.
15. Gasbarrini A, Carloni E, Gasbarrini G, Chisholm S. *H. pylori* and extragastric diseases – other helicobacters. Helicobacter 2004; 9(Suppl 1):57–66.
16. Stopeck A. Links between *Helicobacter pylori* infection, cobalamin deficiency, and pernicious anemia. Arch Intern Med 2000; 160:1229–1230.
17. Chey WD, Moayyedi P. Uninvestigated dyspepsia and non-ulcer dyspepsia – the use of endoscopy and the roles of *Helicobacter pylori* eradication and antisecretory therapy. Aliment Pharmacol Ther 2004; 19(Suppl 1):1–8.
18. Moayyedi P, Malfertheiner P. *H. pylori* in non-malignant disease. Helicobacter 2002; 7(Suppl 1):30–36.
19. Bodger K, Crabtree JE. *Helicobacter pylori* and gastric inflammation. Br Med Bull 1998; 54:139–150.
20. Fox JG, Beck P, Dangler CA et al. Concurrent enteric helminth infection modulates inflammation and gastric immune responses and reduces helicobacter-induced gastric atrophy. Nat Med 2000; 6:536–542.
21. Atherton J, Cao P, Peek RM, Tummuru MKR, Blaser MJ, Cover TC. Mosaicism in vacuolating cytotoxin alleles of *Helicobacter pylori*: association of specific *vacA* types with cytotoxin production and peptic ulceration. J Biol Chem 1995; 270:17771–17777.
22. Crabtree JE, Taylor JD, Wyatt JI et al. Mucosal IgA recognition of *Helicobacter pylori* 120 kDa protein, peptic ulceration, and gastric pathology. Lancet 1991; 338:332–335.
23. Yamaoka Y, Kikuchi S, El-Zimaity HMT et al. Importance of *Helicobacter pylori oipA* in clinical presentation, gastric inflammation, and mucosal interleukin 8 production. Gastroenterology 2002; 123:414–424.
24. Malaty HM, Graham DY, Isaksson I, Engstrand L, Pedersen NL. Co-twin study of the effect of environment and dietary elements on acquisition of *Helicobacter pylori* infection. Am J Epidemiol 1998; 148:793–797.
25. Rothenbacher D, Weyermann M, Bode G, Kulaksiz M, Stahl B, Brenner H. Role of Lewis A and Lewis B blood group antigens in *Helicobacter pylori* infection. Helicobacter 2004; 9:324–329.
26. Moss SF, Legon S, Bishop AE, Polak JM, Calam J. Effect of *Helicobacter pylori* on gastric somatostatin in duodenal ulcer disease. Lancet 1992; 340:930–932.
27. NIH Consensus Conference. *Helicobacter pylori* in peptic ulcer disease. JAMA 1994; 272:65–69.
28. Chan FK, Graham DY. Prevention of non-steroidal anti-inflammatory drug gastrointestinal complications – review and recommendations based on risk assessment. Aliment Pharmacol Ther 2004; 19:1051–1061.
29. Hawkey CJ. *Helicobacter pylori*, NSAIDs and cognitive dissonance. Aliment Pharmacol Ther 1999; 13:695–702.
30. International Agency for Research on Cancer 1994.
31. Correa P. Human gastric carcinogenesis: a multistep and multifactorial process – First American Cancer Society Award Lecture on Cancer Epidemiology and Prevention. Cancer Res 1992; 52: 6735–6740.
32. Blaser MJ, Pérez-Pérez GI, Kleanthous H et al. Infection with *Helicobacter pylori* strains possessing *cagA* associated with an increased risk of developing adenocarcinoma of the stomach. Cancer Res 1995; 55:2111–2115.
33. Peek RM Jr, Blaser MJ. *Helicobacter pylori* and gastrointestinal tract adenocarcinomas. Nat Rev Cancer 2002; 2:28–37.
34. Peterson WL. *Helicobacter pylori* and gastric adenocarcinoma. Aliment Pharmacol Ther 2002; 16(Suppl 1):40–46.
35. Leung WK, Lin SR, Ching JY et al. Factors predicting progression of gastric intestinal metaplasia: results of a randomised trial on *Helicobacter pylori* eradication. Gut 2004; 53:1244–1249.
36. Watanabe T, Tada M, Nagai H, et al. *H. pylori* infection induces gastric cancer in Mongolian gerbils. Gastroenterology 1998; 115:642–648.
37. Hirayama F, Takagi S, Iwao E, et al. Development of poorly differentiated adenocarcinoma and carcinoid due to long-term *Helicobacter pylori* colonization in Mongolian gerbils. J Gastroenterol 1999; 34:450–454.
38. Sugiyama A, Maruta F, Ikeno T, et al. *H. pylori* infection enhances N-methyl-N-nitrosourea-induced stomach carcinogenesis in the Mongolian gerbil. Cancer Res 1998; 58:2067–2069.
39. Fox JG, Sheppard BJ, Dangler CA, et al. Germ-line p53-targeted disruption inhibits *Helicobacter*-induced premalignant lesions and invasive gastric carcinoma through down-regulation of Th 1 proinflammatory responses. Cancer Res 2002; 62:696–702.
40. Wong BC, Lam SK, Wong WM, et al. *H. pylori* eradication to prevent gastric cancer in a high-risk region of China: a randomized controlled trial. JAMA 2004; 291:187–194.
41. Ahmad A, Govil Y, Frank BB. Gastric mucosa-associated lymphoid tissue lymphoma. Am J Gastroenterol 2003; 98:975–986.
42. Lehours P, Menard A, Dupouy S et al. Evaluation of the association of nine *Helicobacter pylori* virulence factors with strains involved in low-grade gastric mucosa-associated lymphoid tissue lymphoma. Infect Immun 2004; 72:880–888.
43. Goddard AF, Logan RP. Diagnostic methods for *Helicobacter pylori* detection and eradication. Br J Clin Pharmacol 2003; 56:273–283.
44. Gatta L, Ricci C, Tampieri A, Vaira D. Non-invasive techniques for the diagnosis of *Helicobacter pylori* infection. Clin Microbiol Infect 2003; 9:489–496.
45. Vaira D, Vakil N, Menegatti M et al. The stool antigen test for detection of *Helicobacter pylori* after eradication therapy. Ann Intern Med 2002; 136:280–287.

46. Kabir S. Detection of *Helicobacter pylori* DNA in feces and saliva by polymerase chain reaction: a review. Helicobacter 2004; 9:115–123.
47. Hjalmarsson S, Sjolund M, Engstrand L. Determining antibiotic resistance in *Helicobacter pylori*. Expert Rev Mol Diagn 2002; 2:267–272.
48. Talley NJ, Newell DG, Ormand JE et al. Serodiagnosis of *Helicobacter pylori*: comparison of enzyme-linked immunosorbent assays. J Clin Microbiol 1991; 29:1635–1639.
49. Perez-Perez GI, Cutler AF, Blaser MJ. Value of serology as a noninvasive method for evaluating the efficacy of treatment of *Helicobacter pylori* infection. Clin Infect Dis 1997; 25:1038–1043.
50. Malfertheiner P, Megraud F, O'Morain C et al. European Helicobacter Pylori Study Group (EHPSG). Current concepts in the management of *Helicobacter pylori* infection – the Maastricht 2-2000 Consensus Report. Aliment Pharmacol Ther 2002; 16:167–180.
51. Ulmer HJ, Beckerling A, Gatz G. Recent use of proton pump inhibitor-based triple therapies for the eradication of *H. pylori*: a broad data review. Helicobacter 2003; 8:95–104.
52. Qasim A, O'Morain CA. Treatment of *Helicobacter pylori* infection and factors influencing eradication. Aliment Pharmacol Ther 2002; 16(Suppl 1):24–30.
53. Broutet N, Tchamgoue S, Pereira E, Lamouliatte H, Salamon R, Megraud F. Risk factors for failure of *Helicobacter pylori* therapy – results of an individual data analysis of 2751 patients. Aliment Pharmacol Ther 2003; 17:99–109.
54. Jenks PJ, Edwards DI. Metronidazole resistance in *Helicobacter pylori*. Int J Antimicrob Agents 2002; 19:1–7.
55. Menard A, Santos A, Megraud F, Oleastro M. PCR-restriction fragment length polymorphism can also detect point mutation A2142C in the 23S rRNA gene, associated with *Helicobacter pylori* resistance to clarithromycin. Antimicrob Agents Chemother 2002; 46:1156–1157 (letter).
56. Hjalmarsson S, Sjolund M, Engstrand L. Determining antibiotic resistance in *Helicobacter pylori*. Expert Rev Mol Diagn 2002; 2:267–272.
57. Holtmann G, Howden CW. Management of peptic ulcer bleeding – the roles of proton pump inhibitors and *Helicobacter pylori* eradication. Aliment Pharmacol Ther 2004; 19(Suppl 1):66–70.
58. Roderick P, Davies R, Raftery J et al. The cost-effectiveness of screening for *Helicobacter pylori* to reduce mortality and morbidity from gastric cancer and peptic ulcer disease: a discrete-event simulation model. Health Technol Assess 2003; 7:1–86.
59. Ford AC, Delaney BC, Forman D, Moayyedi P. Eradication therapy in *Helicobacter pylori* positive peptic ulcer disease: systematic review and economic analysis. Am J Gastroenterol 2004; 99:1833–1855.
60. Gisbert JP, Khorrami S, Carballo F, Calvet X, Gene E, Dominguez-Munoz JE. *H. pylori* eradication therapy vs. antisecretory non-eradication therapy (with or without long-term maintenance antisecretory therapy) for the prevention of recurrent bleeding from peptic ulcer. Cochrane Database Syst Rev 2003; (4)CD004062.
61. Manes G, Menchise A, de Nucci C, Balzano A. Empirical prescribing for dyspepsia: randomised controlled trial of test and treat versus omeprazole treatment. *BMJ* 2003; 326:1118.
62. Chey WD, Moayyedi P. Uninvestigated dyspepsia and non-ulcer dyspepsia – the use of endoscopy and the roles of *Helicobacter pylori* eradication and antisecretory therapy. Aliment Pharmacol Ther 2004; 19(Suppl 1):1–8.
63. Forman D, Graham DY. Impact of *Helicobacter pylori* on society – role for a strategy of "search and eradicate". Aliment Pharmacol Ther 2004; 19(Suppl 1):17–21.
64. Inadomi JM, Sonnenberg A. The impact of peptic ulcer disease and infection with *Helicobacter pylori* on life expectancy. Am J Gastroenterol 1998; 93:1286–1290.

Chapter 35

Peptic ulcer

C J Hawkey and J C Atherton

KEY POINTS
• *Helicobacter pylori* and NSAIDs are the commonest cause of peptic ulceration • Most duodenal ulcers are caused by *H. pylori* • Most gastric ulcers are caused by NSAIDs • The proportion of idiopathic ulcers is small but likely to rise as *H. pylori* prevalence falls • Smoking is an important cofactor for *H. pylori*-induced duodenal ulcers • Virulence factors (CagA, VacA) influence whether colonization leads to ulceration • NSAIDs inhibit the synthesis of gastroprotective prostaglandins • Follow-up endoscopy is indicated for gastric but not duodenal ulcers to exclude cancer or lymphoma • Zollinger-Ellison syndrome, multiple endocrine neoplasia, and systemic mastocytosis are unusual causes of peptic ulceration • One-week triple therapy heals ulcers and eradicates *H. pylori* in over 90% of cases • NSAID toxicity can be reduced by switching to a Coxib OR combining NSAID and proton pump inhibitor (PPI) • Low dose aspirin (75mg/day) carries a risk of peptic ulceration; consider PPI in at-risk groups • Eradication of *H. pylori* in NSAID ulcers is controversial • Most of the mortality due to bleeding peptic ulcer is not due to exsanguination

INTRODUCTION, INCLUDING DEFINITION

Peptic ulcers are localized breaches of the gastric or duodenal mucosa with tissue destruction at least to the depth of the muscularis mucosa (Fig. 35.1). The word 'peptic' reflects a belief (probably misplaced) that peptic activity is involved in pathogenesis. Peptic ulcers include ulcers in the stomach, pylorus, duodenum, or a Meckel's diverticulum, as well as ulcers at sites of gastrointestinal anastomosis (stomal ulcers) and at the gastroesophageal junction (Fig. 35.2). The commonest symptom is pain. The most serious complications are bleeding and perforation.

CAUSES OF PEPTIC ULCERATION

It is only in the past 20 years that the causes of peptic ulcers have been identified and rational management defined. Previous speculations about causation, which resulted in management strategies that were misplaced or of peripheral relevance, continue to contaminate some accounts of peptic ulceration.

Common causes

Most ulcers are directly caused by infection with *Helicobacter pylori* or by nonsteroidal anti-inflammatory drugs (NSAIDs),[1–5] including aspirin[6,7] (Fig. 35.3), which inhibit prostaglandin synthesis and abrogate mucosal defence mechanisms. In developed countries, duodenal ulcers are proportionally caused more commonly by *H. pylori* and gastric ulcers by NSAIDs, but either factor may produce an ulcer at either site. In patients who deny NSAID use and in whom a test for *H. pylori* is negative,[8] *H. pylori* and NSAIDs are still the most likely causes. Tests for *H. pylori* have a low but measurable false-negative rate and NSAIDs purchased directly, and sometimes unknowingly in compound preparations, are easily ignored by doctors and patients.

CAUSES AND RISK FACTORS

COMMON AND UNCOMMON CAUSES OF PEPTIC ULCERATION

Causes of peptic ulcer	Main mechanisms
COMMON	
Helicobacter pylori	Inflammation, toxin, acid
NSAIDs	Compromised mucosal defence
LESS COMMON	
Zollinger-Ellison syndrome	
Multiple endocrine neoplasia	Acid hypersecretion
Systemic mastocytosis	
Duodenal Crohn's disease	Inflammation
Radiation	
Stress ulcers	
Celiac axis stenosis	Ischemia or compromised mucosal defence
Hepatic artery chemotherapy	
CONTROVERSIAL	
Corticosteroids	Enhance risks in NSAID users
Idiopathic	Some cases represent missed *H. pylori* or NSAIDs

Uncommon causes

Uncommon, but significant, causes of peptic ulcers include conditions with *acid hypersecretion* (Zollinger-Ellison syndrome, multiple endocrine neoplasia, and mastocytosis[9]; see Chapter 109) severe *physical stress* such as being in intensive care, and *mucosal ischemia* due to critical celiac axis vascular disease and radiation.

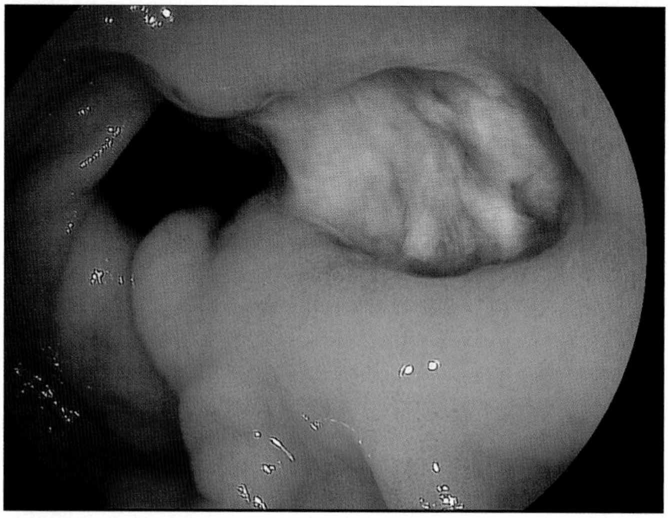

Fig. 35.1 Large pyloric ulcer with red spot (minor bleeding stigma). (Courtesy of Dr Marco Bruno, Academic Medical Center, Amsterdam.)

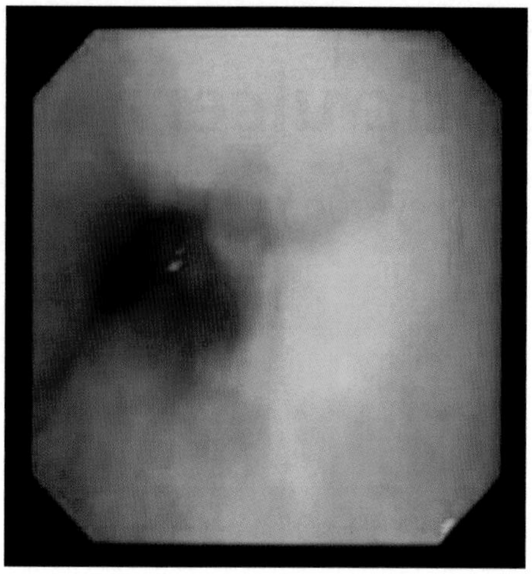

Fig. 35.2 Ulceration of the gastroesophageal junction.

Controversies

There is continuing debate about whether *corticosteroids* alone can cause ulcers,[10,11] although the ability of corticosteroids to enhance NSAID-associated ulcers is well established (see below).[11,12]

Idiopathic ulcers are rare. Most are probably due to falsely negative *H. pylori* tests or sporadic or surreptitious NSAID use. If these causes are confidently excluded, rare conditions such as those described above should be sought. However, a small group of idiopathic peptic ulcers still exist and, because of falling *H. pylori* prevalence, the proportion of peptic ulcers that are idiopathic is likely to be increasing.[8]

EPIDEMIOLOGY

The epidemiology of peptic ulceration reflects that of the main underlying causes (see Chapter 34 for *H. pylori* and Chapter 25 for NSAIDs). The early twentieth century saw a rapid rise in the incidence of duodenal ulceration in westernized societies.[13] This has been attributed to the spread of *H. pylori*, although this seems unlikely as the bacterium appears to have been ubiquitous in the population for centuries. A change in environment appears most likely, and one possibility is the widespread adoption of smoking – an important co-factor for duodenal ulceration in *H. pylori*-colonized people.

The prevalence of both *H. pylori* and peptic ulcer is falling in westernized societies,[13] probably due to improvements in hygiene in the twentieth century[14] (Fig. 35.4). In other parts of the world such as Hong Kong where *H. pylori* remains common, the prevalence of peptic ulcer also remains high. However, in Africa the prevalence of *H. pylori* is high but peptic ulcer is paradoxically uncommon. Other factors, whether differences in unidentified environmental influences or in bacterial pathgenicity, must play a part.

As the prevalence of *H. pylori* infection has fallen, the importance of NSAIDs as a cause of peptic ulceration has increased, and low-dose aspirin is now the fastest growing cause of ulcer complications[15,16] (Fig. 35.5). Newer NSAIDS that are selective for cyclo-oxygenase (COX) 2 and less toxic to the stomach or duodenum should lead to a reduced incidence of ulceration,[17,18] but this is not yet clear.

RISK FACTORS FOR PEPTIC ULCER DISEASE

The influence of risk factors depends largely but not entirely on whether the peptic ulcer is caused by *H. pylori* or NSAIDs.[19–22]

Peptic ulcer is an age-related disease for both *H. pylori* and NSAIDs (see Fig. 35.4). In *H. pylori*-infected patients, smoking enhances the risk considerably, but has no independent influence after eradication. Whether smoking increases the risk of developing an NSAID ulcer is less certain. Family history largely reflects 'shared' *H. pylori* infection, although the increased incidence of blood group O in patients with duodenal ulcer may indicate a minor genetic influence. A previous history of peptic ulcer increases risk for ulcers caused both by *H. pylori* infection and NSAID use. Some recent evidence suggest that risk may persist after NSAID cessation,[21] which might explain some 'idiopathic' ulceration.[8] It is clear that different NSAIDs affect the risk of peptic ulcer to different extents, and that risk is highly dose dependent[23] (Fig. 35.6).

Risk factors in patients using *low-dose aspirin* are less well defined, but rates of ulcer bleeding are higher in patients with

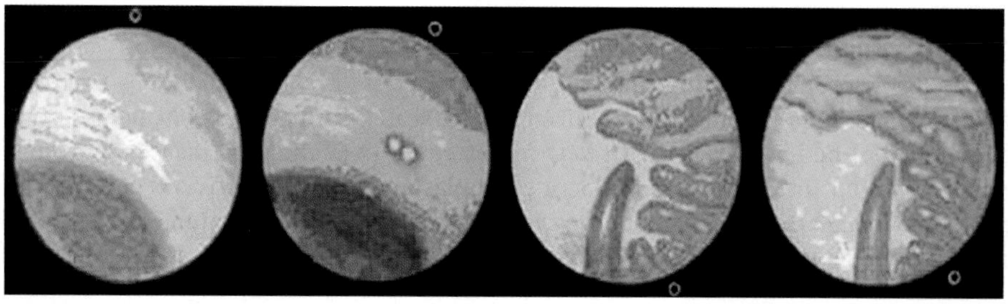

Fig. 35.3 First demonstration of aspirin-induced gastric damage. (Reproduced from Douthwaite & Lintott, *Lancet* 1938.[7])

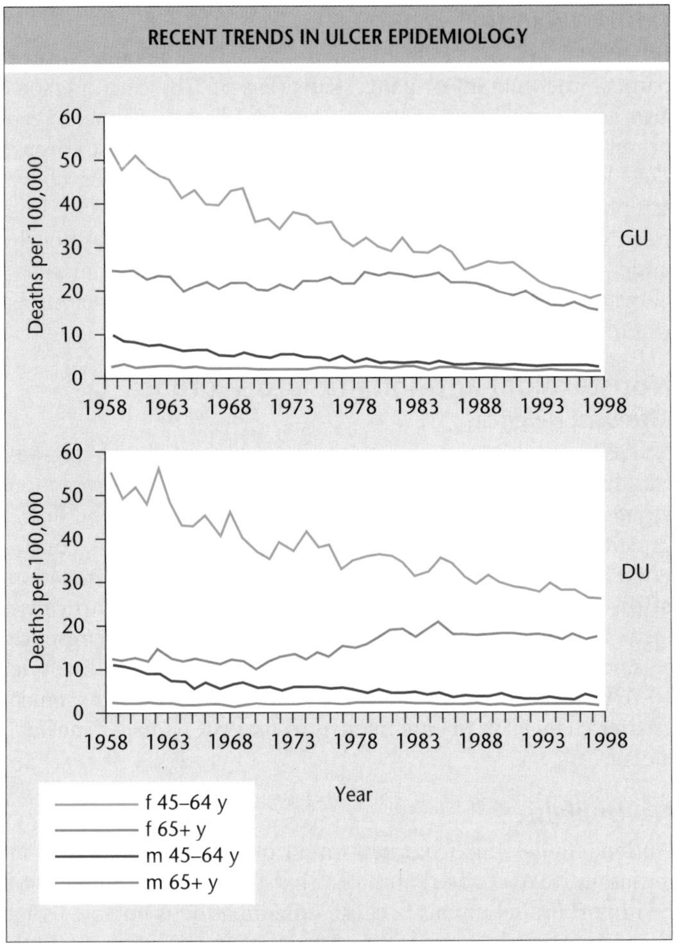

Fig. 35.4 Recent trends in ulcer epidemiology. Top: Deaths from gastric ulcer and unspecified peptic ulcer. Bottom: Deaths from duodenal ulcer. (Reproduced from Higham et al.,[14] with permission.)

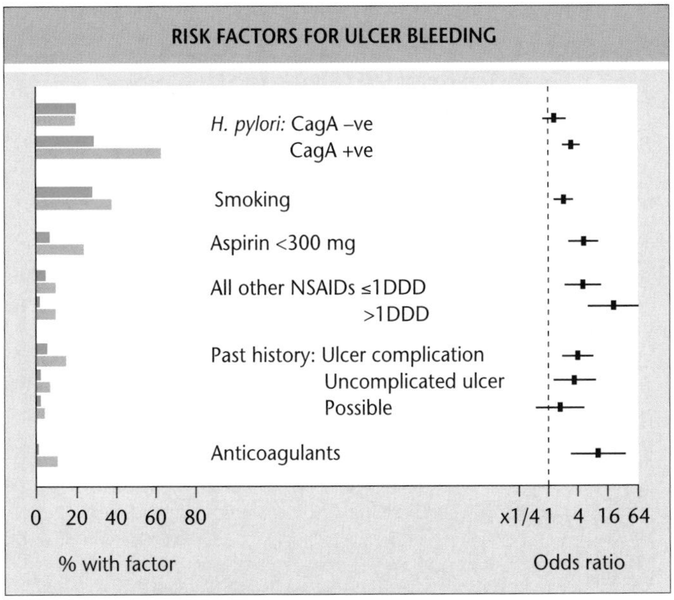

Fig. 35.5 Causes of peptic ulceration. Association of peptic ulcer bleeding with CagA-positive *H. pylori* infection, smoking, aspirin, non-aspirin NSAIDs, past history, and anticoagulants. Left: Proportion of controls (blue) and all cases (red) with the factor. Right: Odds ratio for ulcer bleeding based on data reported by Stack et al.[15]

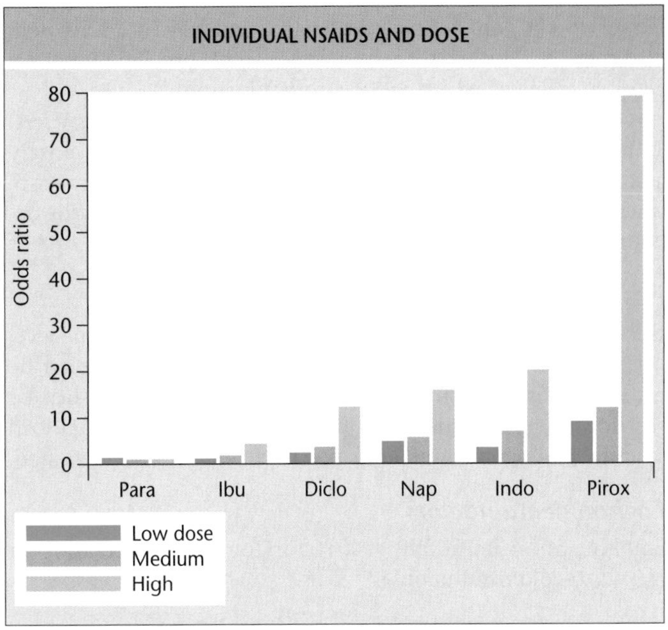

Fig. 35.6 Differences in odds ratio for peptic ulcer bleeding with individual NSAIDs and doses. Note: Confidence intervals were wide (not shown for groups). Para, paracetamol; Ibu, ibuprofen; Diclo, diclofenac; Nap, naproxen; Indo, idomethacin; Pirox, piroxicam.

a past history and in elderly patients.[15] Risk factors for rare causes are unclear, and in some instances (e.g., Zollinger-Ellison syndrome) the underlying disease is a dominant influence.

Disease associations

Peptic ulcer is more common in patients with chronic obstructive lung disease, cirrhosis, coronary artery disease, and renal failure,[14] and in coal miners, possibly because of shared risk factors, including *H. pylori* infection or hypergastrinemia.

PATHOGENESIS

It is a truism that mucosal integrity represents a balance between aggressive and protective factors. *H. pylori* infection and acid are the main aggressive factors. The main protective factors are mucus and bicarbonate secretion, hydrophobicity (waxiness) of epithelial cells, and mucosal blood flow. These are mediated by prostaglandins (and other mediators such as nitric oxide) and abrogated when their synthesis is inhibited by NSAIDs.[3]

H. pylori-associated ulcers

H. pylori colonization is lifelong in the absence of effective treatment,[24] yet only about 15% of infected people develop peptic ulceration in their lifetime. The development of ulceration is due to a combination of bacterial virulence, host genetic susceptibility, and environmental co-factors.

Bacterial virulence

The best understood bacterial virulence factor is the *cag* pathogenicity island (*cag* PAI). *H. pylori* strains possessing this factor induce more inflammation and are more closely associated with peptic ulceration and gastric adenocarcinoma than *cag*-negative strains.[24–26] The *cag* PAI is a collection of genes encoding a bacterial type IV secretion system, a sort of molecular syringe through which at least one protein, CagA, is 'injected' into epithelial cells.[27] Several signaling pathways are activated, resulting in epithelial cell changes and pro-inflammatory cytokine release, which induces inflammation.[28]

A second virulence factor is the vacuolating cytotoxin, VacA. *H. pylori* strains producing more active forms are more closely associated with disease.[29,30] Other factors that have been associated with increased strain pathogenicity include an adhesin, BabA,[31] and an outer membrane inflammatory protein, OipA.[32]

Host susceptibility

Genetic polymorphisms in some cytokine genes increase the level of inflammation induced by *H. pylori*, induce the pan-gastritic pattern of inflammation, and increase the risk of *H. pylori*-associated gastric atrophy and adenocarcinoma.[33] Specific factors that lead to antral predominant inflammation have not yet been identified.

Environmental factors

Smoking is an important risk factor for peptic ulceration in *H. pylori*-colonized people.[19]

Localization of *H. pylori*-associated ulcers

Duodenal ulceration

Duodenal ulcers occur against a background of *H. pylori* colonization with a predominantly antral pattern of gastritis (Fig. 35.7A). Antral inflammation results in reduced somatostatin production by antral D cells and, as somatostatin normally has a negative feedback on gastrin, this results in hypergastrinemia.[34] Gastrin stimulates the healthy gastric corpus to produce more acid. The increased acid load in the duodenum contributes to the formation of gastric metaplasia – a (possibly protective) change in the duodenal mucosa to resemble that in the stomach. *H. pylori*, which can colonize only gastric-type mucosa, can now colonize the duodenum and cause inflammation, damage, and ulceration (Fig. 35.7A).

Gastric ulceration

Gastric ulcers occur in *H. pylori*-colonized people with a corpus-predominant or pangastritis (Fig. 35.7B). Such persons also have hypergastrinemia, but acid production is unchanged or reduced because of the inflamed and damaged gastric corpus. This leads to a cycle of chronic damage with progressive atrophy of gastric glands and further hypochlorhydria. The pathogenesis of gastric ulceration in this environment is poorly understood, but ulcers usually occur in the transitional zone, between antrum and corpus mucosa, often on the lesser curve, where inflammation is usually heavy.

Nonsteroidal anti-inflammatory drugs

Mucosal defence

NSAIDs inhibit the synthesis of gastroduodenal prostaglandins, which are centrally important for mucosal protection via mucus and bicarbonate secretion and mucosal blood flow.[3] Prostaglandins are thought to be dependent on the constitutively expressed COX-1 enzyme (but see below). Abrogation of prostaglandin-dependent mechanisms is sufficient to cause local erosions, which deepen to form ulcers in the presence of acid and pepsin. A central role for pepsin is more likely in NSAID ulcers than in ulcers caused by *H. pylori*, as much greater changes in pH are needed to prevent damage[35] or heal ulcers.[36]

Neutrophils

Animal studies implicate neutrophil plugging of capillaries in initiating NSAID gastric injury,[37] but this appears unlikely to be important in humans because inflammation is notable by its absence. Animal studies also suggest that inhibition of both COX-1 and COX-2 is needed for mucosal injury,[37] but again the relevance to humans is unclear as pure COX-1 inhibitors are not available for human use.

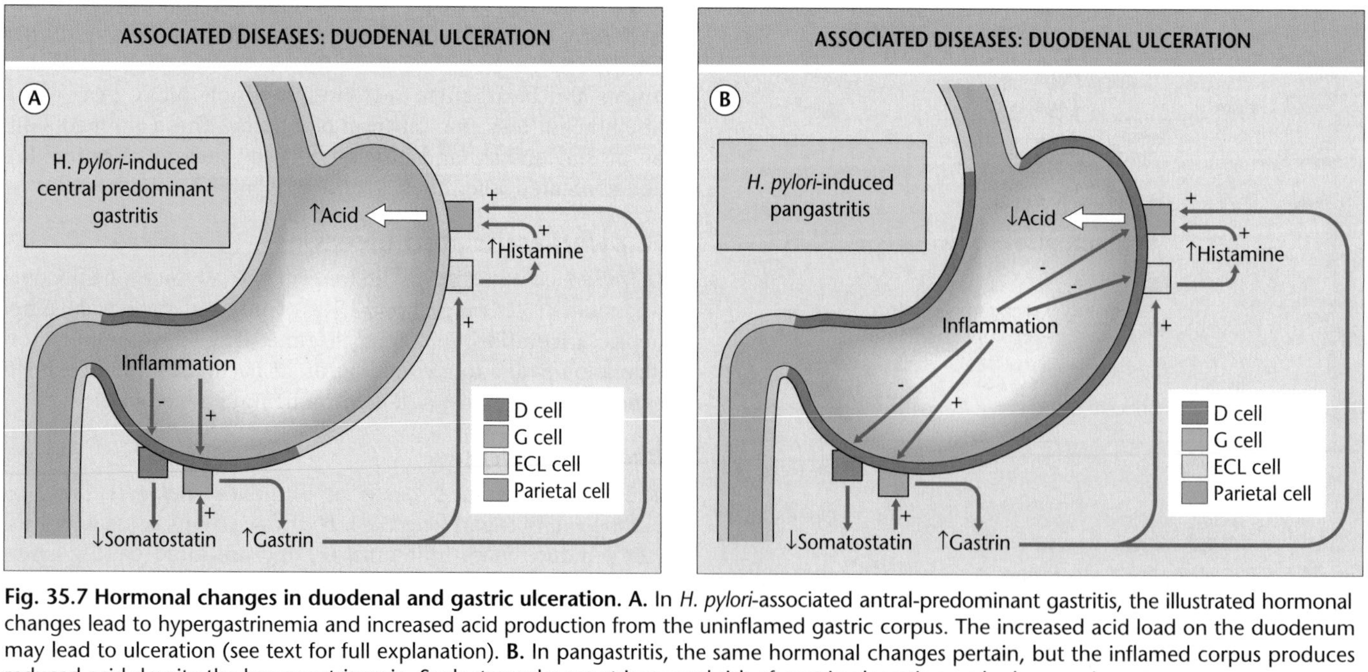

Fig. 35.7 Hormonal changes in duodenal and gastric ulceration. A. In *H. pylori*-associated antral-predominant gastritis, the illustrated hormonal changes lead to hypergastrinemia and increased acid production from the uninflamed gastric corpus. The increased acid load on the duodenum may lead to ulceration (see text for full explanation). **B.** In pangastritis, the same hormonal changes pertain, but the inflamed corpus produces reduced acid despite the hypergastrinemia. Such stomachs are at increased risk of gastric ulceration and adenocarcinoma.

Hemostasis

Aspirin inhibits thromboxane synthesis and platelet aggregation. The extent to which ulceration and impaired hemostasis contribute to ulcer bleeding in patients on low-dose aspirin is undetermined.

Other ulcer types

Acid plays a dominant role in ulcers associated with gastrinomas, whether sporadic or occurring in the multiple endocrine neoplasia (MEN) 1 syndrome, and in systemic mastocytosis, where histamine stimulates acid secretion. Acid output is increased in ulcers designated as idiopathic. Conversely, stress ulcers are associated with mucosal underperfusion and abrogation of defence mechanisms. Inflammatory pathogenic mechanisms in Crohn's disease and radiation are considered in Chapters 54 and 113 respectively.

Pathogenesis of symptoms

Pain is the hallmark symptom of peptic ulceration. The origin and pathogenesis of ulcer pain and ulcer-like pain are poorly understood. The mucosa is normally anesthetic, but contains fibers with the characteristics of acid-receptive nociceptors, which may be activated during mucosal injury and inflammation.[38]

PATHOLOGY

Histologically, for a lesion to be an ulcer it must extend beneath the muscularis mucosa. More superficial lesions are classified as *erosions*. Endoscopically, a rough pragmatic equivalence is applied and erosions are commonly defined as lesions that are less than 3 mm in diameter and/or without discernible depth (Fig. 35.8), whereas other lesions are classified as ulcers. Endoscopists are poor at discriminating NSAID-associated erosions and ulcers from those caused by *H. pylori*.[39] Histologically, erosions show localized superficial mucosal destruction with acute inflammation and local congestion. Acute ulcers are similar but with extension below the muscularis mucosa. Chronic peptic ulcers are additionally characterized by collagenous tissue in the base.

CLINICAL PRESENTATION OF UNCOMPLICATED ULCERS

Duodenal ulceration

The classical symptom of duodenal ulceration caused by *H. pylori* is epigastric pain occurring before meals or overnight, relieved by antacids, milk, food, and acid-suppressing treatments.[40–43]

The pain may radiate to the back, particularly in patients with posterior duodenal ulcers. The pointing sign, in which a patient points to a discrete epigastric point of pain, is moderately predictive of duodenal ulceration if present. Because ulcers naturally form and heal, the pain is classically episodic, typically with clusters of pain lasting for 1–3 months with asymptomatic spells in between. Duodenal ulcer pain is classically described as gnawing or a 'hunger' pain, but the qualitative description of the pain is not very helpful in diagnosis.

Not all presentations are classic. Uncomplicated duodenal ulcers may present with any combination of heartburn, anorexia, weight loss, or vomiting. Skillful symptom elicitation can by itself identify many duodenal ulcers, but will miss many others in patients who may not present with classic symptoms. This has led many to recommend more blanket use of endoscopy, or of test and treat policies (see below).

Gastric ulcer

Patients with gastric ulcer have a less stereotypical presentation. An epigastric location is common, but pointing is less so. Pain is more likely to occur soon after meals and somewhat less likely to be relieved by food. Anorexia, nausea, vomiting, and weight loss are more common than in duodenal ulcer and often lead to a suspicion of gastric cancer.

NSAID-associated ulcers

These are difficult to diagnose on the basis of symptoms. Drug-induced nonulcer dyspepsia is common in NSAID

CLINICAL PRESENTATION

SYMPTOMATOLOGY OF DUODENAL ULCERS

Symptom	Duodenal ulcer (%)	Gastric ulcer (%)	Nonulcer dyspepsia (%)
Pointing sign	13	8%	7%
Epigastric pain	61–86	67	52–73
Clusters of pain episodes	56	16	35
Relieved by food	20–63	2–48	4–32
Occurs at night	50–88	32–43	24–32
Heartburn	27–59	19	28
Relieved by alkali	39–86	36–87	26–75
Radiation to back	20–31	34	24–28
Anorexia	25–36	46–57	26–36
Weight loss	19–45	24–61	18–32
Nausea	49–59	54–70	43–60
Vomiting	25–57	38–73	26–34
Fatty food intolerance	41–72		53

Based on data from references 38–41.

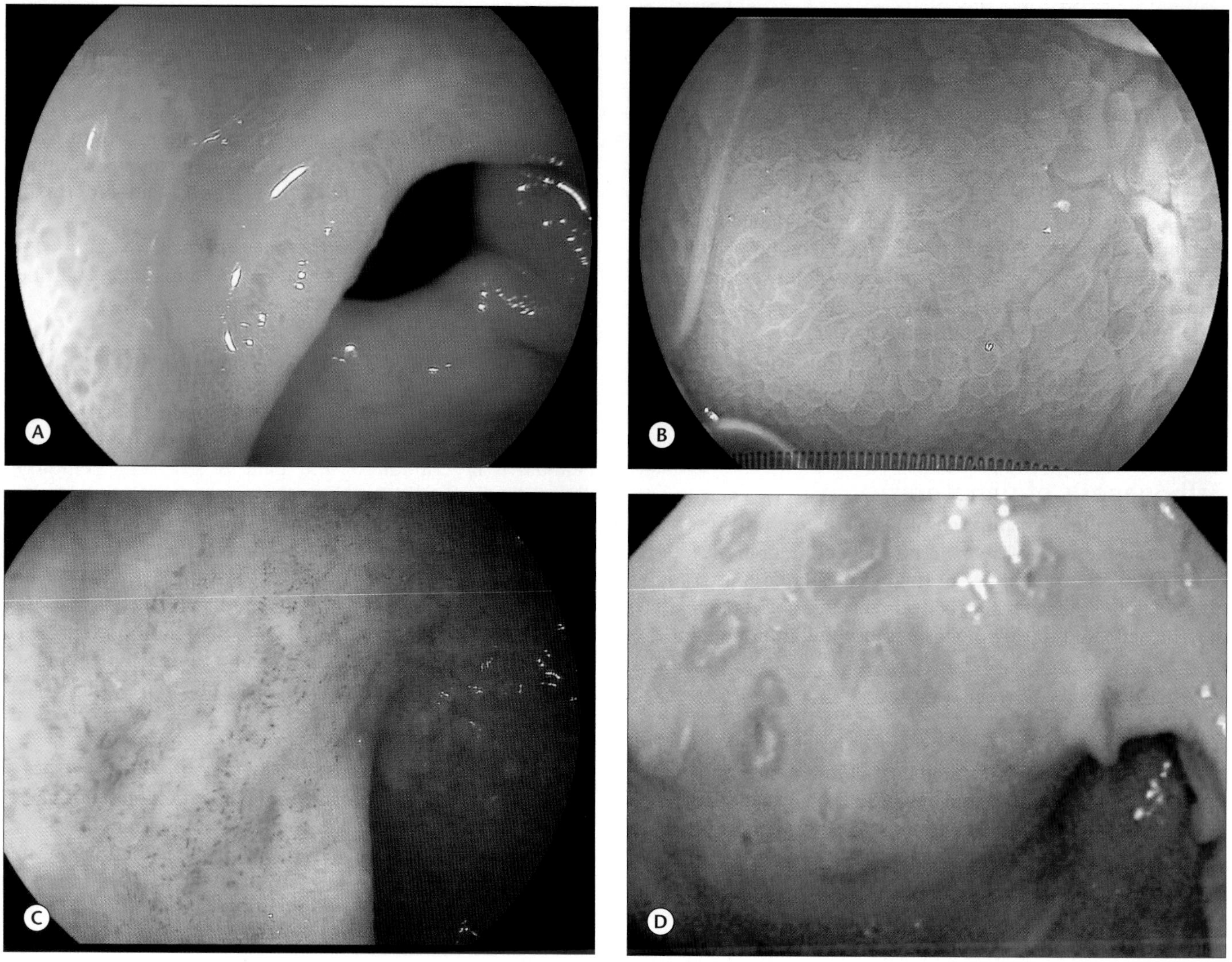

Fig. 35.8 Differences between ulcers and erosions. A. Ulcer with clear depth. **B–D.** Superficial erosions. **B.** Magnifying endoscopy shows erosions in villous duodenal mucosa. (Images A–C, courtesy of Dr Marco Bruno, Academic Medical Center, Amsterdam.)

users, whereas most peptic ulcers are silent, making dyspepsia a poor predictor. Nevertheless, the onset of epigastric pain in an NSAID user is associated with an increased likelihood of finding an endoscopic ulcer or the development of complications.

DIFFERENTIAL DIAGNOSIS

Any cause of chronic recurrent upper abdominal pain (see Chapter 4) enters into the differential diagnosis of peptic ulcer disease.

Diagnostic approach

Several conditions (including functional dyspepsia, gastroesophageal reflux disease, and gastric adenocarcinoma) commonly present with pain or discomfort centered predominantly in the upper abdomen and sometimes accompanied by the other symptoms detailed above. Examination is rarely helpful, and a definite diagnosis can be made only after investigation, usually upper gastrointestinal endoscopy. Because dyspeptic symptoms are so common, some healthcare systems reserve endoscopy for patients with 'alarm symptoms' suggestive of malignancy or other severe pathology.[44]

Empiric management of dyspepsia

In patients with 'simple dyspepsia', causes outside the gastrointestinal tract are excluded as far as possible by history and examination, and stopping any drugs that may be contributing to dyspepsia. In areas of low *H. pylori* prevalence, patients are then managed by testing for *H. pylori* and treating those positive. This 'test and treat' approach effectively treats ulcers (and those without ulcers) even when a firm diagnosis is never made. Where the prevalence of *H. pylori* infection is low, empiric proton pump inhibitor (PPI) treatment is an alternative.[45–48] The various ways of managing dyspepsia are discussed further in Chapter 5.

Diagnostic tests

Where diagnosis is considered necessary, upper gastrointestinal endoscopy (see Chapter 119) is the investigation of choice. It is safe, accurate, and well tolerated by patients under light or no sedation. If possible, patients should avoid acid-suppressing agents for 4 weeks before endoscopy, as these drugs may heal ulcers and esophagitis, leading to a falsely negative endoscopy result. If possible, PPIs, antibiotics, and bismuth compounds should also be avoided for 4 weeks before

DIFFERENTIAL DIAGNOSIS OF PEPTIC ULCER DISEASE

	Trap	Clue
Duodenitis	Pain like duodenal ulcer	Disease continuum? Similar management
Nonulcer dyspepsia	Common	Typically epigastric bloating
Irritable bowel syndrome	Pain from transverse colon felt in upper abdomen	Pain with altered bowel activity; relief from bowel actions
Gastroesophageal reflux	Common	Stereotypical history
Drug-induced dyspepsia	Often like ulcer pain	Relation to drug intake
Gastric cancer	Difficult to distinguish from gastric ulcer	Supraclavicular node in some
Pancreatitis	Atypical presentation may be ulcer-like	Pain 12–36h after a binge in recurrent alcoholic pancreatitis
Biliary disease	Pain can be epigastric	(Prolonged) waves of colic; abdominal tenderness
Pancreatic cancer	Rarely enters differential diagnosis	Liver function testing usually abnormal

CLINICAL TIPS

ALARM SYMPTOMS AND SIGNS PROMPTING URGENT INVESTIGATION

- Hematemesis or malena[a]
- Dysphagia
- Weight loss
- Persistent vomiting
- Abdominal mass
- Anemia due to possible gastrointestinal blood loss

[a]Usually requires urgent hospital admission.

endoscopy as these render biopsy-based tests for *H. pylori* unreliable.

If a duodenal ulcer is found at endoscopy, biopsies should be taken from the gastric antrum to test for *H. pylori* (usually by biopsy urease test and/or histologic examination (see Chapter 34) and from the duodenum if Crohn's disease is suspected. In patients with previous *H. pylori* treatment or multiple antibiotic courses for other conditions, biopsies should also be taken for microbiologic culture and antibiotic sensitivity testing.

Similar tests are indicated for gastric ulceration, but additional biopsies should be taken from the ulcer rim to exclude carcinoma or lymphoma. The usual practice is also to check gastric ulcer healing 6 weeks after treatment is started and take further biopsies if healing is incomplete (although the pick-up rate for cancer if original biopsies are negative is very low).

Barium radiology (see Chapter 125) is less accurate for picking up small ulcers and does not allow gastric biopsies to be taken to test for *H. pylori* or to exclude malignancy.

Diagnosis of the cause of an ulcer

NSAIDs

There are no diagnostic tests for NSAID involvement, although measurement of serum thromboxane concentration has been considered. Diagnosis depends on an accurate history.

Zollinger-Ellison syndrome

A random serum gastrin estimation is a useful screen but can be affected by food and PPIs. A fasting gastrin is more specific. The diagnosis is formally established by showing increased basal gastric acid output and a fasting gastrin level of less than 1000 pg/mL (10-fold increase) with an intragastric pH of 2.0, sometimes backed up by a secretin test (see Chapters 109 and 131).

Multiple endocrine neoplasia

This should be suspected where Zollinger-Ellison syndrome is associated with hyperparathyroidism (see Chapter 109).

Systemic mastocytosis

Systemic mastocytosis should be suspected in the presence of pruritus, urticaria or a characteristic rash (Fig. 35.9). Diagnosis is based on the presence of infiltrates in bone marrow and/or

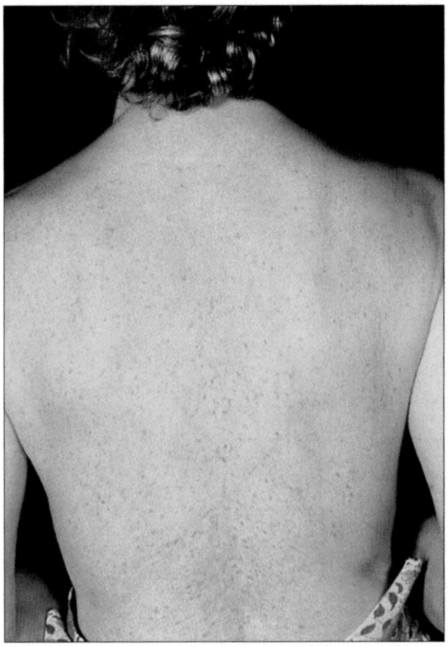

Fig. 35.9 Cutaneous manifestations of systemic mastocytosis (urticaria pigmentosa). Patient presented with duodenal ulceration attributable to acid hypersecretion and diarrhea associated with intestinal involvement.

extracutaneous organs, detection of c-*kit* mutations, raised serum α-tryptase, and expression of CD2 and CD25 in c-*kit*-positive mast cells.[49]

Duodenal Crohn's disease

Duodenal involvement is reported in 0.5–13% of patients with Crohn's disease and recognized to cause duodenal ulcer with typical symptoms.[50] Thus, any patient not taking NSAIDs who is *H. pylori* negative should have duodenal biopsies to exclude Crohn's disease.

Stress ulcer

Ulcer bleeding occurring in the context of current or recent severe illness and/or intensive care should be assumed to be a stress ulcer (see below).

Celiac axis stenosis

The site may be atypical and pain intense. Celiac axis angiography is necessary to establish this diagnosis (see Chapter 67).

TREATMENT AND PREVENTION

H. pylori-associated ulcers

Eradication of H. pylori

H. pylori eradication heals ulcers and prevents recurrence (Fig. 35.10). Modern 1-week triple therapy regimens with twice daily dosing are successful in 90% of cases.[51] Such regimens use a PPI twice daily and two antibiotics, most commonly clarithromycin 500mg and amoxicillin 1g or metronidazole 400mg, all twice daily. Some physicians routinely check treatment success by urea breath test 1month after the end of treatment, but others check only for complicated ulcers or if symptoms recur. When *H. pylori* status is not known, PPIs can be started and antibiotics added once *H. pylori* test results are available. The management of *H. pylori* treatment failures is discussed in Chapter 34.

Ancillary drug treatment

For duodenal ulcers, continuation of acid suppression after the antibiotic course is unnecessary, but some physicians give PPIs for a total of 1month for very large or complicated ulcers. If this is done, checking for *H. pylori* eradication must be delayed for a further month.

For gastric ulcers, which often heal more slowly, PPIs are usually continued until the second check endoscopy. The use of 'ulcer-healing' drugs such as H_2-receptor antagonists, sucralfate, misoprostol, bismuth, and high-dose antacids to heal *H. pylori*-associated ulcers is largely of historic interest, and these drugs are now largely used for other indications (see Chapter 136).

Management of patients taking NSAIDs

Ulcer healing

PPIs accelerate healing compared with standard doses of H_2 antagonists, and appear to overcome the adverse retarding effects of smoking and concurrent NSAID use.[52] Misoprostol heals NSAID-associated ulcers but causes more side effects.

Strategies to reduce risk of ulcer development

For NSAID users, removing the cause of the ulcer, by stopping the drug or switching to one that does not damage the stomach or duodenum, is the equivalent of *H. pylori* eradication. An alternative is to continue the NSAID where needed, at the lowest possible dose, and to give concurrent antiulcer prophylaxis.

Low-toxicity drugs

Ibuprofen at dosages of less than 1200mg per day appears to confer little risk of bleeding peptic ulcer[23] (see Fig. 35.6). Alternatively, and where higher doses are needed, selective COX-2 inhibitors have been shown to reduce the risk of ulcers that are detected endoscopically and clinically.[53–56] Clinical outcomes have been studied in large cohorts of patients (up to 18500) for celecoxib, rofecoxib, and lumiracoxib. The VIGOR and TARGET studies of rofecoxib and lumiracoxib showed a

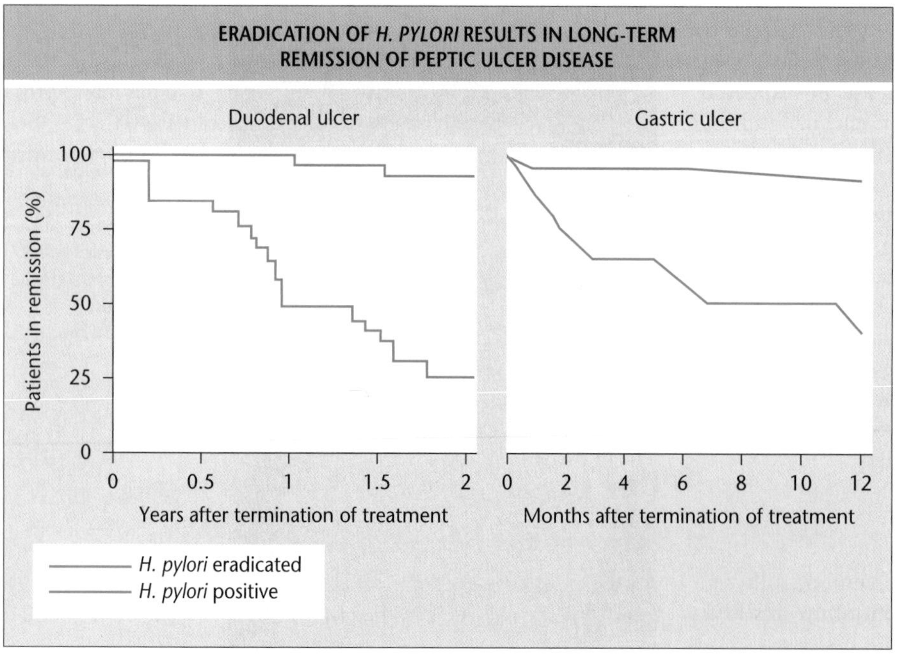

Fig. 35.10 ***Helicobacter pylori*** **eradication.** There is a marked reduction in relapse rates for duodenal and gastric ulcer following *H. pylori* eradication.

TREATMENT AND PREVENTION	
TREATMENT CHOICES	
Coxib	**PPI protection**
No risk factors	Past history
H. pylori (+ eradication)	Low-dose aspirin
Corticosteroids	
Impaired hemostasis	
Old age	Old age

Management in patients with cardiovascular disease is controversial. One coxib (rofecoxib) was associated with an increase in myocardial infarction compared with placebo. It is not clear whether this property is shared by nonselective NSAIDs or other selective coxibs.

reduction in the risk of all ulcers of between 27% (celecoxib) and 57% (rofecoxib), and the TARGET study showed a 79% reduction in ulcer complications for lumiracoxib compared with ibuprofen or naproxen (Fig. 35.11).

Prophylactic co-prescription

Prostaglandin replacement A large 8000-patient "outcomes" study of misoprostol (the MUCOSA Study) showed a 40% reduction in ulcer complications, but with a high level of drug-related adverse events.[57]

PPIs: The effect of acid suppression has been studied endoscopically for a wide range of patients and for clinical outcomes in those who have already presented to hospital with a life-threatening ulcer complication.[24,58–62] PPIs (and high doses of H_2 antagonists) can prevent the development and recurrence of ulcers, and recurrence of ulcer complications, whereas standard doses of H_2 antagonists are not effective in preventing NSAID-associated gastric ulcer development.

COX-2 inhibitors versus NSAIDs and prophylaxis: who should receive what?

Overall, one direct comparison suggests that COX-2 inhibitors and NSAIDs plus prophylaxis are similar when used after presentation with peptic ulcer bleeding.[61] Based on detailed discussion elsewhere,[4] the box on Treatment Choices indicates the patients for which each strategy is appropriate. Coxibs do not avoid risks due to other factors, whereas PPIs are not fully effective against NSAID ulcers. Recent endoscopic data strongly suggest that a coxib plus PPI strategy results in extremely low ulcer rates; although costly, this strategy may be appropriate for very high-risk patients.[63]

H. pylori-positive NSAID ulcers

This is a controversial area. The evidence ranges from showing a benefit for *H. pylori* eradication in patients starting NSAIDs through to greater effectiveness of PPI prophylaxis in patients who remain infected.[64–66] Whatever the truth, it is clear that *H. pylori* eradication alone is not sufficient to protect high-risk patients from developing ulcer complications.

Low-dose aspirin

Importance of dose

A sound epidemiologic study suggests that there is a detectable increase in the risk of ulcer disease with aspirin 75 mg daily, and this rises further with doses of 150 and 300 mg daily.[6] The first and most important steps to improve safety are therefore *restriction of use* to those in whom indications are clearcut, and *restriction of dose* to 75–82.5 mg daily.

Protective strategies

It is possible that *H. pylori* eradication may be sufficiently effective to protect low-dose aspirin users,[60] but until there are further data this cannot be recommended above PPI prophylaxis.[62] If funds allow, patients taking low-dose aspirin should receive PPI prophylaxis if they have any significant risk factor,[11] such as age over 65 years or a past ulcer history. There is some evidence that the cardiovascular disease for which aspirin is

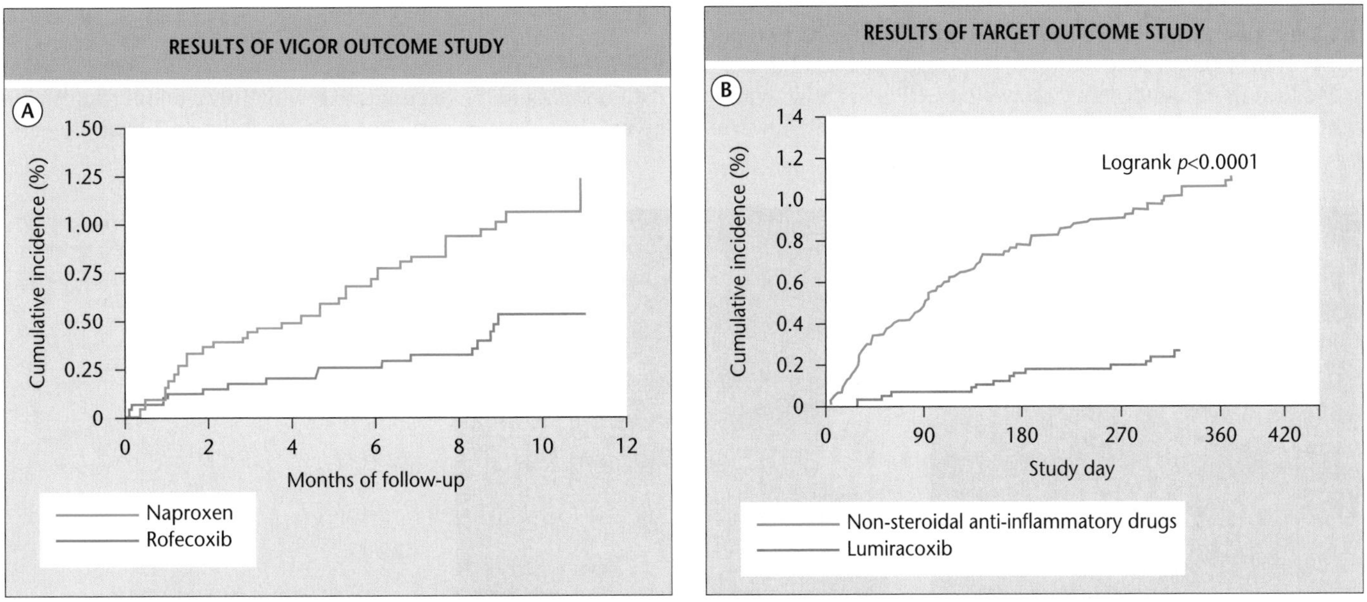

Fig. 35.11 Results of VIGOR and TARGET outcome studies (primary outcomes). Left: VIGOR – perforations, ulcers, and bleeds. Right: TARGET – ulcer complications.

prescribed may itself be a risk factor,[11] and some would argue that a precautionary principle would support PPI prophylaxis for all in whom aspirin is needed.

Patients taking prophylactic aspirin and a non-aspirin NSAID

By competing at the level of the platelet, nonselective NSAIDs such as ibuprofen may substantially interfere with aspirin's ability to inhibit platelet aggregation and thereby prevent coronary heart disease.[67] Low-dose aspirin users should use a coxib for anti-inflammatory effects, to avoid this pharmacodynamic interaction. The clinical evidence is mixed as to the clinical importance of this.[68,69] There have been fears that COX-2 inhibitors may enhance the risk of myocardial infarction, but there is no evidence for this in patients using aspirin.[56] In patients taking aspirin and a coxib, a PPI should be used where the risk of aspirin alone would warrant it.[5]

COMPLICATIONS AND THEIR MANAGEMENT

Bleeding

Epidemiology

Peptic ulcer is the commonest cause of acute upper gastrointestinal bleeding (see Chapter 23), accounting for nearly half of all instances and occurring in approximately 2–5 per 1000 of people aged over 60 years.[5]

Clinical presentation

Hematemesis and/or melena (Fig. 35.12) are usually obvious, especially when accompanied by tachycardia or hypotension, usually leading to emergency hospital admission. Retrospective accounts of 'melena' in well patients only occasionally indicate significant gastrointestinal bleeding.

Diagnosis and management

After resuscitation, patients should undergo endoscopy, both to establish the diagnosis and to institute endoscopic management if the stigmata of hemorrhage are present. As detailed in Chapter 23, endoscopic therapy of bleeding peptic ulcers reduces rebleeding and the need for surgery, and may reduce mortality. The choices are injection therapy with epinephrine (adrenaline) or sclerosant, light- or heat-based coagulation of the vessel, or a combination.

Medical treatment with intravenous PPIs is now widely used.[70,71] Early studies of all comers showed no benefit; however, most (but not all) recent studies of intravenous PPIs following successful endoscopic therapy have shown a reduction in rebleeding (see Chapter 23).

Where *H. pylori* is the cause, eradication results in a substantial reduction in the risk of rebleeding.[72] Patients taking NSAIDs can resume these drugs after healing if they take a PPI, as this has been shown substantially to reduce the readmission rate for ulcer complications over 6 months.[60–62]

Mortality

In a large, comprehensive British survey the mortality rate was 13%.[73] Patients die mainly as a result of pneumonia and the thrombotic complications of bleeding or surgery (deep vein thrombosis and pulmonary embolism, myocardial infarction), rather than exsanguination.

Perforation (see also Chapters 22–24)

Epidemiology

The incidence of ulcer perforation is about 7–10 per 100 000 population per annum.[74] Perforation is still more common in men than in women, and in those with duodenal versus gastric ulcers. There is a diurnal and seasonal variation. Many perforated ulcers are *H. pylori* negative.[75] NSAID use and cigarette smoking are risk factors, but presentation in their absence is quite common. The reported incidence of *H. pylori* infection ranges from 0% to 100%.[76]

Clinical presentation

This is usually stereotypical and obvious, with an abrupt onset of *severe upper abdominal pain*, rapidly spreading through the abdomen, and the development of symptoms and signs of *peritonitis* (see Chapter 98), hypotension, and shock.

Diagnosis

Diagnosis is largely based on history, examination, and plain radiography. Air within the abdominal cavity wall under the diaphragm is seen on plain abdominal and erect chest radiographs in most cases (Fig. 35.13). Endoscopy is avoided because of theoretical risks of increased peritoneal soiling. Water-soluble contrast studies are rarely needed.

Management

Patients should be resuscitated with intravenous fluids and given broad-spectrum antibiotics (e.g., cefuroxime and

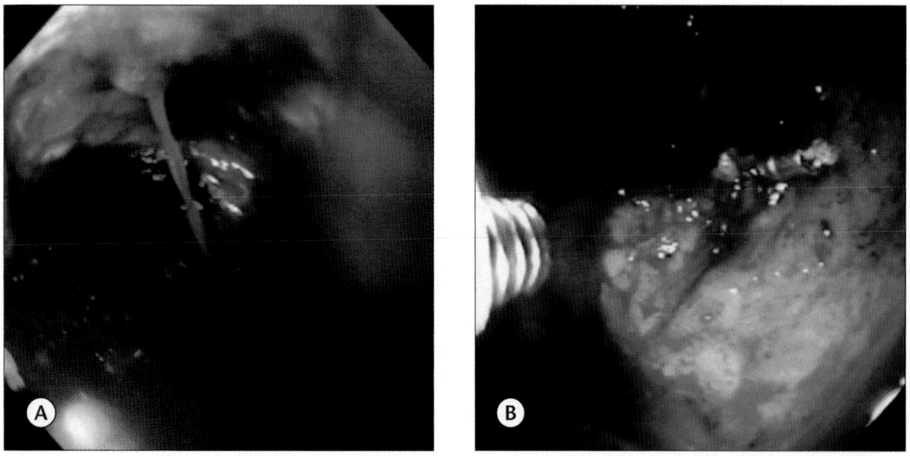

Fig. 35.12 Bleeding ulcer. Arterial bleeding from a visible vessel in an ulcer **(A)** before and **(B)** after control by application of a hemoclip. Courtesy Dr Paul Fortun.

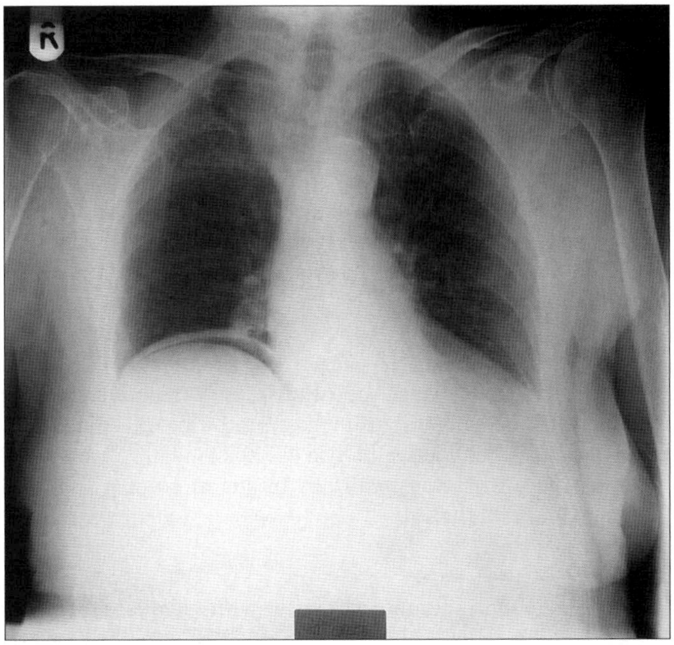

Fig. 35.13 Chest radiograph showing air under the diaphragm in a patient with perforated peptic ulcer.

metronidazole). Laparotomy to close the perforation should be carried out as soon as possible after resuscitation, although in patients with a high operative risk who are improving on conservative treatment, continued nonoperative management may be possible.

Prevention of recurrence

After successful recovery, management to prevent recurrence is standard (*H. pylori* eradication, NSAID avoidance). There are no direct data on the benefits of switching to a COX-2 inhibitor or taking PPI prophylaxis after perforation.

Mortality

The overall mortality rate is about 10%. Risk factors for death are age, co-morbid illness, delayed surgery, preoperative shock, heart rate, and a high serum creatinine level.[77]

Penetration

Posterior perforation may result in digestive penetration into an adjacent organ rather than free penetration. Posterior duodenal ulcer penetration most commonly involves the pancreas, often resulting in different, more severe, pain than is typical. Other organs that may be involved include the left lobe of the liver, common bile duct (choledochoduodenal fistula), colon (gastrocolic fistula), lung, and pericardium. Except where fistulae have formed, treatment is by acid suppression with *H. pylori* eradication or NSAID cessation, as appropriate.

Gastric outlet obstruction

Epidemiology

Gastric outlet obstruction by peptic ulcers is relatively uncommon, probably affecting less than the quoted 2% of patients with ulceration. Obstruction occurs with (pre)pyloric or duodenal ulcers, especially in patients with a long history, and is thought particularly to be associated with NSAID use.

Clinical features

Obstruction should be suspected in patients with an ulcer who develop vomiting, particularly if projectile or occurring daily. Early satiety (60%), upper abdominal pain and distention (87%), and weight loss (65%) are common. A succussion splash is present in 25% or more of patients. Depending on severity, increases in serum urea concentration and electrolyte abnormalities (low K^+, metabolic alkalosis, low Na^+) are common.

Management

Nasogastric aspiration should be performed to empty the stomach prior to endoscopy. Aspiration of more than 200 mL after an overnight fast suggests delayed gastric emptying. At endoscopy, biopsy samples should be taken to exclude malignancy. Endoscopic balloon dilatation (see Chapter 146) and/or treatment with acid suppression can restore gastric emptying. Some patients require surgery by antrectomy and Billroth 1 or 2 procedures.

SURGERY FOR PEPTIC ULCER

Nowadays, surgical intervention is rarely used for gastric or duodenal ulcers, except in the context of complications (see above).

Postoperative syndromes

Peptic ulcer surgery was an unphysiologic intervention that resulted in significant morbidity,[78] including the following.

Dumping syndromes

These are characterized by flushing, palpitations, sweating, light-headedness, tachycardia, postural hypotension, and fatigue.

The *early dumping syndrome* occurs 30–60 min after eating in patients who have had a gastrectomy. Dumping of food into the duodenum is thought to cause rapid fluid shifts, leading to faintness. Excessive release of vasoactive hormones may play a role. Octreotide may have therapeutic value (see Chapter 41).

In the *late dumping syndrome*, dumping of food into the duodenum stimulates excessive insulin secretion resulting in rebound hypoglycemia 2–3 h after a meal.

Postgastrectomy malnutrition

Most patients who have had a gastrectomy lose weight and/or become anemic or malnourished because of a combination of early satiety, impaired control of nutritional digestion and absorption, inadequate production of co-factors such as vitamin B_{12}, and altered iron absorption. Problems develop over years and also include metabolic bone disease (vitamin D) and neuropathy (vitamin B_{12}).

Stomal ulceration

After partial gastrectomy, ulcers may develop at the site of anastomosis and present with pain or sometimes complications. They can be managed with acid-suppressing drugs. The role of *H. pylori* in this situation is unclear, but eradication is wise.

Postgastrectomy neoplasia

Surgery for peptic ulcer is associated with an increased risk of later gastric cancer. This is discussed in Chapter 37.

Postvagotomy syndromes

Truncal vagotomy results in diarrhea in many patients.[78] Pathogenesis is multifactorial and management is symptomatic.

MECKEL'S DIVERTICULUM

This is an ileal diverticulum with acid-secreting heterotopic gastric mucosa that arises because of developmental abnormality in approximately 2% of the population. It can cause ulceration with pain or bleeding, as well as obstruction due to intussusception or volvulus. Diagnosis is often made incidentally during barium radiology. Technetium (^{99m}Tc) pertechnetate, which has an affinity for parietal cells, is the basis of the scan. Treatment is by surgical removal.

STRESS ULCERS

Severe medical stresses such as burns, head injuries, major trauma, sepsis, multisystem organ failure, or ventilation on an intensive care unit are associated with the development of stress ulcers in the stomach or duodenum that may bleed and are associated with a high mortality rate.[79,80] Curling's ulcers are those associated with burns, and Cushing's ulcers with head injury.[81] Stress ulcers are seen less commonly now than previously, possibly due to preventive measures in intensive care. In one large recent study, 31 of 2252 patients (1.4%) on an intensive care unit experienced clinically important bleeding.[82]

Risk factors

A need for ventilation because of respiratory failure is the most important risk factor, increasing the chance of upper gastrointestinal bleeding by 15-fold.[82,83] Coagulopathy has been reported to enhance risk 4-fold, and hypotension is probably a risk factor of similar magnitude. Sepsis, hepatic and renal failure, and glucocorticoids may enhance risk, although the evidence is less secure. Clinically important bleeding is extremely rare in patients with no risk factors.[82,83]

Pathogenesis

The pathogenesis varies according to etiology. Reduced mucosal defence, largely because of poor blood flow that allows increased acid back diffusion, predisposes to stress ulcers in ventilated patients and after severe burns, despite an overall reduction in acid secretion.[79,80] Cushing ulcers differ in being associated with hypergastrinemia and hypersecretion of acid.[81]

Clinical presentation

The most common presentation is with bleeding, manifesting as shock, hematemesis, or melena. This may occur at any time during a stressful illness, but is common at 10–14 days and may therefore present as the patient is improving in other respects. Perforation and penetration are much less common. Some patients may complain of antecedent pain.

Treatment and prevention

Once severe stress ulcer bleeding has occurred, the patient should be managed as for other ulcer bleeding; however, the mortality rate is high. Consequently, attention has focused on prophylaxis.[84,85]

Prophylaxis

The goal of stress ulcer prophylaxis should be to reduce the incidence of clinically significant ulcer bleeding without enhancing drug-related adverse events. The literature is confusing. Some studies have used rather trivial endpoints, and in others a reduction in adverse events has been a dominant feature.[85,86]

H_2-receptor antagonists

A meta-analysis has suggested that these drugs decrease the incidence of clinically important gastrointestinal bleeding (odds ratio 0.44, 95% confidence interval (CI) 0.22–0.88)[84,85] compared with placebo, with nonsignificant trends in comparison with antacids and sucralfate.

Sucralfate

However, the mortality rate was lower with sucralfate than with antacids (odds ratio 0.73, 95% CI 0.54–0.97), and there was a nonsignificant trend compared with H_2-receptor antagonists (odds ratio 0.83, 95% CI 0.62–1.09).[85]

Proton pump inhibitors[87]

PPIs raise pH more effectively than H_2 antagonists, are not prone to tachyphylaxis, and reduce surrogate measures of stress ulceration; however, there are insufficient data to recommend them as yet.[87]

Enteral nutrition

Although enteral nutrition has not been the subject of controlled trials, observational data strongly suggest that it reduces substantially the incidence of clinically important stress ulcer bleeding.

Practical management

The following guidelines, updated from Tryba & Cook,[88] are suggested:

- Stress ulcer prophylaxis should be restricted to patients with risk factors, particularly respiratory failure, coagulopathy, sepsis, shock, burns, head injury, or a history of peptic ulcer disease.
- Enteral nutrition, where given, probably reduces the incidence of ulcer bleeding.
- Where there is good general intensive care management, other specific measures are seldom needed.
- Alternatives are:
  1. Sucralfate 1g six times daily by mouth
  2. Enteral nutrition with sucralfate 1g twice daily during a rest period when enteral nutrition is supended
  3. Ranitidine 50mg by slow intravenous injection, then 125–250mg/kg/h by infusion.

CAMERON'S ULCER

These ulcers typically occur in the neck of a big hiatus hernia, and are believed to arise on an ischemic basis.[89] They may be associated with iron deficiency anemia and can be cured by surgical intervention.[90]

PROGNOSIS AND ADVICE TO PATIENTS WITH PEPTIC ULCER

Patients should be told what their ulcer is due to and to eat a normal diet. They should understand the harmful effects of NSAIDs and the ability of modern medicines to overcome this damage in most cases. Early trials showed a, presumably spontaneous, placebo-healing rate of about 40% over 4 weeks for duodenal ulcers and over 8 weeks for gastric ulcers. However, ulcers that heal spontaneously or in response to acid-suppressing treatment nearly always recur subsequently, unless the cause is removed. After proven eradication of *H. pylori* in patients not taking NSAIDs, the relapse rate falls to less than 5%. Similarly, for patients using NSAIDs who stop these drugs, relapse is rare if they have no other risk factors such as *H. pylori* infection. Switching to a COX-2 inhibitor or using PPI prophylaxis is an alternative. Rebleeding rates with PPI prophylaxis and switch to a COX-2 inhibitor are similar. Recent data suggest that combined use of PPI prophylaxis and a switch to a COX-2 may result in a very low ulcer incidence. However, the use of selective COX-2 inhibitors has become controversial because of possible cardiac risks (see below).

SOURCES OF INFORMATION FOR PATIENTS AND DOCTORS

http://www.nlm.nih.gov/medlineplus/pepticulcer.html
http://www.medinfo.co.uk/conditions/pepticulcer.html
http://www.cdc.gov/ulcer/
http://www.kidshealth.org/parent/medical/digestive/peptic_ulcers
http://www.digestive.niddk.nih.gov/ddiseases/pubs/hpylori/
http://www.digestive.niddk.nih.gov/ddiseases/pubs/nsaids/
http://www.netdoctor.co.uk/diseases/facts/pepticulcertreatment.htm
http://www.gastro.org/clinicalRes/brochures/pud.html
http://www.gastro.org/clinicalRes/brochures/ulcered1.html
http://patients.uptodate.com/topic.asp?file=digestiv/9148
http://www.patient.co.uk/showdoc/23069184/
http://www.patient.co.uk/showdoc/971/

CURRENT CONTROVERSIES

Peptic ulceration is becoming less frequent in developed countries, mirroring falling *H. pylori* prevalence. It is unclear whether developing countries will undergo an epidemic of peptic ulceration with modernization, as occurred in the USA and Europe in the early twentieth century. In developed countries, as the causes of dyspepsia change in frequency and ulcers become less common, endoscopy for simple dyspepsia is becoming less economically viable. A Medical Research Council trial in the UK is addressing which of *H. pylori* 'test and treat' or empirical PPI treatment is better for the initial management of community dyspepsia. Controversy persists about the importance and prevalence of non-*H. pylori* non-NSAID ulcers, including their etiology and optimal management. Although *H. pylori* prevalence is falling, antibiotic resistance is a growing problem and ongoing studies are addressing optimal treatment strategies for resistant strains. In developing countries, *H. pylori*-associated gastric cancer is an enormous public health problem, and research into *H. pylori* vaccination and other population management strategies continues. Although COX-2 inhibitors undoubtedly reduce the risks of ulcer complications, the related questions of whether they may predispose to myocardial infarction and whether use of low-dose aspirin abrogates their benefits have been thrown into sharp focus with the withdrawal of rofecoxib because of an incidence of myocardial infarction that was higher than that of placebo in the APPROVe study. What is unclear is whether this is a unique property of rofecoxib or whether it is shared by other selective COX-2 inhibitors or nonselective NSAIDs, and whether it is due to hypertension, an effect on thrombosis, or another unidentified mechanism.

REFERENCES

1. Chan FK, Leung WK. Peptic-ulcer disease. Lancet 2002; 360:933–941, 2002.
2. Warren JR, Marshall B. Unidentified curved bacilli on gastric epithelium in active chronic gastritis. Lancet 1983; i:1273–1275.
3. Hawkey CJ. Nonsteroidal anti-inflammatory drug gastropathy. Gastroenterology 2000; 119:521–535.
4. Hawkey CJ. Nonsteroidal anti-inflammatory drugs and the gastrointestinal tract: consensus and controversy. Am J Med 2001; 110:1S–100S.
5. Hawkey CJ, Langman MJ. Non-steroidal anti-inflammatory drugs: overall risks and management. Complementary roles for COX-2 inhibitors and proton pump inhibitors. Gut 2003; 52:600–608.
6. Slattery J, Warlow CP, Shorrock CJ, Langman MJ. Risks of gastrointestinal bleeding during secondary prevention of vascular events with aspirin – analysis of gastrointestinal bleeding during the UK-TIA trial. Gut 1995; 37:509–511.
7. Douthwaite AH, Lintott SAM. Gastropic observation of the effect of aspirin and certain other substances on the stomach. Lancet 1938; ii:1222–1225.
8. Quan C, Talley NJ. Management of peptic ulcer disease not related to *Helicobacter pylori* or NSAIDs. Am J Gastroenterol 2002; 97:2950–2961.
9. Arguedas MR, Ferrante D. Systemic mastocytosis and giant gastroduodenal ulcer. Gastrointest Endosc 2001; 54:530–533.
10. Messer J, Reitman D, Sacks HS et al. Association of adrenocorticosteroid therapy and peptic ulcer disease. N Engl J Med 1983; 309:21–24.
11. Weil J, Langman MJ, Wainwright P et al. Peptic ulcer bleeding: accessory risk factors and interactions with non-steroidal anti-inflammatory drugs. Gut 2000; 46:27–31.
12. Piper JM, Ray WA, Daugherty JR et al. Corticosteroid use and peptic ulcer disease: role of nonsteroidal anti-inflammatory drugs. Ann Intern Med 1991; 114:735–740.
13. Susser S. Civilisation and peptic ulcer. Lancet 1962; i:115–118.
14. Higham J, Kang JY, Majeed A. Recent trends in admissions and mortality due to peptic ulcer in England: increasing frequency of hemorrhage among older subjects. Gut 2002; 50:460–464.
15. Stack WA, Atherton JC, Hawkey GM, Logan RFA, Hawkey CJ. Interactions between *Helicobacter pylori* and other risk factors for peptic ulcer bleeding. Aliment Pharmacol Ther 2002; 16:497–506.
16. Pirmohamed M, James S, Meakin S et al. Adverse drug reactions as cause of admission to hospital: prospective analysis of 18820 patients. BMJ 2004; 329:15–19.
17. Tacconelli S, Capone ML, Patrignani P. Clinical pharmacology of novel selective COX-2 inhibitors. Curr Pharm Des 2004; 10:589–601.
18. Brune K, Hinz B. Selective cyclooxygenase-2 inhibitors: similarities and differences. Scand J Rheumatol 2004; 33:1–6.
19. Borody TJ, George LL, Brandl S, Andrews P, Jankiewicz E, Ostapowicz N. Smoking does not contribute to duodenal ulcer relapse after *Helicobacter pylori* eradication. Am J Gastroenterol 1992; 87:1390–1393.
20. Kurata JH, Nogawa AN. Meta-analysis of risk factors for peptic ulcer. Nonsteroidal

antiinflammatory drugs, *Helicobacter pylori*, and smoking. J Clin Gastroenterol 1997; 24:2–17.
21. Hawkey CJ, Laine L, Harper SE, Quan HU, Bolognese JA, Mortensen E. Rofecoxib Osteoarthritis Endoscopy Multinational Study Group. Influence of risk factors on endoscopic and clinical ulcers in patients taking rofecoxib or ibuprofen in two randomized controlled trials. Aliment Pharmacol Ther 2001; 15:1593–1601.
22. Laine L, Bombardier C, Hawkey CJ et al. Stratifying the risk of NSAID-related upper gastrointestinal clinical events: results of a double-blind outcomes study in patients with rheumatoid arthritis. Gastroenterology 2002; 123:1006–1012.
23. Lewis SC, Langman MJ, Laporte JR, Matthews JN, Rawlins MD, Wiholm BE. Dose–response relationships between individual non-aspirin non-steroidal anti-inflammatory drugs (NANSAIDs) and serious upper gastrointestinal bleeding: a meta-analysis based on individual patient data. Br J Clin Pharmacol 2002; 54:320–326.
24. Blaser MJ, Atherton JC. *Helicobacter pylori* persistence: biology and disease. J Clin Invest 2004; 113:321–333.
25. Crabtree JE, Taylor JD, Wyatt JI et al. Mucosal IgA recognition of *Helicobacter pylori* 120 kDa protein, peptic ulceration, and gastric pathology. Lancet 1991; 338:332–335.
26. Blaser MJ, Pérez-Pérez GI, Kleanthous H et al. Infection with *Helicobacter pylori* strains possessing *cagA* associated with an increased risk of developing adenocarcinoma of the stomach. Cancer Res 1995; 55:2111–2115.
27. Odenbreit S, Puls J, Sedlmaier B, Gerland E, Fischer W, Haas R. Translocation of *Helicobacter pylori* CagA into gastric epithelial cells by type IV secretion. Science 2000; 287:1497–1500.
28. Argent RH, Kidd M, Owen RJ, Thomas RJ, Limb MC, Atherton JC. Determinants and consequences of different levels of CagA phosphorylation for clinical isolates of *Helicobacter pylori*. Gastroenterology 2004; 127:514–523.
29. Atherton J, Cao P, Peek RM, Tummuru MKR, Blaser MJ, Cover TC. Mosaicism in vacuolating cytotoxin alleles of *Helicobacter pylori*: association of specific *vacA* types with cytotoxin production and peptic ulceration. J Biol Chem 1995; 270:17771–17777.
30. Letley DP, Rhead JL, Twells RJ, Dove B, Atherton JC. Determinants of non-toxicity in the gastric pathogen *Helicobacter pylori*. J Biol Chem 2003; 278:26734–26741.
31. Gerhard M, Lehn N, Neumayer N et al. Clinical relevance of the *Helicobacter pylori* gene for blood-group antigen-binding adhesion. Proc Natl Acad Sci USA 1999; 96:12778–12783.
32. Yamaoka Y, Kikuchi S, El-Zimaity HMT et al. Importance of *Helicobacter pylori* oipA in clinical presentation, gastric inflammation, and mucosal interleukin 8 production. Gastroenterology 2002; 123:414–424.
33. Macarthur M, Hold GL, El-Omar EM. Inflammation and cancer II. Role of chronic inflammation and cytokine gene polymorphisms in the pathogenesis of gastrointestinal malignancy. Am J Physiol Gastrointest Liver Physiol 2004; 286:G515–G520.
34. Moss SF, Legon S, Bishop AE, Polak JM, Calam J. Effect of *Helicobacter pylori* on gastric somatostatin in duodenal ulcer disease. Lancet 1992; 340:930–932.
35. Elliott SL, Ferris RJ, Giraud AS, Cook GA, Skeljo MV, Yeomans ND. Indomethacin damage to rat gastric mucosa is markedly dependent on luminal pH. Clin Exp Pharmacol Physiol 1996; 23:432–434.
36. Yeomans ND, Tulassay Z, Juhasz L et al. A comparison of omeprazole with ranitidine for ulcers associated with nonsteroidal antiinflammatory drugs. Acid Suppression Trial: Ranitidine versus Omeprazole for NSAID-associated Ulcer Treatment (ASTRONAUT) Study Group. N Engl J Med 1998; 338:719–726.
37. Wallace JL. Pathogenesis of NSAID-induced gastroduodenal mucosal injury. Best Pract Res Clin Gastroenterol 2001; 15:691–703.
38. Hawkey CJ, Jones JIW, Lynn P, Millns P, Kendall D. Novel population of nociceptors requiring low pH stimulation possibly sub-serving dyspepsia. Gut 2002; 51(Suppl III):A43.
39. Hudson N, Eeritt S, Hawkey CJ. Inter-observer variability in assessment of gastric lesions video endoscopy. Gut 1994; 35:1030–1032.
40. Edwards FC, Coghill NF. Clinical manifestations in patients with chronic atrophic gastritis, gastric ulcer and duodenal ulcer. Q J Med 1968; 37:337.
41. Horrocks JC, De Dombal FT. Clinical presentation of patients with "dyspepsia." Detailed symptomatic study of 360 patients. Gut 1978; 19:19–26.
42. Earlam R. Computerized questionnaire analysis of duodenal ulcer symptoms. Gastroenterology 1976; 71:314–317.
43. Rinaldo JA Jr, Scheinok P, Rupe CE. Symptom diagnosis. A mathematical analysis of epigastric pain. Ann Intern Med 1963; 59:145–154.
44. Gillen D, McColl KEL. Does concern about missing malignancy justify endoscopy in uncomplicated dyspepsia in patients aged less than 55? Am J Gastroenterol 1999; 94:75–79.
45. McColl KE, Murray LS, Gillen D et al. Randomised trial of endoscopy with testing for *Helicobacter pylori* compared with non-invasive *H. pylori* testing alone in the management of dyspepsia. *BMJ* 2002; 324:999–1002.
46. Chiba N, Van Zanten SJ, Sinclair P et al. Treating *Helicobacter pylori* infection in primary care patients with uninvestigated dyspepsia: the Canadian adult dyspepsia empiric treatment – *Helicobacter pylori* positive (CADET-*Hp*) randomised controlled trial. *BMJ* 2002; 324:1012–1016.
47. Manes G, Menchise A, de Nucci C, Balzano A. Empirical prescribing for dyspepsia: randomised controlled trial of test and treat versus omeprazole treatment. *BMJ* 2003; 326:1118.
48. Chey WD, Moayyedi P. Uninvestigated dyspepsia and non-ulcer dyspepsia – the use of endoscopy and the roles of *Helicobacter pylori* eradication and antisecretory therapy. Aliment Pharmacol Ther 2004; 19(Suppl 1):1–8.
49. Castells MC. Mastocytosis: classification, diagnosis, and clinical presentation. Allergy Asthma Proc 2004; 25:33–36.
50. van Hogezand RA, Witte AM, Veenendaal RA, Wagtmans MJ, Lamers CB. Proximal Crohn's disease: review of the clinicopathologic features and therapy. Inflamm Bowel Dis 2001; 7:328–337.
51. Lind T, Megraud F, Unge P et al. The MACH2 study: role of omeprazole in eradication of *Helicobacter pylori* with 1-week triple therapies. Gastroenterology 1999; 116:248–253.
52. Walan A, Bader JP, Classen M et al. Effect of omeprazole and ranitidine on ulcer healing and relapse rates in patients with benign gastric ulcer. N Engl J Med 1989; 320:69–75.
53. Bombardier C, Laine L, Reicin A et al. Comparison of upper gastrointestinal toxicity of rofecoxib and naproxen in patients with rheumatoid arthritis. VIGOR Study Group. N Engl J Med 2000; 343:1520–1528.
54. Silverstein F, Simon L, Faich G. Reporting of 6-month vs 12-month data in a clinical trial of celecoxib. JAMA 2002; 286:2399.
55. Schnitzer TJ, Burmester GR, Mysier E et al. Comparison of lumiracoxib with naproxen and ibuprofen in the Therapeutic Arthritis Research and Gastrointestinal Event Trial (TARGET), reduction in ulcer complications: randomised controlled trial. Lancet 2004; 364;665–674.
56. Farkouh ME, Kirshner H, Harrington RA et al. TARGET Study Group. Comparison of lumiracoxib with naproxen and ibuprofen in the Therapeutic Arthritis Research and Gastrointestinal Event Trial (TARGET), cardiovascular outcomes: randomised controlled trial. Lancet 2004; 364:675–684.
57. Silverstein FE, Graham DY, Senior JR et al. Misoprostol reduces serious gastrointestinal complications in patients with rheumatoid arthritis receiving nonsteroidal anti-inflammatory drugs. A randomized, double-blind, placebo-controlled trial. Ann Intern Med 1995; 123:241–249.
58. Taha AS, N Hudson, Hawkey CJ et al. Famotidine for the prevention of gastric and duodenal ulcers caused by nonsteroidal anti-inflammatory drugs. N Engl J Med 1996; 334:1345–1349.
59. Hawkey CJ, Karrasch JA, Szczepanski L et al. Omeprazole compared with misoprostol for ulcers associated with nonsteroidal antiinflammatory drugs. Omeprazole versus Misoprostol for NSAID-induced Ulcer Management (OMNIUM) Study Group. N Engl J Med 1998; 338:727–734.
60. Chan FK, Chung SC, Suen BY et al. Preventing recurrent upper gastrointestinal bleeding in patients with *Helicobacter pylori* infection who are taking low-dose aspirin or naproxen. N Engl J Med 2001; 344:967–973.
61. Chan FK, Hung LC, Suen BY et al. Celecoxib versus diclofenac and omeprazole in reducing the risk of recurrent ulcer bleeding in patients with arthritis. N Engl J Med 2002; 347:2104–2110.
62. Lai KC, Lam SK, Chu KM et al. Lansoprazole for the prevention of recurrences of ulcer complications from long-term low-dose aspirin use. N Engl J Med 2002; 346:2033–2038.
63. Scheiman JM, Yeomans N, Talley N et al. Esomeprazole (20 mg and 40 mg) prevents NSAID associated gastric and duodenal ulcers in increased-risks patients. Gut (in press).
64. Hawkey CJ, Tulassay Z, Szczepanski L et al. Randomised controlled trial of *Helicobacter pylori* eradication in patients on non-steroidal anti-inflammatory drugs: HELP NSAIDs study. Helicobacter Eradication for Lesion Prevention. Lancet 1998; 352: 1016–1021 (Erratum, Lancet 1998; 352:1634).
65. Hawkey CJ. Personal review: *Helicobacter pylori*, NSAIDs and cognitive dissonance. Aliment Pharmacol Ther 1999; 13:695–702.
66. Huang J-Q, Sridhar S, Hunt RH. Role of *Helicobacter pylori* infection and non-steroidal anti-inflammatory drugs in peptic ulcer disease: a meta analysis. Lancet 2002; 359:14–22.
67. Catella-Lawson F, Reilly MP, Kapoor SC et al. Cyclooxygenase inhibitors and the antiplatelet effects of aspirin. N Engl J Med 2001; 345:1809–1817.
68. MacDonald TM, Wei L. Effect of ibuprofen on cardioprotective effect of aspirin. Lancet 2003; 361:573–574.
69. Patel TN, Goldberg KC. Use of aspirin and ibuprofen compared with aspirin alone and

the risk of myocardial infarction.Arch Intern Med 2004; 164:852–856.
70. Palmer KR. Intravenous omeprazole after endoscopic treatment of bleeding peptic ulcers. Gut 2001; 49:610–611.
71. Holtmann G, Howden CW. Management of peptic ulcer bleeding – the roles of proton pump inhibitors and *Helicobacter pylori* eradication. Aliment Pharmacol Ther 2004; 19(Suppl 1):66–70.
72. Gisbert JP, Khorrami S, Carballo F, Calvet X, Gene E, Dominguez-Munoz JE. *H. pylori* eradication therapy vs. antisecretory non-eradication therapy (with or without long-term maintenance antisecretory therapy) for the prevention of recurrent bleeding from peptic ulcer. Cochrane Database Syst Rev 2003; (4)CD004062.
73. Rockall TA, Logan RF, Devlin HB et al. Incidence of and mortality from acute upper gastrointestinal haemorrhage in the United Kingdom. Steering committee and members of the National Audit of Acute Upper Gastrointestinal Haemorrhage. BMJ 1995; 311:222–226.
74. Svanes C. Trends in perforated peptic ulcer: incidence, etiology, treatment, and prognosis. World J Surg 2000; 24:277–283.
75. Reinbach DH, Cruickshank G, McColl KE. Acute perforated duodenal ulcer is not associated with *Helicobacter pylori* infection. Gut 1993; 34:1344–1347.
76. Gisbert JP, Pajares JM. *Helicobacter pylori* infection and perforated peptic ulcer: prevalence of the infection and role of antimicrobial treatment. Helicobacter 2003; 8:159–167.
77. Mishra A, Sharma D, Raina VK. A simplified prognostic scoring system for peptic ulcer perforation in developing countries. Indian J Gastroenterol 2003; 22:49–53.
78. Carvajal SH, Mulvihill SJ. Postgastrectomy syndromes: dumping and diarrhea. Gastroenterol Clin North Am 1994; 23:261–279.
79. Fennerty MB. Pathophysiology of the upper gastrointestinal tract in the critically ill patient: rationale for the therapeutic benefits of acid suppression. Crit Care Med 2002; 30(Suppl):S351–S355.
80. Spirt MJ. Stress-related mucosal disease: risk factors and prophylactic therapy. Clin Ther 2004; 262:197–213.
81. Bowen JC, Fleming WH, Thompson JC. Increased gastrin release following penetrating central nervous system injury. Surgery 1993; 75:720–724.
82. Cook D, Heyland D, Griffith L, Cook R, Marshall J, Pagliarello J. Risk factors for clinically important upper gastrointestinal bleeding in patients requiring mechanical ventilation. Canadian Critical Care Trials Group. Crit Care Med 1999; 27:2812–2817.
83. Cook DJ, Fuller HD, Guyatt GH et al. Risk factors for gastrointestinal bleeding in critically ill patients. Canadian Critical Care Trials Group. N Engl J Med 1994; 339:377–381.
84. MacLaren R, Jarvis CL, Fish DN. Use of enteral nutrition for stress ulcer prophylaxis. Ann Pharmacother 2001; 35:1614–1623.
85. Cook DJ, Reeve BK, Guyatt GH, Raffin TA. Stress ulcer prophylaxis in critically ill patients. JAMA 1996; 275:309–314.
86. Cook D, Heyland D, Marshall J. Canadian Critical Care Trials Group. On the need for observational studies to design and interpret randomized trials in ICU patients: a case study in stress ulcer prophylaxis. Intens Care Med 2001; 27:347–354.
89. Jung R, MacLaren R. Proton-pump inhibitors for stress ulcer prophylaxis in critically ill patients. Ann Pharmacother 2002; 36:1929–1937.
88. Tryba M, Cook D. Current guidelines on stress ulcer prophylaxis. Drugs 1997; 54:581–596.
89. Cameron AJ, Higgins JA. Linear gastric erosion: a lesion associated with large diaphragmatic hernia and chronic blood loss. Gastroenterology 1986; 91:338–342.
90. Johns TNP, Clements EL. The relief of anaemia by repair of hiatus hermia. J Thorac Cardiovasc Surg 1961; 41:737–747.

Chapter 36

Gastritis

Robert M Genta

KEY POINTS

- Inflammation of the gastric mucosa per se does not usually produce symptoms
- *H. pylori* gastritis is the commonest chronic infection in humans
- Atrophic pangastritis is commoner in less industrialized countries and populations with a high incidence of gastric adenocarcinoma
- Antrum-predominant *H. pylori* gastritis carries a 15–20% lifetime risk of peptic ulcer
- Carcinoma and lymphoma may present years after eradication of *H. pylori* infection
- Autoimmune gastritis can cause iron deficiency or pernicious anemia
- Lymphocytic gastritis is associated with celiac disease, *H. pylori* infection, varioliform gastritis, and Ménétrièr's disease
- Chemical gastropathy is caused by NSAIDs or alkaline reflux (bile or pancreatic secretion)

INTRODUCTION AND DEFINITION

The discovery of *Helicobacter pylori* catapulted gastritis onto center stage. Intensive research and a voluminous literature followed. In this chapter the references are not cited in the text but rather grouped and annotated in the reference list to guide the reader to specific areas that are covered.

The term body or gastric body is used here as synonymous with corpus. The main compartments or gland zones of the stomach are in the antrum, the body and fundus, and the cardia. Each zone is characterized histologically by the types of gland present. In the gastric antrum the glands are of the mucous type; in the gastric body and fundus the gland zone is collectively called the oxyntic gland zone, with glands consisting primarily of parietal and chief cells. Histologically the gastric cardia is a narrow band of mucosa juxtaposed to the squamous mucosa of the esophagus at the Z-line. Typical cardiac glands are of the mucous type, similar to those of the gastric antrum, but they often contain oxyntic gland elements.

The histologic gland zones do not necessarily correspond to the gross anatomic landmarks. For example, the oxyntic gland mucosa has also been referred to as the fundic gland mucosa, and thus there may be potential confusion with the anatomic fundus, the dome of the stomach. Cardia tumors, in anatomic terms, usually refer to their location straddling both sides of the gastroesophageal junction, whereas the cardiac gland zone refers to the gastric glands just at and below the squamocolumnar junction.

Gastritis, simply defined as the inflammation of the gastric mucosa, is a condition not a disease. With few exceptions, the inflammation of the gastric mucosa *per se* does not produce signs or symptoms. A subset of patients may have symptoms due to gastritis, but no independent tests are available to make that prediction in an individual patient.

A second group of conditions characterized by gastric mucosal lesions with little or no inflammation were traditionally included in classifications of gastritis, and are now categorized as gastropathies. The term reactive gastropathy, for example, refers to intense epithelial change with little or no inflammation. Congestive gastropathy refers to prominent vascular abnormalities as the dominant feature. Hypertrophic gastropathy refers to just that, namely thickening of the mucosa due to thickening of the foveolae, the glands, or both. In some gastropathies, inflammation may be present but the abnormal thickness is considered the dominant feature structurally and pathogenetically.

CLASSIFICATION

The histologic changes listed in Table 36.1 can be viewed as the foundations for the terminology of gastritis, and some familiarity with them is indispensable to understand both the classification and related manifestations of non-neoplastic gastric conditions. The Updated Sydney System (outlined in Table 36.2) has become the standard classification of gastritis used widely by many gastroenterologists, especially in research studies.

HELICOBACTER PYLORI GASTRITIS (see Chapter 34)

Definition

Chronic active gastritis is the result of specific and nonspecific responses mounted by the gastric mucosa against *H. pylori* infection. 'Chronic' refers to mononuclear cell infiltrates, especially lymphocytes and plasma cells, as well as eosinophils. 'Active' refers to the presence of neutrophils infiltrating the epithelium and lamina propria.

Epidemiology

H. pylori gastritis is the most common chronic infection in humans. It affects between three and four billion people, with a prevalence that varies from less than 20% in industrialized Western regions with ethnically homogeneous populations (e.g., Scandinavia) to more than 80% in developing areas of the world (e.g., parts of South America, equatorial Africa, South-East Asia). Within countries, the most important predictor of high prevalence is low socioeconomic status. Improved socioeconomic conditions have resulted in a decreased prevalence of *H. pylori* in most Western countries and Japan.

TABLE 36.1 HISTOPATHOLOGIC COMPONENTS OF GASTRITIS

Histologic component	Common causes	Significance
Epithelial degeneration	Chemical injury *H. pylori* infection	Direct surface damage
Foveolar hyperplasia	Chemical injury *H. pylori* infection	An adaptive response to increased cellular exfoliation from the surface epithelium
Hyperemia or edema	Chemical injury	Nonspecific acute inflammatory response
Neutrophilic polymorphs	*H. pylori* infection Other infections	Indicates "activity"
Eosinophilic polymorphs	Eosinophilic gastroenteritis Anisakis *H. pylori* infection	Wide range of normal in different populations
Lymphocytes	Chronic gastritis Lymphocytic gastritis (when intraepithelial)	Moderate range of normal amongst individuals
Plasma cells	Chronic gastritis	Moderate range of normal amongst individuals
Lymphoid follicles	*H. pylori* infection	Rare lymphoid aggregates without germinal centers may be found in normal corpus
Atrophy	Long-standing *H. pylori* infection Autoimmune gastritis	
Intestinal metaplasia	Long-standing *H. pylori* infection Autoimmune gastritis If focal, possible chemical injury	
Pyloric metaplasia	Severe corpus atrophy	Usually autoimmune gastritis
Endocrine cell hyperplasia	Atrophy Chronic acid suppression	
Parietal cell alterations	Chronic acid suppression with proton pump inhibitors	

Causes, risk factors, disease associations

Humans are the only important reservoir for *H. pylori. Helicobacter heilmannii*, a pathogen of dogs and cats, is responsible for approximately 1% of human *Helicobacter* infections; its histopathologic aspects and clinical associations are similar to those of *H. pylori* gastritis. Transmission occurs primarily from human to human and is most efficient in childhood, as suggested by the finding that children and their parents are often infected by strains with identical genetic fingerprints.

H. pylori is a spiral, microaerophilic, urease-producing, Gram-negative bacterium. A number of proteins expressed by *H. pylori*, collectively known as pathogenicity factors, have been suspected of an association with particular manifestations of the infection (Table 36.3). However, the virulence of *H. pylori* seems to be largely host dependent, and none of these factors is disease specific.

H. pylori infection is associated with most duodenal and gastric ulcers not related to the use of nonsteroidal anti-inflammatory drugs (NSAIDs) and almost all primary gastric lymphomas of the mucosa-associated lymphoid tissue (MALT). In certain populations a considerable proportion of infected subjects develop atrophic gastritis, a documented precursor of gastric carcinoma.

Pathogenesis and pathology

Studies of the *initial phases* of *H. pylori* infection reveal acute mucosal inflammatory responses that usually involve all gastric compartments (gland zones), and may be accompanied by multiple antral erosions and subepithelial hemorrhages.

The *chronic phase* is characterized by a mixed infiltrate in the lamina propria (usually most intense in its most superficial portions), consisting of lymphocytes, plasma cells, and variable amounts of eosinophils, and by the infiltration of the surface and pit epithelium by neutrophils. The intensity of inflammation is generally greater in the antrum and the cardia than in the gastric body, where it may be minimal despite visible bacterial colonization. This distribution of inflammation characterizes the *antrum-predominant gastritis*, the most common type of gastritis in Western populations. In a proportion of infected subjects the inflammation is equally intense in all gastric compartments. This pattern, known as *pangastritis*, is associated with a progression toward glandular destruction with resulting atrophy and intestinal metaplasia. Atrophic pangastritis is the predominant phenotype in subjects from less industrialized areas of the world and particularly in populations with high incidence of gastric adenocarcinoma.

Lymphoid follicles, an expression of MALT (see Chapter 38), are virtually always found in infected stomachs, and their presence is a reliable indication of active or recently treated *H. pylori* gastritis. Their greatest density is in the region of the *incisura angularis* and the lowest in the proximal body greater curvature.

TABLE 36.2 UPDATED SYDNEY SYSTEM FOR CLASSIFICATION OF GASTRITIS AND GASTROPATHIES

Type of gastritis	Etiologic factors	Other designations
Nonatrophic	*Helicobacter pylori*	Superficial Diffuse antral gastritis Chronic antral gastritis Interstitial – follicular Hypersecretory Type B1
ATROPHIC		
Autoimmune	Autoimmunity Cross-reactivity with *H. pylori* antigens	Type A1 Diffuse corporal Pernicious anemia associated
Multifocal atrophic	*H. pylori*, in association with dietary, environmental, and host factors	Type B1, type AB1 Environmental Metaplastic
SPECIAL FORMS		
Chemical gastropathy	Chemical irritation Bile NSAIDs ?Other agents	Reactive Reflux NSAID Type C1
Radiation	Radiation injury	
Lymphocytic	Idiopathic ?immune mechanisms Gluten Drug (ticlopidine) ?*H. pylori*	Varioliform (endoscopic) Celiac disease associated
Noninfectious granulomatous	Crohn's disease Sarcoidosis Wegener's granulomatosis and other vasculitides Foreign substances Idiopathic	Isolated granulomatous
Eosinophilic	Food sensitivity ?Other allergies	Allergic
Other infectious gastritides	Bacteria (other than *H. pylori*) Viruses Fungi Parasites	Phlegmonous

Clinical presentation

The relationship of chronic *H. pylori* gastritis with dyspepsia (see Chapter 5) remains unclear. *H. pylori* eradication in patients with nonulcer dyspepsia has not been shown conclusively to improve the dyspeptic symptoms. A subset may respond, but prediction of which patients might belong to that subset is not possible at this time.

Subjects with *antrum-predominant H. pylori gastritis* have a lifetime risk for peptic ulcer disease of 15–20% (see Chapter 35). Most subjects who do not develop ulcer disease remain asymptomatic and are believed to have no increased risk for gastric adenocarcinoma (see Chapter 37); those with *pangastritis* also remain asymptomatic, but their gastric mucosa develops progressive destructive and reparative changes that result in expanding areas of glandular loss (atrophy) and replacement of the native gastric mucosa with an intestinal-type epithelium (intestinal metaplasia). Atrophic gastritis is epidemiologically and biologically associated with gastric adenocarcinoma of the intestinal type, and patients with this phenotype account for much of the increased risk of cancer related to *H. pylori* infection. Based on case–control and other retrospective epidemiologic studies, the overall gastric cancer risk for *H. pylori*-infected subjects has been estimated as 3–10-fold that of the uninfected population. *H. pylori* infection is also related to diffuse gastric cancer of the stomach, which accounts for 50% or more of all gastric cancers in some populations. Here there is no diffuse intestinal metaplasia or atrophy and no apparent dysplastic 'soil.' The risk for primary gastric B-cell lymphoma, a rare condition, is in the range of 5–7-fold that of noninfected subjects.

Both carcinoma and lymphoma may be diagnosed years or even decades after *H. pylori* infection has disappeared, possibly because of the combined effects of the hypochlorhydria related to atrophy, an inhospitable gastric environment brought upon by metaplasia and incipient epithelial and lymphoid neoplasia, and possibly incidental antibiotic treatments. Thus, it is likely that retrospective studies seriously underestimate the risk of neoplasia conferred by *H. pylori* infection. Studies taking into account the infecting strain of *H. pylori* (with regard to pathogenicity factors), the phenotype of gastritis, and the time elapsed between detection of the infection and the diagnosis of carcinoma, have raised the estimated risk to 23-fold.

TABLE 36.3 PUTATIVE PATHOGENICITY FACTORS OF *H. PYLORI* AND THEIR ALLEGED ASSOCIATIONS

Putative pathogenicity factor	Characteristics	Associations
VacA (vacuolating cytotoxin)	Genotypes *s*1 (associated with CagA positivity) and *s*2	Not useful for predicting symptoms, presentation, degree of inflammation, or response to therapy
CagA (cytotoxin-associated gene product A)	Product of one of the genes in the *cag* pathogenicity island	Induction of cytokine expression in gastric epithelial cells, with raised mucosal levels of interleukin-8 and marked neutrophil infiltration Increased risk of a symptomatic outcome (peptic ulcer and gastric cancer), but not in all populations No predictive value in individual patients
iceA (induced by contact with epithelium)	Bacterial restriction enzyme	No known biologic or epidemiologic evidence of a role for iceA as a virulence factor in *H. pylori*-related disease
babA (blood group antigen-binding adhesin)	Outer membrane protein, involved in adherence of *H. pylori* to Lewis-b (Leb) blood group antigens on gastric epithelial cells	No individual predictive value Infection with *babA*2 gene, *cagA*+ and *vacA s*1 ('triple-positive strains') may be related to duodenal ulcer risk

Diagnostic methods

Testing for *H. pylori* should be performed only if treatment is intended. The diagnosis can be made by endoscopic biopsy of the gastric mucosa or by noninvasive methods, depending on the clinical setting. Biopsy specimens (ideally at least two from the antrum and two from the gastric body greater curve) are examined for the detection of *H. pylori* and for the diagnosis of gastritis (Fig. 36.1). Many pathologists also use special stains that make it easier to detect the organisms quickly, and in some circumstances to detect them when they are sparse (Figs 36.2 and 36.3). A urease test on an antral biopsy specimen permits the rapid detection of urease activity in the biopsy material, with a sensitivity of 80–100% and a specificity of 92–100%. Culture of *H. pylori* with antibiotic sensitivity testing is not performed routinely for the initial diagnosis of *H. pylori* infection. Some laboratories have high-quality culture facilities for *H. pylori*, and culture may be used if a second course of therapy also fails to eradicate the organisms.

Treatment

The 1998 US Consensus Conference recommended three possible first-line therapy combinations (see Chapter 34):

- A proton pump inhibitor, clarithromycin, and either amoxicillin or metronidazole for 2 weeks
- Ranitidine bismuth citrate, clarithromycin, and amoxicillin, metronidazole, or tetracycline for 2 weeks
- A proton pump inhibitor, bismuth, metronidazole, and tetracycline for 1–2 weeks.

The regimens recommended by the European Maastricht 2-2000 conference are a proton pump inhibitor (or ranitidine bismuth citrate), clarithromycin, and amoxicillin or metronidazole for 7 days. After a first treatment failure (usually due to either poor patient compliance or the development of antibiotic resistance), eradication is more difficult. Therefore, a 10–14-day course is suggested for second-line therapies. One commonly used second-line therapy consists of a proton pump inhibitor, tetracycline, metronidazole, and bismuth citrate.

Indications for therapy

Primary indications for testing and treatment include active peptic ulcer disease, a history of documented peptic ulcer, or gastric MALT lymphoma. Testing of asymptomatic subjects and patients with nonulcer dyspepsia are not recommended, except when there is a documented history of gastric cancer in first-degree relatives. Despite the absence of data, many patients with life-dominating nonulcer dyspepsia are treated if they have evidence of *H. pylori*. In children, testing for *H. pylori* is recommended when the symptoms are severe enough to justify therapy.

In spite of, or perhaps because of, the many recommendations issued by gastroenterologic associations and consensus groups, several issues regarding indications for therapy remain unresolved. In practice, treatment decisions are rarely based on evidence alone; frequently a number of patient- and doctor-driven considerations have the greatest weight in making these choices.

BIOPSY PROTOCOL

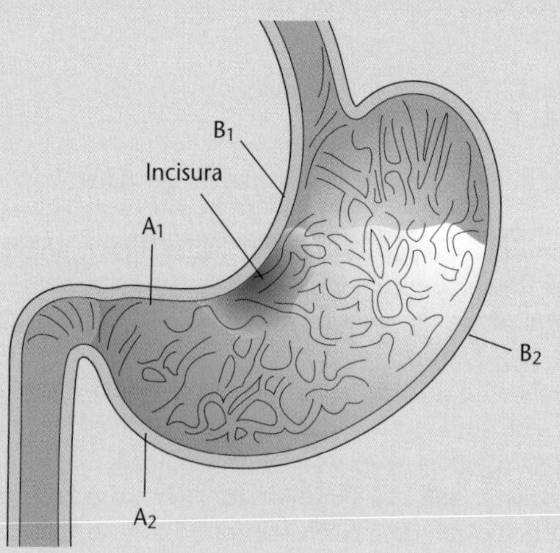

Fig. 36.1 Biopsy protocol. Schematic representation of the biopsy protocol recommended by the Updated Sydney System when the objective is to map the severity and extent of gastritis. A minimum of two specimens is obtained from each of the antrum (A_1 and A_2 – lesser and greater curvature) and the corpus (B_1 and B_2 – lesser and greater curvature). In addition, one biopsy specimen from the incisura angularis (IA) is recommended to detect early atrophic and metaplastic changes, represented in blue.

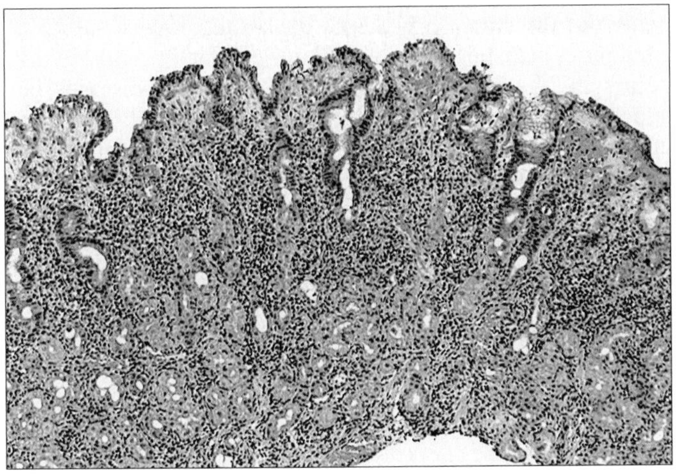

Fig. 36.2 Biopsy of the gastric body showing moderate chronic active gastritis. The dark staining mixed inflammatory infiltrate is concentrated mostly in the upper portions of the mucosa. Various degrees of clear-staining edema and hemorrhage are seen in the subepithelial zone.

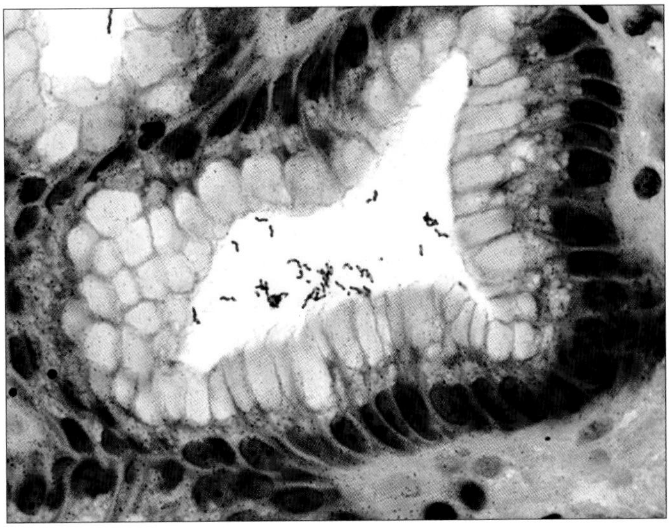

Fig. 36.3 High-power photomicrograph of a gastric pit with numerous *H. pylori*, made visible by a triple stain.

DIAGNOSTIC METHODS			
NONINVASIVE TESTS FOR DETECTION OF *H. PYLORI*			
Test	**Characteristics**	**Advantages**	**Disadvantages**
Urea breath test	Detects current infection, relying on *H. pylori*-derived urease activity in the stomach	Sensitivity and specificity >90% Can be used in children Useful for initial diagnosis and to evaluate treatment	Requires ^{13}C or ^{14}C detection equipment Expensive in some settings
Laboratory-based serologic tests	Detect anti-*H. pylori* IgG in serum	Approved tests have high specificity and sensitivity (≈85–90%) Inexpensive Useful for initial diagnosis	Detect evidence of past infection; no information on current infection Limited usefulness in determining success of therapy (titers diminish slowly after eradication and may remain positive after 1 year) Antigens used are crucial to specificity and may be 'population specific'
Simplified 'in-office' immunoenzymatic tests	Detect anti-*H. pylori* IgG in serum	Inexpensive disposable kits Quick results (10 min) Some tests use whole blood	Detect evidence of past infection; no information on current infection Sensitivity and specificity <90%
Urine tests	Detect anti-*H. pylori* IgG in urine	Inexpensive disposable kits Quick results (20 min) Recently developed tests (e.g., RAPIRUN, URINELISA) have moderate specificity and sensitivity (≈85%)	Not yet completely validated Sensitivity and specificity may be too low for clinical use Low specificity in children
Saliva tests	Detect anti-*H. pylori* IgA or IgG in saliva	Convenient collection of saliva	Low specificity and sensitivity (70–85% reported) Not approved, not readily available
Stool tests	Detect *H. pylori* antigens	Detects current infection Useful for determining eradication (8 weeks after therapy) Excellent specificity and sensitivity (>95%) Inexpensive May become noninvasive test of choice in children	Specimen collection may be inconvenient

AUTOIMMUNE GASTRITIS AND PERNICIOUS ANEMIA

Definition

Autoimmune gastritis is a chronic atrophic gastritis affecting the oxyntic gland mucosa (gastric body and fundus) and commonly associated with circulating serum antiparietal cell and anti-intrinsic factor antibodies and intrinsic factor deficiency. In its endstage it is associated with vitamin B_{12} deficiency. Pernicious anemia is the vitamin B_{12} deficiency associated with chronic atrophic autoimmune gastritis.

Epidemiology

Americans aged 60 years or older have a prevalence of pernicious anemia of 2.7% in women and 1.4% in men. There is a strong family association.

Pathogenesis

In autoimmune gastritis, autoantibodies to parietal cells and to their secretory product, intrinsic factor, are present in the serum and gastric juice. The antigen recognized by parietal cell autoantibodies is gastric H^+/K^+-ATPase, the major protein of the membrane lining the secretory canaliculi of parietal cells, which secrete hydrogen ions in exchange for potassium ions. During the course of the disease, both parietal and chief cells disappear progressively from the oxyntic glands.

The high prevalence of specific familial histocompatibility haplotypes (HLA-B8 and -DR3) in patients with corpus-restricted atrophic gastritis, and its association with other autoimmune conditions, strongly indicate an autoimmune origin. *H. pylori* infection may induce the formation of antibodies that cross-react with parietal-cell antigens and has been proposed as a possible etiologic factor in the pathogenesis of autoimmune gastritis. This correlation, however, remains unproven, and similarly, much stronger biologic, clinical, and epidemiologic evidence is needed before *H. pylori* can be viewed as the cause of autoimmune gastritis.

Pathology

Patients with autoimmune gastritis have an oxyntic gland-restricted chronic atrophic gastritis with an antral mucosa that is usually normal. Mononuclear cell infiltrates (plasma cells and lymphocytes) are found in the lamina propria between the gastric glands and may extend into the submucosa. Infiltrating plasma cells contain autoantibodies to the parietal cell antigen and to intrinsic factor. In the initial phases of the disease, individual parietal cells may be surrounded by lymphocytes or drop out from oxyntic glands. As the disease progresses over a period of two to three decades, the oxyntic mucosa may be completely replaced by pyloric-type (antral type) glands ('pyloric metaplasia') and intestinal metaplasia. At this stage the inflammation becomes less intense. In patients with classic pernicious anemia, residual small nests of parietal and chief cells may persist, but their numbers are greatly reduced. Enterochromaffin-like (ECL) cell hyperplasia is common, and microcarcinoids may be found. Multiple carcinoid tumors, usually benign, as well as hyperplastic polyps are frequent in endstage patients.

Clinical presentation

Most clinical manifestations of autoimmune gastritis become apparent when the parietal cell mass decreases beyond a critical point and the stomach becomes unable to produce sufficient amounts of acid, pepsinogens, and intrinsic factor. Achlorhydria occurs in the most advanced stages of the disease, but hypochlorhydria may also occur in patients with moderate numbers of surviving parietal cells, suggesting that anti-proton pump antibodies or inhibitory lymphokines released by subsets of inflammatory cells may participate in the inhibition of acid secretion. Patients with oxyntic gland atrophy and achlorhydria have hypergastrinemia, which tends to correlate with the severity of the mucosal damage. Injury to chief cells leads to a reduction of pepsin activity in gastric juice and of pepsinogens in blood. Pepsinogen I concentration (<20 ng/mL) is a sensitive and specific indicator of atrophic gastritis.

Patients with advanced autoimmune gastritis may develop either iron deficiency or pernicious anemia. Hypochromic anemia (15% of patients) may be caused by achlorhydria, as gastric acid is important in the absorption of nonheme iron, which in Western diets supplies at least two-thirds of nutritional iron needs. Frank pernicious anemia is usually preceded by gastric chronic atrophic gastritis and reduced or absent acid secretion by approximately a decade, and is generally associated with a histologic pattern of endstage atrophic gastritis. Thus a considerable number of patients with severe atrophic oxyntic gland gastritis may still not fulfill the criteria for the diagnosis of pernicious anemia but are clearly at risk for the development of vitamin B_{12} deficiency.

Disease associations

Autoimmune gastritis is a risk factor for hyperplastic and adenomatous polyps, carcinomas, and endocrine tumors. Polyps, found in 20–40% of patients with pernicious anemia, are mostly sessile, small, and multiple. Most are hyperplastic, but up to 10% may contain dysplastic foci. The risk of gastric carcinoma is believed to be increased 3-fold, and that of gastric carcinoid tumors 13-fold in patients with pernicious anemia. The trophic action of gastrin may be responsible for the evolution of endocrine cells from hyperplasia to neoplasia.

Diagnostic methods

The diagnosis of autoimmune gastritis may not be made because patients (elderly subjects with anemia) are successfully treated by hematologists or general practitioners with iron and vitamin B_{12} supplements, and are never referred to a gastroenterologist for the evaluation of atrophic gastritis, pepsinogen levels, or antiparietal cell antibodies.

The diagnosis can be confirmed by a combination of histopathologic and serologic studies. A set of at least four biopsy specimens from the gastric mid-body on the greater curvature, and two from the antrum, should be available. The coexistence of severe corpus atrophic gastritis (with chronic inflammation, marked or complete depletion of the parietal cell mass, and intestinal and pyloric metaplasia) with a normal antrum is virtually pathognomonic of autoimmune atrophic gastritis. Serum antibodies to gastric parietal cells are found in 90% of patients with pernicious anemia and in about 30% of their nonanemic first-degree relatives. The demonstration of circulating intrinsic factor autoantibodies is almost diagnostic of autoimmune gastritis and is present in approximately 50%. Hypergastrinemia is the result of sparing of the antrum and stimulation of the gastrin-producing G cells by achlorhydria. A low serum pepsinogen I concentration results from destruction of the chief cells.

Treatment

The standard treatment is regular monthly intramuscular injections of at least 100 µg vitamin B_{12} to correct the vitamin deficiency. Hydroxycobalamin 1 mg every 3 months is a common regimen.

OTHER GASTRITIDES

Infectious gastritides due to agents other than *Helicobacter* spp

The acid environment of the normal stomach is inhospitable to most infectious agents. However, in subjects with atrophic gastritis and decreased acid secretion, in patients with impaired immune responses, or as part of systemic infections, a number of viruses, bacteria, and parasites can infect the stomach. These infectious gastritides are normally rare, but some are not uncommon (e.g., cytomegalovirus) in immunocompromised patients. Their most important clinical and pathologic features are summarized in Table 36.4.

Lymphocytic gastritis

This is a distinctive type of pangastritis characterized by the presence of large numbers of mature lymphocytes (CD8) infiltrating the surface and foveolar epithelium. The lamina propria is infiltrated by an often dense population of inflammatory cells in which lymphocytes and plasma cell predominate, although significant numbers of neutrophils and eosinophils are also present.

Epidemiology

Lymphocytic gastritis is uncommon, found in 1–3% of subjects who undergo endoscopy with biopsy sampling.

Causes and pathogenesis

Because virtually all intraepithelial lymphocytes are CD8 suppressor T cells (the same cells that form the intraepithelial infiltrate in celiac disease), an immune mechanism has been proposed. In most cases of lymphocytic gastritis there is no role for *H. pylori*. However, an idiosyncratic response to *H. pylori* has been the development of a hypertrophic gastropathy with lymphocytic gastritis. In some of these cases the thick folds and lymphocytic gastritis disappear with *H. pylori* eradication. Lymphocytic gastritis is primarily of importance because of the company it keeps: approximately one-third of patients with celiac disease have lymphocytic gastritis (see Chapter 44). It may occur as an idiosyncratic reaction to *H. pylori infection*, has been described as the signature lesion of the now rare disorder diffuse varioliform gastritis, and was seen to be present in approximately one-half of patients with Ménétrièr's disease

TABLE 36.4 INFECTIOUS GASTRITIDES CAUSED BY AGENTS OTHER THAN *HELICOBACTER* SPP

Agent	Main characteristics	Pathology
VIRAL		
Rotaviruses, caliciviruses	Stomach may be infected during gastroenteritis	None known
Cytomegalovirus	Children Immunocompromised patients	 Megaloblastic inclusions Mucosal erosions, ulcerations Rarely large-fold gastropathy
BACTERIA		
Various	Overgrowth only in achlorhydric subjects	No detectable changes
Pyogenic bacteria (streptococci, staphylococci, *Escherichia coli*, *Proteus*, and *Hemophilus* spp)	Phlegmonous gastritis Exceedingly rare	Large areas of purulent necrosis involving full thickness of the gastric wall
Mycobacterium tuberculosis	Primary gastric tuberculosis rare Stomach may be involved in disseminated infections	Necrotizing granulomas may be found in gastric mucosa
Treponema pallidum	Gastric involvement in secondary syphilis Rare, more common in patients with HIV infection	Mixed inflammatory infiltrate, mostly plasma cells, and mucosal ulcerations. Swelling of gastric folds with erosions and ulcerations may mimic endoscopic appearance of lymphoma or carcinoma
FUNGI		
Candida spp *Histoplasma capsulatum* Mucoraceae	Only in immunocompromised patients	
PARASITES		
Cryptosporidium spp *Giardia intestinalis* *Strongyloides stercoralis*	Rarely found in stomach; mostly in immunocompromised patients	No inflammatory responses
Anisakidae	"Sushi worm" Many species of edible fishes have larvae of Anisakidae in their muscles. In a small proportion of individuals who eat infected fish, larvae penetrate the gastric wall causing a sudden onset of epigastric pain	Mostly eosinophilic response around penetrating larvae Dead larvae may elicit granulomas

(in one series). It is not uncommonly seen in gastric biopsies where there is no known association.

Diagnostic methods

A substantial increase in intraepithelial lymphocytes, particularly in the gastric body, is accompanied by a spectrum of inflammation in the lamina propria ranging from a minor increase in chronic inflammatory cells with no activity to a marked chronic inflammatory cell infiltration with activity and focal erosions. In most cases the histologic picture can be distinguished from that of *H. pylori* chronic gastritis, in which few intraepithelial lymphocytes are present. The diagnostic threshold for lymphocytic gastritis is generally accepted as more than 25 intraepithelial lymphocytes per 100 epithelial cells, but in most cases the counts are greater than 50.

Granulomatous gastritis

Granulomatous gastritis can be considered as a histopathologic category to which stomachs bearing granulomas are temporarily assigned while the condition responsible for their development is identified. In most cases the morphologic appearance of granulomas does not provide a useful clue to their etiology, except when foreign materials, acid-fast bacilli, or fungal forms are found. Thus, a specific diagnosis can be made only by integrating histopathologic findings with clinical and laboratory information.

Causes and pathogenesis

Granulomatous inflammation in the gastrointestinal mucosa can be found in disseminated *Mycobacterium tuberculosis* (see Chapter 51) and *Histoplasma capsulatum* infections. Primary gastric tuberculosis has been reported mostly from developing countries; it manifests as a large nonhealing ulcer. In gastric anisakiasis, fragments of helminthic cuticles may elicit the formation of foreign body granulomas. Other causes of foreign body granuloma are suture material in patients who have undergone a partial gastrectomy, and food particles that may become engulfed in an ulcer crater. Unusual causes of gastric granuloma include immune-mediated vasculitis syndromes (see Chapter 108) and Wegener's granulomatosis.

The stomach may be involved in patients with Crohn's disease (see Chapter 54) and sarcoidosis. In Crohn's disease, the prevalence of gastric granuloma may be as high as 10%. However, more common in Crohn's disease is a focal non-*H. pylori* gastritis in 30–70% of patients. In sarcoidosis, involvement of the gastrointestinal tract rarely has any clinical importance, although outlet obstruction and bleeding have occasionally been reported. Endoscopic findings may include nodularity; polypoid changes; erosions; ulcers; and segmental, usually distal, rigidity resembling linitis plastica. These gross changes reflect the presence of numerous mucosal granulomas and severe fibrosis.

As the finding of gastric mucosal granulomas may precede the discovery of these diseases in other organs, the careful interpretation of gastric biopsy findings together with appropriate suggestions for further tests may lead to the diagnosis of conditions that might otherwise remain obscure for a long time.

The term 'isolated (or idiopathic) granulomatous gastritis' should be applied only as a temporary diagnostic label to cases of granulomatous gastric inflammation for which no etiology has yet been determined. Even after careful evaluation, a proportion of gastric granulomas will remain unexplained. These lesions are usually asymptomatic; there is no information on their natural history or evolution, and so no treatment can be recommended.

GASTROPATHIES

Reactive or chemical gastropathy (Fig. 36.4)

Also known as 'type C' gastritis, reactive or chemical gastropathy is defined as the constellation of endoscopic and histologic changes caused by chemical injury to the gastric mucosa. The term chemical is used broadly. It refers to the gastric mucosa in some patients who take NSAIDs (see Chapter 25), and also includes patients with alkaline reflux after partial gastrectomy or those with poorly understood motility disorders resulting in the same. The term chemical gastropathy is often confusing to clinicians who can relate it to NSAID injury but do not usually consider injury from alkaline reflux (bile and/or pancreatic juice) to represent a chemical injury.

No relationship has been established between the endoscopic or histologic appearance of the mucosa in patients who take NSAIDs and dyspeptic symptoms. Chemical or reactive gastropathy has been interpreted by some to represent a diffuse lesion in those who take NSAIDs regularly. However, it is only seen in 10–45% of such individuals. However, biopsies at the edges of gastric erosions and ulcers more often reveal the features of reactive or chemical gastropathy, even in settings other than those of NSAID ingestion.

Histopathologic changes associated with reactive gastropathy include epithelial regeneration, foveolar hyperplasia, edema of the lamina propria, and expansion of the smooth muscle fibers into the upper third of the mucosa. However, both the specificity and predictive value of these features are low, and the diagnosis rests on the integration of clinical and histopathologic data. If reactive gastropathy is found unexpectedly in the course of biopsy of normal-appearing gastric mucosa for *H. pylori*, this may remind the physician that the patient is taking NSAIDs.

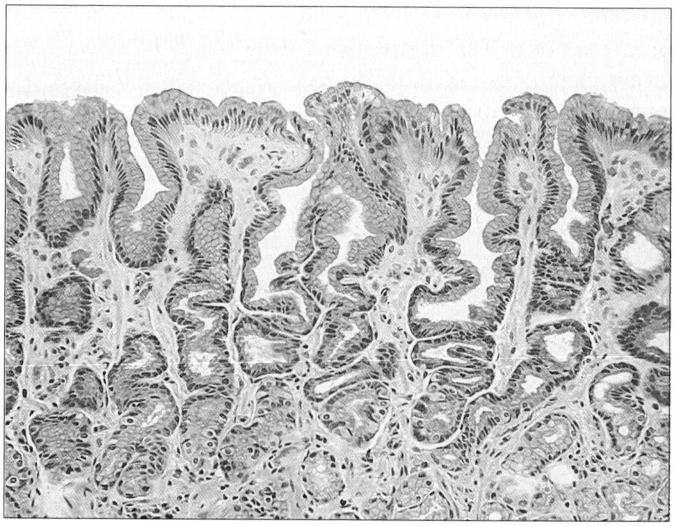

Fig. 36.4 Hyperplastic 'corkscrew' gastric foveolae and absence of inflammation. These features are characteristic of reactive or chemical gastropathy, which is seen in up to 45% of patients on chronic NSAIDs and in alkaline reflux gastropathy.

Hemorrhagic gastropathy

This group of conditions, characterized by subepithelial hemorrhages and erosions, is related to the use of NSAIDs (see Chapter 25), the ingestion of large quantities of alcohol, and severe physical stress (see Chapter 35).

Aspirin or other NSAIDs may induce acute mucosal injury, ranging from edema and hyperemia to multiple erosions and ulcerations. Such lesions may occur without warning symptoms in both first-time NSAIDs users and patients who have taken NSAIDs regularly for years. Except for generic risk factors (older age, female sex, and previous episodes), there are no ways prospectively to identify NSAID users who might be susceptible to severe gastric injury. Similar mucosal lesions, although usually less severe and only rarely evolving to ulcerations, can be caused by the ingestion of large quantities of alcohol.

The most severe degrees of hemorrhagic gastropathy are those induced by stress in critically ill patients. Most patients admitted to an intensive care unit have mucosal lesions, approximately 20% of them with overt bleeding and 2–5% with life-threatening hemorrhage (see Chapter 35).

The pathogenesis of stress-induced hemorrhagic gastropathy is not known, but when the mucosal defense mechanisms lose their integrity luminal acid may exert a damaging effect. Vascular disturbances – in association with stasis, vasoconstriction, and increased vascular permeability – may contribute further to mucosal vulnerability. Aspirin and NSAIDs act by interfering with prostaglandin synthesis. Alcohol causes direct damage to the gastric mucosa, particularly at higher concentrations.

Acute hemorrhagic gastropathy is characterized by a hyperemic edematous mucosa with erosions and active bleeding. As the diagnosis is usually clear from the clinical context, gastric biopsies are rarely obtained. The only exception might be to take biopsies in this setting from patients who are immunocompromised to look for evidence of infection such as cytomegalovirus. In addition, if hemorrhagic gastropathy is encountered without the usual associations, biopsy for a diffuse process like lymphoma should be performed.

Vascular gastropathies

This heterogeneous group of conditions is characterized by alterations in the gastric circulation and their effects on the gastric mucosa. The best defined from the morphologic and pathogenetic viewpoint are the watermelon stomach and portal hypertensive gastropathy.

Watermelon stomach

Watermelon stomach, or gastric antral vascular ectasia, is a condition of unknown etiology frequently associated with gastric atrophy and connective tissue disorders, particularly scleroderma (see Chapter 108), and sometimes portal hypertension. More than 70% of reported cases have occurred in women older than 65 years of age. Occult bleeding with iron deficiency anemia is present in almost 90% of patients, melena or hematemesis in 60%. The picturesque name was inspired by the endoscopic appearance of 'longitudinal antral folds seen converging on the pylorus, containing visible and ecstatic vessels resembling the stripes on a watermelon.' The prominent dilated vessels have also been compared to a large flat mushroom or honeycomb.

Histopathology

The lamina propria is expanded by smooth muscle proliferation and fibrosis, and contains dilated mucosal capillaries increased in cross-sectional area. Fibrin thrombi may be found within the dilated capillaries. Other localized conditions (e.g., gastric hyperplastic inflammatory polyps) may share some of these histopathologic characteristics; therefore, a tissue diagnosis is possible only if there is appropriate endoscopic correlation. Sometimes the degree of dilated capillaries is minimal relative to the striking endoscopic appearance. This may be due to shrinkage of the vessels in biopsies with formalin fixation, and also reflects the fact that the primary and most striking leashes of abnormal vessels are in the submucosa.

Treatment

Endoscopic obliteration of the dilated vessels by electrocoagulation or argon plasma coagulation is effective and has greatly reduced the need for antrectomy. Recurrence and the need for retreatment is not uncommon. Because atrophic oxyntic gland gastritis is a common accompaniment, patients with watermelon stomach should have biopsies taken from the mid-body greater curvature to rule out atrophic gastritis. If present, the patient should be monitored for the development of vitamin B_{12} deficiency.

Portal hypertensive gastropathy

A proportion of patients with cirrhosis of the liver (see Chapter 95) have dilatation of the mucosal vessels, more prominent in the proximal stomach; the prevalence parallels the severity of portal hypertension (see Chapter 96). Bleeding is relatively uncommon and rarely severe, except in patients with severe portal hypertension. The endoscopic appearance of portal hypertensive gastropathy, variously described as snake skin (mosaic), scarlatina rash, and cherry-red spots, is nonspecific and does not correlate well with the degree of portal hypertension.

Because of the understandable reluctance to biopsy the stomach of a patient with apparent portal hypertensive gastropathy, the contribution of histopathology to the diagnosis of portal hypertensive gastropathy is of negligible importance.

Hypertrophic gastropathies

The classic description of hypertrophic gastropathies proposed by Ming is still useful because it serves as a scaffold to be adapted to new entities, recognized, or better understood. The three classic types of hypertrophic gastropathy are:

1 Foveolar hyperplasia with normal or atrophic oxyntic glands
2 Hyperplasia of oxyntic glands with a largely unaffected epithelial cell component
3 A mixed type, in which both epithelial and oxyntic glands show variable degrees of hyperplasia.

Type 1 corresponds to Ménétrièr's disease, type 2 to Zollinger-Ellison syndrome (see Chapters 35 and 109), and type 3 incorporates a variety of conditions that may result from mixed glandular and foveolar hyperplasia, including infections (*H. pylori* infection, cytomegalovirus in children, syphilis) and other diseases of uncertain etiology (lymphocytic gastritis, eosinophilic gastroenteritis, sarcoidosis, and Cronkhite-Canada syndrome).

Ménétrièr's disease

This condition is defined as an idiopathic diffuse enlargement of the gastric folds largely confined to the gastric body and fundus. When well established, the massive foveolar cell hyperplasia is associated with major loss of parietal and chief cells. The amount of inflammation is variable; some patients have multifocal superficial erosions whereas others have polypoid configurations of the hypertrophic mucosa. If chronic active inflammation or lymphocytic infiltration of the epithelium is seen, the large-fold type of *H. pylori* gastritis or lymphocytic gastritis should be considered. Childhood Ménétrièr's disease is due to cytomegalovirus infection. In immunocompromised adults, gastric cytomegalovirus infection may sometimes produce localized hypertrophic gastropathy in the gastric antrum or body.

The hyperplastic foveolar cells secrete large amounts of mucus and fluid, resulting in protein-losing enteropathy; hypochlorhydria is the rule in well established cases.

Ménétrièr's disease is rare. Most patients are men in their fifth or sixth decade who present with weight loss, epigastric and abdominal pain, nausea, and vomiting. The disease evolves over several years or decades, and eventually patients develop severe hypoalbuminemia as a consequence of the chronic protein loss.

The pathogenesis is unknown, but it has been hypothesized that overproduction of transforming growth factor-α (TGFα) might explain several of the disturbances occurring in Ménétrièr's disease. TGFα, a mediator of gastric mucosal homeostasis produced by the gastric mucosa, inhibits acid secretion, stimulates mucosal repair after injury, and augments gastric mucin levels. A monoclonal antibody against the TGFα receptor may hold some promise. A variety of other therapies have been tried without any uniform success. Sometimes total gastrectomy is required because of the relentless hypoalbuminemia and the development of persistent anasarca (edema).

Ménétrièr's disease appears to be associated with an increased risk of gastric adenocarcinoma. Given the rarity of the disorder, it is unlikely that any cogent surveillance strategy will emerge.

Zollinger-Ellison syndrome (see Chapters 35 and 109)

The oxyntic mucosa shows hyperplasia of both the foveolar and the glandular compartment due to the trophic effect of circulating gastrin. This same effect causes proliferation of the ECL cells of the oxyntic mucosa, which may present as diffuse, linear, micronodular, or adenomatoid patterns, with the possible development of carcinoids.

FURTHER READING

Appelmelk BJ, Negrini R, Moran AP, Kuipers EJ. Molecular mimicry between *Helicobacter pylori* and the host. Trends Microbiol 1997; 5:70–73.

Bazzoli F, Cecchini L, Corvaglia L et al. Validation of the ^{13}C-urea breath test for the diagnosis of *Helicobacter pylori* infection in children: a multicenter study. Am J Gastroenterol 2000; 95:646–650.

Bazzoli F, Olivieri L, De Luca L, Pozzato P, Lehours P, Megraud F. Therapy and drug resistance in *Helicobacter pylori* infection. Dig Liver Dis 2000; 32(Suppl 3):S207–S210.

Correa P. Chronic gastritis as a cancer precursor. Scand J Gastroenterol Suppl 1984; 104:131–136.
One of the fundamental articles on the theory known as the Correa cascade, in which the hypothesis that chronic gastritis is the first step of a multistep process leading to gastric cancer is presented.

Dewar EP, Dixon MF, Johnston D. Bile reflux and degree of gastritis after highly selective vagotomy, truncal vagotomy, and partial gastrectomy for duodenal ulcer. World J Surg 1983; 7:743–750.
A seminal study on bile-induced reactive (chemical) gastropathy.

Ectors NL, Dixon MF, Geboes KJ, Rutgeerts PJ, Desmet VJ, Vantrappen GR. Granulomatous gastritis: a morphological and diagnostic approach. Histopathology 1993; 23:55–61.
The most comprehensive study on granulomatous gastritis.

El Zimaity HM, Genta RM, Graham DY. Histological features do not define NSAID-induced gastritis. Hum Pathol 1996; 27:1348–1354.
A detailed analysis of the difficulties associated with the histopathologic diagnosis of chemical gastritis.

Genta RM. A year in the life of the gastric mucosa. Gastroenterology 2000; 119:252–254.
This editorial makes a case for widespread eradication of H. pylori *for the prevention of gastric cancer, lymphoma, and peptic ulcer disease, even when data indicate that a year after cure of the infection there is no regression of either atrophy or intestinal metaplasia.*

Graham DY, Smith JL. Gastroduodenal complications of chronic NSAID therapy. Am J Gastroenterol 1988; 83:1081–1084.

Graham DY, Genta RM, Dixon MF. Gastritis. Philadelphia: Lippincott Williams & Wilkins; 1999.
A comprehensive multiauthored book issued in the wake of the publication of the Updated Sydney System. All types and aspects of gastritis are discussed.

Hocker M, Hohenberger P. *Helicobacter pylori* virulence factors – one part of a big picture. Lancet 2003; 362:1231–1233.
A review of the virulence factors of H. pylori *and their possible associations with different outcomes of gastritis.*

Laine L, Weinstein WM. Histology of alcoholic hemorrhagic "gastritis": a prospective evaluation. Gastroenterology 1988; 94:1254–1262.

Lynch DA, Dixon MF, Axon AT. Diagnostic criteria in lymphocytic gastritis. Gastroenterology 1997; 112:1426–1427.

Primignani M, Carpinelli L, Preatoni P et al. Natural history of portal hypertensive gastropathy in patients with liver cirrhosis. The New Italian Endoscopic Club for the study and treatment of esophageal varices (NIEC). Gastroenterology 2000; 119:181–187.

Schoenfeld P, Kimmey MB, Scheiman J, Bjorkman D, Laine L. Nonsteroidal anti-inflammatory drug-associated gastrointestinal complications – guidelines for prevention and treatment. Aliment Pharmacol Ther 1999; 13:1273–1285.

Solcia E, Rindi G, Fiocca R et al. Distinct patterns of chronic gastritis associated with carcinoid and cancer and their role in tumorigenesis. Yale J Biol Med 1992; 65:793–804.

Suerbaum S, Michetti P. *Helicobacter pylori* infection. N Engl J Med 2002; 347:1175–1186.
A critical review that addresses all aspects of H. pylori *gastritis.*

Talley NJ, Vakil N, Ballard ED, Fennerty MB. Absence of benefit of eradicating *Helicobacter pylori* in patients with nonulcer dyspepsia. N Engl J Med 1999; 341:1106–1111.

Toh BH, Van Driel IR, Gleeson PA. Pernicious anemia. N Engl J Med 1997; 337:1441–1448.
A comprehensive review of autoimmune gastritis and pernicious anemia.

Uemura N, Okamoto S, Yamamoto S et al. *Helicobacter pylori* infection and the development of gastric cancer. N Engl J Med 2001; 345:784–789.

Yamaoka Y, Graham DY. Disease-specific *Helicobacter pylori* virulence factors: the role of *cagA, vacA, iceA, babA2* alone or in combination. In: Hunt RH, Tytgat GN, eds. *Helicobacter pylori.* Basic Mechanisms to Clinical Cure 2000. Dordrecht: Kluwer Academic; 2000:37–42.
A critical discussion of the possibility (or lack thereof) of predicting the evolution of gastritis by determining the virulence factors of the infecting strain of H. pylori.

Chapter 37

Adenocarcinoma (gastric cancer and miscellaneous malignancy)

Alastair W McKinlay and Emad M El-Omar

KEY POINTS

- Gastric cancer remains a common malignancy in many parts of the world but the incidence varies significantly
- Symptomatic presentation is usually a sign of advanced disease
- The 5-year survival rate is less than 10%
- Known predisposing conditions include *Helicobacter pylori*, autoimmune gastritis, and previous gastric surgery
- Diagnosis is usually made by endoscopy
- Surgery remains the mainstay of treatment

INTRODUCTION AND DEFINITION

Napoleon Bonaparte's meteoric career was ended by Wellington in 1815. His death in 1824 was due to gastric cancer. A childhood of poverty, poor diet in his early career, and a strong family history of gastric cancer probably all contributed. It is now clear that *Helicobacter pylori*, acting in the context of host genetic susceptibility, is responsible for most cases of gastric cancer. Napoleon was probably infected by *H. pylori* – a case of the bacterium being mightier than the sword. The interaction between bacterium and host offers a new paradigm for carcinogenesis in the gastrointestinal tract and may serve as a model for other malignancies.

Gastric cancer remains a major global health problem, particularly in Asia and eastern Europe. Sadly, even with modern diagnostic and treatment methods, only 10% of patients are alive at 5 years.[1]

Gastric cancer is a malignant tumor arising in the stomach with evidence of invasive growth, or metastasis to regional lymph glands or distant organs. Some 90% of gastric malignancy is adenocarcinoma, which is broadly subdivided into:

- An intestinal form in which the malignant cells form glandular-like structures. This form is easily detectable at endoscopy and diagnosed on biopsy. The etiology and behavior of the intestinal form of gastric cancer differs for tumors located distally and proximally in the stomach.
- A diffuse form that infiltrates the wall of the stomach and causes relatively little mucosal disturbance, making endoscopic diagnosis more difficult.

Other gastric malignancies occur much less frequently, and include lymphoma (<5%), stromal tumors (<2%), and malignant carcinoid (<1%). This chapter concentrates exclusively on adenocarcinoma.

EPIDEMIOLOGY

Gastric cancer is a major global health problem and remains the world's second commonest malignancy, having been overtaken by lung cancer only in the late 1980s.

The incidence of gastric cancer varies markedly across the world. In northern European countries, North America, Australia, and New Zealand, death rates are now less than 10 per 100 000 and the incidence of gastric carcinoma has shown a substantial decline since the 1940s.

Death rates of 10–20 per 100 000 are found in southern Europe and the Middle East, whereas rates of 20–30 per 100 000 have been reported from South America, India, and eastern Europe. The highest rates, however, are found in Japan, China, and Russia, with cancer death rates of more than 30 per 100 000.[2] The high incidence of the disease in Japan has justified formal screening programs and a very methodical and organized approach to diagnosis. As a result the Japanese have a unique experience of early gastric carcinoma, which appears to have a much better prognosis. In contrast, in the UK and other Western countries, the cancer usually presents at a late stage and the outcome is poor.

Risk factors

Gastric cancer in Europe is increasingly a condition of the elderly, the median age at presentation being 72 years.[3] Since the early 1990s, 25% of new diagnoses have been in patients over the age of 80 years.[4] Males have a higher incidence of gastric cancer and there is also an increased risk in carriers of blood group A,[5] which seems to be associated with a family history of gastric cancer. Germ-line mutations in the E-cadherin (*CDH1*) gene have also been described in young subjects with familial diffuse gastric cancer. This subtype does not seem to be preceded by *H. pylori* infection or inflammation, and with a penetrance approaching 70% may prove difficult to survey endoscopically, prompting some to advocate prophylactic gastrectomy.[6]

Distal versus proximal cancers

Distal gastric adenocarcinoma is commoner in most populations, but is declining in incidence worldwide, particularly in Western countries. Carcinoma of the cardia and fundus (proximal cancers) seems to be increasing in caucasians and its incidence has increased significantly over the past 30 years, with less association with *H. pylori* infection, suggesting that the etiology may be different.

PATHOGENESIS

Significant advances in the understanding of gastric cancer pathogenesis have occurred in the past two decades, increasing

CAUSES AND RISK FACTORS

SIGNIFICANT RISK FACTORS

Conditions associated with hypochlorhydria
- *Helicobacter pylori*-associated gastritis
- Autoimmune gastritis
- Postgastric surgery (>20 years)
- Chronic atrophic gastritis

Chronic mucosal changes
- High-grade dysplasia
- Barrett's esophagus (adenocarcinoma of cardia and distal esophagus)
- Gastric adenoma
- Intestinal metaplasia

Genetic risk factors
- Gastric cancer family history
- Familial adenomatous polyposis coli (FAP)
- Hereditary nonpolyposis coli
- Germline E-cadherin (*CDH1*) mutations
- Proinflammatory cytokine gene polymorphisms

POSSIBLE RISK FACTORS
- Peutz-Jeghers syndrome
- Ménétrier's disease
- Smoking
- Diets low in fresh fruit and vegetables
- Diets high in preserved, pickled, or smoked items
- Alcohol

the number of the well recognized risk factors for this malignancy.

Earlier observations

Pernicious anemia, with its hallmark of autoimmune gastritis leading to atrophy, has long been known to confer an increased risk of gastric cancer. Similarly, it is well established that benign ulcer surgery, such as partial gastrectomy, is also associated with gastric cancer, with a lead-in time of 15–30 years.[7] Following gastric surgery, inflammation of the gastric remnant is common and usually associated with the reflux of bile. Although the histologic appearances are different, both pernicious anemia and the postsurgical stomach share a common pathophysiologic abnormality, namely hypochlorhydria.

H. pylori

The discovery of *H. pylori* by Marshall and Warren in 1983 was a turning point in gastroenterology. Its causative role in peptic ulcer disease was soon recognized and studied extensively, but the link with gastric cancer lagged almost a decade behind and finally culminated in the designation of *H. pylori* as group I (definite) human carcinogen in 1994.[8] It is now clear that *H. pylori* infection induces, in genetically predisposed hosts, a cascade of events that may ultimately lead to gastric neoplasia.

Distal gastric cancer: The key histopathologic stages of this cascade, particularly the intestinal type, have been described by Correa and include:[9]
- *H. pylori*-induced chronic superficial gastritis
- Gastric atrophy
- Intestinal metaplasia
- Dysplasia
- Gastric cancer.

In the diffuse type there is rapid progression from *H. pylori*-induced gastritis to cancer.

Achlorhydria: In both intestinal and diffuse distal gastric cancer, more than 90% of patients are achlorhydric, and this physiologic abnormality precedes the onset of malignancy by decades. It is now known that the increased proliferation induced by chronic inflammation creates a genetically unstable gastric mucosa, which is further compromised by the presence of genotoxic substances generated by inflammatory and bacterial products. The hypochlorhydria contributes to bacterial overgrowth, which further exacerbates the inflammation and leads to the generation of carcinogenic nitrogenous products.

Proximal gastric cancer (cardia cancer): Here the relationship with *H. pylori*, gastric atrophy, and hypochlorhydria is not clear; it appears that this type of gastric cancer does not have the same etiologic or pathophysiologic factors as distal gastric cancer. The pathogenesis remains poorly understood and much progress is still needed. The following discussion applies largely to distal gastric cancer.

Host factors

Cytokine polymorphisms: Several host genetic factors that increase the risk of gastric cancer have been described recently, and include polymorphisms in the proinflammatory cytokines interleukin 1β (IL-1β) and the tumor necrosis factor-α (TNF-α) genes.[10–12] It appears that the effect of these polymorphisms operates early in the disease process and requires the presence of *H. pylori* infection. When *H. pylori* infection challenges the gastric mucosa, a vigorous inflammatory response with a high IL-1β/TNF-α component may appear to be beneficial in driving the infection out, but concomitant inhibition of acid secretion may allow the infection to extend its colonization and damaging inflammation to the corpus mucosa, an area that is usually well protected by secretion of acid.

Acid: A decreased flow of acid may also undermine attempts to flush out mutagenic and genotoxic byproducts of inflammation, causing further damage to the mucosa and the risk of DNA damage. More inflammation in the corpus leads to sustained inhibition of acid secretion and a vicious cycle that accelerates glandular loss and onset of gastric atrophy. This ultimately succeeds in driving the infection out, but at a very high price for the host. The hypochlorhydric milieu is ideal for growth of non-*H. pylori* bacteria, some of which will no doubt contribute to further damage to the mucosa and production of carcinogenic *N*-nitroso-compounds.

Other factors

H. pylori infection in hosts with proinflammatory genetic makeup leads to the development of a hypochlorhydric, atrophic phenotype that increases the risk of distal gastric cancer, but the ultimate neoplastic transformation is clearly dependent on many other genetic and environmental factors.[10,13,14] Progression of severe gastritis or atrophy towards cancer depends on other components of the host genetic constitution acting epistatically, as well as by dietary and other factors in the environment. For example, a high intake of fresh fruits and vegetables containing antioxidants such as vitamin C may retard the progression of atrophy, whereas smoking and a high salt intake may accelerate it. Thus, the route to hypochlorhydria and gastric atrophy varies from patient to patient and is influenced by host genetic, bacterial, and environmental factors (Fig. 37.1). Cardia cancer remains poorly understood and has a different pathogenesis from distal cancer.

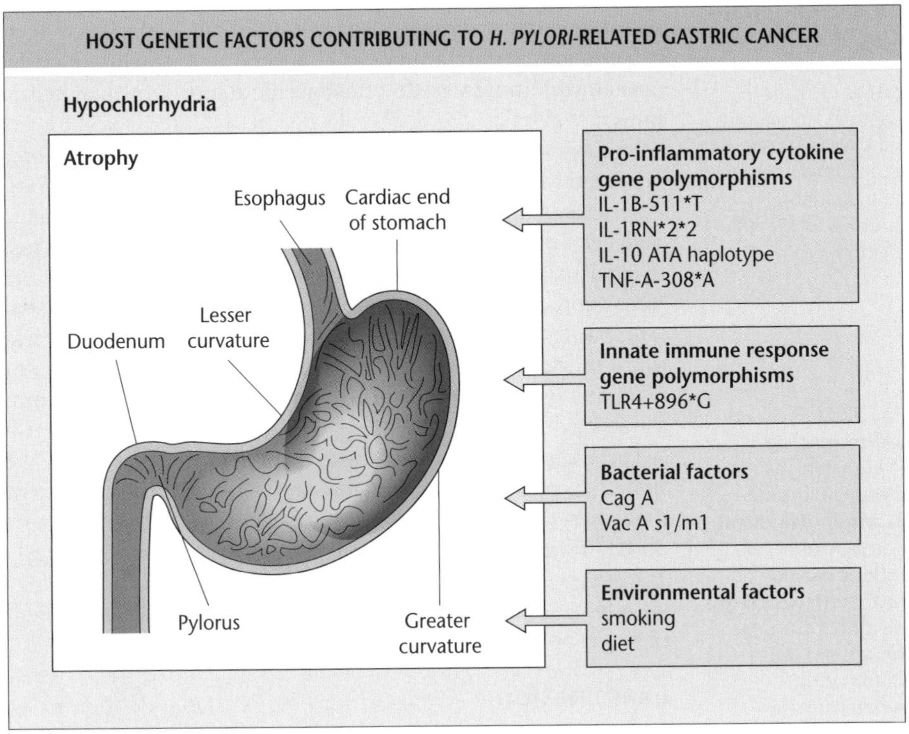

Fig. 37.1 Host genetic factors contributing to *H. pylori*-related gastric cancer.

PATHOLOGY

Some 90% of gastric malignancy is adenocarcinoma, which is usually classified according to the Laurén scheme.[15] This is a simple and still widely used three-tiered system comprising:

- The intestinal type – well differentiated and accounting for approximately half the cases. The malignant cells form glandular-like structures with different degrees of differentiation.
- The diffuse type – poorly differentiated and accounting for one-third of cases. The cells infiltrate through the wall of the stomach giving rise to a rigid 'leather bottle' stomach.
- A mixed or unclassified type.

Early gastric cancer

By definition, early gastric cancer involves only the mucosa and submucosa. Early lesions are typically asymptomatic and in the West are usually found by chance. By contrast in Japan, where the frequency of the disease is sufficiently high to warrant screening, true early gastric carcinoma is seen more frequently and is usually classified according to the Japanese Research Society for Gastric Cancer (JRSCG) scheme:[16]

- Type I lesions are polypoid
- Type II lesions are superficial and are divided into elevated, flat, and depressed forms
- Type III lesions are excavated and usually penetrate through the mucosa into the submucosa, but not through the muscularis propria.

Type I and IIa lesions have a tendency to be better differentiated than type III. The mucosal appearance of early gastric carcinoma is often extremely subtle and requires careful inspection of the stomach (Fig. 37.2).

As gastric carcinoma is less common in western Europe, Australasia, and the United States, endoscopists are probably less familiar with its detection; this may explain the lower rates of diagnosis.[17]

Advanced gastric cancer

Unfortunately most gastric carcinomas are advanced and will have penetrated the submucosa by the time of presentation. The histopathology is usually that of an adenocarcinoma, and may vary from well differentiated to poorly differentiated forms. Tumor cells may contain mucus, giving rise to the so-called 'signet ring' appearance.

Macroscopically, tumors may present as raised nodular areas, often with extensive infiltration of the gastric wall. Presentation with ulceration is also common, however, and macroscopic appearances may be indistinguishable from those of a benign gastric ulcer (Fig. 37.3). For this reason gastric ulcers should always be biopsied. Typically, malignant ulcers tend to be more asymmetric, producing distortion of the rugae and often altering the surrounding mucosal appearance as infiltration occurs (Fig. 37.4). Malignant areas often appear nodular and the tissue is frequently more friable. Endoscopic biopsy of such areas often lacks the characteristic elastic 'tug' of normal gastric tissue. In

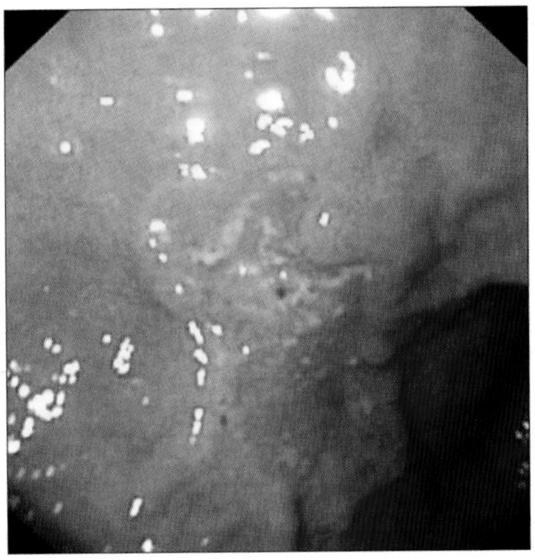

Fig. 37.2 Early gastric cancer, diffuse type. As gastric carcinoma is less common in western Europe, Australasia, and the United States, endoscopists are probably less familiar with its detection; this may explain the lower diagnostic rates.[17] Courtesy of Dr H. Bjorknas.

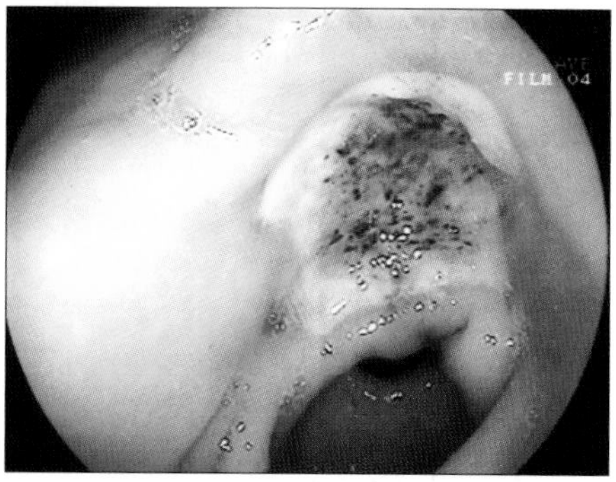

Fig. 37.3 Endoscopic view of a prepyloric ulcer. Biopsy of all gastric ulcers is essential to rule out malignancy. This ulcer turned out to be malignant. Courtesy of Dr A W McKinlay.

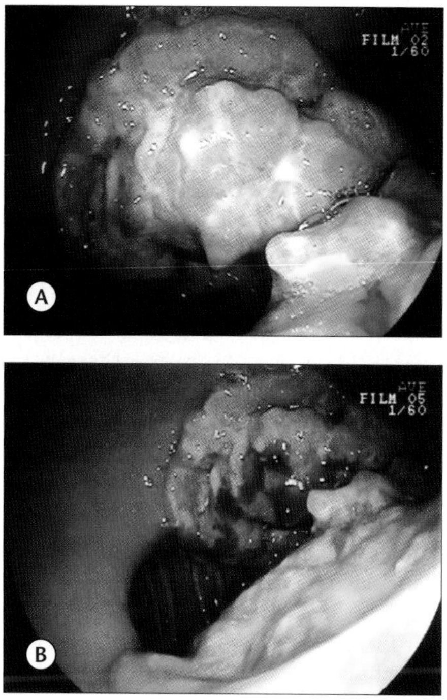

Fig. 37.4A,B Endoscopic view of a gastric adenocarcinoma arising in the distal stomach of a patient with a gastroenterostomy. Malignant tumors can arise in these achlorhydric stomachs many decades after surgery for benign peptic ulcer disease (30 years in this case).

diffuse forms, the anatomy of the stomach may be distorted, making retroflexion and inflation more difficult. At surgery, advanced gastric carcinoma is often palpable, and unfortunately local spread and metastatic dissemination are common.

Local and distant spread

Involvement of the antrum by distal or diffuse gastric cancer may distort the pylorus and lead to gastric outlet obstruction. Proximal gastric cancer commonly involves the esophagogastric junction. Spread to local and regional lymph nodes is common. The omentum and spleen may be involved, as well as organs in close proximity such as the transverse colon, occasionally giving rise to gastrocolic fistula.

Distant spread is most frequently to the liver and lungs (approximately 40%), and to the peritoneum and bone marrow in 10%. Spread to supraclavicular nodes (Virchow's node), left axillary nodes, and even umbilical nodes have all been documented. Peritoneal spread may result in malignant ascites, and ovarian involvement in the form of Krukenberg tumors is recognized.

CLINICAL PRESENTATION

Early gastric carcinoma is asymptomatic in 80% of patients. Some 10% may have peptic ulcer symptoms or nonspecific features such as nausea, anorexia, or early satiety. The majority of cases of early gastric carcinoma outwith Japan are usually found by chance while investigating nonspecific upper intestinal symptoms.[18]

In advanced gastric carcinoma the most common symptoms are weight loss, followed by abdominal pain, nausea and vomiting, anorexia, and dysphagia. Patients may present with anemia and signs of chronic gastrointestinal blood loss, but acute gastrointestinal hemorrhage is a relatively uncommon presentation. Because the symptoms are nonspecific, patients often present late. Some 40% of patients will have had symptoms of less than 3 months' duration, 60% will have been symptomatic for 3 months or longer, and up to 20% may have had symptoms for a year.

The clinical manifestations also depend on the location of the tumor. Tumors in the antrum interfere with gastric emptying or may directly infiltrate the pylorus and present with gastric outlet obstruction, sometimes manifesting as a succussion splash. Tumors of the fundus and body may reach a very large size with no symptoms other than chronic blood loss. Involvement of the esophagogastric junction can produce dysphagia.

Examination

The signs of gastric cancer include a palpable epigastric mass, supraclavicular or axillary lymphadenopathy, and malignant ascites. None of these features is specific to gastric cancer and investigations are usually required.

CLINICAL PRESENTATION

- Upper abdominal discomfort or pain
- New-onset dyspepsia
- Anorexia and early satiety
- Weight loss
- Vomiting (may be unaltered food in gastric outlet obstruction)
- Iron deficiency anemia
- Distant lymphadenopathy (Virchow's node, etc.)
- Metastatic spread – hepatomegaly, malignant ascites, bone pain, pulmonary metastases
- Early gastric cancer is often asymptomatic

CLINICAL TIPS

- Gastric cancer is increasingly a disease of the elderly
- It often presents with vague upper abdominal symptoms or iron deficiency anemia
- The diffuse form of gastric cancer is less common but can be difficult to diagnose at endoscopy
- The presence of concomitant disease is often a crucial determining factor in the decision process for treatment
- Early gastric cancer has a better prognosis but is frequently asymptomatic and is often a chance endoscopic finding
- Surgery remains the treatment of choice when curative treatment is attempted
- Radical surgery is a major undertaking and the patient must be fit enough to survive. A careful assessment of any concomitant disease and the anesthetic risk is required

DIFFERENTIAL DIAGNOSIS

- **Benign peptic ulcer:** The most important differential diagnosis is benign peptic ulceration of the stomach (see Chapters 5 and 35). Although large gastric ulcers may inherently appear alarming, they are more commonly benign than malignant and can occur in the context of nonsteroidal anti-inflammatory drug (NSAID) use. Similarly a gastric cancer may be indistinguishable from a 'benign' ulcer, and temporary 'healing' of malignant ulcers, particularly with proton pump inhibitors, is well recognized. Consequently, it is essential to biopsy gastric ulcers irrespective of whether they appear benign or malignant. Ulcers should be followed to complete healing and re-biopsy undertaken while any mucosal break remains.
- **Lymphoma** accounts for 5% of all malignant gastric tumors and can appear identical to gastric carcinoma (see Chapter 38). Typically patients with maltomas (gastric B-cell lymphoma) may appear less ill than would be expected for the size of the tumor, but again it is important to stress that biopsy is essential.
- **Benign polyps and pseudo-polyps:** True gastric adenomas are relatively rare but gastric polyps and pseudo-polyps are common.
- **Hyperplastic polyps (cystic fundal hyperplasia):** Usually distinguished by being small and by their biopsy appearance. Cystic fundal hyperplasia with multiple small 'polyps' in the fundus and body is also common and usually easily recognized at endoscopy.
- **Inflammatory polyps**
- **Adenomatous polyps**.

DIFFERENTIAL DIAGNOSIS

- Benign gastric (peptic) ulcer
- Gastric lymphoma
- Benign polyps and pseudo-polyps + gastric adenomas and polyps
- Hyperplastic polyps (cystic fundal hyperplasia)
- Gastrointestinal stromal tumors (leiomyoma and leiomyosarcoma)
- Carcinoid tumors
- *Helicobacter* gastritis
- Ménétrier's disease
- Other infiltrating conditions of the stomach + Crohn's disease
- Amyloid
- Sarcoid
- Kaposi's sarcoma

DIAGNOSTIC METHODS

The diagnosis of gastric cancer may be straightforward in advanced cases, but none of the symptoms or signs is unique. For this reason a high index of suspicion is often required in association with a careful history and physical examination, in selecting patients to undergo endoscopy.

Hematology and chemical pathology results may be supportive, but none is diagnostic. A hypochromic, microcytic anemia is a common finding; the fecal occult blood test may be positive, but this test is inaccurate, does not localize the source of blood loss, is therefore rarely diagnostic, and is not recommended. Liver function may be deranged in advanced disease and both the C-reactive protein concentration and erythrocyte sedimentation rate may be raised, but all of these findings can occur in other conditions and are particularly common in elderly patients. For these reasons, when gastric cancer is suspected some form of visualization of the upper gastrointestinal tract is indicated.

DIAGNOSTIC METHODS

ESTABLISHING A DIAGNOSIS
- Upper gastrointestinal endoscopy and biopsy
- Barium meal

METHODS MAINLY FOR STAGING
- Computed tomography
- Ultrasonography
- Endoscopic ultrasonography
- Positron emission tomography

Endoscopy

Upper gastrointestinal endoscopy is the diagnostic approach of choice because it allows the close inspection needed for diagnosis of early gastric carcinoma and endoscopic biopsy of any suspicious lesions. It is more accurate than barium radiology and generally well tolerated, even in elderly patients (see Chapter 119).

Difficulties and challenges

Gastric carcinoma is usually obvious at endoscopy, often as a polypoidal mass. Certain presentations are, however, difficult. These include mimicking a benign gastric ulcer and the presentation of a diffuse gastric carcinoma, because the mucosa itself may appear normal. An experienced endoscopist may note a different 'feel' to the stomach and it may be more difficult to produce adequate air insufflation of the fundus and body, making retroflexion more difficult. However, the changes are often subtle and mucosal biopsies may not be diagnostic because the carcinoma can infiltrate through the submucosal tissues giving rise to the 'leather bottle' appearance. Under these circumstances, a double-contrast barium meal demonstrating abnormal motility, or computed tomography (CT) to confirm the thickened wall, may be helpful.

Postoperative stomach

It is also recognized that examination of the postoperative stomach can present particular difficulties. Malignancy in the postoperative stomach often presents in the seventh and eighth decade. A variety of operative procedures were in common use, including antrectomy and gastroenterostomy (Pólya gastrectomy), antrectomy and primary anastomosis (Billroth 1 partial gastrectomy), vagotomy and pyloroplasty, and vagotomy and gastroenterostomy. It may be very difficult in the presence of a gastroenterostomy to achieve adequate inflation of the stomach; in addition, a bile reflux gastritis is almost invariable and may produce a fragile and mottled mucosa. The appearance of gastric cancer around the margins of a gastroenterostomy can therefore be difficult to find. Multiple biopsies are usually essential for diagnosis, particularly as gastric atrophy and intestinal metaplasia are common findings in older patients. The presence of high-grade dysplasia is always suspicious because it is known to indicate a high risk of malignant transformation, or may occur in areas of the mucosa adjacent to established malignancy.

Double-contrast barium studies

These are occasionally useful for some older or frailer patients, or as second-line investigation (e.g., for suspected linitis plastica with negative histological findings).

Techniques for staging and preoperative assessment

Transcutaneous ultrasonography

This investigation (see also Chapter 124) is useful as part of the staging of a gastric cancer. It may detect lymphadenopathy and is particularly valuable in assessing liver metastases.

Endoscopic ultrasonography

Endoscopic ultrasonography (see Chapter 121) is a more recent development. It provides good definition of the gastric wall (Fig. 37.5) and can also detect lymph nodes adjacent to the stomach; however, it is less useful for imaging distant lymph nodes, liver, or lungs. It has particular value in determining the depth of invasion and defining early gastric carcinoma with its better prognosis.

Similarly, with its ability to determine gastric wall thickness, endoscopic ultrasonography can be useful in detecting diffuse gastric carcinoma.

Chest radiography

X-ray may detect pulmonary metastases, but for more detailed staging CT remains the mainstay.

Computed tomography

CT of the chest is useful for detecting pulmonary metastases, whereas abdominal CT (Fig. 37.6) will detect hepatic metastases and may define perigastric involvement. Lesions less than 5 mm in diameter may not be detected by CT, or may be difficult to define. The primary role is to detect the size of lymph nodes, so that nodes that are involved but not enlarged may not be detected on scanning. CT may detect peritoneal or omental disease and has been reported to have an accuracy of up to 90% in detecting distant metastases.

However, some studies suggest that up to 50% of tumors are understaged and, more importantly, 15% are overstaged. In other words, a proportion of patients who appear to have inoperable disease may actually be operable at the time of surgery. As a result, some surgeons may perform preoperative or intraoperative laparoscopy and/or intraoperative ultrasonography. The most important point, however, is that in the absence of distant metastases a patient who is otherwise fit and capable of undergoing surgery should not be refused an operation on the basis of a single screening modality.

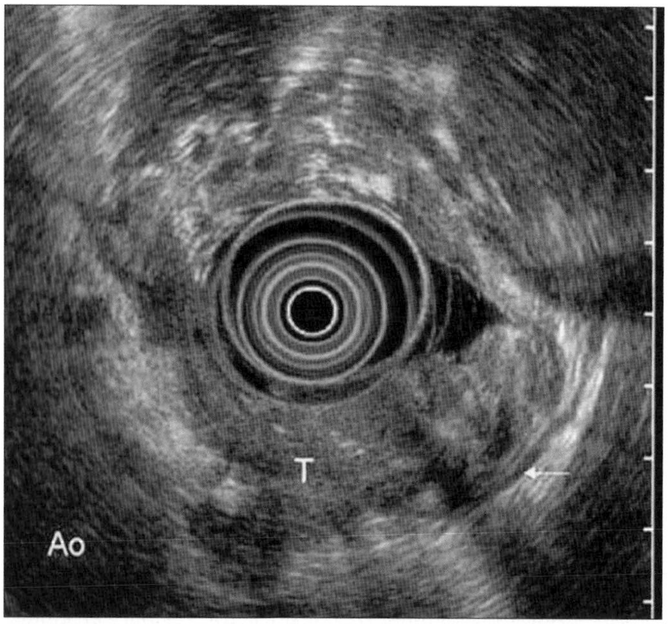

Fig. 37.5 Endoscopic ultrasonography of the gastric wall. The hypoechoic layer corresponding to the muscularis propria has been breached by an irregular hypoechoic tumor (arrow), with complete disruption of the gastric wall layer structure. From Digestive Disease Center, Medical University of South Carolina, with permission.

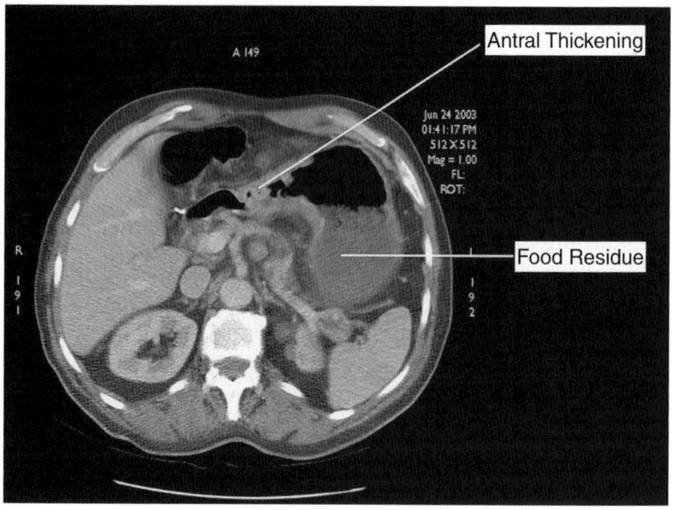

Fig. 37.6 Spiral computed tomogram of an antral adenocarcinoma. The image shows antral wall thickening and partial gastric outlet obstruction with food residue within the stomach. Courtesy of Dr Dympna McAteer.

TNM staging

Traditionally staging is carried out according to the tumor node metastasis (TNM) classification:[19]

- T1 tumors are confined to the mucosa and submucosa.
- T2 tumors penetrate the muscularis propria but not the serosa.
- T3 tumors reach the serosa but without the involvement of other organs.
- T4 tumors have spread beyond the serosa.

Nodal involvement is defined as:

- N0 for no involvement
- N1 for involvement of perigastric nodes within 3 cm of the primary tumor
- N2 for spread to more distant regional nodes.
- N3 involvement is to more distant intra-abdominal lymph glands that are not removable with surgery.

Distant metastases is defined as:

- M0 – no metastases
- M1 – distant metastases.

Five-year survival correlates closely with staging, with true in situ carcinoma having a survival rate of nearly 100%, through to stage 4 disease with a 5-year survival rate of 2%.

TREATMENT AND PREVENTION

The treatment of gastric cancer is dependent on:
- Making an accurate diagnosis
- Careful assessment and staging of the disease
- Consideration of the patient's overall condition including age, nutritional status, and, particularly, whether they have concomitant disease. The latter is probably more important than age per se.

Early gastric cancer

The outlook for patients with true early gastric carcinoma is good; if treated appropriately, many patients are cured. The only proven method of producing long-term survival in patients with gastric cancer is surgery, with complete resection of both macroscopic and microscopic disease. This is a major undertaking, and for this reason alternatives to full resection have been explored for early tumors.[18]

Endoscopic methods: Laser ablation, photodynamic therapy, and, in particular, endoscopic mucosal resection (EMR)[20] have all been proposed for tumors confined to the gastric mucosa and where lymphatic spread appears to be minimal. As soon as tumors encroach into the submucosa, the incidence of lymphatic spread rises and mucosal ablation techniques are unlikely to achieve clearance of the disease. Unfortunately no imaging technique is entirely reliable in assessing the depth of tumor invasion. For this reason, it is essential that, when a mucosal resection technique is undertaken, excessive diathermy should be avoided and the resected mucosa (carefully oriented) sent for detailed histologic examination. If histologic examination shows that the lateral margins of the resected specimen are clear of tumor and the malignancy has not spread into the submucosa, the chance of a cure is likely to be good.

Surgery: Tumors that are ulcerated, however, are thought to pose particular problems with infiltration and there are some suggestions that metastases to regional lymph glands occur early. Accordingly endoscopic mucosal resection should probably not be undertaken in these forms of early gastric cancer unless the patient is so unfit that no other treatment is possible. If histologic examination suggests that any of the criteria have not been fulfilled and there is a possibility that the tumor may have breached the submucosa or spread beyond the resection, then laparotomy and full surgical resection should be performed if the patient is fit.

Advanced gastric cancer

In patients who are thought to have a potentially resectable cancer, a partial or (more usually) total gastrectomy is the operation of choice. Although there is no controversy about removing the primary tumor, there is some debate about the extent of lymphadenectomy that is required. Extended lymph node dissection is thought to produce better control of local disease and a more accurate determination of tumor stage, but appears to have a higher morbidity because of the greater technical difficulty of the operation and the length of surgery. To date no clear survival benefit for patients has emerged.

Work in Japan involving meticulous mapping of lymph nodes has suggested that systematic lymphadenectomy may improve the outcome of patients when compared with historic controls. In Europe, however, two randomized controlled trials comparing systematic lymph node dissection (D2) with localized lymph node dissection (D1) suggested that D2 operations were associated with increased mortality and morbidity, and did not improve long-term outcome.[21,22] In both trials, however, distal splenectomy and pancreatectomy were performed as part of the systematic lymphadenectomy and this contributed to the morbidity. Other centers have demonstrated that D2 dissections can be performed without the need for splenectomy and pancreatectomy, providing a more acceptable morbidity. Prospective audit of D2 gastrectomy has suggested an advantage in patients with stage 2 and 3a tumors, but the majority of patients from Europe and the United States present with more advanced tumors and therefore probably do not receive benefit from the more detailed D2 resection. In Japan, where organized screening is able to identify early gastric carcinomas, the benefits of D2 resection may be higher.

Metastatic gastric cancer

Patients with evidence of distant metastases, or in whom spread has occurred outwith the regional lymph glands, have a very poor prognosis. A radical surgical approach is usually not indicated, although palliative procedures to relieve specific complications such as gastric outlet obstruction or hemorrhage may be required.

Adjuvant treatment

Advanced gastric cancer is associated with a poor survival even after surgery, with 5-year survival rates as low as 10% in some studies. This has led to the development of postoperative (adjuvant) chemotherapy and preoperative (neoadjuvant) therapy. Early trials using chemotherapy or single-dose radiotherapy suggested that there might be some survival advantage.

Neoadjuvant chemotherapy: Treatment is given before surgical resection. In theory, less toxic regimens could be used and might allow tumors to be downstaged from inoperable to potentially resectable.[23] Numerous small studies have been reported, none having more than 59 patients. More recently a large UK Medical Research Council trial 'MAGIC' has reported its preliminary results.[1] Some 503 patients with resectable adenocarcinoma of the stomach (74%), cancer of the lower third of the esophagus (14%), or esophagogastric junction cancer (12%) were randomly assigned to preoperative chemotherapy, followed by surgery, then postoperative chemotherapy or surgery alone. Preliminary results showed that the use of perioperative chemotherapy (compared with surgery alone) was associated with significantly higher curative resection rates (79% versus 69%; $P=0.018$), significantly improved progression-free survival ($P=0.002$), and a strong trend towards better survival (hazard ratio 0.80, 95% confidence interval (CI) 0.63–1.01; $P=0.063$), including median survival (24 versus 19 months) and 2-year survival (48% versus 40%, 95% CI 0–16). Even in this large well organized study, however, the improved survival was a trend rather than a clear advantage, although the results overall imply that perioperative chemotherapy may have a role. The final results of the MAGIC study are currently awaited. There is a need for further large studies, and a number are likely to report in the next few years.[1]

Postoperative chemotherapy: No study to date has shown a significant survival benefit, although meta-analyses suggest a small survival gain. The situation is likely to be clarified as larger studies report. At present, treatment should be carried out by oncologists with an interest in gastrointestinal malignancy, and patients should be part of organized clinical trials or looked after in units that audit their results.[1]

The US intergroup 0116 study of postoperative chemoradiation showed a significant improvement in mean survival over surgery alone (36 versus 27 months) at a cost of significant toxicity.[24] Chemoradiotherapy is used more frequently in North America than in Europe, and further clinical trials are necessary to define its role more clearly. Furthermore, a number of newer chemotherapeutic agents and drug combinations are under trial and it seems likely that the results of chemotherapy will improve in the future.

TREATMENT AND PREVENTION

EARLY GASTRIC CANCER
- Surgical resection
- Endoscopic mucosal resection (nonulcerated lesions)

ADVANCED GASTRIC CANCER
Curative
- Radical surgery – D1 or D2 lymph node resection
- Possibly combined with adjuvant, neoadjuvant chemotherapy or chemoradiotherapy (still subject to trials)

Palliative
- Debulking surgery
- Bypass procedures for gastric outlet obstruction
- Endoscopic laser therapy, or injection with absolute alcohol to debulk
- Stenting of the gastroesophageal junction for dysphagia

COMPLICATIONS AND PALLIATIVE TREATMENT

Curative surgery is not always possible and in patients with complications palliative treatment may be required.

Gastric outlet obstruction

Antral tumors frequently affect gastric emptying. This may be related to direct infiltration of the pylorus by the tumor producing stenosis, although the antrum itself plays an important role in gastric emptying and an infiltrated section with loss of peristalsis may greatly impede emptying of the stomach.

Diagnosis

Delayed gastric emptying produces early satiety, nausea, and vomiting that may be severe and projectile and often contains undigested food. Weight loss is almost invariable. Patients are often anorexic and thin, with a poor nutritional status. Physical examination may reveal a succussion splash.

Plain abdominal radiography will sometimes show an enlarged fluid-filled stomach. At endoscopy the stomach is often filled with fluid despite fasting overnight. A patient with a distended stomach due to outlet obstruction may be at considerable risk of aspirating during endoscopy, particularly as the scope enters the stomach. If there is any doubt, it is prudent to empty the stomach first with a nasogastric tube to minimize this risk. Similarly barium should be given with caution to patients with outlet obstruction.

Treatment

Treatment of malignant outlet obstruction is often difficult. Some patients may respond to balloon dilatation of the pylorus, but the effects are usually transient. Stenting of the pylorus and duodenum is difficult. Even if the pylorus is patent, the patient may still have delayed gastric emptying because of antral involvement, and stenting usually does not help. Prokinetics such as domperidone or metoclopramide may offer some benefit but are likely to become less effective as the disease progresses. Surgical bypass is often required, typically with a gastroenterostomy or sometimes with resection of the tumor and anastomosis if technically possible. If a major surgical procedure cannot be contemplated, a drainage percutaneous endoscopic gastrostomy (PEG) can be considered; in this technique the gastrostomy is used to drain the stomach rather than to feed. Although the insertion of a drainage PEG is often an attractive proposition, it can be technically challenging as it may be difficult to find an area of transillumination if the stomach is very thickened.

Hemorrhage

Severe hemorrhage from gastric cancer is unusual but may occur occasionally if the tumor ulcerates and invades a large blood vessel. The effects are usually obvious with hematemesis or melena, but endoscopy is usually required to confirm the site of bleeding. Sometimes a localized bleeding point may be amenable to laser or heater probe therapy, or the injection of 1:10 000 epinephrine (adrenaline). Bleeding from gastric cancers may involve a large area and may be difficult to stop it in this way.

Chronic blood loss from gastric cancer is common and patients often require transfusion. When the blood loss becomes excessive and the need for transfusion frequent, palliative treatment may be required. Treatment options include laser therapy (see Chapter 143) to shrink the tumor, but in the authors' experience this is often difficult in patients with advanced large tumors and often does not result in decreased blood loss. Similarly, argon plasma coagulation can be tried. The injection of absolute alcohol may also produce necrosis and shrinkage of the tumor. In many patients in whom blood loss is a problem, the tumor is often large and at best only temporary relief is obtained.

Dysphagia and involvement of the gastric cardia

Tumors of the fundus and body may involve the lower esophagus and cardia of the stomach, producing dysphagia.

Diagnosis

This is usually made at endoscopy, or sometimes a barium swallow can be used.

Treatment

Laser coagulation (see Chapter 143) can be successful in re-establishing a lumen and opening a malignant stricture. Balloon dilatation (see Chapter 146) often produces short-term relief, but if a definitive procedure is not possible esophageal stenting (see Chapter 146) through the stricture and into the stomach may restore swallowing.

Metastatic spread to the liver

The appearance of liver metastases is usually a very bad prognostic sign and most patients have very limited survival under these circumstances. The presence of a single metastasis is unusual and resection is rarely undertaken. Occasionally spread to involve the common bile duct can occur and may require stenting.

Malignant ascites

Omental spread may result in malignant ascites. Diagnosis is usually confirmed at ultrasonography and by paracentesis and cytologic examination. Treatment is usually by paracentesis. Sometimes a chemotherapeutic agent such as doxorubicin can be given intraperitoneally.

Poor nutritional status

Advanced gastric cancer often has profound effects on appetite and the ability to take normal-sized meals. Most patients with advanced stomach cancer lose weight and their nutritional status may deteriorate rapidly. Some gastroenterologists, particularly in Europe and the United States, advocate total parenteral nutrition (see Chapter 139) to try to maintain nutritional status. This is controversial. There is no evidence that TPN prolongs life, and effects on the quality of life are difficult to ascertain. TPN is, however, associated with some potentially dangerous complications such as infection and thrombosis. Training a patient to go home on TPN may take several weeks, and support is often required from community nurses. It is suggested that the pros and cons of parenteral nutrition are discussed carefully with the patient on an individual basis; routine use cannot be recommended in patients with gastric cancer.[25]

COMPLICATIONS AND THEIR MANAGEMENT

Complication	Management
Gastric outlet obstruction	Surgery Balloon dilatation and stenting
Hemorrhage	Endoscopic therapy, laser, heat probe, epinephrine (adrenaline) injection Surgery
Dysphagia and involvement of the cardia	Esophageal stenting Surgery Endoscopic laser therapy
Liver metastases	Rarely resected
Malignant ascites	Paracentesis, instillation of doxorubicin
Poor nutritional state	Oral sip feeds and supplements Intravenous feeding in carefully selected patients

General palliative measures

As gastric cancer spreads, patients can experience pain and alteration in bowel habit, particularly constipation. Involvement of the palliative care team can be extremely useful and it is recommended that this be considered early rather than late in the course of treatment.

PROGNOSIS WITH AND WITHOUT TREATMENT

Early gastric cancer

The best results for treating early gastric cancer have come from Japan. Patients with true stage 0 (true carcinoma in situ) and stage 1 disease may have a 5-year survival rate of between 80% and 100%. In stage 2 disease, with spread into the submucosa or with lymph node involvement, the 5-year survival rate is 55%. More advanced cancers are associated with a rapidly diminishing prognosis.[26]

At present surgery is the only treatment that offers the possibility of cure. Patients with potentially curative lesions should be offered surgery. A partial or total gastrectomy is, however, a major undertaking and may involve several weeks in hospital. Patients with more advanced disease who undergo noncurative surgery may therefore lose some of their best quality time recovering from surgery and may not receive a survival advantage as a result of operation. In advanced tumors, therefore, where surgery is unlikely to alter the prognosis, palliative measures and supportive treatment of the patient may offer a longer period of good quality life. As for all aspects of treatment, it is important to discuss these issues with the patient and determine what suits them as an individual.

CONCLUSION

Gastric cancer remains a common and serious malignancy. Ironically, although Napoleon's risk factors and family history are better understood, it remains doubtful whether his gastric cancer would have been found any earlier despite the huge advances in diagnostic methods. It is also doubtful, in the light of the advanced nature of his tumor, whether his chances of cure would have been any greater than 10% even with all the treatment techniques currently available. This highlights the importance of prevention, and this can be achieved only through a better understanding of the pathogenesis of the disease.

SOURCES OF INFORMATION FOR PATIENTS AND DOCTORS

http://www.cancerhelp.org.uk/help/default.asp?page=3887
http://my.webmd.com/hw/cancer/ncicdr0000271446-general-information-about-gastric-cancer.asp

REFERENCES

1. Dickson JLB, Cunningham D. Systemic treatment of gastric cancer. Eur J Gastroenterol Hepatol 2004; 16:255–263.
2. Greenlee RT, Murray T, Bolden S, Wingo PA. Cancer statistics, 2000. CA Cancer J Clin 2000; 50:7–33.
3. Scottish Executive. The Scottish audit of gastric and oesophageal cancer 1997–1999. Edinburgh: Scottish Executive; 2002.
4. Kranenbarg EK, van de Velde CJ. Gastric cancer in the elderly. Eur J Surg Oncol 1998; 24:384–390.
5. Callender S, Langman MJ, Macleod IN, Mosbech J, Nielsen KR. ABO blood groups in patients with gastric carcinoma associated with pernicious anaemia. Gut 1971; 12:465–467.
6. Huntsman DG, Carneiro F, Lewis FR et al. Early gastric cancer in young, asymptomatic carriers of germ-line E-cadherin mutations. N Engl J Med 2001; 344:1904–1909.
7. Tersmette AC, Giardiello FM, Tytgat GN, Offerhaus GJ. Carcinogenesis after remote peptic ulcer surgery: the long-term prognosis of partial gastrectomy. Scand J Gastroenterol Suppl 1995; 212:96–99.
8. International Agency for Research on Cancer. Working group on the evaluation of

carcinogenic risks to humans. *Helicobacter pylori*. In: Schistosomes, liver flukes and *Helicobacter pylori*: views and expert opinions of an IARC working group on the evaluation of carcinogenic risks to humans. Lyons: IARC; 1994:177–240.
9. Correa P. Human gastric carcinogenesis: a multistep and multifactorial process – first American Cancer Society Award Lecture on Cancer Epidemiology and Prevention. Cancer Res 1992; 52:6735–6740.
10. El-Omar EM, Carrington M, Chow WH et al. Interleukin-1 polymorphisms associated with increased risk of gastric cancer. Nature 2000; 404:398–402 (erratum appears in Nature 2001; 412:99).
11. El-Omar EM, Rabkin CS, Gammon MD et al. Increased risk of non-cardia gastric cancer associated with pro-inflammatory cytokine gene polymorphisms. Gastroenterology 2003; 124:1193–1201.
12. Machado JC, Figueiredo C, Canedo P et al. A proinflammatory genetic profile increases the risk for chronic atrophic gastritis and gastric carcinoma. Gastroenterology. 2003; 125:364–371.
13. El-Omar EM, Oien K, El Nujumi A et al. *Helicobacter pylori* infection and chronic gastric acid hyposecretion. Gastroenterology 1997; 113:15–24.
14. El-Omar EM, Chow W, Rabkin CS. Gastric cancer and *H. pylori*: host genetics open the way. Gastroenterology 2001; 121:1002–1004.
15. Laurén P. Histogenesis of intestinal and diffuse types of gastric carcinoma. Scand J Gastroenterol Suppl 1991; 180:160–164.
16. Japanese Research Society for Gastric Cancer. Group classification of gastric biopsy specimens. In: Nishi M, Omori Y, Miwa K, eds. Japanese classification of gastric carcinoma, 1st edn. Tokyo: Kanehara; 1995:73–76.
17. Lauwers GY, Shimizu M, Correa P et al. Evaluation of gastric biopsies for neoplasia: differences between Japanese and Western pathologists. Am J Surg Pathol 1999; 23:511–518.
18. Everett SM, Axon AT. Early gastric cancer in Europe. Gut 1997; 41:142–150.
19. American Joint Commitee on Cancer. Manual for staging of cancer, 4th edn. Philadelphia: JB Lippincott; 1993.
20. Ono H, Kondo H, Gotoda T et al. Endoscopic mucosal resection for treatment of early gastric cancer. Gut 2001; 48:225–229.
21. Bonenkamp JJ, Hermans J, Sasako M, Van de Velde CJH. Extended lymph-node dissection for gastric cancer. N Engl J Med 1999; 340:908–914.
22. Cuschieri A, Weeden S, Fielding J et al. Patient survival after D1 and D2 resections for gastric cancer: long-term results of the MRC randomized surgical trial. Br J Cancer 1999; 79:1522–1530.
23. Sun W, Haller DG. Recent advances in the treatment of gastric cancer. Drugs 2001; 61:1545–1551.
24. Macdonald JS, Smalley SR, Benedetti J et al. Chemoradiotherapy after surgery compared with surgery alone for adenocarcinoma of the stomach or gastroesophageal junction. N Engl J Med 2001; 345:725–730.
25. McKinlay A. Nutritional support in patients with advanced cancer: permission to fall out? Proc Nutr Soc 2004; 63:431–435.
26. Kunisaki C, Shimada H, Nomura M et al. Comparative evaluation of gastric carcinoma staging: Japanese classification versus new American Joint Committee on Cancer/International Union Against Cancer classification. Ann Surg Oncol 2004; 11:203–206.

Chapter 38

Gastric lymphoma

Andrew Wotherspoon and Ahmet Dogan

KEY POINTS

- The commonest types are MALT lymphoma and diffused large B-cell lymphoma (DLBCL)
- Stomach is the commonest gastrointestinal site for lymphoma
- Lymphomas account for 10% of gastric malignancy
- Helicobacter pylori (*HP*) is a class 1 carcinogen in the etiology of MALT lymphoma
- EUS is the most sensitive method for local staging
- 70% of MALT lymphomas respond to *HP* eradication
- Deeper penetration, loco regional lymph node spread and T(11;18) translocation types are less likely to respond to *HP* eradication
- Chemotherapy and radiotherapy are effective treatments
- Lifelong endoscopy follow-up is required

DEFINITION

Primary gastric lymphoma is defined as a lymphoma originating in the stomach. Historically, these were considered to be lymphomas that were confined to the stomach and contiguous lymph nodes. This is now considered to be overly restrictive as it excluded the possibility of gastric lymphoma presenting with more disseminated nodal or extranodal involvement or with bone marrow involvement. Currently, a primary gastric lymphoma would be considered to be a lymphoma where the main bulk of the tumor is confined to the stomach and contiguous nodes.

Many of the subtypes of non-Hodgkin lymphoma (NHL) identified in modern lymphoma classifications may arise within the stomach, including mantle cell lymphoma, follicular lymphoma, and Burkitt's lymphoma. The commonest lymphomas encountered in the stomach are extranodal marginal zone B cell lymphoma of mucosa associated lymphoid tissue-type (MALT lymphoma) and diffuse large B cell lymphomas.

The stomach may also be infiltrated in up to 25% of nodal type lymphomas as part of widespread dissemination.

EPIDEMIOLOGY

The gastrointestinal tract is the commonest site for extranodal lymphoma accounting for 4–18% of NHLs in the Western countries and up to 25% of NHLs in the Middle East. In the Western world, the stomach is the most common site for lymphoma in the gastrointestinal tract accounting for up to 10% of cases of gastric malignancy. In recent years, its incidence has apparently increased, but this may in part be due to increased awareness by histopathologists of the diagnostic characteristics of MALT lymphoma. In the future, the decreased prevalence of *Helicobacter* infection may result in a decrease in the incidence of gastric MALT lymphoma.

Incidence rates are similar in males and females. The majority of patients are over 50 years at presentation, but the age range is wide with occasional cases reported in patients in their second decade of life.

ETIOLOGY/PATHOGENESIS

Helicobacter infection

The normal gastric mucosa is devoid of lymphoid tissue from which a lymphoma can arise. The most frequent cause for acquired organized gastric lymphoid tissue is infection by *Helicobacter pylori* (Hp). Initial reports suggested that up to 90% of gastric MALT lymphoma is associated with Hp infection[1] but other reports have suggested this association may be lower (60–75%). Gastric diffuse large B cell lymphomas are also associated with Hp infection in 50–70% of cases associated with a concurrent MALT component and 25–40% of pure *de novo* cases.[2] A minority of cases are unrelated to Hp.[3]

In the case of gastric MALT lymphoma, serological studies have confirmed the presence of Hp infection predating the development of lymphoma, and serial gastric biopsies in some reported series have shown the clonal evolution of the lymphoma from the lymphoid tissue acquired in Hp-associated gastritis.[4]

In vitro studies have shown that the neoplastic cells from cases of gastric MALT lymphoma proliferate in the presence of Hp organisms.[5] This proliferation is driven by contact with tumor infiltrating T cells associated with the lymphoma, which in turn accumulate in response to the presence of the organism.

Progression to large cell lymphoma in a MALT lymphoma is heralded by the accumulation of neoplastic transformed 'blastic' cells. Eventually, these become confluent to form sheets of cells that are indistinguishable from *de novo* diffuse large B cell lymphomas.

Molecular genetics

Initial molecular studies confirmed the presence of clonal immunoglobulin gene rearrangement in all cases of gastric MALT lymphoma. Several chromosomal translocations have been associated with these lymphomas. The t(11;18)(q21;q21) is the most frequently encountered abnormality in these lymphomas.[6] It is usually seen as the sole abnormality and results in a translocation involving the API2 gene on chromosome 11 and the MALT1 gene on chromosome 18.[7] The API2-MALT1 fusion products have been shown to activate NK-kB, a transcription factor critical in lymphocyte activation and survival.[8, 9]

The presence of this translocation appears to protect against further genetic aberrations and the t(11;18) is almost never encountered in large cell gastric lymphomas.[10]

A rarer chromosomal translocation specifically associated with MALT lymphoma is the t(1;14)(p22;q32). This juxtaposes the BCL-10 gene from chromosome 1 next to the immunoglobulin heavy chain gene. The BCL-10 gene also acts through activation of NF-kB.[11]

Both *de novo* diffuse large B cell lymphomas and MALT lymphomas associated with secondary development of large cell lymphoma are associated with further genetic abnormalities including those involving the p53, p16, BCL-6, and C-MYC genes.[12]

PATHOLOGY

Gastric MALT lymphomas show expansion of the gastric wall by a proliferation of small lymphoid cells. These cells can have variable morphology including small round lymphocytes, cells with irregular nuclei, and scanty cytoplasm (so-called centrocyte-like cells) and cells with a more monocytoid appearance with round nuclei and more abundant clear cytoplasm. Plasmacytoid features are frequently seen and extensive plasma cell differentiation may be seen in some cases. Scattered large B cells are seen in almost all cases. The neoplastic infiltrate starts in the marginal zone around reactive lymphoid follicles and eventually expands to occupy the gastric wall overrunning the pre-existing germinal centers. Infiltration of the glandular epithelium with destruction of the gastric glands is frequently seen.

CLINICAL PRESENTATION

The symptoms most frequently associated with gastric lymphoma are those of dyspepsia, nausea, and vomiting.[13] The dyspepsia may be due in part to the presence of Hp infection and eradication of this organism may result in symptomatic relief even in cases where tumor regression is not seen. Very rarely, gastric lymphoma may present with an epigastric mass.

CLINICAL PRESENTATION OF GASTRIC LYMPHOMA
PRIMARY
Common
Extranodal marginal zone B cell lymphoma (MALT lymphoma)
Diffuse large B cell lymphoma
Rare
Mantle cell lymphoma
Follicular lymphoma
Burkitt's lymphoma
SECONDARY

DIFFERENTIAL DIAGNOSIS

Endoscopically, the differential diagnosis includes *Helicobacter*-associated gastritis, where the mucosal changes are minimal, and gastric adenocarcinoma, where there is a large localized lesion.

Histologically, the differential diagnosis of early MALT lymphoma is with gastritis when the lymphomatous infiltrate is subtle. For overt lymphoma the differential diagnosis is with other small B cell lymphomas. Immunocytochemistry can usually distinguish between MALT lymphomas and mantle cell lymphoma (CD5+; cyclinD1+), follicular lymphoma (CD10+; bcl-6+), and infiltration by B-chronic lymphocytic leukemia (CD5+; CD23+).

The main differential diagnosis for diffuse large B cell lymphomas is with adenocarcinoma. These lesions can be distinguished by stains for mucin or by immunocytochemical studies for cytokeratin and lymphoid-related antigens.

DIFFERENTIAL DIAGNOSIS
CLINICAL/ENDOSCOPIC
For MALT lymphoma
Gastritis
Adenocarcinoma
For diffuse large B cell lymphoma
Adenocarcinoma
HISTOLOGICAL
For MALT lymphoma
Gastritis
Other small B cell lymphomas
Mantle cell lymphoma
Follicular lymphoma
Small lymphocytic lymphoma/B-chronic lymphocytic leukemia
For diffuse large B cell lymphoma
Adenocarcinoma

DIAGNOSTIC METHODS (Fig. 38.1)

Diagnosis of gastric lymphoma is achieved by endoscopic biopsy in the majority of cases. A small proportion of cases will be diagnosed following formal resection of a gastric tumor either following a clinical emergency (perforation or uncontrolled bleeding) or in previously undiagnosed cases thought to be carcinoma. Following a diagnosis of MALT lymphoma a further endoscopy with multiple (8–10) biopsies from the abnormal area is recommended to exclude a large cell component/localized transformation.

Histological examination to determine the proportion of large cells is essential. Determination of t(11;18) status in MALT lymphoma gives important information as to the likelihood of response to Hp eradication alone.

Staging is crucial to management and prognostication. Endoscopic ultrasound is the most sensitive method of assessing depth of penetration of the gastric wall and loco-regional nodal involvement. An examination of the upper airway and a pan-endoscopy is recommended to exclude extragastric involvement. Bone marrow biopsy and all the other usual procedures for staging lymphoma are required to complete staging.[13] The bone marrow is involved in 2–15% of cases.

TREATMENT

A large number of studies have shown that around 70% of MALT lymphomas will respond to eradication of Hp with prolonged (>8–10 years follow-up so far) remission.[13] Time to complete remission is variable with most responding in 1–12 months

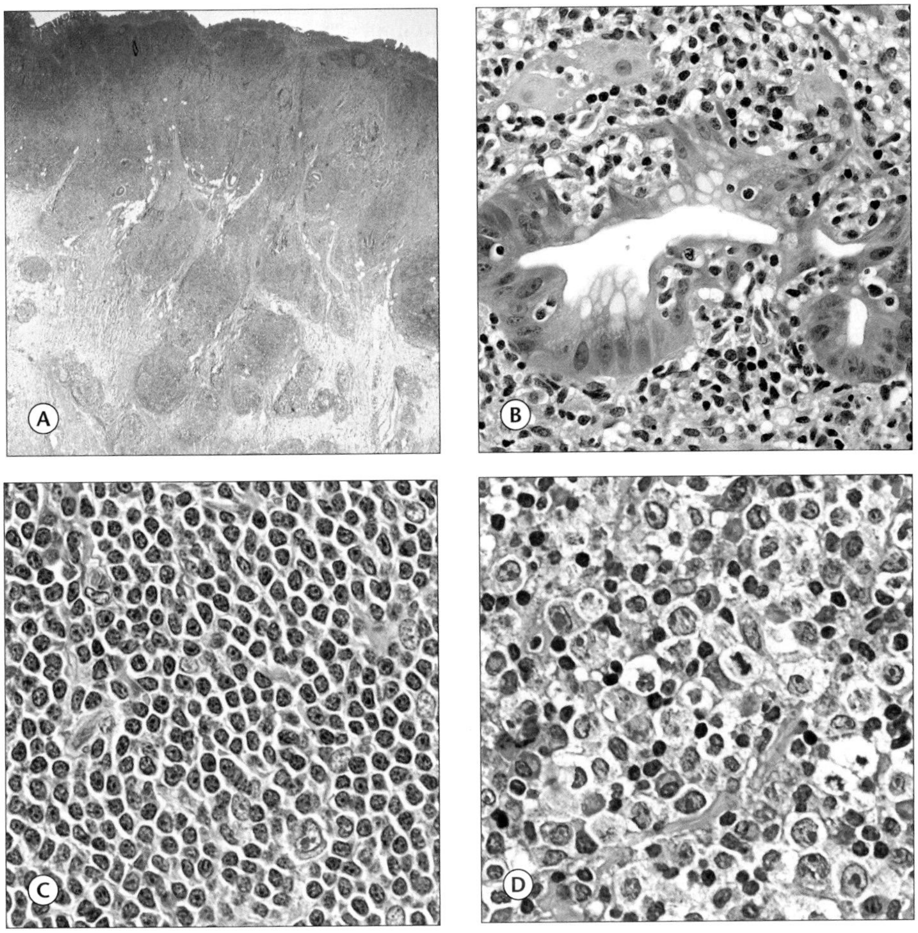

Fig. 38.1 Histological appearance of gastric lymphoma. A. Low-power view of advanced gastric MALT lymphoma showing extensive infiltration of the gastric wall by small blue cells. **B.** High-power view of the mucosal portion showing numerous small lymphocytes infiltrating the crypt epithelium, a characteristic feature of gastric MALT lymphoma. **C.** High-power view of the lymphoid cells invading the submucosa in gastric MALT lymphoma. The vast majority of these cells are small in size and mitotic activity is not seen. **D.** High-power view of a large cell lymphoma of the stomach. The cells are much larger in size compared to (C) and show mitotic activity.

but with some responses only after several years following Hp eradication. The presence of loco-regional lymph node involvement or the t(11;18) is associated with a markedly reduced likelihood of response to Hp alone.[14] Hp-negative lymphomas would not be expected to respond to eradication therapy.

In the past, MALT lymphomas were frequently treated with surgical resection. These lymphomas are multifocal within the stomach and partial gastrectomy will leave micro-lymphomas within the stump.

There have been few randomized clinical trials to assess the most appropriate anti-lymphoma therapy in MALT lymphoma. Mono-agent chemotherapy (e.g., chlorambucil or cyclophosphamide) and radiotherapy are both highly effective.[13] More recently, anti-CD20 antibody therapy (with rituximab) has been shown to have activity in MALT lymphoma.[15]

Diffuse B cell lymphomas needs to be treated with combination chemotherapy. Surgery may be used in combination with chemotherapy for patients with bleeding or incipient perforation.

TREATMENT AND PREVENTION
MALT LYMPHOMA
***Helicobacter* associated**
Helicobacter eradication
***Helicobacter* negative or unresponsive *Helicobacter* associated cases**
Single agent chemotherapy
Radiotherapy
Surgery
Treatment selection dependent on patient characteristics/clinical factors
DIFFUSE LARGE B CELL LYMPHOMA
Multi-agent chemotherapy +/– surgery

COMPLICATIONS AND THEIR MANAGEMENT

Occasionally, tumors may bleed or perforate. This is more frequently seen in diffuse large B cell lymphomas and may require local surgical intervention. Chemotherapy and radiotherapy are associated with treatment-associated side effects. These may be mild and transient. Chemotherapy may induce bone marrow suppression. Both chemotherapy and radiotherapy may be associated with second malignancies. Surgery is associated with a small mortality and variable morbidity and impairment of quality of life. Both mortality and morbidity are increased for total rather than partial gastrectomy.

PROGNOSIS

The major prognostic factors for gastric lymphoma are stage and histological grade (MALT vs diffuse large B cell lymphoma).

MALT lymphoma is a generally indolent disease with slow clinical progression. In the past, difficulties in diagnosis have left cases unrecognized for months or years without significant progression or serious clinical consequences for the patient. There is a risk of transformation into a more aggressive large cell lymphoma.

Up to 70% of cases will achieve remission with anti-Hp therapy. Cases with superficial involvement only are most likely to respond (up to 100%), while deeper penetration of the wall or loco-regional nodal involvement are less likely to. In the past, surgery alone has been associated with a 90% 5-year overall survival but most studies have had insufficient follow-up to detect delayed relapse in the stump. Patients have been treated with a range of conventional anti-lymphoma chemotherapy and radiotherapy regimes with similar results and an 80–95% 5-year survival.[13]

For diffuse large B cell lymphoma, remissions can be achieved in 70–80% of cases with 5-year survival of up to 60% in localized tumors but only 40% for more disseminated (Ann Arbor stage II_2–IV) cases.

Follow-up of patients requires regular endoscopic examination. The frequency of the follow-up remains uncertain but in the early stages response to therapy should be closely monitored. Once complete regression has been achieved, follow-up may be less frequent (annually) but should be life long. A proportion of MALT lymphoma patients may subsequently develop gastric adenocarcinoma, presumably related to previous epithelial cell damage associated with the original Hp infection.

WHAT TO TELL THE PATIENT

Gastric MALT lymphoma is an indolent disease most frequently associated with Hp infection. Laboratory and clinical studies have shown that the majority of such cases will respond to eradication of the organism alone but this is partly dependent on how advanced the tumor is and on some of the characteristics of the tumor cells. The time to regression is variable but may take many months.

If the tumor is unsuitable for Hp eradication therapy or if no response is seen, these tumors can be treated with radiotherapy or chemotherapy. In some cases, surgical excision may be appropriate. The selection of the appropriate therapy is best made following assessment of individual tumor and clinical characteristics.

SOURCES OF INFORMATION FOR PATIENTS AND DOCTORS

http://www.geocities.com/Heartland/Valley/6727/stopNHL/link.html

REFERENCES

1. Wotherspoon AC, Ortiz-Hidalgo C, Falzon MR, Isaacson PG. *Helicobacter pylori*-associated gastritis and primary B-cell gastric lymphoma. Lancet 1991; 338:1175–1176.
2. Eck M, Schmausser B, Greiner A, Muller-Hermelink HK. *Helicobacter pylori* in gastric mucosa-associated lymphoid tissue type lymphoma. Recent Results Cancer Res 2000; 156:9–18.
3. Ye H, Liu H, Raderer M et al. High incidence of t(11;18)(q21;q21) in *Helicobacter pylori*-negative gastric MALT lymphoma. Blood 2003; 101:2547–2550.
4. Nakamura S, Aoyagi K, Furuse M et al. B-cell monoclonality precedes the development of gastric MALT lymphoma in H*Helicobacter pylori*-associated chronic gastritis. Am J Pathol 1998; 152:1271–1279.
5. Hussell T, Isaacson PG, Crabtree JE, Spencer J. The response of cells from low-grade B-cell gastric lymphomas of mucosa-associated lymphoid tissue to *Helicobacter pylori.* Lancet 1993; 342:571–574.
6. Auer IA, Gascoyne RD, Connors JM et al. t(11;18)(q21;q21) is the most common translocation in MALT lymphomas. Ann Oncol 1997; 8:979–985.
7. Dierlamm J, Baens M, Wlodarska I et al. The apoptosis inhibitor gene API2 and a novel 18q gene, MLT, are recurrently rearranged in the t(11;18)(q21;q21)p6 associated with mucosa-associated lymphoid tissue lymphomas. Blood 1999; 93:3601–3609.
8. Uren AG, O'Rourke K, Aravind LA et al. Identification of paracaspases and metacaspases: two ancient families of caspase-like proteins, one of which plays a key role in MALT lymphoma. Mol Cell 2000; 6:961–967.
9. Lucas PC, Yonezumi M, Inohara N et al. Bcl10 and MALT1, independent targets of chromosomal translocation in malt lymphoma, cooperate in a novel NF-kappa B signaling pathway. J Biol Chem 2001; 276:19012–19019.
10. Ott G, Katzenberger T, Greiner A et al. The t(11;18)(q21;q21) chromosome translocation is a frequent and specific aberration in low-grade but not high-grade malignant non-Hodgkin's lymphomas of the mucosa-associated lymphoid tissue (MALT-) type. Cancer Res 1997; 57:3944–3948.
11. Willis TG, Jadayel DM, Du MQ et al. Bcl10 is involved in t(1;14)(p22;q32) of MALT B cell lymphoma and mutated in multiple tumor types. Cell 1999; 96:35–45.
12. Du MQ, Isaccson PG. Gastric MALT lymphoma: from aetiology to treatment. Lancet Oncol 2002; 3:97–104.
13. Zucca E, Bertoni F, Roggero E, Cavalli F. The gastric marginal zone B-cell lymphoma of MALT type. Blood 2000; 96:410–419.
14. Liu H, Ye H, Ruskone-Fourmestraux A et al. T(11;18) is a marker for all stage gastric MALT lymphomas that will not respond to *H. pylori* eradication. Gastroenterology 2002; 122:1286–1294.
15. Conconi A, Martinelli G, Thieblemont C et al. Clinical activity of rituximab in extranodal marginal zone B-cell lymphoma of MALT type. Blood 2003;102:2741–2745.

Chapter 39

Gastrointestinal stromal tumors and gastroduodenal carcinoid tumors

Raquel E Davila and Douglas O Faigel

GASTROINTESTINAL STROMAL TUMORS

KEY POINTS
GASTROINTESTINAL STROMAL TUMORS
• Gastrointestinal stromal tumors (GISTs) are mesenchymal tumors arising from the gastrointestinal wall, mesentery, omentum or retroperitoneum that express the c-kit proto-oncogene protein • This expression of c-kit distinguishes GISTs from other mesenchymal tumors of the gastrointestinal tract including leiomyomas and leiomyosarcomas • In the stomach and duodenum, GISTs usually appear as submucosal mass lesions within the wall

INTRODUCTION

Gastrointestinal stromal tumors (GISTs) are defined as mesenchymal tumors arising from the gastrointestinal wall, mesentery, omentum, or retroperitoneum that express the c-kit proto-oncogene protein, a cell membrane receptor with tyrosine kinase activity.[1] Although GISTs are rare neoplasms of the gastrointestinal tract, they constitute the majority of all gastrointestinal mesenchymal tumors. In the past, GISTs were thought to represent smooth muscle tumors of the gastrointestinal tract and were formerly classified as leiomyomas and leiomyosarcomas. Now GISTs are recognized as a distinct class of mesenchymal tumors that is different from true smooth muscle tumors of the gastrointestinal tract.

EPIDEMIOLOGY

Estimates for annual incidence in the US are in the range of 5000–6000 cases per year.[2] GISTs typically present in older patients with the peak occurrence being in the 5th and 6th decades, and are rare under the age of 40 years. The incidence appears to be equal or slightly higher in men compared to women.

CAUSES, RISK FACTORS, DISEASE ASSOCIATIONS

There are no known environmental risk factors for the development of GISTs. Several families with multiple members with GISTs have been identified and have been found to have germ line mutations in the c-kit gene expressed within their tumors. There may rarely be an association of GISTs with neurofibromatosis.

PATHOGENESIS AND PATHOLOGY

Immunohistochemical analysis of archived tissue specimens of GISTs has demonstrated almost universal expression of the c-kit proto-oncogene protein.[2] The c-kit protein, also known as CD117, is now recognized as a highly sensitive and specific marker for GISTs that differentiates them from other gastrointestinal mesenchymal tumors such as leiomyomas, which do not express CD117. The c-kit receptor ligand is a growth factor known as stem cell factor and, when bound, it leads to activation of the receptor and subsequent phosphorylation of a series of signal transduction molecules that control intracellular processes including gene transcription, cell division, actin reorganization, and chemotaxis.

CD117 is also expressed in a wide variety of cell types including the interstitial cells of Cajal (ICC), which are a complex network of cells within the gastrointestinal muscle layers that serve as a pacemaker system to regulate gut motility. Immunohistochemical studies comparing ICC and GISTs have demonstrated identical patterns of staining of a variety of cell antigens including CD117. Given their structural and immunophenotypic similarities, it has been proposed that GISTs originate from the ICC or may evolve from pluripotential stem cells that differentiate towards a pacemaker cell phenotype.

Several gain-of-function mutations in the c-kit proto-oncogene have been discovered in GISTs.[3] These mutations result in the constitutive activation of the c-kit tyrosine kinase receptor independent of the receptor ligand. This, in turn, leads to uncontrolled cell proliferation and inhibition of normal apoptosis. The development of gain-of-function mutations in the c-kit gene is therefore thought to be critical in the pathogenesis of GISTs. Tumors lacking c-kit mutations may have activation mutations in a related tyrosine kinase, PDGFRα, which also lead to activation of multiple internal cell signaling pathways and tumor development.[4]

Histopathologic appearances: These can be divided into three main categories. Approximately 70–80% of tumors are of the spindle cell type consisting of uniform eosinophilic cells arranged in short fascicles or whorls. In general, the spindle cells have a pale eosinophilic cytoplasm with indistinct cell margins and uniform nuclei ovoid in shape rather than cigar shaped (see Fig. 39.1). The epithelioid type accounts for approximately 20–30% of GISTs and consists of round cells with variable eosinophilic to clear cytoplasm. These tumors also tend to have uniform nuclei, round to ovoid in shape and

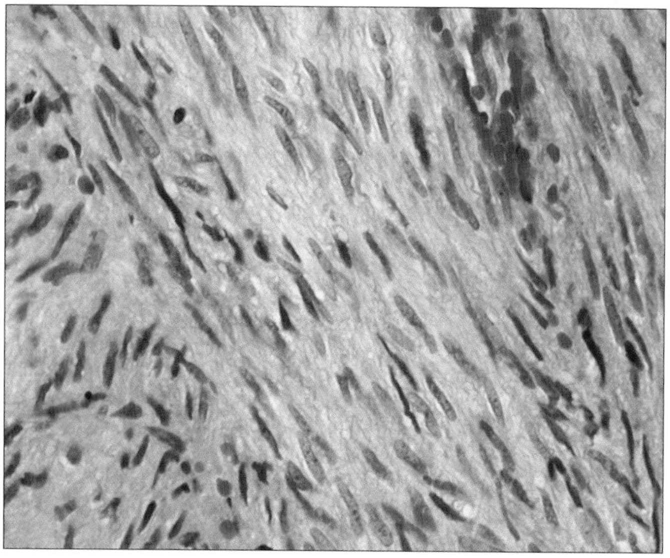

Fig. 39. 1 GIST core biopsy. Photomicrograph of a GIST core biopsy showing multiple spindle cells with eosinophilic cytoplasms and ovoid to elongated nuclei (H&E, orig. mag. ×400).

their architecture can sometimes resemble that of carcinoid tumors. Less than 10% of GISTs can have mixed histology exhibiting separate areas of spindle cell and epithelioid cell types.

Malignant GISTs may declare themselves at the time of presentation by having already spread to adjacent areas or to extraintestinal sites. The pathologic classification of GISTs according to relative risk of malignancy is given in Table 39.1.

CLINICAL PRESENTATION

Approximately 60–70% of GISTs occur in the stomach and 20–30% in the small intestine. Tumors of the small intestine are more frequently found in the jejunum, followed by the ileum and duodenum.

GISTs of the stomach usually present with bleeding, abdominal pain, or more rarely are discovered on physical examination as a palpable mass. Duodenal and further-downstream small bowel GISTs may have a similar presentation with the addition of luminal obstruction as one possible manifestation. The duodenal tumors rarely cause jaundice. Small tumors in asymptomatic patients may be found incidentally during endoscopy or surgery performed for unrelated reasons.

TABLE 39.1 PROPOSED CLASSIFICATION OF GIST BY RELATIVE RISK OF MALIGNANCY

Risk	Tumor size	Mitotic count (per high-power field, HPF)
Very low risk	<2 cm	<5/50 HPF
Low risk	2 cm–5 cm	<5/50 HPF
Intermediate risk	<5 cm	6–10/50 HPF
	5–10 cm	<5/50 HPF
High risk	>5 cm	>5/50 HPF
	>10 cm	Any mitotic rate
	Any size	>10/50 HPF

Based on the National Institutes of Health GIST Workshop convened in April 2001.
Adapted from Fletcher CD et al. Diagnosis of gastrointestinal stromal tumors: a consensus approach. Hum Pathol 2002; 33:459–465.

CLINICAL PRESENTATION

GASTROINTESTINAL STROMAL TUMORS

- Incidental finding
- Acute gastrointestinal hemorrhage
- Abdominal pain
- Palpable mass on physical examination

DIFFERENTIAL DIAGNOSIS

The differential diagnosis of gastric GISTs includes: leiomyomas and schwannomas; other lesions that may appear as a submucosal mass such as duplication cysts, pancreatic rests, lipomas, carcinoids, or hemangiomas; and tumors metastatic to the stomach wall. Similarly, the differential diagnosis of duodenal GIST includes other submucosal mass lesions such as duplication cysts, lipomas, or carcinoids, as well as malignant tumors metastatic to the duodenal wall.

DIFFERENTIAL DIAGNOSIS

GASTROINTESTINAL STROMAL TUMORS

GASTRIC GISTs

Other mesenchymal tumors
- leiomyomas
- schwannomas

Other submucosal mass lesions
- duplication cysts
- pancreatic rests
- lipomas
- carcinoids
- hemangiomas

Metastatic tumors
- lymphoma
- breast cancer
- lung cancer
- melanoma

DUODENAL GISTs

Other submucosal mass lesions
- duplication cysts
- lipomas
- carcinoids

Metastatic tumors
- lymphoma
- melanoma

DIAGNOSTIC METHODS

GISTs encountered in the stomach or duodenum during esophagogastroduodenoscopy usually appear as a submucosal mass lesion or a bulge in the lumen with normal overlying mucosa (Fig. 39.2). Occasionally, an area of umbilication or ulceration can be seen within the overlying mucosa. An accurate diagnosis of GISTs and differentiation from other submucosal lesions usually cannot be achieved by endoscopic evaluation alone. Endoscopic biopsies are generally negative as these tumors are located within the muscularis propria and are not within the reach of biopsy forceps, unless the tumor is ulcerated.

Endoscopic ultrasound (EUS) is critically important in the evaluation and diagnosis of GISTs. Endosonographically, GISTs appear as hypoechoic, solid mass lesions arising from the fourth hypoechoic gastrointestinal wall layer or the muscularis propria (Fig. 39.3). Rarely, GIST can be found within the muscularis mucosae (second wall layer) or in the submucosa (third wall layer). Several EUS features have been found to be predictors of malignancy in tumors. Cystic spaces, echogenic foci, irregular borders, and tumor size >4 cm have all been identified as independent factors associated with malignancy.[5] Alternatively, size = 3 cm, homogeneous echo pattern, and regular borders are EUS features associated with benign GISTs.[6]

EUS-guided fine needle aspiration (EUS-FNA) is a reliable method of obtaining tissue diagnosis. Cytological specimens obtained by EUS-FNA can be analyzed with immunohistochemical stains for CD117, which, if positive, confirm the diagnosis of GISTs. Immunohistochemical staining for other markers including CD34, smooth muscle actin (SMA), desmin, and S100 protein can also be used to distinguish GISTs from other mesenchymal tumors. Approximately 90% of gastric GISTs are positive for CD34 and only 50% of small intestinal tumors are CD34 positive. Unlike leiomyomas, GISTs are negative for desmin and are usually negative for SMA. Leiomyomas are always negative for CD117 and CD34. Schwannomas, another class of gastric mesenchymal tumors, are CD117 and CD34 negative and positive for S100.

If EUS is not available then clinical decisions regarding resection must be made upon the apparent size of the tumors and whether they have caused such complications as bleeding or obstruction.

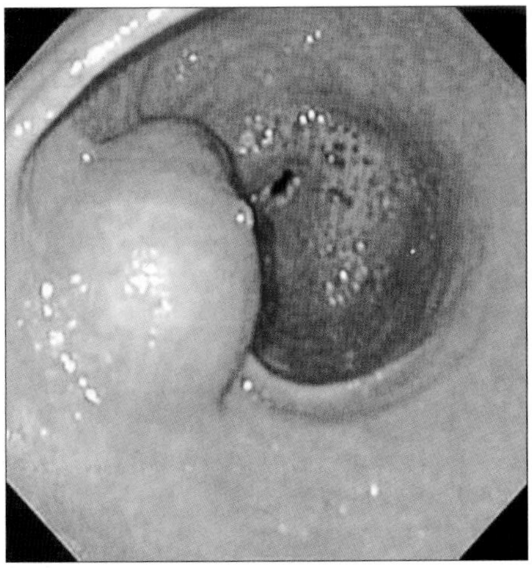

Fig. 39.2 Endoscopic image of GIST. Endoscopic image of a gastric GIST in the antrum appearing as a submucosal lesion with normal overlying mucosa.

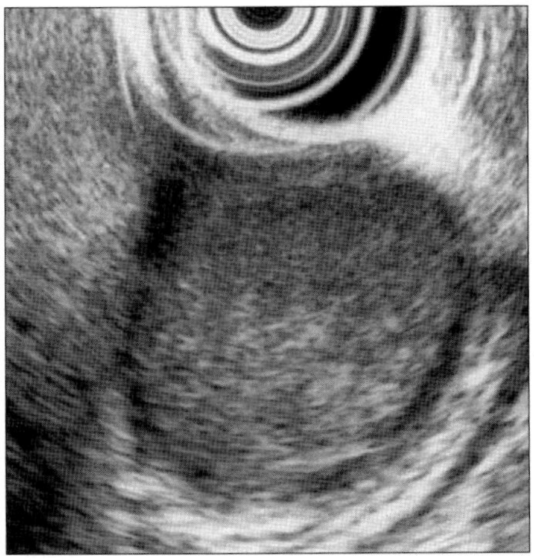

Fig. 39.3 Endosonographic image of GIST. Radial endosonographic image of a gastric GIST seen as a large rounded hypoechoic lesion arising from the muscularis propria (fourth wall layer).

DIAGNOSTIC METHODS
GASTROINTESTINAL STROMAL TUMORS
• An accurate diagnosis usually cannot be made on routine endoscopic evaluation alone • EUS with FNA is important in the evaluation and diagnosis of GISTs • Pathology relies on positive immunohistochemistry with CD117 (the c-kit gene product)

TREATMENT

Surgery is the treatment of choice for isolated GISTs without evidence of metastasis. Surgical resection is indicated for all tumors causing symptoms and those with significant risk of malignant behavior. There are no definitive guidelines for the management of small tumors with suspected low risk of malignancy. Whether these tumors should be removed or undergo close clinical surveillance with repeat EUS is unknown.

Chemotherapy Unresectable or metastatic GISTs can be treated with imatinib mesylate or STI-571 (Gleevec; Novartis Pharmaceuticals, Basel, Switzerland). STI-571 is a synthetic tyrosine kinase inhibitor, which has been demonstrated to bind the c-kit tyrosine kinase in human cell lines and lead to decreased cell proliferation and apoptosis. Clinical trials in the US and Europe using STI-571 in patients with metastatic or unresectable GISTs have demonstrated tumor regression in 54–70% of patients and overall control of disease in 80–90% of patients.[7,8] Disease progression was noted in only 11–13% of patients during treatment. The most common side effects of STI-571 include edema, nausea, diarrhea, myalgias, and fatigue. Tumor hemorrhage is the most serious adverse event seen during treatment, occurring in approximately 5% of patients.

TREATMENT
GASTROINTESTINAL STROMAL TUMORS
• Surgery for isolated tumors of the stomach or duodenum without evidence of metastasis • Medical therapy with imatinib mesylate is used in cases of unresectable or metastatic GISTs

COMPLICATIONS AND THEIR MANAGEMENT

The most common complications of GISTs include gastrointestinal hemorrhage, obstruction, and perforation or rupture. Surgical resection is indicated for uncontrolled gastrointestinal hemorrhage, symptomatic obstruction, and perforation.

PROGNOSIS WITH AND WITHOUT TREATMENT

Prognosis is determined by the malignant potential of the primary tumor. Malignancy is defined by: omental, mesenteric, or peritoneal seeding; invasion of adjacent organs; tumor recurrence after surgical resection; or metastasis to extraintestinal organs or the abdominal wall. In the absence of these findings, isolated tumors are stratified by relative risk of malignancy based on size and mitotic count (Table 39.1). Those tumors with large size (>5 cm) and mitotic count of 5 mitoses per 50 high-power fields are considered to have a higher risk of local recurrence or metastasis.

The 5-year survival of all patients undergoing potential curative resection ranges from 20–78% in the surgical literature. For those patients undergoing surgery, the overall survival appears to be related primarily to tumor size and completeness of resection, with small tumors (<5 cm) and tumors with negative margins demonstrating the best prognosis. Tumor recurrence after surgical resection is common and usually presents locally with tumor involving the regional peritoneum or can present with liver metastasis. Tumor recurrence usually presents within 2 years of surgical resection; however, cases have been reported to occur even 20 years after the initial operation. In those instances, one may question whether another primary was responsible for the presentation with metastases. Patients who develop local recurrence after surgery have an estimated survival of 9–12 months if not treated and a median survival of 15 months after repeat surgical resection. Resection of isolated liver metastases is associated with a 30% 5-year survival.

Patients with recurrence or liver metastasis: Long-term survival following STI-571 is not yet known. The overall survival of patients with metastatic GISTs at the time of presentation is approximately 20 months if not treated. It is still unknown by how much patient survival will be extended with the use of STI-571 in metastatic disease and if continuation of the drug will result in markedly increased survival.

CARCINOID TUMORS OF THE STOMACH AND DUODENUM

KEY POINTS
CARCINOID TUMORS OF THE STOMACH AND DUODENUM

- Carcinoid tumors are neuroendocrine tumors arising from the enterochromaffin cells of the gastrointestinal tract
- In the stomach, most (type 1) occur in association with end-stage atrophic oxyntic gland gastritis and achlorhydria – these have the most benign course
- Some occur with Zollinger-Ellison syndrome and MEN 1 (type 2) and some sporadically (type 3) without associations
- Type 3 carcinoid tumors are the most aggressive

INTRODUCTION

Carcinoid tumors are neuroendocrine tumors arising from the enterochromaffin cells of the gastrointestinal tract. These tumors represent less than 1% of all neoplasms of the stomach and less than one-third of small intestinal neoplasms. The majority of carcinoid tumors of the stomach and duodenum are indolent and asymptomatic. Because of their neuroendocrine origin, carcinoid tumors are characterized by the secretion of a variety of neuropeptides and amines that can lead to clinical symptoms and the carcinoid syndrome (see Chapter 110).

EPIDEMIOLOGY

The true incidence of carcinoid tumors is unknown, as many tumors can be completely asymptomatic. The annual incidence of carcinoids has been estimated to be approximately 2 per 100 000 in the US.[9] Patients usually present within the 2nd to 9th decade of life, with a peak incidence between the 6th and 7th decades. Gastric carcinoid tumors appear to be more common in women than in men; African Americans appear to have a higher incidence of carcinoids compared with Caucasians.[10]

CAUSES, RISK FACTORS, DISEASE ASSOCIATIONS

In an epidemiologic study of 5184 carcinoid tumors from the Swedish Family-Cancer Database, a family history of carcinoids, high socioeconomic status, and birth in a large city were all identified as independent risk factors for carcinoid tumors on regression analysis.[11] Type 1 gastric carcinoids are associated with atrophic oxyntic gland gastritis and approximately half of patients have pernicious anemia. Type 2 gastric carcinoids are associated with Zollinger-Ellison syndrome and multiple endocrine neoplasia (MEN) type 1. Approximately 10–20% of patients with carcinoid tumors are found to have a synchronous adenocarcinoma in the gastrointestinal tract, with the most common site being the colon.

Type 3 gastric carcinoids occur sporadically without any known associated disorder.

PATHOGENESIS AND PATHOLOGY

A cause of carcinoid tumor formation has not been identified. Approximately 75% of gastric carcinoids are associated with chronic atrophic oxyntic gland gastritis and associated hypochlorhydria or achlorhydria, and hypergastrinemia. Gastrin hypersecretion in response to hypo- or achlorhydria is presumed to cause the hyperplasia of the enterochromaffin-like cells in the stomach and lead to carcinoid tumor formation (Type 1 gastric carcinoids).[9]

Between 5% and 10% of gastric carcinoids are associated with the Zollinger-Ellison syndrome and MEN I (see Chapter 109).[9] The hypergastrinemia resulting from a gastrin-secreting tumor in Zollinger-Ellison syndrome has been hypothesized to lead to hyperplasia of the enterochromaffin-like cells and subsequent carcinoid tumor formation in the stomach (type 2 gastric carcinoids). Type 3 sporadic gastric carcinoids tend to be larger in size and have more aggressive behavior compared to the type 1 and 2 tumors.

Carcinoid tumors are trabecular, insular, or glandular. The tumor cells are uniform with pale pink granular cytoplasms and round nuclei with few mitoses. Carcinoid tumor cells are termed enterochromaffin due to their staining properties reflecting cells containing serotonin.

CLINICAL PRESENTATION

Gastric carcinoid tumors are discovered at endoscopy incidentally or in the course of the evaluation of anemia or abdominal pain. Even in the latter circumstances the anemia or abdominal pain may or may not be related to the carcinoid tumors. Duodenal carcinoids may be found incidentally on endoscopy or may present with abdominal pain or obstruction. Carcinoids arising within the major papilla can present with jaundice.

CLINICAL PRESENTATION
CARCINOID TUMORS OF THE STOMACH AND DUODENUM
• Commonly incidental finding on upper endoscopy • Abdominal pain or anemia (may be unrelated) • Intestinal obstruction

DIAGNOSIS/DIFFERENTIAL DIAGNOSIS

The differential diagnosis for carcinoid tumors includes other submucosal lesions such as lipomas, pancreatic rests, metastatic mass lesions to the stomach or duodenal wall, GISTs and other rare gastrointestinal neuroendocrine tumors.

In the setting of a visible submucosal lesion of the stomach or duodenum, a diagnosis of carcinoid can usually be made by endoscopy alone. Endoscopically, carcinoid tumors are round, polypoid yellowish submucosal lesions often with a central erythematous depression or ulceration (Fig. 39.4). Standard endoscopic biopsies are usually sufficient for diagnosis. When gastric carcinoids are suspected, biopsies should also be taken from the midbody greater curve where the oxyntic gland mucosa is normally thickest. If there is extensive atrophic gastritis then the patient should be screened for vitamin B_{12} deficiency.

EUS is a useful tool in the evaluation of these tumors to determine depth of invasion within the stomach or duodenal wall and the presence or absence of associated lymphadenopathy, which would indicate malignancy. On EUS examination, these tumors are hypoechoic and homogenous with smooth margins (Fig. 39.5). The majority of them are located within the submucosa or third wall layer, but they can be seen invading the mucosa or the muscularis propria. The overall accuracy of EUS for determining depth of invasion is 90% and for lymph node metastases is 75%.

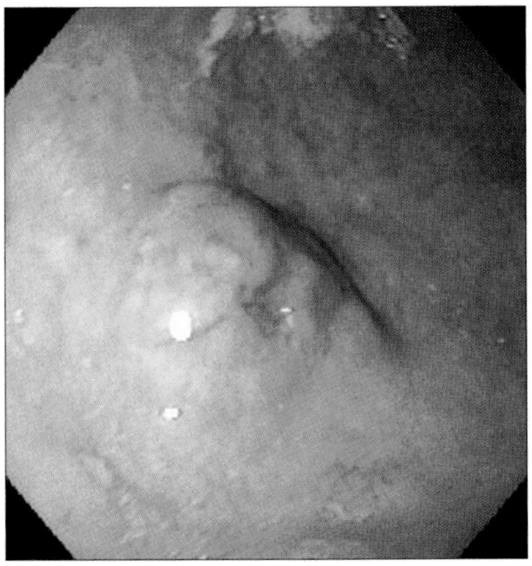

Fig. 39.4 Endoscopic image of gastric carcinoid. Endoscopic image of a gastric carcinoid in the body appearing as a submucosal lesion with umbilication and ulceration.

Nuclear medicine scans with radiolabeled somatostatin analogs can be used to identify the location of primary and metastatic carcinoid tumors and have been reported to have detection rates of 80–90%.

DIFFERENTIAL DIAGNOSIS
CARCINOID TUMORS OF THE STOMACH AND DUODENUM
OTHER SUBMUCOSAL LESIONS OF THE STOMACH AND DUODENUM • Lipomas • Pancreatic rests • Metastatic tumors • GISTs **OTHER NEUROENDOCRINE TUMORS**

DIAGNOSTIC METHODS
CARCINOID TUMORS OF THE STOMACH AND DUODENUM
• Endoscopic biopsy is usually sufficient for making a diagnosis of carcinoid in the stomach or duodenum • EUS is useful in the evaluation of depth of tumor invasion and local lymph node metastasis • Nuclear medicine scans with radiolabeled somatostatin analogs can be used to identify the location of primary and metastatic carcinoid tumors

TREATMENT

Small localized tumors measuring <2 cm that are confined to the submucosa without evidence of invasion of the muscularis propria or lymph node metastasis can be removed endoscopically by endoscopic submucosal/mucosal resection (EMR or

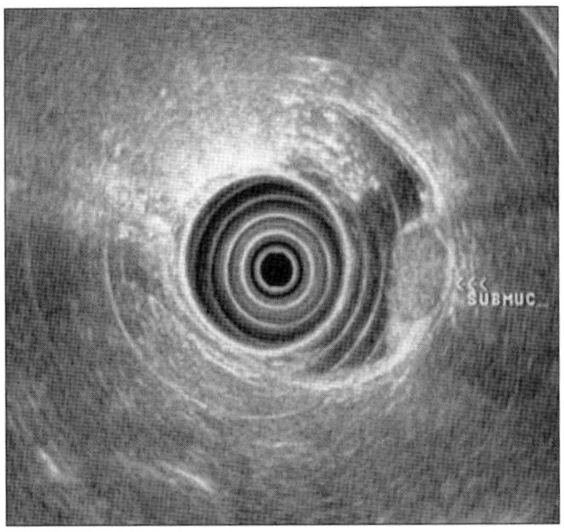

Fig. 39.5 Radial endosonographic image of gastric carcinoid. Radial endosonographic image of a gastric carcinoid seen as a hypoechoic lesion within the submucosa (third wall layer).

ESMR). Close endoscopic follow-up should be performed after endoscopic tumor resection. Tumors measuring ≥2 cm that are localized to the stomach or duodenal wall should be surgically removed. If there are multiple tiny gastric carcinoids then endoscopic follow-up is done to determine whether the lesions progress in size. In the setting of atrophic oxyntic gland gastritis with achlorhydria, they often do not enlarge. Antrectomy has been done in some cases of multiple gastric carcinoids, larger than the pinpoint type. Here the rationale is to reduce the gastrin hypersecretion that drives the ECL cells and hopefully lead to tumor regression. In the majority of instances, however, the usual scenario is either multiple tiny lesions or one or more larger ones that can be removed endoscopically. However, patients with multiple large gastric carcinoids may require total gastrectomy (see Chapter 110).

TREATMENT

CARCINOID TUMORS OF THE STOMACH AND DUODENUM

- Small localized tumors measuring <2 cm that are confined to the submucosa without evidence of invasion of the muscularis propria or lymph node metastasis can be removed endoscopically
- Tumors measuring ≥2 cm that are localized to the stomach or duodenal wall should be surgically removed

COMPLICATIONS AND THEIR MANAGEMENT

Obstruction can be seen with large duodenal tumors. Local fibroblastic (desmoplastic) reaction in the adjacent mesentery to carcinoid tumors can cause the mesentery to buckle and kink the small intestine leading to small bowel obstruction. Tumor spread to the mesentery and local lymph nodes can lead to vascular encasement and wall thickening of local blood vessels that may result in ischemia and bowel infarction. Surgical resection is indicated for small bowel obstruction and may be necessary for small bowel infarction. Large bulky tumors with excessive neuropeptide secretion and those tumors metastatic to the liver can present with the carcinoid syndrome (see Chapter 110).

PROGNOSIS

The overall 5-year survival of patients with gastric carcinoids is 48.6% and for those with small intestinal tumors 55.4%. Prognosis is poor in the setting of regional nodal metastases or distant metastases. Tumor size greater than 2 cm, invasion of the muscularis propria, poorly differentiated histology, and the presence of numerous mitotic figures on histology are findings associated with increased metastatic risk.

REFERENCES

1. Davila RE, Faigel DO. GI stromal tumors. Gastrointest Endosc 2003; 58:80–88.
2. Fletcher CD, Berman JJ, Corless C et al. Diagnosis of gastrointestinal stromal tumors: a consensus approach. Hum Pathol 2002; 33:459–465.
3. Hirota S, Isozaki K, Moriyama Y et al. Gain-of-function mutations of c-kit in human gastrointestinal tumors. Science 1998; 279:577–580.
4. Heinrich MC, Corless CL, Duensing A et al. PDGFRA activating mutations in gastrointestinal stromal tumors. Science 2003; 299:708–710.
5. Chak A, Canto MI, Rosch T et al. Endosonographic differentiation of benign and malignant gastrointestinal stromal cell tumors. Gastrointest Endosc 1997; 45:468–473.
6. Palazzo L, Landi B, Cellier C et al. Endosonographic features predictive of benign and malignant gastrointestinal stromal cell tumours. Gut 2000; 46:88–92.
7. Van Oosterom AT, Judson I, Verweij J et al. Safety and efficacy of imatinib (STI571) in metastatic gastrointestinal stromal tumours: a phase I study. Lancet 2001; 358:1421–1423.
8. Demetri GD, von Mehren M, Blanke CD et al. Efficacy and safety of imatinib mesylate in advanced gastrointestinal stromal tumors. N Engl J Med 2002; 347:472–480.
9. Kulke MH, Mayer RJ. Carcinoid tumors. N Engl J Med 1999; 340:858–868.
10. Modlin IM, Lye KD, Kidd M. A 50-year analysis of 562 gastric carcinoids: small tumor or larger problem? Am J Gastroenterol 2004; 99:23–32.
11. Hemminki K, Li X. Incidence trends and risk factors of carcinoid tumors. A nationwide epidemiologic study from Sweden. Cancer 2001; 92:2204–2210.

Chapter 40

Esophageal motility disorders

Peter J Kahrilas

KEY POINTS
• The best-defined esophageal motility disorders are achalasia, reflux disease, and diffuse esophageal spasm (DES) • Esophageal dysmotility can occur as a secondary phenomenon in systemic diseases including scleroderma, diabetes, malignancy, and Chagas' disease • The only primary esophageal motility disorder with defined neuromuscular pathology is achalasia • Achalasia is rare with an incidence of about 1/100 000 • No population based epidemiology data exist for diffuse esophageal spasm and estimates of its incidence are complicated by inconstant definition • 'Manometric variants' such as nutcracker esophagus, hypertensive lower esophageal sphincter, and nonspecific esophageal motility disorders are of unclear significance

INTRODUCTION

A working, albeit restrictive, definition of an esophageal motility disorder is 'an esophageal disease attributable to neuromuscular dysfunction that causes symptoms referable to the esophagus; most commonly dysphagia, chest pain, or heartburn.' Employing this definition, there are relatively few primary esophageal motility disorders: achalasia, diffuse esophageal spasm, and gastroesophageal reflux disease (see Chapter 29). Esophageal motility disorders can also be secondary phenomena, in which case esophageal dysfunction is part of a more global disease, such as pseudoachalasia, Chagas disease, and scleroderma esophagus. Not included in this discussion are disease entities affecting the pharynx, impairment of which is almost always part of a more global neuromuscular disease process. Thus, the major focus of this chapter will be on the other primary motility disorders, particularly achalasia and diffuse esophageal spasm. Mention will be made of the secondary motility disorders only when important unique features exist.

A number of other conditions (nutcracker esophagus, hypertensive lower esophageal sphincter (LES), ineffective esophageal motility, and non-specific esophageal motility disorders) have been proposed as 'esophageal motility disorders' during the last 25 years. However, the heterogeneity among these patients, absence of specific pathology, and absence of well-defined clinical implications exclude them from the above definition of esophageal motility disorders[1] and suggest that they should be categorized as 'manometric variants.'

UPPER ESOPHAGEAL SPHINCTER DISORDERS

Complex oropharyngeal coordination is necessary for initiation of swallowing. This is impaired by any condition affecting oropharyngeal muscle (e.g., myasthenia gravis) or its innovation (e.g., bulbar palsy, pseudo bulbar palsy, or multiple sclerosis). Resulting dysphagia is characterized by difficulty in initiating swallowing, accompanied by coughing, choking, or nasal regurgitation. Aspiration and pneumonia are important complications. The diagnosis is usually evident but video fluoroscopy can help with difficult cases. Treatment is aimed at the underlying disorder but often placement of a gastrostomy tube enables nutrition to be maintained.

ACHALASIA

Epidemiology

The incidence of achalasia is about 1/100 000 population, affecting both genders equally and usually presenting between 25 and 60 years of age. Because achalasia is a chronic condition, its prevalence greatly exceeds its incidence; prevalence estimates range from 7.1 to 13.4/100 000. Achalasia has been reported in monozygotic twins, siblings, and children of affected parents. However, achalasia has also been reported in only one of a pair of monozygotic twins arguing against a strong genetic determinant. Emphasizing this point, a survey of 1012 first-degree relatives of 159 achalasics identified no affected relatives.[2]

Causes, risk factors, disease associations

No risk factors for achalasia have been identified. Although it was once hypothesized that achalasia was related to herpes zoster or measles virus infections, recent polymerase chain reaction (PCR) data found no evidence of viral particles for herpes, measles, or human papillomavirus.[3] Parkinson's disease and achalasia share many common features neurologically and may be associated.

CAUSES AND RISK FACTORS
• Achalasia is caused by autoimmune destruction of the esophageal myenteric plexus • The neuromuscular pathology responsible for diffuse esophageal spasm is unknown • Scleroderma and other collagen vascular diseases can be associated with connective tissue replacement of the esophageal muscularis propria

Pathogenesis

The neuroanatomic change responsible for achalasia is loss of ganglion cells within the myenteric plexus. Several reports note fewer ganglion cells and ganglion cells surrounded by mononuclear inflammatory cells in the distal esophagus. The degree of ganglion cell loss parallels disease duration with virtual aganglionosis being noted in long-standing cases.

Loss of inhibitory nitrergic neurons which mediate deglutitive inhibition results in impaired LES relaxation, whilst loss of excitatory (cholinergic) neurons accounts for impaired peristalsis. The ultimate cause of ganglion cell degeneration in achalasia is unknown, but evidence suggests an immune-mediated process. Immunohistochemical analyses of the myenteric infiltrate in achalasia patients reveal that the majority of inflammatory cells are cytotoxic T cells.[4] There is also an association with the class II HLA antigens DQW1 151 and DQB1 152.

Pathology

The destruction of ganglion cells in the esophageal wall of patients with achalasia is associated with disintegration of the axoplasm and myelin sheaths within the vagus nerve supplying the esophagus and degenerative changes in the dorsal motor nucleus of the vagus. With long-standing achalasia, the esophageal body undergoes progressive dilatation and sigmoidization with hypertrophy of the LES. However the myocytes themselves are microscopically normal. These changes are less pronounced early in the course of the disease.

Clinical presentation

Clinical manifestations of achalasia include dysphagia, regurgitation, chest pain, weight loss, and aspiration pneumonia. Most patients report solid and liquid food dysphagia. With a dilated esophagus, patients often compensate by drinking a lot while eating, straightening the back, raising their arms, standing, or eating slowly. Strangely, despite the severe dysphagia, significant weight loss is unusual.

Regurgitation occurs when food, fluid, and secretions are retained in the dilated esophagus. The regurgitant is often recognized as food that has been eaten hours, or even days, previously. It tends to be non-bilious, non-acid, and mixed with copious amounts of saliva that has mucoid characteristics, often described as slime by the patient. Some patients induce vomiting to relieve the associated discomfort. Classically, patients will complain of regurgitant on their bed sheets and have often found it necessary to sleep with several pillows or upright in a chair. An estimated 10% of patients with achalasia have bronchopulmonary complications (bronchitis, pneumonia, or lung abscess) from chronic regurgitation and aspiration.

Chest pain is frequent early in the course of achalasia, and is thought to result from esophageal spasm or from the process of esophageal dilatation associated with disease progression. Patients describe a squeezing, pressure-like retrosternal pain, sometimes radiating to the neck, arms, jaw, and back. Paradoxically, many achalasics complain of heartburn. However, an unresolved issue is whether or not this 'heartburn' is related to gastroesophageal reflux or simply the patient's way of perceiving and/or reporting esophageal pain. Treatment of achalasia is less effective in relieving chest pain than it is in relieving dysphagia or regurgitation. However, unlike dysphagia or regurgitation, chest pain may improve spontaneously.

An interesting, but fortunately rare, symptom of achalasia is airway compromise and stridor as a result of the dilated esophagus compressing the membranous trachea. In severe cases, this condition may require emergency treatment.

CLINICAL PRESENTATION

- Most common symptoms: dysphagia, chest pain, and heartburn
- Severe regurgitation, nocturnal aspiration, and pulmonary complications can be the initial presentation of advanced achalasia

CLINICAL TIPS

- Dysphagia for both solid and liquid food is suggestive of a motility disorder whereas uniquely solid food dysphagia suggests mechanical obstruction
- Distal esophageal obstruction or dysfunction is perceived as cervical dysphagia in about 30% of cases
- 'Manometric variants' are frequently detected in patients complaining of chest pain but these should be viewed as epiphenomena rather than etiological
- Reflux, caustic, or infectious esophagitis are much more common causes of chest pain than are achalasia or diffuse esophageal spasm
- Scleroderma esophagus does not necessarily imply coexistent scleroderma or other collagen vascular disease: about 50% of cases are idiopathic

Differential diagnosis

The distinction between vigorous achalasia and diffuse esophageal spasm can be subtle. The differential diagnosis also includes Chagas' disease and pseudoachalasia. These disorders may resemble achalasia so closely that conventional diagnostic tests are misleading. A rare genetic achalasia syndrome, familial adrenal insufficiency with alacrima, has also been described. This is inherited as an autosomal recessive trait that manifests itself with the childhood onset of autonomic nervous system dysfunction including achalasia.

Chagas' disease is endemic in areas of central Brazil, Venezuela, and northern Argentina. Chagas' disease is spread by the bite of the reduvid (kissing) bug, which transmits the culprit protozoan, *Trypanosoma cruzi*. After infection, an acute septicemia develops that varies in severity from being unnoticed to fatal. The chronic phase of the disease develops years later and results from destruction of autonomic ganglion cells throughout the body, including the heart, gut, urinary tract, and respiratory tract. Chronic cardiomyopathy with conduction system disturbances and arrhythmias is the most common cause of death. The digestive tract organs most often affected are the esophagus, duodenum, and colon resulting in megaesophagus, megaduodenum, or megacolon. The diagnosis of Chagas' disease is confirmed by a serologic test utilizing complement fixation or PCR.

Tumor infiltration (especially carcinoma in the gastric fundus) can completely mimic the functional impairment seen with idiopathic achalasia. The resultant 'pseudoachalasia' accounts for up to 5% of suspected cases and is more likely with advanced age, abrupt onset of symptoms (<1 year), and weight loss in excess of 7 kg. Hence, endoscopy should be part of the initial evaluation of achalasia. A clue to the presence of pseudoachalasia is feeling more than slight resistance as the endoscope traverses the gastroesophageal junction. If suspicious of pseudoachalasia, endoscopic biopsy, computerized tomography, magnetic resonance imaging, or endoscopic ultrasound should be considered for further evaluation.

Adenocarcinoma of the stomach accounts for more than half of pseudoachalasia cases with a myriad of other tumors (pancreatic, oat cell, hepatoma, bronchogenic, esophageal squamous cell, prostate, lymphoma) accounting for the remainder. These tumors produce an achalasia syndrome by infiltrating the wall of the esophagus, in essence causing a malignant obstruction at the LES with proximal esophageal dilatation. Similarly, pseudoachalasia can result from esophageal infiltration by amyloid, sphingolipids, eosinophilic gastroenteritis, and sarcoidosis or mechanical obstruction by pancreatic pseudocysts or neurofibromatosis. Although often mentioned in the literature, pseudoachalasia is only rarely due to a paraneoplastic syndrome without direct tumor stenosis of the esophagogastric junction.

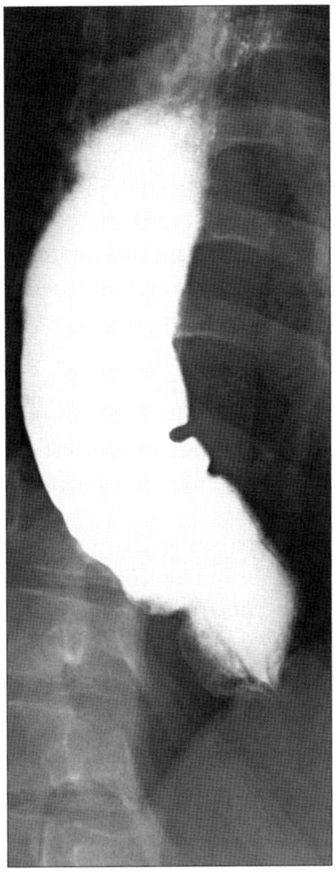

Fig. 40.1 Barium swallow of a patient with achalasia. Barium swallow showing esophageal dilatation, an air–fluid level within the esophagus, and the characteristic distal esophageal tapering in the region of the LES.

DIFFERENTIAL DIAGNOSIS

- Achalasia: diffuse esophageal spasm, Chagas' disease, tumor-mediated pseudoachalasia
- Diffuse esophageal spasm: reflux disease, infectious esophagitis, coronary artery disease, vigorous achalasia
- Chest pain: cardiovascular disease, pulmonary disease, musculoskeletal, reflux esophagitis, infectious esophagitis, caustic (or pill) esophagitis

Diagnostic methods

A barium swallow X-ray or esophageal manometry can demonstrate the physiologic abnormalities of achalasia. The characteristic X-ray is of a dilated intrathoracic esophagus with impaired emptying, an air–fluid level, absence of a gastric air bubble, and an esophagogastric junction that tapers to a point giving the distal esophagus a beak-like appearance (Fig. 40.1). Occasionally, an epiphrenic diverticulum is observed. With long-standing achalasia, the esophagus may assume a sigmoid configuration. In any event, the characteristic radiographic findings depend upon esophageal dilatation that is not always present thereby accounting for radiography's limited sensitivity.

The defining manometric features of achalasia are aperistalsis and incomplete LES relaxation. Impaired LES relaxation by itself (to a nadir value greater than 12 mmHg) has 92% sensitivity and 94% specificity for the detection of achalasia.[5] Nonetheless, atypical cases and cases in which technical difficulties preclude proper placement of the manometric sensor require that additional clinical data also be considered.[6] Some patients exhibit higher amplitude (>60 mmHg) simultaneous repetitive contractions in response to swallows, thereby defining the variant known as vigorous achalasia. Other manometric features (increased resting LES pressure, increased intraesophageal baseline pressure, or isobaric waveforms) provide supportive evidence of achalasia.

Endoscopy is relatively insensitive in the detection of achalasia except in advanced disease. The esophagus may be so full of food as to require lavage or even days of a liquid diet before endoscopy is feasible. With progressive dilatation and stasis, erythema, friability, and superficial ulcerations may be seen. Whitish plaque consistent with *Candida* can be seen; this is usually asymptomatic. The LES has a pinpoint appearance in achalasia and does not open with air insufflation. Nonetheless, the instrument should pass with minimal pressure. Resistance, or a feeling of stiffness as the endoscope crosses the gastroesophageal junction, should raise the suspicion of pseudoachalasia and any mucosal abnormalities should be biopsied.

DIAGNOSTIC METHODS

- Diagnosis entails both demonstrating the functional defect and excluding alternative diagnoses since histopathological diagnosis is usually not possible
- Barium swallow with fluoroscopy or esophageal manometry can demonstrate the functional defects of achalasia, diffuse esophageal spasm, or scleroderma esophagus
- Esophageal manometry is the most sensitive means for detecting achalasia or DES

Treatment and prevention

There is no known way of preventing or reversing achalasia. The main functional abnormality, poor esophageal emptying, is treated by reducing LES pressure so that gravity promotes esophageal emptying. Peristalsis rarely, if ever, returns. LES pressure can be reduced by pharmacologic therapy, forceful dilation, or surgical myotomy. The optimal approach is still debated given the lack of high-quality randomized controlled trials.

Pharmacological therapy

Nitrates or calcium channel blockers administered prior to eating can relieve dysphagia in achalasics by reducing LES pressure. An uncontrolled trial of isosorbide dinitrate (Isordil) reported marked relief of dysphagia but prominent side effects, particularly headaches. Nifedipine (Procardia) 10–30 mg was significantly better than placebo in a group of patients with early achalasia followed for 6–18 months. However, subsequent placebo-controlled crossover trials have found minimal benefit with nifedipine and limiting side effects, especially flushing, dizziness, headaches, peripheral edema, and orthostasis.

Sildenafil decreases LES pressure by blocking the enzyme that destroys cyclic guanosine monophosphate induced by nitric oxide. In a double-blind placebo controlled trial, 50 mg of sildenafil caused a significant decrease in LES pressure and relaxation pressure. No therapeutic trials for achalasia exist.

Botulinum toxin injection

Botulinum toxin is a potent inhibitor of acetylcholine release from nerve endings. In achalasia, 80–100 units of botulinum toxin are injected into the LES with a sclerotherapy catheter. The toxin binds to presynaptic, parasympathetic nerve endings reducing the non-myogenic component of LES pressure. Using this technique, Pasricha reported improved dysphagia in 66% of patients with achalasia for 6 months. However, the botulinum toxin effect is eventually reversed by axonal regeneration and subsequent studies report minimal continued efficacy after 1 year.[7]

Pneumatic dilation

An achalasia dilator is a noncompliant, cylindrical balloon that can be positioned across the LES and inflated to a diameter of at least 3 cm. The only design currently available in the US, the Rigiflex dilator, is positioned fluoroscopically over a guidewire and is available in 3.0, 3.5, and 4.0 cm diameters. A European alternative is the Witzel dilator, a polyethylene balloon mounted onto an endoscope overtube so that the retroflexed endoscope can be used to monitor balloon position during inflation.

A cautious approach to dilation is beginning with relatively low inflation pressures and/or a smaller diameter dilator (3.0–3.5 cm). The reported efficacy of dilation ranges from 32% to 98%.[1] Patients with a poor initial result or rapid recurrence of dysphagia are unlikely to respond to additional dilations but subsequent response to myotomy is not influenced. The major complication of pneumatic dilation is esophageal perforation with a reported incidence ranging from 1% to 5%. Most perforations are quickly evident clinically but cautious practitioners routinely obtain a fluoroscopic examination following pneumatic dilation. If a perforation appears confined, or intramural, conservative management is appropriate. If any substantial perforation has occurred, or if worsening pain and fever occur during observation, surgical repair should be pursued as soon as possible. Patients with perforation from pneumatic dilation that is surgically repaired within 6–8 h have outcomes comparable to patients undergoing elective Heller myotomy.

Heller myotomy

The most common open surgical procedure for achalasia is an anterior myotomy extending from the distal esophagus to the proximal stomach through a thoracotomy. One controlled trial exists comparing pneumatic dilation to myotomy via thoracotomy. That study reported 95% symptom resolution with myotomy versus 51% with dilation,[8] but the study was criticized for the atypically low response rate of pneumatic dilation. Some surgeons routinely perform an antireflux procedure (partial fundoplication) concurrently with the myotomy while others reserve this for patients with an associated hiatal hernia. Regardless, with the availability of proton pump inhibitors, postoperative reflux is usually easily controlled.

The appeal of myotomy is that it is more predictable than pneumatic dilatation. Surgical series report good to excellent results in 62–100% of patients with achalasia. In a recent report of 168 patients with achalasia who underwent thoracoscopic (35 patients) or laparoscopic (133 patients) myotomy accompanied by a partial fundoplication, there were no deaths and only eight patients required another operation.[9] Relief of dysphagia was obtained in 93% who underwent the laparoscopic myotomy and 85% treated with thoracoscopic myotomy. Thus, laparoscopic Heller myotomy has become the preferred surgical procedure for achalasia.

Treatment failures

Occasionally, patients fail to respond to even a well done pneumatic dilation or myotomy. In such refractory cases of achalasia, esophageal resection with gastric pull-up or interposition of a segment of transverse colon may be the only option other than gastrostomy feeding. Indications for this intervention include irresolvable obstructive symptoms, cancer, and perforation during dilation. Although excellent long-term functional results can be achieved, the reported mortality of this surgery is about 4%, consistent with the mortality rate of esophagectomy done for other indications.

Complications and management

In achalasia, esophageal dilatation predisposes to aspiration or stasis esophagitis. Aspiration is best dealt with by effective treatment of achalasia, be that pneumatic dilation or surgery. Prolonged stasis esophagitis is the likely explanation for the association between achalasia and esophageal squamous cell cancer. Tumors develop after years of achalasia, usually in a greatly dilated esophagus. A population-based analysis of the Swedish population suggested that the overall squamous cell cancer risk was increased 17-fold compared to controls.

DIFFUSE ESOPHAGEAL SPASM

Epidemiology

No population-based studies exist on the prevalence of other esophageal motility disorders. Referencing their detection rate to that of achalasia, the prevalence of diffuse esophageal spasm is similar to that of achalasia (or lower if more restrictive diagnostic criteria are utilized) while the prevalence of the 'manometric variants' is up to 10 times greater.[10]

Causes, risk factors, disease associations

The neuromuscular pathology responsible for diffuse esophageal spasm is unknown and no risk factors or associated conditions have been established. Certainly, 'manometric variants' and

> **TREATMENT AND PREVENTION**
>
> - Definitive treatments of achalasia are pneumatic dilation or Heller myotomy
> - Treatment of achalasia with smooth muscle relaxants, most commonly nitrates or calcium channel blockers, can be a useful temporizing measure
> - Botulinum toxin injection into the lower esophageal sphincter can improve symptoms of achalasia in about 60% of cases but the effect rarely lasts more than 1 year
> - Treatment of esophageal spasm is empirical and based on anecdotal reports; anxiolytics, nitrates, and calcium channel blockers have been used

esophageal spasm occur more commonly in patients with gastroesophageal reflux disease, but in such cases it is probably best to think of the reflux disease as the parent entity.

Pathogenesis

Although there is no defined histopathology in spastic disorders of the esophagus, physiologic evidence again implicates myenteric plexus neuronal dysfunction. Vagal impulses mediating peristalsis reach all levels of the smooth muscle esophagus simultaneously, activating myenteric plexus neurons that then act on the muscle. Inhibitory ganglionic neurons hyperpolarize the muscle cells and inhibit contraction while excitatory ones depolarize the cells prompting contraction. At each esophageal locus, the net effect results from the balance between these controlling influences. Experimental evidence suggests that some patients with diffuse esophageal spasm primarily exhibit a defect of inhibitory interneuron function, while in others the defect is of excess excitation.

Pathology

There are few histopathologic studies of diffuse esophageal spasm. The most striking reported pathologic change is diffuse muscular hypertrophy or hyperplasia with thickening of up to 2 cm in the distal two-thirds of the esophagus. However, this finding is neither sensitive nor specific for diffuse esophageal spasm. Similarly, no consistent evidence of neuropathology has been reported.

Clinical presentation

The major symptoms of diffuse esophageal spasm are dysphagia and chest pain. Weight loss is rare. Dysphagia is usually intermittent, sometimes related to swallowing specific substances or liquids at extreme temperature. In some instances, patients experience episodes of esophageal obstruction while eating that persist until relieved by emesis. Esophageal chest pain is very similar to angina; described as crushing or squeezing in character, often radiating to the neck, jaw, arms, or midline of the back. Pain episodes may last from minutes to hours, but swallowing is usually not impaired. The mechanism producing pain is poorly understood.

Differential diagnosis

Unlike angina pectoris, which it can mimic, diffuse esophageal spasm is not life threatening. Features suggesting esophageal vs cardiac pain include pain that is nonexertional, prolonged, interrupts sleep, is meal-related, is relieved with antacids, and is accompanied by heartburn, dysphagia, or regurgitation. However, each of these characteristics still exhibits some overlap with cardiac pain, which should always be carefully considered first. Furthermore, even within the spectrum of esophageal diseases, both chest pain and dysphagia are also characteristic of peptic or infectious esophagitis. Only after these more common entities have been excluded by evaluation and/or treatment should diffuse esophageal spasm be pursued as the etiology of chest pain.

Diagnostic methods

Diffuse esophageal spasm is defined by manometry or barium radiography but the abnormal motor events are usually intermittent and there is no uniform definition. In the unequivocal case, nonperistaltic, high-amplitude, prolonged contractions are seen during manometry and these are associated with the patient experiencing pain (Fig. 40.2). The LES typically functions normally. Radiographically, a 'corkscrew esophagus' (Fig. 40.3), 'rosary bead esophagus,' pseudodiverticula, or curling are indicative of diffuse esophageal spasm. Although diffuse esophageal spasm has no pathognomonic endoscopic features, endoscopy is nonetheless useful to rule out structural lesions and inflammation.

Treatment

Little controlled data exist regarding pharmacological therapy of diffuse esophageal spasm. Uncontrolled trials of small numbers of patients with diffuse esophageal spasm report clinical response to nitrates, calcium channel blockers, hydralazine, botulinum toxin, and anxiolytics. The only controlled trial showing efficacy was with an anxiolytic. Consistent with this, success has also been reported using behavioral modification and biofeedback.

If dysphagia becomes so severe that weight loss is observed or if pain becomes unbearable, surgical therapy consisting of a Heller myotomy across the LES with proximal extension to include the involved area of spasm, or even esophagectomy, should be considered. However, there are no controlled studies of these treatments and their indication is extremely rare.

MISCELLANEOUS MOTILITY DISORDERS (MANOMETRIC VARIANTS)

Presentation

Chest pain is also common in patients who are subsequently found to have one of the 'manometric variants' such as nutcracker esophagus, hypertensive LES, ineffective esophageal motility, and non-specific esophageal motility disorders. Among such individuals, there is a high prevalence of reflux and of psychiatric diagnoses, particularly anxiety and depression.[10] Evidence also suggests a lower visceral pain threshold in this group and symptoms of irritable bowel syndrome may be seen in more than 50% of these patients.[11]

Therapy of these conditions is as poorly defined as are the entities themselves. In view of the unproven value of detecting these conditions, current practice guidelines do not support pursuing them in the evaluation of chest pain patients. Rather, we should not overlook therapy aimed at the most common esophageal disorder, gastroesophageal reflux disease (GERD), or more global conditions such as depression or somatization neurosis that are often coexistent in these patients.

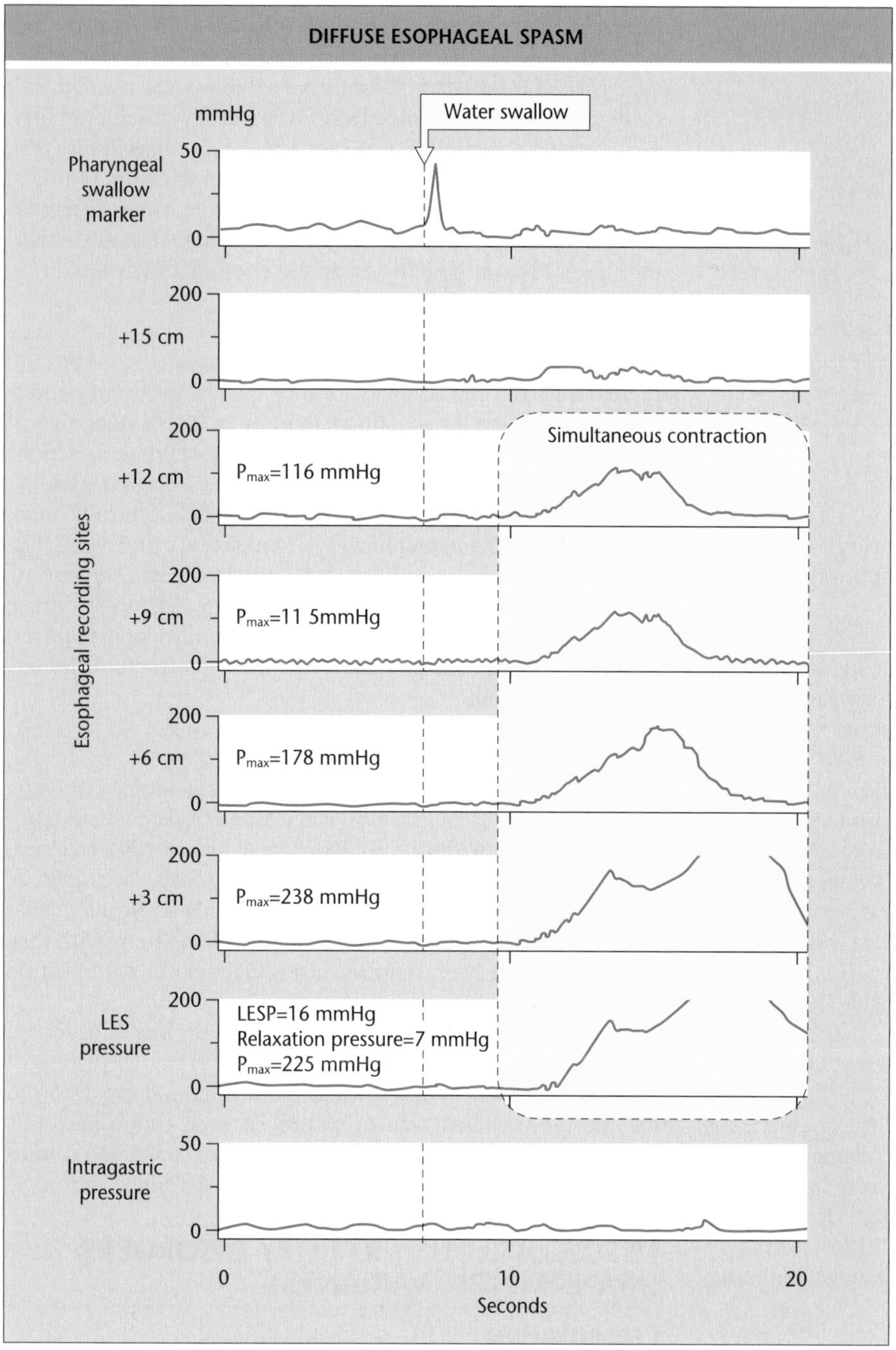

Fig. 40.2 Diffuse esophageal spasm. Esophageal manometric tracing of an unequivocal case of diffuse esophageal spasm. This contractile event was associated with pain.

SCLERODERMA ESOPHAGUS (HYPOTENSIVE LES AND ESOPHAGEAL APERISTALSIS)

Presentation

This was initially described as a manifestation of scleroderma or other collagen vascular diseases. However, this nomenclature ultimately proved unfortunate because an estimated half of qualifying patients do not have an identifiable systemic disease and in such cases reflux disease is the only identifiable association.

Pathology

When scleroderma esophagus occurs as a manifestation of a collagen vascular disease, the histopathological findings are of infiltration and destruction of the esophageal muscularis propria with collagen deposition and fibrosis. The pathogenesis of scleroderma esophagus in the absence of a collagen vascular disease is unknown.

Treatment

Proton pump inhibitors have improved the management of scleroderma esophagus substantially and may reduce the instance of esophageal stricture. Where these strictures occur they can usually be dilated in conjunction with endoscopy.

PROGNOSIS WITH AND WITHOUT TREATMENT

No mortality rate has been established for any of the esophageal motility disorders making their prognosis excellent, regardless

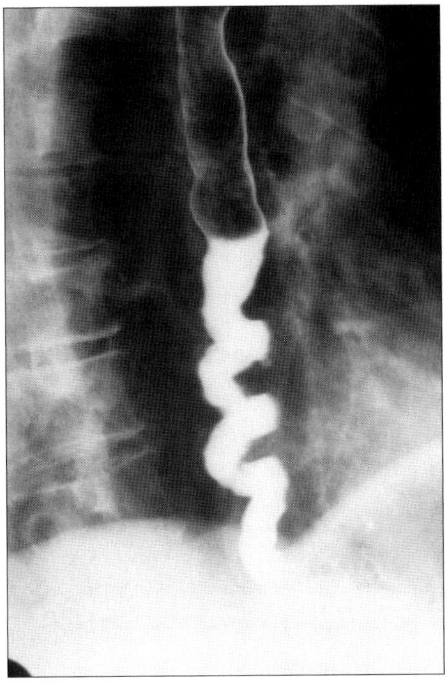

Fig. 40.3 Corkscrew esophagus seen on barium swallow, associated with diffuse esophageal spasm.

of treatment. Nonetheless, it is indisputable that some people have died of complications of achalasia, be they aspiration pneumonia, lung abscesses, or squamous cell cancer of the esophagus. Although no relevant corroborative data exist, the likelihood of incurring these complications is probably reduced by effective therapy.

CURRENT CONTROVERSIES AND THEIR FUTURE RESOLUTION

Because achalasia is rare, the relative merits of dilatation, laparoscopic Heller myotomy, and botulinum toxin injection are still debated. Appropriate diagnostic criteria for diffuse esophageal spasm remain controversial. It is increasingly recognized that reflux and visceral hyperalgesia are more relevant entities in the genesis of chest pain.[11] This controversy may be resolved in the future with careful clinical studies of chest pain patients. Whether 'manometric variants' are of clinical relevance remains very controversial.

CONTROVERSIES

- The rarity of achalasia makes it difficult to perform controlled trials comparing therapies
- Both the diagnostic criteria and therapy of diffuse esophageal spasm are controversial
- Now that the importance of hyperalgesia in the genesis of chest pain is gaining recognition controlled clinical trials should be feasible

SOURCES OF INFORMATION FOR PATIENTS AND DOCTORS

http://www.clevelandclinic.org/gastro/swallowing/patient/achalasia.htm
http://patients.uptodate.com/topic.asp?file=digestiv/4384
http://www.patient.co.uk/DisplayConcepts.asp

REFERENCES

1. Kahrilas PJ. Esophageal motility disorders: current concepts of pathogenesis and treatment. Can J Gastroenterol 2000; 14:221–231.
2. Mayberry JF, Atkinson M. A study of swallowing difficulties in first degree relatives of patients with achalasia. Thorax 1985; 40:391–393.
3. Birgisson S, Galinski MS, Goldblum JR, et al. Achalasia is not associated with measles or known herpes and human papilloma virus. Dig Dis Sci 1997; 42:300–306.
4. Clark SB, Rice TW, Tubbs RR, Richter JE, Goldblum JR. The nature of the myenteric infiltrate in achalasia: an immunohistochemical analysis. Am J Surg Pathol 2000; 24: 1153–1158.
5. Shi G, Ergun GA, Manka M, Kahrilas PJ. Lower esophageal sphincter relaxation characteristics using a sleeve sensor in clinical manometry. Am J Gastroenterol 1998; 93:2373–2379.
6. Hirano I, Tatum RP, Shi G et al. Manometric heterogeneity in patients with idiopathic achalasia. Gastroenterology 2001; 120: 789–798.
7. Annese V, Bassotti G, Coccia G et al. A multicentre randomised study of intrasphincteric botulinum toxin in patients with oesophageal achalasia. GISMAD Achalasia Study Group. Gut 2000; 46:597–600.
8. Csendes A, Braghetto I, Henriquez A, Cortes C. Late results of a prospective randomised study comparing forceful dilatation and oesophagomyotomy in patients with achalasia. Gut 1989; 30:299–304.
9. Patti MG, Pellegrini CA, Horgan S et al. Minimally invasive surgery for achalasia: an 8-year experience with 168 patients. Ann Surg 1999; 230:587–593.
10. Kahrilas PJ, Clouse RE, Hogan WJ. American Gastroenterological Association technical review on the clinical use of esophageal manometry. Gastroenterology 1994; 107:1865–1884.
11. Rao SS, Gregersen H, Hayek B, Summers RW, Christensen J. Unexplained chest pain: the hypersensitive, hyperreactive, and poorly compliant esophagus. Ann Intern Med 1996; 124:950–958.

Chapter 41

Gastric motility disorders

Jan Tack

KEY POINTS

- The stomach and proximal small intestine act in a coordinated fashion to mix and prepare all digested food through the intestine
- The interstitial cells of Cajal and the myenteric plexus play a role in the pacemaker activity of the distal stomach
- Failure of coordinated activity leads to abnormalities such as bacterial overgrowth, gastroparesis, and dumping syndrome
- The symptoms of gastric motility disorders are non specific, e.g. nausea, bloating, early satiety
- Drugs, diabetes, and post surgery are the commonest causes of gastric emptying
- Functional dyspepsia is probably a heterogeneous condition
- Functional tests such as radionuclide gastric emptying tests and breath tests may aid diagnosis but not necessarily treatment
- Not all patients require drug treatment
- Prokinetics, antidepressants, octreotide (dumping syndrome) and psychotherapy are all potential therapeutic modalities

INTRODUCTION

Functional anatomy

The stomach is a hollow organ with different anatomical parts (cardia, fundus, gastric body, antrum, and pylorus) and a sphincter muscle at either end. The proximal stomach (fundus and part of the body), which provides a reservoir for meals, is characterized by a tonic contractile activity, with smooth muscle cells that do not display electrical oscillatory activity.

The distal stomach is characterized by phasic contractile activity, with rhythmic oscillations of the membrane potential in smooth muscle cells at a frequency of 3 cycles/min (slow waves), triggered from an area in the corpus near the greater curvature, the so-called pacemaker region. Slow waves are generated by specialized cells, the interstitial cells of Cajal,[1] that are derived from the neural crest and located near the myenteric plexus, and determine the timing of gastric contractions.

The muscle layers of the stomach comprise an outer longitudinal layer and an inner circular layer, with an additional intermediate oblique muscle layer originating from the gastroesophageal junction in the proximal stomach. The myenteric plexus, which is found between the circular and longitudinal muscle layers in the stomach, has substantial functional autonomy, with limited vagal and sympathetic input. Cell bodies of intrinsic neurons are grouped in ganglia, which increase in number towards the distal antrum.

The vagus nerve is primarily a sensory nerve, conveying information from the nucleus of the solitary tract that is capable of activating motor neurons in the dorsal motor nucleus or nucleus ambiguus. Such vago-vagal reflexes regulate several physiological processes, including gastric emptying. The splanchnic or sympathetic innervation of the stomach originates from spinal segments 6 to 9 and exerts a mainly inhibitory function through the presynaptic inhibition of acetylcholine release from the myenteric plexus.

Physiology of gastric motility

Interdigestive motility

In the fasting state, the proximal gastrointestinal tract displays the migrating motor complex (MMC), a cyclical motor pattern of the stomach and the small intestine that originates from the stomach or proximal small intestine and migrates distally at a speed of 1–4 cm/min (Figs 41.1, 41.2).[2] The MMC consists of three different phases:

- phase I is characterized by the absence of contractile activity;
- phase II displays irregular contractile activity; and
- phase III is a phase of intense contractions at maximal frequency (3/min in the stomach, 12/min in the duodenum).

The average MMC cycle lasts between 90 and 120 min, but there is considerable variability. Phase III contractions act to evacuate indigestible particles from the stomach and small bowel and also effectively clears bacteria from the small bowel.

ANTRODUODENOJEJUNAL CATHETER POSITIONING

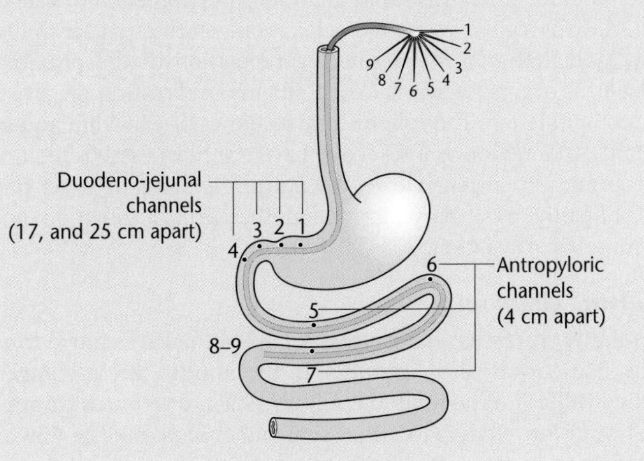

Fig. 41.1 Antroduodenojejunal catheter positioning.

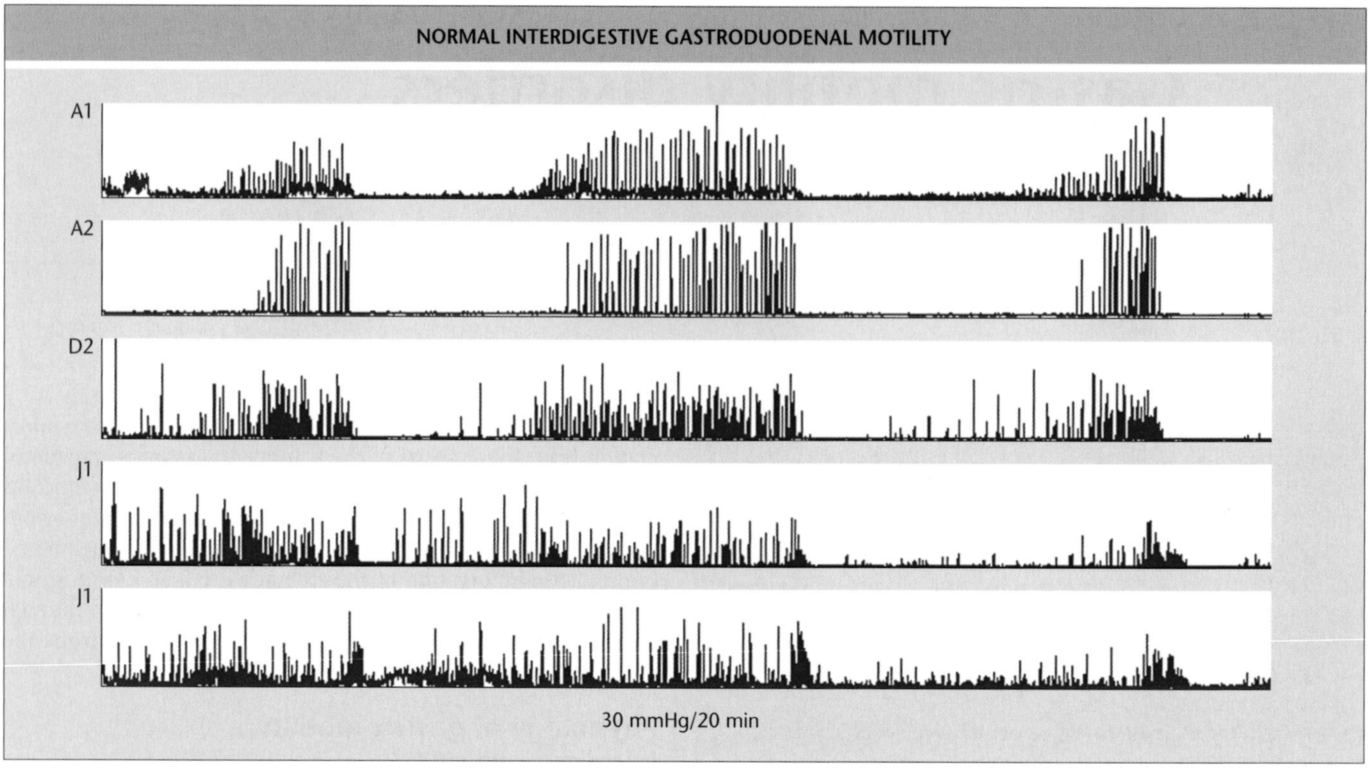

Fig. 41. 2 Normal interdigestive gastroduodenal motility as registered by antroduodenojejunal manometry (A=antral, D=duodenal, and J=jejunal manometry site). The image shows phase 1, 2, and 3 of the MMC migrating aborally.

Gastric reservoir function

When food is ingested, the MMC is suppressed and through the vagus nerve, upper gastrointestinal motility switches to the fed or postprandial pattern. During fasting, muscle fibers of the proximal stomach maintain a vagally mediated tonic contractile activity, which generates gastric fundus tone. During and after ingestion of a meal, a relaxation of the proximal stomach occurs, which provides the meal with a reservoir and enables a gastric volume increase without a rise in pressure.[3] This also allows the stomach to retain food and to allow passage to the duodenum at a rate that matches the duodenal absorptive capacity (Fig. 41.3). Two phases can be distinguished in the gastric reservoir function, and both are vagally mediated. Immediately after deglutition, the lower esophageal sphincter and the proximal stomach relax to allow passage and storage of the food bolus. This rapid inhibitory phenomenon of gastric motility is called receptive relaxation. During gastric filling by food ingestion, a long-lasting relaxation of the proximal stomach occurs, which is called adaptive relaxation or gastric accommodation. The role of tone in the gastric antrum and its ability to function as a reservoir have not been established and according to current views, the antrum is thought to act predominantly as a muscular pump that grinds the food and promotes evacuation.

Gastric emptying

In the postprandial state, circular peristaltic waves move from the mid-corpus to the pylorus. In the antrum, these contractions will grind the food and mix it with gastric juices through retropulsion, leading to propulsion and evacuation. The flow of chyme from the stomach to the duodenum is of a pulsatile nature and is determined by the strength of antral contraction, the degree of pyloric relaxation, and duodenal resistance. The pylorus is also involved in regulation of flow to the small intestine, and helps to discriminate fluid, viscous, and solid gastric contents. When gastric content is fluid, antral contractions occlude the lumen and liquid is easily transferred to the duodenum. In cases of a more viscous or solid gastric content, contractions are not lumen-obliterating, and retropulsion to the proximal stomach serves to mix and grind gastric contents. As the storage capacity of the duodenum is limited compared to the intragastric volume of chyme, duodenal contractions serve to delay further gastric emptying when the duodenum is not empty.

Disorders of gastric motility

Disordered gastric motility occurs whenever the processes of interdigestive motility, gastric reservoir function, or gastric

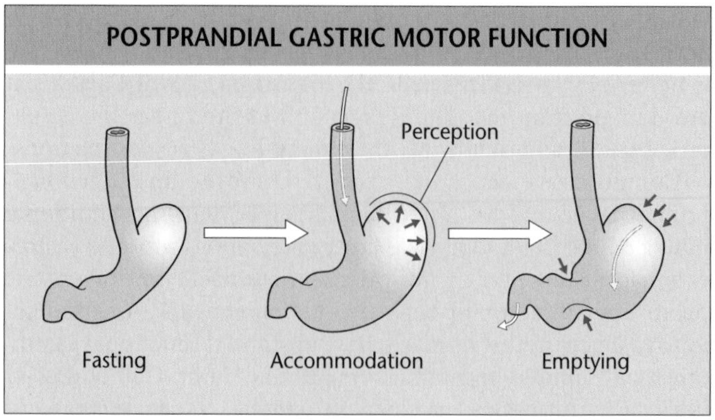

Fig. 41.3 Schematic outline of postprandial gastric motor function.

emptying are not properly controlled. The absence of gastric phase III activity promotes gastric bezoar formation, whereas the absence of small intestinal phase III promotes bacterial overgrowth. Impaired control of gastric accommodation may lead to defective reservoir function and inability to ingest large meals. Disordered gastric emptying control may lead to rapid emptying with duodenal caloric overload and dumping syndrome, or abnormally delayed emptying with prolonged stasis and fermentation of food.

SYMPTOMS

The symptoms that occur in patients with gastric motor disorders are nonspecific, and they consist of poor appetite, postprandial fullness and bloating, nausea, vomiting, epigastric pain, and early satiety (inability to finish a meal of normal size). In more severe cases, this may lead to severe weight loss and ultimately the inability to be fed orally. Depending on the underlying cause, these symptoms may occur intermittently or may be of a continuous nature. The relationship between symptoms and the presence or severity of disordered motility is often very poor and inconsistent.

GASTROPARESIS

Delayed gastric emptying may be caused by a variety of mechanical and nonmechanical causes. Delayed gastric emptying in the absence of mechanical obstruction is called gastroparesis. The most important pathophysiological abnormalities described in subgroups of patients include:

- fundal hypomotility;
- antral hypomotility;
- gastric arrhythmia; and
- lack of antropyloroduodenal coordination.

In addition, excessive negative feedback mechanisms may also delay gastric emptying.

Causes

One-third of cases of gastroparesis are idiopathic.[4] Many drugs can delay gastric emptying, including anticholinergics, opioids, L-dopa, tricyclic antidepressants, and phenothiazines. The most important nondrug causes of gastroparesis are surgery with vagotomy, diabetes mellitus, several metabolic and neurological disorders, and idiopathic gastroparesis.

Vagotomy causes rapid emptying of liquids and delayed emptying of solids. However, when a partial gastrectomy has been carried out in addition to this, a complex situation exists, which may lead to dumping syndrome, bile reflux gastritis, and small intestinal bacterial overgrowth.

Gastroparesis occurs in both type I and type II diabetes, which are usually accompanied by autonomic neuropathy. The reported prevalence varies between 10% and 76%, depending on the patients studied and on the definition of gastroparesis. The gastroparesis involves mainly solids and less frequently liquids. Poor glycemic control may also contribute to delayed emptying, which in its turn impairs glycemic control.

Gastroparesis also occurs in association with less frequent disorders such as anorexia nervosa, renal failure, Parkinson's disease, and chronic intestinal pseudo-obstruction. Delayed gastric emptying often occurs in anorexia nervosa, probably as a consequence of malnutrition and muscular atrophy.

In idiopathic gastroparesis, an acute onset and the presence of antibodies against neurotropic viruses, such as CMV, suggest a possible but unproven viral etiology.

FUNCTIONAL DYSPEPSIA

Functional dyspepsia is defined as the presence of persisting or recurrent pain or discomfort centered in the upper abdomen, in the absence of organic disease that readily explains the symptoms.[5–8] According to recent estimates, functional dyspepsia has a prevalence of 26-29% in the adult population below 65 years of age. Functional dyspepsia is most likely a heterogeneous disorder and, as with gastroparesis, there is currently no reliable diagnostic test.

In a large series, up to 30% of patients were found to have delayed gastric emptying, but the correlation with symptoms was poor.[6] The distinction between functional dyspepsia with delayed gastric emptying and idiopathic gastroparesis has not been clearly defined. The role of *Helicobacter pylori* has been studied, but this is also unclear. Most individual studies failed to demonstrate a beneficial effect of *Helicobacter pylori* eradication and meta-analysis showed any benefit to be limited (see Chapters 5 and 34).

Patients with functional dyspepsia have increased sensitivity to gastric balloon distention. However, the underlying mechanism is not established and the relationship with symptoms is again poor.

Scintigraphic and ultrasonographic studies have demonstrated abnormal preferential accumulation of food in the distal stomach, suggesting defective postprandial accommodation of the proximal stomach and barostat studies show reduced proximal gastric relaxation in response to a meal in up to 40% of patients. This may be associated with early satiety and weight loss[9] and, at least in some, may occur as a consequence of impaired nitrergic nerve function in the proximal stomach,[10] following acute gastroenteritis. Impaired gastric accommodation may be complemented by increased visceral sensitivity, shown in up to 50% of patients. The underlying mechanism is unclear and the relationship with symptoms is limited.

The role of psychosocial factors in functional dyspepsia has not been fully elucidated. Recent studies suggest a complex interaction between psychopathological and physiopathological factors in the dyspeptic symptom complex.[11]

DUMPING SYNDROME

Dumping syndrome is characterized by rapid gastric emptying accompanied by vasomotor and gastrointestinal symptoms. Dumping syndrome occurs mainly after partial or complete gastrectomy but may also be observed after vagotomy, intentional or unintentional, at the time of surgery at the gastroesophageal junction.

Symptoms typically occur after ingestion of a meal. 'Early dumping' occurs in the first hour after meal ingestion and is associated with both abdominal and systemic symptoms (Table 41.1). 'Late dumping' occurs 1–3 h postprandially and is the expression of reactive hypoglycemia. Most patients suffer from early dumping, or a combination of both. Isolated late dumping is rare. Symptoms usually occur within the first weeks after surgery when patients resume their normal diet. Meals rich in carbohydrates and liquid meals are particularly poorly tolerated. Severe dumping may lead to weight loss by fear of food ingestion; extreme cases may lead to malnutrition. Quality of life may be severely impaired.

Symptoms of early dumping are explained in part by the rapid passage of hyperosmolar contents into the small bowel, accompanied by a shift of fluids from the intravascular compartment to the lumen. This induces intestinal distention and the gastrointestinal and vasomotor symptoms listed in Table 41.1. Enhanced release of gastrointestinal hormones, like enteroglucagon, vasoactive intestinal peptide (VIP), peptide YY (PYY), pancreatic polypeptide, and neurotensin are thought to cause the vasodilation that underlies the vasomotor symptoms.

Late dumping occurs 1–3 h postprandially and is characterized by symptoms of hypoglycemia (Table 41.1). Rapid gastric emptying and consequent transient hyperglycemia stimulates a peak of insulin secretion, leading to reactive hypoglycemia when all the sugars have been absorbed. An enhanced release of glucagons-like peptide-1 (GLP-1) is also considered a major contributor to the extreme changes in glycemia levels after (partial) gastrectomy.

DIAGNOSTIC METHODS

Organic disease usually needs to be excluded by upper gastrointestinal endoscopy or radiology and laboratory tests before motility is investigated by functional tests.

Measurement of gastric emptying

The standard method for assessing gastric emptying rate is measurement of gastric emptying of radionuclides. Solid and liquid emptying can be assessed separately or simultaneously. The solid and/or liquid meal is labeled with different radioisotopes, usually ^{99}Tc or ^{111}In. A gamma-camera measures the number of counts in a given region of interest and mathematical processing with curve fitting allows calculation of the half emptying time, lag phase, and % of retention at different time points after the meal (Fig. 41.4). Although not routinely used, the technique also provides information on distribution within the stomach. Disadvantages of this method include the use of radioactive substances, the high cost, and poor level of standardization of meal composition and measuring times between different laboratories.

Breath tests can also be used. The solid or liquid phase of a meal is labeled with a ^{13}C-containing substrate (octanoic acid, acetic acid, glycin, or spirulina).[12] As soon as the labeled substrate leaves the stomach, it is rapidly absorbed and metabolized in the liver to generate $^{13}CO_2$, which appears in the breath.[11] Breath sampling at regular intervals and mathematical processing allows calculation of a gastric emptying curve. The advantages of this test are the use of nonradioactive materials and the ability to perform the test outside a hospital setting. A disadvantage is the absence of standardization of meal and substrate.

Ultrasound allows measurement of gastric antral diameter as a marker of the emptying rate but is time consuming and not suitable for solid meals; therefore, it is mainly used as an experimental tool.

SCINTIGRAPHIC GASTRIC EMPTYING TESTING

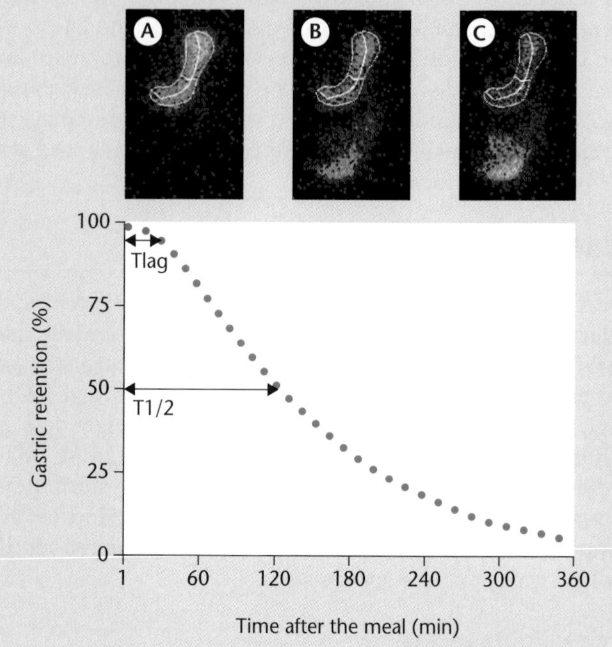

Fig. 41.4 Scintigraphic gastric emptying testing. Images obtained after the ingestion of the radiolabeled meal are analyzed to measure counts in the gastric region of interest at a given time point. This is used to construct an emptying curve. Mathematical processing yields half emptying time, lag time, and % retention at individual time points.

TABLE 41.1 SYMPTOMS ASSOCIATED WITH DUMPING SYNDROME

Early dumping (30–60 min postprandially)		Late dumping (90–240 min postprandially)
Gastrointestinal symptoms	*Vasomotor symptoms*	• Sweating
• Abdominal pain	• Flushing	• Palpitations
• Diarrhea	• Palpitations	• Hunger
• Borborygmi	• Sweating	• Weakness
• Bloating	• Dizziness	• Confusion
• Nausea	• Tachycardia	• Syncope
	• Syncope	• Hypoglycemia
	• Orthostatic hypotension	

Antropyloroduodenal manometry

Antropyloroduodenal manometry allows the investigation of mechanisms involved in the regulation of normal and abnormal gastric emptying (Figs 41.1, 41.2). This is mainly a research tool, with clinical application in the investigation of generalized motility disorders including chronic idiopathic intestinal pseudo-obstruction (CIIP).

Investigational techniques

The gastric barostat consists of a computer-driven pump connected to an oversized balloon, which can be positioned in the proximal or distal stomach. Measurement of volume changes in an isobaric mode allows measurement of changes in gastric tone. Stepwise increments in balloon pressure with assessments of perception allows sensitivity to gastric distention to be quantified (Figs 41.5 and 41.6).[13] Application of barostat measurements is restricted to research.

Cutaneous electrodes allow measurement of electrical activity of the stomach. This so-called electrogastrography (EGG) provides information on frequency and regularity of gastric pacemaker activity, as well as changes in power of the signal after meal ingestion. EGG is an experimental tool.

TREATMENT

General considerations

Not all patients with gastric motility disorders will require drug therapy. Reassurance and explanation of the nature of the disorder takes away the fear of a serious disease in the majority of patients. Although their efficacy is not proven, dietary and lifestyle adjustments are usually recommended.

In the absence of alarm symptoms or risk factors, the optimal indication and timing of endoscopic examination has not been established. Major variables are the cost and availability of endoscopic examination, the population prevalence of *Helicobacter pylori* infection, the cost and efficacy of empirical therapy, and the fear of organic disease in the patient.

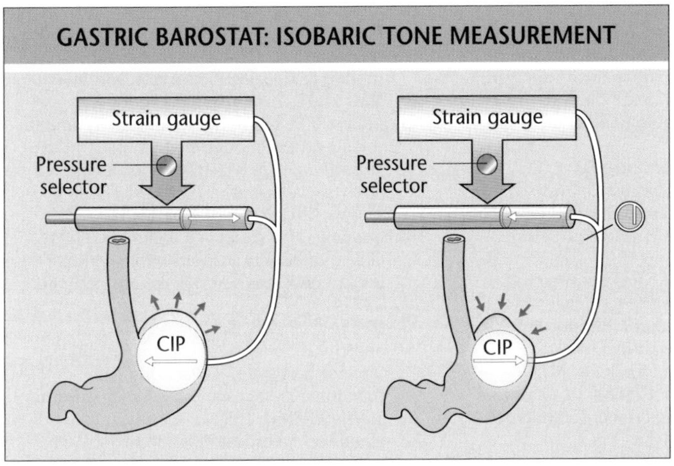

Fig. 41.5 Gastric barostat; isobaric tone measurement. The pressure within the bag is registered and maintained at a predefined set point by adapting intra-balloon volume. During contraction of the proximal stomach, air is withdrawn to maintain constant pressure. During relaxation of the proximal stomach, air is inflated to maintain constant pressure.

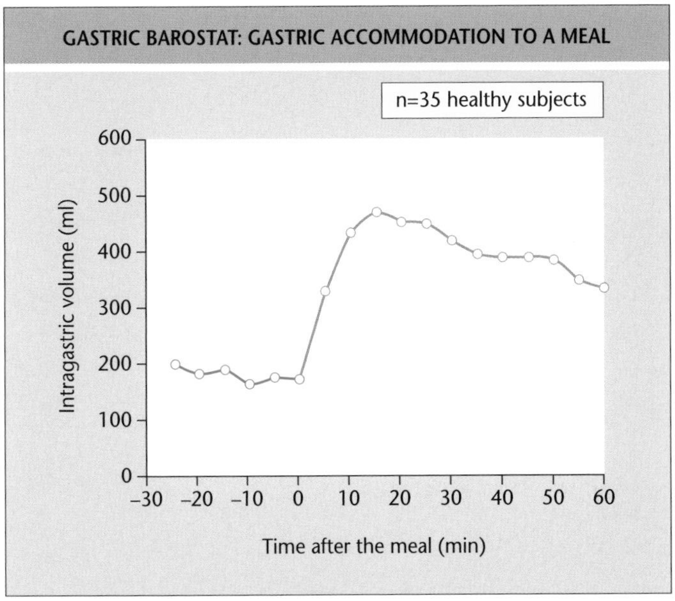

Fig. 41.6 Gastric barostat; measurement of gastric accommodation to a meal. Pooled data of intra-balloon volume before and after the meal in 35 healthy subjects.

Gastroparesis

Clinical suspicion of gastroparesis warrants exclusion of mechanical causes and serum electrolyte imbalances, followed by empirical treatment with the gastroprokinetic drug domperidone (3 × 10 mg).[14] Metoclopramide is an alternative but may cause extrapyramidal side effects. Cisapride is effective in gastroparesis, but not generally available because of an enhanced risk of QT prolongation with cardiac arrhythmias. Short-term studies in diabetic and postsurgical gastroparesis have reported beneficial effects of treatment with the macrolide antibiotic erythromycin (3×250–500 mg),[15] which acts as a motilin receptor agonist and has prokinetic properties. Attempts to develop macrolide prokinetics devoid of antibiotic properties have been disappointing.[16]

Functional dyspepsia

Empirical proton pump inhibitor therapy is now most often the initial approach, but this is probably helpful to identify patients with underlying gastroesophageal reflux disease, rather than treating true dyspepsia.[17] *Helicobacter pylori*, if present, is generally eradicated, but benefit is limited (see Chapters 5 and 34).[18,19] Prokinetics are less widely used now than previously, because of safety or efficacy.[20] Tegaserod, a new prokinetic 5-HT4 agonist, is currently under evaluation for the treatment of functional dyspepsia.

A minority of patients will not benefit from the approach outlined above. In the absence of alarm symptoms or less typical symptoms, the yield of additional diagnostic examinations will be low and this should be avoided. Possible psychiatric comorbidity needs to be considered in more refractory patients. Some may respond to low-dose antidepressants[21] or to psychotherapy.[22,23] Several drugs aimed at decreasing visceral sensitivity or at enhancing gastric accommodation are currently under investigation, but future studies will have to establish their efficacy.

Dumping syndrome

Dietary measures are the first step in the treatment of dumping syndrome. Patients are instructed to spread their daily calorie intake over at least six meals, and to avoid drinking with meals and for the first 2 h postprandially. Rapidly absorbed carbohydrates are eliminated and intake of fat and proteins increased accordingly. Certain food additives like pectin, guar gum, and glucomannan can be used. They form a gel with carbohydrates, thereby slowing absorption and delaying transit time.

Acarbose is a powerful inhibitor of intestinal alpha-glucosidase. Its ingestion slows carbohydrate digestion and blunts postprandial rises in glycemia, hence its application in late dumping. Octreotide is a long-acting synthetic somatostatin analog. It is administered subcutaneously three times daily, or intramuscularly once every 2–4 weeks as a slow-release formulation. Octreotide inhibits gastric emptying of liquids, small bowel transit, release of enteral hormones, and release of insulin as well as slowing monosaccharide absorption.[24] Because of its mode of administration and potential side effect of gallstone formation, octreotide should be reserved for severe cases that do not respond to more conservative measures. In exceptionally difficult-to-manage patients, surgery with creation of a proximal short antiperistaltic intestinal loop can be considered.

SOURCES OF INFORMATION FOR PATIENTS AND DOCTORS

http://www.acg.gi.org/patients/gihealth/gastroparesis.asp
http://www.gpda.net/

REFERENCES

1. Huizinga JD, Thuneberg L, Kluppel M et al. W/kit gene required for interstitial cells of Cajal and for intestinal pacemaker activity. Nature 1995; 373:347–349.
2. Vantrappen G, Janssens J, Hellemans J, Ghoos Y. The interdigestive motor complex of normal subjects and patients with bacterial overgrowth of the small intestine. J Clin Invest 1977; 59:1158–1166.
3. Azpiroz F, Malagelada JR. Vagally mediated gastric relaxation induced by intestinal nutrients in the dog. Am J Physiol 1986; 251:G727–G735.
4. Horowitz M, Su YC, Rayner CK, Jones KL. Gastroparesis: prevalence, clinical significance and treatment. Can J Gastroenterol 2001; 15:805–813.
5. Talley NJ, Stanghellini V, Heading RC et al. Functional gastroduodenal disorders. Gut 1999; 45(Suppl 2):37–42.
6. Stanghellini V, Tosetti C, Paternico A et al. Risk indicators of delayed gastric emptying of solids in patients with functional dyspepsia. Gastroenterology 1996; 110:1036–1042.
7. Talley NJ, Janssens J, Lauritsen K, Racz I, Bolling-Sternevald E. Eradication of *Helicobacter pylori* in functional dyspepsia: randomised double blind placebo controlled trial with 12 months' follow up. The Optimal Regimen Cures Helicobacter Induced Dyspepsia (ORCHID) Study Group. BMJ 1999; 318:833–837.
8. Talley NJ, Vakil N, Ballard ED 2nd, ennerty MB. Absence of benefit of eradicating *Helicobacter pylori* in patients with nonulcer dyspepsia. N Engl J Med 1999; 341:1106–1111.
9. Tack J, Piessevaux H, Coulie B, Caenepeel P, Janssens J. Role of impaired gastric accommodation to a meal in functional dyspepsia. Gastroenterology 1998; 115:1346–1352.
10. Tack J, Demedts I, Dehondt G et al. Clinical and pathophysiological characteristics of acute-onset functional dyspepsia. Gastroenterology 2002; 122:1738–1747.
11. Fischler B, Vandenberghe J, Persoons P et al. Evidence-based subtypes in functional dyspepsia with confirmatory factor analysis: Psychosocial and physiopathological correlates. Gastroenterology 2001; 120:268–276.
12. Ghoos YF, Maes BD, Geypens BJ et al. Measurement of gastric emptying rate of solids by means of a carbon-labeled octanoic acid breath test. Gastroenterology 1993; 104:1640–1647.
13. Azpiroz F, Malagelada J-R. Physiological variations in canine gastric tone measured by an electronic barostat. Am J Physiol 1985; 247:229–237.
14. Veldhuyzen van Zanten SJ, Jones MJ, Verlinden M, Talley NJ. Efficacy of cisapride and domperidone in functional (nonulcer) dyspepsia: a meta-analysis. Am J Gastroenterol 2001; 96:689–696.
15. Janssens J, Peeters TL, Vantrappen G et al. Improvement of gastric emptying in diabetic gastroparesis by erythromycin. Preliminary studies. N Engl J Med 1990; 322:1028–1031.
16. Talley NJ, Verlinden M, Snape W et al. Failure of a motilin receptor agonist (ABT-229) to relieve the symptoms of functional dyspepsia in patients with and without delayed gastric emptying: a randomized double-blind placebo-controlled trial. Aliment Pharmacol Ther 2000; 14:1653–1661.
17. Talley NJ, Meineche-Schmidt V, Paré P et al. Efficacy of omeprazole in functional dyspepsia: double-blind, randomized, placebo-controlled trials (the Bond and Opera studies). Aliment Pharmacol Ther 1998; 12: 1055–1065.
18. Laine L, Schoenfeld P, Fennerty MB. Therapy for *Helicobacter pylori* in patients with nonulcer dyspepsia. A meta-analysis of randomized, controlled trials. Ann Intern Med 2001; 134:361–369.
19. Moayedi P, Soo S, Deeks J et al. Systematic review and economic evaluation of *Helicobacter pylori* eradication treatment for non-ulcer dyspepsia. Dyspepsia Review Group. BMJ 2000; 321:659–664.
20. Sturm A, Holtmann G, Goebell H, Gerken G. Prokinetics in patients with gastroparesis: a systematic analysis. Digestion 1999; 60: 422–427.
21. Mertz H, Fass R, Kodner A. Effect of amitriptyline on symptoms, sleep, and visceral perception in patients with functional dyspepsia. Am J Gastroenterol 1998; 93: 160–165.
22. Hamilton J, Guthrie E, Creed F et al. A randomized controlled trial of psychotherapy in patients with chronic functional dyspepsia. Gastroenterology 2000; 119:661–669.
23. Calvert EL, Houghton LA, Cooper P, Whorwell P. Long-term improvement in functional dyspepsia using hypnotherapy. Gastroenterology 2002; 123:1778–1785.
24. William L, Hani C, Soudah HC et al. Mechanisms by which octreotide ameliorates symptoms in the dumping syndrome. J Pharmacol Exp Ther 1996; 277:1359–1365.

Chapter 42

Food allergy and intolerance

Vicky Chudleigh and John Hunter

KEY POINTS

- True food allergy affects 2% of the population
- IgE mediated sensitization may occur *in utero* or during lactation
- Diagnosis includes history, IgE levels, skin prick and radioallergoabsorbant test (RAST)
- Most food intolerance is not due to allergy or enzyme deficiencies
- Enzyme deficiencies such as lactase deficiencies are common in non-Caucasians
- Colonic fermentation due to overgrowth of facultative anaerobes may be important
- Elemental diets can achieve remission in Crohn's disease in up to 90% of compliant patients
- Dietary management of Crohn's disease requires supervision by an experienced dietician

INTRODUCTION

Food allergy and intolerance is one of the most contentious areas in gastroenterology today. Studies of classical immunology have clearly defined the role of food allergy and IgE antibodies as a cause of anaphylaxis, which may lead to sudden death. Unfortunately, the term 'food allergy' has been incorrectly applied to food reactions that may be related to other gut diseases such as irritable bowel syndrome and Crohn's disease. In fact, the only common ground between food allergy and food intolerance is food itself. The underlying mechanisms are quite distinct. Allergy is immunologically mediated, classically by IgE and possibly also by IgG. The mechanisms leading to food intolerance are several and are not yet completely understood, but they include toxic or irritant effects, enzyme deficiencies, pharmacological effects of chemicals, and malfermentation by intestinal bacteria. Attempts to apply the principles of allergy to food intolerance have led to confusion and subsequent scepticism that food intolerance is a genuine entity.

FOOD ALLERGY

Genuine food allergy is an uncommon problem in gastroenterology. The prevalence of food allergy in the adult population is approximately 2% but most of these patients suffer symptoms in systems other than the gut. The gastrointestinal symptoms of food allergy are abdominal pain, nausea, vomiting and diarrhea within an hour or two of food ingestion. The oropharynx may be affected with tingling and itching around the lips, tongue and mouth, and similar symptoms may precede the onset of acute anaphylaxis, with wheezing, hypotension, and circulatory collapse. This may occur particularly after eating peanuts, nuts, fish, and crustacea. The rapid onset of symptoms after food ingestion usually means that patients are easily able to identify those foods that upset them.[1]

Immunological mechanisms to account for food allergic reactions remain unclear. Two mechanisms currently seem plausible; type I IgE-mediated anaphylactic reactions and possibly T lymphocyte-based type IV reactions which may be seen in gluten sensitivity, gut infections such as giardiasis, and tropical sprue.[2] These conditions are discussed elsewhere.

The cause of food allergy is poorly understood. Specific IgE to food antigens may be detected in newborn infants and sensitization of the fetus to antigens crossing the placenta during the second trimester of pregnancy may be important. Food antigens may also be detected in human breast milk. Allergy is associated with increased Th2 responses in the gut immune system but the reason for this remains unclear.

Morphological changes in the gut in patients with food allergy are inconsistent and unhelpful. Studies, mainly from animal models, suggest that the mucosal mast cell is crucial in the pathogenesis of allergic responses. Food antigens cause degranulation of mast cells coated with specific IgE antibodies, with release of inflammatory agents including histamine, 5-hydroxytryptamine, prostaglandins, and leukotrienes. These cause mucosal edema and increased intestinal permeability, with subepithelial activation of lymphocytes and mast cells. Increased fluid secretion into the gut and smooth muscle spasm produce diarrhea, vomiting, and pain. The importance of the mast cell in food allergy in man is supported by the effectiveness of specific blocking agents such as sodium chromoglycate and H-1 receptor antagonists, which may blunt allergic responses.[3]

The clinical diagnosis of true food allergy is usually straightforward as the rapid onset of symptoms after eating the food concerned makes cause and effect quite clear. Affected individuals are usually atopic and have elevated serum concentrations of IgE. A skin prick test and radioallergoabsorbant test (RAST) may be performed to detect specific IgE antibodies to foods. Results should be interpreted with caution, as false-positive reactions may occur. The patient should be asked to follow a diet from which the foods concerned have been excluded to see if the symptoms clear. If it is considered necessary, double-blind confirmatory challenge tests may be undertaken, although these may sometimes be dangerous, especially if the patient is liable to anaphylactic reactions.

Treatment of true food allergy is usually by avoidance of the offending foods. Direction on dietary exclusion is best supervised by a dietitian. Some patients may wish to try sodium chromoglycate to reduce mast cell degradation and antihistamines or prostaglandin synthetase inhibitors to block the effects of chemicals released, but these drugs are frequently only partially effective, and are of relatively little clinical value. Patients at risk of anaphylactic reactions may carry preloaded syringes containing epinephrine (adrenaline) for self-injection.

FOOD INTOLERANCE

The prevalence of food intolerance is more difficult to determine, as no objective diagnostic test is available. Questionnaire-based studies may overemphasize prevalence of true food intolerance. Self-reported food allergy/intolerance varies significantly across countries ranging from 4.6% in Spain to 19.1% in Australia.[4]

The importance of food intolerance in gastrointestinal disease remains a topic of great controversy and confusion. Whilst there can be no doubt that some patients suffer unpleasant reactions to foods that are reproducible but not mediated through true allergic mechanisms, the importance of this phenomenon remains the source of considerable disagreement. This is partly because the mechanisms of food intolerance (Fig. 42.1) are still poorly understood, but also because ambitious claims have been made as to its importance in a wide range of diseases, sometimes based on sketchy evidence, which have therefore inevitably produced considerable skepticism. Furthermore, food reactions of this sort may come on slowly many hours after food ingestion making the identification of offending foods difficult.

Toxic and irritant effect of foods

Toxic effects of spoiled foods, including vomiting, pain and diarrhea, and pharmacological reactions to food chemicals such as caffeine, ethanol, and monosodium glutamate are usually identified readily from a dietary history. Difficulty most frequently arises with enzyme deficiencies and with those intolerances that have been suggested to arise from colonic malfermentation.

Enzyme deficiencies

Lactase deficiency may be congenital or acquired. Other disaccharide deficiencies (sucrose-isomaltase and trehalase) are rare. In most races, the enzyme lactase, which breaks lactose down to glucose and galactose, disappears from the small bowel mucosa around puberty, and adults frequently suffer diarrhea and flatulence after drinking milk. Northern Caucasians are unusual in this respect as in the majority of subjects, the enzyme persists into adult life so that milk may remain part of their diet. Lactase deficiency is seen in 5% of healthy Caucasians of North European origin. The small bowel mucosa is histologically normal but reduced enzyme activity is demonstrable when it is incubated with lactose as a substrate. The diagnosis may be elegantly confirmed by the hydrogen breath test response to a test dose of 50 g lactose by mouth. Undigested lactose escapes from the small bowel into the colon where it is fermented by the gut bacteria with the release of hydrogen. A rise of >20 p.p.m. within 3 h of lactose ingestion is considered a positive result (Fig. 42.2). Abdominal symptoms may also be provoked.[5]

Patients suffering from hypolactasia present with diarrhea, abdominal pain, and flatulence, which may not obviously be connected with consumption of milk, as lactose is also present in other dairy foods and is widely used as a filler in the food industry. These symptoms may be indistinguishable from those of irritable bowel syndrome (IBS). The incidence of hypolactasia in cases of IBS is approximately 25%. Non-Caucasian patients with apparent IBS should therefore be screened for alactasia. Whether this is justified in white subjects with IBS is less clear as symptoms following milk ingestion may be caused by milk fat or protein as well as by lactose. Low-lactose diets may be ineffective and it is therefore frequently necessary to exclude dairy products completely (milk-free diet) and sometimes other foods as well to control symptoms satisfactorily.[6]

Treatment of hypolactasia involves reduction or complete elimination of lactose-containing foods. Predigestion of lactose

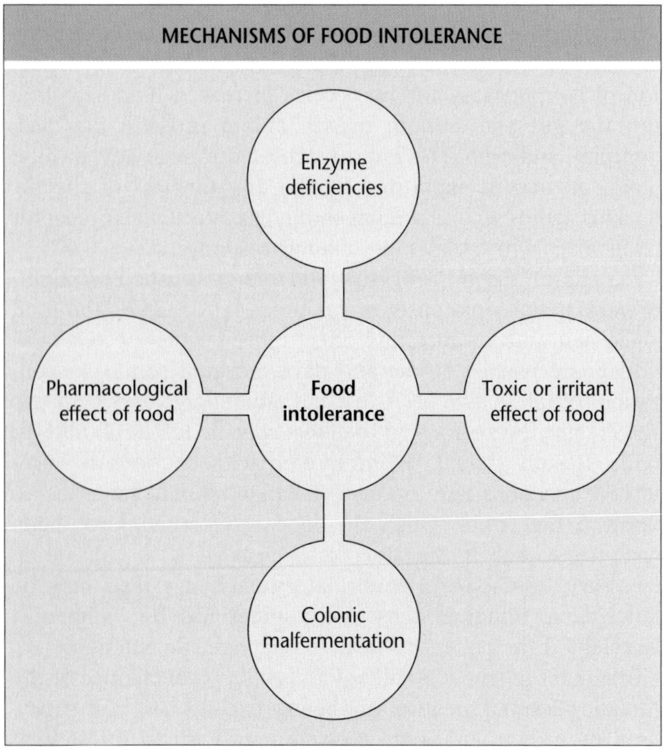

Fig. 42.1 The mechanisms of food intolerance.

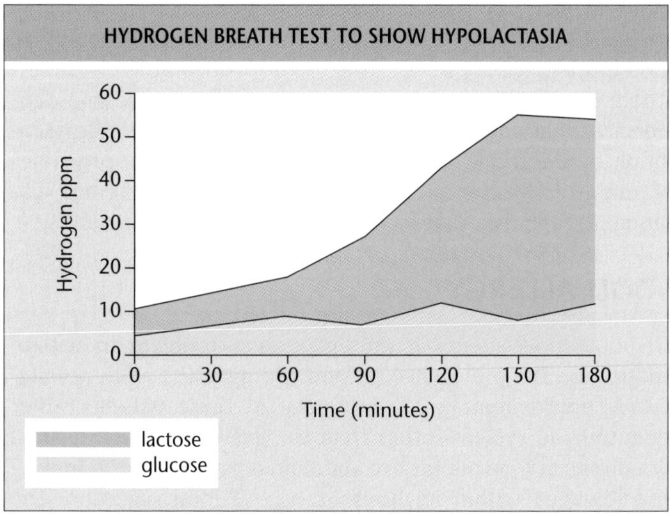

Fig. 42.2 Hydrogen breath test to show hypolactasia. The hydrogen concentration on the breath rises rapidly after 50 g lactose but does not rise after 50 g of glucose.

by the addition of enzyme preparations to milk may be helpful. Attempts to improve colonic fermentation of undigested lactose using preparations of probiotic bacteria remain experimental.

IDIOPATHIC FOOD INTOLERANCE

The majority of genuine food intolerances arise from neither allergy nor enzyme deficiencies. These reactions are usually slow, insidious in onset and may require relatively large helpings of food to trigger them (Fig. 42.3). It has been suggested that they may be due to loss of important bacteria from the colonic flora leading to malfermentation of food residues entering the cecum.

Although patients may complain of headache, joint pains, and fatigue, the prime symptoms of this form of food intolerance are abdominal pain, flatus and an altered bowel habit. No pathological, radiological, or endoscopic abnormalities are detectable on standard investigation and it is therefore difficult to separate these cases from IBS. However, searches for food intolerance in a series of IBS patients have revealed considerable differences. The number of patients with IBS found to have food intolerance has ranged from as little as 6% to as much as 67%.[7] Anxiety is a well recognized factor leading to IBS and to complicate matters further many patients with food intolerances develop secondary anxiety states, especially when their problem does not receive confident management.

Colonic fermentation

Proponents argue that food intolerances are a major factor in the pathogenesis of IBS. Prospective studies show that the risk of developing IBS is greatly increased by events that may damage the colonic flora including bacterial gastroenteritis (relative risk, RR 11.9) and courses of antibiotics (RR 4).[8] Several studies have shown that in IBS the flora is abnormal, with reduced counts of lactobacilli and *Bifidobacter*, together with overgrowth of facultative anaerobes, whose numbers increase after food challenge.[9] Rigorous double-blind challenges have confirmed food intolerances in IBS patients selected by the Rome criteria, sometimes supported by biochemical changes such as increased production of prostaglandin E2 or inflammatory cytokines. Finally, abnormal colonic fermentation with excessive production of hydrogen has been reported in IBS patients. Exclusion diets reduced hydrogen excretion and relieved symptoms (Fig. 42.4).[10]

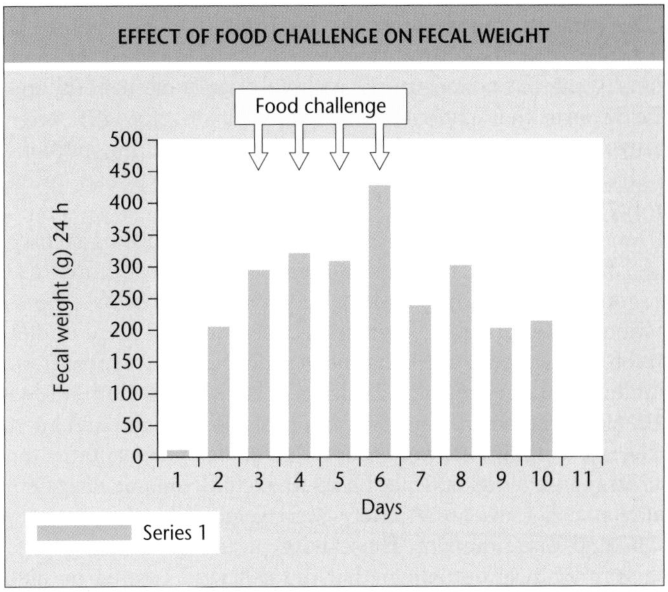

Fig. 42.3 Effect of a double-blind food challenge on fecal weight. Maximum fecal output is not reached until the fourth day of challenge. Reproduced with permission from Hunter JO. Food intolerance and the irritable bowel syndrome. In: Read NW, ed. Irritable bowel syndrome. Oxford: Blackwell Scientific Publications; 1991.

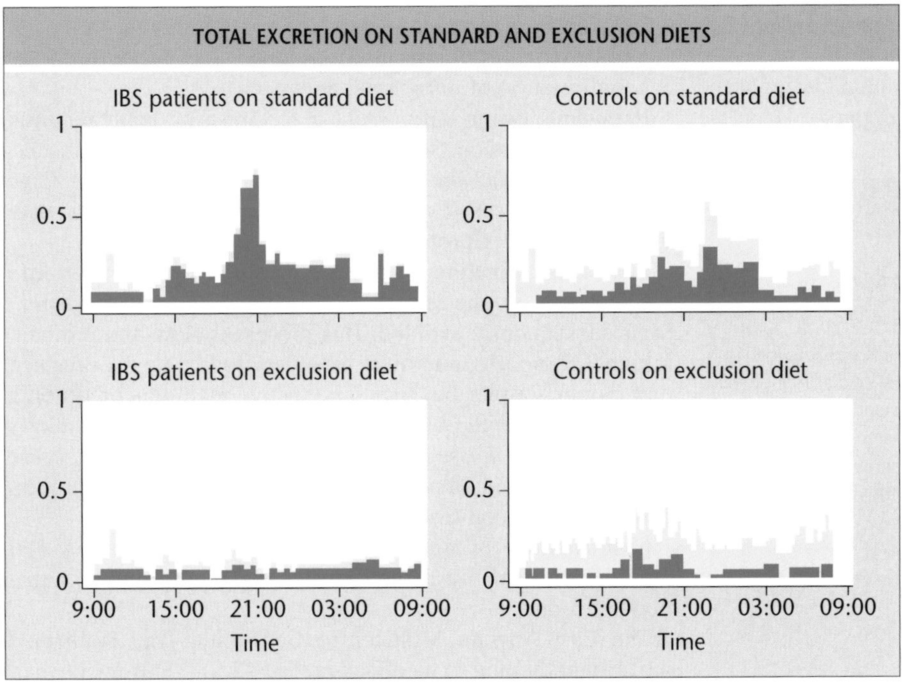

Fig. 42.4 Total excretion on standard and exclusion diets. Area charts showing median rate of total excretion (green: hydrogen; yellow: methane; mL/min (standard temperature and pressure)) at 30 min intervals during 24-h measurement on standard and exclusion diets. From King TS, Elia MA, Hunter JO. Abnormal colonic fermentation in irritable bowel syndrome. The Lancet 1998: 352:1187-1189. Reprinted with permission from Elsevier.

By contrast, others stress the importance of psychological factors in IBS, the all too frequent patients who restrict their diets, sometimes dangerously, with no discernible benefit, and the reports that patients most likely to develop IBS after gastroenteritis are those with evidence of existing psychological stress. Furthermore, treatment with hypnosis often provides excellent results.[11]

Faced with such disagreement, the gastroenterologist may well feel daunted. IBS may be a multifactorial condition, the treatment of which may need to be very different between one patient and another.[12] Nevertheless, the potential value of diet in the management of IBS has been supported by a report from Addenbrookes Hospital, Cambridge, UK, where a dietitian-led IBS clinic was set up. Patients with possible IBS who had been referred by their GPs were sent to the clinic by consultants for screening by blood and stool tests to exclude organic disorders such as celiac disease. Anxiety was excluded by the use of a validated questionnaire. Those with positive tests were sent back to medical outpatients but the rest were treated by diet according to their predominant symptoms (Table 42.1). Sixty-one per cent were satisfactorily treated with no further input by medical staff.[13] In terms of cost-effectiveness, such a clinic compares well with other ways of handling a condition that presents a considerable drain on medical resources, and is a compelling argument for the importance of food intolerances in IBS. Therapeutic dietary manipulation should be guided by a qualified dietitian.[14]

DIETARY MANAGEMENT OF CROHN'S DISEASE

The cause of Crohn's disease (CD) is unknown (see Chapter 54). Nevertheless, it is now recognized that diet may sometimes play a part in its management.

The value of nutritional therapy first became apparent when patients with CD were given total parenteral nutrition (TPN) to correct their nutritional state prior to surgery. Not only did they gain weight but symptoms were relieved and evidence of inflammation subsided. This improvement was initially attributed to bowel rest. The majority of patients, however, rapidly relapsed after returning to a normal diet.

It was later discovered that similar improvements were seen in CD patients receiving enteral feeds and, in particular, pre-digested elemental feeds, where nitrogen was presented as amino acids, starch as maltodextrins, with fat as a single oil, vitamins, minerals, and flavoring. These were initially unpalatable and were given by nasogastric tube, but recent improvements mean that most patients can now take them as sip-feeds. It has been demonstrated that elemental feeds are equally as effective as TPN in inducing remission in CD. As they are considerably cheaper and less invasive they have now largely replaced TPN in the management of CD.[15]

Elemental diets may lead to clinical remission after 2–3 weeks' feeding in as many as 85–90% of compliant patients. Unfortunately, approximately one-third of patients abandon the diet prematurely so that corticosteroids emerge as being superior on an intention-to-treat basis; therefore, attempts have been made to improve their flavor by presenting nitrogen as a single protein (polymeric feeds) or as di- or tripeptides (oligomeric feeds). Neither of these has been convincingly demonstrated to be better, in terms of flavor or effectiveness, than the original elemental preparations. Recent studies suggest that fat may be an important determinant of effectiveness with feeds in which <15% of energy is derived from long-chain triglycerides (LCTs) giving the best results.[16] In compliant patients, however, enteral feeds are equally as effective as corticosteroids.

Although bowel rest was originally believed to explain the effectiveness of enteral feeds in CD it is now clear that these are still beneficial when patients are allowed normal food items as well. Reduction in inflammatory markers precedes any improvement in nutritional status and there is no evidence of food allergy in CD. It has been suggested that food intolerances in CD are, as in IBS, related to changes in colonic bacterial metabolism. Thus fecal bacterial counts fall by over 50% during enteral feeding and stools often turn green because bacteria no longer convert biliverdin to stercobilin. Eighty to a hundred per cent of these bacteria are coated with immunoglobulin in active disease, but this falls significantly after 2 weeks' elemental feeding.[17] Research continues in this field.

TABLE 42.1 SYMPTOMS AND SUGGESTED DIETARY TRIALS

Symptoms	Suggested dietary trial
Constipation (no bloating and wind)	High fiber
Constipation (with bloating and wind)	Low fiber with bulking agent
Diarrhea (no bloating and wind)	1st: low fiber (if diet high fiber) 2nd: exclusion
Diarrhea (with bloating and wind)	1st: low fiber 2nd: exclusion
Alternating constipation/diarrhea (no bloating and wind)	1st: high fiber or bulking agent 2nd: exclusion
Alternating constipation/diarrhea (with bloating and wind)	1st: low fiber with bulking agent 2nd: exclusion

Dietary treatment of Crohn's disease

There are three stages to dietary treatment:

1. remission on enteral feeds;
2. reintroduction of normal foods; and
3. confirmation of nutritional adequacy.

Remission: Two to three weeks of feeding is normally required for clinical remission. Some authorities, especially pediatricians, recommend longer. The optimal length of treatment may emerge with the use of sensitive tests of objective remission, e.g., estimation of fecal calprotectin.

Food reintroduction: Foods are carefully reintroduced into the diet one by one and those provoking any adverse symptoms subsequently avoided. This process is slow and difficult, taking 2–3 months, and must be supervised by an experienced dietitian. A simpler but equally effective regime is based on a low fat fiber limited exclusion diet (LOFFLEX), which allows introduction *en masse* of a number of foods which rarely cause problems. The time of enteral feeding is reduced and the process of subsequent food testing much shortened.

Confirmation of nutritional adequacy: The resulting diet must be checked by a dietitian to ensure the diet is nutritionally sound.

The East Anglian Multicentre Controlled Trial confirmed nutritional therapy to be effective (Fig. 42.5).[18] However, when

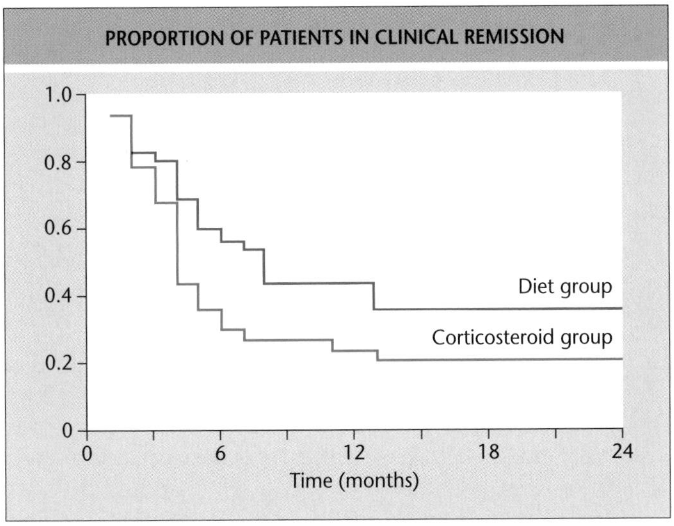

Fig. 42.5 Proportion of patients in clinical remission. East Anglia Multicentre Controlled Trial; proportion of patients in clinical remission p=0.048. Reproduced with permission from Riordan AM, Hunter JO, Woen RE et al. Treatment of active Crohn's disease by exclusion diet: East Anglian Multicentre Controlled Trial. The Lancet 1993; 342: 1131-1134.

failures of enteral feeding and food testing are taken into consideration the overall long-term success rate is only 40–50%. For this reason, many reserve dietary therapy for patients who are unresponsive or develop side effects to corticosteroids. In childhood, however, diet allows normal growth and thus has become the treatment of choice.[19] Other major advantages include the lack of side effects such as osteoporosis[20] and infections and the satisfaction patients derive from achieving control over their disease during long periods of remission.

SOURCES OF INFORMATION FOR PATIENTS AND DOCTORS

http://www.equip.nhs.uk/topics/allergy/foodintol.html

REFERENCES

1. Lessof MH, Wraith DG, Merrett TG, Buisseret PD. Food allergy and intolerance in 100 patients – local and systemic effects. Q J Med 1980; 49:259–271
2. Marsh MN. Intestinal pathogenesis correlates of clinical food allergic disorders. In: Brostoff J, Challacombe SJ, eds. Food allergy and intolerance, 2nd edn. London: Saunders; 2002:267–278.
3. Crowe SE, Perdue MH. Gastrointestinal food hypersensitivity: basic mechanisms of pathophysiology. Gastroenterology 1992; 103:1075–1095.
4. Woods RK, Abramson M, Bailey M, Walters EH. International prevalence of reported food allergy and intolerances. Comparisons arising from the European Community Respiratory Health Survey (ECRHS) 1991-1994. Eur J Clin Nutr 2001; 55: 298–304.
5. Cox TM. Enzyme deficiency. In: Brostoff J, Challacombe SJ, eds. Food allergy and intolerance, 2nd edn. London: Saunders; 2002: 365–385.
6. Parker TJ, Woolner JT, Prevost AT et al. Irritable bowel syndrome: is the search for lactose intolerance justified? Eur J Gastoenterol Hepatol 2001; 13:219–225.
7. Burden S. Dietary treatment of irritable bowel syndrome: current evidence and guidelines for future practice. J Hum Nutr Diet 2001; 14:231–241.
8. Garcia Rodriguez LA, Ruigomez A. Increased risk of irritable bowel syndrome after bacterial gastroenteritis: a cohort study. BMJ 1999; 318:565–566.
9. Madden JAJ, Hunter JO. A review of the role of the gut microflora in irritable bowel syndrome and the effects of probiotics. Br J Nutr 2002; 88:S67–S72.
10. King TS, Elia M, Hunter JO. Abnormal colonic fermentation in irritable bowel syndrome. Lancet 1998; 352:1187–1189.
11. Gonsalkorale WM, Miller V, Afzal A, Whorell PJ. Long term benefits of hypnotherapy for irritable bowel syndrome. Gut 2003; 52:1623–1629.
12. Ragnarsson G, Bodemar G. Division of the irritable bowel syndrome into sub groups on the basis of daily recorded symptoms in two outpatient samples. Scand J Gastroenterol 1999; 34:993–1000.
13. Chudleigh VA, Brennon E, Tarry SA et al. Value of a dietitian led clinic in the management of young patients with irritable bowel syndrome. Gut 2002; 50:A3.
14. Atkinson RJ, Hunter JO. Role of diet and bulking agents in the treatment of IBS. In: Camilleri M, Spiller RC, eds. Irritable bowel syndrome; diagnosis and treatment. Edinburgh: Saunders; 2002:141–150.
15. Goh J, O'Morain CA. Review article: nutrition and inflammatory bowel disease. Aliment Pharmacol Ther 2003; 17:307–320.
16. Bamba T, Shimoyama T, Sasaki M et al. Dietary fat attenuates the benefits of an elemental diet in active Crohn's disease: a randomized, controlled trial. Eur J Gastroenterol Hepatol 2003; 15:151–157.
17. Van der Waaj LA, Kroese FGM, Visser A et al. Increased immunoglobulin-coating of commensal anaerobic bacteria in faeces of patients with inflammatory bowel disease. Eur J Gastro Hepatol 2004; 16:669–674.
18. Riordan AM, Hunter JO, Cowan RE et al. Treatment of active Crohn's disease by exclusion diet: East Anglian multi centre controlled trial. Lancet 1993; 342:1131–1134.
19. Walker-Smith J. The role of enteral feeding in Crohn's disease of childhood. Minerva Pediatr 2000; 52:277–279.
20. Dear KLE, Compston JE, Hunter JO. Treatments for Crohn's disease that minimize steroid doses are associated with a reduced risk of osteoporosis. Clin Nutr 2001; 20:541–546.

Chapter 43

Maldigestion and malabsorption

Arvey I Rogers and Ryan D Madanick

KEY POINTS

- Malabsorption includes impaired digestion and/or absorption
- Carbohydrates, proteins and lipids are absorbed in the duodenum and jejunum
- The ileum can assume the absorptive function of the proximal intestine
- Diagnosis requires a high index of suspicion, confirmatory tests and search for etiology
- Quantitative fecal fat analysis is the gold standard to confirm steatorrhea
- A stool osmotic gap greater than 100 and positive hydrogen breath test are suggestive of carbohydrate malabsorption

INTRODUCTION AND DEFINITION

Malabsorption syndromes include disorders resulting from impaired digestion and/or impaired absorption. Malabsorption is the result of defective nutrient uptake or transport by the intestinal mucosa, whereas maldigestion denotes the impaired breakdown of macronutrients.[1] Etiologies are varied, but there are common presenting signs and symptoms. The first requirement to accurately diagnose a malabsorption syndrome is that it must be suspected on clinical grounds. Suspicion requires confirmation, and once confirmed, its etiology can usually be established.[2] Some understanding of the biochemical and physiologic aspects of the assimilation of dietary foodstuffs (macro- and micronutrients) enhances an appreciation of the various manifestations of malabsorption. We will present the essentials of carbohydrate and fat assimilation and include key points regarding the assimilation of vitamin B_{12}. We will then focus on clinical strategies to approach a patient suspected of having a malabsorption syndrome. The essential aspects of protein assimilation will also be discussed, however protein malabsorption *per se* will not be addressed. Many of the specific disease processes that lead to malabsorption (e.g., celiac sprue, bacterial overgrowth, exocrine pancreatic insufficiency) are discussed more completely in their respective chapters. Bile acid malabsorption will be discussed in detail in Chapter 47 and protein-losing enteropathies will be discussed in Chapter 48.

PHYSIOLOGY OF ASSIMILATION: THE ESSENTIALS

Absorption sites

- Absorption of macro- and micronutrients occurs along a 10-foot length of small intestine (duodenum, jejunum, ileum).
- Carbohydrates, proteins, and lipids are absorbed in the duodenum-jejunum, a process completed at a point 100 cm distal to the ligament of Treitz.
- Calcium, iron, zinc, folic acid, and the fat-soluble vitamins A, D, E, and K are absorbed in the proximal intestine.
- The ileum can assume the absorptive function of macronutrients if the proximal intestinal structure or function is impaired.
- Vitamin B_{12} and bile salts are absorbed in the ileum; the duodenum-jejunum cannot assume this process.

Carbohydrates

Digestion

- Carbohydrates are ingested as polysaccharides (starch), disaccharides (lactose, sucrose), and monosaccharides (glucose, fructose) but absorbed only as monosaccharides.
- Polysaccharides are digested primarily by salivary and pancreatic amylases to branched oligosaccharides, trisaccharides, and disaccharides.
- Brush border enzymes hydrolyze the products of amylase digestion to monosaccharides.

Absorption

- Glucose and galactose absorption occurs by secondary active transport via a sodium-dependent membrane-spanning transporter at the apical membrane of the enterocyte (SGLT1).
- Glucose enters the interstitial space by facilitated diffusion utilizing a basolateral transport protein (GLUT2).
- Fructose is absorbed by facilitated diffusion utilizing an apical transport protein (GLUT5) as well as the basolateral transporter GLUT2.
- Unabsorbed disaccharides are metabolized by colonic bacteria to short chain fatty acids that are absorbed by the colon (colonic salvage).

Proteins

- Sources of protein include ingested food, intestinal juices, and sloughed epithelial cells.
- The chief cells in the stomach produce pepsin, which plays a minor role in initiating digestion and yields amino acids and polypeptides.
- These products of hydrolysis stimulate release of cholecystokinin (CCK) from the duodenum and jejunum.
- CCK stimulates the pancreas to secrete both endopeptidases (trypsin, chymotrypsin, and elastase) and exopeptidases (carboxypeptidase A and B) as inactive precursors (e.g., trypsinogen).

- The brush border enzyme, enterokinase, activates trypsinogen to trypsin, which then autocatalyzes trypsinogen and all other peptidase precursors to their active forms.
- The active peptidases digest the polypeptides to amino acids (AAs) and 4–6 AA residue peptides.
- Brush border peptidases digest the oligopeptides to tri- and dipeptides, some of which are absorbed intact and further digested to AAs by intracellular peptidases.
- AAs are neutral, basic, acidic, and L-isomers, which are absorbed by active, passive, and facilitated diffusion mechanisms.

Lipids

I. Lipolytic stage

- Lipases (lingual, gastric, pancreatic) incompletely digest long-chain triglycerides (TGs) to fatty acids (FAs), monoglycerides (MGs), diglycerides (DGs), and glycerol.
- Lipolysis is enhanced by both bicarbonate (yielding an intestinal pH of 6.8) and the detergent properties of conjugated bile salts.
- Co-lipase facilitates binding of lipase to TG droplets, thus preventing the inhibition of lipase by bile salts.

II. Micellarization stage

- Micellarization is defined as the solubilization of a complex mixture of the products of lipolysis into a micelle.
- It requires conjugated bile salts (CBAs), reaching a critical micellar concentration of >2–3 mM.
- The resulting structure is a mixed micelle, consisting of CBAs, FAs, MGs, and some DGs, capable of solubilizing other fat-soluble substances and facilitating their absorption.
- The mixed micelle facilitates absorption of lipids through the epithelial cell plasma membrane (unstirred water layer).

III. Cellular stage

- Mixed micelles diffuse into the epithelial cell.
- Bile salts remain intraluminal, undergo absorption in the ileum via active transport sodium-dependent mechanisms, return to the liver via the enterohepatic (portal venous) circuit, and complete a recirculation cycle 4–6 times with each meal.
- FAs bind to cellular proteins, are transported to the smooth endoplasmic reticulum where they undergo activation by acetyl CoA, and are esterified with alpha-glycerophosphate or 2-MGs to TG and phospholipid.
- Chylomicrons (TGs, phospholipids, cholesterol esters, apoprotein) undergo synthesis in the Golgi apparatus.

IV. Delivery stage

- Apoprotein B synthesis is essential for the synthesis and transfer of synthesized chylomicrons into the lymphatics.
- Lymphatics are intraintestinal (lamina propria lacteals) and extraintestinal (cisterna chyli, thoracic duct).
- The process of transfer occurs via exocytosis.

Medium chain triglycerides (MCTs)

- MCTs are comprised of FAs of 6–10 carbons in length.
- TGs are hydrolyzed readily by intraluminal pancreatic lipases, but MCTs do not require lipases for assimilation.
- They may be absorbed intact by a duodenojejunal epithelial cell.
- Intracellular MCT lipases can hydrolyze TGs to FAs.
- FAs do not undergo esterification; they are absorbed into the portal circulation bound to albumin.

Vitamin B_{12} (cobalamin)

- Vitamin B_{12} is cleaved from dietary sources by gastric hydrochloric acid secreted by the oxyntic (parietal) cell.
- At gastric pH <3, gastric intrinsic factor (IF) secreted by the oxyntic cell has a poor binding affinity for the vitamin.
- Salivary R-protein is bound to the free vitamin in the stomach and is cleaved from the vitamin by pancreatic trypsin in the small intestine.
- Vitamin B_{12} then undergoes binding to IF in the duodenum.
- The stable B_{12}–IF complex attaches to specific receptor sites on epithelial cells of the terminal ileum.
- Once inside the epithelial cell, the complex is split and the free vitamin is bound to transcobalamin II and circulated via the enterohepatic circulation.

DIFFERENTIAL DIAGNOSIS

The differential diagnosis of malabsorption syndromes is impressive. Broadly, the categories may be recalled with the simple mnemonic 'LIMPS' (luminal disorders, infectious diseases, mucosal disorders, postoperative malabsorption, systemic disorders) (see box).

APPROACHING THE PATIENT WITH SUSPECTED MALABSORPTION

The evaluation of a patient with possible malabsorption proceeds through three logical phases:

1. suspicion of malabsorption (based on signs, symptoms, and laboratory abnormalities);
2. confirmation of the presence of malabsorption; and
3. defining the etiology of the malabsorption.

The following section will focus on a rational approach to a patient whose presentation makes the clinician suspect malabsorption. A thorough 'bedside' evaluation and a limited number of laboratory tests should provide sufficient data to proceed from suspicion to confirmation.

Suspecting malabsorption

'Bedside' evaluation

The clinical manifestations of malabsorption range from covert, mild, subtle symptoms, to overt evidence of severe end-organ damage, depending upon the etiology and stage at presentation. Clinical manifestations may result from:

- the malabsorption itself (e.g., diarrhea);
- the consequences of the substance being malabsorbed (e.g., iron-deficiency anemia with sprue); and
- the underlying etiology (e.g., abdominal pain with chronic pancreatitis).

There is a plethora of signs and symptoms that should alert the clinician to the possibility of malabsorption, and it important to recognize and appreciate the possible significance of these features (Table 43.1). Many of the symptoms are non-specific but provide the clinician with the initial indicators that a malabsorption syndrome may be present.

CAUSES OF MALABSORPTION ('LIMPS')
LUMINAL DISORDERS
• Exocrine pancreatic insufficiency
• Bile acid deficiency
• Zollinger-Ellison syndrome
• Small bowel bacterial overgrowth
INFECTIOUS DISEASES
• Tropical sprue
• Whipple disease
• Parasitic diseases
• Protozoa (giardiasis)
• Tapeworms
• *Mycobacterium avium-intracellulare*
MUCOSAL DISORDERS
• Celiac sprue
• Collagenous sprue
• Lactase insufficiency
• Crohn's disease
• Lymphoma
• Eosinophilic gastroenteritis
• Systemic mastocytosis
• Immunoproliferative small intestinal disease
• Lymphangiectasia
• Radiation enteritis
• Mesenteric vascular disease
• Abetalipoproteinemia
POSTOPERATIVE MALABSORPTION
• After gastric surgery
• After intestinal resection
• After bariatric surgery
SYSTEMIC DISORDERS
• Endocrine disorders
• Diabetic enteropathy
• Hypothyroidism
• Hyperthyroidism
• Addison's disease
• Collagen vascular diseases
• Scleroderma
• Vasculitis
• Amyloidosis
• AIDS enteropathy

Reproduced from Farrell JJ. Overview and diagnosis of malabsorption syndrome. Semin Gastrointest Dis 2002; 13:182–190 with permission of W.B. Saunders.

TABLE 43.1 CLINICAL CLUES TO THE RECOGNITION OF MALABSORPTION

Signs and symptoms	Laboratory abnormalities
GASTROINTESTINAL	**HEMATOLOGIC**
Diarrhea	Microcytic anemia (iron deficiency)
Steatorrhea	Macrocytic anemia (folate, vitamin B_{12} deficiency)
Flatulence	Lymphocytopenia
Bloating, distention	Eosinophilia
Abdominal pain	Hypoprothrombinemia
Glossitis	
Cheilosis	
Stomatitis	**BIOCHEMICAL**
Ascites	Hypokalemia
MUSCULOSKELETAL	Hypocalcemia
Fractures	Hypomagnesemia
Bone pain	Hypophosphatemia
Muscle weakness	Hypoalbuminemia
Tetany	Hypocholesterolemia
Clubbing	Hypotriglyceridemia
NEUROLOGIC	Elevated alkaline phosphatase
Paresthesias	
Peripheral neuropathy	
Night blindness	
Dementia	
DERMATOLOGIC	
Edema	
Acrodermatitis	
Hyperpigmented dermatitis	
Follicular dermatitis	
Koilonychia	
HEMATOLOGIC	
Ecchymoses	
Easy bleeding	
ENDOCRINOLOGIC	
Amenorrhea	
Infertility	
Decreased libido	
CONSTITUTIONAL	
Weakness	
Fatigue	
Weight loss	
Cachexia	

Chronic diarrhea is the most common symptom of malabsorption. However, most diarrheal disorders are not the result of a malabsorption syndrome (see Chapter 10). When diarrhea is the presenting complaint, additional information should be sought to confirm that malabsorption exists. If steatorrhea is present, a patient may complain of visible oil in the toilet water; large, pale stools that float on the surface, or excessively foul-smelling stools. However, most floating stools do so because of gas, not fat, content. Isolated carbohydrate malabsorption may result in increased gas production, which leads to flatulence, bloating, and/or abdominal distention.

Malabsorption syndromes resulting from diffuse intestinal malabsorption may lead to vitamin and other micronutrient deficiencies. The majority of the clinical consequences are manifested in extraintestinal organ systems. Consequently, the patient may not readily provide clinical clues without specific attention to the abnormality. Syndromes of fat malabsorption may result in deficiencies of the fat-soluble vitamins A, D, E, and K. Musculoskeletal symptoms such as tetany, muscle weakness, bone pain, and osteomalacia occur as a consequence of vitamin D deficiency and hypocalcemia. Ecchymoses and easy bleeding can result from the coagulopathy associated with vitamin K deficiency. Vitamin A deficiency may lead to night blindness. Vitamin E deficiency, although rarely symptomatic, can lead to neuropathy and retinopathy. Diffuse intestinal malabsorption can also present with deficiencies of water-soluble vitamins and micronutrients. Cheilosis, glossitis, and stomatitis can result from deficiency of vitamin B complex, vitamin B_{12}, and iron. Iron deficiency also causes microcytic anemia and koilonychia (spoon-shaped nails). Both vitamin B_{12} and folate deficiency can result in macrocytic anemia, whilst vitamin B_{12} (but not folate) deficiency can be associated with neurologic manifestations such as peripheral neuropathy. Dermatologic manifestations can result from micronutrient deficiency, such as perioral acrodermatitis (zinc) or hyperpigmented dermatitis (niacin). Amenorrhea may complicate chronic illness, weight loss, and hypoproteinemia, all of which may be associated with malabsorption. Weight loss (see Chapter 15) in adults and growth retardation in children are additional symptoms and signs that may indicate a malabsorption syndrome (Table 43.1).

When evaluating a patient who presents with unusual, inexplicable, or disparate signs or symptoms, a thorough focused history and physical examination should be performed to elicit additional information that could explain the consequences (clinical observations) and shed further light on the possible etiology of malabsorption. Particularly important points that should be considered routinely, as they may heighten the suspicion for malabsorption, are detailed in Table 43.2. Based on the initial assessment, the clinician should decide if lipid malabsorption (i.e., steatorrhea) is likely, as this judgment will help focus the remainder of the evaluation.

Laboratory evaluation

Although no laboratory finding is specific for malabsorption, routine blood tests can help to amplify the suspicion by identifying metabolic or hematologic consequences of malabsorption. First-line laboratory studies should include a complete blood count and differential, a complete chemistry profile, coagulation studies, and a lipid profile: low cholesterol suggests malabsorption and low serum triglycerides suggests absence of B lipoproteins. Some additional specific (e.g., thyroid-stimulating hormone) and nonspecific (e.g., erythrocyte sedimentation rate (ESR) or C-reactive protein) tests can also be considered in the first-line evaluation as screening tests. However, most specialized laboratory tests should only be ordered if there is a strong likelihood of the disorder in question (e.g., gastrin in Zollinger-Ellison syndrome (see Chapter 39); cortisol levels in suspected Addison's disease, etc.) (Table 43.3).

TABLE 43.2 QUESTIONS AND ANSWERS: IDENTIFYING POTENTIAL ETIOLOGY

Question	Potential etiology
HISTORY OF PRESENT ILLNESS	
Do certain types of food products tend to provoke symptoms:	
Dairy products?	Lactase deficiency
Dietetic candies?	Fructose intolerance
Is abdominal (or back) pain a strong component in the presentation?	Chronic pancreatitis, pancreatic neoplasm, mesenteric vascular disease
Has there been a change in color of urine or stool?	Pancreatic neoplasm, cholestasis
PAST MEDICAL HISTORY	
Is there a previous diagnosis of a malabsorptive disorder?	Crohn's disease, celiac sprue, etc.
Is there a history of:	
Prior gastrointestinal surgery (resection, bypass)?	SBBO, rapid transit, short bowel
Liver disease?	Cirrhosis
Pancreatitis?	Exocrine pancreatic insufficiency
Immune deficiency or suppression?	Infections, AIDS enteropathy, giardiasis
Atherosclerosis or hypercoagulable state?	Mesenteric vascular disease
Diabetes?	Exocrine pancreatic insufficiency, diabetic enteropathy, SBBO
Radiation therapy?	Strictures, fistulae, SBBO
Is there a previous diagnosis that may represent a complication of a malabsorptive disorder, such as:	
Peptic ulcer disease, erosive esophagitis?	Zollinger-Ellison syndrome
Nephrolithiasis?	Crohn's disease
Arthritis?	Whipple's disease
Cardiomyopathy?	Amyloidosis
Is the patient ingesting a medication known to be associated with malabsorption?	Orlistat, acarbose, laxatives
SOCIAL HISTORY	
Is there a history of heavy alcohol use?	Cirrhosis, exocrine pancreatic insufficiency
FAMILY HISTORY	
Is there a family history of a diarrheal disorder?	Crohn's disease, lactase deficiency, celiac sprue

SBBO, small bowel bacterial overgrowth.

Confirming malabsorption

Fat

The initial step in evaluating a patient with suspected lipid malabsorption is confirming the presence of steatorrhea, defined as the excretion of at least 7 g of fat in a 24-h stool collection.[2] A simple screening test is the qualitative Sudan III stain. The test has limited value in patients with mild degrees of steatorrhea, i.e., 7–10 g/24 h. When the patient is ingesting an adequate amount of fat (75–100 g/24 h), the test is expected to be positive in approximately 80–90% of patients with true steatorrhea. False positive tests may occur in patients who ingest mineral oil, excessive nut oils, or use of suppositories containing oils. Therefore, if a strong suspicion for steatorrhea remains, further quantitative evaluation should be performed.

Quantitative fecal fat analysis is the gold standard by which steatorrhea is confirmed.[1] Stool is collected over a 48- to 72-h period while the patient is ingesting 75–100 g of fat per day. Normal values are considered to be less than 7 g of fat per day; however, this normal value may increase by two-fold in the presence of large stool weights of any cause. Unfortunately this test is laborious and does not generally help differentiate between etiologies of the steatorrheal syndrome.

Carbohydrates

The most helpful screening test for isolated disaccharide malabsorption may simply be a well-documented history of dietary intolerance to the implicated disaccharide (i.e., lactose, sucrose).

Stool examination for pH and osmotic gap are indirect tests that may indicate the presence of carbohydrate malabsorption. An acidic fecal pH (under 5.5) results from bacterial fermentation of malabsorbed carbohydrate. Although the sensitivity of the test is questionable at best, the specificity for carbohydrate malabsorption increases as the pH declines.[3] Stool osmotic gap is measured in the fecal supernatant and is calculated as follows based on the assumption that normal stool osmolality is close to that of serum:

$$290\ \text{mosmol/L} - 2\,([Na^+]_{stool} + [K^+]_{stool})$$

An osmotic gap greater than 50-100 mosmol suggests the presence of an unmeasured solute, such as a malabsorbed carbohydrate. It is not however specific for carbohydrate malabsorption since the ingestion of a poorly absorbed ion (e.g., magnesium, sulfate) or compound (e.g., sorbitol, lactulose), whether intentional or unintentional, also yields an elevated stool osmotic gap. Carbohydrate fermentation within the stool collection container may exaggerate the osmotic gap (see Chapter 9).[1]

Hydrogen breath tests (see Chapters 9 and 131) can also demonstrate carbohydrate malabsorption. In patients with carbohydrate malabsorption, an orally administered disaccharide such as lactose remains undigested and passes into the colon, where it is fermented by the colonic bacteria, thus yielding a rise in breath hydrogen at 2–3 h by 20 p.p.m. from baseline.[1,4] In the case of small bowel bacterial overgrowth, lactose can be used but glucose is more specific. With both, the peak will occur within 1 h and will be more prominent than the colonic peak (with lactose). Breath tests may be falsely negative in the approximately 15% of patients who produce methane instead of hydrogen.[4]

D-xylose testing (see Chapter 46)

D-xylose is a pentose sugar that is incompletely absorbed by the small intestine.[5] After ingesting a 25-g dose of D-xylose, the 1- or 2-h serum value should be at least 25 mg/dL, and an adequate 5-h urine collection should yield at least 4 g of the compound. Failure to achieve these levels suggests malabsorption as a result of proximal small bowel disease. False-positive (low values) test results can occur with renal impairment, delayed gastric emptying, small intestinal bacterial overgrowth, surgically induced rapid transit, ascites (from third-spacing), and prokinetic or antimotility drug use.[5]

Vitamin B_{12} (cobalamin)

Cobalamin deficiency is assessed initially by measurement of serum vitamin B_{12}. When this serum test is borderline or equivocal, an elevated serum methylmalonic acid confirms cobalamin deficiency.[6] These tests do not differentiate between malabsorption of the vitamin and inadequate intake. The Schilling test provides both a confirmation of vitamin B_{12} malabsorption as well as a differential assessment of the etiology of the malabsorption. In part I of the Schilling test, 1 µg of radiolabeled vitamin B_{12} is administered orally, and its excretion is measured in a 24-h urine collection. Nonradiolabeled vitamin B_{12} is administered by injection as well in order to saturate the internal hepatic binding sites. At least 7–10% of the administered dose should be recovered in the urine to be considered normal. When part I is abnormal, part II, which involves administration of vitamin B_{12} along with oral intrinsic factor, is performed. In the presence of normal renal function

TABLE 43.3 LABORATORY TESTS TO DEFINE ETIOLOGY

Test	Looking for
BLOOD	
Platelet count[a]	Inflammation, neoplasm
TSH[a]	Hypothyroidism, hyperthyroidism
ESR, C-reactive protein[a]	Crohn's disease, inflammation
Glucose[a]	Diabetic enteropathy, chronic pancreatitis
Liver enzymes, bilirubin[a]	Cirrhosis
Folate	SBBO (elevated folate)
HIV antibody, $CD4^+$ cell count	AIDS enteropathy
Antigliadin, antiendomysial, and tissue transglutaminase antibodies	Celiac disease
Antinuclear antibodies	Connective tissue disorders
Antimitochondrial antibody	Primary biliary cirrhosis
Intrinsic factor antibody	Pernicious anemia
Gastrin	Zollinger-Ellison syndrome
ACTH, cortisol	Addison's disease
Leukocyte differential[a]	
Lymphocytes	Lymphangiectasia (lymphopenia)
Eosinophils	Eosinophilic gastroenteritis (eosinophilia)
STOOL	
Ova and parasites	Parasitic disease
Giardia antigen	Giardiasis
Chymotrypsin, elastase	Chronic pancreatitis

[a]First line tests.
TSH, thyroid-stimulating hormone; ESR, erythrocyte sedimentation rate; HIV, human immunodeficiency virus; ACTH, adrenocorticotropic hormone; SBBO, small bowel bacterial overgrowth; AIDS, acquired immunodeficiency syndrome.

and an adequate urine collection, normal excretion in part II of the test indicates intact ileal absorption of B_{12} and a high likelihood that the patient has pernicious anemia. Persistent abnormalities during part II are the result of ileal dysfunction (e.g., Crohn's disease or terminal ileal resection), small bowel bacterial overgrowth, or exocrine pancreatic insufficiency. The latter two etiologies may be teased out by repeating the test after the administration of antibiotics or pancreatic enzymes, respectively.

Determining the etiology of malabsorption

If steatorrhea or other consequences of malabsorption (e.g., anemia, osteopenia, etc.) are confirmed, an etiology must be pursued. Isolated carbohydrate malabsorption rarely requires sophisticated testing. There is no single algorithm by which to approach each situation, and the sequence of testing is not hard and fast. Some of the tests that assess function (Schilling test, D-xylose test, lactose hydrogen breath test) both confirm malabsorption and help to pinpoint the etiology. A brief discussion of anatomic studies (radiologic, endoscopic, and histologic) and the D-xylose test is given below, followed by a suggested course of evaluation.

Radiologic examinations

A plain abdominal radiograph is frequently unrevealing, but may reveal the pathognomonic finding of pancreatic calcifications in chronic calcific pancreatitis. A small bowel series is a valuable tool in assessing both the anatomy of the small bowel as well as mucosal derangements. Although the negative predictive value of a small bowel series is low, an abnormal study is quite valuable and may guide further diagnostic testing (Table 43.4). The distal small bowel is difficult to assess by other means; thus, a small bowel series may be the only method of detecting lesions in this region. Enteroclysis (see Chapter 125), or small bowel enema, is another radiographic technique for assessing small bowel disease; however, its use is limited by the need for small bowel intubation with a nasoenteric tube. The ileum may also be visualized on barium enema examination performed to include reflux into the terminal ileum. Abdominal CT scanning (see Chapter 126) after the administration of oral contrast may detect intestinal wall thickening or abdominal lymphadenopathy, as could occur in disorders such as Crohn's disease or lymphoma. The gross and ductular anatomy of the pancreas can also be assessed if chronic pancreatitis is a consideration.

Endoscopic and histologic evaluation

Upper gastrointestinal endoscopy or enteroscopy with small bowel biopsy should be performed in most patients in whom a definitive etiology for malabsorption cannot be established by other means. Direct visual examination of the duodenal mucosa may reveal findings that have been missed on radiographic examination, such as aphthous ulcers in Crohn's disease or scalloping of the duodenal folds in celiac sprue. Since gross examination may be unremarkable in several diseases, four to six routine biopsies should be obtained from the region of the ampulla of Vater even with normal-appearing mucosa. It is important to recall that some diseases, such as eosinophilic gastroenteritis, are patchy in nature, so biopsies should be obtained from different portions of the intestine.[7,8] Although some histologic findings such as villous blunting are not highly specific for one particular disease entity, certain findings are sufficiently specific to be diagnostic (Table 43.5). Retrograde terminal ileal endoscopy during colonoscopy should be performed in cases of iron and vitamin B_{12} deficient anemias. Wireless capsule endoscopy (see Chapter 123) is a promising new technology that is increasingly being used to detect diseases with small bowel mucosal abnormalities, such as Crohn's disease, celiac disease, lymphangiectasia, amyloidosis, or small bowel neoplasms.

Problem-solving steatorrhea

There are a number of courses to take to arrive at an etiology for malabsorption. Most importantly, if a diagnosis is strongly

TABLE 43.4 RADIOGRAPHIC FINDINGS ON SMALL BOWEL SERIES

Finding	Interpretation
Decreased small bowel length	Short bowel syndrome
Small bowel diverticula	SBBO
Fistula	Crohn's disease, radiation enteropathy
Hypomotility	SBBO, diabetic enteropathy, scleroderma, amyloid
Dilatation	Celiac sprue, scleroderma, amyloid
Stricture	Crohn's disease, radiation enteropathy
Tumor (with or without ulcers)	Lymphoma
Ulcers	Crohn's disease, NSAID enteropathy
Jejunization of ileum, barium flocculation	Celiac sprue
Thickened folds	Eosinophilic gastroenteritis, giardiasis, Whipple's disease

SBBO, small bowel bacterial overgrowth; NSAID, nonsteroidal anti-inflammatory drug.

TABLE 43.5 DIAGNOSTIC SMALL BOWEL HISTOLOGY

Disease	Pathognomonic histologic findings
GENERALIZED HISTOLOGIC ABNORMALITIES	
Abetalipoproteinemia	Lipid accumulation, vacuolization of enterocytes
Collagenous sprue	Collagen band below atrophic mucosa
Mycobacterium avium-intracellulare	PAS-positive foamy macrophages with acid-fast bacilli
Whipple's disease	PAS-positive foamy macrophages (no acid-fast bacilli)
PATCHY HISTOLOGIC ABNORMALITIES	
Amyloidosis	Congo red-positive deposits
Crohn's disease	Noncaseating granulomas
Eosinophilic gastroenteritis	Eosinophilic infiltration
Lymphangiectasia	Ectatic lymph vessels
Lymphoma	Clonal expansion of lymphocytes
Mastocytosis	Mast cell infiltration
Parasites	Parasites seen

PAS, periodic acid-Schiff.
Reproduced from Högenauer C, Hammer HF. Maldigestion and malabsorption. In: Feldman M, Friedman LS, Sleisinger MH, eds. Sleisinger & Fordtran's gastrointestinal and liver disease, 7th edn. Philadelphia: Saunders; 2002: 1751–1782.

TABLE 43.6 LIPID ASSIMILATION STAGES: KEY FACTORS, DISORDERS, AND PATHOPHYSIOLOGY

Stage	Main organ system(s)	Key factor(s)	Representative disorders	Pathophysiology
I. Lipolytic	Pancreas	Lipase	Chronic pancreatitis Pancreatic cancer ZES Gastric surgery	Impaired lipase production Impaired lipase delivery Inhibition of lipase activity Impaired mixing of fat and lipase (pancreaticocibal asynchrony)
II. Micellarization	Liver and biliary tract	Conjugated bile salts	Chronic liver disease Biliary obstruction SBBO	Impaired bile salt synthesis Impaired bile salt delivery Deconjugation of bile salts
	Terminal ileum	Enterohepatic circulation	Crohn's disease, ileal resection, bypass	Impaired enterohepatic circulation → reduced bile salt pool
III. Cellular	Duodenum and jejunum	Enterocyte (absorbing epithelial cell)	Celiac sprue	Enterocyte inflammation +/– atrophy
			Giardiasis	Physical interference with absorbing unit
			Mesenteric vascular insufficiency	Enterocyte atrophy
		Apolipoprotein B (ApoB); chylomicron	Abetalipoproteinemia	Defective or absent ApoB → impaired chylomicron synthesis
IV. Delivery	Lymphatic circulation	Lymphatic lacteals	Whipple's disease Lymphangiectasia	Lacteal obstruction Ectatic lymphatic channels
		Cisterna chyli	Retroperitoneal fibrosis	Extraintestinal lymphatic obstruction

ZES, Zollinger-Ellison syndrome; SBBO, small bowel bacterial overgrowth.

TABLE 43.7 DEFINING AN ETIOLOGY

Suspected etiology	Confirmatory findings
Chronic pancreatitis	Pancreatic calcifications; pancreatic ductal abnormalities on CT; carbohydrate intolerance, fecal enzyme assays; improvement with enzyme replacement
Celiac sprue	Family history; presence of antigliadin, antiendomysial, and tissue transglutaminase antibodies; abnormal small bowel biopsy; improvement with gluten restriction
Bacterial overgrowth	Gastro- or enteroparesis; jejunal diverticula; enterocolonic fistulae; small bowel obstruction; chronic acid suppression; impaired B_{12} absorption; raised serum folate levels; improvement with antibiotic treatment
Crohn's disease	Prior ileal resection; extensive proximal small bowel disease; fistulae → bacterial overgrowth
Giardiasis	Presence of parasite on small bowel biopsy, string test, or duodenal aspirate; identification of parasite or antigen in stool
Chronic liver disease	Evidence of liver disease on CT, US, or hepatic biopsy
Lactase deficiency [a]	Acid pH on fresh stool; osmotic gap in stool supernatant; predisposing condition; improvement with lactose-free diet
Bile acid (cholerrheic) diarrhea [a]	Prior ileal resection or known ileal disease (<60–90 cm resected or diseased); improvement with bile acid sequestrant treatment (cholestyramine)
Surreptitious laxative use [a]	Fecal supernatant osmotic gap

[a] Nonsteatorrheal malabsorptive syndromes.

considered, the appropriate specific diagnostic studies should be pursued prior to embarking on a potentially costly and exhaustive evaluation.

Once steatorrhea has been confirmed, defining its etiology requires only that the challenged clinician consider which of one or several stages of lipid assimilation has been compromised. Recalling which organ system (and its key factor) facilitates a particular stage sharpens the focus. A limited number of disorders may be the culprits that impair the function of a particular stage (Table 43.6). A focused inquiry into the patient's history will lead the astute clinician to consider possible etiologies. A careful review and interpretation of routine laboratory tests, selected specialized blood studies, and stool examinations, as well as radiologic, endoscopic, and histologic studies will usually enable the identification of a specific etiology. A synthesis of findings that may be helpful in defining an etiology is presented in Table 43.7.

If the diagnosis still remains elusive, two of the previously discussed tests, the D-xylose and Schilling tests, can help determine the location of the pathophysiology. The decision about which to perform first depends on the previous evaluation. If vitamin B_{12} deficiency is present, or if there is a concern for bacterial overgrowth or ileal dysfunction, a Schilling test should be performed first. If the diagnosis still is uncertain, the D-xylose test can then be used to document or disprove the small intestine as the site of malabsorption. If proximal intestinal cellular disease is suspected, endoscopy with a small bowel biopsy is justified. Should all of these tests be normal, then further evaluation of the liver and biliary tract is warranted (Table 43.8).

SOURCES OF INFORMATION FOR PATIENTS AND DOCTORS

http://www.healthinsite.gov.au/topics/Malabsorption_Syndromes
Hypolactasia:
http://www.gastro.org/generalPublic.html

TABLE 43.8 APPLICATION AND INTERPRETATION OF STEATORRHEA TESTS

	DIAGNOSTIC TESTS AND EXPECTED FINDINGS		
STAGE OF LIPID ASSIMILATION	*D-xylose absorption*	*Schilling (B_{12} absorption)*	*Small bowel biopsy (proximal)*
I. Lipolytic	Normal	Normal [a]	Normal
II. Micellarization	Normal (or abnormal with SBBO)	Normal or abnormal [b]	Normal [c]
III. Cellular	Abnormal	Normal	Abnormal
IV. Delivery	Normal	Normal	Abnormal lymphatics

[a] May be abnormal if exocrine pancreatic insufficiency exists and will normalize with pancreatic enzyme supplementation.
[b] Normal with liver or biliary disease; abnormal with ileal dysfunction or small bowel bacterial overgrowth (SBBO), which may normalize with antibiotics.
[c] Minimal inflammatory changes may be seen in some cases of SBBO.

REFERENCES

1. Farrell JJ. Overview and diagnosis of malabsorption syndrome. Semin Gastrointest Dis 2002; 13:182–190.
2. Högenauer C, Hammer HF. Maldigestion and malabsorption. In: Feldman M, Friedman LS, Sleisinger MH, eds. Sleisinger & Fordtran's gastrointestinal and liver disease, 7th edn. Philadelphia: Saunders; 2002:1751–1782.
3. Eherer AJ, Fordtran JS. Fecal osmotic gap and pH in experimental diarrhea of various causes. Gastroenterology 1992; 103:545–551.
4. Romagnuolo J, Schiller D, Bailey RJ. Using breath tests wisely in a gastroenterology practice: an evidence-based review of indications and pitfalls in interpretation. Am J Gastroenterol 2002; 97:1113–1126.
5. Craig RM, Ehrenpreis ED. D-xylose testing. J Clin Gastroenterol 1999; 29:143–150.
6. Elin RJ, Winter WE. Methylmalonic acid: a test whose time has come? Arch Pathol Lab Med 2001; 125:824–827.
7. Talley NJ, Shorter RG, Phillips SF et al. Eosinophilic gastroenteritis: a clinicopathological study of patients with disease of the mucosae, muscle layer, and subserosal tissues. Gut 1990; 31:54–58.
8. Talley NJ. Eosinophilic gastroenteritis. In: Feldman M, Friedman LS, Sleisinger MH, eds. Sleisinger & Fordtran's gastrointestinal and liver disease, 7th edn. Philadelphia: Saunders; 2002:1972–1982.

Chapter 44

Celiac disease

Andrés Cárdenas, Sonal Patel, and Ciarán P Kelly

KEY POINTS

- Celiac disease is a genetically determined small intestinal inflammation provoked by dietary gluten
- There is inappropriate T cell activation in HLA-DQ2- or DQ8-positive individuals
- Tissue transglutamase enzyme is one of the targets of the autoimmune response
- Extraintestinal conditions (neurological, osteopenia) and associated conditions (e.g., type 1 diabetes) are common
- The ileum may be involved in severe disease
- 20% of patients are over 60 years old when they present
- Positive serological tests should be confirmed by D2 and D3 biopsy
- IgA TTG levels reduce by 50% within 2 months of starting dietary treatment and are helpful in monitoring compliance
- Once in remission up to 70 g per day of noncontaminated oats can usually be tolerated
- In refractory cases, review compliance, look for ulcerative jejunoileitis and lymphoma, and consider immunosuppressive treatment

INTRODUCTION

Celiac disease is characterized by malabsorption resulting from inflammatory injury to the small intestinal mucosa following gluten ingestion. In celiac disease, there is clinical and histological improvement when a strict gluten-free diet is followed, and relapse when dietary gluten is reintroduced.[1] Celiac disease is a common disorder affecting 0.3–1% of the population in the Western world, causing considerable morbidity and increased mortality, including that from lymphoma.[2–6] The pathogenesis of celiac disease is related to inappropriate intestinal T cell activation in HLA-DQ2- or DQ8-positive individuals triggered by antigenic cereal peptides from wheat, barley, or rye. There is a wide variety of presentations ranging from asymptomatic enteropathy to severe chronic diarrhea, weight loss, iron deficiency anemia, and nutritional deficiencies. Extraintestinal manifestations of celiac disease such as osteopenia or neurological disorders and associated conditions such as type I diabetes mellitus or hypothyroidism are commonly present. Although newer highly sensitive and specific serologic tests are available for the diagnosis of celiac disease, the demonstration of characteristic histological abnormalities in a biopsy of the small intestine remains the diagnostic gold standard. Treatment consists of lifelong avoidance of dietary gluten to control symptoms and to prevent complications.

EPIDEMIOLOGY AND THE SPECTRUM OF DISEASE

The true prevalence of celiac disease is not well documented because many patients are asymptomatic or have atypical symptoms. A multicenter Italian study identified seven new cases of childhood celiac disease for each known celiac patient, leading to the term the 'celiac iceberg.'[4] Based on a recent Finnish study, the estimated prevalence of celiac disease among school children is at least 1 in 99. This estimate includes asymptomatic cases, which were diagnosed based on serology and histology.[6] There is a high prevalence of celiac disease in people of Northwestern Europe and countries where these people emigrated to, such as North America and Australia where it is estimated to occur in 1:113 to 300 persons.[3–6] Other areas where the incidence is lower include parts of Northwest India, South America, North Africa, and Asia.[7] Most series report a slight female preponderance. The mortality rate in patients not adhering to a strict gluten-free diet exceeds that of the general population mainly due to an increased risk for malignancy.[8] However, treated patients adhering to a strict gluten-free diet have no significant difference in mortality rates when compared to the general population.[9]

Celiac disease classically presents with symptoms of severe chronic diarrhea, nutritional deficiencies, and anemia. Although cases of classical celiac disease still occur, the majority of patients now present with atypical and subtler manifestations such as iron deficiency anemia, short stature, dermatitis herpetiformis, or infertility. Cases of silent celiac disease in which the disease is identified by a serological test in an asymptomatic individual are increasingly common. Refractory celiac disease, defined as symptomatic severe small intestinal villous atrophy mimicking celiac disease but not responding to at least 6 months of a strict gluten-free diet, is a life-threatening complication. This rare condition should only be diagnosed after carefully excluding concealed or inadvertent gluten ingestion, other causes of villous atrophy, and overt intestinal lymphoma.

PATHOGENESIS

The interaction of the water-insoluble protein moiety of wheat gluten, or similar prolamins from the cereal grains barley and rye, with the mucosa of the small intestine in susceptible individuals is critical to the pathogenesis of celiac disease.[10] Although the exact molecular mechanisms by which gluten damages the intestinal mucosa it not completely understood, celiac disease is considered a disease in which there is an inappropriate T cell-mediated immune response that is triggered by an identified environmental agent (gliadin) in genetically predisposed individuals. There is a high concordance in monozygotic twins, and an approximately 10% prevalence among first-degree relatives.[1,2,5,7,10] Celiac disease is associated with specific human leukocyte (HLA) class II DQ haplotypes.[10] HLA class II molecules are glycosylated transmembrane heterodimers (α- and β-chains) organized in three related subregions: DQ, DR, and DP and encoded within the HLA class II region of the major histocompatibility complex on chromosome 6p. The HLA-DQ(α1*501,β1*02) heterodimer, known as HLA-DQ2 is present in over 95% of patients. The related DQ(α1*0301,β1*0302) heterodimer, known as HLA-DQ8 is found in almost all of the remainder. However, celiac disease develops in only a small fraction of the 20–30% of the population that express HLA-DQ2 or HLA-DQ-8.[11] Thus, the presence of the HLA-DQ2 or HLA DQ8 molecules are necessary but not sufficient for disease expression to occur.[12]

Following gluten ingestion the partially digested gliadin peptides are taken up by lamina propria antigen presenting cells. The cereal-derived peptides are then presented on the α/β heterodimer antigen binding grooves of cell surface HLA-DQ2 or DQ8 to sensitized T lymphocytes expressing the α/β T cell receptor (Fig. 44.1).[10,11] The T lymphocytes then activate B lymphocytes to produce immunoglobulins and other T lymphocytes to secrete cytokines such as IFN-γ, IL-4, IL-5, IL-6, IL-10, TNFα, and TGFβ. These cytokines cause damage to

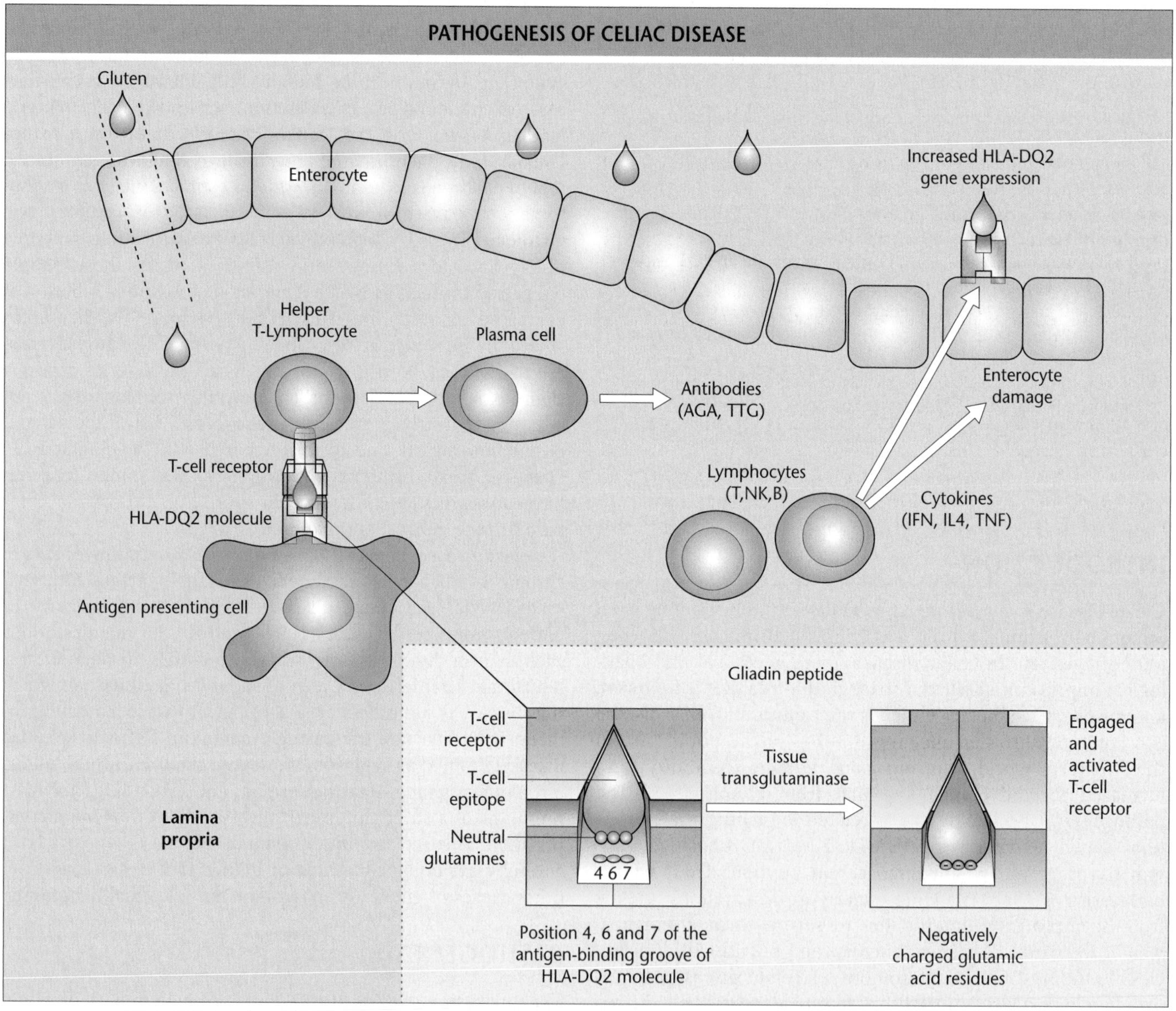

Fig. 44.1 Pathogenesis of celiac disease. Gluten is absorbed and presented in conjunction with HLA-DQ2 or DQ8 cell-surface antigens by antigen-presenting cells. Tissue transglutaminase (TTG) deamidates gliadin peptides, generating negatively charged residues of glutamic acid from neutral glutamines (inset). Because negatively charged residues are preferred in positions 4, 6, and 7 of the antigen-binding groove of HLA-DQ2, deamidated gliadin produces a stronger T cell response. These lymphocytes then activate other lymphocytes to generate cytokines, such as interferon-, interleukin-4, and tumor necrosis factor (TNF), which lead to villous damage and enteritis. Induction of aberrant HLA class II cell-surface antigens on the enterocytes may permit these cells to present additional antigens to the sensitized lymphocytes. Adapted with permission from Farrell R, Kelly C. Current concepts: celiac sprue. New Engl J Med 2002; 346:180-188. Copyright © 2002 Massachusetts Medical Society. All Rights Reserved.

enterocytes, and induce aberrant cell-surface expression of HLA class II molecules on the luminal surface of enterocytes. This event may enable additional, more direct, antigen presentation by epithelial cells to sensitized T lymphocytes. The enzyme tissue transglutaminase is one of the targets of the autoimmune response in celiac disease, and some theories suggest that peptides are incompletely digested because reduced transglutaminase activity plays a central role in initiation of the immune response. The detection of IgA antibodies directed towards tissue transglutaminase (IgA TTG) is a valuable serological marker for the diagnosis of untreated celiac disease.[1,2,5–7,10,12]

HISTOLOGY

Celiac disease primarily affects the mucosa of the small intestine. The mucosal abnormalities are most evident proximally and decrease in severity with distal progression, but in severe disease even the ileum may be involved. The mucosal surface of biopsy specimens from untreated patients with severe lesions reveals a flat mucosa with absence of normal intestinal villi. Histological features include loss of the normal villous structure with a variable reduction in the villous height, i.e., partial or subtotal villous atrophy (Fig. 44.2).[13] The intestinal crypts are hyperplastic, markedly elongated, and open onto a flattened absorptive surface. The total thickness of the mucosa is only slightly reduced in most instances, because crypt hyperplasia compensates for the absence or shortening of the villi. These architectural changes together with the reduction in mature, fully differentiated villous enterocytes decrease both the epithelial surface available and its capacity for digestion and absorption. The cellularity of the lamina propria is increased consisting largely of plasma cells and lymphocytes. The number of IgA-, IgM-, and IgG-producing plasma cells is increased two- to six-fold; but as in normal mucosa, IgA-producing cells predominate. Polymorphonuclear leukocytes, eosinophils, and mast cells may also contribute substantially to the increased cellularity of the lamina propria. Although the number of intraepithelial lymphocytes (IEL) observed per 100 enterocytes is increased in untreated celiac disease, the total number of IEL may not be increased, because the absorptive surface area is markedly reduced.[13,14] In untreated celiac disease, as in the healthy small intestine, lamina propria T cells are predominantly CD4-positive (helper) while the IELs are mainly CD8-positive (suppressor) cells. The density of cells in both compartments returns to normal on a gluten-free diet.[15]

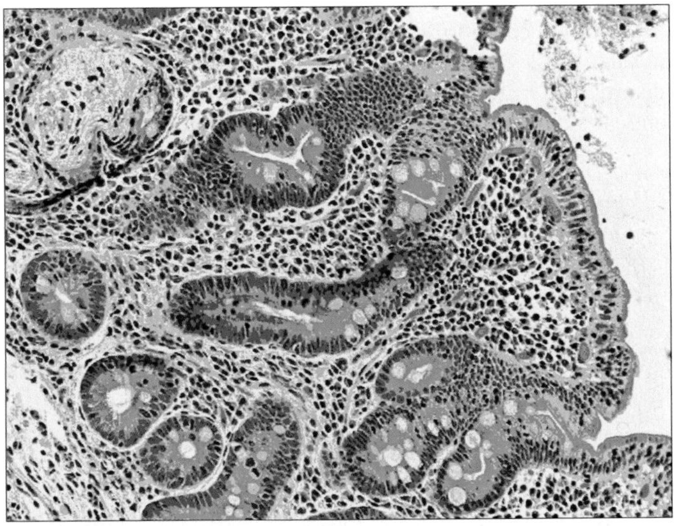

Fig. 44.2 Histological appearance of the duodenal mucosa. There is an increased number of intraepithelial lymphocytes and increased chronic inflammatory cells in the lamina propria. Note the architectural changes of focal epithelial injury and near complete absence of normal intestinal villi. The crypts are markedly elongated and open onto a flattened absorptive surface. (Courtesy of Maria L. Botero, MD, Beth Israel Deaconess Medical Center.)

CLINICAL PRESENTATION

Celiac disease can present with a wide spectrum of gastrointestinal and extraintestinal manifestations (Table 44.1). Hence, celiac disease is easily missed unless it is included in the differential diagnosis of a multitude of symptoms, signs, and laboratory abnormalities. In children, celiac disease usually presents between 4 and 24 months of age with symptoms such as failure to thrive, impaired growth, vomiting, diarrhea, abdominal distention, wasting, hypotonia, anorexia, and irritability. Infants may have difficulty gaining weight, have pubertal delay, and short stature. Other manifestations in childhood include constipation, recurrent abdominal pain, increased liver enzymes, recurrent or severe aphthous stomatitis, arthralgia, and dental

TABLE 44.1 CLINICAL PRESENTATION

Classical features	Other features
Chronic diarrhea	**General**
Iron deficiency anemia	Short stature
Abdominal pain	Delayed puberty
Irritability and depression	Clubbing
Abdominal distention	Edema
Failure to thrive	**Gastrointesinal**
Weight loss	Bloating
Malaise	Recurrent aphthous stomatitis
Anorexia	Steatorrhea
	Flatulence
	Vomiting
	Constipation
	Extraintestinal
	Folate deficiency
	Vitamin K and/or D deficiency
	Persistent hypertransaminasemia
	Thrombocytosis
	Osteomalacia, osteoporosis, fractures
	Dental enamel hypoplasia
	Arthralgia, arthropathy
	Peripheral neuropathy
	Ataxia
	Epilepsy (± cerebral calcification)
	Night blindness
	Female and male infertility
	Recurrent spontaneous abortions
	Poor academic performance
	Follicular keratosis, alopecia, easy bruising

Reproduced with permission from Farrell R, Kelly C. Diagnosis of celiac sprue. Am J Gastroenterol 2001; 96:3237–3246.

enamel defects. Children may also have significant behavioral problems, such as depression, irritability, and poor academic performance.

Some adult patients are of short stature or give a history of undiagnosed diarrhea and abdominal pain in childhood. Nonetheless, symptomatic celiac disease often develops *de novo* in adult life. Celiac disease can also be diagnosed in patients of advanced age; in fact, approximately 20% of cases present after the age of 60 years.[16] Gastrointestinal symptoms can include large-volume or nocturnal diarrhea, flatulence, and weight loss. In many cases, gluten-sensitive enteropathy results in symptomatic lactose intolerance. Steatorrhea is less common and often indicates severe and extensive enteropathy. Dyspepsia and bloating are common and may lead to an erroneous diagnosis of irritable bowel syndrome. The diagnosis of celiac disease in adults is often delayed especially if patients present with multiple, mild, and nonspecific symptoms consistent with irritable bowel syndrome.

Many patients initially present with atypical symptoms and as a result celiac disease is initially undiagnosed or misdiagnosed in over 50% of cases.[17] Adults with celiac disease are more likely to present with extraintestinal symptoms (Table 44.1). Iron deficiency anemia due to malabsorption is the most common clinical presentation for adult celiac disease. Other laboratory abnormalities include macrocytic anemia secondary to folate deficiency, elevated prothrombin time resulting from vitamin K deficiency, and/or vitamin D deficiency leading to hypocalcemia.[18] Osteopenic bone disease develops as a result of impaired calcium absorption due to defective calcium transport, impaired vitamin D absorption, and binding of intraluminal calcium to unabsorbed fatty acids. Patients may present with bone pain and fractures, paresthesias, muscle cramps, and even tetany. Osteoporosis is common in both adults and children with celiac disease.[18] Measurement of bone mineral density is recommended in patients with newly diagnosed celiac disease because osteopenia or osteoporosis are common and indicate a need for calcium and vitamin D supplementation in addition to treatment with a gluten-free diet.[12,18] Women may present with infertility or recurrent spontaneous abortions, and it is common for infertile women with celiac disease to become pregnant after commencing a gluten-free diet.

Ataxia is the most common severe neurological disorder associated with celiac disease and in some patients, progressive gait and limb ataxia may be the only indication of celiac disease.[19] Patients presenting with nonhereditary progressive ataxia are frequently found to have evidence of gluten sensitivity and the disorder is believed to result from immune-mediated spinocerebellar degeneration. Peripheral neuropathy, muscle weakness, and sensory loss may also develop in celiac disease. Although the association of epilepsy and celiac disease is well recognized, the underlying cause is again unknown.[20]

Malignant diseases occur more frequently in patients with untreated celiac disease. Representative and reliable data are difficult to obtain but one recent large study found that the relative risk for malignancy in celiac disease was 30% higher than in the general population.[21] Enteropathy-associated intestinal T cell lymphoma is the most commonly recognized fatal complication of celiac disease. Additional celiac disease-associated malignancies include other non-Hodgkin lymphomas, esophageal and oropharyngeal squamous carcinoma, and small bowel adenocarcinoma.

TABLE 44.2 ASSOCIATED DISEASES AND COMPLICATIONS

Associated conditions	Complications
Definite associations	Refractory sprue (5–10%)
Hyposplenism	Enteropathy-associated T cell lymphoma (2–10%)
Dermatitis herpetiformis	Carcinoma
IgA deficiency	(oropharyngeal, esophageal, small intestinal)
Autoimmune thyroid disease	Ulcerative jejunoileitis
Sjögren's syndrome	Collagenous sprue
Type 1 diabetes mellitus	
Microscopic colitis	
Rheumatoid arthritis	
Down's syndrome	
IgA mesangial nephropathy	
Other reported associations	
Inflammatory bowel disease	
Sarcoidosis	
Congenital heart disease	
Addison's disease	
Systemic lupus erythematosus	
Vasculitis	
Polymyositis	
Autoimmune hepatitis	
Primary biliary cirrhosis	
Recurrent pericarditis	
Cystic fibrosis	
Fibrosing alveolitis	
Lung cavities	
Pulmonary hemosiderosis	
Myasthenia gravis	
Schizophrenia	

Reproduced with permission from Farrell R, Kelly C. Diagnosis of celiac sprue. Am J Gastroenterol 2001; 96:3237-3246.

ASSOCIATED CONDITIONS

Many of the conditions associated with celiac disease are listed in Table 44.2. Dermatitis herpetiformis (DH) (Fig. 44.3), a skin disorder in which intensely pruritic papulovesicular lesions appear symmetrically over the extensor surfaces of the extrem-

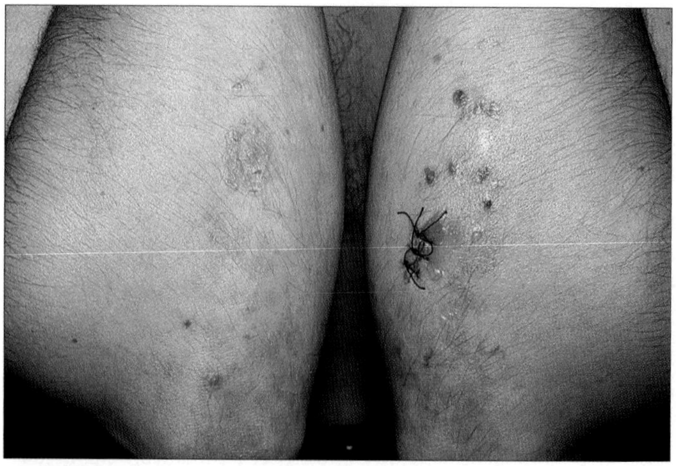

Fig. 44.3 Dermatitis herpetiformis, characterized by itchy vesicular lesions.

ities, buttocks, trunk, neck, and scalp, deserves special mention since it is invariably associated with gluten-sensitive enteropathy. The diagnosis of DH is confirmed by performing immunofluorescence, which shows granular IgA deposits in an area of normal skin unaffected by blistering.[22] Although the skin lesions and pruritus usually respond to drug therapy with dapsone, the treatment of choice for DH and the associated celiac disease is a lifelong, strict gluten-free diet.

The most common autoimmune disorders associated with celiac disease are insulin-dependent diabetes mellitus (IDDM) and autoimmune thyroiditis with hypothyroidism.[23,24] The reported prevalence of celiac disease in patients with IDDM is approximately 4% and vice versa. Chronic diarrhea, other gastrointestinal symptoms, nutritional deficiencies, or unexplained episodes of hypoglycemia should alert the practitioner to the possibility of celiac disease in patients with IDDM. The relationship between celiac disease and other organ-specific autoimmune disorders may simply reflect shared HLA-haplotype associations. However, it has also been suggested that untreated celiac disease may increase the risk for autoimmunity through chronic uncontrolled lamina propria T cell activation.[25]

DIFFERENTIAL DIAGNOSIS/DIAGNOSTIC METHODS

A diagnostic approach to celiac disease is described in Fig. 44.4. The availability of a highly sensitive and specific serological test, the IgA tissue transglutaminase assay, has greatly simplified the approach to making the diagnosis of celiac disease (see below). If the clinical suspicion of celiac disease is low (i.e., episodic mild diarrhea), a negative serological test has a high negative predictive value, which would preclude the need for small bowel biopsy. Because the specificity of the IgA TTG test is high (>95%) the positive predictive values are also high even in low-risk populations.[26] Nonetheless, a positive serological test for celiac disease should be confirmed by biopsy of the small intestine before starting treatment with a gluten-free diet for the remainder of the patient's lifetime. When the index of suspicion is high (e.g., chronic watery diarrhea, family history of celiac disease, iron deficiency anemia), both serology and a small bowel biopsy should be performed. The incidence of IgA deficiency is 16 times greater in patients with celiac disease compared to the general population. This occasionally results in a false-negative IgA TTG test. Thus, measurement of total

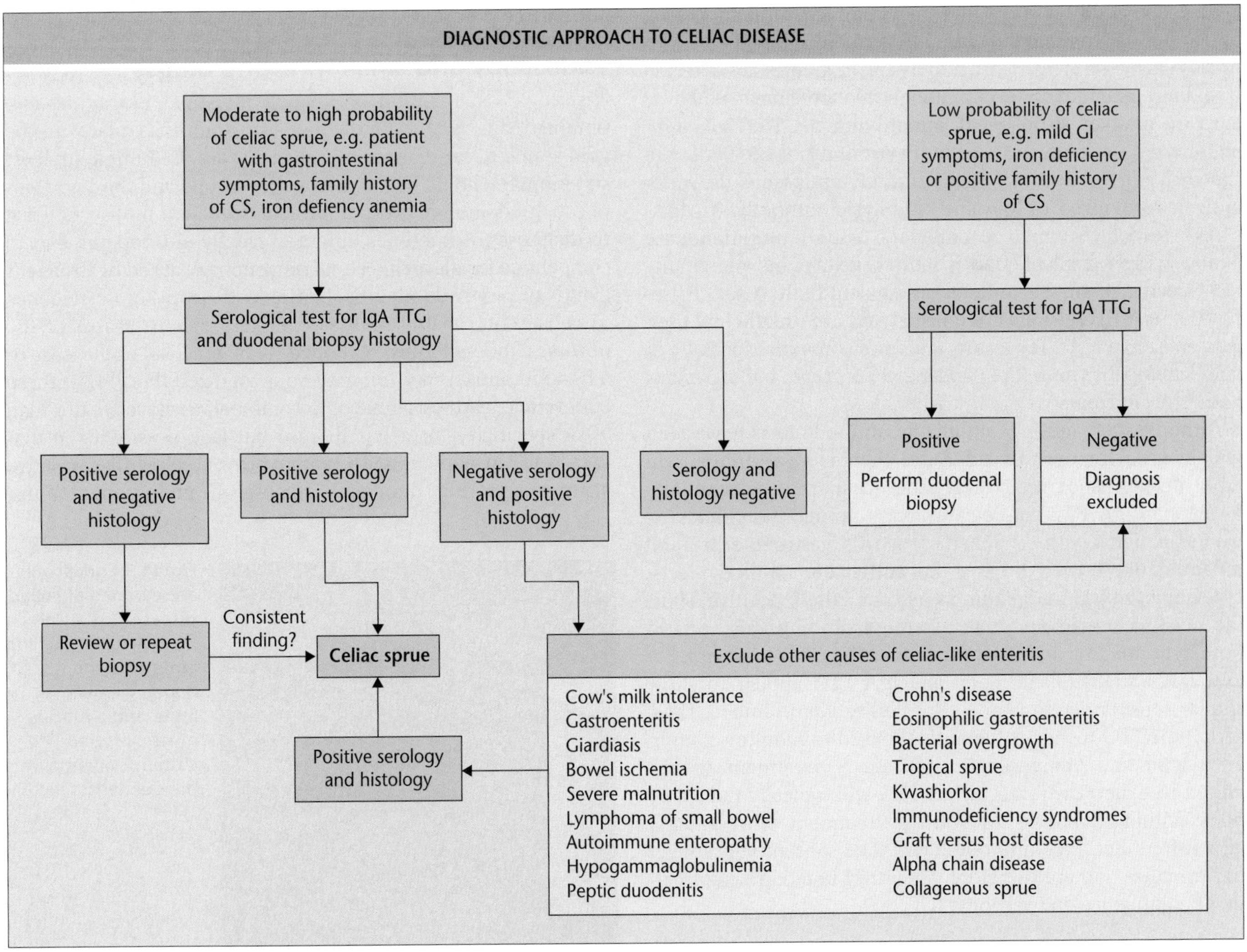

Fig. 44.4 Diagnostic approach to celiac disease. Reproduced with permission from Farrell R, Kelly C. Diagnosis of celiac sprue. Am J Gastroenterol 2001; 96:3237-3246.

TABLE 44.3 SENSITIVITY AND SPECIFICITY OF SEROLOGICAL TESTS IN PATIENTS WITH UNTREATED CELIAC SPRUE

Serological test	Sensitivity (%)[a]	Specificity (%)[a]
IgA human tissue transglutaminase antibodies	93	99
IgA endomysial antibodies	85–98	97–100
IgA guinea pig tissue transglutaminase antibodies	95–98	94–95
IgA antigliadin antibodies	75–90	82–95
IgG antigliadin antibodies	69–85	73–90

[a] Wide variations are reported between different laboratories.
Reproduced with permission from Farrell R, Kelly C. Diagnosis of celiac sprue. Am J Gastroenterol 2001; 96:3237–3246.

serum IgA levels may be useful if a false-negative IgA TTG test result is suspected.[1,2,7,12]

Serologic tests

Serologic tests have revolutionized the diagnostic approach to celiac disease. These tests are useful for diagnosing individuals with suspected disease, evaluating those with atypical or extra-intestinal manifestations, and for monitoring adherence and response to gluten-free diet.[7, 25] Numerous serologic tests are available in addition to IgA TTG including IgA-antiendomysial antibodies, IgA antigliadin antibodies, and IgG antigliadin antibodies (Table 44.3). IgA antiendomysial antibodies are detected by indirect immunofluorescence using sections of human umbilical cord or monkey esophageal smooth muscle. The IgA anti-endomysial antibody tests have a sensitivity of 85–98% and specificity of 97–100%.[27] Tissue transglutaminase is the auto-antigen recognized by the antiendomysial antibody. An IgA-ELISA to detect human recombinant tissue transglutaminase is now widely available and is more sensitive, but marginally less specific, than the antiendomysial antibody assay. False-positive IgA TTG results are unusual and are usually low titer. False-negative IgA TTG results are more common especially in mild enteropathy, in children under 2 years of age, and in patients with IgA deficiency as noted earlier.

Although IgA and IgG antigliadin antibody tests have been widely used for over two decades their clinical utility is in rapid decline since their diagnostic accuracy is substantially lower than IgA TTG serology. In many normal individuals, as well as patients with esophagitis, gastritis, gastroenteritis, and inflammatory bowel disease, the antigliadin antibody tests, especially the IgG antigliadin assays, are falsely positive. Thus, the positive predictive value of antigliadin antibody tests in both symptomatic and asymptomatic subjects is unacceptably low. IgA antigliadin antibody and IgA TTG appear to show similar sensitivities to changes in dietary gluten intake. Thus, serial IgA TTG testing is increasingly used to monitor compliance with and immunologic response to treatment with a gluten-free diet. The levels of IgA TTG will typically reduce by 50% within 2 months of starting treatment with a strict gluten-free diet. IgG antibody levels take substantially longer to normalize and are therefore less useful in monitoring treatment compliance and response.

Other blood tests

Iron, folate, and/or vitamin D deficiency and secondary hyperparathyroidism are often present in patients with untreated celiac disease. Vitamin B_{12} deficiency is less common because celiac disease typically does not affect the ileum. For unclear reasons features of hyposplenism with Howell-Jolly bodies and thrombocytosis are seen in older untreated patients. Untreated celiac disease is often associated with mild elevation of serum transaminase levels, thus celiac disease should always be considered in patients with persistent and unexplained hypertransaminasemia. Liver enzyme levels revert to normal on a gluten-free diet unless there is coexistent liver disease.

Endoscopy and small intestine biopsy

Histologic examination of a small intestinal biopsy, usually obtained during duodenoscopy, still retains its place as the gold standard for diagnosing celiac disease.[26] Multiple (at least six) biopsies should be taken from the second and third portions of the duodenum in order to provide sufficient biopsy material to diagnose a sometimes mild and patchy enteropathy and to compensate for the architectural distortion produced by Brunner's glands or peptic duodenitis. During endoscopy, gross evidence of celiac enteropathy such as complete or partial loss of the normal duodenal folds, scalloped folds, mucosal nodularity, or a fissured, mosaic pattern may be recognized (Fig. 44.5). These endoscopic features, singly or in combination, have greater than 90% specificity for celiac disease but lack sensitivity in that over 40% of patients with biopsy-proven celiac disease have normal-appearing duodenal mucosa at endoscopy.[28] Thus,

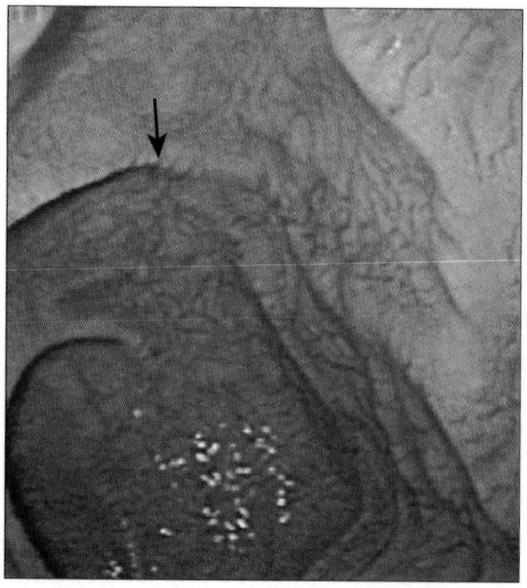

Fig 44.5 Endoscopic appearance of celiac disease. Scalloping (arrow), flattening, and atrophy of the duodenal mucosal folds, and a reticular, mosaic fissured pattern evident over the duodenal mucosa.

biopsy is indicated whenever celiac disease is suspected regardless of the endoscopic appearance of the duodenal mucosa.

The characteristic histological appearance of the small bowel in patients with untreated celiac disease is described above (see also Fig. 44.2). The severity and extent of the histological abnormalities of celiac disease vary; individuals with mild, focal abnormalities confined to the proximal small intestine are likely to have fewer symptoms, less severe malabsorption, and fewer nutritional deficiencies compared to patients with severe celiac enteropathy.

Radiological tests

Small bowel barium X-rays and abdominal computed tomography may be indicated in a small subset of celiac disease patients that do not response to treatment with a strict gluten-free diet or in those with marked weight loss, abdominal pain, a palpable abdominal mass, profound hypoalbuminemia, gastrointestinal bleeding, or obstruction in which complications such as lymphoma or ulcerative jejunoileitis are suspected. Diffuse bone demineralization may be evident on plain films but bone mineral density testing is indicated in newly diagnosed celiac disease to provide a more sensitive and quantitative evaluation of bone mineral content. Osteoporosis or significant osteopenia in a patient with celiac disease indicates the need for oral calcium and/or vitamin D supplementation and monitoring of calcium, vitamin D, PTH concentrations, and bone health.

Repeat biopsy and gluten challenge

Even though an initial small bowel biopsy is required to establish the diagnosis, serologic testing for TTG autoantibodies has dramatically reduced the need for repeat biopsies to confirm mucosal recovery on treatment and/or the recurrence of celiac enteropathy during subsequent gluten challenge. In short, a positive IgA TTG serology in combination with abnormal small bowel histology that is consistent with celiac disease combine to provide an absolute diagnosis of celiac disease that does not require any routine re-evaluation. Nonetheless, a second biopsy may be needed for patients with a poor clinical response to gluten-free diet or in those where the initial diagnosis is less secure.[1,2,7,12,26]

A gluten challenge is indicated when the diagnosis of celiac disease is in doubt during a period of gluten restriction (e.g., patients who began a gluten-free diet without histological confirmation of celiac disease). Gluten challenge should be started with caution, as some patients are exquisitely sensitive to gluten. If a small amount of gluten (a piece of a cracker or bread) is well tolerated, the portion can be doubled every 3 days until the equivalent of four slices of bread is ingested daily and continued for 6–8 weeks or until symptoms develop. At that point serological tests and biopsy are repeated. If serology and biopsy are both negative at 6–8 weeks, these individuals should be monitored for signs and symptoms of celiac disease on a normal diet for at least 6 months, after which serologic tests should again be checked and another small bowel biopsy considered.

TREATMENT AND PREVENTION

The mainstay of therapy for celiac disease is strict adherence to a gluten-free diet. Treatment represents a lifelong commitment, can be expensive, and is socially inconvenient. These characteristics limit compliance for all age groups but particularly for children and teenagers. Consequently, it is very important that the diagnosis is made correctly and unambiguously before recommending treatment. Products that contain wheat gluten or are produced from barley or rye must be avoided. Gluten is present in many dietary items because wheat flour is widely used in processed foods as a thickener and inexpensive filler. Furthermore, gluten-free grain can become contaminated with wheat, if producers use the same equipment to process both gluten-containing and gluten-free foods. As a result, complete elimination of gluten from the diet is a challenge to achieve and maintain. Patient education is of crucial importance and an effective gluten-free diet requires extensive, repeated counseling and instruction of the patient by the physician and a skilled dietician. It also requires a motivated patient who will read labels carefully and critically.

While the long-term safety of oats is still unproven, it is clear that moderate amounts of oats (50–70 g/day) taken for 6–12 months are nontoxic in adults and children with celiac disease or DH.[29] Still, it is important to warn patients that oat products obtained from the grocery store may be contaminated with small amounts of wheat. Accordingly, it is recommended that oats be avoided in all newly diagnosed patients until remission is achieved on a strict gluten-free diet. Then, if the patient understands the difficulties in obtaining noncontaminated oats, up to 2 oz/day from a reliable source can be introduced and continued if well tolerated. Patients with untreated celiac disease often have secondary lactase deficiency and thus need to avoid dairy products initially. After 3–6 months of treatment and mucosal healing dairy products can be reintroduced if tolerated.

The majority of patients (70–75%) improve within 2 weeks of beginning a gluten-free diet.[1] In many, symptomatic improvement is noticed within 48 h, although it may take several weeks or months to achieve full clinical remission. The speed and degree of histological improvement usually lags behind the symptom response and may not be evident for 2 or 3 months. Lack of clinical or histologic response almost always indicates inadequate adherence to the diet. However, it is also important to note that persistent symptoms may be due to coexisting disorders such as irritable bowel syndrome, lactose intolerance, microscopic colitis, or pancreatic insufficiency.

In addition to a gluten-free diet, all patients with clinical evidence of malabsorption should take a gluten-free multivitamin tablet daily. Iron and/or folate supplements are needed to replete body stores in those with deficiencies and anemia. Patients with steatorrhea, hypocalcemia or osteopenic bone disease should also take gluten-free oral calcium and vitamin D supplements. In patients with hyposplenism, prophylactic antibiotics before invasive procedures and pneumococcus vaccination should be considered. In rare instances, intravenous corticosteroid therapy may be required for critically ill patients with acute celiac crisis manifested by severe diarrhea, dehydration, weight loss, acidosis, hypocalcemia, and hypoproteinemia, or the even more rare condition of gliadin shock complicating gluten challenge.

REFRACTORY CELIAC DISEASE

Refractory celiac disease is a diagnosis of exclusion defined as symptomatic severe celiac enteritis that does not respond to at least 6 months of a strict gluten-free diet and is not accounted for by other causes of villous atrophy or by intestinal lymphoma.[30] Recent studies have elucidated the close links between refractory celiac disease and the other life-threatening complications of celiac disease specifically ulcerative jejunoileitis and enteropathy-associated T cell lymphoma.[31] Over half of patients with refractory celiac disease have an abnormal CD3 positive, CD4/CD8 double-negative IEL T cell population. Many also have an intestinal T cell clonal expansion referred to as a cryptic enteropathy associated T cell lymphoma. These cells have destructive properties related to their cytotoxic phenotype, which lead to mucosal ulceration, lymph-node cavitation, and progression to overt lymphoma. Therapy with corticosteroids and other immunosuppressant drugs such as azathioprine or cyclosporine may be beneficial in the short term but death from malnutrition, immunocompromise, and lymphoma is difficult to avert. Although the data are not conclusive, most published studies indicate that strict adherence to a gluten-free diet reduces the risk of all celiac disease-associated malignancies including enteropathy-associated T cell lymphoma.[30,32]

SOURCES OF INFORMATION FOR PATIENTS AND DOCTORS

http://patients.uptodate.com/topic.asp?file=digestiv/4656
http://digestive.niddk.nih.gov/ddiseases/pubs/celiac/
http://www.patient.co.uk/DisplayConcepts.asp
http://www.aafp.org/afp/20021215/2269ph.html

REFERENCES

1. Farrell R, Kelly C. Celiac sprue. N Engl J Med 2002; 346:180–188.
2. Ciclitira PJ, King AL, Fraser JS. AGA technical review on celiac sprue. American Gastroenterological Association. Gastroenterology 2001; 120:1526–1540.
3. Mylotte M, Egan-Mitchell B, McCarthy CF et al. Celiac disease in the West of Ireland. Br Med J 1973; 3:498–499.
4. Catassi C, Fabiani E, Ratsch IM et al. The celiac iceberg in Italy. A multicentre antigliadin antibodies screening for celiac disease in school-age subjects. Acta Paediatr Suppl 1996; 412:29–35.
5. Fasano A, Berti I, Gerarduzzi T. Prevalence of celiac disease in at-risk and not-at-risk groups in the United States: a large multicenter study. Arch Intern Med 2003; 163:286–292.
6. Maki M, Mustalahti K, Kokkonen J et al. Prevalence of celiac disease among children in Finland. N Eng J Med 2002; 348:2517–2524.
7. Fasano A, Catassi C. Current approaches to diagnosis and treatment of celiac disease: an evolving spectrum. Gastroenterology 2001; 120:636–651.
8. Logan RF, Rifkind EA, Turner I et al. Mortality in celiac disease. Gastroenterology 1989; 97: 265–271.
9. Collin P, Reunala T, Pukkala et al. Celiac disease – associated disorders and survival. Gut 1994; 35:1215–1218.
10. Schuppan D. Current concepts of celiac disease pathogenesis. Gastroenterology 2000; 119:234–242.
11. Mowat AM. Celiac disease – a meeting point for genetics, immunology, and protein chemistry. Lancet 2003; 361:1290–1292.
12. Green PH, Jabri B. Celiac disease. Lancet 2003; 362:383–391.
13. Rubin CE, Brandborg LL, Phelps PC et al. Studies of celiac disease: I. The apparent identical and specific nature of the duodenal and proximal jejunal lesion in celiac disease and idiopathic sprue. Gastroenterology 1960; 38:28.
14. Niazi NM, Leigh R, Crowe P, Marsh MN. Morphometric analysis of small intestinal mucosa. I. Methodology, epithelial volume compartments and enumeration of inter-epithelial space lymphocytes. Virchows Arch A Pathol Anat Histopathol 1984; 404:49–60.
15. Jarvinen TT, Kaukinen K, Laurila K et al. Intraepithelial lymphocytes in celiac disease. Am J Gastroenterol 2003; 98:1332–1337.
16. Hankey GL, Holmes GK. Celiac disease in the elderly. Gut 1994; 35:65–67.
17. Loftus C, Murray J. Celiac disease: diagnosis and management. J Clin Outcomes Manag 2002; 9:341–349.
18. Cellier C, Flobert C, Cormier C et al. Severe osteopenia in symptom-free adults with a childhood diagnosis of celiac disease. Lancet 2000; 355:806.
19. Hadjivassiliou M, Grunewald RA, Chattopadhyay AK. Clinical, radiological, neuorophysiological, and neuropathological characteristics of gluten ataxia. Lancet 1998; 352:1582–1585.
20. Cronin CC, Jackson LM, Feighery C et al. Celiac disease and epilepsy. QJM 1998; 91:303–308.
21. Askling J, Linet M, Gridley G et al. Cancer incidence in a population-based cohort of individuals hospitalized with celiac disease or dermatitis herpatiformis. Gastroenterology 2002; 123:1428–1435.
22. Fry L. Dermatitis herpetiformis. Baillières Clin Gastroenterol 1995; 9:371–393.
23. Cronin CC, Feighery A, Ferriss JB et al. High prevalence of celiac disease among patients with insulin-dependent (type I) diabetes mellitus. Am J Gastroenterol 1997; 92:2210–2212.
24. Counsell CE, Taha A, Ruddell WS. Celiac disease and autoimmune thyroid disease. Gut 1994; 35:844–846.
25. Ventura A, Magazzu G, Greco L. Duration of exposure to gluten and risk for autoimmune disorders in patients with celiac disease. Gastroenterology 1999; 117:297–303.
26. Farrell R, Kelly C. Diagnosis of celiac sprue. Am J Gastroenterol 2001; 96:3237–3246.
27. Grodzinsky E, Hed J, Skogh T. IgA antiendomysium antibodies have a high positive predictive value for celiac disease in asymptomatic patients. Allergy 1994; 49:593–597.
28. Oxentenko A, Grisolano S, Murray J et al. The insensitivity of endoscopic markers in celiac disease. Am J Gastroenterol 2002; 97: 933–938.
29. Janatuinen EK, Pikkarainen PH, Kemppainen TA et al. A comparison of diets with and without oats in adults with celiac disease. N Engl J Med 1995; 333:1033–1037.
30. Ryan BM, Kelleher D. Refractory celiac disease. Gastroenterology 2000; 119: 243–251.
31. Cellier C, Delabesse E, Helmer C et al. Refractory sprue, celiac disease, and enteropathy-associated T-cell lymphoma. French Celiac Disease Study Group. Lancet 2000; 356: 203–208.
32. Holmes GK, Prior P, Lane MR et al. Malignancy in celiac disease-effect of a gluten free diet. Gut 1989; 30:333–338.

Chapter 45

Short bowel syndrome

Simon M Gabe and David B A Silk

KEY POINTS

- With < 50 cm small bowel with colon in continuity, or <100 cm small bowel to ileostomy, parenteral nutrition and fluids are usually required
- Functional short bowel syndrome occurs with high output fistulas or stomas despite adequate bowel length
- Preservation of the ileocecal valve may slow small intestinal transit
- Mild short bowel syndrome is manifested by dehydration and hypomagnesemia
- Excessive thirst may lead to increased drinking which exacerbates high output and sodium losses
- Differential causes of high output include bacterial overgrowth and bile salt malabsorption
- Residual bowel length is more informative for future management than length of resected specimen
- Urinary sodium <20 mmol/L indicates volume and/or sodium depletion
- Advances in intestinal transplantation offer hope for the future

INTRODUCTION

The adult small intestine varies considerably in length, ranging from 275 to 850 cm from the duodenojejunal flexure.[1] Short bowel syndrome is a form of intestinal failure (see Chapters 43 and 138), and can be subcategorized as anatomic and functional types (Table 45.1). Anatomic short bowel syndrome occurs after extensive small intestinal resections and also applies to patients with a high-output enterocutaneous fistula. This typically occurs when there is less than 200 cm of remaining small bowel in continuity, and the lack of functioning gut results in diarrhea, weight loss, and nutrient malabsorption. However, it is not until there is less than 50 cm of small bowel with colon in continuity, or 100 cm of small bowel to an end stoma, that patients will be dependent on parenteral fluids with or without parenteral nutrition for survival.[2] The term functional short bowel syndrome applies to patients with a high-output fistula or stoma despite an adequate length of small intestine (Table 45.1). The key determinant is whether a patient can maintain a positive fluid or nutritional balance.

Intestinal failure has a wider definition as it includes the nonfunctioning intestine as well as high-output states. Intestinal failure occurs when there is insufficient functioning gut mass to absorb the nutrients and/or electrolytes necessary for survival.[3] In this situation parenteral administration is necessary.

TABLE 45.1 SHORT BOWEL SYNDROME

Anatomic	Functional
<100 cm small intestine to end stoma or to an enterocutaneous fistula <50 cm small intestine and colon in continuity	>200 cm small intestine with a severe malabsorptive process (refractory sprue, chronic intestinal pseudo-obstruction syndrome, congenital villous hypoplasia)

TABLE 45.2 PREVALENCE AND INCIDENCE OF HOME PARENTERAL NUTRITION[4]

Country	Incidence ($\times 10^{-6}$ population/year)	Prevalence ($\times 10^{-6}$ population)
UK, 2001		9 (point prevalence)
Scotland, 2001		14 (point prevalence)
Wales, 2003		6 (point prevalence)
Europe, 1997	0.4–3	0.7–12.7 (point prevalence)
Denmark, 1999		12.7 (point prevalence)
USA, 1992		40 (annual occurrence)

EPIDEMIOLOGY

There is little information on the epidemiology of short bowel syndrome, but more on home parenteral nutrition (HPN) and intestinal failure for which short bowel syndrome is the predominant indication. The incidence and prevalence of HPN is similar in the UK and Europe, but appears to be substantially higher in the USA (Table 45.2). Some of this can be accounted for by the way that the data are presented, as in Europe the point prevalence is presented, whereas in the USA the annual occurrence is calculated.

In the UK, data on the numbers of patients on HPN has been collected since the first patients were fed in the late 1970s. Since 1995, this function has been performed by the British Artificial Nutrition Survey, a constituent committee of the British Association for Parenteral and Enteral Nutrition. Each annual report has identified an increasing number of patients receiving HPN (Fig. 45.1). Allowing for underreporting, it is estimated that the point prevalence of HPN in the UK is approximately 500 patients, and the period prevalence of HPN over each year may be around 600 patients.[5]

HOME PARENTAL NUTRITION IN THE UK

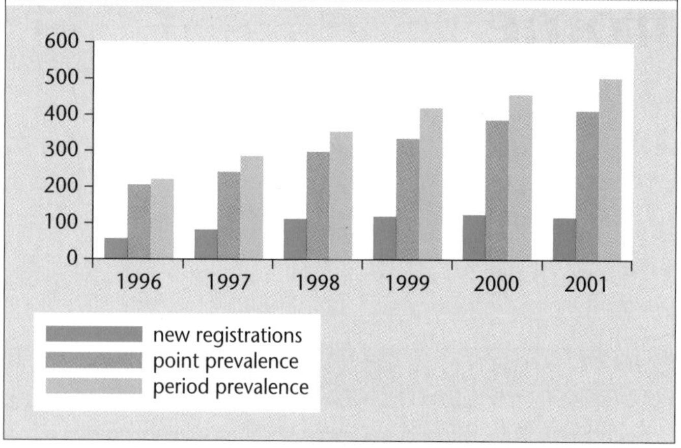

Fig. 45.1 Home parenteral nutrition in the UK. Values for HPN in the UK, showing the number of new registrations, point prevalence, and period prevalence for the years 1996–2001.

THE THREE TYPES OF SHORT-BOWEL SYNDROME

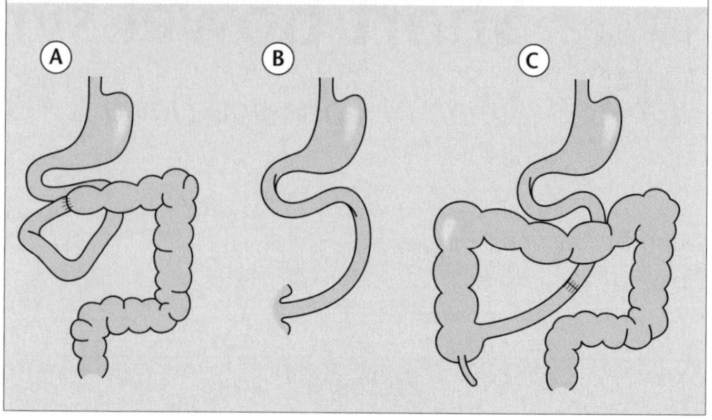

Fig. 45.2 The three types of patient with short bowel syndrome. **A.** Jejunocolic anastomosis. **B.** End jejunostomy. C. Jejunoileal anastomosis. Reproduced from Nightingale J (2001),[3] with permission.

CAUSES, RISK FACTORS, DISEASE ASSOCIATIONS

There are three types of patient with a short bowel (Fig. 45.2): those with a jejunoileal or jejunocolic anastomosis, or an end jejunostomy.[6,7] Patients with a high-output enterocutaneous fistula can be considered in the same group as those with an end jejunostomy.

It is commonly believed that the ileocecal valve slows small intestinal transit so that preservation of the ileocecal valve is beneficial in patients with short bowel syndrome. In fact, the data are conflicting and reports suggesting a benefit due to the presence of the ileocecal valve may reflect the retention of a significant length of terminal ileum.[8] By contrast, the presence of the colon has clearly been shown to be beneficial in patients with short bowel syndrome, given its ability to absorb water, electrolytes, and fatty acids, to slow intestinal transit, and to stimulate intestinal adaptation. Patients with a jejunocolic anastomosis may survive without parenteral nutrition, even with a very short segment of remaining jejunum, and less frequently require fluid and electrolyte supplements.

The causes of short bowel syndrome in adults are shown in Table 45.3. In childhood and infancy, short bowel syndrome is caused by multiple jejunoileal atresia, midgut volvulus, gastroschisis, and necrotizing enterocolitis.[9]

TABLE 45.3 REASONS FOR SHORT BOWEL IN ADULTS IN 1992[6]

Underlying disease	%
Crohn's disease	58
Ischemia	10
Irradiation	10
Ulcerative colitis	6
Volvulus	6
Adhesions	6
Diverticular disease	2
Desmoid tumor	2

CLINICAL PRESENTATION

The classic presentation of short bowel syndrome is the combination of weight loss and dehydration in a patient with a large stoma or fistula output. When mild, this may be indolent and simply present as dehydration (symptomatic and biochemical), usually with hypomagnesemia. When severe, patients are dependent on parenteral fluids to maintain hydration on a daily basis and require additional electrolytes (especially magnesium), calories, protein, and vitamins (i.e., parenteral nutrition). Patients with short bowel syndrome can be subclassified as either net 'absorbers' or net 'secretors.' Adult absorbers generally have at least 100 cm of jejunum and are able to absorb more water and sodium from the diet than taken orally. The stool output is less than 2 L/day, and in general these patients can be managed with oral sodium and water supplements, and parenteral fluids are not needed. In contrast, adult secretors generally have less than 100 cm of jejunum and greater stomal losses (usual stoma output may be 4–8 L/day), resulting in a negative fluid and sodium balance after any food or drink.[7]

CAUSES AND RISK FACTORS

COMMON AND UNCOMMON CAUSES AND RISK FACTORS IN ADULTS

Group	Common	Uncommon
Small intestinal resections Massive intestinal resection Enterocutaneous fistula Bypass surgery	Crohn's disease Infarction (SMA/SMV thrombosis) High output	Postirradiation enteritis Repeated surgery for surgical complications SMA embolus Massive volvulus Desmoid tumour Gastric bypass for obesity

SMA, superior mesenteric artery; SMV, superior mesenteric vein.

CLINICAL PRESENTATION
• Weight loss • Diarrhea – exacerbated by oral intake • Nutrient malabsorption

Dehydration

Patients with short bowel syndrome usually have an insatiable thirst. Drinking gives some immediate relief, but may result in increased output, and net accentuation of any sodium and fluid depletion. Early signs of dehydration include lethargy, tiredness, and headaches. Patients should also be told to note their urine color and frequency.

Cramps

These can be severe and are caused by hypomagnesemia with or without hypocalcemia. Stomal magnesium losses are considerable in patients with short bowel syndrome, resulting in a negative magnesium balance. The hypocalcemia that ensues cannot be corrected without correcting the hypomagnesemia.

Weight loss

Daily fluctuations in weight reflect fluid balance, and this provides a simple and essential gauge in the management of the patient with short bowel syndrome. Changes in weight over weeks reflect nutritional changes, thereby reflecting fat and protein reserves, and must be monitored in these patients.

High stoma or fistula output

Patients often have problems with leakage around the bag or splitting of the bag as a result of a high output. If the output is very high, this is best managed using a high-flow system.

DIFFERENTIAL DIAGNOSIS

The usual cause for a high-output state in a patient who has undergone an intestinal resection and has a stoma is excessive drinking. Such patients are usually told to drink more in the postoperative period when their output is high, but this only aggravates the problem by increasing the output further. Other causes for a high-output state include infection (infective gastroenteritis), small bowel bacterial overgrowth, and a small intestinal stricture, which can present in this way rather than with obstructive symptoms. Bile acid malabsorption may result in profuse diarrhea in patients who have undergone limited ileal resection.

DIAGNOSTIC METHODS

The best method to assess residual small bowel length is direct measurement during surgery. This is performed by measuring 10–30-cm segments along the antimesenteric border, taking care not to overstretch the bowel. Unfortunately surgeons often measure only the resected segment. As there is such a wide variation in normal small bowel length, estimation of the length of the residual segment is not possible.

When no surgical measurement has been performed it is possible to estimate length radiologically using an opisometer to trace along the length of small bowel shown on a small bowel meal radiograph. This technique is relatively accurate if the total small intestinal length is less than 200 cm and the entire small bowel is shown on one film. Recently, plasma citrulline has been developed as a marker of small intestinal length. Citrulline is not derived from food or proteolysis, but synthesized in enterocytes from glutamine; it is not incorporated into body proteins.[10]

An accurate daily fluid balance chart and daily weight are, however, much more informative than a barium meal. If the stoma or fistula output is more than 2 L with weight loss, low urine output, and net negative balance, the patient needs to be treated with a short bowel regimen. Random urine sodium measurement is a further informative but under-utilized test. A value of less than 20 mmol/L indicates volume and/or sodium depletion that needs to be addressed This measure of hypovolemia or sodium depletion occurs in tandem with the early symptoms of dehydration (headaches, thirst, poor concentration, lethargy, dizziness), but well before any abnormalities become apparent from the blood picture.

CLINICAL TIPS
• **Assessment of hydration status** Measure spot urine sodium concentration (aim for >20 mmol/L) • **If output is too high** The patient must be drinking too many hypotonic fluids (limit to <1 L/day) Ensure that the short bowel regimen is being strictly adhered to

TREATMENT

The presentation and long-term outcome of a patient following a small bowel resection can be predicted from knowledge of the remaining small bowel and the presence or absence of functioning colon. Treatment is initially aimed at maintaining fluid balance.

Jejunum–colon anastomosis

These patients are often deceptively well after resection except for diarrhea or steatorrhea. This reflects the ability of the residual colon to absorb fluid and sodium, so maintaining a positive fluid balance (net absorber). However, this does not imply that nutritional balance will also be positive, and over a number of months patients can become severely undernourished.

Jejunostomy

These patients have immediate problems after surgery with a large stoma output that increases further with food and drink. Often patients are told to increase their oral fluid intake to match the output, but this will lead to serious problems with dehydration. The mainstay of treatment is to restrict oral hypotonic fluid intake, introduce a glucose–saline solution (sodium concentration 90–120 mmol/L) to sip through the day, antimotility agents, and drugs to suppress gastric acid production together with the introduction of a high-energy and low-fiber diet. In addition, it is important to avoid drinking when eating food, as this will decrease transit time. An elemental diet is not recommended as it is hyperosmolar and will increase stoma output.

TREATMENT AND PREVENTION
SHORT BOWEL REGIMEN
• **Limit oral fluid intake** 1 L hypotonic fluids (or less) 1 L electrolyte mix • **Optimize drug therapy** Loperamide (up to 4 mg four times daily) Codeine phosphate (up to 60 mg four times daily) Omeprazole (40 mg twice daily) • **Optimal timing of medications** Loperamide and codeine to be taken 30–60 min before meals • **Nutrition** Encourage a high-energy, low-fiber diet

Treatment options in net secretors

Water and sodium losses

If a patient remains in a net negative fluid balance despite optimizing medical therapy (net secretors), parenteral fluids will be necessary. The route of administration may depend on the degree of negative balance.

Subcutaneous fluids

A net negative balance of up to 1 L/day can be managed using subcutaneous fluids self-administered at night. This is a realistic treatment option that is infrequently used and has the advantage of being able to add magnesium (4 mmol/L) into the infusate.

Intravenous electrolytes

A net negative balance of 1 L/day or more will need to be managed with intravenous replacement. In a patient with short bowel syndrome this is a long-term option, and a dedicated Hickman-type (Broviac) catheter should be placed. The care of this catheter must be meticulous and the patient needs to be fully trained to administer their own fluids if they are to have any independence.

Intravenous nutrition

This will be necessary in patients who become malnourished despite optimal medical therapy. Although this will apply to patients with very high stoma outputs, it is not universal. Consequently, it is important to separate fluid balance and nutritional balance in these patients, and to consider these aspects separately.

Magnesium

Magnesium deficiency occurs in patients with short bowel syndrome as a result of increased losses. There is a decreased surface area for magnesium absorption; fatty acids (dietary or from bacterial fermentation of malabsorbed carbohydrate) combine with magnesium, calcium, and zinc, and prevent their absorption; and secondary hyperaldosteronism (due to volume depletion) also increases renal magnesium excretion. A low serum level of magnesium reduces both the secretion and function of parathormone. This in turn decreases renal magnesium absorption and the absorption of magnesium and calcium from the intestine (via 1,25-hydroxycholecalciferol).

The clinical features of magnesium deficiency include fatigue, depression, muscular weakness, ataxia, athetoid movements, cardiac arrhythmias, and, if severe, convulsions. If there is concomitant hypocalcemia, carpopedal spasm and positive Chvostek and Trousseau signs may be seen.

Treatment generally entails rehydration and oral supplements (magnesium oxide contains more elemental magnesium than the other salts). If this is not sufficient to correct magnesium deficiency, 1α-hydroxycholecalciferol (1–9 μg daily) may be given orally or ergocalciferol intramuscularly to improve magnesium balance.[1] Finally, parenteral magnesium may be given intravenously or subcutaneously. An acceptable regimen is 4 mmol magnesium sulfate diluted in 1 L saline given subcutaneously overnight; this has the advantage of correcting any dehydration at the same time. This can be repeated daily if necessary, but if more fluid or magnesium is still required then this is best administered parenterally via a long-term intravenous catheter.

Diet in patients with short bowel syndrome

Protein

Human and experimental studies have shown that the products of luminal protein digestion are absorbed in the form of dipeptides and tripeptides as well as free amino acids. In short bowel syndrome the absorption of exogenous nitrogen is limited by inadequate luminal hydrolysis and reduced membrane absorptive capacity. Use of partial enzymic hydrolysates of protein may be advantageous, particularly in the early phase of management, as small-peptide and mixed diets have been shown to enhance nitrogen absorption compared with a whole protein diet.[11] However, other studies have demonstrated that patients with short bowel syndrome stable on an oral diet will absorb 61–81% of ingested protein, which is further compensated by an adaptive hyperphagia.[12,13] A complementary adaptive process is upregulation of the oligopeptide transporter PEPT1 in the colonic mucosa of patients with colon in continuity.

Carbohydrate and fat

Carbohydrate is avidly absorbed in the proximal small intestine. However, a significant amount still reaches the colon, where colonic fermentation has been estimated to contribute 5–10% of energy requirements in healthy individuals.[14] Thus, patients with small bowel–colon continuity absorb more energy from a low-fat, high-carbohydrate diet,[15] although osmotic diarrhea from unfermented carbohydrate and rarely D-lactic acidosis (produced from starch by colonic bacteria) may result. A high-fat diet should be used in patients with an end jejunostomy as carbohydrate absorption and stoma output are not adversely affected.[16]

Fistuloclysis

Fistuloclysis is the infusion of enteral feed into the distal limb of an enterocutaneous fistula. In 1988, Levy et al.[17] described a similar technique in patients with a defunctioned bowel segment, although in this technique enteral feed was mixed with the proximal stoma output. The Manchester group have the largest experience of this technique and have been able to render patients off parenteral nutrition while awaiting definitive corrective surgery.[18]

Surgery in short bowel syndrome

Surgery for the treatment of short bowel syndrome can be undertaken:

- to restore intestinal continuity
- to lengthen the intestine
- to delay intestinal transit
- to improve its function;
- intestinal transplantation is a final surgical option.

Unlike restoration of continuity, the other surgical procedures are performed only when medical therapy has been optimized and adequate time given for the residual short bowel to adapt (1–2 years). In addition, it should be noted that clinical experience of measures to lengthen the small bowel or improve its function has been confined largely to highly selected groups of patients, mainly in the pediatric population.[19] The outlook for adults undergoing intestinal transplantation is improving as immunosuppressive regimens develop (see Current controversies below).

COMPLICATIONS AND THEIR MANAGEMENT

Acute complications that occur in a patient with short bowel syndrome include:

- dehydration
- electrolyte abnormalities
- malnutrition.

These have all been discussed above. Late complications that may occur in patients who have had a massive small bowel resection include:

- renal stones
- gallstones
- D-lactic acidosis in patients with colon in continuity
- complications associated with long-term parenteral nutrition (e.g., hepatic and venous complications).

Renal stones

Renal stones are frequent in patients with an ileostomy (10–13%) and may be urate or calcium oxalate stones. Hyperoxaluria occurs both in patients with an ileal resection and in those with a short bowel who have had a distal small bowel resection. Increased colonic oxalate absorption occurs because colonic calcium binds preferentially to bile salts, releasing colonic oxalate to be absorbed.

Treatment involves:

- a low-oxalate diet
- cholestyramine to bind bile salts
- citrate to prevent stone formation.

A low-oxalate diet typically excludes cocoa, peanut products, tea, coffee, wheatgerm, rhubarb, beets, collards, spinach, tofu, and soybeans, and restricts citrus drinks, tomatoes, and fruit.

Gallstones

Early anecdotal reports from the 1970s suggested that cholelithiasis and acalculous cholecystitis were more frequent in patients on total parenteral nutrition (TPN). More recently, studies in adults have demonstrated that 23% develop gallbladder disease after 3 months of TPN, increasing to 40% in patients with Crohn's disease or an ileal resection. In children, 43% receiving TPN for a mean duration of 20 months developed gallstones.[2] This is likely to be multifactorial in origin. The disturbance of the enterohepatic circulation of bile salts may play an important role in gallstone formation, but other factors also contribute significantly to gallstone formation, including nucleation rate and gallbladder stasis. Ileal resection will alter the cholesterol : phospholipid ratio within bile as well as bilirubin composition, leading to pigment stone formation. In addition, gallbladder contractility is reduced, together with the intestinal release of cholecystokinin and peptide YY. There is no agreed protocol for the role of cholecystokinin or prophylactic cholecystectomy in patients with a short bowel. Research is also needed on the use of aspirin and ursodeoxycholic acid in the prophylaxis and treatment of gallstones.

D-Lactic acidosis

Some patients with a short bowel and residual colon may have episodes of a syndrome of slurred speech, ataxia, and altered affect. This can occur as a result of fermentation of malabsorbed carbohydrate in the colon to D-lactic acid. The D-lactic acid is absorbed in the colon and can rarely accumulate, resulting in D-lactic acidosis. This should be suspected in a patient with acidosis, a large anion gap, and a normal L-lactic acid concentration in the blood. Treatment involves:

- restriction of monosaccharides and oligosaccharides in favor of polysaccharides to reduce the formation of colonic lactate
- broad-spectrum antibiotics (neomycin or vancomycin) orally.

Complications of parenteral nutrition

Parenteral nutrition is associated with certain complications, including:

- catheter sepsis
- central venous occlusion
- liver failure.

In patients receiving HPN, the central venous catheter infection rate ranges between 0.1 and 0.59 infections per year,[20,21] and is increased in patients on opiate analgesia[22] and in hospitalized patients on short-term parenteral nutrition, who receive nutrition via a temporary multilumen catheter that is also used for drugs and other fluids and is not cared for as meticulously as a dedicated feeding catheter. Generally, treatment should be eradication of infection by administering antibiotics down the catheter rather than catheter removal, unless the patient is in septic shock.

Hepatic alterations, as manifested by abnormal enzyme values and intrahepatic cholestasis, are more common in hospitalized patients receiving parenteral nutrition, probably as a result of a higher caloric load administered, noncyclic administration, concomitant medication, and ongoing sepsis. In patients on HPN, the reported prevalence of this complication varies between 15% and 85%.[23] It is more common in patients with a very short residual small bowel, and the development of hepatic fibrosis also relates to the administration of parenteral lipid at a rate of more than 1 g/kg daily.[24]

PROGNOSIS WITH AND WITHOUT TREATMENT

The survival of patients on HPN is impressive as there is no doubt that many would die without this artificial nutritional support. Data from France demonstrate survival rates of 86% and 75% at 2 and 5 years respectively for patients with benign disease on HPN.[25] Older data from the USA show survival rates of 94% and 80% at 1 and 4 years respectively for all patients on HPN, and 70% at 5 years for patients with benign disease.[26] The survival rates from St Mark's Hospital in Harrow, UK were 85% at 1 year, 68% at 5 years, 66% at 10 years, 48% at 15 years, and 17% at 20 years for all patients (including those with underlying malignancy) started on HPN.[27] Poor prognostic factors[25,27] include:

- active malignancy (relative risk [RR] of death 63)
- systemic sclerosis (RR 5)
- radiation enteritis (RR 4)
- an end enterostomy
- a small bowel length of less than 50 cm
- underlying etiology of mesenteric infarction.[25]

The cause of death in patients on HPN usually relates to the underlying etiology. HPN accounts for 9–22% of deaths (catheter sepsis 5–16%, liver failure 2–6%).[25,28]

CURRENT CONTROVERSIES AND THEIR FUTURE RESOLUTION

Although long-term parenteral nutrition is life-saving in patients with intestinal failure, it is expensive, impairs quality of life, and has serious complications. Treatments aimed at promoting pharmacologic adaptation in order to increase absorption by the remnant bowel have been investigated. Among these, recombinant human growth hormone (GH) appears to promote intestinal adaptation in animals. However, in humans there are conflicting data, with two controlled studies demonstrating no benefit of GH, glutamine, and a high carbohydrate diet,[29,30] and another study demonstrating benefit from GH alone on intestinal absorption.[31] Glucagon-like peptide 2 (GLP-2) has antisecretory, transit modulating, and intestinotrophic properties. Initial studies have shown that treatment with GLP-2 improves intestinal absorption and nutritional status in patients with a short bowel and a jejunostomy;[32] and further studies are currently under way using a longer-acting GLP-2 analog.

The place of intestinal transplantation in the management of patients with short bowel syndrome varies worldwide according to expertise and experience. This is a developing field and survival rates are steadily improving as better immunosuppressive regimens are developed. Patients are usually referred when the prognosis is poor, but it is clear that these patients are also at high risk for transplantation; for survival rates to improve further, patients should be referred at an earlier stage. Current indications for intestinal transplantation for patients with intestinal failure include:[33]

- the loss of two or more central veins
- the development of hepatic fibrosis
- patient preference.

Survival rates are quoted as 75% at 1 year, 54% at 5 years, and 42% at 10 years.[34] Recipients of liver plus intestine had the best long-term prognosis and the lowest risk of graft loss from rejection. Since 1994, survival rates have improved. In the UK, the 1- and 3-year survival rates following intestinal transplantation are now 57% and 43% respectively.[33]

SOURCES OF INFORMATION FOR PATIENTS AND DOCTORS

http://www.icongrouponline.com/health/Short_Bowel_Syndrome.html
http://depts.washington.edu/growing/Assess/SBS.htm

REFERENCES

1. Nightingale JMD. The short bowel. In: Nightingale JMD, ed. Intestinal failure. London: Greenwich Media; 2001:177–198.
2. Scolapio JS. Treatment of short-bowel syndrome. Curr Opin Clin Nutr Metab Care 2001; 4:557–560.
3. Nightingale JMD, ed. Intestinal failure, 1st edn. London: Greenwich Medical Media & Cambridge University Press; 2001.
4. Messing B, Hebuterne X, Nightingale J. Home enteral and parenteral nutrition in adults. In: Nightingale JMD, ed. Intestinal failure. London: Greenwich Medical Media; 2001:407–430.
5. Jones BJ. Home parenteral nutrition in the United Kingdom. Report for the British Association of Parenteral and Enteral Nutrition, 2003:1–16.
6. Nightingale JM, Lennard-Jones JE, Gertner DJ, Wood SR, Bartram CI. Colonic preservation reduces need for parenteral therapy, increases incidence of renal stones, but does not change high prevalence of gall stones in patients with a short bowel. Gut 1992; 33:1493–1497.
7. Carbonnel F, Cosnes J, Chevret S et al. The role of anatomic factors in nutritional autonomy after extensive small bowel resection. JPEN J Parenter Enteral Nutr 1996; 20:275–280.
8. Weber TR, Tracey T Jr, Connors RH. Short-bowel syndrome in children. Quality of life in an era of improved survival. Arch Surg 1991; 126:841–846.
9. Goulet OJ, Revillon Y, Jan D et al. Neonatal short bowel syndrome. J Pediatr 1991; 119: 18–23.
10. Crenn P, Coudray-Lucas C, Cynober L, Messing B. Post-absorptive plasma citrulline concentration: a marker of intestinal failure in humans. Transplant Proc 1998; 30:2528.
11. Cosnes J, Evard D, Beaugerie L, Gendre JP, Le Quintrec Y. Improvement in protein absorption with a small-peptide-based diet in patients with high jejunostomy. Nutrition 1992; 8:406–411.
12. Messing B, Pigot F, Rongier M, Morin MC, Ndeindoum U, Rambaud JC. Intestinal absorption of free oral hyperalimentation in the very short bowel syndrome. Gastroenterology 1991; 100:1502–1508.
13. Woolf GM, Miller C, Kurian R, Jeejeebhoy KN. Nutritional absorption in short bowel syndrome. Evaluation of fluid, calorie, and divalent cation requirements. Dig Dis Sci 1987; 32:8–15.
14. McNeil NI. The contribution of the large intestine to energy supplies in man. Am J Clin Nutr 1984; 39:338–342.
15. Nordgaard I, Hansen BS, Mortensen NJ. Colon as a digestive organ in patients with short bowel. Lancet 1994; 343:373–376.
16. McIntyre PB, Fitchew M, Lennard-Jones JE. Patients with a high jejunostomy do not need a special diet. Gastroenterology 1986; 91:25–33.
17. Levy E, Frileux P, Sandrucci S et al. Continuous enteral nutrition during the early adaptive stage of the short bowel syndrome. Br J Surg 1988; 75:549–553.
18. Teubner A, Farrer K, Ravishankar HR, Shaffer JL, Carlson GL. Fistuloclysis can successfully replace parenteral feeding in acute intestinal failure. Clin Nutr 2003; 22(Suppl 1):S79.
19. Thompson JS. Surgery for patients with a short bowel. In: Nightingale JMD, ed. Intestinal failure. London: Greenwich Medical Media; 2001:515–528.
20. Bozzetti F, Mariani L, Bertinet DB et al. Central venous catheter complications in 447 patients on home parenteral nutrition: an analysis of over 100 000 catheter days. Clin Nutr 2002; 6:475–485.
21. Williams N, Carlson GL, Scott NA, Irving M. Incidence and management of catheter-related sepsis in patients receiving home parenteral nutrition. Br J Surg 1994; 81:392–394.
22. Richards DM, Scott NA, Shaffer JL, Irving M. Opiate and sedative dependence predicts a poor outcome for patients receiving home parenteral nutrition. J Parenter Enteral Nutr 1997; 21:336–338.
23. Luman W, Shaffer J. Prevalence, outcome and associated factors of deranged liver function tests in patients on home parenteral nutrition. Clin Nutr 2002; 21:337–343.
24. Cavicchi M, Beau P, Crenn P, Degott C, Messing B. Prevalence of liver disease and contributing factors in patients receiving home parenteral nutrition for permanent

intestinal failure. Ann Intern Med 2000; 132:525–532.
25. Messing B, Crenn P, Beau P, Boutron-Ruault MC, Rambaud JC, Matuchansky C. Long-term survival and parenteral nutrition dependence in adult patients with the short bowel syndrome. Gastroenterology 1999; 117:1043–1050.
26. Howard L, Malone M. Current status of home parenteral nutrition in the United States. Transplant Proc 1996; 28:2691–2695.
27. Vega R, Polymeros D, Papadia C, Hodgson R, Forbes A, Gabe S. Survival analysis in a cohort of adult patients on home parenteral nutrition. Prognostic factors related to early and overall mortality. Clin Nutr 2003; 22(Suppl 1):S88–S89.
28. Scolapio JS, Flemming CR, Kelly DG, Zinsmeister AR. Survival of home parenteral nutrition-treated patients: 20 years of experience at the Mayo Clinic. Mayo Clin Proc 1999; 74:217–222.
29. Scolapio JS, Camilleri M, Fleming CR et al. Effect of growth hormone, glutamine, and diet on adaptation in short-bowel syndrome: a randomized, controlled study. Gastroenterology 1997; 113:1074–1081.
30. Szkudlarek J, Jeppesen PB, Mortensen PB. Effect of high dose growth hormone with glutamine and no change in diet on intestinal absorption in short bowel patients: a randomised, double blind, crossover, placebo controlled study. Gut 2000; 47:199–205.
31. Seguy D, Vahedi K, Kapel N, Souberbielle JC, Messing B. Low-dose growth hormone in adult home parenteral nutrition-dependent short bowel syndrome patients: a positive study. Gastroenterology 2003; 124:293–302.
32. Jeppesen PB, Hartmann B, Thulesen J et al. Glucagon-like Peptide 2 improves nutrient absorption and nutritional status in short-bowel patients with no colon. Gastroenterology 2001; 120:806–815.
33. Middleton SJ, Pollard S, Friend PJ et al. Adult small intestinal transplantation in England and Wales. Br J Surg 2003; 90:723–727.
34. Abu-Elmagd K, Reyes J, Bond G et al. Clinical intestinal transplantation: a decade of experience at a single center. Ann Surg 2001; 234: 404–416.

Chapter 46

Small intestinal bacterial overgrowth

Rodrigo M Quera and Eamonn M M Quigley

KEY POINTS

- Normal enteric flora facilitate colonic mucosal development and help protect against pathogenic species
- Small intestinal bacterial overgrowth (SIBO) is defined as >10^5 colony-forming units (cfu)/mL bacteria in the proximal small bowel, or >10^3 cfu/mL if isolates are large bowel bacteria or absent from saliva and gastric juice
- The elderly are susceptible due to hypochlorhydria and hypomotility
- Conditions that cause stagnation or recirculation of intestinal contents predispose to small intestinal bacterial overgrowth (SIBO)
- Decreased carbohydrate absorption by enterocyte disaccharidases results in fermentation by colonic bacteria to short-chain fatty acids, causing osmotic diarrhea
- Breath tests are more reliable than jejunal aspiration and culture
- Empiric antibiotic therapy reduces symptoms in 46–90% of patients; breath tests become negative in 20–75%; repeated courses may be required

INTRODUCTION

In the healthy host, enteric bacteria colonize the alimentary tract soon after birth, and the composition of the intestinal microflora remains relatively constant throughout life. In the colon there is a complex ecosystem of approximately 400 bacterial species at a concentration of 10^{12} colony-forming units (cfu)/mL, particularly anaerobes such as bacteroides, porphyromonas, bifidobacteria, lactobacilli, and clostridia.[1] Normal enteric bacteria metabolize unabsorbed dietary sugars into short-chain fatty acids, synthesize some vitamins and facilitate colonic mucosal development. The flora promotes the low-level inflammation characteristic of normal colonic histology and helps to protect the host from colonization by pathogenic species.

Because of peristalsis and the antimicrobial effects of gastric acidity, the stomach and proximal small intestine of healthy subjects contain relatively small numbers of bacteria. Jejunal cultures may not detect any bacteria in as many as 33% of healthy people. When bacterial species are present, they are usually lactobacilli, enterococci, oral streptococci, and other Gram-positive aerobic or facultative anaerobes, reflecting the bacterial flora of the oropharynx. The bacterial counts of coliforms rarely exceed 10^3 cfu/mL in jejunal juice.

In small intestinal overgrowth, both oropharyngeal and colonic-type bacteria such as streptococcus (71%), *Escherichia coli* (69%), staphylococcus (25%), micrococcus (22%), and *Klebsiella* (20%) are common.[2] Small intestinal bacterial overgrowth is usually defined as more than 10^5 cfu bacteria per milliliter in the proximal small bowel.[3,4] Other authors have entertained the diagnosis of small intestinal bacterial overgrowth in the presence of lower colony counts (>10^3 cfu/mL), provided the species of bacteria isolated in the jejunal aspirate is that normally colonizing the large bowel, or the same species is absent from saliva and gastric juice.[4]

EPIDEMIOLOGY

The prevalence of small intestinal bacterial overgrowth is directly dependent on the characteristics of the study population and the diagnostic method employed to detect or define bacterial overgrowth. If a breath test is employed as the diagnostic method, prevalence will vary further depending on the nature and dose of substrate used (Table 46.1). In healthy people, small intestinal bacterial overgrowth has been described in 0–12.5% on the basis of the glucose breath test, in 20–22% by the lactulose breath test, and in 0–35% by the [^{14}C]D-xylose breath test. The elderly may be especially susceptible to small intestinal bacterial overgrowth owing to both a lack of gastric acid and the consumption of a disproportionately large number of drugs that can cause hypomotility. Although small intestinal bacterial overgrowth has been diagnosed in up to 35% of apparently healthy elderly subjects with hypochlorhydria by the [^{14}C]D-xylose breath test, others have described small intestinal bacterial overgrowth as an important cause of occult malabsorption in the elderly.[5]

PATHOGENESIS AND PATHOLOGY

Several host defense mechanisms determine the numbers and types of bacteria found in the small intestine. The most important defensive factors are gastric acid and small intestinal motility. In the stomach, acid kills and suppresses the growth of most organisms that enter from the oropharynx. In the small bowel, the cleansing action of aborad propulsive forces, and especially that of phase III of the interdigestive migrating motor complex (MMC), limits the ability of bacteria to colonize the small intestine. The movement of phase III, which is referred to as the 'intestinal housekeeper,' sweeps the small bowel clean between meals.[6] Other protective factors include the integrity of the intestinal mucosa and its protective mucous layer; the enzymatic activities of intestinal, pancreatic, and biliary secretions; the protective effects of some of the commensal flora, such as lactobacilli; and the mechanical and physiologic properties of the ileocecal valve.[7] Small intestinal dysmotility rather than fasting hypochlorhydria or immunodeficiency is probably

TABLE 46.1 PREVALENCE OF SMALL INTESTINAL BACTERIAL OVERGROWTH IN VARIOUS STUDY POPULATIONS

Reference	Disorder	Diagnostic test	Proportion with small intestinal bacterial overgrowth
Boissieu D J Pediatr 1996; 128:203–207	Children with chronic diarrhea and/or abdominal pain	GBT	34%
Lewindon PJ J Pediatr Child Health 1998; 34:79–82	Children with cystic fibrosis	LBT	32%
Ghoshal U BMC Gastroenterology 2003;3:9–14	Adults with malabsorption	Jejunal aspirate	42%
Castiglione F J Clin Gastroenterol 2000; 31:63–66	Crohn's disease	LBT and methane	23% (30% in patients with previous surgery, 18% in nonoperated patients)
Trespi E Curr Med Res Opin 1999; 15:47–52	Chronic pancreatitis	GBT	34%
Husebye E Gastroenterology 1995; 109:1078–1089	Radiation enteropathy	[^{14}C]d-XBT and GBT	39% detected by XBT (50% of those had negative cultures)
Virally-Monod M Diabetes Metab 1998; 24:530–536	Chronic diarrhea and diabetes mellitus	GBT	43%
Madrid AM Gastr Latinoam 2002; 5:381	Scleroderma	LBT	62.5%
Ronnblom A Eur J Gastroenterol Hepatol 1998; 10:607–610	Myotonic dystrophy	Bile acid breath test	10% had abnormal breath test
Iioven MK Scand J Gastroenterol 1998; 33:63–70	Total gastrectomy	GBT	86% of Roux-en-Y group; 91% of jejunal pouch group
Wigg AJ Gut 2001; 48:206–211	Nonalcoholic steatohepatitis	[^{14}C]d-XBT or LBT	50%
Gunnarsdottir SA Am J Gastroenterol 2003; 98:1362–1370	Liver cirrhosis	Jejunal aspirate	33% of patients with portal hypertension versus 0% of patients with cirrhosis alone
Pimentel M Am J Gastroenterol 2003; 98:412–419	Irritable bowel syndrome	LBT	84%
Tursi A Am J Gastroenterol 2003; 98:839–843	Celiac patients with persistent GI symptoms	LBT	66.7%
Riordan SM Am J Gastroenterol 1997; 92:47–51	Symptomatic elderly	Jejunal aspirate	65%

GBT, glucose breath test; LBT, lactulose breath test; XBT, xylose breath test.

the major contributor to small intestinal bacterial overgrowth in elderly subjects.

Disorders leading to alterations in one or more of these defensive systems may be associated with small intestinal bacterial overgrowth. The most common disorders associated with small intestinal bacterial overgrowth are intestinal dysmotility syndromes and chronic pancreatitis. As dysmotility predisposes to an increase in colonic bacteria in the small intestine, diseases resulting in impaired intestinal motility are likely to have small intestinal bacterial overgrowth as a complication. The cause of small intestinal bacterial overgrowth in chronic pancreatitis is multifactorial and includes a decrease in intestinal motility consequent upon the inflammatory process, the effects of narcotics on gut motility, and intestinal obstruction. Stagnation and/or recirculation of intestinal contents resulting from fistulae, enterostomies, and anastomoses also predispose to small intestinal bacterial overgrowth, thus explaining the frequent association of small intestinal bacterial overgrowth with Crohn's disease, radiation enteropathy, and reconstructive surgery.

Recently, small intestinal bacterial overgrowth has been associated with disorders such as irritable bowel syndrome (IBS),[8] celiac disease,[9] nonalcoholic fatty liver disease, and

DIFFERENTIAL DIAGNOSIS
CLINICAL CONDITIONS ASSOCIATED WITH SMALL INTESTINAL BACTERIAL OVERGROWTH
SMALL INTESTINAL STASIS
• **Anatomic abnormality**
Small intestinal diverticulosis
Surgical (Billroth II, end-to-side anastomosis)
Strictures (Crohn's disease, radiation, surgery)
• **Abnormal small intestinal motility**
Diabetic autonomic neuropathy
Scleroderma
Amyloidosis
Hypothyroidism
Idiopathic intestinal pseudobstruction
Radiation enteritis
Crohn's disease
ABNORMAL COMMUNICATION BETWEEN PROXIMAL AND DISTAL GI TRACT
Gastrocolic or jejunocolic fistula
Ileocecal valve resection
MULTIFACTORIAL
Liver disease
Irritable bowel syndrome
Celiac disease
Chronic pancreatitis
Immune deficiency (e.g., AIDS, severe malnutrition)
End-stage renal disease
The elderly

spontaneous bacterial peritonitis;[4] the true status of these associations remains uncertain. Pimentel et al.,[8] using the lactulose breath test, observed small intestinal bacterial overgrowth in 84% of patients with IBS. Normalization of the lactulose breath test in this group, by use of neomycin, resulted in a significant improvement in IBS symptoms. Furthermore, methane excretion, on breath testing, was highly associated with a constipation-predominant subgroup of IBS. The same group found that their IBS patients with small intestinal bacterial overgrowth exhibited both a lower number and duration of phase III of the MMC on antroduodenal manometry, in comparison to control subjects.

Tursi et al.[9] reported that 67% of their celiac patients with persistent gastrointestinal symptoms following gluten withdrawal had small intestinal bacterial overgrowth when studied using the lactulose breath test; eradication of the bacterial overgrowth led to disappearance of their, admittedly nonspecific, symptoms.

Lastly, studies have reported a relationship between the presence of small intestinal bacterial overgrowth and liver disease, as well as some of its complications. Gunnarsdottir et al.[10] found that their cirrhotic patients with portal hypertension had a higher prevalence of small intestinal bacterial overgrowth, diagnosed on the basis of culture of a jejunal aspirate, than those without portal hypertension.

In contrast to prior studies, which used the glucose breath test, Bauer et al.[4] did not find an association between small intestinal bacterial overgrowth, diagnosed by jejunal aspirate, and the risk of developing spontaneous bacterial peritonitis.

SMALL INTESTINAL DIVERTICULA

Small intestinal bacterial overgrowth is associated with small intestinal diverticulosis. *This generally differs from colonic diverticula in being wide-necked.*

Duodenal diverticula have been reported in 2–5% of patients undergoing barium studies of the upper gastrointestinal tract and in 7% of patients undergoing endoscopic retrograde cholangiopancreatography. They occur in equal numbers of men and women, and are most commonly found in patients over 40 years of age. Their pathogenesis is unclear and some may be at the site of previous ulceration. Diverticular stasis and bacterial contamination predispose to pigment stones. The etiology of diverticula is not clearly defined, but the 'locus minoris resistentiae' theory remains the most widely accepted. The majority of duodenal diverticula are extraluminal (i.e., acquired as a result of mucosal herniation through the defect related to the entrance of the major vessels), and are associated with the development of pigment stones, as a result of stasis within the diverticulum, and bacterial contamination of the biliary tree. In contrast, intraluminal diverticula result from defective recanalization of the duodenal lumen during fetal development and are associated with malformations of the intestinal tract. Fewer than 10% are symptomatic and only 1% require definitive treatment.

Diverticula in the jejunum occur in 0.07–2% of the population; they tend to be large and multiple, whereas those in the ileum are small and single. These features explain the observation that symptoms and complications, such as small intestinal bacterial overgrowth, have been reported in 10–40% and 6–40% of jejunal and ileal diverticula respectively. Jejunal diverticula are twice as frequent in men and are observed predominantly among those aged over 60 years. Morphologic studies suggest that disorders of intestinal motility such as progressive systemic sclerosis, visceral myopathies, and neuropathies play an important role in the formation of the small bowel diverticula.[11] Abnormalities of the MMC such as clustered contractions during phase II and a reduced frequency of phase III have been found in some patients.

Complications of jejunal diverticula include small intestinal bacterial overgrowth (3–12%) secondary to stasis, which can, in turn, lead to malabsorption and/or inflammation of the diverticula. Diverticulitis in small intestinal diverticula is, however, rare (2–3%), probably related to the more liquid composition of the jejunal and ileal contents and the broad-mouthed nature of the diverticula, which allows more ready recirculation of intestinal contents in comparison to colonic diverticula. If diverticulitis occurs it may lead to perforation and abscess formation within the mesentery. Gastrointestinal bleeding (4–5%), volvulus, pseudo-obstruction (10–25%), intussusception, and ileoabdominal fistula have also been reported. Asymptomatic jejunoileal diverticula should be managed conservatively; when symptoms are severe and persistent, or complications develop, resection of the affected bowel segment is indicated.

EFFECTS OF SMALL INTESTINAL BACTERIAL OVERGROWTH ON THE GASTROINTESTINAL TRACT

Bacterial colonization damages the small intestine via protease release, generation of oxygen radicals, release of enterotoxins, and the secondary effects of cobalamin deficiency and production of deconjugated bile acids such as lithocholic acid.

Carbohydrate malabsorption results from a combination of carbohydrate degradation by bacteria and a loss of the activity of brush border disaccharidases resulting from enterocyte damage. The resultant unabsorbed carbohydrates are then available for metabolism by small bowel and colonic bacteria to short-chain organic acids. The latter increase the osmolarity of intestinal fluid, thereby contributing to diarrhea. Furthermore, mucosal injury interferes with carbohydrate uptake.

Protein malnutrition is also multifactorial and results from intraluminal utilization of dietary protein by bacteria, impaired absorption, and the development of a protein-losing enteropathy. In one-third of patients, small intestinal bacterial overgrowth is severe enough to cause deficiencies of vitamins, such as vitamin B_{12} and fat-soluble vitamins (A, D, and E).

Although the gross histologic features of the small bowel are usually normal, bacterial overgrowth may be associated with a reduction in villus height, crypt depth, and mucosal thickness, an increase in the number of intraepithelial lymphocytes, and focal areas of ulceration and erosion.

These changes are reversible following successful antibiotic treatment. Anaerobic or facultatively anaerobic species contain proteases that are capable of removing components of the intestinal surface membrane and may be involved in the etiology of disaccharidase deficiency in small intestinal bacterial overgrowth. In the ileum, xanthine oxidase-generated oxidants are important in the pathogenesis of endotoxin-induced mucosal injury. Luminal concentrations of immunoglobulin (Ig) A_2, IgM, and interleukin-6, but not interferon-gamma or tumor necrosis factor-alpha, are significantly increased in the proximal small intestine of subjects with small intestinal bacterial overgrowth, particularly when the overgrowth includes colonic-type bacteria.[12]

Other possible consequences of small intestinal bacterial overgrowth

Although the gut plays a role in the development of sepsis and multiple organ failure syndromes, recent studies have shown that gut-derived bacteremia appears to be an insufficient stimulus for the systemic inflammatory responses typically seen in the context of severe and prolonged catabolic stress.[13] The gut flora has also been implicated in the pathogenesis of steatohepatitis and related liver pathology in the context of alcohol abuse, obesity, jejunoileal bypass, intestinal failure, and other causes.

CLINICAL PRESENTATION

The clinical manifestations of bacterial overgrowth vary greatly and depend on the severity of small intestinal bacterial overgrowth, as well as on the underlying cause.

Although symptoms may be nonspecific, some, such as the combination of diarrhea, steatorrhea, postprandial bloating, and vitamin deficiency, may be regarded as highly suggestive of small intestinal bacterial overgrowth. However, in many instances, symptoms related to small intestinal bacterial overgrowth are nonspecific and are readily confused with those related to IBS, functional dyspepsia, celiac disease, and Crohn's disease.

Laboratory investigations may reveal anemia, which is usually macrocytic because of malabsorption of vitamin B_{12} as a result of the binding and incorporation of this vitamin into the bacteria. Levels of both folate and vitamin K are, however, usually normal or raised in the context of small intestinal bacterial overgrowth as a result of bacterial synthesis of these vitamins. Microcytic anemia can result from bleeding from ulcers or erosions, if present. In advanced cases, micronutrient deficiency and evidence of malnutrition may also be present.

CLINICAL PRESENTATION

SYMPTOMS
Abdominal discomfort
Bloating
Flatulence
Diarrhea OR steatorrhea
Nausea
Weight loss
Neuropathy

CLINICAL FINDINGS
Fat and carbohydrate malabsorption
Vitamin deficiencies – Cobalamin (vitamine B_{12}) and fat-soluble vitamins (A, D, E, K)
Hypoproteinemia and hypoalbuminemia
Iron deficiency

DIAGNOSTIC METHODS

The diagnosis should be entertained in any patient with a clinical condition known to be associated with small intestinal bacterial overgrowth and who has gastrointestinal symptoms compatible with bacterial overgrowth (Fig. 46.1). Controversy continues to surround the diagnosis of bacterial overgrowth; several invasive and noninvasive diagnostic methods of differing sensitivity and specificity are available.

DIAGNOSTIC METHODS

Test	Sensitivity (%)	Specificity (%)	Ease of performance
Culture of jejunal aspirate	100	100	Poor
Culture of small bowel biopsy	90.3	100	Poor
[^{14}C]-D-xylose breath test	14.3–95	100	Excellent
Glucose breath test	6–93	78–100	Excellent
Lactulose breath test	6–68	44–70	Excellent
Rice breath hydrogen	33–81	67–91	Excellent
G–L chromatography of jejunal fluid[a]	56	100	Poor
Bile acid breath test	33–70	60–76	Excellent

[a] Gas–liquid chromatography for volatile fatty acids.

Aspiration and direct culture of jejunal contents is regarded by many as the gold standard for the diagnosis of small intestinal bacterial overgrowth.[14] However, this method has several limitations, including the potential for contamination by oropharyngeal bacteria during the procedure itself, the observation that bacterial overgrowth may be patchy and thus

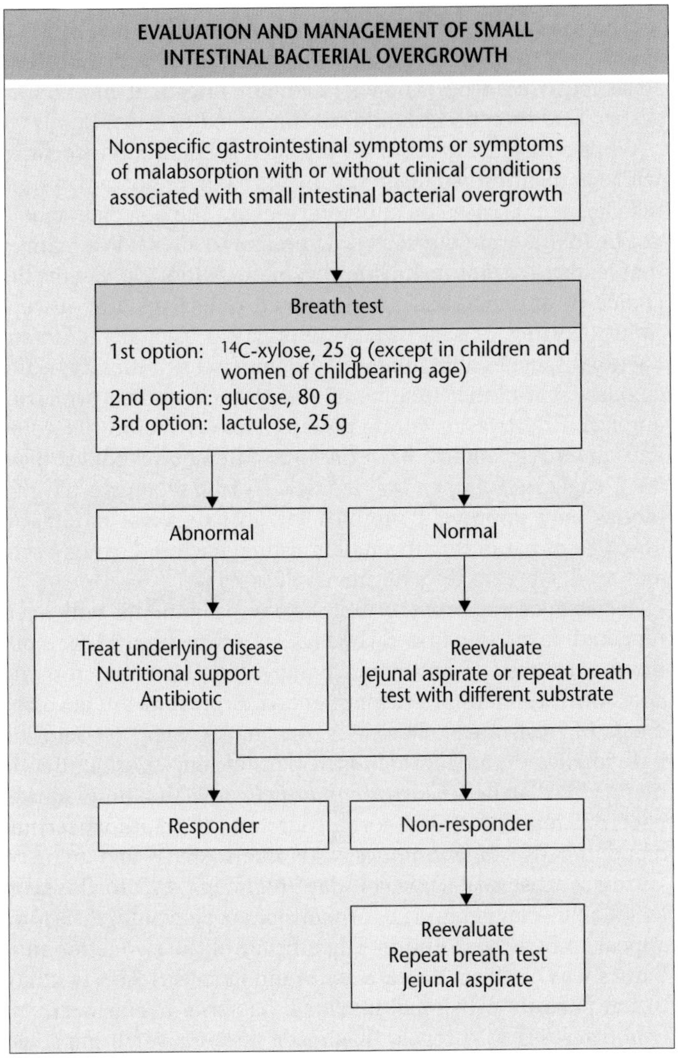

Fig. 46.1 Evaluation and management of small intestinal bacterial overgrowth.

missed by a single aspiration, and the possibility that overgrowth may involve only the more distal portions of the small bowel that are out of reach for conventional intubation techniques. Furthermore, the culture of anaerobic organisms requires meticulous microbiologic technique and an unknown proportion of the gut flora are not culturable by available methods. Studies have revealed a significant correlation between the closed and open-ended tube systems in both quantitative and qualitative terms. Therefore, contamination arising from the open sampling system appears to be of limited importance in the diagnosis of small intestinal bacterial overgrowth. Overall, the reproducibility of jejunal aspiration and culture has been reported to be as low as 38%, in comparison to 92% for breath tests. In addition, aspiration methods may be regarded as cumbersome and invasive for a patient with nonspecific symptoms. For this reason, a variety of different noninvasive diagnostic tests have been devised for the diagnosis of small intestinal bacterial overgrowth.[15]

Breath tests (see also Chapter 131): The principle behind these tests is the administration of a dose of carbohydrate (D-xylose, lactulose, or glucose) that, when metabolized by the contaminating flora, leads to the production of hydrogen, which is absorbed and ultimately excreted in the breath. Because hydrogen production is a normal phenomenon, patient preparation is vital for test accuracy. Therefore, the ingestion of certain foods such as bread, fiber, and pasta, cigarette smoking, oral bacteria, and lung disease can affect diagnostic accuracy. In these tests, the diagnosis of small intestinal bacterial overgrowth is established when the concentration of hydrogen exhaled increases by more than 10 parts per million (ppm) over baseline on two consecutive samplings, or when the fasting breath hydrogen level exceeds 20 ppm. This latter finding is especially prevalent among patients with untreated celiac disease. Fermentation of residual carbohydrate by oropharyngeal bacteria may also contribute to raised levels of hydrogen and thus to an overestimation of the fasting breath hydrogen level. Rinsing the mouth with a chlorhexidine-containing mouthwash prior to breath collection can solve this problem.

The **reliability** of breath tests has been criticized; their interpretation may be especially problematic in the context of disorders associated with impaired gastric emptying (false-negative results) or rapid intestinal transit (false-positive results). Furthermore, studies have demonstrated that between 15% and 27% of the population will not produce hydrogen in these circumstances; breath tests reliant on the measurement of hydrogen alone may, therefore, provide a significant number of false-negative results. The combination of measurements of both hydrogen and methane, which are both end-products of anaerobic bacterial metabolism in the intestine, may avoid this problem.

Xylose, given a dose of 1 g, is predominantly catabolized by Gram-negative organisms and, as such, is an excellent substrate for the diagnosis of small intestinal bacterial overgrowth. The sensitivity and specificity of the xylose breath test appears to be better than that of other breath tests. As the administration of ^{14}C is associated with radiation exposure, the [^{13}C]xylose breath test, using a stable isotope, has been used as an alternative in children and women of childbearing age.

The **lactulose breath test**, on the other hand, is safe, easy to perform, and applicable to children and women of childbearing age. As lactulose is not absorbed in the normal small intestine, normal individuals should produce a peak at 2–3 h (Fig. 46.2A), reflecting the arrival of the substrate into the colon – assuming that the colonic flora is intact. In small intestinal bacterial overgrowth, another peak occurs within 1 h of ingestion, and is less prominent than the colonic peak (Fig. 46.2B). Double peaks do not always signify small intestinal bacterial overgrowth, and may also result from rapid orocecal transit, resulting in the premature delivery of the fermentable substrate to cecal bacteria.

For this reason, the combination of a lactulose breath test with transit scintigraphy may increase the specificity of the former to 100%; sensitivity remains low at 39%, however. Moreover, 'flat' responses to lactulose may be found in those with altered bacterial flora (from antibiotic administration or diarrheal diseases), motility disorders, or prominent methane production. Patients should wait a least 1 week after completion of antibiotic therapy before presenting for a lactulose breath test.

Glucose breath test: As glucose is rapidly absorbed from the proximal small bowel, only proximal overgrowth can be detected by this test. The fact that any peak is abnormal in this test is its main advantage over those using nonabsorbable substrates such as lactulose.[15]

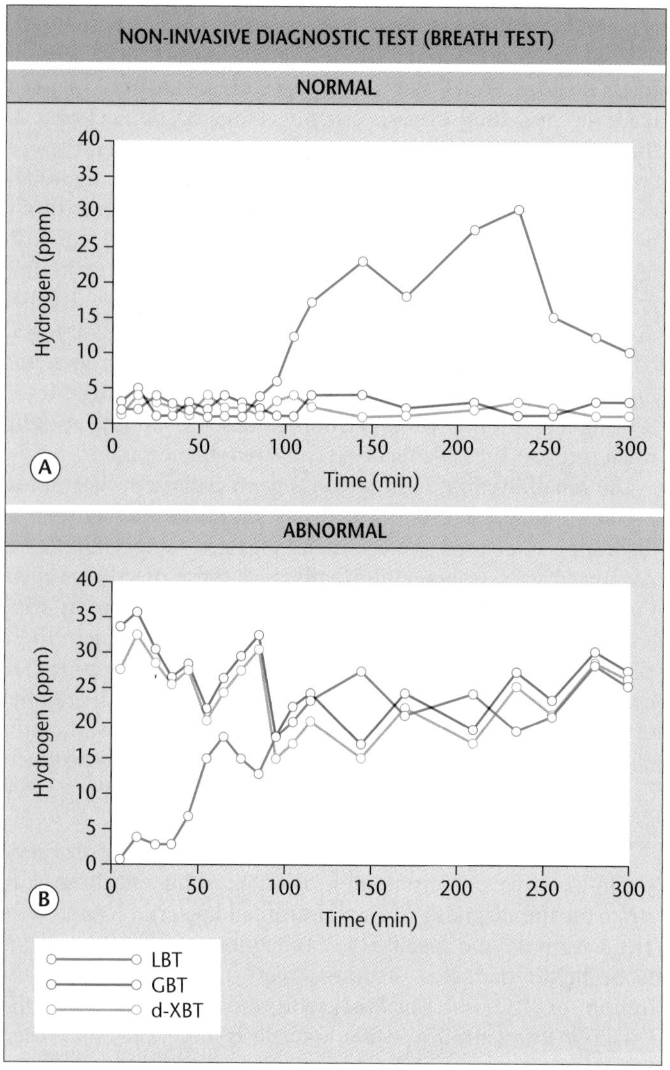

Fig. 46.2 Noninvasive diagnostic test (breath test). Normal (A) and abnormal (B) d-xylose breath test (d-XBT), glucose hydrogen breath test (GBT), and lactulose breath test (LBT)

In patients with vitamin B_{12} deficiency, small intestinal bacterial overgrowth may be diagnosed by performing the final stage of the Schilling test; in this instance, antibiotic administration normalizes the absorption of vitamin B_{12}.

TREATMENT

Although small intestinal bacterial overgrowth may be found in up to 35% of healthy subjects, the combination of compatible gastrointestinal symptoms and a positive result from a test for bacterial overgrowth should lead to a decision to treat (see Fig. 46.1).

There are three components to the treatment of small intestinal bacterial overgrowth:

- treating the underlying disease
- eradicating overgrowth
- addressing any associated nutritional deficiencies

Clearly, the primary goal should be the treatment or correction of any underlying disease or defect, when possible. Unfortunately, several of the clinical conditions associated with small intestinal bacterial overgrowth, such as visceral myopathies and multiple jejunal diverticula, are not readily reversible. It stands to reason that medications associated with intestinal stasis, such as drugs known to inhibit intestinal motility or gastric acid secretion, should be eliminated or substituted.

When surgical correction of the clinical condition associated with small intestinal bacterial overgrowth is not an option, management is based on antibiotic therapy. The objective should not be to eradicate the bacterial flora but to alter it in a manner that leads to symptomatic improvement. Although, ideally, the choice of antimicrobial agents should reflect in vitro susceptibility testing, this is usually impractical as many different bacterial species, with different antibiotic sensitivities, typically coexist. Antibiotic treatment therefore remains primarily empiric. Effective antibiotic therapy must cover both aerobic and anaerobic enteric bacteria, and different schedules have been suggested. In general, a single 7–10-day course of antibiotics may improve symptoms for up to several months in 46–90% of patients with small intestinal bacterial overgrowth, and render breath tests negative in 20–75%.

Because of recurrent symptoms, some patients will need repeated (e.g., the first 5–10 days of every month) or continuous courses of antibiotic therapy. For the latter, rotating antibiotic regimens are recommended to prevent the development of resistance. Decisions on management should be individualized and consider such risks of long-term antibiotic therapy as diarrhea, *Clostridium difficile* infection, intolerance, bacterial resistance, and costs. Therefore, the authors recommend the use of antibiotics with low toxicity and reduced systemic absorption. Seven-day regimens of norfloxacin, amoxicillin–clavulanic acid, or metronidazole would, therefore, appear to be a good option. The efficacy of the two latter antibiotics was confirmed in a recent randomized crossover study of ten patients with small intestinal bacterial overgrowth.[16] It is not necessary to repeat diagnostic tests for small intestinal bacterial overgrowth following antibiotic therapy, should gastrointestinal symptoms respond.

TREATMENT AND PREVENTION
ANTIBIOTIC THERAPY FOR SMALL INTESTINAL BACTERIAL OVERGROWTH
Ciprofloxacin (250 mg BID)
Norfloxacin (800 mg/day)
Metronidazole (250 mg TID)
Trimethoprim–sulfamethoxazole (1 double strength BID)
Doxycycline (100 mg BID)
Amoxicillin–clavulanic acid (500 mg TID)
Tetracycline (250 mg QID)
Chloramphenicol (250 mg QID)
Neomycin (500 mg BID)

Although recent studies have reported some effects for 'probiotic' microbial supplements in the treatment and evolution of some gastrointestinal diseases such as inflammatory bowel diseases and IBS, results in patients with small intestinal bacterial overgrowth have been inconclusive. The value of adding prokinetic agents such as cisapride and erythromycin is uncertain. Moreover, cisapride has been withdrawn in many countries because of cardiovascular side effects. As octreotide stimulates propagative phase III activity in the small intestine, low doses (50 mg per day) have been advocated for patients who do not respond to antibiotics, cannot tolerate them, or develop antibiotic-related complications. Nonabsorbable purgative solutions may improve gastrointestinal symptoms in children with short bowel syndrome and small intestinal bacterial overgrowth.

Nutritional support is an important component of the management of small intestinal bacterial overgrowth. Dietary modifications may include a lactose-free diet, replacement of vitamin deficiencies (especially fat-soluble vitamins), and correction of deficiencies in nutrients such as calcium, magnesium, and vitamin B_{12}. As mucosal damage may persist for some time after the eradication of bacterial overgrowth, nutritional support may be required over a prolonged period of time.

SUMMARY

Small intestinal bacterial overgrowth is characterized by nutrient malabsorption associated with excessive numbers of bacteria in the proximal small intestine. The diagnosis of bacterial overgrowth continues to represent a diagnostic challenge; there is no widespread agreement with regard to the optimal diagnostic test. Small intestinal bacterial overgrowth occurs when there are alterations in intestinal anatomy or gastrointestinal motility, or a lack of gastric acid secretion. The nature of the association, if any, between small intestinal bacterial overgrowth and IBS and celiac disease remains to be defined. Treatment of small intestinal bacterial overgrowth usually relies on the eradication of bacterial overgrowth by empiric antibiotic therapy, the provision of nutritional support, as required, and, when possible, the correction of any reversible underlying or predisposing condition.

SOURCES OF INFORMATION FOR PATIENTS AND DOCTORS

http://www.emedicine.com/med/topic198.htm

REFERENCES

1. Simon GL, Gorbach SL. The human intestinal microflora. Dig Dis Sci 1986; 31:147–162.
2. Bouknik Y, Alain S, Attar A. Bacterial populations contaminating the upper gut in patients with small intestinal overgrowth syndrome. Am J Gastroenterol 1999; 94:1327–1331.
3. Toskes PP. Bacterial overgrowth of the gastrointestinal tract. Adv Intern Med 1993; 38:387–407.
4. Bauer T, Steinbrückner B, Brinkmann F et al. Small intestinal bacterial overgrowth in patients with cirrhosis: prevalence and relation with spontaneous bacterial peritonitis. Am J Gastroenterol 2001; 96:2962–2967.
5. McEvoy A, Dutton J, James OF. Bacterial contamination of the small intestine is an important cause of occult malabsorption in the elderly. BMJ 1983; 287:789–793.
6. Vantrappen G, Janssens J, Coremans G et al. Gastrointestinal motility disorders. Dig Dis Sci 1986; 31:5S–25S.
7. Khloloussy AM, Yang Y, Bonacquisti K et al. The competence and bacteriologic effect of the telescoped intestinal valve after small bowel resection. Am Surg 1986; 52:555–559.
8. Pimentel M, Chow EJ, Lin HC. Normalization of lactulose breath testing correlates with symptom improvement in irritable bowel syndrome: a double-blind, randomized, placebo-controlled study. Am J Gastroenterol 2003; 98:412–419.
9. Tursi A, Brandimarte G, Giorgetti G. High prevalence of small intestinal bacterial overgrowth in celiac patients with perseverance of gastrointestinal symptoms after gluten withdrawal. Am J Gastroenterol 2003; 98:839–843.
10. Gunnarsdottir S, Sadik R, Shev S et al. Small intestinal motility disturbances and bacterial overgrowth in patients with liver cirrhosis and portal hypertension. Am J Gastroenterol 2003; 98:1362–1370.
11. Krishnamurthy S, Kelly MM, Rohrmann CA et al. Jejunal diverticulosis: a heterogeneous disorder caused by a variety of abnormalities of smooth muscle or myenteric plexus. Gastroenterology 1983; 85:538–547.
12. Riordan SM, McIver CJ, Wakefield D et al. Mucosal cytokine production in small-intestinal bacterial overgrowth. Scand J Gastroenterol 1996; 31:977–984.
13. Alberdi J, Laughlin R, Lichen WU. Influence of the critically ill state on host–pathogen interactions within the intestine: gut-derived sepsis redefined. Crit Care Med 2003; 31:598–607.
14. Corazza GR, Menozzi MG, Strocchi A et al. The diagnosis of small bowel bacterial overgrowth. Gastroenterology 1990; 98:302–309.
15. Romagnuolo J, Schiller D, Bailey R. Using breath tests wisely in a gastroenterology practice: an evidence-based review of indications and pitfalls in interpretation. Am J Gastroenterol 2002; 97:1113–1126.
16. Attar A, Flourié B, Rambaud JC et al. Antibiotic efficacy in small intestinal bacterial overgrowth-related chronic diarrhea: a crossover, randomized trial. Gastroenterology 1999; 117:794–797.

Chapter 47

Bile acid malabsorption

Matthias Stelzner and Sum P Lee

KEY POINTS
• Terminal ileum is the only site capable of congregated bile acids • Bacterial overgrowth causes deconjugation and impaired absorption • Bile acid malabsorption (BAM) results in fat malabsorption, renal oxalate stones, and cholesterol gallstones • The commonest cause of secondary BAM is ileum resection • The mainstay of treatment is cholestyramine and loperamide • The synthetic conjugation bile acid cholysarcosine shows promise as a future therapy

INTRODUCTION

Bile acids are steroid molecules that are synthesized from cholesterol in the liver. They are then conjugated through their carboxyl group with glycine or taurine and secreted into the bile, and travel with the biliary flow into the duodenum. Hepatic conjugation of bile acids is very efficient and only 1% appears in the bile in unconjugated form. The chemical transformation renders the molecules more polar by increasing the hydrophilicity. Conjugated bile acids are more soluble in the acidic environment of the duodenum and readily form mixed micelles that help to solubilize fatty acids in the intestinal lumen.[1] The fatty acids can then be absorbed at the mucosal surface. The small percentage of unconjugated bile acids can be reabsorbed in the jejunum and ileum by diffusion. These deconjugated molecules return to the liver via the portal vein, are reconjugated, and again secreted into the bile.

In contrast, conjugated bile acid molecules are only poorly absorbed due to their larger size and higher polarity. They therefore travel with the ingesta through the jejunum before being taken up in the ileum. This allows for thorough mixing and optimal fat absorption. This absorption occurs via an energy-consuming transport mechanism. At the center of this uptake process is the ileal bile acid transporter (IBAT). This transport protein was cloned by Wong and coworkers in 1994[2] and is expressed in large quantities only on the mucosal surface of terminal ileum and in lower amounts in the renal tubule and the intrahepatic bile ducts. The uptake process is highly efficient and less than half a gram of bile acids per day is normally lost into the colon. IBAT transports conjugated bile acids across the apical membrane of the ileal enterocyte. They are then shuttled into the portal vein and return to the liver. The bile acid pool consists of 2–4 g of bile acids, which are cycled in this 'enterohepatic circulation' 5–10 times each day.[1] Inhibition of the passive absorption of bile acids, significant deconjugation, e.g., due to bacterial overgrowth in the small bowel, or any disturbance of the active uptake process in the ileum will result in bile acid malabsorption. Bile acid malabsorption leads to a spillover of significant amounts of conjugated and deconjugated bile acids into the colon and results in secretory diarrhea. In addition, bile acid malabsorption has indirect effects. Resultant malabsorption of fat and increased cecal permeability increases intestinal oxalate absorption and leads to an increased risk of urolithiasis[3] and the diminished bile acid pool is thought to increase the risk for the formation of cholesterol gallstones.[4]

CAUSES

Bile acid malabsorption may be idiopathic (Table 47.1), but the most common cause of secondary bile acid malabsorption is surgical resection of the ileum, often carried out because of Crohn's ileitis or as part of urologic procedures (e.g., bladder reconstruction, ileal conduit). There are reports of pediatric patients with an autosomal recessive inborn form of bile acid malabsorption due to mutations of the IBAT gene.[5] Such mutations impair the expression of functional IBAT transport proteins resulting in cholegenic diarrhea. However, other data suggest that forms of bile acid malabsorption with adult onset are not linked to gene mutations.[6] The decrease in IBAT activity may occur due to regulatory processes that are as yet unknown. Some disease conditions result in bile acid malabsorption in spite of an increase in IBAT activity. For example, Stelzner and coworkers showed that CFTR-knockout mice with cystic fibrosis display a fourfold upregulation of IBAT activity and IBAT protein expression, although cystic fibrosis is clinically associated with bile acid malabsorption.[7] These data indicate that other luminal factors, e.g., the mucin layer on the surface of the mucosa, may play a causative role in bile acid malabsorption.

TABLE 47.1 CAUSES OF SECONDARY BILE ACID MALABSORPTION
Crohn's ileitis
AIDS enteropathy
Cystic fibrosis
Hyperthyroidism
Radiation enteritis
Ileal resection (e.g., for ileitis, tumor, bladder reconstruction)
Vagotomy
Cholecystectomy
Small intestinal bacterial overgrowth syndrome

SYMPTOMS

Diarrhea is the leading symptom associated with bile acid malabsorption. Some patients also develop cholelithiasis and may present with symptoms suggestive of gallstone disease. A syndrome of taurine deficiency leading to growth retardation and weight loss has been described in children suffering from bile acid malabsorption.[8]

DIAGNOSTIC METHODS

While the cause of bile acid malabsorption is often obvious in patients who have undergone ileal resections or abdominal radiation therapy, others may require tests to make the diagnosis. The largest patient group requiring such work-up usually includes patients with unclear chronic diarrhea. A thorough gastroenterologic work-up with enteroscopy colonoscopy and ileoscopy is often the best first step to finding morphologic changes. The determination of 24-h fecal bile acid excretions can confirm abnormal bile acid losses. Insufficient intestinal absorption of bile acids can be demonstrated by a ^{14}C-cholylglycine breath test. In this test, nonabsorbed radioactive cholylglycine enters the colon and is then rapidly deconjugated by colonic bacteria. The ^{14}C-glycine is metabolized and $^{14}CO_2$ is measured in the breath. However, this test may be falsely positive in conditions with bacterial overgrowth in the small intestine. Another option, the selenium-75-homocholic acid taurine (SeHCAT) test, is simple and more reliable than the breath test. SeHCAT, a synthetic bile acid, is administered orally and gamma radiation over the abdomen is quantified repeatedly during the following 7 days.

DIAGNOSTIC METHODS
• General gastroenterologic work-up (incl. enteroscopy, colonoscopy, and ileoscopy) • 24-h fecal bile acid excretion • Serum concentrations of bile acid precursors • ^{14}C-Cholylglycine breath test • Selenium-75-homocholic acid taurine (SeHCAT) test[a] • Schilling test with added intrinsic factor (as indirect test for bile acid malabsorption)

[a] In many units, this is the main specific test used.

Like natural bile acids, SeHCAT will remain in the enterohepatic circulation for a long time, unless significant losses into the feces occur due to ileal malabsorption. Although widely used elsewhere, this test is not currently available in the USA. Consequently, in contrast to Europe and other regions, bile acid metabolism is rarely studied in the USA outside a research setting.[9] Here, most patients receive a trial of bile acid binders, and if this is successful the diarrhea is considered to be due to bile acid malabsorption. Occasionally, a Schilling test with added intrinsic factor is performed since it is widely available and can provide evidence for ileal dysfunction; this is viewed as an indirect test for bile acid malabsorption. Potentially more convenient serum tests have been proposed but are not in widespread use. For example, serum concentrations of 7α-hydroxy-4-cholesten-3-one, an intermediate of bile acid synthesis, represent a good measure for bile acid production. It is elevated in patients with bile acid malabsorption and correlates well with SeHCAT tests.

TREATMENT

Agents that bind bile acids such as cholestyramine or colestipol have long been the mainstay of symptomatic treatment for bile acid malabsorption (Table 47.2). Adsorption of bile acids to these resins removes bile acids from the aqueous phase of the ingesta and abolishes their secretory effects in the colon. As an adjunct, agents that decrease small intestinal transit time, such as loperamide 2–4 mg 1–3 times a day, may be helpful in cases where rapid transit is found to be a contributing factor to bile acid malabsorption in the ileum. In recent years, some groups have reported beneficial effects on fat and bile acid malabsorption when the synthetic conjugated bile acid cholylsarcosine is administered to patients with short bowel syndrome and remaining colon.[10] These patients often have significant fat and bile acid malabsorption and a major deficit in circulating bile acids. While patients with an ileostomy may be treated effectively with naturally occurring bile acids, those with a colon segment will develop severe secretory diarrhea. Cholylsarcosine has the advantage over naturally occurring bile acids in that it is resistant to deconjugation and subsequent dehydroxylation by colonic bacteria; therefore, it can help with fat absorption but has no secretory side effects. The cloning of the ileal bile acid transporter IBAT has generated the possibility of mucosal gene therapy for the treatment of congenital ileal bile acid malabsorption, but its clinical application is likely to be many years in the future.

SOURCES OF INFORMATION FOR PATIENTS AND DOCTORS

http://patients.uptodate.com/topic.asp?file=digestiv/4974

TABLE 47.2 THERAPEUTIC OPTIONS FOR BILE ACID MALABSORPTION
Agents that bind bile acids (cholestyramine, colestipol)
Antibiotics (if due to bacterial overgrowth)
Small bowel resection (e.g., bacterial overgrowth due to jejunal diverticulum)
Constipating agents, e.g., loperamide
Natural or synthetic bile acids

REFERENCES

1. Hofmann AF. Biliary secretion and excretion. The hepatobiliary component of the enterohepatic circulation of bile acids. In: Johnson LR, ed. Physiology of the gastrointestinal tract. New York: Raven Press; 1994:1555–1576.
2. Wong MH, Oelkers P, Craddock AL, Dawson PA. Expression cloning and characterization of the hamster ileal sodium-dependent bile acid transporter. J Biol Chem 1994; 269:1340–1347.
3. Smith LH, Fromm H, Hofmann AF. Acquired hyperoxaluria, nephrolithiasis, and intestinal disease. N Engl J Med 1972; 286:1371–1375.
4. Farkkila MA. Biliary cholesterol and lithogeneity of bile in patients after ileal resection. Surgery 1988; 104:18–25.
5. Oelkers P, Kirby LC, Heubi JE, Dawson PA. Primary bile acid malabsorption caused by mutations in the ileal sodium-dependent bile acid transporter gene (SLC10A2). J Clin Invest 1997; 99:1880–1887.
6. Montagnani M, Love MW, Rossel P, Dawson PA, Qvist P. Absence of dysfunctional ileal sodium-bile acid cotransporter gene mutations in patients with adult-onset idiopathic bile acid malabsorption. Scand J Gastroenterol 2001; 36:1077–1080.
7. Stelzner M, Somasundaram S. Ileal bile acid transporter (IBAT) function and density are increased in mice with cystic fibrosis. Gastroenterology 1999; 116:A:G4060.
8. O'Brien S, Mulcahy H, Fenlon H, O'Broin A, Casey M, Burke A. Intestinal bile acid malabsorption in cystic fibrosis. Gut 1993; 34: 1137–1141.
9. Eusufzai S, Axelson M, Angelin B, Einarsson K. Serum 7 alpha-hydroxy-4-cholesten-3-one concentrations in the evaluation of bile acid malabsorption in patients with diarrhoea: correlation to SeHCAT test. Gut 1993; 34: 698–701.
10. Heydorn S, Jeppesen PB, Mortensen PB. Bile acid replacement therapy with cholylsarcosine for short-bowel syndrome. Scand J Gastroenterol 1999; 34:818–823.

Chapter 48

Protein-losing disorders of the gastrointestinal tract

Simon Murch

KEY POINTS

- Protein-losing enteropathy (PLE) is due to loss of epithelial barrier function or raised venous/lymphatic pressure
- The cause of PLE may be diffuse (e.g. IBD) or focal (e.g. Ménétrier's disease)
- Kwashiorkor is the commonest and most lethal cause
- The end result, hypoalbuminemia, mimics nephrotic syndrome; renal losses should be excluded from the differential diagnosis
- Symptoms are due to protein loss and underlying vitamin and mineral deficiencies
- Investigations should be guided by the patient's age and general assessment but may include albumin, globulins, renal functions, OGD, gastroscopy, colonoscopy, barium follow through, and hydrogen breath test
- Prognosis is determined by whether treatment can be directed at the underlying cause

INTRODUCTION

Many conditions can cause excess leakage of protein from the gastrointestinal tract. Such protein loss can be severe and life threatening, and in conditions such as inflammatory bowel disease can reach 20g or more daily.[1] Protein-losing enteropathy (PLE) can occur as part of a more generalized impairment of intestinal function, and may be accompanied by secretory diarrhea and malabsorption. In other conditions, particularly if caused by raised hydrostatic pressure within the lymphatic system, protein losses may be predominant, and only fat absorption compromised.

The source of protein loss may be restricted to the stomach, associated with giant hypertrophy of the gastric rugae (Ménétrier's disease), or may be due to either focal or diffuse pathology within the small intestine or colon. The causes of excess enteric protein loss can broadly be divided into two groups, due either to loss of barrier function of the epithelium and its basement membrane, or to raised pressure within the lymphatics or mesenteric veins.

The prognosis of acute enteric protein-losing states is generally good, unless part of a broader pathological process. By contrast, chronic protein-losing conditions of more than moderate severity can have a poor prognosis.

EPIDEMIOLOGY

There are a large number of potential causes of protein-losing enteropathy, and the epidemiology of these underlying causes will largely determine local incidence (Table 48.1).

The most common cause of excess enteric protein loss worldwide is tropical enteropathy and particularly kwashiorkor, which kill millions of children annually (see below). In the developed world, inflammatory bowel disease remains one of the most common causes of persistent intestinal protein loss. Malnutrition itself may predispose to increased enteric protein loss, and

TABLE 48.1 CAUSES OF EXCESSIVE INTESTINAL PROTEIN LOSS

LYMPHATIC OBSTRUCTION
- Congenital – lymphangiectasia; this may be focal or extensive, and may be associated with lymphedema of the legs
- Acquired, e.g., tuberculosis, retroperitoneal fibrosis, Whipple's disease, sarcoidosis, lymphoma, radiotherapy, endometriosis

EXCESSIVE MESENTERIC VENOUS PRESSURE
- Constrictive pericarditis, congestive cardiac failure
- Malrotation
- Cyanotic congenital cardiac disease following Fontan surgery

LOSS OF THE GUT EPITHELIAL BARRIER

(a) Ulcerating lesions
- Gastric, duodenal, or esophageal ulceration
- IBD – Crohn's disease, ulcerative colitis, indeterminate colitis
- Atypical colitides – lymphocytic colitis, collagenous colitis
- Pseudomembranous colitis
- Graft-versus-host disease
- Amyloidosis
- Malignancy – mucosal tumors or carcinoid syndrome
- Kaposi's sarcoma
- Ulcerative jejuno-ileitis

(b) Nonulcerating lesions

Congenital (rare)
- Heparan sulfate deficiency
- Congenital disorders of glycosylation

Acquired (common)
- Tropical enteropathy and kwashiorkor (most common worldwide cause)
- Giant hypertrophic gastritis (Ménétrier's disease)
- Enteropathies, e.g., celiac disease, autoimmune enteropathy, cystic fibrosis
- Mucosal eosinophilia, e.g., food allergic enteropathy, eosinophilic gastroenteropathy
- Connective tissue disorders – notably SLE
- Immune-mediated disorders – Henoch-Schönlein purpura, angioedema
- AIDS
- Whipple's disease
- Bacterial overgrowth, sometimes associated with dysmotility
- Parasites, e.g. strongyloides, trichuris

cases of kwashiorkor occur each year amongst elderly hospitalized patients within the developed world.

One recently noted cause of severe PLE, which is notable for providing insights into its pathophysiology, occurs following the Fontan operation, performed for congenital heart disease with single ventricle.

PATHOGENESIS AND PATHOLOGY

The causes of excess enteric protein loss relate either to excess hydrostatic pressure within the lymphatics or mesenteric veins, or to loss of albumin restriction within the lamina propria by the epithelial barrier. Excess leakage across the epithelium, in the absence of an increased hydrostatic gradient, is not due to simple increase in permeability, except in cases where there is extensive ulceration.

Two conditions associated with severe PLE give insights into the relative role of lymphatic and venous back-pressure in inducing PLE. **Lymphangiectasia** occurs due to physical obstruction of lymphatic drainage, and causes severe persistent protein leakage, together with loss of lymphocytes into the lumen, inducing hypoalbuminemia and lymphopenia. This may be congenital or acquired, and the features are similar. Excess lymphatic pressure alone is thus sufficient to induce PLE. However, the extent of protein loss may be modulated to some extent, particularly in pediatric patients, by intake of fats, which are absorbed via the lymphatics. High intake of long-chain triglycerides worsens both intestinal protein leakage and loss of lymphocytes. Substitution of medium chain triglycerides, which are absorbed directly into the portal vein without requiring lymphatic drainage, may reduce but not prevent protein loss.

By contrast to lymphatic obstruction, **raised mesenteric venous pressure** may predispose to enteric protein loss, but may require additional impairment of the epithelial barrier. In the severe PLE that occurs in up to 4–10% of patients after Fontan surgery, raised mesenteric vascular pressure is necessary but insufficient on its own to induce protein leakage. The PLE usually begins some time after surgery, with no detectable change in right atrial pressure, but once established, the PLE is often relentless. Cardiac transplantation has however been curative. It is currently unknown why some cases develop this and not others, and the relationship to pressure is quite variable. It is likely that the epithelial barrier to protein leak may be impaired, for as yet unknown reasons, in those who go on to develop PLE.

The **epithelial barrier** to albumin leakage is not simply based on pore size, and the relationship between protein and electrolyte leakage across epithelia is not linear. It is likely that electrostatic charge plays a particularly important role in restricting albumin within the mucosa (Fig. 48.1). There is evidence from renal and vascular physiology that the major regulator of albumin flux across membranes is the negative electrostatic charge provided by glycosaminoglycans (GAGs) such as heparan sulfate, due to interaction with arginyl residues in the albumin molecule.[2–4] Thus, simple neutralization of the constitutive negative charge on endothelial monolayers or the glomerular basement membrane induces a major increase in albumin leakage.[3,4] Loss of glomerular basement membrane GAG expression contributes significantly to minimal lesion nephrotic syndrome, while congenital absence of basement membrane heparan sulfate proteoglycans causes the rare condition of congenital nephrotic syndrome.[5]

Similar electrostatic restriction may be important in gastrointestinal physiology.[6] There is strong expression of heparan sulfate proteoglycans (HSPG) on the basolateral surface of small intestinal enterocytes and on colonocytes.[7] Congenital absence of enterocyte HSPG expression has been identified in infants who suffer severe PLE from birth, despite histologically normal small intestinal biopsies.[7] Further evidence suggesting that enterocyte heparan sulfate expression may be critical was provided by the finding of intracellular heparan sulfate mislocalization during episodes of severe PLE in a child with a congenital disorder of n-glycosylation (CDG-1c).[8] Thus, in addition to impaired biosynthesis of HSPG, a separate pathway of potential rele-

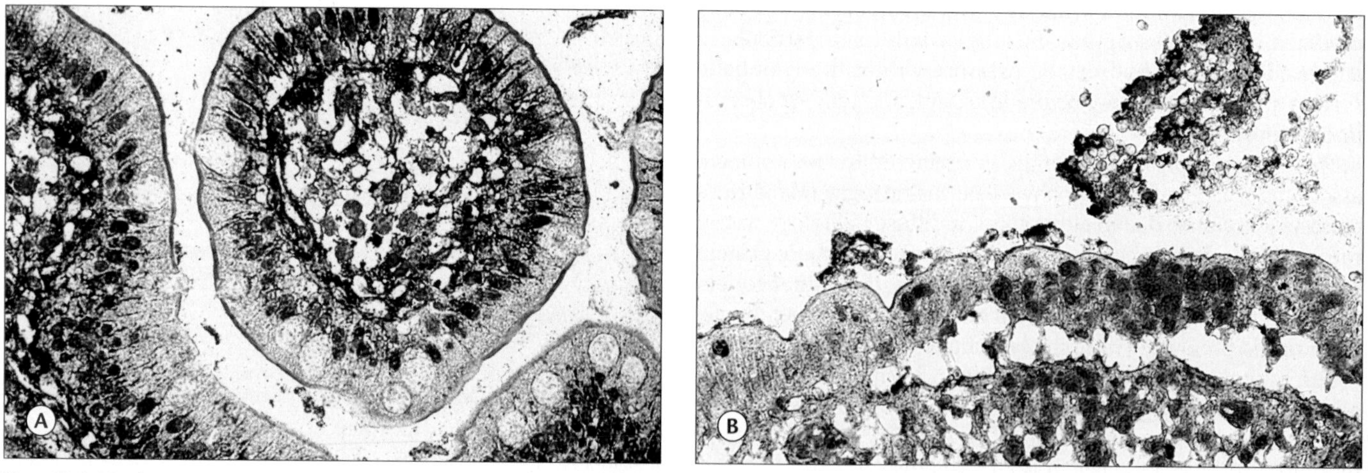

Fig. 48.1 Mechanism of enteric protein loss. A possible common mechanism of enteric protein loss – reduction of epithelial heparan sulfate proteoglycan expression. These negatively charged glycosaminoglycans restrict albumin movement across membranes of all kinds, by electrostatic attraction. When they are degraded by matrix-degrading metalloproteases, the consequence is unrestricted albumin movement. **A.** Dense heparan sulfate expression (black) on subepithelial basement membrane and between enterocytes in normal terminal ileum. Macrophages are shown by immunohistochemistry in red. Similar findings are seen throughout the gut. **B.** Complete loss of basement membrane and epithelial heparan sulfate, with epithelial lifting in active Crohn's disease, associated with dense macrophage infiltration. There will be little restriction of albumin in these circumstances.

vance to PLE would appear to be n-glycosylation. Inadequate n-glycosylation prevents normal protein folding, leading to sequestration of epithelial heparan sulfate proteoglycans such as syndecan-1 within the endoplasmic reticulum, rather than localizing to the basolateral epithelial surface.

In **inflammatory conditions** such as inflammatory bowel disease (IBD), there is a different mechanism by which epithelial HSPGs are reduced. Here, there is inflammatory degradation of HSPG glycan chains by matrix-degrading metalloproteases (MMPs). MMPs are themselves inhibited by naturally occurring antagonists, the tissue inhibitors of metalloproteases (TIMPs). Sulfated GAGs are widely disrupted in IBD,[9] related to excess mucosal MMP expression, without concomitant increase in TIMP response.[10] Amongst the potential inducers of this enhanced MMP response, the cytokines TNF-α and IL-1 appear to be of pivotal importance,[11] and immune-mediated breakdown of sulfated GAGs in organ culture is prevented by TNF blockade.[12] Activated T cells are known to produce MMPs, and thus conditions associated with increased infiltration of activated intraepithelial lymphocytes may also manifest albumin leakage.

Thus, a final outcome of inadequate epithelial HSPG expression may rarely occur due to congenital absence, but more commonly may develop due to inadequate n-glycosylation or to inflammatory degradation by MMPs and other glycanases. These phenomena are likely to occur in a variety of conditions. It is possible that the relatively high incidence of protein-losing enteropathy in SLE may relate to the anti-heparan sulfate autoantibodies that may occur. If there is an additional cause of raised mesenteric vascular or lymphatic pressure, this may exacerbate the tendency to leak protein. Conversely, if pressure is raised in the veins or lymphatics, protein leakage may depend on the adequacy of the epithelial barrier.

CLINICAL PRESENTATION

This will depend upon the underlying cause, and the primary initial manifestations of PLE may depend on the underlying disease. These diseases broadly group into intestinal, such as Crohn's disease, cardiac diseases causing raised inferior vena caval pressure, and multisystem diseases such as SLE or amyloidosis.

Regardless of underlying cause, the effects of uncompensated intestinal protein loss will be those of hypoalbuminemia, and may therefore mimic nephrotic syndrome. Thus, the first sign may be swelling of the legs or other dependent areas due to peripheral edema, which occurs due to loss of plasma oncotic pressure. In more severe cases, facial and periorbital edema may be seen, and anasarca may develop. Secondary complications include peritonitis or venous thrombosis.

Physical examination may simply show peripheral edema of variable severity, or may elicit signs of the underlying medical condition. In cases where the PLE is due to structural abnormalities within the lymphatic system (lymphangiectasia), there may be evidence of lymphedema in one or both of the lower limbs. This may be severe.

DIFFERENTIAL DIAGNOSIS

The major differential diagnosis in the initial establishment of a protein-losing enteropathy is protein loss from the renal tract, and thus it is important to perform urinalysis for protein in all cases, and formal timed quantitation of urinary protein loss if initial screening is positive.

In infants presenting with severe PLE, an inherited cause is more likely than in older children. Lymphedema of the lower limbs would suggest lymphangiectasia, and this diagnosis would be supported by findings of lymphopenia. If there is also facial dysmorphism, then the rare Hennekam syndrome should be considered, but transferrin glycosylation should also be checked to exclude a congenital disorder of glycosylation (CDG). Cystic fibrosis and intestinal malrotation can both present atypically, as apparently isolated infantile PLE. Enterocyte heparan sulfate deficiency is very rare, but should be considered in cases where there is no evidence of lymphangiectasia and gastric, duodenal, and colonic biopsies are normal. Excess protein leak can occur in infants and children with celiac disease or food-sensitive enteropathy, and mucosal biopsy is an important part of the investigation of the hypoalbuminemic infant with no urinary protein leak. There are several rare infantile IBD syndromes, which may induce widespread ulceration, while older children may develop classic IBD. Henoch-Schönlein purpura is an important cause of acute enteric protein loss in childhood, and may sometimes occur without the classic accompanying skin rash. While Ménétrier's disease of the stomach is rare in childhood, quite extensive gastric ulceration can occur after viral infections, particularly influenza. *Helicobacter pylori* infection is rarely associated with severe protein loss in childhood.

In adult life, there is a wide variety of medical conditions that can cause enteric protein loss (Table 48.1). It is important to identify the site of protein loss and to look for potential underlying causes. Determination of whether this is primarily an intestinal disorder is a major aim of investigation. In particular, it is important to exclude cardiac abnormalities and to consider the possibility of a multisystem disease such as SLE. A full travel history should be taken and inflammatory markers checked. As Ménétrier's syndrome is a relatively common cause of intestinal protein loss in adults, endoscopy is an important component of investigation and should be performed early. This should be combined with colonoscopy to exclude ulcerating colonic lesions.

> **CLINICAL PRESENTATION**
>
> - Nephrotic syndrome-like presentation of hypoalbuminemia
>   - peripheral or facial edema, ascites, occasionally anasarca
>   - potential secondary peritonitis, venous thrombosis
> - Symptoms due to associated malabsorption
> - Immunodeficiency, if associated enteric lymphocyte loss (lymphangiectasia)
> - Symptoms of underlying condition, e.g., cardiac, inflammatory, metabolic

DIAGNOSTIC METHODS

There are two main objectives of investigation, the first being to confirm and localize excess enteric protein loss and the second to determine a potentially treatable underlying cause.

The hallmark finding on initial investigation is a reduction in serum albumin and globulins. There may be apparent relative preservation of globulins if there is an underlying inflammatory cause. The detection of excess α_1-antitrypsin in stools provides formal confirmation of excess protein loss, but this may be misleadingly negative in states of profound hypoproteinemia and artifactually negative in hyperacidity syndromes due to its luminal degradation. Radiolabeled albumin can also be administered intravenously, and then detected within stools.

In almost all cases, the role of endoscopy and colonoscopy is important, and multiple biopsies should be performed even if appearances are macroscopically normal. The detection of lymphatic dilatation within the villous core does not necessarily confirm primary lymphangiectasia, and degrees of dilatation may be seen in very hypoalbuminemic patients without structural lymphatic damage. Barium follow-through should be considered to exclude malrotation, particularly in younger patients, while computerized tomography may suggest the need for lymphangiography to demonstrate lymphangiectasia. Hydrogen breath testing should be performed to exclude small bowel bacterial overgrowth.

In cases of ongoing PLE without clear underlying diagnosis, echocardiography should be considered, and Doppler studies of mesenteric vascular flow may give some insight into vascular resistance within this compartment. Lymphangiography can be a technically challenging procedure, but may sometimes demonstrate focal lymphangiectasia amenable to resection.

The spectrum of ancillary investigations may be dictated by the age of the patient and the results of more general assessment. However, milder variants of some conditions considered essentially pediatric, notably cystic fibrosis and congenital disorders of glycosylation, are being increasingly recognized in previously undiagnosed adults. By contrast, some conditions previously thought to be found almost exclusively in adults, such as Whipple's disease, amyloidosis (see Chapter 114), and eosinophilic gastroenteropathy (see Chapter 57), are being seen more commonly in childhood.

TREATMENT AND PREVENTION

In cases of secondary PLE, recognition and treatment of the underlying cause is essential. Such treatment may vary from simply a gluten-free diet in celiac disease to complex immunosuppressive therapy in intractable IBD or other immunopathologies, and has even included cardiac transplantation in individual cases of intractable PLE of cardiac origin.

Few medications have been shown to be specifically beneficial in protein-losing gastrointestinal states. Heparin therapy, using full molecular weight heparin, can induce significant improvement in some cases, at doses lower than are required for systemic anticoagulation. Octreotide is sometimes helpful in cases of severe PLE, particularly if associated with secretory diarrhea. Even in the absence of a defined mucosal inflammatory state, some cases do respond to empirical use of corticosteroids, at least in the short term, and the use of these and other immunosuppressants should clearly be considered in cases of intractable or life-threatening PLE.

TREATMENT AND PREVENTION

1. Treatment of underlying cause
   - Enteropathy – appropriate dietary exclusion, immunosuppression, etc.
   - Cardiac lesions – reduce right atrial pressure, relieve pericardial constriction
   - Lymphatic obstruction – surgical resection if localized lesion
2. Augment barrier to protein leakage
   - Heparin therapy may reduce protein loss
3. Treat hypoalbuminemia as necessary
   - Fluid intake restriction
   - Avoid excess intravenous fluid therapy
   - 20% albumin infusion with diuretic cover
4. Minimize complications
   - Use medium-chain triglycerides for main fat source if lymphatic obstruction
   - Give antibiotic cover if immunodeficient with ascites, e.g., splenectomy
   - Check micronutrient and fat-soluble vitamin status
5. Prevention
   - Avoid inappropriate malnutrition states (this is not restricted to the developing world, and occurs frequently in chronically hospitalized, postsurgical, and elderly patients)

PROGNOSIS WITH AND WITHOUT TREATMENT

The prognosis of enteric protein loss depends largely on the underlying condition, and the extent of PLE. In states of very high protein loss, the outcome can be very poor. Thus, small bowel transplantation has now been carried out in cases of severe congenital lymphangiectasia. In other primary conditions such as SLE, or following Fontan operation, the development of significant enteric protein loss can be a complication of very adverse significance. In other cases, the loss of protein may be transient and easily dealt with. The current lack of effective therapies for intestinal protein loss contributes to the poor prognosis in many cases.

KWASHIORKOR

The term kwashiorkor (meaning 'deprived child') was first suggested in Ghana by Cicely Williams in 1933. Because of its importance worldwide, kwashiorkor is highlighted here.

Kwashiorkor is a complication of protein energy malnutrition caused by a deficiency of protein in the presence of adequate energy (in contrast to marasmus, with combined protein and energy deficiency). In addition, loss of albumin from the bowel as a result of gastroenteritis or measles enteropathy contributes to its development. It is typically seen in developing countries where there is a scarcity of foods containing protein in weaning infants following the birth of a sibling.

In industrialized societies, kwashiorkor-like secondary protein energy malnutrition is seen in hypermetabolic acute illnesses such as trauma, burns, and sepsis.

The **consequences** of severe malnutrition in childhood are widespread: impaired intellectual development, frequent

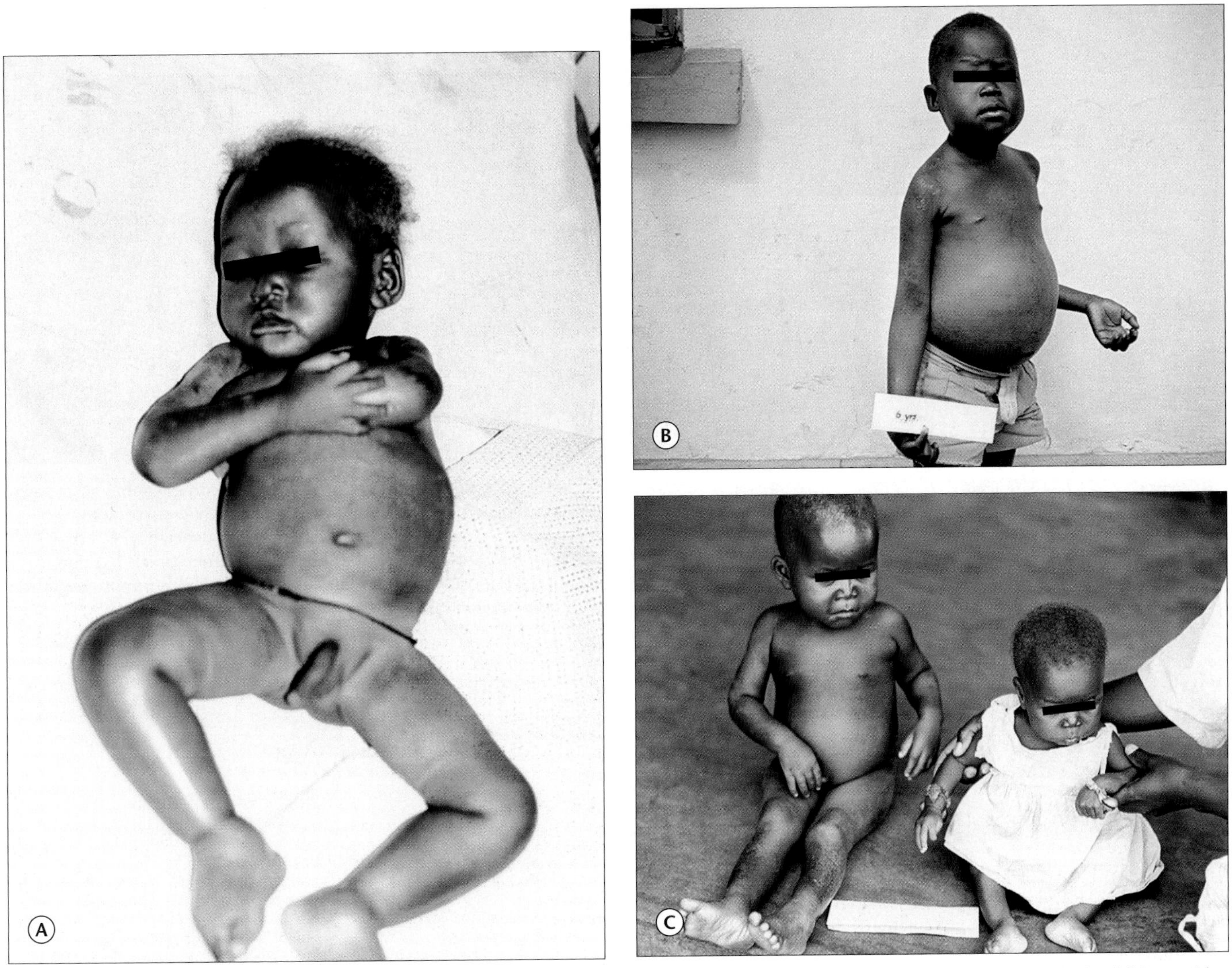

Fig. 48.2 Kwashiorkor in Ugandan children. The most common worldwide cause of death due to enteric protein loss occurs in children with tropical enteropathy and kwashiorkor. **A.** Characteristic peripheral edema and ascites in an infant. **B.** A 6-year-old with ascites and facial edema. C. The arrival of a younger sibling often precipitates kwashiorkor, as breast-feeding of the older child ceases and the diet becomes deficient in protein. Photographs courtesy of Dr Jake Mackinnon.

infections such as diarrhea, malaria and tuberculosis, growth retardation, nutrient deficiencies, and metabolic disturbance leading to edema and ascites due to hypoalbuminemia.

Early symptoms are typical for malnutrition: fatigue, lethargy, irritability, progressing to loss of muscle mass, growth retardation, generalized edema, and impaired immunity. Other signs include abdominal distention due to ascites, skin changes (dermatitis, vitiligo), and thinning of hair (Fig. 48.2). There is a very high incidence of complications (Fig. 48.3), and death is common.

After prolonged starvation, starting oral feeding can present problems, especially if the caloric density is too high at first. Food must be reintroduced slowly – carbohydrates first to supply energy, followed by protein. Vitamin and mineral supplements are essential. Lactose intolerance is common and lactase supplements will need to be given if patients are to benefit from milk products. Treatment early in the course of kwashiorkor generally produces good results; in its late stages, treatment will improve the child's general health, but he or she may be left with permanent physical problems and intellectual disabilities.

SOURCES OF INFORMATION FOR PATIENTS AND DOCTORS

http://www.emedicine.com/med/topic1926.htm
http://www.wfp.org/
http://www.nlm.nih.gov/medlineplus/ency/article/001604.htm

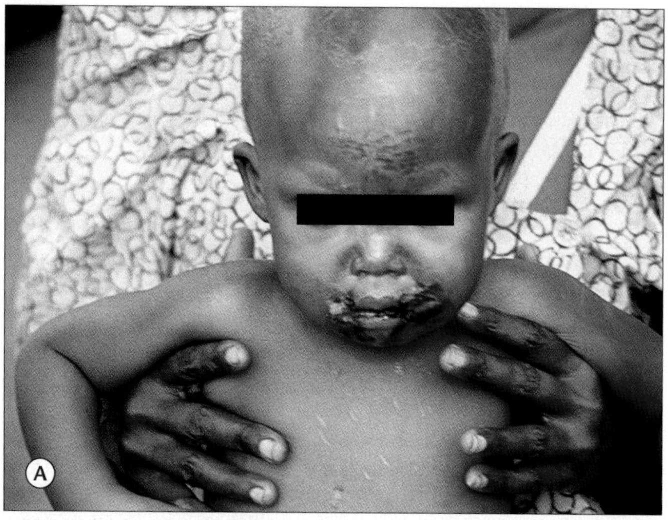

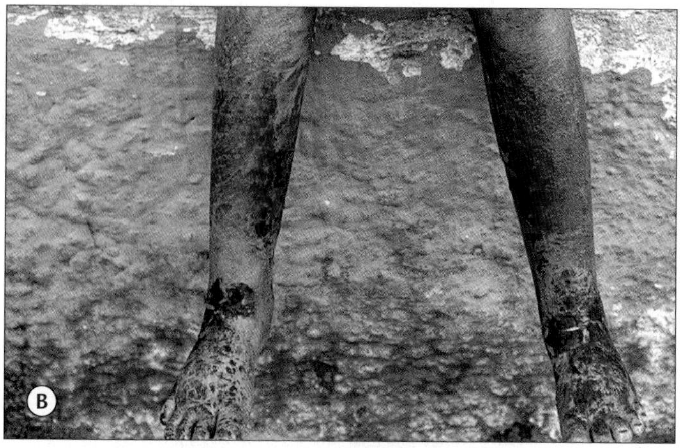

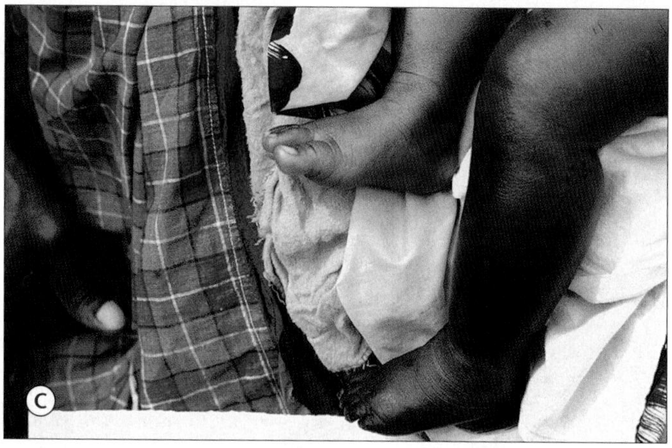

Fig. 48.3 Potential complications. Potential complications of protein-losing enteropathy seen in African children with kwashiorkor. **A.** Secondary vitamin deficiencies: pyridoxine deficiency. **B.** Leg ulceration in adult with kwashiorkor. **C.** Gangrene of left leg due to arterial thrombosis in infant with kwashiorkor. Photographs courtesy of Dr Jake Mackinnon.

REFERENCES

1. Beeken WL, Busch HJ, Sylwester DL. Intestinal protein loss in Crohn's disease. Gastroenterology 1972; 62:207–215.
2. Powers MR, Blumenstock FA, Cooper JA, Malik AB. Role of albumin arginyl sites in albumin-induced reduction of endothelial hydraulic conductivity. J Cell Physiol 1989; 141:558–564.
3. Jeansson M, Haraldsson B. Glomerular size and charge selectivity in the mouse after exposure to glucosaminoglycan-degrading enzymes. J Am Soc Nephrol 2003; 14:1756–1765.
4. Comper WD, Laurent TC. Physiological function of connective tissue polysaccharides. Physiol Rev 1978; 58:255–315.
5. Vernier RL, Klein DJ, Sisson SP et al. Heparan sulfate-rich anionic sites in the human glomerular basement membrane. Decreased concentration in congenital nephrotic syndrome. N Engl J Med 1983; 309:1001–1009.
6. Bode L, Eklund E, Murch S, Freeze H. A link between protein-losing enteropathy and loss of heparan sulfate proteoglycans. Glycobiology 2003; 13:819 (abstract).
7. Murch SH, Winyard PJD, Koletzko S et al. Congenital enterocyte heparan sulphate deficiency is associated with massive albumin loss, secretory diarrhoea and malnutrition. Lancet 1996; 347:1299–1301.
8. Westphal V, Murch S, Kim S et al. A congenital disorder of glycosylation (CDG-Ic) impairs heparan sulfate proteoglycan accumulation in small intestine epithelial cells and contributes to protein-losing enteropathy. Am J Pathol 2000; 157:1917–1925.
9. Murch SH, MacDonald TT, Walker-Smith JA et al. Disruption of sulphated glycosaminoglycans in intestinal inflammation. Lancet 1993; 341: 711–714.
10. Heuschkel RB, MacDonald TT, Monteleone G et al. Imbalance of stromelysin-1 and TIMP-1 in the mucosal lesions of children with inflammatory bowel disease. Gut 2000; 47:57–62.
11. Klein NJ, Shennan GI, Heyderman RS, Levin M. Alteration in glycosaminoglycan metabolism and surface charge on human umbilical vein endothelial cells induced by cytokines, endotoxin and neutrophils. J Cell Sci 1992; 102:821–832.
12. Pender SLF, Fell JME, Chamow SM, Ashkenazi A, MacDonald TT. A p55 TNF receptor immunoadhesin prevents T cell-mediated intestinal injury by inhibiting matrix metalloproteinase production. J Immunol 1998, 160: 4098–4103.

Chapter 49

Infective diarrhea

Michael J G Farthing and Anna Casburn-Jones

KEY POINTS

- Diarrheal illnesses kill 3 million pre-school children per year
- In the industrialized world, overseas travel, antibiotic use and food handling are important factors
- Severity of clinical infection depends on the interaction of host and pathogen factors
- Diarrhea is caused by both increased intestinal secretion and decreased absorption
- Early histological features may help distinguish infective diarrhea from IBD

INTRODUCTION AND DEFINITION

Infections of the gastrointestinal tract are the most common intestinal disorders. They have their major impact in the developing world and are still responsible for the deaths of up to three million preschool children each year. The seventh cholera pandemic continues to take lives in the Indian subcontinent, Africa, and Latin America. Despite industrialization, wealth, and public health interventions to ensure water quality and sewage disposal, intestinal infections still have a major impact in the Western world, including both food-borne and waterborne infections.[1] The increase in food-borne disease is related to a number of factors including the widespread contamination of poultry flocks with *Salmonella* and *Camplyobacter* species and the use of raw or partially cooked foods such as eggs. Large outbreaks of waterborne disease have been reported in Europe and North America, commonly due to the protozoa *Cryptosporidium parvum* and *Giardia intestinalis*.

The importance of an infective cause of colitis is now widely recognized following the steady increase in reports of *Salmonella* and *Campylobacter jejuni* infections in the UK (Fig. 49.1). In addition there have been a series of major outbreaks of enterohemorrhagic *Escherichia coli* (EHEC) infection with a reported mortality rate of 1–2% and a relatively high incidence of serious complications such as the hemolytic–uremic syndrome. The increase in foreign travel has further contributed to the importance of infectious colitis in individuals living in the industrialized world,[2] as has the increasing use of broad-spectrum antibiotics and associated antibiotic-related diarrhea and pseudomembraneous colitis due to infection with *Clostridium difficile*.

Diarrhea is usually defined as an increase in stool frequency (more than three stools in 24h) almost invariably associated with an increase in stool liquidity. Acute infectious diarrhea usually resolves within 5–10 days; persistent diarrhea is defined as diarrhea that has continued for more than 14 days. Dysentery is diarrhea associated with blood and accompanied by fever. An increase in bowel frequency also occurs in some functional bowel disorders such as irritable bowel syndrome, although in this case stool weight does not exceed the generally accepted upper limit of 200g per 24h.

EPIDEMIOLOGY

Reservoirs

The major reservoirs of human enteropathogens are food, water, and other humans. Certain infective agents are carried by animals that act as a reservoir for human infection; these conditions are known as zoonoses (Table 49.1). Almost any of the major bacterial, viral, and protozoal enteropathogens can enter the alimentary tract using food or drink as a vehicle. A recent example was a major outbreak of *Cyclospora cayetanensis* infection following ingestion of contaminated raspberries. Domestic water supplies, swimming pools, sea water, and inland freshwater lakes and rivers also harbor enteropathogens; this may occur through contamination by animal and sometimes human feces, and by inadequate disposal of raw sewage. Despite adequate chlorination and acceptable coliform counts, the cysts of *Giardia* and *Cryptosporidium* can survive in municipal water supplies.

Transmission

Intestinal infections are generally transmitted by the fecal–oral route. In humans this occurs either through ingestion of contaminated food or fluids or by direct person-to-person contact. The latter is particularly important when only small infective doses are required to initiate infection such as in shigellosis. *Vibrio cholerae* and other noncholera vibrios are transmitted by contaminated water, shellfish, and other seafood, and by person-to-person contact. Direct transmission of *Giardia* is

TABLE 49.1 ZOONOTIC INFECTIONS OF THE ALIMENTARY TRACT

- **Bacteria**
  - *Salmonella* spp.
  - *Campylobacter jejuni*
  - Enterohemorrhagic *Escherichia coli*
  - *Yersinia enterocolitica*
- **Protozoa**
  - *Giardia intestinalis*
  - *Cryptosporidium parvum*
  - *Balantidium coli*

CAUSES AND RISK FACTORS

MICROBIAL PATHOGENS RESPONSIBLE FOR FOODBORNE DIARRHEAL DISEASE

Organism	Source	Incubation period (h)	Symptoms	Recovery
GUT COLONIZATION				
Salmonella spp.	Eggs, poultry	12–48	Diarrhea, blood, pain, vomiting, fever	2–14 days
Campylobacter jejuni	Milk, poultry	48–168	As above	7–21 days
EHEC	Beef	24–168	As above	7–21 days
V. parahaemolyticus	Seafood	2–48	As above (blood less common)	2–30 days
Y. enterocolitica	Milk, pork	2–144	Diarrhea, fever, pain	1–3 days
Clostridium perfringens	Spores in food, especially meat	8–22	Diarrhea, pain	1–3 days
PREFORMED TOXINS				
Staphylococcus aureus	Transmitted to food by humans	2–6	Nausea, vomiting, pain (diarrhea)	Few hours
Bacillus cereus	Spores in food, reheated rice	1–2	As above	Few hours
Clostridium botulinum	Spores in home-bottled or home-canned food	18–36	Transient diarrhea, paralysis	10–14 days

EHEC, enterohemorrhagic *E. coli*.

common in day-care centers when young children are in close contact. Intimate sexual contact, notably oroanal sex, is commonly associated with transmission of enteropathogens. Viruses, such as the norovirus (previously known as small round structured viruses of the Norwalk family), can be spread by aerosol, especially as vomiting is an important early symptom of the illness. This probably explains why this infection spreads so rapidly through cruise ships, hotels, and hospital wards.[3]

Infective dose

The infective dose is an important determinant of whether clinical infection occurs following ingestion of an enteropathogen. For *V. cholerae* the standard infective dose is high at around 10^9 vibrios, but may fall to 10^3 in individuals with low gastric acidity. For *Shigella* the dose is low at 10^{1-2} organisms, with a similar number of cysts being required to initiate infection with *Giardia*.

Seasonality

Seasonality is recognized to occur in a number of intestinal infections. In cholera, for example, infection is more common in the warmer, wetter months of the year, whereas rotavirus diarrhea in the northern hemisphere peaks in the winter months. Enteric adenovirus infections, however, occur at similar frequencies throughout the year.

LABORATORY REPORTING OF GI PATHOGENS IN ENGLAND AND WALES

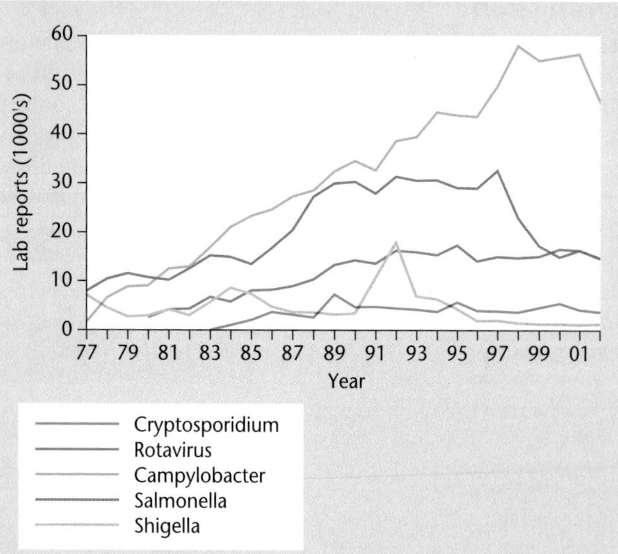

Fig. 49.1 Laboratory reporting of gastrointestinal pathogens in England and Wales. Annual reporting of intestinal infective agents by the Health Protection Agency (formerly the Public Health Laboratory Service).

CAUSES, RISK FACTORS, DISEASE ASSOCIATIONS

Causes

Infective diarrhea presents as a variety of clinical patterns, the recognition of which may assist clinical diagnosis and early management. The three major patterns are: (1) acute watery diarrhea; (2) bloody diarrhea (dysentery), usually due to an infective colitis; and (3) persistent diarrhea, sometimes with steatorrhea and evidence of an enteropathy. However, there is considerable overlap between these clinical patterns with some organisms such as *Shigella* sp. and *Campylobacter jejuni* presenting initially as acute watery diarrhea but then progressing to a dysenteric illness with fever and bloody diarrhea. Similarly, giardiasis may start as acute watery diarrhea but eventually become persistent with features of malabsorption.

Host and environmental risk factors

There are a number of important clinical settings in which the risk of intestinal infection is increased.

Age

Individuals at the extremes of the age spectrum are more susceptible to the acquisition of infection and are at greater risk of its consequences. This probably relates to increased exposure in infants and young children, although breastfed infants

CAUSES AND RISK FACTORS

CAUSES OF INFECTIOUS DIARRHEA BY CLINICAL PATTERN

Enteropathogen	Acute watery diarrhea	Dysentery	Persistent diarrhea
VIRUSES			
Rotavirus	+	–	–
Enteric adenovirus (types 40, 41)	+	–	–
Calicivirus	+	–	–
Astrovirus	+	–	–
Cytomegalovirus	+	+	+
BACTERIA			
Vibrio cholerae and other vibrios	+	–	–
Enterotoxigenic *E. coli* (ETEC)	+	–	–
Enteropathogenic *E. coli* (EPEC)	+	–	+
Enteroaggregative *E. coli* (EAggEC)	+	–	+
Enteroinvasive *E. coli* (EIEC)	+	+	–
Enterohemorraghic *E. coli* (EHEC)	+	+	–
Shigella spp.	+	+	+
Salmonella spp.	+	+	+
Campylobacter spp.	+	+	+
Yersinia spp.	+	+	+
Clostridium difficile	+	+	+
Mycobacterium tuberculosis	–	+	+
PROTOZOA			
Giardia intestinalis	+	–	+
Cryptosporidium parvum	+	–	+
Microsporidia	+	–	+
Isospora belli	+	–	+
Cyclospora cayetanensis	+	–	+
Entamoeba histolytica	+	+	+
Balantidium coli	+	+	+
HELMINTHS			
Strongyloides stercoralis	–	–	+
Schistosoma spp.	–	+	+

are protected. Immune defence is suboptimal at both extremes of age.

Travel (see also Chapter 50)

Gastrointestinal infection affects 30–50% of travelers from Western countries to the developing world and is commonly due to infection of the small intestine with enterotoxigenic *E. coli* (ETEC), but can also be caused by a variety of other microorganisms (Table 49.2).[4,5] The impact of travelers' diarrhea is usually viewed solely from the point of view of the tourist. However, there are important implications for business travelers, the military (as was clearly identified during the first Gulf War), and for tourism-dependent economies of countries in the developing world.

Food poisoning

Food-borne infection is an important source of intestinal diarrheal disease. Although many episodes of food poisoning are due to true infection of the small intestine, others such as staphylococcal food poisoning relate to the ingestion of a preformed toxin.

TABLE 49.2 PREVALENCE OF MICROBIAL ENTEROPATHOGENS IN TRAVELERS' DIARRHEA

Enteropathogens	Reported isolation rates (%)
BACTERIA	
ETEC	20–75
Salmonella spp.	0–16
Shigella spp.	0–30
Campylobacter jejuni	1–11
Aeromonas and *Plesiomonas* spp.	1–57
Vibrio parahaemolyticus	1–16
EIEC	5–7
PROTOZOA	
Giardia intestinalis	0–9
Entamoeba histolytica	0–9
Cryptosporidium parvum	1–10
Microsporidia, Cyclospora	Uncertain
HELMINTHS	
Viruses	
Rotavirus	0–36
Norovirus	
MULTIPLE PATHOGENS	9–22
NO PATHOGEN ISOLATED	15–55

ETEC, enterotoxigenic *E. coli.*

Disease associations

Immunodeficiency and HIV/AIDS (see also Chapter 111)

Immunocompromise has long been recognized as an important risk factor for intestinal infection, but with the advent of HIV infection a unique spectrum of opportunistic infectious intestinal disease has become apparent. Many of these infections can be life-threatening when there is a background of profound immune deficiency (Table 49.3). The prevalence of these infections has, however, decreased dramatically in regions of the world that are able to afford highly active antiretroviral therapy. Protozoal infections such as *Giardia* are more common in congenital forms of immune deficiency, such as in defective immunoglobulin production.

The use of immunosuppressive drugs for the treatment of cancer and to prevent organ rejection following transplantation renders these individuals at increased risk of intestinal infection. Of particular importance is the helminth *Strongyloides stercoralis*, which under such conditions can produce the hyperinfection syndrome that has a high mortality rate.

Impaired nonimmune host defence

The gastric acid barrier has been recognized to be an important impediment to the acquisition of intestinal infection. Cholera and giardiasis are particular examples where gastric acid appears to be important in preventing infection. With the development of potent acid suppressive agents such as the H_2-receptor antagonists and the proton pump inhibitors, it is now clear that these drugs do increase the risk of intestinal infection, particularly in older age groups in which the overall increased risk may approach 10-fold.[6,7]

TABLE 49.3 ENTEROPATHOGENS RESPONSIBLE FOR HIV-RELATED DIARRHEA

- **Protozoa**
  Cryptosporidium parvum
  Microsporidium spp.
  Giardia intestinalis
  Isospora belli
  Cyclospora cayetanensis
- **Bacteria**
  Salmonella spp.
  Shigella spp.
  Campylobacter spp.
  Vibrio parahaemolyticus
  Clostridium difficile
  Mycobacterium avium complex
- **Viruses**
  Cytomegalovirus

MECHANISMS FOR AC/GC ACTIVATION AND CHLORIDE ION SELECTION

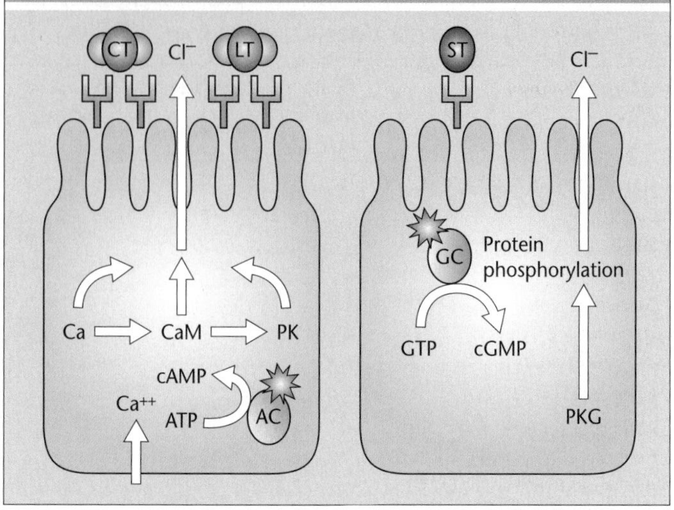

Fig. 49.2 Mechanisms for AC/GC activation and chloride ion secretion. Intracellular mechanisms by which bacterial enterotoxins – cholera toxin (CT), *Escherichia coli* heat-labile toxin (LT), and heat-stable toxin (ST) – activate adenylate cyclase (AC) and guanylate cyclase (GC), and through a series of second messengers such as calcium–calmodulin (CA, CaM) and protein kinases (PK) promote chloride ion secretion. cAMP, cyclic adenosine monophosphate; cGMP, cyclic guanosine monophosphate; PKG, protein kinase G.

PATHOGENESIS

Diarrhea occurs during intestinal infection as a result of two major disturbances of normal intestinal physiology: (1) increased intestinal secretion of fluid and electrolytes, predominantly in the small intestine; and (2) decreased absorption of fluid, electrolytes, and sometimes nutrients, disturbances that can involve both the small intestine and the colon.

Increased intestinal secretion

Intestinal secretory processes in infective diarrhea are generally activated by secretory enterotoxins. Cholera toxin (CT) is the prototype enterotoxin.[8,9] The A_1 subunit of CT activates the catalytic unit of the enzyme adenylate cyclase (Fig. 49.2). This results in an increase in intracellular cyclic adenosine monophosphate, which through a series of intermediate steps results in opening of the transmembrane chloride channel protein in the apical membrane of the enterocyte. Chloride ions leave the enterocyte, closely followed by sodium ions (to preserve electroneutrality) and fluid, which follows passively down the osmotic gradient.

ETEC produces heat-labile toxins (LT-1 and LT-2), a group of proteins that are closely related – structurally, functionally, and immunologically – to CT and, like CT, activate adenylate cyclase. ETEC also produces a low molecular weight, heat-stable enterotoxin (ST). ST differs from LT and CT in that it activates guanylate cyclase, which is directly linked to a specific ST receptor on the enterocyte. Heat-stable toxins are also produced by other enteric pathogens including *Yersinia enterocolitica*, *V. cholerae* non-O1 and enteroaggregative *E. coli* that produces enteroaggregative *E. coli* heat-stable toxin 1 (EAST-1).

Enterotoxin-related secretory diarrhea may be partly mediated by a variety of endogenous secretagogues, including prostaglandins, 5-hydroxytryptamine (5-HT), and substance P. Neuronal pathways have been shown to be involved in amplification of the effects of enterotoxins.[10] CT, for example, has been shown to release 5-HT from enterochromaffin cells; this is thought to activate the afferent limb of a neuronal reflex. The effector limb of the neuronal reflux probably completes the neuronal pathway by releasing the secretory neurotransmitter vasoactive intestinal polypeptide (VIP). Interneurons are thought to propagate the secretory effects of CT distally in the small intestine. LT and ST also appear to activate neural secretory reflexes, although 5-HT is not involved in the secretory mechanism of either toxin.[11]

Decreased intestinal absorption (see also Chapter 43)

Impaired intestinal absorption is the other major mechanism by which enteropathogens cause diarrhea and is generally accompanied by macroscopic or microscopic injury to the intestine. Diarrhea due to decreased absorption can be related to: (1) impaired fluid, electrolyte, and nutrient absorption in the small intestine; (2) osmotic diarrhea due to the appearance of incompletely absorbed nutrients in the colon; and (3) impaired water and sodium retrieval by the colon due to direct involvement of colonic absorptive processes. Intestinal absorption is dependent not only on intact epithelial transport processes but also on there being adequate time for digestion and contact with the epithelium. Thus, reductions in small intestinal and whole gut transit times may result in impaired intestinal absorption.

Intestinal injury can occur at many levels, ranging from discrete damage to the microvillus membrane, such as that which occurs during the attachment process of enteropathogenic *E. coli* (EPEC) and *Cryptosporidium parvum*, to the mucosal inflammatory response to invasive pathogens such as *Shigella* sp., *Salmonella* sp., and *Entamoeba histolytica*, usually involving the release of cytolethal cytotoxins and resulting in epithelial cell loss and ulceration. Epithelial injury in the small intestine and colon occurs in association with a variety of enteropathogens including bacteria, parasites, and viruses. Rotavirus, for example, directly invades the epithelial cells in the mid and upper portion of the villus with rapid epithelial cell death and acute villus atrophy.[12] Invasive enteropathogens also produce an acute inflammatory response within the mucosa, with recruitment of pro-inflammatory mediators such as prostaglandins and leukotrienes, thereby not only impairing intestinal absorption but also initiating a pro-secretory state in the intestine. Many invasive enteropathogens also promote the synthesis and release of chemokines, such as interleukin 8 (IL-8), by intestinal epithelial cells. IL-8 is a potent chemoattractant for polymorphonuclear leukocytes, which enhance the inflammatory cascade and produce further mucosal and epithelial damage by release of reactive oxygen species.

Although it is helpful to consider the pathophysiology of infectious diarrhea under two broad headings, there are often situations in which these two pathophysiologic disturbances coexist.

PATHOLOGY

Small intestine

In the enterotoxin-mediated diarrheas there is no macroscopic or microscopic injury to the intestine. However, there is a spectrum of pathology in the small intestine ranging from the mildest microvillus disruption (*G. intestinalis, C. parvum*, and EPEC adherence with pedestal formation) to overt enteropathy. In the latter there can be mild to severe partial villus atrophy (*G. intestinalis, C. parvum*, and the intracellular protozoa, *Microsporidium*, *Cyclospora*, and *Isospora*).[13] Villus atrophy is almost invariably associated with increased numbers of mucosal and intraepithelial lymphocytes. The invasive enteropathogens such as *Salmonella* and *Yersinia* species commonly produce an ileitis that manifests as a nonspecific inflammatory response in the mucosa and submucosa. *Yersinia* can produce classic aphthoid ulcers in the terminal ileum.

Colon

Invasive colonic enteropathogens commonly produce a macroscopic colitis. In addition to a loss of vascular pattern and erythema there may be discrete ulceration. The histologic appearances of colonic mucosa in the later stages of infection with invasive enteropathogens such as *Salmonella* spp., *Shigella* spp., and *Campylobacter jejuni* are often indistinguishable from those of nonspecific inflammatory bowel disease. However, if biopsies are taken within the first 24–72 h, features that might suggest infectious colitis include mucosal edema, straightening of the glands, and an acute inflammatory infiltrate including polymorphonuclear leukocytes, which can sometimes be seen penetrating the epithelium.[14] In *C. difficile* infection there may be the typical appearances of pseudomembranous colitis; histologically there is an acute inflammatory infiltrate combined with the typical 'erupting volcano' lesion, which is the histologic counterpart of pseudomembrane. Some organisms can be identified in mucosal biopsies, including the trophozoites of *E. histolytica*, ova of *Schistosoma* sp., *C. parvum*, and the 'owl's eye' inclusion bodies indicative of cytomegalovirus infection.

CLINICAL PRESENTATIONS

Acute watery diarrhea (see also Chapter 9)

Rotavirus infection, the most common cause of acute diarrhea in infants and young children, is often preceded by a brief prodromal illness with fever and mild respiratory symptoms, followed by vomiting and diarrhea. If fluid and electrolyte losses are not replaced promptly, dehydration and metabolic acidosis soon follow. The degree of dehydration can be assessed clinically by noting skin tone and tissue turgor, intraocular tension, and, in young infants, depression of the anterior fontanelle. In addition, there may be dryness of mucous membranes. As the degree of dehydration increases, there is impairment of consciousness ultimately leading to stupor and coma. Typically the illness lasts about 7 days. Adenovirus results in a more prolonged illness with pronounced respiratory symptoms.

Acute watery diarrhea in adults is usually bacterial in origin, most commonly due to ETEC in travelers or one of the foodborne pathogens in the indigenous population of industrialized countries. ETEC usually begins after a short incubation period and on average lasts 3–5 days. Watery diarrhea is often accompanied by anorexia, nausea, vomiting, abdominal cramps, bloating, and low-grade fever. In adults, severe dehydration is uncommon, although this may become clinically important in infants and young children and in the elderly.[15] Mild cholera may be indistinguishable from other agents that produce acute watery diarrhea. However, when severe, diarrhea begins abruptly, with stool volume rates of up to 1 L/h. Fecal output is highest in the first 24–48 h but, provided stool losses are matched by either oral or intravenous fluid and electrolyte replacement, stool volumes decline progressively over a 5-day period. Fever is usually absent, but vomiting is common in the early stages of the illness.

Bloody diarrhea, dysentery, and colitis

(see also Chapter 9)

The organisms responsible for acute bloody diarrhea are the invasive bacterial enteropathogens (*Shigella* spp., *Salmonella* spp., *Campylobacter jejuni*, and EHEC) and the protozoan *E. histolytica*. There is often a prodromal illness of low-grade fever, headache, anorexia, and lassitude. The incubation period is variable, and can range from 1 to 7 days. After an initial period of watery diarrhea, stool volume may actually decrease with the appearance of blood and mucus in the stools. Moderate or severe, cramping, lower abdominal pain is an important feature of a dysenteric illness, as is tenesmus and rectal prolapse, particularly in children with shigellosis. There may be fever and mild abdominal distention with some tenderness over the colon.

Clinically it is difficult to distinguish acute infectious colitis from nonspecific inflammatory bowel disease. Any form of severe colitis can give rise to abdominal tenderness, distention, and in some cases reduced bowel sounds due to ileus. Proctosigmoidoscopy should form part of the initial clinical assessment and may confirm the presence of colitis. Although some forms of infective proctitis do have specific features that might favour a diagnosis of infection (Table 49.4), ulceration in the rectum can occur in infection and in nonspecific inflammatory bowel disease; pseudomembrane may be a feature of ischemic colitis as well as *C. difficile* infection. In addition, the endoscopic appearances in the rectum may be normal in many forms of infective colitis that may be limited to the right colon.

Persistent diarrhea

In adults, *G. intestinalis* is the most common cause of persistent diarrhea, often associated with anorexia, abdominal bloating, substantial weight loss, and overt steatorrhea. The other intracellular protozoa are also relatively common causes of persistent diarrhea, particularly in the immunocomprised (see Table 49.3). In children, EPEC is an important organism to consider. Any cause of persistent diarrhea in infants and young children can result in failure to thrive and growth retardation. *Strongyloides stercoralis* infection may also cause chronic diarrhea and

TABLE 49.4 ENDOSCOPIC APPEARANCES OF THE RECTUM IN INFECTIVE PROCTITIS

Endoscopic appearances	Microbiologic diagnosis
'Colitis,' but may be normal	Salmonellosis Shigellosis Campylobacteriosis Yersiniosis Tuberculosis *Clostridium difficile* infection Amebiasis
Deep ulcers	Amebiasis Tuberculosis Syphilis
Pseudomembrane	*C. difficile* infection
Vesicles	Herpes simplex virus
Beads of pus	Gonorrhea

malabsorption, although this is more common in the hyperinfection syndrome. Amebic colitis can persist in a relatively indolent manner without there being overt blood loss.

DIFFERENTIAL DIAGNOSIS

Acute watery diarrhea

Noninfectious causes of watery diarrhea include drugs, bile salt malabsorption, and the neuroendocrine diarrheas (VIPoma, carcinoid syndrome, medullary carcinoma of the thyroid). Laxative abuse and sorbitol ingestion should also be considered.

Bloody diarrhea and colitis

Diarrhea with blood presents a major diagnostic challenge for the clinician because of the importance of distinguishing infection from nonspecific inflammatory bowel disease and other inflammatory conditions of the colon. The clinical differentiation of infection from these other conditions is usually not easy, although infective colitis generally has a relatively abrupt onset and cramping lower abdominal pain often emerges as the most disruptive symptom, which is usually not the case in ulcerative colitis. Physical examination rarely distinguishes between infection and nonspecific inflammatory bowel disease unless there are obvious perianal stigmata of Crohn's disease, or other typical extraintestinal manifestations of inflammatory bowel disease such as erythema nodosum, aphthous ulceration, pyoderma gangrenosum, and arthralgia. However, joint symptoms may accompany infection due to certain invasive enteropathogens and may form part of a Reiter's syndrome.

The presence of physical signs suggestive of HIV infection include cutaneous Kaposi's sarcoma, choroidoretinitis, hairy leukoplakia, and oral candidiasis.

Persistent diarrhea

There is a long list of conditions that cause persistent diarrhea, including small bowel disorders such as celiac disease and other enteropathies, bacterial overgrowth, lactose intolerance, and inflammatory bowel disease. Pancreatic insufficiency in all its many forms will also result in chronic diarrhea and malabsorption. Many drugs and the neuroendocrine diarrheas are also part of the differential diagnosis. Occasionally patients may fabricate diarrhea by adding water or urine, so-called factitious diarrhea.

DIAGNOSTIC METHODS

Although the majority of episodes of acute infective diarrhea resolve without the need for identifying a specific etiologic agent, persistent diarrhea and bloody diarrhea usually always require further investigation. This is particularly important in severely ill patients when delay in starting appropriate treatment might significantly alter the outcome. Confident exclusion of an infective etiology is rarely achieved in less than 24–48 h and, although imprecise, clinical assessment is important for guiding management during this early phase of the illness. Routine laboratory investigations are of limited diagnostic value because anemia, a raised neutrophil count, and evidence of an inflammatory process with a raised erythrocyte sedimentation rate, C-reactive protein, and platelet count occur in infective colitis and nonspecific inflammatory bowel disease. The cornerstone of evidence-based management is identification of the etiologic agent; this ultimately relies on a microbiologic approach.

Microbiology

Microscopy

Light microscopic examination of three sequential fecal specimens continues to be important for the identification of all enteropathogenic protozoa. It is essential to examine fresh specimens if there is a requirement to identify the free-living forms (trophozoites) in giardiasis and amebiasis as these organisms lose their motility at room temperature and rapidly disintegrate; protozoal cysts, oocysts, and sporocysts are more robust and survive storage. *Balantidium coli* is a large motile ciliate and can sometimes be seen with a hand lens. Fecal microscopy is also of potential value in identifying the ova of *Schistosoma* spp., and a skilled parasitologist can identify the various subspecies by ova morphology.

Culture

Stool culture will usually isolate the classic invasive enteropathogens provided that appropriate culture conditions are employed. However, it is unusual for a bacterial enteropathogen to be identified in less than 24–48 h, and for the slower growing organism such as *Yersinia enterocolitica* and *Campylobacter jejuni* information may not be forthcoming for 3–5 days. DNA-based technology, usually directed towards specific virulence factors of these enteropathogens, offers the opportunity to make a rapid, highly specific diagnosis. These techniques are widely used in research laboratories to investigate the role of potential virulence factors in pathogenesis and will ultimately be incorporated into clinical practice.

Blood culture should be performed in ill patients with fever and other systemic symptoms. Invasive organisms that produce an enteric fever-like illness, including *Salmonella* spp., *C. jejuni*, and *Y. entercolitica*, can be detected by this approach.

Serology

Serology is of limited value in the diagnosis of intestinal infection.[16,17] However, in amebic colitis, serology is positive in 80–90% of patients and is an important screening test alongside fecal microscopy if amebiasis is an important diagnostic possibility. Serology can detect *Y. enterocolitica* infection, although results are not usually positive for at least 10–14 days after the onset of the illness, and therefore the results may become available only as the diarrhea resolves. Enzyme-linked immunosorbent assays are now available for the diagnosis of strongyloidiasis and schistosomiasis, and should be regarded as first-line screening tests for travelers returning from endemic areas. They are of little value in the indigenous population once an infection has been diagnosed and treated, because antibodies may persist for months or even years after the initial infection.

Abdominal imaging

Imaging of the intestine has a limited place in establishing the diagnosis of intestinal infection but may be useful in defining the severity and extent of infective colitis and in the detection of any complications.

Endoscopy

If rigid sigmoidoscopy reveals the presence of colitis in the rectum, it is usually unnecessary to pursue this further with a more extensive examination of the colon and distal ileum. A rectal biopsy should, however, be taken for histologic examination. If the rectum is normal, it is usually appropriate to examine the proximal colon endoscopically. However, the endoscopic differentiation between acute infectious colitis and other forms of colitis is difficult. Appearances of *Shigella*, *Salmonella*, and *Campylobacter* infections are macroscopically indistinguishable from nonspecific inflammatory bowel diseases. These infections may produce a predominantly right-sided colitis that macroscopically resembles ulcerative colitis. However, an experienced endoscopist may be able to identify the typical amebic ulcers, which are shallow lesions with undermined edges often covered with a yellow exudate. The intervening mucosa appears normal, and this distinguishes it from ulcerative colitis and other invasive bacterial infections of the colon. However, the diagnosis must be confirmed by microscopic examination of ulcer slough for trophozoites.

The presence of pseudomembranes in the colon – appearing as pale, white-yellow excrescences on the epithelium that, when removed, leave an area of spontaneous bleeding separated by areas of normal mucosa – is generally indicative of *C. difficile* infection, although pseudomembrane is not specific for this condition and may occur in ischemia. Multiple colonic biopsies should always be taken, as in some instances it may be possible to detect the presence of an enteropathogen directly in tissue (*E. histolytica*, *Schistosoma* spp., and cytomegalovirus).

Radiology and ultrasonography

A supine plain abdominal radiograph can be invaluable in assessing the severity and extent of infectious colitis. A gas-filled colon devoid of feces is consistent with total colitis; loss of haustration and colonic dilatation is indicative of severe inflammation. The examination is also useful for detecting free air in the abdominal cavity, a sign of colonic perforation. Ultrasonography may reveal bowel wall thickening in invasive ileocolitis and enlarged lymph nodes in yersiniosis and abdominal tuberculosis. The examination may also be invaluable in detecting complications of intestinal infections such as amebic liver abscess.

TREATMENT AND PREVENTION

Fluid and electrolyte replacement

Fluid and electrolyte replacement via the oral route is usually sufficient except when losses are very severe or there is associated profound vomiting. Dehydration occurs more quickly in infants and young children, and therefore early administration of an oral rehydration solution is advised to prevent dehydration and acidosis.[15] In severe dehydration in infants and young children, intravenous fluids are advisable. Food should be commenced as soon as the individual wishes to eat and drink normally. Breastfeeding should be continued in infants. In most cases in adults formal oral rehydration is usually not required, but it is recommended that they should increase oral fluids such as salty soups (sodium) and fruit juices (potassium), and take carbohydrates (salty crackers, rice, bread, pasta, potatoes), to provide glucose for glucose–sodium co-transport.

Antidiarrheal therapy

Antimotility agents

The most commonly used antimotility agent is loperamide. These agents act by increasing intestinal transit time and enhancing the potential for reabsorption of fluid and electrolytes. Loperamide may have some antisecretory activity. The efficacy of loperamide has been evaluated in a variety of clinical trials, not all of which have shown it to be superior to placebo,[18] although it is probably most effective when combined with an antibiotic.[19] Antimotility agents are not recommended for children and young infants owing to concerns about respiratory depression. Antimotility agents are generally not recommended in dysentery because of the risk of colonic dilatation, but they are safe when used in conjunction with an antibiotic.[19] Antimotility agents have also been thought to increase the fecal carriage of gut enteropathogens, but there is little evidence that this is the case.

Antisecretory agents

There is an ongoing search for the agents that will directly inhibit secretory processes.[20] An important approach has been the development of an enkephalinase inhibitor, racecadotril, which has pro-absorptive activity via its ability to potentiate endogenous enkephalins in the intestine.[21] This is an effective agent for reducing stool weight and bowel frequency; it can be used safely in children and does not cause rebound constipation, which can be a problem with antimotility agents.[22]

The thiazolidinone moieties that inhibit the cystic fibrosis transmembrane regulator protein may also hold promise for the future as the basis for drug development.[23] This protein is integral to the chloride channel on the apical membrane of the intestinal epithelial cell that is an essential component of the secretory process. Further clinical evaluation is required to determine whether this is or will be a valuable addition to the management of secretory diarrhea. SP303, a naturally occurring polyphenolic polymer with chloride channel blocking activity, has been shown to have antisecretory actions, and in a double-blind randomized controlled trial reduced the duration of travelers' diarrhea by 29%.[24] Further studies are required to determine whether this agent will find a place in the treatment regimens for this condition.

It is now well established that the enteric nervous system (ENS) is involved in the promotion of intestinal secretion. A number of neurotransmitters have been identified in the ENS; many are thought to be involved in intestinal secretion and are therefore potential pharmacologic targets for the treatment of watery diarrhea.[25]

Antimicrobial therapy

Antibiotic therapy for infectious diarrhea is controversial. Mild illnesses probably do not need antibiotic treatment, although there are infections in which treatment is recommended: dysenteric shigellosis, cholera, pseudomembranous enterocolitis, and some protozoal infections. There are several diseases for which the indications are less clear but treatment is usually recommended: infection with the noncholera vibrios, prolonged or protracted infection with *Yersinia*, early in the course of campylobacteriosis, *Aeromonas*, and *Plesiomonas* infections, and outbreaks of EPEC diarrhea in nurseries. Patients should be treated if they are debilitated, particularly with malignancy, immunosuppressed, have an abnormal cardiovascular system, have valvular, vascular, or orthopedic prostheses, have hemolytic anemia (especially if salmonellosis is involved), or are extremely young or old. Treatment is also advised for those with prolonged symptoms and those who relapse.

Acute watery diarrhea

Antibiotic therapy is controversial unless the illness is severe or due to cholera. Indiscriminate use of antibiotics may

TREATMENT AND PREVENTION

ANTIMICROBIAL THERAPY FOR ACUTE INFECTIOUS DIARRHEA

Organism	Efficacy of antimicrobial therapy	Drug of choice	Alternative choice
BACTERIA			
Vibrio cholerae	Proven	Tetracycline 500 mg qds for 3 days Ciprofloxacin 1000 mg single dose	TMP-SMX, doxycyline, norfloxacin, ciprofloxacin: 3 days
ETEC	Proven	Ciprofloxacin 500 mg bd for 3–5 days Norfloxacin 400 mg bd for 3–5 days	Ciprofloxacin 500 mg single dose
EPEC	Possible		
EIEC	Possible	?Same as for Shigella spp.	
EHEC	Controversial	See text	
Shigella spp.	Proven efficacy in dysenteric shigellosis	TMP-SMX 2 tablets bd for 5 days[a] Ciprofloxacin 500 mg bd for 5 days Other quinolones: norfloxacin, fleroxacin, cinoxacin	Short-term quinolone Cefixime 400 mg daily for 5–7 days *or* other third-generation cephalosporins Nalidixic acid 1 g qds for 5–7 days
Salmonella spp.	Doubtful efficacy in enterocolitis Proven efficacy in severe salmonellosis (dysentery, fever)	Ciprofloxacin 500 mg bd for 10–14 days Third-generation cephalosporins for 10–14 days **Carrier state:** Norfloxacin 400 mg bd for 28 days	TMP-SMX, ampicillin, amoxicillin
Campylobacter spp.	Possible efficacy in Campylobacter enteritis Proven efficacy in Campylobacter dysentery or sepsis	Erythromycin 250–500 mg qds for 7 days	Ciprofloxacin 500 mg bd for 5–7 days Azithromycin 500 mg od for 3 days
Yersinia spp.	Doubtful efficacy in Yersinia enteritis Proven efficacy in Yersinia septicemia	Ciprofloxacin 500 mg bd for 7–10 days	Tetracycline 250 mg qds for 7–10 days
Clostridium difficile	Proven	Metronidazole 400 mg tds for 7–10 days	Vancomycin 125 mg qds for 7–10 days Fusidic acid, teicoplanin
PROTOZOA			
Cryptosporidium parvum	Proven	Nitazoxanide 500 mg bd for 3–14 days	
Isospora belli	Proven		
Cyclospora cayetanensis	Proven		
Entamoeba histolytica	Proven	Metronidazole 750 mg tds for 5 days Diloxanide furoate 500 mg tds for 10 days	Paromomycin 25–35 mg/kg tds for 7–10 days
Balantidium coli	Proven	Metronidazole 400 mg tds for 10 days	Tetracycline 500 mg qds for 10 days

Antimicrobial therapy is not indicated for acute viral diarrhea such as that due to rotavirus, enteric adenoviruses, and small round structured viruses.
[a] TMP-SMX (trimethoprim–sulfamethoxazole) is of limited value because of resistance patterns.
Modified from Casburn-Jones AC, Farthing MJG. Management of infectious diarrhoea. Gut 2004; 53:296–305, with permission.

TREATMENT AND PREVENTION

ANTIMICROBIAL THERAPY FOR PERSISTENT INFECTIOUS DIARRHEA

Enteropathogen	Antimicrobial therapy	Alternative(s)
PROTOZOA		
Giardia intestinalis	Metronidazole 400 mg tds for 7–10 days	Tinidazole 2 g single dose
Cryptosporidium parvum	Nitazoxanide 500 mg bd for 3–14 days	?Albendazole 400 mg bd for 7–14 days
Cyclospora cayetanensis	TMP-SMX 2 tablets bd for 7 days	
Isospora belli	TMP-SMX 2 tablets qds for 10 days	
MICROSPORIDIA		
Encephalitozoon intestinalis	?Albendazole 400 mg bd for 14–28 days	?Furazolidone 100 mg qds for 20 days
Enterocytozoon bieneusi	?Atovaquone	
Entamoeba histolytica	Metronidazole 750 mg tds for 5 days Diloxanide furoate 500 mg tds for 10 days	
Balantidium coli	Metronidazole 400 mg tds for 10 days	
HELMINTHS		
Strongyloides stercoralis	Ivermectin 200 μg/kg/day for 2 days	Albendazole 400 mg od for 3 days
Schistosoma spp.	Praziquantel 2–3 doses on day 1	Ivermectin 100–200 μg/kg od for 2 days
S. mansoni, S. haematobium	Praziquantel 40 mg/kg/day	
S. japonicum	Praziquantel 60 mg/kg/day	
VIRUS		
Cytomegalovirus	Ganciclovir 5 mg/kg bd for 14–21 days	Foscarnet 60 mg/kg tds for 14–21 days Maintenance therapy required

Modified from Casburn-Jones AC, Farthing MJG. Management of infectious diarrhoea. Gut 2004; 53:296–305.

contribute to the emergence of antibiotic resistance and exposes the individual to severe unwanted side effects such as the Stevens-Johnson syndrome or pseudomembranous colitis. However, in travelers' diarrhea antimicrobial therapy is unequivocally effective and is recommended for severe infections or when the individual is unable to tolerate a diarrheal illness because of work or other commitments. Quinolone antibiotics are now the treatment of choice; standard doses for 3–5 days can reduce the severity and duration of illness by at least 50%,[26] but single-dose regimens have similar efficacy.[27] Recently there has been renewed interest in a nonabsorbed locally active antibiotic, rifaximin, for the treatment of traveler's diarrhea. This drug has been shown to be as effective as ciprofloxacin but with the potential advantage of only minimal systemic absorption.[28]

Dysentery

Antibiotics are recommended for the treatment of dysentery due to most organisms.[29] However, antibiotic therapy for *Campylobacter* and EHEC infection remains controversial. In *Campylobacter* infection there is good evidence that antibiotics do not alter the natural course of the illness if they are started more than 4 days after the onset of symptoms. Antimicrobial therapy in EHEC infection remains controversial for two reasons: (1) antibiotics do not significantly improve outcome, especially if started well after infection was established;[30] and (2) there is anecdotal evidence that antibiotics can promote the development of hemolytic–uremic syndrome. Antibiotics are thought to increase the lysis of organisms and the release of shiga-like toxin (verotoxin) and endotoxin.

Persistent diarrhea

Most of the enteropathogens that cause persistent diarrhea are amenable to antimicrobial therapy.[29] *Cryptosporidium parvum* is, however, difficult to treat and is resistant to most antimicrobial agents. Paromomycin has been shown to have some efficacy in one open study[31] but a more recent randomized controlled trial has indicated that this drug is no better than placebo.[32] Recent studies have shown that high-dose albendazole or nitazoxanide may be the most efficacious agents in cryptosporidiosis.[33,34] Microsporidia are also difficult to treat and have variable sensitivity to many agents. Albendazole is effective in treating *Encephalitozoon intestinalis* but not very effective in treating *Enterocytozoon bieneusi*. *C. cayetanensis* infection can be treated effectively with trimethoprim–sulfamethoxazole.

Probiotics

In 1985, Gorbach and colleagues identified a lactobacillus as a result of screening bacteria in fermented milk products thought to be beneficial to human health.[35] This lactobacillus species was acid and bile resistant, adhered to human intestinal epithelial cells, and had growth characteristics necessary for commercial development. This strain, identified as *Lactobacillus* GG, is one of several probiotics, a nonpathogenic organism, used to improve intestinal microbial balance. Following this discovery, multiple candidate microorganisms have been developed, but *Lactobacillus* GG remains the most common strain to be tested in controlled trials. In a multicenter trial *Lactobacillus* GG was shown to reduce the duration of rotavirus episodes but had no effect on bacterial diarrheas.[36] A recent meta-analysis supports the view that probiotics can shorten the duration of acute diarrheal illness in children by 1 day.[37] Although this meta-analysis also suggests that probiotics benefit antibiotic-associated diarrhea, further studies are required to provide a definitive answer.

Prevention

Primary prevention of gastrointestinal infection can be achieved by interruption of the fecal–oral transmission route. This involves ensuring the availability of high-quality drinking water, adequate sanitation to ensure the safe disposal of feces, and clear guidelines on personal hygiene to minimize person-to-person transmission. In addition, guidelines and legislation are required to ensure the highest standards in animal husbandry, food production, and subsequent food handling, with regular surveillance procedures to ensure that these standards are maintained. In the UK this is now the responsibility of the Foods Standards Agency.

Chemoprophylaxis

Broad-spectrum antibiotics taken at approximately half the therapeutic dose can prevent certain intestinal infections, particularly cholera (tetracycline) and travelers' diarrhea (fluoroquinolones). Their use in the latter, however, is not generally recommended because of concerns about adverse effects and emerging drug resistance. The nonantibiotic preparation bismuth subsalicylate is an alternative, but is less effective than antibiotics.

Probiotics

The concept that the gut can be colonized with harmless bacteria that will protect against the harmful effects of enteropathogens has been around for more than a century, since the time of Louis Pasteur. The evidence for their efficacy as a prophylactic remains controversial but some studies have clearly demonstrated a protective effect against rotavirus infection in children. This is a rapidly developing field and it is likely that genetically modified organisms with improved efficacy will be available in the future.

Immunoprophylaxis

Although parenteral vaccines for cholera and typhoid have been available for many years, their efficacy is low. The major thrust of vaccine development in recent years has focused on oral vaccines to ensure that there is the capacity for a local protective immune response in the gut. A whole cell–B-subunit oral cholera vaccine has been subjected to extensive field trials and shown to be moderately effective. More recently, a genetically engineered live oral cholera vaccine has been developed which appears to be as effective after a single dose. These cholera vaccines also have some protective effects against travelers' diarrhea caused by other organisms, and the whole cell–B-subunit vaccine is currently marketed in some countries for travelers' diarrhea. Although there have been successful attempts to develop vaccines against rotavirus infection, particularly a tetravalent rhesus assortant vaccine, the program has been seriously curtailed by the occurrence of an important adverse effect, namely intussusception. Vaccines for *Shigella* and *Salmonella* are also under development.

COMPLICATIONS AND THEIR MANAGEMENT

Dehydration and acidosis

Although the majority of deaths worldwide from intestinal infection are still due to dehydration and acidosis, this aspect of the illness should always be possible to manage by oral or intravenous rehydration. In recent years it has become increasingly clear that death also occurs as a result of the complications of infection, particularly those due to the invasive enteropathogens.

Hemolytic–uremic syndrome

Shigella dysenteriae type 1 infection has been known for several decades to cause hemolytic–uremic syndrome, and it is now well established that this is also responsible for a substantial proportion of the mortality associated with EHEC infection. Hemolytic–uremic syndrome, which consists of a triad of features – acute renal failure, thrombocytopenia, and microangiopathic hemolytic anemia – is also described with *Salmonella typhi*, *Campylobacter jejuni*, and *Yersinia pseudotuberculosis* infections. It occurs in about 6% of patients with EHEC infection and carries a mortality rate of 3–5%.[38]

Nonseptic arthritis and Reiter's syndrome

These symptoms are commonly associated with several invasive organisms including *Salmonella* spp., *Shigella* spp., *Y. enterocolitica*, and *C. jejuni*. More than 70% of patients who develop nonseptic arthritis are HLA-B27 positive. Nonseptic arthritis may be associated with iritis and conjunctivitis, which may occur in up to 90% of patients with arthritis following shigellosis and in up to 25% of those with *Salmonella*, *Campylobacter*, or *Yersinia* infections. The term Reiter's syndrome is reserved for the classic triad of symptoms consisting of arthritis, urethritis, and conjunctivitis. Again, HLA-B27 positivity strongly predicts the likelihood of developing Reiter's syndrome and is indicative of its severity.

Guillain-Barré syndrome

There is now a clear link between *C. jejuni* infection and the Guillain-Barré syndrome.[39] If the syndrome follows *Campylobacter* infection, it appears to be predominantly a motor disorder and has a particularly poor outcome with an increased risk of requiring ventilatory support and of having severe disability at 1 year.

Septic arthritis

Purulent synovitis during enteric infection is relatively rare, occurring in 0.2–2.5% of individuals with *Salmonella* infection. Infection is usually monoarticular, involving the large joints. Symptoms begin within 2 weeks of the gastrointestinal symptoms, but may occur as late as 7 weeks. There is no association with HLA-B27.

Chronic carrier state

rolonged carriage is well recognized in *Salmonella* infection, articularly in the presence of renal stones or gallstones. radication can be achieved in more than 80% of cases by dministration of amoxicillin or a quinolone for 4–6 weeks at tandard doses.

rritable bowel syndrome

here is now good evidence that acute intestinal infection can ad on to irritable bowel syndrome following clearance of e enteropathogen.[39] It has been proposed that this may be elated to subclinical 'inflammation' and an increase in 5-HT-ontaining enterochromaffin cells. Management is the same as r other causes of irritable bowel syndrome.

PROGNOSIS WITH AND WITHOUT TREATMENT

Many acute intestinal infections are self-limiting and will esolve without specific treatment. Even infections such as holera and intestinal amebiasis that benefit from antibiotic herapy will resolve without treatment, provided supportive herapy is given. Antibiotic therapy, however, is vital when here is evidence of bacteremia and systemic complications. imilarly, patients with impaired immunity are also less likely o clear infections naturally and thus it is wise to give antibiotic therapy early in the course of the illness. It is this group hat is most likely to succumb to an intestinal infection. Death s also more likely in infants and young children, but is generlly avoidable provided that fluid and electrolyte losses are eplaced promptly. The hemolytic–uremic syndrome has a signficant mortality when associated with *Shigella dysenteriae* nd EHEC infection.

WHAT TO TELL PATIENTS

Avoidance

Travelers should be made aware of the risk factors associated vith intestinal infection and given advice about an avoidance trategy. 'Boil it, cook it, peel it, or forget it.'[40] This is clearly lescribed on a number of travel health websites. Immunoompromised patients should be aware of their susceptibility and take avoidance measures at all times, whether or not they are traveling.

Self-therapy

Individuals should be made aware of the importance of early oral rehydration during an attack of acute infectious diarrhea. Some travelers may want advice on the use of an antibiotic should they develop diarrhea during a trip abroad in which they could not afford to be unwell for 2–3 days.[41]

The time to seek medical advice

When diarrhea persists for more than 2–3 weeks it is entirely reasonable for a patient to seek medical advice. The same would apply to patients experiencing bloody diarrhea, especially when associated with high fever. Patients with immune deficiency should have a particularly low threshold for seeking self-referral.

CURRENT CONTROVERSIES AND THEIR FUTURE RESOLUTION

- The role of antibiotic therapy in a number of infective diarrheas – more high-quality randomized controlled trials are needed.
- The role of probiotics in the prevention and treatment of infective diarrhea – more high-quality clinical trials with established probiotic preparations and the development of new agents with enhanced capacity to colonize the human intestine are necessary.
- The role of antisecretory drugs in the management of watery diarrhea – further clinical trials of established agents and a search for agents that will target novel sites in the enterocyte and the enteric nervous system are required.

SOURCES OF INFORMATION FOR PATIENTS AND DOCTORS

Adults:
http://www.patient.co.uk/showdoc/23069066/
Children:
http://www.patient.co.uk/showdoc/23069067/

REFERENCES

1. Wheeler JG, Sethi D, Cowden JM et al. Study of infectious intestinal disease in England: rates in the community, presenting to general practice, and reported to national surveillance. BMJ 1999; 318:1046–1050.
2. Handszuh H, Waters SR. Travel and tourism patterns. In: DuPont HL, Steffen R, eds. Textbook of travel medicine & health. Hamilton: Decker, 1997:20–26.
3. Lopman B, Vennema H, Kohli E et al. Increase in viral gastroenteritis outbreaks in Europe and epidemic spread of new norovirus variant. Lancet 2004; 363:682–688.
4. Farthing MJG, DuPont HL, Guandalini S et al. Treatment and prevention of travellers' diarrhoea. Gastroenterol Internat 1992; 5:162–175.
5. DuPont HL, Ericsson CD. Prevention and treatment of traveler's diarrhea. N Engl J Med 1993; 328:1821–1827.
6. Neal KR, Brij SO, Slack RCB et al. Recent treatment with H_2 antagonists and antibiotics for gastric surgery as risk factors for *Salmonella* infection. BMJ 1994; 308:176.
7. Neal KR, Scott HM, Slack RCB. Omeprazole as a risk factor for *Campylobacter* gastroenteritis: case control study. BMJ 1996; 312:414–415.
8. Rao MC. Molecular mechanisms of bacterial toxins. In: Farthing MJG, Keusch GT, eds. Enteric infection. London: Chapman & Hall; 1989:87–104.
9. Field M, Fao M, Chang EB. Intestinal electrolyte transport and diarrheal disease. N Engl J Med 1989; 321:879–883.
10. Jodal M. Neuronal influence on intestinal transport. J Intern Med 1990; 228:125–132.
11. Turvill JL, Mourad FH, Farthing MJG. Crucial role for 5-HT in cholera toxin but not *Escherichia coli* heat-labile enterotoxin-intestinal secretion in rats. Gastroenterology 1998; 115:883–890.
12. Salim AFM, Phillips AD, Walker-Smith JA, Farthing MJG. Sequential changes in small intestinal structure and function during rotavirus infection in neonatal rats. Gut 1995; 36:231–238.
13. Farthing MJG, Kelly MP, Veitch AM. Recently recognised microbial enteropathies and HIV infection. J Antimicrob Chemother 1996; 37:61–70.
14. Nostrant TT, Kumar NB, Appelman HD. Histopathology differentiates acute self-limited colitis from ulcerative colitis. Gastroenterology 1987; 92:318–328.
15. Farthing MJG. Dehydration and rehydration in children. In: Arnaud MJ, ed. Hydration throughout life. Paris: John Libbey Eurotext; 1998:159–173.

16. Farthing MJG, Goka AKJ, Butcher PD, Arvind AS. Serodiagnosis of giardiasis. Serodiag Immunother 1987; 1:233–238.
17. Arvind AS, Shetty N, Farthing MJG. Serodiagnosis of amoebiasis. Serodiag Immunother 1988; 2:79–84.
18. Kaplan MA, Prior MJ, McKonly KI et al. A multicentre randomised controlled trial of a liquid loperamide product versus placebo in the treatment of acute diarrhoea in children. Clin Pediatr 1999; 38:579–591.
19. Murphy GS, Bodhidatta L, Echeverria P et al. Ciprofloxacin and loperamide in the treatment of bacillary dysentery. Ann Intern Med 1993; 118:582–586.
20. Farthing MJG, Casburn-Jones A, Banks MR. Getting control of intestinal secretion: thoughts for 2003. Dig Liv Dis 2003; 35:378–385.
21. Farthing MJG. Enkephalinase inhibition: a rational approach to anti-secretory therapy for acute diarrhoea. Aliment Pharmacol Ther 1999; 13(Suppl 6):1–2.
22. Cezard JP, Duhamel JF, Meyer M et al, Efficacy and tolerability of racecadotril in acute diarrhea in children. Gastroenterology 2001; 120:799–805.
23. Ma T, Thiagarajah JR, Yang H et al. Thiazilinone CFTR inhibitor identified by high throughput screening blocks cholera toxin-induced intestinal fluid secretion. J Clin Invest 2002; 110:1651–1658.
24. DiCesare D, DuPont HL, Mathewson JJ et al. A double-blind, randomized, placebo-controlled study of SP 303 (Provir) in the symptomatic treatment of acute diarrhea among travelers to Jamaica and Mexico. Am J Gastroenterol 2002; 97:2585–2588.
25. Farthing MJ. Novel targets for the control of secretory diarrhoea. Gut 2002; 50(Suppl 3):III 15–18.
26. Mattila L, Peltola H, Siitonen A et al. Short-term treatment of traveler's diarrhea with norfloxacin: a double-blind, placebo-controlled study during two sessions. Clin Infect Dis 1993; 17:779–782.
27. Salam I, Katelaris P, Leigh-Smith S et al. A randomised placebo-controlled trial of single dose ciprofloxacin in treatment of travellers' diarrhoea. Lancet 1994; 344:1537–1539.
28. DuPont HL, Jiang Z-D, Ericsson CD et al. Rifaximin versus ciprofloxacin for the treatment of traveler's diarrhea: a randomised, double-blind clinical trial. Clin Infect Dis 2001; 33:1807–1815.
29. Casburn-Jones AC, Farthing MJG. Management of infectious diarrhoea. Gut 2004; 53:296–305.
30. Prouix F, Turgeon JPJ, Delage G et al. Randomized, controlled trial of antibiotic therapy for *Escherichia coli* O157-H7 enteritis. J Pediatr 1992; 121:299–303.
31. Bissuel F, Cotte L, Rabodonirina M, Rougier P, Piens MA, Trepo C. Paromomycin: an effective treatment fpr cryptosporidial diarrhea in patients with AIDS. Clin Infect Dis 1994; 18: 447–449.
32. Hewitt RG, Tiannoutsos CT, Higgs ES et al. Paromomycin: no more effective than placebo for treatment of cryptosporidiosis in patients with advanced immunodeficiency virus infection. AIDS Clinical Trial Group. Clin Infect Dis 2000; 31:1084–1092.
33. Bailey JM, Erramouspe J. Nitazoxanide treatment for giardiasis and cryptosporidiosis in children. Ann Pharmacother 2004; 38:634–640.
34. Farthing MJG. Clinical aspects of human cryptosporidiosis. Contrib Microbiol 2000; 6:50–74.
35. Gorbach SL. The discovery of *Lactobacillus* GG. Nutrition Today 1996; 31:2S–4S.
36. Guandalini S, Kirjavainen PV, Zikri MA et al. *Lactobacillus* GG administered in oral rehydration solution to children with acute diarrhoea: a multicenter European trial. J Pediatr Gastroenterol Nutr 2000; 30:54–60.
37. Huang JS, Bousvaros A, Lee JW, Diaz A, Davidson EJ. Efficacy of probiotic use in acute diarrhea in children: a meta-analysis. Dig Dis Sci 2002; 47:2625–2634.
38. Boyce TG, Swerdlow DL, Griffin PM. *Escherichia coli* O157:H7 and the hemolytic–uremic syndrome. N Engl J Med 1995; 333:364–368.
39. Spiller RC. Postinfectious irritable bowel syndrome. Gastroenterology 2003; 124:1662–1671.
40. Kozicki M, Steffen R, Schar M. "Boil it, cook it, peel it, or forget it": does this rule prevent travelers' diarrhea? Int J Epidemiol 1985; 14:169–172.
41. Casburn-Jones AC, Farthing MJ. Traveler's diarrhea. J Gastroenterol Hepatol 2004; 19:610–618.

Chapter 50

Travelers' diarrhea

Andrew W DuPont and Herbert L DuPont

KEY POINTS

- Defined as ≥ 3 unformed stools in 24 hours with abdominal discomfort or cramps or vomiting
- Travel from low to high risk geographical areas carries a 40% risk
- Protective immunity develops within months of living in endemic areas
- Susceptibility to some pathogens, e.g. enterotoxigenic *E. coli*, is probably genetically determined
- Ciprofloxacin-resistant campylobacter is an increasing worldwide problem
- Vomiting as a primary symptom suggests viral gastroenteritis or food-borne intoxication
- Bismuth and loperamide are helpful symptomatically
- Care with choice of food and drinks are the key to prevention

INTRODUCTION

Traveler's diarrhea is typically defined as a clinically important illness with at least three unformed stools over a 24-h period with one or more additional signs or symptoms of enteric infection, such as abdominal discomfort and cramps, nausea, and vomiting, in a person traveling from an industrialized region to a tropical or semitropical region.

EPIDEMIOLOGY

Annually more than 600 million people travel outside their country, with more than 50 million visiting tropical and subtropical regions hyperendemic for diarrhea. The world can be divided broadly into three levels of diarrhea risk to the international traveler.[1] The low-risk areas include northern Europe, the United States, Canada, Japan, Australia, and New Zealand, with diarrhea occurring in 2–4% of those visiting these regions. Those traveling from the low-risk areas to high-risk regions of Latin America, southern Asia, and much of Africa have an approximately 40% chance of developing illness. Countries of the northern Mediterranean, the Caribbean, Russia, and China comprise a third category of intermediate risk where travelers experience rates of illness varying from 10% to 20%.

Protective immunity develops within months of living in endemic areas, presumably through repeated exposure to enteric pathogens found in food, with the most striking immunity developing against the major cause of illness in many settings – enterotoxigenic *Escherichia coli*. The finding of short-term immunity in international travelers has given hope for control of disease through immunoprophylactic approaches.

CAUSES, RISK FACTORS, DISEASE ASSOCIATIONS

Illness rates are increased in adventure travelers, missionaries, Peace Corps volunteers, and others working or living close to the local population and staying in inexpensive hotels or camps, or living with the local population. Age of the traveler influences the rate of acquisition of diarrhea,[1,2] with two peaks of increased rate: travelers aged 0–2 years and those less than 30 years of age (see Chapters 9 and 49).

It has been well established that food is the major source of enteric infection among international travelers.[3,4] There is clearly an association with illness rates and the location of food consumption, with lowest rates when food is self-prepared in apartments and higher rates when it is eaten in the homes of local people or in public restaurants.

Foods and beverages can be categorized as high or low risk based on several principles. Contamination of food and beverages may be diminished or eliminated by heating to at least 59°C (food that is steaming hot). Recontamination becomes a problem when food is cooked too early before consumption, as is commonly seen for hamburgers. Other generally safe foods include those that are dry (bread), those that have been peeled (fruit), and food with a high sugar content (jellies, honey, and syrup) or low pH if refrigerated between use.[4]

Some international travelers are able to remain well during periods of risk, whereas others with a similar travel experience and risk factors may be affected repeatedly. Genetic factors appear to explain a proportion of illness susceptibility variation among travelers to high-risk areas. Blood type O predisposes persons to Norwalk virus gastroenteritis and to cholera, which constitutes an unexplained genetic association with enteric infectious diseases. The occurrence of diarrhea due to the two major pathogens in this setting, enterotoxigenic *E. coli* (ETEC) and enteroaggregative *E. coli* (EAEC), appears to show genetic associations. ETEC receptors in the small bowel, which are required for enteric infection, are genetically acquired in susceptible piglets.[5] It is likely in humans that ETEC receptors are present or absent on a genetic basis, explaining relative susceptibility to this pathogen. In EAEC diarrhea the major mediator of the inflammatory diarrhea appears to be release of intestinal interleukin-8 (IL-8).[6] We have recently shown that among US travelers to Mexico, where EAEC diarrhea commonly occurs, susceptibility to this form of diarrhea is determined by genetic polymorphism in the promoter region of the *IL-8* gene.[7]

For more than a century investigators have supported the idea that decreased gastric acidity predisposes to enteric infection by bacterial pathogens, although the association remains largely unstudied for travelers. It appears intuitive that travelers with hypochlorhydria or achlorhydria would be at increased risk for diarrhea when traveling to the tropics, although the association may not be as strong as once thought.

PATHOGENESIS AND PATHOLOGY

Etiologic agents

The major causes of diarrhea among international travelers to high-risk tropical and subtropical areas are a variety of bacterial pathogens, explaining approximately 80% of illness (Table 50.1). The diarrheagenic *E. coli* (ETEC, EAEC, and enteroinvasive *E. coli*) explain over 50% of illness in most areas.[8,9] ETEC strains contain up to three important virulence characteristics, including an attachment ligand called colonization factor antigens as well as two toxins – cholera-like heat-labile toxin (LT) and a low molecular weight and inflammatory heat-stable toxin (ST). All ETEC strains produce one of the following: LT only; ST only; and ST plus LT. The more pathogenic strains are positive for ST only, or for ST plus LT (see Chapter 49). Other important bacterial agents include *Shigella*, *Salmonella*, *Campylobacter*, *Aeromonas*, and *Plesiomonas* species. Parasitic pathogens explain less than 5% of cases and viruses about 10%.[8] *Cyclospora* has been shown to be an important cause of spring or early summertime diarrhea in travelers to Nepal, and *Giardia* and *Cyclospora* have been commonly identified in travelers to Russia, particularly St Petersburg. In Thailand, ciprofloxacin-resistant *Campylobacter* is an important cause of diarrhea in international visitors.[10] Resistant *Campylobacter* is an important cause of diarrhea with worldwide occurrence, and should be considered as the major cause of fluoroquinolone-unresponsive travelers' diarrhea regardless of region.

CLINICAL PRESENTATION

More than 80% of travelers with diarrhea will experience watery diarrhea without significant fever that, left untreated, typically consists of passage of 13 unformed stools over a 5-day interval. Those affected characteristically experience abdominal cramps and pain that is temporarily debilitating (see also Chapters 9 and 49). In less than 10% of travelers with diarrhea, febrile dysentery (bloody stools) may occur and is most often due to strains of *Shigella*, *Campylobacter*, *Salmonella*, noncholera vibrios, and *Aeromonas*. In approximately 10% of cases, vomiting is the predominant symptom, likely due to infection with viruses or ingestion of the preformed toxin of *Staphylococcus* or *Bacillus cereus*. Travelers' diarrhea regularly forces a change in itinerary, confining 20–46% to bed for 1 day or more. Between 4% and 17% will seek care from a local physician and nearly 0.2% require local hospitalization.

In 10% of patients, diarrhea lasts for more than a week, and in 2–10% it persists for more than 1 month.[11] In an important subset of those with travelers' diarrhea, a chronic illness develops that is compatible with post-infectious irritable bowel syndrome,[12] and in a small number inflammatory bowel disease may be precipitated or unmasked. Other potential causes of protracted illness include disaccharide deficiency and small bowel overgrowth, as well as Brainerd diarrhea, a chronic diarrheal illness that may last for years and can often be traced to the consumption of raw (unpasteurized) milk or untreated surface water.

TABLE 50.1 GEOGRAPHIC CONSIDERATIONS IN THE MICROBIAL ETIOLOGY OF TRAVELERS' DIARRHEA

Geographic area	Characteristic etiology
All regions of the tropical and semitropical developing world	Bacterial enteropathogens, especially ETEC and EAEC
Thailand	Ciprofloxacin-resistant *Campylobacter*
Russia (St Petersburg)	*Giardia* and *Cryptosporidium*
Nepal (spring, early summer)	*Cyclospora*

ETEC, enterotoxigenic *Escherichia coli*; EAEC, enteroaggregative *E. coli*.

DIFFERENTIAL DIAGNOSIS

In most cases of travelers' diarrhea a bacterial pathogen should be suspected. When vomiting is the primary symptom of the illness, viral gastroenteritis or food-borne intoxication are most likely explanations of illness. For those with persistent illness, parasitic agents and post-infectious irritable bowel syndrome should be considered as possible causes of illness.

DIAGNOSTIC METHODS

Laboratory testing should be done for a limited number of indications including persistent diarrhea (see Chapter 49), fluoroquinolone-resistant illness, or when the traveler has a serious underlying medical condition, such as acquired immune deficiency syndrome (AIDS).

In cases of prolonged symptoms in which stool studies have been unrevealing (e.g., negative tests for parasites including *Giardia* and *Cryptosporidium* antigens) and a dietary association has not been found (e.g., lactose intolerance), endoscopic and/or radiographic studies may be indicated. Endoscopic evaluation of the small bowel with aspiration or biopsy can help to diagnose parasitic infections; proctosigmoidoscopy can be used to evaluate for persistent colonic infection; and barium studies may be useful to rule out inflammatory bowel disease in the appropriate setting.

TREATMENT AND PREVENTION

Symptomatic treatment will help to control the passage of unformed stools and allow travelers to function when they develop illness.[13] Bismuth subsalicylate works through its antisecretory properties and will decrease the number of stools passed by 40%. The antimotility drug loperamide is more effective, reducing the number of stools passed by 60%, but may produce objectionable post-treatment constipation. Novel antisecretory drugs may safely offer a more physiologic relief of symptoms and may in the future become standard treatment for the symptoms of travelers' diarrhea.

Antibacterial drugs with activity against prevalent bacterial pathogens will successfully shorten illness by 1–2 days compared with untreated or placebo-treated illness,[13] and can be used in a single dose for most patients.[14] When trimethoprim resistance became widespread, the fluoroquinolones became standard therapy. Levofloxacin offers advantages over ciprofloxacin as it can be given once a day. Azithromycin is as effective as the fluoroquinolones in shortening the duration of diarrhea after the initiation of therapy and has the advantages of being effective against ciprofloxacin-resistant *Campylobacter*; it can be given safely to children and potentially pregnant women with illness. These absorbable drugs, including fluoroquinolones and azithromycin, are effective in treating most cases of travelers' diarrhea with a single dose. Where available, rifaximin may be the drug of choice for nonfebrile, nondysenteric illness. Rifaximin is as effective as ciprofloxacin in treating travelers' diarrhea.[15]

TREATMENT AND PREVENTION

ANTIBACTERIAL THERAPY OF ACUTE TRAVELERS' DIARRHEA IN ADULTS

Antibacterial agent	Dose and duration	Comments[a]
Ciprofloxacin	500 mg bid for 3 days	Not to be used in pregnant women or children; *Campylobacter* resistance is a growing problem
Levofloxacin	500 mg once; can repeat next morning if not well and repeat the second day if needed	Not to be used in pregnant women or children; advantage is single daily dose
Azithromycin	500 mg once; can repeat next morning if not well and repeat the second day if needed	Safe in all patients; can be used in children and pregnant women
Rifaximin	200 mg tid or 400 mg bid for 3 days	Safe in all patients; can be used in children

[a]All drugs shorten illness by more than 1 day compared with placebo.

The key to prevention of travelers' diarrhea is careful food and beverage selection. This approach, while potentially successful, is often not followed.[10] Drugs can be used to prevent the illness. Bismuth subsalicylate will prevent 65% of the disease that would occur without daily use. A fluoroquinolone is more effective, preventing approximately 80% of the disease that would otherwise occur. Use of prophylaxis with systemically absorbed antimicrobials is currently not recommended for all travelers in view of potential side effects of the drugs and concern about the development of general resistance. The poorly absorbed drug rifaximin has been used in a recent clinical trial and has great promise in prevention of travelers' diarrhea (DuPont HL, et al – unpublished data).

COMPLICATIONS AND PROGNOSIS

Travelers' diarrhea is a nonfatal condition. Although the diarrhea may be severe, the major concern other than short-term disability is the production of postinfectious chronic illness, most importantly post-infectious irritable bowel syndrome. These patients should be investigated and treated.

FUTURE CONSIDERATIONS

Rates of diarrhea during international travel have not changed since studies were initiated 50 years ago. Local governments should be encouraged to work with restaurants, hotels, and tour operators to improve the hygienic conditions of international travelers. If this is not possible, the restaurants and hotels should work independently to create safe havens where persons can remain disease-free while in the area of risk. Preventive medications and vaccines are likely to have important future roles in reducing rates of illness among international travelers.

SOURCES OF INFORMATION FOR PATIENTS AND DOCTORS

http://www.traveldoctor.co.uk/diarrhoea.htm
http://www.masta.org/travel-health/disease-risks.asp?group=3&dis_id=17
http://www.irishhealth.com/?level=4&con=248

REFERENCES

1. DuPont HL. Traveler's diarrhea. In: Blaser MJ, Smith PD, Ravdin JI, Greenberg HB, Guerrant RL, eds. Infections of the gastrointestinal tract, 2nd edn. Philadelphia: Lippincott Williams & Wilkins; 2002:253–265.
2. Pitzinger B, Steffen R, Tschopp A. Incidence and clinical features of travelers' diarrhea in infants and children. Pediatr Infect Dis J 1991; 10:719–723.
3. Wood LV, Ferguson LE, Hogan P et al. Incidence of bacterial enteropathogens in foods from Mexico. Appl Environ Microbiol 1983; 46:813–816.
4. Adachi JA, Mathewson JJ, Jiang Z-D et al. Enteric pathogens in Mexican sauces of popular restaurants in Guadalajara, Mexico and in Houston, Texas. Ann Intern Med 2002; 136: 884–887.
5. Rutter JM, Burrows MR, Sellwood R, Gibbons RA. A genetic basis for resistance to enteric disease caused by *E. coli*. Nature 1975; 257: 135–136.
6. Greenberg DE, Jiang ZD, Steffen R et al. Markers of inflammation in bacterial diarrhea among travelers with a focus on enteroaggregative *Escherichia coli* pathogenicity. J Infect Dis 2002; 185:944–949.
7. Jiang ZD, Okhuysen PC, Guo DC et al. Genetic susceptibility to enteroaggregative *Escherichia coli* diarrhea – polymorphism in interleukin-8 promoter region. J Infect Dis 2003; 188: 506–511.
8. Jiang Z-D, Lowe B, Verenker MP et al. Prevalence of enteric pathogens among international travelers with diarrhea acquired in Kenya (Mombasa), India (Goa), or Jamaica (Montego Bay). J Infect Dis 2002; 185:497–502.
9. Adachi JA, Jiang Z-D, Mathewson JJ et al. Enteroaggretative *Escherichia coli* as a major etiologic agent in traveler's diarrhea in 3 regions of the world. Clin Infect Dis 2001; 32: 1706–1709.
10. Kushner RA, Trofa AF, Thomas RJ et al. Use of azithromycin for the treatment of Campylobacter enteritis in travelers to Thailand, an area where ciprofloxacin resistance is prevalent. Clin Infect Dis 1995; 21:536–541.
11. DuPont HL, Capsuto EG. Persistent diarrhea in travelers. Clin Infect Dis 1996; 22:124–128.
12. Okhuysen PC, Jiang Z-D, Carlin L, et al. Post-diarrhea chronic intestinal symptoms and irritable bowel syndrome in North American travelers to Mexico. Amer J Gastroenterol 2004; 99:1774–1778.
13. DuPont HL, Ericsson CD. Prevention and treatment of traveler's diarrhea. N Engl J Med 1993; 328:1821–1826.
14. Salam I, Katelaris P, Leigh-Smith S, Farthing MJG. Randomized trial of single-dose ciprofloxacin for travelers' diarrhea. Lancet 1994; 344:1537–1539.
15. DuPont HL, Jiang Z-D, Ericsson CD et al. Rifaximin versus ciprofloxacin for the treatment of traveler's diarrhea: a randomized, double-blind clinical trial. Clin Infect Dis 2001; 33:1807–1815.

Chapter 51

Abdominal tuberculosis

Bhupinder Anand

KEY POINTS

- Abdominal infection is more common with cavitating lung lesions than fibrotic lung lesions
- The ileocecum is the most commonly affected site
- Ulcerative, hyperplastic (resembling Crohn's disease) and sclerotic forms are recognized in the intestine
- Peripheral lymphadenopathy (fixed or matted) is a helpful diagnostic clue
- Only 30% have an abnormal chest x-ray
- Standard treatment consists of an induction phase for two months (rifampicin, isoniazid, pyrazinamide and ethambutol) followed by a continuation phase for four months (rifampicin and isoniazid)
- MAC infection in immunocompromised patients frequently involves the gastrointestinal tract

INTRODUCTION

Abdominal tuberculosis refers to disease of the gastrointestinal tract, lymph nodes, peritoneum, and intra-abdominal organs such as liver and spleen (Table 51.1). Many patients have associated pulmonary tuberculosis; abdominal infection occurs more frequently with cavitating lung disease compared with predominantly fibrotic lesions.

EPIDEMIOLOGY

Nearly a third of the world's population (2 billion people) are infected with *Mycobacterium tuberculosis*. The WHO predicts continued increase in tuberculosis in underdeveloped countries, with 12 million new cases by 2005.[1] By contrast in the West, after the resurgence of tuberculosis in the 1980s due to the AIDS epidemic, new infections have declined to the lowest level in 50 years.

PATHOGENESIS

Mycobacterium tuberculosis is responsible for nearly all cases of abdominal tuberculosis; other mycobacteria (see below) are encountered infrequently. The tubercle bacillus reaches the gastrointestinal tract by several routes: swallowed sputum from pulmonary infection, food, adjacent tissues (pelvic organs), lymphatic spread, and bloodstream. In immunocompetent individuals, the infection is localized by the influx of specific lymphocytes and monocytes. If the immune response is inadequate, the disease progresses locally and systemically by lymphohematogenous dissemination.

TABLE 51.1 CLASSIFICATION OF ABDOMINAL TUBERCULOSIS

GASTROINTESTINAL
- Ulcerative (ulcers: single, multiple, diffuse)
- Hypertrophic (mass lesion)
- Fibrotic (stricture formation)

PERITONEAL
- Ascites (localized, generalized)
- Fibrotic or dry form (peritoneal adhesions, rolled up omentum)
- Mixed form

NODAL
- Mesenteric adenitis
- Mesenteric abscess

VISCERAL DISEASE
- Liver, spleen, urinary tract, genital organs

PATHOLOGY

Intestinal tuberculosis

The sites of involvement in order of decreasing frequency are: ileocecum, colon, jejunum, rectum and anal canal, duodenum, stomach, and esophagus. Three pathological forms are described; these are not mutually exclusive and can be seen in the same patient (Table 51.1).

Ulcerative variety

Mucosal ulcers cover a variable length of the bowel, with normal intervening mucosa.[2] The ulcers are placed transversely and if the entire circumference is involved, the lumen becomes narrowed in a 'napkin-ring'-like contraction. The ulcers are superficial and do not penetrate the muscularis mucosa. The corresponding mesenteric surface has increased fat content and enlarged lymph nodes. Histology reveals granulation tissue, with neutrophils and microabscesses. The characteristic tuberculous granulomas, consisting of lymphocytes, plasma cells, and Langhans' giant cells are seen in the ulcer bed. Rarely, colonic tuberculosis may present as diffuse disease, resembling ulcerative colitis.

Hyperplastic lesion

The bowel wall is thickened, measuring up to 3 cm in width. The mucosal surface has a cobblestone pattern, with numerous pseudopolyps. The bowel assumes a tubular form with narrowing of the lumen. The hypertrophic variety typically affects the ileocecal region. The intestinal lesion together with the increased mesenteric fat and enlarged lymph nodes may form an abdominal mass. Histology shows exuberant granulomatous tissue extending from the mucosa to the serosa, accompanied by hypertrophy of the muscularis layer.

Sclerotic form

Areas of marked narrowing of the bowel characterize the sclerotic form. There may be a single stricture or multiple strictures over a large segment of the intestine. The proximal bowel is dilated and enteroliths are noted at the stricture site. Histology shows diffuse fibrosis extending from the submucosa to the serosa. Granulation tissue is limited to the bowel segment adjacent to the strictured areas.

Peritoneal tuberculosis

Ascites is the most frequent presentation of peritoneal disease. Typically, grayish white 'miliary' nodules are scattered over the peritoneum. Fibrous bands or adhesions are common. The adhesions are mostly thin, but when thick and dense they divide the peritoneal cavity into compartments, with formation of loculated ascites. In some cases, the fibrotic response is so exuberant that the peritoneal cavity is completely obliterated, encasing the intestines like a cocoon. The omentum may become thickened, presenting as a transversely placed mass ('rolled up' omentum). Histology of the miliary nodules usually shows caseating necrosis and tuberculous granulomas.

Nodal tuberculosis

Isolated involvement of mesenteric nodes is uncommon. Enlarged lymph nodes may cause extrinsic compression and narrowing of the bowel lumen. Inflamed nodes can produce traction diverticula, seen mostly in the esophagus and colon.

TABLE 51.2 CHARACTERISTIC SYMPTOMS AND SIGNS OF ABDOMINAL TUBERCULOSIS

SYMPTOMS
- Systemic: fever, night sweats, weight loss, menstrual abnormalities
- Abdominal
  Pain: right iliac fossa, diffuse
  Change in bowel habit
  Subacute intestinal obstruction: episodic colicky pain, distention, borborygmi
  Malabsorption: diarrhea, bulky stools
- Organ specific
  Esophagus: dysphagia
  Stomach and duodenum: ulcer-like pain, gastric outlet obstruction
  Colon: ulcerative colitis-like picture – diarrhea with blood and mucus

SIGNS
- General: sick appearing, febrile, emaciated patient
- Peripheral lymphadenopathy
  Cervical, inguinal, axillary
  Nodes often fused ('matted'), fixed to tissues, sinus tracks
- Abdomen
  Distention:
    localized (mass, loculated ascites)
    generalized (intestinal obstruction, ascites)
  Intestinal obstruction: visible peristalsis, borborygmi
  Mass lesions: ileocecal mass, rolled up omentum, hepatosplenomegaly, nodal mass
  Doughy feel: diffuse peritoneal involvement
  Fistulae: cutaneous, perianal, internal

CLINICAL PRESENTATION (Table 51.2)

The peak presentation is between 30 and 50 years of age. There is no gender difference in the West but women outnumber men 2:1 in developing countries.

Systemic symptoms

Fever, malaise, anorexia, and weight loss occur frequently.[3] Fever is low grade, with an evening spike. Sweating can be profuse, often drenching clothes and bed sheets. Pulmonary symptoms are present in patients with lung disease. Menstrual abnormalities including amenorrhea are seen in 20% of women. Women may become sterile because of disease of the pelvic organs.

Abdominal symptoms

The characteristic symptom is abdominal pain. The pain is localized to the site of the disease, usually the right iliac fossa but can be diffuse and nonspecific. Typically, patients experience episodes of subacute intestinal obstruction with colicky pain, distention, and borborygmi, relieved to some extent by vomiting. The bowel habit is erratic, with episodes of diarrhea and constipation. Patients may have symptoms related to disease at a specific site: dysphagia in esophageal involvement, ulcer-like pain, and gastric outlet obstruction in duodenal disease, and diarrhea with blood in diffuse colonic involvement.

Physical Examination (Table 51.2)

Patients appear sick and emaciated. A low-grade temperature is noted. Peripheral lymphadenopathy should be carefully sought as it provides an easy source of diagnosis. Diseased nodes frequently fuse together ('matted') and form adhesions with surrounding tissues; as a result, they appear 'fixed' on examination and sinus tracks may form through the overlying skin. A palpable mass in the right iliac fossa is typical, but masses may be felt at other sites including the epigastrium (rolled up omentum). Visible peristalsis is noted in subacute bowel obstruction. Tenderness is localized to the site of disease. Diffuse tenderness with a 'doughy' feel is suggestive of peritoneal involvement. Presence of an uneven abdominal distention indicates loculated ascites. Fecal fistulae, and perianal fistulae and fissures may be noted. Enlargement of liver and spleen indicates involvement of these organs.

DIFFERENTIAL DIAGNOSIS

Lymphoma, carcinoma, and ameboma can mimic the abnormalities in tuberculosis. However, the condition most difficult to differentiate from tuberculosis is Crohn's disease (Table 51.3). Both involve any part of the gastrointestinal tract, produce skip lesions, have a predilection for the ileocecal area, and histology shows inflammatory cells with granulomas.

DIAGNOSTIC METHODS (Table 51.4)

Identification of *M. tuberculosis* provides a precise diagnosis. However, the organism is usually difficult to detect and a definitive diagnosis is possible only in a minority of individuals. Therefore, a therapeutic trial is justified in endemic countries.

TABLE 51.3 CHARACTERISTICS OF INTESTINAL TUBERCULOSIS AND CROHN'S DISEASE

Characteristic	Tuberculosis	Crohn's disease
Epidemiology	Developing countries	Developed countries
Clinical findings		
Intestinal obstruction	50%	<10%
Diarrhea	30%	>80%
Fistulae	<10%	30%
Anal lesions	<5%	30%
Extraintestinal lesions	<5%	30%
Pathology		
Ulcers	Superficial, transverse	Deep, longitudinal
Granulomas	Confluent	Discrete
Caseation, AFB	Present	Never
Investigations		
Positive tuberculin test	90%	Never
Abnormal chest X-ray	30%	Never
Treatment		
Steroid use	Worsening of disease	Beneficial response
Clinical course	Cured with treatment	Relapses despite treatment

AFB, acid-fast bacilli.

Indirect tests

A high sedimentation rate is a common but nonspecific finding. An abnormal chest X-ray is helpful (seen in 30% patients). A positive tuberculin response is an excellent screening test in nonendemic countries, but is of little use in endemic areas because of high positive rates in healthy individuals and after BCG inoculation. Moreover, the test is difficult to interpret,[4] and false-negative results are common in immunesuppressed conditions like AIDS. Serological tests (based on specific antibody response) are not used as they fail to differentiate active disease from past infection, and from other mycobacterial infections.

TABLE 51.4 DIAGNOSTIC TESTS IN ABDOMINAL TUBERCULOSIS

LABORATORY TESTS
- Elevated sedimentation rate (nonspecific finding)
- Positive tuberculin test (low specificity in endemic countries)
- Serological tests (not reliable)

IMAGING STUDIES
- Abnormal chest X-ray: very helpful if sputum is AFB +ve
- Flat films: dilated bowel loops, air–fluid levels, calcified nodes
- Barium study: assessment of location and extent of bowel disease; fistulae and sinus tracts
- Ultrasound/CT scan: assessment of free fluid, nodal disease, bowel wall thickness, mass lesions, disease of pelvic organs

ENDOSCOPY AND BIOPSY
- Evaluation of diseased area
- Histopathology: granulomas, caseation necrosis, staining for AFB
- Culture for *M. tuberculosis*

ASCITIC FLUID ANALYSIS
- Exudate, high lymphocyte count
- AFB and culture (low yield)
- Elevated adenosine deaminase (high yield)

LAPAROSCOPY
- Peritoneum: thickened, irregular, dull appearance
- Adhesions
- Miliary nodules: high positive yield at histology

AFB, acid-fast bacilli.

Imaging studies

Plain X-rays show dilated bowel loops, air–fluid levels, and calcified nodes. Barium study, best performed by enteroclysis, is useful in establishing the location and extent of bowel involvement, and identification of fistulae. The classic radiological features are: contracted terminal ileum with a wide, open ileocecal valve (Fleischner sign) and a narrow ileum opening into a contracted cecum (Sterlin's sign) (Fig. 51.1). However, overlapping small bowel loops may interfere with an accurate assessment, especially in the presence of bowel adhesions.

Ultrasonography is very sensitive in detecting small quantities of fluid. Other abnormalities noted are: fibrous strands; enlarged nodes with hypoechoic centers (secondary to caseation necrosis); and alternating pattern of echogenic and echo-free layers (club sandwich appearance) produced by diseased bowel loops with intervening fluid collection.[5]

Computerized tomography (Fig. 51.2) provides better assessment of bowel wall thickness and mass lesions, enlarged nodes that have low-density centers with peripheral enhancement after contrast injection, diffuse or localized fluid collection, and abnormality of pelvic organs.[6]

Endoscopy and biopsy

Diseased areas that are within reach should be examined with an endoscope.[7] Biopsy specimens should be used for histopathology, acid-fast bacilli (AFB) staining, and culture. Aspira-

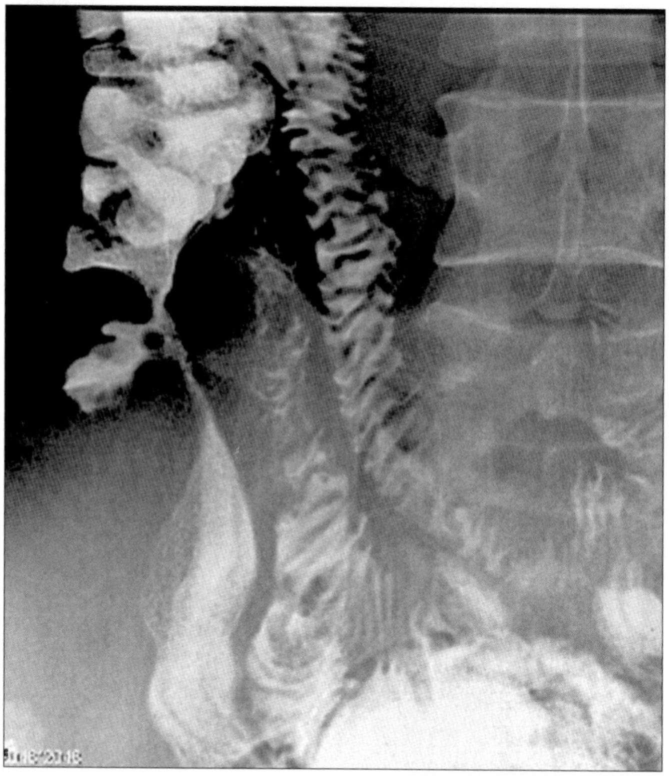

Fig. 51.1 Narrow ileum opening into a contracted cecum (Sterlin's sign). Courtesy of Drs Nirmal Kumar and Veena Chaudhary, Maulana Azad Medical College, New Delhi, India.

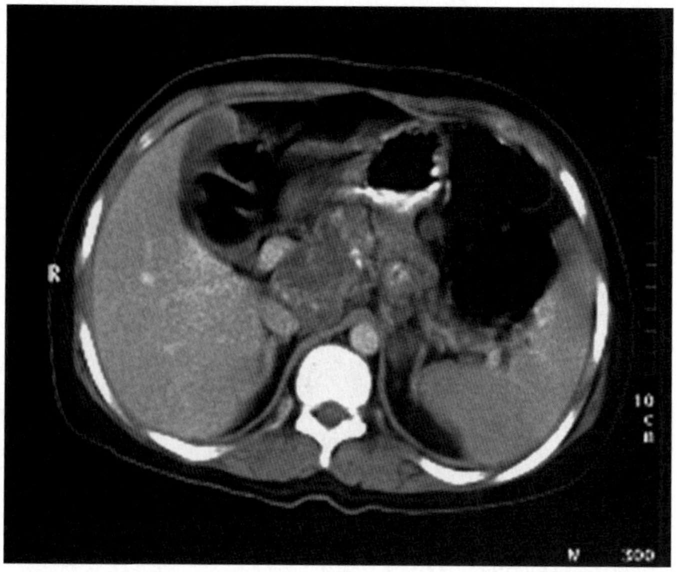

Fig. 51.2 CT scan showing enlarged retroperitoneal lymph nodes. Courtesy of Drs Nirmal Kumar and Veena Chaudhary, Maulana Azad Medical College, New Delhi, India.

tion cytology improves the yield in nodular lesions. Overall, a definitive diagnosis by endoscopy is made in one-third of patients. Another advantage of endoscopy is that conditions such as lymphoma and carcinoma can be excluded.

Tuberculous ascites

The ascitic fluid has a high-protein content (exudate), with a predominant lymphocytic response. A positive culture is obtained in <20% and AFB are detected infrequently (<5%). Ascitic fluid adenosine deaminase, an enzyme released by stimulated T cells, has high diagnostic sensitivity (94%) and specificity (92%).[8] At laparoscopy, the peritoneum is thickened and is covered with miliary nodules.[9] Biopsy of nodules confirms the diagnosis in 90% of patients.

TREATMENT AND PREVENTION

Medical therapy consists of an 'induction phase' of four drugs: isoniazid, rifampin, pyrazinamide, and ethambutol or streptomycin administered daily for 2 months (Table 51.5). The patient is then switched to the 'continuation phase' with two drugs: isoniazid and rifampin daily for 4 months. There is much evidence that twice weekly directly observed therapy (DOT) is equally effective. While a 6-month course is acceptable in drug-sensitive infection, a three-drug 'continuation phase' (containing ethambutol) over longer duration (9–12 months) should be used in countries with a high prevalence of drug-resistant tuberculosis.

Adverse reactions

The most common drug-related adverse reaction is hepatitis, seen more frequently (four times) with combined isoniazid and rifampin than isoniazid alone. Fulminant hepatitis can occur in susceptible individuals, often within 2 weeks of starting treatment. When hepatitis occurs both drugs should be discontinued until transaminases become normal. Isoniazid is restarted in increasing doses under close monitoring of transaminase levels. Treatment should continue for 18–24 months along with a second drug other than rifampin.

COMPLICATIONS AND THEIR MANAGEMENT

The most common complication is acute intestinal obstruction. Less frequent complications include perforation, malabsorption, fistulae, and bleeding from penetrating ulcer. Emergency surgery is required for complications such as free perforation, complete intestinal obstruction, and acute bleeding. The most common indication for elective surgery is failure of medical therapy, usually for strictures. Other indications are: bowel adhesions, abdominal abscess secondary to localized perforation, and fistulae. The current surgical approach to intestinal strictures is stricturoplasty. Peritoneal adhesions are treated by adhesiolysis and placement of reabsorbable cellulose membranes over the peritoneal surface.

PROGNOSIS

Most patients respond well to treatment. Systemic symptoms subside within weeks, while the mucosal abnormalities take longer to disappear. Eventually, 70% of patients have resolution of the radiologic abnormality.[10] Noncompliance and emergence of resistant bacteria are the primary reasons for treatment failure. Every effort should be made to obtain culture and drug sensitivity before initiating therapy. Patients with resistant bacteria should receive at least three drugs and treatment should be given for 12–24 months. Lack of clinical response should prompt repeat susceptibility testing. Since compliance is critical, DOT should be attempted in every patient. Moreover, all patients should be tested for HIV.

TABLE 51.5 MEDICAL TREATMENT OF TUBERCULOSIS

Drug	Daily dose	Adverse effects	Action
Isoniazid (x3 ULN)	5 mg/kg	Hepatitis	Stop if liver enzymes elevated (x3 ULN)
		Peripheral neuropathy	Prophylactic vitamin B6
		Interaction with phenytoin and carbamazepine	
Rifampin	10 mg/kg	Hepatitis	Same as for isoniazid
		Thrombocytopenia	Monitor blood counts
		Skin rash	
		Several drug interactions	
Pyrazinamide	15–30 mg/kg	Hepatitis	Same as for isoniazid
		Gout	Monitor uric acid
		Skin rash	
		Avoid in pregnancy	
Ethambutol	15–25 mg/kg	Optic neuritis, color blindness	Baseline visual check; F/U as needed
Streptomycin	15 mg/kg	Ototoxicity	Baseline audiography; F/U as needed
		Nephrotoxicity	Baseline renal tests; F/U as needed

ULN, upper limit of normal; F/U, follow-up.

WHAT TO TELL PATIENTS

Tuberculosis can involve any part of the intestinal tract. The main defect is narrowing of the intestines resulting in abdominal pain, distention, and vomiting. Other symptoms are: fever, sweating, and decrease in appetite and weight. Treatment consists of multiple drugs, which have to be taken for several months. Tuberculosis is a curable disease if treatment is started early. Poor compliance results in emergence of resistant bacteria, which are difficult to eradicate.

CURRENT CONTROVERSIES AND THEIR FUTURE RESOLUTION

Mycobacterium tuberculosis is a difficult organism to culture. The traditional method (Lowenstein-Jensen media) takes 6 weeks to confirm the diagnosis. The use of liquid broth (Bectec system) has reduced this to 2 weeks. Current research is directed at producing more rapid diagnostic tests utilizing nucleic acid amplification techniques.[11,12] One test uses a DNA probe (GenProbe) to target mycobacterial RNA. Another employs the polymerase chain reaction to amplify bacterial DNA. It is hoped that these tests will soon become sufficiently reproducible for routine clinical use.

OTHER MYCOBACTERIAL INFECTIONS

The family Mycobacteriaceae is divided into two groups: tuberculous and nontuberculous mycobacteria (Table 51.6).

Tuberculous forms include *M. tuberculosis* complex, which contains *M. tuberculosis*, *M. bovis*, and *M. africanum*. *Mycobacterium bovis* was once a common cause of infection but has been largely eradicated because of pasteurization of milk and stringent control measures in dairy herds. However, *M. bovis* infection is still reported from developed and developing countries. Active disease is mostly seen in immunosuppressed individuals. The main sites of involvement are the lungs and genitourinary tract.[13] Treatment is similar to *M. tuberculosis*, except for pyrazinamide, which is ineffective. *Mycobacterium africanum* is a rare cause of disease, seen exclusively in Africa.

Nontuberculous mycobacteria ('atypical mycobacteria') are ubiquitous in the environment. There are nearly 50 species

TABLE 51.6 CLASSIFICATION AND CLINICAL SYNDROMES OF MYCOBACTERIAL SPECIES

Organism	Clinical syndromes
TUBERCULOUS SPECIES	
Mycobacterium complex	
• *M. tuberculosis*	Localized or disseminated
• *M. bovis*	Lung, genitourinary, disseminated
• *M. africanum*	Rare, exclusive to Africa
Mycobacterium lepra	Leprosy
NONTUBERCULOUS SPECIES	
Rapidly growing	
• *M. fortuitum* group	Lung, skin, soft tissues, catheter-related infections
• *M. chelonei/abscessus* group	Lung, bone, nodes, skin, soft tissues
Slowly growing	
• *M. avium* complex	Lung, disseminated (mostly HIV +ve)
• *M. kansasii*	Lung, bone, disseminated (mostly HIV +ve)
• *M. xenopi*	Lung
• *M. scrofulaceum*	Lung, nodes, bones
• *M. haemophilum*	Skin, soft tissues, bone
Intermediately growing	
• *M. marinum*	Skin (swimming pool), bone

that cause disease. The most important is *M. avium* complex (MAC), which includes *M. avium* and *M. intracellulare*. Pulmonary infection can occur in healthy individuals resulting in productive cough, hemoptysis, fever, and weight loss. Children often present with lymphadenitis. The enlarged nodes are nontender and usually localized to one area. Disseminated MAC infection, seen in AIDS patients with CD4 $<100/mm^3$, is associated with fever, sweats, weight loss, diarrhea, and hepatosplenomegaly. The gastrointestinal tract is frequently involved and shows blunted villi containing histiocytes loaded with AFB. Treatment consists of three drugs: clarithromycin (500 mg b.i.d) or azithromycin (500 mg/day), ethambutol (15 mg/kg/day), and rifabutin (300 mg/day). Patients with CD4 $\leq 50/mm^3$ should receive prophylaxis with clarithromycin or azithromycin.

SOURCES OF INFORMATION FOR PATIENTS AND DOCTORS

http://www.emedicine.com/radio/topic885.htm

REFERENCES

1. Global Tuberculosis Program. In: Global tuberculosis control. WHO report 1998. Geneva: World Health Organization, 1998:237.
2. Tandon HD, Prakash A. Pathology of intestinal tuberculosis and its distinction from Crohn's disease. Gut 1972; 13:260–269.
3. Marshall JB. Tuberculosis of the gastrointestinal tract and peritoneum. Am J Gastroenterol 1993; 88:989–999.
4. Kendig EL Jr, Kirkpatrick BV, Carter WH, Hill FA, Caldwell K, Enteistle M. Underreading of the tuberculin skin test reaction. Chest 1998; 113:1175–1177.
5. Kedar RP, Shah PP, Shivde RS, Malde HM. Sonographic findings in gastrointestinal and peritoneal tuberculosis. Clin Radiol 1994; 49:24–29.
6. Hulnick DH, Megibow AJ, Naidich DP et al. Abdominal tuberculosis: CT evaluation. Radiology 1985; 157:199-204.
7. Singh V, Kumar P, Kamal J et al. Clinico-colonoscopic profile of colonic tuberculosis. Am J Gastroenterol 1996; 91:565-568.
8. Burgess LJ, Swanepoel CG, Taljaard JJF. The use of adenosine deaminase as a diagnostic tool for peritoneal tuberculosis. Tuberculosis 2001; 81:243-248.
9. Bhargava DK, Shriniwas, Chopra P et al. Peritoneal tuberculosis: Laparoscopic patterns and its diagnostic accuracy. Am J Gastroenterol 1992; 87:109-112.
10. Anand BS, Nanda R. Sachdev GK. Response of tuberculous stricture to antituberculous treatment. Gut 1988; 29:62-69.
11. Clarridge JE, Shawar RM, Shinnick TM, Plikaytis BB. Large-scale use of polymerase chain reaction for detection of *Mycobacterial tuberculosis* in a routine mycobacteriology laboratory. J Clin Microbiol 1993; 31: 2049–2056.
12. Nucleic acid amplification tests for tuberculosis. Morb Mortal Wkly Rep 1996; 45:950–951.
13. Grange JM. *Mycobacterium bovis* infection in human beings. Tuberculosis 2001; 81:71–77.

Chapter 52

Parasites

Paul Kelly

KEY POINTS

- The expression of disease in parasitic infection is determined by the interaction between the host and pathogen
- Dose of infection, route of infection, and lifecycle influence pathogenicity
- The dynamics of transmission affect the scale of outbreaks/epidemics
- Dysentery (bloody diarrhea) is caused by intestinal protozoa, e.g. *entamoeba histolytica*
- Helminth infections give rise to T-helper type 2 responses
- Immunocompromised patients (e.g. AIDS) are susceptible to coccidia and microsporidia infections
- Diagnosis requires specific tests and liaison with the laboratory

INTRODUCTION

The term 'parasite' refers to an organism that exists in a parasitic relationship with a host, so strictly speaking pathogenic bacteria are also parasitic. However, in medicine, the term parasite usually refers to eukaryotic organisms, i.e., protozoa, helminths, and the insect ectoparasites. In gastroenterology and hepatology, the important parasites are protozoans (Tables 52.1 and 52.2) and helminths (Table 52.3).

EPIDEMIOLOGY

Parasitic infections are predominantly problems of tropical populations, and the numbers of people afflicted by each infection are enormous. However, the great majority of these infections cause no adverse consequences and the majority of infected people have no symptoms. For example, the intestinal protozoans that infect man listed in Table 52.1, which are undoubtedly pathogenic, cause disease only in a minority of carriers.

The spectrum of clinical features and natural history of these infections is wide, from asymptomatic infection to fulminant life-threatening disease. It is not possible to explain why one individual has mild and another severe clinical features, but there are some important determinants of outcome that have been established.

Host factors

Immune status has a dramatic effect on the clinical features of infection. For example, prior exposure to *Cryptosporidium parvum* leads to protective acquired immunity, and in tropical populations, infection in childhood protects against cryptosporidiosis in adult life. Cryptosporidiosis in adults is usually transient or even asymptomatic, but if T cell function is impaired (as in AIDS), cryptosporidiosis can be very severe (see below). Patients with IgA deficiency are more susceptible to giardiasis, and the infection is difficult to eradicate. Nutritional status is also likely to be important, but few specific examples have been described.

Pathogen factors

The genotype of the pathogen may be a critical determinant of outcome, as in amebiasis. There is now consensus that the genetics of the parasite is so important in *Entamoeba* spp. that the old species *Entamoeba histolytica* has been divided into two new species, *Entamoeba histolytica* and *Entamoeba dispar*, which can be distinguished only by genetic tests; the latter species is never pathogenic.[1] This means that the epidemiology of this organism needs to be completely rewritten.

Exposure factors

The dominant factor here is dose. The higher the dose ingested, the more severe the symptoms and the faster the onset of symptoms. Note that as a general rule the infective dose is lower for invasive organisms (e.g. 10–100 for *Shigella dysenteriae*) than for toxigenic organisms (e.g. at least 1 000 000 for *Vibrio cholerae*).

Transmission

The route of transmission of parasites varies greatly. The oocysts or spores of protozoa (Fig. 52.1) are transmitted by the feco-oral route, often in contaminated water or food, or by direct contact from diarrheal stools of infected individuals to the hands of those looking after them. However, the transmission of helminths is much more complex, being dependent on the parasite life cycle, which may involve a secondary host. In simple terms, there are five broad groups of helminths:

1. Eggs are ingested orally and hatch in the human intestine (e.g., *Enterobius, Trichuris, Echinococcus, Hymenolepis, Fasciola*).
2. Hatching in the intestine is followed by tissue penetration, blood-borne transport, migration up the bronchial tree, and swallowing before maturation in the intestine (e.g., *Ascaris*).
3. Eggs hatch outside the human host, mature in the soil and penetrate the skin when in contact with the ground (e.g., both hookworm species, *Strongyloides*).
4. Eggs hatch outside, penetrate another host (e.g., snail), and then mature before penetrating the skin of the human host while swimming (e.g., schistosomes).
5. Eggs hatch in an intermediate host and penetrate into its tissues before being eaten in meat (e.g., *Taenia*) or fish (e.g., *Diphyllobothrium, Clonorchis*).

TABLE 52.1 CLINICALLY IMPORTANT PROTOZOA

Organism	Classification	Drug and dose	Duration
ORGANISMS CAUSING BLOODY DIARRHEA (DYSENTERY)			
Entamoeba histolytica	Ameba	Metronidazole 800 mg t.i.d.	5–10 days
		Diloxanide 500 mg t.i.d.	10 days
Balantidium coli	Ciliate	Tetracycline 500 mg t.i.d.	10 days
		Metronidazole 800 mg t.i.d.	10 days
ORGANISMS CAUSING WATERY AND PERSISTENT DIARRHEA			
Giardia intestinalis	Flagellate	Tinidazole 2 g (single dose)	–
Cryptosporidium parvum	Coccidian	Nitazoxanide 500 mg b.d.	3 days
Isospora belli	Coccidian	Co-trimoxazole 960 mg q.i.d.	10 days
Cyclospora cayatenensis	Coccidian	Co-trimoxazole 960 mg q.i.d.	10 days
Enterocytozoon bieneusi	Microsporidian	Albendazole 400 mg b.d.	28 days
Encephalitozoon intestinalis	Microsporidian	Albendazole 400 mg b.d.	28 days
ORGANISMS OF UNCERTAIN PATHOGENICITY OR RARE			
Dientamoeba fragilis	Flagellate	Metronidazole 800 mg t.i.d.	10 days
Blastocystis hominis	Unclassified	Metronidazole 800 mg t.i.d.	10 days
Sarcocystis hominis	Coccidian	Co-trimoxazole 960 mg q.i.d.	10 days

Doses given are adult doses. For children's doses see Cook (2003)[2] and Schlossberg (2000).[11]

TABLE 52.2 NONPATHOGENIC PROTOZOA FOUND IN FECAL SAMPLES

Organism	Classification
Entamoeba dispar	Ameba
Entamoeba coli	Ameba
Entamoeba hartmanni	Ameba
Endolimax nana	Ameba
Iodamoeba butschlii	Ameba
Trichomonas hominis	Flagellate
Chilomastix mesnili	Flagellate
Embadomonas intestinalis	Flagellate
Enteromonas hominis	Flagellate

These organisms are regarded as nonpathogenic. However, in occasional cases these may be the only findings in a patient with persistent symptoms, in which a therapeutic trial may be considered. All the above would be treated with tinidazole 2 g daily for 3 days.

For a fuller discussion of life cycles and transmission, the reader is referred to the References.[2,3]

The dynamics of transmission also vary. Those protozoa that are transmitted in water (e.g., *C. parvum*) can produce massive outbreaks of infection.[4] This is also true of food-borne outbreaks of *Cyclospora cayatenensis*[5] (one outbreak was transmitted by raspberries). Epidemics would be rare in schistosomiasis, which relies on a complex two-host transmission cycle and the potential for epidemic spread is therefore reduced, but large foci of intense but stable transmission can occur, for example in the Nile delta.

PATHOGENESIS AND PATHOLOGY/CLINICAL PRESENTATION

Protozoa

The pathology caused by intestinal protozoa is of two types. Members of the first group, *Entamoeba histolytica* and *Balantidium coli*, cause severe colonic inflammation and ulceration, leading to dysentery (bloody diarrhea). This may rarely progress to colonic dilatation, and ultimately to perforation in a very small minority of cases.[1] This process is analogous to the colonic dilatation seen in ulcerative colitis. The inflammation and ulceration in amebiasis is generated by the impressive array of cytolytic enzymes synthesized by the organism in the colonic environment.

Members of the second group of intestinal protozoa cause less dramatic intestinal damage. While *Giardia intestinalis* is an extracellular pathogen (Fig. 52.2A) that causes diarrhea by an as yet uncertain combination of pathological processes, the coccidia and microsporidia inhabit an intracellular niche in the epithelial cells of the small intestine (Fig. 52.2B). The enteropathy caused by the coccidia is subtle and it seems likely that the pathological effects are mediated by cytoskeletal damage and by cell–cell signaling.

Helminths

The pathogenesis of disease caused by helminths is complex and varied, and relates closely to clinical features. These parasites live in an ecological niche in the human host and most infections are well tolerated. Disease is produced by the presence of large numbers of parasites. Helminth infections give rise to a T helper cell type 2 response, and sometimes it is this response that mediates disease.

Nematodes

Ascaris lumbricoides lives in the lumen of the intestine and causes little harm. In heavy infections, the bulk of worms may cause vague abdominal pains and obstruct the intestine or the bile duct.

Hookworms burrow into the intestinal mucosa and attach themselves by means of teeth to enable them to draw blood, which is their primary nutrition. In cases of infection with large numbers, the total loss of blood may cause iron deficiency anemia.

TABLE 52.3 HUMAN INTESTINAL HELMINTH INFECTIONS

Classification	Organism	Drug of choice
Nematodes	*Ascaris lumbricoides* (roundworm)	Mebendazole
	Necator americanus (hookworm)	Albendazole
	Ancylostoma duodenale (hookworm)	Albendazole
	Strongyloides stercoralis	Tiabendazole
	Trichuris trichiura (whipworm)	Mebendazole
	Enterobius vermicularis (threadworm)	Mebendazole
Trematodes (flukes)	*Schistosoma mansoni*	Praziquantel
	Schistosoma japonicum	Praziquantel
	Fasciola hepatica	Praziquantel
	Fasciolopsis buski	Praziquantel
	Clonorchis sinensis	Praziquantel
	Opisthorchis viverrini	Praziquantel
Cestodes (tapeworms)	*Taenia saginata*	Praziquantel
	Taenia solium	Praziquantel
	Echinococcus granulosus	Albendazole
	Hymenolepis nana	Praziquantel
	Diphyllobothrium latum	Praziquantel

This list includes only the most commonly encountered parasites of the digestive system; it is not exhaustive and in certain geographical areas other rare helminths may reach high prevalence. For duration of treatment courses see text.

Strongyloides penetrates right into the mucosa and gives rise to an inflammatory response and enteropathy. However, in certain immunocompromised states (not AIDS, interestingly) hyperinfection can occur when larvae penetrate into the bloodstream and cause infection of remote tissues, leading to haemorrhagic bronchopneumonia, for example.

Trichuris trichiura causes chronic dysentery, which is mediated by a T helper cell type 2 immune-mediated pathology.[6]

Trematodes

In all cases, adult trematodes (Table 52.3) live outside the gut lumen. In the case of *Schistosoma mansoni* and *S. japonicum*, the adult flukes reside in the mesenteric veins, and the excreted eggs exit through the inflamed intestinal mucosa (Fig. 52.2C) to be passed out in the feces. The passage of some eggs up the portal vein leads to Symmer's fibrosis in the hepatic portal radicals (Fig. 52.3), ultimately leading to portal hypertension.

In the case of the liver flukes (*Fasciola, Fasciolopsis, Clonorchis, Opisthorchis*), the adults live in the biliary tree causing chronic inflammation. This chronic inflammation may lead to stricturing and ultimately to cholangiocarcinoma, which reaches the proportions of a public health problem in certain parts of South East Asia.

Cestodes

The cestodes (see Table 52.3) generally cause very little intestinal damage. However, *Echinococcus granulosus* may escape from the intestine and hydatid cysts may develop in liver (80%)

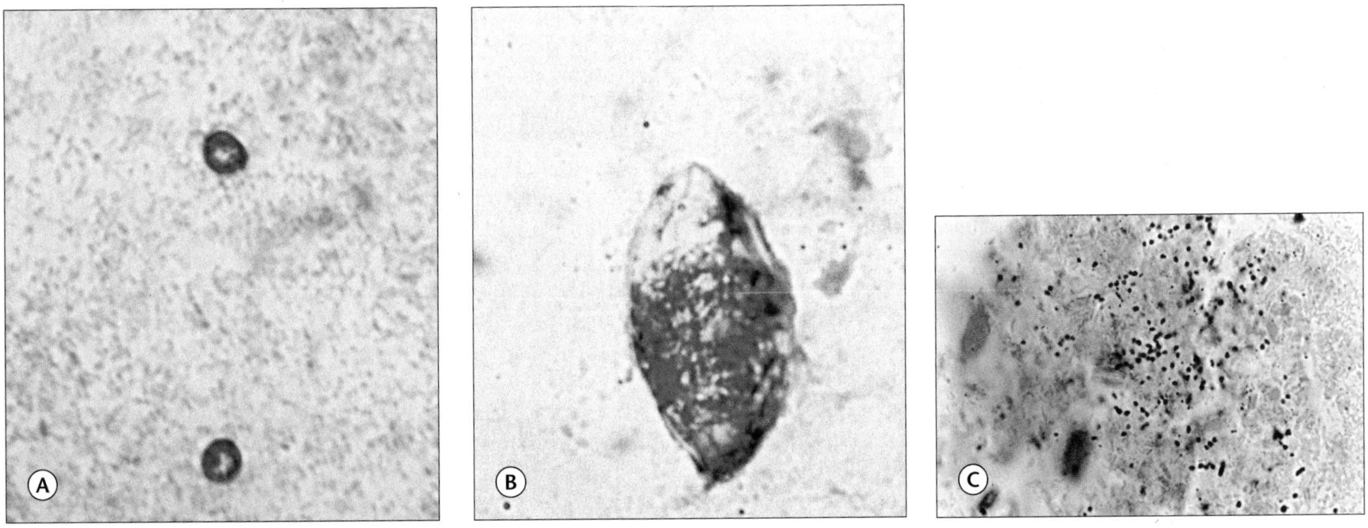

Fig. 52.1 Coccidia and microsporidia seen in stool samples. Diagnostic images of (A) oocysts of *Cryptosporidium parvum,* which are 5 μm in diameter, and (B) an oocyst of *Isospora belli,* 30 x 10 μm, both stained using the modified Ziehl-Neelsen stain. Spores of microsporidia (C) are much smaller (1–1.5 μm long depending on species) and stain with modified trichrome stains.

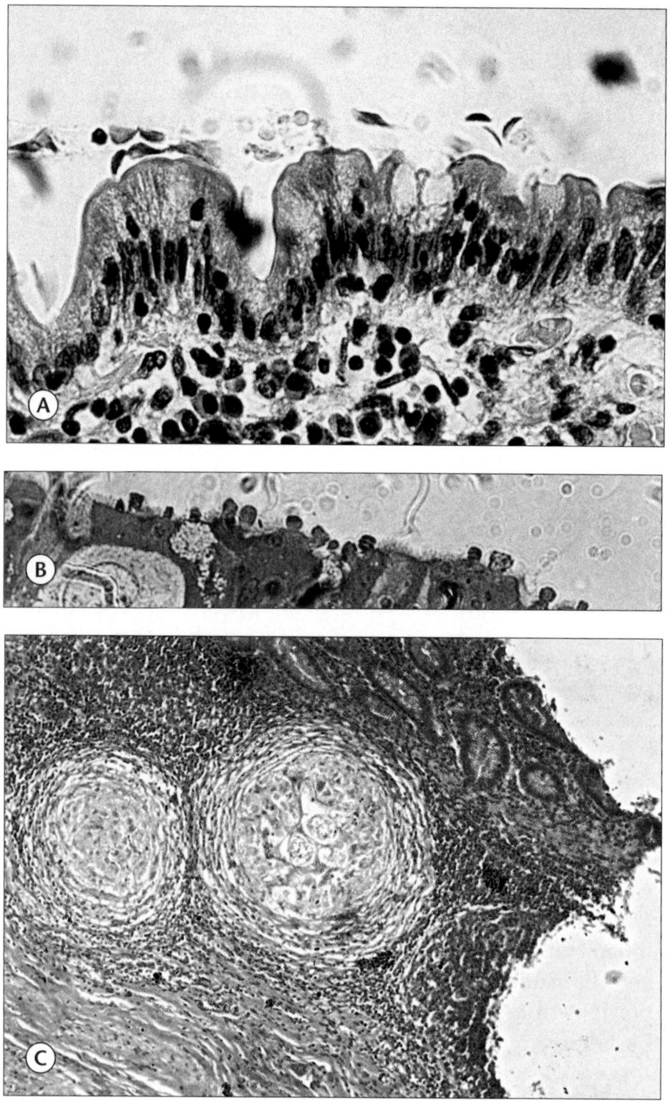

Fig. 52.2 Parasites seen in the intestine. Histological sections of **(A)** duodenum showing trophozoites of *Giardia intestinalis,* which appear as cross-sections of curved disks in this hematoxylin and eosin (H&E) stained section, **(B)** jejunum showing trophozoites of *C. parvum* in the brush border in this toluidine blue stained section, and **(C)** ova of *Schistosoma mansoni* in granulomata in a rectal biopsy, stained with H&E.

or lung (20%). These cysts are fluid-filled cavities lined by a membrane full of scolices of the worms.[2,3] The clinical features of the hydatids are caused by pressure effects, but if the cysts rupture, for example into the abdominal cavity, multiple daughter cysts may be seeded, multiplying the clinical problems considerably.

CLINICAL PRESENTATION

Protozoa

Diarrhea caused by parasites may be predominantly bloody (dysentery), with or without fever, or nonbloody (Table 52.1). Fulminant amebic colitis may occur, and has a high morbidity and mortality.[1] Nonbloody diarrhea is more likely to be persistent (i.e., of 14 days duration or more) when due to protozoa than when due to bacteria or viruses.

In immunocompromised or malnourished patients, infections with coccidia and microsporidia may cause much more dramatic clinical features. For example, in AIDS patients with cryptosporidiosis, the severity of diarrhea is largely dependent on CD4 count (a marker of the severity of immunosuppression in AIDS).[7] Diarrhea due to isosporiasis or microsporidiosis is rare in immunocompetent adults. In children in tropical countries, cryptosporidiosis may present as malnutrition,[8] and it is associated with increased mortality.[9] Cryptosporidiosis and microsporidiosis in AIDS patients may present with a low-grade cholangitis that is radiologically indistinguishable from sclerosing cholangitis (see Chapter 78).

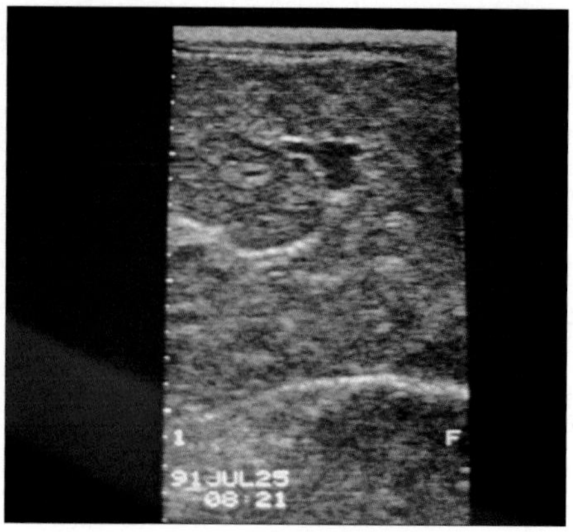

Fig. 52.3 Ultrasound scan of a liver showing Symmer's pipe-stem fibrosis. This appearance can usually be distinguished from multiple metastases by the fact that the hyperechoic zones all contain portal radicals.

Helminths

Most helminth infections do not give rise to symptoms. Nematode infections cause vague abdominal pains when infection is heavy, but each infection may have specific features. *Ascaris* may cause obstruction of the intestine, biliary tree (giving rise to cholangitis or jaundice), or pancreatic duct (pancreatitis). Hookworms are an important cause of iron deficiency anemia in many parts of the tropics.

Strongyloides hyperinfection syndrome (see above) presents with fever, eosinophilia, hemoptysis, dyspnea, and respiratory failure, and is a medical emergency in patients receiving immunosuppressive chemotherapy (interestingly, it does not often complicate AIDS).

Enterobius infection commonly presents with pruritus ani in children.

Strongyloides stercoralis and *Trichuris trichiura* infection may result in diarrhea, but otherwise helminths rarely cause this symptom.

Trematodes

Schistosomiasis presents with the clinical sequelae of portal hypertension, and this is the commonest cause of severe gastrointestinal hemorrhage in my practice in Lusaka, Zambia. Liver flukes, on the other hand, cause pathology within the biliary tree, and present with jaundice, generalized pruritus, or cholangiocarcinoma.

Cestodes

Cestodes rarely cause symptoms, except for three interesting clinical problems:

1. hydatid disease (which usually presents with hepatic enlargement and/or pain) due to *Echinococcus granulosus*;
2. *Cysticercosis*, which occurs when autoinfection with *Taenia solium* gives rise to tissue cysticerci (these commonly occur in the brain, leading to convulsions); and

3. megaloblastic anemia due to vitamin B_{12} deficiency, caused by infection with *Diphyllobothrium latum*, which competes for the vitamin.

DIFFERENTIAL DIAGNOSIS

Each of the clinical manifestations of parasitic disease described above needs to be distinguished from other possible causes. Several important examples are:

1. In travelers, bloody diarrhea (dysentery) could be due to amebiasis, shigellosis (see Chapter 50), or inflammatory bowel disease. The most useful test is amebic serology. However, in the case of colonic dilatation and impending perforation, surgical management may be required.[1]
2. Persistent diarrhea of protozoal origin cannot be distinguished from other causes and requires focused investigation (see below). Testing for HIV is an important part of the diagnostic process, especially in people who have traveled or resided in many parts of Africa or Asia.
3. Variceal bleeding requires full evaluation. In people from endemic areas for schistosomiasis, stool examinations, rectal biopsy, and serology must be carried out as a diagnosis of schistosomiasis has important implications. Not only is treatment simple and effective for schistosomiasis, but also hepatic cell function is relatively well preserved so shunt procedures are less likely to lead to encephalopathy.[10]

DIAGNOSTIC METHODS

The foundation of diagnosis of these parasitic infections is stool examination in a good laboratory. In this day and age, it is not sufficient to request 'ova, cysts, and parasites'. If the patient is immunocompromised, stains for cryptosporidia and microsporidia specifically should be requested. The laboratory will then perform modified Ziehl-Neelsen and trichrome stains, which will reveal coccidia and microsporidia. Stool for diagnosis of amebiasis should be fresh and needs to be handled in a particular way, so the laboratory should be phoned first. Otherwise, most parasites are revealed by routine techniques, bearing in mind that stool microscopy is not a sensitive technique so a minimum of three samples must be examined.

Serology is useful in diagnosis of amebiasis, schistosomiasis, strongyloidiasis, and hydatid disease. Molecular techniques have not yet found a place in routine diagnosis of any of these infections as sensitivity is not yet as high as initial hopes suggested. Rectal biopsy gives useful information in diagnosis of amebiasis, schistosomiasis, balantidiasis, and trichuriasis. In investigation of persistent diarrhea, duodenal, or jejunal biopsy may be very informative in revealing coccidian infections or giardiasis. Ultrasound examination is the most useful single test in diagnosis of hydatid disease.

TREATMENT AND PREVENTION

Drugs available for treatment of parasites are generally now safe and simple to administer (Tables 52.1 and 52.3). The coccidia are the most challenging group as eradication is difficult to achieve, especially in the immunocompromised patient.

Protozoa (Table 52.1)

For amebiasis, metronidazole is followed by diloxanide furoate to achieve permanent eradication of cysts. Surgery may occasionally be required.[1] Giardiasis can usually be eradicated by single-dose tinidazole, but refractory cases may require more prolonged courses.[11] In AIDS patients, isosporiasis requires life-long secondary prophylaxis after completion of treatment, at a dose of 960 mg three times a week. Treatment of cryptosporidiosis in AIDS patients is difficult, but immunocompetent patients benefit from a 3-day course of nitazoxanide.[12] In AIDS patients, the dose should be 1 g b.d. for 4 weeks, but the outcome is uncertain. Of the two species of microsporidia, only *Encephalitozoon* responds predictably to albendazole.

Nematodes (Table 52.3)

For nematode infections, mebendazole is given as a single dose, albendazole and tiabendazole are given twice daily for 3 days. Praziquantel is given as a single dose of 60 mg/kg, divided into three doses over the course of a single day. For hydatid disease, albendazole is given in a dose of 10 mg/kg daily for 8 weeks, and percutaneous drainage is then required.[13]

SOURCES OF INFORMATION FOR PATIENTS AND DOCTORS

http://www.biosci.ohio-state.edu/~parasite/home.html

REFERENCES

1. Stanley SL. Amoebiasis. Lancet 2003; 361:1025–1034.
2. Cook G, ed. Manson's tropical diseases, 2nd edn. London: Saunders; 2003.
3. Topley and Wilson's medical microbiology, vol. 5: Parasitology, 10th edn. London: Hodder Arnold; 2005.
4. MacKenzie WR, Hoxie NJ, Proctor ME et al. A massive outbreak in Milwaukee of Cryptosporidium infection transmitted through the public water supply. New Engl J Med 1994; 331:161–167.
5. Ortega YR, Sterling CR, Gilman RH. *Cyclospora cayetanensis*. Adv Parasitol 1998; 40:399–418.
6. Cooper ES, Spencer J, Whyte-Alleng CAM et al. Immediate hypersensitivity in colon of children with chronic *Trichuris trichiura* dysentery. Lancet 1991; 338:1104–1107.
7. Blanshard C, Jackson AM, Shanson DC, Francis N, Gazzard B. Cryptosporidiosis in HIV seropositive patients. Q J Med 1992; 85:813–823.
8. Molbak K, Andersen M, Aaby P et al. *Cryptosporidium* infection in infancy as a cause of malnutrition: a community study from Guinea-Bissau, West Africa. Am J Clin Nutr 1997; 65:149–152.
9. Amadi BC, Kelly P, Mwiya M et al. Intestinal and systemic infection, HIV and mortality in Zambian children with persistent diarrhoea and malnutrition. J Ped Gastroenterol Nutr 2001; 32:550–554.
10. Ezzat FA, Abu-Elmagd KM, Aly M et al. Selective shunt versus nonshunt surgery for management of both schistosomal and non-schistosomal variceal bleeders. Ann Surg 1990; 212:97–108.
11. Schlossberg D, ed. Current therapy of infectious disease, 2nd edn. St Louis: Mosby; 2000.
12. Amadi BC, Mwiya M, Musuku J et al. Effect of nitazoxanide on morbidity and mortality in Zambian children with cryptosporidiosis: a randomised controlled trial. Lancet 2002; 360:1375–1380.
13. Khuroo MS, Wani NA, Javid G et al. Percutaneous drainage compared with surgery for hepatic hydatid cysts. New Engl J Med 1997; 337:881–887.

Chapter 53

Ulcerative colitis

Fergus Shanahan

KEY POINTS
• Ulcerative colitis – a chronic relapsing inflammatory disease confined to the colonic mucosa • The first controlled clinical therapeutic trial of corticosteroids in ulcerative colitis half a century ago highlighted evidence-based gastroenterology • Despite remarkable advances, ulcerative colitis remains a significant burden on healthcare resources and a cause of much individual suffering • Ulcerative colitis has changed face over time; once considered rare, it is now a major gastroenterologic problem in the developed world with changing demographics

INTRODUCTION

Ulcerative colitis is a chronic relapsing and remitting inflammatory disease of the colorectal mucosa. Along with Crohn's disease, these two major forms of inflammatory bowel disease represent distinct syndromes with overlapping features. Unlike Crohn's disease, where the inflammatory process is transmural and may affect any part of the alimentary tract, uncomplicated ulcerative colitis is confined to the mucosa and restricted to the large bowel. Together, these differences in disease distribution account for much of the differences in disease progression and risk of complications between the two disorders. Both forms of inflammatory bowel disease are responsible for much personal suffering that is occasionally disabling; they impose a significant burden on healthcare resources and have important economic implications including work absenteeism.

Ulcerative colitis was one of the first areas in clinical medicine to enter the arena of what is now popularly referred to as evidence-based medicine. Half a century ago, Sidney Truelove and colleagues conducted one of the first double-blind controlled clinical trials in gastroenterology in showing the efficacy of corticosteroids in ulcerative colitis.[1] Although corticosteroids remain a cornerstone treatment for moderate to severe ulcerative colitis, improved understanding of the pathogenesis of the disorder and continued application of evidence-based approaches have expanded medical and surgical therapeutic options. In addition to the influence of scientific advances on diagnostics and therapy, few disorders have changed face over time to such a degree as with ulcerative colitis. Once considered rare, ulcerative colitis has become a major gastroenterologic problem in the developed world. Traditionally accepted risk factors such as Jewish ethnicity and high socioeconomic status are either less evident today or are being challenged along with several other earlier epidemiologic observations (Table 53.1). Changes include an apparent shift in disease distribution with proportionately more patients presenting with proctitis rather than pancolitis than in the past.[2]

As discussed later, much of the changing face of ulcerative colitis probably reflects environmental and lifestyle changes associated with modern industrialized societies. However, the most important change may relate to doctor–patient relationships. For example, comparisons of current with earlier editions of classic textbooks of internal medicine reflect the changing attitudes of clinicians towards patients with ulcerative colitis. Unsubstantiated linkages of patients' personality or behavioral traits with susceptibility to colitis have been replaced with objectivity and compassion.

EPIDEMIOLOGY

Ulcerative colitis has become a worldwide problem. While improvements in diagnostic techniques have contributed to increased detection rates, there appears to have been a real increase in incidence in many countries over the past 50 years; in some areas this has reached a plateau. Although more common in the Western world than in Africa, Asia, or South America, the incidence seems to increase as countries become developed and industrialized. In developing countries, the appearance and rising incidence of ulcerative colitis tends to precede that of Crohn's disease. After an interval of one to two decades, the latter then follows a similar trend.[2,3] A north–south geographic gradient has appeared in many reports, but this appears to be becoming less distinct. More important than geographic latitude, may be variations in socioeconomic development and urban/

TABLE 53.1 THE CHANGING FACE OF ULCERATIVE COLITIS

Historically accepted feature	Changing patterns
Incidence higher than Crohn's disease	The opposite has emerged in some recent studies from Europe
Incidence follows a north–south gradient	This has become less evident
Male to female ratio	The male to female ratio has changed over several decades with slight male predominance at present
Ethnicity, e.g., Jewish background is a good predictor of risk for colitis	This is no longer true and is subject to numerous confounding variables

Based on data from Ekbom.[2,3]

rural differences; there is about a twofold higher incidence for ulcerative colitis in urban areas. Features of a modern lifestyle associated with developed or industrialized nation status are summarized in Table 53.2.

Ethnic variations in the epidemiology of ulcerative colitis were once thought to represent good predictors of risk but this is no longer the case. Although ulcerative colitis appears to be more common in Jews, this appears to apply to a subset, i.e., those of Ashkenazi descent. Confounding variables such as socioeconomic status and migration between geographic areas of high and low prevalence have diminished the apparent impact of ethnicity.

Reported incidences for ulcerative colitis from North America and northern Europe have been in the range of 10–20 new cases per 100 000 population (associated prevalence rates are about 150–250/100 000). Age-specific incidence rates for ulcerative colitis are usually described as bimodal with a major peak age of onset at 20–40 years and a later minor peak occurring after the age of 60 years. The male/female ratio for ulcerative colitis appears to have shifted from a female toward a marginal male predominance, particularly in patients with proctitis. The opposite trend appears to apply to Crohn's disease and might be influenced by smoking patterns.

Smoking is the most consistent polarizing influence on inflammatory bowel disease, conferring protection against ulcerative colitis, in contrast to an increased risk for Crohn's disease. Indeed, patients with ulcerative colitis often relate the onset to recent cessation of cigarette smoking. The mechanism of these intriguing effects is unclear although smoking has been shown to influence mucosal immunity, colonic mucus production and motility.[4]

Another consistent observation has been the apparent protective effect of appendectomy against development of ulcerative colitis. Patients with ulcerative colitis are significantly less likely to have had appendectomy compared with controls, particularly if the procedure has been performed before the age of 20.[5] One interpretation of this might be that appendectomy has a direct protective effect in reducing the risk of ulcerative colitis. This has been supported by evidence from an animal model of colitis (T cell receptor-α knockout mice) where resection of the cecal patch at 1 month of age attenuates subsequent development of colitis.[6] This interpretation has also prompted some investigators to perform appendectomy as a form of treatment. Alternatively, appendicitis rather than appendectomy *per se* might be inversely associated with ulcerative colitis. This is suggested by a large population-based study where the risk of colitis was not reduced in cases where a nondiseased appendix was resected.[7] A third interpretation might be that the factors that predispose to development of ulcerative colitis also protect against appendicitis.

TABLE 53.2 FACTORS THAT MAY INCREASE THE RISK OF ULCERATIVE COLITIS

Changing lifestyle and environment linked with socioeconomic development that may confer increased risk of ulcerative colitis
- Improved sanitation and hygiene
- Refrigeration
- Reduced consumption of fermented food products
- Decline in prevalence of *H. pylori* infection
- Decline in endemic parasitism
- Life on concrete – reduced exposure to soil microbes
- Increased antibiotic usage
- Vaccinations
- Smaller family size
- Delayed or altered pattern of exposure to childhood mucosal infections

CAUSES, RISK FACTORS, DISEASE ASSOCIATIONS

A simple explanation for the cause of ulcerative colitis has not emerged; a single cause and effect relation seems unlikely. As with most chronic inflammatory disorders, ulcerative colitis probably represents an interaction amongst genetic predisposing factors, environmental influences, and endogenous modifiers. The outcome is activation of the intestinal immune system and a continual cycle of inflammation and healing (Fig. 53.1). In common with chronic inflammatory disorders in other organs, ulcerative colitis may be a heterogeneous syndrome, comprised of different conditions with different causes but with a similar final common pathway of tissue injury.

Genetic factors

A large body of evidence indicates that ulcerative colitis and Crohn's disease are genetically related forms of inflammatory bowel disease in which some genetic predisposing factors are shared but others are specific to either condition.[8] However, patterns of familial aggregation and concordance rates for monozygotic twins consistently show that a genetic influence is not as strong in ulcerative colitis (6–14%) as it is in Crohn's disease (44–50%).

In ulcerative colitis, particular attention has been directed at the human leukocyte antigen (HLA) region on chromosome 6. Genes in this region code for molecules involved in immunoregulation and antigen presentation – the major histocompatibility

PATHOGENESIS: CONTRIBUTORY ELEMENTS

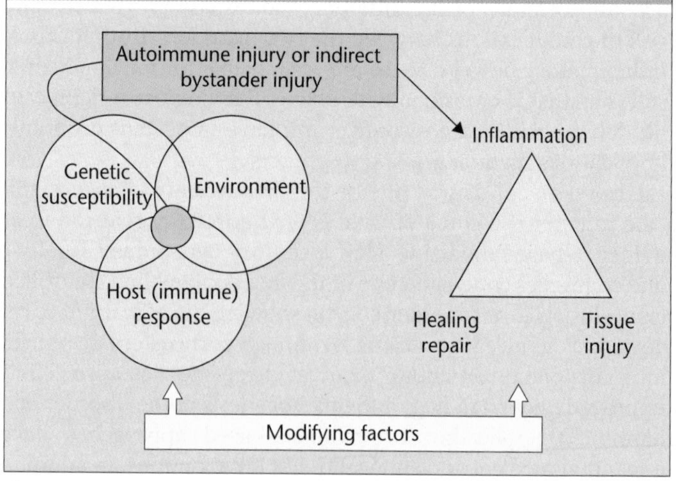

Fig. 53.1 Contributory elements in the pathogenesis of ulcerative colitis. The immunoinflammatory response mediates tissue damage either by indirect innocent bystander injury or by direct autoimmune reactivity. Genetic susceptibility and environmental modifiers may act either at the level of the immune response or at the end organ. More than one gene is involved and several environmental modifiers have been implicated including the colonic flora, cigarette smoking, and nonsteroidal anti-inflammatory drugs.

complex (MHC). The most consistent HLA/MHC associations with disease susceptibility have been with Class II MHC alleles, particularly DRB1*0103, DRB1*1502, and DRB1*0401.[9] The DRB1*0103 allele has been linked with extensive and severe disease with progression to colectomy. There is also some evidence to suggest that disease limited to the distal colon might be associated with homozygosity for the common TNF promotor haplotype. In addition, it appears that extracolonic manifestations such as erythema nodosum may be linked with polymorphisms in the TNF promoter.[9] Thus, in addition to disease susceptibility genes, other genetic modifiers determine disease phenotype.

Outside the HLA region, several other genes appear to influence susceptibility, phenotype, or responsiveness to therapy for ulcerative colitis. An association with a polymorphism of the interleukin-1 receptor antagonist (IL-1RA) gene on chromosome 2 has been found by some, but not all investigators. While most candidate genes investigated have been related to the immunoinflammatory response, some genetic factors almost certainly operate at the level of the target organ. In this respect, reports of a linkage with polymorphisms of genes coding for intestinal mucin and for the multi-drug resistance gene (MDR1), which influences epithelial transport and barrier function, are intriguing, but need confirmation.[8,9]

Environmental factors

The importance of nongenetic or environmental factors in ulcerative colitis is indicated by the relatively low concordance rate in monozygotic twins (6–14%). Similar epidemiologic patterns and temporal trends in disease frequency suggest that some environmental risk factors for inflammatory bowel disease are probably common to Crohn's disease and ulcerative colitis. In contrast, as discussed earlier, other environmental influences such as appendectomy in early life and smoking are either specific to colitis or have opposing effects on the two forms of inflammatory bowel disease. There is some evidence that nonsteroidal anti-inflammatory drugs (NSAIDs) may trigger exacerbation or the onset of ulcerative colitis. Reduced mucosal cytoprotective eicosanoids seems a likely mechanism, although selective cyclo-oxygenase-1 (COX-1) and COX-2 inhibitors have both been implicated.[4]

The pattern of exposure to environmental microbes, particularly in early life, may be the most important exogenous factor influencing risk of developing inflammatory bowel disease. Elements of a modern lifestyle in developed societies (Table 53.2) have altered the pattern of microbial exposure. This has important implications for the development and education of the immune system. Development of the mucosal immune system is incomplete at birth and continual fine-tuning of cytokine responses and T cell repertoires occurs throughout childhood and adolescence. Since the function of the immune system is to sense microbial danger within the environment, immune education requires appropriate exposure to indigenous colonizing flora in early life and to episodic infections, both of which prime and condition the intestinal immune response.[10,11] As with any sensory organ, inappropriate or inadequate stimulatory input may lead to dysfunction and errors of immune perception.

The most persuasive evidence implicating the indigenous flora, or components thereof, in the pathogenesis of ulcerative colitis is from animal models of colitis. A diversity of defects, either at the level of mucosal barrier function or at the level of immunoregulation, has been associated with the development of colitis in experimental animals.[12] Irrespective of the underlying genetic defect in these models, the colitis does not occur in a germ-free environment and only develops after colonization with commensal bacterial flora. This suggests the flora either has a permissive role by priming the development of the immunoinflammatory response or has a more direct pro-inflammatory effect. In humans, there is some evidence for a loss of immunologic tolerance to the flora with the development of autoreactive antibodies that are cross-reactive with components of the flora and epithelial and nonepithelial antigens. None of these autoimmune phenomena has been shown to mediate tissue damage but have been explored for diagnostic purposes (see below). Whether some patients with ulcerative colitis have a defect in innate immunity to the flora, as demonstrated in a subset of patients with Crohn's disease and CARD15/NOD2 mutations, is unclear.

While many clinical and experimental observations support the concept that ulcerative colitis is causally related to direct exposure to alimentary bacterial and other antigens, some observations are difficult to reconcile in this context. Firstly, the striking demarcation of disease distribution in subtotal colitis does not conform to the limits of bacterial exposure. Secondly, ulcerative colitis has been reported to occur in an autotransplanted colonic neovagina where there is no exposure to alimentary antigens.[13] This might be explained by intermucosal traffic of immune cells, cross-reactivity with vaginal microbes, or may represent a subset of disease that is not due to direct microbial exposure.

Endogenous modifiers

Endogenous outcome modifiers include the brain–gut axis, placebo response, coping skills, and positive and negative emotional factors including psychologic stress.[4,14] Although logistically difficult to quantify and study in humans, the role of stress has been demonstrated well in animals with experimental colitis. Stress-induced reactivation of colitis has been adoptively transferred and is dependent on T cells. It appears that stress may adversely affect mucosal barrier function and promote uptake of bacterial antigens, which activate previously sensitized mucosal T cells.

Disease associations

Extraintestinal disease associations and manifestations may occur in up to 5–10% of patients.[15] Some are true disease associations, whereas other conditions are complications or manifestations secondary to the inflammatory activity or are side effects of its treatment (Table 53.3). Those involving the joints (peripheral arthritis and spondyloarthropathy), skin (erythema nodosum, pyoderma gangrenosum), eye (uveitis, episcleritis), and liver (sclerosing cholangitis) are the most common.

Articular disease is the most common extracolonic manifestation/disease association of ulcerative colitis. This includes axial arthropathies (ankylosing spondylitis and isolated sacroiliitis) and peripheral arthropathies. The former are unrelated to the inflammatory activity in the colon, whereas the latter consist of two patterns: pauciarticular, which affects large joints (<5 joints) and is usually self-limiting and associated with colitis activity (type 1); and polyarticular (>5 joints), affects a wide range of joints but particularly the metacarpophalangeal joints and is independent of colitis activity (type 2). Both forms of peripheral arthropathy are nonerosive. Recently, distinct HLA gene associations have been differentially linked with each pattern of arthropathy associated with ulcerative colitis.[9]

TABLE 53.3 EXTRAINTESTINAL DISEASE ASSOCIATIONS AND MANIFESTATIONS/COMPLICATIONS

Organ or system	Manifestation or complication	Disease association
General/constitutional[a]	Weight loss, anemia, malaise Growth retardation Hypercoagulation syndromes Amyloidosis	
Skin and buccal mucosa		Erythema nodosum[a] Pyoderma gangrenosum Oral apthous ulcers
Musculoskeletal	Osteopenia[a] Avascular necrosis[a,b]	Spondyloarthropathy Peripheral arthritis[a]
Liver and biliary tract		Sclerosing cholangitis
Ocular		Uveitis/iritis[a] Episcleritis[a] Conjunctivitis[a]
Pulmonary		Varied and nonspecific including drug-induced

[a] Tends to be related to activity of the colitis.
[b] This has traditionally been linked with steroid therapy but there are several reports of avascular necrosis occurring without steroid exposure and may be related to hypercoagulability.

The most common skin manifestation is erythema nodosum, which is related to the activity of the colitis. In most cases, it occurs at the time of diagnosis or prior to presentation. In up to one-third of cases it may be recurrent. Pyoderma gangrenosum is a more serious, albeit less common, problem. Unlike erythema nodosum, its clinical course is frequently independent of the activity of the colitis. The lesions are characteristically painful, beginning as one or more lumps usually on the lower limbs, which develop into pustules that break down and leave a necrotic center with undermined violaceous edges. Because the lesions exhibit pathergy (i.e., may be extended by trauma), surgical debridement should be avoided. In contrast, to erythema nodosum, pyoderma gangrenosum tends to be indolent if not aggressively treated with immunosuppression.

Ocular involvement presents with an acute painful red eye and is usually linked with active colitis and involves the anterior chamber (iritis, episcleritis, scleritis, and uveitis). HLA genes such as B27 appear to have an important role in predisposing to these conditions in patients with ulcerative colitis.

Abnormalities in liver tests are common in patients with ulcerative colitis and may be due to various factors such as sepsis, malnutrition, treatment with parenteral nutrition, adverse drug effects, and transfusion-associated viral infections. However, clinically significant liver disease is far less common and present in about 5%. In contrast to most other extraintestinal manifestations/associations, liver disease is more common in ulcerative colitis than in Crohn's disease. Primary sclerosing cholangitis is by far the most common clinically significant liver disease associated with ulcerative colitis. In some patients, it may precede the onset of colitis. It is unrelated to colitis activity, is unaffected by colectomy and may even occur years after colectomy. There is an increased risk not only of cholangiocarcinoma but also of colorectal cancer in patients with ulcerative colitis who have sclerosing cholangitis. Although a miscellany of other nonspecific liver disorders have been associated with inflammatory bowel disease, including autoimmune hepatitis, such diagnoses should be made with caution and only if sclerosing cholangitis has been excluded and if cholangiography is normal.

CAUSES AND RISK FACTORS

Etiology: a convergence of genetic susceptibility, environmental modifiers and immune-mediated tissue injury

Pathogenesis – major theories

1. An organ-specific autoimmune disease with immune reactivity against the colonic mucosa; the bacterial flora are required but play a permissive role priming the development of the mucosal immune response
2. An abnormal immune reactivity against components of the colonic flora in which the mucosa is subject to innocent bystander injury
3. A heterogeneous syndrome or group of conditions with different causes but with a final common pathway of tissue damage

DISEASE MODIFIERS

VARIABLE	COMMENT
Industrialized society	A complex array of lifestyle and environmental factors
Smoking	Impact differs from that in Crohn's disease Ulcerative colitis is uncommon in smokers A history of recent cessation of smoking is common prior to onset or relapse
Enteric infections	Occasionally precipitate relapse
Appendectomy	Apparently protective against risk of developing colitis
Stress	Unproven adverse effect in humans but persuasive evidence in animal models
Drugs	Relapses have occasionally been linked with usage of antibiotics and NSAIDs

PATHOGENESIS

The colonic mucosa is a functional barrier between the internal milieu and a living mass of antigenic bacteria within the lumen. Antigenic presence maintains the mucosal immune system in a state of controlled physiologic inflammation. This requires precise regulation to avoid excessive reactivity to the indigenous flora, whilst remaining on standby for responsiveness against episodic challenge with pathogens. Tissue injury and colitis are an expected outcome if breakdown of mucosal immunoregulation occurs with excessive inflammatory responses to innocuous bacterial antigens or if there is failure to turn off appropriate immune responses after resolution of infection with a pathogen.

The normal mucosal cytokine response to commensal bacteria and dietary antigens is thought to be biased toward a type 1 (T_H1) cytokine pathway in humans.[16] This contrasts with data from murine studies where the normal default pathway for mucosal immune responses follows type 2 and/or type 3 cytokine production (by T_H2 and T_H3 cells). T_H1 responses are dependent on IL-12 and include IL-1, IL-6, TNF-α, and interferon-γ (IFN-γ), whereas T_H2 cytokines include interleukin (IL)-4, IL-5, and IL-10, which drive the production of IgA. T_H3 cells produce transforming growth factor-β (TGF-β), which induces B cells to switch to the IgA isotype and maintains oral tolerance.[10] The balance of mucosal cytokines is probably variable and influenced by genetic and environmental factors, including the composition of the luminal flora. In ulcerative colitis, the cytokine profile does not fit clearly into the T_H1/T_H2 dichotomy but appears to be a modified T_H2 response, whereas in Crohn's disease there is an excessive T_H1 cytokine response.

The control of cytokine production and immune activation involves transcription factors that bind to the gene promoter regions. Of these, nuclear factor-kappa B (NF-κB) is a pivotal regulator of pro-inflammatory cytokines within the mucosal epithelium and immune system. Mucosal expression of NF-κB is enhanced in patients with ulcerative colitis, and its activation is influenced by cytokines such as TNF-α thereby creating the basis of a positive feedback or amplification loop. NF-κB is also activated by bacterial signals from the lumen via Toll-like receptors (TLRs), which are pattern recognition receptors on the surface of enterocytes and on antigen presenting cells of the immune system. Increased epithelial expression of TLR4, which recognizes bacterial lipopolysaccharide, has been described in ulcerative colitis. The molecular basis of host–flora interactions including a search for polymorphisms of TLRs that might predispose to inappropriate responses to lumenal bacteria in ulcerative colitis is now a focal area of research.[11,17]

Enhanced humoral immunity is more evident in ulcerative colitis than Crohn's disease.[18] Mucosal plasma cells from patients with ulcerative colitis produce high levels of immunoglobulins, and in contrast with those from controls or patients with Crohn's disease preferentially produce IgG1 subclass antibodies that can activate complement. In addition, a variety of autoantibodies, including anticolon and antineutrophil cytoplasmic antibodies (ANCA), are detectable in the sera of most patients. Deposits of complement and IgG1 antiepithelial antibodies directed against epithelial tropomyosins are detectable within the epithelium in ulcerative colitis but the autoantibodies do not otherwise have pathogenic potential. They probably reflect disturbed immunoregulation and appear to be cross-reactive between self- and bacterial antigens.

In both forms of inflammatory bowel disease, the downstream effects of unrestrained T cell activation and cytokine release are similar. Upregulation of vascular adhesion molecules facilitate recruitment of additional effector cells causing amplification of the inflammatory response and the generation of activated matrix metalloproteinases, such as stromolysin-1, which mediate tissue destruction (Figure 53.2). Thus, irrespective of whether the initiating mechanism of immune activation is autosensitization or microbial stimulation or both, the final common pathway of tissue damage involves transmigration of neutrophils and other acute inflammatory cells from the vasculature through the mucosa and into the lumen. The molecular basis of both the transendothelial and transepithelial migration are multi-step

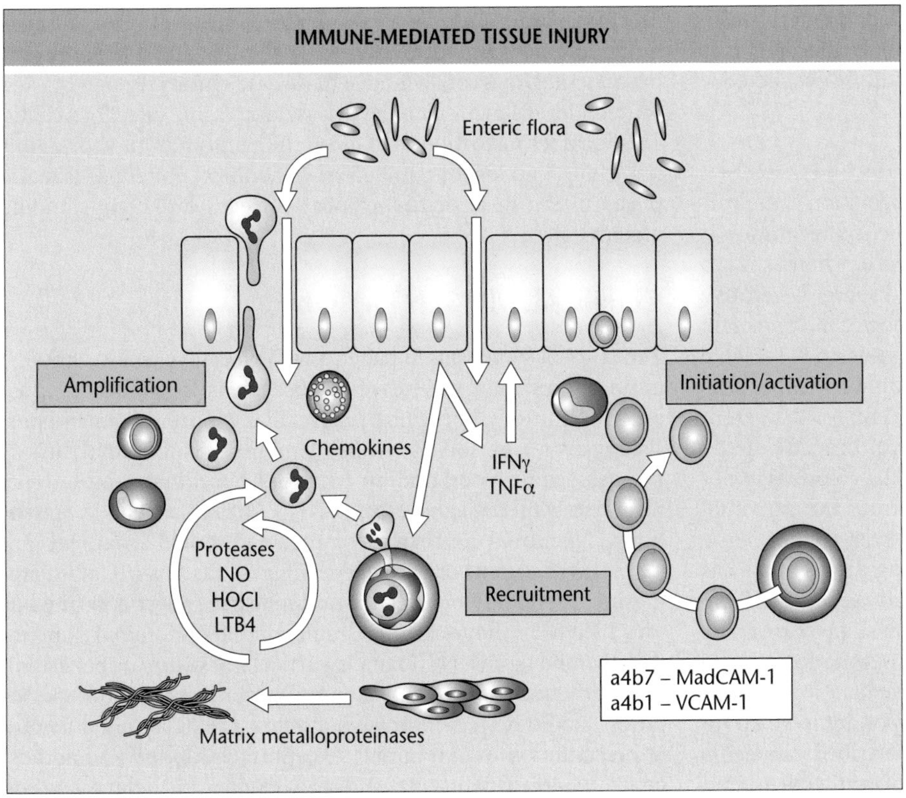

Fig. 53.2 Immune-mediated tissue injury in ulcerative colitis.

processes requiring cell–cell contacts using a series of adhesion molecules that are upregulated under the influence of cytokines. Further amplification of the inflammatory process occurs due to disruption of mucosal barrier function by the transepithelial migration of neutrophils, enhancing ingress of bacterial-derived chemotactic peptides and antigens. Tissue injury is mediated in a non-specific fashion by release of inflammatory mediators released by the transmigrating cells. These include reactive oxygen metabolites and matrix metalloproteinases. Some neutrophil-derived mediators such as leukotriene B4 (LTB4), which is the most potent chemotactic factor within the inflamed mucosa, cause additional amplification of the inflammatory response by increasing inflammatory cell recruitment and activation.[18]

Pathophysiology of symptoms

Diarrhea in ulcerative colitis is multifactorial. Inflammation may inhibit fluid absorption and/or increase secretion. Mechanisms of reduced absorption include: (1) decreased colonic surface area with epithelial denudation in severe cases; (2) neural and hormonal inhibition of salt absorption; (3) increased motor activity and transit in some cases; and (4) increased osmolar load from nutrient malabsorption such as impaired colonic salvage of carbohydrate. In contrast, increased secretion is due to inflammation-derived secretagogues including arachadonic acid metabolites, leakage of plasma from denuded mucosa, and loss of barrier function. Bowel frequency and urgency in colitis are due not only to increased stool volume (diarrhea) but may also arise because of irritability and reduced compliance of the inflamed rectum. It is noteworthy that despite increased stool frequency, proximal colonic transit may be reduced (proximal constipation) particularly in patients with proctitis or left-sided colitis. Bleeding is secondary to the adverse effects of inflammation on the mucosal microvasculature. Mucosal capillaries become engorged, leaky, and occasionally thrombosed. Bleeding is almost always present when ulcerative colitis is severe enough to cause diarrhea, and, if absent, another diagnosis should be suspected. Similarly, resolution of inflammation should lead to control of bleeding; if it does not, an alternative source of blood loss should be suspected.

PATHOLOGY

Despite its name, inflammation rather than ulceration is the cardinal feature of ulcerative colitis. Indeed, mucosal ulceration is usually evident only in severe advanced disease, whereas it is a defining feature of early lesions in Crohn's disease. Ulcerative colitis is a disease of the colorectal mucosa; it begins in the rectum at the anal verge and characteristically extends to a variable degree proximally in a diffuse continuous manner without skip areas. Progression or regression of the upper limit of the extent of the colitis is variable and unpredictable over time. When the disease is limited to the rectum or left side of the colon, its upper limit is often remarkably well demarcated from the proximal noninflamed mucosa. It is noteworthy, however, that in some patients, particularly those with long-standing disease that has been treated, the degree of inflammation may appear variable and give a false impression of patchiness or skip lesions.[19] A mistaken diagnosis of Crohn's disease in this situation can be avoided if biopsies are taken that confirm the histologic continuity of the inflammatory process. It is also important to be aware that a 'cecal patch' of inflammation has been described in patients with ulcerative colitis; this appears as an area of erythema around the appendiceal orifice. In patients with distal colitis, it does not imply Crohn's colitis.

Macroscopically or endoscopically, the mucosa in acutely active ulcerative colitis appears hyperemic, granular, and friable – bleeding easily when touched. As the condition becomes more severe, punctate ulceration appears and may become confluent and leave islands of inflammatory tissue. When the clinical course is one of frequent severe recurrences with extensive ulceration, 'pseudopolyps' (more correctly termed inflammatory polyps) and mucosal bridging may develop due to undermining of the mucosa by confluency of ulceration. When the colitis is inactive or 'burnt out,' inflammatory polyps persist and the intervening mucosa is smooth and atrophic. While these inflammatory polyps do not have the neoplastic implications of true adenomatous polyps, they make accurate dysplasia surveillance more difficult. Unlike Crohn's disease, fibrosis is not a prominent feature of the healing phase of ulcerative colitis. Over time, shortening of the colon and a reduction in diameter are due to thickening and contracture of its muscle layer. This is usually best illustrated by barium enema, which confirms the colonic foreshortening along with loss of haustral folds, an increase in retrorectal space, and, rarely, the appearance of benign nonfibrotic strictures.

Because ulcerative colitis is primarily a mucosal disease, its histologic features can be fully assessed using endoscopic biopsies. Cardinal features of acute disease include vascular congestion, edema, goblet cell mucin depletion, crypt abscess formation, and inflammatory cell infiltration of the lamina propria. Crypt abscesses are collections of neutrophils that have migrated across the crypt epithelium into the lumen. They also occur in infectious colitides and in Crohn's colitis. The inflammatory infiltrate in the lamina propria consists mainly of plasma cells and lymphocytes with a moderate increase in eosinophils and mast cells. Ulceration, if it occurs, is superficial and only becomes penetrating to the propria muscularis when the disease is fulminant or if toxic megacolon occurs. As disease activity subsides, crypt abscesses and mucin depletion resolves. Inflammatory cell infiltrates diminish more slowly. Regenerative changes within the epithelium become prominent. However, evidence of disease chronicity persists and is useful for distinguishing the disease from acute infectious colitis. This includes distortion of gland architecture such as shortening, branching, and loss of parallelism. In addition, Paneth cells metaplasia in the base of the crypts is a feature of long-standing ulcerative colitis.

CLINICAL PRESENTATION

The onset of symptoms in patients with ulcerative colitis, although more abrupt than with Crohn's disease, is frequently gradual and intermittent, becoming progressively more severe and persistent over a period of weeks or months. Bloody diarrhea or the passage of blood and mucus are the cardinal symptoms of ulcerative colitis and are present in over 90% of patients at presentation. Nocturnal diarrhea is common and should always prompt suspicion of organic disease. Depending on the severity of inflammation, there may be urgency and tenesmus (best described as 'dry heaves in the rectum'). Cramping and abdominal pain are usually mild or absent. If pain is particularly severe or persistent, an alternative diagnosis or a complication such as microperforation should be considered. Weight loss is usually not a feature at presentation or is minimal, except in childhood and adolescence where weight gain and growth may be delayed. When inflammation is confined to the rectum (proctitis), patients often complain of passing fresh blood and mucus and may have constipation. It is common for such patients to have an empty distal colon and rectum combined with fecal loading of the proximal colon.

CLINICAL PRESENTATION

COLITIS
Bloody diarrhea
Peri-defecatory abdominal cramping

PROCTITIS
Urgency of defecation
Tenesmus
Mucous discharge, pruritus ani
Proximal constipation and fecal loading in some patients

SYSTEMIC FEATURES
Fatigue, malaise, arthralgia, fever, and weight loss (mild, depending on severity)

EXTRAINTESTINAL MANIFESTATIONS
Rarely, may occur before the onset of colonic symptoms

Physical examination is usually unremarkable when the disease is mild or moderate. Systemic signs are absent and general health is usually maintained, particularly in patients with proctitis. Even patients with severe disease or pancolitis may appear deceptively healthy. Abdominal examination may be normal or exhibit mild tenderness over the sigmoid colon. Rectal examination is usually normal except for the presence of blood. Unlike Crohn's disease, perianal lesions are not a characteristic feature of ulcerative colitis. If they arise, they are nonspecific and secondary to diarrhea, and include excoriation, superficial abscess formation, hemorrhoids, mucosal prolapse, and superficial fissures. Fistula formation is rare and should raise suspicion of Crohn's disease.

With increasing severity of disease, anemia, fever, tachycardia, and fluid depletion become apparent (Table 53.4). Further deterioration with the development of severe persistent abdominal pain or distention may signal the development of a complication such as toxic megacolon or perforation.

Laboratory markers of the presence of severe inflammation include a raised erythrocyte sedimentation rate (ESR) or C-reactive protein, leukocytosis and thrombocytosis, and anemia. Hypokalemia, hypoalbuminemia, and elevated urea suggest severe pancolitis with fluid and electrolyte depletion.

Various activity indices have been devised to quantify disease severity. It is important to appreciate that these relate only to the degree of clinical activity at a given time and do not take into account the disease distribution or the clinical course of disease over time or the responsiveness to therapy. The Truelove and Witts classification (Table 53.4) is a classic and is still used in reporting clinical trials. However, few clinicians routinely use this or any formal activity index in daily practice. An example of a simple activity index that is convenient because it does not require any laboratory values and includes key questions that are used routinely by clinicians in assessing disease severity is shown in Table 53.5.[20]

CLINICAL TIPS

- Despite its name, ulcerative colitis is seldom an ulcerating disease; ulcers arise in advanced severe/fulminant disease
- The appearance of relative rectal sparing or patchy disease distribution in patients with long-standing treated ulcerative colitis is not a reason to change the diagnosis to Crohn's disease
- Common causes of treatment failure include inadequate dosing with aminosalicylates or corticosteroids and/or insufficient duration of steroid treatment
- Patient satisfaction and compliance with topical enema therapy is far superior if foam rather than liquid preparations are prescribed
- **The forgotten order** – stop all antispasmodics and antidiarrheals in patients with acute colitis to reduce risk of toxic megacolon
- Treatment with purine analogs requires at least 3 months before clinical efficacy is manifest – continuation with steroid therapy in the interim is required

Extracolonic disease associations

Occasionally, patients with ulcerative colitis may present with one of the extracolonic disease associations and, in some cases, one or more of these manifestations my precede the onset of colitis by several years. However, it is noteworthy that some patients may not complain of colonic symptoms but have endoscopic and histologic evidence of inflammatory activity.

TABLE 53.4 TRUELOVE AND WITTS CLASSIFICATION OF CLINICAL SEVERITY OF ULCERATIVE COLITIS

Variable	Mild[a]	Severe	Fulminant
Bowel frequency	<4/day	>6	>10
Blood in stool	Intermittent	Frequent	Continuous
Temperature (°C)	Normal	>37.5	>37.5
Pulse	Normal	>90	>90
Hemoglobin	Normal	<75% baseline	Transfusion required
ESR (mm/h)	<30	>30	>30
Plain film X-ray		Colonic air, edema, thumbprinting	Colonic dilatation
Physical signs		Abdominal tenderness	Distention and tenderness

[a] Moderate disease severity includes features of both mild and severe disease.

TABLE 53.5 CLINICAL ASSESSMENT OF ULCERATIVE COLITIS ACTIVITY BASED ON HISTORY AND NOT REQUIRING DETAILED PHYSICAL EXAMINATION OR LABORATORY TESTS

Symptom	Variable	Score
Stool frequency	1–3	0
	4–6	1
	7–9	2
	>9	3
Nocturnal frequency	1–3	1
	4–6	2
Urgency of defecation	Hurry	1
	Immediately	2
	Incontinence	3
Blood in stool	Trace	1
	Occasionally frank	2
	Usually frank	3
General well being	Very well	0
	Slightly below par	1
	Poor	2
	Very poor	3
	Terrible	4
Extracolonic manifestations[a]		1 per manifestation

[a] Includes arthritis, pyoderma gangrenosum, erythema nodosum, uveitis.
A score of >3–5 is consistent with active disease.

DIFFERENTIAL DIAGNOSIS

No single clinical, endoscopic, histologic, or other marker is diagnostic of ulcerative colitis. The diagnosis requires consideration of the composite clinical picture over time. In effect, the diagnosis rests upon: (1) a clinical picture compatible with colitis, usually bloody diarrhea or blood and mucus; (2) exclusion of other disorders, which are mainly infectious colitides that mimic acute ulcerative colitis; and (3) demonstration of chronicity. While a wide range of conditions might present with blood per rectum or with diarrhea, these symptoms seldom occur alone in ulcerative colitis: in practice, the differential diagnosis can be resolved firstly into the distinction between ulcerative colitis and acute infectious colitis; and secondly the distinction between ulcerative colitis and colonic Crohn's disease.

Ulcerative colitis versus acute infectious colitis

At first presentation, the most important differential diagnosis to be excluded is acute infectious colitis. This is particularly true when the inflammation is confined to the rectosigmoid. When the duration of symptoms exceeds 3 weeks, a first presentation of ulcerative colitis is more likely than an infectious etiology. However, a specific infectious pathogen cannot be detected in all cases of acute self-limited colitides and a negative stool examination for pathogens or parasites does not necessarily imply a diagnosis of ulcerative colitis. In such circumstances, the histopathologic features of rectal biopsy may be helpful. Distorted crypt architecture favors a diagnosis of chronic ulcerative colitis over acute infectious colitis. Plasmacytosis in the lamina propria extending to the mucosal base (basilar plasmacytosis) is another marker of the chronic condition over a self-limited colitis. Regardless of the findings in the acute phase of the illness, the best differential approach is patient follow-up and observation of the clinical course of colitis over time.

Ulcerative colitis versus colonic Crohn's disease

Differentiating Crohn's disease from ulcerative colitis is usually not difficult; the presence of small bowel disease immediately rules out ulcerative colitis. Difficulty arises only when Crohn's disease is confined to the colon, which occurs in up to 25% of patients with Crohn's disease (Figure 53.3). In most of these cases, the combined endoscopic, histopathologic, and radiologic features are sufficiently characteristic to permit a differential diagnosis, but in 5–10% of cases the colitis is indeterminate. Patchy, asymmetrical involvement and rectal sparing, with or without histopathologic evidence of granulomas, is consistent with Crohn's disease. Although granulomas may be found in 60% of resected specimens, they are found in only about 20% of patients with Crohn's disease in endoscopic series. Furthermore, while diffuse continuous involvement is characteristic of ulcerative colitis, some degree of patchiness is expected when the condition becomes chronic and after treatment.[19] Therefore, the colonoscopic examination performed at the time of first presentation is the most helpful in distinguishing ulcerative colitis from Crohn's colitis. However, in some patients, the differential diagnosis is impossible and even examination of the surgically resected colon may not be definitive because the inflammatory process frequently becomes transmural if the condition becomes fulminant or progresses to toxic megacolon.

DIAGNOSTIC METHODS

Diagnosis is based on the composite clinical picture and not on the basis of endoscopy, histology, or any other single disease marker. Colonoscopy is the mainstay of diagnosis. Plain abdominal

ENDOSCOPIC, HISTOLOGIC AND SEROLOGIC FEATURES

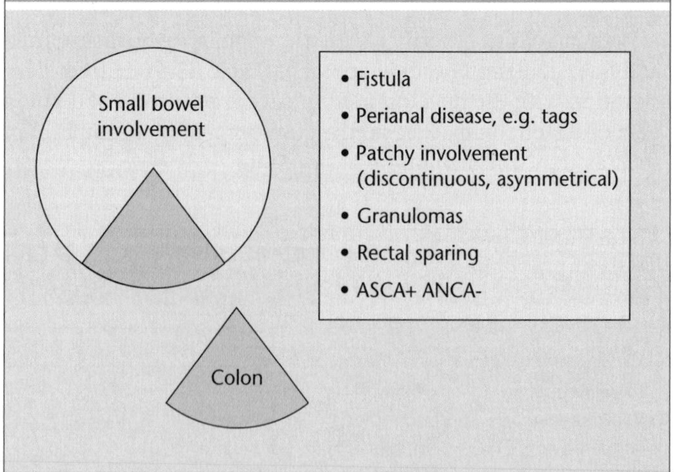

Small bowel involvement
Colon
• Fistula
• Perianal disease, e.g. tags
• Patchy involvement (discontinuous, asymmetrical)
• Granulomas
• Rectal sparing
• ASCA+ ANCA-

Fig. 53.3 Endoscopic, histologic, and serologic features. Endoscopic, histologic, and serologic features of colitis suggesting Crohn's versus ulcerative colitis in patients with indeterminate colitis. However, it is noteworthy that the endoscopic appearances may become patchy after treatment and granulomas are present in only a minority of endoscopic series of Crohn's colitis. In addition, the sensitivity and accuracy of serology (ANCA and ASCA) is insufficient to be recommended for routine use.

DIFFERENTIAL DIAGNOSIS
CAUSES OF BLOODY DIARRHEA THAT MIMIC ULCERATIVE COLITIS
INFLAMMATORY Crohn's colitis Behçet's colitis
INFECTIOUS COLITIDES (EXAMPLES) *Campylobacter* *Salmonella* *Shigella* *Clostridium difficile* Enterohemorrhagic *Escherichia coli*
SEXUALLY TRANSMITTED PROCTITIDES Cytomegalovirus Herpes simplex Chlamydia
NEOPLASTIC Colorectal cancer
VASCULAR Ischemic colitis
IATROGENIC Irradiation Nonsteroidal anti-inflammatory drugs

DIAGNOSTIC BASELINE METHODS
BLOOD TESTS (FOR MARKERS OF SYSTEMIC IMPACT AND SEVERITY OF INFLAMMATION) Raised ESR and C-reactive protein Thrombocytosis and leukocytosis Presence or absence of anemia Hypoalbuminemia (marker of chronicity and severity) Liver enzymes (to screen for co-morbidity)
STOOL EXAMINATION (TO RULE OUT INFECTIOUS COLITIDES) Microscopy for ova/parasites Culture *C. difficile* toxin
SEROLOGY (SELECTED PATIENTS) Serum pANCA, ASCA (optional – not for routine use) HIV, amebiasis (selected patients)
CONVENTIONAL RADIOLOGY Plain film of abdomen (to monitor for colonic dilatation) Chest X-ray (if TB suspected or immunosuppressive contemplated) Barium enema (neither necessary nor desirable in most patients) Barium small bowel study (only if Crohn's suspected)
ENDOSCOPY This is the mainstay of diagnosis, particularly the initial examination of the untreated patient; diffuse continuous pattern of erythema, granularity, and friability with exudate – followed by ulceration in advanced severe cases. After treatment, the appearances may become patchy

radiology of the abdomen provides useful information regarding the extent of colonic involvement and the presence of right-sided fecal loading in patients with proctitis. It is particularly useful in monitoring patients for the development of toxic megacolon. While a barium enema may show characteristic appearances, barium studies are no longer necessary for the diagnosis of ulcerative colitis and should be avoided in acute severe disease to avoid increasing the risk of toxic megacolon.

The immunologic disturbances in patients with inflammatory bowel disease include various serum antibody markers such as perinuclear antineutrophil cytoplasmic antibodies (pANCA) and anti-*Saccharomyces cerevisiae* antibodies (ASCA).[21] Since these two antibody markers are differentially and oppositely expressed in ulcerative colitis and Crohn's disease, their role in differential diagnosis has been investigated. Detection of pANCA in ulcerative colitis and ASCA in Crohn's disease has a high degree of specificity for these conditions respectively, but sensitivity is modest in both cases (55–65%). When combined testing for both markers is performed, diagnostic accuracy in terms of specificity and positive predictive value increases to greater than 95% but sensitivity decreases by about 10%. However, in patients with Crohn's disease confined to the colon, the prevalence of ASCA is relatively low and the sensitivity of ASCA positivity alone or in combination with ANCA negativity was only 45% and 32%, respectively, in one study.[22] Thus, serologic testing for ANCA and ASCA is least helpful in the subset of patients where the differential diagnosis is most problematic (i.e., Crohn's confined to colon vs ulcerative colitis).[20] Furthermore, up to 15% of patients with Crohn's disease of the colon have been reported to be ANCA positive. Finally, a prospective study of ANCA and ASCA in patients with indeterminate colitis showed that serology was unhelpful in over half of the patients and its accuracy otherwise was insufficient to justify routine use of serology.[23]

TREATMENT AND PREVENTION

There is no specific, curative treatment for ulcerative colitis – the emphasis is on supportive measures and judicious use of potentially toxic anti-inflammatory and immunosuppressive drugs on an individualized basis. The objectives of therapy are to improve quality of life, to reduce the risk of disease-related complications, and to avoid the need for surgery. The single most important aspect of disease management is access for the patient to a physician who is interested in the disease, compassionate, and committed to long-term care.

General measures

As with every chronic illness, patient education is a pivotal component of successful long-term management. This includes guidance on the nature of the disease and reasonable expectations for therapy. In some cases, stress may exacerbate colitis and perhaps trigger relapse. Advice from a counselor, particularly for patients without strong family support, may improve ability to cope with the uncertainties of the disease.

A well-balanced diet with minimal restrictions is encouraged. This is particularly important in children and adolescents with colitis. Emphasis is placed on maintaining adequate caloric intake and avoidance of excessive weight loss or malnutrition. A requirement for specific dietary supplements should be anticipated. These include iron for patients at risk of developing depleted iron stores and anemia due to chronic blood loss. Calcium is indicated to offset risk of metabolic bone disease in patients receiving corticosteroid therapy. A pragmatic exercise program such as a regular walking routine has also been shown to help prevent bone thinning in those taking corticosteroids. Consensus guidelines on management of inflammatory bowel disease-related osteoporosis have been published.[24,25] In addition, the health benefit of dietary supplementation with folic acid is increasingly recognized and recommended by several clinicians.

For hospitalized patients with active severe disease, consideration should be given to use of preventive measures against thromboembolic disease. This may include wearing support stockings or the use of low molecular weight heparin. Active inflammatory bowel disease is associated with a procoagulant state and thromboembolism is an important cause of mortality in this young age group.[26,27]

Induction of remission

The current status of commonly used drugs for both the induction and maintenance of remission in ulcerative colitis is summarized in Table 53.6 and is contrasted with their roles in Crohn's disease. The characteristics of these drugs are covered in Chapter 54; considerations regarding their usage will be summarized here. While treatment should be individualized, a general strategy for drug usage is shown in Figure 53.4.

For patients with mild-to-moderate ulcerative colitis, aminosalicylates remain the cornerstone treatment of active disease and for maintenance of remission.[28] Efficacy is dose-dependent; consequently, patients should receive maximum tolerated doses before resorting to the use of systemic steroids (Figure 53.5).[4,29] For patients with distal or left-sided disease, topical aminosalicylate enemas alone or in combination with oral aminosalicylates are as good or better than steroid enemas. Budesonide retention enemas have some advantage over prednisolone enemas because of low systemic activity due to high first-pass hepatic metabolism. Therefore, prolonged usage is less likely to impair endogenous cortisol responsiveness.[4,30] In practice, the choice of topical therapy is often based on patient preference for foam enema preparations over liquid formulations because the former are easier to retain within the bowel.

Once the clinical assessment indicates that the colitis is moderately severe, there is nothing to be gained from postponing corticosteroid medication. The goal of treatment is to prevent progression to severe or fulminant disease and to achieve reduced inflammatory activity and remission. Corticosteroids should be prescribed at high dosage (e.g., 40 mg/day prednisolone) to bring the condition under control and tapered as the clinical course permits. The tapering regimen should be individualized but typically is not linear and may be by weekly decrements of 5 mg/day while tapering from 40 mg/day to 20 mg/day, and thereafter by 2.5 mg/day decrements weekly. It should be noted that the most troublesome symptoms of patients with pancolitis may be due to proctitis (tenesmus, urgency, and bleeding). For such patients, the addition of a topical corticosteroid foam enema may hasten relief and enable the systemic steroids to be tapered more rapidly.

Patients presenting with acute severe or fulminant ulcerative colitis require admission to hospital for treatment and observation. The emphasis is on careful clinical assessment and vigilance for emergence of toxic megacolon. There is no place for full colonoscopy or barium enema at this stage of the disease; these procedures are not necessary, can be deferred, and may precipitate toxic megacolon. Surgical consultation should be obtained at the outset and a joint physician/surgeon team approach is important. The four components of management are intravenous fluid and electrolyte replacement, broad-spectrum antibiotic

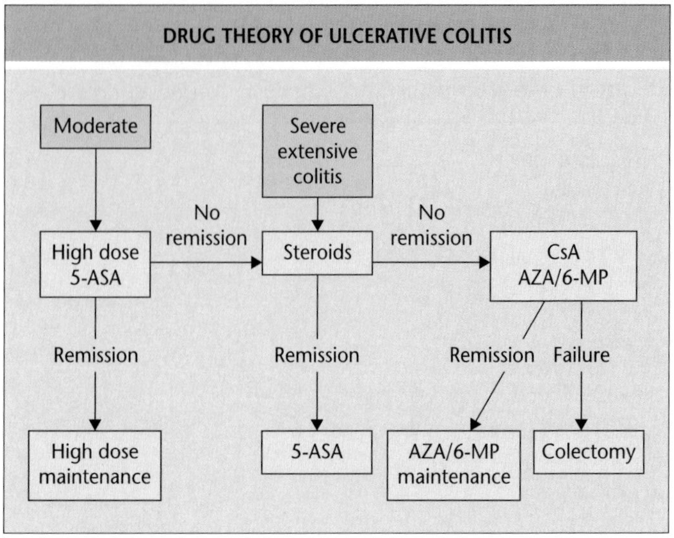

Fig. 53.4 Algorithm for drug therapy of ulcerative colitis. Based on data from Rutgeerts.[28]

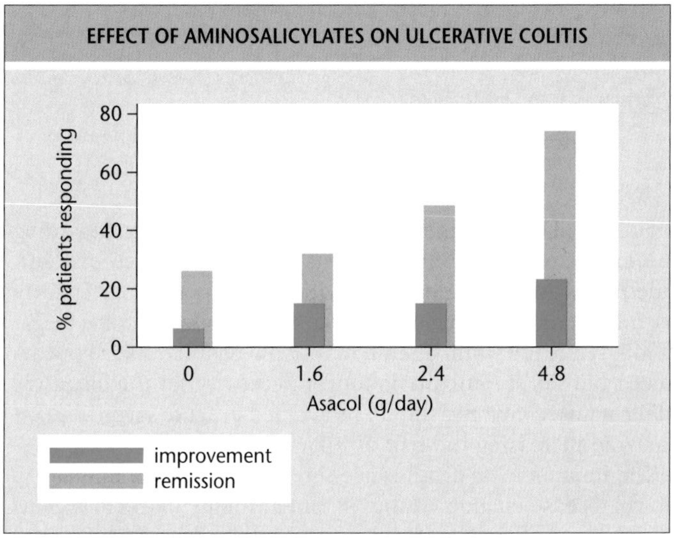

Fig. 53.5 Effect of aminosalicylates on ulcerative colitis. Dose-dependent influence of aminosalicylates on ulcerative colitis. Compiled from data in Schroeder K et al. N Engl J Med 1987; 317:1625-1629 and Sninsky et al. (1991).[29]

TABLE 53.6 DRUGS USED FOR INDUCTION AND MAINTENANCE OF REMISSION

	Ulcerative colitis		Crohn's disease	
	Acute	*Maintenance*	*Acute*	*Maintenance*
Aminosalicylates	+	+	+	–
Corticosteroids	+	–	+	–
Purine analogs	–	+	–	–
Methotrexate	–	–	+	–
Cyclosporine	+	–	–	–
Anti-TNF-α (infliximab)	–	–	+	+

+, established role; –, no conclusive role.

coverage, intravenous corticosteroids, and discontinuation of all opiate or anticholinergic, antispasmodic or antidiarrheal drugs because they are risk factors for toxic megacolon. Aminosalicylates are not likely to have a significant therapeutic effect at this advanced stage of the disease. Nutrition should continue to be given by the enteral route; parenteral nutrition should be avoided, if possible, because it is usually unnecessary and because of the risk of complications including central vein thrombosis and sepsis. Prophylaxis against thromboembolism should be instituted.

Irrespective of the extent of colitis, an important subset of patients is resistant to aminosalicylates and corticosteroids (up to 16% in one study).[31] For severe disease, intravenous cyclosporine is an effective option either alone or in conjunction with steroids. Although initial reports used a relatively high dose (4 mg/kg/day) of cyclosporine, it is clear that lower doses (2 mg/kg/day) are equally effective.[32] Cyclosporine should only be used by experienced clinicians in referral centers where blood levels can be monitored. Prophylaxis against *Pneumocystis carinii* with co-trimoxazole should be considered.[4] The advantage of cyclosporine is its rapid action. However, because of its potential toxicity, the drug cannot be recommended as a routine oral therapy over a long term.[33] It is noteworthy that of the patients with severe disease treated with cyclosporine and in whom a colectomy is initially avoided, at least half will require colectomy within the following year. In the transition to long-term therapy, consideration should be given to switching to azathioprine/6-mercaptopurine in those patients who respond to steroids and/or cyclosporine in the acute phase.

Surgical intervention should not be delayed if there is failure of medical therapy or clinical deterioration despite aggressive medical therapy. Persistent pain (other than cramping associated with defecation) is a particularly worrisome development as is any evidence for colonic dilatation on abdominal X-ray films. In addition, a requirement for blood transfusion is a sinister development. Indeed, for acutely ill patients, surgery is often the conservative approach and may be safer than prolonged immunosuppressive therapy.

Maintenance therapy

The long-term goal is to keep patients in remission and to minimize frequency of relapses. The efficacy of medical therapy is judged in terms of quality of life and ability to work and function socially. Assessment of disease activity at regular follow-up visits is primarily on a symptomatic basis and not on endoscopic or biopsy findings. Patients should not be subjected to repeated radiologic or endoscopic procedures just 'to see how things are.'

Most patients with ulcerative colitis can be successfully maintained with aminosalicylates and intermittent brief courses of corticosteroids.[33] Controlled clinical trials have confirmed the efficacy of sulfasalazine and the aminosalicylates in prevention of relapses. However, corticosteroids are indicated only for breakthrough symptoms and have no role as a maintenance therapy.

Evidence from controlled studies of the prophylactic efficacy of azathioprine or 6-mercaptopurine in ulcerative colitis is sparse, but these drugs remain the treatment of choice for patients who fail to respond to aminosalicylates and corticosteroids.[33] The starting dose for 6-mercaptopurine is 50 mg/day and may be adjusted to 1.5 mg/kg/day in 25 mg/day increments depending on clinical response after 3–6 months. The dose for azathioprine is about twice that for 6-mercaptopurine. The rate-limiting enzyme for catabolism of these purine analog drugs is thiopurine methyltransferase (TPMT), which is variably expressed due to genetic polymorphism. Therefore, assessment of TPMT genotype in advance of prescribing purine analogs has been recommended, where available,[21,34,35] so that rare (<1%) homozygotes with low or absent levels of the enzyme can be identified for whom the drug should be contraindicated. In addition, heterozygotes (10%) with intermediate levels of enzyme activity may require dosage adjustment. The use of enzyme and metabolite levels to monitor drug therapy has also been proposed but studies have been conflicting. Irrespective of whether these assays are used, they do not preclude the need for regular blood counts to monitor for delayed bone marrow suppression. Patients should be advised to have a monthly full blood count.

There is no supporting evidence for methotrexate as a maintenance therapy in ulcerative colitis, although this requires further study.[33,36] However, cyclosporine, which is an effective inductive agent for severe colitis, cannot be recommended as a maintenance therapy because of its toxicity.[33]

Emerging therapeutic strategies

A wide range of immunosuppressive drugs including mycophenolate mofetil and other agents has been studied in ulcerative colitis with varying results. Controlled trials are awaited. Results with other agents including heparin, nicotine, fish oils, leukopheresis, antibiotics, and leukotriene inhibitors have so far not lived up to the initial promising expectations in controlled trials.[4] While infliximab has been reported to be effective in a small number of cases, it is less effective in ulcerative colitis than in Crohn's disease and its use should be restricted to investigational protocols.[21,33] Some new strategies are particularly exciting and include the use of growth factors such as epidermal growth factor[37] and monoclonal antibodies to block the homing of effector lymphocytes to the inflamed mucosa. Indeed, it seems likely that the next biologic therapy to move from the research bench to the bedside will be based on antagonizing alpha-4 integrins (Fig. 53.2).[38]

An alternative therapeutic strategy is to target the microbial environment within the colon.[21,39] The rationale for using probiotics is based on the notion that inflammatory bowel disease is due to an abnormal host immune response to some but not all components of the indigenous colonic bacteria. Accordingly, bacteria such as lactobacilli and bifidobacteria that lack proinflammatory potential have been successfully used as probiotics in experimental rodent models of enterocolitis. Other bacteria including *E. coli* Nissle 1917, a non-pathogenic coliform, have also been reported to have efficacy equivalent to that of mesalazine as a maintenance therapy in human ulcerative colitis.[33] Additional controlled trials of probiotic strategies are underway.

Surgical management

There are three main groups of indications for colectomy in ulcerative colitis. First, emergency colectomy is indicated for acute fulminating course or toxic megacolon. Second, elective colectomy becomes a serious consideration for patients in whom medical therapy has either failed to restore an acceptable quality of life or in whom there is unacceptable drug toxicity, such as a requirement for continual steroids despite optimal aminosalicylate and immunosuppressive drug therapy. Third, detection of either low-grade or high-grade dysplasia, particularly if confirmed by a second pathologist, is an indication for colectomy.

In emergency situations, a subtotal colectomy with ileostomy is often the procedure of choice. This can be converted to a total colectomy with permanent ileostomy by resecting the rectal stump at a later time, once the patient has recovered physically and emotionally. Alternatively, the option to proceed at a later stage to surgical creation of an ileal pouch and subsequent pouch–anal anastomosis may be exercised. The choice of procedure will depend on several individual variables including the age of the patient, co-morbidity, coping skills, and ability to psychosocially adjust to stoma care. Where possible, in elective situations, patients should be counseled well in advance and given realistic expectations. An experienced stoma therapist should outline stoma care. It is important that patients understand there can be no guarantee regarding the distinction between ulcerative colitis and Crohn's disease in advance of surgery. They should also appreciate that any continent pouch procedure may fail and require repeat surgery; complications may necessitate complete surgical revision, possibly ending with a standard ileostomy.

Pouchitis

The cumulative frequency of developing pouchitis after colectomy with ileal pouch–anal anastomosis (IPAA) increases with duration of follow-up and may be up to 50% after 10 years. The condition is in a sense a human experimental model of ulcerative colitis in a colonized pouch, and should be considered as a recurrence of ulcerative colitis.[40] Pouchitis is largely confined to patients who have IPAA performed for ulcerative colitis and is much less common in those having it performed for familial adenomatous polyposis. The mainstay of treatment for pouchitis is antibiotics. Many patients will respond to metronidazole 200–400 mg three times daily for 1–2 weeks or longer. Alternatives to metronidazole include ciprofloxacin or similar broad-spectrum agents. Some patients may require the addition of aminosalicylates, topical steroids, or even immunosuppressive drugs. However, the most promising preventive therapy that has emerged is the use of probiotics following induction of remission with antibiotics. Controlled trials of probiotic therapy have shown that this is a safe and effective strategy deserving further study.[41,42]

TREATMENT: INDUCTIVE AND MAINTENANCE

GENERAL AND SUPPORTIVE
- Patient education and psychosocial support
- Specialist multidisciplinary hospital care
- Diet and nutrition (particularly in childhood and adolescence)
- Osteopenia prophylaxis
- Thromboembolism prophylaxis for immobilized patients
- Drugs to avoid (e.g., anticholinergics in acute colitis, antibiotics, and NSAIDs unless specifically indicated)

ANTI-INFLAMMATORY OR IMMUNOMODULATORY DRUG THERAPY
- Aminosalicylates (topical or oral)
- Corticosteroids (topical or systemic)
- Purine analogs (6-mercaptopurine, azathioprine)
- Cyclosporine

SURGERY
- Total colectomy with end ileostomy
- Colectomy with ileal pouch–anal anastomosis (IPAA)

COMPLICATIONS AND THEIR MANAGEMENT

Toxic megacolon

Toxic megacolon is a medical emergency. It may occur as a complication of any form of severe colitis.[43] Occasionally, it is the presenting feature. Risk factors for development of this complication include the use of anticholinergics, opiates, hypokalemia, and barium enema or colonoscopic procedures in the setting of fulminant disease. Dilatation may involve the entire colon but appears maximal in the transverse colon radiographically. This is because air tends to rise in the upright position. In affected areas, the inflammatory process, which is usually confined to the mucosa, extends into the muscle layer, perhaps due to bacterial overgrowth. There is bowel wall thinning and paralysis of motor function. The texture of the bowel wall has been likened to wet tissue paper; perforation with systemic sepsis poses a major threat with a mortality rate up to 30%. The cardinal symptoms of toxic dilatation are abdominal tenderness, guarding, tympany, and reduced or absent bowel sounds. Diagnosis is confirmed by plain abdominal radiograph; a continuous column of colonic air usually precedes onset of dilatation. Loss of haustral markings and an irregular luminal border may be visible with nodular defects indicating islands of inflammatory necrotic mucosa alternating with areas of ulceration. Gas shadows within the wall of the colon are a particularly ominous sign. It is important to recognize that the patient's clinical status may change over a period of hours from toxic dilatation to perforation and shock. Immediate treatment includes discontinuation of any precipitating drug, correction of fluid and electrolyte imbalances, and broad-spectum antibiotics. Colonic decompression may be achieved with a soft rectal tube and a long nasoenteral tube. Colonic gas can also be redistributed by intermittent repositioning of the patient from supine to prone position. However, unless prompt resolution occurs with these strategies, emergency colectomy should be performed.

Colitis-associated cancer

The risk of developing colorectal cancer in ulcerative colitis increases with disease duration, severity, and extent of disease,[44,45] and also appears to be adversely influenced by the presence of sclerosing cholangitis,[46] a positive family history of sporadic colorectal cancer,[47] and backwash ileitis.[48]

The pathogenesis of colitis-associated carcinogenesis differs from that of sporadic colorectal cancer.[49,50] While the two forms of cancer share many molecular abnormalities, the timing or sequence of molecular events distinguishes the two neoplastic pathways. For example, abnormalities of the p53 tumor suppressor gene are a relatively early event in chronic colitis, occasionally preceding dysplasia, but are observed late in pathogenic sequence of sporadic colorectal carcinoma. In addition, mutation or deletion of the *APC* tumor suppressor gene tends to be late and uncommon in colitis-associated cancer, but an early event in sporadic colon cancer. The two neoplastic processes also differ in relation to expression of cell cycle regulatory proteins. Multiple mechanisms appear to predispose to colitis-associated cancer. The increased frequency of mutant p53 in chronic colitis has been shown to be related to oxidative stress in the presence of reactive oxygen and nitrogen species. The p53 pathway is also modulated by cytokines. Functional inactivation of p53 has been linked with the actions of macrophage migration inhibitory factor (MIF). This could lead to an antiapoptosis feedback loop in inflamed tissue and reduce the host cell response to genetic damage and predispose to accumulation of oncogenic mutations.[49]

While prophylactic colectomy is the only certain method of avoiding progression to colorectal cancer, this is seldom an attractive option. Therefore, the management of cancer risk in patients with colitis depends on surveillance colonoscopy. Surveillance colonoscopy has not been shown to reduce mortality from colitis-associated cancer and a randomized controlled trial has not yet been performed.

Several problems associated with surveillance endoscopy as currently practiced have been highlighted.[51,52] First, there is poor understanding on the part of most gastroenterologists of the true meaning of the term dysplasia. Many gastroenterologists do not appreciate that dysplasia means neoplasia confined to the epithelium and is not preneoplasia. Second, there is a lack of consistency and consensus on the optimal number of biopsies taken at endoscopy. This influences sampling error. For example, it has been estimated that 65 biopsies are required to have a 95% confidence of finding the highest grade of neoplasm (dysplasia or cancer), and 33 biopsies are required to find the highest degree of dysplasia.[53] Third, even if pathologists receive adequate biopsy material, their inter-observer agreement for diagnosing low-grade dysplasia is only about 60% for experienced, specialized pathologists. It is, therefore, not surprising that gastroenterologists have inconsistent approaches to the management of low-grade dysplasia. This is disturbing because a confirmed finding of low-grade dysplasia is a strong predictor of progression to invasive cancer and early colectomy should be a serious consideration.[54] Fourth, if clinicians wait for the development of high-grade dysplasia before recommending colectomy, it may be too late to prevent invasive cancer. The progression of low-grade to high-grade dysplasia is not evident in all cases and once high-grade dysplasia is detected, an invasive cancer will already be present in up to 30% of cases, in many of which it will be advanced (Dukes C).[51,52]

Developments that promise to improve the accuracy of surveillance colonoscopy in identifying those patients at particular risk of colitis-associated cancer include the introduction of magnifying or high-resolution endoscopy coupled with mucosal dye staining (chromoendoscopy).[52] Early reports have been encouraging and prospective outcome studies are awaited. In addition, a more fundamental understanding of the molecular events underlying the inflammation-dysplasia-cancer sequence promises to facilitate the development of a molecular profile of the genetic alterations in the colonic epithelia conferring increased risk of cancer.[50]

Since colitis-associated cancer appears to be a result of chronic inflammation, it is plausible to conclude that effective therapy can reduce the risk of cancer. There is retrospective evidence that aminosalicylates may act as a form of chemoprophylaxis against colitis-associated cancer.[55] However, results are inconclusive and population-based data have cast some doubt on the protective role of aminosalicylates against cancer.[56] In the absence of definitive data, the use of aminosalicylates is a logical preventive strategy that could reasonably be combined with other preventive strategies, such as the use of folic acid and calcium supplements with putative chemopreventive effects.

PROGNOSIS

The clinical course of ulcerative colitis in individual patients is impossible to predict but its relapsing nature is revealed by population-based studies showing a 1-year risk of relapse of around 50%, even in patients receiving maintenance aminosalicylates. Follow-up studies of patients with ulcerative colitis have shown that only half the patients are in remission at any one time. In untreated patients, the relapse rate is 50–70% over 1 year, as estimated from the placebo-treated groups in clinical trials of aminosalicylate therapy.[33] The likelihood of surgery becoming a necessity for any patient is much more difficult to estimate because of so many individual variables and because it is almost certainly changing with the increasing use of more effective drugs including immunosuppressive agents.

The clinical course of patients in the placebo-controlled limb of clinical therapeutic trials may reveal lessons regarding the clinical course of ulcerative colitis. In one analysis, the mean placebo response for clinical symptoms was similar to that for more objective measures such as endoscopy and histology (25–30%). More importantly, the only factor that appeared to influence the placebo response was the number of doctor–patient contacts.[57] This is circumstantial support for regular follow-up but is not necessarily at variance with the concept of guiding patients to help themselves.[58] Thus, guided self-management of ulcerative colitis has some advantages for patients but should not be a substitute for regular contact with a committed experienced clinician.

While early studies indicated a reduced life expectancy in patients with ulcerative colitis creating difficulties for patients seeking life insurance, recent studies have been less pessimistic. Some, but not all population-based studies have since shown either improved or equivalent survival for ulcerative colitis relative to the general population. Interpretation of the data may be confounded by subtle variables in methods and design.[59] It appears that while survival has improved, some clinical subsets of ulcerative colitis such as pancolitis and older age may still have reduced life expectancy. Indeed, it has been speculated that a higher mortality rate from cancers or infections might be the price paid for avoiding colectomy.[59]

WHAT TO TELL PATIENTS

Perhaps the most important thing to tell patients is that they should take some responsibility for their own management. A minimal expectation should be that patients know precisely the names and dosages of their medications and have a reasonable understanding and perspective on the risks, benefits, and alternatives of the different drug strategies. As with any chronic disease, patients who are well informed at the outset are likely to comply with medical advice and not seek cures by doctor-hopping. Removing fear of the unknown by frank discussion of prognosis and worst-case scenarios is important for some patients. It may also be helpful to let patients observe the colonoscopic appearances of themselves while in relapse and remission so that they have a tangible rather than abstract understanding of the disease process. With regard to the risk of developing colon cancer, patients and physicians need to know that the risk increases with time but the ability of the clinician to detect it by colonoscopic surveillance is limited and may not change over time. Patients need to be aware of the difficulty in distinguishing Crohn's disease from ulcerative colitis and that an absolute guarantee cannot be given in advance of surgery.

For patients who wish to join or make contact with support groups and sources of patient-oriented information, the following sources are recommended: in the United States, the Crohn's and Colitis Foundation of America (http://www.ccfa.org/); in Europe the European Federation of Crohn's and Ulcerative Colitis Associations (EFCCA, http://www.efcca.org/); and similar national organizations are easy to access by the internet in other continents.

CURRENT CONTROVERSIES AND THEIR FUTURE RESOLUTION

The biotechnology and gene technology boom has made it possible to develop drug strategies that mimic or antagonize any mediator or receptor involved in the inflammatory cascade. Thus, drug development is no longer a problem, but prediction of individual responsiveness and the development of biomarkers including pharmacogenomics to facilitate individualized treatment are now required and are being pursued.

Most drug strategies are directed towards suppression of the host inflammatory or immune response. In this respect, it is likely that the next group of immunomodulators to be introduced to the clinic will be those that antagonize mucosal homing of lymphocytes by monoclonal inhibition of α-4 integrins. However, the role of the bacterial flora in relation to the pathogenesis of colitis, which may be permissive or stimulatory, will drive research into the therapeutic manipulation of the enteric microbial microenvironment with prebiotics and probiotics.

For patients who avoid colectomy with improved medical therapy, there is an acute need to resolve the deficiencies of current dysplasia practices. New molecular markers for identifying those at increased risk of neoplasia are likely to emerge, and devices such as chromoendoscopy may improve targeting of endoscopic biopsy material.

Irrespective of advances in molecular medicine and diagnostics, the traditional principles of good patient care are unlikely to be replaced. The science of the art of the doctor–patient relationship can still be a fruitful area of research. For example, if the mechanisms underlying the placebo response were understood, and if the conditions favoring enhancement of the response could be harnessed, the outcome for most patients could be improved substantially.

SOURCES OF INFORMATION FOR PATIENTS AND DOCTORS

http://patients.uptodate.com/topic.asp?file=digestiv/10728
http://www.clevelandclinic.org/gastro/ibd/patient/colitis.htm
http://www.patient.co.uk/showdoc/23068968/
http://www.patient.co.uk/showdoc/611/
http://www.gastro.org/generalPublic.html
http://www.nacc.org.uk/content/home.asp

REFERENCES

1. Truelove SC, Witts LT. Cortisone in ulcerative colitis: a final report on a therapeutic trial. Br Med J 1955; 2:1041–1048.
2. Ekbom A. The changing face of Crohn's disease and ulcerative colitis. In: Targan S, Shanahan F, Karp LC, eds. Inflammatory bowel disease: from bench to bedside, 2nd edn. Dordrecht: Kluwer Academic Publishers; 2003:5–20.
3. Ekbom A. The epidemiology of IBD. Inflamm Bowel Dis 2004;10 (Suppl 1):S32–S34.
4. Farrell RJ, Peppercorn MA. Ulcerative colitis. Lancet 2002; 359:331–340.
5. Koutroubakis IE, Vlachonikolis IG, Kouroumalis EA. Role of appendicitis and appendectomy in the pathogenesis of ulcerative colitis: a critical review. Inflamm Bowel Dis 2002; 8:277–286.
6. Mizoguch A, Misoguchi E, Chiba C, Bhan AK. Role of the appendix in the development of inflammatory bowel disease in TCR-alpha mutant mice. J Exp Med 1996; 184:707–715.
7. Andersson RE, Olaison G, Tysk C, Ekbom A. Appendectomy and protection against ulcerative colitis. N Engl J Med 2001; 344:808–814.
8. Taylor KD, Rotter JI, Yang H. Genetics of inflammatory bowel disease. In: Targan SR, Shanahan F, Karp LC, eds. Inflammatory bowel disease: from bench to bedside, 2nd edn. Dordrecht: Kluwer Academic Publishers; 2003:21–65.
9. Ahmad T, Marshall S, Jewell D. Genotype-based phenotyping heralds a new taxonomy for inflammatory bowel disease. Curr Opin Gastroenterol 2003; 19:327–335.
10. Shanahan F. Mechanisms of immunologic sensation of intestinal contents. Am J Physiol (Gastrointest Liver Physiol) 2000; 278:G191–G196.
11. Shanahan F. The host-microbe interface within the gut. Best Practice Res Clin Gastroenterol 2002; 16:915–931.
12. Strober W, Fuss IJ, Blumberg RS. The immunology of mucosal models of inflammation. Annu Rev Immunol 2002; 20:495–549.
13. Froese DP, Haggitt RC, Friend WG. Ulcerative colitis in the autotransplanted neovagina. Gastroenterology 1991; 100:1749–1752.
14. Mayer EA. Psychological stress and colitis. Gut 2000; 46:595–596.
15. Orchard T. Extraintestinal complications of inflammatory bowel disease. Curr Gastroenterol Rep 2003; 5:512–517.
16. MacDonald TT, Monteleone G. Interleukin-12 and Th1 immune responses in human Peyer's patches. Trends Immunol 2001; 22:244–247.
17. Shanahan F. Host–flora interactions in inflammatory bowel disease. Inflamm Bowel Dis 2004; 10 (Suppl 1): S16–S24.
18. Shanahan F. Pathogenesis of ulcerative colitis. Lancet 1993; 342:407–411.
19. Bernstein CN, Shanahan F, Weinstein WM. Patchiness of mucosal inflammation in treated ulcerative colitis. A prospective study. Gastrointest Endosc 1995; 42:232–237.
20. Walmsley RS, Ayres RCS, Pounder RE, Allen RN. A simple clinical colitis activity index. Gut 1998; 43:29–32.
21. Shanahan F. Inflammatory bowel disease: immunodiagnostics, immunotherapeutics and ecotherapeutics. Gastroenterology 2001; 120:622–635.
22. Quinton J-F, Sendid B, Reumaux D et al. Anti-*Saccharomyces cerevisiae* mannan antibodies combined with antineutrophil cytoplasmic autoantibodies in inflammatory bowel disease: prevalence and diagnostic role. Gut 1998; 42:788–791.
23. Joossens S, Reinisch W, Vermeire S et al. The value of serologic markers in indeterminate colitis: a prospective follow-up study. Gastroenterology 2002; 122:1242–1247.
24. American Gastroenterological Association. Medical position statement: guidelines on osteoporosis in gastrointestinal diseases. Gastroenterology 2003; 124:791–794.
25. Bernstein CN, Leslie WD, Leboff MS. AGA technical review on osteoporosis in gastrointestinal diseases. Gastroenterology 2003; 124:795–841.
26. Miehsler W, Reinisch W, Valic E et al. Is inflammatory bowel disease an independent and disease specific risk factor for thromboembolism? Gut 2004; 53:542–548.
27. Jackson LM, O'Gorman PJ, O'Connell J et al. Thrombosis in inflammatory bowel disease: clinical setting, procoagulant profile and factor V Leiden. Q J Med 1997; 90:183–188.
28. Rutgeerts P. Modern therapy for inflammatory bowel disease. Scand J Gastroenterol 2003; 38 (Suppl) 237:30–33.
29. Sninsky CA, Cort DH, Shanahan F et al. Oral Mesalamine (Asacol) for mildly to moderately active ulcerative colitis. Ann Intern Med 1991; 115:350–355.
30. Navarro F, Hanauer SB. Treatment of inflammatory bowel disease: safety and tolerability issues. Am J Gastroenterol 2003; 98 (Suppl):S18–S23.
31. Faubion WA Jr, Loftus EV Jr, Harmsen WS, Zinsmeister AR, Sandborn WJ. The natural history of corticosteroid therapy for

inflammatory bowel disease: a population-based study. Gastroenterology 2001; 121:255–260.
32. Van Assche G, D'Haens G, Noman M et al. Randomized, double-blind comparison of 4 mg/kg versus 2 mg/kg intravenous cyclosporine in severe ulcerative colitis. Gastroenterology 2003; 125:1025–1031.
33. Feagan BG. Maintenance therapy for inflammatory bowel disease. Am J Gastroenterol 2003; 98 (Suppl):S6–S17.
34. Dubinsky MC, Lamothe S, Yang HY et al. Pharmacogenomics and metabolite measurement of 6-mercaptopurine therapy in inflammatory bowel disease. Gastroenterology 2000; 118:705–713.
35. Colombel JF, Ferrari N, Debuysere H et al. Genotypic analysis of thiopurine S-methyltransferase in patients with Crohn's disease and severe myelosuppression during azathioprine therapy. Gastroenterology 2000; 118:1025–1030.
36. Schröder O, Stein J. Low dose methotrexate in inflammatory bowel disease: current status and future directions. Am J Gastroenterol 2003; 98:530–537.
37. Sinha A, Nightingale J, West KP, Berlanga-Acosta J, Playford RJ. Epidermal growth factor enemas with oral mesalamine for mild-to-moderate left-sided ulcerative colitis or proctitis. N Engl J Med 2003; 349:350–357.
38. Sandborn WJ, Yednock TA. Novel approaches to treating inflammatory bowel disease: targeting alpha-4 integrin. Am J Gastroenterol 2003; 98:2372–2382.
39. Shanahan F. Probiotics in inflammatory bowel disease: is there a scientific rationale? Inflamm Bowel Dis 2000; 6:107–115.
40. Sandborn WJ. Pouchitis following ileal pouch–anal anastomosis: definition, pathogenesis, and treatment. Gastroenterology 1994; 107:1856–1860.
41. Gionchietti P, Rizzello F, Venturi A et al. Oral bacteriotherapy as maintenance treatment in patients with chronic pouchitis: a double blind, placebo-controlled trial. Gastroenterology 2000; 119:305–309.
42. Mimura T, Rizzello F, Helwig U et al. Once daily high dose probiotic therapy (VSL#3) for maintaining remission in recurrent or refractory pouchitis. Gut 2004; 53:108–114.
43. Sheth SG, LaMont JT. Toxic megacolon. Lancet 1998; 351:509–513.
44. Rutter M, Saunders B, Wilkinson K et al. Severity of inflammation is a risk factor for colorectal neoplasia in ulcerative colitis. Gastroenterology 2004; 126:451–459.
45. Eaden JA, Abrams KR, Mayberry JF. The risk of colorectal cancer in ulcerative colitis: a meta-analysis. Gut 2001; 48:526–535.
46. Shetty K, Rybicki L, Brzezinski A, Carey WD, Lashner BA. The risk for cancer or dysplasia in ulcerative colitis patients with primary sclerosing cholangitis. Am J Gastroenterol 1999; 94:1643–1649.
47. Nuako KW, Ahlquist DA, Mahoney DW et al. Familial predisposition for colorectal cancer in chronic ulcerative colitis: A case control study. Gastroenterology 1998; 115:1079–1083.
48. Heuschen UA, Hinz U, Allemeyer EH et al. Backwash ileitis is strongly associated with colorectal carcinoma in ulcerative colitis. Gastroenterology 2001; 120:841–847.
49. Shanahan F. Relation between colitis and colon cancer. Lancet 2001; 357:246–247.
50. Brentnall TA. Molecular underpinnings of cancer in ulcerative colitis. Curr Opin Gastroenterol 2003; 19:64–68.
51. Shanahan F. Colitis-associated cancer – time for new strategies. Aliment Pharmacol Ther 2003; 18 (Suppl 2):6–9.
52. Bernstein CN. The color of dysplasia in UC. Gastroenterology 2003; 124:1135–1138.
53. Rubin CE, Haggitt RC, Burmer GC et al. DNA aneuploidy in colonic biopsies predicts future development of dysplasia in ulcerative colitis. Gastroenterology 1992; 103:1611–1620.
54. Ullman T, Croog V, Harpaz N, Sachar D, Itzkowitz S. Progression of flat low-grade dysplasia to advanced neoplasia in patients with ulcerative colitis. Gastroenterology 2003; 125: 1311–1319.
55. Eaden J, Abrams K, Ekbom A, Jackson E, Mayberry J. Colorectal cancer prevention in ulcerative colitis: a case-control study. Aliment Pharmacol Ther 2000; 14:145–153.
56. Bernstein CN, Blanchard JF, Metge C, Yogendran M. Does the use of 5-aminosalicylates in inflammatory bowel disease prevent the development of colorectal cancer? Am J Gastroenterol 2003; 98:2784–2788.
57. Ilnychyj A, Shanahan F, Anton PA, Cheang M, Bernstein CN. The placebo response in ulcerative colitis. Gastroenterology 1997; 112:1854–1858.
58. Robinson A, Thompson DG, Wilkin D et al. Guided self-management and patient-directed follow-up of ulcerative colitis: a randomised trial. Lancet 2001; 358:976–981.
59. Loftus Jr EV. Mortality in inflammatory bowel disease. Gastroenterology 2003; 125: 1881–1895.

Chapter 54

Crohn's disease

Severine Vermeire and Paul Rutgeerts

KEY POINTS

- Development of Crohn's disease appears to be an interaction of genetic and environmental factors
- Crohn's disease appears to be a manifestation of loss of tolerance to normal intestinal flora
- Mutations or polymorphisms in the *CARD15* gene impair handling of bacterial flora
- Biological markers may be helpful in distinguishing ulcerative colitis from Crohn's disease in the 10–15% with indeterminate colitis
- Heterozygotes for thiopurine methyltransferase deficiency should be started at 50% of the standard dose of azathioprine
- Antibiotics show similar efficacy to steroids in the treatment of Crohn's disease
- TNFα is a key molecule in the inflammatory cascade, presenting a target for therapy

INTRODUCTION AND DEFINITION

Crohn's disease (CD) is a chronic inflammatory disease of the gastrointestinal tract that develops mostly in young people between the ages of 15 and 25 years. Common symptoms include diarrhea, abdominal cramps, and weight loss. The exact cause of the disease is still unknown but current data suggest that the gut flora triggers sustained inflammation in a genetically susceptible host.[1] In this chapter, an overview on the different aspects of CD is given, including the epidemiology, pathogenesis, clinical presentation, (differential) diagnosis, complications, and treatment.

EPIDEMIOLOGY

Discovery

Although clinical descriptions of diarrhea and blood loss go back thousands of years, clear descriptions of ulceration and enteritis date only from the nineteenth century. Doctors at Mount Sinai Hospital in New York had shown interest in tuberculosis-like ileocecal enteritis without the presence of tubercle bacilli. On December 11th 1931, Dr Burril Crohn wrote to the American Gastroenterological Association:

> 'I have an important scientific contribution I would like to present before the American Gastroenterological Association. I have discovered, I believe, a new intestinal disease, which we have named Terminal Ileitis. I would like to present the facts before the Association in connection with the general subject of Benign Granulomata of the Intestinal Tract...'

Burril Crohn, together with his colleagues Ginzburg and Oppenheimer, presented their findings in May 1932 to the American Gastroenterological Association. The report was followed later that year by the landmark article entitled 'Regional ileitis: a pathologic and clinical entity,' by the same authors.[2]

Changes with time

Almost 75 years later, the exact cause of CD remains unknown, although the incidence is higher, having risen between the 1950s and 1970s.[3] In Copenhagen, Denmark, the incidence rose from 1 to 4.1 per 100 000 per year between 1962 and 1987.[4] With a prevalence of 1–2 per 1000, the disease has become an important entity in North America and western Europe.[3,5,6] The incidence of CD now averages 5–6 per 100 000 population and has been increasing worldwide, although the increase has been slowing in highly affected countries.[3] The onset of the disease occurs most often in the second or the third decade of life, but a second and smaller peak is seen between 50 and 60 years.

Geographic variations

Geographically, there is a north–south gradient in many countries of the northern hemisphere.[7] In Europe, age-adjusted incidence rates of 10 cases per 100 000 have been reported for Norway[8] versus 0.9 per 100 000 for Spain[9] and 3.4 per 100 000 in Italy.[10] There is also something of an west–east gradient, with low incidence rates in Japan. This west–east gradient may reflect differences in lifestyle, although important ethnic differences are observed.[3] The highest risk occurs in Ashkenazi Jews, who are reported to have a 2–8-fold greater risk, followed by North American and northern European Caucasian people. African-Americans and Asians carry the lowest risk. Other ethnic groups, such as the Roma gypsies in Hungary, have a considerably lower prevalence than the average surrounding population. The increased risk for certain ethnic groups to develop inflammatory bowel disease (IBD) is not altered dramatically when they move to different continents (and hence being submitted to different environment) where the risk is much lower; this points towards genetic factors.

Inheritance

Family studies have further underscored the genetic etiology of the disease. They have shown the risk for a patient with IBD of having a first-degree relative who suffers from the same disease to be around 10%.[11–13] Hence first-degree relatives of patients with CD are 10 times more likely also to develop the disease. Familial aggregation data further suggest the λ_s (relative risk of disease for a sibling of an affected individual) to be around

15–30 for CD[5–7] (Table 54.1). Important direct evidence for genetic factors comes from twin studies (Table 54.2). Three published twin studies have shown that concordance rates in monozygotic twins are much higher than those in dizygotic twins (33% versus 4%).[13–16] However, as the concordance is not 100%, nongenetic, environmental factors must also be involved.

CAUSES, RISK FACTORS, DISEASE ASSOCIATIONS

CD is a chronic inflammatory disease with a complex and multifactorial etiology. The current hypothesis is that a normal luminal flora drives an inappropriate activation of the mucosal immune system in a genetically susceptible host and that this activation is triggered by yet unknown environmental factors. To date, very few risk factors have been identified; smoking is probably the best known.[3,17] Smokers have not only an increased risk for the development of CD (Table 54.3), they also present with more severe disease in comparison with nonsmoking patients and have a higher relapse rate for the disease after surgery.[17,18] Despite these well described associations, the mechanism by which cigarette smoking affects CD is not known.

Several studies have shown that high levels of hygiene in childhood predispose to CD,[3] an observation that could plausibly explain the rise in incidence during the twentieth century. Most studies have found breast-feeding to be protective, an observation that might imply importance for early immune programming. Diet has been proposed to be an important etiologic factor. Patients with CD are more likely to eat a diet high in unrefined carbohydrates, but whether this is causal or consequential is unclear.

Infectious agents have been put forward as risk factors, and one of the most discussed putative agents has been *Mycobacterium avium* subspecies *paratuberculosis* (*M. avium*). *M. avium* is an acid-fast bacillus that causes Johne's disease (enteritis) in cattle. Whether it can cause CD is controversial and any mode of transmission is unclear, but some evidence suggests that humans may become infected via contaminated milk.[19]

TABLE 54.1 FAMILY STUDIES IN IBD, IMPLICATING THE RELATIVE RISK TO A SIBLING

Reference	Relative risk of CD
Orholm et al[12]	10
Satsangi et al[13]	15–35
Peeters et al[11]	13

TABLE 54.2 CONCORDANCE FOR CD IN TWIN STUDIES

Reference	Concordance	
	Monozygotic twins	Dizygotic twins
Tysk et al[14]	8/18 (44%)	1/26 (4%)
Thompson et al[15]	5/25 (20%)	3/46 (7%)
Orholm et al[16]	5/10 (50%)	0/27

CD has been associated with other immune-mediated disorders such as psoriasis, ankylosing spondylitis, multiple sclerosis, and arthritis. In addition, associations with rare genetic diseases such as the Hermansky-Pudlak syndrome and Turner's syndrome have been described.

PATHOGENESIS

The current idea about the pathophysiology of IBD is that the intestinal flora, in conjunction with yet unidentified environmental factors, triggers and drives an aberrant immune response in a genetically susceptible host, resulting in chronic inflammation of the gut (Fig. 54.1).

Genetics

CD is a polygenic disease that has some, but not all, susceptibility genes in common with ulcerative colitis (UC); some genes are present in one individual, and yet other mutations are found in other individuals – a model of genetic heterogeneity. Worldwide efforts in IBD genetics have led to the identification of eight to ten candidate genomic regions (Fig. 54.2). The first gene underlying CD susceptibility was identified in 2001.[20–22] The gene encodes a cytoplasmic protein designated NOD2 – renamed CARD15 (caspase activation and recruitment domain) – and is expressed in monocytes, macrophages, dendritic cells, epithelial cells, and Paneth cells. The CARD15 protein is important in the intracellular recognition of bacterial products by the carboxy-terminal leucine-rich repeat (LRR) region. The bacterial motif peptidoglycan muramyl dipeptide (MDP) has been identified as the essential structure recognized by CARD15. The presence of this bacterial component has been reported to lead to apoptosis at the site of bacterial invasion and to activation of the nuclear factor (NF)-κB signaling pathway, via the N-terminal CARDs.

Three variants of the *CARD15* gene, consisting of single nucleotide polymorphisms (SNPs), have been associated with CD. Two of these SNPs lead to a change in one amino acid (missense mutations; Arg702Trp and Gly908Arg). The third polymorphism (Leu1007insC), which consists of the insertion of one base pair, introduces a premature stop codon and leads

CROHN'S DISEASE: CURRENT PATHOGENIC MODEL

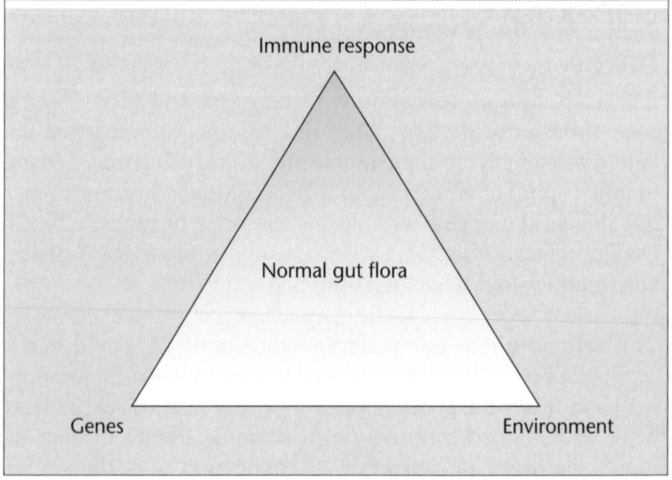

Fig. 54.1 Current pathogenic model of Crohn's disease.

TABLE 54.3 EFFECT OF SMOKING ON RISK OF CROHN'S DISEASE

Reference	Year	Study period	Site of disease	Data collection	Length of follow-up	Outcome: Non smokers	Outcome: Smokers	Outcome: Ex-smokers	Statistical analysis
Sutherland et al.[94]	1990	1966–1983	SB+IC+LB	Questionnaire	Mean 10–8 years	Reoperation rate			
						(*n*=85)	(*n*=89)		
						5 years 29%	5 years 36%		*P*=0.007
						10 years 41%	10 years 70%		RR 2.1
Lindberg et al.[95]	1992	No record	SB+IC+LB	Questionnaire	10 years	Reoperation rate 10 years postop.			
						(*n*=81)	(*n*=54)		
						26%	42% (heavy smokers: >10/day)		P=0.015 RR 1.79
Cottone et al.[96]	1994	1973–1991	SB+IC+LB	Questionnaire	Mean 8–2 years	(*n*=53)	(*n*=110)	(*n*=19)	
						Clinical recurrence[a] rate 6 years postop.			
						40%	73%	59%	*P*=0.006[c] RR 1.4
						Reoperation rate 6 years postop.			
						8%	24%	21%	*P*=0.005[c] RR 2.0
						Endoscopic recurrence rate 1 year postop.			
						35%	70%	27%	*P*=0.002[c] RR 4.3
Breuer-Katschinski et al.[97]	1996	1989–1992	SB+IC+LB	Questionnaire	No record	Reoperation rate			
						(*n*=143)	(*n*=144)		
						5 years 26%	5 years 43%		*P*<0.00
						10 years 33%	10 years 64%		RR 3.1
Cosnes et al.[98]	1996	1974–1995	SB+IC+LB	Personal interview	No record	Crude reoperation rate			
						(*n*=89)	(*n*=115)		
						22%	30%		n.s.
Timmer et al.[99]	1998	1990–1993	SB+IC+LB	Personal interview	48 weeks	Relapse[b] rate 48 weeks postop.			
						(*n*=53)	(*n*=59)	(*n*=40)	
						30%	53%	35%	*P*=0.02[c] RR 2.1
Medina et al.[100]	1998	No record	SB+IC+LB	No record	No record	Crude symptomatic recurrence rate			
						(*n*=14)	(*n*=26)		
						86%	50%		n.s.
Yamamoto & Keighley[101]	1999	1975–1990	IC alone	Personal interview and questionnaire	Median 8–1 years	Reoperation rate			
						(*n*=79)	(*n*=62)		
						5 years 19%	5 years 35%		*P*=0.007
						10 years 36%	10 years 55%		RR 2.3
Yamamoto et al.[102]	1999	1960–1996	LB alone	Personal interview and questionnaire	Median 18–6 years	Reoperation rate			
						(*n*=36)	(*n*=33)		
						5 years 11%	5 years 25%		
						10 years 15%	10 years 46%		*P*=0.005
						15 years 18%	15 years 52%		RR 3.0

SB, small bowel; IC, ileocecal; LB, large bowel; CDAI, Crohn's Disease Activity Index; RR, relative risk; n.s. not significant. [a]CDAI > 150; [b]CDAI > 150 or increase of CDAI > 60; [c]smokers *versus* non-smokers.

to a truncated protein lacking the distal 33 amino acids of the LRR region. These mutations occur in or around the LRRs, suggesting that they alter the capacity to respond to bacterial components. CARD15 expression in HEK 293T cells resulted in a diminished responsiveness to lipopolysaccharide for the frameshift mutation compared with the full-length construct, and also both other variants have a common signaling defect in response to bacterial components. The prevalence of *CARD15* variants ranges from 35% to 45%, with exceptions for Japanese and African-American populations with CD. In Europe, the prevalence is also significantly lower in the Scandinavian population. *CARD15* variants have been associated with ileal disease location, young age at onset, and possibly fibrostenosing disease, and are estimated to account for 30–40% of cases of CD with ileal involvement.[22]

The relative risk of developing the disease when carrying one mutation is 2–3, but increases dramatically, to 20–40, in those with two mutations (compound heterozygotes or homozygotes). With a prevalence of CD in western Europe of 0.1–0.2%, it can be deduced from these relative risks that the probability of developing the disease is 2–8% in individuals carrying two mutations. However, even with the above-mentioned genotype

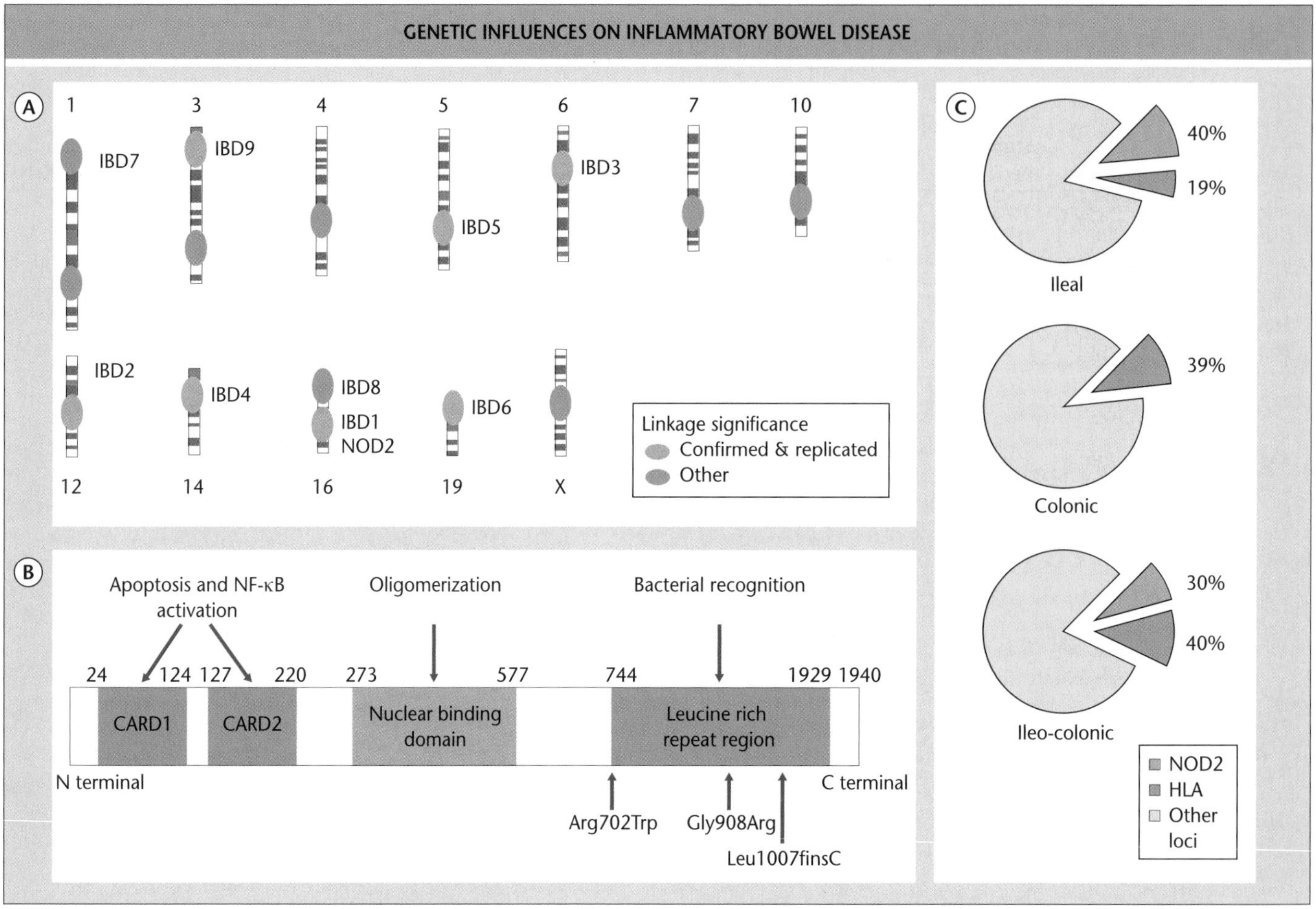

Fig. 54.2 Genetic influences on inflammatory bowel disease. A. Candidate genomic regions. **B.** Structure of the *NOD2* gene and sites of polymorphism. **C.** Proportional contribution of *NOD2* polymorphisms to Crohn's disease at different sites. (Adapted from Ahmad T et al.[22])

relative risks, the penetrance is modest: less than 10% of all persons carrying two *CARD15* risk alleles will develop CD. This means that other genes and environmental stimuli are needed for disease expression.

The mechanisms by which *CARD15* mutations lead to CD are not fully understood. Impaired handling of bacterial flora, altered activation of NF-κB, and, possibly, deficient production of the endogenous antibiotic defensin are possible. Other genetic influences may be mediated differently. For example, patients with CD and their first-degree relatives have been shown to have increased mucosal permeability.

Immunology

Acute inflammation in the gut of patients with CD is characterized by infiltration of granulocytes and mononuclear cells, and by epithelial cell necrosis.[23] The chronic phase of the transmural inflammation is frequently accompanied by fibrosis and bowel strictures. The mucosal inflammation in established CD is dominated by CD4+ lymphocytes with a type 1 helper T cell (Th1) phenotype (see Fig. 54.1), characterized by the production of interferon-γ and interleukin (IL) 2. Th1 cytokines activate macrophages, which in turn produce IL-12, IL-18, and macrophage migration inhibitory factor, which further stimulate Th1 cells in a self-sustaining cycle. Just as importantly, activated macrophages produce a potent mix of cytokines, which amplify the inflammatory reaction. These cytokines include tumor necrosis factor (TNF), IL-1, IL-6, chemokines, and growth factors, as well as metabolites of arachidonic acid (e.g., prostaglandins and leukotrienes) and reactive oxygen metabolites such as nitric oxide. A central signaling molecule in macrophages is the transcription factor NF-κB. Inflammation in CD is characterized by increased expression of adhesion molecules on endothelial cells and leukocytes. This is responsible for further recruitment of additional leukocytes from the vascular space to sites of disease activity, and is important in maintaining inflammation.

There is increasing evidence that these inflammatory events are due to loss of tolerance against bacterial antigens. An important mechanism of tolerance induction is cell apoptosis, the physiologic process of programmed cell death. This balance between T-cell death and survival is essential to maintain immune homeostasis. In CD, there appears to be a resistance to apoptotic stimuli and this is further underscored by Bcl-2/Bax ratio in the inflamed mucosa, and decreased Bax expression with a high $Bclx_1$/Bax ratio in isolated mucosal T cells.[24] Monocytes/macrophages are also important in providing the first line of intestinal defence, and abnormal apoptosis of monocytes/macrophages may be relevant to the pathogenesis of IBD.

Bacteria

Observations derived from patients suffering from CD or UC, and from experimental animal models of colitis, show that the gut microflora is involved in the etiopathogenesis of IBD. CD lesions are located mainly in regions of the gut colonized by large numbers of bacteria (ileum, colon), and diversion of the fecal stream from inflamed sites often results in clinical improvement in the patient and prevents postoperative recurrence of CD.[25] Moreover, infusion of intestinal contents into excluded ileum of patients with CD reinduced inflammation.[26] An increased association of luminal bacteria with the mucous layer of patients with IBD compared with controls has been reported. Antibiotic therapy results in transient clinical improvement of CD, and treatment with metronidazole prevents recurrence of CD after surgery to some extent,[27] although the possibility that metronidazole acts by other mechanisms cannot be excluded.

Results from experiments on germ-free rodents with a dysfunctional immune system (gene knockout or transgenic animals), in which intestinal inflammation is absent, have indicated that bacteria are indispensable contributors to the pathogenesis of the chronic intestinal inflammation. Despite many attempts, specific pathogens have not been identified as the cause of IBD. *Mycobacterium paratuberculosis*, *Listeria monocytogenes*, and measles virus have been candidate pathogens, but data have been inconclusive so far. The hypothesis that a gut flora of 'abnormal composition' might be present has also not been proven, but this is extremely difficult to study. Molecular methods will allow the composition of the intestinal microflora to be revealed.

Bacterial antigens

There is evidence that patients with IBD have a loss of tolerance to specific bacterial and possibly also autoantigens.[28] They display antibodies against oligomannan epitope (anti-*Saccharomyces cerevisiae* antibody; ASCA), against outer membrane protein C of *Escherichia coli* (anti-OmpC), and against an epitope of *Pseudomonas fluorescens* (anti-I2) in CD. In UC an antibody response is found against nuclear antigens (perinuclear anti-neutrophil cytoplasmic antibody; p-ANCA), and for both CD and UC there is an antibody response to pancreas proteins (pancreatic antibodies (PAB)). The epitopes for the different antibodies have either not been identified or it is not clear what the significance of the antibodies is. The oligomannan to which ASCA is elicited are present not only in the membrane of *S. cerevisiae* but also in yeasts and mycobacteria.[29] The antigen eliciting p-ANCA in UC has also not been identified, although Terjung et al[30] suggested that p-ANCA recognizes a 50-kDa nuclear envelope protein of neutrophils and myeloid cell lines. It is of key importance to identify the antigens to which serologic responses are directed, and to detect other specific serologic responses to bacterial epitopes or autoantigens in patients with CD and UC.

PATHOLOGY

Inflammation in CD is patchy and focal, at both the histologic and the macroscopic level. Discontinuous bowel involvement with interspersed uninvolved segments (skip lesions) is typical of CD. The earliest lesion of CD is aphthous ulceration (Fig. 54.3A). Macroscopically, tiny ulcers are surrounded by a halo of erythema. Histologically, inflammation is focal. Microfistulization from aphthous ulcers is then associated with deeper inflammation that may be associated with cobblestoning (Fig. 54.3C). Inflammation typically extends beyond the mucosa and through to the serosa (Fig. 54.4). Increasing fistulization may result in macroscopic tracks between loops of bowel to adjacent organs, or to the skin. Noncaseating granulomas, which are highly suggestive but not absolutely diagnostic of CD, have been reported in 15–70% of patients (Fig. 54.5).

CLINICAL PRESENTATION

CD may typically affect the entire gastrointestinal tract from the mouth to the anus in a discontinuous and transmural way, with a preference for the terminal ileum and right colon. Clinical symptoms of CD vary, but classically the most common symptoms have been:

- *Diarrhea* – This may arise by a number of mechanisms including colonic involvement, bile acid malabsorption (especially after terminal ileal resection), and small bowel malabsorption.
- *Weight loss* – may variously be due to inflammatory cachexia, malabsorption, and anorexia (Fig. 54.6).
- *Abdominal pain* – most often located in the right lower quadrant (implying terminal ileal involvement).
- *Perianal disease* – Nowadays, one of the first symptoms may also relate to perianal disease, and 20–80% of patients with CD show anal involvement with abscesses, fistulae, or fissures (Fig. 54.7). These account for considerable morbidity.[31]

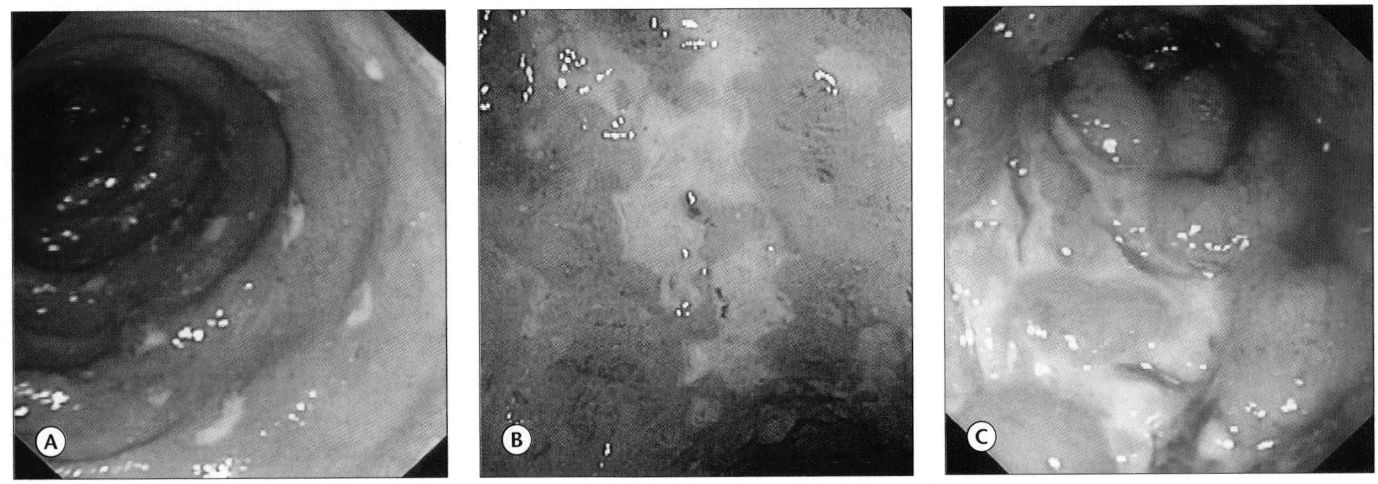

Fig. 54.3 Mucosal ulceration in Crohn's disease. A. Aphthous ulcers as the first manifestation of Crohn's disease. **B.** Longitudinal ulcers in the colon, typical of Crohn's disease. **C.** Serpiginous ulcers interspersed by nodular thickening – the typical cobblestone pattern.

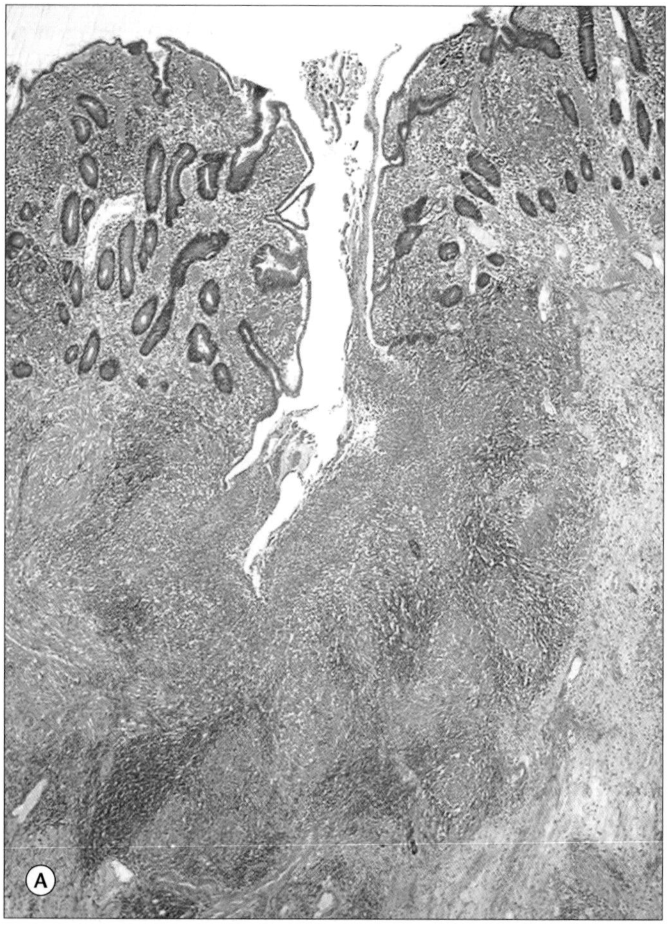

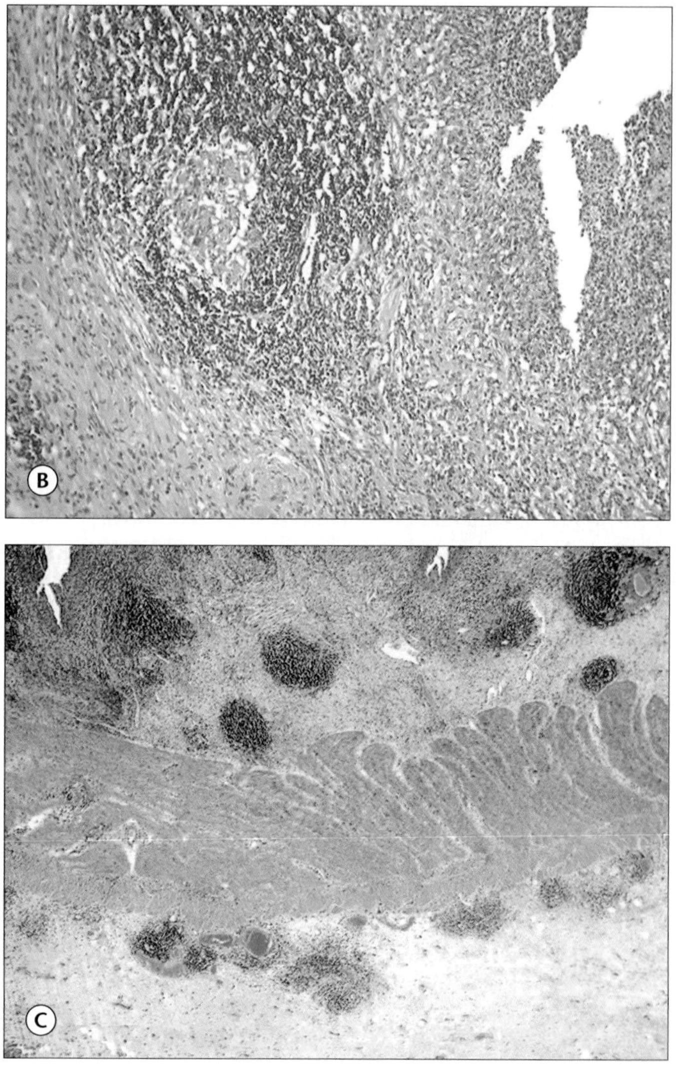

Fig. 54.4 Histologic features in Crohn's disease. A. Mucosal ulceration with microfissuring, and transmural inflammation with numerous lymphoid aggregates. **B.** Microfissure with adjacent granuloma. **C.** String of lymphoid aggregates on either side of muscularis propria in both mucosa and serosa. Courtesy of Dr Philip Kaye, University Hospital, Nottingham.

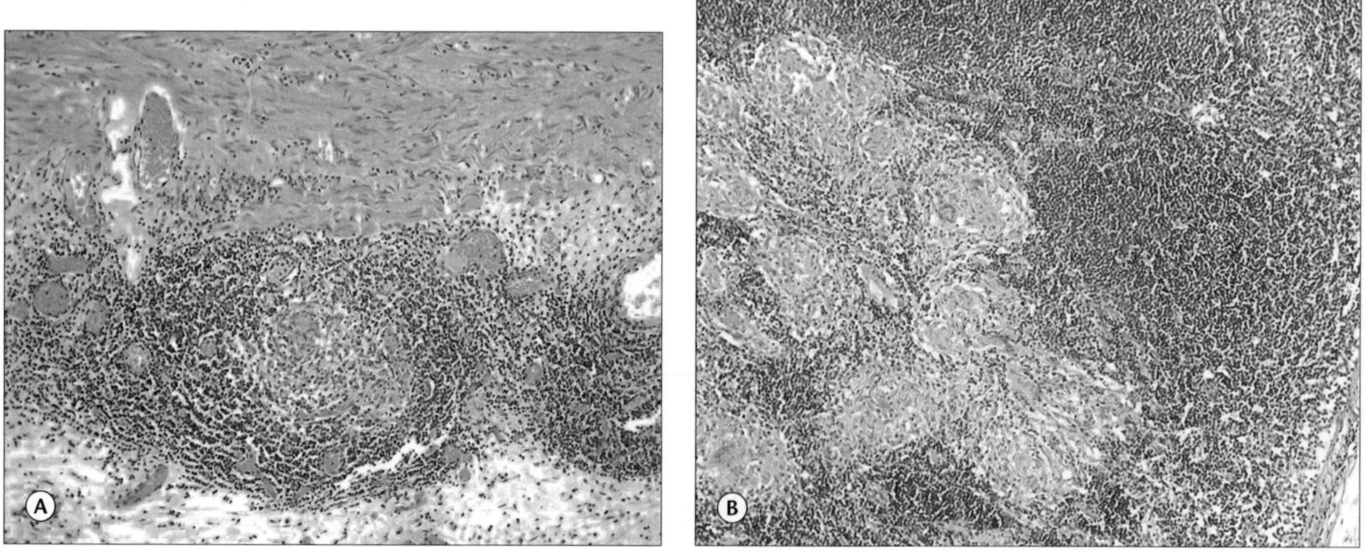

Fig. 54.5 Granuloma in Crohn's disease. A. In serosa. **B.** In draining lymph node. Courtesy of Dr Philip Kaye, University Hospital, Nottingham.

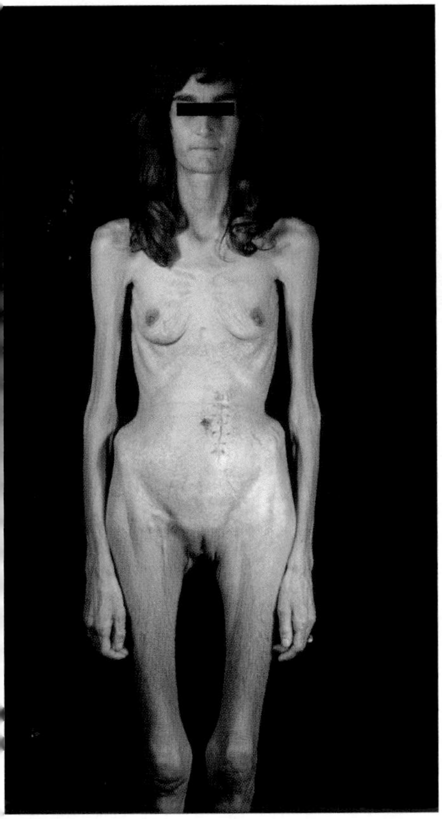

Fig. 54.6 Patient with extensive small bowel Crohn's disease and extreme weight loss.

CD may present with more general symptoms, such as fatigue, weight loss, anemia, or pyrexia of unknown origin.

Symptoms by site

The clinical features of CD disease can thus be very variable, but in most cases are predictable from the site of disease:

- *Mouth* – Oral CD is characterized by aphthous ulceration, often on a background of mucosal edema greater than that seen with simple mouth ulcers.
- *Esophagus* – This is rare but may cause dysphagia or pain.
- *Stomach and duodenum* – Asymptomatic gastric involvement is not uncommon. Duodenal involvement may result in typical ulcer symptoms. Stricturing may result in symptoms of gastric outlet obstruction.
- *Small bowel* – Diffuse extensive mucosa involvement can lead to malabsorption (see Chapter 43), protein-losing enteropathy (see Chapter 48), diarrhea (see Chapter 9), and sometimes steatorrhea. Segmental thickening or stricturing results in painful obstructive symptoms and may lead to bacterial overgrowth.
- *Ileocecal involvement* – Symptoms of obstruction due to inflammatory swelling or stricturing are common, with postprandial bloating, pain, and borborygmi, particularly after consumption of fibrous vegetables or fruit. Transmural inflammation and local sepsis result in matting of local loops of bowel and a palpable inflammatory mass.
- *Colon* – Typically colonic involvement results in diarrhea that, in contrast to the case in UC, is seldom bloody and more often associated with abdominal pain.
- *Perianal disease* – This is common and may precede other manifestations. Fistulous discharge may alternate with abscess formation (Fig. 54.7).

The disease may behave in different ways in different individuals. Symptoms of postprandial abdominal pain, abdominal distention, or nausea should raise the suspicion of a stricture. Strictures are characterized by narrowing of the lumen and thickening of the bowel wall, with or without prestenotic dilatation (Fig. 54.8). Other symptoms, such as fecal loss per vagina or pneumaturia, imply the presence of fistulae to the vagina or bladder respectively. Fistulae to the abdominal wall may result in a purulent or feculent discharge (Fig. 54.9). Fistulae between loops of bowel may present with early passage of undigested food and otherwise unexplained weight loss.

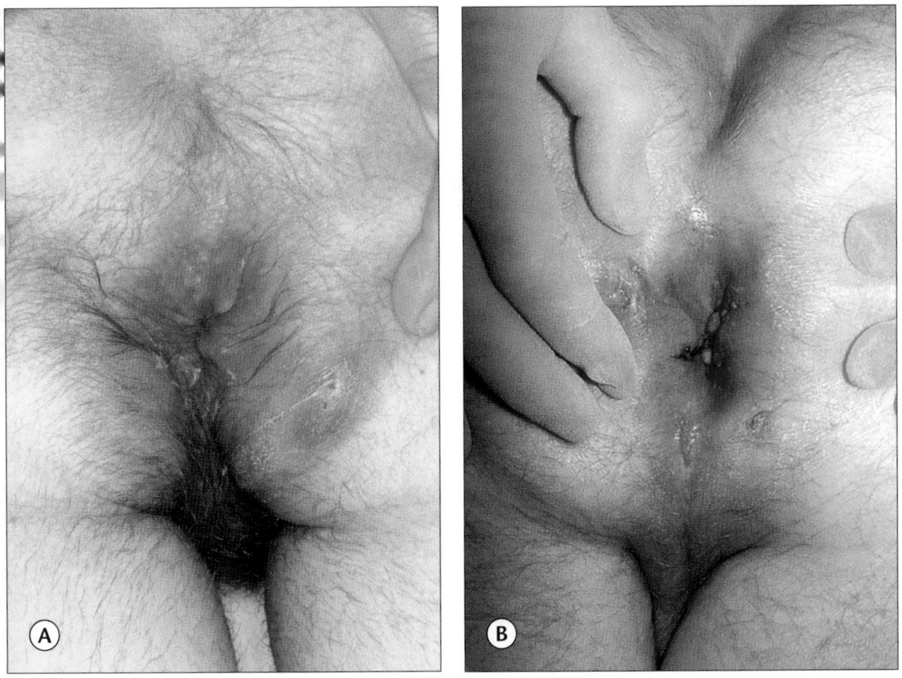

Fig. 54.7 Two examples of perianal Crohn's disease.

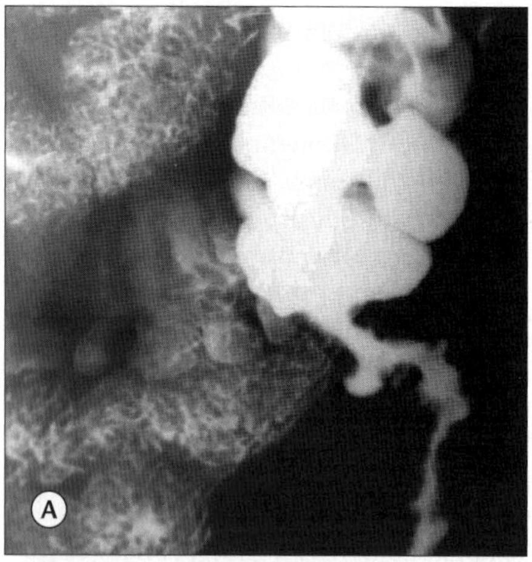

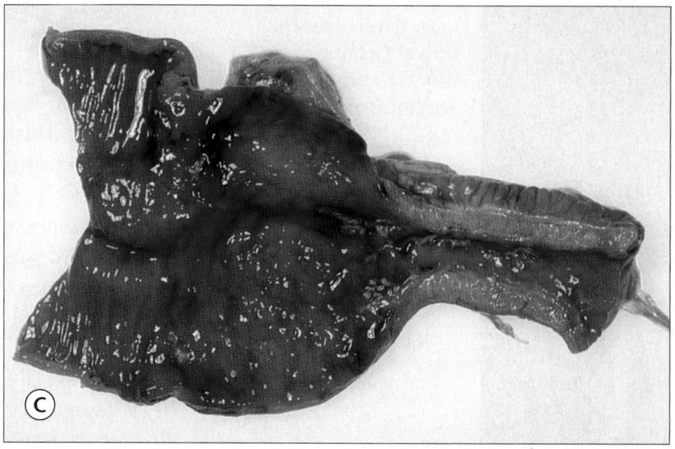

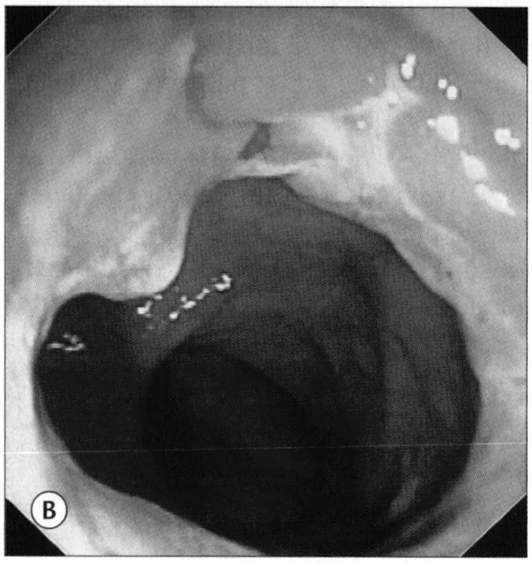

Fig. 54.8 Fibrostenotic Crohn's disease. A. Small-bowel follow-through of a Crohn's patient showing extensive involvement of the ileum with stenosis. **B.** Crohn's disease colonic stricture. **C.** Resected specimen showing fibrostenosis with proximal dilatation.

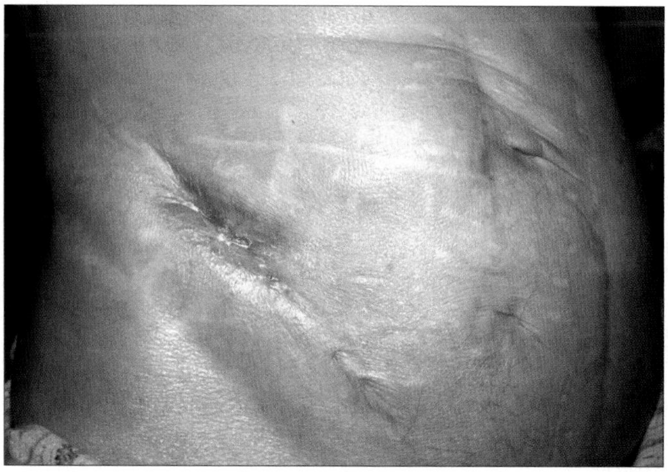

Fig. 54.9 Active and healed enterocutaneous fistulae.

Extraintestinal manifestations of Crohn's disease

Up to 40% of patients with CD suffer from extraintestinal symptoms (Table 54.4, Fig. 54.10). Some, such as erythema nodosum, iritis, or peripheral arthritis, occur intermittently at times of disease activity. Typically, the activity-related arthritis involves two or three medium-sized joints. Other extraintestinal symptoms, such as ankylosing spondylitis or sclerosing cholangitis, represent disease associations unaffected by changes in CD activity. Others, such as gallstones or renal stones, are a metabolic consequence of CD or its treatment. Bile acid loss from malabsorption due to terminal ileal involvement or resection predisposes to gallstone formation. The consequently increased absorption of oxalate predisposes to renal stones.

Extraintestinal manifestations of IBD are of importance because they may represent the only symptom index of disease activity. Moreover, they do not only follow intestinal symptoms, but sometimes precede them by years. Where extraintestinal

TABLE 54.4 EXTRAINTESTINAL MANIFESTATIONS OF IBD

Organ or system	Condition
Skin	Erythema nodosum[a]
	Pyoderma gangrenosum[a,b]
Joint	Peripheral arthritis[a]
	Sacroiliitis
	Ankylosing spondylitis
Eye	Iritis, uveitis, and episcleritis[a]
Biliary	Gallstones
	Sclerosing cholangitis[b]
	Cholangiocarcinoma[b]
Renal	Stones
	Amyloid

[a]Varies with bowel activity.
[b]More common in ulcerative colitis.

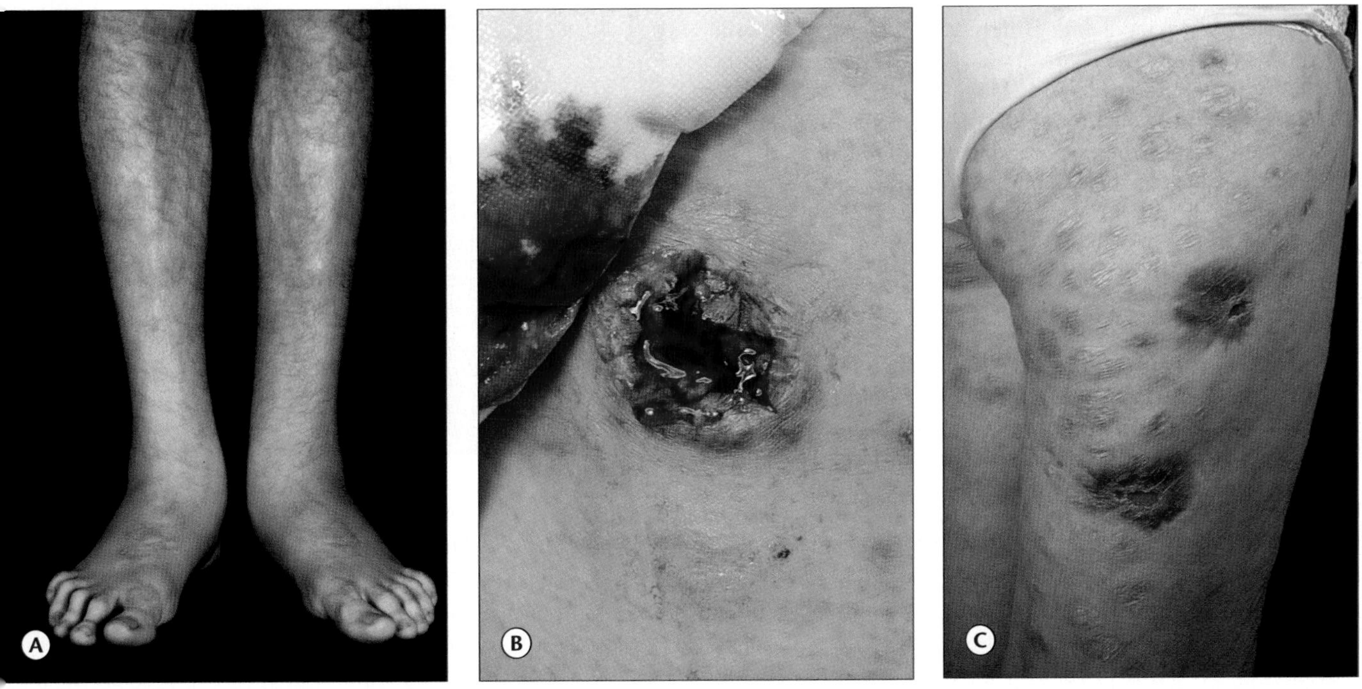

ig. 54.10 **Some skin manifestations of Crohn's disease. A.** Erythema nodosum. **B.** Active pyoderma gangrenosum. **C.** Active pyoderma with nultiple healed lesions. Activity of pyoderma gangrenosum generally follows bowel activity, but not always.

nanifestations reflect overall disease activity, treatment of the ntestinal inflammation – either medical or surgical – usually helps in the resolution of these complications.

Special situations

Pediatric disease

CD commonly presents in children and adolescents. Active disease mpairs physical growth, and this may be the first symptom to come to light. Otherwise, children and adolescents suffer symptoms similar to those in adults, although the consequences of CD for personal and sexual development may dominate the effect that CD has in this age group.

Pregnancy

Overall, there appears to be little pregnancy-related variation n CD activity, but individual women may display an individually stereotyped pattern of remission or relapse with successive pregnancies. CD reduces fertility, implying that many women need to continue full treatment during conception. Active disease probably increases the rate of spontaneous abortion, premature labour, and stillbirth. Limited evidence suggests that most drugs are not harmful to the baby, and certainly appear to pose less threat than active disease. Male patients should, of course, cease sulfasalazine as this drug produces sperm abnormalities.

Proposed classifications

Given the heterogeneous presentation of CD, several classification systems have been proposed over the years. The most recent classification, also known as the Vienna classification, resulted from an international working party of the World Congress of Gastroenterology in 1998,[32] and includes:

- Age at diagnosis – below 40 years (A1), equal to or above 40 years (A2).
- Location – terminal ileum (L1), colon (L2), ileocolon (L3), upper gastrointestinal (L4)
- Behavior – nonstricturing, nonpenetrating (B1), stricturing (B2), penetrating (B3).

However, in clinical practice, it is not always easy to classify patients into one of the categories.

DIFFERENTIAL DIAGNOSIS

Initial diagnosis

Although CD causes many symptoms, the diagnosis is usually not difficult to make. Gastrointestinal symptoms normally call attention to the part of the gastrointestinal tract involved, and endoscopy or radiology will show changes compatible with CD. Under these circumstances, the challenge is often to establish that it is CD rather than another pathology that is responsible for inflammation.

Systemic manifestations

Differential diagnosis is more difficult when the presentation is with predominantly nongastrointestinal symptoms. CD should enter into consideration in patients with pyrexia of unknown origin, failure to thrive or loss of weight (see Chapter 15), abdominal pain (see Chapter 22), intra-abdominal abscess (see Chapter 117), anemia,[33] or extraintestinal manifestations such as erythema nodosum. Penetrating CD in the ileocecal region may mimic appendicitis and/or cause iliopsoas irritation, infection, or abscess characterized clinically by pain on hip extension.

Acute infection

The clinical picture of CD, certainly in the presence of an acute onset, is very similar to an acute infectious episode. *Yersinia* infection may resemble CD, given its preferential location in the terminal ileum. Differential diagnosis also includes other colitides (vascular, drug induced, or toxic), and a check should always be made for a history of travelling, drug and medication intake, and sexual habits. Differential diagnosis with other disorders, such as lymphocytic or collagenous colitis, is another possibility. In its chronic phase, CD is characterized by histologic lesions very similar to those seen in intestinal tuberculosis. Mycobacteria (especially *M. paratuberculosis*) remain one of the putative causal agents of CD, and antimycobacterial therapies have been tried.[34]

Distinction from other colitides

Differential diagnosis between CD and UC (see Chapter 53) can usually be made based on clinical, radiologic, endoscopic, and histologic determinations. CD may affect any part of the gastrointestinal tract (most commonly the terminal ileum) and is characterized by the presence of discontinuous transmural inflammation, whereas UC affects only the large bowel in a continuous way and is restricted to the mucosa. Both diseases may be complicated by extraintestinal manifestations (skin, eyes, joint) or colorectal malignancy. Microscopic colitis (see Chapter 56) and infectious colitides can sometimes be difficult to distinguish, especially where inflammation is patchy. A precise classification for about 10–15% of patients presenting with colonic inflammation remains difficult in practice. These patients are categorized as having 'indeterminate colitis' (see Chapter 55).

DIAGNOSTIC METHODS

The diagnosis of CD is based on a combination of symptoms, radiologic examination, endoscopy, and histologic criteria. Laboratory findings consistent with CD include a raised platelet count[35] or erythrocyte sedimentation rate, and increased levels of acute-phase proteins (particularly C-reactive protein), anemia due to iron, vitamin B_{12}, or folate deficiency, or chronic disease.[33] Hypoalbuminemia associated with protein-losing enteropathy, and deficiencies of vitamins and minerals, are fairly common.

The inflammation in CD typically affects the entire gastrointestinal tract. Colonoscopy is a frequent diagnostic maneuver.[36] Intestinal CD is most frequently located in the terminal ileum, and in patients with colonic involvement the rectum is often spared, making colonoscopy more appropriate than limited sigmoidoscopy. Discontinuous inflammation and aphthous or longitudinal ulcers are often seen as the first manifestation (see Fig. 54.3A,B). At a later stage, serpiginous ulcers interspersed by nodular thickening (the so-called cobblestone pattern) occur (see Fig. 54.3C). A CD Endoscopic Index of Severity (CDEIS) has been devised that has prognostic significance and is used principally in research.[37] Growing evidence suggests that capsule endoscopy (see Chapter 123) may be more sensitive (but perhaps less specific) than radiology in the diagnosis of CD of the small bowel (Fig. 54.11), but more data are needed.[38]

Histologic changes include an abnormal mucosal architecture and increased cellularity of the lamina propria with infiltration of neutrophils (see Fig. 54.4). However, the histologic hallmark of CD is the granuloma, which is seldom found in UC.[39] A granuloma is defined as a collection of monocytes/macrophages and other inflammatory cells with or without giant cells, and is reported in 15–70% of patients. In contrast to tuberculosis, central necrosis and caseation are very rare, and should raise the suspicion of tuberculosis.

Small-bowel follow-through (SBFT) remains an important radiologic examination for assessing the extent of small bowel involvement and for detecting fistulous tracks or strictures (see Fig. 54.8). SBFT should be performed at least once, usually at the time of diagnosis, in every patient.

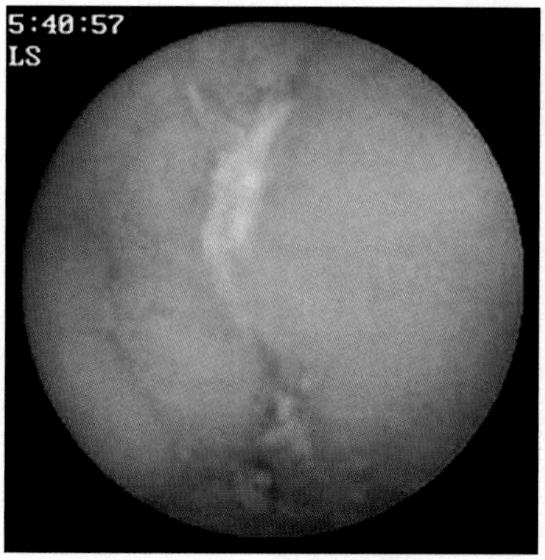

Fig. 54.11 Capsule endoscopy of small bowel Crohn's disease. Courtesy of Paul Swain.

CD is further associated with antibody responses to a variety of (bacterial) antigens,[28,30,40–42] although their meaning and clinical value remain unclear. However, their high specificity (95–99%) means that their use may be warranted where distinction between CD or UC is not clear. In terms of phenotypic expression, ASCA, OmpC and I2 have been associated with ileal and fibrostenosing or internal perforating disease, whereas p-ANCA is associated with UC-like CD.[41,42]

TREATMENT AND PREVENTION

Medical treatment

Patients with CD require extensive treatment because of the chronic relapsing nature of the disease. Medical management includes a combination of 5-aminosalicylates (5-ASAs), systemic corticosteroids, budesonide, immunosuppressive agents, antibiotic treatment, and novel biologic therapies such as anti-tumor necrosis factor α (anti-TNFα) antibodies (infliximab). Therapy can be divided into agents that are effective for induction and maintenance of remission:

- *Induction of remission* – Drugs that have been shown to be effective in randomized controlled trials include sulfasalazine, antibiotics, budesonide, oral corticosteroids, and infliximab.
- *Maintenance of remission* – Patients who relapse within 6–12 months after discontinuation of induction therapy should be given induction therapy again but should also receive maintenance therapy with an immunosuppressive agent (azathioprine, 6-mercaptopurine, or methotrexate) or infliximab (Fig. 54.12).

The degree of disease activity also plays a role: salicylates and antibiotics are effective in mild to moderate disease, whereas steroids and infliximab are preserved for more severe active disease.

5-Aminosalicylates

Although 5-ASAs are widely used in the treatment of CD, the scientific evidence supporting this practice is poor. High doses of mesalamine (4 g/day) are effective in mild to moderate CD, although not all studies have shown consistent results. A meta-analysis of 15 randomized controlled trials of mesalamine maintenance therapy involving a total of 2097 patients showed that mesalamine significantly reduced the risk of symptomatic relapse

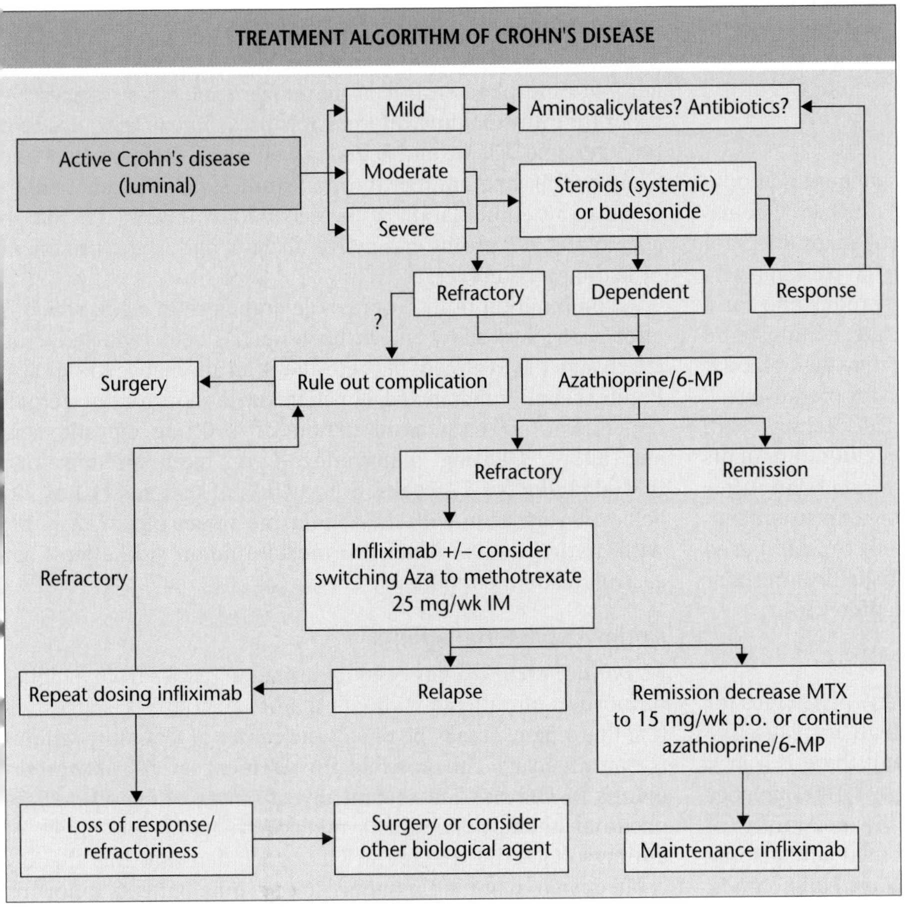

Fig. 54.12 Treatment algorithm of Crohn's disease.

in 13%, but only in the postsurgical setting and in patients with ileitis and with prolonged disease duration.[43] In the medical setting, the benefit was not significant. However, in practice, 5-ASA compounds are often started as initial therapy in newly diagnosed mild to moderate CD. See also Chapter 136.

Corticosteroids

Prednisone and prednisolone have an efficacy in active disease that is superior to placebo, antibiotics, and 5-ASA. Corticosteroids inhibit T-cell activation and proinflammatory cytokine production. However, in a prospective trial by Munkholm et al,[44] 36% of patients with CD were steroid dependent and 20% steroid resistant after 1 year. Corticosteroids are further associated with a multitude of side effects, both short term (gastrointestinal intolerance and dyspepsia, moon facies, acne, hypertension, hyperglycemia, depression, and psychosis) and long term (osteoporosis, cataract, growth failure). Budesonide, a synthetic glucocorticosteroid, provides the efficacy of a corticosteroid without the corticosteroid toxicity. It has a high ratio of topical to systemic activity owing its extensive first-pass metabolism in the liver. In a study by Rutgeerts et al,[45] prednisone 40 mg/day was as effective as budesonide 9 mg/day in inducing remission. These findings have been confirmed in at least two subsequent studies.[46,47]

Azathioprine and 6-mercaptopurine

Azathioprine and its metabolite 6-mercaptopurine (6-MP) offer a therapeutic advantage over placebo in the maintenance of remission in CD. In the Candy & Wright study of 1995, 63 patients with active CD treated with prednisolone were randomized to either azathioprine (2.5 mg/kg) or placebo.[48] At 15 months, 42% of patients receiving azathioprine were in remission, compared with 7% of those receiving placebo (P=0.001). Azathioprine is, however, associated with a number of side effects, including bone marrow toxicity, pancreatitis and hepatotoxicity (see Chapter 136). A number of these adverse events are related to the metabolism of azathioprine by the enzyme thiopurine methyltransferase (TPMT). The activity of TPMT is genetically regulated and several polymorphisms have been described within the gene.[49] Approximately 11% of the population is heterozygous for the common TPMT polymorphisms and around 1 in 300 is a homozygous mutant. Heterozygotes show decreased activity of TPMT, and homozygotes have almost absent TPMT activity.[50] A deficiency of TPMT is associated with an increased risk of bone marrow suppression and neutropenia.[51] Dosage recommendations for azathioprine and 6-MP vary with the patient's genotype. In patients with the wild-type genotype, a standard dose (2–2.5 mg/kg daily for azathioprine and 1–1.25 mg/kg daily for 6-MP) may be started.[52] Patients who are homozygous mutants, however, are know to develop early pancytopenia following the introduction of azathioprine. Azathioprine is not recommended in these patients. Heterozygous patients should be started at 50–60% of the dose. Close monitoring of the blood count is important – and mandatory if the genotype is not known. Hepatotoxicity is another adverse event of the metabolism of azathioprine and is related to the metabolite 6-MP.[53] Other side effects of azathioprine, such as pancreatitis, fever, myalgia, and arthralgia, are type I hypersensitivity reactions. In the unlikely event of such an adverse event, azathioprine should be stopped; rechallenge is not recommended.

Methotrexate

The folate antagonist methotrexate is used as an immunomodulator in CD and other inflammatory conditions such as rheumatoid arthritis. A double-blind placebo-controlled multicenter study of weekly injections of methotrexate in patients who had chronically active CD despite receiving prednisone for a minimum of 3 months showed that methotrexate, administered at a dose of 25 mg once weekly, was more effective than placebo in improving symptoms and reducing the need for prednisone.[54] A follow-up trial showed that maintenance therapy with methotrexate (15 mg intramuscularly, once weekly) in patients with chronically active CD who entered remission after 4–6 months of treatment with 25 mg methotrexate was beneficial compared with placebo.[55] Methotrexate is typically used as a second-line immunosuppressive drug for patients unresponsive to or intolerant of azathioprine (see Chapter 136).

Antibiotics

Antibiotics have been used empirically by many physicians for many years in the treatment of CD, although no causative microorganism has been identified for CD and there is a lack of controlled trials to validate this approach.[56] This includes antimycobacterial strategies[34,57] based on the possibility of mycobacterial infection. In addition, as well as their antibacterial action, some antibiotics, such as metronidazole and quinolones, have potential immunosuppressive properties. Enteric bacteria play a role in the pathogenesis of certain complications of CD, including abscesses and fistulae, and antibiotics are used successfully for these complications. The most commonly used antibiotics are metronidazole and ciprofloxacin.

Metronidazole

This is an imidazole compound with activity against protozoa and most Gram-negative and Gram-positive anaerobic bacteria. Several uncontrolled trials, as well as clinical experience, suggest the drug is efficacious for perianal complications of CD, but no controlled trials have been published to support this.[58–60] Metronidazole is sometimes also used where a secondary infective component is suspected elsewhere in the gastrointestinal tract (e.g., with complex matted distal ileum or suspected enteroenteric fistulization), started at a dose of 20 mg/kg (typically 400 mg three times daily) (see Chapter 136). The dose can be halved once improvement or remission has been achieved. Side effects occur in 1–20% of patients and most often include nausea, gastrointestinal intolerance, neurotoxicity, and metallic taste. Metronidazole is usually given in courses lasting up to 3 months to patients with active perianal disease. Long-term treatment can give rise to peripheral neuropathy, characterized by paresthesias in the extremities. The adverse effects are reversible with discontinuation of the drug, although the neuropathy may sometimes continue after metronidazole is stopped. The antibiotic seems to be safe, although some mutations and teratogenicity have been reported in animal studies. Available evidence suggests that the metronidazole does not affect fetal outcome adversely. However, caution is warranted and, until more data are available, the drug should be discontinued in women who want to become pregnant.

Ciprofloxacin

This is a quinolone with a selective action against *E. coli* and aerobic Enterobacteria; it is therefore a selective suppressive agent for intestinal microflora. Ciprofloxacin has been used for both perianal disease and ileitis, as well as UC and pouchitis (see Chapter 53). In a number of open studies, ciprofloxacin either alone or in combination with metronidazole was effective in controlling symptoms and active disease, and in the treatment of fistulae and abscesses.[61,62]

A combination of metronidazole and ciprofloxacin, which is effective against many enteric bacteria, has been reported to be effective in the treatment of acute CD as an alternative to steroids. Prantera et al[62] randomized 41 patients with refractory or steroid-dependent CD to a combination of 1000 mg ciprofloxacin and either 1000 mg metronidazole or methylprednisolone 0.70–1 mg/kg for 12 weeks. Some 45% of patients (10 of 22) achieved remission with metronidazole versus 63% (12 of 19) with methylprednisolone. The most common side effects are gastrointestinal complaints.

Antimycobacterial agents

M. paratuberculosis has been identified in tissues from a higher proportion of patients with CD than from controls, suggesting that this organism may be one of the causes of CD, although this is controversial. The possible involvement of *M. paratuberculosis* in CD has led several investigators to use antimycobacterial therapy. A recent meta-analysis of the effect of antimycobacterial therapy in CD concluded that this therapy is effective in maintaining remission in some patients following a course of corticosteroids combined with antimycobacterial therapy to induce remission.[57] Treatment of CD with antimycobacterial therapy does not seem to be effective without a course of corticosteroids to induce remission.

Probiotics

There are many different preparations of probiotic lactobacilli, and some evidence showing that they are of value in CD, although this is not conclusive.[56]

Biologic therapy

Anti-TNFα antibodies

The management of IBD entered a new era at the beginning of the 1990s with the development of biologic therapies that selectively block the inflammatory cascade.[63,64] Biologic therapies have been developed thanks to an increasing knowledge regarding disease pathogenesis, and their production has been precipitated by the techniques of molecular biology. One of the first biologic treatments, and the most important to date, involves chimeric antibodies to TNFα: infliximab (Remicade®). TNFα plays a central role in the inflammatory reaction observed in IBD. Infliximab is a mouse–human chimeric monoclonal IgG1 antibody against TNFα. It is prescribed in the USA and Europe for the treatment of active therapy-resistant CD[65,66] and for active fistulizing CD.[67,68] Response rates of 75–80% are reached after a single infusion of infliximab 5 mg/kg, with up to 50% of patients entering clinical remission. The underlying reasons for the lack of response seen in 25% of patients are not known, and efforts are being made into identifying factors predictive of response or failure.[69–71] Most patients relapse 8–12 weeks after initial infusion. Retreatment with infliximab every 8 weeks was shown to maintain clinical benefit.[66,72] In trials, some clinical benefit was obtained even in those who failed a three-injection induction course[72,73] In the ACCENT 2 study of infliximab maintenance treatment for fistulizing CD, about two-thirds responded initially (greater than 50% reduction in the number of draining fistulae), and of these 62% who received placebo maintenance experienced a loss of response after a median of 14 weeks compared with 42% of those given maintenance treatment (median time to loss of response greater than 40 weeks).[68] Infliximab is also capable of inducing colonic mucosal healing assessed on the CDEIS.[38] Use in children has been limited, but two studies suggest likely benefit.

TNFα is a key molecule in the inflammatory cascade, so it is not surprising that blocking it leads to an increase in the number of infectious events. The most frequently reported side effect is upper respiratory tract infection. In addition, a reactivation of latent tuberculosis has been seen. American and European guidelines for the use of infliximab now recommend that all patients undergo chest radiography and, in some countries, a skin PPD test before infliximab in administered.[74] Infliximab is further contraindicated for moderate to severe heart failure, and caution should be exercised when administering infliximab to patients with mild heart failure.[75] Although infliximab may induce antinuclear antibodies in almost 50% of patients, these autoantibodies are not associated with clinical manifestations of drug-induced lupus.[76]

Antibodies to infliximab

The presence of murine elements is associated with a risk of immunogenicity. In a prospective study of 125 infliximab-treated patients, 61% developed antibodies to infliximab (ATI), previously know as human antichimeric antibodies (HACA), after the fifth infusion.[77] ATI are more likely to develop when infliximab is given sporadically, and especially after 12–18 months or more. ATI are clearly associated with infusion reactions and loss of response to the drug.

Acute infusion reactions are anaphylactoid and accompanied by dyspnea, chest tightness, urticaria, and headache. They should be treated with antihistamines, steroids, or epinephrine (adrenaline), and can be reduced in patients known to suffer them or to be at risk by prior use of immunosuppressives, including steroids.

Delayed hypersensitivity usually occurs several days after the infusion in a patient who typically has not had infliximab for at least a year. Symptoms are of myalgia and atrophy, fever, rash, pruritus and urticaria, edema, sore throat, and dysphagia. These can be reduced with immunosuppression and intravenous steroids.[77] Infliximab-treated patients should therefore receive concomitant immunosuppression with azathioprine, 6-MP, or methotrexate.

Other anti-TNF therapies

The TNFα receptor proteins, etanercept and onercept, which have been successful in the treatment of rheumatoid disease, do not seem to be effective in CD.[78]

To avoid the problem of immunogenicity, more humanized anti-TNF antibodies have been developed. Adalimumab (Humira®) is a fully human antihuman TNFα monoclonal antibody. Given the absence of murine elements, it could have advantages over infliximab in terms of immunogenicity. Results of large trials on efficacy and safety are currently ongoing.

Other biologic therapies under assessment are shown in Table 54.5.[79–82]

Adhesion molecules

Adhesion molecules play a role in the trafficking of leukocytes in normal and inflamed gut. They are also involved in local lymphocyte stimulation and antigen presentation within the intestinal mucosa. In IBD, most of the adhesion factors are upregulated. Therapeutic compounds directed against trafficking of lymphocytes toward the gut mucosa have been developed as a novel class of drugs in the treatment of CD. α4 Integrins are important mediators of leukocyte migration across the vascular endothelium. They form heterodimers with subunits β7 and β1, and interact with vascular cell adhesion molecule 1 (VCAM-1) and mucosal addressin cell adhesion molecule 1 (MadCAM-1) respectively. In this way they are involved in the recruitment of leukocytes to the place of inflammation. The anti-α4 integrin antibody natalizumab (Antegren®) is a humanized mouse monoclonal antibody containing approximately 5% mouse-derived protein. The ENACT study randomized 905 patients to natalizumab 300 mg at weeks 0, 4, and 8, or to placebo. At 12 weeks, 42% of patients with severe luminal CD characterized by a raised CRP level entered into remission, compared with 29% of placebo-treated patients.[83] LDP-02 is a humanized monoclonal antibody to anti-α4β7 integrin. A double-blind placebo-controlled dose-finding trial in 185 patients with active CD showed that LDP-02, administered at 2.0 mg/kg, is biologically active.[84]

Surgical treatment

Surgery should be reserved for patients in whom medical treatment fails to control the inflammation, or for complications as

TABLE 54.5 BIOLOGIC THERAPIES FOR CROHN'S DISEASE UNDER ASSESSMENT

Drug name	Property	Molecular target	Functional target
Adalimumab	Neutralizing antibody	TNFα	Immune activation
Visilizumab	Neutralizing antibody	CD3	Immune initiation
Basiliximab	Neutralizing antibody	CD25	Steroid resistance
Sargramostin	GM-CSF analog	GM-CSF receptor	Mucosal barrier
Natalizumab	Anti-adhesion molecule	α4 integrin	
LDP-02	Anti-adhesion molecule	α4β7 integrin	

GM-CSF, granulocyte–macrophage colony-stimulating factor.

strictures, abcesses, or fistulae. Sands et al[85] showed that 20% of patients with CD require surgery within 3 years of their diagnosis, and almost 5% had already had major surgery at the time of diagnosis. The most common risk factor for surgery is smoking, whereas isolated colonic involvement is seen as a negative risk factor for early surgery. The most common operations used in CD (see Chapter 151) are listed in Table 54.6. Temporary or permanent defunctioning may be used for downstream disease, and as an adjunct to surgery for fistulae, where standard surgical procedures are accompanied by challenging individual dissections. Perianal abscesses may require drainage, but the surgical approach to perianal disease should be conservative because of poor healing. Postoperative recurrence at sites of anastomosis, often fibrostenotic, is common and in some patients appears to occur with accelerated rapidity. There is some evidence that prophylactic immunosuppression with azathioprine or 6-MP after surgery reduces the relapse rate.

Given that the disease may recur after surgery, bowel-saving operations should be performed to prevent short bowel syndrome (SBS). Operative techniques have changed significantly over the past few years, and novel techniques as strictureplasty are much less invasive and may prevent SBS. Therapy for recurrent anorectal CD follows the same rules, and proctectomy remains the last option. In addition, emergency surgery in recurrent CD follows the same rules as in elective surgery.

Nutritional therapy

Ensuring adequate nutrition and replacement, or prevention of specific deficiencies, is of central importance in the management of CD. In addition, there is some evidence that nutritional therapy reduces disease activity, although not as effectively as with glucocorticoids.[86] Enteral diet therapy is used, particularly for children. There is some limited evidence that specific dietary exclusions might be of value (see Chapter 42).

Helminths

Recently, the possibility that nematode infection could result in improvements in IBD by inducing a global Th1 to Th2 immunologic response has been investigated. These studies have been triggered by the observation that CD is characterized by a Th1 response and that IBD is rare in countries where nematode infection is prevalent. As yet, the data are uncontrolled, requiring evaluation in randomized clinical trials.[87]

COMPLICATIONS AND THEIR MANAGEMENT

Fibrostenosis

Inflammation of the bowel of patients with CD does not only result in ulceration but may also lead to fibrostenosis after healing.[88] Intestinal fibrostenosis is a frequent and debilitating complication of CD, resulting in small bowel obstruction that requires surgery (strictureplasty or resection). Repeated bowel resection may potentially result in SBS. Colonic strictures can be managed by endoscopic dilatation, with some success.[89] More than one-third of Crohn's patients have a clear stenosing disease phenotype, often in the absence of luminal inflammatory symptoms. Recent genetic studies on *CARD15/NOD2* have shown that patients carrying two *CARD15* mutations have a 7.44-fold increased risk of stricturing disease, and this increased to a 17-fold increased risk in the case of two *CARD15* variants and the presence of ileal involvement.[88]

Short bowel syndrome

Patients with CD are at high risk for postoperative recurrence (60% after 15 years) and often undergo multiple operations. SBS is defined as a remaining bowel length of less than 180 cm with associated malabsorption. Several factors, including aggressive resectional therapy, but also surgical complications and errors in initial diagnosis, may contribute to the development of SBS. Therefore, bowel-saving operations should be performed whenever possible. (See also Chapters 45, 138, and 139.)

Colorectal cancer (see Chapter 60)

Colorectal cancer (CRC) remains a feared complication of colitis. Although the risk is probably highest for total UC, it has become clear that less extensive colitis and Crohn's colitis also increase the risk. IBD cancers are preceded by dysplasia, and

TABLE 54.6 MOST COMMON OPERATIONS USED FOR PATIENTS WITH CROHN'S DISEASE

Site	Indication	Operation
Gastroduodenal	Outlet obstruction	Gastrojejunostomy Duodenal strictureplasty
Small intestine	Obstruction	Strictureplasty Segmental resection
Ileocecal	Obstruction or pain	Ileal resection or right hemicolectomy Resection and ileostomy
Colonic	Obstruction Pain Other symptoms not controlled medically	Colonic resection and ileostomy Colonic resection and ileorectal anastomosis Segmental resection
Anorectal	Uncontrolled by medical treatment	Temporary defunctioning colostomy Colonic resection and ileostomy Colonic resection and ileorectal anastomosis
	Recurrent abscess formation	Seton stitch

the relative risk increases by 0.5–1.0% per annum, and starts typically about 10 years after diagnosis. Currently, the main preventive strategy is a secondary one: surveillance colonoscopy after 8 years of disease duration. CRC tends to occur at the site of overt disease and develops at an earlier age (mean 50 years) than in sporadic non-IBD-associated CRC (70 years). Cancer should also be suspected in a *de novo* stricture of the colon, as this is associated with a 5–10-fold increased risk of colonic cancer.

The increased risk of colonic cancer exists in patients with CD even when disease is confined to the small bowel, and patients also have an increased risk of developing extraintestinal and reticuloendothelial tumors, as well as anovulval and malignant melanoma. The treatment of CRC includes segmental resection, total proctocolectomy, subtotal colectomy, and palliative procedures. The prognosis is no worse after operation than that of sporadic non-IBD-associated colonic cancer. There have been recent reports that 5-ASA given in a dose of 1.2 g/day may reduce the risk of colonic carcinoma. Other studies have suggested a role for folate and ursochol as chemopreventive agents.

Adenocarcinoma of the small bowel is extremely rare, compared with adenocarcinoma of the large bowel. Although only few small bowel cancers have been reported in patients with CD, the number is significantly increased in relation to the expected number.[90] Most small bowel cancers in CD are adenocarcinomas. They present at a younger age, more diffusely, and more distally than *de novo* cancers, usually making them undiagnosable at a curable early stage; indeed, two-thirds present with intestinal obstruction.

Fistulae

Fistulae consist of an abnormal communication between the lumen of the gut and the mesentery and/or another organ or the abdominal wall or skin. Symptoms such as fecal loss per vagina or pneumaturia (bladder fistula) imply the presence of a fistula. Fistulae also occur between bowel and skin (enterocutaneous), and between any two segments of bowel, sometimes resulting in malnutrition and eating-induced diarrhea (e.g., duodenocolic or ileosigmoid fistula).

Before the introduction of infliximab, antibiotics were the only nonsurgical treatment for fistulae, and often needed to be given over a very long period of time, leading to adverse effects and noncompliance. The introduction of infliximab has dramatically improved the management of fistulizing CD.[56] However, despite closure of draining external orifices after infliximab therapy, fistulous tracks with varying degrees of residual inflammation may persist, and may cause recurrent fistulae and pelvic abscesses[91] (Fig. 54.13). Whether complete fistula fibrosis occurs over time with repeated infliximab infusions is not known, and is subject of current studies.

Abscess formation

In some patients, penetrating transmural disease and fistulization may result in local abscess formation (see Chapter 117). Frank perforation is unusual. If an abscess is suspected, the patient should be started on broad-spectrum antibiotics and the abscess identified by computed tomography (CT), usually accompanied by attempts at CT-guided percutaneous drainage. If this is not possible or the patient is ill with signs of local inflammation (e.g., iliopsoas irritation), surgical exploration and drainage should be carried out.

Bleeding

Although the diarrhea of CD is characteristically nonbloody, rapid bleeding is recognized as an uncommon but occasionally life-threatening complication.

Malnutrition

Patients with CD become malnourished (see Fig. 54.6) for many reasons, including anorexia (see Chapter 14), vomiting, malabsorption (see Chapter 43), protein-losing enteropathy (see Chapter 48), small bowel bacterial overgrowth (see Chapter 46), and intestinal bypass because of fistula formation. Vitamin supplementation and caloric support are of central importance in CD. Enteral nutrition is preferred to parenteral where possible, because of both its enterotropic and therapeutic effects.

BONE DISEASE

Patients with CD are prone to osteopenic bone disease and osteoporosis.[92] Persistent inflammation, malnutrition, and use of corticosteroids are all contributory. Many would give calcium and vitamin D with steroids prophylactically (although there is no firm evidence of benefit). Patients with established osteoporosis, diagnosed by dual X-ray absorptiometry (DEXA) scanning, can be treated with bisphosphonates.

PROGNOSIS AND WHAT TO TELL PATIENTS

CD typically involves relapse and remission between relatively good and relatively poor health. Most patients are likely to require surgery at some time. Typical estimates are that up to 57% of patients require at least one surgical resection and that on average approximately 15 years elapse between resections, although the disease is very variable. When planning a family, patients need to know that there is a strong genetic component. They should also know that smoking cessation substantially

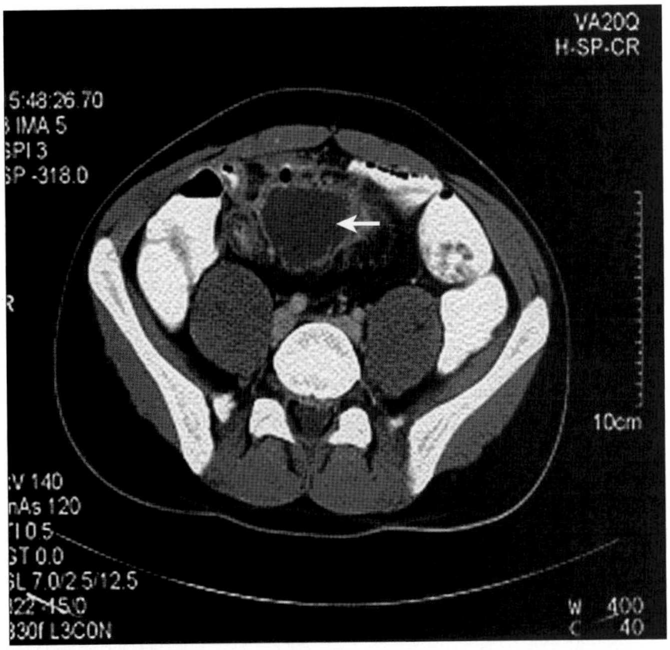

Fig. 54.13 Computed tomogram of a Crohn's patient showing a large abscess (arrow).

reduces activity and symptom burden. Patients with CD have been shown to have a somewhat reduced life expectancy throughout the course of the disease. Some of this may, however, be attributable to the cardiovascular consequences of smoking.[93]

SOURCES OF INFORMATION FOR PATIENTS AND DOCTORS

http://www.angelfire.com/ga/crohns/
http://www.patient.co.uk/showdoc/23068969/
http://www.patient.co.uk/showdoc/222/
http://www.gastro.org/generalPublic.html
http://www.nacc.org.uk/content/home.asp

REFERENCES

1. Podolsky DK. Inflammatory bowel disease. N Engl J Med 2002; 347:417–429.
2. Crohn BB, Ginzburg L, Oppenheimer GD. Regional ileitis: a pathologic and clinical entity. JAMA 1932; 99:1323–1328.
3. Loftus EV Jr, Sandborn WJ. Epidemiology of inflammatory bowel disease. Gastroenterol Clin North Am 2002; 31:1–20.
4. Munkholm P, Langholz E, Nielsen OH, Kreiner S, Binder V. Incidence and prevalence of Crohn's disease in the county of Copenhagen, 1962–87: a sixfold increase in incidence. Scand J Gastroenterol 1992; 27:609–614.
5. Loftus EV Jr, Silverstein MD, Sandborn WJ, Tremaine WJ, Harmsen WS, Zinsmeister AR. Crohn's disease in Olmsted County, Minnesota, 1940–1993: incidence, prevalence, and survival. Gastroenterology 1998; 114:1161–1168.
6. Loftus EV Jr, Schoenfeld P, Sandborn WJ. The epidemiology and natural history of Crohn's disease in population-based patient cohorts from North America: a systematic review. Aliment Pharmacol Ther 2002; 16:51–60.
7. Shivananda S, Lennard-Jones J, Logan R et al. Incidence of inflammatory bowel disease across Europe: is there a difference between north and south? Results of the European Collaborative Study on Inflammatory Bowel Disease (EC-IBD). Gut 1996; 39:690–697.
8. Moum B, Ekbom A, Vatn MH et al. Inflammatory bowl disease: re-evaluation of the diagnosis in a prespective population based study in south eastern Norway. Gut 1997; 40:328–332.
9. Martinez-Salmeron JF, Rodrigo M, de Teresa J et al. Epidemiology of inflammatory bowel disease in the Province of Granada, Spain: a retrospective study from 1979 to 1988. Gut 1993; 34:1207–1209.
10. Ranzi T, Bodini P, Zambelli A et al. Epidemiological aspects of inflammatory bowel disease in a north Italian population: a 4-year prospective study. Eur J Gastroenterol Hepatol 1996; 8:657–661.
11. Peeters M, Nevens H, Baert F et al. Familial aggregation in Crohn's disease: increased age adjusted risk and concordance in clinical characteristics. Gastroenterology 1996; 111:597–603.
12. Orholm M, Munkholm P, Langholz E et al. Familial occurrence of inflammatory bowel disease. N Engl J Med 1991; 324:84–88.
13. Satsangi J, Grootscholten C, Holt H, Jewell DP. Clinical patterns of familial inflammatory bowel disease. Gut 1996; 38:738–741.
14. Tysk C, Lindberg E, Jarnerot G et al. Ulcerative colitis and Crohn's disease in an unselected population of monozygotic and dizygotic twins. A study of heritability and the influence of smoking. Gut 1988; 29:990–996.
15. Thompson NP, Driscoll R, Pounder RE et al. Genetic versus environment in inflammatory bowel disease: results of a British twin study. BMJ 1996; 312:95–96.
16. Orholm M, Binder V, Sorensen TI et al. Concordance of inflammatory bowel disease among Danish twins. Results of a nationwide study. Scand J Gastroenterol 2000; 35:1075–1081.
17. Thomas GA, Rhodes J, Green JT, Richardson C. Role of smoking in inflammatory bowel disease: implications for therapy. Postgrad Med J 2000; 76:273–279.
18. Cosnes J, Beaugerie L, Carbonnel F, Gendre JP. Smoking cessation and the course of Crohn's disease: an intervention study. Gastroenterology 2001; 120:1093–1099.
19. Greenstein RJ. Is Crohn's disease caused by a mycobacterium? Comparisons with leprosy, tuberculosis, and Johne's disease. Lancet Infect Dis 2003; 3:507–514.
20. Hugot JP, Chamaillard M, Zouali H et al. Association of CARD15 leucine-rich repeat variants with susceptibility to Crohn's disease. Nature 2001; 411:599–603.
21. Ogura Y, Bonen DK, Inohara N et al. A frameshift mutation in *CARD15* associated with susceptibility to Crohn's disease. Nature 2001; 411:603–606.
22. Ahmad T, Tamboli CP, Jewell D, Colombel JF. Clinical relevance of advances in genetics and pharmacogenetics of IBD. Gastroenterology 2004; 126:1533–1549.
23. Neurath MF. Mucosal immunity in Crohn's disease. Inflamm Bowel Dis 2004; 10(Suppl 1):S29–S31.
24. Ina K, Itoh J, Fukushima K, Kusugami K et al. Resistance of Crohn's disease T cells to multiple apoptotic signals is associated with a Bcl-2/Bax mucosal imbalance. J Immunol 1999; 163:1081–1090.
25. Rutgeerts P, Geboes K, Peeters M et al. Effect of faecal stream diversion on recurrence of Crohn's disease in the neoterminal ileum. Lancet 1991; 338:771–774.
26. D'Haens GR, Geboes K, Peeters M, Baert F, Penninckx F, Rutgeerts P. Early lesions of recurrent Crohn's disease caused by infusion of intestinal contents in excluded ileum. Gastroenterology 1998; 114:262–267.
27. Rutgeerts P, Hiele M, Geboes K et al. Controlled trial of metronidazole treatment for prevention of Crohn's recurrence after ileal resection. Gastroenterology 1995; 108:1617–1621.
28. Landers CJ, Cohavy O, Misra R et al. Selected loss of tolerance evidenced by Crohn's disease-associated immune responses to auto- and microbial antigens. Gastroenterology 2002; 123:689–699.
29. Sendid B, Colombel JF, Jacquinot PM et al. Specific antibody response to oligomannosidic epitopes in Crohn's disease. Clin Diag Lab Immunol 1996; 3:219–226.
30. Terjung B, Spengler U, Sauerbruch T, Worman HJ. "Atypical p-ANCA" in IBD and hepatobiliary disorders react with a 50-kilodalton nuclear envelope protein of neutrophils and myeloid cell lines. Gastroenterology 2000; 119:310–322.
31. Singh B, Mortensen NJMcC, Jewell DP, George B. Perianal Crohn's disease. Br J Surg 2004; 91:801–814.
32. Gasche C, Scholmerich J, Brynskov J et al. A simple classification of Crohn's disease: report of the Working Party for the World Congresses of Gastroenterology, Vienna 1998. Inflamm Bowel Dis 2000; 6:8–15.
33. Wilson A, Reyes E, Ofman J. Prevalence and outcomes of anemia in inflammatory bowel disease: a systematic review of the literature. Am J Med 2004; 116(Suppl 7A):44S–49S.
34. Afdhal NH, Long A, Lennon J et al. Controlled trial of antimycobacterial therapy in Crohn's disease. Clofazimine versus placebo. Dig Dis Sci 1991; 36:449–453.
35. Danese S, Motte Cd Cde L, Fiocchi C. Platelets in inflammatory bowel disease: clinical, pathogenic, and therapeutic implications. Am J Gastroenterol 2004; 99:938–945.
36. Hommes DW, van Deventer SJ. Endoscopy in inflammatory bowel diseases. Gastroenterology 2004; 126:1561–1573.
37. D'haens G, Van Deventer S, Van Hogezand R et al. Endoscopic and histological healing with infliximab anti-tumor necrosis factor antibodies in Crohn's disease: a European multicenter trial. Gastroenterology 1999; 116:1029–1034.
38. Eliakim R, Adler SN. Capsule video endoscopy in Crohn's disease – the European experience. Gastrointest Endosc Clin N Am 2004; 14:129–137.
39. Kleer CG, Appelman HD. Surgical pathology of Crohn's disease. Am J Surg Pathol 1998; 22:983–989.
40. Vermeire S, Peeters M, Vlietinck R et al. Anti-*Saccharomyces cerevisiae* antibodies (ASCA), phenotypes of IBD, and intestinal permeability: a study in IBD families. Inflamm Bowel Dis 2001; 7:8–15.
41. Vasiliauskas EA, Plevy SE, Landers CJ et al. Perinuclear antineutrophil cytoplasmic antibodies in patients with Crohn's disease define a clinical subgroup. Gastroenterology 1996; 110:1810–1819.
42. Mow WS, Vasiliauskas EA, Lin YC et al. Association of antibody responses to microbial antigens and complications of small bowel Crohn's disease. Gastroenterology 2004; 126:414–424.
43. Camma C, Giunta M, Rosselli M, Cottone M. Mesalamine in the maintenance treatment of Crohn's disease: a meta-analysis adjusted for confounding variables. Gastroenterology 1997; 115:1465–1473.

44. Munkholm P, Langholz E, Davidsen M, Binder V. Frequency of glucocorticoid resistance and dependency in Crohn's disease. Gut 1994; 35:360–362.
45. Rutgeerts P, Lofberg R, Malchow H et al. A comparison of budesonide with prednisolone for active Crohn's disease. N Engl J Med 1994; 331:842–845.
46. Campieri M, Ferguson A, Doe W, Persson T, Nilsson LG. Oral budesonide is as effective as oral prednisolone in active Crohn's disease. The Global Budesonide Study Group. Gut 1997; 41:209–214.
47. Bar-Meir S, Chowers Y, Lavy A et al. Budesonide versus prednisone in the treatment of active Crohn's disease. The Israeli Budesonide Study Group. Gastroenterology 1998; 115:835–840.
48. Candy S, Wright J, Gerber M, Adams G, Gerig M, Goodman R. A controlled double blind study of azathioprine in the management of Crohn's disease. Gut 1995; 37:674–678.
49. Weinshilboum RM, Sladek SL. Mercaptopurine pharmacogenetics: monogenic inheritance of erythrocyte thiopurine methyltransferase activity. Am J Hum Genet 1980; 32:651–662.
50. Yates CR, Krynetski EY, Loennechen T et al. Molecular diagnosis of thiopurine *S*-methyltransferase deficiency: genetic basis for azathioprine and mercaptopurine intolerance. Ann Intern Med 1997; 126:608–614.
51. Colombel JF, Ferrari N, Debuysere H et al. Genotypic analysis of thiopurine *S*-methyltransferase in patients with Crohn's disease and severe myelosuppression during azathioprine therapy. Gastroenterology 2000; 118:1025–1030.
52. Dubinsky MC, Lamothe S, Yang HY et al. Pharmacogenomics and metabolite measurement for 6-mercaptopurine therapy in inflammatory bowel disease. Gastroenterology 2000; 118:705–713.
53. Dubinsky MC, Yang H, Hassard PV et al. 6-MP metabolite profiles provide a biochemical explanation for 6-MP resistance in patients with inflammatory bowel disease. Gastroenterology 2002; 122:904–915.
54. Feagan BG, Rochon J, Fedorak RN et al. Methotrexate for the treatment of Crohn's disease. The North American Crohn's Study Group Investigators. N Engl J Med 1995; 332:292–297.
55. Feagan BG, Fedorak RN, Irvine EJ et al. A comparison of methotrexate with placebo for the maintenance of remission in Crohn's disease. North American Crohn's Study Group Investigators. N Engl J Med 2000; 342:1627–1632.
56. Sartor RB. Therapeutic manipulation of the enteric microflora in inflammatory bowel diseases: antibiotics, probiotics, and prebiotics. Gastroenterology 2004; 126:1620–1633.
57. Borgaonkar MR, MacIntosh GD, Fardy JM. A meta-analysis of antimycobacterial therapy for Crohn's disease. Am J Gastroenterol 2000; 95:725–729.
58. Bernstein LH, Frank MS, Brandt LJ et al. Healing of perineal Crohn's disease with metronidazole. Gastroenterology 1980; 79:357–365.
59. Rosen A, Ursing B, Alm T et al. A comparative study of metronidazole and sulfasalazine for active Crohn's disease: the Cooperative Crohn's Disease Study in Sweden. I. Design and methodological considerations. Gastroenterology 1982; 83:541–549.
60. Sutherland L, Singleton J, Sessions J et al. Double blind, placebo controlled trial of metronidazole in Crohn's disease. Gut 1991; 32:1071–1075.
61. Turunen U, Färkkilä V, Valtonen V et al. Long-term outcome of ciprofloxacin treatment in severe perianal or fistulous Crohn's disease. Gastroenterology 1993; 104:A793.
62. Prantera C, Zannoni F, Scribano ML et al. An antibiotic regimen for the treatment of active Crohn's disease: a randomized, controlled trial of metronidazole plus ciprofloxacin. Am J Gastroenterol 1996; 91:328–332.
63. Rutgeerts P, Van Assche G, Vermeire S. Optimizing anti-TNF treatment in inflammatory bowel disease. Gastroenterology 2004; 126:1593–1610.
64. Egan LJ, Sandborn WJ. Advances in the treatment of Crohn's disease. Gastroenterology 2004; 126:1574–1581.
65. Targan SR, Hanauer SB, van Deventer SJ et al. A short-term study of chimeric monoclonal antibody cA2 to tumor necrosis factor alpha for Crohn's disease. Crohn's Disease cA2 Study Group. N Engl J Med 1997; 337:1029–1035.
66. Hanauer SB, Feagan BG, Lichtenstein GR et al. Maintenance infliximab for Crohn's disease: the ACCENT I randomised trial. Lancet 2002; 359:1541–1549.
67. Present DH, Rutgeerts P, Targan S et al. Infliximab for the treatment of fistulas in patients with Crohn's disease. N Engl J Med 1999; 340:1398–1405.
68. Sands BE, Anderson FH, Bernstein CN et al. Infliximab maintenance therapy for fistulizing Crohn's disease. N Engl J Med 2004; 350:876–885.
69. Parsi MA, Achkar JP, Richardson S et al. Predictors of response to infliximab in patients with Crohn's disease. Gastroenterology 2002; 123:707–713.
70. Vermeire S, Louis E, Carbonez A et al. Logistic regression of clinical parameters influencing response to infliximab. Am J Gastroenterol 2002; 97:2357–2363.
71. Arnott ID, McNeill G, Satsangi J. An analysis of factors influencing short-term and sustained response to infliximab treatment for Crohn's disease. Aliment Pharmacol Ther 2003; 17:1451–1457.
72. Rutgeerts P, D'Haens G, Targan S et al. Efficacy and safety of retreatment with anti-tumor necrosis factor antibody (infliximab) to maintain remission in Crohn's disease. Gastroenterology 1999; 117:761–769.
73. Rutgeerts P, Feagan BG, Lichtenstein GR et al. Comparison of scheduled and episodic treatment strategies of infliximab in Crohn's disease. Gastroenterology 2004; 126:402–413.
74. Keane J, Gershon S, Wise RP et al. Tuberculosis associated with infliximab, a tumor necrosis factor alpha-neutralizing agent. N Engl J Med 2001; 345:1098–1104.
75. Chung ES, Packer M, Lo KH et al. Randomized, double-blind, placebo-controlled, pilot trial of infliximab, a chimeric monoclonal antibody to tumor necrosis factor-alpha, in patients with moderate-to-severe heart failure: results of the Anti-TNF Therapy Against Congestive Heart Failure (ATTACH) trial. Circulation 2003; 107:3133–3140.
76. Vermeire S, Noman M, Van Assche G et al. Autoimmunity associated with anti-tumor necrosis factor alpha treatment in Crohn's disease: a prospective cohort study. Gastroenterology 2003; 125:32–39.
77. Baert F, Noman M, Vermeire S et al. Influence of immunogenicity on the long-term efficacy of infliximab in Crohn's disease. N Engl J Med 2003; 348:601–608.
78. Sandborn WJ, Hanauer SB. Infliximab in the treatment of Crohn's disease: a user's guide for clinicians. Am J Gastroenterol 2002; 97:2962–2972.
79. Sandborn WJ, Hanauer SB, Loftus Jr EV et al. An open-label study of the human anti-TNF monoclonal antibody adalimumab in subjects with prior loss of response or intolerance to infliximab for Crohn's disease. Gastroenterology 2004; 126(Suppl 2):435.
80. Plevy S, Salzberg B, van Assche G et al. A humanized anti-CD3 monoclonal antibody, visilizuman, for treatment of severe steroid-refractory ulcerative colitis: results of a phase 1 study. Gastroenterology 2004; 126(Suppl 2):579.
81. Creed T, Probert C, Dayan C, Hearing S. Basiliximab (anti-CD25) for the treatment of steroid resistant ulcerative colitis. Gastroenterology 2004; 126(Suppl 2):581.
82. Korzenik J, Dieckgraefe B, Valentine JF. Duration of sargramostim effects in patients with moderately-to-severely active Crohn's disease (CD): follow-up results from a randomized, double-blind, placebo controlled trial. Gastroenterology 2004; 126(Suppl 2):582.
83. Rutgeerts P, Colombel J, Enns R et al. Subanalysis from a phase 3 study on the evaluation of natalizumab in active Crohn's disease. Gut 2003; 52(Suppl):A239.
84. Ghosh S, Goldin E, Gordon FH et al. Natalizumab for active Crohn's disease. N Engl J Med 2003; 348:24–32.
85. Sands BE, Arsenault JE, Rosen MJ et al. Risk of early surgery for Crohn's disease: implications for early treatment strategies. Am J Gastroenterol 2003; 98:2712–2718.
86. Griffiths AM, Ohlsson A, Sherman PM et al. Meta-analysis of enteral nutrition as a primary treatment of active Crohn's disease. Gastroenterology 1995; 108:1056–1067.
87. Hunter MM, McKay DM. Helminths as therapeutic agents for inflammatory bowel disease. Aliment Pharmacol Ther 2004; 19:167–177.
88. Brant SR, Picco MF, Achkar JP et al. Defining complex contributions of *NOD2/CARD15* gene mutations, age at onset, and tobacco use on Crohn's disease phenotypes. Inflamm Bowel Dis 2003; 9:281–289.
89. Erkelens GW, van Deventer SJ. Endoscopic treatment of strictures in Crohn's disease. Best Pract Res Clin Gastroenterol 2004; 18:201–207.
90. Munkholm P. The incidence and prevalence of colorectal cancer in inflammatory bowel disease. Aliment Pharmacol Ther 2003;18(Suppl 2):1–5.
91. Van Assche G, Vanbeckevoort D, Bielen D et al. Magnetic resonance imaging of the effects of infliximab on perianal fistulizing Crohn's disease. Am J Gastroenterol 2003; 98:332–339.
92. Harpavat M, Keljo DJ, Regueiro MD. Metabolic bone disease in inflammatory bowel disease. J Clin Gastroenterol 2004; 38:218–224.
93. Card T, Hubbard R, Logan RF. Mortality in inflammatory bowel disease: a population-based cohort study. Gastroenterology 2003; 125:1583–1590.
94. Sutherland LR, Ramcharan S, Bryant H, Fick G. Effect of cigarette smoking on recurrence of Crohn's disease. Gastroenterology 1990; 98:1123–1128.
95. Lindberg E, Jarnerot G, Huitfeldt B. Smoking in Crohn's disease: effect on localisation and clinical course. Gut 1992; 33:779–782.
96. Cottone M, Rosselli M, Orlando A et al. Smoking habits and recurrence in Crohn's

disease. Gastroenterology 1994; 106:643–648.
97. Breuer-Katschinski BD, Hollander N, Goebell H. Effect of cigarette smoking on the course of Crohn's disease. Eur J Gastroenterol Hepatol 1996; 8:225–228.
98. Cosnes J, Carbonnel F, Beaugerie L, Le Quintrec Y, Gendre JP. Effects of cigarette smoking on the long-term course of Crohn's disease. Gastroenterology 1996; 110:424–431.
99. Timmer A, Sutherland LR, Martin F. Oral contraceptive use and smoking are risk factors for relapse in Crohn's disease. The Canadian Mesalamine for Remission of Crohn's Disease Study Group. Gastroenterology 1998; 114:1143–1150.
100. Medina C, Vergara M, Casellas F, Lara F, Naval J, Malagelada JR. Influence of the smoking habit in the surgery of inflammatory bowel disease. Rev Enferm Dig 1998; 90:771–778.
101. Yamamoto T, Keighley MR. The association of cigarete smoking with a high risk of recurrence after ileocolonic resection for ileocecal Crohn's disease. Surg Today 1999 29:579–580.
102. Yamamoto T, Allan RN, Keighley MR. Smoking is a predictive factor for outcome after colectomy and ileorectal anastomosis in patients with Crohn's colitis. Br J Surg 1999; 86:1069–1070.

Chapter 55

Indeterminate colitis

Konstantinos A Papadakis and Stephan R Targan

KEY POINTS

- In 10–20% of colonic IBD a clear distinction between ulcerative colitis (UC) and Crohn's disease (CD) cannot be made
- Indeterminate colitis probably represents a distinct entity within the heterogeneous spectrum of IBD
- Indeterminate colitis can be classified histologically as active and patchy transmucosal chronic inflammation with minimal or moderate architectural distortion and an absence of diagnostic features for either CD (such as granulomas) or UC
- The identification of small bowel lesions on capsule endoscopy may allow more patients with indeterminate colitis to be reclassified as having CD
- Serologic markers may be helpful – anti-*Saccharomyces cerevisiae* antibody (ASCA)-positive, perinuclear antineutrophil cytoplasmic antibody (pANCA)-negative indeterminate colitis predicts evolution to CD in 80% of patients; ASCA-negative, pANCA-positive indeterminate colitis predicts UC in 64%
- Attempts to distinguish between UC and CD become important when considering restorative proctocolectomy (ileal pouch–anal anastomosis) as the subsequent development of CD is associated with a poor long-term outcome and pouch failure

INTRODUCTION AND DEFINITION

Inflammatory bowel disease (IBD) has been traditionally classified into two distinct disease entities: ulcerative colitis (UC) and Crohn's disease (CD). The diagnosis of UC and CD relies on a series of clinical, radiographic, endoscopic, and histopathologic criteria. In UC the mucosal inflammation is limited to the superficial layers of the colon (mucosa and submucosa), whereas in CD, which can affect any part of the gastrointestinal tract, the inflammatory process is patchy, transmural, and often associated with granuloma formation.[1] In 10–20% of patients with IBD with isolated colonic involvement, however, a clear distinction between UC and CD cannot be made with certainty. These cases have been referred to as 'unclassified colitis' or 'indeterminate colitis'.[1,2]

Indeterminate colitis was originally used by pathologists to describe the colitis observed in surgical specimens that could not be accurately classified as UC or CD.[2,3] This was therefore a provisional classification prior to establishing a definitive diagnosis.[4] In the modern era the term indeterminate colitis has been extended in the precolectomy evaluation of patients with chronic IBD to characterize the type of colitis that cannot be definitively classified as UC or CD. Some authorities argue that indeterminate colitis represents a distinct clinical entity, whereas others believe that it is simply a problem of classification at the time of evaluation.[4,5]

Recent advances in our understanding of the pathogenesis of mucosal inflammation in animal models and humans suggest that IBD represents a heterogeneous group of diseases based on clinical, subclinical, and genetic characteristics (Fig. 55.1). For example, *CARD15* (*NOD2*) variants have been shown to be associated not only with CD but also with younger age of disease onset, ileal involvement, and a tendency to develop strictures.[6] This notion of disease heterogeneity has been further supported by the development of several animal models of IBD with distinct phenotypes and immunologic features following selective manipulation of a variety of genes, including those of proinflammatory or immunoregulatory cytokines.[1] Given this premise and its extrapolation to human disease, indeterminate colitis may in fact be a distinct manifestation within the IBD spectrum.

INCIDENCE, NATURAL HISTORY, DIAGNOSTIC EVALUATION, AND TREATMENT

Between 5% and 23% of the initial diagnoses of IBD are classified as indeterminate colitis with an incidence of approximately 2.4 per 100000.[5,7–9] Indeterminate colitis has been associated with a higher risk of colorectal cancer development and increased mortality compared with UC.[10] In addition, the cumulative incidence of colectomy in patients with indeterminate colitis in a population-based study was four times higher than in patients with definite UC.[10] Although many patients with indeterminate colitis will be reclassified as having CD or UC on long-term follow-up evaluation, a significant proportion of them will still carry the diagnosis of indeterminate colitis.[8]

PATHOGENESIS AND PATHOLOGY

The pathogenesis of indeterminate colitis is similar to that of UC or CD. Inappropriate activation of the mucosal immune system in response to commensal bacterial antigens of the colon initiates a cascade of events leading to mucosal inflammation and epithelial cell dysfunction.[1,6] The pathology of indeterminate colitis has been described in surgical specimens and includes macroscopic features such as total severe colitis, segmental disease with rectal sparing, and variation in disease severity in different parts of the colon. The microscopic features may include fissuring ulcers, mucosal islands with a regular epithelium, preserved goblet cells, and mild inflammation and transmural inflammation associated with severe ulceration.[2,11] Granulomas and transmural lymphoid aggregates are not present. However, given the limitations of the precolectomy evaluation of mucosal biopsies in patients with indeterminate

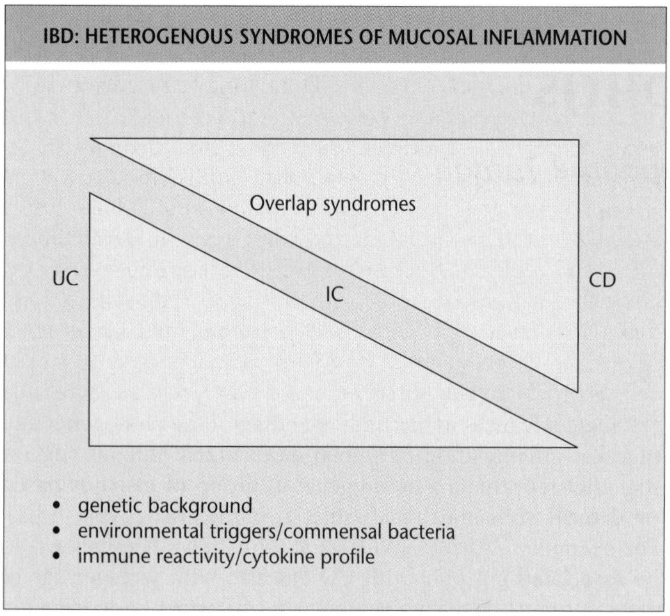

Fig. 55.1 IBD represents heterogeneous syndromes of mucosal inflammation. At the extreme ends of the spectrum, classic cases of ulcerative colitis (UC) and Crohn's disease (CD) are seen. The phenotypic expression of these diseases is influenced by the genetic background of the individual, the environmental triggers of the disease, the mucosal cytokine profile, and specific immune reactivity to luminal bacterial flora, which could be interrelated. IC, indeterminate colitis.

colitis (inability to evaluate for transmural lymphoid aggregates and granulomas in the deeper layers of the bowel and the potential effect of prior treatment), the physician should often rely on the evaluation of multiple biopsy specimens from the ileum and colon in combination with endoscopy to establish a definitive diagnosis.[2] The absence of diagnostic features of CD in the biopsy specimens (such as granulomas) in repeated histopathologic evaluations of the ileum and colon would indicate that the patient has indeterminate colitis. A recent study classified patients as having indeterminate colitis if they had isolated colitis, endoscopy was inconclusive, and microscopy indicated 'active and patchy transmucosal chronic inflammation with minimal or moderate architectural distortion and an absence of diagnostic features for either CD or UC.'[12]

CLINICAL PRESENTATION

The typical clinical presentation of indeterminate colitis includes symptoms related to colitis such as abdominal pain, diarrhea, rectal bleeding, and tenesmus. Systemic manifestations are frequently observed, such as fever, weight loss, and anemia.

DIFFERENTIAL DIAGNOSIS

By definition, indeterminate colitis refers to chronic idiopathic colitis that cannot be differentiated from UC and CD at the initial presentation. Distinction from UC or CD becomes clinically important in medically refractory cases when surgery is contemplated.[13–15]

In patients with indeterminate colitis the probability of having a diagnosis of CD on follow-up evaluation was increased in patients with fever at their initial presentation, segmental endoscopic lesions, or extraintestinal complications, and in current smokers, whereas the probability of having a diagnosis of UC was increased in patients who had not undergone appendectomy before diagnosis.[9] The development of new endoscopic modalities such as the wireless capsule has assisted in the diagnostic evaluation of patients with indeterminate colitis. A subset of such patients, despite normal radiographic studies of the small bowel, will be found to have small bowel lesions characteristic of CD.

Serologic testing in patients with an initial diagnosis of indeterminate colitis may be helpful in categorizing the disease and predict the follow-up diagnosis.[1,12] The most extensively studied serologic markers in IBD include perinuclear antineutrophil cytoplasmic antibody (pANCA) and anti-*Saccharomyces cerevisiae* antibody (ASCA). As subclinical indicators of immune dysregulation, these markers can be used in IBD to stratify patients based on clinical, immunologic, and genetic characteristics. pANCA is detected in the serum of 60–70% of patients with UC and in 10–20% of patients with CD. ASCA is present in 50–70% of patients with CD and in 6–14% of patients with UC. ASCA is rarely expressed in individuals who do not have IBD and thus is highly specific for CD.[1] In a recent prospective study, pANCA and ASCA were studied in 97 patients with indeterminate colitis. ASCA-positive pANCA-negative indeterminate colitis predicted evolution to CD in 80% of the patients.[12] ASCA-negative pANCA-positive indeterminate colitis predicted UC in 64% of patients, whereas this combination was 100% predictive of UC or 'UC-like CD.' The latter represents cases of CD with left-sided colonic involvement, which resemble UC both clinically and endoscopically. Interestingly, almost half of patients with indeterminate colitis were negative for both of these serologic markers, and most of these patients (85%) continued to carry the diagnosis of indeterminate colitis on follow-up evaluation (mean follow-up 10 years).[12] The immune reactivity to other bacterial antigens such as OmpC, I2, and CBir (flagellin) are likely to improve further the classification of patients with indeterminate colitis.

TREATMENT AND PREVENTION

Randomized controlled trials of medical therapies in IBD have included only well documented cases of UC or CD. As many patients with indeterminate colitis will eventually be found to have either UC or CD, any therapy that is effective in both diseases may prove useful in the treatment of indeterminate colitis.[5] The goals of medical treatment in indeterminate colitis are the same as those for other forms of IBD, namely induction and maintenance of remission.[16]

Aminosalicylates: The mainstay of medical treatment for mild to moderately active indeterminate colitis includes the use of 5-aminosalicylates (5-ASAs). There are three delivery systems for oral aminosalicylates and several topical (rectal) formulations. The oral formulations include azo-bond conjugates (sulfasalazine, olsalazine, and balsalazide), pH-dependent mesalazine with varied Eudragit (USP) coatings (Asacol®, Salofalk®, and Claversal®), and time/pH release formulations of mesalazine encapsulated into ethylcellulose beads (Pentasa®).[16] As indeterminate colitis usually involves the entire colon, combined administration of oral and topical 5-ASA may have an additive therapeutic effect.

Corticosteroids and immunosuppressives: In patients with indeterminate colitis who fail to respond to 5-ASA treatment, or those with severe disease, corticosteroids are often required to induce remission. However, corticosteroids have no maintenance benefit in patients with CD or UC, and should not be used long term in patients with indeterminate colitis either.[16] In cases where indeterminate colitis becomes steroid-dependent, immunomodulatory treatment with 6-mercaptopurine (6-MP) or azathioprine (AZA) should be initiated.[16] In patients who are intolerant to 6-MP or AZA, or fail to respond adequately, methotrexate can be tried. This drug has been shown to be effective for the induction and maintenance of remission in steroid-dependent chronic active CD, but is less effective in UC. However, its efficacy in indeterminate colitis is unknown. Novel treatments that target inflammatory mediators (e.g., tumor necrosis factor-α; TNF-α), such as the human–chimeric monoclonal antibody directed against TNF-α, infliximab (Remicade®), have been found to be highly effective for the treatment of inflammatory and fistulizing CD, but less so for the treatment of UC. In a series of patients with medically refractory indeterminate colitis, infliximab was effective in 67% of patients, several of whom avoided colectomy.[17] Ciclosporin may also be effective in patients with indeterminate colitis who have failed to respond to corticosteroid treatment, similar to patients with UC.[5] The use of 6-MP or AZA is required for maintenance of remission in these patients.

As discussed above, the risk of major surgery is increased several-fold in patients with indeterminate colitis compared with those with UC. Ileal anal–pouch anastomosis (IPAA) has been considered the gold standard surgical treatment for UC and is generally contraindicated in patients with CD owing to the high incidence of complications, including pelvic abscess, fistula, and pouch failure, which may require pouch excision.[13] The major decision regarding surgical treatment of indeterminate colitis is whether to perform restorative proctocolectomy (IPAA) or total colectomy with ileostomy or, in patients with rectal sparing, subtotal colectomy with ileorectal anastomosis.[15] The outcome of patients operated on for indeterminate colitis with IPAA who did not develop CD in long-term follow-up is reportedly as good as in those operated on for UC, although other studies have reported a higher incidence of complications in patients operated on for indeterminate colitis. This discrepancy may be related to differences in the definition of indeterminate colitis used in different studies. Nevertheless, the development of CD following IPAA for either UC or indeterminate colitis is associated with a poor long-term outcome.[5] Extensive evaluation of patients with an upper gastrointestinal series/small bowel follow-through or even wireless capsule endoscopy should be performed to rule out CD of the small bowel before performing an IPAA. IBD serologies may be helpful in predicting the potential development of complications following IPAA for indeterminate colitis, but long-term follow-up studies are needed to assess their utility in this setting.[1]

CONCLUSION

Indeterminate colitis was originally reported in colectomy specimens to describe inflammatory processes that could not be classified definitively as either UC or CD. Recently, the term has been extended to include cases of chronic IBD without small bowel inflammation and inconclusive diagnostic features of either UC or CD. Although long-term follow-up may change the diagnosis to either UC or CD, a significant number of patients will still have indeterminate colitis. The heterogeneity of IBD supports the idea that, although indeterminate colitis may represent a problem of classification at the time of initial evaluation in some patients, others may truly represent a distinct disease entity. Medical therapies are similar to those used for the treatment of UC, and sometimes CD. Surgical treatment may be needed in those patients with severe treatment-resistant disease.

REFERENCES

1. Papadakis KA, Targan SR. Serologic testing in inflammatory bowel disease: its value in indeterminate colitis. Curr Gastroenterol Rep 1999; 1:482–485.
2. Geboes K, De Hertogh G. Indeterminate colitis. Inflamm Bowel Dis 2003; 9:324–331.
3. Price AB. Overlap in the spectrum of nonspecific inflammatory bowel disease –"colitis indeterminate." J Clin Pathol 1978; 31:567–577.
4. Odze R. Diagnostic problems and advances in inflammatory bowel disease. Mod Pathol 2003; 16:347–358.
5. MacDermott RP. Indeterminate colitis. In: Bayless T, Hanauer S, eds. Advanced therapy of inflammatory bowel disease. Lewiston, NY: BC Decker; 2001:157–160.
6. Ahmad T, Tamboli CP, Jewell D, Colombel JF. Clinical relevance of advances in genetics and pharmacogenetics of IBD. Gastroenterology 2004; 126:1533–1549.
7. Stewenius J, Adnerhill I, Ekelund G et al. Ulcerative colitis and indeterminate colitis in the city of Malmö, Sweden. A 25-year incidence study. Scand J Gastroenterol 1995; 30:38–43.
8. Wells AD, McMillan I, Price AB, Ritchie JK, Nicholls RJ. Natural history of indeterminate colitis. Br J Surg 1991; 78:179–181.
9. Meucci G, Bortoli A, Riccioli FA et al. Frequency and clinical evolution of indeterminate colitis: a retrospective multi-centre study in northern Italy. GSMII (Gruppo di Studio per le Malattie Inflammatorie Intestinali). Eur J Gastroenterol Hepatol 1999; 11:909–913.
10. Stewenius J, Adnerhill I, Anderson H et al. Incidence of colorectal cancer and all cause mortality in non-selected patients with ulcerative colitis and indeterminate colitis in Malmö, Sweden. Int J Colorectal Dis 1995; 10:117–122.
11. Geboes K. Crohn's disease, ulcerative colitis or indeterminate colitis – how important is it to differentiate? Acta Gastroenterol Belg 2001; 64:197–200.
12. Joossens S, Reinisch W, Vermeire S et al. The value of serologic markers in indeterminate colitis: a prospective follow-up study. Gastroenterology 2002; 122:1242–1247.
13. Wolff BG. Is ileoanal the proper operation for indeterminate colitis: the case for. Inflamm Bowel Dis 2002; 8:362–365; discussion 368–369.
14. McIntyre PB, Pemberton JH, Wolff BG, Dozois RR, Beart RW Jr. Indeterminate colitis. Long-term outcome in patients after ileal pouch–anal anastomosis. Dis Colon Rectum 1995; 38:51–54.
15. Lindsey I, Warren BF, Mortensen NJMcC. Indeterminate colitis: surgical approaches. In: Bayless T, Hanauer S, eds. Advanced therapy of inflammatory bowel disease. Lewiston, NY: BC Decker; 2001:241–244.
16. Hanauer SB. Update on medical management of inflammatory bowel disease: ulcerative colitis. Rev Gastroenterol Dis 2001; 1:169–176.
17. Papadakis KA, Treyzon L, Abreu MT, Targan SR, Vasiliauskas EA. Infliximab for the treatment of medically refractory indeterminate colitis. Aliment Pharmacol Ther 2003; 18:741–747.

Chapter 56

Microscopic colitis

C J J Mulder, I M Harkema, and J W R Meijer

KEY POINTS

- Microscopic colitis includes both lymphocytic colitis and collagenous colitis
- In collagenous colitis there is a thick (10 μm), sub epithelial collagen deposition between the basement membranes throughout the colon with lymphocytic infiltrates in the lamina propria
- In lymphocytic colitis this collagen band is absent, and the lymphocytic infiltration more marked
- Clinical features are chronic watery diarrhea without blood, abdominal pain, normal blood tests, and no signs of malabsorption
- Microbiology, radiology and endoscopy findings are normal
- Remission in pregnancy, antibody markers, response to steroids and azathioprine, and association with other diseases favor an autoimmune etiology
- Collagenous colitis shares features with NSAID- and lansoprazole-induced colitis
- Proximal and distal biopsies are required due to the patchy nature of the disease
- Empirical treatments include bismuth subsalicylate, anti-diarrheals, ASAs, corticosteroids, azathioprine, and octreotide

INTRODUCTION

Microscopic colitis is an umbrella term applicable to both lymphocytic colitis and collagenous colitis.[1–3] The first case of collagenous colitis was published in 1976 by Lindström, who described a new entity in which chronic watery diarrhea was associated with a thick subepithelial collagen deposition in biopsy samples of endoscopically normal colonic mucosa.[1] The term lymphocytic colitis was proposed in 1989, recognizing cases with more lymphocytic inflammation than so-called classic collagen bands on histologic evaluation.[3] These entities are now generally recognized, and microscopic colitis has become a common condition of unknown cause affecting the large bowel in particular.[4]

The clinical features of microscopic colitis are:

- chronic watery diarrhea without blood
- abdominal pain
- normal blood test results
- no signs of malabsorption
- normal microbiologic, radiologic, and endoscopic findings.

Histopathologic examination reveals thickening of the subepithelial collagen layer beneath the basement membrane throughout the colon with lymphocytic infiltrates in the lamina propria. The pathogenesis and significance of these findings are still unknown.

Therapeutic options are based mainly on case reports. However, in recent literature budesonide and azathioprine seem promising. In some cases, the symptoms resolve spontaneously.

EPIDEMIOLOGY

Patients with collagenous colitis are usually middle-aged women, with a female : male ratio of 3–20 : 1.[4,5] Most are in the fifth or sixth decade of life, although the age range is 10–90 years, with a mean of about 55 years.[5–7] The incidence of collagenous colitis is estimated as between 0.2 and 2.3 per 10^5 population.[4]

For lymphocytic colitis there is a less pronounced predominance of women: 1.6–3 : 1.[6] The peak onset for lymphocytic colitis is similarly in the fifth or sixth decade, with the same age range as for collagenous colitis and a mean of about 57 years.[5,6] The differences in incidence probably reflects the differences in definition of these conditions. Familial clustering of collagenous colitis has been recognized.[5,8,9] Smoking seems to protect against microscopic colitis, as for ulcerative colitis.

PATHOGENESIS

The cause of microscopic colitis is unknown. There are three main possibilities: autoimmune disease, involvement of a luminal agent, and fibroblast dysfunction.

Autoimmune disease

There are many features that suggest microscopic colitis might be an autoimmune disease. The female predominance, association with other autoimmune diseases, and the response to steroids underscore this hypothesis. Remission has been reported during pregnancy.[7] A luminal agent or an immunologic reaction to an endogenous antigen produced by enterocytes might trigger the disease.[7] Immunoglobulin (Ig) M concentration is increased by 40% in patients with collagenous colitis.[10] Positive antinuclear antibodies were found in 30–50%[5,6] and peripheral antineutrophil cytoplasmic antibody (P-ANCA) in 10–14% of patients.[5]

Up to 40% of patients have one or more associated autoimmune diseases (Table 56.1).[6] Celiac disease has been reported in 6–40% of patients with microscopic colitis,[6,11] thyroid disease in up to 20%,[6,12] diabetes mellitus in 10%, and rheumatoid arthritis in 2.5%. Other autoimmune diseases have been reported, such as CREST syndrome, Sjögren's syndrome, psoriasis, Raynaud's phenomenon, dermatomyositis, polymyalgia rheumatica, Wegener's granulomatosis, Behçet's syndrome, and systemic lupus erythematosus.[6] Levels of intraepithelial lymphocytes are increased in patients with collagenous colitis.

TABLE 56.1 REPORTED ASSOCIATIONS OF MICROSCOPIC COLITIS AND OTHER AUTOIMMUNE DISEASES

Disease	Association (%)	Reference
Celiac disease	6–10	6 &11
Thyroid disease	≤20	6 &12
Diabetes mellitus	≤10	6
Rheumatoid arthritis	≤2.5	6

From Mulder CJ, et al. Microscopic colitis. Romanian Journal of Gastroenterology 2004; 13:113–117.

These lymphocytes are predominantly $CD8^+$ T lymphocytes with the αβ heterodimer, whereas the lymphocytes in the lamina propria are dominated by $CD4^+$ T lymphocytes. However, the distribution of $CD8^+$ T lymphocytes in the epithelium versus $CD4^+$ T lymphocytes in the lamina propria is the same as in normal intestinal mucosa.

Luminal agent

The observation that diversion of the fecal stream can normalize or reduce the histopathologic changes in collagenous colitis support the hypothesis that a luminal agent injures the epithelial barrier, stimulating the formation of a new subepithelial collagen barrier.[13] The luminal agent might be phagocytosed by macrophages and then presented to immunocompetent cells, stimulating immune and inflammatory responses and fibroblast proliferation, and possibly more collagen deposits. No agent has been identified; *Yersinia enterocolitica* has been suggested,[14] and the resolution of collagenous colitis after antibiotic treatment supports the microbiologic hypothesis.[15] Nitric oxide and plasma nitrate and nitrite levels are increased in patients with collagenous colitis, but whether the source is inflamed mucosa or bacterial is unclear.[5,16]

Nonsteroidal anti-inflammatory drugs (NSAIDs) and lansoprazole are the best known drug causes of microscopic colitis,[4,17,18] and some suggest that NSAID-associated colitis should be classified as a distinct entity,[18] with histopathologic features of collagenous colitis and hypoproteinemia. This might be caused by NSAID-induced protein-losing enteropathy. The watery stool can even contain mucus and/or blood. Ulcerations and perforations have been described.[18] NSAIDs inhibit the synthesis of prostaglandins, especially of PGE_2, and stimulate the production of collagen.[17] Withdrawal of NSAIDs is usually followed by improvement of the clinical and histological abnormalities.[6]

Lansoprazole-induced microscopic colitis shows histopathologic abnormalities as seen in collagenous colitis and lymphocytic colitis. The mechanism is unexplained. Toxic or immunologic factors may be involved. Symptoms are watery stool and mild abdominal pain. These complaints can occur in up to 5% of lansoprazole users.[19] Discontinuing the drug resolves the complaints and the histological appearance normalizes.[20] Similar case reports have been made for other proton pump inhibitors, but these observations have not been confirmed by others.[20,21] Other agents associated with microscopic colitis are ticlopidine (lymphocytic colitis),[22] cimetidine,[23] ranitidine (lymphocytic colitis and collagenous colitis),[24] Cyclo 3 Fort (lymphocytic colitis),[5,25] carbamazepine (lymphocytic colitis),[26] simvastatin,[27] vinca alkaloid (lymphocytic colitis),[28] Tardyferon (lymphocytic colitis),[29] and a case of acarbose (lymphocytic colitis).[30]

Fibroblast dysfunction

A dysfunction in synthesis of the fibroblast has been reported. Decreased levels of interstitial collagenase (matrix metalloproteinase-1; MMP-1) and increased expression of tissue inhibitor of MMP-1 (TIMP-1) have been found in patients with microscopic colitis, suggesting that reduced matrix degradation and not overactivation of matrix synthesis leads to subepithelial accumulation of matrix proteins such as collagen type III and, especially, type IV and tenascin. These findings indicate that inadequate local fibrinolysis is a major cause of collagen accumulation in collagenous colitis.[31,32]

The basement membrane consists of collagen type IV. In collagenous colitis, the collagen layer beneath the basement membrane consists of collagen types I, III, IV, and VI. Collagens I and III are thought to be important in tissue repair.[7,17] However, type VI collagen might be considered to be a pathologic collagen deposition.[17]

CLINICAL PRESENTATION

The onset of microscopic colitis is insidious in 60% of cases and (sub)acute in 40%. The main symptoms are:

- watery diarrhea (4–10 stools per day)
- nocturnal diarrhea
- fecal urgency
- bloating
- abdominal pain
- abdominal distention with relief by flatulence.

Sometimes symptoms are intermittent. Weight loss is quite common. Dehydration is uncommon. When sticky feces are found, celiac disease should be suspected. In contrast, persistent diarrhea in treated celiacs indicates a strong likelihood of microscopic colitis.

The course of microscopic colitis is relapsing and benign.[6] Sometimes, patients are socially disabled caused by frequent diarrhea. Although the majority of patients are females, the symptoms and progression are similar in men and women.

Laboratory findings may show a mildly raised erythrocyte sedimentation rate, a normocytemic anemia, and occasionally abnormalities in serum levels of IgG, C3 or C4.[33] Differences in HLA haplotype between patients with collagenous colitis and those with lymphocytic colitis have been suggested. In lymphocytic colitis there is an increase in the HLA-A1 and a decrease in the HLA-A3 haplotype, whereas in collagenous colitis there are no differences between patients and controls;[7] however, data are limited. Microbiologic findings remain negative. Steatorrhea and increased excretion of fecal leukocytes are reported in more than 50% of patients.[5] P-ANCA and other autoimmunologic factors are found, implicating a link with autoimmune diseases. For diagnosis, colonoscopy is preferred over sigmoidoscopy because of the patchy distribution and proximal predominance of the collagenous layer. Little correlation has been found in diagnostic accuracy between sigmoidoscopy and colonoscopy.[5,34,35] Radiology is not helpful in recognizing microscopic colitis.

DIAGNOSTIC METHODS

Diagnosis is based on the classic symptoms of chronic watery diarrhea without blood, abdominal pain, normal blood test results, no signs of small bowel malabsorption, and normal microbiologic, radiologic, and endoscopic findings. The pathophysiology of the watery diarrhea has been investigated, paying particular attention to the disturbed electrolyte and water transport in collagenous colitis.[36] The mechanisms for diarrhea in microscopic colitis include:

- malabsorption of fluid due to impaired transport and collagenous bands
- secretory diarrhea due to anion (chloride) secretion
- 'leak flux-induced diarrhea' due to an impaired epithelial barrier secondary to lymphocyte infiltration and thickening of the collagenous band (similar to findings for *Yersinia* colitis),[36] and to a passive backleak of ions and water into the intestinal lumen. This is probably related to decreased function of the tight junctions.[36]

The definitive diagnosis of microscopic colitis relies on histologic examination of biopsies taken from the colon, characterized by:

1. A diffuse thickening of the collagen layer beneath the basement membrane in a patchy manner throughout the colon in collagenous colitis but absent in lymphocytic colitis, with lymphocytic infiltration in the lamina propria in collagenous colitis and more pronounced in lymphocytic colitis. The presence of more than 10 intraepithelial lymphocytes per 100 epithelial cells seems specific and helpful for the diagnosis of collagenous colitis and/or lymphocytic colitis.[6] The thickness of the subepithelial layer in normal individuals varies from 0 to 3 μm.[1] A thickness of 10 μm or more has been accepted as establishing the diagnosis of collagenous colitis. A collagen thickness exceeding 45 μm might be an epithelial barrier.[36,37] Stool weight correlates with severity of mucosal inflammation and not with collagen thickness.[5]
2. The inflammation in the lamina propria is dominated by lymphocytes and plasma cells. Eosinophils and mast cells may be found, but neutrophils are rarely observed.[7] Cryptitis and crypt abscesses do not exclude the diagnosis of microscopic colitis.[38]
3. The epithelial cells appear to be flattened and vacuolized. Intraepithelial lymphocyte infiltration is present, but is more prominent in lymphocytic colitis.
4. Subtle endoscopic changes, such as mucosal edema, erythema, or mucosal paleness, have been described in up to 30% of cases. Detachment of the surface epithelium can occur. Hemorrhagic mucosal laceration after insufflation has been recognized in patients with collagenous colitis and a thick collagen layer.[39]

Biopsies of macroscopically normal mucosa are mandatory in patients with diarrhea.[4]

Changes elsewhere in the gut

Case reports have been made of subepithelial collagen deposits in the duodenal and ileal mucosa of patients with collagenous colitis, so-called collagenous enterocolitis.[7] Collagenous gastritis in combination with collagenous colitis has been reported.[17,40] Collagenous and lymphocytic gastritis seem to be strongly associated with celiac disease in up to 40% of the patients.[41] Considering the benign course of the disease with no evidence of premalignant potential, there appears to be no need for routine follow-up colonoscopy.[5,37,42]

Treatment

Treatment of microscopic colitis is empiric, via a stepwise approach:

1. The first and most important step is to ban all NSAIDs and other colitis-inducing medications.[5] Additional medication is mostly symptomatic, for example bismuth subsalicylate, antidiarrheals (loperamide, dephenoxylate, atropine), and a high-fiber diet. Although bismuth is effective and well tolerated, its use in western Europe is limited because it is not readily available.[43]
2. 5-Aminosalicylic acid (5-ASA) agents might be helpful (45% response);[4,44] Bonner et al. found a short-term response in 17 (77%) of 22 patients taking an average 5-ASA dose of 1500 mg over a 6-week period.[44]
3. (Topical) corticosteroids, immunosuppressives such as azathioprine, and octreotide may be useful.
4. As a last resort, surgery can be considered. In the authors' experience, surgery has never been necessary.

In some studies, 40% of the subjects had complete resolution of symptoms without therapy.[6] Loperamide, dephenoxylate, and bismuth subsalicylate were effective treatments and were well tolerated.[6] Some patients develop disabling pouchitis after surgery.

TREATMENT AND PREVENTION

REPORTED TREATMENT OPTIONS FOR MICROSCOPIC COLITIS

Drug	Dosage (mg)	Response (%)	Reference
5-ASA	1500	80	4, 44
Corticosteroid	40–60	–	11
Budesonide	9	–	31, 32, 45
Azathioprine	2 mg/kg	–	47, 48

From Mulder CJ, et al. Microscopic colitis. Romanian Journal of Gastroenterology 2004; 13:113–117.

For most patients, the usually benign course of microscopic colitis does not justify prolonged use of steroids. Budesonide is a topical steroid with high lipophilicity, leading to both a high receptor-binding affinity and a high first-pass effect in the liver. The clinical efficiency of budesonide in inflammatory bowel disease is not significantly different to that of prednisolone, but it has fewer significant side effects.[31] Budesonide has effects on both the inflammatory mucosal changes and the thickness of the collagen band.[32,45] The recommended dosage for these patients is 9 mg budesonide for the duration of the course of treatment.[32,43,46]

Azathioprine and methotrexate should be considered in steroid-dependent and steroid-refractory patients,[47,48] or as a steroid-sparing agent. Data for these drug treatments are limited. Azathioprine seems to be successful in a dose of 2 mg/kg daily.[47] The long-term follow-up results are promising, with high response rates.[44] In a minority of patients the diarrhea remains severe despite treatment. In these patients a diverting ileostomy with or without a colectomy is effective, interestingly showing normal ileostomic volumes after surgery.[5] The data are similar for collagenous colitis and lymphocytic colitis. Abdo et al.[49] investigated several clinical and histologic predictors of response in the treatment of collagenous colitis. They found that the age of onset was significant: older patients were most likely to be controlled with antidiarrheal agents or no medication. The younger patients needed more medication. NSAID use at the time of presentation was associated with a greater need for 5-ASA and steroid therapy.[4,49] Interestingly, cessation of NSAIDs did not affect the course in 60% of patients. In addition, the degree of inflammation of the lamina propria may be used as a predictor. The more intense the inflammation, the more likely the patient is to fail on symptomatic treatment.[49]

SOURCES OF INFORMATION FOR PATIENTS AND DOCTORS

http://digestive.niddk.nih.gov/ddiseases/pubs/collagenouscolitis/
http://www.emedicine.com/med/topic1351.htm
http://www.finerhealth.com/Educational_Info/Microscopic_Colitis/ FAQ/

REFERENCES

1. Lindström CG. Collagenous colitis: with watery diarrhoea – a new entity? Pathol Eur 1976; 11:87–89.
2. Read NW, Krejs GJ, Read MG et al. Chronic diarrhoea of unknown origin. Gastroenterology 1980; 78:264–267.
3. Lazenby AJ, Yardley JH, Giardiello FM et al. Lymphocytic ("microscopic") colitis: a comparative histopathologic study with particular reference to collagenous colitis. Hum Pathol 1989; 20:18–28.
4. Kitchen PA, Levi AJ, Domizio P, Talbot IC, Forbes A, Price AB and the London Inflammatory Bowel Disease Forum. Microscopic colitis: the tip of the iceberg? Eur J Gastroenterol Hepatol 2002; 14:1199–1204.
5. Tremaine WJ. Collagenous colitis and lymphocytic colitis. J Clin Gastroenterol 2000; 30: 245–249.
6. Pardi DS, Ramnath VR, Loftus EV Jr, Tremaine WJ, Sandborn WJ. Lymphocytic colitis: clinical features, treatment, and outcomes. Am J Gastroenterol 2002; 97:2829–2833.
7. Bohr JA. Review of collagenous colitis. Scand J Gastroenterol 1998; 33:2–9.
8. Thomson A, Kaye G. Further report of familial occurrence of collagenous colitis. Scand J Gastroenterol 2002; 37:1116.
9. Jarnerot G, Hertervig E, Granno C et al. Familial occurrence of microscopic colitis: a report on five families. Scand J Gastroenterol 2001; 36:959–962.
10. Bohr J, Tysk C, Yang P, Danielsson D, Jarnerot G. Autoantibodies and immunoglobulins in collagenous colitis. Gut 1996; 39:73–76.
11. Rostami K, Meijer JWR, Mulder CJJ. Collagenous colitis – an epiphenomenon of autoimmune disorders? Rom J Gastroenterol 2000; 9:87–90.
12. Cindoruk M, Tuncer C, Dursun A et al. Increased colonic intraepithelial lymphocytes in patients with Hashimoto's thyroiditis. J Clin Gastroenterol 2002; 34:237–239.
13. Jarnerot G, Bohr J, Tysk C, Eriksson S. Faecal stream diversion in patients with collagenous colitis. Gut 1996; 38:154–155.
14. Bohr J, Nordfelth R, Jarnerot G, Tysk C. *Yersinia* species in collagenous colitis: a serologic study. Scand J Gastroenterol 2002; 37:711–714.
15. Narayani RI, Burton MP, Young GS. Resolution of collagenous colitis after treatment of *Helicobacter pylori*. Am J Gastroenterol 2002; 97:498–499.
16. Lundberg JO, Herulf M, Olesen M et al. Increased nitric oxide production in collagenous and lymphocytic colitis. Eur J Clin Invest 1997; 27:869–871.
17. Castellano VM, Munoz MT, Colina F, Nevado M, Casis B, Solis-Herruzo JA. Collagenous gastrobulbitis and collagenous colitis. Case report and review of the literature. Scand J Gastroenterol 1999; 34:632–638.
18. Yagi K, Nakamura A, Sekine A, Watanabe H. Nonsteroidal anti-inflammatory drug-associated colitis with a history of collagenous colitis. Endoscopy 2001; 33:629–632.
19. Freston JW. Long-term acid control and proton pump inhibitors: interactions and safety issues in perspective. Am J Gastroenterol 1997; 92: 51S–55S.
20. Thomson RD, Lestina LS, Bensen SP et al. Lanzoprazole-associated microscopic colitis: a case series. Am J Gastroenterol 2002; 97: 2908–2913.
21. Wilcox, Gilbert M. Collagenous colitis associated with lansoprazole. J Clin Gastroenterol 2002; 34:164–166.
22. Berrebi D, Sautet A, Flejou JF et al. Ticlopidine induced colitis: a histological study including apoptosis. J Clin Pathol 1998; 22:280–283.
23. Duncan HD, Talbot IC, Silk DB. Collagenous colitis and cimetidine. Eur J Gastroenterol Hepatol 1997; 9:819–820.
24. Beaugerie L, Patey N, Brousse N. Ranitidine, diarrhea, and lymphocytic colitis. Gut 1995; 37:708–711.
25. Beaugerie L, Luboinski J, Brousse N et al. Drug induced lymphocytic colitis. Gut 1994; 35:426–428.
26. Mahajan L, Wyllie R, Goldblum J. Lymphocytic colitis in a pedriatric patient: a possible adverse reaction to carbamazepine. Am J Gastroenterol 1997; 92:2126–2127.
27. Chagnon JP, Cerf M. Simvastatin-induced protein-losing enteropathy. Am J Gastroenterol 1992; 87:257.
28. Chauveau E, Prignet JM, Carloz E et al. Lymphocytic colitis likely attributable to use of vinburnine (Cervoxan). Gastroenterol Clin Biol 1998; 22:362.
29. Bouchet-Laneuw F, Deplaix P, Dumollard JM et al. Chronic diarrhea following of ingestion of Tardyferon associated with lymphocytic colitis. Gastroenterol Clin Biol 1997; 21:83–84.
30. Piche T, Raimondi V, Schneider S et al. Acarbose and lymphocytic colitis. Lancet 2000; 356:1246.
31. Tromm A, Griga T, Mollmann HW et al. Budesonide for the treatment of collagenous colitis: first results of a pilot trial. Am J Gastroenterol 1999; 94:1871–1875.
32. Miehlke S, Haymer P, Bethke B et al. Budesonide treatment for collagenous colitis: a randomized, double-blind, placebo-controlled, multicenter trial. Gastroenterology 2002; 123:978–984.
33. Bohr J, Tysk C, Eriksson S et al. Collagenous colitis: a retrospective study of clinical presentation and treatment in 163 patients. Gut 1996; 39:846–851.
34. Shah DI et al. Usefulness of colonoscopy with biopsy in the evaluation of patients with chronic diarrhea. Am J Gastroenterol 2001; 96:1091–1095.
35. Matteoni C, Wang N, Goldblum JR et al. Flexible sigmoidoscopy for the detection of microscopic colitis. Am J Gastroenterol 2000; 108:416–418.
36. Bürgel N, Bojarski C, Mankertz J et al. Mechanisms of diarrhea in collagenous colitis. Gastroenterology 2002; 123:433–443.
37. Bonderup OK, Folkersen BH, Gjersoe P, Teglbjaerg PS. Collagenous colitis: a long-term follow-up study. Eur J Gastroenterol Hepatol 1999; 11:493–495.
38. Jessurun J, Yardley JH, Giardiello FM et al. Chronic colitis with thickening of the subepithelial layer (collagenous colitis) histopathologic findings in 15 patients. Hum Pathol 1987; 18:839–848.
39. Cruz-Correa M, Milligan F, Giardiello FM et al. Collagenous colitis with mucosal tears on endoscopic insufflation: a unique presentation. Gut 2002; 51:600.
40. Vesoulis Z, Lozanski G, Ravichandran P, Esber E. Collagenous gastritis: a case report, morphologic evaluation, and review. Mod Pathol 2000; 13:591–596.
41. Stancu M, De Petris G, Palumbo TP, Lev R. Collagenous gastritis associated with lymphocytic gastritis and celiac disease. Arch Pathol Lab Med 2001; 125:1579–1584.
42. Chan JL, Tersmette AC, Offerhaus GJ et al. Cancer risk in collagenous colitis. Inflamm Bowel Dis 1999; 5:40–43.
43. Baert F, Schmit A, D'Haens G et al. Budesonide in collagenous colitis: a double-blind, placebo-controlled trial with histological follow up. Gastroenterology 2002; 122:20–25.
44. Bonner GF, Petras RE, Cheung DM et al. Short- and long-term follow-up of treatment for lymphocytic and collagenous colitis. Inflamm Bowel Dis 2000; 6:85–91.
45. Bonderup OK, Hansen JB, Birket-Smith L et al. Budesonide treatment of collagenous colitis: a randomised, double blind, placebo controlled trial with morphometric analysis. Gut 2003; 52:248–251.
46. Bonderup OK et al. Budesonide treatment of collagenous colitis: a randomized, double blind, placebo-controlled trial. Gut 2001; 49(Suppl III):A1906.
47. Vennamaneni SR, Bonner GF. Use of azathioprine or 6-mercaptopurine for treatment of steroid-dependent lymphocytic and collagenous colitis. Am J Gastroenterol 2001; 96: 2798–2799.
48. Pardi DS, Loftus EV Jr, Tremaine WJ, Sandborn WJ. Treatment of refractory microscopic colitis with azathioprine and 6-mercaptopurine. Gastroenterology 2001; 120:1483–1484.
49. Abdo A, Raboud J, Freeman HJ et al. Clinical and histological predictors of response to medical therapy in collagenous colitis. Am J Gastroenterol 2002; 97:1164–1168.

Chapter 57

Eosinophilic esophago-gastroenteritis

Jon A Vanderhoof and Rosemary J Young

KEY POINTS

- Eotaxin, IL-3, IL-5, and GM-CSF factor all have a role in stimulating eosinophils
- A personal or family history of atopy is common
- Eosinophilic gastroenteritis is manifested by a peripheral eosinophilia, diarrhea, and malabsorption
- Diagnosis based on history of gastrointestinal symptoms, histologic evidence of eosinophil infiltration (greater than 20/HPF), and exclusion of parasite infection
- Eosinophils in submucosal, muscular, or serosal layers is considered abnormal
- Peripheral eosinophilia, hypoalbuminemia, and raised IgE, ESR and fecal α-1antitrypsin are diagnostic clues
- Intermittent courses of corticosteroids are the mainstay of treatment
- Cromolyn sodium and montelukast are possible therapies
- Eosinophilic esophagitis is increasingly recognized in patients with dysphagia unresponsive to PPIs

INTRODUCTION

The true extent of eosinophilic disease in the gut is largely unknown but it appears to affect all age groups. The clearly defined syndrome of classic eosinophilic gastroenteritis has been well understood for a number of years. More recently, it has been appreciated that eosinophilic diseases of the gut also cause syndromes of infant diarrhea and of esophagitis and constipation in adults. Therapies utilizing anti-inflammatory agents such as corticosteroids are effective in many instances. Some patients have various manifestations of dietary allergies resulting in more precisely defined eosinophilic disorders, which may be treated through avoidance of specific allergens.

PATHOGENIC PROCESSES

Eosinophils are thought to be recruited in excess numbers by eotaxin, a chemoattractant produced by irritation in the epithelial cells.[1] The mechanism that stimulates eosinophil formation is not well understood but interleukin (IL)-3, IL-5, and granulocyte-macrophage colony-stimulating factor (GM-CSF) are thought to be involved.[2] The activated eosinophils generate the cytotoxic products causing tissue damage and subsequent development of symptoms.

CLASSIC EOSINOPHILIC GASTROENTERITIS

This consists of eosinophilic inflammatory changes anywhere in the gastrointestinal tract, often accompanied by peripheral eosinophilia, and often with diarrhea and malabsorption. Infiltration of the deeper layers of the gut results in additional symptoms of abdominal pain and serosal inflammation may result in ascites. In many cases, there is a family history of allergic disorders but the true cause is somewhat obscure.

Classic eosinophilic gastroenteritis often begins with mild and variable symptoms making the diagnosis difficult. Severity of the symptoms often increases over time and may even become debilitating, regardless of treatment. Some patients exhibit symptoms only in response to certain trigger factors such as food, while others have seasonal exacerbations. Typically, patients with eosinophilic duodenitis or enteritis have abdominal pain with or without diarrhea. Eosinophilic colitis may present with abdominal pain and diarrhea.

Diagnosis

The diagnosis of eosinophilic gastroenteritis is based on the presence of gastrointestinal symptoms, the demonstration of eosinophilic infiltration in gastrointestinal biopsies, and the exclusion of parasitic infections (see Chapter 52). The differential diagnosis of eosinophilic gastroenteritis also includes early inflammatory bowel disease (see Chapters 53–55), connective tissue diseases, immunological disorders, and adverse effects of drugs.

Generally, visual endoscopic findings of the upper and lower gastrointestinal tract are normal. Small numbers of eosinophils are normally present in the lamina propria of the gastrointestinal tract to protect against parasitic and minor allergic irritants. Grading the severity of eosinophilic gastroenteritis has been attempted and it is generally agreed that greater than 20 eosinophils per high-powered field are required for a histological diagnosis.[3,4] Although there is no general agreement on what increased level constitutes a pathological condition, the presence of any eosinophils in submucosa, muscular, or serosal layers is considered abnormal.

The gastric antrum is often involved in eosinophilic gastroenteritis but eosinophilic infiltrates can be patchy in nature and necessitates multiple biopsy specimens for appropriate identification. If the small bowel and colonic biopsies reveal increased eosinophilic inflammatory changes, increased mononuclear cells, neutrophils, and intraepithelial lymphocytes may also be noted. Endoscopic visualization often reveals increased lymphoid hyperplasia.[5] Superficial biopsy specimens lacking the muscular and serosal layers may obscure diagnostic findings as well and, therefore, a full thickness biopsy may occasionally be needed.[6]

Peripheral eosinophilia, an elevated immunoglobulin E (IgE) and sedimentation rate, hypoalbuminemia, and increased fecal α-1 antitrypsin may assist in the diagnosis of eosinophilic gastroenteritis. Radiologic findings are uncommon but in severe cases, esophageal narrowing and antral stenosis may be identified on barium studies.[7] Ultrasonography may also demonstrate gastrointestinal wall thickening and/or ascites.[8]

Treatment

Since the etiology of eosinophilic gastroenteritis is not known, treatment of the condition primarily relies on management of symptoms. Avoidance of certain foods is rarely helpful in widespread eosinophilic disease. Anti-inflammatory medications are therefore generally utilized. If symptoms are severe, initiation of high-dose systemic corticosteroid therapy may often be required; subsequent maintenance with less potent anti-inflammatory agents and diet therapy may be useful. Repeat administration of systemic steroids may be required if symptoms return. Other medications specifically targeting control of eosinophils have been explored. Case reports of cromolyn sodium and more recently montelukast have demonstrated success.[9–12] Ketotifen, which inhibits secretion of mast cell mediators such as histamine, and suplatast tosilate, a selective T-helper-2 cytokine IL-4 and IL-5 inhibitor, have been used in some cases of eosinophilic gastroenteritis with success.[11,12] Acid suppression may be used for patients with upper gastrointestinal symptoms. Treatment of other symptoms such as nausea may include medications such as ondansetron or prokinetic agents such as metaclopramide.

ALLERGIC ENTEROCOLITIS IN INFANCY

Pathogenesis

In infants, allergic enterocolitis is becoming more commonly appreciated. Between 2% and 7% of infants appear to be allergic to cows' milk protein, most of these through a non-IgE-mediated mechanism characterized by inflammatory changes in the small bowel or colon, often with increased peripheral eosinophilia.[13] About half of the babies who are allergic to milk also turn out to be allergic to soy. Some have been shown to be allergic to fragments of cows' milk protein in extensively hydrolyzed infant formulas and even to the cows' milk protein fragments present in breast milk.[14–16] Allergic infants seem to be more common in families with a strong history of food allergy. Atopic dermatitis often accompanies the inflammatory changes in the gut.

Epidemiology

The true incidence of cows' milk protein intolerance in babies is often difficult to determine because the presentation is extremely subtle and few, if any, laboratory parameters can reliably diagnose the condition. Likewise, response to dietary challenge is often delayed for a period of days to weeks and the therapeutic response to removal of cows' milk protein from the diet is slow, often taking up to 2–3 weeks for the inflammatory changes to clear and symptoms to totally resolve.

Clinical features

Symptoms in these infants are typical of many gastrointestinal problems. Blood streaked stools or bloody diarrhea is the symptom most easily identified and characteristic because of the inflammatory process in the colon.[17] More subtle inflammatory conditions may present with mild diarrhea and, often, irritability or colicky-like symptoms.[18] Because of poor oral intake, these infants often manifest poor growth. Symptoms vary based upon the location of the mucosal injury. Infants with predominantly small bowel disease will present with diarrhea, malabsorption, and poor intake. Chronic irritability is common and, because of delayed gastric emptying, gastroesophageal reflux is also common. In infants with predominantly large bowel inflammatory changes, bloody stools containing large quantities of mucus are more typical.

Older infants and children who react to cows' milk protein often do so through an IgE-mediated mechanism. In this situation, symptoms are often quite abrupt in onset and, likewise resolve quickly if the antigen is removed.[19] Foods other than cow's milk protein may also be involved. Cutaneous and systemic manifestations are likewise common. These children may experience anaphylaxis, trouble in breathing, or develop severe skin manifestations. In infants with non-IgE-mediated allergic enterocolitis, IgE testing to a specific antigen either by skin test or RAST test is not of significant benefit.[18]

Treatment

Although soy protein formulas are often used as the initial therapeutic modality in such infants, many of these infants will relapse after a few days or weeks on soy with recurrence of symptoms and reappearance of histologic inflammatory changes.[20] Most will effectively resolve on protein hydrolysate formulas provided the proteins in the formulas are extensively hydrolyzed.[21] Partially hydrolyzed infant formulas are not beneficial and should be avoided in such infants.[15] Occasionally, the use of an amino acid-based infant formula is required for a small number of such infants.[22] Breast-fed infants are typically treated by eliminating cows' milk and occasionally certain other common dietary antigens from the mother's diet.[23]

ALLERGIC CONSTIPATION

Clinico-pathological features

Recently, the association with constipation and milk allergy has been reported by Iacono et al.[24] Numerous reports have confirmed this association.[25–28] The clinical characteristics of this syndrome include severe constipation with extreme difficulty in expelling stool, as well as unresponsiveness to traditional medical management. The history of formula intolerance in an infant often precedes the clinical syndrome.[25] Abdominal pain accompanies the constipation and is frequently periumbilical and poorly described. Colonic lymphoid hyperplasia and focal tissue eosinophilia may be present in small bowel biopsies as well.

Treatment

Following a short course of laxative therapy, prolonged dietary restriction is required. Treatment with a cows' milk protein-free diet often relieves both the symptoms and the histological abnormalities.[25]

ALLERGIC ESOPHAGITIS

Clinico-pathological features

The syndrome of allergic esophagitis has also been recently appreciated. These patients may present at any age from early childhood to adulthood. While symptoms of gastroesophageal reflux including heartburn may be present, the more typical presentation is one of dysphagia.[29] Frequently, recurrent food impaction in the esophagus occurs. The disorder should be suspected in the presence of poor response to aggressive treatment with proton pump inhibitors. Endoscopy often reveals concentric rings or trachealization typical of esophageal spasm (Fig. 57.1). Small white patches of exudate (clusters of eosinophils) have been noted in eosinophilic infiltration of the esophagus.[6] Biopsies reveal dense eosinophilic infiltrate within the esophageal epithelium (Fig. 57.2).

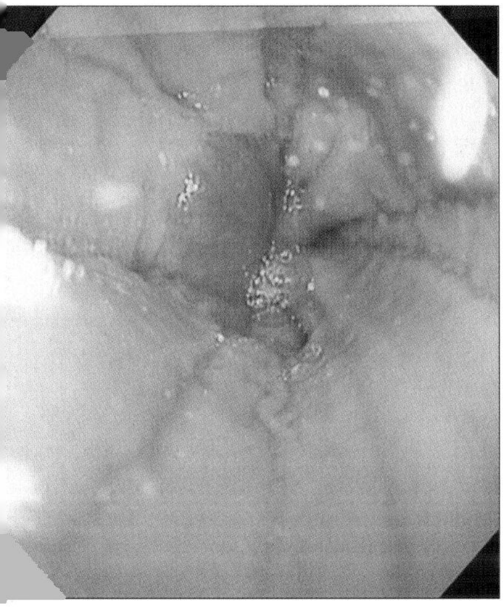

Fig. 57.1 Endoscopy. Concentric rings and white exudates in a 29-year-old male with dysphagia. Histology confirmed eosinophilic esophagitis. Image courtesy of Dr Paul Fortun.

Treatment

If symptoms are severe, systemic steroid therapy may be required followed by less potent anti-inflammatory medications and dietary restrictions. The older the patient, the less likely will be the response to dietary therapy as a sole treatment. Most recently, the benefit of fluticasone, an inhalable corticosteroid that is swallowed, has been shown to be of particular benefit for eosinophilic esophagitis thus avoiding systemic steroid side effects.[30, 31]

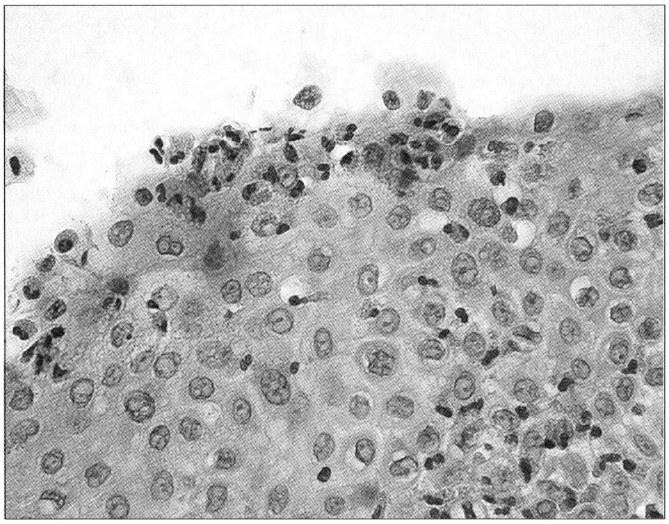

Fig. 57.2 Esophageal squamous epithelium. Esophageal squamous epithelium infiltrated by abundant eosinophils with bright orange granules (H&E ×200). This biopsy is from a 16-year-old boy who presented with food impaction. Image courtesy of Dr Philip Kaye.

CONCLUSION

Eosinophilic disorders of the gastrointestinal tract are rarely known to be fatal and, although previously considered to be rare, seem to be on the increase; this is probably due to greater awareness of the condition and better diagnostic methodologies. Although treatment traditionally responds to immunosuppression with corticosteroids, current knowledge of the pathophysiological mechanisms has led to the use of alternative therapies including restrictive diet and pharmacologic agents targeted at decreasing the eosinophilic response. Placebo-controlled trials are lacking primarily due to small patient numbers and highly variable symptoms but are needed.

SOURCES OF INFORMATION FOR DOCTORS AND PATIENTS

http://www.emedicine.com/med/topic688.htm
http://answers.google.com/answers/threadview?id=423853

REFERENCES

1. Bischoff SC. Mucosal allergy: role of mast cells and eosinophil granulocytes in the gut. Baillières Clin Gastroenterol 1996; 10:443–459.
2. Rankin SM, Conroy DM, Williams TJ. Eotaxin and eosinophil recruitment: implications for human disease. Mol Med Today 2000; 6:20–27.
3. Talley NJ, Shorter RG, Phillips SF, Zinsmeister AR. Eosinophilic gastroenteritis: a clinicopathological study of patients with disease of the mucosa, muscle layer, and subserosal tissues. Gut 1990; 31:54–58.
4. Whitington PF, Whitington GL. Eosinophilic gastroenteropathy in childhood. J Pediatr Gastroenterol Nutr 1988; 7:379–385.
5. Bellanti JA, Zeligs BJ, Malka-Rais J, Sabra A. Abnormalities of Th1 function in non-IgE food allergy, celiac disease, and ileal lymphonodular hyperplasia: a new relationship? Ann Allergy Asthma Immunol 2003; 90(Suppl 3):84–89.
6. Khan S, Orenstein SR. Eosinophilic gastroenteritis: epidemiology, diagnosis and management. Paediatr Drugs 2002; 4:563–570.
7. Blackshaw AJ, Levison DA. Eosinophilic infiltrates of the gastrointestinal tract. J Clin Pathol 1986; 39:1–7.
8. Stevoff C, Rao SA, Parsons W, et al. EUS and histopathologic correlates in eosinophilic esophagitis. Gastrointest Endosc 2001; 54:373–377.
9. Perez-Millan A, Martin-Lorente JL, Lopez-Morante A, et al. Subserosal eosinophilic gastroenteritis treated efficaciously with sodium cromoglycate. Dig Dis Sci 1997; 42:342–344.
10. Vanderhoof JA, Young RJ, Hanner TL, Kettlehut B. Montelukast: use in pediatric patients with eosinophilic gastrointestinal disease. J Pediatr Gastroenterol Nutr 2003; 36:293–294.
11. Melamed I, Feanny SJ, Sherman PM, Roifman CM. Benefit of ketotifen in patients with eosinophilic gastroenteritis. Am J Med 1991; 90:310–314.
12. Shirai T, Hashimoto D, Suzuki K, et al. Successful treatment of eosinophilic gastroenteritis with suplatast tosilate. J Allergy Clin Immunol 2001; 107:924–925.
13. Host A. Frequency of cow's milk allergy in childhood. Ann Allergy Asthma Immunol 2002; 89(Suppl 1):33–37.
14. Rozenfeld P, Docena GH, Anon MC, Fossati CA. Detection and identification of a soy protein component that cross-reacts with caseins from cow's milk. Clin Exp Immunol 2002; 130:49–58.
15. Vanderhoof JA, Murray ND, Kaufman SS, et al. Intolerance to protein hydrolysate infant formulas: an underrecognized cause of gastrointestinal symptoms in infants. J Pediatr 1997; 131:741–744.
16. Pumberger W, Pomberger G, Geissler W. Proctocolitis in breast fed infants: a

contribution to differential diagnosis of haematochezia in early childhood. Postgrad Med J 2001; 77:252–254.
17. Fox VL. Gastrointestinal bleeding in infancy and childhood. Gastroenterol Clin North Am 2000; 29:37–66, v.
18. Sicherer SH. Clinical aspects of gastrointestinal food allergy in childhood. Pediatrics 2003; 111:1609–1616.
19. Kaplan MS. Complications in children with a severe allergy to cow milk. Ann Allergy 1993; 71:529–532.
20. Chandra RK. Five-year follow-up of high-risk infants with family history of allergy who were exclusively breast-fed or fed partial whey hydrolysate, soy, and conventional cow's milk formulas. J Pediatr Gastroenterol Nutr 1997; 24:380–388.
21. Vanderhoof JA. Chronic diarrhea. Pediatr Rev 1998; 19:418–422.
22. de Boissieu D, Dupont C. Allergy to extensively hydrolyzed cow's milk proteins in infants: safety and duration of amino acid-based formula. J Pediatr 2002; 141:271–273.
23. Arshad SH. Food allergen avoidance in primary prevention of food allergy. Allergy 2001; 56 (Suppl 67):113–116.
24. Iacono G et al. Intolerance of cow's milk and chronic constipation in children. N Engl J Med 1998; 339:1100–1104.
25. Vanderhoof JA et al. Allergic constipation: association with infantile milk allergy. Clin Pediatr (Phila) 2001; 40:399–402.
26. Daher S et al. Cow's milk protein intolerance and chronic constipation in children. Pediatr Allergy Immunol 2001; 12:339–342.
27. Carroccio A et al. Evidence of very delayed clinical reactions to cow's milk in cow's milk intolerant patients. Allergy 2000; 55:574–57
28. Shah N, Lindley K, Milla P. Cow's milk and chronic constipation in children. N Engl J Med; 1999; 340:891–892.
29. Khan S, Orenstein SR, Di Lorenzo C, et al. Eosinophilic esophagitis: strictures, impaction dysphagia. Dig Dis Sci 2003; 48:22–29.
30. Faubion WA Jr, Perrault J, Burgart LJ, et al. Treatment of eosinophilic esophagitis with inhaled corticosteroids. J Pediatr Gastroenter Nutr 1998; 27:90–93.
31. Teitelbaum JE, Fox VL, Twarog FJ, et al. Eosinophilic esophagitis in children: immunopathological analysis and response to fluticasone propionate. Gastroenterology 2002; 122:1216–1225.

Chapter 58

Pseudomembranous colitis

Elizabeth Broussard and Christina Surawicz

KEY POINTS
• *Clostridium difficile* is the commonest enteric nosocomial infection in the US • Most antibiotics are implicated but clindamycin, cephalosporins and amoxicillin are the commonest culprits • Fulminant colitis occurs in 2–3% of affected patients • Assays for toxin A and toxin B are reliable tests • Metronidazole is the first-line drug of choice • Preventative measures are essential

INTRODUCTION

Pseudomembranous colitis (PMC) is defined as severe inflammation in the colon secondary to overgrowth of the organism *Clostridium difficile* with production of toxin A and toxin B; this usually occurs in the setting of antibiotic therapy, but sporadic cases can occur. *Clostridium difficile* is a Gram-positive, anaerobic spore-forming bacillus. *Clostridium difficile*-associated disease has become increasingly common as antibiotic usage has increased.

EPIDEMIOLOGY

Clostridium difficile is the leading cause of enteric nosocomial infection in US hospitals, with an estimated 3 million new cases of diarrhea and colitis annually, and affecting up to 10% of patients hospitalized for greater than 2 days.[1] The prevalence of PMC, the most severe form of *C. difficile* colitis, ranges from 0.1 to 10.1% of inpatients that receive penicillins or cephalosporins.[2] The major mode of transmission is patient-to-patient transmission, but transient carriage on healthcare workers' hands, stethoscopes, and clothing has also been documented, as well as contamination of commodes, neonatal bathing tubs, telephones, and rectal thermometers.[3,4]

CAUSES, RISK FACTORS, DISEASE ASSOCIATIONS

Advanced age and exposure to antibiotics are the major risk factors. Almost all antibiotics have been implicated with *C. difficile* diarrhea and colitis, but the most frequent culprits include clindamycin, cephalosporins, ampicillin, and amoxicillin.[5]

PATHOGENESIS AND PATHOLOGY

The pathophysiology of PMC follows a sequence of events, beginning with the disturbance of normal colonic microflora, exposure to and colonization by *C. difficile*, production of toxin and toxin-mediated inflammation and injury, and colonic damage. Interaction with host factors such as age, immunologic status, and coexisting disease also affect the course of this disease.[6] Table 58.1 outlines the effects of the toxins on the enterocyte.

PMC ranges in severity from inflammatory changes confined to superficial epithelium, to severe, intense necrosis of the full thickness of the mucosa with formation of a confluent layer of pseudomembrane (Fig. 58.1).

CLINICAL PRESENTATION

The incubation period can be as short as 1–5 days after starting antibiotics, or up to 1–5 weeks after antibiotics are discontinued. Patients present with watery diarrhea, abdominal cramps, anorexia, and fevers. When severe, marked leukocytosis and hypoalbuminemia occurs in up to 25% of patients.[2] Complications can include fulminant colitis in 2–3% of patients, colonic perforation, toxic megacolon, severe loss of intravascular volume, and electrolyte disturbances, prolonged ileus, and even death.

TABLE 58.1 OVERVIEW OF ENTEROTOXICITY FOR *CLOSTRIDIUM DIFFICILE* TOXINS

Direct toxin effects on the enterocyte	Subsequent effects in lamina propria
↓	↓
Binding of toxin to receptors	Release of cytokines from enterocytes
↓	↓
Internalization	Activation of mast cells, afferent neurons
↓	↓
Inactivation of Rho	Activation of afferent neurons
↓	↓
Disaggregation of actin filaments	Release of mast cell products, substance p
↓	↓
Cell rounding	Regulation of adhesion molecules on vascular epithelium
↓	↓
Impairment of tight junctions	Recruitment of neutrophils
↓	↓
DIARRHEA AND INFLAMMATION	

Reproduced with permission from LaMont JT. Updates on *Clostridium difficile*. Paris: Springer-Verlag; 1996:73–82.[7]

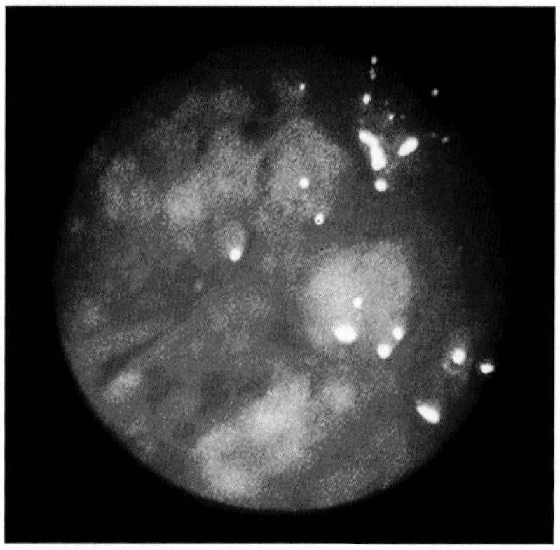

Fig. 58.1 Endoscopic appearance of PMC.

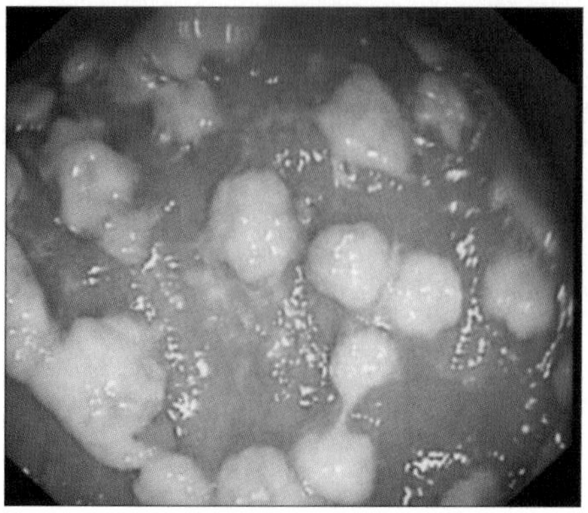

Fig. 58.2 PMC localized to the sigmoid colon. Severe pseudomembranous colitis localized to the sigmoid colon secondary to treatment with cephalosporin. *Clostridium difficile* toxin was detected in the stool. Photo courtesy of Dr Paul Fortun.

DIFFERENTIAL DIAGNOSIS

The differential diagnosis includes antibiotic-associated diarrhea, ischemic colitis, diarrhea caused by other enteric pathogens such as *Campylobacter jejuni, Clostridium perfringens, Salmonella, Shigella, Escherichia coli* 0157:H7 and *Yersinia*, adverse reactions to medications other than antibiotics such as chemotherapy and typhlitis (especially in patients receiving chemotherapy with Gram-positive cocci on stool specimen), inflammatory bowel disease, and intra-abdominal sepsis.

DIAGNOSTIC METHODS

Most pathogenic strains of *C. difficile* produce toxins A and B so a toxin assay is a reliable diagnostic test. Toxin assays detect toxins capable of causing a cytopathic effect in tissue culture cell lines, and can detect the presence of toxin B with a sensitivity and specificity of 95–100%. This method requires specialized facilities, costs about $30 to $40 per kit, and requires 24–48 h to produce results.

Enzyme-linked immunoassay (EIA) test kits detect *C. difficile* toxins A and B by using a monoclonal antibody, are relatively inexpensive, and are easier to perform than cytotoxicity tests, producing results in 2–6 h with good specificity but lower sensitivity than cytotoxin assay.[8]

A negative test, however, does not eliminate the possibility of disease, and if clinically indicated, the test should be repeated, or another test should be performed, and empiric therapy with antibiotics should be started.

Endoscopic examination is not necessary unless the diagnosis remains in doubt or rapid diagnosis is necessary. If endoscopic examination is performed, the presence of pseudomembranes is virtually pathognomonic for PMC. Pseudomembranes appear as off-white or yellow plaques, raised, 0.2–2.0 cm in diameter alternating with normal appearing mucosa, often with full thickness bowel wall edema and hyperemia (Fig. 58.2).

TREATMENT AND PREVENTION

The initial treatment is to stop the suspected culprit antibiotic; if that is not feasible, the antibiotic regimen should be switched to one less likely to exacerbate diarrhea,[9] preferably one that has a narrower spectrum of antibacterial activity. Pharmacological treatment should be initiated in all but the mildest cases. Metronidazole (500 mg p.o. t.i.d.) and vancomycin (125 mg p.o. q.i.d.) are equally effective in treating *C. difficile* infection, but metronidazole is the drug of choice.[10] It is far less expensive and does not select for vancomycin-resistant enterococci. However, in the critically ill patient, vancomycin may be recommended as first-line therapy,[11] especially if there has been no response to metronidazole. Patients that do not tolerate oral therapy can be treated with intravenous metronidazole, but this is much less effective.

Patients should not be considered therapeutic failures until they have completed 6 days of treatment, and treatment continued for 10 days is more likely to be successful. Some cases do take longer for improvement. Testing for cure by checking toxin assays after treatment is not recommended, as these results do not accurately predict relapse.[8,12,13]

Prevention is directly related to modes of transmission, and involves the use of disposable gloves, single-use disposable rectal thermometers, and hand washing using chlorhexidine and disinfection of patient environment with agents that kill *C. difficile* spores such as hypochlorous acid (Table 58.2).[14,15]

COMPLICATIONS AND THEIR MANAGEMENT

Recurrent *C. difficile* diarrhea occurs in 15–20% of patients, most often within 1–2 weeks of stopping therapy, but can appear as late as 4–6 weeks.[16] The treatment of a first relapse is the same as for initial treatment, and if symptoms persist, a second course with metronidazole or vancomycin for 10–14 days is given with tapering and pulsing the drug for several weeks after the initial 10 days.

TABLE 58.2 PRACTICE GUIDELINES FOR PREVENTION OF *CLOSTRIDIUM DIFFICILE* DIARRHEA

- Limit use of antimicrobial drugs
- Wash hands between contact with all patients
- Use enteric (stool) isolation precautions for patients with *C. difficile* diarrhea
- Wear gloves when contacting patients with *C. difficile* diarrhea/colitis or their environment
- Disinfect objects contaminated with *C. difficile* with sodium hypochlorite, alkaline glutaraldehyde, or ethylene oxide
- Educate the medical, nursing, and other appropriate staff members about the disease and its epidemiology

Reproduced from Fekety RF. Am J Gastroenterol 1997; 92:739–750.[16]

Patients with toxic megacolon who have failed medical therapy and have impending or known bowel perforation need surgical intervention with subtotal colectomy and ileostomy. The mortality rate is high, ranging from 32% to 50%,[17–19] which reflects the severity of illness in this patient population.

PROGNOSIS WITH AND WITHOUT TREATMENT

In cases of PMC that are diagnosed and where antibiotics are stopped, recovery occurs within 7 days. If the diagnosis is delayed and the culprit antibiotics are continued, then PMC can last up to 3 weeks. Mortality can be as high as 75% without treatment, as fulminant colitis and perforation have been associated with delayed diagnosis. Toxic megacolon necessitates surgical intervention in 65% to 71% of cases, with a mortality rate as high as 35%.[17–19]

SOURCES OF INFORMATION FOR PATIENTS AND DOCTORS

http://cchs-dl.slis.ua.edu/patientinfo/infectious/byorganism/bacterial/gram-positive/clostridial/antibiotic-associatedcolitis.htm

REFERENCES

1. McFarland LV, Mulligan ME, Kwok RY, Stamm WE. Nosocomial acquisition of *Clostridium difficile* infection. N Engl J Med 1989; 320:204–210.
2. Olson MM, Shanholtzer CJ, Lee JT, Gerding DN. Ten years of prospective *Clostridium difficile*-associated disease surveillance and treatment at the Minneapolis VA Medical Center, 1982–1991. Infect Control Hosp Epidemiol 1994; 15:371–381.
3. Kim KH, Fekety R, Batts DH et al. Isolation of *C. difficile* from the environment and contacts of patients with antibiotic-induced colitis. J Infect Dis 1981; 143:42–44.
4. Fekety R, Kim KH, Brown D et al. Epidemiology of AAC: Isolation of *C. difficile* from the hospital environment. Am J Med 1981; 70:906–908.
5. Hecht JR, Olinger EJ. *Clostridium difficile* colitis secondary to intravenous vancomycin. Dig Dis Sci 1989; 34:148–149.
6. Kyne L, Farrell RJ, Kelly CP. *Clostridium difficile*. Gastroenterol Clin 2001; 30:3.
7. LaMont JT. Recent advances in the structure and function of *Clostridium difficile* toxins. In: Rambaud JC, LaMont JT, eds. Updates on *Clostridium difficile*. Paris: Springer-Verlag; 1996:73–82.
8. McFarland LV. *Clostridium difficile*-associated disease. In: Surawicz CM, Owens RL, eds. Gastrointestinal and hepatic infections. Philadelphia: W.B. Saunders; 1995.
9. Kelly CP, Pothoulakis C, LaMont JT. *Clostridium difficile* colitis. N Engl J Med 1994; 330: 257–262.
10. Bartlett JG. AAPMC. Hosp Pract (Off Ed). 1981; 16:85–95.
11. Fekety, RF. Guidelines for the diagnosis and management of *Clostridium difficile*-associated diarrhea and colitis. Am J Gastroenterol 1997; 92:739–750.
12. Samore MH, DeGirolami PC, Tlucko A et al. *Clostridium difficile* colonization and diarrhea at a tertiary care hospital. Clin Infect Dis 1994; 18:181–187.
13. Cleary RK. *Clostridium difficile*-associated diarrhea and colitis: Clinical manifestations, diagnosis and treatment. Dis Colon Rectum 1998; 41:1435–1449.
14. Pierce PF, Wilson R, Silva J et al. AAPMC: An epidemiologic investigation of a cluster of cases. J Infect Dis 1982; 145:269–274.
15. Brooks SE, Veal RO, Kramer M et al. Reduction in the incidence of *Clostridium difficile*-associated diarrhea in an acute care hospital and a skilled nursing facility following replacement of electronic thermometers with single-use disposables. Infect Control Hosp Epidemiol 1992; 13:98–103.
16. Fekety RF. Guidelines for the diagnosis and management of *Clostridium difficile*-associated diarrhea and colitis. Am J Gastroenterol 1997; 92:739–750.
17. Bradbury AW, Barrett S. Surgical aspects of *Clostridium difficile* colitis. Br J Surg 1997; 84:150–159.
18. Morris JB, Zollinger RM, Stellato TA. Role of surgery in antibiotic-induced pseudomembranous colitis. Am J Surg 1990; 160:535–539.
19. Lipsett PA, Samantaray DK, Tam ML et al. Pseudomembranous colitis: a surgical disease. Surgery 1994; 116:491–496.

Chapter 59

Ischemia/ischemic colitis

Vaman S Jakribettuu and Joel S Levine

KEY POINTS

- Ischemic colitis is the most common form of intestinal ischemia
- The majority of cases are caused by nonocclusive mesenteric ischemia
- The splenic flexure and rectosigmoid watershed regions are often affected
- Associated with aortic surgery, congestive heart failure, cocaine use, coagulopathies, and colonic obstruction
- Most often the only symptoms are crampy lower abdominal pain and hematochezia
- Persistent fever, distention, ileus, and peritoneal signs may indicate bowel infarction
- Diagnosis depends on a high degree of clinical suspicion
- Colonoscopy is the most helpful test, but should be used cautiously as overdistention of the colon can worsen ischemia
- Differential diagnosis includes infectious colitis, inflammatory bowel disease, and diverticulitis
- Management is mainly supportive for mild cases; antibiotics and surgery for clinically severe cases of colonic infarction

INTRODUCTION AND DEFINITION

Colonic ischemia is different in many respects from the less common small bowel mesenteric ischemia or infarction. Ischemic colitis is most frequently found in the elderly; a clear precipitating factor may not be defined; and most cases are nonocclusive without embolism or thrombosis.[1] Angiography is rarely helpful in either diagnosis or management. In a majority, the condition resolves with conservative management, but if colonic infarction occurs other co-morbidities may portend a poor outcome.

EPIDEMIOLOGY

More than 90% of reported patients are over the age of 60 years. Women account for approximately two-thirds of the cases, perhaps because of the use of estrogens. Colonic ischemia accounts for 3–9% of acute lower gastrointestinal bleeding, and for 10% of all emergency surgery for distal colonic peritonitis.[2]

CAUSES, RISK FACTORS, DISEASE ASSOCIATIONS

The majority of patients with ischemic colitis have nonocclusive mesenteric ischemia; many are elderly with associated congestive heart failure. A specific inciting cardiovascular event may not be identified. At presentation, some of these patients may have previously unsuspected arrhythmias, atherosclerosis, or heart failure.[3]

Ischemic colitis in the elderly is associated with congestive heart failure, any event associated with hypotension, cardiac surgery, aortic aneurysm repair (7% of elective, 60% of emergent), some medications (digitalis, estrogens, pseudoephedrine, vasopressin, sumatriptan, alosteron), systemic conditions such as vasculitides and coagulopathies, and obstructing lesions of the colon such as diverticulitis or colonic cancer.

Ischemic colitis due to mesenteric vein thrombosis may be associated with an underlying coagulopathy or cardiac source.

In ischemic colitis in younger people, related conditions include connective tissue disorders (e.g., polyarteritis nodosa, systemic lupus erythematosus), cocaine and methamphetamine use, oral contraceptives and pregnancy, strenuous physical exertion (long distance runners), sickle cell disease, and coagulopathies.[4]

CAUSES AND RISK FACTORS

- Nonocclusive mesenteric ischemia associated with congestive heart failure or hypotension
- Embolism from aortic plaques, atrial or valvular thrombi, or atrial myxoma
- Thrombosis in the setting of protein C and S deficiency, antithrombin III deficiency, oral contraceptive use, factor V Leiden mutation, or polycythemia vera
- Postsurgical complication of abdominal aortic aneurysm repair or aortoiliac bypass
- Associated with drugs such as digitalis, cocaine, metamphetamines, vasopressin, pseudoephedrine, sumatriptan, estrogens, and alosteron
- Strangulated hernia or volvulus
- Miscellaneous associations such as connective tissue disorders, sickle cell disease, vasculitis, trauma, long distance running, and pregnancy

PATHOGENESIS AND PATHOLOGY

Most of the colon's blood supply comes from branches of the superior mesenteric artery (SMA) and the inferior mesenteric artery (IMA). Branches of the internal iliac artery supply the rectum, with abundant collaterals between the three vascular systems. The two watershed regions are the splenic flexure (SMA and IMA) and the rectosigmoid (IMA and internal iliac). They have fewer collaterals and thus are more susceptible to ischemia from decreased mucosal blood flow.

The right colon is affected in 8% of cases, transverse in 15%, splenic flexure in 23%, descending colon in 23%, sigmoid in 23%, and rectum in 24%.[5] Nonocclusive injuries involve longer discontinuous segments, whereas atheromatous embolism (uncommon) involves smaller isolated segments.

Grossly there may be mucosal erythema and edema that may evolve into reddish-purple lobular mucosal swellings, difficult to distinguish from a colonic neoplasm. Ultimately the mucosa may slough and leave large linear ulcerations and a cobblestone appearance. Gangrenous bowel may appear green to black. Sometimes the picture is indistinguishable from a diffuse or patchily distributed colitis.

Reversible colopathy involves the superficial half of the mucosa with submucosal hemorrhage and superficial crypt loss. Ischemic colitis is one of the recognized causes of pseudomembranous colitis. Transient colitis may involve full-thickness mucosal ulceration with evidence of mucosal regeneration. Fulminant colitis shows complete mucosal loss with complete crypt destruction, and chronic ulcerating ischemic colitis may mimic inflammatory bowel disease. Fibrosis may eventually lead to stricture formation.

Gangrene is associated with transmural destruction of the mucosa and muscularis propria, with eventual perforation through the serosa.

Many endoscopic and histologic changes, especially those at the milder end of the spectrum, may resemble other disorders, such as inflammatory bowel disease, solitary rectal ulcer, antibiotic-associated pseudomembranous colitis, and infectious colitis.

CLINICAL PRESENTATION

Most patients present with acute onset, variably severe, crampy lower abdominal pain, rectal bleeding, or bloody diarrhea. Infarction should be suspected with severe constant pain and disproportionately little abdominal tenderness to palpation. Blood loss is usually mild, but if significant bleeding occurs the other 'usual suspects' for severe hematochezia need to be considered.

The clinical spectrum of ischemic colitis includes reversible colopathy, transient colitis, chronic ulcerating ischemic colitis, stricture formation, gangrene, and fulminant colitis. Most patients without aortic surgery have benign, self-limiting ischemic colitis. The symptoms subside in 24–48 h, and lesions heal by 1–2 weeks. Peritoneal signs, if present, are usually transient, but if they persist for more than a few hours colonic infarction is suspect. Colonic infarction can present as an acute abdomen and should prompt consideration for immediate laparotomy.

Uncommonly patients have chronic ulcerating ischemic colitis characterized by recurrent fevers, bloody diarrhea, and sepsis. Occasionally it also causes a protein-losing colopathy. Colonic strictures do not usually manifest with obstructive symptoms.

Ischemic colitis may be found proximal to obstructing lesions that include cancer,[6] diverticulitis, fecal impaction, and radiation strictures.

DIFFERENTIAL DIAGNOSIS

The diagnosis may be delayed in severely ill postoperative patients, who may not be able to communicate their pain. Pain from acute ischemic injury of the small bowel is mainly periumbilical and constant, with infrequent bloody diarrhea; pain in ischemic colitis is milder and localized usually to the left lower quadrant. Identifiable precipitating events with ischemic colitis are uncommon; bloody diarrhea is common, yet patients at the outset do not appear to be seriously ill.

Ischemic colitis needs to be differentiated from other conditions. Careful drug and medication history with screens for illegal drugs, when appropriate, is important. In all patients, stool studies should be sent to rule out infectious colitis. Clinical presentation and follow-up with complete resolution in 2 weeks helps to differentiate ischemic colitis from Crohn's disease or ulcerative colitis. Sometimes ischemic colitis presents as a chronic ulcerating or inflammatory disease, difficult to differentiate from inflammatory bowel disease.

CLINICAL PRESENTATION

- A reversible colopathy with submucosal or intramural hemorrhage and few symptoms
- Most commonly encountered as a transient colitis with crampy lower abdominal pain, hematochezia, and urgent desire to defecate, usually improving in 24–48 h
- A chronic ulcerating ischemic colitis that may be asymptomatic or have recurrent fevers and bloody diarrhea, sepsis, and protein-losing colopathy
- A stricture from a previous ischemic episode – may be asymptomatic or cause constipation and colonic obstruction
- Fulminant universal colitis with generalized abdominal pain, peritoneal signs, fever, distention, megacolon, and ileus
- Colonic gangrene and infarction with severe constant abdominal pain and peritoneal signs, fever, and ileus

DIFFERENTIAL DIAGNOSIS

- **Common**
  Acute infectious colitis – *Campylobacter, Shigella, Salmonella, E. coli* 0157:H7, *Clostridium difficile*
  Inflammatory bowel disease
  Acute small bowel mesenteric ischemia
  Radiation colitis
  Diverticulitis
- **Uncommon**
  Solitary rectal ulcer
  Colonic cancer
  Hydrogen peroxide enemas
  Glutaraldehyde left on an inadequately rinsed colonoscope

DIAGNOSTIC METHODS

Ischemic colitis should be considered in all patients with acute-onset, crampy abdominal pain with blood in the stool. At presentation, plain radiography of the abdomen is crucial. It is often nondiagnostic early on, but severe changes of thumbprinting and *Pneumatosis* may be identified in 30%;[7] colonic dilatation is a more ominous potential finding. Computed tomograms early in the course of the disease may be normal or show nonspecific segmental bowel thickening. Gas in the mesenteric veins and *Pneumatosis* are seen in more advanced disease (Fig. 59.1).

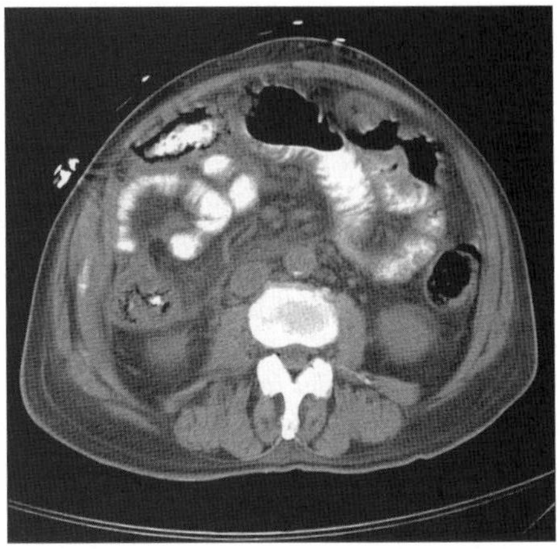

Fig. 59.1 Computed tomogram of the abdomen. Scan illustrates *Pneumatosis coli* at the hepatic flexure.

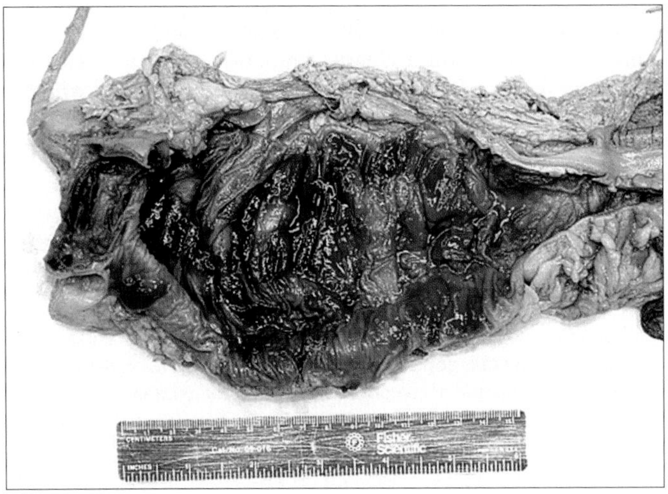

Fig. 59.3 Ischemia and infarction. Ischemia and infarction of the cecum at autopsy in a patient with embolism to the superior mesenteric artery.

Careful (minimal air insufflation) colonoscopy is the preferred diagnostic test. Overdistention of the colon may further reduce colonic blood flow.[1] Insufflation with carbon dioxide, a rapidly absorbed vasodilator, has been touted for some time as preferable to room air in high-risk colonoscopy. In the authors' unit, carbon dioxide is not used. When an apparent ischemic segment is encountered, biopsies are taken and the procedure is aborted. Biopsies should include the edge of the ulceration and 1 cm of noninvolved tissue. Sometimes the ulcerated mucosa does not reveal its source of injury, but the adjacent mucosa may reveal histologic 'footprints' of ischemia. Usually, pale or cyanotic and edematous mucosa with ulcerations (Fig. 59.2), petechial bleeding, and bluish hemorrhagic nodules are seen on endoscopy. The distribution of these lesions is segmental and there is an abrupt transition from injured to normal mucosa. Although black mucosa should suggest gangrene, colonoscopy is not helpful in distinguishing ischemic from infarcted bowel (Fig. 59.3).

Angiography is rarely useful in this primarily nonocclusive disease with circulation affected at the arteriolar level. In most patients, blood flow has returned to normal by the time of clinical presentation. Magnetic resonance angiography and duplex ultrasonography may detect a high-grade arterial stenosis,[8] yet such a stenosis may have nothing to do with the clinical presentation.

If the patient is very ill, with or without a clear diagnosis, exploratory surgery should be strongly considered. Delayed diagnosis and development of sepsis, acidosis, or pneumoperitoneum increase the morbidity and mortality associated with surgical resection.

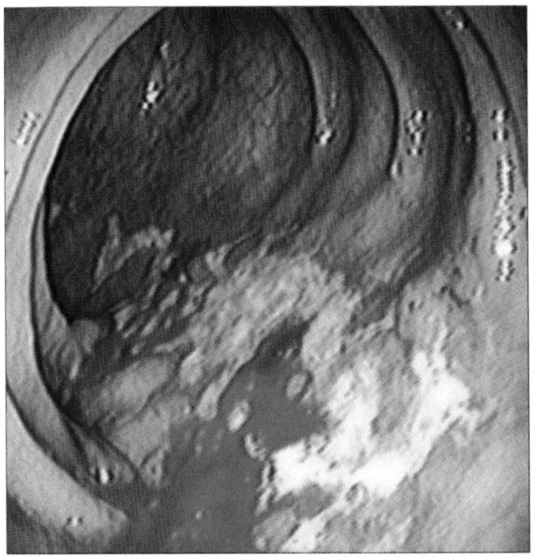

Fig. 59.2 Localized ischemic ulcer. Localized ischemic ulcer of the splenic flexure in a patient with nonocclusive mesenteric ischemia; resolution was complete without therapy.

Laparoscopy is better tolerated than laparotomy for the diagnosis of ischemic colitis in an elderly population. Laparoscopy is also helpful after surgical resection for a second look, to assess viability of the bowel. Intraperitoneal pressures should not exceed 10–15 mmHg with laparoscopy, as the pneumoperitoneum may further reduce blood flow to the colon.[9]

TREATMENT AND PREVENTION

Supportive measures are directed at reducing the progression to infarction. Oxygen is started, potentially causal drugs are withdrawn, and intravenous fluids are given to ensure adequate colonic perfusion. Correction of anemia, arrhythmia, or congestive heart failure is undertaken. Avoidance of oral intake is desirable until the course is defined, and nasogastric tube suction is required if ileus is present.

Empiric antibiotic coverage is given in moderate to severe cases, theoretically to reduce bacterial translocation across the damaged colon. Patients need to be monitored for persistent fever, bleeding or diarrhea, leukocytosis, acidosis, and peritoneal signs. Regular plain films of the abdomen and periodic CT imaging should be used to follow slowly resolving cases. Emergent surgery is indicated if the patient's condition deteriorates, infarction becomes evident, or there is massive hemorrhage, recurrent fevers, or sepsis. Toxic megacolon is associated with significant (50–70%) rates of operative mortality and morbidity in this setting.[10] A second-look operation in 12–24 h may be needed to see whether there is ischemic change beyond the original resection margins.

In patients undergoing aortoiliac surgery, recognition of postoperative ischemic colitis is important, because prompt intervention may be required.[11] Routine sigmoidoscopy has not been shown to improve survival.[12]

Ischemic colitis from *mesenteric vein thrombosis* should be assessed for underlying hypercoagulable states. Anticoagulation therapy is started and continued for at least 6 months if there is an underlying coagulopathy or a cardiac source.[13] In those unusual patients with a clearly defined cause (e.g., vasculitis, polycythemia, embolism), therapy is directed at the primary disease.

TREATMENT AND PREVENTION
• Reversible colopathy and transient colitis – supportive management that may include intravenous fluids, stopping potentially causal drugs, bowel rest, and antibiotics if the symptoms are moderate to severe; nasogastric decompression for ileus; optimization of cardiopulmonary function including oxygen supplementation; and monitor carefully for peritoneal signs • Chronic ulcerating ischemic colitis – if persistently symptomatic, surgery with segmental colectomy • Ischemic colonic stricture – no treatment if asymptomatic, but if symptomatic endoscopic colon dilatation or surgery with segmental colectomy • Fulminant universal colitis – surgery if there is no clear improvement with medical management • Colonic gangrene – surgery

COMPLICATIONS AND THEIR MANAGEMENT

Patients need to be monitored for clinical worsening and signs of peritonitis. The team management approach should include an early surgical consultation.

A minority develop chronic ischemic colitis associated with features that may include recurrent abdominal pain, bacteremia, bloody diarrhea, sepsis, strictures, weight loss, and protein-losing enteropathy. Such patients may need segmental resection. Strictures may be symptomatically improved with endoscopic balloon dilatation. Inflammatory bowel disease must be excluded because corticosteroid therapy in ischemic colitis may lead to perforation.

PROGNOSIS WITH AND WITHOUT TREATMENT

Most patients resolve completely with supportive care. Many patients never have another episode of ischemia. Anticoagulation has no role in the common patient with nonocclusive disease. With colonic infarction and gangrene, the mortality rate in the elderly with multiple co-morbid conditions may approach 50–75% with surgery, and is universally fatal with nonsurgical management.

REFERENCES

1. Greenwald DA, Brandt LJ, Reinus JF. Ischemic bowel disease in the elderly. Gastroenterol Clin North Am 2001; 30:445–475.
2. Biondo S, Pares D, Rague JM et al. Emergency operations for nondiverticular perforations of the left colon. Am J Surg 2002; 183:256–260.
3. Collett, Even C, Bouin M et al. Prevalence of electrocardiographic and echocardiographic abnormalities in ambulatory ischemic colitis. Dig Dis Sci 2000; 45:23–25.
4. Preventza OA, Lazarides K, Sawyer MD. Ischemic colitis in young adults; a single-institution experience. J Gastrointest Surg 2001; 5:388–392.
5. Price AB. Ischemic colitis. In: Williams GT, ed. Current topics in pathology: gastrointestinal pathology. New York: Springer; 1990:81: 229–246.
6. Glotzer DJ, Roth SI, Welch CE. Colonic ulceration proximal to obstructing carcinoma. Surgery 1964; 56:950–956.
7. Smerud MJ, Johnson CD, Stephens DH. Diagnosis of bowel infarction: comparision of plain films and CT scans in 23 cases. AJR Am J Roentgenol 1990; 154:99–103.
8. Ernst O, Asnar V, Sergent G et al. Comparing contrast-enhanced breath-hold MR angiography and conventional angiography in the evaluation of mesenteric circulation. AJR Am J Roentgenol 2000; 174:433–439.
9. Kleinhaus S, Sammartano R, Boley SJ. Effects of laparoscopy on mesenteric blood flow. Arch Surg 1978; 113:867–869.
10. Longo WE, Ward D, Vernava AM et al. Outcome of patients with total colonic ischemia. Dis Colon Rectum 1997; 40:1448–1454.
11. Van Damme H, Creemers E, Limet R. Ischaemic colitis following aortoiliac surgery. Acta Chir Belg 2000; 100:21–27.
12. Houe T, Thorboll JE, Sigild U et al. Can colonoscopy diagnose transmural ischaemic colitis after abdominal aortic surgery? An evidence-based approach. Eur J Vasc Endovasc Surg 2000; 19:304.
13. American Gastroenterological Association. Medical position statement: guidelines on intestinal ischemia. Gastroenterology 2000; 118:951–953.

Chapter 60A

Biology and genetics of colorectal cancer

Lisa Strate, Eric Pieramici and Dennis Ahnen

KEY POINTS

- Familial adenomatous polyposis and hereditary nonpolyposis colorectal cancer carry a 100% and 80% lifetime risk, respectively, of developing colorectal cancer
- 20–30% of colorectal cancers are due to an interaction between genetic susceptibility and environmental carcinogens
- Loss of APC function is the initiating and rate-limiting step in most adenoma development
- Mutations in DNS mismatch repair (MMR) are central to the pathogenesis of hereditary nonpolyposis colorectal cancer
- Progression along the adenoma-carcinoma sequence is due to accumulated mutations in growth regulation genes
- Sporadic MSI-high tumors may evolve via a hyperplastic polyp-serrated adenoma-adenocarcinoma pathway
- Tumors arise at a greater rate than would be expected by chance mutations due to chromosomal and genomic instability
- Molecular profiling of tumors may predict prognosis and treatment response

INTRODUCTION

Remarkably rapid advances are being made in our understanding of the genetic and biologic basis of colorectal cancer. Several unique characteristics make colorectal cancer a useful system in which to study tumor development. Almost all colonic cancers arise from discernible precursor lesions – adenomatous polyps – which are both prevalent and endoscopically accessible. In addition, several distinctive hereditary colorectal cancer syndromes have played important roles in defining the principal genetic mutations and pathways underlying the pathogenesis of most colorectal cancers. The identification of the genes responsible for hereditary cancers has significantly improved the care of patients and families with these disorders. Understanding the molecular events in colorectal carcinogenesis also promises to impact on the prevention and management of all colorectal cancers.

INHERITED SUSCEPTIBILITY TO COLORECTAL CANCER

Inherited syndromes: A small fraction (2–10%) of all colorectal cancers can be attributed to defined inherited syndromes,[1] the two most common being familial adenomatous polyposis (FAP) and hereditary nonpolyposis colorectal cancer (HNPCC) (Table 60a.1). In these autosomal dominantly transmitted disorders, one mutated allele of a high penetrance cancer susceptibility gene is inherited in the germline, resulting in a striking predisposition to colorectal cancer. The lifetime risk of colonic cancer is nearly 100% in patients with FAP, and is as high as 80% in patients with HNPCC. The hamartomatous polyposis syndromes, Peutz-Jeghers and juvenile polyposis, also predispose to colorectal cancer but are thought to account for less than 1% of the total colorectal cancer risk. The prevalence of the recently described autosomal recessive MutY homolog (MYH) polyposis syndrome is not yet defined.

Familial tendency: In a much larger proportion of colorectal cancers (20–30%), the tendency to develop cancer exhibits familial clustering, but inheritance patterns are not mendelian.[2] Although the genetic basis for common familial colorectal cancers is largely unknown, most are thought to derive from the inheritance of mild to moderately penetrant alleles that enhance susceptibility to environmental carcinogenic exposures. Therefore, in contrast to the defined hereditary syndromes, the risk of cancer is less predictable and is significantly influenced by environmental factors. As a rule, first-degree relatives of persons with colorectal cancer exhibit a 2–3-fold increased risk of this malignancy compared to average-risk populations. The presence of an additional first-degree relative with colorectal cancer, or a first-degree relative diagnosed at a young age (less than 50 years), further increases this risk. In addition, close relatives of persons with adenomatous polyps are predisposed to colorectal cancer, especially if an adenoma is diagnosed before the age of 50 years or exhibits advanced histology.[3]

Sporadic cancers: The majority (60–80%) of colorectal cancers do not appear to be inherited, and are thus referred to as sporadic. It is currently thought that in the absence of an inherited mutation a colonic cell must incur multiple mutations and/or epigenetic alterations such as hypermethylation in one copy of an oncogene or in both copies of a tumor suppressor or DNA repair gene in order to progress through the process of colonic tumorigenesis. Genetic redundancy provides a buffer, ensuring that the lifetime risk of developing and dying from colorectal cancer in the general population is relatively low (about 5% and 2.5% respectively). This risk is, however, significantly modulated by environmental factors.

GENETIC PRINCIPLES OF COLORECTAL CARCINOGENESIS

Adenoma–carcinoma sequence

Several lines of evidence suggest that the vast majority of colonic tumors arise from pre-existing adenomas (Figs 60A.1 and 60A.2). The potential for progressive dysplasia and malignant transformation increases as a polyp grows in size, and adenomatous and malignant tissue can often be found within

TABLE 60A.1 INHERITED RISKS OF COLORECTAL CANCER

Risk group	Proportion of all CRC	Lifetime risk of CRC
Sporadic cancer, general population	60–80%	5%
Familial cancers	20–30%	
One first-degree relative with CRC		2–3-fold increase
Two first-degree relatives with CRC		3–4-fold increase
One second- or third-degree relative with CRC		1.5-fold increase
Two second- or third-degree relatives with CRC		2–3-fold increase
One first-degree relative with adenoma		2-fold increase
One first-degree relative with adenoma, age <60 years		2–3-fold increase
Hereditary syndromes	2–8%	
Hereditary nonpolyposis colonic cancer	1–6%	80%
Familial adenomatous polyposis	1%	100%
Hamartomatous polyposis syndromes	<1%	2–50%

CRC, colorectal cancer.
Adapted and reprinted with permission from Burt RW, Ahnen DJ. Genetics of colon cancer. In: Yamada T, ed. Gastroenterology Updates, vol. 3. Philadelphia: JB Lippincott; 1998:1–16.

the same lesion. Moreover, a strong correlation exists between the prevalence of adenomas and carcinomas, and the incidence of colorectal cancer is reduced following endoscopic removal of adenomas. At the molecular level, adenomas are known to contain genetic alterations also found in carcinomas, and specific mutations tend to correlate with the histopathologic stages of tumor progression.

Multistep carcinogenesis

The progression from adenoma to carcinoma is thought to be the result of a progressive accumulation of mutations in critical growth regulation genes. This multistep model of colonic carcinogenesis evolved from the pioneering work of Vogelstein and colleagues,[4] who analyzed the genetic alterations in various histopathologic stages from adenoma to carcinoma, and observed that certain mutations appeared to occur in a preferred sequence. Inactivated forms of a critical tumor suppressor gene *APC* (*a*denomatous *p*olyposis *c*oli) were found in the majority of early adenomas, whereas a mutated oncogene (*Ras*) was found in approximately half of larger adenomas. Adenomas with severe dysplasia tended to carry alterations in the cancer-suppressing gene *DCC* (*d*eleted in *c*olonic *c*ancer), although other genes also located on chromosome 18q are now thought to be more important targets. Finally, 75% of advanced carcinomas contained inactivating mutations of the tumor suppressor gene *p53*. Although this multistep model has defined our understanding of colonic carcinogenesis, it cannot fully explain the complexity and heterogeneity of this disease and the model has been expanded to include a number of alternative genetic pathways for colorectal cancer (Fig. 60A.3).

Genetic instability

Estimates of the mutation rate observed in normal cells suggest that they are insufficient for tumor development under the multistep model. Therefore, genetic instability is another essential principle of colorectal carcinogenesis. Two general types of genetic instability occur during the process of colonic carcinogenesis: chromosomal and microsatellite instability. Most human colonic cancers demonstrate chromosomal instability (CIN), characterized by frequent allelic losses (loss of heterozygosity), aneuploidy (abnormal chromosome number), and chromosomal amplifications and translocations. Defects in genes involved in chromosomal segregation are thought to underlie the development of CIN. Microsatellite instability, on the other hand, can be due to defective DNA mismatch repair mechanisms and leads to the rapid accumulation of errors in the nucleotide sequence. The resulting hallmark of tumors derived from this mechanism is the insertion or deletion of short repetitive DNA sequences known as microsatellites. While conceptually chromosomal and microsatellite instability appear to represent distinct genetic mechanisms to colonic carcinogenesis, they may not be entirely independent or inclusive. In many sporadic cancers these forms of genetic instability overlap, and some cancers appear to develop through molecular mechanisms that are not typical of either pathway.

GENETIC PATHWAYS INVOLVED IN COLONIC CARCINOGENESIS

Two principal genetic pathways by which the multistep process of colonic carcinogenesis occurs have been identified: the *tumor suppressor pathway*, which typically is driven by chromosomal instability, and the *microsatellite instability pathway* caused by the absence of DNA mismatch repair activity. These pathways are distinctive in their causative genetic events, forms of genetic instability, and associated hereditary syndromes.

Tumor suppressor/chromosomal instability pathway

The tumor suppressor/chromosomal instability pathway is the predominant genetic pathway defective in colorectal carcinogenesis. The majority of sporadic colonic cancers, as well as tumors arising in FAP, are believed to develop via defects in this pathway. Mutations in tumor suppressor genes play central roles, but proto-oncogenes also participate. Defective tumor suppression is believed to lead to increased chromosomal instability, and vice versa. Cancers that develop from this pathway tend to be more commonly aneuploid, and are characterized by frequent allelic loss as well as chromosomal amplifications and translocations.

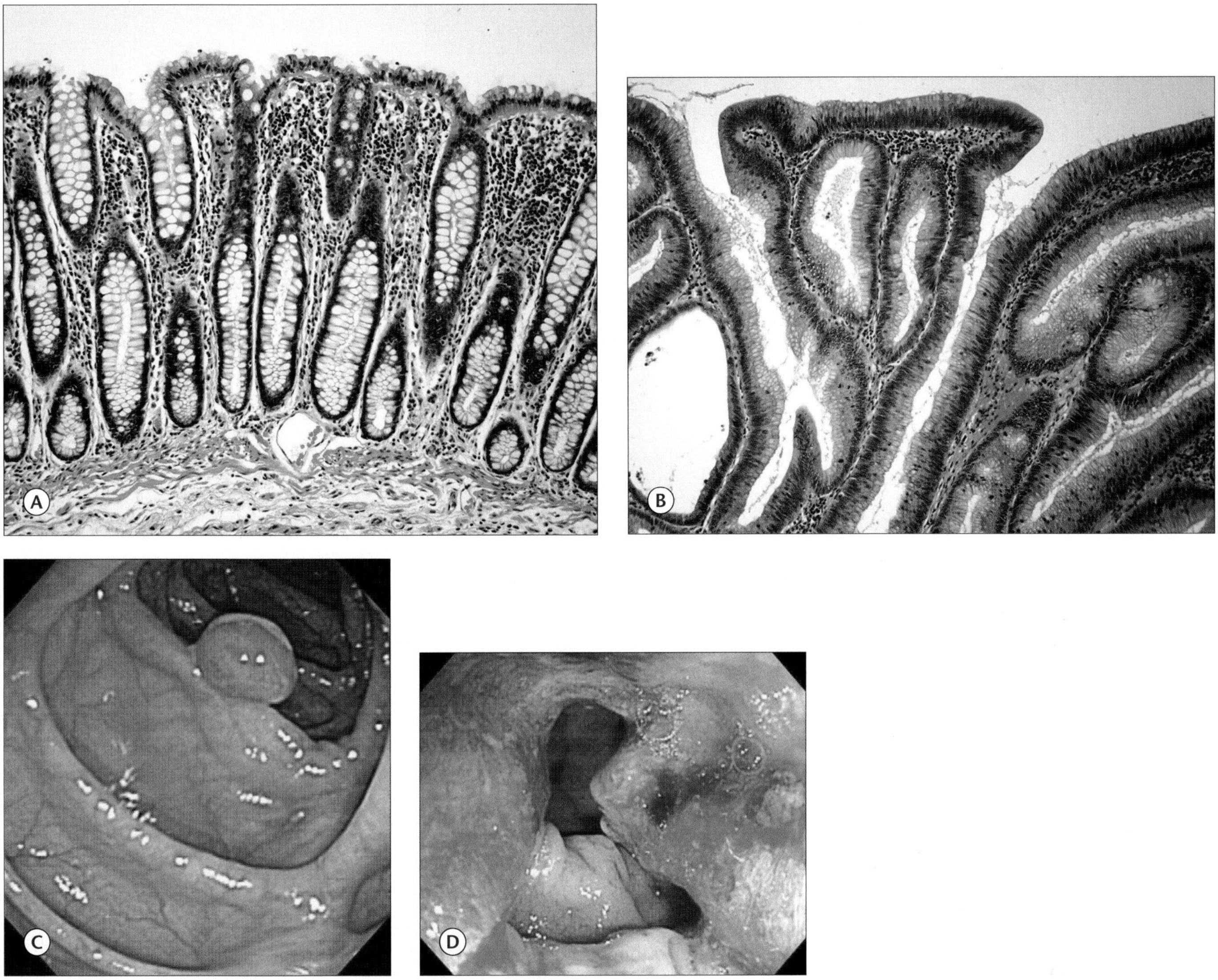

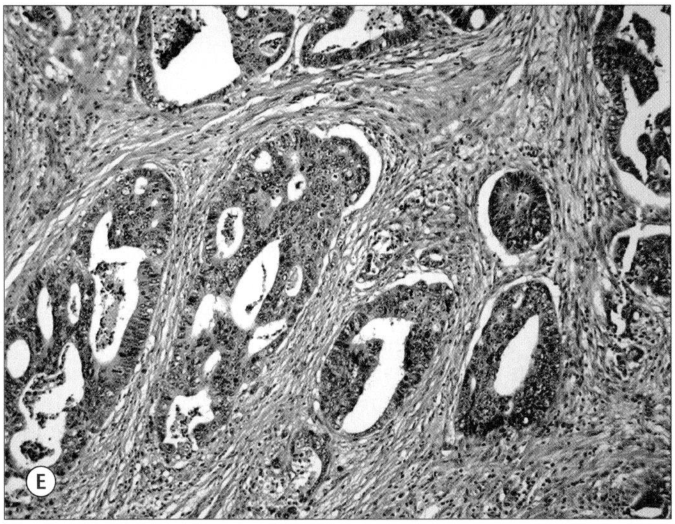

Fig. 60A.1 Histologic and endoscopic appearance of lesions in the adenoma to carcinoma sequence. A. Normal colonic epithelium. **B,C.** Adenoma. **D,E.** Colonic adenocarcinoma.
Histologic images courtesy of Jonathan N. Glickman.

Tumor suppressor genes (Table 60A.2) often encode proteins that normally restrain cell proliferation or mediate programmed cell death. One wild-type allele of a tumor suppressor gene is generally sufficient to maintain normal cell function, so that loss or inactivation of both alleles is thought to be necessary for neoplastic transformation. Hereditary cancer syndromes are often caused by germline inactivating mutations in tumor suppressor genes. In these disorders, one mutant allele is transmitted in the germline, and hence is present in every cell. Somatic loss or mutation of the remaining wild-type allele in a single cell will therefore remove a critical regulator of cell growth. In sporadic cancers, one tumor suppressor allele typi-

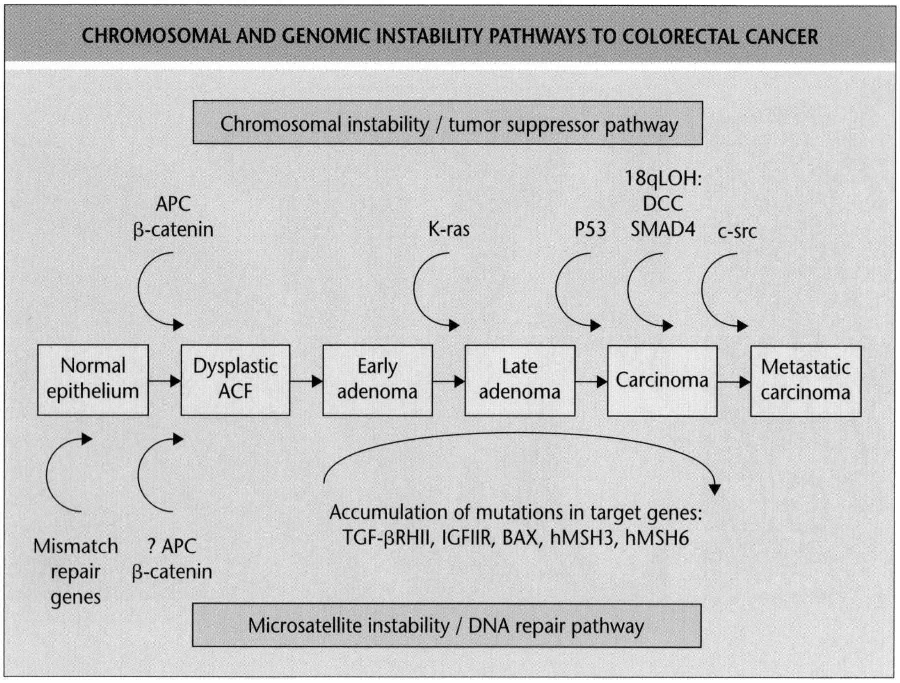

Fig. 60A.2 Chromosomal and microsatellite instability pathways to colorectal cancer. Dysplastic aberrant crypt foci (ACF) are the earliest recognized precursors to colonic cancer and are thought to give rise to adenomas then carcinomas. The chromosomal instability/ tumor suppressor pathway is the predominant pathway accounting for 60–85% of sporadic colonic cancers, as well as cancers in FAP kindreds. Tumors arising in this pathway demonstrate chromosomal instability characterized by aneuploidy (abnormal chromosome number), allelic losses (loss of heterozygosity), and chromosomal amplifications and translocations. Mutations in the tumor suppressor gene, *APC* (adenomatous polyposis coli) are thought to be the rate-limiting step in the chromosomal instability pathway. The sequence of subsequent genetic events driving tumor progression via this pathway is shown. Mutations in DNA repair genes underlie the pathogenesis of tumors arising in the microsatellite instability pathway. Mutations or epigenetic silencing of the DNA mismatch repair (*MMR*) genes account for HNPCC-related tumors, and 15–20% of sporadic colonic cancers. Inactivation of both alleles of a *MMR* gene is thought to be the initial event in this pathway, and leads to genomic instability via the accumulation of sequence errors throughout the genome. The growth regulatory genes noted above appear to be particularly susceptible to these errors. The timing of other genetic events is unknown. Likewise, the role of APC and β-catenin in the MMR pathway remains uncertain. The hallmark of tumors with defective MMR is microsatellite instability (see text for details).

cally succumbs to an inactivating mutation, after which the cell may become homozygous for the mutant allele by a process referred to as 'loss of heterozygosity' (LOH) or the remaining allele may be inactivated by gene silencing via promoter methylation. The hypothesis that inherited defects in one allele and a single somatic inactivation of the other allele caused familial forms of cancer, whereas sporadic cancers of the same organ required two separate somatic mutations of the gene, was originally proposed for hereditary retinoblastoma by Knudson.[5] This hypothesis explained why familial forms of cancer typically occur at younger ages and are more often multiple when compared to sporadic cancers of the same organ.

APC

The *APC* (*a*denomatous *p*olyposis *c*oli) gene is the best characterized tumor suppressor gene in colonic adenomas and cancers. Loss of the normal APC function is central to the process of colorectal carcinogenesis. Inactivating mutations of *APC* are thought to be the initial and rate-limiting step governing the progression from normal epithelial maturation to adenoma. Germline mutations in *APC* were originally described as the causative lesion in FAP.[6,7] Patients with FAP develop hundreds to thousands of adenomas, some of which will inevitably progress to cancer. Somatic mutations of the *APC* gene were subsequently identified in the majority of sporadic colonic cancers (60–80%). Adenomas and even aberrant crypt foci also harbor a high rate of *APC* defects.

The normal APC protein has several diverse functions related to cell growth and differentiation. APC plays a key regulatory role in the Wnt (Wingless-Int) cell signaling pathway, which is involved in many evolutionarily conserved developmental and growth processes, in large part through its regulation of the protein β-catenin. The abnormal function of these proteins and pathways leads to upregulated transcription of multiple growth-related genes. APC also appears to participate in cell–cell adhesion, cell migration, cell morphogenesis, and chromosomal segregation.

A germline truncating mutation in *APC* is found in approximately 80% of patients with classic clinical manifestations of FAP, and detection of shortened APC proteins forms the basis of one of the primary screening tests for FAP.[8] The position of the mutation within the *APC* gene has some influence on the severity of disease and the occurrence of some extraintestinal manifestations. Classic FAP is seen in families with mutations near the center of the gene, whereas an attenuated form of FAP in which fewer adenomas and a lower penetrance of colorectal cancer occurs has been found in patients with *APC* mutations near either end of the gene. However, the variability in the frequency of extraintestinal manifestations (osteomas, fibromas, sebaceous cysts, and desmoid tumors) within families that contain the exact same *APC* germline mutation suggests the importance of modifier genes in determining the clinical phenotype.

p53

The *p53* tumor suppressor gene on chromosome 17p appears to be mutated in the majority of human cancer types, including colorectal cancers. The p53 protein regulates the transcription of numerous growth regulatory target genes. These genes affect a variety of cell processes including cell cycle arrest and apoptosis. In colonic carcinogenesis, one *p53* allele is typically inactivated by somatic mutation followed by LOH of the remaining wild-type allele. Mutations in *p53* occur in at least 75% of colorectal cancers, but are uncommon in early adenomas, suggesting that such mutations are a later event in sporadic colorectal carcinogenesis.[4]

DCC

The *DCC* (*d*eleted in *c*olonic *c*ancer) gene is a candidate tumor suppressor gene on chromosome 18q that encodes a molecule homologous to other cell adhesion molecules that appear to regulate growth pathways and apoptosis. Although loss of wild-type *DCC* was initially thought to be a late event in tumor development and to portend a poor prognosis, recent evidence suggests that *DCC* may be an innocent bystander. Other tumor suppressor genes on 18q including *SMAD2* and *SMAD4* are probably responsible for the apparent importance of the *DCC* locus in colorectal carcinogenesis.

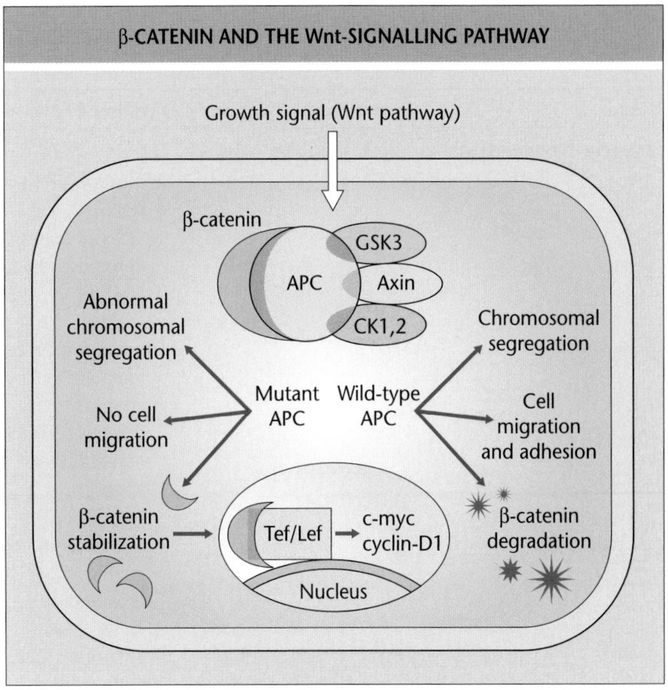

Fig. 60A.3 APC, β-catenin and the Wnt-signaling pathway. The normal (wild-type) APC protein in conjunction with glycogen synthase kinsase-3β (GSK-3β), axin, and casein kinase (CK) 1 or 2 phosphorolates β-catenin and targets it for degradation. The result is controlled levels of proliferation and apoptosis. In addition, the APC protein interacts with α, β, and γ catenin, and with E-cadherin, to direct cell migration and adhesion. APC also interacts with microtubules to maintain chromosomal stability. Inactivating mutations of APC (or β-catenin) disrupt these processes. If β-catenin is not normally degraded, it accumulates and binds to the Tcf/Lef transcription factors, activating target genes in the Wnt-signaling pathway including c-*myc*, *cyclin D1*, and *peroxisome proliferator-activated receptor-γ* (*PPAR-γ*). In addition, cell migration and chromosomal segregation are disrupted because of loss of these normal APC protein functions.

Proto-oncogenes

Proto-oncogenes are genes that normally participate in cell growth or differentiation but, when mutated or aberrantly expressed, result in unregulated cell growth and tumor development (i.e., oncogenesis). In contrast to tumor suppressor genes, oncogenes act in a dominant fashion because only one mutant allele may be required for neoplastic transformation. The K-*ras* gene on the short arm of chromosome 12 has been implicated as a principal proto-oncogene in colorectal carcinogenesis. Mutations in K-*ras* are identified in approximately half of large adenomas and carcinomas,[4] and are independently associated with villus histology and high-grade dysplasia, suggesting that K-*ras* participates in an intermediate stage of carcinogenesis.

Microsatellite instability pathways

The microsatellite instability or 'mutator' pathway represents the second major genetic mechanism contributing to colorectal carcinogenesis (Fig. 60A.3). Mutations in DNA mismatch repair (*MMR*) genes give rise to microsatellite instability and to hereditary non-polyposis colorectal cancer (HNPCC).

DNA mismatch repair

At least ten MMR proteins can participate in the essential process of recognizing, removing, and repairing errors in nucleotide pairing that occur during DNA replication (Fig. 60A.4). These genes include *hMLH1*, *hMLH2*, *hMSH3*, *hMSH6*, *hPMS1*, and *hPMS2*. *MMR* genes have been conceptualized as 'caretaker' genes in deference to their critical role in maintaining genomic integrity. Inactivation of *MMR* genes lead to the accumulation of small uncorrected sequence errors that occur preferentially in short stretches of DNA termed microsatellites. These microsatellite repeats are particularly susceptible to slippage during the normal course of replication, resulting in gain or loss of base pairs. These errors occur throughout the genome, but when they affect critical growth regulatory genes they predispose cells to neoplastic transformation.

Microsatellite instability: In somatic cells, the integrity of the MMR pathway can be ascertained by examining the degree to which microsatellites contain uncorrected errors, and thus become 'unstable.' Such microsatellite instability (MSI) is the hallmark of tumors with defective MMR. A consensus panel of five microsatellite markers is often used to define the presence of MSI in tumors. Tumors with instability at two or more of these markers are classified as 'MSI high'. About 95% of colon cancers in HNPCC demonstrate a high level of MSI, and therefore this test can be used in some clinical settings to screen for this disorder. However, MSI testing may be less sensitive for patients with *hMSH6* mutations.

TABLE 60A.2 GENES IMPLICATED IN COLORECTAL CARCINOGENESIS

Gene	Chromosome location	Presumed function	Associated inherited syndrome	Comment
TUMOR SUPPRESSOR				
APC	5q21	Regulation of B-catenin/Wnt signaling; cell migration; cell–cell adhesion; chromosome segregation	Familial adenomatous polyposis	Somatic mutations in 60–80% of sporadic colonic cancers; thought to be the rate-limiting step in tumor initiation
p53	17p13	Transcription factor; regulates cell cycle and apoptosis	Li-Fraumeni syndrome	Mutations occur late in colorectal carcinogenesis
DCC	18q21	Cell adhesion molecule, regulates cell migration, apoptosis		Mutations occur late in carcinogenesis, and may indicate a poor prognosis
TGFβIIR		TGF-β receptor component; inhibition of cell proliferation	HNPCC-like syndrome with late-onset tumors	Mutations occur late at carcinoma stage; found in most MSI-high tumors
SMAD2	18q21	Transcription factor in TGF-β pathway		Mutations found in 10% of colorectal cancers
SMAD4	18q21	Transcription factor in TGF-β pathway	Juvenile polyposis	Mutations found in 25% of colorectal cancers
STK11/LKB1	19p	Serine/threonine protein kinase	Peutz-Jeghers syndrome	
PTEN	10q23	Phosphoinositide 3-phosphatase; tyrosine phosphatase	Cowden's disease, sporadic cases of juvenile polyposis	Possible target of MMR dysfunction
ONCOGENES				
K-*ras*	12p	Guanosine triphosphate hydrolase (GTPase); activation of growth pathways		Participates in an intermediate stage of carcinogenesis
CTNNB1 (B-catenin)	3p22	Signal transduction protein; upregulates growth-related genes; cell–cell adhesion	50% of colonic cancers lacking *APC* mutations, but no inherited syndrome identified	Found in 50% of tumors lacking *APC* mutations (a small fraction of all sporadic tumors)
c-*src*	20q11	Tyrosine kinase		Mutations found only in metastatic tumors
DNA mismatch repair			Hereditary nonpolyposis colorectal cancer	
hMSH2	2p16	Recognizes mismatches	30% of HNPCC cases	
hMLH1	3p21	Excises mismatches	30% of HNPCC cases	
hPMS1	2q32		Rare	
hPMS2	7p22	Excises mismatches	Rare	
hMSH6	2p16	Binds to hMSH2 and single base-pair mismatches	Variant form of HNPCC	
hMSH3	5q11	Binds to hMSH2 and longer base-pair mismatches		
Base excision repair				
MYH	1p	DNA glycosylase, helps repair oxidative DNA damage	Recessive inheritance of multiple adenomas	May account for 30% of multiple adenoma cases lacking dominant inheritance

Mutations in *MMR* genes underlie the pathogenesis of HNPCC, and are also found in 10–15% of sporadic colonic cancers.[9] Germline mutations in two of the DNA repair genes – *hMLH1* and *hMSH2* – are detected in up to 60% of classic HNPCC families,[10] accounting for more than 90% of genetically defined cases of HNPCC. In HNPCC, one mutant allele is inherited and the MMR phenotype becomes manifest when the other allele is inactivated through LOH, promoter methylation or somatic mutation. In contrast, somatic mutations of DNA repair genes are uncommon in MSI-high sporadic colonic cancers. In

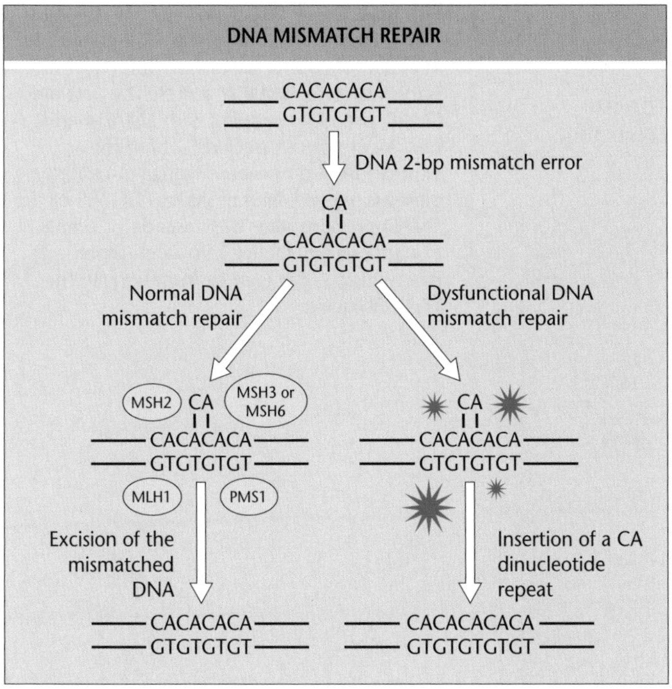

Fig. 60A.4 DNA mismatch repair. During DNA replication, a slippage error occurs in a microsatellite sequence. This results in the insertion of a CA dinucleotide repeat and a mismatched loop of DNA. In the presence of normal DNA mismatch repair (MMR), this error is corrected. If MMR is dysfunctional, due to inactivation of both alleles of one of the DNA *MMR* genes, the error is not corrected and the resulting strand contains an additional CA repeat. The insertion or deletion of short DNA repeats is termed microsatellite instability (MSI) and is the hallmark of MMR deficiency. In addition to correcting loops of mismatched DNA, the MMR system also corrects single base-pair (bp) mismatches (not shown). To repair single base-pair mismatches, MSH2 joins with MSH6 instead of either MSH3 or MSH6, and then forms a heterodimeric complex with MLH1 and PMS1.

these cancers, methylation of *hMLH1* is the most frequently identified mechanism of inactivation of DNA repair genes. This inactivation is an 'epigenetic' process resulting in gene silencing.

Distribution: In comparison to colorectal cancers arising via defects in the tumor suppressor pathway, the MSI-high tumors that occur in HNPCC show a predilection for the proximal colon, have diploid DNA content, undergo a more rapid progression from adenomas to carcinoma, are poorly differentiated, and paradoxically have a better prognosis. It is possible that the hypermutable state of these tumors may form the basis of many of these characteristics. Initially, the rapid accumulation of mutations in growth control genes could accelerate tumor progression. However, the rapid mutation rate also may concurrently inactivate genes required for tumor survival and progression.

Cancer evolution: Some evidence suggests that the sequence of genetic events in the MMR carcinogenic pathway is partially analogous to that seen in the tumor suppressor pathway. Mutations in the *APC* and β-catenin genes (*CTNNB1*) are frequently identified in MSI-high tumors, but mutations in other growth control genes (K-*ras*, *p53*) are found less consistently. Alternatively, genes containing microsatellites within their coding regions are particularly vulnerable to replication errors, and mutations in these genes may account for much of the tumor progression via the MMR pathway. Several such genes have been identified, including the transforming growth factor-βII receptor gene (TGF-βRII), a potent inhibitor of colonic cell proliferation (Fig. 60A.5). TGF-βRII mutations are found in the majority of MSI-high colonic cancers, and are associated with progression to carcinoma. Mutations in *SMAD* genes, which are critical signaling molecules in the TGF-β pathway, have also been commonly identified in MSI-high colorectal cancers. Other MSI target genes include the insulin-like growth factor-II receptor gene (*IGFIIR*), the apoptosis (cell death) regulator gene *BAX*, and even the MMR genes, *hMSH3* and *hMSH6* themselves. Genomic instability due to defects in the MMR system can thus have effects on numerous growth regulatory genes and it is the effects of mutations in these secondary genes that drive this colonic carcinogenesis pathway.

DNA base excision repair

Germline mutations in the *MYH* gene, one of the DNA *BER* genes, have been recently described to predispose to colonic adenomas and cancer. The DNA *BER* system is responsible for the repair of oxidative DNA damage, which is a major source of cellular mutations. Reactive oxygen species are a normal byproduct of aerobic cellular metabolism and are thought to be a major source of oxidative DNA damage detected in normal cells. The *BER* pathway protects cells from oxidative DNA damage by a sequential multistep process involving three main proteins: MutT homolog (MTH1), 8-oxo-guanosine glycosylase (OGG1), and MYH (Fig. 60A.6). Germline mutations in *MYH* have recently been shown to cause a colonic adenomatous polyposis syndrome.[11–14] To date, no pathogenic germline mutations have been identified in the other *BER* genes (*OGG1* or *MTH1*).

MYH-associated polyposis

The initial observation that germline mutations in one of the *BER* genes could cause colonic adenomas came from findings in adenomas from members of a family with multiple adenomatous polyps despite no germline mutations in the *APC* or *HNPCC* genes.[15] *Bi-allelic* germline mutations in the *MYH* gene were found in these affected family members, and studies in other similar families confirmed these findings leading to the designation of an autosomal recessive polyposis syndrome that has been called MYH-associated polyposis (MAP).[11–14] Inactivation of both copies of the *MYH* gene thus leads to a form of genomic instability. Colonic adenomas are thought to occur, at least in part, by failure of *BER* of DNA damage in critical regions of both *APC* alleles, and in the K-*ras* gene in MAP tumors. MAP tumors resemble HNPCC tumors in their gross genetic features, such as diploid DNA content and less frequent LOH.

Unlike autosomal dominant FAP or HNPCC, MAP is an autosomal recessive syndrome. In light of this, clinicians and genetic counselors now need to analyze pedigrees for evidence of autosomal recessive patterns of colorectal cancer inheritance, and consider *MYH* gene mutations in patients with polyposis but no family history of vertical transmission. Siblings of patients with MAP have a 25% risk of having also inherited both germline mutations and will require appropriate genetic counseling, screening, and treatment. It is estimated that up to 1% of caucasians are heterozygous for one inactivating germline mutation in the *MYH* gene, thus the frequency of MAP in this group could be as high as 1 per 10 000. Currently it is thought that MAP may

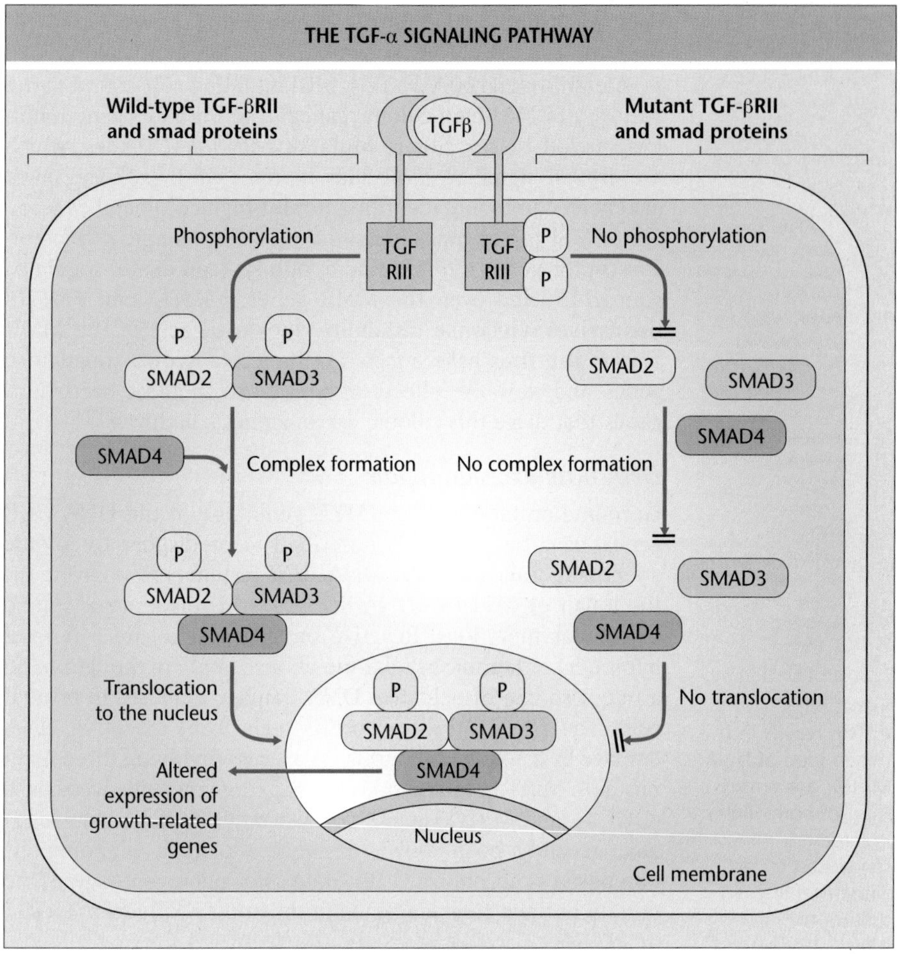

Fig. 60A.5 The TGF-β signaling pathway. TGF-β binds to the receptors TGF-βRI and RII. TGF-βRII phosphorylates TGF-βRI, which then phosphorylates SMAD2 and 3. The activated SMAD proteins complex with SMAD4 and translocate to the nucleus, where the expression of a number of growth-related genes is altered. Mutations in TGF-βRII or the SMAD proteins alter this cascade of events. In particular, defective mismatch repair mechanisms may lead to mutations in the TGF-βRII gene.

account for about 15–30% of individuals with multiple (30–500) adenomas without an autosomal dominant pattern of inheritance or a germline *APC* gene mutation. Ongoing research will help further to define the age of onset of adenomatous polyposis and colorectal cancer, the timing of colonic screening and surveillance, associated tumors (if any), and treatment options for patients with MAP.

Alternative pathways

A number of alternative pathways to colorectal carcinogenesis have been proposed. These pathways include cancers developing in the setting of inflammatory bowel disease, serrated adenomas, flat adenomas, and hamartomatous polyps.

Inflammatory bowel disease (IBD): Patients with IBD are known to have an increased incidence of colorectal carcinoma. Chronic inflammation and regeneration may predispose colonic epithelial cells to somatic mutations. Oxidative stress has been shown to inactivate the MMR system and may be responsible for the microsatellite instability seen in some chronically inflamed tissues. The precursor lesions in IBD are usually diffuse flat lesions that progress from low- to high-grade dysplasia. Distinguishing genetic features include early aneuploidy, *p53* mutations, low-frequency MSI, and a relatively low frequency of mutations in *APC* and K-*ras*.[16]

Serrated polyps encompass a range of morphologies including nondysplastic aberrant crypt foci, hyperplastic polyps, serrated adenomas, and mixed hyperplastic adenomatous polyps. Epigenetic gene silencing through promoter hypermethylation and MSI has been frequently noted across this continuum. In addition, MSI-high sporadic colorectal cancers have been found adjacent to serrated adenomas and in patients with hyperplastic polyps, raising the possibility that sporadic MSI-high cancers may evolve via a distinct hyperplastic polyp-serrated adenoma– adenocarcinoma pathway.[17] Hyperplastic polyposis, a familial disorder characterized by multiple, large, and predominantly right-sided hyperplastic polyps and a modest predisposition to colorectal cancer, may be the paradigm for this pathway.

Hamartomatosis polyposis syndromes: These include juvenile polyposis and Peutz-Jeghers syndrome. Patients have an increased susceptibility to colonic and small bowel cancers. The genetic mutations underlying these disorders are distinct from other familial and sporadic colorectal cancers described above.[18] A direct hamartoma-to-carcinoma sequence has not been defined and the cancers in this setting are thought to arise from areas of adenomatous change that occur within the hamartomas.

Recent attention has also been called to **flat carcinomas** and their possible relation to flat adenomas. In contrast to typical adenomas, flat adenomas can demonstrate a high degree of dysplasia in relatively small lesions, and likely evolve through distinct molecular mechanisms.

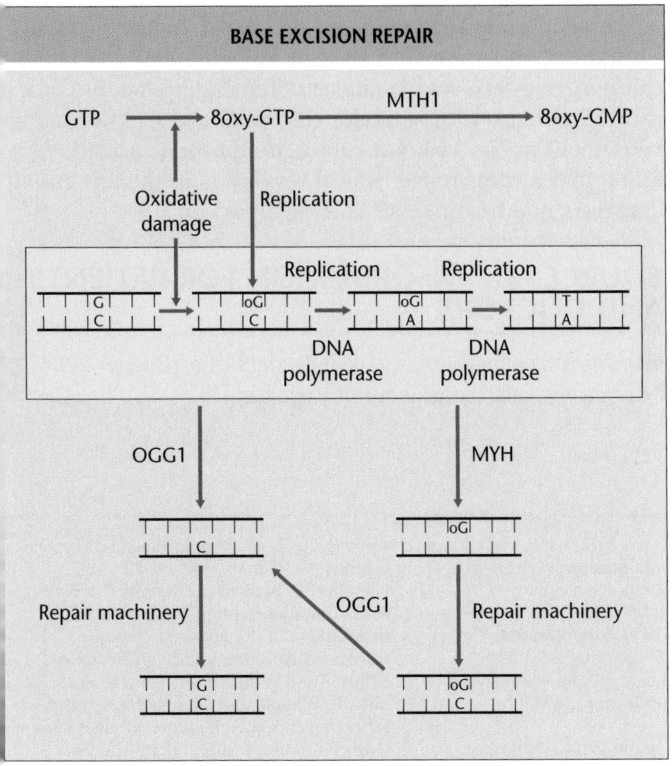

Fig. 60A.6 Base excision repair. Oxidative DNA damage can convert guanine (G) to 8-oxy-guanine (oG) within DNA or in the nucleotide pool. If not removed, 8-oxy-G can mispair with adenine, and if this is not repaired the adenine will pair with thymidine at the next cell division leading to G–C to T–A transversions. MTH1 is a nucleoside triphosphatase that removes 8-oxy-guanosine triphosphate (GTP) from the nucleotide pool, thus reducing the likelihood of 8-oxy-G incorporation during DNA replication.[1] 8-Oxo-guanosine glycosylase (OGG1) excises 8-oxy-G from 8-oxy-G:C base mispairs that do occur, thus restoring the normal G:C base pair. MYH (MutY homolog) is an adenine-specific DNA glycosylase that can recognize and excise adenines mismatched with 8-oxo-G, allowing the 8-oxo-G:C mispair to be restored and subsequently repaired by OGG1.

CLINICAL IMPLICATIONS

Our current understanding of the genetic basis of colorectal cancer has the potential to influence patient care at multiple levels, including screening, prevention, prognostication, and treatment.

Diagnosis: Commercially available genetic tests have allowed the identification of individuals who have inherited the gene for one of the familial colorectal cancer syndromes (FAP, HNPCC, MAP, the hamartomatous syndromes). Genetic testing has allowed targeted surveillance and treatment programs for gene carriers, and importantly has identified at-risk family members who have not inherited the mutation and therefore are not at increased cancer risk.

Prognosis: The genetic profile of established colorectal cancers has also been found to provide useful clinical information.[19–21] Microsatellite-unstable tumors have been reported to have a better prognosis than and to be less responsive to 5-fluorouracil chemotherapy than microsatellite-stable tumors. Other molecular markers (K-*ras*, *p53*, and *DCC* mutations) have been reported to predict both outcome and response to certain chemotherapeutic agents. Thus molecular profiling of colorectal cancers may prove useful in determining prognosis and for the selection of treatment regimens.

Treatment: Knowledge of the molecular pathways that control tumor growth provide multiple targets for the development of novel chemotherapeutic agents to be used in selected cancers based upon their molecular profile. For example, the high frequency of K-*ras* mutations in colorectal cancer has led to studies of agents, such as farnesyltransferase inhibitors, that prevent the translocation of Ras proteins to their site of action at the plasma membrane. Very active drug discovery programs that take advantage of the understanding of the genetic alterations that appear to drive the process of colonic carcinogenesis are under way. Similarly, gene therapy based on the understanding of the genetics of colorectal cancer offers hope for the future.

Screening: The knowledge of specific mutations that occur in adenomas and cancers has led to attempts to detect these same mutations in fecal DNA as a screening test for colorectal neoplasia. This approach holds promise for noninvasive 'somatic genetic' colorectal cancer screening in both average-risk and high-risk populations.

CURRENT CONTROVERSIES AND OUTLOOK FOR THE FUTURE

Although our basic understanding of the molecular basis of colorectal carcinogenesis has grown rapidly over the past 15 years, the clinical impact of this knowledge has lagged behind. If the process of colonic carcinogenesis is driven by mutations or mutation-like events, the genetic profile of adenomas and cancers should be more predictive of the natural history, prognosis, and likelihood of response to therapy than the histologic appearance of the cancer. Although there are studies suggesting that specific somatic mutations (*ras*, *DCC*, *p53*) are independently related to prognosis, none of these has become a routine part of the pathologic assessment of colorectal cancers. As noted above, it has been reported that MSI may be prognostic in young patients with colorectal cancer and that it may predict likelihood of response to adjuvant chemotherapy.[20] MSI testing may become the first genetic marker routinely used in the evaluation of colorectal cancers.

As yet unanswered questions include determining the relationship between the proposed molecular pathways, clarifying the existence of alternate pathways, and defining the precise role of many cancer susceptibility genes. The data for the importance of epigenetic methylation in colonic carcinogenesis is increasing, but it remains to be determined how important a primary methylator pathway to colorectal cancer is compared to the chromosomal and genomic instability pathways.

There are likely other genes that are important in familial colonic cancer. About 30% of families that meet the Amsterdam criteria for HNPCC do not have a mutation in the known DNA repair genes. Some of this is due to technical issues preventing the detection of large *MMR* gene deletions by current techniques, but there are likely other genes responsible for a HNPCC-like syndrome. The recent reports that the autosomal recessive colonic polyposis syndrome MYH-associated polyposis accounts for about a substantial proportion (20–30%) of *APC* mutation-negative patients with more than 30 adenomas raises the question of what genetic predispositions account for the remainder.

Many mutations have been identified in colonic neoplasia, but just because a mutation in a specific gene occurs does not necessarily mean that it is driving the process. Some mutations are likely epiphenomena of the chromosomal and genomic instability that occurs in colonic neoplasia, and others are critically important in driving the process. Defining these differences is important if we are to use molecular profiling information to guide drug development and treatment strategies.

The relationships between environmental factors and both genetic events and genetic predisposition remain important areas of investigation. For example, low folate intake has been reported to be associated with a higher risk of K-*ras* mutant adenomas, and interactions between folate intake and polymorphisms of the methylene tetrahydrofolate reductase gene have been reported.

The genetic understanding of colorectal cancer has had a substantial impact on the care of patients with the familial colorectal cancers, yet the impact of the findings on the clinical care of patients with sporadic colorectal cancer has thus far been modest. The task is to translate the basic science revolution into a comparable clinical revolution in the prevention, diagnosis, and treatment of colorectal cancer.

SOURCES OF INFORMATION FOR PATIENTS AND DOCTORS

http://www.cancerhelp.org.uk/help/default.asp?page=2786
http://www.gastro.org/generalPublic.html

REFERENCES

1. Aaltonen LA, Salovaara R, Kristo P et al. Incidence of hereditary nonpolyposis colorectal cancer and the feasibility of molecular screening for the disease. N Engl J Med 1998; 21:1481–1487.
2. Burt RW. Colon cancer screening. Gastroenterology 2000; 119:837–853.
3. Winawer SJ, Zauber AG, Gerdes H et al. Risk of colorectal cancer in the families of patients with adenomatous polyps. National Polyp Study Workgroup. N Engl J Med 1996; 334:82–87.
4. Vogelstein B, Fearon ER, Hamilton SR et al. Genetic alterations during colorectal-tumor development. N Engl J Med 1988; 319: 525–532.
5. Knudson AG Jr. Hereditary cancer, oncogenes, and antioncogenes. Cancer Res 1985; 45:1437–1443.
6. Nishisho I, Nakamura Y, Miyoshi Y et al. Mutations of chromosome 5q21 genes in FAP and colorectal cancer patients. Science 1991; 253:665–669.
7. Groden J, Thliveris A, Samowitz W et al. Identification and characterization of the familial adenomatous polyposis coli gene. Cell 1991; 66:589–600.
8. Powell SM, Petersen GM, Krush AJ et al. Molecular diagnosis of familial adenomatous polyposis. N Engl J Med 1993; 329: 1982–1987.
9. Samowitz WS, Curtin K, Lin HH et al. The colon cancer burden of genetically defined hereditary nonpolyposis colon cancer. Gastroenterology 2001; 121:830–838.
10. Syngal S, Fox EA, Li C et al. Interpretation of genetic test results for hereditary nonpolyposis colorectal cancer: implications for clinical predisposition testing. JAMA 1999; 282:247–253.
11. Enholm S, Hienonen T, Suomalainen A et al. Proportion and phenotype of MYH-associated colorectal neoplasia in a population-based series of Finnish colorectal cancer patients. Am J Pathol 2003; 163:827–832.
12. Halford SE, Rowan AJ, Lipton L et al. Germline mutations but not somatic changes at the *MYH* locus contribute to the pathogenesis of unselected colorectal cancers. Am J Pathol 2003; 162:1545–1548.
13. Sampson JR, Dolwani S, Jones S, Eccles D, Ellis A, Evans DG, et al. Autosomal recessive colorectal adenomatous polyposis due to inherited mutations of MYH. Lancet 2003;362(9377):39–41.
14. Sieber OM, Lipton L, Crabtree M et al. Multiple colorectal adenomas, classic adenomatous polyposis, and germ-line mutations in *MYH*. N Engl J Med 2003; 348:791–799.
15. Al-Tassan N, Chmiel NH, Maynard J et al. Inherited variants of *MYH* associated with somatic G:C→T:A mutations in colorectal tumors. Nat Genet 2002; 30:227–232.
16. Chaubert P, Benhattar J, Saraga E, Costa J. K-*ras* mutations and *p53* alterations in neoplastic and nonneoplastic lesions associated with longstanding ulcerative colitis. Am J Pathol 1994; 144:767–775.
17. Jass JR, Whitehall VL, Young J, Leggett BA. Emerging concepts in colorectal neoplasia. Gastroenterology 2002; 123:862–876.
18. Howe JR, Bair JL, Sayed MG et al. Germline mutations of the gene encoding bone morphogenetic protein receptor 1A in juvenile polyposis. Nat Genet 2001; 28:184–187.
19. Ahnen DJ, Feigl P, Quan G et al. Ki-*ras* mutation and *p53* overexpression predict the clinical behavior of colorectal cancer: a Southwest Oncology Group study. Cancer Res 1998; 58:1149–1158.
20. Gryfe R, Kim H, Hsieh ET et al. Tumor microsatellite instability and clinical outcome in young patients with colorectal cancer. N Engl J Med 2000; 342:69–77.
21. Carethers JM, Smith EJ, Behling CA et al. Use of 5-fluorouracil and survival in patients with microsatellite-unstable colorectal cancer. Gastroenterology 2004; 126:394–401.

Chapter 60B

Colorectal cancer: screening and surveillance

John H Bond

KEY POINTS

- The goals of screening are to detect early cancers before they metastasize, and resect advanced adenomas to prevent cancer
- Colorectal cancer has a long preclinical phase during which curable asymptomatic neoplasia can be detected
- Advanced adenomas (greater than 1 cm, with villous tissue or high-grade dysplasia) are the target of screening
- Annual fecal occult blood tests achieve a 30–45% reduction in the colorectal cancer mortality rate
- Screening with flexible sigmoidoscopy reduces mortality for colorectal cancer by 60–80%. Screening by colonoscopy and polypectomy can reduce cancer incidence by up to 90%
- Virtual colonoscopy and testing of stool DNA may be future screening options

INTRODUCTION

Colorectal cancer screening has been defined as the use of a simple indirect test applied to the asymptomatic average-risk population to identify those most likely to have colorectal neoplasia, in whom one can justify the use of a more definitive diagnostic evaluation (Fig. 60B.1). The term surveillance refers to the periodic performance of definitive examinations (usually colonoscopy) in people who are at above-average risk because they have had previous resection of adenomatous polyps or cancer.

Colorectal cancer fulfills the criteria of the International Union Against Cancer for a malignancy that warrants a screening approach. First, it is an important health problem in the USA and most European countries. It is the second leading cause of cancer death in the USA, with an estimated 146 940 new cases in 2004 causing 56 730 deaths.[1] Although the age-related incidence of colorectal cancer and polyps is higher in men than in women, both sexes have almost an equal lifetime risk because women have a longer average life expectancy. Second, the disease has a relatively long preclinical phase during which screening can detect curable asymptomatic neoplasia. Most colorectal cancers arise in benign adenomatous polyps that develop and grow slowly over many years before they turn cancerous. Third, early colorectal neoplasia can be treated successfully. Most advanced adenomas can be completely resected during colonoscopy, and the 5-year postsurgical survival rate of early stage cancers approaches 90%. Lastly, we have several safe, acceptable, and cost-effective screening tests for this disease.

Evidence-based guidelines separately developed and revised over the past 10 years by the US Preventive Services Task Force, a consortium of five US gastroenterologic societies, and by the American Cancer Society, strongly recommend that physicians screen their average-risk patients over the age of 50 years for colorectal cancer.[2–4] The guidelines also recommend that, before beginning screening, each patient should be evaluated for any other risks of colorectal cancer that might indicate the need for earlier or more intense screening or surveillance. If an indirect screening test is positive, appropriate diagnostic evaluation is essential. If screening is negative, repeat screening should be carried out at appropriate intervals for the method used. This chapter presents the current screening guideline recommendations and discusses the advantages and limitations of each screening approach. It also outlines surveillance recommendations for patients who have undergone colonoscopic polypectomy or curative resection of colorectal cancer.

OBJECTIVES OF COLORECTAL CANCER SCREENING

There are two primary objectives of screening. The first is to detect cancers before they have metastasized. Large case series show that the 5-year survival rate for such Dukes' A and B cancers (stages I and II) exceeds 85%.[5] As these early cancers rarely cause symptoms, they must be detected by screening. This applies as much to those whose cancers do not generally develop from polyps, including hereditary nonpolyposis colorectal cancer (HNPCC) or inflammatory bowel disease, as it does to those whose cancers arise from polyps. The second main objective of screening is cancer prevention. As almost all colorectal cancers originate in benign adenomatous polyps (adenomas), the detection and removal of premalignant adenomas prevents cancer. Studies such as the US National Polyp Study and the Minnesota Fecal Occult Blood Screening Trial have demonstrated that screening that leads to resection of advanced adenomas significantly decreases the subsequent incidence of cancer.[6,7] Thus, screening reduces not only cancer mortality, but through prevention it also decreases cancer-related morbidity and treatment costs.

ADVANCED ADENOMA AS A PRIMARY TARGET OF SCREENING

The prevalence of small (less than 1 cm) tubular adenomas in people aged over 50 years in Western countries exceeds 30%.[8] These small adenomas, however, have a very low malignant potential because only a few develop the additional acquired

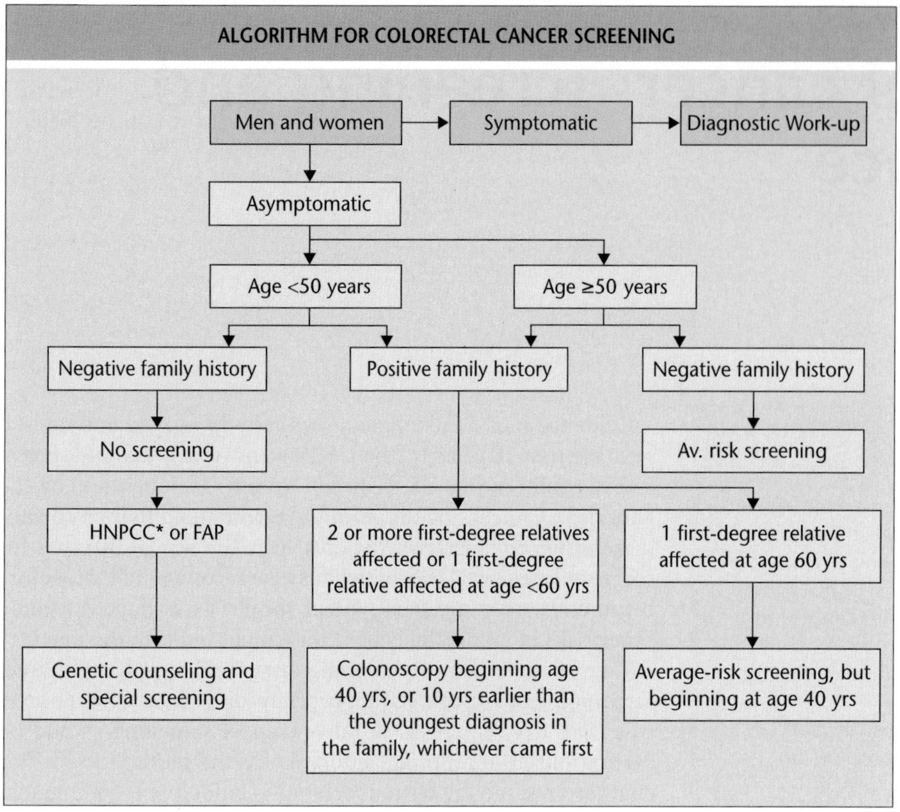

Fig. 60B.1 Algorithm for colorectal cancer screening. *, Either colorectal cancer or adenomatous polyp. FAP, familial adenomatous polyposis; HNPCC, hereditary nonpolyposis colorectal cancer. Reproduced with permission from Winawer S, Fletcher R, Rex D, et al. Colorectal cancer screening and surveillance: clinical guidelines and rationale based on new evidence. Gastroenterology 2003; 124: 544–560. © American Gastroenterological Association.

molecular genetic alterations that cause them to grow, develop advanced histologic features, and eventually turn cancerous. As defined by the US National Polyp Study, advanced adenomas are those that are more than 1 cm in size or contain villous tissue or high-grade dysplasia. These advanced adenomas are much less common than small tubular adenomas, but they are more likely to progress to cancer if not detected by screening. Recent colonoscopy screening experiences indicate that the prevalence of advanced adenomas in women and men is about 6% and 10% respectively. Clinicians now are being urged to shift their efforts away from detecting small tubular adenomas, toward strategies that reliably detect advanced adenomas.[9] Long-term postpolypectomy studies have shown that patients who have had resection of only one or two small tubular adenomas have no measurably increased risk of developing metachronous colorectal cancer.[8] However, those with large (greater than 1 cm) or multiple (more than three) adenomas, or adenomas with villous changes or high-grade dysplasia, have a risk of subsequent cancer that is increased 3–6-fold. Thus, the two main goals of screening are to detect early cancers before they metastasize and to resect advanced adenomas, thereby preventing cancer. The choice of a screening option should, in large part, depend on how well it accomplishes these two goals.

RISK STRATIFICATION FOR COLORECTAL CANCER

Most people are at average risk for colorectal cancer because they have reached the age at which the prevalence of cancer and advanced adenomas is sufficient to justify screening. Based on age–incidence curves, the guidelines recommend that screening of average-risk men and women begin at the age of 50 years. A recent colonoscopy screening study performed in people aged 40–49 years confirmed the very low prevalence of advanced neoplasia in average-risk people under the age of 50 years.[10] Patients with a personal or family history of colorectal neoplasia, and those with longstanding inflammatory bowel disease (ulcerative colitis or Crohn's colitis), may have an above-average risk of colorectal cancer that often begins at a younger age. For patients at risk of HNPCC (Table 60B.1), colonoscopy should

CAUSES AND RISK FACTORS

FAMILIAL RISK OF COLONIC CANCER

Familial setting	Approximate lifetime risk of colonic cancer
General population risk in the USA	6%
One first-degree relative with colonic cancer[a]	2–3-fold increased
Two first-degree relatives with colonic cancer[a]	Increased 3–4-fold
First-degree relative with colonic cancer diagnosed at ≤50 years	Increased 3–4-fold
One second- or third-degree relative with colonic cancer[b,c]	Increased about 1.5-fold
Two second-degree relatives with colonic cancer[b]	Increased about 2–3-fold
One first-degree relative with adenomatous polyp[a]	Increased about 2-fold

[a]First-degree relatives include parents, siblings, and children.
[b]Second-degree relatives include grandparents, aunts, and uncles.
[c]Third-degree relatives include great-grandparents and cousins.
Reprinted with permission from Burt RW. Colon cancer screening. Gastroenterology 2000; 119:837–853. © American Gastroenterological Association.

TABLE 60B.1 CLINICAL CRITERIA FOR HNPCC

AMSTERDAM CRITERIA (FOR CLINICAL IDENTIFICATION OF HNPCC)
At least three relatives with colorectal cancer plus all of the following:
- One affected patient is a first-degree relative of the other two
- Two or more successive generations affected
- One or more affected relative received colorectal cancer diagnosis at age <50 years
- FAP excluded
- Tumors verified by pathologic examination

AMSTERDAM II CRITERIA (FOR CLINICAL IDENTIFICATION OF HNPCC, MODIFIED TO TAKE ACCOUNT OF THE INCREASED OCCURRENCE OF CANCER OTHER THAN OF THE COLON AND RECTUM)
At least three relatives with a *HNPCC-associated cancer (colorectal cancer and cancer of the endometrium, small bowel, ureter, or renal pelvis)*[a] plus all of the following:
- One affected patient is a first-degree relative of the other two
- Two or more successive generations affected
- One or more affected relative received colorectal cancer diagnosis at age <50 years
- FAP excluded *in any case of colorectal cancer*[a]
- Tumors verified by pathologic examination

BETHESDA GUIDELINES (FOR IDENTIFICATION OF PATIENTS WITH COLORECTAL TUMORS WHO SHOULD UNDERGO TESTING FOR MICROSATELLITE INSTABILITY)

B1 Individuals with cancer in families that meet the Amsterdam Criteria
B2 Individuals with two HNPCC-related tumors, including synchronous and metachronous colorectal cancer or associated extracolonic cancer (endometrium, ovarian, gastric, hepatobiliary, or small bowel cancer or transitional cell carcinoma of the renal pelvis or ureter)
B3 Individuals with colorectal cancer and a first-degree relative with colorectal cancer or HNPCC-related extracolonic cancer or a colorectal adenoma; one of the cancers diagnosed at age <45 years,[b] and the adenoma diagnosed at age <40 years
B4 Individuals with colorectal cancer or endometrial cancer diagnosed at age <45 years[b]
B5 Individuals with right-sided colorectal cancer with an undifferentiated pattern (solid, cribriform) on histopathology, diagnosed at age <45 years[b] (solid or cribriform), defined as poorly differentiated for undifferentiated carcinoma composed of irregular, solid sheets of large eosinophilic cells and containing small gland-like spaces
B6 Individuals with signet ring cell type colorectal cancer diagnosed at age <45 years[b] (composed of more than 50% signet ring cells)
B7 Individuals with adenomas diagnosed at age <40years

[a]Differences between Amsterdam and Amsterdam II Criteria are shown in italics.
[b]Modified Bethesda Criteria replace the age of '<45 years' for colorectal cancer diagnosis in B3, B4, B5, and B6 to '<50 years.'
Adapted and reprinted with permission from Raedle J, Trojan J, Brieger A, et al. Bethesda Guidelines: relation to microsatellite instability and MLH1 promoter methylation in patients with colorectal cancer. Ann Intern Med 2001; 135:566–576.

be carried out every 1–2 years beginning at age 20–25 years or 10 years earlier than the youngest familial occurrence of colonic cancer. Relatives of people with a known inherited mismatch repair gene mutation should be offered genetic testing.

Precise evidence to guide management in inflammatory bowel disease is lacking, but a case–control study has suggested better survival in patients with ulcerative colitis who are in a surveillance program.[3] The risk is highest with total ulcerative colitis, and colonoscopy to determine extent at 10 years and colonoscopic surveillance every 1–2 years thereafter is commonly used. Risk is also increased in patients with less extensive ulcerative colitis and in those with Crohn's colitis; surveillance practice varies from country to country. When high-grade dysplasia or a dysplasia-associated lesion or mass is found, colectomy should normally be offered. With low-grade dysplasia, particularly in the presence of inflammation, repeat colonoscopy after 3–6 months is appropriate, but persistent multifocal low-grade dysplasia should prompt consideration of colectomy.[3] A careful family and personal history looking for these special risk factors should be taken before initiating any of the screening options.

GUIDELINE OPTIONS FOR SCREENING

Unlike screening for other major malignancies in which a single screening test usually is recommended, the evidence-based colorectal cancer screening guidelines present a menu of five different options, any one of which is considered satisfactory. These options are listed in Table 60B.2. The guidelines emphasize that each of these five options has unique advantages and limitations that should be considered by each healthcare delivery system, and perhaps by each patient. Then, in a 'shared decision process' the patient could be given an opportunity to help choose how he or she wishes to be screened.

ADVANTAGES AND LIMITATIONS OF THE FIVE SCREENING OPTIONS

Fecal occult blood test

The fecal occult blood test (FOBT) is the only screening option that has been proven to be effective in prospective randomized controlled trials. Five such trials involving nearly 350 000 participants have been performed, two in the USA and three in Europe. The Minnesota FOBT Trial was the first of these to publish definitive endpoint results. Beginning in 1993, the trial reported a reduction in colorectal cancer mortality rate of 33% and 21%, respectively, for annual and biennial FOBT screening using rehydrated Hemoccult tests (Beckman-Coulter, Palo Alto, CA, USA), followed by colonoscopy for those with a positive screen.[5,11] Participants who complied with all recommended rounds of annual screening experienced a 45% colorectal cancer mortality rate reduction. This, therefore, is the benefit that patients reasonably can expect if they comply with annual FOBT screening. Follow-up in the Minnesota trial also demonstrated a significant reduction in colorectal cancer incidence, presumably the result of detection of advanced adenomatous polyps.[7] Three of the other trials (New York, UK, and

TABLE 60B.2 COLORECTAL CANCER SCREENING GUIDELINES: ACCEPTABLE SCREENING OPTIONS FOR ASYMPTOMATIC, AVERAGE-RISK MEN AND WOMEN AGED 50 YEARS OR MORE[2–4]

- Annual screening with fecal occult blood tests (FOBTs)
- Flexible sigmoidoscopy screening every 5 years
- The combination of annual FOBTs and flexible sigmoidoscopy every 5 years
- Double-contrast barium enema every 5 years
- Direct colonoscopy screening every 10 years

Denmark) later also reported consistent reductions in colorectal cancer mortality as a result of FOBT screening.[12]

Screening with FOBTs has a number of practical advantages. A program of annual screening using a reasonably sensitive FOBT – HemoccultSensa guaiac cards (Beckman-Coulter) or one of the newer immunochemical FOBTs – followed by colonoscopy when stool blood is found, detects most colorectal cancers and many advanced adenomas. A modeling decision analysis that was performed as part of the GI Consortium Screening guideline preparation showed that, even if an individual FOBT screen sensitivity for cancer is only 40%, the program sensitivity for annual screening over 5 years is 85%.[3] A 60% and 80% individual screen sensitivity translates into a 93% and 98% program sensitivity, respectively. A detailed analysis of actual data from the Minnesota trial determined that the sensitivity of the rehydrated Hemoccult test for detecting colorectal cancers, for both one-time testing and the program of repetitive annual testing, exceeded 90%. This method of screening has a very low upfront cost, significantly reduces both colorectal cancer mortality and incidence, and is feasible, widely available, and acceptable to patients. Disadvantages of FOBT screening include the need for frequent screening, low sensitivity for polyps, especially smaller ones, and a relatively high false-positivity rate for advanced neoplasia. Some argue, however, that, unlike the case with indirect screening tests for other cancers, a false-positive FOBT is not completely without some benefit to the patient. At worst, it initiates a colonoscopy – a highly definitive diagnostic test that many are now proposing for direct screening anyway. A negative colonoscopy finding provides considerable reassurance about future colorectal cancer risk, and obviates the need for any further screening for at least 10 years, according to the guidelines.

Flexible sigmoidoscopy

Screening with flexible sigmoidoscopy also has a number of important advantages. It detects the majority of colorectal cancers and advanced adenomas, as most are located in the left colon within reach of the 60-cm instrument. A recent analysis from the VA Multicenter Colonoscopy Screening Study showed that a single screening flexible sigmoidoscopy would detect 70–80% of all advanced colorectal neoplasia provided that patients found to have a left-sided neoplasm then underwent full colonoscopy.[13] When performed by experienced examiners, flexible sigmoidoscopy is highly accurate (few false positives or false negatives), safe, and well tolerated. The examination is inexpensive and can be performed in a few minutes after a simple bowel cleansing preparation. Screening sigmoidoscopy has been shown in cohort and case–control studies to reduce mortality from colorectal cancers located within its reach by 60–80%. Some of these studies also indicate that the protective effect of a single screening examination may last up to 9 years, so infrequent screening is possible.

Fecal occult blood test and flexible sigmoidoscopy

Combining annual FOB testing and flexible sigmoidoscopy every 5 years appears to be an especially effective screening approach because it largely corrects the limitations of performing either option alone. The FOBT misses many polyps, and has been shown in three of the long-term trials to be relatively insensitive for cancers located in the rectosigmoid colon and rectum. Repeated annually, however, the FOBT will detect most colorectal cancers before they become incurable. Flexible sigmoidoscopy is highly accurate in the left colon, where most cancers and advanced adenomatous polyps occur, but misses 20–30% of proximal advanced neoplasias in patients who do not also have a synchronous left-sided neoplasm. If both a FOBT and flexible sigmoidoscopy are recommended at a given time, the FOBT always should be done first. A positive test is an indication for colonoscopy and obviates the need for the screening flexible sigmoidoscopy.

Barium enema

Although double-contrast barium enema (DCBE) is included in the menus of guideline options, it is used infrequently for screening in the USA and has never been directly studied for this purpose. Furthermore, DCBE has been shown to be relatively insensitive for detecting advanced neoplasia. A retrospective study by Rex et al[14] in 20 centers in Indiana showed that about 15% of colorectal cancers are missed by barium enema examination, compared with a miss rate for colonoscopy of 3–5%. The US National Polyp Study performed back-to-back DCBE and colonoscopy on 580 patients and found that the sensitivity for detecting large adenomas (greater than 1 cm) was only 48%.[15] Because of its lower sensitivity for cancer and polyps, when DCBE is used for screening the guidelines recommend a screening interval of 5 years.

Colonoscopy

Although virtually unimaginable only 5–10 years ago, direct colonoscopy screening has now become the overwhelming preference of gastroenterologists and many others throughout the Western world. This option is somewhat of a perturbation of the classic World Health Organization definition of a screening test, as defined in the introduction to this chapter. Instead of performing a simple, acceptable, inexpensive, and indirect test to identify those in the average-risk population who might benefit from further evaluation, we instead have moved upfront to the performance of a complex, expensive, and somewhat invasive, definitive diagnostic and therapeutic examination. Direct screening colonoscopy, however, now is championed by many physician and patient groups because it accurately detects almost all cancers and advanced adenomas, and allows for resection of almost all polyps during a single sitting with a single bowel-cleansing preparation. Although no prospective randomized trials showing the efficacy of colonoscopy screening have yet been published, it clearly is the most reliable way of accomplishing both of the major objectives of screening–cancer prevention through polyp resection and reduced mortality through the diagnosis of early-stage cancers. Because of colonoscopy's high negative predictive value and the long natural history of the adenoma–carcinoma sequence, infrequent screening every 10 years is currently recommended by the guidelines.

A number of recent reports have demonstrated that, when performed by well trained experienced endoscopists, colonoscopy screening is feasible, acceptable, and safe. The VA Multicenter Colonoscopy Screening Trial performed screening colonoscopy on 3196 patients in 13 VA centers. Examinations were complete to the cecum in 97.7% of patients; there were no perforations, and the overall rate of major complications (mostly bleeding after polypectomy) was only 0.3%.[16] To date, more than 6000 screening colonoscopies have been reported in the literature, with no deaths. Compelling indirect evidence suggests that this approach is highly effective at reducing both the incidence and mortality of colorectal cancer. For example, colonoscopy and polypectomy in the US National Polyp Study reduced colorectal cancer incidence by up to 90%; a number of case–control studies strongly suggest efficacy; and the large FOBT trials ultimately effected their reduction of cancer incidence and mortality, mostly by doing colonoscopy for those with fecal occult blood. Potential limitations of screening colonoscopy include issues of risk, cost, patient acceptability, and capacity. Conscious sedation with its attendant risk, cost, and inconvenience is usually required for screening colonoscopy. There appears also to be a considerable indirect cost of performing screening colonoscopy. A single screening examination requires the better part of 2 days to complete the bowel purging preparation, the examination itself, and subsequent recovery. When time lost from work for the patient and his or her accompanying 'responsible adult' plus transportation costs and other attendant expenses are considered, the indirect cost of a screening colonoscopy is substantial. Although screening colonoscopy has been shown to be very safe when performed by experienced physicians, there are concerns about both the accuracy and risk of this option when it is carried out in increasing numbers by less experienced examiners.

COLONOSCOPY DEMAND VERSUS CAPACITY

In many countries, including the USA, the great demand for screening colonoscopy shows signs of overwhelming the capacity to perform these examinations. Many endoscopy centers are reporting long waiting times for a screening colonoscopy, and this threatens to diminish the attractiveness and practicality of this option. An important issue that is now being addressed by a number of interested groups is whether or not adequate capacity exists to perform screening colonoscopy for all those over the age of 50 years. Rex and Lieberman[17] reported that in 1999 about 4.4 million colonoscopies were performed in the USA. Using reasonable estimates of compliance, and current levels of screening, they estimated that widespread implementation of screening colonoscopy will require about 2.6 million additional examinations per year. It is unlikely that this increased demand will be satisfied in the near future by training more endoscopists. They suggested, however, that some of this new demand might be met by increasing colonoscopy productivity, by decreasing the number of screening flexible sigmoidoscopies performed by gastrointestinal specialists, and by decreasing the number of colonoscopies that currently are being performed either for too-frequent postpolypectomy surveillance or for signs and symptoms that have a low positive predictive value for detecting clinically significant neoplasia. Data from the US Clinical Outcomes Research Initiative (CORI) indicate that about 10% of colonoscopy procedures now are performed for vague symptoms of abdominal pain, bloating, and change in bowel habits.[18] However, the proportion of patients with these symptoms without bleeding who have neoplasia is similar to that of asymptomatic populations.

COST-EFFECTIVENESS OF SCREENING

Mathematical modeling analyses using reasonable assumptions and current charge and cost data have concluded that screening for colorectal cancer is highly cost-effective compared with other preventive interventions commonly used today.[19] Most of these analyses concluded that all of the guideline screening options are cost-effective and none can be favored based on this parameter alone. These economists concluded that colorectal cancer screening represents a very good investment for high-risk countries such as the USA. In one analysis, Lieberman[20] concluded that, if the cost of colonoscopy could be reasonably constrained, screening for colorectal cancer might become cost saving. In most health delivery systems, the cost of caring for a patient with advanced cancer far exceeds that of screening, polypectomy, or surgery for an early-stage cancer. Lieberman's study also calculated the cost of not doing screening. This cost, incurred by failing to find advanced adenomas and prevent cancer, or by failing to find cancers at an early, curable stage, averaged $670–1000 (US) per potential patient screened per 10 years.[20]

EMERGING NEW SCREENING TESTS

Two new methods of screening for colorectal neoplasia – virtual colonoscopy and DNA-based stool tests – have recently been introduced clinically, and these may be added to the menu of screening options in the future. Virtual colonoscopy (computed tomographic (CT) colography) combines thin-section rapid helical CT scanning with sophisticated computer software capable of rendering two- and three-dimensional images of the large bowel. Using a conventional workstation, a radiologist can conduct a thorough examination of the colon images looking for polyps and cancer. Advantages of virtual colonoscopy compared with conventional optical colonoscopy are a shorter examination time, no need for sedation, and few if any complications. Precise localization of lesions is possible, both sides of the bowel wall and bowel folds can be examined, and the proximal colon can be cleared of lesions when there is an obstructing left-sided cancer or colonoscopy is incomplete. Disadvantages of virtual colonoscopy include the need for thorough bowel cleansing and for uncomfortable gas distention of the colon, lower accuracy in some studies for small and flat lesions, interference with readings by bowel spasm and retained debris, and the fact that the examination is diagnostic only (cannot remove polyps). Earlier comparison studies in selected patients indicated that virtual colonoscopy was less accurate than colonoscopy, especially for the detection of medium-sized and small polyps. However, a recent large study performed in three US military hospitals by Pickhardt et al,[21] in a low-prevalence, largely average-risk population of 1233 asymptomatic adults, showed comparable sensitivity of virtual and optical colonoscopy for polyps greater than 6 mm in diameter. If other centers are able to adopt the techniques used in this remarkable study to achieve similar results, and if issues of cost and patient acceptability are satisfactorily addressed, virtual colonoscopy will likely soon be added to the guideline menu of screening options.

Human DNA can be isolated from stool and analyzed for the presence of genetic abnormalities that are characteristic of advanced colorectal adenomas and cancers. A stool test now is being marketed that checks for a battery of these genetic abnormalities. Using this 'PreGen-Plus test' (Exact Sciences, Marlborough, MA, USA), a double-blind multicenter study compared results in 2507 patients with a standard one-time

Hemoccult II FOBT screen. Sensitivity of the DNA test and the FOBT for cancer was 52% and 13%, respectively (presentation, annual meeting of the American College of Gastroenterology, October 2003). Specificity for both tests was 95%, indicating few false positives. A second large multicenter trial in average-risk patients is in progress, and the manufacturer is continuing development of the test to increase sensitivity. Many predict that this method will also be added to the menu of screening options, perhaps in combination with other methods.

GUIDELINE RECOMMENDATIONS FOR POSTPOLYPECTOMY SURVEILLANCE

Patients who have had colonoscopic resection of one or more adenomatous polyps may have an increased risk of recurrent advanced adenomas and subsequent cancer. Depending on their estimated level of risk, they might therefore benefit from follow-up colonoscopic surveillance. Current guideline recommendations for postpolypectomy follow-up surveillance are based largely on data from the US National Polyp Study.[22] In this seven-center trial directed by Winawer, 1418 patients with at least one newly diagnosed colorectal adenoma had polyps resected colonoscopically and their colon cleared of all synchronous lesions. Eligible patients then were randomized to two equal groups, one to have follow-up colonoscopy at 1 year and then every 3 years, the second to have colonoscopy only every 3 years. There was a high rate (32–42%) of 'recurrent' (many were likely missed initially) adenomas detected 3 years after the initial polypectomy. Most of these, however, were small tubular adenomas with little immediate clinical importance. Only 3.3% of patients in each group were found to have advanced adenomas. The study concluded that a 1-year follow-up colonoscopy was not indicated. The chance of having an advanced adenoma at follow-up was increased if a patient's index adenomas were multiple (more than 3), large (greater than 1 cm), or if they had a first-degree relative with colorectal cancer. Patients with only one or two small tubular adenomas without a family history of colorectal cancer had a very low incidence of metachronous advanced adenomas at 3 years. Other large polyp trials have suggested that villus histology and high-grade dysplasia are also predictors of recurrence of advanced adenoma.[23,24]

Postpolypectomy recommendations are listed in Table 60B.3. Current guidelines recommend that clinicians tailor postpolypectomy surveillance to a careful assessment of each patient's risk for developing metachronous advanced adenomas.[3,25] Patients with colorectal adenomas can be stratified into high- and low-risk groups. After the colon has been cleared of all synchronous adenomas, repeat colonoscopy is recommended in 3 years for patients who are at high risk. These include those who have large (greater than 1 cm) or multiple (more than three) adenomas, or an adenoma with villus change or high-grade dysplasia, and all those over the age of 60 years with a parent with colorectal cancer. After a negative finding at 3-year colonoscopy, subsequent surveillance can be extended to 5-year intervals. Patients with a low risk of metachronous advanced adenomas include those who have only one or two small (less than 1 cm) simple tubular adenomas and no significant family history of colorectal cancer. For these low-risk patients, the first postpolypectomy follow-up colonoscopy can be safely delayed for at least 5 years; in patients with advanced

TABLE 60B.3 POSTPOLYPECTOMY SURVEILLANCE RECOMMENDATIONS[3,25]

- Complete colonoscopy should be performed at time of polypectomy to clear the colon of all synchronous neoplasia.
- Repeat colonoscopy to check for metachronous adenomas should be performed in 3 years in patients at high risk of developing metachronous advanced adenomas. This includes those who at baseline examination have multiple (three or more) adenomas, a large (≥1 cm) adenoma, an adenoma with villous histology or high-grade dysplasia, or a significant family history of colorectal cancer.
- Repeat colonoscopy to check for metachronous adenomas should be performed in 5 years for most patients at low risk of developing advanced adenomas. This includes those who at baseline examination have only one or two small tubular adenomas (<1 cm) and no family history of colorectal cancer.
- Selected patients at low risk of metachronous advanced adenomas may not require follow-up surveillance because of advanced age or co-morbidity.
- After one negative follow-up colonoscopy, subsequent surveillance intervals may be increased to 5 years.
- Surveillance should be discontinued when, because of advanced age or co-morbidity, it seems unlikely that it will benefit the patient.

age or significant co-morbidity, no follow-up may be indicated. Because many clinicians perform postpolypectomy surveillance more frequently than needed, widespread adoption of these evidence-based guideline recommendations will substantially lower the cost of postpolypectomy surveillance. In his cost-effectiveness analysis of colorectal cancer screening, Lieberman[20] concluded that, because screening detects many unsuspected adenomatous polyps, traditional postpolypectomy surveillance comprises 19–34% of the total cost of any screening program. If surveillance were done correctly and focused only on the detection of advanced adenomas, this percentage cost could be reduced by more than 40%.

SURVEILLANCE AFTER SURGICAL RESECTION OF COLORECTAL CANCER

The objectives of surveillance following curative surgical resection of a colorectal cancer are to detect treatable recurrences, missed synchronous cancers or adenomas, and new metachronous neoplasia. Except in a few selected patients, curative treatment of recurrent colorectal cancer is rarely possible; in addition, palliation for irresectable recurrent cancer is not very effective and is not much improved by finding irresectable recurrences before they cause symptoms.[26] Anastomotic (suture-line) recurrences of cancers of the abdominal colon (above the rectum) are very rare. A recent meta-analysis by Renahan et al[27] of five follow-up studies involving 1026 patients undergoing colorectal cancer resection showed an average incidence of anastomotic recurrence of only 3.2%. Resection of these recurrences rarely results in long-term survival. Thus, nearly all recurrences of proximal colonic cancer occur outside the bowel and cannot be detected by colonoscopy. Local recurrences in the area of an anastomosis do, of course, occur after anterior resection of Dukes' B or C rectosigmoid cancers. Because these recurrences may be amenable to radiation, or occasionally to a second surgical resection, affected patients should be followed more closely with flexible sigmoidoscopy –

every 3–6 months for a period of 2 years. In reality, therefore, the main objectives of follow-up surveillance in the majority of patients are to detect curable synchronous and metachronous advanced adenomatous polyps and cancers. The incidence of synchronous colorectal cancers and advanced adenomas in patients with a known cancer is reported to be 2–7% and 8–15%, respectively. Metachronous cancers and advanced adenomas develop with similar frequency.

Outcome studies indicate that traditional intensive surveillance programs for patients with colorectal cancer are ineffective, do not often detect curable cancer recurrences, and rarely alter management.[28] Schoemaker et al[29] prospectively randomized 325 patients who underwent curative resection of colorectal cancer to either intensive or standard follow-up programs. Intensive follow-up consisted of yearly colonoscopy and computed tomography of the liver, chest radiography, and clinical visits with simple blood and stool screening tests. Standard follow-up consisted of clinical visits and simple blood and stool screening tests only. On completion of 5-year follow-up, there was no significant difference in survival between the two groups. Yearly colonoscopy failed to detect any asymptomatic local recurrences. These investigators concluded that intensive surveillance will not improve survival from colorectal cancer when added to symptom and simple screening test review.

The following is a rational follow-up plan for patients after curative resection of colorectal cancer (Table 60B.4). Compared with traditional follow-up practices still used in many centers, this program consists of more accurate studies performed less frequently, directed primarily at reducing mortality from the disease. Colonoscopy should be performed during the perioperative period to clear the colon of synchronous neoplasia, preferably before surgery so that cancers and large polyps may be included in the resection. If not feasible before surgery because of an obstructing left colonic cancer, clearing colonoscopy is done 3–6 months after surgery if no distant metastases are found at operation. Because a few interval cancers are found within a year or two of surgery in most large series, some experts and some surgical guidelines recommend that an additional 'clearing' colonoscopy be performed 1 year after surgery. Postoperative visits are scheduled as needed to educate the patient about symptoms of early recurrence, check for postsurgical problems, and provide medical and emotional support. Repeat surveillance colonoscopy is performed in 3 years, and then, depending on findings, every 3–5 years to detect metachronous neoplasia. Surveillance flexible sigmoidoscopy every 3–6 months is reserved for selected patients undergoing sphincter-sparing low anterior resection of rectal or rectosigmoid cancers.

Long-term survival has been reported in selected patients undergoing surgical resection of solitary hepatic and, less commonly, pulmonary metastases.[28] Some report that about 20–30% of patients undergoing curative resection of colorectal cancer will develop isolated hepatic metastases; about 25% of these will ultimately be resectable, with a 5-year survival rate of about 25%. Thus, the total number of patients who have a favorable outcome is very small, and this may not justify routine intensive surveillance for all cases. Instead, selected patients who are in good enough health to tolerate major hepatic or pulmonary resection, and who have colorectal cancer with a substantial likelihood of metastasis (stages II or III), might be offered special intensive surveillance. Because the majority of solitary metastases occur in the first 2 years after initial surgery, this surveillance should usually not be prolonged much beyond that time interval. Surveillance for this select group, which comprises only about 20% of cases, generally includes serial chest radiography every 3–6 months, serum carcinoembryonic antigen determinations every 2–3 months, and abdominal CT scans every 6–12 months. Liver function chemistries are insufficiently sensitive to be of value.

TABLE 60B.4 SURVEILLANCE RECOMMENDATIONS AFTER CURATIVE SURGICAL RESECTION OF COLORECTAL CANCER[3,28]

- Colonoscopy should be performed during the perioperative period to clear the colon of synchronous neoplasia.
- Some guidelines recommend a second clearing colonoscopy at 1 year.
- Postoperative visits are scheduled as needed to support the patient.
- Repeat colonoscopy to detect metachronous neoplasia at 3 years, then every 3–5 years depending on findings.
- Discontinue colonoscopic surveillance when, because of advanced age or co-morbidity, it seems unlikely that it will benefit the patient.
- Perform carcinoembryonic antigen measurements every 2–3 months, chest radiography every 3–6 months, and abdominal computed tomography every 6–12 months, for 2–3 years in selected patients.

SUMMARY

Colorectal cancer is a disease that is highly suited for a screening approach. The two objectives of screening are detection of early cancer and prevention of cancer through the detection and resection of advanced adenomatous polyps. Evidence-based guidelines recommend one of five screening options for average-risk asymptomatic people over the age of 50 years. Each option has unique advantages and limitations that need to be considered by both health delivery systems and patients when choosing how to be screened. All screening options have been shown to be cost-effective. Although direct colonoscopy screening is considered the preferred option by many, a number of barriers exist including limited capacity in most countries with a high risk of colorectal cancer. Virtual colonoscopy and DNA-based stool tests have been introduced and may soon be added to the menu of screening options. After colonoscopic polypectomy, most patients should be offered colonoscopic surveillance tailored to the features of each case. Surveillance after curative resection of a colorectal cancer is designed mainly to detect all synchronous and metachronous advanced adenomas before a metachronous cancer can develop.

REFERENCES

1. Jemal A, Tiwari RC, Murray T et al. Cancer statistics, 2004. CA Cancer J Clin 2004; 54:8–29.
2. Pigone M, Rich M, Teutsch SM et al. Screening for colorectal cancer in adults at average risk: summary of the evidence for the US Preventive Services Task Force. Ann Intern Med 2002; 137:132–141.
3. Winawer SJ, Fletcher RH, Rex D et al. Colorectal cancer screening and surveillance: clinical guidelines and rationale based on new evidence. Gastroenterology 2003; 124:544–560.
4. Smith RA, von Eschenbach AC, Wender R et al. American Cancer Society guidelines for the early detection of cancer: update of early detection guidelines for prostate, colorectal, and endometrial cancers. CA Cancer J Clin 2001; 51:38–75.
5. Mandel JS, Bond JH, Church TR et al. Reducing mortality from colorectal cancer by screening for fecal occult blood. N Engl J Med 1993; 328:1365–1371.
6. Bond JH. Clinical evidence for the adenoma–carcinoma sequence, and the management of patients with colorectal adenomas. Semin Gastrointest Dis 2000; 11:176–184.
7. Winawer SJ, Zauber AG, Ho MN et al. Prevention of colorectal cancer by colonoscopic polypectomy: The National Polyp Study Workgroup. N Engl J Med 1993; 329:1977–1981.
8. Mandel JS, Church TR, Ederer F, Bond JH. The effect of fecal occult-blood screening on the incidence of colorectal cancer. N Engl J Med 2000; 343:1603–1607.
9. Winawer SJ, Zauber AG. The advanced adenoma as the primary target of screening. Gastrointest Endosc Clin N Am 2002; 12:1–10.
10. Imperiale TF, Wagner DR, Lin CY et al. Results of screening colonoscopy among persons 40 to 49 years of age. N Engl J Med 2002; 346:1781–1785.
11. Mandel JS, Church TR, Ederer F, Bond JH. Colorectal cancer mortality: effectiveness of biennial screening for fecal occult blood. J Natl Cancer Inst 1999; 91:434–437.
12. Bond JH. Fecal occult blood test screening for colorectal cancer. Gastrointest Endosc Clin N Am 2002; 12:11–22.
13. Lieberman DA, Weiss DG, for the VA Cooperative Study Group 380. One-time screening for colorectal cancer with combined fecal occult blood testing and examination of the distal colon. N Engl J Med 2001; 345:555–560.
14. Rex DK, Rahmani EY, Haseman JH et al. Relative sensitivity of colonoscopy and barium enema for detection of colorectal cancer in clinical practice. Gastroenterology 1997; 112:17–23.
15. Winawer SJ, Stewart ET, Zauber AG et al. A comparison of colonoscopy and double-contrast barium enema for surveillance after polypectomy. N Engl J Med 2000; 342:1766–1772.
16. Nelson DB, McQuaid KR, Bond JH et al. Procedural success and complications of large-scale screening colonoscopy. Gastrointest Endosc 2002; 55:307–314.
17. Rex DK, Lieberman DA. Feasibility of colonoscopy screening: discussion of issues and recommendations regarding implementation. Gastrointest Endosc 2001; 54:662–667.
18. Lieberman DA, deGarmo PL, Fleischer DE et al. Colonic neoplasia in patients with nonspecific GI symptoms. Gastrointest Endosc 2000; 51:647–651.
19. Wagner J, Tunis S, Brown M et al. The cost effectiveness of colorectal cancer screening in average risk adults. In: Young G, Rozen P, Levin B, eds. Prevention and early detection of colorectal cancer. Philadelphia: WB Saunders; 1996:321–356.
20. Lieberman DA. Cost-effectiveness model for colon cancer screening. Gastroenterology 1995; 109:1781–1790.
21. Pickhardt, PJ, Choi JR, Hwang I et al. Computed tomographic virtual colonoscopy to screen for colorectal neoplasia in asymptomatic adults. N Engl J Med 2003; 349:2191–2200.
22. Winawer SJ, Zauber AG, O'Brien MJ et al. Randomized comparison of surveillance intervals after colonoscopic removal of newly diagnosed adenomatous polyps. N Engl J Med 1993; 328:901–906.
23. Van Stolk RU, Beck GJ, Baron JA et al. Adenoma characteristics at first colonoscopy as predictors of adenoma recurrence and characteristics at follow-up. Gastroenterology 1998; 115:13–18.
24. Kairasp C, Noshirwani MD, van Stolk RU et al. Adenoma size and number are predictive of adenoma recurrence: implications for surveillance colonoscopy. Gastrointest Endosc 2000; 51:422–427.
25. Bond JH, for the Practice Parameters Committee of the American College of Gastroenterology. Polyp guideline: diagnosis, treatment, and surveillance for patients with colorectal polyps. Am J Gastroenterol 2000; 95:3053–3063.
26. Rossini FP, Waye JD. Colonoscopy after colon cancer resection. In: Waye JD, Rex DK, Williams CB, eds. Colonoscopy: principles and practice. Malden, MA: Blackwell; 2003:468–477.
27. Renahan AG, Egger M, Saunders MP, O'Dwyer ST. Impact on survival of intensive follow-up after curative resection for colorectal cancer: systematic review and meta-analysis of randomized trials. BMJ 2002; 324:813–819.
28. Bond JH. The postoperative colon. In: Raskin JB, Nord HJ, eds. Colonoscopy: principles and techniques. New York: Igaku-Shoin; 1995:227–240.
29. Schoemaker D, Black R, Giles L, Toouli J. Yearly colonoscopy, liver CT and chest radiography do not influence 5-year survival of colorectal cancer patients. Gastroenterology 1998; 114:7–14.

Chapter 60C

Polyps and polyposis

Douglas J Robertson and John A Baron

KEY POINTS

- A polyp is any raised lesion emanating from the normally flat colonic mucosa
- Polyps are important because some may develop into cancer
- The most important neoplastic polyp is the adenoma

NTRODUCTION

. colorectal polyp is any raised lesion emanating from the ormally flat mucosa of the colon or rectum. These lesions ıay be either sessile (without a stalk) or pedunculated (on a talk or stem) (Fig. 60C.1). Polyps are clinically important ecause some may develop into cancer; historically polyps ave been classified by their potential for such malignant transormation. The most common neoplastic polyps are adenomas; on-neoplastic polyps include hyperplastic polyps and hamarɔmas. Some hyperplastic polyps may have malignant potenial (see below).

Because of their high prevalence and premalignant potential, denomas are clinically the most important polyps. Nonetheless, ecent insights suggest that the classical 'adenoma-carcinoma' equence may not explain all large bowel malignancy.[1]

:PIDEMIOLOGY

n adults, colorectal polyps are extremely common: autopsy tudies suggest a prevalence that may approach 50%. Histoɔgically, the majority (up to 90%) of these lesions are lentified as either adenomas or hyperplastic polyps.

Adenoma-carcinoma sequence: Most colorectal cancers evelop from adenomas. Adenomas are visible masses or bumps f dysplastic epithelium, i.e., all adenomas are dysplastic.)ysplasia is a neoplastic change without invasion across the asement membrane into the lamina propria. Countries with igh colorectal cancer rates also seem to have a high prevalence f adenomas. Like colorectal cancer, the prevalence of adenomas ıcreases with age, and the distribution of adenomas within he large bowel is similar to that for carcinoma. Both autopsy nd colonoscopy studies demonstrate that larger and more ysplastic adenomas are more often found distal to the splenic exure than in the proximal colon, a distribution that parallels hat of colorectal cancer.[2] Further evidence for the adenomaarcinoma sequence derives from the finding of foci of invaive carcinoma with adenomas, the occurrence of adenomatous issue at the margin of carcinomas, and the broad similarity of genetic changes in adenomas and carcinomas (though of course more pronounced in the latter).

CAUSES, RISK FACTORS

Environmental factors: Investigations of the association between dietary patterns and adenoma risk have been inconsistent. Observational studies of intake of vegetables, fruits, fiber, and fat have shown no consistent pattern of association.[3] Moreover, with the exception of calcium supplementation,[4] clinical trials of dietary interventions have been negative.

Nonetheless, certain lifestyle factors do appear to be important. Exercise is inversely associated with risk, particularly with regards to colon adenoma formation in men,[5] and obesity may be a risk factor. Current smoking has repeatedly been associated with increased risk; studies of the effect of alcohol consumption are less consistent.[6]

A final important environmental exposure is medication use. Nonsteroidal anti-inflammatory drugs (including aspirin) are inversely associated with adenoma risk.[7] This association has been documented in well-carried out observational studies[8] and confirmed in clinical trials of these agents (see 'Treatment and prevention' below).

Genetic factors: These also certainly play a role in adenoma formation. For example, first-degree relatives of patients with adenomas are at increased risk for colorectal cancer, and there are several well-recognized genetic syndromes associated with colorectal adenomas (see Chapter 60A).

CAUSES AND RISK FACTORS

- Polyps are common, occurring in up to 50% of adult patients
- At endoscopy, adenomas and hyperplastic polyps are the most common types of polyps encountered
- The epidemiology of adenomas mirrors that of colorectal cancer
- Risk factors for adenomas include both environmental and genetic exposures
- Important environmental exposures include exercise, smoking, and medications (e.g., NSAIDs)

PATHOGENESIS

Normal colorectal mucosa is characterized by constant cellular proliferation that results in replacement of the surface epithelium every 4–6 days. During carcinogenesis, the pattern of cell kinetics appears to be altered. The overall proliferative activity is both increased and active mitotic activity (normally limited

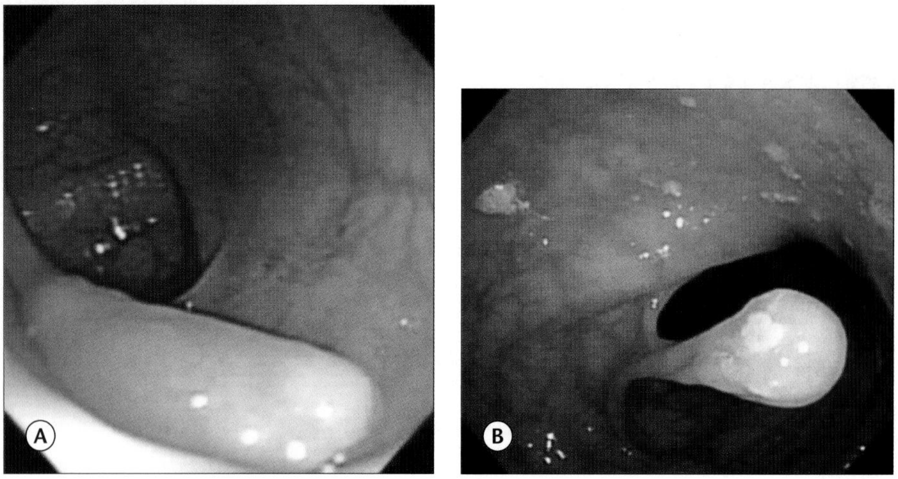

Fig. 60C.1 Colorectal polyps. A. Sessile polyp. **B.** Pedunculated polyp.

to the base of the crypt) extends toward the lumen leading to an increase in the surface epithelium undergoing continued turnover. The increased epithelial proliferation appears to be accompanied by impairment of normal programed cell death (apoptosis). The genetic processes that drive the transition from normal epithelium through adenoma to cancer are also now more fully understood. The biological and genetic changes leading to cancer development are detailed in Chapter 60A.

Traditionally, hyperplastic polyps have not been considered to have malignant potential; however this view may be too simplistic. It is now believed that there is a 'serrated pathway' to colorectal cancer that may involve some types of hyperplastic appearing polyps. The increasing recognition of these lesions and their potential to develop into cancer has led to an on-going re-evaluation of the role of hyperplastic-appearing polyps in carcinogenesis.

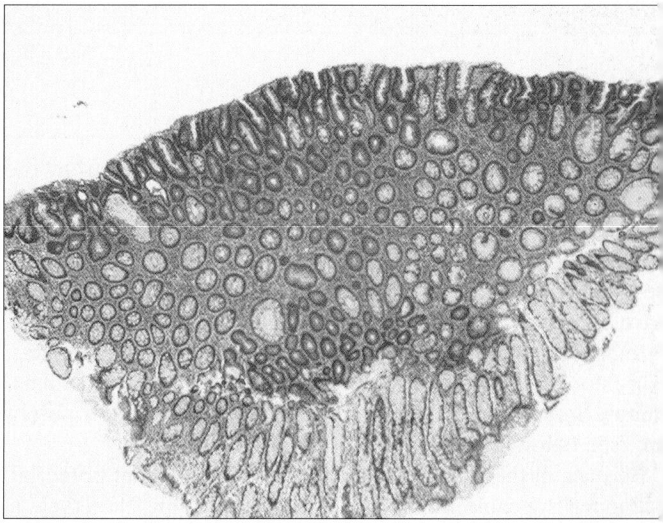

Fig. 60C.2 Tubular adenoma. (Note the normal-appearing glands at the bottom of the figure.)

PATHOLOGY

Subtypes: Adenomas can be classified as tubular, villous, or tubulovillous depending on their histologic features. Most (80%) adenomas are tubular, composed of simple branching epithelia as characterized in Fig. 60C.2. Villous adenomas account for between 5% and 15% of adenomas. Microscopically, the mucosa of villous adenomas has a 'frond-like' appearance similar to that of a normal small bowel biopsy (Fig. 60C.3). By definition, an adenoma must have at least 75% villous architecture to be considered a villous adenoma. Tubulovillous adenomas also compose between 5% and 15% of adenomas and have features of both lesions. Specifically, these lesions have a villous component that ranges from 25% to 75%.

Dysplasia: As indicated previously all adenomas are composed of dysplastic epithelium. Within the epithelium there is nuclear crowding and hyperchromasia. Adenomas with high-grade dysplasia are characterized by marked cellular atypia (resembling carcinomatous change), with the area of adenomatous change limited to the epithelium. If severe dysplasia penetrates its basement membrane into the lamina propria then intramucosal cancer is present. If the dysplastic epithelium penetrates the muscularis mucosae into the submucosa, then by definition the lesion is an invasive adenocarcinoma. Invasion into the submucosa defines invasive cancer, not the grade of dysplasia.

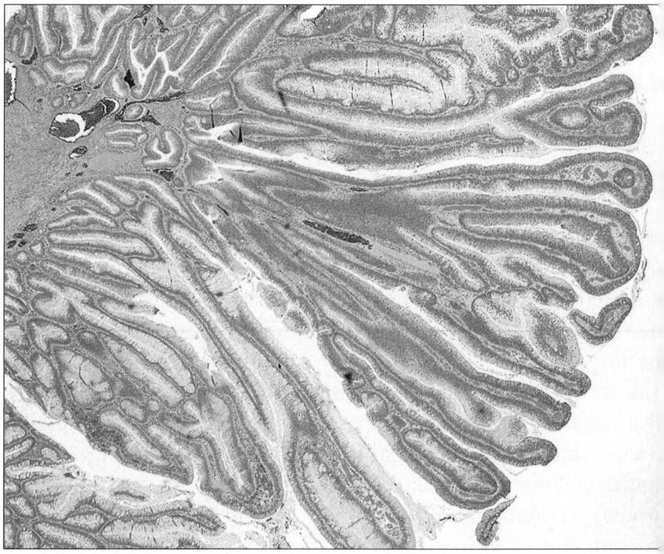

Fig. 60C.3 Villous adenoma.

Hyperplastic polyps: In contrast to the adenoma, these are composed of well-differentiated epithelium without dysplasia. Histologically, there are focal areas of crypt elongation, but the epithelium itself is preserved with abundant cytoplasm, normal appearing and basally positioned nuclei, and normal nuclear cytoplasmic ratio. The crypt distortion leads to a classic starfish appearance of the mucosa on cross-section (see Fig. 60C.4) or serrated appearance in longitudinal sections.

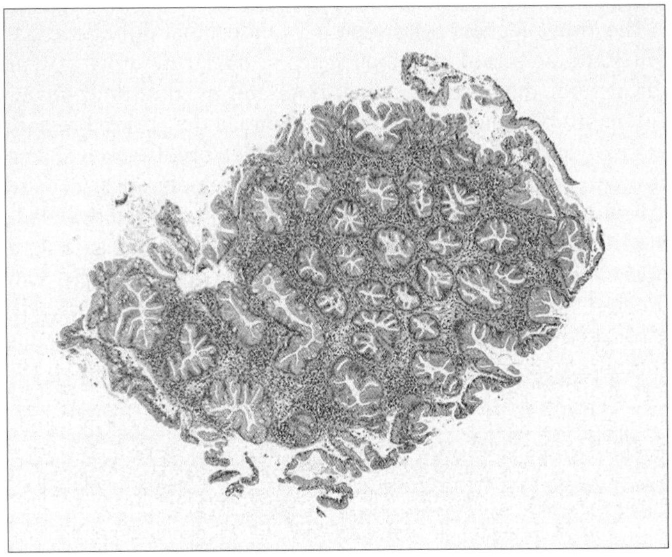

Fig. 60C.4 Hyperplastic polyp.

CLINICAL PRESENTATION

Most patients have only a few sporadic lesions during their lifetime. When polyps present clinically at a young age or in great numbers (hundreds or even thousands) then particular (often genetic) clinical conditions should be considered (see Table 60C.1).

Familial adenomatous polyposis (FAP) is the best recognized of these syndromes. Its prevalence is estimated at 1 in 5000 to 1 in 7500, occurring equally in men and women. By definition, subjects with FAP have at least 100 colorectal adenomas, but those with fully developed disease can have thousands of lesions. Generally, adenomas first appear in the teenage years, but can present even earlier. Without colectomy, development of colorectal cancer is inevitable, often by the fourth decade of life.[9] A milder variant of the syndrome ('attenuated FAP') is also recognized. Affected patients develop fewer polyps (average of 30) that are more often distributed in the right colon. Those with this condition are likely to develop colorectal cancer by their mid 50s. Two other recognized variants of FAP include Gardner's syndrome and Turcot's syndrome. Patients with Gardner's syndrome suffer from both polyposis and a host of extracolonic manifestations including osteomas, mandibular and jaw lesions, and dental and ocular abnormalities (e.g., congenital hypertrophy of the retinal pigment epithelium, CHRPE). Turcot's syndrome includes those with both polyposis and intracranial tumors. FAP is inherited in an autosomal dominant pattern, although about 20% of cases appear to be new genetic mutations. The disease is caused by a germline mutation in the adenomatous polyposis coli (APC) gene located on chromosome 5q (see Chapter 60A).

Hereditary nonpolyposis colorectal cancer (HNPCC): Like FAP, this is also inherited in an autosomal dominant pattern. Affected patients suffer from a germline mutation in mismatch repair genes, particularly hMSH2 (chromosome 2p) and hMLH1 (chromosome 3p). Those affected develop adenomas at a younger age than the sporadic patient; the adenomas also tend to be larger and more frequently with villous histology and/or high-grade dysplasia. Not surprisingly, colorectal cancer also develops at an earlier age (average 40–45 years) than in the general population.

Two other uncommon conditions that can present with multiple polyps at an early age are juvenile polyposis and the Peutz-Jeghers syndrome. In both these conditions, the polyps are hamartomas, not adenomas. A hamartoma is a tumor containing an overgrowth of mature cells (generally stromal) with a disordered architecture and organization.

Juvenile polyps are characterized by a predominant stroma, cystic crypts, and a lamina propria lacking smooth muscle. The lesions are so named because most occur in children less than 10 years of age. The polyps tend to be single and pedunculated, and frequently come to clinical attention because of their propensity to bleed. Sporadic cases are not associated with an increased risk of malignancy. However, in some cases, juvenile polyps can occur in a familial setting (familial juvenile polyposis). Here, juvenile polyps occur throughout the gastrointestinal tract and there is an increased risk of both upper and lower gastrointestinal tract tumors.

TABLE 60C.1 POLYPOSIS SYNDROMES

Syndrome	Polyp type	Polyp number	Polyp location	Genetic basis
FAP	Adenoma	100s –1000s	Colon > small bowel	APC gene (5q)
HNPCC	Adenoma	Similar to sporadic	Colon	hMSH2 (2p) hMLH1 (3p)
Familial juvenile polyposis	Hamartoma	50–200	Colon > small bowel	SMAD-4 (18q) BMPR1A (10q)
Peutz-Jehgers syndrome	Hamartoma	Variable	Small bowel > colon	LKB1/STK (19p)
Hyperplastic polyposis	Hyperplastic polyp	More than 30	Colon	Allelic loss of chromosome 1p

The **Peutz-Jeghers syndrome** is an autosomal dominant disorder characterized by the presence of hamartomatous polyps throughout the gastrointestinal tract and by abnormal mucocutaneous pigmentation, most commonly in the perioral region. Pathologically, the polyps contain crowded crypts and a sparse stroma characterized by prominence of smooth muscle. Like juvenile polyps, Peutz-Jeghers polyps can present with bleeding or (when present in the small bowel) can serve as a lead point for obstruction. While not common, these polyps can undergo malignant transformation. The syndrome is clearly associated with an increased risk of both colorectal and extracolonic carcinomas.

CLINICAL PRESENTATION
• Polyps generally are asymptomatic and present sporadically during adulthood • The presence of large number of polyps and/or polyps presenting in those younger than 40 years of age should raise suspicion for the presence of polyposis syndromes (see Table 60C.1)

DIFFERENTIAL DIAGNOSIS

While it is the endoscopist who identifies polyps in the colon and rectum, it is the pathologist who determines the nature of those lesions. Most lesions removed will either be simple adenomas (e.g., tubular or villous) or hyperplastic polyps, but there are a number of other types that will occasionally be encountered.

Serrated adenomas (Fig. 60C.5): These have many features of classical hyperplastic polyps (mucin-rich, well-differentiated epithelium, serrated microscopic morphology), but have important differences from them. Unlike hyperplastic polyps, these lesions exhibit abnormal proliferation, dilated crypts, and subtle nuclear atypia. While such lesions are uncommon, they seem to have malignant potential that may exceed that of the 'routine' adenoma. For example, these polyps often contain areas of high-grade dysplasia (up to 40%).

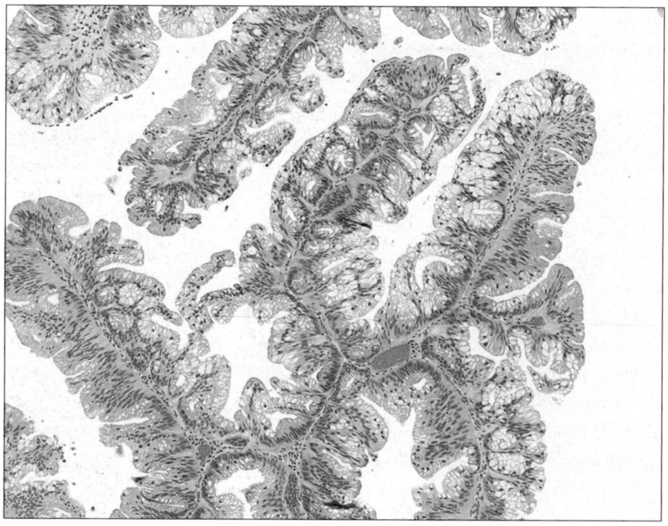

Fig. 60C.5 Serrated adenoma.

Flat adenoma: While most neoplastic polyps (adenomas, serrated adenomas) are raised lesions, this is a discrete area of adenomatous tissue that is only minimally raised above the mucosal surface either in a flat or convex pattern. By definition the growth of this lesion above the muscularis is no more than twice the thickness of the normal mucosa. Visualization of these lesions may be improved with the use of special magnifying endoscopes in combination with dye spraying of the mucosa.

Other non-neoplastic polyps

As in all parts of the gut, biopsies of putative polyps sometimes reveal only normal mucosa. Although some pathologists collaborate with the endoscopist to give these a name such as mucosal polyps, mucosal tags, polypoid folds, it is best if they just report the mucosa as normal. Inflammatory polyps are seen most commonly in the setting of inflammatory bowel disease (IBD). Inflammatory 'pseudopolyps' represent residual normal mucosa that appears elevated because the surrounding mucosa is denuded by inflammatory disease or healing takes place in a 'pinched' fashion leaving one area in the center raised. True raised mucosal lesions can also occur, composed of granulation tissue. These polyps are not precancerous, but they can be difficult to distinguish from malignant or premalignant colorectal lesions that occur in IBD patients. These inflammatory polyps are also described in some infectious colitides, including amebiasis, tuberculosis, and schistosomiasis. Finally, hamartomatous polyps can also be identified (see above).

DIAGNOSTIC METHODS

Most adenomas are small, slow growing (averaging 0.5 mm/year), and clinically asymptomatic. Complaints of rectal bleeding or anemia unrelated to these mucosal lesions often prompt colonic evaluation, at which time they may be discovered by 'serendipity.' Adenomas are also detected as a direct result of colorectal cancer screening programs (see Chapter 60B).

Colonoscopy is clearly the most sensitive and specific modality currently available to detect polyps (see Chapters 120 and 125). While it is the gold standard for polyp identification and removal, it is not perfect. A study of back-to-back tandem colonoscopy reported a miss rate for adenomas larger than 1 cm of 6%.[10]

Radiological alternatives to colonoscopy include double-contrast barium enema and virtual colonoscopy (high-resolution helical CT scan). The comparison of barium enema with colonoscopy has been published.[11] Further refinement and standardization of both the technology and technique for virtual colonoscopy (colography) will be required before it could reliably substitute for conventional colonoscopy (see Chapters 120, 125, and 130).[12,13]

TREATMENT AND PREVENTION

At the time of endoscopy, small polyps (less than 5 mm) can be excised via biopsy forceps, with or without monopolar cautery. Larger lesions can be removed using a snare device. Electrocautery decreases the risk of immediate bleeding and extends the polyp resection margin (via local tissue injury in the area of the 'burn'), but its use increases the risk of delayed bleeding and perforation. Consequently, smaller lesions and those located in the thin-walled cecum are preferably removed without it.

arge and/or flat lesions can be raised off the submucosa with line to increase the margin of safety for resection of these olyps. Every effort should be made to retrieve all polypoid aterial removed at endoscopy for subsequent pathologic eview.

Surveillance: Those with a history of adenoma formation are t increased risk for recurrence and thus require surveillance xams. Follow-up intervals are based on the number and type f adenomas previously removed. For patients with only a w simple tubular adenomas a 5-year interval is generally ecommended. For those with multiple (≥3) adenomas or more dvanced histology (e.g., villous) a 3-year follow-up examination suggested. An even shorter interval might be appropriate in atients with many polyps or with worrisome lesions.[14]

Chemoprevention: While adenoma removal is the current tandard for colorectal cancer prevention, colonoscopy is not ithout risk and surveillance programs are not without cost. s an alternative, strategies of chemoprevention (i.e., the use f drugs to prevent colorectal neoplasia) are under active nvestigation. In well-executed randomized trials, fiber supplementation showed no effect on reducing adenoma recurrence n those with a history of polyps.[15,16] A significant reduction n adenoma formation was found in large placebo controlled rials of aspirin[17] and calcium.[4] Nonetheless, aspirin use may ot be cost effective for most patients.[18]

TREATMENT AND PREVENTION

- At the time of colonoscopy, polyps can be removed with biopsy or snare devices utilized with or without electrocautery
- Removal of large or flat adenomas may be facilitated by saline solution-assisted polypectomy
- Chemoprevention is the use of drugs to prevent colorectal neoplasia
- Both aspirin and calcium have been shown to decrease adenoma recurrence in those with a history of prior adenoma removal, though clinical guidelines for use have not been established

PROGNOSIS WITH AND WITHOUT TREATMENT

It is generally accepted that if left *in situ*, some small adenomas will progress to cancer. However, the frequency with which this occurs and the effectiveness of polypectomy in reducing cancer risk is less certain. There have been both retrospective and prospective studies examining the natural history of the adenoma. Taken together, they suggest that only a fraction (perhaps 5%) of polyps are destined to progress through to cancer and in most cases this growth is slow. It has been estimated that large polyps progress to cancer at a rate of about 1% per year.[19]

The benefit of adenoma removal in cancer prevention has been evaluated in observational studies. Case–control studies of sigmoidoscopy[20,21] or colonoscopy[22] suggest a reduction in colorectal cancer mortality in the range of 50–80%. However, these observations are subject to a host of biases. In the absence of randomized controlled trials, the precise benefit of adenoma removal in cancer prevention remains unknown.

WHAT TO TELL PATIENTS

Polyps are bumps or growths that arise from the wall of the colon. The risk for developing polyps increases with age. Broadly speaking, there are two different types of growths. 'Hyperplastic polyps' are generally small and usually do not progress to cancer. 'Adenomatous polyps' are not cancer, but if left inside the colon for many years, they can grow and develop into cancer.

Because of their small size and slow growth, polyps rarely cause symptoms. Very often polyps are identified as the result of screening performed to prevent colon cancer. The best test for removing polyps is 'colonoscopy.' For this test, patients are generally sedated. A tube is then placed through the rectum and the lining of the whole large bowel is visualized. In most cases, any polyps seen during that test can be removed so that they no longer pose any threat to become cancer.

CURRENT CONTROVERSIES AND THEIR FUTURE RESOLUTION

Clinically, adenoma removal remains central to efforts at cancer prevention. Currently, significant resources are expended repeating surveillance colonoscopy in those with a history of adenoma. A better understanding of the natural history of patients who have undergone adenoma resection is likely to lead to further tailoring of surveillance recommendations. As alternative modalities (e.g., virtual colonoscopy (colography)) are refined, they may also play a role in the follow-up of these patients.

While the adenoma-carcinoma sequence clearly explains much of the colorectal cancer burden, there is increasing recognition that alternative pathways (e.g., through serrated polyps) are also important. Hopefully, molecular epidemiological studies will clarify these issues of cancer progression.

SOURCES OF INFORMATION FOR PATIENTS AND DOCTORS

There are a number of excellent resources for patients wanting to learn more about polyps, colon cancer, and tests to prevent colon cancer:

http://www.nlm.nih.gov/medlineplus/colorectalcancer.html (information on cancer screening tests and on latest research pertaining to colorectal cancer).

http://digestive.niddk.nih.gov/ddiseases/pubs/colonpolyps_ez/ (nice monograph on polyps, their significance, and treatment).

http://www.gastro.org/clinicalRes/brochures/fact-cc.html

http://www.cancerlinksusa.com/colorectal/tx_patient/tx_stage.htm

http://personalweb.sunset.net/~mansell/polyp.htm

http://www.patient.co.uk/showdoc/27000573/

For physicians wanting to learn more about polyposis syndromes and available genetic testing: http://www.genetests.org/

REFERENCES

1. Jass JR, Whitehall VL, Young J, Leggett BA. Emerging concepts in colorectal neoplasia. Gastroenterology 2002; 123:862–876.
2. Matek W, Hermanek P, Demling L. Is the adenoma-carcinoma sequence contradicted by the differing location of colorectal adenomas and carcinomas? Endoscopy 1986; 18:17–19.
3. Kim YI. AGA technical review: impact of dietary fiber on colon cancer occurrence. Gastroenterology 2000; 118:1235–1257.
4. Baron JA, Beach M, Mandel JS et al. Calcium supplements for the prevention of colorectal adenomas. Calcium Polyp Prevention Study Group [see comments]. N Engl J Med 1999; 340:101–107.
5. Sandler RS, Pritchard ML, Bangdiwala SI. Physical activity and the risk of colorectal adenomas. Epidemiology 1995; 6:602–606.
6. Lieberman DA, Prindiville S, Weiss DG, Willett W. Risk factors for advanced colonic neoplasia and hyperplastic polyps in asymptomatic individuals. JAMA 2003; 290:2959–2967.
7. Garcia Rodriguez LA, Huerta-Alvarez C. Reduced incidence of colorectal adenoma among long-term users of nonsteroidal antiinflammatory drugs: a pooled analysis of published studies and a new population-based study. Epidemiology 2000; 11:376–381.
8. Sandler RS, Galanko JC, Murray SC, Helm JF, Woosley JT. Aspirin and nonsteroidal anti-inflammatory agents and risk for colorectal adenomas. Gastroenterology 1998; 114:441–447.
9. Lynch HT, de la Chapelle A. Hereditary colorectal cancer. N Engl J Med 2003; 348:919–932.
10. Rex DK, Cutler CS, Lemmel GT et al. Colonoscopic miss rates of adenomas determined by back-to-back colonoscopies. Gastroenterology 1997; 112:24–28.
11. Winawer SJ, Stewart ET, Zauber AG et al. A comparison of colonoscopy and double-contrast barium enema for surveillance after polypectomy. National Polyp Study Work Group. N Engl J Med 2000; 342:1766–1772.
12. Cotton PB, Durkalski VL, Pineau BC et al. Computed tomographic colonography (virtual colonoscopy): a multicenter comparison with standard colonoscopy for detection of colorectal neoplasia. JAMA 2004; 291:1713–1719.
13. Pickhardt PJ, Choi JR, Hwang I et al. Computed tomographic virtual colonoscopy to screen for colorectal neoplasia in asymptomatic adults. N Engl J Med 2003; 349:2191–2200.
14. Winawer S, Fletcher R, Rex D et al. Colorectal cancer screening and surveillance: clinical guidelines and rationale – update based on new evidence. Gastroenterology 2003; 124:544–560.
15. Alberts DS, Martinez ME, Roe DJ et al. Lack of effect of a high-fiber cereal supplement on the recurrence of colorectal adenomas. Phoenix Colon Cancer Prevention Physicians' Network. N Engl J Med 2000; 342:1156–1162.
16. Schatzkin A, Lanza E, Corle D et al. Lack of effect of a low-fat, high-fiber diet on the recurrence of colorectal adenomas. Polyp Prevention Trial Study Group. N Engl J Med 2000; 342:1149–1155.
17. Baron JA, Cole BF, Sandler RS et al. A randomized trial of aspirin to prevent colorectal adenomas. N Engl J Med 2003; 348:891–899.
18. Suleiman S, Rex DK, Sonnenberg A. Chemoprevention of colorectal cancer by aspirin: a cost-effectiveness analysis. Gastroenterology 2002; 122:78–84.
19. Stryker SJ, Wolff BG, Culp CE et al. Natural history of untreated colonic polyps. Gastroenterology 1987; 93:1009–1013.
20. Newcomb PA, Storer BE, Morimoto LM, Templeton A, Potter JD. Long-term efficacy of sigmoidoscopy in the reduction of colorectal cancer incidence. J Natl Cancer Inst 2003; 95:622–625.
21. Selby JV, Friedman GD, Quesenberry CP, Jr, Weiss NS. A case–control study of screening sigmoidoscopy and mortality from colorectal cancer [see comments]. N Engl J Med 1992; 326:653–657.
22. Muller AD, Sonnenberg A. Prevention of colorectal cancer by flexible endoscopy and polypectomy. A case–control study of 32,702 veterans. Ann Intern Med 1995; 123:904–910.

Chapter 60D

Colorectal cancer: a multidisciplinary approach

R S Midgley, A Merrie, D J Kerr, and N Mortensen

KEY POINTS
• The proportion of patients with colorectal cancer diagnosed at an earlier, treatable stage is increasing • The treatment algorithm needs to be tailored to the natural history and molecular biology of the specific cancer being assessed • Most chemotherapy regimens have a narrow therapeutic window • 5-FU has been the mainstay of colorectal cancer chemotherapy for 4 decades; combination of novel agents will probably lead to improved effectiveness • 5-FU is only active in the S phase of the cell cycle, therefore continuous infusion may be more effective against cycling cells than bolus regimens • Both preoperative radiotherapy and total mesorectal incision have reduced local recurrence rates in rectal cancer • Immunotherapy and gene therapy offer hope for future advances in management

CAUSES AND RISK FACTORS
RISK AND PROTECTIVE FACTORS FOR COLORECTAL CANCER
RISK FACTORS
Unavoidable
Male sex
Increased age
Genetic predisposition (see Chapter 60A)
Inflammatory bowel disease
Previous history of CRC or polyps
Avoidable
Decreased dietary fiber
Increased dietary saturated fat
Increased weight or obesity
Decreased physical activity
PROTECTIVE FACTORS
Hormone replacement therapy
Regular NSAID use

INTRODUCTION

Colorectal cancer (CRC) is a significant cause of morbidity and mortality in the Western World. In North America, western Europe, Australasia, and Japan the incidence exceeds 40 per 100 000 of the population in males and 25–30 per 100 000 in females. Significantly, in Africa and Central and South America the incidence is typically less than 5 per 100 000. Some of this discrepancy in incidence may be explained by genetic variability, as described in Chapter 60A, but it is likely to be due largely to differences in diet (low in fiber, high in fat) and the increasingly sedentary lifestyles observed in the West.

Many patients presenting with CRC are symptomatic, although the number of patients who are asymptomatic and whose cancers are detected by screening is increasing with the gradual introduction of formal screening programs (see Chapter 60B). The most common symptoms that patients describe are rectal bleeding, a change in bowel habit, pain, and occasionally a palpable mass or fatigue secondary to anemia; the latter two symptoms are more common in patients with right-sided tumors.

There has been a clearcut shift towards earlier diagnosis of colorectal cancer. In France one cancer registry showed that, in 1976, 40% of patients had stage I or stage II disease at diagnosis, whereas this figure had risen to 57% by 1991. Over the same period, the percentage of patients with stage IV (advanced) disease decreased from 34% to 22%.[1] This stage migration has probably contributed to the increase in overall survival observed for this disease since 1980. For most countries in Europe, the 5-year survival rate from colorectal cancer has increased from 40% to approximately 55% in the past 20 years.

However, a number of other factors that will be described in this chapter have contributed significantly to the observed improvement in prognosis for CRC. Surgical advances and the evolution of effective postoperative care have reduced perioperative mortality and the likelihood of local recurrence. Preoperative radiotherapy for rectal cancer has also diminished local recurrence rates. Chemotherapy administered after surgery appears to have an impact on the risk of metastatic disease and also on overall survival of patients with colonic tumors.

OVERVIEW: WHAT HAPPENS WHEN A PATIENT IS DIAGNOSED WITH COLORECTAL CANCER?

When a patient is diagnosed with colorectal cancer, they should be staged to assess local and distant disease (Table 60D.1). For colonic tumors this usually means colonoscopy with biopsy and computed tomography (CT) of the chest, abdomen, and pelvis. Rectal tumors, particularly those in the lower two-thirds of the rectum, should also be assessed by pelvic magnetic resonance imaging (MRI) or endoscopic ultrasonography (EUS), as precise local staging is necessary to determine the appropriate first-line treatment. Ideally, the results of staging investigations should then be discussed at a multidisciplinary meet-

TABLE 60D.1 STAGING AND SURVIVAL OF PATIENTS WITH COLORECTAL CANCER

TNM system				Approx. 5-year survival rate (%)	Dukes' classification
Stage	Tumor	Lymph nodes	Metastasis		
0	T0	N0	M0		
I	T1	N0	M0	97	A
I	T2	N0	M0	90	
II	T3	N0	M0	78	B
II	T4	N0	M0	63	
III	Any T	N1	M0	56–66	C
III	Any T	N2	M0	26–37	
IV	Any T	Any N	M1	1	D

T1, tumor invades submucosa; T2, tumor invades muscularis propria; T3, tumor invades through muscularis propria into subserosa, or into nonperitonealized pericolis or perirectal tissues; T4, tumor directly invades other organs or structures, and/or perforates visceral peritoneum; N0, no regional lymph node metastasis; N1, metastasis in one to three regional lymph nodes; N2, metastasis in four or more regional lymph nodes; M0, no distant mestastasis; M1, distant metastasis.

ing. Meetings of such teams allow face-to-face contact between surgeons, radiation oncologists, radiologists, pathologists, and specialist nurses, streamlining the patient's care and standardizing protocols for each clinical situation based on best available evidence.

Figure 60D.1 (A and B) shows how the pertinent factors are considered for each patient and how the decision about the treatment pathway is made. For example, if the patient were fit and well with a tumor in the colon, surgery to remove the primary tumor would be the first line of treatment followed by assessment of operative histology and consideration of adjuvant chemotherapy. Conversely, for a patient who has a tumor in the mid third of the rectum that extends into the mesorectum, and an associated large lymph node, downstaging chemoradiotherapy prior to surgery would be sensible in order to increase the chances of a clear (R0) resection margin.

COLONIC AND RECTAL TUMORS: THE ANATOMIC, THERAPEUTIC, AND MOLECULAR DISTINCTION

Rectal tumors, probably because of their anatomic location and difficulty in achieving clear planes of resection at surgery, tend to recur locally within the pelvis. Conversely, colonic tumors tend to seed early to distant sites, leading to liver and lung metastases. These differences have determined the pattern of therapy for the two sites of disease. Whereas patients with colonic tumors tend to undergo excision followed by chemotherapy to prevent distant recurrence, those with rectal tumors often have preoperative radiotherapy or chemoradiotherapy, followed by resection to prevent local recurrence.

Colonic and rectal tumors may also differ at the molecular level. Colorectal carcinogenesis is a multistep pathway[2] (see Chapter 60C). Two proteins that are central to this tumorigenic pathway are p53 and APC (the adenomatous polyposis coli protein). One study has suggested that tumors of colonic and rectal origin differ in terms of the relative importance of these proteins.[3] The *APC* mutations may be less important in rectal cancer. Furthermore, the p53 pathway appeared more important in the rectal tumors. Expression of mutated *p53* was more consistent in rectal tumors (64% versus 29% for colonic tumors) and there was a correlation between positive mutated *p53* expression and worse disease-free survival ($P=0.008$). No such expression or outcome correlation existed for the colonic tumors.[3] It could be that this difference in disease-free survival for patients with rectal tumors that were *p53* mutation positive or negative reflected the relative radiation resistance or sensitivity of the two groups. It is clear then that there is evidence to suggest that treating colonic and rectal tumors as distinct entities in terms of therapy is appropriate.

SURGERY FOR COLORECTAL CANCER

Assessment

Surgery with curative intent is aimed at removing the tumor and the corresponding lymphatic drainage to allow accurate staging, and is the primary form of treatment for CRC. All patients being considered for surgery should have a histologic diagnosis, imaging of the colon, and staging for metastatic disease prior to discussion at a multidisciplinary meeting. Imaging of the colon can be accomplished using a variety of techniques, discussed elsewhere in this book (see Chapters 120, 125 and 129). Staging for metastatic disease involves imaging the liver and lungs, and can also be accomplished by a variety of techniques: ultrasonography, CT, MRI, and positron emission tomography (PET). Accuracy of detection of liver metastases is optimal with MRI or intraoperative ultrasonography, but CT remains an accurate and readily available imaging technique.

Local staging of rectal cancer has undergone revolutionary changes. Current best practice is for all rectal cancers to be assessed with MRI with a body coil, or with EUS to assess the extent of tumor spread, clearance of surgical margins, and, more recently, lymph node involvement (Fig. 60D.2). This determines the need for and type of preoperative adjuvant treatment. Formal assessment also includes careful physical examination including rigid sigmoidoscopy to determine the position of the tumor in relation to the anal sphincters, and assessment of function of the anal sphincters. This may need to be done under anesthesia to enable an accurate assessment; if there is concern about anal sphincter function, preoperative assessment of anal physiology may be useful.

SURGERY FOR COLONIC CANCER

Segmental resection of the colon is based on lymphovascular drainage. The principles of anatomic dissection apply to both colonic and rectal surgery, with sharp dissection in the planes of embryologic fusion. This is usually done in an open surgical fashion; however, the laparoscopic approach is gaining acceptance for some patients, and a discussion of the technique and comparison with the open technique is given in Chapter 152. Surgery for obstructing CRC carries a high mortality rate. The development of self-expanding colorectal stents shows promise in relieving acute obstruction to allow surgery to be performed in an elective setting after appropriate staging and assessment.[4]

SURGERY FOR RECTAL CANCER

A high local recurrence rate in patients with rectal cancer (25%) was traditionally the driving force behind the use of preoperative and postoperative radiotherapy, as discussed above. However, the adoption of anatomic rectal excision, best known as total mesorectal excision (TME), has seen these recurrence rates drop to under 10%.[5,6] Rarely has a change in surgical practice produced such a significant improvement in outcome. TME is a careful extrafascial excision of the rectum and mesorectum down to the pelvic floor, thereby excising the tumor and surrounding lymphatic drainage en bloc. Although there has been much debate about semantics and terminology, essentially TME is used for low and middle rectal cancers. For high rectal cancers, 5 cm of mesorectum distal to the tumor is taken to ensure adequate clearance within the mesorectum.

Low anterior resection is the preferred treatment of choice for low rectal cancers, except for tumors with inadequate distal clearance (<2 cm) and in cases where the sphincter mechanism

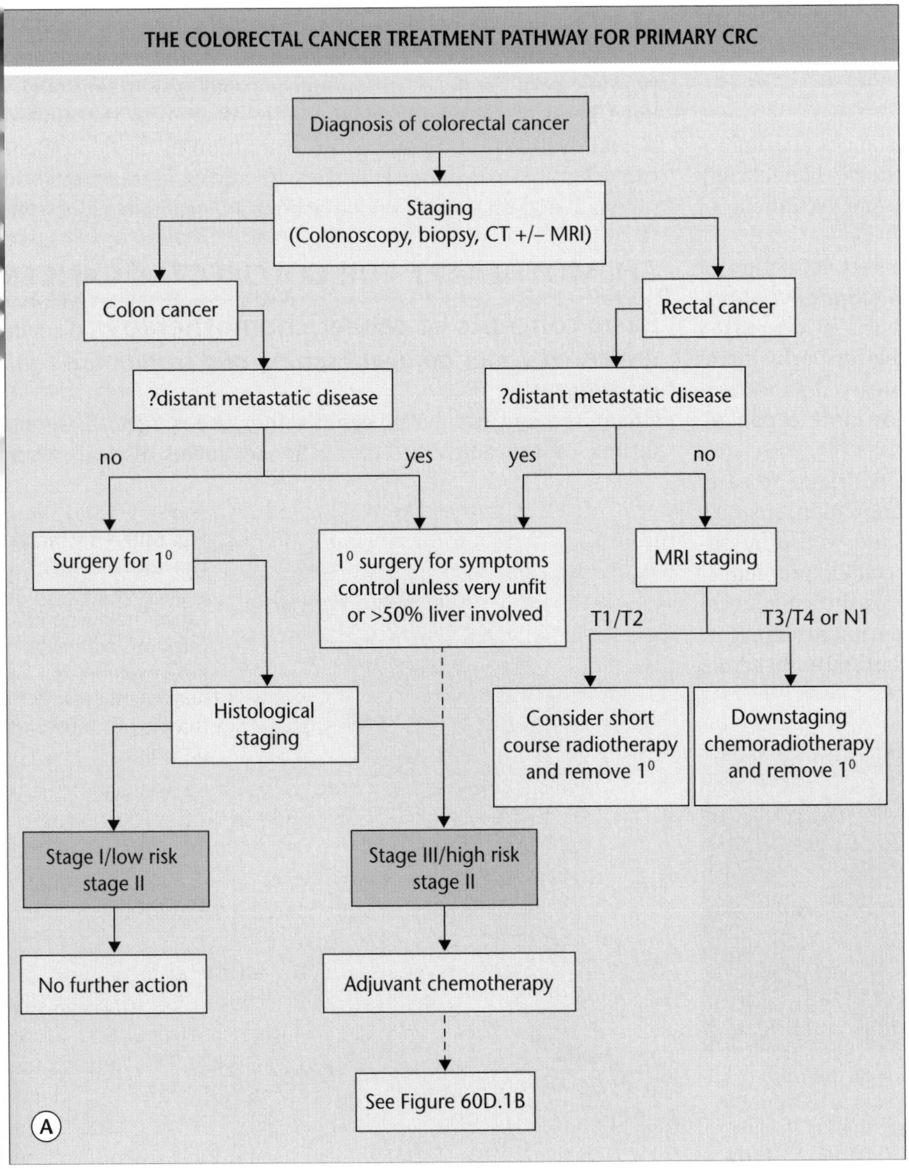

Fig. 60D.1 Multidisciplinary decision-making approach to patients with colorectal cancer. **A.** Treatment pathway for primary CRC. **B.** Treatment pathway when distant metastatic disease is present at diagnosis.

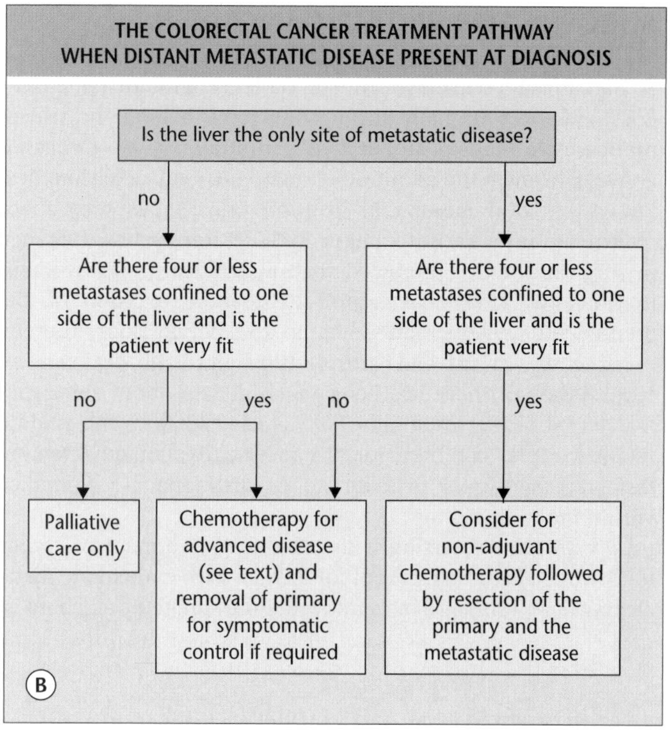

THE COLORECTAL CANCER TREATMENT PATHWAY WHEN DISTANT METASTATIC DISEASE PRESENT AT DIAGNOSIS
Is the liver the only site of metastatic disease?
no
yes
Are there four or less metastases confined to one side of the liver and is the patient very fit
Are there four or less metastases confined to one side of the liver and is the patient very fit
no
yes
no
yes
Palliative care only
Chemotherapy for advanced disease (see text) and removal of primary for symptomatic control if required
Consider for non-adjuvant chemotherapy followed by resection of the primary and the metastatic disease
B

Fig. 60D.1—Cont'd B. Treatment pathway when distant metastatic disease is present at diagnosis.

is not adequate for continence. In these instances abdomino-perineal excision remains the treatment of choice. Increasingly adjuvant chemoradiotherapy is utilized in the treatment of these patients.

Use of a short-term colonic J pouch: For reconstruction of low anterior resections, this has been shown to improve short-term postoperative neorectal function with a decreased anastomotic leak rate due to theoretically better perfusion at the anastomosis. The pouch should be no bigger than 5 cm at the level of the pelvic floor; if it is longer or more cephalad, impaired evacuation can occur.

Local excision of rectal cancer is generally restricted to early rectal cancers that are mobile on clinical examination, stage T1 on endoanal ultrasonography (Fig. 60D.3) and well differentiated on biopsy, or in less fit patients. The major problem is that prediction of lymph node involvement is difficult. Local excision can be done via transanal endoscopic microsurgery or by per anal disc excision. The principles in both are the same:

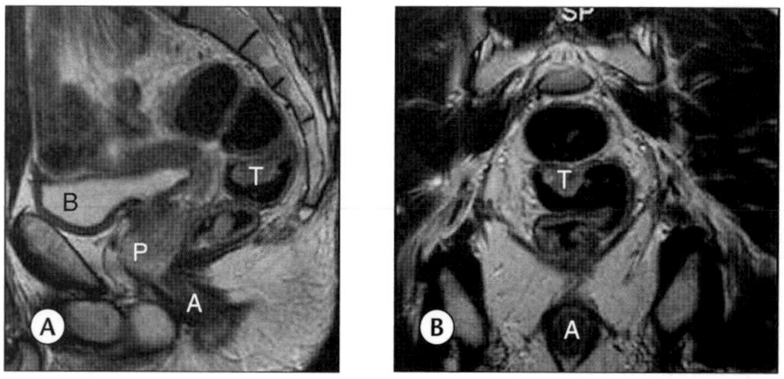

Fig. 60D.2 Pelvic MRI demonstrating a T2 tumor of the mid rectum. A. Sagittal section. **B.** Coronal section. This is a T2 tumor as it can be seen involving, but not invading through, the full thickness of the bowel wall. A, anus; B, bladder; P, prostate; T, tumor; S, sacrum.

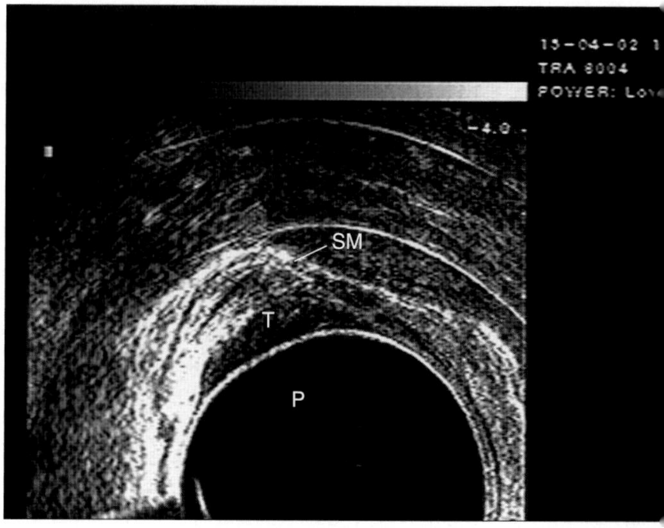

Fig. 60D.3 Endoanal ultrasound scan demonstrating a T1 rectal cancer. P, endorectal ultrasound probe; T, T1 tumor; SM, submucosa.

to excise the lesion in a full-thickness manner with a cuff of normal surrounding tissue (Fig. 60D.4).

Impotence and retrograde ejaculation in men are recognized complications of pelvic surgery. The adoption of the TME approach and a better understanding of the anatomy and physiology of the pelvic autonomic nervous system (Fig. 60D.5) have been accompanied by a parallel decline in the rates of sexual dysfunction. Spontaneous resolution of these problems can occur up to 1 year after surgery; in addition, treatment with sildenafil and drugs with similar actions are generally successful.

CHEMOTHERAPY FOR COLORECTAL CANCER

Basic concepts of cancer chemotherapy

Advanced versus adjuvant setting and traditional trial paradigms

Chemotherapy can be given in either the advanced disease setting or the adjuvant setting. In advanced disease, where

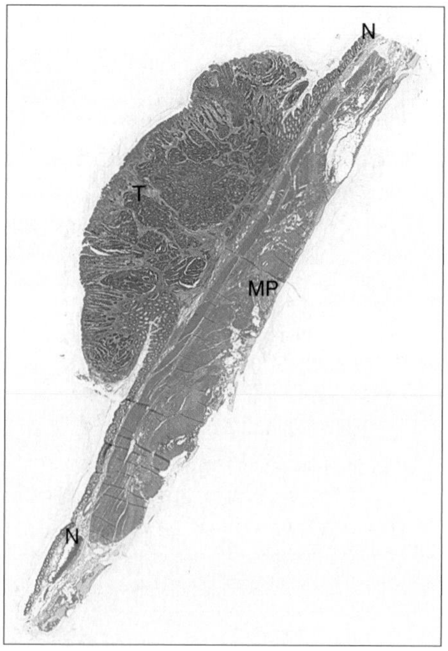

Fig. 60D.4 T1 rectal cancer. Histologic section of a T1 rectal cancer following full-thickness complete local excision. N, normal mucosa; T, T1 tumor; MP, muscularis propria.

AUTONOMIC NERVES AND ANATOMY OF THE MALE PELVIS

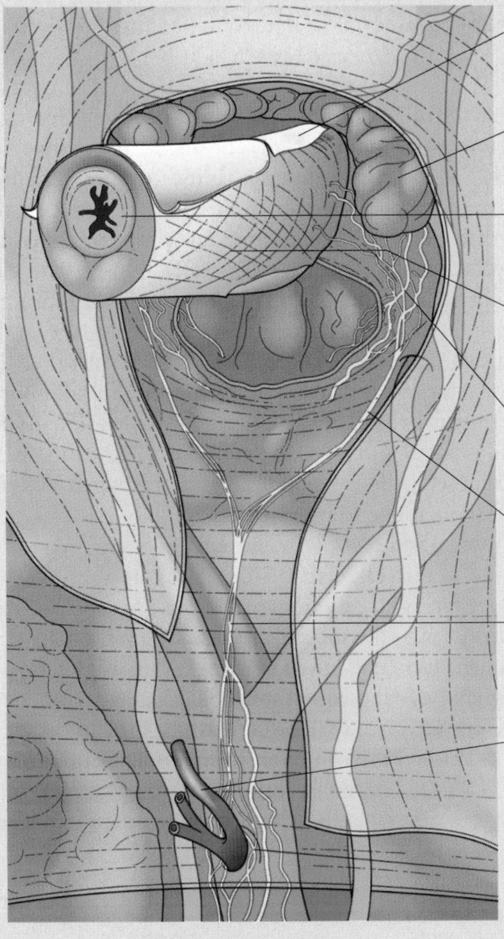

Fig. 60D.5 Pelvic anatomy. Dissection in the extrafascial (total mesorectal excision) plane, with autonomic nerves and seminal vesicles exposed. Reproduced with permission of and acknowledgment to Mr Ian Bissett, University of Auckland, New Zealand.

there is distant metastasis or inoperable local recurrence, chemotherapy is administered to palliate symptoms or to prolong life with no expectation of cure. In the adjuvant setting, chemotherapy is administered to patients after potentially curative surgery in an attempt to decrease the risk of recurrence and death from the disease. Therefore the goal is cure for a proportion of the patients treated. The different objectives in these two scenarios determine the balance between toxicity and quality of life that clinicians and patients are prepared to accept from such therapy. When novel chemotherapeutic agents are being assessed, they are first tested in the advanced disease setting where a rough assessment of their efficacy in terms of tumor response rates, as well as their toxicity, can be made. The agents go through phase I, phase II, and then randomized phase III trials (comparison with the 'gold standard' treatment) in patients with advanced disease, and finally they are tested in the adjuvant arena (Fig. 60D.6). The process from first clinical trial to being accepted for use in the adjuvant setting to prevent recurrence of disease takes somewhere between 12 and 15 years.

Important pharmacologic concepts in chemotherapy

Cytotoxic drugs tend to have steep dose–response curves: the higher the plasma level that can be achieved, the greater the chance of response. Furthermore, the drugs generally have a narrow therapeutic window, which means there is little difference in the plasma concentration required to bring about tumor cytotoxicity and that which induces significant toxicity to normal tissues. In general, chemotherapy doses are calculated according to the patient's individual body surface area (determined by their height and weight), although there are a number of genetic polymorphisms and differences in renal or hepatic physiology that can cause deficiencies in the metabolism of cytotoxic drugs, leading to greatly enhanced toxicity. Oncologists grade patients' toxicity on a scale from 1 to 4. Generally toxicity equal to or greater than grade 3 or repeated episodes of grade 2 toxicity necessitates dose reduction for future cycles of chemotherapy (Table 60D.2).

Routes of administration

Although historically chemotherapy has always been given intravenously, attempts are being made to formulate drugs that are predictably absorbed through the bowel mucosa. This has huge implications on patient acceptability and cost of administration.

TABLE 60D.2 NATIONAL CANCER INSTITUTE COMMON TOXICITY CRITERIA FOR SOME COMMON CHEMOTHERAPY TOXICITIES

	Grade 1	Grade 2	Grade 3	Grade 4
Mucositis	Soreness or erythema	Erythema, ulcers – can eat solids	Erythema, ulcers – liquid diet only	Alimentation not possible
Nausea	Able to eat reasonable intake	Can eat but decreased intake	No significant intake	
Vomiting	1 episode in 24 h	2–5 episodes in 24 h	6–10 episodes in 24 h	>10 episodes or requiring parenteral nutrition
Diarrhea	Increase of 2–3 stools per day compared to pre-treatment	Increase of 4–6 stools or nocturnal stools	Increase of 7–9 stools per day or malabsorption	Increase of 10 or more stools per day or grossly bloody stools, dehydration
Fatigue	Increased fatigue – able to conduct normal activities	Moderate difficulty performing some activities	Severe loss of ability to perform some activities	Bedridden or disabling
Neutropenia ($\times 10^9$/L)	1.5–1.9	1.0–1.4	0.5–0.9	<0.5

THE TRADITIONAL TRIAL PARADIGM FOR NOVEL ANTI-CANCER AGENTS

Phase I
Dose finding and toxicity assessment Number of arms: 1 Setting: advance disease Numbers: 10 to 20

Phase II
First efficacy testing Number of arms: 1 or 2 Setting: advance disease Numbers: 10 to 50 (more if two arms)

Phase III
Efficacy testing against gold standard Measured by response rate Number of arms: 2 or more Setting: Advance disease first Numbers: 100s

Phase III Adjuvant
Efficacy testing against gold standard Measured by disease-free and overall survival differences Number of arms: 2 or more Setting: adjuvant after removal of primary Numbers: many 100s or 1000s

Fig. 60D.6 Traditional trial paradigm for novel anticancer agents.

Regional delivery of chemotherapy via the hepatic artery

The majority of metastatic CRC is confined to the liver. Also, it has been known for many years that micrometastases within the liver derive their blood supply from the hepatic artery, whereas normal hepatocytes derive their supply predominantly from the portal vein. Furthermore, a number of chemotherapy drugs are largely metabolized during their first pass through the liver. Hence relatively high doses of drug can be administered directly to the liver, while still keeping systemic exposure low.[8] Randomized trials comparing hepatic arterial infusion with systemic therapy have given conflicting results, but many have suffered from poor trial design. Most have confirmed a higher response rate, but evidence of improved survival has been lacking.

Chemotherapy for advanced colorectal cancer: the evidence

When considering chemotherapy for advanced CRC the risks and benefits must be weighed carefully. A randomized trial more than 10 years ago established that chemotherapy with 5-fluorouracil (5-FU)-based regimens improved median survival from 5 to 10 months when compared with best supportive care for patients with metastatic CRC. There was also evidence of an improvement in quality of life in responding patients. The major dose-limiting toxicities of the common CRC chemotherapy regimens are mucositis with soreness of the mouth, diarrhea (usually by drugs such as loperamide or diphenoxylate), plantar-palmar erythema, and mild myelosuppression (usually manifesting as a fall in neutrophil count).

5-Fluorouracil

5-FU has been the mainstay of CRC chemotherapy for over 40 years. It is an antimetabolite and a pro-drug. It is converted into its active form, fluorodeoxyuridine monophosphate (FdUMP), within the cell. This metabolite binds to the enzyme thymidylate synthase, blocking its action and preventing pyrimidine, and therefore DNA, synthesis (Fig. 60D.7). 5-FU can also be falsely incorporated into RNA, interfering with protein synthesis. An interesting feature of 5-FU metabolism is the presence of a degree of genetic polymorphism governing the enzyme that inactivates FdUMP, dihydropyrimidine dehydrogenase (DPD). Approximately 1–2% of the caucasian population exhibits severely depressed levels of DPD, and these individuals demonstrate exaggerated and prolonged plasma levels of FdUMP, leading to augmented toxicity such as prolonged neutropenia and complete alopecia.

As one of the major effects of 5-FU is disruption of DNA replication, the drug is largely active in the S phase of the cell cycle. Given the small fraction of cells in S phase at any one time, it was suggested that infusional regimens might have a greater 'hit' against cycling cells than bolus regimens. Indeed a meta-analysis in advanced CRC, comparing infusional 5-FU against bolus 5-FU treatment (given on five consecutive days every 4 weeks – Mayo regimen), found that infusional therapy delivered a higher response rate and prolonged progression-

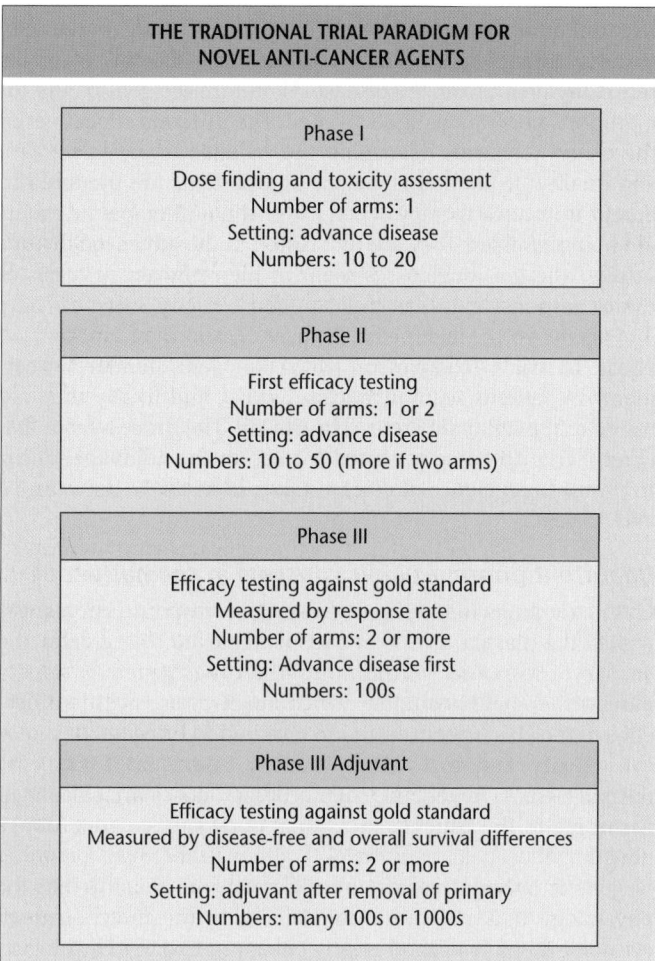

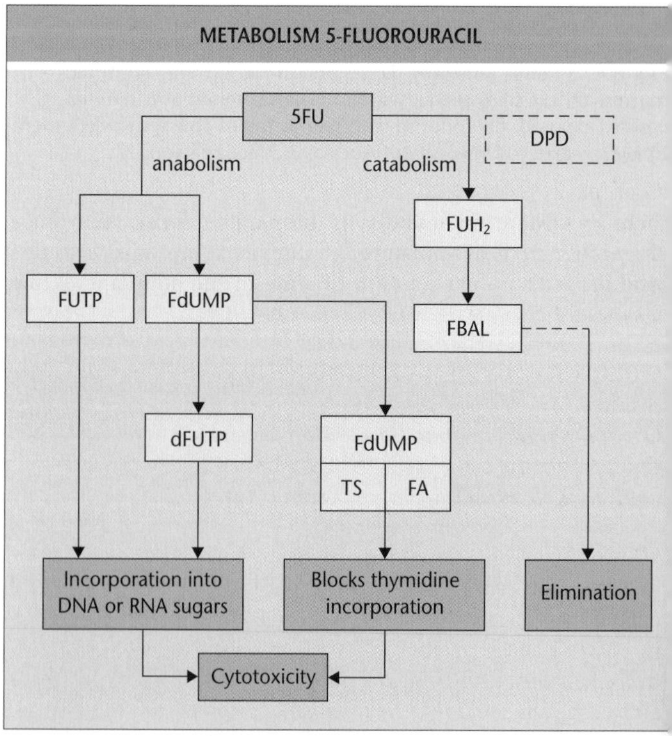

Fig. 60D.7 Metabolism of 5-fluorouracil (5FU). DPD, dihydropyridine dehydrogenase; FUH_2, dihydrofluorouracil; FBAL, fluoro-β-alanine; FdUMP, fluorodeoxyuridine monophosphate; dFUTP, fluorodeoxyuridine triphosphate; FUTP, fluorouridine triphosphate; TS, thymidine synthase; FA, folinic acid.

free survival but only a negligible improvement in median survival. Infusional 5-FU regimens are now the standard of care in Europe and in many parts of the United States. However, with infusional regimens it must be remembered that, unless patients want to be confined to hospital for the duration of their chemotherapy, central line insertion, with all the incumbent risks of infection and thrombophlebitis, is a prerequisite for such therapy.

Folinic acid (FA) is given with 5-FU as it provides a further mechanism to augment the efficacy of 5-FU. The addition of FA increases the pool of reduced folate in the cell and stabilizes the FdUMP–thymidylate synthase complex. Studies have shown that the addition of FA to 5-FU in bolus regimens doubles the response rate.

Novel agents

Irinotecan

Irinotecan, also known as CPT-11, is a potent inhibitor of topoisomerase I, an enzyme essential for DNA supercoiling. Randomized studies have shown that in patients whose advanced CRC has become resistant to treatment with 5-FU response rates of up to 15% are achievable with single-agent irinotecan, resulting in a statistically significant overall survival benefit when compared to best supportive care alone.

The use of irinotecan in the first-line setting was initially avoided because of concerns about its toxicity. Irinotecan can be a difficult drug for patients to tolerate, with approximately one-quarter to one-third of patients suffering grade 3 or 4 diarrhea. Neutropenia, nausea, and alopecia are also reported frequently. However, with greater experience of the drug and an evolving ability to deal with the toxicities, there has been increasing interest in the use of irinotecan in combination with 5-FU as first-line palliative CRC therapy. Randomized phase III studies have now shown that triple therapy with infusional 5FU–FA–irinotecan gives better response rates, increased median time to progression, and increased median survival compared with single- or double-agent combinations.

Oxaliplatin

Oxaliplatin is a third-generation platinum compound that induces DNA cross-linkages and apoptotic cell death. Unlike the related agents cisplatin and carboplatin, it does have activity against human CRC. There is evidence that oxaliplatin acts in a synergistic way with 5-FU, the combination achieving response rates of up to 50% when used in first-line therapy. Infusional 5-FU plus oxaliplatin as first-line treatment for advanced CRC resulted in a doubled response rate compared with 5-FU alone.[9] Oxaliplatin has no renal and minimal hematologic toxicity. It does, however, cause a particular dysesthesia precipitated by cold, as well as a cumulative sensory neuropathy.

Oral 5-fluorouracil analogs

Tablet equivalents of 5-FU, such as uracil–ftorafur (UFT) or capecitabine, have been the subject of four multicenter trials in patients with advanced CRC comparing oral UFT plus FA or capecitabine with intravenous 5-FU. These studies demonstrated approximately equal efficacy and similar median survival times. There was less mucositis, neutropenia, and alopecia but more hand–foot syndrome (erythema desquamation of the palms and soles) with oral agent administration.

Combination of novel agents will probably be the next logical step in the path towards improved effectiveness. Early unpublished data from the co-administration of capecitabine and irinotecan suggest that this might be a particularly promising combination.

Chemotherapy for advanced CRC: what is the standard of care?

There is general consensus in Europe and the United States that combination chemotherapy should become the standard of care in the therapy of advanced CRC. However, the specific sequencing with respect to oxaliplatin and irinotecan is still a point of contention. One large study compared the delivery of 5-FU–FA–oxaliplatin in combination for first-line therapy, followed by 5-FU–FA–irinotecan on progression, with the reverse sequence. There was no difference in overall survival; however, in both arms median survival was in excess of 20 months, which compares very favourably to historic controls.[10]

The present United Kingdom National Institute for Clinical Excellence guidelines allow for infusional 5FU–FA only as the first-line treatment, with single-agent irinotecan on progression. Capecitabine can be substituted for infusional 5-FU if it is considered that the oral drug would be better tolerated by the patient. Although capecitabine is a more expensive drug than 5-FU, there are many cost savings with respect to line complications and chemotherapy nurse administration time. For patients with potentially resectable metastases confined to the liver, a first-line combination of 5FU–FA–oxaliplatin is recommended. This is based on a large French series in which patients initially deemed to have borderline irresectable liver disease were given this combination and one in eight patients was converted to resectability.

Adjuvant chemotherapy for colorectal cancer: the evidence

Despite the best efforts of the surgeon in the 80% of colorectal tumors that are deemed operatively curable, 50% of these patients will subsequently relapse and die from their disease. This is as a result of occult tumor cells that are present at the time of the operation, either locally, in the lymph nodes, or at distant sites (spread by hematogenous routes), but are too small to detect by available radiologic techniques. Adjuvant chemotherapy is administered in an attempt to eradicate the cells before they become large functional tumor masses.

Adjuvant chemotherapy: Its role in increasing the chance of cure from CRC is now well established, but it has taken many years to prove the extent of the benefit. In 1990 results showed a 33% lower odds of death and 41% reduced risk of recurrence amongst patients with Dukes' C colonic cancer who received adjuvant 5-FU–levamisole after surgery compared with surgery alone.[11] Levamisole has been superseded by FA, as in the advanced setting. Subsequent large prospective randomized trials showed convincing evidence of improved 3-year disease-free survival and overall survival in patients treated with 5-FU–FA, with a 25–30% decrease in the odds of dying from colonic cancer (or an absolute improvement in survival rate of 5–6%) compared with surgery-alone controls. Based upon this it is now advised that, on current evidence, 6 months' bolus treatment with the combination of 5-FU–FA should be accepted as standard adjuvant therapy for patients with stage III (Dukes' C) colonic cancer. However, the use of infusional 5-FU, plus the addition of the novel agents such as irinotecan and oxaliplatin, is now being assessed in the large adjuvant trials. Furthermore, oral capecitabine administered for 6 months may be superior to bolus 5-FU–FA in the adjuvant treatment of stage III CRC with respect to recurrence-free survival.[12]

Chemotherapy in stage II (Dukes' B) colonic cancer: Its role is less certain. Adjuvant therapy in this setting is not at present recommended as standard practice in Europe. However, data from the Quasar trial in patients with stage II colonic cancer randomized to chemotherapy or surgery alone suggest a small but statistically significant improvement in the overall survival in the chemotherapy-treated patients. It is possible that there will be a subset of stage II patients who have specific poor prognostic factors (perforation, obstruction, T4 tumors) that will derive most benefit from adjuvant therapy. This will be a question addressed in future trials. In the United States the consensus is a little different, and many patients with stage II disease are receiving adjuvant chemotherapy. Indeed, a number of cancer physicians are already advocating the use of infusional rather than bolus regimens in this setting.

Adjuvant chemotherapy for rectal tumors is another contentious issue. Because of the anatomic constraints within the pelvis, local recurrence rather than distant metastasis has historically been the main problem and the major determinant of outcome. Based on this, the role of the oncologist has been largely restricted to radiotherapy, although chemoradiotherapy may have a role for patients whose rectal tumors are likely to be difficult to remove with clear margins (see below).

RADIOTHERAPY AND CHEMORADIOTHERAPY FOR RECTAL CANCER

Radiotherapy as an adjuvant treatment to surgery in the treatment of rectal cancer has been assessed in a series of trials and proven benefit has been established. The postoperative radiotherapy approach has been largely superseded by preoperative radiotherapy, either with a short (1 week) course of radiotherapy or the more traditional longer course.[13] Both regimens allow for a decrease in dose requirements, decreased small bowel irradiation, significantly decreased local recurrence rates by up to 50%, and, in some studies, an increase in overall survival has been suggested.

Chemoradiation: The integration of chemotherapy with the preoperative regimen appears to prime the tissue for radiotherapy effect, allowing increased tumor downstaging, with complete pathologic response in some tumors (Fig. 60D.8). With continual improvement in preoperative imaging, nodal status can now be accurately predicted on MRI,[14] enabling patients who may benefit from chemotherapy to be identified early and offered chemoradiotherapy, often in conjunction with postoperative chemotherapy. There is no rigid consensus about which patients should receive preoperative radiotherapy. The initial dramatic results shown with preoperative radiotherapy probably reflect the historic unacceptably high local recurrence rates that were prevalent prior to the widespread adoption of anatomic rectal surgical techniques (discussed below). Despite improvements in surgery to a general high standard, however, studies still demonstrate that the administration of preoperative radiotherapy does further decrease local recurrence rates. However, this is a proportional effect, so the benefit to patients with early tumors that have a low rate of local recurrence is not great.[15] It is accepted that patients with T4 tumors and tumors with invasion within 2 mm of the enveloping fascia of the mesorectum (fascia propria) on imaging benefit from long-course preoperative (chemo)radiotherapy, and it is generally accepted that patients with T3 tumors, tumors with MRI evidence of lymph node metastases, tumors in the most distal 5 cm of the rectum, and anterior tumors in men also benefit from radiotherapy.

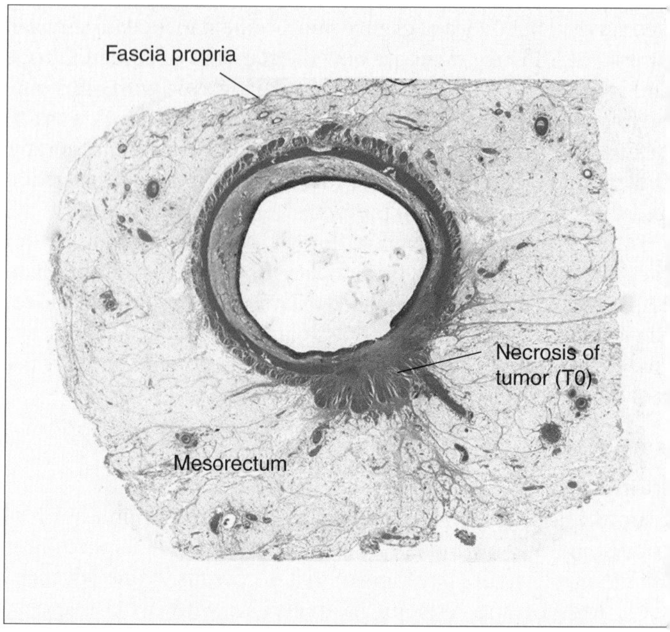

Fig. 60D.8 Histology showing complete response. Full-mount histologic section of rectal cancer showing complete regression following chemoradiotherapy – histologic stage T0.

PATHOLOGY AND PROGNOSIS OF COLORECTAL CANCER

Many factors impact on the prognosis of patients with CRC. Accurate clinicopathologic staging remains the mainstay for decision-making with regard to further adjuvant treatment. The histologic staging is of paramount importance; detailed assessment of the resected specimen enables precise staging to be done (Fig. 60D.9).

Particular to rectal cancer is assessment of the circumferential margin; this is the TME resection margin. Involvement or encroachment of this by tumor is highly predictive of the development of local recurrence.[16] Several staging systems for CRC exist of which the tumor node metastasis (TNM) system, summarized in Table 60D.1, is the most comprehensive. This is reviewed regularly and takes into account factors such as the circumferential resection margin. Also, systematic reviews have consistently demonstrated that higher patient volumes and increased specialization of individual surgeons are associated with improved survival and decreased morbidity.[17]

FOLLOW-UP OF PATIENTS WITH COLORECTAL CANCER

Evidence is accumulating to suggest that intensive follow-up, including liver imaging, is associated with a decrease in mortality rate. Therefore, consideration must be given to intensive follow-up of high-risk patients.[18]

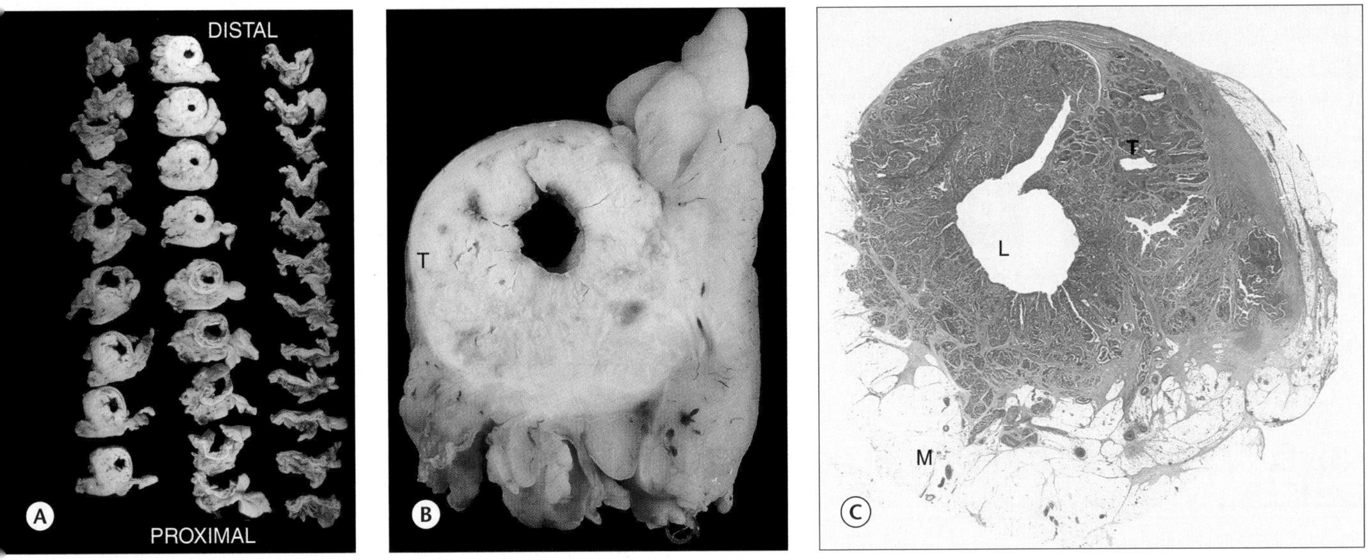

Fig. 60D.9 Histologic staging. A. Multiple gross transverse sections taken from a formalin-fixed specimen of an extended right hemicolectomy for a transverse colonic cancer. **B.** Appearance of a gross transverse section of the tumor; this is circumferential and obstructing, and stage T3 as it has invaded beyond the bowel wall. **C.** Full-mount histologic appearance of the cancer – histologic grade pT3 N0 M1 (stage III). L, lumen; M, mesocolon; T, tumor.

RECURRENCE OF COLORECTAL CANCER

Most episodes of recurrence present within 2 years; the most common site is in the liver (33%), followed by lung (20%) and then local recurrence (20%), which is mainly in the pelvis. Rectal cancer is more likely than colonic cancer to present with local recurrence. The chance of local recurrence is influenced by several factors including tumor stage, surgical technique, and the use of adjuvant (chemo)radiotherapy.

Treatment of local recurrence is difficult. After thorough imaging with MRI and/or PET, radiotherapy followed by excision, which may include sacrectomy and pelvic exenteration, can yield acceptable long-term results in patients who have complete excision of the disease. However, careful patient selection is required.

SURGERY FOR METASTATIC DISEASE

CRC liver metastases are present in 18% of patients at diagnosis (Table 60D.3). The natural history without any intervention is poor, with an average life expectancy of 5–10 months. The short-term outlook is better in unilobular and solitary metastases, with a 1-year survival rate of up to 77% and a 3-year survival rate of 23%. Imaging for hepatic metastases is best performed using triphasic helical CT, with scans performed before the administration of arterial contrast and during arterial and portal venous phases, and repeated after a delay.

Chemotherapy: This can be offered to many patients with hepatic metastatic disease to palliate symptoms and prolong life (see above). However, hepatic resection is the only potentially curative modality for isolated hepatic disease. Outcome is influenced largely by patient selection. Median survival of the order of 25–45% at 5 years can be achieved and is determined by a variety of factors: deferred presentation after primary resection, no extrahepatic disease, resectable pattern of metastases (not necessarily solitary), sufficient hepatic reserve, and a fit patient. Imaging (including MRI of the liver and CT of the chest and abdomen) is usually performed prior to consideration of resection, and liver function tumor markers are assessed. All patients should be discussed at a multidisciplinary meeting.

Liver failure can be a major complication following resection and is related to age, extent of resection, remnant size and quality, presence of chronic liver disease, and steatosis. For those patients who survive the operation without undue complications, consideration is now being made of "adjuvant" systemic or hepatic arterial chemotherapy. Although this is not advocated in Europe because of a perceived lack of adequate randomized evidence, it is practised by a number of centers in North America.

Other modalities have been assessed in the therapy of isolated liver metastases; both radiofrequency ablation and cryotherapy can be useful in conjunction with resection; preoperative embolization stimulates growth of the hepatic remnant; and hepatic artery chemotherapy can be administered.

Surgery for pulmonary metastases is also worth considering. Development of lung lesions in a resectable pattern is less common than with liver metastases. However, for patients with limited disease, a 5-year survival rate of up to 25% can be obtained.

TABLE 60D.3 RECURRENCE OF RECTAL CANCER RELATED TO TECHNIQUE AND ADJUVANT TREATMENT

Technique	Recurrence (%)
Conventional surgery	25
Postop. radiotherapy	15–20
Preop. radiotherapy	10–15
Total mesorectal excision	10
Preop. radiotherapy	2–5

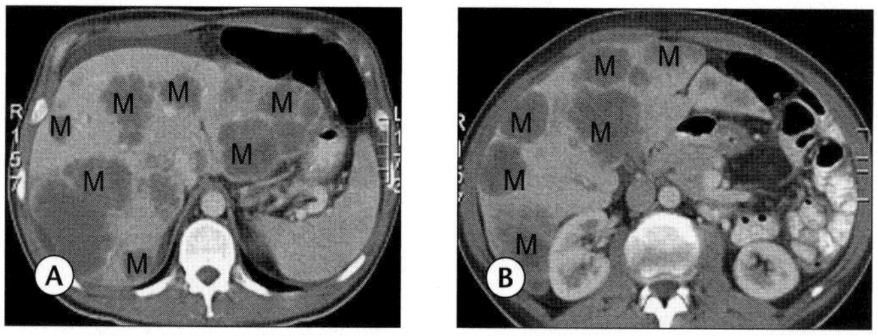

Fig. 60D.10 Computed tomogram showing bilobar hepatic metastases from colorectal cancer. Axial sections from oral (**A**) and intravenous (**B**) contrast-enhanced scans (portal venous phase). M, metastases.

NOVEL STRATEGIES TO TREAT COLORECTAL CANCER

There are other new exciting therapies predicated upon basic science advances that are now entering the clinical arena. These include those that have phase III supporting evidence in advanced disease such as bevacizumab (Avastin), a monoclonal antibody that targets the vascular endothelial growth factor (VEGF) receptor. However, there are more "translational approaches" that really do bridge the gap between basic medical science and clinical treatment, such as immunotherapy and gene therapy. These treatments are likely to have greatest impact in the curable adjuvant setting, where tumor burden is low. Clearly larger-scale treatment trials for any new therapies are required before they can be used in clinical practice.

Immunotherapy

Immunotherapy in CRC can involve rather nonspecific stimulation of the host immune system through administration of BCG or cytokines, or more directed strategies such as anti-idiotypic monoclonal antibodies, or the use of virus vaccines. Early trials of vaccines constructed with vaccinia virus or fowlpox virus backbones flanking inserted tumor-associated antigen genes such as *CEA* and *MUC1* have been completed. Disease stabilization and minimal toxicity have been documented. Furthermore, in vitro post-vaccination testing of peripheral blood lymphocytes found specific lytic activity against carcinoembryonic antigen (CEA)-expressing tumor cells.

Gene therapy

Cancer gene therapy encompasses a myriad of genetic manipulation strategies including the insertion of genes encoding cytokines, expression of tumor suppressor genes to abort excessive proliferation, and insertion of drug resistance genes into healthy cells to allow aggressive cytotoxic therapy. However, phase I trials are now under way using an innovative technique termed virus-directed enzyme pro-drug therapy (VDEPT). This involves insertion of genes into cells that are capable of metabolizing pro-drugs. Retroviral vectors linking the *CEA* promoter to the structural gene for the bacterial enzyme cytosine deaminase have been formulated. The cytosine deaminase metabolizes the pro-drug 5-fluorocytosine to 5-FU, but transduction should occur only in CEA-expressing cells (i.e. CRC cells). The objective is to confer selectivity of the cytotoxic agent, allowing a 10 000-fold higher concentration of the 5-FU in the tumor and in neighboring bystander cells than in the systemic circulation.

CONCLUSIONS

The field of colorectal oncology is ever-expanding and serves as a superb model of how dedicated cooperation between many specialist groups – medical oncologists, radiotherapists, surgeons, and basic scientists – can rapidly advance understanding and improve treatment outcomes. Much of the advancement in terms of cure for CRC is likely to be based on the success of streamlined care between these professional groups.

REFERENCES

1. Faivre-Finn C, Bouvier AM, Mitry E et al. Chemotherapy for colon cancer in a well-defined French population: Is it under- or over-prescribed? Aliment Pharmacol Ther 2002; 16:353–359.
2. Fearon ER, Hamilton SR, Vogelstein B. Clonal analysis of human colorectal tumors. Science 1987; 238:193–197.
3. Kapiteijn E, Liefers GJ, Los LC et al. Mechanisms of oncogenesis in colon versus rectal cancer. J Pathol 2001; 195:171–178.
4. Khot UP, Lang AW, Murali K, Parker MC. Systematic review of the efficacy and safety of colorectal stents. Br J Surg 2002; 89:1096–1102.
5. Heald RJ, Husband EM, Ryall RDH. The mesorectum in rectal cancer surgery – the clue to pelvic recurrence? Br J Surg 1982; 69:613–616.
6. McCall JL, Cox MA, Wattchow DA. Analysis of local recurrence rates after surgery alone for rectal cancer. Int J Colorectal Dis 1995; 10:126–132.
7. Keating JP. Sexual function after rectal excision. Aust N Z J Surg 2004; 74:248–259.
8. Kerr DJ, McArdle CS, Ledermann J et al. Intrahepatic arterial versus intravenous fluorouracil and folinic acid for colorectal cancer liver metastases: a multicentre randomised trial. Lancet 2003; 361:368–373.
9. de Gramont A, Figer A, Seymour M et al. Leucovorin and fluorouracil with or without oxaliplatin as first-line treatment in advanced colorectal cancer. J Clin Oncol 2000; 18:2938–2947.
10. Douillard JY, Sobrero A, Carnaghi C et al. Metastatic colorectal cancer: integrating irinotecan into combination and sequential chemotherapy. Ann Oncol 2003; 14(Suppl 2):7–12.
11. Moertel CG, Fleming TR, Macdonald JS et al. Levamisole and fluorouracil for adjuvant therapy of resected colon carcinoma. N Engl J Med 1990; 322:352–358.
12. McKendrick JJ, Cassidy J, Chakrapee-Sirisuk G et al. Capecitabine is resource-saving compared with IV bolus 5FU/LV in adjuvant chemotherapy for Dukes' C colon cancer patients: Medical resource utilization data from a large phase III trial (X-ACT). Proc ASCO 2004; 23:265 (Abstract).
13. Colorectal Cancer Collaborative Group. Adjuvant radiotherapy for rectal cancer: a systematic overview of 8507 patients from 22 randomised trials. Lancet 2001; 358:1291–1304.
14. Brown G, Radcliffe AG, Newcombe RG et al. Preoperative assessment of prognostic factors in rectal cancer using high-resolution magnetic resonance imaging. Br J Surg 2003; 90:355–364.
15. Kapiteijn E, Marijnen CA, Nagtegaal ID et al. Dutch Colorectal Cancer Group. Preoperative radiotherapy combined with total mesorectal excision for resectable rectal cancer. N Engl J Med 2001; 345:638–646.
16. Quirke P, Durdey P, Dixon MF, Williams NS. Local recurrence of rectal adenocarcinoma due to inadequate surgical resection. Lancet 1986; ii: 996–999.
17. Hodgson DC, Fuchs CS, Ayanian JZ. Impact of patient and provider characteristics on the treatment and outcomes of colorectal cancer. J Natl Cancer Inst 2001; 93:501–515.
18. Jeffery GM, Hickey BE, Hider P. Follow-up strategies for patients treated for non-metastatic colorectal cancer (Cochrane Review). In: The Cochrane Library, 2004, Issue 3. Chichester, UK: John Wiley.

Chapter 61

Other gastrointestinal tumors

Sushovan Guha

KEY POINTS

- Uncommon gastrointestinal malignancy with preponderance of benign tumors
- Associated with multiple hereditary conditions and synchronous tumors in colon, breast, endometrium, and prostate
- Association with celiac and Crohn's disease
- Unclear etio-pathogenesis, but molecular changes in adenocarcinoma are similar to colon carcinoma
- Mostly present with nonspecific symptoms and signs
- Imaging work-up commonly elusive, diagnosis mostly intraoperative

INTRODUCTION

Small bowel (SB) tumors are extremely elusive and pose a unique challenge to clinicians across medical specialties. Table 61.1 depicts the classification of small intestinal neoplasms into primary benign and malignant epithelial, neuroendocrine, mesenchymal, lymphoproliferative, and metastatic lesions. The most common primary malignant SB neoplasms in Western countries are adenocarcinomas, followed by carcinoid tumors (see Chapters 109 and 110), SB lymphomas, and gastrointestinal stromal tumors (GISTs) (see Chapter 39).[1]

EPIDEMIOLOGY

The small intestine represents 75% of the length and 90% of the surface area of the alimentary tract, yet it accounts for <3% of all gastrointestinal (GI) neoplasms and <0.4% of all cancers in the US.[2] An estimated 5260 new cases of small intestinal cancer were diagnosed in the US in 2003, with an estimated 1130 deaths reported in the same year.[3] A preponderance of benign tumors are seen at autopsies, the most frequent being adenomas and mesenchymal tumors.

Malignant SB tumors represent the majority of those detected during surgery. Adenocarcinomas and carcinoid tumors are the most common SB malignancies, with an annual incidence of 3.8 and 3.7 cases, respectively, per million people in the US, followed by GIST (1.3/million) and lymphomas (1.1/million).[3] There is a slight male predominance, and the mean age at presentation is 57 years. Patients with SB lymphomas are usually diagnosed a decade earlier. SB malignancies are associated with several heritable conditions that affect the GI tract (Table 61.2). The incidence of SB adenocarcinoma and malignant carcinoids is greater in African-Americans than in Caucasians. In addition, up to 25% of affected patients have synchronous cancers involving the colon, endometrium, breast, and prostate.

TABLE 61.1 CLASSIFICATION OF SMALL BOWEL NEOPLASMS

PRIMARY

Benign

- Adenoma – nonampullary small bowel, ampullary/periampullary
- Neuroendocrine – carcinoid, G-cell, D-cell, EC-cell, gangliocytic paraganglioma
- Mesenchymal – stromal (GIST), neurogenic (neurofibroma), smooth muscle (leiomyoma), lipocyte (lipoma), desmoid, vascular (hemangioma)
- Lymphoproliferative – nodular lymphoid hyperplasia

Malignant

- Adenocarcinoma – nonampullary small bowel and ampullary
- Neuroendocrine – carcinoid
- Mesenchymal – stromal (GIST), autonomic nerve (plexosarcoma), smooth muscle (leiomyosarcoma), lipocyte (liposarcoma), malignant fibrous histiocytoma, Kaposi's sarcoma, angiosarcoma
- Lymphoproliferative
  B-cell lymphoma:
  - Mucosa-associated lymphoid tissue (MALT) type – marginal zone, Immunoproliferative small intestinal disease (IPSID)
  - Mantle cell lymphoma
  - Other types (large B-cell, lymphocytic, follicular center)
  - Immunodeficiency related – AIDS, CVID with hypogammaglobulinemia, selective IgA deficiency, post-transplant

  T-cell lymphoma:
  - Enteropathy associated T-cell (EATL)
  - Adult T-cell leukemia/lymphoma
  - HTLV-1

METASTATIC

- Malignant melanoma
- Bronchogenic carcinoma – large cell carcinoma
- Breast carcinoma
- Gastric signet-ring cell carcinoma

PATHOGENESIS

The reason for the low incidence of small intestinal carcinogenesis, in comparison with the colon, remains obscure.[4,5] The unique microenvironment has been proposed in a global sense to explain the decreased susceptibility but no specific factors have been identified.[2,5]

The pathogenesis of specific types of SB tumors including carcinoids and GISTs is discussed in Chapters 110 and 39, respectively. Little is known regarding the pathogenesis of primary small intestinal lymphoma. While the majority appears to have no overt predisposing cause, analogous to *Helicobacter pylori* in the stomach, nevertheless, there are

TABLE 61.2 CLINICAL CONDITIONS PREDISPOSING TO SB NEOPLASMS

Clinical conditions	Type of SB lesion
Familial adenomatous polyposis (FAP)	Adenoma, adenocarcinoma
Gardner's syndrome	Adenoma, adenocarcinoma
Peutz-Jeghers syndrome	Adenocarcinoma
Hereditary nonpolyposis colorectal cancer (HNPCC)	Adenocarcinoma
Crohn's disease	Adenocarcinoma, lymphoma (B-cell)
Ileostomy and ileal conduits	Adenocarcinoma
Ileo-pouch anal anastomosis (IPAA)	Adenoma, adenocarcinoma
Celiac disease	Lymphoma (T-cell), adenocarcinoma
Chronic infection/antigenic stimulation	Immunoproliferative small intestinal disease (IPSID)
Immunodeficiency diseases CVID with hypogammaglobulinemia Selective IgA deficiency X-linked AIDS	Lymphoma (B-cell and rarely T-cell)
Von Recklinghausen's disease	Paraganglioma
Multiple endocrine neoplasia 2b (MEN 2b)	Ganglioneuroma

OTHER RISK FACTORS FOR SB NEOPLASMS

- Male gender
- Increasing age
- African-American ethnicity
- High-fat diet

well-defined clinicopathologic associations including chronic antigenic stimulation from chronic infections that may shed some light on the pathogenesis of small intestinal lymphoma.

PREDISPOSING CONDITIONS

The primary role of the gastroenterologist with respect to SB neoplasms is to identify patients who are at an increased risk. A number of disease states are associated with an increased incidence of SB neoplasms as illustrated in Table 61.2.[1,5]

At least 70% of patients with familial adenomatous polyposis (FAP) will develop adenomas in the region of the ampulla of Vater (see Chapter 60C). However, only about 5–8% will develop duodenal adenocarcinoma. Predictors of cancer risk include number, size, histology, and degree of dysplasia (modified Spigelman's score).[6] Rarely, patients with hereditary nonpolyposis colon cancer (HNPCC) (see Chapter 60A) present with SB adenocarcinoma. Patients with Peutz-Jeghers syndrome develop hamartomas of the SB (see Chapter 60C), with symptoms including bleeding, obstruction, or intussusception. Although these hamartomas are presumably non-neoplastic, the risk of adenocarcinoma appears after the development of focal dysplastic (adenomatous) changes.

Patients with celiac disease (see Chapter 44) have an increased risk for enteropathy-associated T-cell lymphomas (EATL) as well as adenocarcinoma. Because the risk for both of these malignancies appears to be very small (<1%), there is no established role for surveillance with any imaging modality; neither is there in Crohn's disease-associated adenocarcinoma or lymphoma.

CLINICAL PRESENTATION

Mostly, patients present with nonspecific symptoms and signs including intermittent abdominal pain, intussusception, occult bleeding, anemia, weight loss, palpable abdominal mass, or SB obstruction. Perforation and gross bleeding are rare. In Table 61.3, clinical presentations and common locations of some selected SB neoplasms are presented. Patients with malignant SB neoplasms more often have GI symptoms, compared to those with benign tumors, which are usually discovered at autopsy. However, the clinical presentation alone does not distinguish between benign and malignant lesions.[1]

When the different subtypes of SB malignancy are considered together (Table 61.4), 65% present with intermittent abdominal pain that is typically dull, crampy, and radiates to the back, 50% of patients present with anorexia and weight loss, while only 25% will present with signs and symptoms of bowel obstruction. Bowel perforation, which occurs in fewer than 10% of patients, is most common amongst those with lymphoma or sarcoma.

Of the four most common specific types of SB tumors, GIST, gut/pancreatic endocrine tumors, and carcinoid syndrome are discussed in Chapters 39, 109, and 110, respectively.

Adenocarcinoma

Adenocarcinoma (nonampullary) is the most common primary malignant tumor of the small intestine in Western countries, accounting for approximately 30–50% of all primary malig-

TABLE 61.3 CLINICAL PRESENTATIONS AND COMMON LOCATIONS OF PRIMARY SB NEOPLASMS

Symptom/sign	Location	Type
Jaundice + GI bleeding	Ampulla	Adenoma, adenocarcinoma
Occult GI bleeding, anemia	Duodenum	Adenoma, adenocarcinoma
Flushing + diarrhea	Ileum, jejunum	Carcinoid-mid gut (metastatic)
Intestinal obstruction	Jejunum, ileum	Lipoma
Intussusception + melanin pigmentation	Jejunum, ileum	Peutz-Jeghers syndrome
GI bleeding, perforation	Jejunum, ileum	Gastrointestinal stromal tumor (GIST)
Fever + diarrhea + weight loss	Ileum, jejunum	Lymphoma

Reproduced from Abu-Hamda EM et al. Small bowel tumors. Curr Gastro Rep 2003; 5:386–393 with permission from Current Medicine.

TABLE 61.4 OVERALL FREQUENCY OF SYMPTOMS

Symptom/sign	Frequency (%)
Abdominal pain	42–83
Weight loss	23–87
Anemia	18–75
GI bleeding	13–68
Intestinal obstruction	16–65
Abdominal mass	19–29
Jaundice	18–30
Anorexia	18–25

Reproduced from Abu-Hamda EM et al. Small bowel tumors. Curr Gastro Rep 2003; 5:386–393 with permission from Current Medicine.

nant SB tumors. These tumors are mainly located in proximal duodenum and jejunum, except in the setting of Crohn's disease where they occur in the ileum. The proximal location of most SB adenocarcinomas may reflect the presence of higher concentrations of bile (and/or pancreatic juice), previously linked to increased risk for adenocarcinoma.[7] Peak incidence is in the 7th decade of life, with a male preponderance.

Unlike ampullary and periampullary carcinomas, which are usually circumscribed and polypoid, SB adenocarcinomas are usually large, annular, constricting, and centrally ulcerated masses with circumferential involvement of the bowel wall. Microscopically, these tumors are very similar to their colonic counterparts, but with a higher proportion of poorly differentiated tumors. These tumors are also similar in their development to adenomatous polyps and shared genetic susceptibility.[1,6] Most of the duodenal adenocarcinomas become symptomatic much earlier than other SB tumors. Yet, most SB carcinomas are already metastatic at the time of diagnosis. Unlike the large bowel, SB mucosa contains lymphatics that course through the villi extending near the luminal surface, and invasion of mucosal tumor into these lymphatics may account for this tendency of early metastasis.[8]

Small bowel lymphoma

Primary SB lymphoma is the third most common primary malignant neoplasm of the small intestine and accounts for 15–20% of all malignant SB tumors. Although the GI tract is the most common extranodal site for lymphomas, it accounts for only approximately 5–20% of all lymphomas and is quite uncommon in Western countries. The SB is the second most common site of primary GI lymphoma after the stomach.[8]

Several types of SB lymphomas exist, and the particular type is largely dependent upon the geographic location. The majority are B-cell non-Hodgkin's lymphomas (NHL). The B-cell NHL can be divided into two major categories, immunoproliferative and non-immunoproliferative SB disease.[8] Immunoproliferative small intestinal disease (IPSID) is extremely rare in the US. IPSID is found primarily in the Middle East, Mediterranean countries, and North Africa, where it is endemic and affects young adults of lower socioeconomic status. Nonimmunoproliferative SB disease encompasses several subtypes. One subtype is the intestinal mucosa-associated lymphoid tissue (MALT) lymphoma, also called extranodal marginal zone B-cell lymphoma, which is most commonly seen in middle-aged men. Most patients with intestinal MALT lymphoma present with a single exophytic mass, commonly located in the distal ileum and causing symptoms of intestinal obstruction, perforation, or GI bleeding. In contrast to the stomach, where MALT lymphomas are usually low grade, those of the intestine are frequently high grade.[8] Unlike gastric MALT lymphoma (see Chapter 38), no association between *Helicobacter pylori* infection and intestinal MALT lymphoma has been established. Those rare cases of T-cell NHL are usually EATL associated with underlying celiac disease.

CLINICAL TIPS

- Suspect SB tumors in elderly male with African-American ethnicity and predisposing conditions including FAP, HNPCC, and Peutz-Jegher's syndrome
- Suspect SB tumors in patients with refractory celiac disease (on gluten-free diet) or development of treatment-resistant symptomatic Crohn's disease strictures
- Negative initial work-up (EGD, colonoscopy, and CT) for abdominal pain, weight loss, anemia, SB obstruction, and GI bleeding should trigger high suspicion of SB neoplasms
- Perform SBFT, push enteroscopy, laparoscopy, or laparotomy with biopsy if indicated
- In pediatric patients with suspected intussusception, perform US and look for 'target' sign
- In FAP and Peutz-Jegher's syndrome, close surveillance required
- Surgery is the main therapy and adjuvant chemotherapy + radiotherapy may benefit in SB lymphoma

DIFFERENTIAL DIAGNOSIS

The differential diagnosis depends on the predominant clinical symptoms/signs at the initial presentation. These consist of: (1) common causes of SB obstruction – adhesions or strictures, endometriosis, congenital pancreatic rest, splenosis, and enteric duplication cysts; (2) abdominal pain causes (see Chapter 4) – peptic ulcer disease, cholelithiasis, pancreatitis, functional bowel disorder to diverticular disease, appendicitis, and endometriosis; and (3) anemia and obscure causes of bleeding (see Chapter 16) – peptic, NSAID/medication induced erosions and ulcers, and vascular lesions (e.g., vascular ectasia and Dieulafoy's lesion).[5]

DIAGNOSTIC METHODS

Most of the patients with SB tumors present with nonspecific symptoms/signs and the diagnosis is significantly delayed, in the order of 7–12 months.[1] The clinical presentation usually dictates the order of imaging, and endoscopic and surgical modalities used for diagnosis as shown in Table 61.5 (see Chapters 39 and 110 for the specific diagnosis of GISTs and carcinoid syndrome, respectively).

Plain abdominal X-rays may show SB obstruction or free air, prompting an exploratory laparotomy. Patients with chronic symptoms of abdominal pain, nausea, vomiting, weight loss, and signs of gastrointestinal bleeding usually have undergone an unrevealing work-up (colonoscopy, upper endoscopy, and computed tomography (CT) of the abdomen).

TABLE 61.5 DIAGNOSTIC MODALITIES OF SUSPECTED SB NEOPLASMS

Diagnostic tests	Utility
RADIOLOGY	
Abdominal X-rays	±
Small bowel follow-through (SBFT)	+
Enteroclysis	++
Ultrasound (US)	+
CT scan	++
MRI	++
Angiography	+
MRI + enteroclysis	+++
ENDOSCOPY	
Esophagogastroduodenoscopy (EGD)	+
Push enteroscopy	+++
Sonde enteroscopy	++
Intraoperative enteroscopy	++++
Colonoscopy with ileoscopy	++
Endoscopic ultrasound (EUS)	Ampullary lesions
Wireless capsule endoscopy	++
NUCLEAR MEDICINE	
Octreotide scintigraphy	Neuroendocrine tumors
Gallium-67 scan	±
SURGERY	
Explorative laparotomy	++++
Laparoscopy	+++

See Chapters 39, 110, 119, 125.

An **upper gastrointestinal series** with SB follow-through (UGI-SBFT) and enteroclysis remains the most common method to evaluate SB intraluminal pathology distal to the ligament of Trietz (see Chapter 125). The sensitivity of UGI-SBFT is usually <50–60%.[9] SB enteroclysis, which requires duodenal intubation and injection of barium and methylcellulose directly into the SB, reveals a sensitivity of >90% in the majority of studies.[9] It is the most useful preoperative diagnostic modality in patients suspected of having proximal SB tumors. Abdominal CT may provide information on the local invasiveness as well as the metastatic spread of the disease.[10] There is no role for transcutaneous abdominal ultrasonography (US) (see Chapter 124) in the evaluation of patients with suspected SB tumors except in pediatric patients with suspected intussusception, where the classic 'target sign' can be seen.[9]

Upper endoscopy with a side-viewing duodenoscope is well suited for the identification of duodenal tumors, and may have a therapeutic role in selected instances.[5] 'Push' enteroscopy without an overtube (using a pediatric colonoscope or specialized enteroscope) may allow visualization of the proximal 50–100 cm of jejunum. In contrast, extended SB enteroscopy using a 120-degree, forward-viewing, 2560-mm, balloon-tipped endoscope (Sonde enteroscopy) can allow visualization of up to 70% of the SB mucosa. The Sonde technique, while not widely available, relies upon small bowel peristalsis to advance the endoscope; in one report, it permitted successful intubation of the terminal ileum in 77% of cases within 8 h.[1] Wireless capsule endoscopy may visualize SB mucosa for sources of obscure GI bleeding/anemia, and recurrent abdominal pain. However, it is contraindicated in the presence of strictures identified in prior imaging studies.[11]

Explorative laparotomy and laparoscopy are often required to evaluate patients suspected of having SB tumors when most of the imaging work-up is inconclusive and also to obtain adequate tissue samples in case of suspected SB lymphoma.[1]

MANAGEMENT AND PROGNOSIS

The management of SB tumors, outlined in Table 61.6, depends on several variables: the histologic subtype, whether it is malignant or benign, the stage of the tumor if it is malignant, and its location within the SB.

The management of benign lesions of the SB largely depends on their size, location, and malignant potential. Tubular adenomas may be cured with simple endoscopic polypectomy or local resection. Adenomas with villous features can be managed in a similar fashion as long as the resected specimen does not contain invasive carcinoma. The management of duodenal adenomas in FAP is more complex (see Chapter 60C). The majority of patients can be managed expectantly. This involves surveillance by upper endoscopy with a side-viewing duodenoscope for optimal assessment of the ampulla. Endoscopic treatment of duodenal adenomas has a role in FAP, including cautery, bipolar probe, argon plasma coagulation (APC) or Nd-YAG laser, endoscopic mucosal resection (EMR), and endoscopic ampullectomy, all of which may be used for nonfamilial adenomas as well (see Chapter 146).[1,5]

Patients with Peutz-Jeghers syndrome should undergo upper endoscopy and biopsy of hamartomas to look for adenomatous foci in the polyps, UGI-SBFT, and enteroclysis, or possibly wireless capsule endoscopy (WCE) to evaluate the entire SB.[12] Polyps >5 mm should be endoscopically resected if they are accessible. Those >15 mm or symptomatic should be considered for laparotomy with intraoperative enteroscopy and polypectomy because bleeding and intussusception are common.[12]

Patients with celiac disease who become symptomatic after years of quiescent disease while strictly adhering to a gluten-free diet should be thoroughly investigated for an SB cancer.

TABLE 61.6 MANAGEMENT OF SB NEOPLASMS

KEY POINTS
- Location
- Histological grading (Grade 1–4 and Grade X)
- Clinical classification ($cT_{0\text{-}4}$, $_xN_{0\text{-}1}$, $_xM_{0\text{-}1}$, $_x$) and staging (Stage 0–IV)

BENIGN NEOPLASMS
- Endoscopy (see Chapter 146): cautery and polypectomy, endoscopic mucosal resection (EMR), endoscopic ampullectomy, intraoperative enteroscopy with polypectomy
- Surgery: laparoscopy and laparotomy

MALIGNANT NEOPLASMS
- Surgery: Whipple, segmental/wedge resections, right hemicolectomy, and lymph node dissection
- Adjuvant chemotherapy: 5-fluorouracil/folinic acid (5-FU/FA), mitomycin C, adriamycin, and irinotecan
- Adjuvant chemotherapy (lymphoma): CHOP or BACOP hybrid regimens
- Adjuvant chemotherapy + radiotherapy: CHOP-based regimens + whole abdomen (WAR), involved-field (IF), or intensity modulated radiotherapy (IMRT) – sequentially, alternately, or concomitantly

In patients with Crohn's disease, development of a symptomatic SB stricture that does not respond to steroids and immunosuppressive drugs should be considered for surgical resection to rule out any malignancy.[1]

Surgery is the mainstay of therapy for all SB tumors, although the type of operation and the histologic subtype, stage, and location of the tumor dictate the need for adjuvant therapy. Overall, the prognosis is poor with the 5-year survival rate between 20% and 38%.[13]

Adenocarcinoma

Duodenal tumors involving the 1st and 2nd portions usually lead to a Whipple resection. Tumors in the 3rd and 4th portions of the duodenum usually require a wider segmental resection, although a Whipple procedure may be done additionally. Jejunal and proximal ileal adenocarcinomas are treated with segmental resection, including mesentery and associated lymph nodes. Tumors involving the terminal ileum are treated like right-sided colonic tumors, with right hemicolectomy and lymph node dissection.[1]

The role of adjuvant chemotherapy in this subgroup of patients is clearly undefined. There are no proven benefits of 5-fluorouracil/folinic acid (5-FU/FA), mitomycin C, and adriamycin in metastatic disease. A novel camptothecin analog, irinotecan, is being evaluated in clinical trials for adjuvant chemotherapy and metastatic disease. Thus, chemotherapy cannot be recommended in these patients outside of clinical trials. SB adenocarcinoma is relatively resistant to radiotherapy.[5]

Lymphoma

SB lymphoma is rarely diagnosed before surgery. Complete resection of the primary tumor and a wedge resection of mesentery should be performed along with extensive lymph node resection. Adjuvant chemotherapy, radiotherapy, or both may improve survival.

REFERENCES

1. Abu-Hamda EM, Hattab EM, Lynch PM. Small bowel tumors. Curr Gastroenterol Rep 2003; 5:386–393.
2. Neugut AI, Jacobson JS, Suh S, Mukherjee R, Arber N. The epidemiology of cancer of the small bowel. Cancer Epidemiol Biomarkers Prev 1998; 7:243–251.
3. Jemal A, Clegg LX, Ward E et al. Annual report to the nation on the status of cancer, 1975–2001, with a special feature regarding survival. Cancer 2004; 101:3–27.
4. Lowenfels AB. Why are small-bowel tumours so rare? Lancet 1973; 1(7793):24–26.
5. Gill SS, Heuman DM, Mihas AA. Small intestinal neoplasms. J Clin Gastroenterol 2001; 33:267–282.
6. Spigelman AD, Talbot IC, Penna C et al. Evidence for adenoma-carcinoma sequence in the duodenum of patients with familial adenomatous polyposis. The Leeds Castle Polyposis Group (Upper Gastrointestinal Committee). J Clin Pathol 1994; 47:709–710.
7. Lowenfels AB. Does bile promote extra-colonic cancer? Lancet 1978; 2(8083):239–241.
8. Riddell RH, Petras RE, Williams GT, Sobin LH. Tumors of the intestines. Washington, DC: Armed Forces Institute of Pathology; 2003.
9. Nolan DJ. Imaging of the small intestine. Schweiz Med Wochenschr 1998; 128:109–114.
10. Horton KM, Fishman EK. Multidetector-row computed tomography and 3-dimensional computed tomography imaging of small bowel neoplasms: current concept in diagnosis. J Comput Assist Tomogr 2004; 28:106–116.
11. Eliakim R. Wireless capsule video endoscopy: Three years of experience. World J Gastroenterol 2004; 10:1238–1239.
12. McGarrity TJ, Kulin HE, Zaino RJ. Peutz-Jeghers syndrome. Am J Gastroenterol 2000; 95:596–604.
13. Howe JR, Karnell LH, Menck HR, Scott-Conner C. The American College of Surgeons Commission on Cancer and the American Cancer Society. Adenocarcinoma of the small bowel: review of the National Cancer Data Base, 1985–1995. Cancer 1999; 86:2693–2706.

Chapter 62

Obstruction and volvulus

R Bhardwaj and M C Parker

KEY POINTS

- It is clinically important to differentiate between functional and mechanical obstruction, and to determine the site of mechanical obstruction
- Significant disturbance in electrolytes and fluid balance often occurs
- If the ileocecal valve is incompetent, gas may reflux into the small bowel, making distinction between large and small bowel obstruction difficult
- In pseudo-obstruction, a cecal diameter of 9–12 cm signifies a risk of perforation
- Splenic flexure cancers are particularly prone to obstruction
- Endoluminal stenting provides palliation in malignant colonic obstruction where surgery is not possible

INTRODUCTION

The management of bowel obstruction involves differentiation between functional and mechanical obstruction. In the latter case, an accurate determination of the level of obstruction is required to facilitate efficient clinical resolution. This chapter focuses on established concepts in the surgical management of pseudo-obstruction, malignant and benign colonic obstruction, small bowel obstruction and volvulus. The role of novel minimally interventional strategies, including percutaneous and endoscopic techniques, is discussed.

CAUSES OF INTESTINAL OBSTRUCTION

Small and large bowel obstructions have different etiologies (Tables 62.1 and 62.2). Small bowel obstruction is most commonly caused by adhesions or herniae (although the incidence is declining), whereas colonic malignancy, sigmoid diverticulitis, or volvulus of the sigmoid colon or cecum are the main causes of large bowel obstruction. Crohn's disease can cause both small and large bowel obstruction. Although malignancy (intrinsic and peritoneal deposits) is a much less common cause of small rather than large bowel obstruction, it is by no means insignificant. Motility disturbances, particularly ileus (most commonly postoperative), have functionally the same consequences as mechanical obstruction and enter into the differential diagnosis. There is a gradient from acute/total motility disturbance through to chronic/subtotal conditions (see Chapter 66).

PATHOPHYSIOLOGY

Clinical evidence of obstruction arises through a combination of mechanical obstruction (whether luminal, in the bowel wall, or extrinsic), inadequate propulsion, and often an ischemic component.

TABLE 62.1 SMALL BOWEL OBSTRUCTION

Category	Mechanism	Cause	Example
Mechanical	Extrinsic	**Adhesions**	*Postoperative*, congenital
		Hernia	External more common than internal
		Serosal involvement	Endometriosis
	Intrinsic/extrinsic	*Malignancy*	Carcinoma, polyps, mesenteric deposits
	Intrinsic	Inflammatory	*Crohn's disease*, tuberculosis, radiation
		Chemical	Meckel's diverticulum, caustic injury
	Intraluminal		Gallstone ileus, intussusception, foreign body, parasites (*Strongyloides*)
Vascular	Infarction	Acute occlusion	Mesenteric embolus
	Ischemia	Chronic insufficiency	Superior mesenteric artery syndrome
Nonmechanical	**Ileus**	Multiple	*Postoperative*
		Inflammatory	*Peritonitis*
		Neurogenic	Spinal cord injury ± hematoma, pancreatitis, renal colic, splanchnic nerve irritation
		Metabolic	Electrolyte disorders (hypokalemia), uremia, diabetes mellitus
		Pharmacologic	Anticholinergics, tricyclics, phenothiazines, narcotics
		Thoracic disease	Pnemonia, pleurisy, rib fracture, myocardial infarction
		Idiopathic	Intestinal pseudo-obstruction

The commonest causes are shown in bold type, with next most common in italics.

TABLE 62.2 LARGE BOWEL OBSTRUCTION

Category	Mechanism	Cause	Example
Mechanical	Intrinsic	**Malignancy**	**Carcinoma**, polyps, mesenteric deposits
		Inflammatory	**Sigmoid diverticulitis**, Crohn's disease, tuberculosis, radiation
	Extrinsic	**Volvulus**	*Sigmoid, cecal*, transverse/splenic
		Serosal involvement	Endometriosis
Vascular	Ischemia	Chronic insufficiency	Inferior mesenteric artery stenosis/occlusion/embolus, venous thrombosis
Nonmechanical	Colonic motility disorder	Inflammatory	*Peritonitis*, toxic dilatation (ulcerative and other colitides)
		Neurogenic	Spinal cord injury ± hematoma, splanchnic nerve irritation
		Metabolic	Electrolyte disorders (hypokalemia)
		Pharmacologic	Anticholinergics, tricyclics, phenothiazines, narcotics
		Idiopathic	Colonic pseudo-obstruction

The commonest causes are shown in bold type, with next most common in italics.

CLINICAL FEATURES

History

Intestinal obstruction is characterized by abdominal pain, which is often severe and episodic. This is followed by distention, nausea, and vomiting. Vomitus may be substantial and occur early if obstruction is proximal. Conversely, an inability to pass flatus or feces may point to distal obstruction.

Examination

The abdomen becomes distended. Partial obstruction is characterized by loud explosive bowel sounds which may become progressively more high pitched and eventually cease. At this point the differential diagnosis is ileus. Pain is more common with obstruction than ileus, but severe pain should raise the possibility of local perforation or inflammation. Examination may reveal the cause (e.g., hernial obstruction).

Initial management

Patients with obstruction often have substantial fluid disturbance, which requires evaluation and correction. Radiology plays a key role in the management of patients with obstruction.

RADIOLOGIC DETERMINATION OF BOWEL OBSTRUCTION

Clinical evaluation of the patient usually precedes upright chest and supine abdominal radiography. The detection of free air can be enhanced with a lateral decubitus film.

In the assessment of small bowel obstruction, plain radiographic signs may include distention of small bowel, the presence of fluid levels, and an empty colon, although none of these is diagnostic. Water-soluble contrast radiology is safe and easy to use and interpret. Small bowel enteroclysis is more sensitive than the standard oral small bowel examination, as contrast flow rates are better controlled and there is less dilution of the contrast. Compared with the per-oral technique, it does not rely on waiting for the stomach to empty, although there may be technical difficulty in intubating the duodenum. Comparison of abdominal computed tomography (CT) with plain radiography in the evaluation of small bowel obstruction shows comparable sensitivity, although CT is more specific. CT also allows better determination of closed-loop obstruction and may identify coexisting intra-abdominal pathology such as malignancy or a focus of inflammation. To determine mechanical obstruction, both CT and contrast studies identify a transition between proximally dilated and distally collapsed bowel. *Strangulation of small bowel* is difficult to interpret clinically; plain radiologic signs include edematous bowel wall, pneumatosis and gas in the portal vein; CT signs may include ascites, asymmetric enhancement of bowel loops, circumferential thickening of the bowel wall, pneumatosis intestinalis, and hemorrhage into the mesentery.

Colonic obstruction may reveal itself with dilated, gas-filled colonic loops proximal to the obstruction, with diminished or absent gas patterns distally on plain radiography. In the presence of a competent ileocecal valve, colonic distention ensues rapidly. However, if the ileocecal valve is incompetent, gas may flow into the small bowel. The actual site of obstruction may not correlate with the plain radiographic appearance. A water-soluble enema is recommended in order to differentiate mechanical from colonic pseudo-obstruction (Ogilvie's syndrome) (Fig. 62.1). In demonstrating mechanical obstruction, CT may be used in isolation, or may augment the single-contrast enema as it aids identification of both the etiology of the obstructing lesion and concurrent pathology such as distant metastases in patients with malignant obstruction. In the latter scenario this may influence therapeutic intervention. A cecal diameter of 9–12 cm is a traditional measure of impending colonic ischemia and perforation. In cases where contrast enemas are contraindicated, such as toxic megacolon, CT is of particular benefit.

Exciting advances are being reported with the use of magnetic resonance imaging (MRI) as an investigative modality. Beall et al[1] reported a correct diagnosis of small and large bowel obstruction of 95% with MRI compared to 71% with CT in a series of 44 patients. Causes included fibrous adhesions, malignancy, Crohn's disease, intra-abdominal abscesses, herniae, lymphoma, intussusception, and an anastomotic stricture.

PSEUDO-OBSTRUCTION

Acute colonic pseudo-obstruction (Ogilvie's syndrome) refers to marked dilatation of the colon without an identifiable obstructing lesion (see Chapter 66). The condition is related to recent surgery, trauma, severe illness, or medication. Evaluation in the *critically ill patient* includes the exclusion of

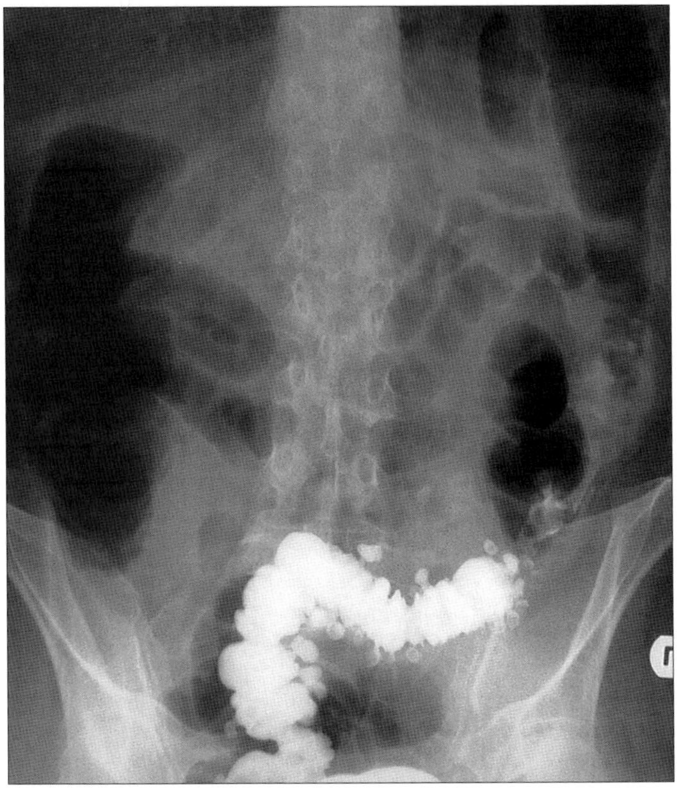

Fig. 62.1 Obstructing sigmoid lesion. 'Cut off' of water-soluble contrast medium with an obstructing sigmoid lesion. Note the incidental diverticulosis.

mechanical obstruction, other causes of toxic megacolon, and observing the patient's clinical state for signs of colonic ischemia and perforation. The precise cecal diameter, as measured on a plain radiography or CT, that indicates impending colonic perforation varies from patient to patient. Although work by Lowman & Davis in 1956[2] showed that in 19 surgically treated patients who had cecal perforation or 'impending' perforation cecal diameters were above 9 cm, Vanek & Al-Salti[3] reviewed 400 cases and highlighted that perforation or ischemia was not seen unless the cecum was at least 12 cm in diameter.

Treatment includes correction of underlying causes, cessation of drugs that decrease colonic motility, and specific drug treatment such as neostigmine or other prokinetic agents.

MALIGNANT OBSTRUCTION

Clinical features

Colorectal carcinoma accounts for the majority of cases of large bowel obstruction, with one-third of colonic cancers presenting with obstruction. Approximately half of *splenic flexure* tumors obstruct, compared with approximately one-quarter of left colonic tumors and up to one-third of right-sided lesions. However, few rectosigmoid cancers present with obstruction. The rapidity of onset of symptoms may reflect the level of obstruction. *Cecal or ascending colonic obstruction* may present with colicky abdominal pain, abdominal distention, and vomiting indicative of small bowel dilatation. In the presence of a competent ileocecal valve, cecal distention may occur rapidly. With *left-sided colonic obstruction* absolute constipation may be a predominant feature; pain, colonic distention, and vomiting may be late presenting features.

Clinical examination may identify a palpable *abdominal or rectal mass* indicative of a malignant lesion, and hepatomegaly which may reflect metastases. An assessment of the patient's co-morbidity is essential to plan intervention. The patient may be too frail initially to undergo operative intervention without adequate resuscitation and physiologic optimization. Although a single-contrast water-soluble enema can demonstrate complete obstruction, CT can do this as well, and may also demonstrate metastatic spread, which may influence management.

Treatment

When surgery is undertaken, the presence of local and distant disease will influence whether the procedure is regarded as curative or palliative, although the latter does not necessarily negate resection of the tumor. For *right-sided and transverse colon* lesions a single-stage procedure such as a right hemicolectomy or an extended right hemicolectomy is recommended. This would remove the obstructing carcinoma and the proximally dilated segment of colon. A primary anastomosis is usually feasible, but high leak rates in anastomoses constructed in the emergency situation (10%) have prompted some authors to suggest that exteriorization of the divided bowel may be suitable in cases where anastomotic healing may be in doubt. Carcinomas of the *transverse colon* often necessitate resection of part of the greater omentum, and those near or at the splenic flexure may prove difficult to remove as mobilization of the splenic flexure is required.

The management of *left-sided colonic neoplasms* has evolved as a compromise of surgical speed, and effective cure must be made. The formation of a transverse colostomy, whilst relieving the obstruction and allowing recovery, does not deal with the primary disease; it is associated with death in approximately one-tenth of patients, and in a quarter of cases the patient's co-morbidity does not allow for further surgery. This procedure does have the advantage that when definitive resection occurs, as part of a three-stage procedure, a defunctioning stoma to protect the anastomosis after resection has already been constructed. The final stage involves closing the stoma. A *two-stage procedure* – resection and formation of a proximal end-colostomy (Hartmann's procedure), with closure of the rectal stump or with the creation of a mucous fistula and subsequent reversal – allows a simple solution. The combined mortality rate is 10%. The main advantage of the two-stage over the three-stage procedure is a reduced hospital stay. Although some patients do not proceed to reversal, the timing of the reversal is important as re-anastomosis after a delay of 6 months is not associated with anastomotic leakage.

There are two surgical options when a *single-stage procedure* is undertaken. The first involves an oncologic resection of the tumor, on-table colonic irrigation, and primary anastomosis. If there is any doubt over the creation of an anastomosis, exteriorization of the colon may be performed. The second option involves resection of the entire colon proximal to the obstructing tumor and creation of an ileosigmoid or ileorectal anastomosis. This has the advantage of removing synchronous tumors that may be present. The SCOTIA Study Group conducted a randomized prospective evaluation of single-stage treatment for malignant left-sided colonic obstruction in 91 patients, comparing subtotal colectomy in 47 patients with segmental resection following intraoperative resection in 44.[4] This study showed no significant difference in rates of operative mortality, hospital stay, anastomotic leakage, or wound sepsis.

Endoluminal stenting provides a safe option in those who are initially medically unfit to tolerate an operative procedure, as stenting provides immediate relief of an acute obstructive lesion prior to planned curative resection (bridge to surgery); stenting is also effective for palliation of advanced colorectal cancer, avoiding a stoma. An ideal colonic stent is one that can be inserted easily transrectally, can negotiate the colonic folds, be comfortably deployed, allow a sufficient channel for fecal material to pass, and remain in position (Fig. 62.2). Khot et al[5] conducted a detailed systematic review of the literature on the use of self-expanding metal stents from 1990 to January 2001 and revealed 58 publications, with analysis of outcomes possible in 29 papers. This review detailed that of 598 patients selected the intended treatment for 336 (56%) was palliative and 262 (44%) were treated with the intention of surgical intervention at a later date. In the whole group clinical success was reported in 525 patients (88%). Importantly, of 233 patients selected for surgery and stented successfully, 212 (91%) went on to have a successful one-stage surgical resection of the colonic segment. Saida et al,[6] in a comparison of long-term prognosis of emergency surgery in 40 patients versus stenting as a preoperative 'bridge to surgery' in 44 patients, showed leak rates of 11% versus 3% and a 5-year survival rate of 44% versus 40%.[6]

In the UK, recent cost analyses demonstrated that stenting reduces costs by £685 per patient. In the palliative setting, use of colorectal stents is associated with a lower morbidity than surgery for patients who are terminally ill, and allows for maintenance of a quality of life in patients during their remaining lifespan.

Other modes of therapy, such as cryotherapy, electrocoagulation, photodynamic therapy, and ablation with a neodymium–yttrium aluminum garnet (Nd-YAG) laser, have been advocated. However, these are usually suitable only for distal rectal tumors and often need to be repeated.

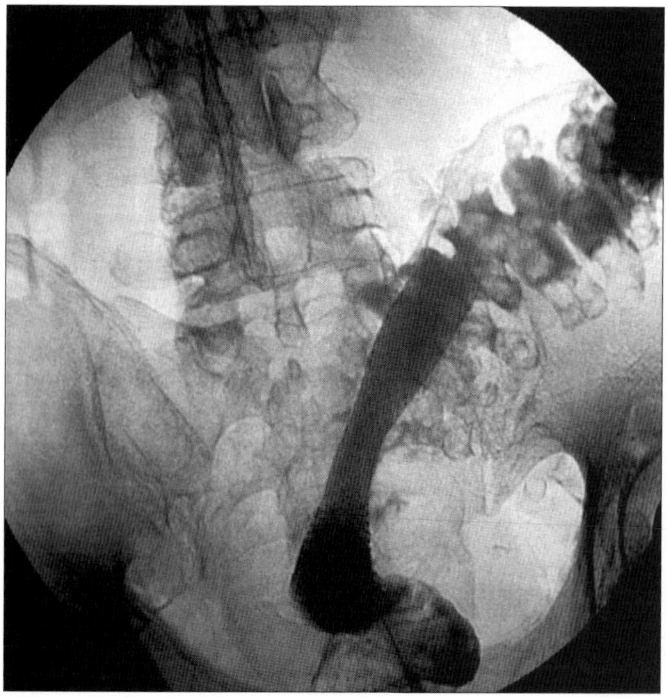

Fig. 62.2 Self-expanding stent. Insertion of a self-expanding metal stent to relieve an obstructing sigmoid carcinoma.

OBSTRUCTION DUE TO DIVERTICULAR DISEASE

Obstruction with diverticular disease often occurs as a result of the complications of severe inflammation. McConnell et al[7] found that women were more likely to present with obstruction; in a series of 934 patients requiring surgical resection for diverticular disease, 61 had obstructive symptoms. Assessment may be made on clinical grounds alone, but usually involves hematologic analysis, urinalysis, and plain radiography. A water-soluble enema permits identification of complete obstruction, with extravasation of the contrast in cases of perforation, although CT with oral, rectal, or intravenous contrast is often required to identify accurately the local inflammatory complications, such as abscesses or fistula formation. Resection and diversion is a safe surgical option with obstruction due to diverticulitis, although primary anastomosis with on-table lavage is an alternative where there is minimal contamination of the peritoneal cavity.

SMALL BOWEL OBSTRUCTION: ADHESIONS

Fevang et al[8] studied factors that influenced complications and death after operation for small bowel obstruction in 877 patients, involving 975 operations over a 30-year period. Adhesions accounted for 526 procedures (54%), incarcerated hernias for 293 (30%), and small bowel volvulus for 30 (3%). Other causes included Crohn's disease, radiation injury, gallstones, and foreign body obstruction. Logistic regression analysis showed that advanced age, co-morbidity, nonviable strangulation, and a treatment delay of more than 24 h increased the death rate. Parker et al[9] conducted a 10-year follow-up of 12584 patients who underwent lower abdominal surgery in 1986. In the study period, 430 abdominal interventions for direct adhesion-related disease were identified, 200 of which were for small bowel obstruction. The authors raised concerns over the costs and staffing-related effort expended on the treatment of adhesions, and advocated the use of new adhesion prevention strategies.

VOLVULUS

Volvulus is the torsion of a segment of bowel and mesentery. The reported incidence in Western societies ranges from 1.4 to 1.7 per 100000. Patients may present with recurrent abdominal pain, and in the emergency situation severe abdominal pain with distention. The sigmoid colon is commonly affected (Fig. 62.3), followed in descending order of frequency by the cecum, splenic flexure, and transverse colon. Once the colonic segment torts, distention occurs in the obstructed loop with subsequent ischemia, gangrene, and perforation. The diagnosis is often made on clinical grounds with plain radiography, although water-soluble enemas and CT are useful. With sigmoid volvulus, a loop arising from the left iliac fossa, the 'omega loop' sign, may be identified on plain abdominal radiography, and the 'coffee bean' sign is demonstrable in the right iliac fossa with cecal volvulus. Fluid levels within the obstructed loop and thickened bowel loops may also be noted.

In the case of a nonviable sigmoid colon, either a Hartmann's procedure, a Paul Mikulicz procedure, or primary anastomosis with on-table colonic lavage is appropriate. Conservative management strategies for sigmoid volvulus with a viable sigmoid

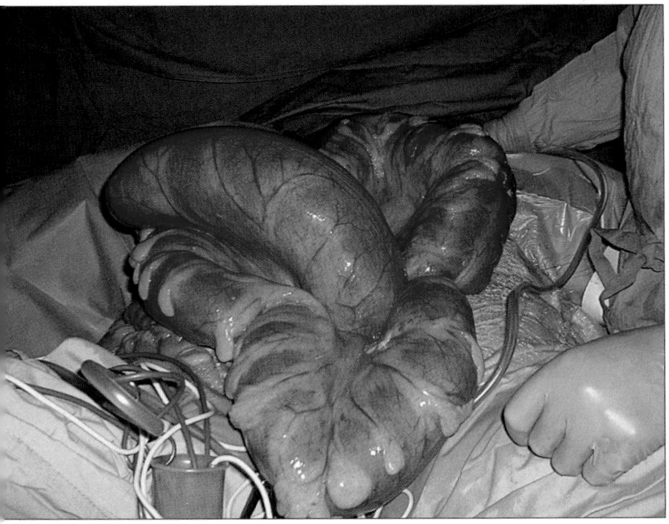

Fig. 62.3 **Acute volvulus.** Grossly distended sigmoid colon resulting from acute volvulus. Courtesy of Mr P J Webb, Medway Maritime Hospital, Gillingham, UK.

colon, such as drainage tube or colonoscopic decompression, are more suited to elderly patients and those with severe concurrent disease as recurrence rates are high. Even when a delayed surgical procedure was advocated after initial decompression, Chung et al[10] reported that of 14 (48%) of 29 patients who refused surgery after endoscopic decompression, 12 (86%) developed recurrent volvulus in a median time of 2.8 months. With recurrent sigmoid volvulus in patients unfit for major surgery, percutaneous endoscopic fixation of the sigmoid colon has been advocated with good outcomes.[11] Operative detorsion and sigmoid fixation, although simple, has been found to have recurrence rates of up to 50%. In order to reduce this, extraperitonealization of the sigmoid colon is practised by some; this may also be performed laparoscopically. Owing to the paucity of randomized trials to demonstrate the superiority of a particular operative technique in treating sigmoid volvulus, Kuzu et al[12] reported on primary resection with or without anastomosis in 106 consecutive patients, 57 of whom had primary colonic anastomosis. Four of the 57 patients (7%) with primary anastomoses had wound dehiscence, and 7 of the total 107 died. These results compared favourably with a review of 880 cases from 1952 to 2000 identified by the authors. Alternatives to sigmoid resection in patients with a nongangrenous sigmoid colon include mesosigmoidoplasty, which aims to reduce the ability of the long and narrow sigmoid mesocolon to rotate around its axis. Bach et al[13] proposed a modification of the technique in which, rather than just the peritoneal cover being adjusted, all layers of the sigmoid colon were shortened and widened. Ten of 12 patients who underwent this procedure required no further intervention, and during a short follow-up of 4–8 months there were no complaints of abdominal pain.

Colonoscopic treatment of cecal volvulus is not recommended because recurrence rates are high. Cecopexy and cecostomy should be reserved for elderly and frail patients. Cecal resection and anastomosis is the preferred option.

The 'ileosigmoid knot,' first described by Parker in 1845, is a form of sigmoid volvulus in which the ileum wraps itself around the base of the sigmoid and causes a closed-loop obstruction of both the ileum and colon. Operative intervention is mandatory as endoscopic attempts to correct the abnormality are usually unsuccessful. Although resection of both involved bowel segments is often required, there is some merit in unwrapping of the torted segments if viable bowel is present. If a segment of small bowel necessitates resection, anastomosis of the ileal ends is safe, and the recent trend is to resect the sigmoid colon and construct a primary anastomosis. Raveenthiran[14] described the successful surgical management of an ileosigmoid knot in seven patients treated over a 6-year period from 1994. In all cases the sigmoid colon was gangrenous. After initial deflation of the distended bowel loops, the knot was unraveled in five patients. In all patients a primary ileoileal and/or colocolic anastomosis was constructed, although in one patient an ileocolic anastomosis was necessary as the resected small bowel was close to the ileocecal valve.

CONCLUSION

Advances in imaging, critical care, and endoscopic and laparoscopic strategies have enabled clinicians to target specific treatments for the treatment of both small and large bowel obstruction. Rapid differentiation between mechanical and functional obstruction is crucial. Operative intervention is not always indicated, but when surgery is necessary a balance between resolution of the underlying disease process and further therapy is required. This is particularly the case in patients with malignant colonic obstruction and repeated adhesiolysis.

REFERENCES

1. Beall DP, Fortman BJ, Lawler BC et al. Imaging bowel obstruction: a comparison between fast magnetic resonance imaging and helical computed tomography. Clin Radiol 2002; 57:719–724.
2. Davis L, Lowman RM. An evaluation of cecal size in impending perforation of the cecum. Surg Gynecol Obstet 1956; 103:711–718.
3. Vanek VW, Al-Salti M. Acute pseudo-obstruction of the colon (Ogilvie's syndrome). An analysis of 400 cases. Dis Colon Rectum 1986; 29:203–210.
4. The SCOTIA Study Group. Single-stage treatment for malignant left-sided colonic obstruction: a prospective randomized clinical trial comparing subtotal colectomy with segmental resection following intraoperative irrigation. Br J Surg 1995; 82:1622–1627.
5. Khot UP, Lang AW, Murali K, Parker MC. Systematic review of the efficacy and safety of colorectal stents. Br J Surg 2002; 89:1096–1102.
6. Saida Y, Sumiyama Y, Nagao J et al. Long-term prognosis of preoperative "bridge to surgery" expandable metallic stent insertion for obstructive colorectal cancer: comparison with emergency operation. Dis Colon Rectum 2003; 46(Suppl):S44–S49.
7. McConnell EJ, Tessier DJ, Wolff BG. Population-based incidence of complicated diverticular disease of the sigmoid colon based on gender and age. Dis Colon Rectum 2003; 46:1110–1114.
8. Fevang BT, Fevang J, Stangeland L, Soreide O, Svanes K, Viste A. Complications and death after surgical treatment of small bowel obstruction: a 35-year institutional experience. Ann Surg 2000; 231:529–537.
9. Parker MC, Ellis H, Moran BJ et al. Postoperative adhesions: ten-year follow-up of 12584 patients undergoing lower abdominal surgery. Dis Colon Rectum 2001; 44:822–829.
10. Chung YF, Eu KW, Nyam DC et al. Minimizing recurrence after sigmoid volvulus. Br J Surg 1999; 86:231–233.
11. Daniels IR, Lamparelli MJ, Chave H, Simson JN. Recurrent sigmoid volvulus treated by percutaneous endoscopic colostomy. Br J Surg 2000; 87:1419.

12. Kuzu MA, Aslar AK, Soran A et al. Emergent resection for acute sigmoid volvulus: results of 106 consecutive cases. Dis Colon Rectum 2002; 45:1085–1090.

13. Bach O, Rudloff U, Post S. Modification of mesosigmoidoplasty for nongangrenous sigmoid volvulus. World J Surg 2003; 27:1329–1332.

14. Raveenthiran V. The ileosigmoid knot: new observations and changing trends. Dis Colon Rectum 2001; 44:1196–1200.

Chapter 63

Constipation and constipation syndromes

Arnold Wald

KEY POINTS

- Risk factors for functional constipation include female gender, increased age, and sedentary life style but not decreased dietary fiber or fluid intake
- Chronic use of stimulant laxatives is not harmful to the colon
- Colonic inertia appears to be a disorder of the enteric nervous system in the colon
- The most useful tests for constipation which responds poorly to conservative measures are colonic transit of markers, rectal balloon expulsion and anorectal manometry
- Symptoms of constipation such as infrequent defecation and defecatory difficulties do not predict pathophysiology: diagnostic testing is the same regardless of predominant symptoms
- Daily defecation is not the goal of therapy; 98% of the population defecate from three times per week to three times per day
- Megacolon and megarectum require a treatment approach that differs from constipation with normal colon diameter
- Colon function does not deteriorate with aging; otherwise healthy constipated elderly patients should be evaluated similar to younger adults
- Pelvic floor dyssynergia is an acquired disorder of defecation that may respond to behavioral interventions such as biofeedback
- Partial surgical resections to shorten colons rarely succeed; for colonic inertia, subtotal colectomy is a surgical procedure of proven efficacy only if abnormalities of anorectal and gastrointestinal motility are excluded

INTRODUCTION

Constipation is prevalent in both children and adults in Western countries and is a common complaint in clinical practice. As with many functional disorders, constipation is often mild and may be managed by the patient with over-the-counter laxatives and fiber supplements. However, more severe constipation may become debilitating and unresponsive to simple interventions, resulting in medical consultation.

The definitions of constipation vary among laypersons and physicians. The previous narrow definition of bowel infrequency has been broadened to encompass difficult defecation, a concept that is highly subjective and hard to quantify. A consensus definition of constipation[1] is now frequently used in clinical research and may serve as a guide for practitioners (Table 63.1). A modification of this concept is fewer than three spontaneous and complete bowel movements per week.[2]

TABLE 63.1 ROME II CRITERIA FOR CONSTIPATION[1]

ADULTS

Two or more of the following for at least 12 weeks (not necessarily consecutive) in the preceding 12 months:

- straining during >25% of bowel movements
- lumpy or hard stools for >25% of bowel movements
- sensation of incomplete evacuation for >25% of bowel movements
- sensation of anorectal blockage for >25% of bowel movements
- manual maneuvers to facilitate >25% of bowel movements (e.g., digital evacuation or support of the pelvic floor)
- <3 bowel movements per week

Loose stools not present, and there are insufficient criteria for irritable bowel syndrome

INFANTS AND CHILDREN

- Pebble-like, hard stools for a majority of bowel movements for at least 2 weeks
- Firm stools ≤2 times per week for at least 2 weeks
- No evidence of structural, endocrine, or metabolic disease

EPIDEMIOLOGY

Estimates of the prevalence of constipation in the general population vary according to how constipation is defined. If a frequency of defecation less than three times per week is used, prevalence rates are generally no more than 4%. If definitions include difficulties with defecation or self perceived constipation, rates are as high as 28%, with considerable variability among countries.[3,4] In all populations, constipation is more frequent in women, in children, and in the elderly.[5]

In the US, more than US$800 million are spent on laxatives yearly. Constipation accounted for about 20 000 hospitalizations and 2.5 million office visits per year from 1958 to 1986,[5] most of these to primary care physicians.

CAUSES, RISK FACTORS, DISEASE ASSOCIATIONS

Risk factors associated with constipation include low income, low educational levels, physical inactivity, depression, low caloric intake, and perhaps nationality.[5] Contrary to general belief, low dietary fiber and fluid intake have not been associated with constipation, although fiber supplements may benefit many constipated patients.

Constipation may occur because of a primary motor disorder, in association with a large number of diseases, or as a side effect of many drugs. Those diseases include metabolic or endocrine disorders and neurogenic disorders that affect the gastrointestinal tract.[6,7] Chronic illnesses leading to physical and mental impairments can produce or exaggerate constipation due to inactivity or physical immobility, medications, and dietary inadequacies. Generalized weakness or striated muscle diseases may result in poor expulsion efforts.

CAUSES AND RISK FACTORS

SECONDARY CAUSES OF FUNCTIONAL CONSTIPATION

METABOLIC AND ENDOCRINE DISORDERS
- Diabetes mellitus
- Hypothyroidism
- Hypercalcemia, hypokalemia
- Pregnancy
- Porphyria
- Panhypopituitarism
- Pheochromocytoma

NEUROGENIC DISORDERS

Peripheral:
- Hirschsprung's disease
- Chagas' disease
- Neurofibromatosis
- Ganglioneuromatosis
- Autonomic neuropathy
- Hypoganglionosis
- Intestinal pseudo-obstruction

Central:
- Multiple sclerosis
- Spinal cord lesions
- Parkinson's disease
- Shy-Drager syndrome
- Trauma to nervi erigentes
- Cerebrovascular accidents

COLLAGEN VASCULAR AND MUSCLE DISORDERS
- Systemic sclerosis
- Amyloidosis
- Dermatomyositis
- Myotonic dystrophy

PATHOGENESIS AND CLINICAL PRESENTATIONS OF IDIOPATHIC FUNCTIONAL CONSTIPATION

Constipation in children

Chronic constipation in childhood is multifactorial in origin. Although behavioral problems may occur, idiopathic constipation in children is not synonymous with psychogenic constipation. Severe constipation in children may be associated with fecal impaction, megarectum or megacolon, and fecal soiling. Many constipated children exhibit slow transit in the distal colon and rectum, which suggests either withholding behavior or anorectal dysfunction. Although they may complain that they do not sense an urge to defecate, demonstration of rectal sensory impairment has been inconsistent.

SOME DRUGS ASSOCIATED WITH CONSTIPATION

ANALGESICS
- Nonsteroidal anti-inflammatory agents

ANTICHOLINERGICS
- Antispasmodics
- Antidepressants
- Antipsychotics
- Antiparkinsonian drugs (some)

CATION-CONTAINING AGENTS
- Iron supplements
- Aluminum (antacids, sucralfate)
- Metallic intoxication (arsenic, lead, mercury)

OTHER AGENTS
- Opiates
- Antihypertensives
- Ganglionic blockers
- Vinca alkaloids
- Anticonvulsants
- Calcium channel blockers
- $5HT_3$ antagonists

Relaxation of the internal anal sphincter is usually normal and its absence suggests Hirschsprung's disease. Many constipated children with fecal soiling fail to relax the puborectalis and external sphincter muscles when asked to defecate. This may be a learned behavior acquired at an earlier age, for example, if attempts to evacuate a large fecal bolus were associated with discomfort or an anal fissure. Theoretically, this could lead to further retention of stool, continuing the vicious cycle of events.

Constipation in adults

Chronic constipation in adults is more prevalent in women, abdominal pain is uncommon, and megacolon is rare. Patients may complain of infrequent defecation, excessive straining when defecating, or both. Patients may be distinguished by studies of colonic transit and anorectal function.

Most patients who consult for constipation associated with infrequent defecation have normal colonic transit.[8,9] In the absence of abdominal pain, they do not meet diagnostic criteria for irritable bowel syndrome. Some patients with normal transit constipation demonstrate abnormalities of anorectal sensory and motor function; the relationship of these findings to the patients' complaints is unclear.

Slow colonic transit: The remaining patients with severe constipation exhibit slow colonic transit (see also Chapter 66). Theoretically, slow colonic transit may occur as a result of decreased propulsion (hypomotility) or increased distal motility and retropulsion of markers (hypermotility). Colonic inertia is defined as the delayed passage of radiopaque markers through the proximal colon (Fig. 63.1 and Fig. 63.2) and the term is generally reserved for cases in which transit in the proximal colon is delayed without evidence of retropulsion of markers from the left colon. In addition, there should be no evidence of anorectal dysfunction that could result in secondary colonic stasis.

Baseline colonic motility in these patients is similar to nonconstipated controls but there is little or no increase of motor activity after meals or administration of bisacodyl. A number

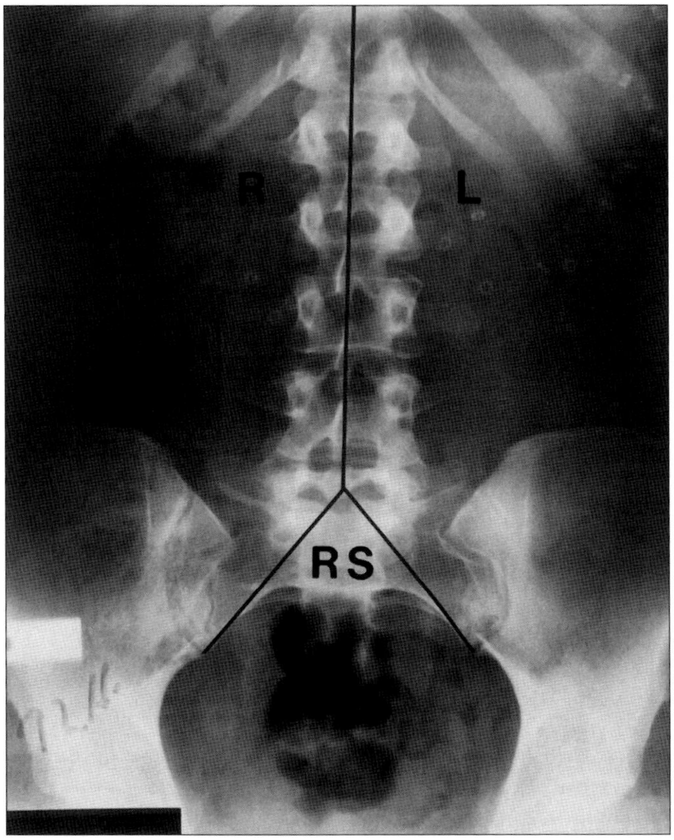

Fig. 63.1 Abdominal radiograph obtained during colonic transit study. The colon is divided into the right, left, and rectosigmoid (RS) regions by lines drawn through bone landmarks. The number of radiopaque markers in each region is quantitated over time, ceasing when 80% has been expelled or 7 days have elapsed. Reproduced with permission from Wald A. Constipation. In Yamada T, ed. Atlas of gastroenterology. Philadelphia: Lippincott Williams & Wilkins; 1999.

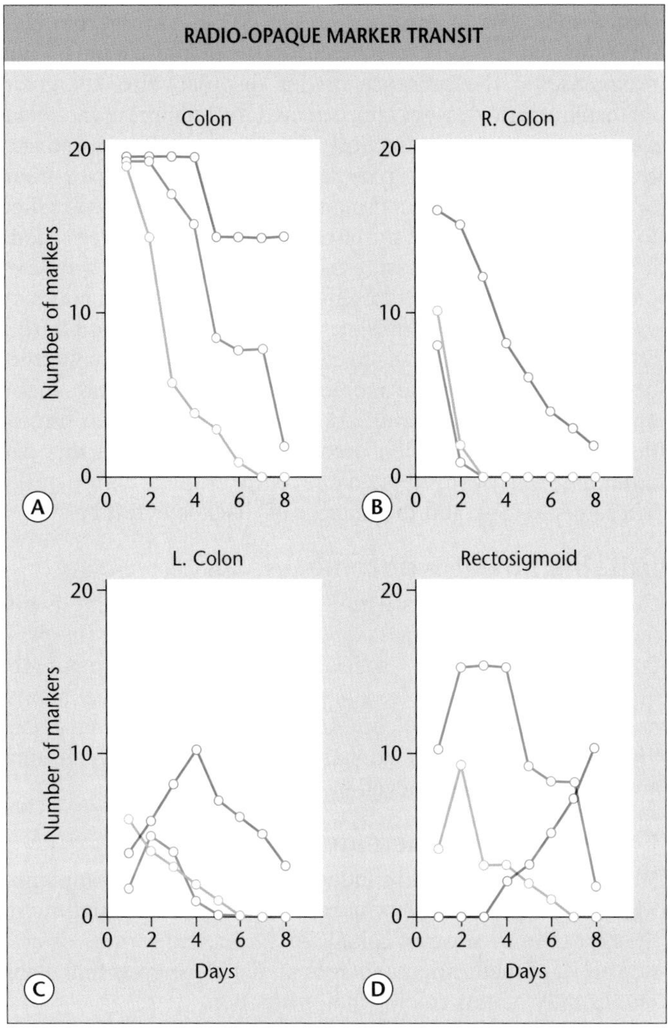

Fig. 63.2 Patterns of radiopaque marker transit through the colon. Twenty markers were swallowed by patients and daily abdominal radiographs (maximum of 8) were obtained. In normal individuals (green), markers are rapidly passed from the colon so that at least 80% are passed by the fifth day. In patients with colonic inertia (red), passage of markers is delayed in the proximal colon (right and left) with delayed entry into the rectosigmoid segment. In those patients with outlet delay (blue), there is normal transit through the proximal colon but delayed transit through the rectosigmoid segment. Reproduced from Wald A. Colonic transit and anorectal manometry in chronic idiopathic constipation. Arch Int Med 1996; 146:1713–1716.

of histologic abnormalities and abnormalities of the contractile properties of colonic smooth muscle have been demonstrated in resected colon specimens from patients with colonic inertia, though the relevance of these findings is unclear.[10,11,12] Some patients with severe colonic inertia also have generalized gastrointestinal dysmotility.

Outlet delay: Another category of idiopathic slow transit constipation is termed outlet delay in which markers progress normally through the proximal colon but collect in the rectum (see Fig. 63.2). This pattern has also been described in Hirschsprung's disease, fecal impaction, megarectum,[13] and other disorders associated with muscular hypotonicity. These disorders may be grouped under the heading of disorders of defecation,[14] or pelvic floor dysfunction (Table 63.2).

Management: Normal defecation involves the coordinated relaxation of the internal anal sphincter, puborectalis, and external anal sphincter muscles together with increased intra-abdominal pressure and colonic motor activity, which propels stool towards the rectum. In some patients, ineffective defecation appears to be associated with failure to relax, or inappropriate contraction of, the puborectalis and external anal sphincter muscles.[15] This narrows the anorectal angle and increases the pressures of the anal canal so that evacuation is less effective. Because relaxation of these muscles involves cortical inhibition of the spinal reflex during defecation, this pattern may repre-

TABLE 63.2 FUNCTIONAL DISORDERS OF DEFECATION

Mechanisms	Disorders
Weak propulsion	Megarectum Pain syndromes Neuromuscular diseases
Misdirection of propulsion	Rectocele (occasional)
Failure of IAS relaxation	Hirschsprung's disease
Failure of muscle relaxation	Pelvic floor dyssynergia

IAS, internal anal sphincter.

sent a conscious or unconscious act. It can also be modified in some patients using biofeedback and muscle retraining programs.[16,17] The presence of this disorder, also known as rectosphincteric dyssynergia, can be detected during the rectal examination, as the contraction of the puborectalis and external anal sphincter muscles can be palpated when asking the patient to strain. During anorectal manometry, if the patient is asked to expel the manometer, the characteristic normal pattern is one in which intrarectal pressure increases and external sphincter pressure decreases; in rectosphincteric dyssynergia, in contrast, external sphincter pressures increase or remain constant during attempted expulsion of the manometer (Fig. 63.3). Finally, with barium defecography the anorectal angle either does not widen or actually narrows during attempts to expel the barium, so that little or no expulsion occurs. The prevalence of this disorder has been overestimated due to the artificial nature of the laboratory setting and the manner of diagnostic testing.[18]

Irritable bowel syndrome (see also Chapter 64)

Constipation in patients with irritable bowel syndrome is differentiated from functional constipation primarily by the presence of abdominal pain, especially in the lower abdomen.[1] Not uncommonly, patients also complain of irregular bowel habits, abdominal bloating, flatulence, and upper gastrointestinal symptoms. In contrast to functional constipation, such symptoms are not consistently relieved by bowel evacuation.

Constipation in the elderly

Many constipated elderly individuals had similar complaints when they were younger while others develop constipation for the first time because of colonic or systemic disorders or as a side effect of medications. There is no data to suggest that aging significantly affects colonic motor function.

Fecal impaction may be a significant problem in elderly individuals who are institutionalized. Mental confusion, immobility, or inadequate toilet arrangements may cause such persons to ignore the urge to defecate, and the fecal bolus may become too large or uncomfortable to pass. The development of megarectum often leads to blunting of rectal and anal sensation that persists even after disimpaction.[13] This predisposes such patients to reaccumulation of feces unless a scrupulous toileting program or periodic evacuation is instituted. Fecal impaction is the most common cause of spurious diarrhea and of fecal incontinence in the institutionalized elderly.

Megarectum and megacolon

Although few patients with constipation have megacolon or megarectum, most patients with a dilated colon or rectum have constipation. Idiopathic megacolon may be divided into primary (congenital) megacolon and secondary (acquired) disease. Both are thought to be associated with myogenic or neurogenic dysfunction. Patients have increased rectal compliance and elasticity, blunted rectal sensation, and increased threshold of and decreased depth of internal anal sphincter relaxation.[13]

Megarectum may be associated with fecal impaction and soiling, which most often occurs in children and in the physically and mentally impaired elderly. In addition, megarectum can occur in Hirschsprung's disease, lesions of the lumbosacral cord, and in patients with poor toileting routines. The reversibility of sensory and motor abnormalities associated with megarectum with therapy has not been established in adults, and abnormalities may persist long after successful treatment.

DIAGNOSTIC METHODS

Physical examination

Physical examination includes a careful neurologic examination and abdominal palpation for evidence of bowel distention, retained stool, or previous surgical procedures.

Anorectal examinations should evaluate for evidence of perineal disease or deformity, abnormal location of the anal orifice and atrophy of the gluteal muscles. Digital examination can elicit the pain of an anal fissure, detect stenosis of the anal canal or rectum, assess tone and strength of the anal canal, or detect a rectal mass or fecal impaction. While the patient strains, the physician should look for the presence of rectosphincteric dyssynergia, an anterior rectocele, perineal descent, or rectal prolapse. Perineal sensation and reflex contraction of the anal canal after pinprick of the perianal area ('anal wink') test neurologic function of the perineal areas.

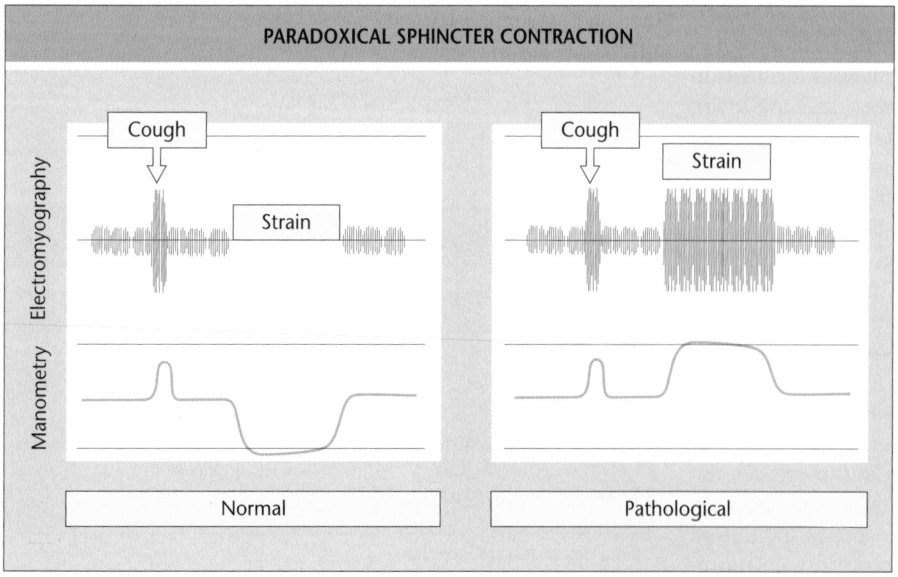

Fig. 63.3 Paradoxical sphincter contraction. Manometric and EMG patterns of anal sphincter responses to normal expulsion effort (left) and dyssynergia (right). In normal subjects, cough elicits increased EMG activity and external anal sphincter pressures whereas straining results in inhibited EMG activity and sphincter relaxation. With dyssynergia, EMG activity and anal sphincter pressures increase with straining, leading to increased resistance to evacuation of stool from the rectum.

Studies of colonic and anorectal structure

Flexible sigmoidoscopy or colonoscopy may identify lesions that narrow or occlude the bowel and can detect melanosis coli, a brown-black discoloration of the bowel mucosa that is associated with chronic use of anthraquinone laxatives.[19]

Barium or gastrografin radiographs are an important complement to colonoscopy to detect organic causes and also to diagnose megacolon and megarectum. However, radiographs provide limited information about colonic motor function in patients with chronic constipation.[7]

Barium radiographs show the characteristic denervated bowel segment with proximal dilation of the colon in classic Hirschsprung's disease (Fig. 63.4A). Bowel cleansing should not be ordered, so that the characteristic changes will be accentuated.[20] Plain films of the abdomen can evaluate stool retention in the colon, suggest megacolon, and monitor the adequacy of bowel cleansing of patients.

Rectal biopsies are useful in patients with suspected Hirschsprung's disease to identify the characteristic loss of myenteric neurons. Suction biopsy samples should be obtained at least 3 cm above the internal anal sphincter; samples obtained with endoscopic forceps are thought to be too superficial to be of clinical utility.

DIAGNOSTIC METHODS

Tests	Information provided
Colonoscopy	Intralumenal structure
Radiographs	Obstruction Megabowel Hirschsprung's disease Fecal loading
Rectal biopsies	Enteric elements Acetylcholinesterase stain
Colonic transit	Regional and total transit
Balloon expulsion	Screens for outlet obstruction
Anorectal manometry[a]	Rectal sensation, compliance Internal sphincter relaxation Expulsion pattern
Defecography[a]	Megarectum Expulsion dynamics Structural abnormalities

[a] Best performed at tertiary care centers.

Studies of colonic and anorectal function

Function tests are reserved for patients with severe constipation who fail to respond to relatively simple therapeutic measures. They are useful in defining subgroups of constipation in order to select potentially useful therapeutic strategies.

Colonic transit studies

A colonic transit study is useful in severe constipation that is unresponsive to simple therapy.[8] The patient consumes a high-fiber diet (10–30 g/day) while abstaining from laxatives, enemas, and medications that may affect bowel function. Radiopaque markers are swallowed and their transit through the colon is monitored by abdominal radiographs. Markers are counted in the right, left, and rectosigmoid colons, as defined by certain bone landmarks (Fig. 63.1) and are totaled to obtain segmental and total transit times. Various protocols exist, which are shown in Table 63.3.

Anorectal manometry

Anorectal motility studies provide useful information in some patients with severe constipation.[20] The most useful parameters are rectal sensation, pressure volume curves, relaxation of the internal anal sphincter, and defecatory patterns during attempted expulsion of the apparatus. Patients with irritable bowel syndrome often tolerate distention poorly, in contrast to patients with megarectum who have greater compliance. The presence of internal anal sphincter relaxation excludes Hirschsprung's disease (Fig. 63.4B); in the presence of megarectum, it is important to use larger volumes of rectal distention and to evacuate the rectum to avoid an inappropriate diagnosis of aganglionosis.[20,21]

Manometry is also used to characterize anorectal patterns during attempted expulsion. Intrarectal pressures give some indication of intra-abdominal pressures generated during expulsion, whereas pressure and or EMG recordings in the anal canal indicate relaxation or inappropriate contraction of the external anal sphincter.[15,21]

Studies of defecation

These studies may be useful in patients who complain of excessive straining during defecation or who employ digital manipulation to facilitate evacuation.

Expulsion of a water-filled balloon provides some information about expulsion but no information about anatomic changes or relations in the anorectum.[22] It has never been evaluated systematically, but can be used as a simple office screening test for defecatory dysfunction.[8]

Defecography is a technique in which barium thickened to a consistency that approximates stool is introduced into the rectum. Evacuation of the barium is monitored by fluoroscopy. Anorectal structures, including the anorectal angle, are assessed at rest and during defecation; also, rectoceles and intussusceptions may be apparent during defecation. However, emptying is semiquantitative and subjective; interobserver reproducibility is poor even in experienced hands. This technique is not recommended for making definitive therapeutic decisions.[21]

TABLE 63.3 COLONIC TRANSIT STUDIES

	Hinton	Arhan	Metcalf	Consensus
Day 1	24 Markers	24 Markers	24 Markers	24 Markers
Day 2	X-Ray	24 Markers	24 Markers	
Day 3	X-Ray	24 Markers	24 Markers	
Day 4	X-Ray	X-Ray	Markers	
Day 5	X-Ray	X-Ray	24 Markers	
Day 6		X-Ray	24 Markers	
Day 7		X-Ray	X-Ray	X-Ray
Day 8		X-Ray		
Transit (T)	–	$T = n_1+n_2...$	$T = n_4+n_7$	$T = n_7$
Normal	<20% retention	<70 h	<70 h	<70 h

T is expressed in hours (h).
n_4 = number of markers on day 4.

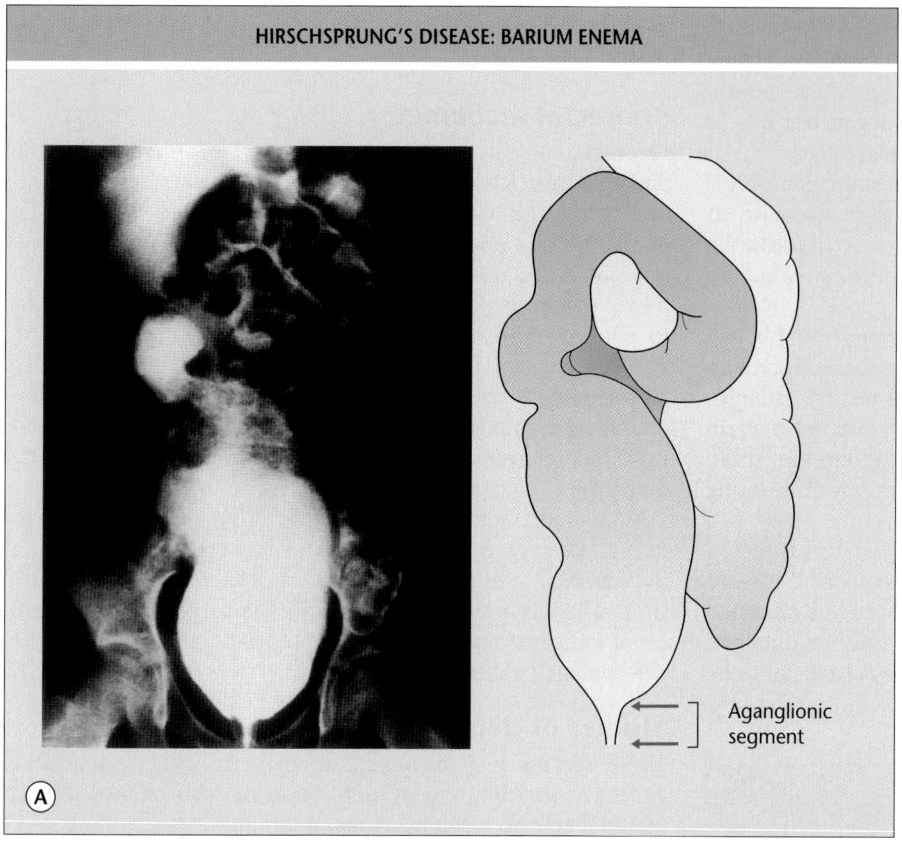

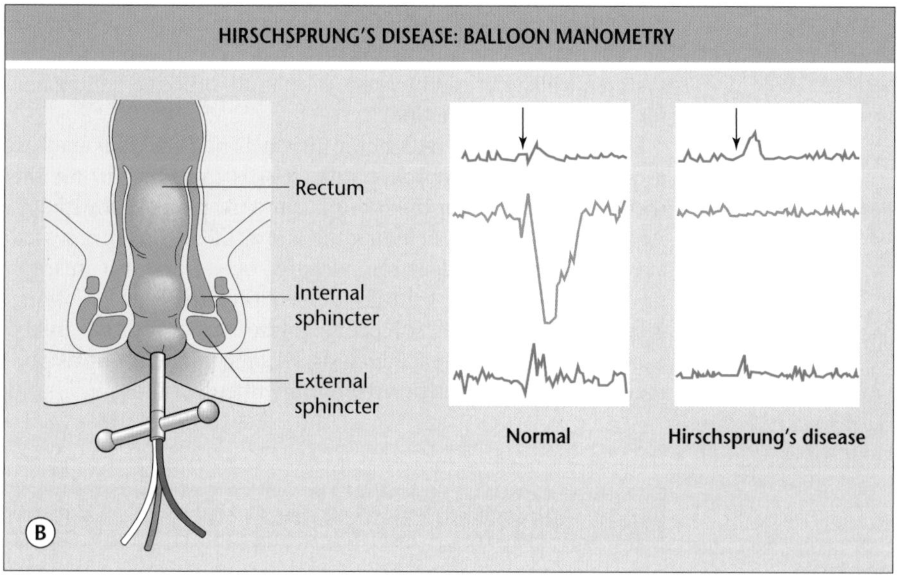

Fig. 63.4 Hirschsprung's disease.
A. Hirschsprung's disease: barium enema. An 11-year-old boy with involvement of only the distal 1–2 cm of rectum (i.e., short segment disease). It is important to remove the insertion catheter used to instill barium to avoid missing short segment disease.
B. Hirschsprung's disease: balloon manometry. Internal anal sphincter responses to rectal distention in a patient with Hirschsprung's disease are compared with those in a normal subject using a balloon manometer. In contrast to normal reflexive relaxation of the internal anal sphincter to rectal distention (arrows), no such relaxation occurs in patients with Hirschsprung's disease. Thus, the presence of internal anal sphincter relaxation in a constipated patient excludes Hirschsprung's disease from consideration. From Schuster Atlas of Gastrointestinal Motility, 2nd ed. A Wald, Manometry, BC Decker Inc.

DIAGNOSTIC STRATEGIES

Most chronically constipated patients do not require diagnostic studies beyond a careful history and physical examination.

The evaluation of chronic severe constipation begins with carefully defining the complaint and choosing studies that are most likely to yield diagnostic information concerning that complaint. As symptoms do not discriminate among physiological subgroups of patients with severe idiopathic constipation, the work-up is similar regardless of presenting symptoms (Fig. 63.5).

A 2-week, prospectively obtained bowel diary and measurement of colonic transit time is the single most useful diagnostic study to obtain. For the patient who complains of excessive defecatory straining, both colonic transit and anorectal studies should be done. Normal studies may reassure both physician and patient that colorectal function is not seriously impaired.

Patients with colonic inertia or outlet delay usually respond poorly to medical therapy. Anorectal manometry and balloon expulsion should be performed to identify coexistent defecatory dysfunctions. Studies of upper gastrointestinal motor

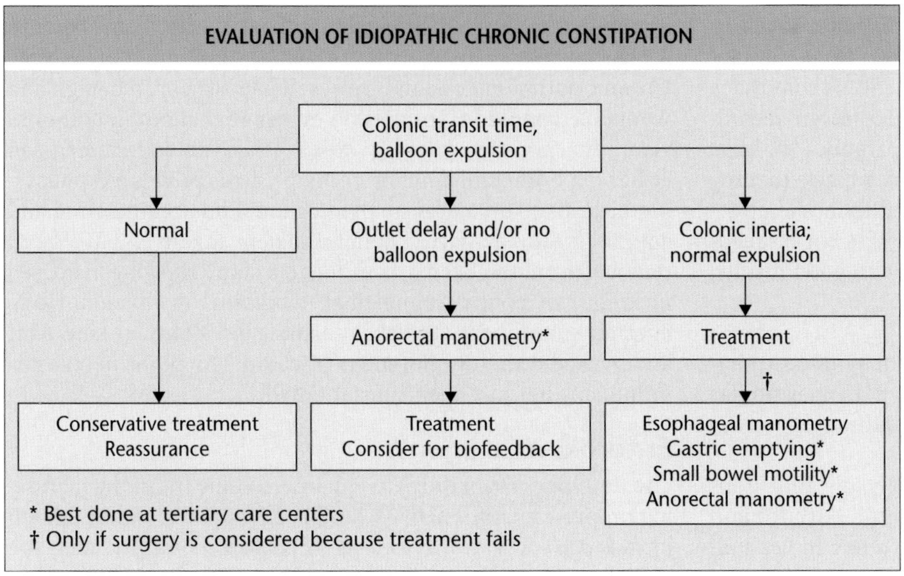

Fig. 63.5 Office evaluation of idiopathic chronic constipation.

function to look for evidence of gastrointestinal pseudo-obstruction are indicated if surgery is being considered.

TREATMENT AND PREVENTION

Dietary approaches

Dietary adjustments are the first line of intervention for most adults with constipation. Increased dietary fiber increases stool weight and frequency of defecation and decreases gastrointestinal transit time in nonconstipated persons. Although constipated patients in general do not consume less fiber than nonconstipated persons, many do respond to increases in fiber intake to between 20 and 30g per day.

Fiber components are not equivalent in their ability to modify stool characteristics and bowel habit. The bulking effect of fibers is related to their water retention capabilities, mechanical factors, effects on colonic microbial ecology, and interaction with intralumenal contents (Fig. 63.6). Some fibers serve to increase stool bulk by proliferation of bacteria and production of gases that are trapped in the stool. Microbial breakdown products such as short-chain fatty acids also may stimulate colonic motility. The net effect is increased stool bulk and shortened colonic transit in many individuals.

Fiber should be introduced cautiously in patients with constipation-predominant irritable bowel syndrome, to avoid undue cramping and bloating.[1] Fecal impactions should be removed before initiating fiber supplementation. Patients with obstructive lesions in the gastrointestinal tract should not be given fiber supplements. Fiber is not indicated in patients with megacolon or megarectum (see below).

Behavioral approaches

Habit training has been successful in constipated children and many patients with neurogenic constipation. The goal is to achieve regular evacuation to prevent buildup of stool and fecal soiling.

Initially, the patient must be disimpacted and the colon evacuated effectively with twice-daily enemas for several days, drinking a balanced electrolyte solution containing polyethylene glycol or occasionally by the use of gastrografin enemas. Occasionally, a patient may have to be hospitalized if cleansing cannot be achieved at home.

After bowel cleansing, polyethylene glycol is given in amounts to produce at least one stool every other day. The patient is instructed to use the bathroom after breakfast or dinner to take advantage of meal-stimulated increases in colonic motility. If there is failure to defecate after 2 days, a stimulant or osmotic laxative is given to prevent recurrence of fecal impaction. After regular bowel habits are restored, weaning from laxatives may be attempted.

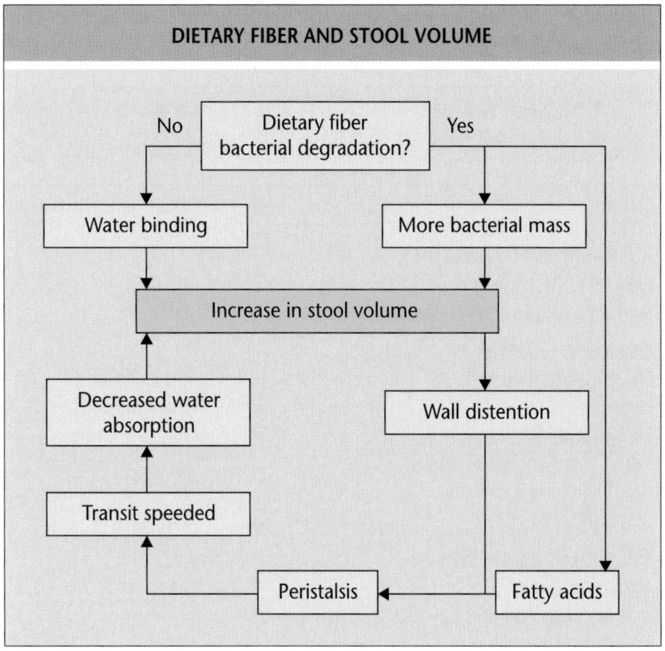

Fig. 63.6 Dietary fiber and stool volume. Fiber may be divided into soluble (degradable) and nonsoluble forms. Unabsorbed fiber that reaches the colon may increase stool volume by binding water or by serving as fuel for colonic bacteria. In addition to serving as fuel for colonocytes, short-chain fatty acids, produced by bacteria, increase colonic peristalsis to speed transit and further decrease water absorption.

Another behavioral approach is the use of biofeedback to correct inappropriate contraction of the pelvic floor muscles and external anal sphincter during defecation.[16,17] Studies have used anal electromyographic (EMG) or sphincter pressure recordings during attempted expulsion of the apparatus.[20] A large controlled study in children found that biofeedback therapy resulted in success rates no higher than conventional therapy.[23] Sizeable studies have not been reported in adults but biofeedback is used in many tertiary centers, often with good results.

Laxatives (Table 63.4)

The bulk-forming laxatives comprise natural or synthetic polysaccharides or cellulose derivatives that act in a manner similar to that of dietary fiber. They are used daily and titrated to maximum effectiveness.

Osmotic agents include polyethylene glycol and nonabsorbable sugars such as lactulose and sorbitol. Sorbitol and lactulose are degraded by colonic bacteria to low-molecular-weight acids that increase stool acidity and osmolarity and lead to accumulation of fluid in the colon. Doses should be adjusted to reduce abdominal bloating and flatulence and modulate defecation. Polyethylene glycol solutions have proven effective for periods of up to 6 months when given on a daily basis.[24] Of these agents, sorbitol is the most cost effective and polyethylene glycol is least likely to produce bloating and flatulence.

Magnesium-containing laxatives contain poorly absorbed cations and anions that exert an osmotic effect to increase intralumenal water content. Because an appreciable amount of magnesium may be absorbed, they should be avoided in patients with renal insufficiency because of the danger of magnesium toxicity.

Stimulant laxatives include anthraquinones and diphenylmethanes. Anthraquinone laxatives increase fluid and electrolyte accumulation in the distal ileum and colon after conversion to a pharmacologically active state by intestinal microorganisms. Chronic anthraquinone use causes melanosis coli, a benign and reversible condition. There is no evidence that anthraquinones given in clinically relevant doses cause enteric damage in either experimental animals or man.[19] Bisacodyl is a diphenylmethane that stimulates small intestine fluid accumulation and colonic motor activity. Phenolphthalein laxatives have been removed from the US markets due to a study showing increased incidence of nongastrointestinal neoplasms in rodents. However, in subsequent studies a relationship between stimulant laxatives and the development of colonic or other neoplasms in humans has not been substantiated.[19]

TABLE 63.4 PREFERRED LAXATIVES FOR THE MANAGEMENT OF CONSTIPATION

Laxative	Usual adult dose[a]
BULK-FORMING LAXATIVES	
Natural (e.g., psyllium)	7 g/day
Synthetic (e.g., methylcellulose, polycarbophil)	4–6 g/day
OSMOTIC LAXATIVES	
Polyethylene glycol	8–25 g/day
Lactulose	15–30 mL/day
Sorbitol (70%)	15–30 mL/day
Saline laxatives:	
magnesium hydroxide	2400 mg (30 mL)
magnesium citrate	200 mL
STIMULANT LAXATIVES	
Anthraquinones	
Aloe (casanthranol)	30–60 mg
Cascara sagrada	2–5 mL
Senna	17–34 mg
Diphenylmethanes	
Bisacodyl	30 mg 10-mg suppository

[a] Oral except where indicated otherwise.

Enterokinetic agents

The development of drugs to enhance colonic transit by increasing propulsive motor activity has been hampered by our limited knowledge of various aspects of colonic motility and the pathophysiology of severe idiopathic constipation. Cholinergic agents such as bethanechol, cholinesterase inhibitors such as neostigmine, and metoclopramide have had little success. Studies using cisapride have shown disparate results and in the US use is severely restricted by the Food and Drug Administration (FDA) due to potential cardiac toxicity. Some patients with severe constipation have been treated successfully with misoprostol, with and without polyethylene glycol.[25] A small study reported that colchicine (0.6 mg three times daily) was effective in refractory slow transit constipation.[26] Further studies are needed to assess the possible efficacy of these agents in severely constipated individuals.

There has been intense interest in 5-hydroxytryptamine (5-HT) agonists that stimulate intestinal motility, in part by facilitating enteric cholinergic transmission. Tegaserod, a partial $5HT_4$ receptor agonist, has been approved for women with constipation predominant irritable bowel syndrome and is modestly effective in some women with chronic constipation.[27]

Surgical treatment

With several exceptions, the indications for surgical intervention in managing patients with chronic constipation are somewhat controversial. The indications and contraindications for surgery are discussed below.

Hirschsprung's disease

The goal of surgical treatment for Hirschsprung's disease is to remove or bypass the aganglionic segment. Surgical techniques vary depending on patient age, extent of disease, and surgical expertise. Anorectal myectomy as an initial approach to adult Hirschsprung's disease has been advocated because of its low morbidity and technical ease of performance. However, it is difficult to identify patients who require a myectomy only from those who will benefit from both myectomy and anterior resection. Within the last decade, open surgical correction of Hirschsprung's disease has been replaced by a laparoscopic approach in a number of centers.

Colonic inertia

In selected patients with severely incapacitating colonic inertia, subtotal colectomy with ileorectal anastomosis can ameliorate incapacitating symptoms.[14] Limited resection of the colon generally produces unsatisfactory results. Studies should be perormed before surgery to establish normal esophageal, gastric, small intestine, and anorectal function. Patients who have evidence of a more extensive dysmotility disorder will have less satisfactory results. Anorectal dysfunction is a contraindication to ileorectal anastomosis. There is a substantial complication rate and bloating and abdominal pain are unlikely to improve with surgery.[28]

Rectocele

The indications for surgical repair of a rectocele are not well defined; the size of the rectocele does not seem to influence the outcome and surgery does not always improve symptoms. Optimally, one should demonstrate improved defecation when pressure is placed on the posterior wall of the vagina during defecation before a repair is entertained.

Outcomes of surgical repairs for rectoceles are difficult to evaluate because reported symptoms are heterogeneous and preoperative investigations and surgical techniques are variable. There are no controlled studies comparing posterior colporrhaphy, transanal repair, and repair with mesh augmentations, all of which seek to relieve symptoms and restore anatomy.

Idiopathic megarectum and megacolon

Surgery may be considered in patients with megarectum or megacolon if medical treatment fails.[29] It is crucial that patients be categorized accurately because colonic abnormalities determine surgical options. In patients with a moderately dilated colon, subtotal colectomy with ileorectal anastomosis offers the best results. If the entire colon and rectum are dilated, proctocolectomy with ileoanal anastomosis is an alternative if anal sphincter function is normal; if not, ileostomy should be performed.

Rectal intussusception and prolapse

Surgical therapy consists of various resuspension procedures and abdominal rectopexy with sigmoid resection. However, most patients who undergo surgery experience no improvement in their defecatory problems. As with rectoceles, rectal intussusceptions are not uncommon in nonconstipated individuals, and their presence in constipated patients should not imply causation.

Rectosphincteric dyssynergia

Surgery for this disorder is contraindicated because patients receive no benefits from posterior or lateral division of the puborectalis muscle, and fecal incontinence commonly occurs after surgery.

Antegrade colonic enemas

Antegrade colonic irrigation via reversed appendicostomy was developed for the treatment of pediatric fecal incontinence and later was applied to severe constipation in children and adults. The premise of antegrade colonic enemas (ACE) is that they produce complete colonic emptying to prevent fecal soiling. The best success rates have been achieved in children with Hirschsprung's disease, anorectal anomalies, and spina bifida. Fewer studies have assessed this procedure in the adult population. The ACE procedure may be associated with a high burden of complications and surgical revisions[14] including intestinal obstruction, cecal torsion, and perforation during catheterization.

CLINICAL TIPS

1. In patients with fecal impaction, treatment will fail unless the colon is completely evacuated. Monitor with abdominal X-ray if necessary.
2. If fecal impaction is suspected and digital rectal examination is negative, obtain a simple abdominal X-ray to look for high impaction.
3. Use gastrografin to assess general colon structure and to assist in colon evacuation; barium is not necessary and could harden with retention in severe constipation.
4. Use a high-fiber diet cautiously in patients with constipation and irritable bowel syndrome; it generally worsens symptoms.
5. Magnesium salts and polyethylene glycol are generally better tolerated in severe constipation than are lactulose and sorbitol. This is because gas production is not an issue.
6. Use stimulant laxatives only if there is no defecation after 3 days; use osmotic laxatives and fiber daily and titrate to desired outcome.
7. Recommend a rectocele repair cautiously in constipated women and only when digital compression of the bulge into the vagina greatly improves defecation.
8. Do not recommend segmental resection of the colon to shorten the bowel or remove loops of colon in constipated patients.
9. Do not recommend subtotal colectomy for colonic inertia if abdominal pain is a significant complaint.

FALLACIES AND MISCONCEPTIONS

1. Chronic constipation with excessive residence time of stools in the colon leads to autointoxication.
2. A colon that is 'too long' (dolichocolon) may cause constipation and should be shortened.
3. Chronic use of stimulant laxatives (anthraquinones and diphenylmethanes) is harmful to the colon and may cause cathartic colon.
4. Colonic function normally deteriorates with aging.
5. The most common cause of chronic constipation is decreased dietary fiber and fluid intake.
6. Treatment of chronic megacolon is the same as for chronic constipation without megacolon.
7. Chronic use of laxatives may lead to dependency, tolerance, and less responsive constipation.
8. The efficacy of most laxatives in current use is supported by strong clinical evidence.

SOURCES OF INFORMATION FOR PATIENTS AND DOCTORS

MedicineNet.com: Constipation – good review; ignore the advertisements

International Foundation for Functional Gastrointestinal Disorders: www.iffgd.org

The Merck Manual of Medical Information; 2nd Home Edition. R Berkow, ed. West Point PA: Merck & Co.; 2003:Chapter 129 (also www.merck.com/pubs).

http://www.gastro.org/clinicalRes/brochures/constipation.html

CURRENT CONTROVERSIES AND THEIR FUTURE RESOLUTION

The concept of disordered defecation was a major conceptual advance but current tests are not optimal. In part, this is because they do not mimic defecation and they are conducted in a laboratory setting, which may inhibit a very private function. The use of dynamic pelvic MRI may lead to a better understanding of the dynamic anatomic changes during continence and defecation. Most critical is to determine the prevalence and clinical significance of pelvic floor dyssynergia and the role of biofeedback to treat this defecation disorder. With the demonstrated failure of biofeedback to improve upon conservative therapy in constipated children, the results of an ongoing study of biofeedback in constipated adults are eagerly awaited.

We still have an incomplete understanding of colonic motor function and how it is regulated. Serotonin agonists appear to be of modest efficacy in constipation syndromes. Research to discover important pharmacologic targets to accelerate colon transit is needed. We also need larger controlled studies of existing laxatives to demonstrate their efficacy and limitations as well as trials comparing laxatives with enterokinetic agents in order to provide cost effective guidelines for patients, physicians, and organized health service providers.

REFERENCES

1. Thompson WG, Longstreth GF, Drossman DA et al. Functional bowel disorders and functional abdominal pain. Gut 1999; 45(Suppl 11):43–45.
2. Stewart WF, Liberman JN, Sandler RS et al. Epidemiology of constipation (EPOC) study in the United States: relation of clinical subtypes to sociodemographic features. Am J Gastroenterol 1999; 94:3530–3540.
3. Stanghellini V, Reyniers G, Beerse LP. A European survey of constipation and related behavior in the general population. Gastroenterology 2000; 118:720A.
4. Pare P, Ferrazzi S, Thompson WG, Irvine EJ, Rance L. An epidemiological survey of constipation in Canada: definitions, rates, demographics and predictors of health care seeking. Am J Gastroenterol 2001; 96:3130–3137.
5. Sonnenberg A, Koch TR. Physician visits in the United States for constipation: 1958–1986. Dig Dis Sci 1989; 34:606–611.
6. Lennard-Jones JE. Constipation. In: Feldman M, Friedman LS, Sleisenger MH eds. Gastrointestinal and Liver Disease: pathophysiology/diagnosis/management, 7th ed. Philadelphia: WB Saunders; 2002:181–210.
7. Wald A. Constipation. Med Clin North Am 2000; 84:1231–1246.
8. Locke GR, Pemberton JH, Phillips SF. AGA technical review on constipation. Gastroenterology 2000; 119:1766–1778.
9. Lembo A, Camilleri M. Chronic constipation. New Eng J Med 2003; 349:1360–1368.
10. He CL, Burgart L, Wang L et al. Decreased interstitial cells of Cajal volume in patients with slow transit constipation. Gastroenterology 2000; 118:14–21.
11. Wedel T, Roblick UJ, Ott V et al. Oligoneuronal hypoganglionosis in patients with idiopathic slow transit constipation. Dis Colon Rectum 2002; 45:54–62.
12. Slater BJ, Varma JS, Gillespie JI. Abnormalities in the contractile properties of colonic smooth muscle in idiopathic slow transit constipation. Br J Surg 1997; 84:181–184.
13. Chiarioni G, Bassotti G, Germani V et al. Idiopathic megarectum in adults: an assessment of manometric and radiologic variables. Dig Dis Sci 1995; 40:2286–2292.
14. Cheung O, Wald A. Management of pelvic floor disorders. Aliment Pharmacol Ther 2004; 19: 481–495.
15. Rao SS, Welcher KD, Leistikow JS. Obstructive defecation: a failure of rectoanal incoordination. Am J Gastroenterol 1998; 93:1042–1050.
16. Enck P. Biofeedback training in disordered defecation: a critical review. Dig Dis Sci 1993; 38:1953–1960.
17. Dailianas A, Skandalis N, Rimikis MN et al. Pelvic floor study in patients with obstructive defecation: Influence of biofeedback. J Clin Gastroenterol 2000; 30:176–180.
18. Voderholzer WA, Neuhaus DA, Klauser AG et al. Paradoxical sphincter contraction is rarely indicative of anismus. Gut 1997; 41:258–262.
19. Wald A. Is chronic use of stimulant laxatives harmful to the colon? J Clin Gastroenterol 2003; 36:386–389.
20. Wald A. Manometry. In: Schuster Atlas of Gastrointestinal Motility. Schuster M, Crowell M, Koch K, eds. 2nd ed. Hamilton BC: Decker; 2002:289–303.
21. Diamant NE, Kamm MA, Wald A, Whitehead WE. AGA technical review on anorectal testing techniques. Gastroenterology 1999; 116:735–760.
22. Minguez M, Herreros B, Sanchiz V et al. Predictive value of the balloon expulsion test for excluding the diagnosis of pelvic floor dyssynergia in constipation. Gastroenterology 2004; 126:57–62.
23. Van der Plas RN, Benninga MA, Buller HA et al. Biofeedback training in treatment of childhood constipation: a randomized controlled study. Lancet 1996; 348:776–780.
24. Corazziari E, Badiali D, Bazzocchi G et al. Long-term efficacy, safety and tolerability of low daily doses of isosmotic polyethylene glycol balanced solution (PMF-100) in treatment of functional chronic constipation. Gut 2000; 46:522–526.
25. Roarty TP, Weber F, Soykan I, McCallum RW. Misoprostol in the treatment of chronic refractory constipation: results of a long-term open label trial. Aliment Pharmacol Ther 1997; 11: 1059–1166.
26. Verne GN, Davis RH, Robinson ME et al. Treatment of chronic constipation with colchicine: randomized double bind placebo controlled crossover trial. Am J Gastroenterol 2003; 98: 1112–1116.
27. Johanson JF, Wald A, Tougas G et al. Effect of Tegaserod in chronic constipation: A randomized, double-blind controlled trial. Clin Gastroenterol Hepatol 2004; 2:796–805.
28. Knowles CH, Scott M, Lumiss PJ. Outcome of colectomy for slow transit constipation. Ann Surg 1999; 230:627.
29. O'Siulleabain CB, Anderson JH, McKee RF, Finlay IG. Strategy for the surgical management of patients with idiopathic megarectum and megacolon. Brit J Surg 2001; 88:1392–1396.

Chapter 64

Irritable bowel syndrome

Robin Spiller

KEY POINTS
• Irritable bowel syndrome (IBS) accounts for 2% of all GP consultations and 40% of all gastroenterology outpatient referrals • Rome criteria can be used to diagnose IBS with confidence if alarm features are absent • Key presenting symptoms are fluctuating abdominal pain or discomfort often relieved by defecation and associated with altered bowel frequency and consistency • Currently there are no diagnostic laboratory tests for IBS • Treatment consists of psychological, dietary, and pharmacological interventions • Antispasmodics and antidepressants are the most commonly used drugs at present, although several serotonergic modulating agents are starting to be used throughout the world

INTRODUCTION

Irritable bowel syndrome (IBS) is one of the commonest conditions seen in gastroenterologic practice. It is characterized by recurrent chronic abdominal pain and discomfort associated with disordered bowel habit. The bowel habit can vary between constipation and diarrhea, often with disordered defecation and associated bloating. This plethora of sometimes contradictory symptoms led to confusion and inconsistency in the literature until an international coordinating committee produced the Rome Criteria. These criteria have been revised and the current version, known as the Rome II criteria, has been widely adopted in both surveys and scientific studies.

ROME II DIAGNOSTIC CRITERIA FOR IBS[1]
At least 12 weeks or more, which need not be consecutive, in the preceding 12 months of abdominal discomfort or pain having two out of the following three features: 1. relieved with defecation and/or 2. onset associated with a change in frequency of stool and/or 3. onset associated with a change in form/appearance of stool Other features that were part of the more complex Rome I criteria are no longer required for the diagnosis but are often present, including: 1. abnormal stool frequency 2. abnormal stool form 3. abnormal passage of stool (straining, urgency, or feeling of incomplete evacuation) 4. passage of mucus 5. bloating or feeling of abdominal distention

Though not life threatening, these symptoms cause considerable anxiety resulting in frequent healthcare consultations. Recent studies suggest that around 4% of all consultations in primary care are for functional diseases and of these more than half are for IBS,[2] whilst IBS patients account for around 40% of the workload in gastroenterology specialist practice. Experienced primary care physicians are quite good at diagnosing IBS without using the Rome Criteria (see Chapter 13), but using non-GI features instead. Factors that predict a diagnosis of IBS in primary care include multiple previous consultations for non-GI symptoms, previous medically unexplained symptoms, and fear of cancer, which was found in 46% of such patients. The other important predictor was a history of symptoms >2 years.[2]

FACTORS FAVORING A DIAGNOSIS OF IBS VERSUS OTHER DIAGNOSES IN PRIMARY CARE[2]
DOCTOR'S OBSERVATIONS: Polysymptomatic Multiple previous consultations for non-GI symptoms Previous medically unexplained symptoms Symptoms > 6 months
PATIENT'S OBSERVATIONS Fear of cancer Stress aggravates Dissatisfied with consultation

EPIDEMIOLOGY

Both in outpatients and in the general population IBS is one of the commonest disorders. Incidence varies, depending on the precise criteria used.[3] Using the Rome I or II criteria gives an incidence of between 5% and 10% with a female predominance. Recent large surveys suggest a peak in incidence in the 20s and 30s with a decline thereafter (Fig. 64.1).[4] The condition is found throughout the world in both urban and rural environments and in the tropics as well as in the temperate zones. In the UK, consultation rates are around 14 per thousand person years for females and 4 per thousand for males. This equates to more than 850 000 consultations per annum, an average of 1.6 contacts per year. The total number of visits by IBS patients to primary care clinics was around double this when non-GI consultations were included. Indeed, it is characteristic of IBS patients that they consult more for non-GI symptoms than non-IBS patients.[5] The US Householder survey indicated an average of 4 physician visits per year and 13 missed days of work.

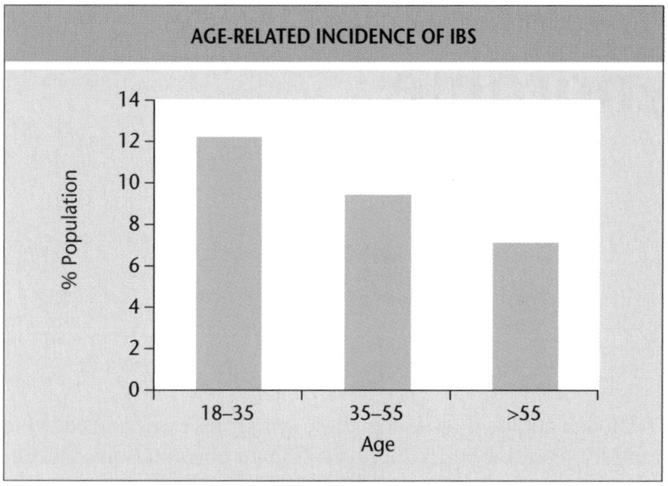

Fig. 64.1 Age-related incidence of IBS. The proportion of the population reporting IBS symptoms in this telephone survey of over 40 000 Europeans shows a progressive fall from age 18-55 years. Redrawn from Hungin et al. Aliment Pharmacol Ther 2003; 17:643-650.

Health care burden

The estimated direct costs of IBS in the USA in 1998 were over 1.6 billion dollars while in the UK it was much less at around 46 million pounds. Although IBS management is relatively cheap owing to lack of effective drugs, the ensuing time off work ensures that the indirect costs are high. Quality of life assessments such as the SF36 indicate that IBS sufferers have considerable impairment in quality of life, both in physical and emotional zones. Indeed, the impairment in social and emotional functioning was comparable with depression (not surprising considering the frequent overlap between the two syndromes), while the impairment in physical function was on average worse than in both diabetes and hypertension.

Predictors of healthcare utilization

The determinants of consultation for IBS, which in turn determine costs, have been extensively studied. Health anxiety, female sex, and physical and sexual abuse in childhood increase the risks of consultation. Increasing age also increases the probability of consultation for IBS, as it does for other symptoms. Ethnicity also plays a role and in the USA, whites are more likely than blacks to seek care. Cultural factors are important: in the Asian subcontinent, in some communities, men are more likely to seek care than women. The factors listed above are, however, less important than the perceived severity of symptoms which is, in most studies, the strongest predictor of healthcare seeking. Studies in tropical countries have shown a prevalence of IBS similar to that in the West. In some tropical countries, particularly India and China, the predominant bowel habit is diarrhea rather than constipation, but this not always the case.

CAUSES AND RISK FACTORS

Since the condition is quite heterogeneous it is no surprise to learn that there is no single cause. The condition appears to be determined by multiple brain and gut factors. These include anxiety, visceral hypersensitivity, and disordered GI physiology, both secretion and motility. Anxiety, depression, and somatization are commoner in patients attending outpatient clinics with IBS compared with normal controls but the difference is much less when IBS sufferers who are not patients are studied in the community. The best estimate of risk factors comes from the General Practice Research Database (GPRD) in the UK, which is a prospective survey of over 580 000 British primary care records. The annual incidence of new diagnoses of IBS in this unselected population is around 0.4%, with female sex and a history of bacterial food poisoning being the strongest predictors of developing IBS during the next year.[6] There are a number of non-GI symptoms that are commonly associated with IBS and hence are helpful in making the diagnosis. These include headache, dysuria, dyspareunia, backache, and lethargy.[7] A substantial proportion of people with fibromyalgia also suffer from IBS as do those with functional dyspepsia.

PATHOGENESIS

The three key factors are visceral hypersensitivity, psychological abnormalities including anxiety, depression and somatization and abnormal gut motility. IBS may start after infectious gastroenteritis,[8] which may induce abnormalities of sensation and motor function, but in most IBS cases the cause of these abnormalities is unknown.

Visceral hypersensitivity

It is a common experience that performing a sigmoidoscopy with air insufflation often causes excessive pain and discomfort in a patient with IBS compared with other patients. This has been formalized using a balloon placed in the rectum and distended to fixed pressures. With such a technique, IBS patients demonstrate greater pain at lower pressures and volumes (Fig. 64.2).[9] They also report an abnormally extensive somatic referral, with pain felt not only in the anal region where normal subjects experience it, but also in the abdomen (Fig. 64.3). Thus, normal cutaneous stimuli induced by contact of clothes are interpreted as painful. This phenomenon, allodynia, is typical of hypersensitivity induced by inflammation or chronic stimulation of spinal

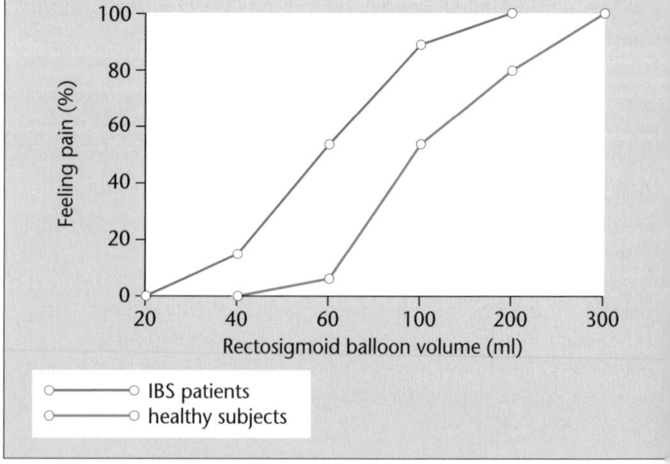

Fig. 64.2 Increased sensitivity to rectal distention in IBS versus controls. The volume of the rectal sigmoid balloon needed to induce a sensation of pain was decreased in IBS patients compared with controls. From Ritchie J. Gut 1973; 14:125-132. Reproduced with permission from the BMJ Publishing Group.

SOMATIC REFERRAL OF VISCERAL PAIN

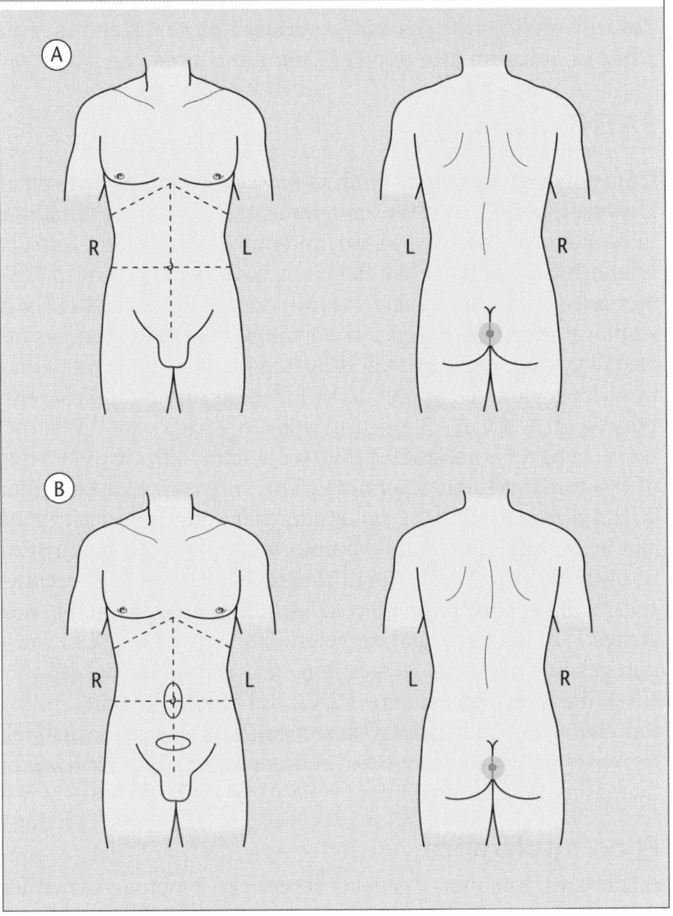

Fig. 64.3 Increased somatic referral of visceral pain in IBS. These diagrams represent areas where pain was inferred during rectal distention. While control subjects experienced pain peri-anally only, most IBS patients experienced in addition central or suprapubic abdominal pain. Reprinted from Gastroenterology, Mertz H, Naliboff B, Munakata J, Niazi N, Mayer EA. Altered rectal perception is a biological marker of patients with irritable bowel syndrome, 1995; 109:40–52, with permission from the American Gastroenterological Association.

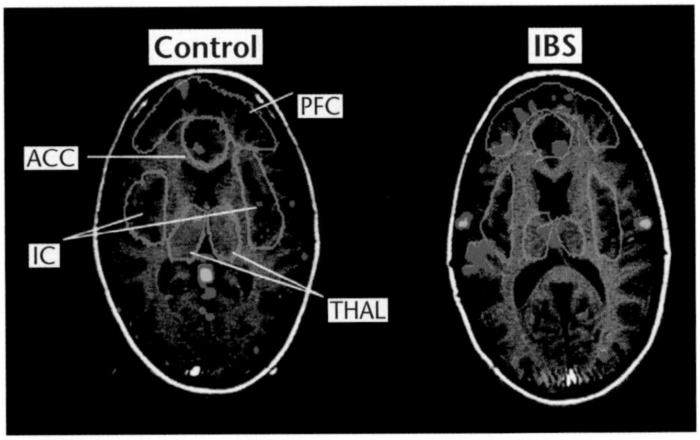

Fig. 64.4 Abnormal central processing of visceral stimuli in IBS. These functional magnetic resonance images (FMRI) show increased cerebral blood flow in IBS patients during rectal distention compared with controls. The increase was particularly noted in the anterior cingulated cortex (ACC), thalamus (THAL), prefrontal cortex (PFC), and insular cortex (IC). The anterior cingulate is the area of the brain activated by anticipation of pain and some activation can be seen equally during true or sham distentions. Reprinted from Gastroenterology, Mertz H et al. Regional cerebral activation in irritable bowel syndrome and control subjects with painful and nonpainful rectal distention, 2000; 118:842–848, with permission from the American Gastroenterological Association.

pain pathways and reflects neural plasticity whereby chronic stimulation of visceral nociceptive C fibers facilitates neurotransmission in adjoining nerves from somatic tissue.

Cerebral influences are also important. Visceral hypersensitivity in some patients is due to anticipation of discomfort and even sham distentions can induce the perception of pain. Even those IBS patients who do not initially show hypersensitivity can be induced to show it by repetitive painful distention of the sigmoid colon. Whereas under these circumstances normal volunteers show a degree of habituation, IBS patients show a fall in threshold or 'wind up.' Brain imaging using functional magnetic resonance and positron emission tomography (PET) scanning has shown increased activation of the anterior cingulate and impaired activation of brainstem nuclei in IBS (Fig. 64.4). These changes are noted both during actual and sham distentions and again represent an anticipation of discomfort.[10] Recent evidence suggests the possibility of defective anti-nociceptive mechanisms whereby pain perception is inhibited by neural activity in descending tracts originating in the mid brain. These descending anti-nociceptive pathways, which reduce the response of spinal nerves to nociceptive stimuli, include both serotonergic and noradrenergic nerves whose activities are decreased in depression. This may partially explain why antidepressants are among the most effective treatments for IBS even in the absence of overt depression. Some of their benefit may be by enhancing these anti-nociceptive pathways.

Anxiety, depression, and somatization

There is an increasing excess of anxious and hypochondriacal individuals in the IBS populations as one moves up the referral pyramid, from the community setting through primary care to secondary and even tertiary care. The proportion of patients with an overt psychiatric diagnosis peaks in tertiary care, with a lifetime incidence of a psychiatric diagnosis as high as 60% compared with 2% in community samples of IBS and 1% of normal controls (Fig. 64.5).[11] An enrichment of anxious patients in secondary care is guaranteed by the referral process. Those that are not reassured in primary care are likely to insist on referral to secondary care, thereby increasing the proportion of anxious individuals.

Many psychological characteristics are heavily influenced by childhood experiences. Abuse of either a sexual or physical nature is commoner in a range of painful conditions like IBS or fibromyalgia, and animal experiments suggest that emotional trauma in early life can induce long-lasting visceral hypersensitivity.[12]

Disordered motility

Bowel habits in the normal population vary widely with gender, diet, and exercise all playing a part. IBS patients with predominant diarrhea have transit times that are at the lower limit of normal while those complaining of constipation tend to have transit time at the upper limit of normal (Fig. 64.6). The stool weights tend to be inversely proportional to transit time but in both cases the IBS values lie within the normal range. Variability in bowel habit is however greater in IBS. Though not part of the definition, many subjects experience exacerbation

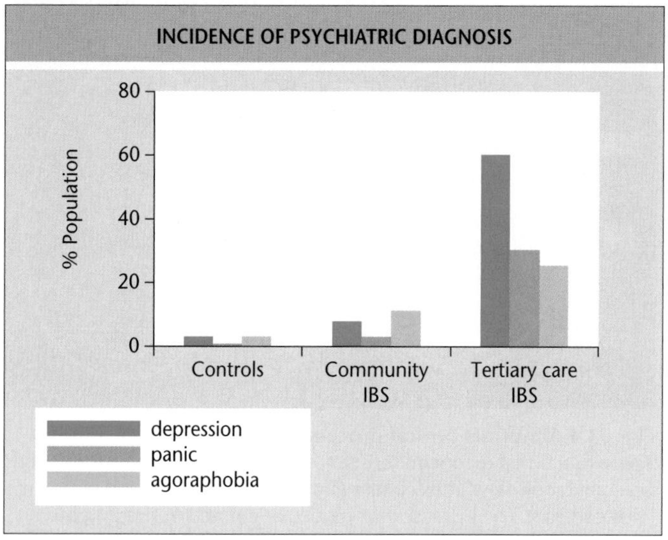

Fig. 64.5 Incidence of lifetime psychiatric diagnosis in IBS. Percentage of patients with a lifetime diagnosis of depression, panic, and agoraphobia, showing that while IBS patients in the community have a modest increase in psychiatric diagnosis, those in tertiary care have a much more substantial increase with nearly 60% experiencing a lifetime diagnosis of depression. Redrawn from Walker EA et al. Gen Hosp Psychiat 1996; 18:220-229.

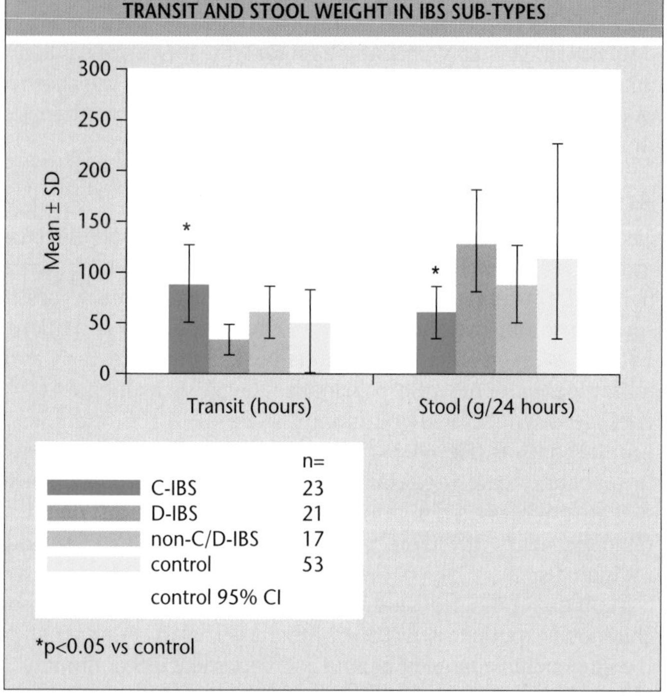

Fig. 64.6 Whole gut transit and stool weight in subtypes of IBS. Graph shows that patients with constipation-predominant IBS (C-IBS) have longer transit and smaller stool weights than those with diarrhea-predominant IBS (D-IBS); even in normal subjects there is considerable variability. Redrawn from Cann PA et al. Gut 1983; 24:405-411.

of pain and urgent bowel movements after eating. This gastrocolonic response to feeding is part of normal physiology but can be exaggerated in IBS. Some studies have shown enhanced response to cholecystokinin (CCK), with excessive propulsive activity.

One of the normal functions of GI motor patterns is to rapidly expel swallowed air and gas derived from colonic fermentation of food residues. While the normal gut can deal with an infusion of gas of up to 30 ml/min without excessive distention, IBS patients retain more gas and experience more distention, even when an infusion rate of just 12 ml/min is used.[13]

PATHOLOGY

Conventional radiology and microscopy in IBS is normal. However, several studies have indicated subtle abnormalities in both motor patterns, transit, and mucosal histology. Those in whom IBS develops after infection have been shown to have increased lymphocytes and entero-endocrine cells. Others have similarly shown increases not only in lymphocyte numbers but also in cytokine mRNA indicating ongoing low-grade inflammation (for review see Spiller 2003[8]). Recent surveys indicate that between 6% and 17% of cases arise in such a way.[14] Whether there are as yet unrecognized mucosal abnormalities in other types of IBS remains to be determined. The importance of low-grade inflammation in IBS is as yet unknown but visceral sensitization can be readily induced in laboratory animals by inflammation of both biological and chemical nature. Inflammation releases sensitizing agents in the mucosa including prostaglandins, substance P, bradykinin, and nerve growth factor. These can cause upregulation of a range of receptors such as the vanilloid receptor VR-1, the purinergic receptor, P2X3, and ASIC3, the acid-sensitive ion channel. Upregulating these ligand-gated cation channels increases neuronal excitability and neurotransmitter release by increasing both intracellular cyclic-AMP and calcium.

Food intolerance

A substantial number of patients experience symptoms only when they eat certain foods and they can avoid these by elimination diets. The best example is lactose intolerance found in 1 in 10 of the Caucasian population but as many as 90% of Orientals. Most patients learn to associate milk ingestion with symptoms; hence, they avoid milk and do not present with IBS. However, there is a subgroup that does not recognize their lactose intolerance and may benefit from being put on a restricted lactose intake. Another common dietary intolerance is that for wheat, which is a substantial part of the Western diet. In wheat intolerant individuals, around 15% of wheat starch is malabsorbed and therefore enters the colon where it is fermented to various products depending on the precise bacterial flora. Restricting wheat may alleviate bloating, flatulence, and abdominal discomfort.

CLINICAL PRESENTATION

The commonest reason for consultation is abdominal pain, which is typically described as severe, often colicky, exacerbated by eating, and relieved by defecation. The release by defecation is variable and not always consistent. The pain is typically central or lower abdominal and bilateral. It is generally indicated by a circular movement of the outstretched hand and not precisely localized. Radiation to the back and perianal region is not uncommon. The bowel habit varies and in most series a third of the patients are predominantly constipated, a third have predominantly diarrhea, and a third alternate between diarrhea and constipation. During a constipated phase patients pass small hard stools, often straining with some difficulty. They may also notice mucus with the stool. Loose stools are often associated with urgency and even incontinence. Other patients with an alternating habit may pass solid stool first thing in the morning and then pass increasingly liquid stool over the next few hours. This pattern is probably an exaggeration of the normal reflex emptying of the colon after overnight quiescence. Other patients may describe days of constipation alternating with days of diarrhea. Bloating is a very common complaint even in otherwise healthy people. It is part of normal physiology for the abdomen to distend during the day and to flatten on lying down at night. This is partly due to changes in muscle tone but is mostly due to changes in the contents of the gut, with increases in secretions and/or gas after larger meals, which are often eaten in the evening. IBS patients appear to show an exacerbation of this normal phenomenon and for the same amount of distention experience more symptoms in keeping with visceral hypersensitivity.

Non-GI symptoms

IBS patients typically suffer from many other medically unexplained conditions including chronic backache, headache, and fibromyalgia and in some, irritable bladder. Common features include sleep disturbance, health anxiety, somatization, and often lack of a close personal contact with whom to share anxieties and concerns. These symptoms may respond to low-dose antidepressants.

DIFFERENTIAL DIAGNOSIS

The differential diagnosis of abdominal pain and constipation is limited once intestinal obstruction is excluded. By contrast abdominal pain and diarrhea has many causes.

Apart from Crohn's disease, most of the conditions that present with abdominal pain and diarrhea are for the most part associated with only mild discomfort often relieved by defecation. However, they can all be mistaken for IBS. Since the incidence of colonic cancer and diverticular disease rises steeply after age 50 years, most guidelines suggest that when new symptoms develop after this age the colon should be imaged. However, this cut off has never been validated and given the fact that IBS is several orders of magnitude more common than colon cancer it is likely that this may be erring on the side of caution.

A diagnosis can be made with some security providing the Rome criteria are satisfied in the absence of alarm symptoms (see Fig. 64.7).[15] The diagnosis is made more secure by a history of more than 2 years. A normal blood count also increases the reliability of the diagnosis. Associated features that support the diagnosis include bloating, sense of incomplete evacuation, passage of mucous pr or straining at stool. Other factors that may be helpful include previous multiple presentations with medically unexplained conditions, somatization, and failure of reassurance by primary care practitioners.

ALARM SYMPTOMS

The following symptoms are not part of IBS and warrant further investigation:
- Weight loss
- Rectal bleeding
- Nocturnal pain
- Anemia
- Abnormal physical findings
- Fever

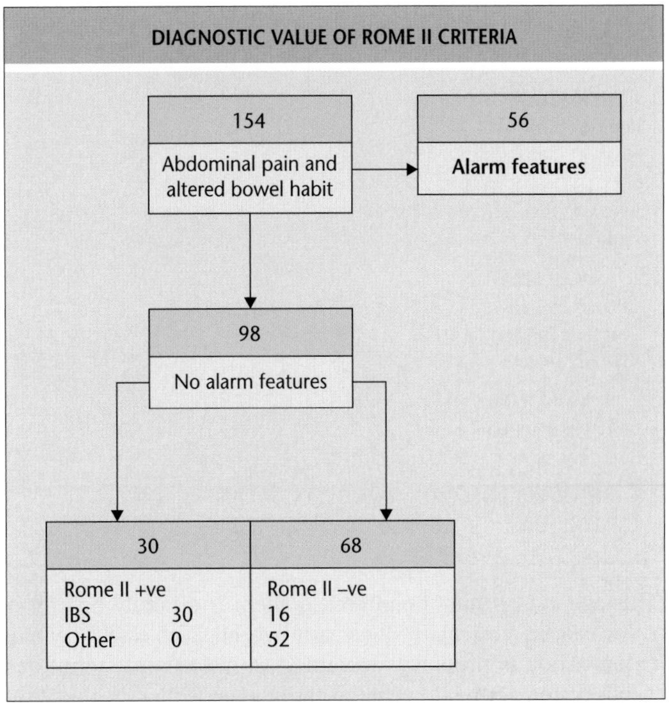

Fig. 64.7 Diagnostic value of Rome II criteria. In this prospective study of 154 patients with possible IBS, 56 were excluded because of alarm features. Of the 98 with no alarm features who met the Rome II criteria, 30 were finally diagnosed with IBS after full evaluation. A further 16 IBS patients were diagnosed after full evaluation with the remaining 68 giving a sensitivity of 65% in the specificity of 100% or diagnosing IBS in the absence of alarm features. Redrawn from Vanner et al. American Journal of Gastroenterol 1999; 94:2912-2917.

DIFFERENTIAL DIAGNOSIS

ABDOMINAL PAIN AND DIARRHEA
- Crohn's disease
- Hypolactasia
- Celiac disease
- Tropical sprue
- Small bowel contamination
- Giardiasis
- Colonic cancer
- Diverticular disease
- Microscopic colitis
- Bile salt malabsorption

DIAGNOSTIC METHODS

In primary care, provided the Rome criteria are met in the absence of alarm features, the diagnosis is reasonably secure on clinical grounds since the a priori probabilities strongly favor IBS. However, in secondary care, patients will have been referred because of some diagnostic uncertainty, which may alter the probabilities, particularly in those with diarrhea. For these patients, some screening tests are indicated.

Positive results in these screening tests are in practice rare (usually <5%) but are probably cost effective, since for some (e.g., celiac patients) this will lead to a lifelong cure. In subjects over the age of 45 years with a short history, imaging of the colon should be carried out to avoid mistaking colon cancer for IBS.

SCREENING TESTS FOR PATIENTS WITH DIARRHEA-PREDOMINANT IBS.
1. HEMATOLOGY
Hemoglobin
MCV
ESR
Serum vitamin B_{12}, red cell folate
Ferritin
2. BIOCHEMISTRY
Calcium and albumin
Liver function tests
Thyroid function
3. IMMUNOLOGY
Endomysial antibodies
C reactive protein (CRP)
4. STOOL MICROSCOPY – OVA CYSTS, PARASITES, AND FAT GLOBULES

This age cut-off may be altered if there is a family history of colon cancer, particularly at an early age, in which case, screening colonoscopy is probably warranted even without symptoms. Anxiety and depression can be easily assessed by means of the Hospital Anxiety and Depression Scale.[16] High scores should lead to consideration of psychological treatments, which will often improve bowel symptoms.

TREATMENT AND PREVENTION

Treatments can be considered under the following headings: dietary, psychological, and pharmacological.

Dietary treatment

Identification of lactose intolerance and adoption of a low-lactose diet can be effective treatment, although this has been somewhat disappointing in the UK, probably because most patients in whom lactose intolerance is the cause of their symptoms will have recognized this and will not consult a doctor. Furthermore, many IBS patients do not take enough lactose to induce symptoms and hence restricting lactose intake produces no benefit. A variety of other exclusion diets have been described. The principle is to exclude common dietary offenders such as wheat, dairy products, citrus fruits, chocolate, nuts, and onions. If symptoms resolve then each food item can be added back to the diet and over a number of months the culprit responsible for symptoms can be identified and excluded. This can be successful in some leading to sustained (>12 months) improvements in over half the patients.[17] Unfortunately unless adequately supervised this can lead to nutritionally inadequate diets, as some patients exclude progressively more and more items in a vain attempt to limit symptoms. Other diets have been described which specifically exclude sources of poorly absorbed fermentable polysaccharide. These diets have been shown to not only reduce 24 hour H_2 and CH_4 production, but also to alter the fermentation profile of colonic organisms.[18]

Psychological treatment

Since anxiety and depression are common associated features, treatment of these may be warranted on their own merits. Where excessive anxiety exists, treatment of this may result in resolution of bowel symptoms.

A range of psychological treatments has been shown to be of benefit including psychotherapy, cognitive behavioral therapy, hypnotherapy, and relaxation therapy but many of the trials are methodologically suspect.[19] Controlled trials are difficult since the placebo effect of any therapy in IBS is high and adequate controls for psychological therapy are difficult to devise. Controlled trials of both behavioral and relaxation therapy showed symptoms improved after both but this was equal in both treatment and placebo groups.[20] By contrast both psychotherapy[21] and hypnotherapy[22] have been shown in large placebo-controlled trials to produce long lasting benefit in otherwise resistant patients. Hypnotherapy has a particular advantage in that patients can be taught to self administer treatment, which can be used indefinitely at no additional cost.

Pharmacological treatment

Anxiolytics and antidepressants

IBS patients are typically rather intolerant of drugs and may require very small doses of antidepressants. Thus, while the full therapeutic dose of amitriptyline is 150 mg at night, IBS patients may typically manage on as little as 10–25 mg up to 3 times daily. Amitriptyline has a number of advantages over more selective serotonin re-uptake inhibitors (SSRIs) in that it also has antihistaminic effects, which give it a mild sedative effect. This is particularly helpful for agitation and insomnia, which is common in IBS of all types and undoubtedly contributes to the lethargy and fatigue frequently associated with IBS. A recent meta-analysis of a range of different tricyclics[23] suggested that the number needed to treat (NNT) to achieve one responder over and above that achieved by placebo was 3.2. This is comparable to the NNT for common treatments for allergic rhinitis, migraine, or hypertension but much larger than the NNT for proton pump inhibitors when treating reflux esophagitis (NNT=1.2).

Antispasmodics

Although many trials of antispasmodics have been of inadequate power and design meta-analysis and clinical experience suggest there may be a benefit, the NNT being 4.5. The commonest one prescribed in the UK is mebeverine, which has the merit of being extremely safe and cheap. It is a smooth muscle relaxant that can reduce the muscular contractions[24] that may underlie symptoms in some IBS patients.

Opiates

Opiates act as analgesics by stimulating central descending antinociceptive pathways and also inhibiting pain pathways at the level of the spinal cord. They also inhibit intestinal secretions and propulsive motor patterns and improve diarrheal symptoms. Codeine is a highly effective antidiarrheal agent but poorly tolerated because of central effects such as nausea and sedation. Loperamide is a μ-opioid receptor agonist that does not cross the blood–brain barrier and is hence largely free of CNS side effects. It improves diarrhea but has less effect on pain.[25]

Serotonin antagonists

5-HT_3 antagonists were developed initially for the treatment of chemotherapy-induced nausea and vomiting caused by massive 5-hydroxytryptamine (5-HT) release. These drugs (ondansetron and granisetron) are dramatically effective and safe. They also slow intestinal transit and a second-generation 5-HT_3 receptor antagonist, alosetron, designed to be gut selective with minimal entral nervous system effects was highly successful in treating liarrhea-predominant IBS. It slows colonic transit, increases tool consistency, and reduces IBS symptoms (Fig. 64.8), the NNT oeing 5.5.[26] Unfortunately, after >450 000 prescriptions it was bruptly withdrawn owing to rare serious adverse effects. These ncluded severe constipation in a substantial proportion of oatients, rarely inducing ileus and intestinal obstruction. While his side effect can be seen as merely an extension of its desired herapeutic effect, which could have been controlled by more areful prescribing, the other rare (1 in 700) side effect of schemic colitis was unexplained. In all cases, this was transient, elf-limiting, and benign, with only a small proportion of patients equiring hospitalization. Nevertheless, these two adverse effects ed to the drug's withdrawal, though it is now available under pecial license in the US. In spite of this, alosetron did demontrate the effectiveness of 5-HT_3 antagonists in the treatment of diarrhea IBS. On its withdrawal there was a substantial ampaign by patients to return it to the market, which suggests t was truly effective in some. Similar agents are under developnent and can be expected to be equally successful for IBS oatients in whom diarrhea is a feature.

5-HT_4 agonists

Pharmacological studies show that 5-HT_4 agonists stimulate oeristalsis and intestinal secretions. Constipated patients have educed frequency of propulsive motor patterns and serotonin gonists acting on the 5-HT_4 receptor have been shown to accelerate colonic transit, increase stool frequency (Fig. 64.9), and mprove symptoms in IBS patients where constipation is the oredominant symptom.

COMPLICATIONS

BS does not develop into other diseases and as such there are no true complications. However, IBS patients are often not diagnosed as such and their symptoms may be misinterpreted as hronic cholecystitis, pelvic inflammatory disease, and a range

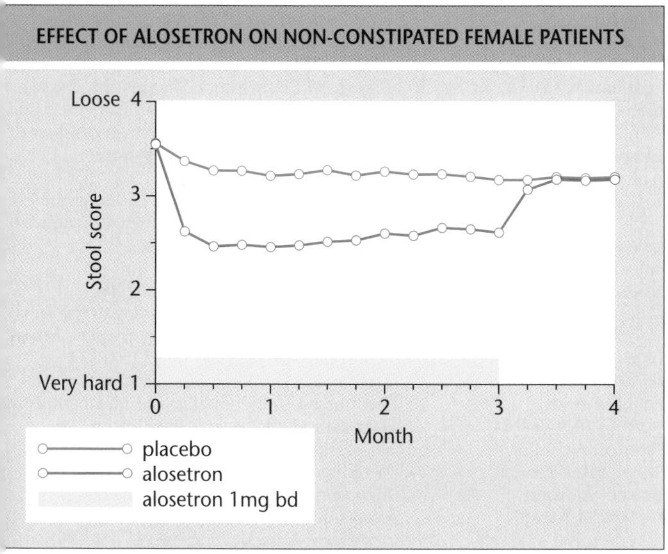

ig. 64.8 Normalization of stool form by alosetron. Alosetron 1 mg .d. in 647 nonconstipated females with IBS induced a normalization f stool form, which lasted throughout the 3 months ($p<0.001$). eproduced from Camilleri M et al. Arch Intern Med 2001; 61:1733-1740.

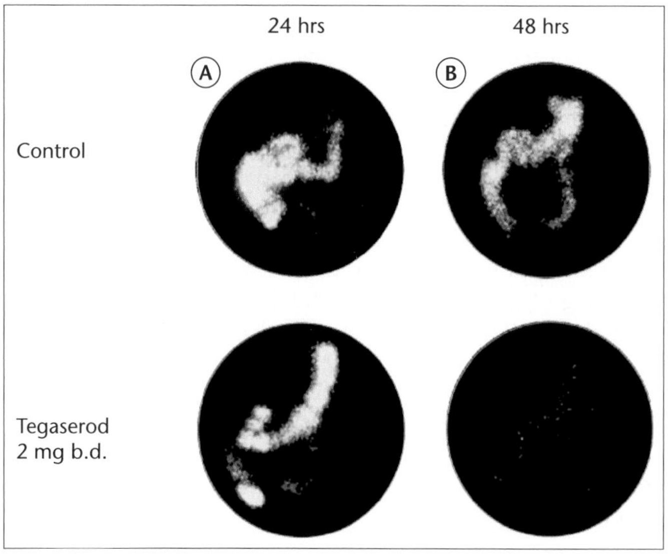

Fig. 64.9 The effect of a 5-HT_4 agonist on colonic transit. At 24-h, isotope in the Tegaserod-treated patient is filling the tranverse colon **(A)** while at 48 h it has virtually all been expelled **(B)**. In contrast, in the control conditions at 48 h, the isotope is seen outlining the entire colon, thus showing the accelerating effect of Tegaserod on colonic transit. Reprinted from Gastroenterology, Prather CM et al. Tegaserod accelerates orocecal transit in patients with constipation-predominant irritable bowel syndrome, 2000; 118:463–468, with permission from the American Gastroenterological Association.

of other conditions, which can all result in unnecessary abdominal surgery.[27] The same study also showed that patients with unrecognized IBS who attended gynecological clinics fared worse and were more likely to still be symptomatic at the end of 1 year follow-up. Therefore, it is important that the condition is recognized and that the patient sees a single physician who can prevent them being repeatedly referred to different surgeons with the attendant risk of further unnecessary surgery.

PROGNOSIS

IBS is a diagnosis that can be made with some confidence and in which the diagnosis is rarely revised. The prognosis for survival is therefore excellent; however, IBS remains a chronic cause of substantial impairment of quality of life, which may last for many decades. Regrettably, there are no large prospective studies so data on long-term prognosis is weak and largely based on cross-sectional studies. One small prospective survey of post-infective IBS found that over a 6-year period around 40% of patients had recovered.[28] Other small studies have suggested that chronic ongoing life stressors or the presence of psychiatric disorders reduce the chances of resolution of symptoms, which certainly fits with clinical experience.

WHAT TO TELL THE PATIENTS

Reassurance

Patients need reassurance that the physician is confident of the diagnosis from the symptoms and a brief normal examination and that it is unlikely that an alternative diagnosis has been missed. They also need to know that if any investigations are ordered, they are expected to be normal. This is important to avoid an endless series of negative tests, which leads the patient to believe that their condition is not understood. They should be told that the condition is chronic but benign.

Explanation of symptoms

Some attempt should be made to explain the symptoms in a way the patient can understand. That the pain can arise from distention of the gut or forceful contractions is readily acceptable as is the concept that their guts may be hypersensitive. Introducing the idea that hypersensitivity may be due to abnormal processing of visceral stimuli by the brain allows one to then explain how antidepressants might help by enhancing descending pain inhibiting pathways. The idea that abnormal contractions might be due to dietary intolerances allows one to explore the possible precipitation of symptoms by certain foods.

SOURCES OF INFORMATION FOR PATIENTS AND DOCTORS

There are many self-help groups, which produce material of variable usefulness. Good examples include www.ibsandhealth.com/public/resources/resources.html, which has links to many other reputable sites as does www.ibsnetwork.org.uk/ and www.ibsgroup.org. However, many sites on the web are of less value, either being hospital advertisements or attempts to sell unproven therapies.

Some useful websites include:
http://www.patient.co.uk/showdoc/23068776/
http://www.patient.co.uk/showdoc/386/
http://www.gastro.org/generalPublic.html
http://digestive.niddk.nih.gov/ddiseases/pubs/ibs/
http://www.aboutibs.org
http://www.ibsgroup.org
http://www.panix.com/~ibs/
Spanish:
http://www.gastro.org/generalPublic.html

CURRENT CONTROVERSIES AND THEIR FUTURE RESOLUTION

While all agree that IBS has both central and peripheral components the precise balance is a matter of much debate, as is the issue of whether it is more helpful to subdivide IBS by predominant bowel habit. Substantial efforts are being made to understand the pharmacology of visceral pain with the aim of targeting treatment to specifically inhibit relevant pathways. These efforts have particularly focused on receptors that are upregulated by inflammation such as purinergic (P2X3), vanilloid (VR-1), and acid-sensitive ion channels (ASIC3) in the expectation that these might be specific for IBS with an inflammatory basis. Abnormalities in 5-HT metabolism in the mucosa of the various subtypes of IBS have been described with decreased release in constipated IBS patients and increased release in diarrhea-predominant IBS beginning after infectious gastroenteritis.[29] The significance of this and whether it could be used to predict which patients will respond to 5HT antagonists/agonists is an active area of research as new serotonin-modulating drugs come on to the market. All current IBS trials have comparatively large NNTs suggesting that there is considerable need for objective markers to identify subtypes who will respond to specific therapies in the future.

REFERENCES

1. Thompson WG, Longstreth GF, Drossman DA et al. Functional bowel disorders and functional abdominal pain. Gut 1999; 45 (Suppl 2):II43–II47.
2. Thompson WG, Heaton KW, Smyth GT, Smyth C. Irritable bowel syndrome in general practice: prevalence, characteristics, and referral. Gut 2000; 46:78–82.
3. Jones J, Boorman J, Cann P et al. British Society of Gastroenterology guidelines for the management of the irritable bowel syndrome. Gut 2000; 47(Suppl 2):ii1–19.
4. Hungin AP, Whorwell PJ, Tack J, Mearin F. The prevalence, patterns and impact of irritable bowel syndrome: an international survey of 40,000 subjects. Aliment Pharmacol Ther 2003; 17:643–650.
5. Wells NE, Hahn BA, Whorwell PJ. Clinical economics review: irritable bowel syndrome. Aliment Pharmacol Ther 1997; 11:1019–1030.
6. Rodriguez LA, Ruigomez A. Increased risk of irritable bowel syndrome after bacterial gastroenteritis: cohort study. BMJ 1999; 318:565–566.
7. Whorwell PJ, McCallum M, Creed F, Roberts CT. Non-colonic features of irritable bowel syndrome. Gut 1986; 27:37–40.
8. Spiller RC. Postinfectious irritable bowel syndrome. Gastroenterology 2003; 124:1662–1671.
9. Mertz H, Naliboff B, Munakata J, Niazi N, Mayer EA. Altered rectal perception is a biological marker of patients with irritable bowel syndrome. Gastroenterology 1995; 109:40–52.
10. Mertz H, Morgan V, Tanner G et al. Regional cerebral activation in irritable bowel syndrome and control subjects with painful and non-painful rectal distention. Gastroenterology 2000; 118:842–848.
11. Walker EA, Gelfand MD, Gelfand AN, Creed F, Katon WJ. The relationship of current psychiatric disorder to functional disability and distress in patients with inflammatory bowel disease [see comments]. Gen Hosp Psychiatry 1996; 18:220–229.
12. Mayer EA, Collins SM. Evolving pathophysiologic models of functional gastrointestinal disorders. Gastroenterology 2002; 122:2032–2048.
13. Serra J, Azpiroz F, Malagelada JR. Impaired transit and tolerance of intestinal gas in the irritable bowel syndrome. Gut 2001; 48:14–19.
14. Longstreth GF, Hawkey CJ, Mayer EA et al. Characteristics of patients with irritable bowel syndrome recruited from three sources: implications for clinical trials. Aliment Pharmacol Ther 2001; 15:959–964.
15. Vanner SJ, Depew WT, Paterson WG et al. Predictive value of the Rome criteria for diagnosing the irritable bowel syndrome. Am J Gastroenterol 1999; 94:2912–2917.
16. Zigmond AS, Snaith RP. The hospital anxiety and depression scale. Acta Psychiatr Scand 1983; 67:361–370.
17. Nanda R, James R, Smith H, Dudley CK, Jewell DP. Food intolerance and the irritable bowel syndrome. Gut 1989; 30:1099–1104.
18. King TS, Elia M, Hunter JO. Abnormal colonic fermentation in irritable bowel syndrome. Lancet 1998; 352:1187–1189.
19. Talley NJ, Owen BK, Boyce P, Paterson K. Psychological treatments for irritable bowel syndrome: a critique of controlled treatment trials. Am J Gastroenterol 1996; 91:277–283.
20. Blanchard EB, Schwarz SP, Suls JM, Gerardi MA, Scharff L, Greene B et al. Two controlled evaluations of multicomponent psychological treatment of irritable bowel syndrome. Behav Res Ther 1992; 30:175–189.
21. Guthrie E, Creed F, Dawson D, Tomenson B. A controlled trial of psychological treatment for the irritable bowel syndrome. Gastroenterology 1991; 100:450–457.
22. Whorwell PJ, Prior A, Faragher EB. Controlled trial of hypnotherapy in the treatment of severe refractory irritable-bowel syndrome. Lancet 1984; 2:1232–1234.
23. Jackson JL, O'Malley PG, Tomkins G et al. Treatment of functional gastrointestinal disorders with antidepressant medications: a meta-analysis. Am J Med 2000; 108:65–72.
24. Washington N, Ridley P, Thomas C et al. Mebeverine decreases mass movements and stool frequency in lactulose-induced diarrhoea. Aliment Pharmacol Ther 1998; 12:583–588.
25. Jailwala J, Imperiale TF, Kroenke K. Pharmacologic treatment of the irritable bowel syndrome: a systematic review of randomized, controlled trials. Ann Intern Med 2000; 133:136–147.

6. Camilleri M, Chey WY, Mayer EA et al. A randomized controlled clinical trial of the serotonin type 3 receptor antagonist alosetron in women with diarrhea-predominant irritable bowel syndrome. Arch Intern Med 2001; 161:1733–1740.
7. Prior A, Whorwell PJ. Gynaecological consultation in patients with the irritable bowel syndrome. Gut 1989; 30:996–998.
8. Neal KR, Barker L, Spiller RC. Prognosis in post-infective irritable bowel syndrome: a six year follow up study. Gut 2002; 51:410–413.
29. Dunlop SP, Coleman N, Perkins AC, Singh G, Marsden CA, Spiller RC. Decreased post-prandial 5HT in constipation predominant irritable bowel syndrome. Gastroenterology 2003; 124:A136.
30. Cann PA, Read NW, Brown C. Irritable bowel syndrome: Relationship of disorders in the transit of a single solid meal to symptom patterns. Gut 1983; 24:405–411.
31. Prather CM, Camilleri M, Zinsmeister AR, McKinzie S, Thomforde G. Tegaserod accelerates orocecal transit in patients with constipation-predominant irritable bowel syndrome. Gastroenterology 2000; 118:463–468.

Chapter 65

Diverticular disease of the colon

Harry T Papaconstantinou and Clifford L Simmang

KEY POINTS

- Diverticula of the colon are most commonly false diverticula (pulsion pseudodiverticula)
- The incidence of diverticular disease of the colon in the US is 50% for patients over the age of 60, and increases with age
- There is an inverse relationship between dietary fiber intake and diverticular disease
- Nearly 80% of patients have diverticulosis, a mild or asymptomatic form of this disease
- Diverticulitis occurs in 10–25% of patients with diverticular disease
- Uncomplicated diverticulitis can be managed medically in 70–85% of patients
- Diverticular bleeding occurs in 5% of patients and stops spontaneously in 70–80%
- Surgery is reserved for complicated diverticulitis, recurrent diverticulitis, and persistent diverticular bleeding
- Complete resection of the diseased bowel results in low recurrence rates

NTRODUCTION

)iverticular disease of the colon is the most common disease ffecting the large bowel in industrialized nations. The earliest athologic description of colonic mucosal herniations is attrib- ted to Jean Cruveilhier in 1849.[1] However, this disease has rogressively become more prevalent with geographic vari- bility, and has been termed a 'disease of the 20th century' vith a virtual epidemic in Western civilization.[2]

The spectrum of diverticular disease of the colon ranges from iverticulosis to acute diverticulitis and bleeding. Clinical mani- estations range from asymptomatic and mild irregularities in efecatory function to severe intra-abdominal inflammation and ectal bleeding. In the US, the incidence of diverticular disease f the colon is 50% in patients over 60 years, yet only 20% evelop symptoms and only a small portion require surgery.[3,4]

:PIDEMIOLOGY

'he epidemiology of diverticular disease is closely associated vith diet, geographic location, and age. Clinical reports of diver- icular disease were uncommon until the twentieth century. 'he incidence of diverticular disease in Westernized countries ose sharply as diet changed to include more refined carbohy- rate, fat, and protein with the introduction of roller mills, efrigeration, and canning.

The geographic distribution of diverticulosis is closely linked) dietary fiber intake. It is prevalent in Western countries with a low-fiber diet, less common in South America, and exceedingly rare in Africa and the Orient where a high-fiber diet prevails.[5] The anatomic distribution of colonic diverticula also varies with geographic location. In industrialized regions with a Western diet (North America, Europe, and Australia), up to 90% of diverticula are left sided.[4] Right-sided diverticula are more common in the Orient, and appear to have fewer clinical complications than left-sided disease.[6]

The true prevalence of colonic diverticula is not known since the majority of patients are asymptomatic. However, it is clear that colonic diverticulosis increases with age and is rare before the age of 30 years. Rates vary from less than 10% in patients under 40 years of age to an estimated 50–66% over age 80 years.[4] Males and females are affected similarly.

CAUSES, RISK FACTORS, DISEASE ASSOCIATIONS

The major causes and risk factors for development of diverticulosis are closely linked to intake of dietary fiber and age. Prospective studies have shown an inverse relationship between dietary fiber and the presence of colonic diverticula. Vegetarians who consume twice as much fiber as nonvegetarians exhibit a 12% rate of diverticulosis compared to 33% in nonvegetarians.[7] A large prospective cohort study in the US showed a significant reduction in the relative risk for diverticula with increased fiber intake.[8] Dietary fiber increases stool weight, decreases whole-gut transit time and intraluminal pressure, therefore requiring less 'effort' by the bowel to propel the contents.[9] Structural and functional aspects of the colon render it susceptible to the development of diverticula and are reviewed in the section on pathophysiology. Diverticulosis associated with hypermotility is characterized by muscular thickening and increased intraluminal pressures that causes herniation through anatomic weak points in the colon. Early reports suggest that irritable bowel syndrome is associated with diverticulosis, but the etiologic link is unlikely.[10] Conversely, some patients with simple multiple diverticula throughout the colon have normal colonic musculature and pressures, implying weakness of the colonic wall from aging or illness as the mechanism. It is of interest that connective tissue disorders such as Ehlers-Danlos syndrome and Marfan's syndrome are associated with colonic diverticulosis at a precocious age.[11,12]

PATHOGENESIS AND PATHOLOGY

Diverticular disease of the colon has a characteristic macroscopic appearance that includes a grossly thickened muscular wall, mucosal infoldings into the lumen, and, of course, the characteristic mucosal outpouchings (Fig. 65.1). The pathogenesis of diverticular disease is multifactorial and includes anatomic features intrinsic to the colon, alterations in colonic wall with aging, motor dysfunction, abnormal increases in intraluminal pressure, and dietary fiber.[13] These factors contribute to the development of diverticulosis in an ill-defined interrelationship.

Pathology

Diverticula are sac-like protrusions from the wall of a hollow organ like the colon, and are classically defined as true or false depending on the layers involved. A true diverticulum involves all the layers of the colon including the mucosa, submucosa, and muscular layers. These are congenital anomalies that are rarely found in the colon. False diverticula are the most common type in the colon, and consist of herniations of the mucosa and submucosa through the muscular coat of the colon (Fig. 65.2). These are acquired and termed pulsion pseudodiverticula because they are pushed out by intraluminal pressure.

Diverticula develop in rows between the mesenteric and the two antimesenteric teniae. The point of greatest muscular weakness is where the intramural vasa recta penetrate the circular muscle to the submucosa (Fig. 65.3). In sigmoid diverticulosis, the muscle layers are greatly increased in thickness, which results in shortening of the teniae and a narrowed colonic lumen; a deformity called myochosis. Muscle contractions obliterate the lumen of the colon and divide the bowel into isolated segments. This muscular thickening is attributed to the presence of increased elastin deposition, specifically within the teniae.[14] Elastosis of the teniae contributes to sacculation, while the tensile strength in the remaining bowel wall decreases with age, and increases susceptibility to diverticula.

Pathogenesis

The pathogenesis of diverticulosis is a result of colonic functional abnormalities. Painter suggested that the interplay of hypersegmentation resulting in increased intraluminal pressure and the low-bulk Western diet is the primary cause of diverticular disease.[15] Segmentation allows the motor work of th colon to be transmitted to the bowel wall rather than promotin fecal transit, and results in intraluminal pressures in excess c 90 mmHg. It is postulated that the formation of these isolate colonic segments in myochosis patients generates very hig pressures and results in mucosal herniation (Fig. 65.4). Othe

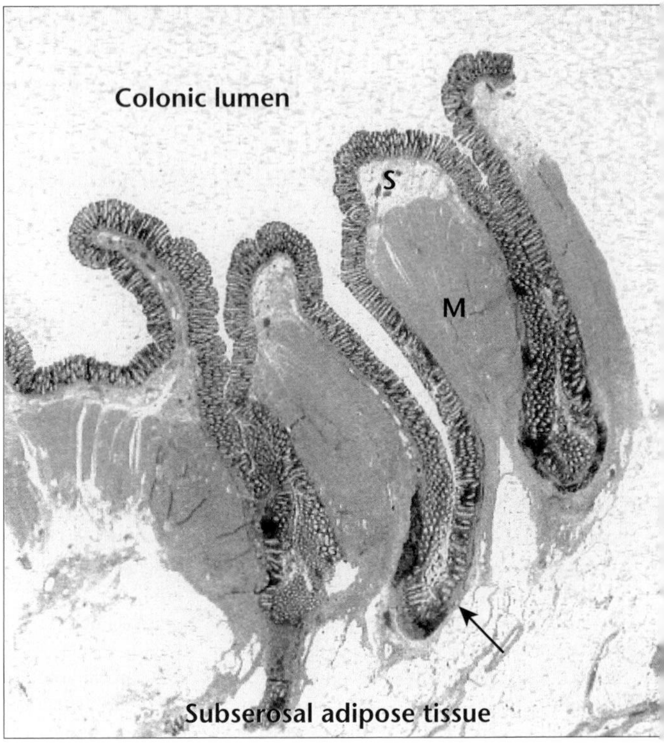

Fig. 65.2 Diverticulum of the colon. Photograph of a colonic diverticulum at low power (H&E stain, 2×). Colonic lumen and subserosal adipose tissue are labeled for orientation. The black arrow points to the diverticulum, and shows the colonic mucosa (blue stain) and submucosa (S) herniated through the muscularis propria (M). Photograph courtesy of S Tunc Gokaslan MD, Department of Pathology, The University of Texas Southwestern Medical Center.

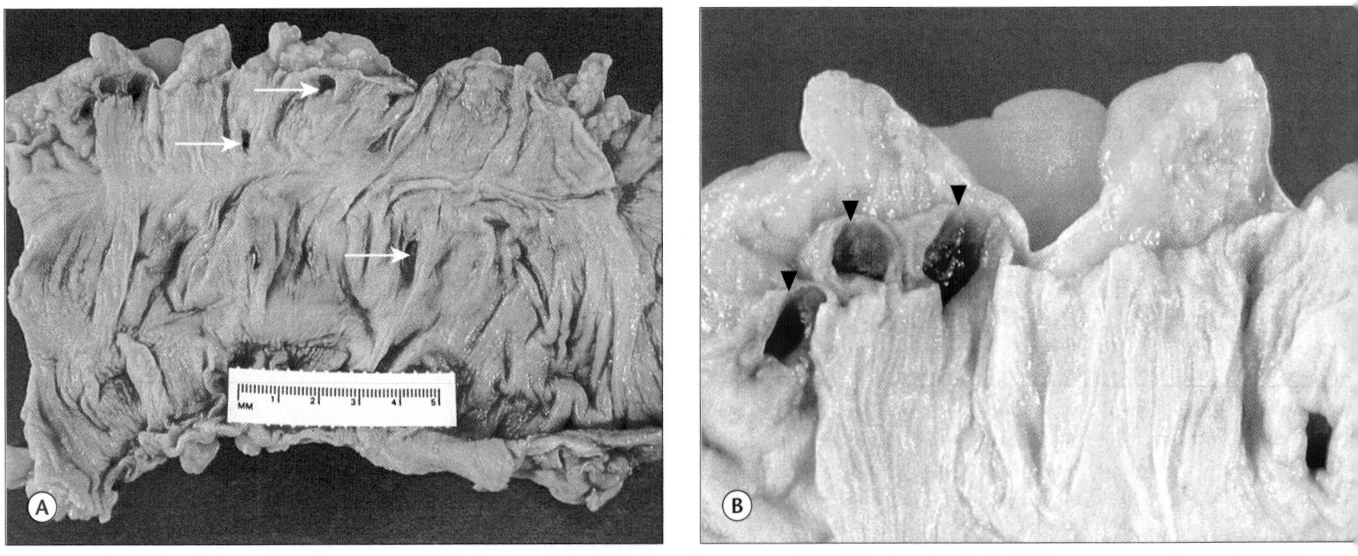

Fig. 65.1 Diverticulosis of the colon. A. A surgical specimen of a colon from a patient with diverticulosis. White arrows point to the orifice of the colonic diverticula. **B.** Close up photograph of diverticula. Black arrowheads point to herniated mucosa and serosa that is devoid of muscularis. Photograph courtesy of S Tunc Gokaslan MD, Department of Pathology, The University of Texas Southwestern Medical Center.

ANATOMY OF THE COLONIC WALL

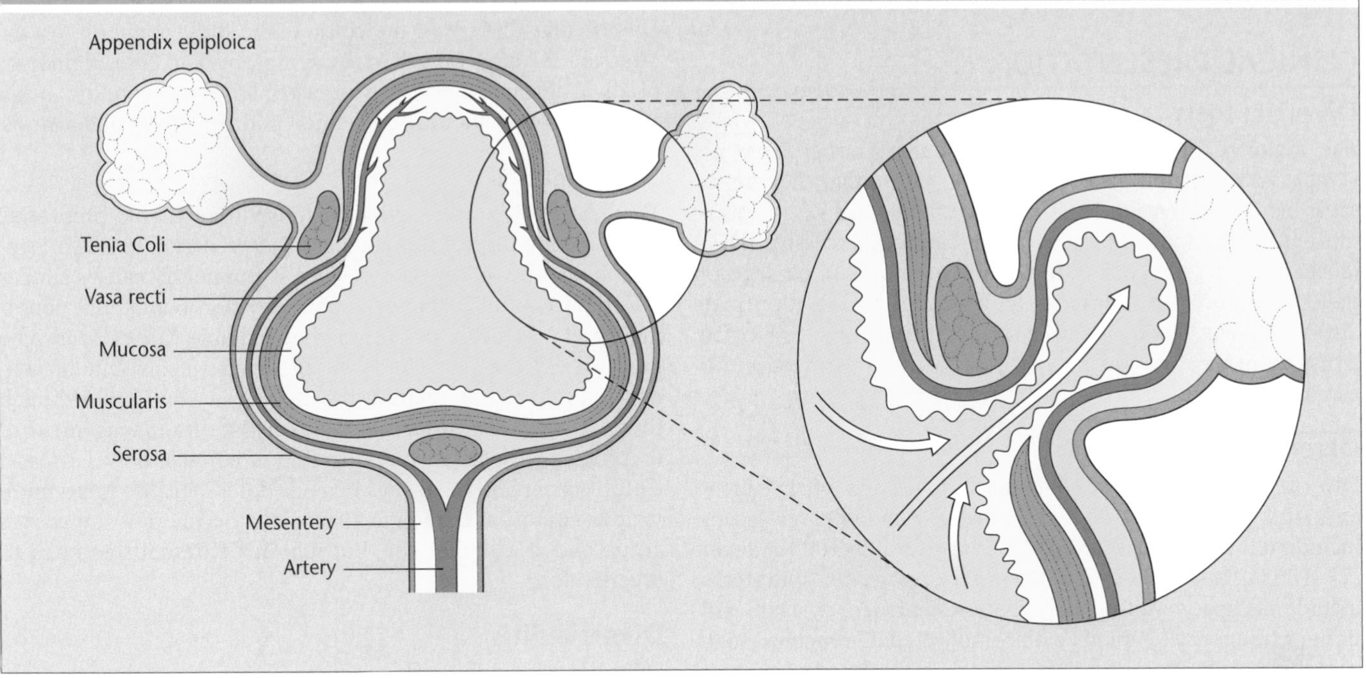

Fig. 65.3 Development of a colonic diverticulum. The diagram shows an axial cross-section representation of the colon anatomy. The point of greatest muscular weakness is where the vasa recti penetrate the circular muscle to the submucosa. Note the location of the artery to the diverticulum.

SEGMENTATION THEORY OF COLONIC DIVERTICULA PATHOGENESIS

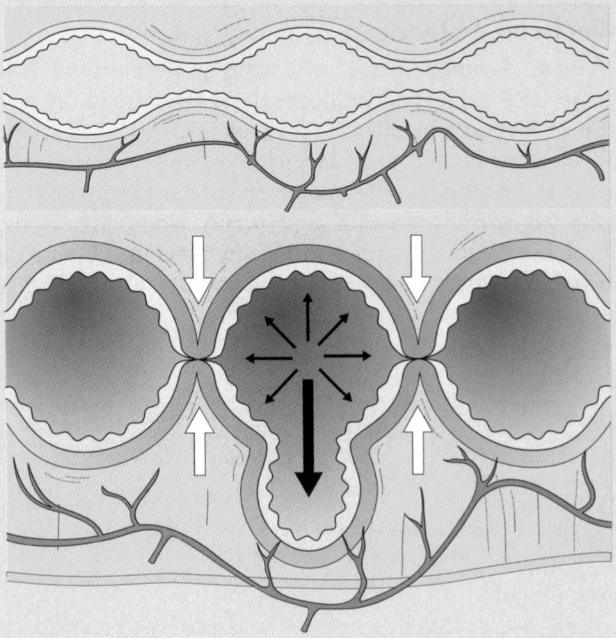

Fig. 65.4 Segmentation theory of colonic diverticula pathogenesis. Myochosis of the sigmoid colon results in a thickened muscular layer with shortening of the teniae. Muscle contractions (white arrows) obliterate the colonic lumen resulting in isolated segments. High pressure within the segments (small black arrows) promotes mucosal herniation (large black arrow) through weak points within the colonic lumen.

studies have yielded confusing data ranging from alterations in colonic motor activity to lack of uniform increases in intraluminal pressure in diverticular disease patients, which supports the concept that diverticular disease of the colon represents a spectrum of underlying causes.[4,10,13]

Diverticulitis refers to inflammation associated with diverticula that result from chronic obstruction and abrasion of the mucosa in the neck of the diverticulum by inspissated stool or fecalith.[4,14] This inflammatory process then proceeds to perforation, the extent and localization of which determine clinical behavior. Uncomplicated diverticulitis refers to microperforations that remain locally contained by pericolonic fat, mesentery, or adjacent organs. This extramural pericolonic process results in a localized phlegmon or abscess. Repeated episodes cause a pericolic fibrotic reaction with segmental narrowing and stricture formation. Macroperforations result in complicated diverticulitis with either free perforation and generalized peritonitis or a walled off pericolonic abscess. Free perforations with bacterial and fecal peritonitis can be life threatening, but fortunately are uncommon. Diverticular abscesses can erode into adjacent organs and develop fistulas with the bladder, vagina, small bowel, and skin.

Diverticular bleeding is a complication of diverticulosis. The anatomic relationship between the herniated sac and the arterial supply plays an important part in diverticular bleeding (Fig. 65.3).[4,16] The mucosal vessels arising from the main circumferential arterial supply course along the neck and are displaced along the dome of the diverticulum. Chronic injury to the vasa recta adjacent to the diverticular lumen results in intimal thickening with fragmentation of the internal elastic lamina, thinning of the media, and bleeding. Bleeding is more common in right-sided diverticula, and may be related to a larger lumen, which exposes more of the vasa recta to potential disruption.

CLINICAL PRESENTATION

Diverticulosis

The majority of patients with diverticulosis either have no symptoms or symptoms of such minor nature that they never seek medical attention.[4,10] Minor symptoms are often intermittent and include abdominal pain, bloating, excessive flatulence, and irregular defecation. Nausea, anorexia, passage of pellet-like stool, or attacks of diarrhea and constipation may also be present. Some patients with diverticulosis have reported a history of narrow-caliber stool, and further investigation for carcinoma is necessary.

Diverticulitis

Diverticulitis is the most common complication of diverticulosis and occurs in 10–25% of patients.[3] Common symptoms include left lower quadrant abdominal pain (93–100%), fever (57–100%), and leukocytosis (69–83%). Associated symptoms include nausea, vomiting, constipation, diarrhea, dysuria, and urinary frequency.[4] Patients with complicated diverticulitis may report pneumaturia or feculent vaginal discharge suggestive of fistula formation. Free perforation into the abdominal cavity results in diffuse fecal peritonitis with acute peritoneal signs and abdominal wall rigidity.

The most common physical examination finding is tenderness in the left lower quadrant. Signs of localized peritoneal inflammation may be present with involuntary guarding and localized rebound tenderness. A tender mass representing a phlegmon may occasionally be palpated. Rectal examination often reveals pelvic tenderness and occasionally a mass.

Diverticular bleeding

Massive bleeding from colonic diverticula occurs in 5% of patients with diverticular disease.[16] Patients often present with profuse rectal bleeding and usually have no antecedent history of diverticular disease. Abdominal pain and other symptoms are usually absent. Painless brisk hematochezia can quickly lead to hypotension; therefore, prompt aggressive resuscitation is required with concurrent organized evaluation.

DIFFERENTIAL DIAGNOSIS

Diverticular disease of the colon is the most common disease affecting the large bowel. Many symptoms and clinical finding of diverticular disease are nonspecific, and therefore other colonic diseases should be included in the differential diagnosis.

Diverticulosis

There is a wide differential diagnosis for patients presenting with uncomplicated diverticular disease. Irritable bowel syndrome should be considered since it frequently causes similar intestinal symptoms, but evaluation reveals no anatomic abnormality. It has been suggested that irritable bowel syndrome may precede the development of diverticulosis, but no evidence of a causal relationship has been found.[17] Although these two disease processes may coexist, the management of diverticular disease is similar to that of irritable bowel disease. Colon cancer should always be considered because it is a more serious condition than diverticulosis, it occurs in a similar age group and at a similar site, but requires different treatment to diverticulosis.

Diverticulitis

Diverticulitis is the inflammation of a colonic diverticulum, often with local perforation. Conditions that mimic this disease process should be considered. The most common misdiagnosis is acute appendicitis. Other considerations should include perforated colon cancer, inflammatory bowel disease, infectious colitis, gynecologic pathology, and urinary tract infections. Specific considerations such as age, persistence of symptoms, medical history, comorbidities, and travel history may help guide the diagnosis. Further evaluation is required for definitive diagnosis.

Diverticular bleeding

The most common causes of lower gastrointestinal bleeding are diverticula and angiodysplasia. Diverticulosis is the cause of bleeding in 20–40% of patients.[4,16] Pain associated with bleeding should raise suspicion for inflammatory bowel disease and ischemic colitis. Colon and rectal carcinoma should always be considered, although occult blood loss is more typical. Less common causes of bleeding include hemorrhoids and polyps, which rarely cause massive rectal bleeding and hematochezia.

CLINICAL PRESENTATION

ASYMPTOMATIC OR NONSPECIFIC SYMPTOMS (75–80%)
Diverticulosis
- Found incidentally on radiographs and colonoscopy
- Intermittent abdominal pain, bloating, excessive flatulence, and irregular defecation

SYMPTOMATIC (20–25%)
Diverticulitis (15–20%)
- Acute abdominal pain (usually left lower quadrant)
- Tenderness and guarding on palpation (± palpable mass)
- Fever, malaise, anorexia, nausea, and/or vomiting
- Leukocytosis

Diverticular bleeding (5–7%)
- Painless, brisk hematochezia

DIFFERENTIAL DIAGNOSIS

DIVERTICULOSIS
- Common – irritable bowel syndrome
- Other – colon and rectal carcinoma

DIVERTICULITIS
- Common – appendicitis, inflammatory bowel disease, urinary tract infections
- Other – ischemic colitis, infectious colitis, perforated colon cancer

DIVERTICULAR BLEEDING
- Common – angiodysplasia, inflammatory bowel disease, and colon and rectal carcinoma
- Other – rectal ulcer, and ischemic colitis, hemorrhoids, and polyps

DIAGNOSTIC METHODS

Diagnostic modalities used to identify diverticular disease of the colon depend on the presentation of the patient, and include routine blood tests, radiologic imaging, and colonoscopy.

Diverticulosis

In patients with diverticulosis, plain abdominal radiographs are normal and contribute little to diagnosis. Colonic evaluation is performed to rule out carcinoma and confirm diverticulosis. Double-contrast barium enema is commonly used to determine extent and severity of the disease (Fig. 65.5A). Radiographic findings include colonic spasm, sacculations, and retained contrast material within diverticula. However, the accuracy of barium enema in diagnosing concomitant lesions has been reported to be as low as 50%,[18] and may be a result of obscured visualization from redundant colon or adherent stool.

Colonoscopy is of particular value in excluding carcinoma by direct visualization (Fig. 65.5B). A review of the literature found that of 125 patients with complicated diverticular disease, colonoscopy identified an associated carcinoma in 17% and additional diagnosis in 32%,[19] particularly with rectal bleeding.

Diverticulitis

Initial laboratory studies include a complete blood count (polymorphonuclear leucocytosis), and erect and supine abdominal radiographs. Urinalysis may reveal pyuria if the inflammatory process is adjacent to the ureters or bladder. The presence of bacteria in the urine sample is suggestive of a colovesical fistula, and culture may show multiple enteric organisms. If the clinical picture is clear, the diagnosis can be made on the basis of laboratory and clinical criteria.

If in doubt, noninvasive imaging studies such as a computed tomography (CT) scan and ultrasonography may be useful. A CT scan with intravenous and oral contrast medium is a more accurate technique.[20,21] CT can reliably detect the location of inflammation and provides valuable additional information such as the presence of abscess and thickened colonic wall (Fig. 65.6), ureteral obstruction, or a fistula formation. Air in the bladder of a patient who has not had urinary tract manipulation is diagnostic of a fistula from the intestinal tract. If an abscess is present, percutaneous catheter drainage under CT or ultrasonic guidance is a valuable therapeutic procedure.

Diverticular bleeding

Nuclear scanning techniques using technetium 99m sulfur colloid and technetium-tagged red blood cells may be useful in patients with diverticular bleeding.[22] These bleeding scans detect very low bleeding rates (0.1 mL/min) and can be performed repeatedly to identify intermittent bleeding (Fig. 65.7), but additional angiography is usually required if surgery is planned.

Emergency angiography has become the procedure of choice for patients with brisk bleeding. Angiography is both specific and

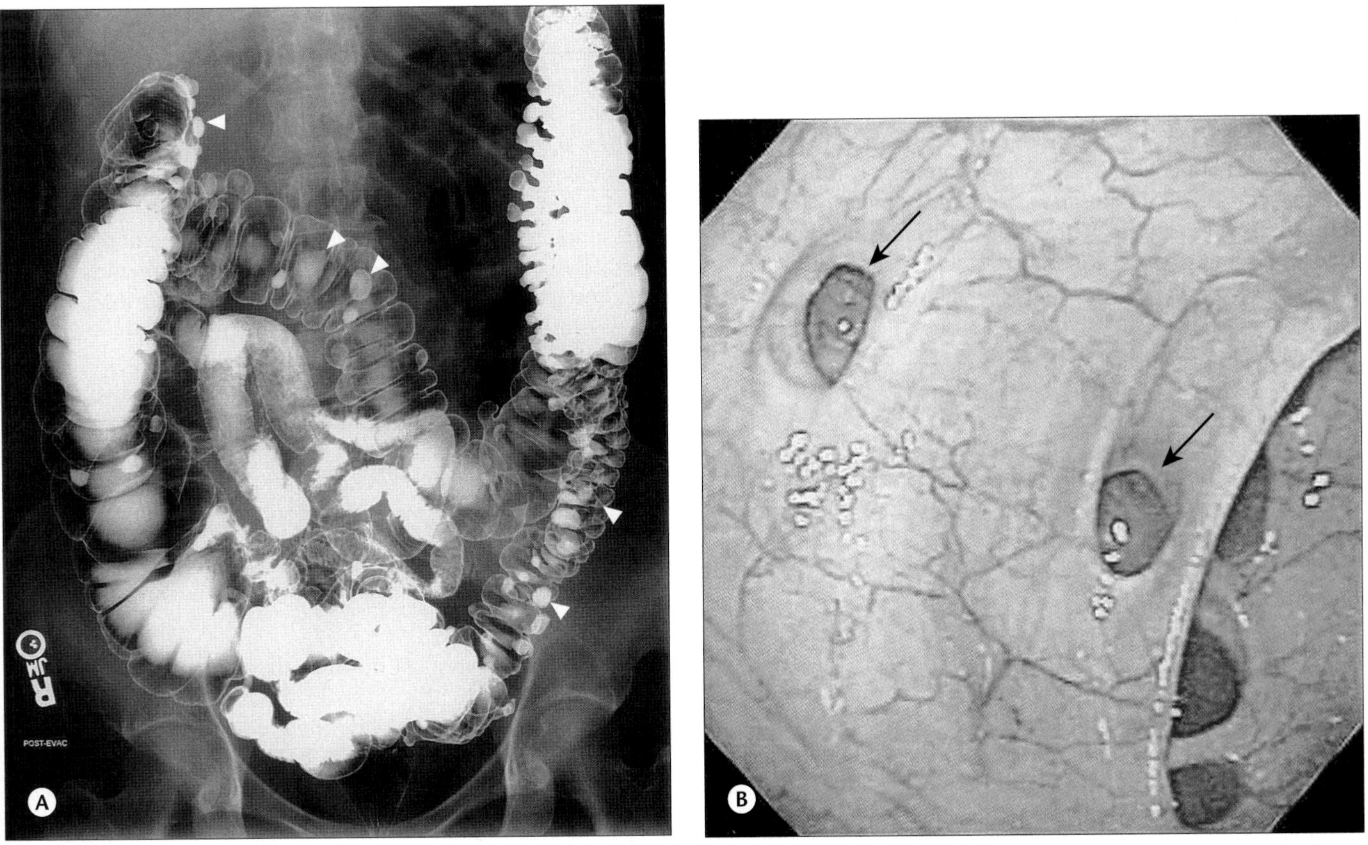

Fig. 65.5 Most common diagnostic studies for diverticular disease of the colon. A. Double contrast barium enema showing a patient with pancolonic diverticulosis. The white arrowheads point to retained contrast material within the diverticula. Note the marked redundancy and overlapping of the sigmoid colon that is obscuring intraluminal definition. **B.** Colonoscopy picture of a patient with diverticulosis. Black arrows point to diverticula orifice. Note the presence of more diverticula behind the mucosal fold.

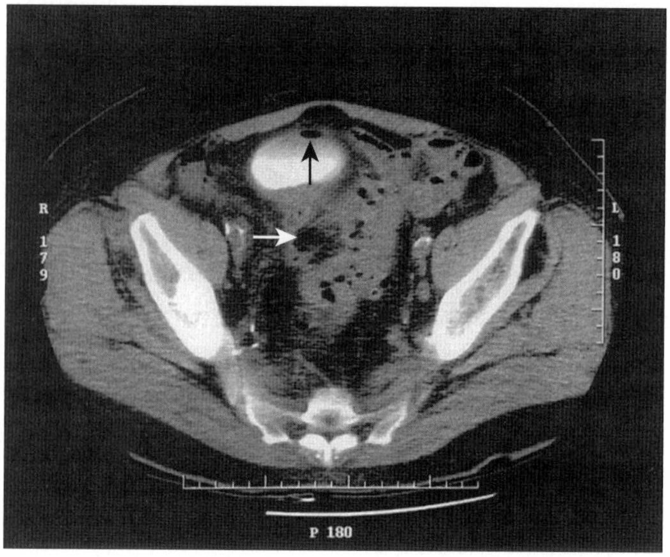

Fig. 65.6 CT scan demonstrating diverticulitis of the sigmoid colon. The peridiverticular abscess (white arrow) is adjacent to the bladder. The air bubble in the bladder (black arrow) is diagnostic of a colovesicular fistula.

DIAGNOSTIC METHODS

DIVERTICULOSIS
- Double-contrast barium enema best determines the extent of disease
- Colonoscopy is the gold standard for evaluating the colon and differentiating diverticular disease from carcinoma

DIVERTICULITIS
- Complete blood count is performed to determine the white blood cell count
- Abdominal X-ray may show free air or an ileus pattern
- CT scan is the test of choice to confirm the diagnosis of diverticulitis

DIVERTICULAR BLEEDING
- Angiography is the test of choice for brisk diverticular bleeding (0.5–1.0 mL/min), and provides diagnostic and therapeutic capabilities
- Technetium-tagged red blood cell scan can detect very low bleeding rates (0.1 mL/min) and can be performed repeatedly to identify intermittent bleeding
- Colonoscopy intervention is useful when the bleeding site can be visualized

highly sensitive if the bleeding rate is at least 0.5–1.0 mL/min.[23] A blush of contrast extravasating from the vasculature into the colonic lumen signifies a positive scan. The superior mesenteric artery is studied first since the incidence of acute bleeding is highest from the right side of the colon, and is followed by injection of the inferior mesenteric artery and celiac axis. The specificity is high if the study is positive. Other findings may include tumors, diffuse mucosal bleeding, or characteristic signs of angiodysplasia including delayed venous emptying, vascular tufts, or an early filling vein.

Colonoscopy should be considered in patients with a positive bleeding scan but negative arteriogram without localization of the bleeding site. Bleeding sites have been identified by colonoscopy in up to 89% of patients with lower gastrointestinal bleeding.[24] Bowel lavage, often via the oral route, is usually necessary to clear the colon of retained blood.

TREATMENT AND PREVENTION

Diverticulosis

Epidemiology studies have suggested that the ingestion of 30 g of bran is associated with a reduced development of diverticular disease.[8] Commercial products such as psyllium provide an alternative treatment to dietary fiber. Surgery for diverticulosis is not indicated and should be reserved for complicated diverticular disease.

Diverticulitis

The severity of the inflammatory and infectious process determines the treatment for diverticulitis.[4,10,21] Patients with minimal symptoms and signs of inflammation can be treated on an outpatient basis with a clear liquid diet and broad-spectrum oral antibiotics (ciprofloxacin and metronidazole) for 7–10 days. Opiate analgesics should be avoided since they increase intraluminal colonic pressure.

Signs of significant inflammation indicate that the patient should be hospitalized for bowel rest, intravenous fluid resuscitation, and broad-spectrum intravenous antibiotics directed at colonic microflora, particularly *Escherichia coli* and *Bacteroides fragilis*.[10,21] The most common antibiotics used are ampicillin/sulbactam, metronidazole plus a cephalosporin, or piperacillin/tazobactam. Most patients improve in the first 48–72 h. As inflammation resolves, diet is resumed and the patient is discharged to complete a 7- to 10-day course of oral antibiotics. Investigative studies such as barium enema or colonoscopy should be performed 4–6 weeks after resolution of symptoms to document diverticular disease and exclude the presence of carcinoma.

After successful recovery from the first episode of simple uncomplicated diverticulitis, surgery is seldom indicated because only 20–30% of patients have a recurrent episode.[3] A high-fiber diet supplemented with psyllium is recommended. Surgery should be considered after a second attack of diverticulitis since the probability of a third episode is greater than 50%.[21] Elective resection should be performed approximately 4–6 weeks after resolution of the inflammation.

Patients who have their first episode of acute diverticulitis before age 50 years are more likely to develop chronic or recurrent disease.[25] Young patients exhibit a more complicated diverticulitis requiring urgent surgery in 50–75%, compared to only 15–30% in older patients.[26] Therefore, for young patients who have successfully completed treatment for a first episode of diverticulitis, elective surgery is strongly recommended.

Surgery

Although several surgical options are available, the extent of resection should be the same in all patients. The abnormal thickened bowel should be completely resected from soft normal colonic tissue proximally to below the confluence of the teniae on the proximal rectum distally. This ensures complete resection of the diseased bowel. Elective resection for recurrent uncomplicated diverticulitis should involve a one-stage procedure with resection and primary anastamosis.[21] The laparoscopic approach is becoming more frequently accepted for surgical treatment of diverticular disease.

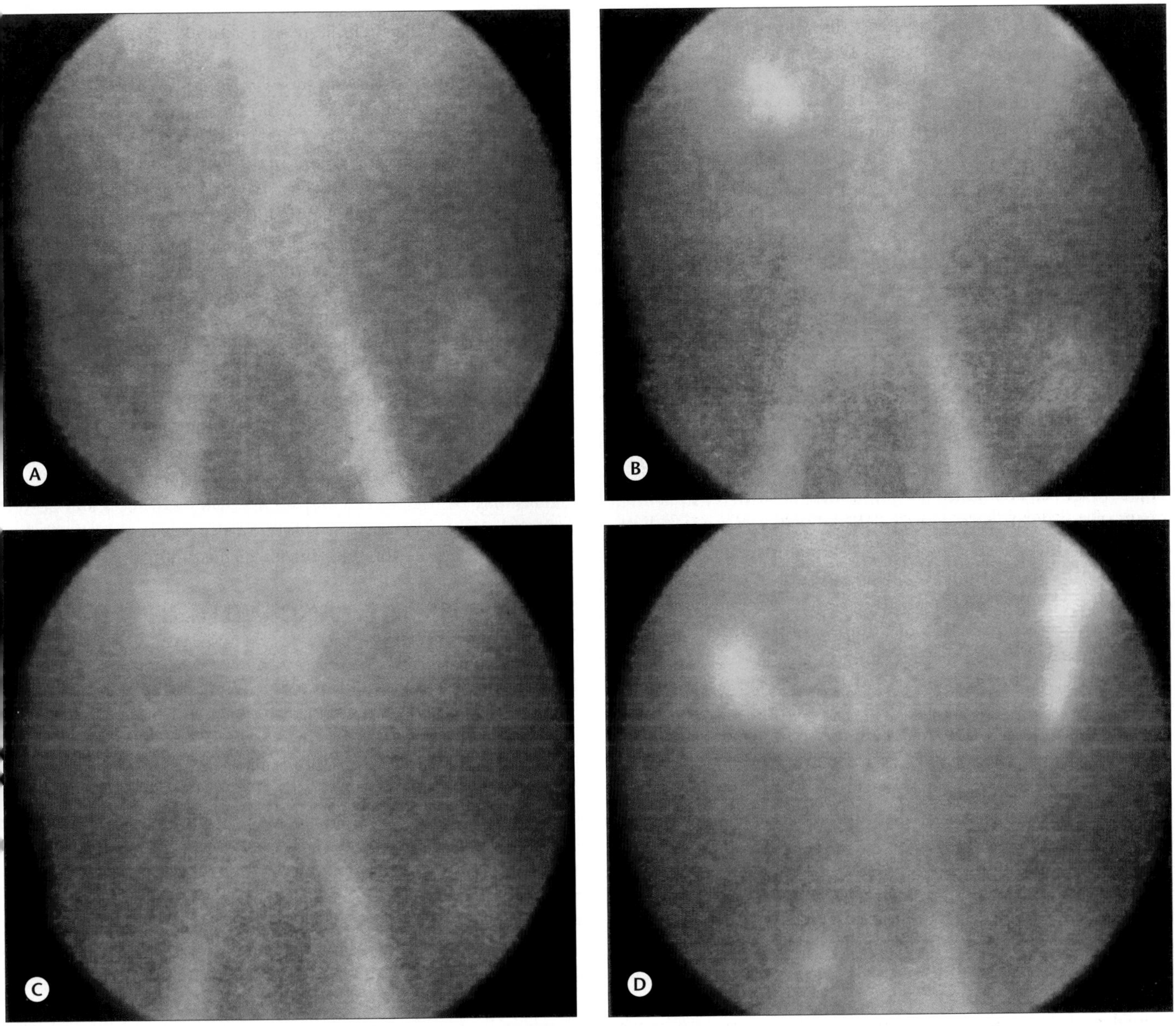

Fig. 65.7 Tagged red blood cell scan demonstrating diverticular bleeding site in the area of the hepatic flexure. Films taken 0–45 min after injection and are shown in anterior view. A. Initial film shows visualization of the aorta and iliac vessels. B. Extravasation is demonstrated early at the hepatic flexure. C, D. Subsequent images show transit of radionuclide into the transverse colon, splenic flexure, and descending colon.

Diverticular bleeding

Seventy to eighty per cent of patients with diverticular hemorrhage resolve spontaneously.[16] Initial therapy is directed to supportive care and includes volume resuscitation and correction of coagulation abnormalities.[27] Patients with hypotension, ongoing transfusion requirements, significant comorbidities, or the elderly may require prompt intervention and should be monitored in the intensive care unit. Angiography may provide the diagnosis and location of the bleeding site, and offers the therapeutic option of selective embolization. Some use local infusion of vasopressin. Pitfalls include a high rebleeding rate, reduced coronary artery perfusion, cardiac arrhythmias, and colonic infarct.[23,28] Increased mortality rates in patients who fail angiographic treatment are probably due to the delay in surgical treatment; therefore, angiographic intervention should be reserved for patients with prohibitive surgical risk.

TREATMENT AND PREVENTION

DIVERTICULOSIS

- High-fiber diet (20–30 g per day)
- Antispasmodic medications

DIVERTICULITIS

- Bowel rest
- Broad-spectrum antibiotics (i.v. or p.o.)
- Analgesics
- Surgery is reserved for complicated or recurrent diverticulitis

DIVERTICULAR BLEEDING

- Most bleeding stops spontaneously (70–80%)
- Supportive care, volume resuscitation, and correction of coagulation abnormalities
- Surgery is indicated for recurrent (2 or more episodes) or persistent bleeding (requiring >6 units blood transfusion)

Colonoscopic intervention is useful when the bleeding site can be visualized, and success has been reported with electrocoagulation and adrenaline (epinephrine) injections.[29] If endoscopic therapy fails, localization of the bleeding site by colonoscopy is extremely valuable for surgical planning. Surgery is indicated for patients with recurrent and persistent bleeding.[27] The most important factor in both safety and efficacy is preoperative localization of the bleeding site. Resection of the angiographically defined colonic segment results in a rebleeding rate of 6%.[23] When localization studies fail to define the bleeding site, subtotal colectomy with ileoproctostomy should be considered since blind resection has a 30% rebleeding rate.

COMPLICATIONS AND THEIR MANAGEMENT

Peritonitis

Generalized peritonitis requires prompt surgical referral and laparotomy. Intra-abdominal findings are classified as purulent peritonitis or feculent peritonitis, which carry a mortality rate of 6% and 35%, respectively.[30,31] Colonic resection is limited to the perforated segment. The distal colon is stapled and proximal end-colostomy formed. A second stage resection and reversal of colostomy with anastomosis is performed between 6 weeks and 3 months later.

Abscess

Diverticular abscess is the most common complication of diverticulitis, and is either a localized abscess in the pericolic or intramesenteric region, or a pelvic abscess. Initial management consists of intravenous broad-spectrum antibiotics and bowel rest. An undrained abscess should be considered if clinical improvement fails to occur in 48–72 h. CT-guided percutaneous catheter drainage of the abscess is recommended, and is usually successful in converting an emergent situation to a semi-elective one.[21,32] The patient is maintained on antibiotics and bowel rest, and total parenteral nutrition is initiated for nutritional support. The catheter may be injected to determine the presence of a fistula. A persistent fistula necessitates early resection and should be planned 10–14 days after drainage of the abscess cavity. If a fistula is not present, the patient is started on a liquid diet and the catheter pulled if no new drainage is noted. Elective resection is performed 3 months later to allow the inflammation to subside.

Fistulas

Diverticular fistulas develop when an associated abscess erodes into an adjacent organ. Fistulas have been reported in 5–33% of patients requiring surgery for diverticular disease. Diverticulitis and sigmoid carcinoma are the two most common causes of colovesical fistula.[33] CT scan identifies colovesical fistulas by demonstrating air in the bladder. Cystoscopy, cystography, and barium enema can be useful diagnostically. Colonoscopy should be performed to exclude carcinoma, since curative surgical treatment requires a wider resection. Other diverticulitis-associated fistulas include colocutaneous, colovaginal, and coloenteric.

Emergency surgical intervention is seldom required for fistulas caused by diverticulitis.[34] Initial management is directed to identify and control sepsis. The general principle of treating fistulas is to remove the offending organ of origin. A preoperative bowel preparation allows a one-stage resection. Preoperative placement of ureteral stents facilitates identification of the ureters, and may prevent ureteral injury when mobilizing the sigmoid colon. The adherent colon is pinched off of the bladder, and the bladder opening is closed in two layers. After the diseased bowel is resected and a primary anastomosis constructed, omentum is used to separate the anastomosis from the previous fistula site. A cystogram is performed after 7 days, and if there is no leak from the bladder the Foley catheter can be removed. During resection of colovaginal fistulas the apex of the vaginal vault may or may not be closed, as closure is often unnecessary. An omental interposition should be considered. Coloenteric fistulas may be managed with primary closure of the small bowel surrounding the fistula if it is soft and supple; otherwise, segmental bowel resection with primary anastomosis is performed.

PROGNOSIS WITH AND WITHOUT TREATMENT

Uncomplicated diverticulitis can be managed medically in 70–85% of patients.[4,10] Surgery is seldom indicated after recovery from the first episode of simple uncomplicated diverticulitis because only 20–30% of patients have a recurrent episode.[3,21] Elective surgery is indicated after a second episode of diverticulitis since subsequent episodes are estimated at 50%. Diverticulitis in patients younger than age 45 is the exception, and surgery is strongly recommended after the first episode due to the more aggressive type of disease.[21,25,26] Complete resection of the diseased bowel has resulted in low recurrence rates.

Diverticular bleeding is an infrequent manifestation of colonic diverticular disease that occurs in about 5% of patients. Bleeding stops spontaneously in 70–80% of patients.[16] The incidence of rebleeding has been estimated at 20–30%, with a readmission rate for further bleeding episodes at 5% per year. Surgery is best performed when bleeding sites have been located, and appropriate segmental colectomy yields low recurrence rates.[23,27] When bleeding is not localized, subtotal colectomy with ileorectal anastomosis is required since segmental colectomy results in a 30% recurrence.

SOURCES OF INFORMATION FOR PATIENTS AND DOCTORS

http://patients.uptodate.com/topic.asp?file=digestiv/6237
http://cchs-dl.slis.ua.edu/patientinfo/gastroenterology/lower/diverticular.htm
http://www.patient.co.uk/showdoc/40000224/
http://www.patient.co.uk/showdoc/23363635/
http://www.patient.co.uk/showdoc/23068723/

REFERENCES

1. Cruveilhier J. Traité d'anatomie pathologique générale. Paris: J.B. Baillière. 1849; 1:593.
2. Painter NS, Burkitt DP. Diverticular disease of the colon, a 20th century problem. Clin Gastroenterol 1975; 4:3–21.
3. Young-Fadok TM, Roberts PL, Spencer MP, Wolf BG. Colonic diverticular disease. Curr Probl Surg 2000; 37:457–514.
4. Stollman NH, Raskin JB. Diagnosis and management of diverticular disease of the colon in adults. Am J Gastroenterol 1999; 94:3110–3121.
5. Jun S, Stollman N. Epidemiology of diverticular disease. Best Pract Res Clin Gastroenterol 2002; 16:529–542.
6. Nakaji S, Danjo K, Munakata A et al. Comparison of etiology of right-sided diverticula in Japan with that of left-sided diverticula in the West. Int J Colorectal Dis 2002; 17:365–373.
7. Gear JS, Ware A, Furdson P et al. Symptomless diverticular disease and intake of dietary fibre. Lancet 1979; 1:511–514.
8. Aldoori WH, Giovannucci EL, Rockett HR et al. A prospective study of dietary fiber types and symptomatic diverticular disease in men. J Nutr 1998; 128:714–719.
9. Cranston D, McWhinnie D, Collin J. Dietary fiber and gastrointestinal disease. Br J Surg 1988; 75:508–512.
10. Place RJ, Simmang CL. Diverticular disease. Best Pract Res Clin Gastroenterol 2002; 16:135–148.
11. Beighton PH, Murdoch JL, Votteler T. Gastrointestinal complications of the Ehlers-Danlos syndrome. Gut 1969; 10:1004–1008.
12. Eliashar R, Eliashar R, Sichel JY, Biron A, Dano I. Multiple gastrointestinal complications in Marfan syndrome. Postgrad Med J 1998; 74:495–497.
13. Bassotti G, Chistolini F, Morelli A. Pathophysiological aspects of diverticular disease of the colon and role of large bowel motility. World J Gastroenterol 2003; 9:2140–2142.
14. Ludeman L, Warren BF, Shepherd NA. The pathology of diverticular disease. Best Pract Res Clin Gastroenterol 2002; 16:543–562.
15. Painter NS. The cause of diverticular disease of the colon, its symptoms and its complications. Review and hypothesis. J Royal Coll Surg Edinb 1985; 30:118–122.
16. Breen E, Murray JJ. Pathophysiology and natural history of lower gastrointestinal bleeding. Semin Colon Rectal Surg 1997; 8:128–138.
17. Simpson J, Scholefield JH, Spiller RC. Origin of symptoms in diverticular disease. Br J Surg 2003; 90:899–908.
18. Boulos PB, Karamanolis DG, Salmon PR, Clark CG. Is colonoscopy necessary in diverticular disease? Lancet 1984; 1:95–96.
19. Hunt RH. The role of colonoscopy in complicated diverticular disease. A review. Acta Chir Belg 1979; 78:349–353.
20. Labs JD, Sarr MG, Fishman EK, Siegelman SS, Cameron JL. Complications of acute diverticulitis of the colon: improved early diagnosis with computerized tomography. Am J Surg 1988; 155:331–336.
21. Schoetz DJ. Diverticular disease of the colon. Dis Colon Rectum 1999; 42:703–709.
22. O'Neill BB, Gosnell JE, Lull RJ et al. Cinematic nuclear scintigraphy reliably directs surgical intervention for patients with gastrointestinal bleeding. Arch Surg 2000; 135:1076–1082.
23. Browder W, Cerise EJ, Litwin MS. Impact of emergency angiography in massive lower gastrointestinal bleeding. Ann Surg 1986; 204:530–536.
24. Ohyama T, Sakurai Y, Ito M, Daito K, Sezai S, Sato Y. Analysis of urgent colonoscopy for lower gastrointestinal tract bleeding. Digestion 2000; 61:189–192.
25. McConnell EJ, Tessier DJ, Wolff BG. Population-based incidence of complicated diverticular disease of the sigmoid colon based on gender and age. Dis Colon Rectum 2003; 46:1110–1114.
26. Konvolinka CW. Acute diverticulitis under age forty. Am J Surg 1994; 167:562–565.
27. Zuccaro G. Practice guidelines. Management of the adult patient with acute lower gastrointestinal bleeding. Am J Gastroenterol 1998; 93:1202–1208.
28. Bandi R, Shetty PC, Sharma RP, Burke TH, Burke MW, Kastan D. Superselective arterial embolization for the treatment of lower gastrointestinal hemorrhage. J Vasc Interv Radiol 2001; 12:1399–1405.
29. Jensen DM, Machicado GA, Jutabha R, Kovacs TO. Urgent colonoscopy for the diagnosis and treatment of severe diverticular hemorrhage. N Engl J Med 2000; 342:78–82.
30. Krukowski ZH, Matheson NA. Emergency surgery for diverticular disease complicated by generalized and faecal peritonitis: a review. Br J Surg 1984; 71:921–927.
31. Tudor RG, Keighley MRB. The options in surgical treatment of diverticular disease. Surg Annu 1987; 19:135–149.
32. Stabile BE, Puccio E, vanSonnenberg E, Neff CC. Preoperative percutaneous drainage of diverticular abscesses. Am J Surg 1990; 159:99–104.
33. Larsen A, Bjerklund Johansen TE, Solheim BM, Urnes T. Diagnosis and treatment of enterovesical fistula. Eur Urol 1996; 29:318–321.
34. Woods RJ, Lavery IC, Fazio VW, Jagelman DG, Weakley FL. Internal fistulas in diverticular disease. Dis Colon Rectum 1988; 31:591–596.

Chapter 66

Colonic dysmotility

Eamonn M M Quigley

KEY POINTS

- Our understanding of colonic motor activity in man is poor
- In many clinical situations, the role of colonic dysmotility is assumed or implied rather than proven
- Few tests of colonic motor function have been validated for use in clinical practice; simple tests of colon transit are of most use clinically
- Acute and chronic megacolon are the most common disorders of colonic motility and are usually related to underlying disease
- Acute megacolon may resolve spontaneously; therapy, if needed, should begin with neostigmine, with colonoscopy reserved for nonresponders
- Surgery may be required for intractable symptoms in patients with chronic megacolon

INTRODUCTION

Because of the relative inaccessibility and the difficulties posed by the presence of solid or semisolid fecal material, our understanding of colonic motility lags far behind that of the other organs of the gastrointestinal tract. This is in spite of the crucial roles of the colon in absorption, salvage of carbohydrates and bile acids, storage and defecation.[1]

Sarna[2] stressed three important differences between the colon and the small intestine, which may well contribute to its unique motor properties:

- the colon is never empty;
- its contents are more viscous than in any other part of the gut; and
- it plays a critical role in defecation.

Initially, studies of colonic motor function focused on phasic contractile activity.[1] Because of the challenges posed by the prolonged recordings that are necessary to describe normal phasic motor patterns in this organ, there is surprisingly little information on colonic motility in man, in health or in disease.

While consensus is lacking in this area, it seems reasonable to summarize the current status of our knowledge of colonic motor patterns by stating that colonic motility, in man, presents alternating periods of activity and quiescence. Some have described some recognizable patterns in the active periods: individual phasic contractions, propagating contractions, propagating bursts or clusters of contractions and, most recognizable of all, high-amplitude propagating contractions (HAPCs). The latter are more prevalent in children than in adults, are associated with the mass movement of fecal material over segments of the colon, and may be accompanied by the passage of flatus or the urge to defecate. HAPCs typically propagate from the cecum or ascending colon to the sigmoid colon at a velocity of 1 cm/min. They may be induced by the administration of laxatives such as cascara and bisacodyl. Given the distinctive nature of this motor phenomenon and the fact that it can be induced, as described, it has served as a marker of the integrity of colonic motor function in disease states. While there is a surprising degree of between-study variability in this area, most studies have indicated that colonic motility is affected by:

- food intake (the so-called gastrocolonic reflex, whose intensity is influenced considerably by the location of the recording sensor, being more intense in the sigmoid colon);
- diurnal variation;
- exercise; and
- stress.

In comparison to the small intestine, the colon is more susceptible to the influences of the autonomic and central nervous systems, a fitting arrangement given our necessity to regulate the time and place of voluntary defecation.

The advent of such techniques as the barostat has permitted the examination of patterns of tonic contractile activity in the colon and has revealed the importance of fluctuations in tone in colonic homeostasis.[1] In the colon, tone is low during sleep, rises on waking, and increases further following meal ingestion or the instillation of short-chain fatty acids. Between-study variations, related, in part, to technical and protocol issues again limit our ability to draw firm conclusions in this area.

Studies of colonic sensation have focused, in particular, on the role of visceral hypersensitivity and/or hyperalgesia in irritable bowel syndrome. Here again, the barostat has proven to be a valuable tool in generating reproducible and clinically relevant levels of distention in the rectum and colon. Distention studies have revealed the poorly localized nature of colonic discomfort and pain. Stimuli in the rectum, for example, give rise in some subjects to symptoms that are localized by the patient to various parts of the abdomen.

Our understanding of the colon's motor and sensory physiology remains far from complete and has certainly not reached the stage where it can represent a firm foundation on which we can progress to an appreciation of the significance of disturbed motor function in disease.

The spectrum of colonic dysmotility disorders

It will be obvious from the above that our approach to colonic dysmotility, in clinical practice, will not be based on syndromes clearly delineated by the presence of distinctive, reproducible, and abnormal phasic and/or tonic motor patterns. In many instances, the roles of colonic motility, in a clinical disorder, remain speculative at best. In others, it is assumed from the nature of the clinical presentation, radiographic findings, or colonic neuropathology. Rarely, is there a convergence of clinical presentation, motor pattern(s), and underlying pathology. Any classification of colonic dysmotility will therefore be incomplete, poorly defined, and subject to change as the true nature of any one these disorders is revealed.

The simplest and most clinically useful classification of colonic dysmotility is into:

- acute colonic pseudo-obstruction (including Ogilvie's syndrome); and
- chronic motor disorders.

These may be further subdivided on the basis of etiology and clinical presentation as detailed in Table 66.1.

TABLE 66.1 CLASSIFICATION
ACUTE
• Ogilvie's syndrome
• Toxic megacolon
CHRONIC
• Congenital (e.g., Hirschsprung's disease, congenital neuropathy, or myopathy)
• Acquired
– Primary colonic disorders (e.g., slow transit constipation)
– Colonic involvement in intestinal motor disorders (e.g., Chagas' disease, enteric myopathy, enteric neuropathy, neurofibromatosis)
– Autonomic neuropathy (e.g., diabetes)
– CNS disease (e.g., Parkinson's disease, multiple sclerosis, spinal cord injury)
– Iatrogenic
– Chronic idiopathic megacolon
– Undefined (IBS, diverticulosis)

ACUTE MEGACOLON

Causes

Acute megacolon may be a manifestation of a variety of disorders. Toxic megacolon, for example, is a dreaded complication of ulcerative colitis and other colitides including inflammatory, infectious and ischemic. Acute colonic pseudo-obstruction, or Ogilvie's syndrome, is defined as an acute dilatation of the colon without evidence of mechanical obstruction distal to the dilated segment.[3] Ogilvie's syndrome is associated with an underlying medical condition or the postoperative state in over 90% of cases (Table 66.2). Risk factors for the development of Ogilvie's syndrome in individual patients following surgery include:

- advanced age;
- obesity;
- immobility; and
- use of patient-controlled analgesia.

TABLE 66.2 SOME CAUSES OF ACUTE MEGACOLON
SURGICAL
• Hip surgery
• Intra-abdominal surgery
• Spinal surgery
MEDICAL
• Acute myocardial infarction
• Cardiac failure
• Parkinson's disease
• Burns
• Pancreatitis
• Peritonitis
• Retroperitoneal disorders
• Medications
– Tricyclics
– Opiates
– Clonidine
• Herpes virus infections

Clinical presentation

Progressive abdominal distention is the clinical hallmark of this condition; in the postoperative state distention is typically evident by the fourth postoperative day. Lower abdominal pain and nausea and vomiting are present in 60–80% and 50%, respectively. Although the vast majority of patients with Ogilvie's syndrome are completely constipated, megacolon can develop in individuals who continue to pass both stool and flatus. Only 40% of patients will have hypoactive or absent bowel sounds. The overall risk of perforation in Ogilvie's syndrome is low (3%) but mortality following perforation, in this context, may be as high as 50%. Cecal diameter is valuable in predicting risk of perforation; a diameter in excess of 9 cm is abnormal and when greater than 12 cm indicates a significant risk of perforation.

Differential diagnosis

In the patient with acute megacolon, the main differential diagnoses to be considered are:

1. toxic megacolon; and
2. acute colonic obstruction due to:
   - carcinoma
   - stricture
   - volvulus
   - intussusception

Toxic megacolon should be obvious from the patient's history and clinical presentation and obstruction may be suspected by the prominence of pain in the symptomatology, as well as by clinical and radiographic findings. It is important to note that, on X-ray, haustral markings are preserved in Ogilvie's syndrome, in contrast to both toxic megacolon and obstruction.

Diagnostic methods

Plain abdominal X-ray may be the only essential investigation. Typically, there is dilatation of the cecum and ascending and transverse colon with less gaseous distention in the left colon (Fig. 66.1). If obstruction needs to be ruled out computerized abdominal tomography may, nowadays, be the best option with barium enema and colonoscopy as alternatives. If colonoscopy is contemplated the endoscopist needs to be mindful of the risk of a cecal perforation due to the closed loop phenomenon, if obstruction is complete.

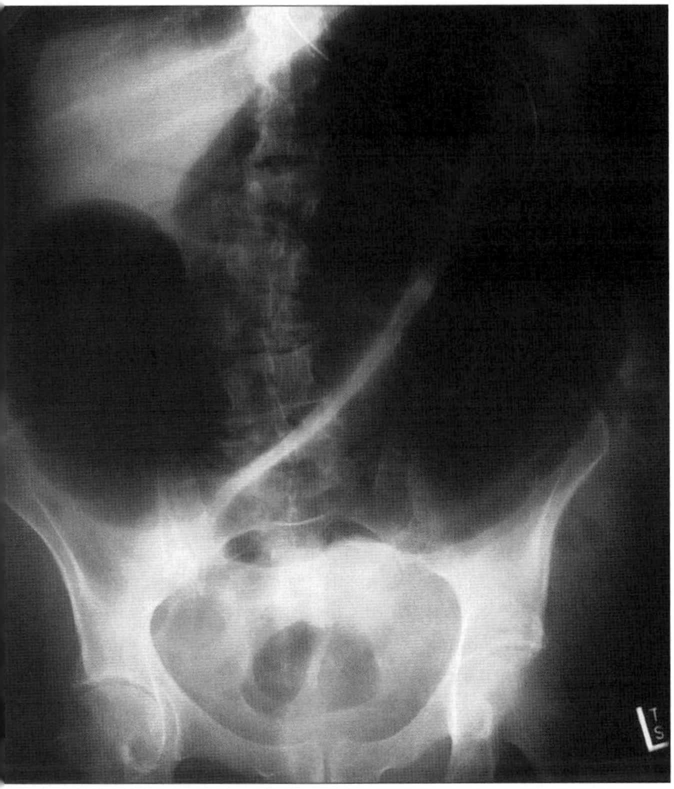

Fig. 66.1 Ogilvie's syndrome. Plain abdominal radiograph – note prominent dilatation of right and transverse colon with preservation of haustrae.

DIAGNOSTIC METHODS
• Plain abdominal radiographs • Computerized tomography, barium enema, or colonoscopy to define obstruction • Colon transit study: radiopaque markers scintigraphy • Manometry • Barostat

Treatment and prevention

The first step in the management of acute megacolon is to search for and, where possible, treat any underlying disorder. Many cases will resolve spontaneously as the associated primary disorder improves; patient positioning may also promote resolution. In resistant cases, therapy should begin with a pharmacological approach.

Cholinergic agonists are effective: Ponec and colleagues administered neostigmine in a dose of 2 mg intravenously to 11 patients with acute colonic pseudo-obstruction and compared their outcome to that of 10 who received intravenous saline.[4] Ten of the 11 patients who received neostigmine had prompt colonic decompression compared with none of the 10 patients who received placebo. The median time for response was 4 min. Two patients who had an initial response to neostigmine required colonoscopic decompression for recurrence of colonic distention; one eventually underwent subtotal colectomy. In contrast, seven patients in the placebo group and the one patient in the neostigmine group without an initial response received open-label neostigmine; all achieved colonic decompression.

TREATMENT AND PREVENTION
ACUTE MEGACOLON • Observation and treatment of primary disorder • Neostigmine • Decompressive colonoscopy • Cecostomy **CHRONIC MEGACOLON** • Management of associated constipation • Surgery

Mechanical approaches

Colonoscopy has played an important role in the management of patients with megacolon and significant cecal distention to prevent perforation, but is not without risk[5–7] By definition, the colon will not be prepared in these patients, making the procedure technically difficult. An overall success rate in achieving a reduction in cecal diameter of approximately 70% has been reported but the recurrence rate has been as high as 40%. Some have advocated the placement of a decompression tube at the time of colonoscopy and have reported that this reduces the recurrence rate. This involves the placement of a guidewire through the biopsy channel of the colonoscope with the subsequent insertion of the decompression tube over the guidewire, under fluoroscopic control, following withdrawal of the colonoscope. Colonoscopy should be reserved for those who fail conservative therapy in view of its risks in Ogilvie's syndrome.

Surgical intervention and the placement of a tube cecostomy, in particular, may become necessary in the patient with megacolon who appears at high risk of perforation and has failed pharmacological and colonoscopic attempts at decompression. Clearly, surgery will also be necessary in those who unfortunately progress to ischemia or perforation. In all of these situations, surgery has been associated with high morbidity and mortality rates. Prevention of acute megacolon will be based on the avoidance, where possible, of those circumstances that may precipitate this event; particular attention should be paid to medications known to induce hypomotility.

CHRONIC MOTOR DISORDERS

Among the spectrum of chronic colonic motor disorders are included a vast array of disorders from the well described, such as colonic varieties of Hirschsprung's disease, to the vague, such as irritable bowel syndrome (IBS) or diverticulosis, where the role of dysmotility is putative, at best.

Causes, risk factors, disease associations

Among the primary colonic motor disorders, Hirschsprung's disease is, perhaps, the best characterized. The primary pathological abnormality is a complete loss of ganglion cells in the submucosal and myenteric plexi in the affected region and their replacement by hypertrophied nerve trunks. The molecular basis for this developmental failure is now understood. A number of mutations associated with the development of this disease have now been defined. These lead to a failure of migration of neurons from the neural crest to the colon and to the loss of inhibitory, nitric oxide-containing neurons, in particular.[8]

In Chagas' disease, chronic infection with the trypanosome *T. cruzi* leads to a similar loss of inhibitory neurons in various parts of the gastrointestinal tract, including the anorectum and colon, and to the development of megacolon (Fig. 66.2). The precise pathogenesis of neural injury is unclear and some have suggested that this may have an autoimmune rather than a direct toxic etiology.[9]

Old age is recognized to be associated with greater risk of constipation; whether this, in turn, reflects age-related changes in colonic function is an issue that remains to be resolved. Indeed, constipation in the elderly can usually be explained on the basis of coexistent disease, increased and prolonged intake of constipating drugs, reduced intake of dietary fiber, and/or relatively low levels of physical exercise.[10] The evidence to support age itself as an independent risk factor for constipation or abnormal colonic motor function is conflicting. Some work indicates significant prolongation of colonic transit time whilst other studies show no significant change with advancing age. The conflicting results of these studies cannot be readily attributed to differences in methodology, since colonic transit time was usually measured by the radiopaque marker technique. One must be cautious not to equate colonic transit time with colonic motility, since normal colonic motility also encompasses nonpropulsive contractions. The latter, however, are difficult to study objectively.

Colonic motor dysfunction is common in neurological disorders. Constipation and defecatory dysfunction are common and potentially disabling symptoms in Parkinson's disease.[11] Orocecal and colonic transit times are significantly increased in patients with idiopathic Parkinson's disease, but are unchanged in non-idiopathic Parkinsonism. Anorectal dysfunction is also prevalent in these patients and may respond to the administration of potent dopaminergic agents.[12] The pathophysiology of colonic dysfunction in Parkinson's disease remains to be defined; loss of CNS control, autonomic dysfunction, and some anti-parkinsonian therapies could all contribute. However, recent evidence of a deficit in dopaminergic neurones in the myenteric and submucosal plexi in the colons of patients with megacolon suggests that peripheral abnormalities in the enteric nervous system may also be relevant.[13] Constipation and megacolon are also recognized complications of spinal cord injury and multiple sclerosis (Fig. 66.3).

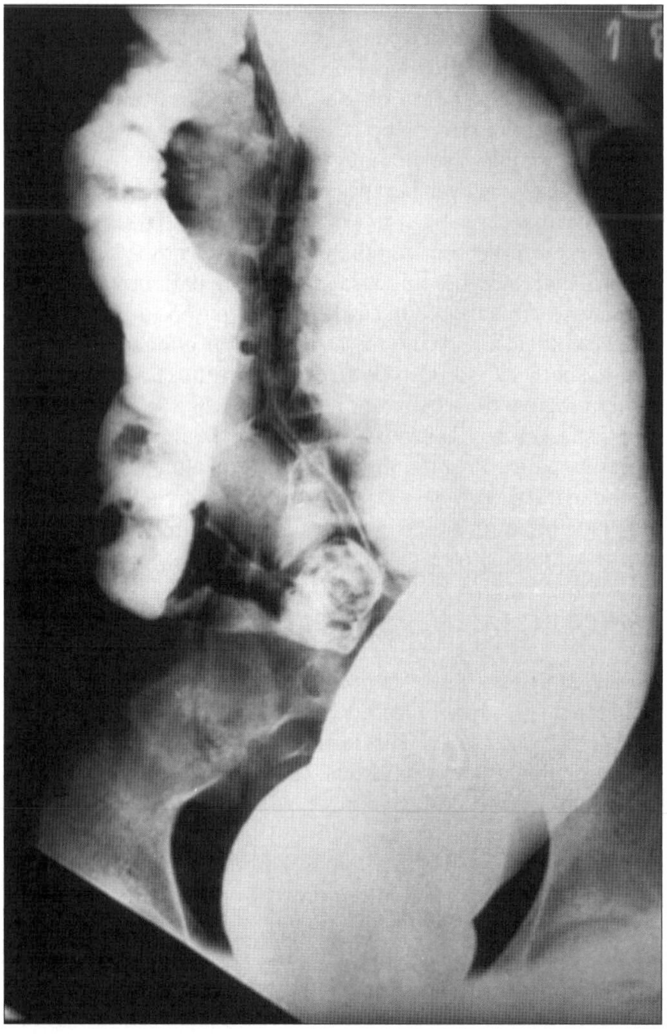

Fig. 66.2 Megacolon and megarectum in Chagas's disease.

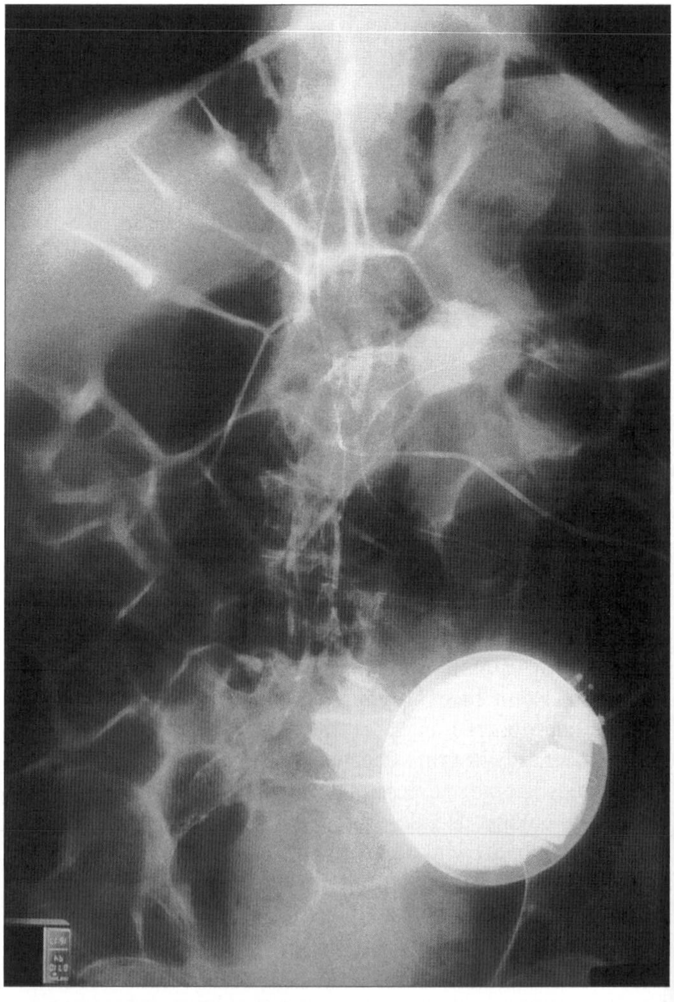

Fig. 66.3 Megacolon in multiple sclerosis and paraplegia. Megacolon in a patient with multiple sclerosis and paraplegia; note the presence of an implanted system for the delivery of baclofen.

Whole gut transit time (WGTT) is significantly increased in depression and WGTT is significantly correlated with the severity of depression.[14] Among elderly people with constipation, colonic transit time is significantly correlated with the presence of psychopathological symptoms (including depression) and their severity. One large-scale retrospective survey of the medical records of 4 million patients discharged from US Veterans hospitals has shown that Alzheimer's disease was associated with significantly increased risk of constipation, megacolon, volvulus and intestinal impaction, when compared with patients without neurological or psychiatric disease.[15]

Given the sensitivity of the colon to autonomic input in health, colonic dysmotility and delayed transit and megacolon, in particular, are to be expected among patients with autonomic dysfunction, regardless of cause. Indeed, increased colonic transit time is a feature of diabetes mellitus with abnormal autonomic function and there is an association, in such patients, between delayed colonic transit and use of laxatives for constipation. The longer the duration of diabetes, the longer the colonic transit time.[16]

The principal gastrointestinal symptom related to hypothyroidism is constipation. However, the relationship of this symptom to colonic motor function remains unclear, studies of colon transit, for example, producing conflicting results.

Pathogenesis and pathology

Hirschsprung's disease and Chagas' disease provide the most clear-cut illustrations of clinical-pathological correlation in the field of colonic dysmotility. Neuronal intestinal dysplasia, a disorder sometimes associated with Hirschsprung's disease, which features neural hyperplasia, has been described in up to 30% of children with pseudo-obstruction; the criteria for the diagnosis of this entity have, however, been questioned.

Neuropathological abnormalities have been described in patients with Parkinson's disease,[13] neurofibromatosis,[17] and multiple endocrine neoplasia type IIb[18]; the relationship between these findings and symptomatology in these disorders remains to be defined. The description of enteric neural changes in the myenteric plexus of the colon among patients who had chronically used anthroquinone-type laxatives led to the assumption that these agents were neurotoxic. More recent studies among patients with chronic idiopathic, slow-transit constipation suggest that such changes may be linked to constipation *per se* and not to the use of laxatives.

Clinical presentation

Chronic colonic pseudo-obstruction and megacolon

Chronic dilatation of the colon may be associated with any of the disorders that may result in acute intestinal pseudo-obstruction.[19] These may be idiopathic or secondary. Idiopathic examples may, in turn, be hereditary or acquired. Hirschsprung's disease provides a good example of an inherited idiopathic enteric neuropathy that can predominantly affect the colon, in contrast to most other causes of chronic intestinal pseudo-obstruction, which tend to diffusely affect the entire gastrointestinal tract. Secondary forms of pseudo-obstruction are far more common and have been described in association with:

- connective tissue disorders;
- neurological disorders (Fig. 66.3);
- skeletal muscle diseases;
- metabolic disorders; and
- drugs and toxins.

Chronic pseudo-obstruction is usually separated into those disorders that predominately involve intestinal muscle (the myopathies) and those that predominately affect the enteric nervous system or the autonomic nerves that supply the gut (the neuropathies). One of the most common examples of an intestinal myopathy is scleroderma. Myopathic disorders lead to a marked reduction in the amplitude of individual contractions, though patterns of organization are retained. In contrast, neuropathies feature the retention of the amplitude of individual contractions (as the enteric muscle is intact) but motor activity is disorganized to a greater or lesser extent. There have been few direct comparisons of manometric findings and enteric neuro- or myopathology and these have all focused on the small intestine, not on the colon. Appropriate histopathological examination of gut muscle and nerve should be performed on full-thickness sections of the intestine, following specialized fixation and staining by an experienced pathologist.[20] Only a few centers in the world can fulfill any one let alone all of these requirements.

In some instances, chronic megacolon may occur in the absence of any discernible cause: idiopathic megacolon (Fig. 66.4). In such instances megacolon usually occurs in a background of chronic constipation and is assumed to represent the expression of a degenerative disorder of intestinal nerve and/or muscle, though the exact nature of the basic defect remains to be defined.[21]

The role of dysmotility in idiopathic constipation, irritable bowel syndrome, and other functional gastrointestinal disorders

Chronic idiopathic constipation is traditionally divided into:

- slow-transit constipation; and
- 'outlet-type' constipation or defecatory dysfunction.

While defecatory dysfunction is thought to be due to dysfunction at the level of the pelvic floor (see Chapter 10) and is therefore not a colonic motor disorder *per se*, slow-transit constipation is presumed to reflect a primary disorder of colonic motility. In support of this presumption, these patients who, by definition, have slow colonic transit, have been shown to demonstrate a variety of motor abnormalities on mano-

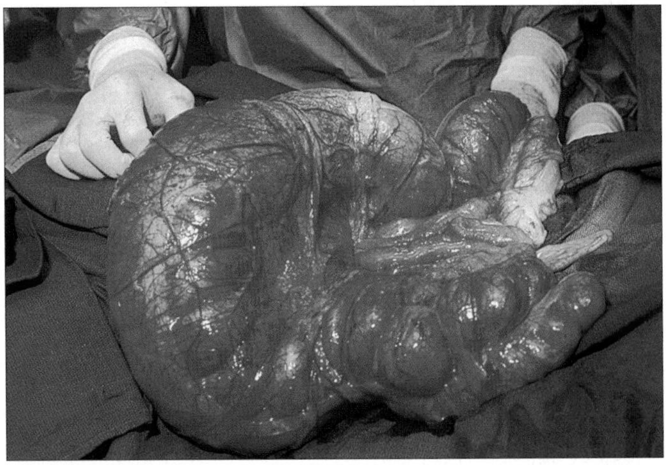

Fig. 66.4 Idiopathic chronic megacolon. Appearances of the colon at the time of colectomy for chronic intractable megacolon.

metric studies of the colon. These patients demonstrate a reduced frequency and amplitude of HAPCs and an impaired colonic motor response to food and exercise.

Various electromyographic abnormalities have been documented among patients with functional diarrhea but the main focus of colonic motility studies, whether electromyographic or manometric, has been on patients with IBS. While a variety of abnormal electromyographic and motor patterns have been described in the past, the specificity of any of these for IBS remains unclear[22] and interest has shifted to the role of colorectal sensation in the pathogenesis of symptoms in IBS[23] (see Chapter 64). The role, if any, of dysmotility in diverticulosis (see Chapter 65) is also unclear.

Differential diagnosis

With regard to chronic megacolon, subacute or chronic obstruction related to carcinoma and stricture again looms large in the differential diagnosis. In the patient with chronic colonic motor dysfunction without megacolon, symptom overlap is to be expected with IBS; the presence of symptoms, signs, or radiographic or manometric evidence of a generalized motor abnormality should suggest chronic megacolon rather than IBS.

Diagnostic methods

As with acute megacolon, plain abdominal radiography is very useful. The radiopaque marker technique is the simplest and most clinically useful approach to the diagnosis of delayed transit in the patient with constipation. Transit may also be studied using scintigraphy; this technique will also provide estimates of transit within various regions of the colon. There is currently no role for either electromyographic or manometric studies in the evaluation of patients with suspected disorders of colonic motor function. While the definition of rectal sensory thresholds using the barostat has been shown to be highly correlated with the diagnosis of IBS,[23] this technique has not gained a place in the clinical armamentarium.

Treatment and prevention

Chronic megacolon and chronic dysmotility

The management of Hirschsprung's disease and of megacolon related to Chagas' disease (Fig. 66.2) is primarily surgical and the approach will depend on the extent of the aganglionic segment. There are few prospective studies of any intervention in the management of other varieties of megacolon; again the main option is colectomy (Fig. 66.4), which may be indicated on the basis of intractable symptoms and risk of perforation.

SOURCES OF INFORMATION FOR PATIENTS AND DOCTORS

http://www.clevelandclinic.org/gastro/motility/patient/pseudo.htm
http://www.bchealthguide.org/kbase/nord/nord452.htm
http://www.aboutkidsgi.org/cip.html

REFERENCES

1. Quigley EMM. Colonic motility and colonic motor function. In: Pemberton JH, Swash M, Henry MM, eds. The pelvic floor, its function and disorders. Philadelphia: W.B. Saunders; 2003:84–93.
2. Sarna SK. Physiology and pathophysiology of colonic motor activity (in two parts). Dig Dis Sci 1991; 36:827–862, 998–1018.
3. Quigley EMM. Acute intestinal pseudo-obstruction. CTO Gastroenterol 2000; 3:273–285.
4. Ponec RJ, Saunders MD, Kimmey MB. Neostigmine for the treatment of acute colonic pseudo-obstruction. New Eng J Med 1999; 341:137–141.
5. Strodel WE, Brothers T. Colonoscopic decompression of pseudo-obstruction and volvulus. Surg Clin North Am 1989; 69:1327–1335.
6. Rex DK. Colonoscopy and acute colonic pseudo-obstruction. Gastrointest Endosc Clin North Am 1997; 7:499–508.
7. Laine L. Management of acute colonic pseudo-obstruction. N Eng J Med 1999; 341:192–193.
8. Milla PJ. Endothelins, pseudo-obstruction and Hirschsprung's disease. Gut 1998; 44:148–152.
9. Goin JC, Serin-Borda L, Bilder CR et al. Functional implications of circulating muscarinic cholinergic receptor autoantibodies in Chagasic patients with achalasia. Gastroenterology 1999; 117:798–805.
10. O'Mahony D, O'Leary P, Quigley EMM. Aging and intestinal motility: a review of factors that affect intestinal motility in the aged. Drugs Aging 2002; 19:515–527.
11. Quigley EM. Gastrointestinal dysfunction in Parkinson's disease. Semin Neurol 1996; 16:245–250.
12. Edwards LL, Quigley EM, Harned RK, Hofman R, Pfeiffer RF. Characterization of swallowing and defecation in Parkinson's disease. Am J Gastroenterol 1994; 89:15–25.
13. Singaram C, Ashraf W, Guamnitz EA et al. Dopaminergic defect of enteric nervous system in Parkinson's disease patients with chronic constipation. Lancet 1995; 346:861–864.
14. Gorard DA, Gomborone JE, Libby GW, Farthing MJ. Intestinal transit in anxiety and depression. Gut 1996; 39;551–555.
15. Sonnenberg A, Tsou VT, Muller AD. The 'institutional colon': a frequent colonic dysmotility in psychiatric and neurologic disease. Am J Gastroenterol 1994; 89:62–66.
16. Maleki D, Camilleri M, Burton DD et al. Pilot study of pathophysiology of constipation among community diabetics. Dig Dis Sci 1998; 43:2373–2378.
17. Kim HR, Kim YJ. Neurofibromatosis of the colon and rectum combined with other manifestations of von Recklinghausen's disease: report of a case. Dis Colon Rectum 1998; 41:1187–1192.
18. Grobmyer SR, Guillem JG, O'Riordain DS et al. Colonic manifestations of multiple endocrine neoplasia type 2B: report of four cases. Dis Colon Rectum 1999; 42:1216–1219.
19. Quigley EMM. Chronic intestinal pseudo-obstruction. CTO Gastroenterol 1999; 2:239–250.
20. Quigley EMM. Enteric neuropathology: recent advances and implications for clinical practice. The Gastroenterologist 1997; 5:233–241.
21. Gattuso JM, Kamm MA, Talbot IC. Pathology of idiopathic megarectum and megacolon. Gut 1997; 41:252–257.
22. McKee DP, Quigley EMM. Intestinal motility in irritable bowel syndrome: Is IBS a motility disorder? Part 1: Definition of IBS and colonic motility. Dig Dis Sci 1993; 38:1761–1772.
23. Bouin M, Plourde V, Boivin M et al. Rectal distension testing in patients with the irritable bowel syndrome: sensitivity, specificity, and predictive values of pain sensory thresholds. Gastroenterology 2002; 122:1771–1777.

Chapter 67

Splanchnic vascular disorders

J Hajo van Bockel, Robert H Geelkerken, and Jeroen J Kolkman

KEY POINTS

- The intestine receives between 10–20% of resting and up to 35% of postprandial cardiac output
- The gut has abundant collateral circulation with the celiac artery, superior mesenteric artery and inferior mesenteric artery sharing a common embryonic origin
- Chronic mesenteria is characterized by postprandial upper abdominal pain (within an hour of eating), an epigastric bruit, and weight loss – less than half of patients will have this typical presentation
- A high index of suspicion is required for diagnosis
- Duplex ultrasound and MRI are useful in risk investigation modalities
- Gastric tonometry shows promise as an investigation tool
- Percutaneous transluminal angioplasty is gaining favor over invasive surgery

INTRODUCTION

Splanchnic vascular disorders encompass a spectrum of acute and chronic occlusive and aneurysmal disorders affecting the vessels of the abdominal viscera. Of these relatively uncommon disorders, splanchnic ischemia occurs most frequently. Vascular disorders of the splanchnic circulation are mostly asymptomatic but occasionally catastrophic. Therefore, early diagnosis and treatment has important clinical implications. Prospective randomized studies on the diagnosis and treatment are not available, therefore current opinions on assessing chronic occlusive splanchnic disorders will be discussed.

EPIDEMIOLOGY

Chronic splanchnic disease is characterized by significant stenosis in the celiac artery, the superior mesenteric artery, and/or the inferior mesenteric artery, which is often symptomless. Atherosclerosis is responsible for these stenoses in more than 95% of cases. In populations with manifestations of atherosclerotic diseases, the incidence of chronic splanchnic disease ranges between 8% and 70%. In patients over 65 years of age, 18% had a greater than 50% narrowing of more than one splanchnic artery.[1] The presence of chronic splanchnic disease may have important clinical implications, as the presence of significant stenoses in more than one splanchnic artery is considered to be a risk factor for acute splanchnic infarction.[2,3] Until properly documented studies of the natural history of chronic splanchnic disease have been performed, it must be assumed that the stenoses will progress.

ANATOMY AND PATHOPHYSIOLOGY

Blood begins to circulate by the end of the third week in the human embryo. The celiac, superior mesenteric, and the inferior mesenteric artery share a common embryonic origin, the ventral group of the left dorsal aorta. Potentially there is an abundant collateral pathway with other vascular beds. Certain clear patterns in the arterial blood supply of the intestine can be distinguished, however variations are frequent. The celiac artery usually arises from the aorta at the level of the 12th thoracic vertebra and supplies part of the foregut, namely the distal esophagus, the stomach, part of the duodenum, the liver, part of the pancreas, and the biliary apparatus. The superior mesenteric artery arises from the aorta at the level of the first lumbar vertebra, just distal to the origin of the celiac trunk. In 7% of cases a common celiacomesenteric trunk is formed. The superior mesenteric artery supplies the midgut, namely the small intestine from the duodenum, the ascending colon and the major portion of the transverse colon. The inferior mesenteric artery originates from the aorta at the level of the third lumbar vertebra. It supplies parts of the transverse colon, the descending colon, the sigmoid, and parts of the rectum. An abundant and extremely variable collateral circulation exists between the celiac, the superior mesenteric, and the inferior mesenteric artery.

The peripheral arteries of the small intestine enter the serosal surface of the gut at the mesenteric border and immediately form several branches. Some of these branches extend around both sides of the intestine to anastomose at the opposite border. Other serosal branches pierce the muscularis externa to form an extensive vascular plexus in the submucosa. From this submucosal plexus, one group of arterioles pierces the smooth muscle at the base of the mucosa and forms a capillary network that delivers blood to the villi. The microcirculation of each intestinal villus is supplied by a central nutrient arteriole. These arterioles branch near the tip of the villus into a subepithelial network of capillaries and venules, in which the flow is in the opposite direction to the flow in the nutrient arteriole. This villous microvasculature system permits arteriovenous shunting of oxygen, resulting in lower oxygen tension at the tip of the villus than at the base. Ischemic damage to the intestinal mucosa begins at the tip of the villi and extends toward the base if the ischemia is prolonged. Colonic blood flow is less than that of the small intestine, although the intramural blood flow distribution is quite similar.

CLINICAL PRESENTATION

Chronic splanchnic syndrome or chronic mesenteric ischemia

Classically, chronic splanchnic syndrome results from stenotic and occlusive disease of splanchnic arteries, which prevents the increased blood flow necessary for satisfying the metabolic demands of the bowel that arise from increased motility, secretion, and absorption after meals. The intestine receives 10–20% of resting and up to 35% of postprandial cardiac output and 70% of this volume supplies the mucosa. This autoregulation can be compromised by stimulation of the sympathetic nervous system, circulating catecholamines, and certain medications such as digoxin.

An ischemic basis for the pain is widely accepted although the pathophysiological mechanism that is responsible for the pain has not been elucidated clearly. In spite of the relatively high prevalence of splanchnic disease, the incidence of chronic splanchnic syndrome appears to be low. Three-quarters of the patients are female. The apparent low incidence may be due to a low index of suspicion since most patients present atypically with longstanding vague abdominal symptoms. The classical syndrome is characterized by upper abdominal pain that is usually provoked by eating, an epigastric bruit, loss of weight, and hemodynamically significant stenosis in at least two of the splanchnic arteries. The typical postprandial pain occurs within the first hour after eating and diminishes within 2h. The complete classical triad is seen in less then half of the patients. In cases of extended chronic splanchnic syndrome, weight loss appears to be an important characteristic and is assumed to be caused by a decrease in the size of the patient's meal owing to postprandial pain rather than malabsorption or its content.

Celiac axis compression syndrome

Isolated occlusive disease of the celiac trunk may be caused by the compression of this vessel by the arcuate ligament of the diaphragm, the so-called 'celiac axis compression syndrome' or 'median arcuate ligament syndrome' (Fig. 67.1A,B). The existence of this syndrome is still controversial.[4] Gastric tonometry may be a promising tool to identify patients with abdominal symptoms and solitary celiac artery stenosis who might benefit from revascularization.[5] In a cohort of 50 patients with abdominal symptoms and solitary celiac artery occlusive disease we diagnosed celiac artery compression syndrome in 31 patients on the basis of positive gastric exercise tonometry. After revascularization 71% of the patients were free of symptoms. In all cases this was associated with normalized postprocedure tonometry and patent vessels.

DIFFERENTIAL DIAGNOSIS

There should be a high index of suspicion for the diagnosis of splanchnic ischemia in patients with chronic abdominal pain, especially if it occurs postprandially and/or in smokers.

If the more common causes of abdominal symptoms have been excluded, chronic splanchnic syndrome should be considered in the absence of a bruit or even in the absence of weight loss in patients with chronic abdominal symptoms, given one or more significant stenoses of the splanchnic arteries and a positive gastric exercise tonometry.

DIAGNOSTIC METHODS

Duplex ultrasound

Duplex ultrasound is the most widely used screening tool fo detection of splanchnic arterial stenosis. The physiologica differences between patients and inherent technical difficultie make splanchnic duplex ultrasound (US) results difficult t interpret. The influence of respiration, meal, exercise, anatomi variations, and collateral circulation on commonly used duple US parameters is not fully clarified. In experienced hands successful visualization of the celiac artery and the superic mesenteric artery (SMA) duplex can be obtained in 80–95% and in these cases US is a reliable screening test of chroni splanchnic disease. Using either the end diastolic velocit (EDV) or the peak systolic velocity (PSV) discrimination ca be made between patients with normal or stenotic vessels Moneta et al. reported cutoff values for PSV and EDV in th celiac artery of 200 cm/s and 55 cm/s, and in the SMA c 275 cm/s and 45 cm/s, respectively.[6] The optimal cutoff value depend on patient selection, expiration measurements, an whether the test is for diagnostic or screening purposes. Ther is poor correlation of anatomical information and abdomina symptoms. Consequently, if duplex US clearly demonstrate significant stenosis in the celiac artery and SMA origins thi may not be sufficient evidence for the existence of chroni splanchnic syndrome.

Magnetic resonance angiography (MRA)

Rapid developments in MRA technology have enabled non invasive visualization of the main visceral arteries. With th introduction of contrast-enhanced MRA, it has become possibl to obtain multiple thin slices in the coronal or frontal plane allowing for visualization of the celiac, the superior mesenteric and the inferior mesenteric artery in a single breath-hold o 20 ± 25 s. Owing to the acquisition of a three-dimensional dat set, the data can be reconstructed in any desired plane usin maximum-intensity-projections (MIP) or surface-renderin techniques. The orifices of the splanchnic vessels can therefor always be visualized with MRA. In a small study of 14 patient with correlative angiograms overall sensitivity and specificit of MRA was 100% and 95%, respectively.[7]

Functional magnetic resonance imaging (fMRI)

MRA can only depict the morphological appearance of th splanchnic vessels but it does not provide physiological evi dence for the symptoms of the patients. With fMRI functiona information on splanchnic blood flow can also be obtained Flow velocities and total flow volumes can be measured in th mesenteric vessels using two-dimensional cine phase contras velocity mapping. We have shown that portal venous flow meas urements are accurate and can be performed with low intra- and inter-subject variability.[8] fMRI has also been used to measure the oxygen saturation of hemoglobin in the blood. The principle behind MR oximetry is that deoxyhemoglobin in erythrocytes is paramagnetic, but oxyhemoglobin (HbO_2) is not. As blood flow decreases, oxygen extraction will increase to maintain the level of oxygen uptake.[9]

Combined approach

Combining morphological evaluation of the splanchnic vessels by MRA with a functional test (either by measurement of flow

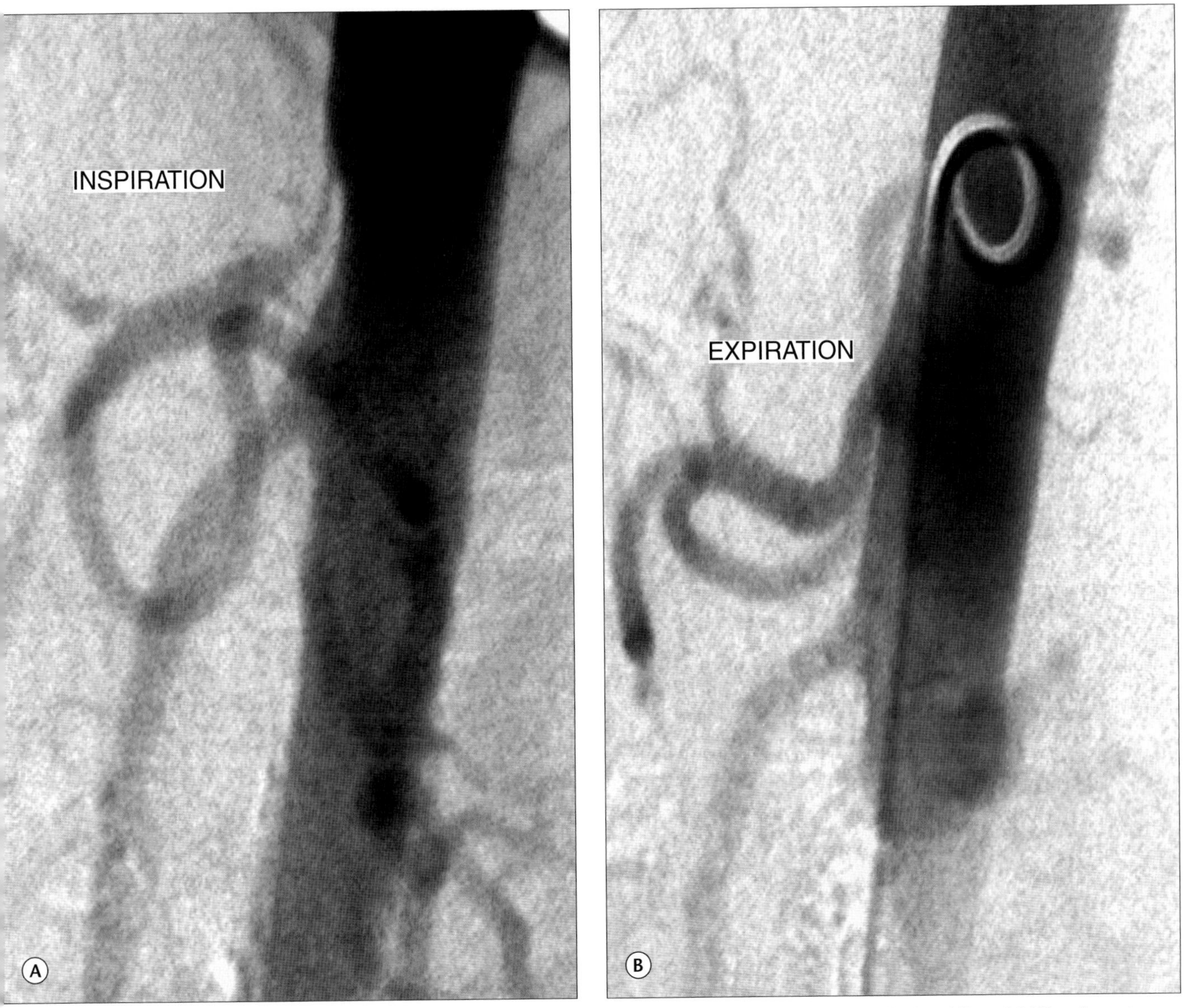

Fig. 67.1 Lateral aortal angiography in celiac artery compression syndrome. Normal celiac artery in inspiration **(A)** and 95% celiac artery stenoses in expiration **(B)**, when the celiac artery is pulled up towards the median arcuate ligament.

or %HbO_2) in a single session may become important in the detection of patients with chronic splanchnic syndrome.

Tonometry is based on a general characteristic of ischemic tissues in which lack of oxygen results in increased production of acids, which are buffered locally leading to increased PCO_2 (Fig. 67.2). Because CO_2 is a small molecule it rapidly diffuses over different membrane layers, the PCO_2 in the gastrointestinal lumen will equal the PCO_2 in the gastrointestinal mucosa. Mucosal ischemia is therefore invariably associated with increased gastrointestinal PCO_2. The latter can be measured using a balloon-tipped catheter, the tonometer, which is attached to a modified capnograph, the Tonocap. An increased PCO_2 gradient between the systemic circulation and the gastrointestinal mucosa indicates mucosal CO_2 production and therefore ischemia.[10] We have now performed over 300 gastric exercise tonometry tests in patients suspected of gastrointestinal ischemia; sensitivity and specificity approach 80% and 75%, respectively. Using jejunal tonometry we were able to show isolated small bowel ischemia in patients with superior mesenteric artery stenosis. Exercise tonometry can distinguish the asymptomatic chronic splanchnic artery disease from the symptomatic chronic splanchnic syndrome.[11]

Biplanar selective splanchnic angiography is still the gold standard for assessment of vascular anatomy and stenoses in the splanchnic vessels (Fig. 67.3A,B). The investigation consists of an anterior-posterior aortic abdominal aortogram, a lateral aortogram during maximal inspiration and expiration, and a selective angiography of all three splanchnic vessels. Collaterals already appearing on an aortic overview indicate origin stenosis and can therefore be considered as pathologic collaterals. With subsequent selective angiography detailed information on the vascular anatomy, stenoses, variations, and collateral anatomy can be obtained. This information is essential in preparation for an optimal revascularization strategy in view of the wide anatomic variations of the splanchnic circulation.

A reliable diagnosis of chronic splanchnic syndrome, based on a proven causal relationship between the occlusive disease and the symptoms, can be very difficult. A multidisciplinary approach including the gastroenterologist, vascular surgeon,

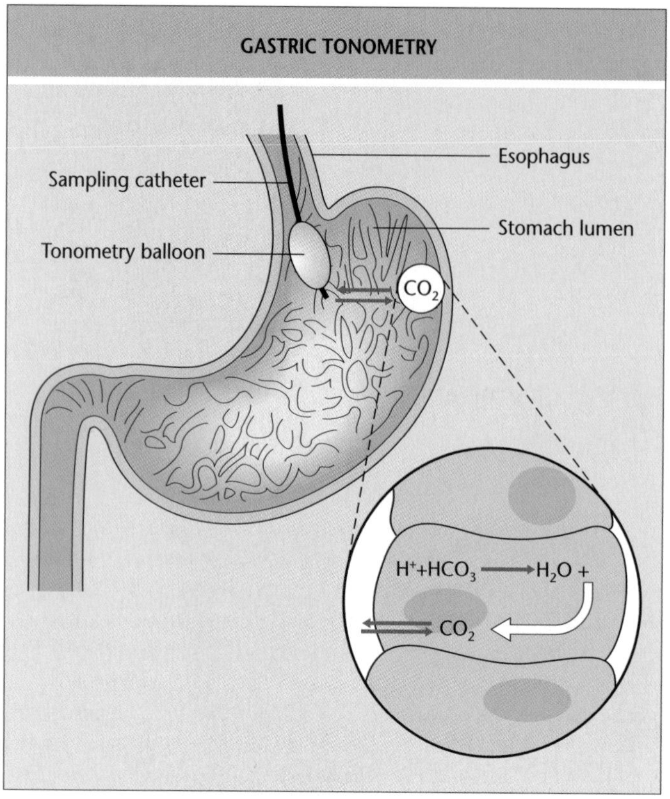

Fig. 67.2 Scheme of gastric tonometry.

and interventional radiologist can be of value in interpretation of symptoms and tests, and agreeing a management plan.

TREATMENT AND PREVENTION

Before considering intervention, information on the natural history of the disease is required. Theoretically, the options for intervention in symptomatic patients are conservative medical treatment, surgical reconstruction, and angioplasty. Unfortunately, information on the natural history of splanchnic occlusive disease and ischemia is scarce. Most lesions of the celiac artery and SMA are ostial stenoses and occlusions caused by atherosclerosis, and progression to occlusion can be anticipated. This has recently been confirmed by serial duplex evaluation as having a progression rate of approximately 20% per year. There is no evidence available supporting the conservative medical treatment of chronic splanchnic syndrome. Suggested treatments are: eat small meals, use omeprazole to diminish the oxygen demand of the gastric mucosa, refrain from smoking, and use vasodilative drugs to diminish vasospasm. The objective effect of all these therapies is unknown.

A variety of surgical and endovascular techniques, such as reimplantation, transarterial and transaortic endarterectomy, antegrade and retrograde aortovisceral bypass using vein or arterial autograft bypasses and prosthetic bypasses, have been advocated for repairing the splanchnic vessels (Fig. 67.4A–C). The conclusions of many reports are flawed by variety in patient

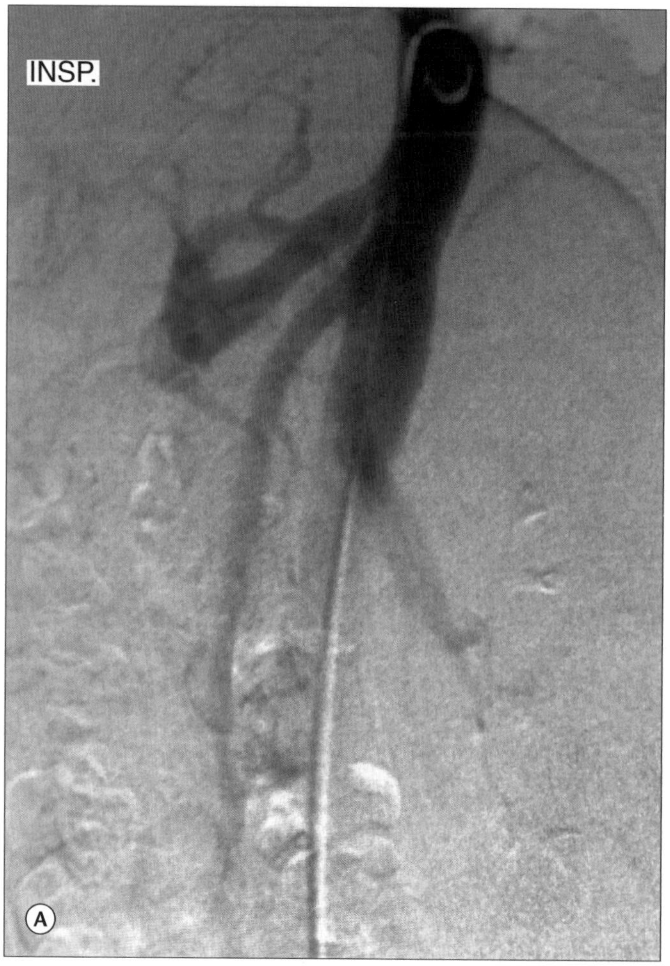

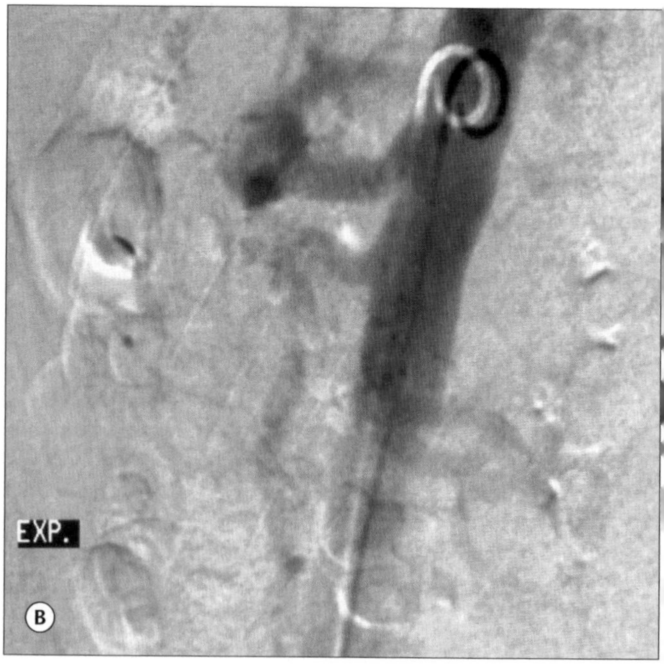

Fig. 67.3 Lateral aortal angiography. Normal celiac artery and superior mesenteric artery in inspiration **(A)** and 70% stenoses in expiration **(B)**.

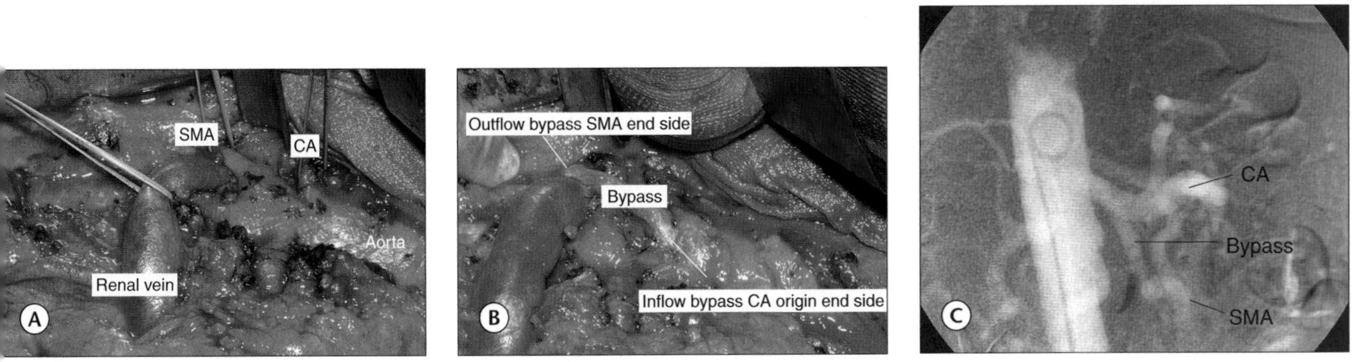

Fig. 67.4 *In vivo* view of the celiac and proximal part of superior mesenteric artery after left retroperitoneal visceral rotation **(A)**, and *in vivo* autologous bypass to celiac and superior mesenteric artery **(B)**. Postreconstruction lateral aortal angiography **(C)**.

selection, a relatively short follow-up, and insufficient documentation of the patency of the reconstructions. Consequently, the evidence for the various methods and techniques used in the diagnosis and treatment of chronic splanchnic ischemia is usually based on the preference and experience of the authors rather than being evidence based. The in-hospital mortality is reported in most series to be below 5%. Patency objectively determined by angiography and/or duplex ultrasound and calculated by the life table method is rarely reported. McMillan et al.[12] presented their results as such and reported patency between 89% and 93% at 36 months and 89% at 72 months. Kihara et al.[13] reported a 73% patency rate at 24 months. Repair of only one of the occluded splanchnic arteries may relieve the symptoms of chronic splanchnic syndrome.[14] However, the best long-term results are reported from surgical repair of more than one artery.[15] Recurrent splanchnic ischemia after a failed revascularization is common. Schneider et al.[16] reported from one of the centers with the largest experience a prevalence rate of up to a third of patients. Recurrent ischemia was associated with younger age, greater weight loss, and modification of surgical technique at the time of initial operation. Multiple techniques were used in the first or second reoperations. Postoperative mortality and complication rates were 6.7% for the first and 33% for the second reoperation. Symptoms recurred in six out of 22 patients (27.3%) after the first reoperation; three of the six were cured or improved after additional reoperations. The life table symptom-free survival was 63% at 5 years.

Encouraging early results using angioplasty with stenting (Fig. 67.5A–C) suggest that this type of intervention may relieve symptoms in selected patients with a higher surgical risk.[17] Percutaneous transluminal angioplasty is gaining favor, with reports of similar patency achieved compared to surgery but with lower mortality.[18] This may come at the cost of a higher incidence of recurrent symptoms.[19]

The surgical treatment of celiac artery compression syndrome consists of decompression of the celiac artery at the diaphragm

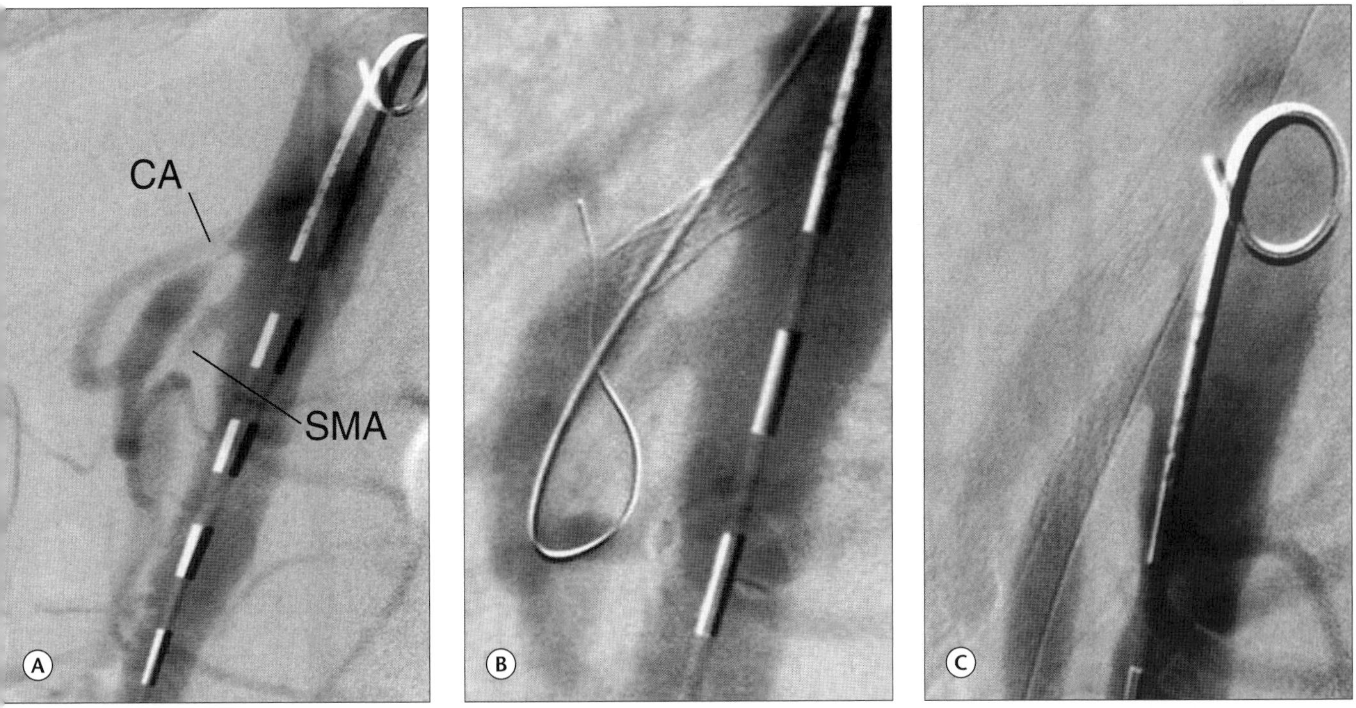

Fig. 67.5 Lateral aortal angiography. Two-vessel chronic splanchnic syndrome. **A.** Severe stenoses in celiac and superior mesenteric artery. Bridge® stents in the celiac **(B)** and the superior mesenteric artery **(C)**.

by a careful division of the crural fibers and nerve tissue. Intra-operative duplex is essential in these patients because long-standing compression can cause localized and severe celiac artery damage that should be treated by a vascular reconstruction. The less favorable outcome in some series may indeed be explained by operative techniques that consisted of release only, and did not ascertain vessel patency. In our recent series 5 out of 21 patients showed no improvement of symptoms afte celiac artery release or reconstruction. Four of these patient had restenosis of the celiac artery. In celiac artery compressio syndrome stent placement is not indicated because repeate pressure from the arcuate ligament with each respiratory cycl can damage the stents. The stents actually fractured 1–2 yea after their placement.

REFERENCES

1. Roobottom CA, Dubbins PA. Significant disease of the celiac and superior mesenteric arteries in asymptomatic patients: predictive value of Doppler sonography. Am J Roentgenol 1993; 161:985–988.
2. Connolly JE, Kwaan JHM. Prophylactic revascularization of the gut. Ann Surg 1979; 190:514–521.
3. Thomas JH, Blake K, Pierce GE, Hermreck AS, Seigel E. The clinical course of asymptomatic mesenteric arterial stenosis [see comments]. J Vasc Surg 1998; 27:840–844.
4. Holland AJ, Ibach EG. Long-term review of coeliac axis compression syndrome. Ann R Coll Surg Engl 1996; 78:470–472.
5. Faries PL, Narula A, Veith FJ et al. The use of gastric tonometry in the assessment of celiac artery compression syndrome. Ann Vasc Surg 2000; 14:20–23.
6. Moneta GL, Lee RW, Yeager RA, Taylor LM, Jr, Porter JM. Mesenteric duplex scanning: a blinded prospective study. J Vasc Surg 1993; 17:79–84.
7. Carlos RC, Stanley JC, Stafford-Johnson D, Prince MR. Interobserver variability in the evaluation of chronic mesenteric ischemia with gadolinium-enhanced MR angiography. Acad Radiol 2001; 8:879–887.
8. Lycklama A, Nijeholt GJ, Burggraaf K et al. Variability of splanchnic blood flow measurements using MR velocity mapping under fasting and post-prandial conditions – comparison with echo-Doppler [see comments]. J Hepatol 1997; 26:298–304.
9. Li KC, Dalman RL, Ch'en IY et al. Chronic mesenteric ischemia: use of in vivo MR imaging measurements of blood oxygen saturation in the superior mesenteric vein for diagnosis. Radiology 1997; 204:71–77.
10. Kolkman JJ, Otte JA, Groeneveld AB. Gastrointestinal luminal PCO_2 tonometry: an update on physiology, methodology and clinical applications. Br J Anaesth 2000; 84:74–86.
11. Otte JA, Oostveen E, Geelkerken RH, Groeneveld AB, Kolkman JJ. Exercise induces gastric ischemia in healthy volunteers: a tonometry study. J Appl Physiol 2001; 91:866–871.
12. McMillan WD, McCarthy WJ, Bresticker MR et al. Mesenteric artery bypass: objective patency determination. J Vasc Surg 1995; 21:729–740.
13. Kihara TK, Blebea J, Anderson KM, Friedman D, Atnip RG. Risk factors and outcomes following revascularization for chronic mesenteric ischemia. Ann Vasc Surg 1999; 13:37–44.
14. Christensen MG, Lorentzen JE, Schroeder TV. Revascularisation of atherosclerotic mesenteric arteries: experience in 90 consecutive patients [see comments]. Eur J Vasc Surg 1994; 8:297–302.
15. Geelkerken RH, Van Bockel JH, De Roos WK Hermans J, Terpstra JL. Chronic mesenteric vascular syndrome. Results of reconstructive surgery. Arch Surg 1991; 126:1101–1106.
16. Schneider DB, Schneider PA, Reilly LM, Ehrenfeld WK, Messina LM, Stoney RJ. Reoperation for recurrent chronic visceral ischemia. J Vasc Surg 1998; 27:276–284.
17. van Wanroij JL, van Petersen AS, Huisman AB et al. Endovascular treatment of chronic splanchnic syndrome. Eur J Vasc Endovasc Surg 2004; 28:193–200.
18. Nyman U, Ivancev K, Lindh M, Uher P. Endovascular treatment of chronic mesenteri ischemia: report of five cases. Cardiovasc Intervent Radiol 1998; 21:305–313.
19. Kasirajan K, O'Hara PJ, Gray BH, Hertzer NR, Clair DG, Greenberg RK et al. Chronic mesenteric ischemia: Open surgery versus percutaneous angioplasty and stenting. J Vas Surg 2001; 33:63–71.

Chapter 68

Drug-induced damage to the small and large intestine

Ingvar Bjarnason, Ken Takeuchi, Laurence Maiden, and Samuel N Adler

KEY POINTS

- NSAID enteropathy is probably more common than gastropathy, and small bowel bleeding is probably as common as gastric bleeding
- 50–60% of patients receiving NSAIDs develop NSAID enteropathy within a few weeks of treatment
- Aspirin is rarely associated with small bowel damage
- NSAID-induced diaphragm strictures may be missed by barium studies
- The commonest manifestations of NSAID enteropathy are anemia and hypoalbuminemia
- Treatment may involve drug cessation, metronidazole, sulfasalazine, or misoprostol

INTRODUCTION

The gastrointestinal tract is a frequent site for adverse drug reactions. This may be by virtue of the fact that most prescribed and over-the-counter preparations are administered orally, exposing both the stomach and small bowel to high concentrations of drugs. Yet parenteral administration is not without intestinal complications, e.g., peptic ulceration from topical nonsteroidal anti-inflammatory gels or debilitating diarrhea following intravenous systemic chemotherapy. Many drugs will cause some unwanted side effects (e.g., nausea, diarrhea) at serum or plasma concentrations within their therapeutic range. It is important to differentiate between:

1. predictable side effects, i.e., resulting from a known pharmacological action of the drug;
2. those causing or aggravating underlying pathology;
3. those with no identifiable cause (idiosyncratic reaction); and
4. dose-related toxicity, especially if there is a narrow therapeutic range, e.g., lithium.

In this chapter we describe important drug-induced diseases of the small and large intestines.

SMALL INTESTINAL DISEASE

There is no widely accepted classification for drug-induced intestinal disease. The most common types of drug-induced problems are due to their propensity to cause mucosal damage and interfere with absorption and motility.

Mucosal damage

Various drugs can cause mucosal damage to the small bowel. The damage is characterized by inflammation often associated with malabsorption, bleeding, and protein loss which may progress to ulceration, which is in turn associated with serious complications such as perforation, overt bleeding, and strictures. Table 68.1 shows the drugs that are most commonly associated with de novo small bowel damage.

Nonsteroidal anti-inflammatory drugs (NSAIDs) are the prototype for this kind of damage and deserve a more detailed description because of the frequency of this complication.

NSAID enteropathy (see Chapter 25)

Conventional NSAIDs that inhibit cyclooxygenase (COX) 1 and 2 frequently cause damage through the gastrointestinal tract.[1,2] The stomach is often adversely affected (NSAID gastropathy),[3] but NSAID enteropathy is equally if not more prevalent than the gastropathy[4] and is associated with almost identical serious outcomes.[5] NSAID enteropathy remains underdiagnosed because of the lack of specific diagnostic tests, but causes much morbidity and at times is a source of mortality in patients on long-term NSAIDs.

Pathogenesis

Almost all the information on the pathogenesis of NSAID enteropathy comes from studies in rodents.[6] We can take the prevailing and simplistic view (and many do!) that NSAID-induced COX-1 inhibition accounts for most of the damage because this leads to very low levels of mucosal prostaglandins that are otherwise essential for the maintenance of intestinal integrity.[7] Alternatively, we can explore the pathogenesis further

TABLE 68.1 DRUGS CAUSING SMALL INTESTINAL MUCOSAL ULCERATION AND HEMORRHAGE

- NSAIDs
- Potassium
- Cocaine
- Chemotherapeutic agents:
  - Actinomycin D
  - Bleomycin
  - Cytosine
  - Arabinoside
  - Doxorubicin
  - 5-fluorouracil
  - Methotrexate
  - Vincristine
- Oral contraceptive pills
- Gold
- Arsenic

in view of ongoing research and the situation is rather more complex.[6,8] The single most important point is that selective COX-1 inhibition or absence (COX-1 knockout animals) appears to have no pathophysiological consequences, and does not lead to gastrointestinal damage.[2,9,10] Rather, NSAIDs initiate small bowel damage by a combination of different biochemical actions. This may involve:

1. dual COX-1 and COX-2 inhibition;
2. COX-1 inhibition plus the topical effect (defined as nonprostaglandin-mediated effect which requires direct contact of the drug from the lumenal side of the mucosa); and
3. possibly COX-2 inhibition and the topical effect (without a concomitant decrease in total mucosal prostaglandin levels).

At present it seems as though the primary pathophysiologic consequence of COX-1 inhibition (and decreased prostaglandins) is a compromise in the microcirculation to the mucosa with impaired oxygenation.[11] COX-2 inhibition may compromise inflammatory responses and resolution and the topical effect may impair the intestinal barrier function because of an interaction with surface membrane lipid[12] or an effect to uncouple mitochondrial oxidative phosphorylation.[13] The above combinations appear to initiate the damage on a cellular level, which then leads to the same phenotypic small bowel damage. How this occurs is a matter of substantial controversy. One suggestion is that the small bowel damage is relayed through increased intestinal permeability.[4] This shifts the balance between the luminal aggressors and mucosal defense in favor of the former, which allows commensal luminal bacteria access to the mucosa. This elicits a neutrophil response (a defining feature of NSAID enteropathy is the acute inflammation). The neutrophils are activated on contact with the bacteria and undergo a respiratory burst and degranulation, both of which damage the surrounding tissue. Concomitant compromised microcirculation (due to inhibition of COX-1) contributes further to the damage.

Prevalence and diagnosis

Fifty to sixty per cent of patients receiving conventional NSAIDs develop small bowel inflammation (NSAID enteropathy) within a few weeks of ingestion.[4] The prevalence and severity of the inflammation is similar with all the acidic NSAIDs, apart from aspirin, which is rarely associated with small bowel damage.[14] NSAID enteropathy is usually low grade and certainly an order of magnitude less than seen in active inflammatory bowel disease. It is predominantly mid–small intestine in location which poses a problem for diagnosis, as it is so inaccessible. It is possible to document the presence of this inflammation by demonstrating increased intestinal permeability or with surrogate markers of intestinal inflammation (using ^{111}indium-labeled white cell fecal excretion or fecal calprotectin concentrations),[15,16] but these markers of damage are not specific for NSAID-induced damage. The inflammation is out of reach of the push enteroscope. Sonde enteroscopy, a prolonged (10h) and uncomfortable procedure, allows visualization of the whole of the small intestine and shows lesions in over 50% of patients on NSAIDs and may be diagnostic.[17]

Video capsule endoscopy has permitted a noninvasive and more accurate diagnosis of NSAID enteropathy. Patients swallow a small camera after an overnight fast. The video capsule takes approximately 50 000 pictures during its intestinal transit. These images are transmitted to an external receiver and analyzed.[18] NSAID enteropathy has a range of appearances. Firstly, there may be scattered petechiae with or without evidence of intralumenal blood. Secondly, there are distinct mucosal lesions compromising ulcers and erosions collectively known as 'mucosal breaks.' These mucosal breaks (Fig. 68.1) are sometimes seen to bleed as the capsule irritates them mechanically. In some patients on conventional NSAIDs there is evidence of semilunar diaphragms (Fig. 68.2). These represent the early developmental phase of 'diaphragm disease,' one of the serious outcomes of

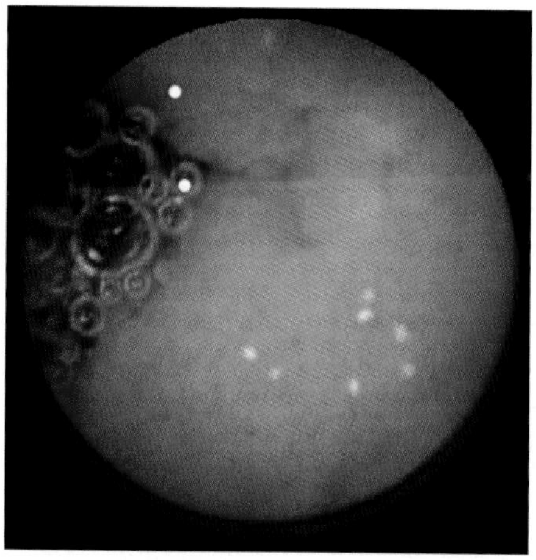

Fig. 68.1 Video capsule endoscopy. Video capsule endoscopic image in a patient on NSAIDs who presented with abdominal pain and a mild anemia. There is a clear-cut small bowel ulcer with a white-yellow base.

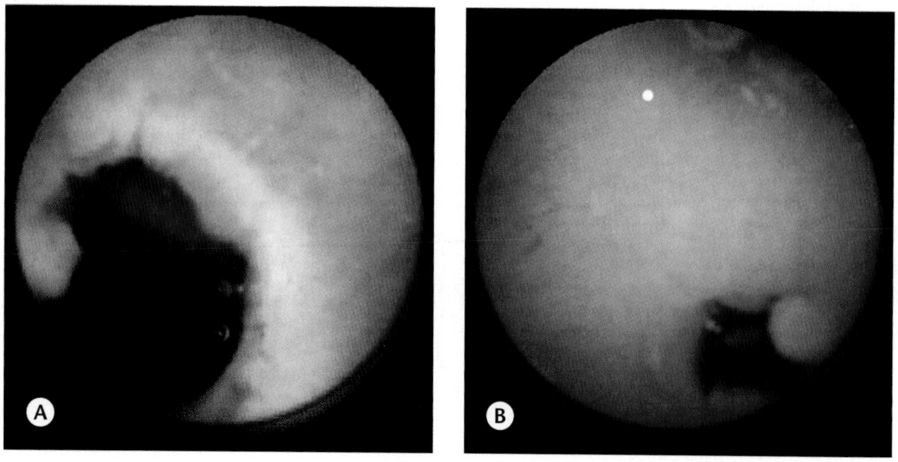

Fig. 68.2 Video capsule endoscopy of 'diaphragm' strictures. Video capsule endoscopic images of 'diaphragm' strictures that are pathognomonic for NSAID-induced damage. **A.** A semilunar white diaphragm represents an earlier stage of fully developed NSAID-induced 'diaphragm' disease. **B.** A fully developed 'diaphragm' stricture of the small bowel in the 5 o'clock position. These usually present with symptoms of intermittent subacute small bowel obstruction.

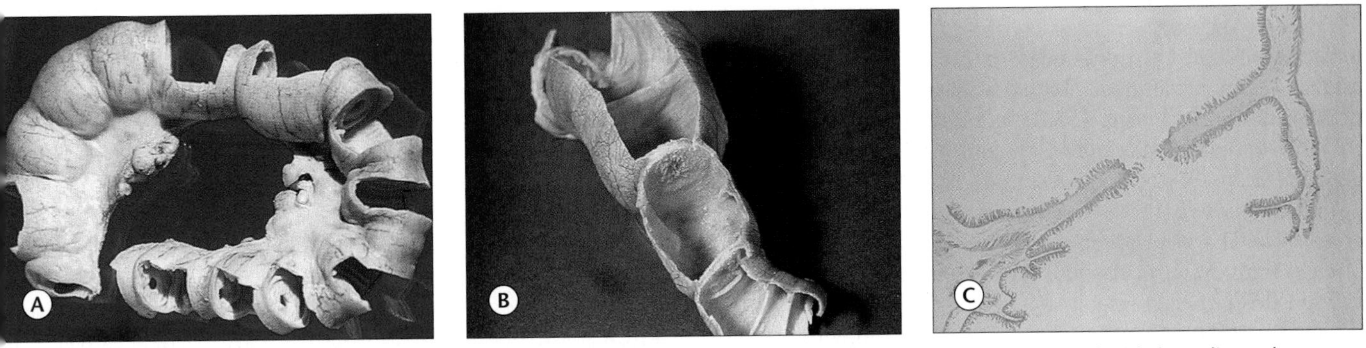

Fig. 68.3 'Diaphragm' disease of the small bowel. The surgical resection specimens in parts A and B were inflated with formalin under pressure. **A.** Patient on long-term NSAIDs presented with symptoms of subacute small bowel obstruction and underwent laparotomy. A segment of small bowel was resected. The exterior shows regular and multiple dimples and when opened up these represent the 'diaphragms' with marked luminal compromise. **B.** Surgical resection specimen from a patient on NSAIDs who presented with complete obstruction. There is prestenotic dilation of the bowel to a concentric 'diaphragm' that has closed the lumen to a pinhole. **C.** Characteristic histopathology of NSAID-induced 'diaphragm' disease of the small bowel. The diaphragm is composed of mucosal fibrosis with minimal acute inflammation at the lesion tip. The muscularis propria is not seen within the diaphragm (which would be pathognomonic of congenital developmental abnormalities).

NSAID enteropathy (Fig. 68.3).[19] Even when strictures and ulcers are present there is usually insufficient distortion for these to be detected by barium studies.

Complications

NSAID enteropathy, despite being associated with erosions and ulcers, is probably asymptomatic. Many clinicians do not therefore perceive this as a clinical problem. However, the consequences of this pathology can lead to problems of anemia due to long-standing blood loss. Protein loss also occurs but is usually not manifest clinically because of compensation by the liver to increase synthesis. The serious events of perforation, overt bleeding, and strictures mandate case-specific treatment.[4]

Bleeding

Figure 68.4 shows that virtually all patients with NSAID enteropathy bleed and there is a significant correlation between the inflammation and bleeding. This bleeding is mild ranging from 1 to 8 mL/day, which by itself is insufficient to lead to an iron deficiency anemia.[20] However, in patients with active rheumatoid arthritis who may have an impaired appetite, hypochlorhydria (due to co-treatment with proton pump inhibitors, etc.), or malabsorption of iron the low-grade bleeding may be an important contributory factor for the development of iron deficiency anemia. The iron deficiency is difficult to diagnose (may require bone marrow examination) as the blood film appearances (hypochromic microcytosis) are overshadowed by the features seen in the anemia of chronic disease (normochromic macrocytosis). Many rheumatologists have a rule of thumb to initiate iron supplementation in their rheumatoid patients when the hemoglobin level falls below 10 g/L. Nevertheless, many patients undergo endo- and colonoscopy to reduce the possibility of intestinal malignancy being missed. Although it has been possible to diagnose small intestinal bleeding with Sonde enteroscopy, video capsule endoscopy is now the preferred technique to provide a positive diagnosis.

Protein loss

Most of the patients with NSAID enteropathy have a mild protein-losing enteropathy. This is of no clinical significance in the majority of patients as the liver has a substantial reserve capacity to produce albumin. However, about 10% of hospitalized patients with rheumatoid arthritis have symptomatic (peripheral edema, congestive heart failure, and even ascites) hypoalbuminemia as a complication of NSAID enteropathy, in which case targeted treatment for the enteropathy is called for.

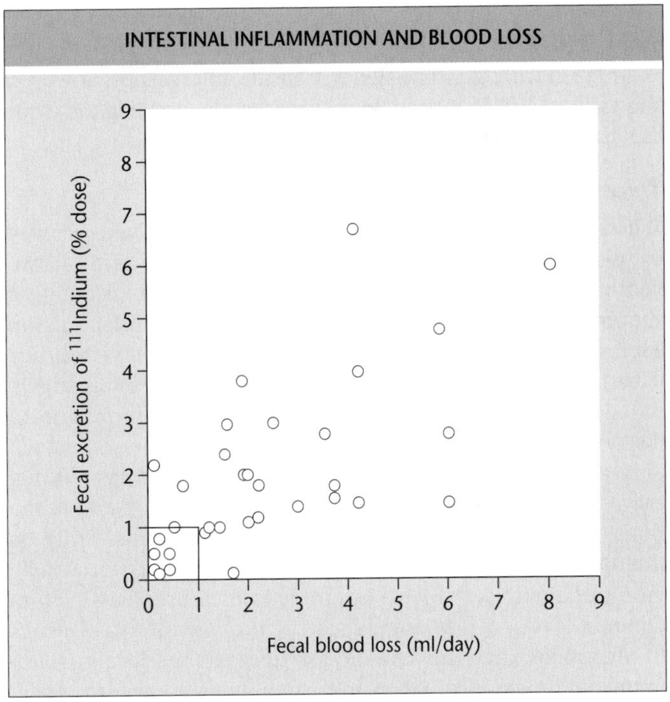

Fig. 68.4 Intestinal inflammation and blood loss. Patients with rheumatoid and osteoarthritis on long-term NSAIDs underwent simultaneous study to assess intestinal inflammation (indium 111-labeled white cell fecal excretion) and blood loss (chromium 51 labeling of red cells). There is a significant correlation between the intestinal inflammatory activity and the intestinal bleeding. Patients with no inflammation (white cell excretion of less than 1%) do not bleed excessively (normal blood loss of less than 1 mL/day).

Serious outcomes

Serious outcomes are defined as overt bleeding, perforation, and strictures usually originating from ulcers. The prevalence of these complications in NSAID-induced gastro- and enteropathy are very similar, namely 60% and 40%, respectively, with absolute annual prevalence rates of 1–2%.[5]

Clinically, overt rectal bleeding is well described from discrete small bowel ulcers in patients with NSAID enteropathy, but is relatively rare. If small bowel bleeding is defined as a sudden drop of hemoglobin by 2 g/L in a person on NSAIDs who has undergone normal endo- and colonoscopy then bleeding from the small bowel is as common as the overt gastric bleedings associated with NSAID gastropathy.

Small bowel perforation, presenting as an acute abdomen, is also perceived as a rare complication of NSAID enteropathy, but requires immediate surgery. It is also worrying that a large autopsy study showed that some patients on NSAIDs had an unexpected (undiagnosed) perforated small bowel ulcer that had contributed to their death.[21]

'Diaphragm' disease of the small bowel is a pathognomonic lesion associated with NSAID enteropathy.[4,22] These are multiple (ranging from 3 to 100), concentric, thin (2–3 mm), fibrous septa that may narrow the lumen to a pinhole (Fig. 68.3). The strictures are usually found in the mid-small bowel although an increasing number is being described at colonoscopy (cecum and right colon) in patients on sustained release formulations of NSAIDs. Most patients with 'diaphragm' strictures have had recurrent iron deficiency anemia and at times hypoalbuminemia, suggestive of a severe NSAID enteropathy.[19] They present with symptoms of intermittent sub-acute small bowel obstruction, i.e., postprandial pain, nausea, and vomiting. Prior to the capsule enteroscopy the diagnosis had to be made on clinical grounds, as conventional small bowel barium studies do not show these with any consistency. Capsule enteroscopy, however, shows the early lesions of semilunar diaphragms (Fig. 68.3) or the classical fully developed stricture (Fig. 68.2B)

Treatment

When NSAID enteropathy leads to problematic iron deficiency or hypoalbuminemia this should be treated according to conventional lines, iron supplementation, etc., but consideration should also be given to treating the intestinal inflammation itself. As yet there are only uncontrolled comparative efficacy trials for NSAID enteropathy.[4] The following algorithm is largely based on personal experience. The first line approach is to discontinue NSAIDs if possible. Treatment with metronidazole (any anaerobic antimicrobial is likely to be effective) 400 mg twice a day for 4–6 weeks reduces the inflammation and at the same time bleeding and protein loss, even if patients continue their NSAID intake.[23] The effectiveness of the treatment can be monitored with serial fecal calprotectin measurements. Serum albumin levels, if low, usually start improving after 2–3 weeks of treatment, but the benefit for hemoglobin levels is not immediately evident unless iron supplements are also given. Where patients wish to continue their NSAIDs we consider treatment with sulfasalazine 1 g three times a day for the long term. Alternatively, misoprostol (200 μg 3–4 times a day) can be given to heal or prevent the enteropathy.

Consideration of prescribing COX-2 selective agents should be made at an early stage. These drugs have been shown to be free of small intestinal side effects when taken in the short term. This is a good predictor of long-term safety although the long-term small bowel tolerability of these agents has not been specifically assessed in man.[24]

The serious consequences of NSAID enteropathy (overt bleeding, perforation, and strictures) need to be dealt with as a matter of urgency. The clinically overt bleeding often requires blood transfusion and surgery is rarely avoided.

Small bowel perforation, if detected, is an indication for laparotomy. The decision to proceed to surgery in patients with 'diaphragm disease' is now, with the increasing use of capsule enteroscopy, relatively straightforward. When surgery is undertaken the operation of choice is a stricturoplasty rather than resection because the strictures are so numerous in many cases.

Summary

Conventional acidic NSAIDs frequently cause small bowel inflammation. Investigation of NSAID enteropathy provides a blueprint for the investigation of the other drug-induced small bowel damage. Apart from the clinical consequences listed above one of the underestimated consequences of NSAID enteropathy is the financial cost of investigation, which may involve imaging of the whole of the gastrointestinal tract.

OTHER (NON-NSAID) DRUG-INDUCED INJURY OF THE SMALL AND LARGE INTESTINE

Certain preparations of potassium chloride were a common cause for small bowel damage in the past. These preparations ran the risk of adhering to the small bowel mucosa with local release of high concentrations of potassium, sufficient to cause vasoconstriction, ischemia, and ulcers.[25] Potassium salts are now formulated in such a way as to minimize the risk of this damage, e.g., a controlled-release wax matrix system. Oral contraceptive pills have been reported to cause mesenteric venous and arterial thrombosis, which, again, lead to ischemia and necrosis of the small bowel. Chemotherapeutic agents affect cells with a rapid turnover, including those of the gastrointestinal tract. Those listed in Table 68.1 can cause erosive enteritis, features of which include pain, bleeding, ileus, diarrhea, and vomiting.

A variety of drugs can give rise to intestinal bleeding (see Table 68.2). The risk of bleeding is dependent on a number of factors that include drug dose, clotting parameters, concomitant medications, and comorbid disorders. Warfarin in particular is notorious for causing overt gastrointestinal bleeding. In half of such cases the bleeding site will be in the small bowel. Rarely, these drugs cause intramucosal hematomas that can present with obstructive symptoms.

TABLE 68.2 DRUGS CAUSING MUCOSAL HEMORRHAGE

- Anticoagulants
- Antiplatelet drugs
- Thrombolytic drugs
- Glycogen IIb/IIIa inhibitors
- Levodopa

Malabsorption

Drugs may have a direct effect on intestinal mucosa causing a generalized impairment of absorption or they may interact with particular absorption pathways leading to selective malabsorption. Table 68.3 lists the drugs more commonly associated with this pathology.

Most of the drugs that cause mucosal damage and malabsorption interfere with cell mitoses and may cause subtotal or partial villous atrophy. This may manifest as an iron deficiency anemia, low serum folates, or even hypocalcemia. Fat malabsorption presenting as mild steatorrhea may also be a common presenting feature.

Motility

Motility of the small bowel may be influenced by drugs but to a lesser extent than the colon (see Chapter 66). Table 68.4 shows drugs that are commonly associated with motility problems of both the small and large intestine.

Increased motility of the small bowel may result in diarrhea (see Chapter 9), although clinically it may be difficult to tell whether such symptoms are, in fact, attributable to small or large intestinal pathology. Increased motility may be the result of interference with the normal fluid and electrolyte balance of the gut. Magnesium salts predictably cause an osmotic diarrhea as do the laxatives lactulose and polyethylene glycol. Digoxin inhibits the sodium-potassium pump involved in the active transport of water and electrolytes across the cell membrane and occasionally leads to problematic diarrhea.

A drug-induced neuropathy may produce profuse diarrhea similar to that seen in diabetic autonomic neuropathy; vincristine has been associated with such a phenomenon.

Drugs may also reduce motility. Occasionally, this may be so severe as to cause a paralytic ileus (see Chapter 66). Tricyclic antidepressants and loperamide are good examples of such a drug reaction. The antimuscarinic, antiparkinsonian drugs such as benzhexol, benzatropine, and orphenadrine frequently inhibit motility contributing to severe constipation (see Chapter 63) whereas the dopaminergic, antiparkinsonian drugs selegiline and entacapone may cause either diarrhea or constipation. Interestingly, levodopa appears to have no adverse effect on gut motility. Usually, cessation of the drug results in resolution of the dysmotility. However, this may not be practicable, in particular with the constipation seen in Parkinson's disease and patients are frequently prescribed drugs to combat constipation.

TABLE 68.3 DRUGS CAUSING MALABSORPTION

MUCOSAL DAMAGE
- Allopurinol
- Colchicine
- Methotrexate
- Methyldopa
- Neomycin
- NSAIDs

INTERACTION
- Tetracycline chelates calcium
- Cholestyramine binds iron and vitamin B_{12}
- Thiazides impair Na^+ transport
- Aluminum and magnesium hydroxides precipitate calcium and phosphate ions

TABLE 68.4 DRUGS AFFECTING INTESTINAL MOTILITY

Increased motility (diarrhea)	Decreased motility (constipation)
GASTROINTESTINAL DRUGS	**ANTICHOLINERGIC PHARMACOLOGY**
Laxatives	Anticholinergic drugs
Magnesium antacids	Tricyclic antidepressants
Misoprostol	Antiparkinsonian drugs
Proton pump inhibitors	Atropine
5-amino salicylates	Hyoscine
CARDIAC DRUGS	**OTHER DRUGS**
Beta blockers	Opiate drugs
Digitalis	Vincristine
Quinidine	Sucralfate
Procainamide	Aluminum/calcium antacids
Diuretics	Calcium channel blockers
ACE inhibitors	Cholestyramine
Hydralazine	
LIPID-LOWERING DRUGS	
Clofibrate	
Gemfibrozil	
Statins	
NEUROPSYCHIATRIC DRUGS	
Lithium	
Fluoxetine	
Sodium valproate	
Ethosuximide	
MISCELLANEOUS	
NSAIDs	
Thyroxine	
Colchicine	
Theophylline	
Chemotherapeutic agents	

LARGE INTESTINAL DISEASE

Drug-induced colonic disease is not as common as that of the small bowel, presumably as most drugs are completely absorbed before reaching the colon. There are isolated case reports of drugs causing colitis but motility problems may be more common.

Colitis

Antibiotics may commonly cause diarrhea but a more serious adverse effect is pseudomembranous colitis (see Chapter 58). Originally attributed to clindamycin, although virtually any antibiotic can cause it, pseudomembranous colitis is the result of *Clostridium difficile* overgrowth of the colon when such broad-spectrum antibiotics have killed the normal flora. *Clostridium difficile* produces a toxin that induces damage to the gut mucosa leading to the colitis. The antibiotics more commonly associated with pseudomembranous colitis are listed in Table 68.5. Apart from NSAIDs, which have already been discussed and frequently cause proctitis when give as a suppository (and may cause strictures), drug-induced colitis is rarely seen in clinical practice. Drug-induced colitis can usually be distinguished from

TABLE 68.5 DRUGS THAT CAUSE COLITIS

ANTIBIOTICS
Amoxicillin
Ampicillin
Clindamycin
Erythromycin
Cephalosporins
DRUGS CAUSING ISCHEMIC COLITIS
Oral contraceptive pill
Chemotherapeutic agents – 5 fluorouracil, cisplatin
Danazol
Vasopressin
Clindamycin
MISCELLANEOUS
NSAIDs
Methyldopa
Penicillamine
Gold (oral)

classical inflammatory bowel disease (ulcerative colitis and Crohn's disease) by endoscopic and histologic features and by elimination of suspect drugs.

Dysmotility

Many of the agents shown in Table 68.4 that affect the small bowel, giving rise to diarrhea or constipation, also affect the colon. Of note, however, is the excessive use of laxatives. Apart from the diarrhea that may be provoked by their use (or misuse), anthraquinones such as senna can damage the myenteric plexus of the colon when used chronically. This atonic (cathartic) colon can result in constipation often resulting in the use of further purgatives. Long-term anthraquinone use can also lead to melanosis coli.

CONCLUSION

A number of commonly used drugs are associated with gastrointestinal side effects that may cause symptoms suggestive of serious underlying disease. In many cases it is sufficient to discontinue the drug and switch to another drug with a similar action. When the drugs have caused structural damage it may also be necessary to treat the inflammation or ulcers. With the increased use of drugs in the aging population and increasing tendency for prescribing multiple drugs in the long term, it is likely that the side effects discussed in this chapter will become more frequent.

REFERENCES

1. Wallace JL, McKnight, Reuter BK, Vergnolle N. Dual inhibition of both cyclooxygenase (COX)-1 and COX-2 is required for NSAID-induced erosion formation. Gastroenterology 2000; 119:704–714.
2. Sigthorsson G, Simpson RJ, Walley M et al. COX-1 and 2, intestinal integrity and pathogenesis of NSAID enteropathy in mice. Gastroenterology 2002; 122:1913–1923.
3. Hawkey CJ. Nonsteroidal anti-inflammatory drug gastropathy. Gastroenterology 2000; 119:521–535.
4. Bjarnason I, Hayllar J, Macpherson AJ, Russell AS. Side effects of nonsteroidal anti-inflammatory drugs on the small and large intestine. Gastroenterology 1993; 104:1832–1847.
5. Laine L, Connors LG, Reicin A et al. Serious lower gastrointestinal clinical events with nonselective NSAID or coxib use. Gastroenterology 2003; 124:288–292.
6. Whittle BJR. Unwanted effects of aspirin and related agents on the gastrointestinal tract. In: Vane JR, Botting RM, eds. Aspirin and other salicylates. London: Chapman & Hall Medical; 1992:465–509.
7. Hawkey CJ. COX-2 inhibitors. Lancet 1999; 353:301–314.
8. Somasundaram S, Hayllar J, Rafi S, Wrigglesworth J, Macpherson A, Bjarnason I. The biochemical basis of NSAID-induced damage to the gastrointestinal tract: A review and a hypothesis. Scand J Gastroenterol 1995; 30:289–299.
9. Langenbach R, Morham SG, Tiano HF et al. Prostaglandin synthase 1 gene disruption in mice reduced arachidonic acid-induced inflammation and indomethacin-induced gastric ulceration. Cell 1995; 83:483–492.
10. Morham SG, Langenbach R, Loftin CD et al. Prostaglandin synthase 2 gene disruption causes severe renal pathology in the mouse. Cell 1995; 83:473–482.
11. Wallace JL. Nonsteroidal anti-inflammatory drugs and gastroenteropathy: the second hundred years. Gastroenterology 1997; 112:1000–1016.
12. Lichtenberger LM, Wang Z-M, Romero JJ et al. Non-steroidal anti-inflammatory drugs (NSAIDs) associate with zwitterionic phospholipids: Insight into the mechanism and reversal of NSAID-induced gastrointestinal injury. Nature Medicine 1995; 1:154–158.
13. Mahmud T, Rafi SS, Scott DL, Wrigglesworth JM, Bjarnason I. Nonsteroidal antiinflammatory drugs and uncoupling of mitochondrial oxidative phosphorylation. Arth Rheum 1996; 39:1998–2003.
14. Sigthorsson G, Tibble J, Hayllar J et al. Intestinal permeability and inflammation in patients on NSAIDs. Gut 1998; 43:506–511.
15. Bjarnason I, Zanelli G, Smith T et al. Nonsteroidal antiinflammatory drug-induced intestinal inflammation in humans. Gastroenterology 1987; 93:480–489.
16. Tibble J, Sigthorsson G, Foster R et al. Faecal calprotectin: A simple method for the diagnosis of NSAID-induced enteropathy. Gut 1999; 45:362–366.
17. Morris AJ, Madhok R, Sturrock RD, Capell HA, Mackenzie JF. Enteroscopic diagnosis of small bowel ulceration in patients receiving non-steroidal antiinflammatory drugs. Lancet 1991; 337:520.
18. Eli C, Remke S, May A et al. The first prospective controlled trial comparing wireless capsule enteroscopy with push enteroscopy in chronic gastrointestinal bleeding. Endoscopy 2002; 34:685–689.
19. Bjarnason I, Zanelli G, Smethurst P et al. Clinico-pathological features of nonsteroidal antiinflammatory drug-induced small intestinal strictures. Gastroenterology 1988; 94:1070–1074.
20. Hayllar J, Price AB, Smith T et al. Nonsteroidal antiinflammatory drug-induced small intestinal inflammation and blood loss: effect of sulphasalazine and other disease modifying drugs. Arthr Rheum 1994; 37:1146–1150.
21. Allison MC, Howatson AG, Torrance CJ, Lee FD, Russell RI. Gastrointestinal damage associated with the use of nonsteroidal anti-inflammatory drugs. N Engl J Med 1992; 327:749–754.
22. Lang J, Price AB, Levi AJ, Burk M, Gumpel JM, Bjarnason I. Diaphragm disease: the pathology of non-steroidal anti-inflammatory drug-induced small intestinal strictures. J Clin Path 1988; 41:516–526.
23. Bjarnason I, Hayllar J, Smethurst P et al. Metronidazole reduces inflammation and blood loss in NSAID enteropathy. Gut 1992; 33:1204–1208.
24. Shah AA, Thjodleifsson B, Murray FE et al. A randomised, double blind, double dummy, crossover study of the effects of nimesulide and naproxen on the gastrointestinal tract and an in vivo assessment of their selectivity for cyclooxygenase 1 and 2. Gut 2001; 48:339–348.
25. Leijonmark CE, Raf L. Ulceration of the small bowel due to slow-release potassium tablets. Acta Chir Scand 1985; 151:273–278.

Chapter 69

Acute appendicitis

Åke Andrén-Sandberg and Hartvig Körner

KEY POINTS

- The appendix may have a role as a lymphoid organ in childhood, but seems to perform no vital purpose in adults
- Etiology probably involves a viral infection, lymphoid reaction, outflow obstruction and ischemia.
- In most cases acute appendicitis is a clinical diagnosis
- In equivocal cases of suspected acute appendicitis, CT and ultrasound may be helpful
- There is little difference between open and laparoscopic appendectomy in terms of outcome

INTRODUCTION AND DEFINITION

Acute appendicitis is one of the most common causes of an 'acute abdomen' in the Western World, and is prevalent elsewhere.[1–6] The diagnosis relies heavily on an accurate history and physical examination. About half of the patients have a history and examination findings consistent with 'typical acute appendicitis,' but symptoms and signs in the remainder can be fickle and elusive. Acute appendicitis is a possible differential diagnosis in almost all patients with acute abdominal symptoms, so that a negative laparotomy and cases of missed appendicitis are both common. The risk of two primary adverse outcomes must be balanced in the management of presumed appendicitis – perforation, due to delayed preoperative diagnosis and misdiagnosis, resulting in removal of a normal appendix. Despite the growing body of evidence supporting the accuracy of modern imaging techniques in detecting appendicitis – computed tomography, ultrasonography, and laparoscopy – misdiagnosis remains a common problem.

EPIDEMIOLOGY

Acute appendicitis accounts for about 25% of hospital admissions for acute abdominal pain.[3] The lifetime cumulative risk of having an appendectomy in the USA is 7% for females and 9% males, based on figures published in 1990. In Sweden the incidence of appendicitis at the beginning of the 1990s was 116 per 100 000 population per year.

More than 50 000 appendectomies are performed yearly in the UK and over 250 000 in the USA.[1–6] At least 10 000 000 appendices are estimated to have been removed in the USA during the last 100 years.[3] In Japan, appendectomy accounts for 5% of all surgical procedures. In Scotland, with a population of about 5 million inhabitants, the number of appendectomies in 1994 was 4846 (i.e., about one operation per 1000 persons); these figures can be compared with the number of hip replacements (4394), coronary artery bypass grafts (4020), and hemorrhoid surgery (4226).[3]

In England in 1992, data from 8651 appendectomies showed an annual appendectomy rate per surgeon of 42, with a mean patient stay in hospital of 4.1 days after surgery. The hospital costs in the USA for acute appendicitis at the beginning of the 1990s were calculated to be US$1.5 billion per year.[3]

FUNCTION OF APPENDIX VERMIFORMIS

Leonardo da Vinci considered that the appendix, being capable of dilatation and contraction, served to protect the cecum from rupture by too great an accumulation of 'superfluous wind.' While many other functions have been proposed for the appendix in humans over the centuries, none has become universally accepted – today, da Vinci's proposal is regarded as a curiosity. Moreover, the appendix is not necessary for digestion in humans, and no functional impairment seems to arise following its removal.

The consensus is that the appendix is a vestigial organ. In carnivores, including members of the *Canis* (dog, wolf) and *Felis* (lion, tiger) species, the appendix is absent. On the other hand, the cecum in herbivores is long and well developed. In omnivores, including wombats, apes, and humans, a portion of the terminal cecum is small in diameter and has a prominent lymphoid component, which is peculiar to these species, and the appendix in these species is susceptible to specific pathologic processes and atrophic changes.

The human appendix secretes up to 2 mL/day of clear fluid containing mucin, amylase, and proteolytic enzymes (mostly produced by bacteria). There is a 10-cmH_2O pressure gradient between the appendix (15–20 cmH_2O) and the cecum (basal intraluminal cecal pressure of around 5 cmH_2O), causing fluid to flow from the appendix to the cecum. Foodstuff is conversely unlikely to enter, whilst the small output of enzymes will have little effect on any foodstuffs in the cecum. Therefore, a food-processing function in humans seems unlikely.

According to the law of Laplace, there is a rapid increase of intraluminal pressure because of the restricted ability of the appendiceal wall to stretch. Stagnant secretion of as little as 0.5 mL leads to an increase of pressure of approximately 45 mmHg. This may explain the possibility of perforation of the appendix within a few hours of onset of acute inflammation.

Although the appendix is richly innervated and contains numerous neuroendocrine cells, there is no reason to believe that it has any selective endocrine function, although this may partly explain the increased predilection of carcinoids for the appendix compared with other parts of the gut.

Several factors suggest a role for the appendix as a lymphoid organ of some significance, at least in childhood. First, its strategic placement gives early access to antigens entering the large intestine. Second, the appendix may not be necessary once humoral immunity has been established (its lymphoid atrophy after early adulthood having no measurable effect on immunologic function). Third, the appendix has a large concentration of lymphoid tissue compared to that in the rest of the colon. It has been estimated that this amount is equal to that in the ascending, transverse, and descending colon put together. The human appendix possesses many of the morphologic and topographic features of gut-associated lymphoid tissue (GALT). Despite these features, proof of a significant immune function in adults is lacking.

ANATOMY

The vermiform appendix and the cecum develop from the cecal bud, which arises from the antimesenteric border of the caudal limb of midgut loop around the beginning of the sixth week of development of the human embryo, when the fetus is 10–12 cm in length. The appendix remains at the tip of the cecum until birth, but owing to unequal growth of the cecum (the lateral wall growing faster than the medial), stretching and elongation of the colon, it descends to its final position. Due to malrotation of different degrees, the appendix can be found in unusual sites (e.g., subhepatic or intracecal).

The appendix has the same basic structures as the colon: serosa, muscularis propria (with an outer and thinner layer consisting of longitudinal fibers, and an inner and thicker layer consisting chiefly of ringlike fibres), submucosa, muscularis mucosae, and large intestinal-type mucosa. The average length of the appendix is 9 cm, but there is a wide range (2–25 cm). The normal luminal diameter is 1–3 mm, but may vary slightly along the length of the organ. The average luminal capacity of the vermiform appendix is only about 1 mL. The appendix reaches its maximum transverse diameter by 4 years of age and then gradually becomes narrower. The change is parallel with the decrease in lymphoid tissue in the wall and the increasing fibrosis, which is clearly evident by 40 years of age.

ETIOLOGY OF ACUTE APPENDICITIS

There have been many putative etiologies for appendicitis, but the issue remains unresolved. It is likely that the etiology is multifactorial or that individual cases need more than one factor to produce full-blown disease. At the end of the nineteenth century, the cause of appendicitis was commonly thought to be associated with the presence of a fecolith or foreign body within the lumen of the appendix, causing damage to the appendiceal mucosa and subsequent invasion of bacteria. The contemporary view is that appendicitis starts with an obstruction, such as a banal viral infection causing a lymphoid reaction. The resultant outflow obstruction of the narrow lumen raises the luminal pressure, leading to mucosal ischemia and bacterial infection.[7]

Epidemiologic studies strongly indicate a hereditary influence on acute appendicitis. This is unhelpful in the clinical situation, as 1 in 13 people suffers from acute appendicitis during their lifetime, so most people can recall one or more relatives who have had appendicitis.

DIAGNOSTIC METHODS

In most cases, acute appendicitis remains a clinical diagnosis[1–6] based on:

- Careful history taking
- Careful physical examination
- Repeated physical examination.

Measurement of leukocytes and C-reactive protein (CRP) levels has some value.[2–4,8] The longer duration of the disease the better the predictive value of these measurements. Over the course of the day the clinical picture often becomes clearer. Importantly, after 24 h of abdominal symptoms, a normal CRP concentration and leukocyte count exclude acute appendicitis with 98% accuracy.[4]

DIFFERENT SYMPTOMS WITH DIFFERENT DIAGNOSTIC VALUE

Although no single aspect of the clinical presentation accurately predicts the presence of the disease, a combination of various signs and symptoms may support the diagnosis (Table 69.1). The three signs and symptoms that are usually regarded as the most predictive of acute appendicitis are:

- Pain in the right lower quadrant
- Abdominal rigidity
- Migration of pain from the periumbilical region to the right lower quadrant.

The duration of pain, defined as the time from onset of symptoms to presentation, is also an important predictor, as patients with appendicitis have a significantly shorter duration of pain than those with other disorders.[9]

IMAGING STUDIES

Both ultrasonography and computed tomography (CT) may be helpful in the diagnosis of acute appendicitis.[10–15] Typical CT findings are distention and thickening of the wall of the appendix and periappendicular inflammation (Fig. 69.1).

TABLE 69.1 SENSITIVITY AND SPECIFICITY OF CLINICAL FINDINGS COMMONLY DISCUSSED WHEN DIAGNOSING ACUTE APPENDICITIS

Symptoms and signs	Sensitivity (%)	Specificity (%)
Right lower quadrant pain	81	53
Nausea	56–68	37–40
Vomiting	49–51	45–69
Onset of pain before vomiting	100	64
Anorexia	84	66
Fever	67	69
Guarding	39–74	57–84
Rebound tenderness	63	69
Indirect tenderness (Perman-Rovsing's sign)	68	58

Adapted with permission from Paulson EK, Kalady MF, Pappas TN. Clinical practice. Suspected appendicitis. New England Journal of Medicine 348(3): 236–242.

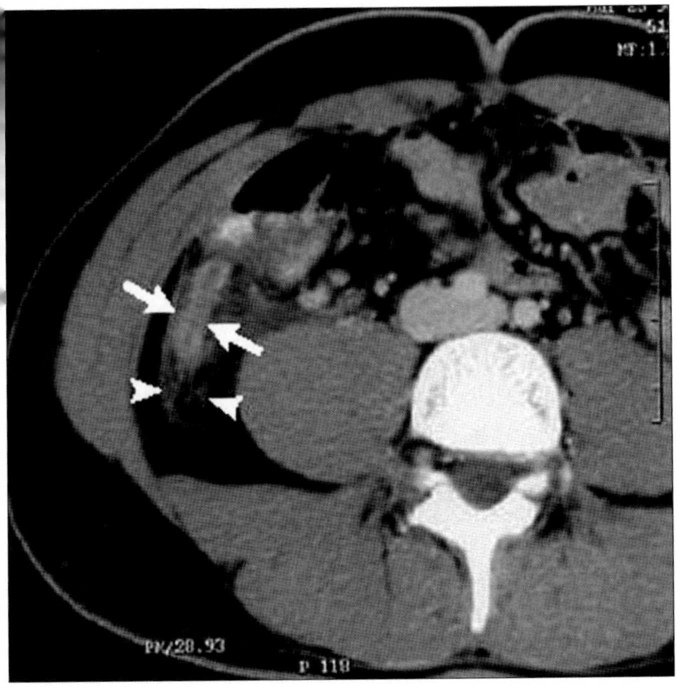

Fig. 69.1 Typical changes of acute appendicitis. Abdominal CT showing dilated thick-walled fluid-filled appendix with inflammatory changes in adjacent fat. From Paulson EK, Kalady MF, Pappas TN. Clinical practice. Suspected appendicitis. New England Journal of Medicine 348(3): 236–242. Copyright © 2003 Massachusetts Medical Society. All rights reserved.

The ability to make a differential diagnoses is also helpful. However, in about 50% of cases the diagnosis can be made without imaging studies; there is a risk that these studies may serve only to delay diagnosis – and there is objective evidence that this is so.[16–18]

Overall the following points should be kept in mind:

- Early cases are difficult to diagnose with CT and ultrasonography.
- Some 50% of all cases of appendicitis require a laparotomy due to peritonitis, whatever the imaging studies suggest.
- CT has 98% sensitivity and 99% specificity after 24 h of symptoms if performed and evaluated correctly.
- The value of ultrasonography is dependent on the ultrasonographer; if performed by an expert, it may be as good as CT (and is easier available, cheaper, and gives no radiation).
- Magnetic resonance imaging is not well evaluated for this indication.
- There is a risk that CT could delay diagnosis, depending on availability.
- The best protocol when performing CT for diagnosing appendicitis is still under discussion.
- Imaging studies should be carried out only in equivocal cases.

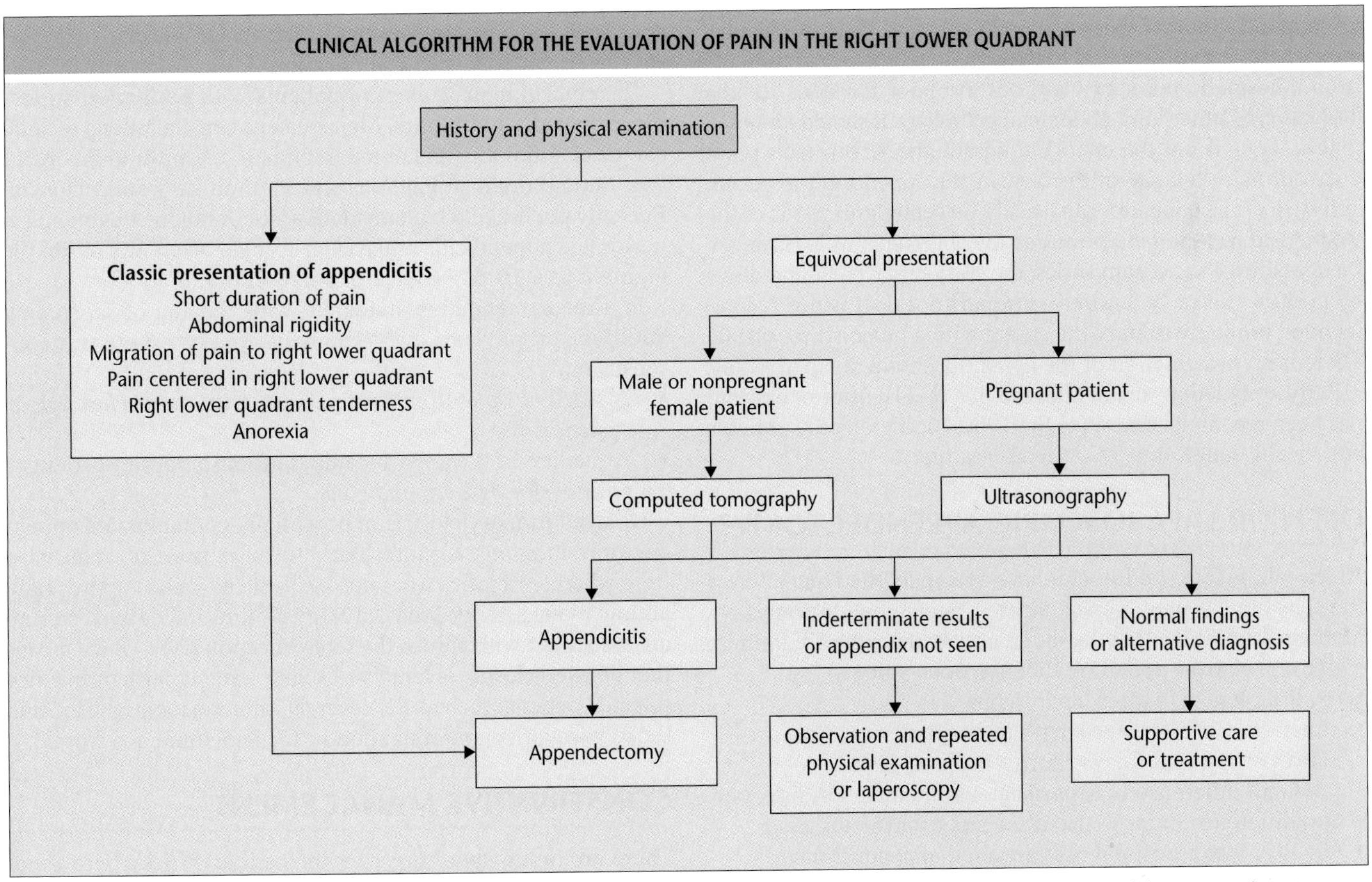

Fig. 69.2 Clinical algorithm for the evaluation of pain in the right lower quadrant. This algorithm is for patients with suspected acute appendicitis. If gynecologic disease is suspected, a pelvic and endovaginal ultrasonographic examination should be considered. From Paulson EK, Kalady MF, Pappas TN. Clinical practice. Suspected appendicitis. New England Journal of Medicine 348(3): 236–242. Copyright © 2003 Massachusetts Medical Society. All rights reserved.

MANAGEMENT PROTOCOL

These considerations are summarised in Figure 69.2.

INTERPRETATION OF A 'NEGATIVE' LAPAROTOMY

A 'negative' laparotomy at appendectomy usually means that a healthy appendix is found. However, the scientific evaluation of this situation should include the final diagnosis. If the appendix appears healthy, but at the same time another treatable condition is found (e.g., small bowel obstruction, extrauterine pregnancy, malignancy), this could be regarded as a 'positive' laparotomy, rather than operative findings of lymphadenitis. However, it is clearly undesirable to operate when, in retrospect, no operation was necessary as surgery may result in unnecessary morbidity (e.g., adhesions, female infertility) and mortality. Therefore, outcomes should be classified into two groups: those requiring an acute operation and those who would have had a better outcome without surgery.

THE OPERATION

In 1950, most patients with acute appendicitis were operated on under spinal anesthesia, but this has largely been replaced by general anesthesia, allowing better relaxation of the abdominal muscles and a smaller incision. The operation can also be performed under local anesthesia and laparoscopically.

Numerous types of incision have been described and proposed for appendectomy. Oblique muscle-splitting right fossa iliac incisions give a good access to the appendix and are acceptable from a cosmetic point of view, but are poor incisions for the evaluation of other intra-abdominal pathology. It should be noted that in many if not the majority of patients, McBurney's point does not mark the site of the base of the appendix. The cecum and base of the appendix can usually be gently pulled out of the wound and resection made outside the abdominal wall. However, the mobility of the cecum varies; the cecum may be bound down by peritoneum or be entirely retroperitoneal. It is not recommended routinely to bury the stump with a purse-string suture. There is no invagination of the appendix stump at laparoscopy.

Early ambulation (i.e., within the first 8–24 h after operation) has been recommended since the 1950s, and today the patients are usually sent home 24–36 h after surgery.

OPEN OR LAPAROSCOPIC APPENDECTOMY?

At least 42 randomized studies have been published that address the question of open versus laparoscopic appendectomy.[19–21] Meta-analyses show that the differences in outcome are limited:

- 16 min shorter operating time for open surgery
- A little less pain after laparoscopy
- Less than 15 h shorter length of hospital stay after laparoscopy, and 6 days shorter recovery time
- A small difference in superficial wound infection rate, but no difference in incidence of intraperitoneal abscesses
- 0–20% lower hospital cost for open appendectomy.

This means that both procedures are acceptable and the choice between them must be made on other grounds, such as:

- If there is no appendicitis, laparoscopy allows better inspection of abdominal cavity.
- Laparoscopy has advantages in overweight patients.
- Laparoscopy allows diagnosis of gynecologic infections such as salpingitis.
- Laparoscopy might give a better cosmetic result, but the differences are small.
- Whether laparoscopy reduces the risk of postoperative infertility is not known.
- Whether postoperative ileus is lessened by laparoscopy is not known.
- Organization and education in laparoscopy may be a limiting factor.

Ultimately the decision may be based on local hospital factors rather than evidence-based medicine.

PREOPERATIVE, PEROPERATIVE, AND POSTOPERATIVE ANTIBIOTICS

The risk of postoperative infection following appendectomy is directly proportional to the degree of appendiceal inflammation. This varies from less than 2% with normal appendices to 50% in perforated appendices. The appendectomy panorama ranges from clean (appendectomy à froid) to heavily contaminated.

The types of organism identified in inflamed appendices vary between geographic regions. The predominant microbial flora associated with acute appendicitis in the Western World are *Escherichia*, *Klebsiella*, *Proteus*, and *Bacteroides* (i.e., 'colonic flora'). The increasing sophistication of bacteriologic identification has not significantly changed the spectrum of bacteria cultured from acutely inflamed appendices. The prime therapeutic concern is the possible presence of mixed aerobic and anaerobic species in patients with complications.

The clinical management of patients with perforated appendicitis includes antibiotics. Management considerations include choice of antibiotics and duration of their administration, operative timing, drain utilization, and method of wound closure. Recently published recommendations for antibiotic treatment for perforated appendicitis range from a single-agent oral antibiotic regimen to a 10-day course of parenteral antibiotics.[22]

In a recommendation statement with the aim of shortening antibiotic prophylaxis and therapy in surgery[23] there was consensus on:

- A single-dose antibiotic in patients with *nonperforated appendicitis*
- A median of 3 (range 1–5) days of antibiotics in patients with *perforated appendicitis*.

Delayed primary closure of potentially contaminated appendectomy incisions is more likely to have been of value at a time when antibiotics were not available or lacked appropriate antimicrobial activity. Today, primary closure and delayed closure are associated with almost the same infection rates, which means that delayed closure is largely obsolete, except perhaps in a few selected patients such as the severely immunocompromised and those with gross contamination in the subcutaneous wound.

CONSERVATIVE MANAGEMENT

There are times when surgery is impossible or risky because of the patient's status or the nonavailability of facilities (including during space flight).[24] For such patients, the wider use of broad-spectrum antibiotics without acute surgical intervention has been proposed, but must still be regarded as an experimental treatment. There are no prospective randomized trials to date that have evaluated the use of antibiotics without early appendectomy.

INTERVAL APPENDECTOMY AND APPENDECTOMY EN PASSANT

Delayed appendectomy in patients with chronic appendicitis or antibiotic-treated acute appendicitis is controversial. In past times there was a consensus that these patients should undergo elective resection of the appendix after about 3 months. Today, this recommendation must be challenged.

Interval appendectomy following symptoms compatible with appendicitis was originally recommended more than 50 years ago to prevent subsequent presentation with a perforated appendix or other serious complications of appendicitis. This issue is still discussed, but most surgeons today omit interval appendectomy. The debate hinges on the recurrence of acute appendicitis versus the morbidity of the elective interval procedure. The recurrence rate of appendicitis in patients who have undergone initial conservative management of appendiceal mass ranges from 3% to 21%.

There have been few recent studies on the issue on appendectomy en passant, and as diagnostic methods and treatments improve over time, this question is of less interest. There is no scientific evidence to support the removal of an apparently healthy appendix at any laparotomy – but neither is there strong evidence for rejecting the practice if it can be done without morbidity for the patient. If the use of the appendix as a reconstructive adjunct for appendicostomy in children with neurologically associated constipation becomes more common in the future, this conclusion may be changed.

SOURCES OF INFORMATION FOR PATIENTS AND DOCTORS

http://www.patient.co.uk/showdoc/1035/
http://health.yahoo.com/health/ency/adam/000256/overview

REFERENCES

1. Simpson J, Speake W. Acute appendicitis. Clin Evidence 2002; 7:386–391.
2. Paulson EK, Kalady MF, Pappas TN. Clinical practice. Suspected appendicitis. N Engl J Med 2003; 348:236–242.
3. Andren-Sandberg A, Korner H. Quantitative and qualitative aspects of diagnosing acute appendicitis. Scand J Surg 2004; 93:4–9.
4. Andersson RE. Meta-analysis of the clinical and laboratory diagnosis of appendicitis. Br J Surg 2004; 91:28–37.
5. Ziegler MM. The diagnosis of appendicitis: an evolving paradigm. Pediatrics 2004; 113:130–132.
6. Shelton T, McKinlay R, Schwartz RW. Acute appendicitis: current diagnosis and treatment. Curr Surg 2003; 60:502–505.
7. Carr NJ. The pathology of acute appendicitis. Ann Diagn Pathol 2000; 4:46–58.
8. Snyder BK, Hayden SR. Accuracy of leukocyte count in the diagnosis of acute appendicitis. Ann Emerg Med 1999; 33:565–574.
9. Kraemer M, Franke C, Ohmann C, Yang Q. Acute Abdominal Pain Study Group. Acute appendicitis in late adulthood: incidence, presentation, and outcome. Results of a prospective multicenter acute abdominal pain study and a review of the literature. Langenbecks Arch Surg 2000; 385:470–481.
10. Rao PM, Rhea JT, Novelline RA, Mostafavi AA, McCabe CJ. Effect of computed tomography of the appendix on treatment of patients and use of hospital resources. N Engl J Med 1998; 338:141–146.
11. Naoum JJ, Mileski WJ, Daller JA et al. The use of abdominal computed tomography scan decreases the frequency of misdiagnosis in cases of suspected appendicitis. Am J Surg 2002; 184:587–589.
12. Raptopoulos V, Katsou G, Rosen MP, Siewert B, Goldberg SN, Kruskal JB. Acute appendicitis: effect of increased use of CT on selecting patients earlier. Radiology 2003; 226:521–526.
13. Wijetunga R, Doust B, Bigg-Wither G. The CT diagnosis of acute appendicitis. Semin Ultrasound CT MR 2003; 24:101–106.
14. Lee JH. Sonography of acute appendicitis. Semin Ultrasound CT MR 2003; 24:83–90.
15. Pena BM, Taylor GA, Fishman SJ, Mandl KD. Effect of an imaging protocol on clinical outcomes among pediatric patients with appendicitis. Pediatrics 2002; 110:1088–1093.
16. Lee SL, Walsh AJ, Ho HS. Computed tomography and ultrasonography do not improve and may delay the diagnosis and treatment of acute appendicitis. Arch Surg 2001; 136:556–562.
17. Weyant MJ, Eachempati SR, Maluccio MA, Barie PS. Is imaging necessary for the diagnosis of acute appendicitis? Adv Surg 2003; 37:327–345.
18. Perez J, Barone JE, Wilbanks TO, Jorgensson D, Corvo PR. Liberal use of computed tomography scanning does not improve diagnostic accuracy in appendicitis. Am J Surg 2003; 185:194–197.
19. Sauerland S, Lefering R, Neugebauer EA. Laparoscopic versus open surgery for suspected appendicitis. Cochrane Database Syst Rev 2002; (1)CD001546.
20. McKinlay R, Mastrangelo MJ Jr. Current status of laparoscopic appendectomy. Curr Surg 2003; 60:506–512.
21. Vernon AH, Georgeson KE, Harmon CM. Pediatric laparoscopic appendectomy for acute appendicitis. Surg Endosc 2004; 18:75–79.
22. Gleisner AL, Argenta R, Pimentel M et al. Infective complications according to duration of antibiotic treatment in acute abdomen. Int J Infect Dis 2004; 8:155–162.
23. Andersen BR, Kallehave FL, Andersen HK. Antibiotics versus placebo for prevention of postoperative infection after appendicectomy. In: The Cochrane Library, 2004, Issue 4. Chichester: John Wiley.
24. Campbell MR, Johnston SL III, Marshburn T, Kane J, Lugg D. Nonoperative treatment of suspected appendicitis in remote medical care environments: implications for future spaceflight medical care. Journal of the Am Coll Surg 2004; 198:822–830.

Chapter 70

Anorectal diseases

Steven D Wexner and Giovanna M da Silva

HEMORRHOIDAL DISEASE

KEY POINTS
HEMORRHOIDS
• Hemorrhoids are cushions of vascular tissue normally present in the anal canal • 'Hemorrhoids' is a term that is used for a variety of anorectal conditions • Hemorrhoidal bleeding may mask a malignant lesion, particularly in younger patients

Introduction

Hemorrhoids are cushions of submucosal tissue composed of blood vessels, smooth muscle fibers, and supporting connective tissue. They are normally present in the anal canal, where they have a potential role in evacuation and continence. The term 'hemorrhoids' is also applied in situations when these cushions become symptomatic. Hemorrhoidal symptoms may mask malignancy; therefore, a complete colonic investigation is warranted in patients at risk of neoplasia or with unusual symptoms.

Epidemiology and risk factors

It is estimated that hemorrhoids affect 10 million people in the US, corresponding to a prevalence rate of 4.4%. In both genders, the peak in prevalence ranges from 45 to 65 years of age. Despite evidence that constipation is not associated with hemorrhoids, hard, bulky stools are more likely to prolapse the cushions out of the anal canal. Diarrhea has been commonly associated with hemorrhoids; other predisposing factors include heredity, erect posture, pregnancy, and conditions associated with increased anal sphincter pressure.

Pathogenesis and pathology

The pathogenesis of hemorrhoids is unclear, although many theories have been postulated over the years. In theory, any factor that causes weakening of the supporting tissue such as age and lax connective tissue can lead to hemorrhoids. The most currently accepted theory is that hemorrhoids occur due to caudad slippage of the anal cushions and anal mucosa due to fragmentation of the supporting tissues (Treitz' and Park's ligaments). The prolapse can then hinder the venous flow leading to dilation of the anal cushions, in turn exposing them to vascular complications such as edema, congestion, thrombosis, and bleeding; soiling and leakage are symptoms associated with the prolapse itself.

Hemorrhoids can be anatomically and clinically classified as internal, external, or combined. Internal hemorrhoids are located proximal to the dentate line and are covered by columnar mucosa or transitional epithelium. They are classified by degree of prolapse: in first degree, there is only bleeding without prolapse; in second degree, prolapse is present on straining but spontaneously reduces; in third degree, the prolapse requires manual reduction; and in fourth degree, the prolapse is irreducible (Fig. 70.1). In these situations, gangrene of the hemorrhoidal tissue may develop, a condition known as 'strangulated' hemorrhoids (Fig. 70.2).

Thrombosed external hemorrhoids are usually associated with trauma and straining. They present as a tender blue colored mass at the anal verge. The late sequela of thrombosis is a skin tag, which although asymptomatic may make perianal hygiene more difficult.

Clinical presentation

Internal hemorrhoids usually manifest as bright red rectal bleeding associated with bowel movements, and prolapsed hemorrhoids with symptoms of discomfort, rectal pressure, feeling of incomplete evacuation, and mucous discharge. Pain is not a common feature unless thrombosis or 'strangulation' occurs, which requires emergent surgery. Similarly, although discomfort, pruritus ani, and perianal skin irritation may coexist in patients with enlarged internal hemorrhoids, the hemorrhoids may not be the etiology of these symptoms.

External hemorrhoids are usually asymptomatic unless a thrombosis develops, presenting with edema of the perianal region and severe pain that can persist for several days. Spontaneous resolution may occur with necrosis of the overlying skin and evacuation of the clots.

Differential diagnosis

DIFFERENTIAL DIAGNOSIS
HEMORRHOIDS
• Bleeding: fissure, polyp, inflammatory bowel disease, rectal cancer, anal cancer • Prolapse: rectal prolapse (procidentia), polyp, anal papilla, anal tag, anal cancer • Itching/discharge: anal papilla, fistula, condyloma, rectal prolapse, fecal incontinence, perianal dermatoses • Pain: abscess, fissure

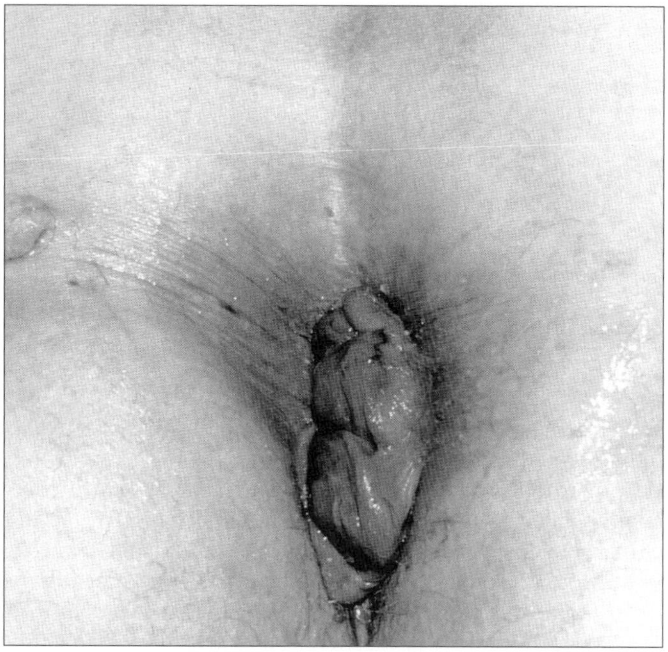

Fig. 70.1 Prolapsing internal hemorrhoids. Radial folds of prolapsing internal hemorrhoids with an internal component.

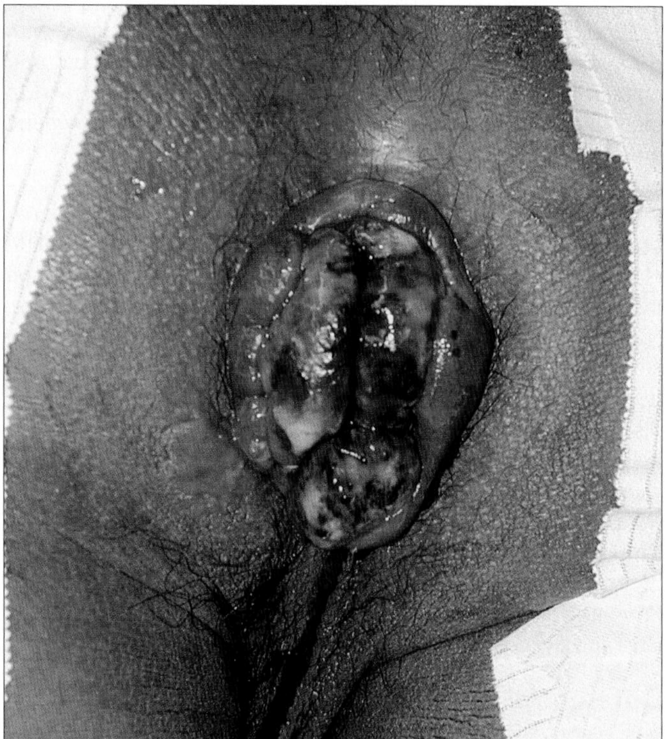

Fig. 70.2 Strangulated hemorrhoids. (Courtesy of Dr Laurence Sands, University of Miami, Miami, FL.)

As previously mentioned, it is crucial to exclude more insidious sources of bleeding in patients at risk for malignancy or with unusual symptoms. Other sources of bleeding include neoplasia, inflammatory bowel disease, anal cancer, and anal fissure. Prolapsed hemorrhoids may be confused with rectal prolapse, rectal polyps, or hypertrophied papillae; the presence of multiple skin tags may suggest Crohn's disease. Typically, the tags in Crohn's disease have a bluish purple discoloration. When pain is present, fissure and perianal abscess must be considered, especially the often difficult to diagnose intersphincteric abscess.

Treatment and prevention

TREATMENT
HEMORRHOIDS
• First degree – conservative treatment • Second/third degree – rubber band ligation, sclerotherapy, photocoagulation, cryotherapy, diathermy; consider PPH procedure for prolapsing hemorrhoids • Third/fourth degree or acute – PPH (preferable) or hemorrhoidectomy

Conservative treatment of hemorrhoids includes dietary modification with high-fiber diet (20–30 g/day) using commercial psyllium fiber supplements, accompanied by generous water intake in order to promote soft, but formed, regular bowel movements. This measure is the mainstay of treatment, and is usually sufficient for patients with first-degree hemorrhoids. Other helpful measures include warm sitz baths (10 min) to relax the anal sphincter; topical medications such as 1% hydrocortisone and suppositories may provide short-term relieve from discomfort, although there is a lack of evidence to support their widespread use.

Patients with second- or third-degree hemorrhoids as well as patients with first-degree disease who do not respond to conservative measures are good candidates for rubber band ligation, sclerotherapy, photocoagulation, cryotherapy, and diathermy.[1] They work by fixating the sliding cushions back onto the muscle wall, either by directly initiating tissue fibrosis or by tissue destruction with subsequent scarring and fibrosis. Large series comparing the efficacy of all treatment modalities are not available. However, a meta-analysis has demonstrated that rubber-band ligation is superior to sclerotherapy or infrared coagulation, providing cure in 79% of patients, although it is associated with more postprocedural discomfort. This technique has been the most common office technique used in the US, whereas traditionally sclerotherapy was preferred in the UK.

Surgery is the definitive treatment and remains the best option for some patients with third- and fourth-degree hemorrhoids and as well as those people who failed previous therapy. Surgery can be done by standard excisional hemorrhoidectomy or by stapled anopexy. The procedure for prolapse and hemorrhoids (PPH) uses a circular device that delivers a double row of staples. Over 10 randomized trials done in Europe[2] and one multicenter trial including 13 institutions in the US[3] report significantly less postoperative pain compared to standard hemorrhoidectomy with PPH, which should therefore be the first-line treatment for patients with hemorrhoids requiring surgery. External hemorrhoids should be initially managed by conservative means and hemorrhoidectomy or PPH performed if no improvement is achieved.

Prognosis with and without treatment

Hemorrhoidal bleeding may cause anemia and prolapse may progressively increase if left untreated and fourth-degree hemorrhoids may eventually strangulate. The majority of the hemorrhoidal symptoms are usually relieved after successful treatment. Recurrence may warrant the next phase of treatment. Ultimately, symptoms should permanently abate after adequate therapy with or without surgery.

ANAL FISSURE

KEY POINTS
IDIOPATHIC ANAL FISSURE
• Anal fissure is a very painful tear in the anal canal • It is usually located in the midline position • Eccentric or multiple fissures suggest other diseases

Introduction

Anal fissure is a painful linear tear that extends from just cephalad to the dentate line to the margin of the anus, usually located in the posterior midline. Anterior fissures are more common in women than men, and eccentric or multiple fissures may prompt evaluation for Crohn's disease.

Epidemiology and risk factors

Fissure-in-ano is a very common problem, the precise incidence and prevalence of which are unknown. It transcends all age groups, but is particularly seen in young and otherwise healthy adults, and has a similar incidence in men and women. Most commonly, anal fissure is initiated by trauma to the anal canal, usually with the passage of hard stool, but it can also occur with diarrhea. It has been described in 11% of patients after childbirth, especially those fissures associated with trauma. Previous anal surgery such as hemorrhoidectomy may lead to scarring and stenosis with consequent loss of mucosal elasticity and development of a fissure.

Pathogenesis

There are several theories for the pathogenesis of the anal fissure and its common location in the midline position. One theory is that the anterior and posterior midline position are weak areas of the anal canal and, subsequently, more prone to tearing during the passage of hard or explosive stool. Another theory is that the anal mucosa in the midline region is tethered to the sphincter muscle, and therefore resistant to stretching during evacuation. Finally, anal fissure has been associated with internal sphincter hypertonia and consequent anal spasm. Increased anal pressure reduces blood flow leading to ischemia, especially in the posterior region where there is a paucity of arterioles. Therefore, for many years treatment has focused on reducing internal sphincter pressure.

Pathology

Acute fissure presents with a flat edge and filmy white base, which is the connective tissue of the submucosal and longitudinal muscle fibers. A chronic fissure has raised edges and a deeper base with exposure of the internal sphincter, which may be fibrotic (Fig. 70.3). There often is an associated 'sentinel' skin tag at the distal portion of the fissure, and a hypertrophied papilla at the proximal portion.

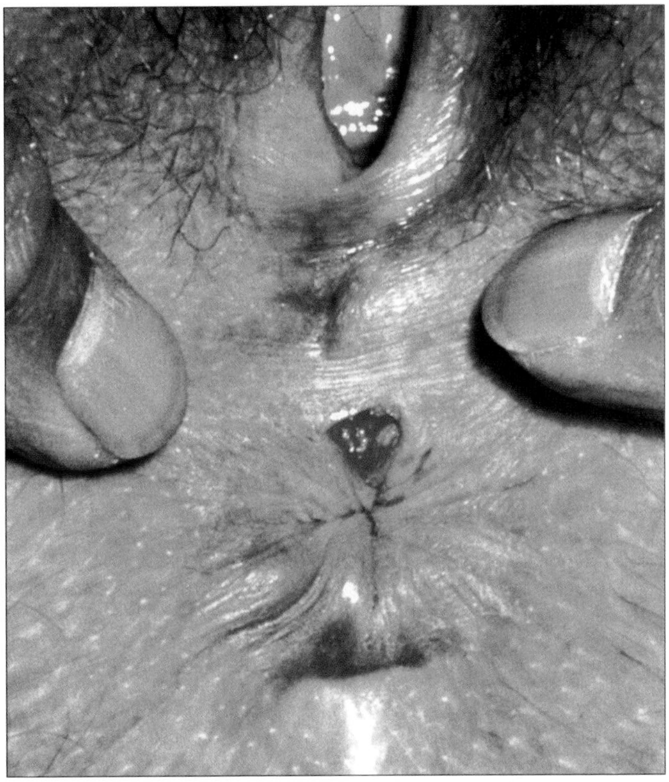

Fig. 70.3 Anal fissure.

Clinical presentation

Anal fissure typically presents with severe intense pain after defecation, which can be described as knifelike, cutting, or tearing in character and may last for hours after bowel movement. Patients usually observe bright red rectal bleeding on the toilet paper upon wiping. They may also complain of pruritus, swelling, prolapse, and discharge. Patients with longer duration of symptoms of drainage and pruritus should be investigated for associated fistula.

Differential diagnosis

DIFFERENTIAL DIAGNOSIS
IDIOPATHIC ANAL FISSURE
• Crohn's disease • Syphilis • Tuberculosis • Leukemia • Malignancy • HIV • Lymphogranuloma venereum

While idiopathic fissures are located in the midline position, atypical fissures can be lateral, multiple, large, and irregular. These fissures can be associated with Crohn's disease or tuberculosis, leukemia, anal carcinoma, cytomegalovirus, and sexually transmitted diseases, especially syphilis. These fissures are broad and painless and are generally associated with edematous external skin tags. The differential diagnosis is important as sphincterotomy performed on patients with Crohn's or other conditions may not heal and may worsen both the disease and fecal incontinence. If an anal fissure is seen by gently spreading the buttocks, the remainder of the exam is usually deferred to avoid causing pain and the fissure is treated. An additional evaluation can be performed after the fissure has healed.

Treatment and prevention

TREATMENT
NONSPECIFIC ANAL FISSURE
CONSERVATIVE • High-fiber diet • Increased oral intake • Sitz baths **MEDICAL** • Nitric oxide – 0.2% nitroglycerin • Calcium channel blockers – nifedipine, diltiazem • Botulinum toxin **SURGICAL** • Sphincterotomy: lateral – open, closed posterior multiple

Patients with acute anal fissure usually respond to conservative treatment such as dietary modifications with psyllium bulking agents, increased water intake, and warm sitz baths.

Pharmacological treatment: Several medications that promote pharmacological sphincterotomy have been recently explored and used for patients with chronic fissure. These medications include topical nitric oxide (0.2% glyceryl trinitrate – GTN, nitroglycerin), botulinum toxin, calcium channel blockers (nifedipine, diltiazem), and alpha-adrenoceptor antagonists. The GTN ointment is used in a concentration of 0.2%, and is applied in the anal canal two or three times daily for at least 6 weeks. Larger trials in the literature have demonstrated a success rate of 30–73%.[4] Transient headache is a major side effect of this treatment occurring in 20–40% of cases, and is more commonly seen at higher concentrations of the compound.

Botulinum toxin is another option usually indicated for patients who are unresponsive to or have contraindications for GTN treatment. The exact dosage of the medication is debatable, however doses as high as 30 U injected in the internal sphincter seem to offer the best results, with a success rate of up to 96%.[5] Temporary fecal incontinence has been reported in from 0 to 12% of cases after this treatment.

Nifedipine can be administered orally or topically. A randomized trial comparing oral vs. topical diltiazem found a healing rate of 38% in patients receiving oral administration and 65% for patients using topical treatment; no adverse events were seen in patients who received topical therapy.[6] Flushing is the most common adverse effect associated with oral administration (66%). The alpha-adrenoceptor antagonist may play an important role in the future, however it is still currently at the developmental stage.

Surgical sphincterotomy is reserved for patients who relapse or fail these newer nonsurgical methods. It is associated with a healing rate of 90–95% but incontinence may occur in up to 35% of patients. Sphincterotomy can be performed in the lateral, posterior, or multiple quadrants and can be performed open or closed.

Prognosis with or without treatment

Fifty to ninety per cent of conservatively treated fissures are expected to heal, especially if soft regular bowel movements are maintained. Pharmacological therapies require longer treatment duration but avoid the risk of postoperative incontinence. Conversely, surgery offers the best results, but is associated with the greatest risk for incontinence. Although that risk is small it is still devastating given the benign nature of the disease.

ANORECTAL ABSCESS AND FISTULA-IN-ANO

KEY POINTS
ANORECTAL ABSCESS
• Anorectal abscess manifests with pain, swelling, and fever • Patients with supralevator or intersphincteric abscesses may have rectal pain without external signs of infection • Treatment of abscess is incision and drainage; antibiotics may be adjuvant but are not a substitute for surgical drainage

Introduction

Anorectal abscess and fistula-in-ano represent different stages of the same disease spectrum. Abscess is the acute phase of infection of the potential spaces around the rectum and/or anus.

Epidemiology

The estimated annual incidence of anal abscess ranges between 68 000 and 96 000 in the US.[7]

Pathogenesis and pathology

The majority of the anorectal abscesses are caused by anal crypt gland blockage, resulting in anal gland infection, which extends to the perirectal spaces. According to the extension to the potential perirectal spaces, anorectal abscesses can be classified as perianal, intersphincteric, ischiorectal, or supralevator (Fig. 70.4). A horseshoe abscess originates from the deep postanal space communicating to the right and left ischiorectal spaces.

Anorectal abscess

Clinical presentation

The classic symptoms of anal abscess are pain, swelling, and fever. Inspection will reveal erythema and swelling. However patients with an intersphincteric or supralevator abscess may lack external manifestation. Symptoms of severe rectal pain accompanied by urinary symptoms such as dysuria, retention or inability to void suggest these locations.

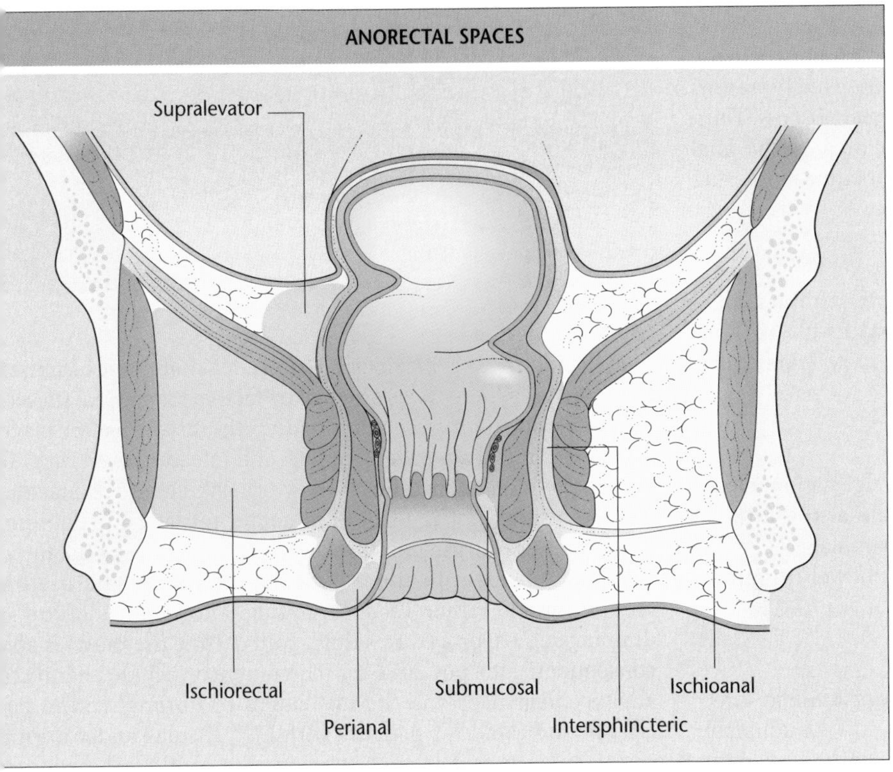

Fig. 70.4 Anorectal spaces. Reprinted from Beck DE, Wexner SD, eds. Fundamentals of Anorectal Surgery 2/e. London: WB Saunders; 1998, with permission from Elsevier.

Differential diagnosis

DIFFERENTIAL DIAGNOSIS
NONSPECIFIC ANORECTAL ABSCESS AND FISTULA
• Inflammatory bowel disease – Crohn's disease • Infection – tuberculosis, actinomycosis, lymphogranuloma venereum • Trauma – impalement, foreign body, iatrogenic • Malignancy – carcinoma, leukemia, lymphoma

Both anorectal abscess and fistula-in-ano must be distinguished from conditions associated with specific diseases such as inflammatory bowel disease, infection, trauma, carcinoma, and radiation. In these situations, an appropriate investigation is warranted. Treatment and surgical outcomes differ for each of these conditions.

Treatment

The treatment of an anorectal abscess is incision and drainage. With the exception of simple perianal and ischiorectal abscesses, the surgery is performed in the operating room under adequate anesthesia. A cruciate incision is made and the edges of the skin are excised to allow adequate drainage. Intersphincteric abscesses require unroofing of the abscess cavity, which in these cases involves partial internal sphincterotomy. Care must be taken not to drain a supralevator abscess originating in the pelvis through the levator plate, because a complex suprasphincteric fistula may develop.

Owing to the increased risk for incontinence, the question of performing a definitive procedure (fistulotomy) at the time of abscess drainage remains controversial. In the US, most surgeons perform fistulotomy during a separate visit.[6] This preference is predicated upon the logic that a fistula may never develop and thus the potential morbidity of a fistulotomy can be avoided in many patients.

Prognosis with and without treatment

If left untreated, anorectal abscess may result in necrotizing infection and even death. Such an infection occurs if there is a delay in the diagnosis, or if the abscess is inadequately drained, especially in patients with diabetes or immunosuppressive conditions. After primary abscess drainage, 11–50% of patients may develop a fistula while in 10–37% the abscess may recur. Recurrence is more likely to occur with complex fistula, and with failure to recognize the internal opening. Reevaluation of these patients until the wounds are completely healed is essential in the prevention of premature wound closure and recurrence.

Fistula-in-ano

KEY POINTS
FISTULA IN ANO
• Fistula-in-ano usually results from incomplete healing of a drained abscess • Correct identification of all tracts and both internal and external openings is essential for successful treatment • Division of the sphincter muscle should be performed with knowledge of the anatomy of the fistula, as incontinence is the major complication of fistulotomy

Introduction

Fistula is defined as an abnormal communication between any two epithelium-lined surfaces. Fistula-in-ano usually results from incomplete healing of a drained anorectal abscess. Thus, the primary opening is the cryptoglandular area of the anal canal at the dentate line and the secondary opening is the skin where the abscess was drained.

Epidemiology

In 1979, the national Center of Health Statistics in the United States recorded 24 000 individuals with anal fistula as their primary diagnosis in American hospitals. The male:female ratio was roughly 2:1.

Clinical presentation

Patients may complain of drainage, pain with defecation, bleeding (due to the presence of granulation tissue at the internal opening), swelling, or decrease in pain with drainage of pus. If the fistula is secondary to intestinal disease, bowel symptoms are usually present.

Pathogenesis and pathology

Most fistulas are thought to arise due to cryptoglandular infection. According to the relationship of the tract to the sphincter musculature and levator ani, fistulas are classified as intersphincteric, trans-sphincteric, extrasphincteric, and suprasphincteric (Fig. 70.5). When the cause of the fistula is unclear anal ultrasound with hydrogen peroxide enhancement can be very helpful.[8]

Treatment

Treatment of nonspecific fistula in ano is surgical. The goal of treatment is to cure the fistula, avoid recurrence, and preserve continence. Therefore, identification of the primary opening and all side tracts with division of the least amount of muscl while opening these tracts are the key factors for surgical succes

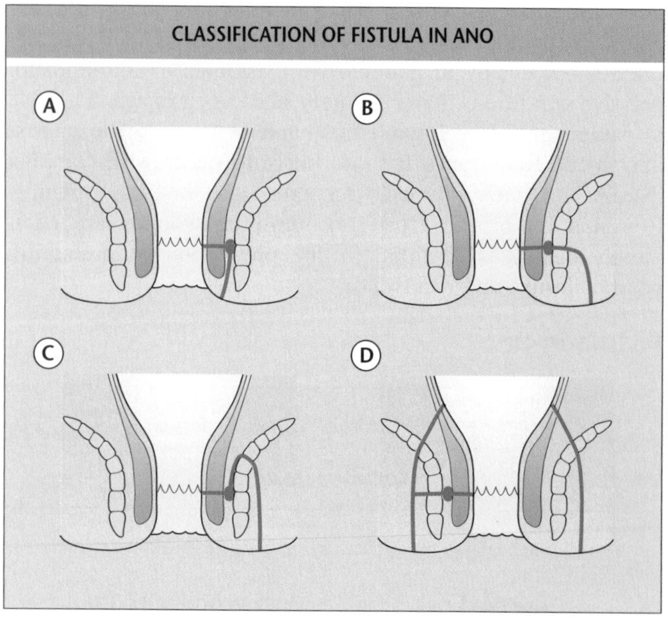

Fig. 70.5 Classification of fistula in ano. A. Intersphincteric; **B.** trans-sphincteric; **C.** suprasphincteric; **D.** extrasphincteric. Adapted from Vasilevski CA. Fistula in ano and abscess. In: Beck DE, Wexner SD, eds. Fundamentals of anorectal surgery, 2nd edn. London: W.B. Saunders; 1998, with permission from Elsevier.

TREATMENT
ANAL FISTULA
• Fistulotomy • Seton placement – cutting or draining • Endorectal advancement flap • Injection of fibrin glue

Treatment options include dividing the fistula, seton placement, endorectal advancement flap, and injection of fibrin glu For simple intersphincteric and low transphincteric fistulas th involve a small portion of the sphincter muscle, a fistulotom with curettage of the granulation tissue is usually optimal.

Crohn's disease: In these patients, setons may be used a chronic drains rather than as cutting setons. In addition t draining setons, procedures that avoid cutting the muscles an consequently, the potential for incontinence, include endorect advancement flaps and the instillation of fibrin glue. The fla may be indicated for patients with high fistulas and a norm rectal mucosa and is successful in up to 60% of patients. Fibrin glue can be used alone or in combination with othe techniques. The use of the glue alone has been shown to hel avoid extensive surgery in 33% of patients.[10] A skin fla advanced into the anus, like an anoplasty, may be used for lo fistula although a keyhole deformity may result.

Prognosis with and without treatment

Once established, fistulas rarely spontaneously heal. If no addressed, there is a potential risk, albeit small, of subsequen cancer development. The most common morbidity associate with surgery is fecal incontinence, especially if fistulotomy i performed.

RECTAL PROLAPSE

KEY FACTS
RECTAL PROLAPSE
• Rectal prolapse is a full thickness protrusion of the rectum through the anal sphincters • Surgical procedure selection depends on the individual patient

Introduction

Rectal prolapse is a full thickness protrusion of the rectum through the anal sphincters. It is an uncommon pathology, th exact incidence of which is unknown. Prolapse tends to occu more in children, with an equal gender distribution and i postmenopausal females.

Risk factors, associated diseases

A higher incidence of prolapse has been observed in patient with mental illness, nulliparous women, and patients with a ng history of constipation and difficult evacuation. In children, has been associated with cystic fibrosis, whooping cough, nd developmental disorders such as meningomyelocele and pina bifida. Additionally, malnutrition and diarrheal states econdary to parasitic infections can lead to rectal prolapse uring childhood, which is usually self-limited.

athogenesis and pathology

t is hypothesized that rectal prolapse begins as an internal ntussusception of the rectum, which with time and increasing axity of the tissues, develops into a full thickness protrusion hrough the anal sphincter. Therefore, the current primary referable treatment is to mobilize the rectum in the presacral pace and then fix it at the superior part of the sacrum near to he promontory level. Because these patients usually have a edundant sigmoid colon associated with constipation, resection of the sigmoid is also performed.

linical presentation

he earliest complaint is usually the protrusion of tissue through he anus, initially during bowel movements and later with any hysical activity. Other symptoms include irregular bowel habits, iscomfort, sensation of incomplete evacuation, and tenesmus. hronic prolapse can lead to ulceration, bleeding, and mucous ischarge. Patients may also complain of both chronic constipation with straining and progressive fecal incontinence commensurate with the duration of the prolapse. Patients may ave associated pathologies of the pelvic floor such as urinary ncontinence or vaginal prolapse.

ifferential diagnosis

The main differential diagnoses of rectal prolapse are mucosal rolapse or prolapsed internal hemorrhoids. Distinguishing eatures of rectal prolapse include the presence of concentric ings of mucosa with the anus in a normal anatomic position, he presence of a sulcus between the anus and the protruding tissue, and palpation of a double rectal wall in the complete rectal prolapse. Biopsies may be necessary to differentiate metaplastic changes in a chronically prolapsed tissue from a polypoid neoplasm. When prolapse cannot be easily distinguished from prolapsing hemorrhoids the patient can be asked to sit on the commode and try to feign evacuation. Assessment of the patient in this position can be helpful in the diagnosis.

Treatment

TREATMENT
RECTAL PROLAPSE
• Good-risk patients – resection rectopexy • Elderly and poor surgical risk patients – perineal rectosigmoidectomy with levatorplasty

In adults, the treatment of rectal prolapse is surgery. The aim is to control the prolapse, restore continence, and correct constipation. Whether a perineal or a transabdominal repair is indicated depends mainly on the patient's medical condition. The most common procedures and their indication are shown in an algorithm form in Fig. 70.6. Although the best operation remains a controversial subject, laparoscopic rectopexy with or without resection has gained wide acceptance, with low morbidity and low recurrence rates, with the added advantages of less pain, shorter hospital stay, and earlier return to work, compared to the open approach.[11]

Perineal procedures are associated with higher recurrence rates than abdominal procedures.[12] However, they have lower morbidity and therefore are indicated for poor-risk and elderly patients. In children, the prolapse usually spontaneously resolves, and surgery is rarely indicated.

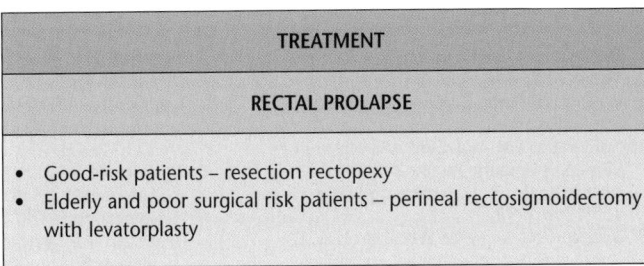

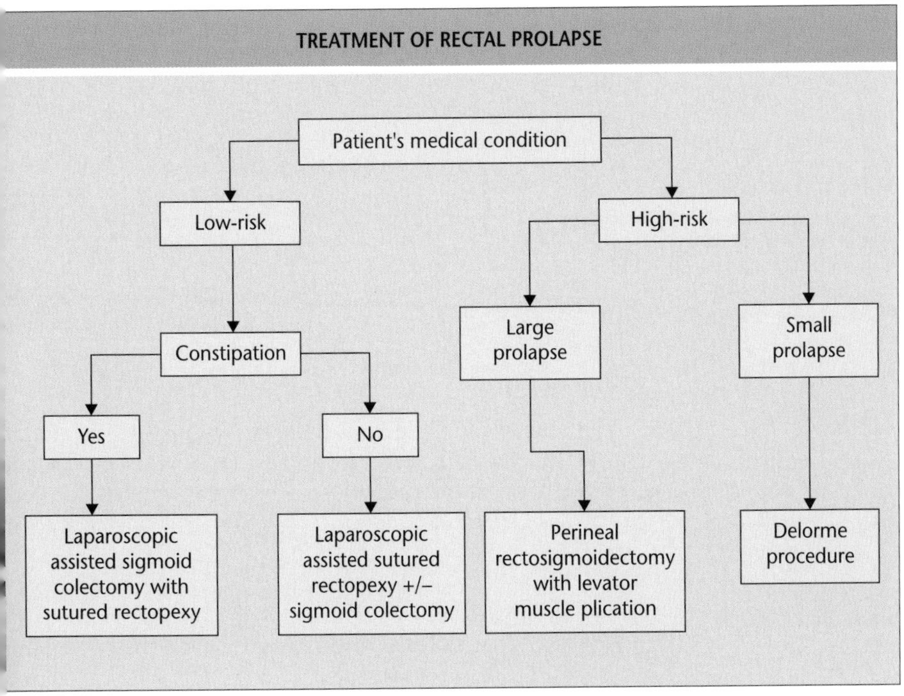

Fig. 70.6 Treatment of rectal prolapse. Suggested algorithm for treatment of rectal prolapse.

Prognosis with and without treatment

Without treatment, rectal prolapse may progressively increase, leading to poor hygiene and adversely impacting patients' quality of life. Furthermore, the prolapse may ulcerate leading to bleeding or 'strangulation' necessitating an emergency operation. Potential surgical complications include constipation, sexual dysfunction, and recurrent prolapse. Finally, 46–93% of patients may experience improvement in fecal incontinence after correction of the prolapse.

SOURCES OF INFORMATION FOR PATIENTS AND DOCTORS

http://www.gastro.org/generalPublic.html

REFERENCES

1. Beck D. Hemorrhoidal disease. In: Beck D, Wexner SD, eds. Fundamentals of anorectal surgery, 2nd edn. London: W.B. Saunders; 1998:261–277.
2. Sutherland LM, Burchard AK, Matsuda K et al. A systematic review of stapled hemorrhoidectomy. Arch Surg 2002; 137:1395–1406.
3. Senagore A, Singer M, Abcarian H et al. A prospective, randomized, controlled, multicenter trial comparing stapled hemorrhoidopexy and Ferguson hemorrhoidectomy: One year results. Presented at the ASCRS meeting, New Orleans, LA, June 21–26, 2003.
4. Utzig MJ, Kroesen AJ, Buhr HJ. Concepts in pathogenesis and treatment of chronic anal fissure – a review of the literature. Am J Gastroenterol 2003; 98:968–974.
5. Brisinda G, Maria G, Sganga G et al. Effectiveness of higher doses of botulinum toxin to induce healing in patients with chronic anal fissures. Surgery 2002; 131:179–184.
6. Jonas M, Neal KR, Abercrombie JF, Scholefield JH. A randomized trial of oral vs. topical diltiazem for chronic anal fissures. Dis Colon Rectum 2001; 44:1074–1078.
7. Nelson R. Anorectal abscess fistula: what do we know? Surg Clin North Am 2002; 82:1139–1151, v–vi (Review).
8. Cheong DM, Nogueras JJ, Wexner SD et al. Anal endosonography for recurrent anal fistulas: image enhancement with hydrogen peroxide. Dis Colon Rectum 1993; 36:1158–1160.
9. Sonoda T, Hull T, Piedmonte MR, Fazio VW. Outcomes of primary repair of anorectal and rectovaginal fistulas using the endorectal advancement flap. Dis Colon Rectum 2002; 45:1622–1628.
10. Zmora O, Mizrahi N, Rotholtz N et al. Fibrin glue sealing in the treatment of perineal fistulas. Dis Colon Rectum 2003; 46:584–589.
11. Kairaluoma MV, Viljakka MT, Kellokumpu IH. Open vs. laparoscopic surgery for rectal prolapse: a case-controlled study assessing short-term outcome. Dis Colon Rectum 2003; 46:353–360.
12. Boccasanta P, Rosati R, Venturi M et al. Surgical treatment of complete rectal prolapse: results of abdominal and perineal approaches. J Laparoendosc Adv Surg Tech A 1999; 9:235–238.

Chapter 71

Acute pancreatitis

Clement W Imrie

KEY POINTS

- Most acute pancreatitis is caused by (often small) gallstones or heavy alcohol intake
- Pancreatitis causing multiorgan failure carries a mortality rate of over 50%
- Hereditary pancreatitis predisposes to pancreatic cancer
- The Marshall prognostic grade can predict poor outcome and need for ventilator support
- Systems, such as the APACHE II and Glasgow scales that grade severity, allow standardization for research but lack positive predictive value in individual patients
- Correction of hypoxaemia and hypovolemia is essential in the context of the systemic inflammatory response syndrome
- On balance, evidence supports the use of prophylactic antibiotics
- Nutritional support is important – nasoenteral feeding is preferable to intravenous nutrition
- Skilled early endoscopic sphincterotomy may improve prognosis where there is evidence of biliary obstruction

INTRODUCTION AND DEFINITION

Acute pancreatitis is an autodigestive process whereby activation of pancreatic enzymes causes pancreatic damage with a local and systemic inflammatory response.

Acute pancreatitis usually presents with sudden-onset upper abdominal pain and vomiting. This is of such severity that most patients are admitted to hospital, often under the care of surgical teams because of the clinical presentation and differential diagnosis. Initial management is uniformly agreed to be conservative therapy based on:

- Correction of hypovolemia
- Treatment of pain
- Provision of oxygen.

Nearly all the deaths within the first 7–14 days are associated with multiorgan dysfunction syndrome (MODS) in which respiratory compromise or failure is the major determinant of outcome.[1] While most patients have a benign course that is easily treated with intravenous fluids, analgesics, and oxygen therapy, approximately 15% either present to hospital with organ compromise or develop this within 72 h. Patients who do not improve fairly rapidly with support measures have persistent or deteriorating MODS and a high mortality rate in the region of 50%.[2,3] Such patients frequently demonstrate pancreatic necrosis of 30% or more of the pancreatic volume on contrast-enhanced computed tomography (CT) (Fig. 77.1). It is unusual for patients who develop later local complications such as infection in or around the pancreatic necrosis to have no sign of early systemic organ dysfunction.

INCIDENCE AND ETIOLOGY

All population studies of patients with acute pancreatitis indicate a steadily increasing incidence of this fairly common cause for emergency hospital admission. There is a range from around 11 to 40 per 100 000 population, with the higher values being found in Scandinavia and Scotland. The mortality rate from acute pancreatitis is fairly consistently around 7–8%, with a slight, but significant, reduction in case mortality in the most recent decades.[1] Gallstones represent the most common etiology, although in Finland alcohol abuse is the cause in 70–80% of cases. Where great care is taken to identify gallstone disease, the incidence of this etiology is approximately 65%. These two common etiologies in prospective studies account for 75–90% of all patients. Other causes include:

- Ampullary tumors
- Viral infections (especially mumps and coxsackie B)
- Hyperparathyroidism
- Hyperlipoproteinemia
- Blunt abdominal trauma.

Surgical or endoscopic procedures at the ampulla of Vater (endoscopic retrograde cholangiopancreatitis; ERCP) and re-exposure to certain drugs (e.g., azathioprine, steroids, and asparaginase) can be important. Many isolated case reports suggest that at least 50 drugs have been implicated in causing acute pancreatitis, although thorough checks for a biliary or viral etiology have rarely been made, thus placing a question mark over some of these alleged associations. In certain areas of the world the presence of *Ascaris*, or liver flukes, in the biliary tree cause acute pancreatitis, and the Trinidad scorpion bite is an unusual focal geographic etiology.

It is worthwhile remembering that more than one etiologic factor may be present in an individual patient and that it is small gallstones that cause most acute pancreatitis. Current detection methods such as standard ultrasonography do not detect stones of 4 mm or less, and it is stones of this size that are implicated most frequently in transient obstruction at the ampulla of Vater. Only endoscopic ultrasonography (EUS) can accurately detect very small stones. This mechanism of disease was elegantly shown originally in Argentina,[4] but thereafter verified in studies in the USA and UK by fecal sieving of initial bowel movements after the onset of acute pancreatitis with subsequent matching of stones with a similar chemical composition in cholecystectomy specimens.

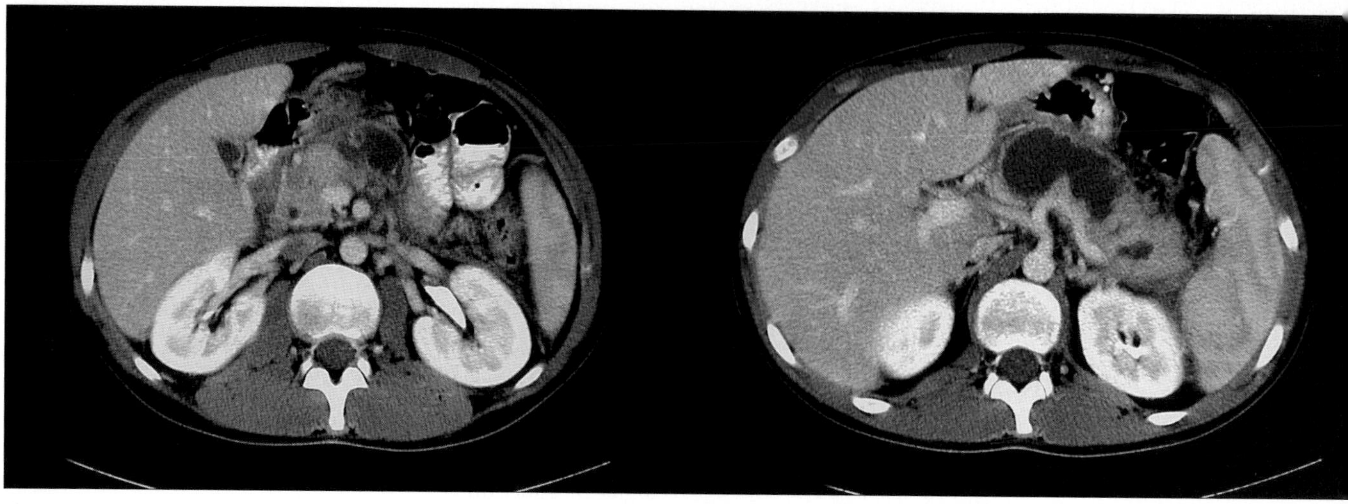

Fig. 71.1 Pancreatic necrosis. Computed tomograms demonstrating approximately 50% necrosis of pancreatic volume (mainly body and tai in an 18-year-old patient who survived, despite this early event. The black areas of pancreas are necrotic.

Sphincter of Oddi dyskinesia and the presence of mal-union of the pancreatic ducts (pancreas divisum) are also associated with acute pancreatitis, although it should be noted that only a small proportion of patients with pancreas divisum develop acute pancreatitis, possibly caused by poor outflow of the accessory duct system.

Hereditary pancreatitis usually presents in patients under the age of 20 years and has been shown to be associated with mutations of the trypsinogen gene *R122H*, *N291*, and *A16V*. Other genetic associations are with the cystic fibrosis gene (*CFTR*) and trypsin inhibitor (*SPINK1*). It is highly probable that other genetic abnormalities will be demonstrated to be associated with acute pancreatitis. In the hereditary acute pancreatitis, patients progress to chronic pancreatitis and, not infrequently, to pancreatic cancer.[5]

CLINICAL PRESENTATION AND DIAGNOSIS

Acute pancreatitis usually presents with severe acute epigastric pain, often radiating to the back, with associated nausea, vomiting, and fever. The diagnosis is usually made when these symptoms occur with levels of blood amylase and/or lipase raised three times above the upper limit of normal. It is important to remember that the patient may have such severe pain that it is difficult for them to differentiate between lower chest and upper abdominal pain. Clinically it can also be difficult to differentiate acute pancreatitis from:

- Perforated duodenal ulcer
- Ischemic gut
- Dissecting aortic aneurysm
- Ectopic pregnancy (no lipase elevation)

All of these conditions can be associated with increased levels of amylase and lipase. In the case of perforated duodenal ulcer, small bowel ischemia, and obstruction, it is the escape of intraluminal enzymes into the peritoneal cavity that causes the increased enzyme levels, and the fallopian tubes are rich in amylase, hence the rise in ectopic pregnancy. Most frequently in the developed world, CT will clarify diagnostic uncertainty. Elsewhere, peritoneal aspiration can be helpful as early infection is rare in acute pancreatitis.

The approximately 3% of patients with an associated hyperlipoproteinemia usually have an alcohol abuse problem and consequent secondary hyperlipoproteinemia; primary hype lipoproteinemia is rarely encountered.[6] In each group mea urement of blood amylase concentration can be difficult, ar urinary amylase or blood lipase measurements are more reliabl The pathogenesis of acute pancreatitis in pregnancy is usual related to gallstones, and occasionally cholecystectomy in mi trimester or endoscopic sphincterotomy without radiolog screening is indicated.

ASSESSMENT OF SEVERITY

At the Atlanta conference in 1992,[7] the following definitio were made.

- *Acute pancreatitis* – an acute inflammatory process of th pancreas, with variable involvement of other regional tissues or remote organ systems.
- *Mild acute pancreatitis* – associated with minimal organ dysfunction and an uneventful recovery. The predominan feature is interstitial edema of the gland.
- *Severe* acute pancreatitis – associated with organ failure and/or local complications such as necrosis (with infection pseudocyst, or abscess. Most often this is an expression o the development of pancreatic necrosis, although patient with edematous pancreatitis may manifest clinical feature of a severe attack.

There is no single marker of severity in acute pancreatiti The most important recent development has been the recogn tion[8] that many patients with clinically severe AP have marke of organ failure at presentation leading to use of prognosti grading methods such as the Marshall system (Table 71.1) Patients with a Marshall score of 2 or more with no improve ment in the first 48 h are those with the poorest outcome an need for respiratory intensive care treatment.[2,3]

Scoring systems: Predicted disease severity based on mult factorial scoring systems such as the Acute Physiology An Chronic Health Evaluation (APACHE) II[10] or Glasgow Scorin System[11] (Table 71.2) do not have very accurate predictiv ability for individual patients. Their main value is in the iden tification of similar groups of patients in order to establis comparability of studies from different parts of the world Optimum positive predictive value of the Glasgow system is i the region of 65%, whereas sensitivity is only 70%. The ag

TABLE 71.1 MODIFIED MARSHALL SCORE (EXCLUDING HEPATIC INDEX)

	SCORE				
	0	1	2	3	4
ystolic blood pressure	>90	<90 Responds to fluid	<90 Poor IV fluid response	<90 (pH <7.3)	<90 (pH <7.2)
o_2/Po_2	>400	301–400	201–300	101–200	<101
lasgow Coma Score	15	13–14	10–12	6–9	<6
atelet count ($\times 10^9$/L)	>120	81–120	51–80	21–50	<21
reatinine (μmol/L)	<134	134–169	170–310	311–439	<439

o_2, fraction of inspired oxygen; Po_2, partial pressure of oxygen.

TABLE 71.2 GLASGOW SCORING SYSTEM FOR SEVERE ACUTE PANCREATITIS[11]

ge	>55 years
/hite blood cell count	$>15\times10^9$/L
lucose	>10 mmol/L (no diabetic history)
rea	>16 mmol/L
ao_2	<60 mmHg (8 kPa)
alcium	<2.0 mmol/L
lbumin	<32 g/L
actate dehydrogenase	>600 IU/L

ao_2, arterial oxygen saturation.

d chronic health evaluation aspects of APACHE II mean at a minimum cutoff score of 8 is required to classify severe ute pancreatitis, whereas many studies have employed a ore of 6.

Obesity (body mass index $>30\,kg/m^2$) is associated with a orer outcome, and the combination of APACHE II and obesity s been used to improve both markers of severity. Obese patients ve a poor respiratory reserve and a greater volume of fat ound the pancreas to be digested, both of which are addi- nal risk factors. Early chest radiologic abnormalities such as eural effusion are associated with a poor outcome, and a later e in the level of the acute-phase reactant C-reactive protein RP) exceeding 150 mg/L can be used to monitor resolution or ntinuation of the disease process. It is rare for patients with ild acute pancreatitis to have a levels above 150 mg/L, whereas vels in those with the most severe forms of disease frequently ceed 200 mg/L, with a practical cutoff being 150 mg/L.[12]

Contrast-enhanced CT can identify areas of malperfusion of e pancreas (Fig. 71.1); there is a close correlation with macro- opic necrosis. The greater the volume of tissue necrosis, the eater the risk of infection of necrotic pancreas.

Amyloid A[13] and pro-calcitonin[14] as well as urinary trypsinogen tivation peptide may become more employed as single arkers of disease severity in the clinical setting. In the future serum interleukin-6 may also prove useful if a cheap, faster assay is available.

MANAGEMENT

Repetitive clinical assessment

Good clinicians repeatedly reassess their emergency patients who are particularly ill, and those with the most severe forms of acute pancreatitis warrant frequent clinical, hematologic, and biochemical assessment. The presence of a systemic inflammatory response syndrome (SIRS) identifies patients at increased risk of organ dysfunction, particularly when three or four of the SIRS criteria are present or persist beyond 48 h:

- Fever
- Tachycardia
- Tachypnea
- Leukocytosis.

Hypoxemia, especially when poorly reversed by the provision of humidified oxygen, is the main marker of major respiratory compromise and the need for intensive care therapy. In the Atlanta Classification of Disease Severity[7] there is no appreciation of the dynamics of organ failure. Thus any patient with a single recorded instance of hypoxemia of less than 60 mmHg (8 kPa) is rated as having severe disease. Clinical studies have now established that transient hypoxemia is associated with neither high mortality nor major morbidity.[2,3] Sustained MODS or a deteriorating picture is found in the sickest patients.

The place of prophylactic antibiotic therapy

Background

The target of antibiotic therapy is to minimize the risk of necrotic pancreatic and peripancreatic tissue becoming infected. There is general agreement that patients with sterile necrosis run a more benign clinical course than those who develop infection, and that infected patients frequently require interventional radiologic or surgical therapy.[15]

Recommendations

Current clinical practice in most specialist world centers appears to be split in a roughly 2 to 1 ratio in favor of using prophylactic antibiotics in the treatment of patients with necrotizing acute pancreatitis. Modern cephalosporins, carbopenem drugs, or quinolones are appropriate choices.

Evidence

There have been many randomized controlled studies of antibiotic therapy in patients with objectively graded severe acute pancreatitis, but these have been small because of stringent entry criteria (e.g., the presence of at least 30% volume necrosis on CT).[16] Nevertheless, as Table 71.3 indicates, there is a trend towards slightly lower mortality and morbidity rates with antibiotic treatment.

The choice of antibiotic has been influenced by studies showing that the penetration of modern cephalosporins and carbopenem drugs into pancreatic tissue is good, whereas that of aminoglycosides is poor.[17] However, whilst Gram-negative organisms predominated in data in the 1993 seminal paper by Pederzoli et al.,[18] this has changed so that Gram-positive cocci and fungal infections are now very important.

In the imipenem study of Pederzoli et al.[18] there was a lower rate of pancreatic infection in the antibiotic group but the mortality difference was marginal. Only in the Helsinki study[19] was there a significant difference in the mortality rate. This study was probably the least satisfactory in scientific terms in that almost 70% of patients in the placebo group received antibiotics within 72–96 h and two of the patients who received placebo died very rapidly from MODS. The median age of patients in this study was around 40 years, and almost all patients had alcohol-related disease. The studies of both Delcenserie et al.[20] and Schwarz et al.[21] contained fewer than 30 patients. One of the conclusions of the study of Isenmann et al.[16] was that it may be justifiable to treat patients conservatively and to withhold antibiotics until a specific infective agent has been identified. It would be desirable to have a much larger study to attempt to answer the question of whether prophylactic antibiotics confer benefit in the management of severe acute pancreatitis.

Nasoenteral feeding

Background

Until 1996 patients were managed by a drip-and-suck regimen with intravenous fluids with or without intravenous nutrition and nasogastric aspiration, in the unproven belief that any oral intake would stimulate the inflamed gland and cause an exacerbation of the disease process. Opinion has changed substantially, and at present approximately one-third of experts believe that early nasoenteral feeding should be standard treatment, with any antibiotic therapy withheld until specific cultures have be obtained.

Recommendations

There is a reasonable cohort of evidence that nasojejunal feedi is cheaper and safer than intravenous nutrition. Strictly speakir we have no proof that it is an improvement on a simple 'nil mouth' policy.

Evidence

Two early studies from Belgium and the USA showed that nea all patients with severe acute pancreatitis could be successfu fed nasoenterically with lower morbidity and cost.[22,23] A prospe tive randomized study from Greece[24] also showed substanti cost savings and a lower incidence of hyperglycemia and infe tive complications with nasojejunal compared with intraveno feeding in patients with severe acute pancreatitis (Table 71.4 Thirty of the patients had a gallstone etiology. The mean Glasgo prognostic score was 4, the APACHE II score was over 11. and the mean CRP level close to 300 mg/L. Average stay in inte sive care was 12 days and total hospital stay approximate 40 days. The caloric intake was approximately 70% of da requirement within 3 days of starting nasoenteric feeding. O'Kee and his team from Virginia found that a hypocaloric nasoente intake also achieved similar clinical outcome to intravenous nut tion at an estimated saving of 2300 US dollars per patient. Others with similar experience from Hungary[26] and the UK[27] al favor nasoenteral feeding.

Specific additional claims for the benefits of early nasoente feeding have been made, based on a study of 34 patients ra domized to either nasoenteral or intravenous nutrition; Winds et al.[28] reported that nasoenteral feeding resulted in an enhanc antioxidant capacity (compared with a decrease with intr venous nutrition), a lower SIRS response after 1 week, a unchanged IgM anticore endotoxin antibodies (compared wi a substantial rise with intravenous nutrition). The only tw deaths occurred in the intravenously fed group. However, on 13 of the 34 patients had objective evidence of severe diseas Moreover, the only study to compare enteral feeding with simple 'nil by mouth' policy in 26 patients with severe acu pancreatitis found no differences in markers of the inflammato response or gut permeability.[29]

Nevertheless, there has been a rapid change in thinking wi the increased utilization of nasojejunal feeding early in the disea process of severe acute pancreatitis in most European cente

TABLE 71.3 STUDIES OF PROPHYLACTIC ANTIBIOTIC THERAPY

Reference	Year	No. of patients	Drugs	Deaths[a]
Pederzoli et al.[18]	1993	74	Imipenem : placebo	3 : 4
Sainio et al.[19]	1995	60	Cefuroxime : placebo	1 : 7
Delcenserie et al.[20]	1996	23	Ceftazidime + amikacin + metronidazole : placebo	1 : 3
Schwarz et al.[21]	1997	26	Ofloxacin + metronidazole : placebo	0 : 2
Isenmann et al.[16]	2004	105	Ciprofloxacin + metronidazole : placebo	2 : 4

[a] Ratio of placebo : antibiotic.

TABLE 71.4 CLINICAL DETAILS AND TREATMENT COMPLICATIONS IN 38 PATIENTS WITH SEVERE ACUTE PANCREATITIS RECEIVING NASOJEJUNAL OR PARENTERAL FEEDING (KALFARENTZOS ET AL.[24])

	Enteral feeding (n=18)	Parenteral feeding (TPN) (n=20)
Clinical details		
Sex ratio (M:F)	8:10	7:13
Mean age (years)	63.0	67.2
Gallstones	14	16
Alcohol-related	3	2
APACHE II score	12.7	11.8
Maximum CRP (mg/L)	290	335
Complications		
Infected necrosis	1	4
Pancreatic abscess	1	0
Pseudocyst	0	1
Catheter sepsis	0	2
Glucose >200 mg	4	9
Systemic sepsis	5	10
Daily cost (GBP)	30	100

APACHE, Acute Physiologoy And Chronic Health Evaluation; CRP, C-reactive protein; GBP, Great Britain pounds.

The location of catheters beyond the duodenojejunal flexure can be tricky and time consuming when awaiting the natural migration of a tube distally, such that most groups place their guidewires and tubes endoscopically believing they must be into the jejunum to minimize the release of cholecystokinin.

Nasogastric feeding

Eatock et al.[30] found that effective feeding was possible in 22 of 26 consecutive patients using fine-bore nasogastic tubes; 70% of normal caloric intake was achieved within 48–72 h, with neither exacerbation of pain nor increase in markers of disease severity such as CRP. In a subsequent study[31] comparing early nasogastric versus nasojejunal feeding in a further 49 consecutive patients with severe acute pancreatitis, the same authors found no significant clinical difference between the two nasoenteric routes. Careful comparison of the records of APACHE II score, CRP level, analgesic requirement, and pain score also showed no difference between the two groups.

Early endoscopic sphincterotomy

Background

Endoscopic sphincterotomy was developed for patients with evidence of common bile duct stones. Although most stones held up in the ampulla of Vater are only transient, some can impact for a longer time and, in addition to acute pancreatitis, ascending cholangitis may be present.

Recommendations

Where the initial ultrasonographic assessment and liver function test results indicate a biliary pathology, early endoscopic sphincterotomy may be beneficial provided it is carried out by an expert. Delay in attempting ERCP can result in duodenal wall edema, making ampullary identification difficult.

Evidence

Table 71.5 summarizes the randomized studies of endoscopic sphincterotomy in patients with severe acute pancreatitis that have been fully published. Two showed benefit. In one UK study of 121 patients with gallstone acute pancreatitis of varying severity, there was little procedure-associated morbidity, perhaps because the procedure was carried out by the same endoscopist in every patient.[32] In 53 patients with objective criteria of severe acute pancreatitis there were lower mortality and morbidity rates (Table 71.5). A study of 127 patients from Hong Kong similarly found a lower mortality rate, but also a marked reduction in biliary sepsis with endoscopic sphincterotomy.[33] Extensive experience from a single center in Poland reported 280 consecutive patients with acute pancreatitis who were allocated to endoscopic sphincterotomy when a specific hospital team was on call. The other group without access to early sphincterotomy had higher mortality and morbidity rates, as well as a greater incidence of recurrent acute pancreatitis. These data have so far been presented only in abstract form.[34]

In contrast, a multicenter German study of 238 patients found no evidence of benefit.[35] However, this study involved multiple operators, with some centers recruiting fewer than two patients per year. Patients with a bilirubin level in excess of 90 μmol/L (arguably the group with most to gain) were excluded from the study, and the mortality rate in the predicted severe acute pancreatitis group was considerably higher than that in the UK[32] and Hong Kong[33] studies. Not all patients were clearly categorized for severity, and less than 50% of the treatment group had a sphincterotomy (Table 71.5) because the protocol allowed it only when bile duct stones were identified at the time of ERCP.

Specific anti-inflammatory therapies

Attempts over the past 30 years to find a specific therapy have proved disappointing. Antiprotease therapy (aprotinin and gabexate mesilate), somatostatin and its analog octreotide, and the platelet-activating factor antagonist lexipafant have all failed

TABLE 71.5 RANDOMIZED STUDIES OF EARLY ENDOSCOPIC SPHINCTEROTOMY IN ACUTE PANCREATITIS

Reference	No. of patients	Complications	Deaths
Neoptolemos et al.[31] (1988)			
Early ES (<72 h)	25[a]	6	1
Standard therapy	28[a]	17	5
Fan et al.[32] (1993)			
Early ES (<24 h)	64	10	1
Standard therapy	63	21	5
Folsch et al.[34] (1997)			
Early ES (only 46%)	126	38	14
Standard therapy	112	40	7

[a] All patients met objective criteria of severe acute pancreatitis.
ES, endoscopic sphincterotomy.

when put to the test of randomized double-blind study. Peritoneal lavage also failed to improve mortality and morbidity rates in two randomized studies of patients in the UK and Sweden.

LATER COMPLICATIONS OF ACUTE PANCREATITIS

Infected necrosis

It has been well established for many years that the greater the volume of necrotic pancreatic tissue the greater the likelihood of infection. The data also indicate that patients with sterile necrosis do not warrant endoscopic, radiologic, or surgically oriented intervention to remove the necrotic tissue. However, the presence of infection in and around necrotic tissue is an indication for intervention. Until the mid-1990s this was usually an open surgical procedure employing various approaches, with the main target of removing necrotic tissue and thereafter establishing multiple drainage tubes to enable peritoneal lavage of the infected necrotic area.

More recently a variety of less invasive approaches have been reported, reflecting a realization of the dangers of open surgery in sick patients with organ failure. Techniques include:

- Radiologically guided percutaneous drainage[36]
- Endoscopic transgastric lavage and drainage[37,38]
- Minimally invasive retroperitoneal surgical approaches.[39,40]

The variety of approaches is a reflection of different skills present in certain specialist units; comparative studies are few and unreliable. In the analysis of published figures it is critically important to have a clear index of the proportion in organ failure at the start of treatment as this is the single most important factor in determining mortality and morbidity. In general, it is wise to advocate the least invasive procedures to ensure a fitter patient, in case repeated attempts or open surgery are required.

Pancreatic abscess

Localized abscess formation as the result of acute pancreatitis is usually relatively easy to deal with. In a proportion of patients, a sterile pancreatic pseudocyst has been converted to an abscess either by natural events, or iatrogenically as a result of endoscopic or percutaneous intervention. Abscess drainage, either b external percutaneous routes or by lavage or internal drainag at the time of a surgical procedure, is a useful way to tackle th problem.

Pancreatic pseudocyst (see Chapter 74)

Open surgery to achieve internal drainage to the stomach c duodenum used to be standard but has been replaced by less inva sive approaches. Where the pseudocyst communicates directl with the disrupted pancreatic duct system, a stent along th pancreatic duct can result in fairly rapid internal drainage; like wise EUS-guided drainage into the stomach or duodenum is useful modern approach. Figure 71.2 provides an example of very large pseudocyst that was not adjacent to the stomach c duodenum and required drainage into a Roux loop of jejunun highlighting the occasional continuing need for an open surgica approach.

Splenic and portal vein thrombosis

With the increasing utilization of both CT and magnetic reso nance imaging, it has become clearer that patients with sever acute pancreatitis frequently develop splenic vein thrombos that may extend into the portal vein. Sustained portal hype tension can be encountered in these patients, and the exact inc dence of this type of complication has not been fully documente

Gastrointestinal hemorrhage

This is an occasional problem in severe acute pancreatitis du to stress-induced duodenal ulcer or, less commonly, late develop ing gastric varices or pseudoaneurysms of the vessels in th area of necrosis. Bleeding may also occur into a pancreati pseudocyst or into the area of inflammation in the most sever disease when a major vessel is disrupted by the necrotic proces Optimal treatment usually involves the use of interventiona radiology to occlude the relevant vessels.

Diabetes mellitus

This occurs in less than 5% of patients with acute pancreatiti Those with necrosis of large volumes of the pancreas are at pa ticular risk. During the acute phase of management of sever acute pancreatitis, hyperglycemia may be a considerable problen

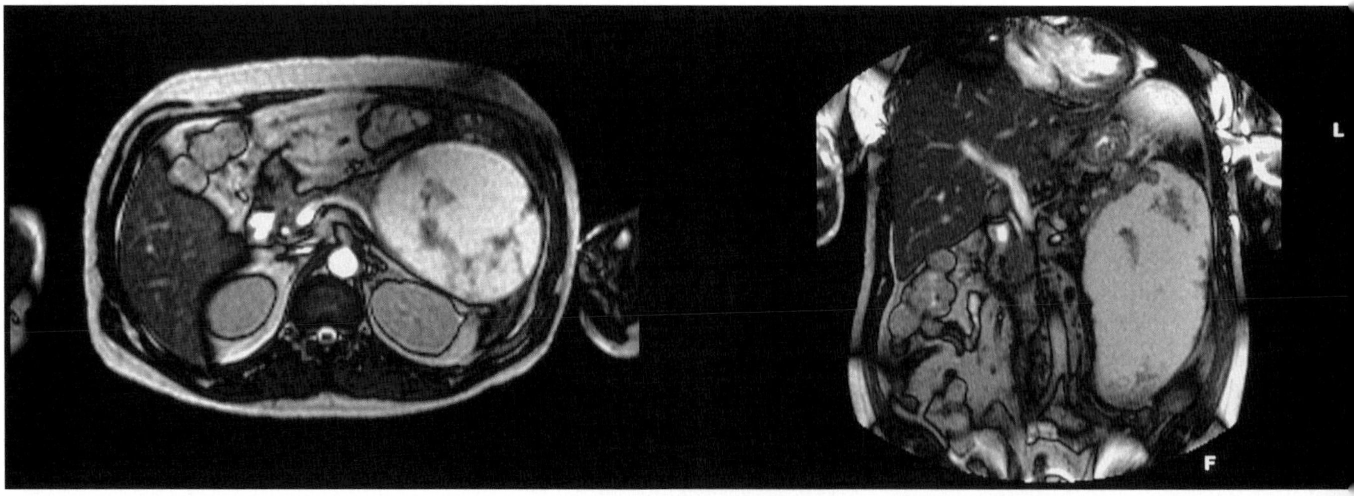

Fig. 71. 2 Pancreatic pseudocyst. Magnetic resonance cholangiopancreatography of transverse and coronal sections of a very large pancreati pseudocyst unattached to the stomach or duodenum. Cystojejunostomy Roux loop drainage at open operation was a success.

other intensive care situations, tight control of blood sugar vels (4.0–6.1 mmol/L) has been shown to result in a better ıtcome, and this approach should be carefully employed in ill ıtients with acute pancreatitis.

egmental chronic pancreatitis

ıajor damage to the main pancreatic duct in a single attack of ute pancreatitis can result in stricture formation, with the oximal duct system draining poorly and ultimately that area the pancreas being subject to chronic pancreatitis, unless ents or surgical duct drainage are employed.

ROGNOSIS

mild pancreatitis the prognosis is favorable, with a mortality te of less than 5%, but this increases up to 50% in severe ute pancreatitis, especially in the context of adult respiratory stress syndrome, shock, or infection of necrotic pancreas.

/HAT TO TELL PATIENTS

ıtients should be warned to seek medical help if they develop mptoms suggestive of recurrent pancreatis: abdominal pain, ıusea, vomiting, and fever. Alcoholic patients should be lvised of the high risk of recurrence and risk of progression chronic pancreatitis (5% of chronic alcoholics).

In patients with gallstones and mild acute pancreatitis, the risk of further attacks should be minimized by cholecystectomy, ideally in the same admission. In the elderly or unfit, endoscopic sphincterotomy is a safer alternative.[41]

The exact timing of these prophylactic measures in severe acute pancreatitis will vary with individual cases.

SOURCES OF INFORMATION FOR PATIENTS AND DOCTORS

http://patients.uptodate.com/topic.asp?file=digestiv/2957
http://cchs-dl.slis.ua.edu/patientinfo/gastroenterology/pancreas/pancreatitis/acute.htm
http://www.patient.co.uk/showdoc/23364025
http://www.gastro.org/clinicalRes/brochures/pancreatitis.html
http://www.gastro.org/generalPublic.html
http://www.pancreasfoundation.org
http://www.nlm.nih.gov/medlineplus/pancreaticdiseases.html
http://digestive.niddk.nih.gov/ddiseases/pubs/pancreatitis/
http://www.vetinfo.com/dpancrea.html
www.pancreatitis.org.uk/
http://www.pancreaticdisease.com/
http://www.patient.co.uk/showdoc/479/
http://www.patient.co.uk/showdoc.asp?doc=23069113

EFERENCES

. McKay CJ, Evans S, Sinclair M et al. High early mortality from acute pancreatitis in Scotland 1984–1995. Br J Surg 1999; 86:1302–1305.
. Buter A, Imrie CW, Carter CR et al. Dynamic nature of early organ dysfunction determines outcome in acute pancreatitis. Br J Surg 2002; 89:298–302.
. Johnson CD, Abu-Hilal M. Persistent organ failure during the first week as a marker of fatal outcome in acute pancreatitis. Gut 2004; 53:1340–1344.
. Acosta JM, Ledesma CL. Gallstone migration as a cause of acute pancreatitis. N Engl J Med 1974; 290:484–487.
. Whitcomb DC. Hereditary pancreatitis; new insights into acute and chronic pancreatitis. Gut 1999; 45:317–322.
. Dickson AP, O'Neill J, Imrie CW. Hyperlipidaemia, alcohol abuse and acute pancreatitis. Br J Surg 1984; 74:685–688.
. Bradley EL. A clinically based classification system for acute pancreatitis. Summary of the International Symposium on Acute Pancreatitis, Atlanta, September 11–13, 1992. Arch Surg 1993; 128:586–590.
. Johnson CD, Kingsnorth AN, Imrie CW et al. Double blind, randomised placebo controlled study of a platelet activating factor antagonist lexipafant in the treatment and prevention of organ failure in predicted severe acute pancreatitis. Gut 2001; 48:62–69.
. Marshall JC, Cook DJ, Christou NV et al. Multiple organ dysfunction score, a reliable descriptor of a complex clinical outcome. Crit Care Med 1995; 23:83–92.
. Knaus WA, Wagner DP, Draper EA et al. APACHE II: final form and national validation results of a severity of disease classification system. Crit Care Med 1984; 12:213–224.
11. Blamey SL, Imrie CW, O'Neill J et al. Prognostic factors in acute pancreatitis. Gut 1984; 25:1340–1346.
12. Wilson C, Heads A, Shenkin A, Imrie CW. C-reactive protein, antiproteases and complement factors as objective markers of severity in acute pancreatitis. Br J Surg 1989; 76:177–181.
13. Mayer JM, Raraty M, Slavin J et al. Serum amyloid A is a better early predictor of severity than C-reactive protein in acute pancreatitis. Br J Surg 2002; 89:163–171.
14. Rau B, Steinbach CHG, Gansauge F et al. The potential role of procalcitonin and interleukin-8 in the prediction of infected necrosis in acute pancreatitis. Gut 1997; 41:832–840.
15. Buchler MW, Gloor B, Muller CA et al. Acute necrotising pancreatitis: treatment strategy according to the status of infection. Ann Surg 2000; 232:619–626.
16. Isenmann R, Runzi M, Kron M et al. Ciprofloxacin/metronidazole in patients with severe acute pancreatitis – results of a double blind placebo controlled multicentre trial. Gastroenterology 2004; 126:997–1003.
17. Buchler M, Malfertheiner P, Friess H et al. Human pancreatic tissue concentrations of bactericidal antibiotics. Gastroenterology 1992; 103:1902–1908.
18. Pederzoli P, Bassi C, Vesentini S et al. A randomised multicenter clinical trial of antibiotic prophylaxis of septic complications in acute necrotizing pancreatitis with imipenem. Surg Gynecol Obstet 1993; 176:480–483.
19. Sainio V, Kemppainen E, Puolakkainen P et al. Early antibiotic treatment in acute necrotising pancreatitis. Lancet 1995; 346:663–667.
20. Delcenserie R, Yzett T, Ducroix JP. Prophylactic antibiotics in treatment of severe acute alcoholic pancreatitis. Pancreas 1996; 13:198–201.
21. Schwarz M, Isenmann R, Meyer H et al. Antibiotika bei nekrotisierender pankreatitis. Ergepnisse einer kontrollierten studie. Deutsch Med Wschr 1997; 122:356–361.
22. Nakad A, Piessevaux H, Marot JC et al. Is early enteral nutrition in acute pancreatitis dangerous? About 20 patients fed by an endoscopically placed nasogastrojejunal tube. Pancreas 1998; 17:187–193.
23. McClave SA, Greene LM, Snider HL et al. Comparison of the safety of early enteral versus parenteral nutrition in mild acute pancreatitis. JPEN Parenter Enteral Nutr 1997; 21:14–20.
24. Kalfarentzos F, Kehagias J, Mead N et al. Enteral nutrition is superior to parenteral nutrition in severe acute pancreatitis: results of a randomised prospective trial. Br J Surg 1997; 84:1665–1669.
25. Abou-Assi S, Craig K, O'Keefe SJ. Hypocaloric jejunal feeding is better than total parenteral nutrition in acute pancreatitis: results of a randomised comparative study. Am J Gastroenterol 2002; 97:2255–2262.
26. Olah A, Pardavi G, Belagyi T et al. Early nasojejunal feeding in acute pancreatitis is associated with a lower complication rate. Nutrition 2002; 18:259–262.
27. Gupta R, Patel K, Calder PC et al. A randomised clinical trial to assess the effect of total enteral and total parenteral nutritional support on metabolic, inflammatory and oxidative markers in patients with predicted severe acute pancreatitis. (APACHE II > or =6). Pancreatology 2003; 3:406–413.
28. Windsor AC, Kanwar S, Li AG et al. Compared with parenteral nutrition, enteral

feeding attenutates the acute phase response and improves disease severity in acute pancreatitis. Gut 1998; 42:431–435.
29. Powell JJ, Murchison JT, Fearon KC et al. Randomized controlled trial of the effect of early enteral nutrition on markers of the inflammatory response in predicted severe acute pancreatitis. Br J Surg 2000; 87:1375–1381.
30. Eatock FC, Brombacher GD, Steven A et al. Nasogastric feeding in severe acute pancreatitis may be practical and safe. Int J Pancreatol 2000; 28:23–30.
31. Eatock FC, Chong P, Menezes N, et al. A randomized study of early nasogastric versus nasojejunal feeding in severe acute pancreatitis. Am J Gastroenterol 2005; 100:432–439.
32. Neoptolemos JP, Carr-Locke D, London NJM. Controlled trial of urgent ERCP and endoscopic sphincterotomy versus conservative treatment for acute pancreatitis due to gallstones. Lancet 1988; ii:989–993.
33. Fan ST, Lai ECS, Mok FPT et al. Early treatment of acute biliary pancreatitis by endoscopic papillotomy. N Engl J Med 1993; 203:228–232.
34. Nowak A, Nowakowska-Dulawa E, Marek TA. Final results of the prospective randomised controlled study of endoscopic sphincterotomy versus conventional management in acute biliary pancreatitis. Gastroenterology 1995; 108(Suppl):A380 (Abstract).
35. Folsch UR, Mitsch ER, Ludt KE et al. Early ERCP and papillotomy compared with conservative treatment for acute biliary pancreatitis. N Engl J Med 1997; 336:237–242.
36. Freeny PC, Hauptmann E, Althaus SJ et al. Percutanous CT guided catheter drainage of infected acute necrotising pancreatitis. Techniques and results. AJR Am J Roentgenol 1998; 1970:969–975.
37. Baron TH, Thaggard WG, Morgan DE. Endoscopic therapy for organised pancreati necrosis. Gastroenterology 1996; 111:755–764.
38. Seifert H, Wehrmann T, Schmitt T et al. Retroperitoneal endoscopic debridement fo infected peripancreatic necrosis. Lancet 20 356:653–655.
39. Carter CR, McKay CJ, Imrie CW. Percutaneous necrosectomy and sinus tract endoscopy in the management of infected pancreatic necrosis: an initial experience. Ann Surg 2000; 232:175–180.
40. Connor S, Ghaneh P, Raraty M et al. Minimally invasive retroperitoneal pancrea necrosectomy. Dig Surg 2003; 20:270–277.
41. Uhl W, Warshaw A, Imrie C et al. IAP guidelines for the surgical management of acute pancreatitis. Pancreatology 2002; 2:565–573.

Chapter 72

Chronic pancreatitis

P O Berberat, Z Dambrauskas, M W Büchler, and H Friess

KEY POINTS

- Excessive alcohol consumption is the main cause of chronic pancreatitis in the Western world
- The incidence of chronic pancreatitis is increasing
- Males are affected more often than females
- Pain is the leading symptom of chronic pancreatitis. Continuous or severe intermittent pain is often resistant to medical treatment, and surgical intervention required for long-term relief
- The disease is associated with various degrees of exocrine (maldigestion) and endocrine (diabetes mellitus) insufficiency
- Chronic pancreatitis is a complex disease, and an interdisciplinary approach from gastroenterologists and surgeons is required for optimal treatment

INTRODUCTION

Chronic pancreatitis is an inflammatory disease of the pancreas characterized by dysplastic ducts, foci of proliferating ductal cells, acinar cell degeneration, marked fibrosis, and often associated with severe pain. Consequently, patients with chronic pancreatitis exhibit variable degrees of pancreatic exocrine and endocrine dysfunction. Chronic pancreatitis is a complex disease, afflicting heavy drinkers in majority of cases, but is also associated with several other causes. Although much is known about the etiologic background of the disease, there is still a large group of patients, perhaps 20–25% of the total, in whom the exact cause of the disease is unknown.[1]

EPIDEMIOLOGY

There are few population-based estimates of frequency. Three studies from Germany, Denmark, and the USA show similar frequency rates, with 6–10 cases per 100 000 population per year. Over time the incidence of chronic pancreatitis has been increasing, as a result of the higher consumption of alcohol. Not surprisingly, because of the relationship of chronic pancreatitis with alcohol consumption, overall more males than females are affected (ratio 3 : 1). Idiopathic and hyperlipidemia-induced pancreatitis are more prevalent in females. Moreover, there are significant differences influenced by race, as the frequency of chronic pancreatitis is greater amongst people of Asian and African descent and in populations native to India and Africa. The reasons for this are not yet known.

A large collaborative report showed that the mean age of the onset of chronic pancreatitis, in all subsets, is approximately 44.6 years. In idiopathic chronic pancreatitis, a bimodal age distribution has been reported, designated as an early-onset form (median age 19.2 years) and late-onset form (median age 56.2 years), whereas hereditary pancreatitis already begins in adolescence.[2]

CAUSES, RISK FACTORS, DISEASE ASSOCIATIONS

Excessive alcohol consumption is considered to be the main etiologic cause of chronic pancreatitis, accounting for more than 70% of all cases. It seems that the mean ethanol intake and the duration of consumption correlates with the risk of developing chronic pancreatitis. In spite of this, however, only a minority of heavy drinkers actually develop chronic pancreatitis, and those who drink moderately have also presented with the disease. These data suggest that other factors, such as genetic predisposition or nutrition, may influence the development of alcoholic pancreatitis.

CAUSES AND RISK FACTORS

- Excessive alcohol consumption
- Idiopathic
- Hypertriglyceridemia
- Hypercalcemia
- Hyperthyroidism
- Uremia
- Hereditary/genetic diseases and syndromes
- Pancreas divisum, anulare, stenosis of the papilla of Vater, and other anatomic abnormalities
- Autoimmune diseases
- Nutritional factors (tropical pancreatitis)

In approximately 20% of patients the disease has to be classified as *idiopathic chronic pancreatitis*, because an explicit etiologic factor cannot be identified. However, the discovery of mutations in genes for the cationic trypsinogen gene (*PRSS1*) and the pancreatic secretory trypsin inhibitor (*SPINK1*) demonstrated that genetic alterations in the cytoprotective mechanism of the pancreas lead to chronic pancreatitis. This and the recognition of other gene mutations, such as the cystic fibrosis transmembrane conductance regulator (*CFTR*) mutation in patients with idiopathic chronic pancreatitis, has heightened the awareness and importance of hereditary factors in this disease.

Rare causes of chronic pancreatitis include hypercalcemia, hyperthyroidism, uremia, hypoproteinemia, and drugs such as phenacetin.

In addition, pancreas divisum, pancreas anulare, and stenosis of the ampulla of Vater, tumors, or trauma are also rare causes of chronic obstructive pancreatitis. Tropical pancreatitis, found in Asia and Africa, develops independently of alcohol intake, and is influenced instead by nutritional factors, leading to early endocrine insufficiency. Some infectious agents have been established as a cause of chronic pancreatitis with reasonable certainty, i.e. echinococcus, coxsackie virus, cytomegalovirus, mumps, HIV, and microsporidia. Many autoimmune diseases may also be associated with chronic pancreatitis, but only Sjögren's syndrome is clearly related with this disease.[3,4]

PATHOGENESIS OF DISEASE

The pathogenesis of chronic pancreatitis remains controversial. For years, three main concepts were proposed:

1. Changes in the *composition of pancreatic juice*, secondary to alcohol overconsumption, leading to increased viscosity and formation of protein plugs, and subsequently obstructing pancreatic ducts
2. The direct *toxic effect of alcohol* and its metabolites on pancreatic acinar and ductal cells
3. Direct damage of the pancreatic parenchyma by increase levels of *free radicals* as a result of reduced hepatic detoxification.

However, none of these classic pathophysiologic concepts ca explain the morphologic, functional, and clinical picture c chronic pancreatitis conclusively.

Recent advances in modern cell and molecular biology hav revealed new distinct mechanisms (Fig. 72.1):

- *Growth factors* – many growth factors are overexpressed in human chronic pancreatitis. Transgenic mice that overexpress important growth factors, such as transforming growth factor (TGF) β and TGF-α, develop severe pancreatic fibrosis and histologic features also seen in humans with chronic pancreatitis.
- *Stellate cells* – recent evidence suggests that pancreatic fibrosis requires the differentiation and stimulation of specific cells called pancreatic stellate cells. It is thought that recurrent acinar cell injuries, caused by oxidative stress (e.g., alcohol, ischemia), and other factors (Fig. 72.1) result in cytokine and chemokine release from acinar cells and the activation of resident macrophages. These macrophages, in turn, suppress acute inflammation by releasing TGF-β and other cytokines, which stimulate stellate cells to produce collagen, and thereby promote fibrosis.

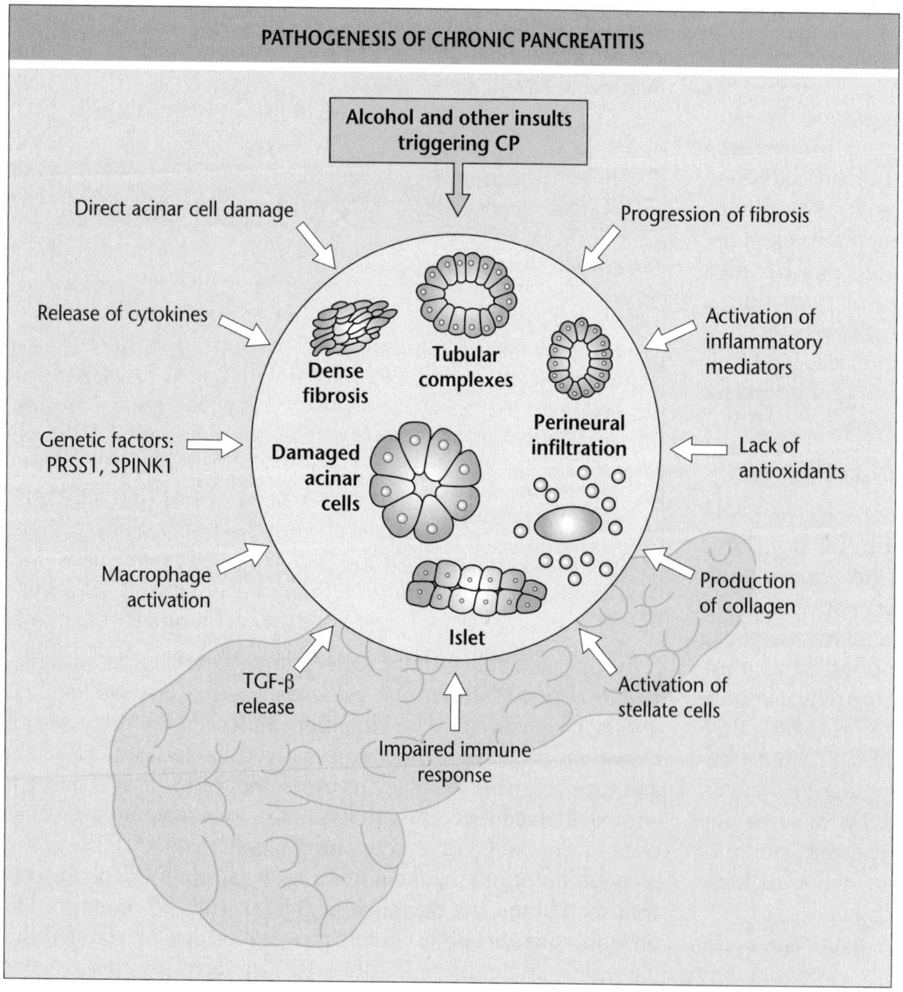

Fig. 72.1 Pathogenesis of chronic pancreatitis.

Other inflammatory mediators – potent proteolytic enzyme systems, such as urokinase-dependent plasminogen activation, and inflammatory mediators, such as phospholipase A_2, also seem to be involved in the pathobiology of chronic pancreatitis.

Immune functions – recent data suggest that decreased regulatory CD4 T cells and uncontrolled activation of CD8 T lymphocytes result in T cell-mediated cytotoxicity.[5,6]

ATHOGENESIS OF SYMPTOMS

Pain – strong interactions between damaged pancreatic parenchymal cells, immunocytes, and proliferating nerves may result in pain. The pathogenesis of pain is probably multifactorial, perhaps explaining why patients do not respond similarly to the same treatment modality.[7]

Malabsorption is due to deficiency of pancreatic enzymes.

Diabetes mellitus – similarly, damage to islet cells leads to diabetes because of reduced insulin secretion.

ATHOLOGY

ı chronic pancreatitis the pancreas usually has a firm appear-nce with signs of calcification; duct obstruction by protein ugs or small calculi are occasionally seen. Histologic evalu-tion of the tissue reveals dense fibrosis and destruction of cinar tissue; often only islets remain relatively unchanged. igns of chronic inflammation, such as infiltration by mono-uclear cells, and marked atrophy of the exocrine pancreas are haracteristic of chronic pancreatitis (Fig. 72.2).

LINICAL PRESENTATION

lost patients with chronic pancreatitis have pain in the upper bdomen, which may radiate to the back. Exceptions include minority of older patients with senile chronic pancreatitis, and a subset of patients with tropical pancreatitis who present at first with diabetes mellitus and may be pain-free. The pain of chronic pancreatitis can be very severe and continuous, but is more often intermittent, and occurs in attacks that are usually not sufficiently severe to require immediate treatment in hospital. Therefore, two types of pancreatic pain have been described:

- Type A pain refers to recurrent episodic pain, suggestive of acute exacerbation of chronic pancreatitis
- Type B pain refers to continuous pain.

A few patients with chronic pancreatitis are pain free.

Enzyme deficiency due to pancreatic damage results in maldigestion and impaired absorption of food, especially fats. Weight loss is characteristic of chronic pancreatitis. Patients may notice bulky, smelly stools due to too much fat (steatorrhea). Occasionally, an 'oil slick' can be seen on the toilet water. Loss of insulin production may result in diabetes. Symptoms related to complications of pseudocyst include jaundice due to extrahepatic bile duct obstruction and signs of duodenal obstruction.[8–10]

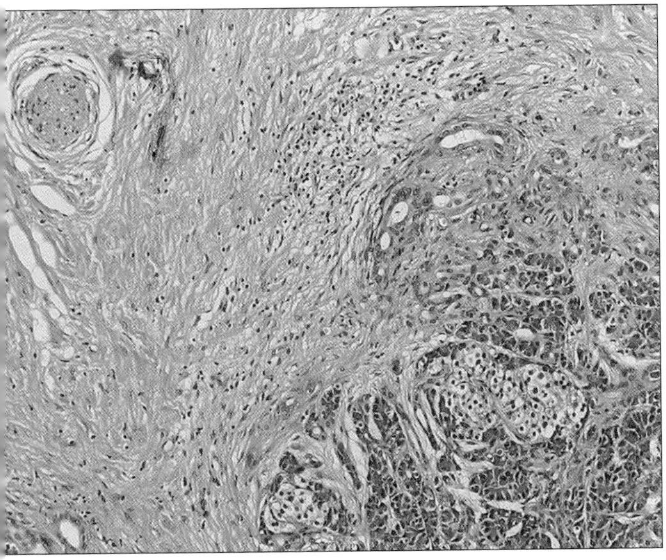

ig. 72.2 Histologic appearance of chronic pancreatitis. Section hows dense fibrosis, proliferating ducts, infiltration of mononuclear ells, and destruction of acinar tissue.

CLINICAL PRESENTATION

- Abdominal pain
  Greatest in upper abdomen
  Lasts from hours to days, eventually continuous
  Exacerbated by eating, drinking, alcohol
  Radiates to the back
- Nausea and vomiting
- Maldigestion and steatorrhea (fatty stools)
- Weight loss
- Signs of diabetes mellitus
- Jaundice and pale or clay-colored stools may also be associated with this condition

DIFFERENTIAL DIAGNOSIS

The diagnosis of chronic pancreatitis in an advanced case is obvious, with typical symptoms such as upper abdominal pain, weight loss, steatorrhea, diabetes mellitus, history of alcohol use, and age approximately 45 years. However, these features are seen only when the disease has been present for many years. In the initial stage of the disease, symptoms are often very nonspecific, and therefore establishment of the diagnosis is difficult. Most patients present with pain only. Similar pain can be caused by cancer of the pancreas (although this is not usually intermittent), stones in the gallbladder and bile duct (biliary colic), or severe types of gastric or duodenal ulcer. All of these conditions have to be considered and appropriate diagnostic tests applied.

DIFFERENTIAL DIAGNOSIS

- Pancreatic carcinoma
- Cystic pancreatic tumor
- Stones in gallbladder and bile duct
- Gastric or duodenal ulcer

DIAGNOSTIC METHODS

Function tests

Poor function of the pancreas can be revealed by testing endocrine (glucose tolerance tests, blood insulin and C-peptide levels) and exocrine secretory capacity. Unfortunately most tests for pancreatic exocrine function have good sensitivity and specificity only when severe pancreatic insufficiency is present (after loss of 90% of the secretory capacity of the pancreas). The secretin–cerulein stimulation test may diagnose already mild disease and could be considered as the 'golden standard' procedure. However, as this procedure is invasive, very unpleasant for the patient, and expensive, it presents many clinical disadvantages. An alternative method that is preferred today is the measurement of pancreatic enzymes in the stool, such as elastase-1 and chymotrypsin. Further indirect tests, which verify maldigestion and help to optimize enzyme treatment, are the quantitative fecal fat test, the pancreolauryl test, and various breath tests. Amylase and lipase blood level measurements are nonspecific and are not useful as diagnostic tests.

Imaging

Pancreatic calcification is detected on plain abdominal films in 25–59% of patients in later stages of chronic pancreatitis. However, the first-line noninvasive diagnostic investigations are transabdominal ultrasonography and computed tomography (CT).

The main findings to note on *transabdominal ultrasonography* are changes in the size, shape, contour, or echotexture of the gland, calcifications, and ductal dilatation. Dilatation of the main pancreatic duct above a diameter of 2 mm, in addition to any kind of extrapancreatic complication, can be revealed by transabdominal ultrasonography.

Endoscopic ultrasonography (EUS) detects more subtle and earlier changes of chronic pancreatitis (sensitivity 80%, specificity 86%). At the same time, this procedure also offers therapeutic options, such as EUS-guided fine-needle aspiration, pancreatic pseudocyst drainage, and celiac plexus neurolysis.[11,12]

CT is a highly accurate method for identification of more or less the same alterations that can be seen with ultrasonography, such as enlargement and irregularity of the pancreas, areas of scarring, dilated biliary ducts, and stones (sensitivity 50–90%, specificity 50–85%). Vascular complications of chronic pancreatitis are best visualized on contrast-enhanced CT, b may be also shown by duplex ultrasonography or *magnet resonance cholangiopancreatography* (MRCP).

A sensitivity and specificity of more than 90% can b attained by endoscopic retrograde cholangiopancreatograph (ERCP). However, as many as 10% of patients with chron pancreatitis may have no pathologic findings on ERCP, an the main disadvantage of ERCP is the risk of complication If papillotomy is performed, the complication rate increases u to 5–10% (without papillotomy, 1.5%), and the risk of deat is around 0.5%. However, ERCP offers the possibility to pe form therapeutic procedures such as dilatation and stentin which is a real advantage. Pancreatic juices can be collecte within the pancreas for laboratory analysis, and tissue spec mens can be taken when there is any suspicion of canc (Fig. 72.3).

DIAGNOSTIC METHODS

PANCREATIC FUNCTION TESTS
- Fecal elastase-1
- Fecal chymotrypsin
- Pancreolauryl test
- Secretin–cerulein stimulation test (gold standard)

IMAGING
- Ultrasonography
- Endosonography
- CT of abdomen (pancreatic pseudocyst, pancreatic duct dilatation)
- Endoscopic retrograde cholangiopancreatography (ERCP) (irregular dilatation of main pancreatic duct, pruning of pancreatic duct branches)
- Magnetic resonance cholangiopancreatography (MRCP)

TREATMENT AND PREVENTION

The treatment of patients with chronic pancreatitis revolve around:

- control of pain
- management of diabetes mellitus
- management of steatorrhea.

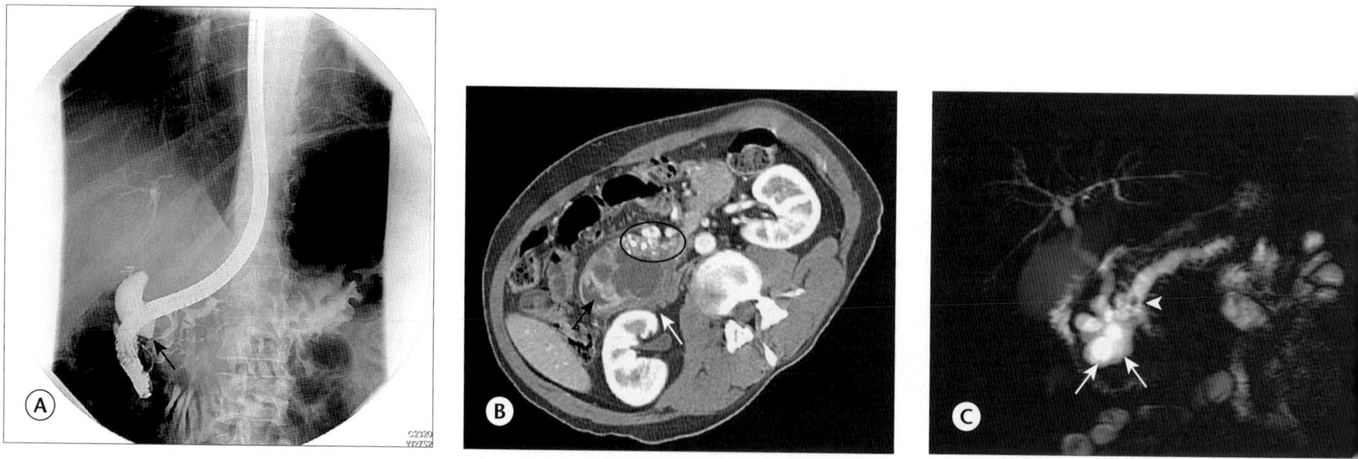

Fig. 72.3 Imaging in chronic pancreatitis. A. ERCP – stenosis of the head of the pancreatic duct (arrow). **B.** CT – cystic lesion (arrows) in the head of the pancreas with multiple calcification (circle) in the head and body. **C.** MRCP – cystic lesion (arrows) in the head, and duct dilatation (arrowhead).

CLINICAL TIPS

DIAGNOSIS OF CHRONIC PANCREATITIS
- Endosonography detects earliest parenchymal changes
- Ductal changes can be detected early through ERCP
- CT scanning is widely available and shows complications
- MRCP has the potential to be the "all-in-one" (including standard scan, MRCP, angiography) for the future

TREATMENT OF CHRONIC PANCREATITIS
- Pancreatic enzymes to treat maldigestion
- Stenting of the bile and pancreatic duct once only – then consider surgery
- Surgical therapy should be considered when complications occur

COMPLICATIONS
- Pseudocysts are the most common complication
- Endoscopic drainage may be the first line of pseudocyst treatment
- Inflammatory pancreatic mass needs surgery

General measures and malabsorption

About 80% of patients with chronic pancreatitis can be managed by dietary recommendations and pancreatic enzyme supplementation. Reduction of steatorrhea and supplementation of calories are the main goals of nutritional therapy. Total abstinence from alcohol and frequent low-fat meals are the basis of dietary recommendations. The diet should be rich in carbohydrates (if diabetes mellitus is not present) and proteins (up to 1.0–1.5 g/day). Weight loss and/or steatorrhea (15 g/day) are indications for supplementation of pancreatic enzymes. Furthermore, malabsorption of proteins and carbohydrates, dyspepsia, meteorism, and diarrhea have also been taken as indications for the substitution of exocrine pancreatic function. Although evidence for the efficacy of pancreatic enzyme replacement is restricted to two randomized trials, their wide use, ease of administration, and lack of any significant side effects make them a first choice in the medical treatment of pain.

Pain

Medical measures

Pain is the most common and the most difficult problem. Pain may be treated interventionally or surgically, but medical treatment is generally the first-line therapy in patients with painful chronic pancreatitis. The guidance for analgesic treatment is based on the recommendations of the World Health Organization. For initial pain relief, non-narcotic analgesics and non-steroidal anti-inflammatory drugs (NSAIDs) are recommended. Opioid analgesics should be prescribed for severe pain on an 'as and when' required basis, but attention should be given to avoid addiction, which is a common problem for people with chronic pancreatitis, especially alcoholic pancreatitis. Some patients with chronic pancreatitis suffer from depression, which lowers the visceral pain threshold. Therefore, antidepressants may have a positive additive effect in pain control. Overall, medical treatment seems to have potential benefit in 40–70% of patients with chronic pancreatitis and pain.

Endoscopic therapy

The next line of treatment for pain and the relief of other associated symptoms should be endoscopic therapy, when feasible. However, the prerequisite is a dilated main pancreatic duct and/or ductal obstruction by stones or stricture. The modalities include pancreatic sphincterotomy, stenting, and possibly lithotripsy to break large calculi. If endoscopic treatment fails, surgical therapy should be considered.

Surgical intervention

There are a number of indications for surgical interventions in chronic pancreatitis, but the most common is intractable pain (Table 72.1). Two main types of surgical treatment are applied today: procedures that involve drainage and those that involve resection (Fig. 72.4; see Table 72.3).

- *Drainage procedures* – pancreaticojejunostomy (Pusteow and Partington–Rochelle procedures). These have the goals of reducing intrapancreatic pressure by draining the pancreatic juice and preserving pancreatic tissue to avoid loss of pancreatic function.
- *Procedures involving resection* – pancreaticoduodenectomy (Whipple operation or left resection). These are indicated in cases of a contracted duct, when the pancreatic head is enlarged, or when a pancreatic carcinoma is suspected.
- *Procedures that combine resection and duct drainage* – (duodenum-preserving pancreatic head resection, Frey operation, Bern operation). These are generally very effective in pain relief, with long-term success rates in the range of 90%, along with good preservation of pancreatic function.

Prevention

Avoidance of heavy alcohol consumption dramatically reduces the risk of developing chronic pancreatitis.[13–15]

COMPLICATIONS AND THEIR MANAGEMENT

Selecting the appropriate procedure for the treatment of complications associated with chronic pancreatitis depends on the anatomic situation and morphologic findings, in addition to the individual patient's symptoms, quality of life, and pancreatic function. The most important complications are pseudocysts, biliary strictures, splenic vein thrombosis, and ascites.

Pseudocysts (see also Chapter 74)

The pseudocyst is the most common local complication of chronic pancreatitis. Pseudocysts are either retention cysts or cysts that develop following acute exacerbation of chronic

TABLE 72.1 INDICATIONS FOR SURGICAL THERAPY IN CHRONIC PANCREATITIS

- Chronic pain:
  Inadequate response to medical and/or endoscopic treatment
- Complications of neighboring structures:
  Duodenal obstruction
  Common bile and/or pancreatic duct obstruction
  Portal and/or splenic vein obstruction
- Mass lesion in pancreatic head and suspected pancreatic cancer
- Effects of ductal rupture
- Persistent or symptomatic pseudocyst
- Pancreatic fistula unresponsive to other therapy
- Pancreatic ascites unresponsive to medical therapy

TREATMENT AND PREVENTION

CONSERVATIVE TREATMENT
- Pain control
- Diet
- Pancreatic enzyme replacement
- Management of diabetes mellitus
- Endoscopic therapy (sphincterotomy, stenting, and lithotripsy)

SURGICAL TREATMENT
- Longitudinal pancreaticojejunostomy (Pusteow and Partington–Rochelle procedures)
- Pancreaticoduodenectomy (Whipple operation, classic and pylorus-preserving)
- Duodenum-preserving pancreatic head resection (Beger operation)
- Longitudinal pancreaticojejunostomy and local pancreatic head excision (Frey operation)
- Central pancreatic head resection (Bern operation)

PREVENTION
- Avoidance of exacerbating factors (abstinence from alcohol consumption and avoidance of fatty foods)

pancreatitis. Pseudocysts develop in approximately 10–25% of all patients with chronic pancreatitis, and may be the cause of persistent pain. Most pseudocysts regress spontaneously over time.

Where treatment is needed, pancreatic cysts and pseudocysts are usually managed by transcutaneous puncture or endoscopic drainage of the collections. Today, three different endoscopic procedures are used to drain pseudocysts:

COMPLICATIONS AND THEIR MANAGEMENT

- Pseudocyst and fistula formation
- Biliary (10–30%) and duodenal (10–25%) obstruction
- Glucose intolerance
- Pancreatic carcinoma
- Narcotic addiction (secondary to chronic pain)

- transgastric drainage
- transduodenal approaches
- the newer procedure of placement of a pigtail endoprosthesis through the papilla into the cyst.[16]

Biliary stricture

Biliary strictures may also occur as a complication. Stenosis c the common bile duct is usually treated by a single attempt a endoscopic stenting, especially in patients with acute cholestasi (before carrying out biliodigestive surgery). Plastic or Wallstent show good short- and medium-term results. Ascending cholan gitis is the main complication with all stents, and long-terr follow-up data are lacking. If jaundice recurs, definitive surgica therapy should be performed, especially in young patients.

Other complications

Splenic vein thrombosis is another important complication and is seen in approximately 10% of patients with chroni pancreatitis. It may lead to the development of gastric funda varices, which can bleed.

SURGICAL THERAPY OF CHRONIC PANCREATITIS

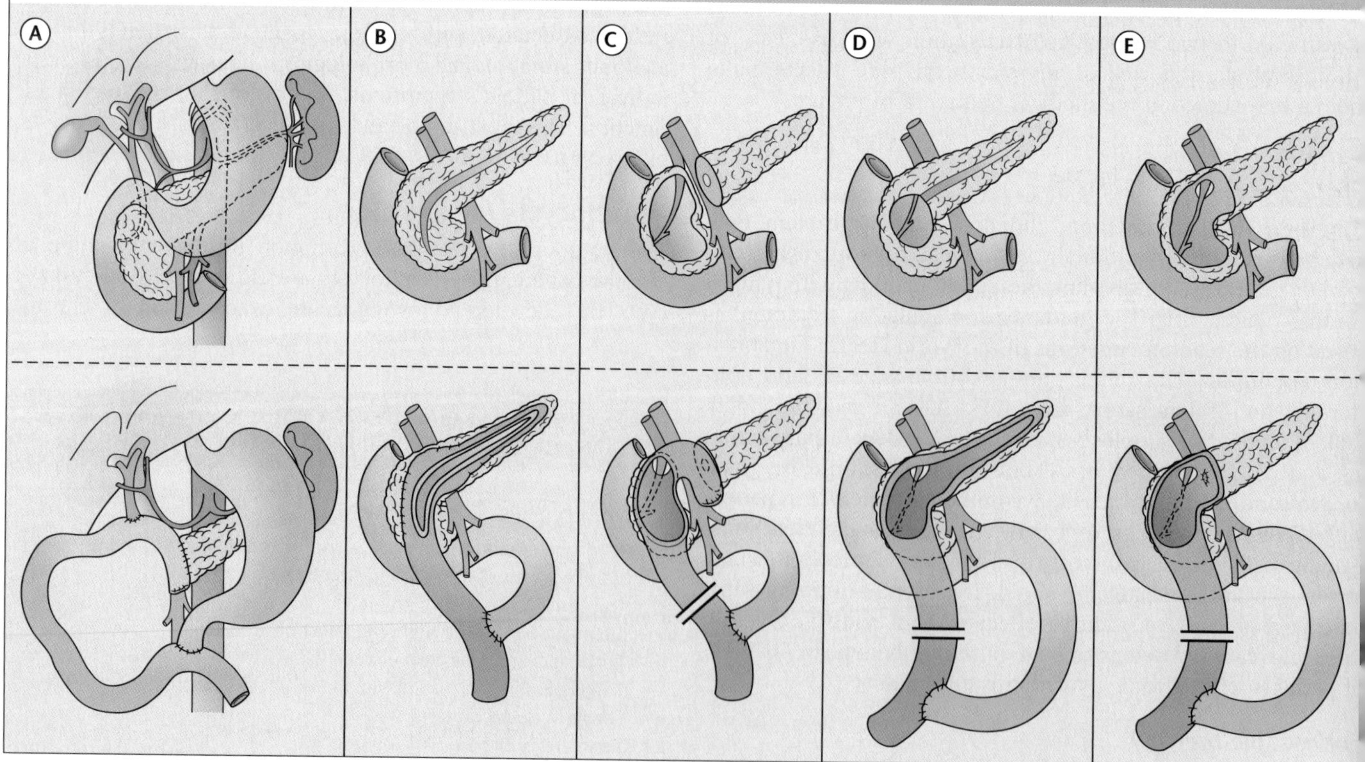

Fig. 72.4 Surgical therapy of chronic pancreatitis. The five main procedures performed: (A) pylorus-preserving Whipple procedure; (B) pancreaticojejunostomy (Pusteow); (C) duodenum-preserving pancreatic head resection (Beger operation); (D) Frey operation; (E) Bern operation (new modification of the Beger operation).

Pancreatic ascites may develop following rupture of the ain pancreatic duct, but this is an uncommon complication of ıronic pancreatitis.

The chronic inflammatory and *fibrosing process* may extend adjacent organs, causing lumen narrowing of the duodenum, e distal stomach, or transverse colon.

ROGNOSIS

hronic pancreatitis is a serious disease that may lead to isability and death. Although it is an incurable, progressive ondition, the severity, frequency, and nature of symptoms can ary. Some people, especially those who stop alcohol conımption entirely, have very mild or occasional symptoms that re easily managed with medication. Other people, especially ose who continue to consume alcohol, can experience disabling, aily pain that may require frequent hospitalization. Chronic ancreatitis is a risk factor in the development of pancreatic ancer[17] (Table 72.2).

OURCES OF INFORMATION FOR PATIENTS ND DOCTORS

ww.chirurgieinfo.com
ww.pancreasfoundation.org
ww.pancreas.org
ww.maraleah.com/chronicpancreatitis.htm
ww.pitt.edu/~super1/lecture/lec3841/index.htm
ww.pankreasinfo.com
ttp://patients.uptodate.com/topic.asp?file=digestiv/5269
ttp://www.patient.co.uk/showdoc/23069114/
ttp://www.patient.co.uk/showdoc/23364026/
ttp://cchs-dl.slis.ua.edu/patientinfo/gastroenterology/pancreas/pancreatitis/chronic.htm
ttp://www.gastro.org/clinicalRes/brochures/pancreatitis.html
ttp://www.gastro.org/generalPublic.html

URRENT CONTROVERSIES AND THEIR UTURE RESOLUTION

enetics

Iutations of three major genes (*PRSS1*, *PST1/SPINK1*, and *FTR*) are associated with an increased risk of acute and chronic pancreatitis. Genetic testing is most useful for persons with family members who have already been found to exhibit a particular pancreatitis-associated mutation. In the future, increased knowledge of genetic causes of pancreatitis may help us to understand why some people are at risk for alcohol pancreatitis and others are not.

Classification system

To test and compare different therapeutic options for chronic pancreatitis, a widely accepted and easy applicable classification system is needed.

Antioxidants

Recent data show that patients with chronic pancreatitis have very low blood levels of antioxidants, which may predispose them to free radical-mediated tissue injury. Some authors have shown that supplementation with antioxidants significantly decreases pain as well as analgesic requirements in patients with alcoholic and tropical pancreatitis. Further studies are required to confirm these findings.

Controlled trials

The review of the literature demonstrates a considerable lack of evidence from randomized clinical trials with regard to the interventional treatment of chronic pancreatitis. Currently five level I evidence-based trials comparing surgical procedures are available (Table 72.3). With evolving new technologies, future randomized trials should also compare interventional endoscopic, laparoscopic, and radiologic treatment with surgery, and possibly medical treatment strategies with surgical concepts.[18]

CONTROVERSIES, FALLACIES, FUTURE DEVELOPMENTS

- Genetics – identify patients at risk of developing alcoholic pancreatitis
- Improvements in the classification of chronic pancreatitis
- New medical treatment for the pain of pancreatitis (especially antioxidants)
- Comparison of interventional, endoscopic, laparoscopic, and radiologic treatment with surgery

TABLE 72.2 PROGNOSIS WITH AND WITHOUT TREATMENT

Treatment	Pain relief	Exocrine insufficiency	Endocrine insufficiency	Complications
Natural course	Pain course of 10–20 years	100%	80–90%	50%
Medical treatment	Symptomatic	Reduction in maldigestion (enzymes)	Control of diabetes (insulin)	No effect
Endoscopic treatment	Selected patients	No effect	No effect	Removal of stricture; drainage of pseudocysts
Surgical treatment	85–95%	No effect	No effect or impairment	Removal stricture; drainage of pseudocysts

TABLE 72.3 EVIDENCE-BASED LEVEL I RANDOMIZED CONTROLLED TRIALS FOR SURGICAL THERAPY OF CHRONIC PANCREATITIS

Trial	Result	Reference
Classic Whipple versus DPPHR (Beger)	DPPHR gave better pain reduction, greater weight gain, better glucose tolerance	Klempa I et al. Chirurg 1995; 66:350–359
Pylorus-preserving Whipple versus DPPHR (Beger)	Less delayed gastric emptying after DPPHR, less pain and better weight gain	Buechler MW et al. Am J Surg 1995; 169:65–70
Pylorus-preserving Whipple versus LPJ-LPHE (Frey)	Same for pain relief and control of complications; LPJ-LPHE resulted in better quality of life	Izbicki JR et al. Ann Surg 1995; 221:350–358
DPPHR (Beger) versus LPJ-LPHE (Frey)	Same for pain relief, quality of life, control of complications, exocrine and endocrine function	Izbicki JR et al. Ann Surg 1998; 228:771–779

DPPHR, duodenum-preserving pancreatic head resection; LPJ-LPHE, longitudinal pancreaticojejunostomy and local pancreatic head excision.

REFERENCES

1. Tandon RK, Sato N, Garg PK. Chronic pancreatitis: Asia–Pacific consensus report. J Gastroenterol Hepatol 2002; 17:508–518.
2. Banks PA. Epidemiology, natural history, and predictors of disease outcome in acute and chronic pancreatitis. Gastrointest Endosc 2002; 56(Suppl):S226–S230.
3. Whitcomb DC. Genetic predisposition to alcoholic chronic pancreatitis. Pancreas 2003; 27:321–326.
4. Strate T, Knoefel WT, Yekebas E, Izbicki JR. Chronic pancreatitis: etiology, pathogenesis, diagnosis, and treatment. Int J Colorectal Dis 2003; 18:97–106.
5. Friess H, Kleeff J, Buchler MW. Molecular pathophysiology of chronic pancreatitis – an update. J Gastrointest Surg 2003; 7:943–945.
6. Charnley RM. Hereditary pancreatitis. World J Gastroenterol 2003; 9:1–4.
7. Hayakawa T, Naruse S, Kitagawa M, Ishiguro H, Jin CX, Kondo T. Clinical evidence of pathogenesis in chronic pancreatitis. J Hepatobiliary Pancreat Surg 2002; 9:669–674.
8. Mitchell RM, Byrne MF, Baillie J. Pancreatitis. Lancet 2003; 361:1447–1455.
9. Petersen JM, Forsmark CE. Chronic pancreatitis and maldigestion. Semin Gastrointest Dis 2002; 13:191–199.
10. Farrell JJ. Overview and diagnosis of malabsorption syndrome. Semin Gastrointest Dis 2002; 13:182–190.
11. Caletti G, Fusaroli P. Endoscopic ultrasonography. Endoscopy 2001; 33:158–166.
12. Robinson PJ, Sheridan MB. Pancreatitis: computed tomography and magnetic resonance imaging. Eur Radiol 2000; 10:401–408.
13. Singh VV, Toskes PP. Medical therapy for chronic pancreatitis pain. Curr Gastroenterol Rep 2003; 5:110–116.
14. Khalid A, Whitcomb DC. Conservative treatment of chronic pancreatitis. Eur J Gastroenterol Hepatol 2002; 14:943–949.
15. Schafer M, Mullhaupt B, Clavien PA. Evidence-based pancreatic head resection for pancreatic cancer and chronic pancreatitis. Ann Surg 2002; 236:137–148.
16. Bhattacharya D, Ammori BJ. Minimally invasive approaches to the management of pancreatic pseudocysts: review of the literature. Surg Laparosc Endosc Percutan Tech 2003; 13:141–148.
17. Whitcomb DC, Pogue-Geile K. Pancreatitis a risk for pancreatic cancer. Gastroenterol Clin North Am 2002; 31:663–678.
18. Rolston RK, Kant JA. Genetic testing in acute and chronic pancreatitis. Curr Gastroenterol Rep 2001; 3:115–120.

Chapter 73

Pancreatic exocrine tumors

Paula Ghaneh and John P Neoptolemos

KEY POINTS

PANCREATIC EXOCRINE CANCER

- Pancreatic adenocarcinoma is one of the most difficult cancers to treat
- One of the commonest causes of cancer death in the western world
- Overall survival 0.4–5.0%
- Surgical mortality and morbidity significantly improved particularly in specialist centers
- Adjuvant chemotherapy improves survival
- Novel therapies may improve outlook for these patients
- Secondary screening programs needed for high-risk groups

NTRODUCTION

ancreatic ductal adenocarcinoma remains one of the most ifficult cancers to treat. It is the commonest cancer affecting he exocrine pancreas and is the 4th to 5th leading cause of ancer-related death in the Western world, characterized by an ncidence:mortality ratio approaching unity. The most recent igures from the International Agency for Research on Cancer IARC) estimated that in the year 2000 there would be 17 000 new cases of pancreatic cancer and 213 000 deaths rom the disease worldwide.[1] Pancreatic cancer has a median urvival of 3–6 months without treatment, which increases to round 20 months with surgical resection and adjuvant treatnent. Unfortunately, the late presentation and aggressive tumor iology of this disease mean that only a minority of patients an undergo potentially curative surgery. Those patients who ndergo pancreatic resection demonstrate a median survival of 10–18 months and a 5-year survival rate of 17–24%. The late resentation is responsible in part for the poor long-term urvival rate of 0.4–5.0%.[2] There have been major improvenents in operative mortality and morbidity in the past decade hrough the development of specialist regional centers and ncouraging evidence of improved long-term survival with the use of adjuvant chemotherapy as shown in the European Society of Pancreatic Cancer (ESPAC)-1 trial. In parallel with these clinical advances, recent remarkable progress has been made in understanding the key molecular events in pancreatic cancer. It is hoped that this knowledge will provide the basis for novel and effective diagnostic and therapeutic approaches n the near future.

EPIDEMIOLOGY

Exocrine pancreatic cancer is one of the top 10 causes of cancer death in the western world. The incidence of pancreatic cancer has increased dramatically over the last century: in the USA, there are over 30 000 deaths per year (over 5% of all cancer mortality) and over 40 000 deaths per year in Europe. The lifetime risk of developing pancreatic cancer in developed countries is 1%. From these figures pancreatic cancer represents 3% of all cancers, and 5% of all cancer deaths. This increase is now tending to level off in men, but is still slowly rising among women, possibly as a result of a higher incidence of tobacco smoking. In the UK, the age-standardized incidence is 10.1 per 100 000 population for men and 8.4 per 100 000 for women.

The incidence of pancreatic cancer increases with each decade resulting in four-fifths of cases occurring between the ages of 60 and 80 years. The highest rates for pancreatic cancer are seen in the Western world including Sweden, Denmark, Austria, the UK, New Zealand, and the USA and range from 12 to 20 per 100 000. The lowest rates are reported in Nigeria, Kuwait, Singapore, and regions of India with rates of 0.7 to 2.1 per 100 000 population.

ETIOLOGY

The biggest risk factors for pancreatic cancer are increasing age, smoking, chronic pancreatitis, hereditary pancreatitis, and an inherited predisposition for pancreatic cancer. Chronic pancreatitis is now recognized as a risk factor, with some series finding a 5–15-fold risk.[3] It has been observed that patients may have chronic pancreatitis for at least 20 years before the development of pancreatic cancer. These patients tend to have severe disease, increased calcification of the gland, and a higher rate of complications.

The risk of developing cancer is even higher with hereditary pancreatitis (HP) with estimates of a 70- to 100-fold increase in risk.[4] This is a rare disorder inherited as an autosomal dominant condition with an estimated 80% penetrance and an equal gender incidence. The gene responsible was identified as the cationic trypsinogen gene (mapped to chromosome 7q35). Mutations that affect this gene have a causative role in the disease and result in a gain-of-function of the digestive enzyme trypsin. Continuing inflammation may continue to provide a persistent mitogenic stimulus that facilitates neoplastic transformation.

There are many germ line diseases that are associated with pancreatic cancer (Table 73.1), such as familial atypical

CAUSES AND RISK FACTORS

- Increasing age
- Smoking
- Chronic pancreatitis
- Hereditary pancreatitis
- Familial pancreatic cancer
- Familial excess of pancreatic cancer (FEPC)

RECOMMENDATIONS

- Continued health education to avoid tobacco consumption should lower the risk of developing pancreatic cancer
- Continued health education to avoid excess alcohol consumption should lower the risk of developing chronic pancreatitis
- All patients with an increased inherited risk of pancreatic cancer should be referred to a specialist center offering specialist clinical advice and genetic counseling, and where appropriate genetic testing such as for BRCA2 mutations

multiple mole melanoma (FAMMM) and cystic fibrosis. Pancreatic cancer is the second most common cancer in the FAMMM syndrome and is particularly significant in patients and families with a p16 mutation. Pancreatic cancer is also seen in some breast cancer families with BRCA1 and BRCA2 mutations. The cumulative risk of pancreas cancer to age 75 years in BRCA2 carriers is 7%, and BRCA2 may account for as many as 5% of all cases of pancreatic cancer. As a group these inherited disorders probably account for approximately 10% of the total cancer burden. They can be referred to as the umbrella term of familial excess of pancreatic cancer (FEPC).

Familial pancreatic cancer is a rare disease and the mode of inheritance is unclear. The European Registry of Hereditary Pancreatitis and Familial Pancreatic Cancer (EUROPAC) has been established to provide a database of these families for long-term follow-up with the intention of identifying individuals at risk and developing a screening program in the future. Familial cancer is an autosomal dominant condition with an as yet unidentified causative mutation. Diagnostic criteria are: two or more first-degree relatives with pancreatic ductal adenocarcinoma (PDAC); one first-degree relative with early on pancreatic cancer (age less than 50 years at diagnosis); or tw or more second-degree relatives with pancreatic cancer, one whom has early onset pancreatic cancer. In families with least two first-degree relatives affected by pancreatic canc the relative risk may be increased 18- to 57-fold depending the number of pre-existing affected relatives.

Other factors including diabetes mellitus, previous surge *Helicobacter pylori* infection, pernicious anemia, vir infections, coffee drinking, and a western diet have weak unclear roles in the causation of pancreatic cancer.

TABLE 73.1 HEREDITARY CANCER SYNDROMES AFFECTING THE PANCREAS

Syndrome	Gene defect/affected chromosome
Hereditary nonpolyposis colon cancer (HNPCC)	Defective DNA mismatch repair enzymes
Familial atypical multiple mole melanoma (FAMMM)	p16
Familial breast cancer	BRCA2
Ataxia telangiectasia	ATM
von Hippel-Lindau disease	VHL
Hereditary pancreatitis	PRSS1
Familial pancreatic cancer	4q32–34 ?
Li-Fraumeni syndrome	p53
Cystic fibrosis	7q31
Familial adenomatous polyposis (FAP)	5q12–21
Peutz-Jeghers syndrome	STK11

PATHOGENESIS

Histological

The histological pathogenesis of pancreatic cancer follows stepwise progression with a number of distinct stages th represent increasing malignant potential. PDAC is believed arise from the ductal epithelium of the pancreas, althou work in a hamster model has shown evidence that the cell origin may derive from the endocrine portion of the pancrea or even multipotent stem cells. The earliest change is one squamous (transitional) metaplasia. The next lesion is desi nated 'pancreatic intraepithelial neoplasia' or 'PanIN.'[5] This h three subtypes, PanIN-1 (further classified as PanIN-1A ar PanIN-1B), PanIN-2, and PanIN-3, dependent on the degr of cytologic and architectural atypia present (Fig. 73.1). It important to note that the malignant potential of the early 1 lesion is unknown. It is only when the basement membrane breached or satellites of tumor deposits are seen that the dia nosis of malignancy can be made. Associated with the develo ment of the invasive phenotype is a dense collagenous reactic termed 'desmoplasia.' Study of the molecular changes prese in each of these stages, and comparing the changes betwee stages allows a temporal blueprint of molecular changes to b described.

Molecular pathogenesis

The molecular pathogenesis of pancreatic cancer involves a accumulation of genetic and molecular changes[6] that result i a malignant phenotype with invasive potential. Studies i sporadic pancreatic cancer have revealed activation of ke oncogenes such as K-ras and inactivation of important tumc suppressor genes such as p53, p16, and SMAD4 in a large prc portion of cases. The frequency of K-ras mutation in pancreati cancer is the highest of any cancer and occurs in 75–100% c series. The K-ras protein is involved in signal transduction c extracellular mitogenic stimuli, thus promoting cell growth an proliferation. The mutation results in constant K-ras signaling which cannot be switched off. Loss of normal tumor suppres sor function in high numbers of pancreatic cancers results i uncontrolled cell growth and failure of programed cell death Abnormalities in growth factors and growth factor receptoi also contribute to the malignant phenotype. Disruption of th normal regulation of the extracellular matrix involving th matrix metalloproteinases (MMPs) and tissue inhibitors o matrix metalloproteinases (TIMPs) and increase in the expres sion of angiogenic factors such as vascular endothelial growt factor (VEGF) and platelet-derived endothelial cell growt factor (PDECGF) also contribute to the invasive potential o tumor cells. K-ras mutation subtype has been shown to b

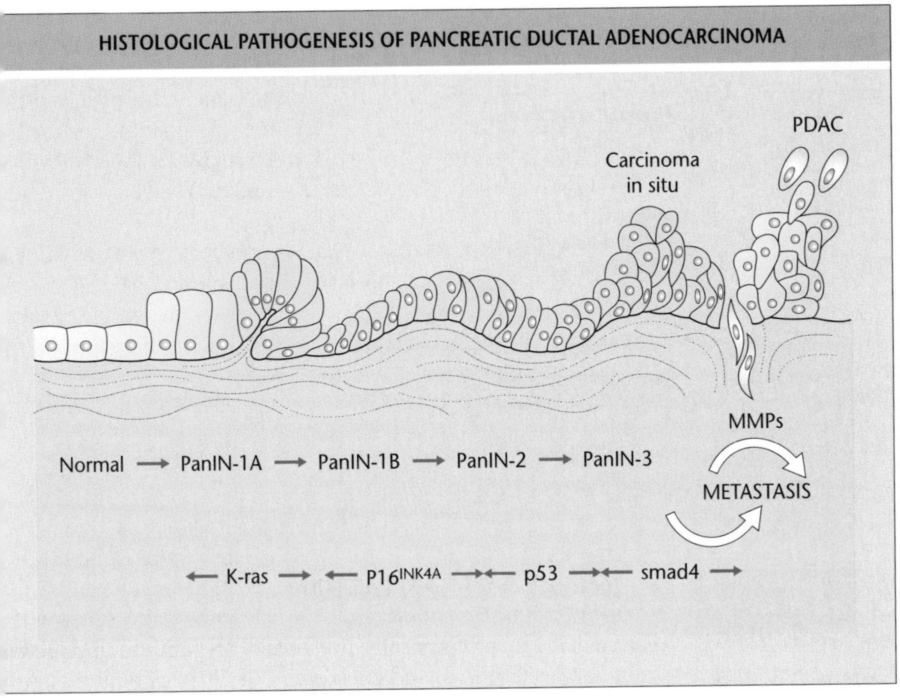

Fig. 73.1 Histological pathogenesis of pancreatic ductal adenocarcinoma. PDCA, pancreatic ductal adenocarcinoma; MMPs, matrix metalloproteinases.

significantly related to survival but inactivation of tumor suppressor genes p16, p53, and p21 and expression of apoptotic genes bax and bcl-2 have not been found to be of any prognostic significance.[7] Expression of wild-type p53, however, may predict responsiveness to chemotherapy. It is hoped that these molecular markers may have a clinically useful prognostic role in patient management in the future and the molecular understanding for pancreatic cancer is the basis for emerging gene therapy trials.

PATHOLOGY

Ductal adenocarcinoma is the most common malignant tumor of the pancreas. Sixty-five per cent are located within the head, 15% in the body, 10% in the tail, and 10% are multifocal. Tumors of the head tend to present earlier with obstructive jaundice. Tumors of the body and tail tend to present later and are associated with a worse prognosis. Microscopically, over 80% of exocrine pancreatic cancers show ductal differentiation and are termed ductal adenocarcinomas. There is often an intense desmoplastic reaction in the stroma surrounding these tumors. Pancreatic ductal adenocarcinoma must be distinguished from carcinomas of the intrapancreatic bile duct, ampulla of Vater, or duodenal mucosa as these tumors have a much better prognosis.

There are some uncommon types of tumor that are considered to be variants of pancreatic ductal adenocarcinoma. These account for a small percentage of the total number of malignant tumors of the pancreas (Table 73.2). Histological grading is outlined in Table 73.3. In addition to histological confirmation of the disease, the International Union Against Cancer (UICC) classification enables a standard staging exercise for tumors. For pancreatic tumors the TNM categories are shown in Table 73.4. The regional lymph nodes are shown in Fig. 73.2.

The pathological classification, i.e., pT, pN, and pM, should correspond to the clinical T, N, and M categories. The stage grouping based on the UICC TNM classification (Table 73.5) has been shown to be a factor in predicting patient survival. Stages I and II are associated with better long-term survival.

TABLE 73.2 HISTOLOGICAL VARIANTS OF MALIGNANT TUMORS OF THE EXOCRINE PANCREAS

Histological type	Frequency	Features
Ductal adenocarcinoma	82%	Long-term survival rare
Anaplastic	5%	Worse prognosis than ductal
Mucinous cystadenocarcinoma	3%	Better prognosis than ductal
Acinar cell	2%	Poor prognosis
Mucinous noncystic	2%	–
Adenosquamous	2%	Poor prognosis
Small cell	1%	Extremely poor prognosis
Squamous cell carcinoma	<1%	More aggressive than ductal
Intraductal papillary-mucinous	<1%	More favorable prognosis then ductal
Serous cystadenocarcinoma	Rare	Prognosis similar to ductal
Pancreatoblastoma	Rare	Childhood tumor

TABLE 73.3 HISTOLOGICAL GRADING OF DUCTAL ADENOCARCINOMA OF THE PANCREAS

Tumor grade	Glandular differentiation	Mucin production	Mitoses (per 10 high-power fields)	Nuclear anaplasia
1	Well-differentiated duct-like glands	Intensive	1–5	Little polymorphism, some polar arrangement
2	Moderately differentiated duct-like and tubular	Irregular	6–10	Some polymorphism
3	Poorly differentiated glands, mucoepidermoid and pleomorphic structures	Abortive	>10	Marked polymorphism, increased nuclear size

TABLE 73.4 UICC TNM CLINICAL CLASSIFICATION OF PANCREATIC DUCTAL ADENOCARCINOMA

T – PRIMARY TUMOR	
TX	Primary tumor cannot be assessed
T0	No evidence of primary tumor
Tis	Carcinoma *in situ*
T1	Tumor limited to the pancreas, 2 cm or less in greatest diameter
T2	Tumor limited to the pancreas, more than 2 cm in greatest diameter
T3	Tumor extends directly into any of the following: duodenum, bile duct, peripancreatic tissues
T4	Tumor extends directly into any of the following: stomach, spleen, colon, adjacent large vessels
N – REGIONAL LYMPH NODES	
NX	Regional lymph nodes cannot be assessed
N0	No regional lymph node metastasis
N1	Regional lymph node metastasis
N1a	Metastasis in a single regional lymph node
N1b	Metastasis in multiple regional lymph nodes
M – DISTANT METASTASIS	
MX	Distant metastasis cannot be assessed
M0	No distant metastasis
M1	Distant metastasis

TABLE 73.5 STAGE GROUPING FOR PANCREATIC DUCTAL ADENOCARCINOMA

Stage	T	N	M
Stage 0	Tis	N0	M0
Stage I	T1	N0	M0
	T2		
Stage II	T3	N0	M0
Stage III	T1	N1	M0
	T2		
	T3		
Stage IVA	T4	Any N	M0
Stage IVB	Any T	Any N	M1

CLINICAL PRESENTATION

Pancreatic cancer classically presents with painless obstructive jaundice, weight loss, and back pain (70–90% of patients). Any one of these symptoms should be investigated in the older patient. The initial symptoms are usually nonspecific leading to delayed diagnosis. Other presentations include late onset diabetes mellitus without obesity, acute or chronic pancreatitis, acute cholangitis, duodenal obstruction, deep venous thrombosis, and thrombophlebitis migrans (as described by Trousseau based on his own pancreatic cancer). Signs may include jaundice, hepatomegaly, palpable gallbladder (Courvoisier's sign – 40%), cachexia, Troisier's sign (involved Virchow's node), an abdominal mass, and ascites. Persistent back pain and/or partial relief of pain by sitting upright usually indicates unresectable disease.

CLINICAL PRESENTATION

- Symptoms
- Painless jaundice
- Weight loss
- Back pain
- Late onset diabetes mellitus
- Acute/chronic pancreatitis
- Acute cholangitis
- Duodenal obstruction
- Deep vein thrombosis
- Signs
- Jaundice
- Hepatomegaly
- Palpable gallbladder (Courvoisier's sign)
- Cachexia
- Troisier's sign (Virchow's node)
- Abdominal mass
- Ascites

DIFFERENTIAL DIAGNOSIS

The differential diagnosis depends on the clinical presentation of the patient. In the presence of jaundice, intrahepatic causes,

LOCO-REGIONAL LYMPH NODE REMOVAL

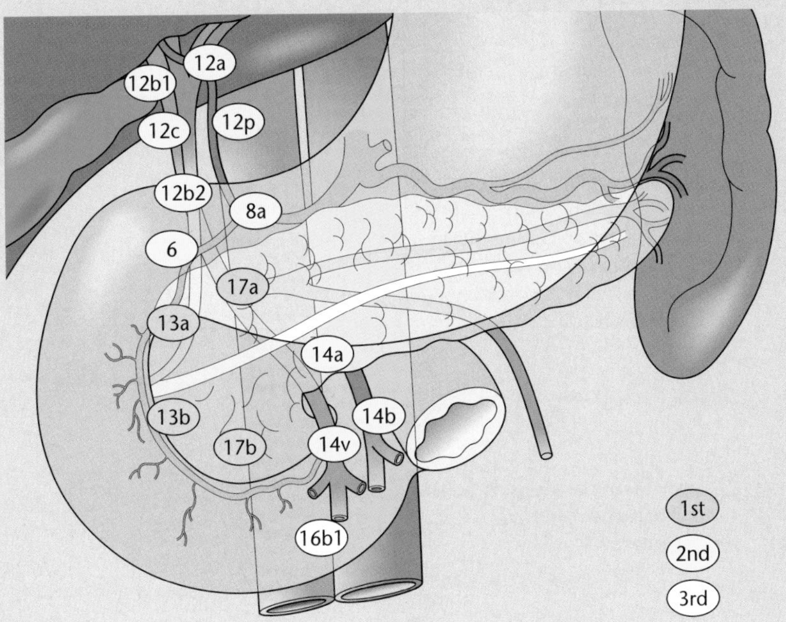

Fig. 73.2 Loco-regional lymph node removal. Loco-regional lymph nodes removed during a standard KW-PPD based on the Japanese numbering system. Reproduced with permission from the University of Liverpool.

cholangiocarcinoma, and benign causes such as gallstone disease or Mirizzi syndrome may be considered. An abdominal mass in the epigastrium needs to be differentiated from a hepatic, gastric, or omental mass. The main diagnostic dilemma is that between pancreatic cancer and chronic pancreatitis both of which may present with very similar symptoms and indeed may coexist. The diagnosis relies on improved imaging modalities as well as clinical acumen.

DIFFERENTIAL DIAGNOSIS OF A PANCREATIC MASS
• Duodenal carcinoma • Ampullary carcinoma • Cholangiocarcinoma • Neuroendocrine tumor • Endocrine tumor • Chronic pancreatitis • Cystadenoma • Anaplastic cancer • Mucinous cystadenocarcinoma • Acinar cell • Mucinous noncystic • Adenosquamous • Small cell • Squamous cell carcinoma • Intraductal papillary-mucinous • Serous cystadenocarcinoma • Pancreatoblastoma • Metastatic tumor • Tuberculous mass • Lymphoma

DIAGNOSTIC METHODS

Initial investigations include blood tests for anemia, clotting profile, liver function tests, and serum CA19.9. At present, there is no single ideal diagnostic modality for pancreatic cancer. Advances in technology have meant that the sensitivity for detecting smaller lesions is improving and also identification of extrapancreatic spread of disease.

DIAGNOSTIC METHODS
• Transabdominal ultrasound • Contrast-enhanced computerized tomography (CE-CT) scan • Spiral CT scan • Magnetic resonance imaging scan (MRI) • Magnetic resonance cholangiopancreatography (MRCP) • Positron emission tomography (PET) scan • Endoscopic ultrasound (EUS) • Endoscopic cholangiopancreatography (ERCP) • Laparoscopy • Laparoscopic ultrasound

Noninvasive imaging techniques

Transabdominal ultrasound is usually the initial investigation and can detect most tumors >2 cm in size, dilatation of the biliary and main pancreatic ducts, and possible extrapancreatic spread, notably liver metastases. Diagnostic accuracy reaches 75% with this method (Table 73.6). A contrast-enhanced computed tomography (CT) scan is the single most useful imaging

TABLE 73.6 IMAGING MODALITIES IN PANCREATIC CANCER

Imaging modality	Advantages	Comments
Conventional CT	Accuracy of staging a resectable tumor 80–85% Accuracy in diagnosing pancreatic cancer 97%	Misses small liver and peritoneal metastasis
Spiral CT	Accuracy of predicting T stage 77–90% Accuracy of predicting N stage 54–68% Accuracy of predicting M stage 75–79% Positive predictive value (Ppv) 92% Almost 100% accurate in predicting unresectable disease Allows 3D reconstruction of anatomy equivalent to arteriography Specificity in predicting unresectability 96% Sensitivity 53–94%; specificity 25–83%	Pancreatic resolution >5 mm Liver resolution >1 cm Dual phase spiral CT: sensitivity 92%, specificity 100%, and accuracy 95% in detecting pancreatic cancer
Endoscopic ultrasound	Sensitivity 95%, specificity 80%, positive predictive value 95%, and negative predictive value 80% for malignant masses Can be combined with FNA to obtain biopsy Sensitivity 86–96%	Less effective at assessing nodal involvement and liver metastasis
MRI	Similar results to spiral dual phase CT Useful for patients that cannot receive intravenous contrast	Less easy to interpret than CT
MRCP	As good as ERCP	
Laparoscopy	Allows direct exploration in patients with equivocal imaging findings Combined with spiral CT increases resectability rates to 91%, reduces unnecessary laparotomies	Depends on management strategy
Laparoscopic ultrasound	Predicts resectability in >90%	
Pancreatic duct ultrasound	Sensitivity of 100% and spec 92% Accuracy 90%	Marginal advantage over laparoscopy alone
Intravascular ultrasound	Possible to delineate venous involvement	Unproven technique
PET	Can differentiate inflammatory conditions Sen 27/31 (87%); Spec 2/2 (50%) Sen 22/31 (71%); Spec 7/11 (64%)	False positives are a problem

procedure[8] and can achieve diagnostic rates of 97% for pancreatic cancer (Fig. 73.3). The accuracy for predicting unresectable lesions is 90%, but the accuracy of predicting resectable lesions is much less (80–85%). False negatives prior to laparotomy are mainly due to small hepatic metastases <1 cm and small peritoneal deposits. Spiral contrast-enhanced computerized tomography (CE-CT) has almost 100% accuracy in predicting unresectable disease, and allows three-dimensional reconstruction of anatomy. Magnetic resonance imaging (MRI) allows for similar results to spiral CE-CT and is useful for patients who cannot receive intravenous contrast. Positron emission tomography (PET) can differentiate inflammatory conditions from tumors and the accuracy continues to improve, although there is cross-over with chronic pancreatitis. Presently, the sensitivity is only 71–87% with specificity of around 64–80%.

Magnetic resonance cholangiopancreatography (MRCP) can also provide images of the biliary and pancreatic duct systems similar to endoscopic retrograde cholangiopancreatography (ERCP).

Invasive imaging techniques

Endoscopic cholangiopancreatography (ERCP) can be used to visualize the biliary tree and pancreatic duct and is both diagnostic and therapeutic. Stents can be placed to relieve obstruction and biopsies or brush cytology can be carried out for diagnosis. Percutaneous transhepatic cholangiography (PTC) may be used to visualize the biliary tree and relieve jaundice in patients who cannot undergo ERCP due to difficult anatomy or previous surgery. Endoscopic ultrasound (EUS) is increasingly being used (Fig. 73.4) and demonstrates a sensitivity of 95% and specificity of 80% with a positive predictive value of 95% and negative predictive value of 80% for malignant masses. EUS can be combined with fine needle aspiration (FNA) to obtain biopsy with a sensitivity of 86–96%.

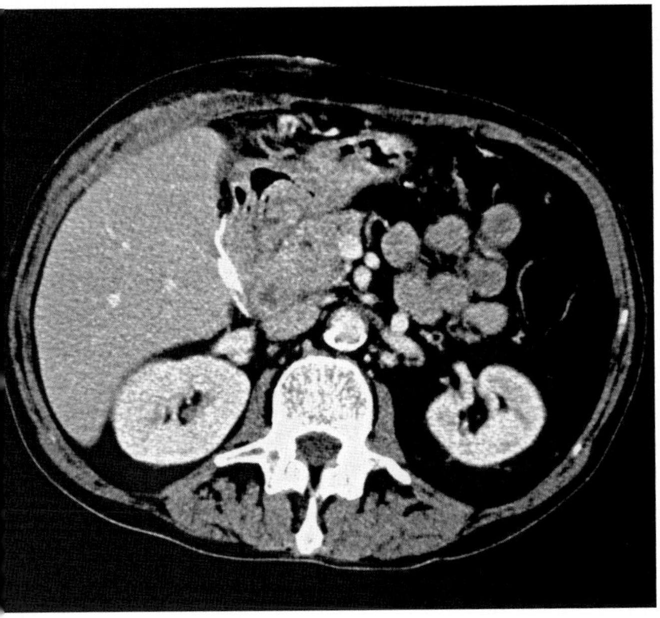

ig. 73.3 CT scan of pancreatic tumor.

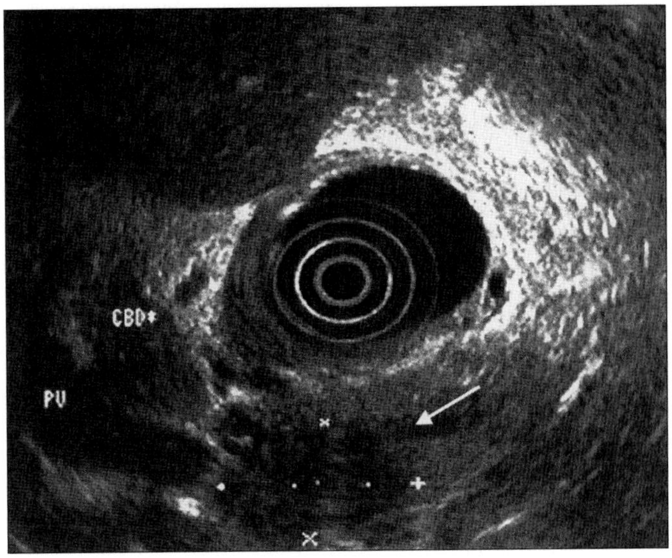

Fig. 73.4 Endoscopic ultrasound (EUS) of pancreatic tumor (arrow). CBD, main bile duct; PV, portal vein. Courtesy of Dr M Lombard, Royal Liverpool University Hospital.

he drawbacks of EUS are that it is less effective at assessing odal involvement and cannot adequately assess distant isease such as liver metastases. At the present time, ERCP hould be reserved for therapeutic intervention and EUS for iagnosis.

Laparoscopy allows direct exploration in patients with equivo-al imaging findings and biopsies may be taken under direct ision. Combined with spiral CT it increases resectability rates o 91% reducing unnecessary laparotomies. Washout for peri-oneal cytology may also be performed. Peritoneal cytology as been shown to be positive in 58% of patients who may ave unresectable tumors or have a limited postoperative sur-ival. Laparoscopic ultrasound (LUS) enables intraoperative canning of the liver and pancreas to be performed and pre-icts resectability in >90%.

Percutaneous FNA biopsy may be used to obtain a diagnosis n patients who are deemed inoperable on imaging.

The majority of centers use a combination of spiral CE-CT vith EUS or ERCP or MRCP and also routine or selective use f laparoscopy combined with LUS. Vascular involvement of he superior mesenteric vessels is of major importance when assessing resectability and current imaging protocols are aimed at improving this factor.

TREATMENT AND PREVENTION

The management of a patient with suspected pancreatic cancer requires the immediate input of a pancreas cancer specialist nurse and the involvement of the regional pancreas tumor multidisciplinary team (Fig. 73.5).

Selection and staging

Once the pancreatic cancer has been identified, the patient needs to be carefully assessed for fitness for major surgery and the tumor staged preoperatively for resectability (Table 73.7). Vascular involvement is of major importance when assessing resectability and the imaging protocols outlined above attempt to improve diagnostic resolution. The presentation and radiological findings of chronic pancreatitis are often similar to those of pancreatic cancer. Up to 5–10% of patients undergoing pancreatectomy for presumed cancer will be found to have chronic pancreatitis on histology. Similarly, up to 5% of patients under-

TABLE 73.7 INDICATORS OF RESECTABILITY IN PANCREATIC CANCER

Factors contraindicating resection	Factors that do not contraindicate resection
Liver, peritoneal, or other metastasis	Continuous invasion of duodenum, stomach, or colon
Distant lymph node metastasis	Lymph node metastasis within the operative field
Major venous encasement (>2 cm in length, >50% circumference involvement)	Venous impingement or minimal invasion of superior mesenteric vein-hepatic portal vein (SMV-HPV)
Superior mesenteric, celiac, or hepatic artery encasement	GDA encasement
Severe co-morbid illness	Age of patient
Cirrhosis with portal hypertension	

GDA, gastroduodenal artery

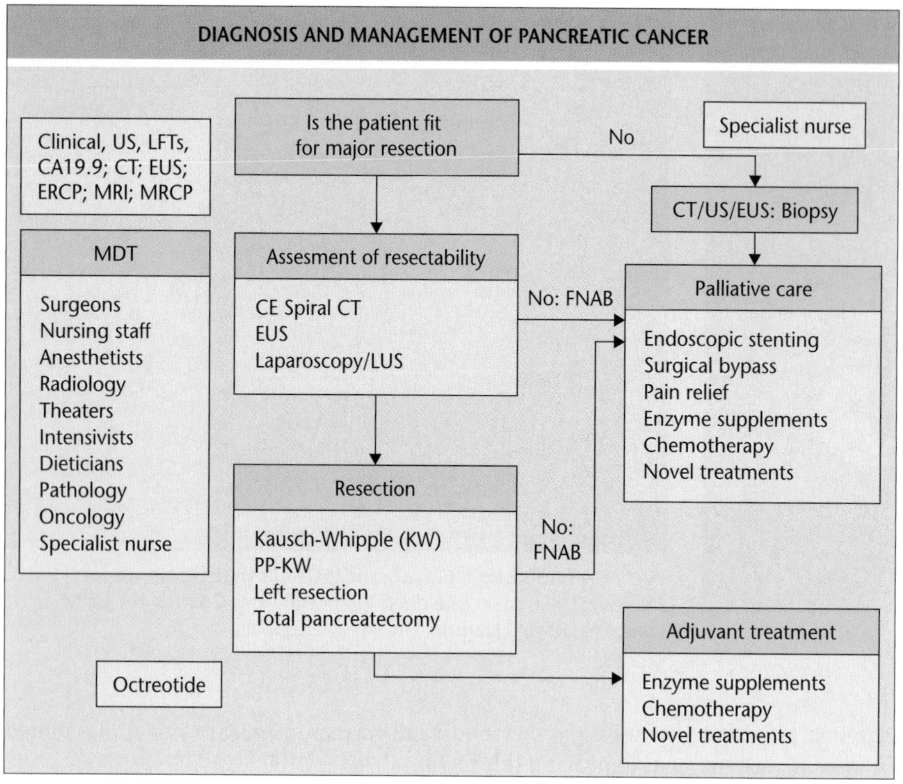

Fig. 73.5 Algorithm for the management of pancreatic cancer. MDT, multidisciplinary team.

going surgery for chronic pancreatitis will be found to have cancer on histology. Further developments in preoperative staging methods should reduce this diagnostic dilemma.

Inoperable disease

Patients who have confirmed metastases and/or invasion of local major blood vessels are deemed unresectable and their treatment is directed at symptom control and maintaining their quality of life.

Pain

Intractable pain is a major problem for these patients and often necessitates the use of high-dose opiate analgesia. Alternative approaches include intraoperative neurolytic celiac plexus block. Percutaneous CT-guided neurolytic celiac plexus block shows reasonable results in patients with cancers in the head of the pancreas but not in those with cancers in the body and tail of the pancreas. EUS can be used to perform a celiac plexus block. Bilateral or unilateral thoracoscopic splanchnicectomy[9] has been used to relieve pain in these patients with variable results.

Weight loss

Weight loss can be a marked feature of pancreatic cancer that to a large extent, at least initially, is due to pancreatic exocrine insufficiency from obstruction of the main pancreatic duct and subsequent fibrosis of the distal gland. Pancreatic exocrine insufficiency may also contribute to abdominal pain and bloating. It is therefore essential that patients receive pancreatic enzyme supplements to alleviate these symptoms.

Biliary and duodenal obstruction

Relief of obstructive jaundice is required in these patients. Biliary stenting using ERCP is the preferred option with the combined PTC-endoscopy approach employed only if the former is technically not possible. Recurrent jaundice is a relatively common complication of stenting because of stent occlusion or migration and approximately 20% of stented patients develop gastric outlet obstruction requiring further intervention. Self-expanding metal stents have greatly reduced the risk of acute cholangitis and obstruction. Metal stents are however very expensive compared to plastic ones and evidence supports the use of metal stents for patients with a good prognosis (locally advanced primary tumor <3 cm) and plastic ones for those patients with metastases and tumors >3 cm in diameter. The life of a plastic stent is approximately 3 months. Expandable metal stents may also be deployed endoscopically for duodenal obstruction with an immediate success rate of 67–87% with complications in up to 25% including perforation, fistula, and bleeding. Recurrent obstruction occurs in up to 23% due to stent migration or fracture.

Surgical bypass can be used to relieve jaundice and duodenal obstruction preferably using a Roux-en-Y loop choledochojejunostomy and gastrojejunostomy. In trials comparing endoscopic stenting and surgical bypass procedures, acute cholangitis and bile leaks are more common in bypass procedures. However, there is a case for surgery to reduce the number of rehospitalizations to treat recurrent jaundice. The authors' current practice is to avoid open surgery if possible or to perform biliary and gastric bypass if surgery is indicated to avoid late onset gastric outlet obstruction.[10]

Operable disease

All surgically fit patients with potentially resectable disease should proceed to exploration in a regional center. In the UK, only between 2.6% and 4.0% of patients with pancreatic cancer undergo resection in district general hospitals. In comparison, e resection rates are much higher in regional pancreatic units 0% in the authors' institution).

urgical techniques

here is no clear evidence that pre-operative endoscopic stent- g is either of benefit or harmful in terms of surgical outcome ut it may facilitate logistical planning of staging and treat- ent. Metal stents should be avoided in patients who have mors that may be resectable because of the tissue reaction ey invoke, although resection is still technically possible.

Ideally, the aim of surgery is to achieve an R0 resection omplete clearance of macroscopic tumor with clear resection argins, even if there are lymph node metastases) if possible. 1 resections (complete clearance of macroscopic tumor with ositive resection margins) may be confirmed after histological nalysis of resection margins including circumferential ones. R2 sections result in incomplete resection of macroscopic tumor.

The vast majority of tumors occur in the head of the pan- reas, hence the standard operation for tumors of the head f the pancreas is the Kausch-Whipple partial pancreato- uodenectomy (KW-PPD). This operation was first successfully erformed by Walter Kausch in Berlin in 1909[11] and later opularized by Allan Whipple in 1935.[12] The procedure emoves the head, neck, and uncinate process of the pancreas, ne duodenum, the distal stomach, and the gallbladder, a small art of the proximal jejunum, and the biliary tree distal to the nction of the choledochus and cystic duct, all performed en- loc to include the loco-regional lymph nodes. The standard ethod of reconstruction includes a pancreaticojejunostomy, a epaticojejunostomy, and a gastrojejunostomy (Fig. 73.6A,B). here are various methods of reconstruction involving the ancreatic anastomosis. Our unit favors the duct to mucosa ancreatojejunostomy.

A popular modification is the pylorus preserving partial ancreatoduodenectomy (PP-PPD) (Fig. 73.7), first described y Watson in 1944 and subsequently reintroduced in the 970s. This involves the formation of a duodenojejunostomy s part of the reconstruction. There have been numerous studies hat have confirmed the effectiveness of this approach for tumor learance and there is also no difference between PP-PPD and W-PPD in terms of delayed gastric emptying in the post- perative period.

Patients with tumors of the pancreatic body or tail undergo eft pancreatectomy usually with en bloc resection of the spleen nd hilar lymph nodes. There is no role for total pancreatec- omy unless this is the only means by which an R0 resection an be achieved. The role of extended lymphadenectomy versus tandard lymphadenectomy (as part of a KW-PPD or PP-PPD) as not been established. There appears to be no survival benefit ssociated with it at the present time. The perioperative use of he somatostatin analog octreotide has been shown to reduce the ncidence of postoperative morbidity, thus the use of octreotide r somatostatin is strongly recommended in the perioperative eriod as part of a systematic approach to pancreatic resection.

Pancreatic surgery is technically demanding and so the best esults are achieved using meticulous surgery by practiced sur- eons in specialist units.[13] There has been a significant decline n operative mortality for pancreatic resection, which is now 5% in specialist units. These low mortality rates reflect a high hroughput of patients rather than a particular surgeon being factor.

TREATMENT

UNRESECTABLE
- Endoscopic biliary stent
- Endoscopic duodenal stent
- Percutaneous biliary stent
- Palliative bypass surgery
- Pancreatic enzyme supplements
- Analgesia
- Celiac plexus block
- Thoracoscopic splanchnicectomy

RESECTABLE
- Preoperative stent
- Kausch-Whipple pancreatoduodenectomy (KW-PPD)
- Pylorus preserving pancreatoduodenectomy (PP-PPD)
- Total pancreatectomy
- Left pancreatectomy
- Adjuvant therapy

COMPLICATIONS OF SURGERY

Surgery-related postoperative morbidity has also decreased in recent years, but it still ranges from 20% to 54%.[14] Many of the postoperative complications respond to medical treatment and radiological and endoscopic intervention.

Medical complications

Medical complications include those arising from the respiratory system (atelectasis, pneumonia, respiratory insufficiency), cardiovascular system (angina, myocardial infarction, arrhythmias, stroke, deep venous thrombosis, and pulmonary embolism), renal system (acute renal failure), as well as hepatic and metabolic disturbances, urinary tract infection, and central line infection.

Surgical complications

The main complications are fistulae, delayed gastric emptying, bleeding, and intra-abdominal abscess. The re-operation rate is 4–9% with high re-operative mortality rates of 23–67%.

Pancreatic fistulae

The reported incidence of pancreatic fistulae or leak ranges from 2% to 24%. A leak can manifest as a pancreatocutaneous fistula, a peripancreatic collection or abscess, or as delayed gastric emptying. The mortality from a major pancreatic leak is up to 28%. In the absence of peritonitis, sepsis, or hemorrhage, conservative management (drain *in situ* or percutaneous drain placement using abdominal CT) should be employed. Total parenteral nutrition and somatostatin analogs serve as the standard treatment. Laparotomy is indicated if there is hemorrhage or if there is a high output fistula with severe sepsis. The recommended procedure is completion pancreatectomy or closure of the jejunal and pancreatic stumps and placement of suction-irrigation drains.

Intra-abdominal abscess

Intra-abdominal abscess following pancreatic resection occurs in 1–12% of patients. The preferred management of intra-abdominal collections is CT-guided percutaneous drainage with appropriate intravenous antibiotics.

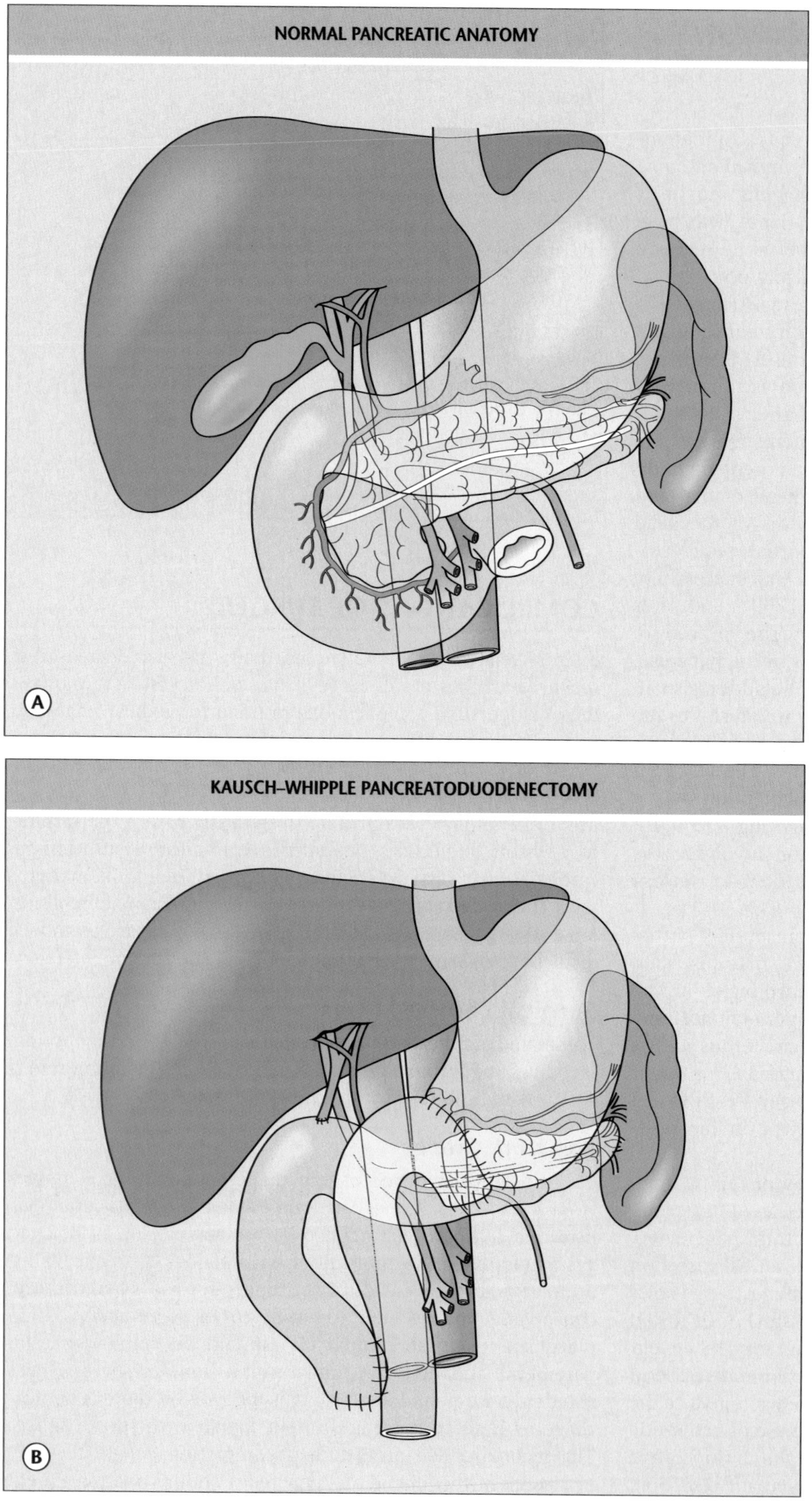

Fig. 73.6 A. Normal pancreatic anatomy. **B.** Kausch-Whipple pancreatoduodenectomy. Reproduced with permission from the University of Liverpool.

Hemorrhage

Postoperative hemorrhage occurs in 2–15% of patients following pancreatic resection. Endoscopy must be carried out to identify gastrointestinal suture line bleeding and is usually managed conservatively. Selective angiography can be used if bleeding persists; if this is not possible or fails then laparotomy is indicated with enterotomies to inspect the anastomoses.

Secondary hemorrhage (usually around 2 weeks following surgery) is commonly related to an anastomotic leak and secondary erosion of the retroperitoneal vasculature or

PYLORUS PRESERVING PANCREATODUODENECTOMY

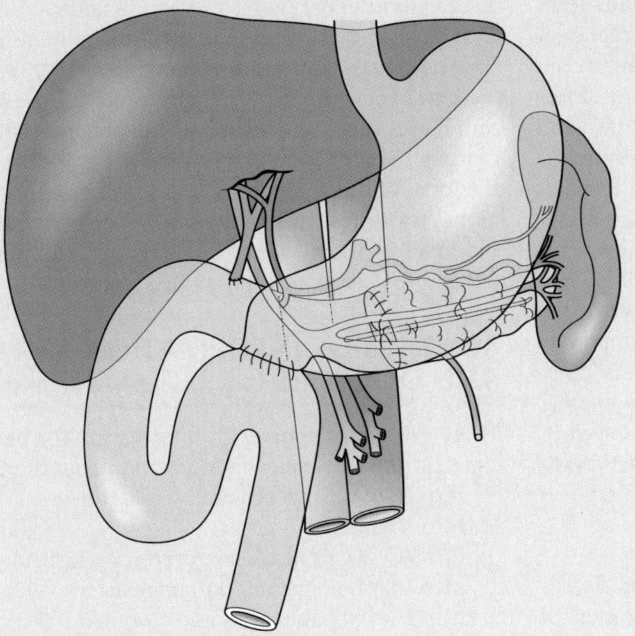

Fig. 73.7 Pylorus preserving pancreatoduodenectomy. Reproduced with permission from the University of Liverpool.

pseudoaneurysm, with a mortality of 15–58%. Key investigations include contrast-enhanced CT, endoscopy, and selective angiography, then selective embolization if a bleeding point can be identified, with a success rate of 63–79%.

Delayed gastric emptying

Delayed gastric emptying is reported to be present in 4% to 37% of patients after resection of the head of the pancreas. The etiology of delayed gastric emptying is not entirely clear but includes anastomotic edema and damage to the fragile vascular supply of the gastroduodenal neuroendocrine axis.

Supportive measures include the use of erythromycin, metoclopramide, and cyclizine. Gastric function normalizes at 2–4 weeks following pancreatoduodenectomy. Although delayed gastric emptying almost invariably resolves with conservative treatment, operative correction is occasionally required.

Other uncommon major complications

Acute cholangitis indicates partial obstruction due to edema of the anastamosis or is associated with a local complication. Acute pancreatitis is rare and usually resolves with conservative management, but bleeding or infection may ensue which may require surgical intervention. Small bowel obstruction is also managed conservatively but ischemia and necrosis may occur so that vigilance is required. Hepatic portal vein thrombosis is rare but if detected early percutaneous transhepatic thrombectomy should be performed. Chylous ascites is probably commoner than suggested by reports from series and can be troublesome – infection may ensue causing an abscess. External drainage of the ascites is necessary and may need to be supplemented with nil by mouth, total parenteral nutrition, and octreotide.

COMPLICATIONS OF SURGERY	
Pancreatic fistula	10.4%
Delayed gastric emptying	9.9%
Bleeding	4.8%
Wound infection	4.8%
Intra-abdominal abscess	3.8%
Mortality rate	1–5%
Re-operation rate	4–9%
Re-operative mortality rate	23–67%

PROGNOSIS AND ONCOLOGICAL THERAPY

Unresectable disease

In unresectable pancreatic cancer, clinical staging and performance status are the two most important prognostic factors. The median survival is 4–8 months with locally advanced disease and 3–5 months with metastatic disease.

Chemotherapy and/or radiotherapy have been used to improve the prognosis of these patients. Unfortunately, pancreatic ductal adenocarcinoma is highly resistant to conventional methods of cytotoxic treatment. There are few chemotherapeutic agents that have been shown to have reproducible response rates of more than 15%. 5-Fluorouracil (5-FU) is an inhibitor of thymidylate synthetase, which is essential for synthesis of DNA nucleotides, and has been the most widely used agent in advanced pancreatic cancer with a median survival of around 5–6 months. Randomized studies have suggested a role for chemotherapy but the survival time is limited.[15] Recently, there has been some emphasis on clinical benefit response. This is significantly increased with the use of gemcitabine (a nucleoside analog). Current trials are now comparing various combinations of gemcitabine (which has been shown to marginally increase survival compared with 5-FU in one trial)[16] with other agents. Radiotherapy has been widely used for the treatment of pancreatic cancer, particularly in the US, but there are no trial data to show there is any benefit over chemotherapy alone. The rationale for combination chemoradiation and follow-on chemotherapy is to produce good local control and systemic destruction of disease. However the absence of phase III trials to test the benefits of newer forms of chemoradiotherapy either alone or in combination in advanced pancreatic cancer prevents an accurate estimate of any treatment benefit. Regional delivery of therapeutic agents can be used to deliver high doses to the tumor bed but further studies are needed. Pancreatic lymphoma is important in the differential diagnosis because it is more chemosensitive than pancreatic cancer.

Advances in molecular biology have allowed the development of targeted treatments for PDAC and these are being evaluated in preclinical and clinical trials.

Resectable disease

Survival following pancreatic resection ranges from 5-year survival rates of 10–24% with median survival times of 12–18 months.[17] There is no significant difference in survival comparing standard and extended (or radical) resection. The lack of survival benefit associated with radical resection may be due in part to the pattern of recurrence following surgery. The majority of patients will go on to develop disease recurrence, which is usually at the resection site, the peritoneum and the liver. The majority of tumor recurrences have been shown to occur within 2 years of surgery.

Following pancreatic resection, the most important independent prognostic markers are lymph node status, tumor size, and tumor grade.[18] Resection margin status appears to be a major determinant of prognosis with R1 tumors having a significantly worse outcome but this is not an independent factor.[19] Rather, R1 tumors represent a biologically more aggressive phenotype equivalent to high grade and lymph node positive tumors. Additional prognostic and therapeutic response information may be obtained from the molecular profile of the tumor. The investigation of biological molecular prognostic and response markers is presently intense but their practical application has yet to be established. Levels of the carbohydrate antigen CA19-9 may allow response to therapy to be identified early and guide further treatment. It is likely that in the future these markers will play an important role in determining prognosis and specific types of therapeutic intervention.

Even with optimum surgical intervention, the survival data for patients with pancreatic cancer is poor; the pattern of disease progression and recurrence are clear indications for the use of additional treatment modalities. The evidence for any individual modality has been weak because of the lack of randomized trials with adequate power.[20] Neoadjuvant therapy has been advocated to increase resection rates and reduce positive resection margins; randomized trials are lacking.

A significant step forward was made recently with the publication of the results of the European Study Group for Pancreatic Cancer trial 1 (ESPAC-1).[18] This pivotal study recruited 541 patients from 11 countries and compared 5-FU-based chemotherapy, chemoradiotherapy, a combination of the two and no treatment. The key findings were:

1. Chemotherapy had a survival benefit.
2. Chemoradiotherapy had no survival benefit.
3. There was great improvement in quality of life irrespective of the type and use of adjuvant therapy.

Similar effects were observed in patients with R1 resection margins. These findings are highly significant and will direct the focus of future studies to the use of chemotherapeutic agents alone. To address this issue patients are now being recruited for the ESPAC-3 trial where patients are randomized to receive either 5-FU or gemcitabine postsurgery.

SOURCES OF INFORMATION FOR PATIENTS AND DOCTORS

There are major sources of information for patients and clinicians on the Internet, the following being the most useful:

http://www.cancerbacup.org.uk/Home
http://pancreas.org/
http://www.liv.ac.uk/surgery/europac.html
http://pathology.jhu.edu/pancreas/
http://www.pancreaticcancer.org.uk/
http://www.liv.ac.uk/surgery/cantrials.html
http://www.liv.ac.uk/surgery/europac.html
http://www.cancerhelp.org.uk/help/default.asp?page=279

Patient information booklets concerning pancreatic cancer and its diagnosis and treatment are available from Solvay Healthcare Limited, Southampton, UK and there are a number of textbooks on the subject, e.g, Beger et al.[21]

CONCLUSIONS

Pancreatic cancer still remains a formidable disease to diagnose and treat. Surgical approaches have become more standardized and are safer, with much improvement in both morbidity and mortality in specialized centers. Diagnosis has improved using conventional imaging methods and appropriate treatment decisions can be made because of these improvements. Palliative treatment is improving including the use of endoscopic stent placement, effective pain relief, and pancreatic enzyme supplementation. Chemotherapy regimens can prolong survival in patients with advanced disease without sacrificing their quality of life. At the present time, only pancreatic resection can improve survival significantly. A further survival benefit may be achievable using adjuvant chemotherapy but not radiochemotherapy. The molecular mechanisms, which are responsible for pancreatic cancer, may represent hope for the future with respect to earlier diagnosis and targeted treatments, using novel genetic and biological approaches. No surgeon should be undertaking pancreatic cancer surgery unless 30 or more resections per year are being performed within a regional pancreas tumor center.

In the past, there has been a nihilistic approach to patients with pancreatic cancer, but we are now entering a very encouraging phase in the diagnosis and treatment of pancreatic cancer. The information and resources now available can result in a reasoned approach to the treatment of patients with pancreatic cancer to ensure the best outcome with an optimum quality of life.

CONTROVERSIES

- Secondary screening for pancreatic cancer in high-risk cases should only be part of an investigational program
- Specialist pancreatic centers
- Neo-adjuvant therapies should only be administered as part of a clinical trial
- Adjuvant chemoradiation has not been shown to improve survival in the absence of maintenance chemotherapy
- Adjuvant 5-FU based chemotherapy may prolong life and improve quality of life, but needs to be more clearly defined through further clinical trials and cannot be recommended as standard treatment
- Future developments
- Novel molecular therapies
- Improved molecular diagnosis
- Improved molecular prognosis

REFERENCES

1. Parkin DM, Bray FI, Devesa SS. Cancer burden in the year 2000. The global picture. Eur J Cancer 2001; 37 (Suppl 8):4–66.
2. Bramhall SR, Allum WH, Jones AG et al. Treatment and survival in 13,560 patients with pancreatic cancer, and incidence of the disease, in the West Midlands: an epidemiological study. Br J Surg 1995; 82:111–115.
3. Lowenfels AB, Maisonneuve P, Cavallini G et al. Pancreatitis and the risk of pancreatic cancer. International Pancreatitis Study Group. N Engl J Med 1993; 328:1433–1437.
4. Howes N, Wong T, Greenhalf W et al. Pancreatic cancer risk in hereditary pancreatitis in Europe. Digestion 2000; 61:300.
5. Kern S, Hruban R, Hollingsworth MA et al. A white paper: the product of a pancreas cancer think tank. Cancer 2001; 61:4923–4932.
6. Magee CJ, Greenhalf W, Howes N et al. Molecular pathogenesis of pancreatic ductal adenocarcinoma and clinical implications. Surg Oncol 2001; 10:1–23.
7. Kawesha A, Ghaneh P, Andren-Sandberg A et al. K-ras oncogene subtype mutations are associated with survival but not expression of p53, p16 (ink4a), p21 (WAF-1), Cyclin D1, erbB-2 and erbB-3 in resected pancreatic ductal adenocarcinoma. Int J Cancer 2000; 89:469–474
8. Mertz HR, Sechopoulos P, Delbeke D et al. EUS, PET, and CT scanning for evaluation of pancreatic adenocarcinoma. Gastrointest Endosc 2000; 52:367–371.
9. Leksowski K. Thoracoscopic splanchnicectomy for control of intractable pain due to advanced pancreatic cancer. Surg Endosc 2001; 15: 129–131.
10. Lillemoe KD, Cameron JL, Hardacre JM et al. Is prophylactic gastrojejunostomy indicated for unresectable periampullary cancer? A prospective randomized trial. Ann Surg 1999; 230: 322–328; discussion 328–330.
11. Kausch W. Carcinom der papilla duodeni und seine radikale entfernung. Beitr Klin Chir 1912; 78:439–486.
12. Whipple AO, Parsons WB, Mullens CR et al. Treatment of carcinoma of the ampulla of vater. Ann Surg 1935; 102:763–769.
13. Neoptolemos JP, Russell RC, Bramhall S et al. Low mortality following resection for pancreatic and periampullary tumours in 1026 patients: UK survey of specialist pancreatic units. UK Pancreatic Cancer Group. Br J Surg 1997; 84:1370–1376.
14. Halloran CM, Ghaneh P, Bosonnet L et al. Complications of pancreatic cancer resection. Dig Surg 2002; 19:138–146.
15. Shore S, Raraty MG, Ghaneh P, Neoptolemos JP. Review article: chemotherapy for pancreatic cancer. Aliment Pharmacol Ther 2003; 18: 1049–1069.
16. Burris HA 3rd, Moore MJ, Andersen J et al. Improvements in survival and clinical benefit with gemcitabine as first-line therapy for patients with advanced pancreas cancer: a randomized trial. J Clin Oncol 1997; 15:2403–2413.
17. Magee CJ, Ghaneh P, Neoptolemos JP. Surgical and medical therapy for pancreatic carcinoma. Best Pract Res Clin Gastroenterol 2002; 16:435–455.
18. Neoptolemos JP, Dunn JA, Stocken DD et al. Adjuvant chemoradiotherapy and chemotherapy in resectable pancreatic cancer: a randomised controlled trial. Lancet 2001; 358:1576–1585.
19. Neoptolemos JP, Moffitt DD, Dunn JA et al. The influence of resection margins on survival for patients with pancreatic cancer treated by adjuvant chemoradiation and/or chemotherapy within the ESPAC-1 randomized controlled trial. Ann Surg 2001; 238:758–768.
20. Klinkenbijl JH, Jeekel J, Sahmoud T et al. Adjuvant radiotherapy and 5-fluorouracil after curative resection of cancer of the pancreas and periampullary region: phase III trial of the EORTC gastrointestinal tract cancer cooperative group. Ann Surg 1999; 230:776–782; discussion 782–784.
21. Beger HG, Warshaw AL, Büchler MW et al. The pancreas. London: Blackwell Science; 1998.

Chapter 74

Cysts of the pancreas

William R Brugge

KEY POINTS

- Pancreatic cysts can be classified into serous (benign), mucinous (premalignant or malignant) and inflammatory (pseudocysts)
- Pancreatic cysts are common (up to 20% of general hospital population in screening MRI studies)
- Serous cyst adenomas are associated with mutations in the VHL gene, mucinous tumours with K-RAS oncogene and P53 mutations
- Serous neoplasms are usually microcystic, mucinous are macrocystic
- Benign legions are rarely painful
- Presence of calcification or history of pancreatitis is suggestive of a pseudocyst
- CT, MR, and more recently EUS plus FNA are useful in evaluating cysts
- Surgery for premalignant lesions is determined by symptoms, risk of malignancy, and surgical risk of patient
- Pseudocysts can be managed by surgery, endoscopic drainage, or radiologic drainage (CT/EUS)

INTRODUCTION

Cystic lesions of the pancreas are composed of a broad range of neoplastic cysts and inflammatory pseudocysts. The neoplastic cysts span the spectrum of malignancy, from frankly malignant to premalignant lesions, and benign cystadenomas. With the widespread use of abdominal imaging, the lesions are increasingly identified in early stages of asymptomatic patients.

There are three basic types of pancreatic cystic lesions, serous, mucinous, and inflammatory[1] (Table 74.1). Serous cysts are considered to be benign lesions without malignant potential. In contrast, mucinous cystic lesions are considered to be premalignant or frankly malignant. Inflammatory cystic lesions are composed of peri-pancreatic fluid collections that occur during episodes of acute pancreatitis or in association with chronic pancreatitis.

TABLE 74.1 TYPES OF CYSTIC LESIONS

- Serous (benign without malignant potential)
- Mucinous (premalignant or malignant)
- Inflammatory (fluid collections, pseudocysts)

EPIDEMIOLOGY

Prevalence

The prevalence of pancreatic cysts has been examined with autopsy studies and imaging. Based on a small number of studies, the prevalence of true pancreatic cysts found at autopsies in Japan was approximately 73 in 300 (24.3%) cases.[2] The frequency of cystic lesions was related to age and the lesions were evenly distributed throughout the pancreas. The epithelium of the cysts ranged from: normal epithelium (47.5%); papillary hyperplasia without atypia (32.8%); atypical hyperplasia (16.4%); carcinoma in situ (3.4%); and invasive carcinoma (0%). The malignant epithelium was more commonly found in small cystic lesions, rather than large lesions.

Screening magnetic resonance imaging (MRI) studies in a general hospital population in the US have demonstrated a similar prevalence rate of pancreatic cysts, about 15–20% in a general hospital population in the US.[3] MRI images of the pancreas in 1444 patients demonstrated 283 (19.6%) patients with at least one pancreatic cyst.

Clinical epidemiology

Serous cystadenomas have been estimated to account for about 25% of all cystic tumors of the pancreas, but the true incidence is difficult to determine.[4] Serous cystadenomas were not recognized as a separate entity until 1978 when the unique histologic and biologic features that distinguish them from mucinous cystic tumors were described. Since then, estimates of their incidence have varied. Using surgical pathology studies, it has been estimated that serous cystadenomas account for about 1–2% of all exocrine pancreatic neoplasms.

Serous cystadenomas occur only in adults and are more commonly found in men. In reported cases, patients have ranged in age from 18 to 91 years, with a median age in the seventh decade of life. Traditionally, about a third of tumors are discovered as incidental findings during abdominal imaging or surgery or at autopsy.

Mucinous cystic neoplasms account for approximately 2–5% of all exocrine pancreatic tumors and are more common than serous cystadenomas. Women are affected far more commonly than men (9:1 female:male ratio), with a mean age at diagnosis in the fifth decade.

Intraductal papillary mucinous neoplasms are closely associated with mucinous cystic neoplasms. Their true incidence is uncertain, but estimates range from 1% to 8% of all pancreatic tumors. Intraductal papillary mucinous neoplasms affect men and women equally or men predominantly, depending on the reported series, and they tend to occur in an older age group than mucinous cystic neoplasms.

CAUSES, RISK FACTORS, DISEASE ASSOCIATIONS

There are few known causes or risk factors for cystic neoplasms of the pancreas. Von Hippel-Lindau (VHL) disease is the best-described genetic, inherited disorder associated with cystic lesions.[5] In the largest series to date, a French group prospectively evaluated 158 patients with VHL. Pancreatic involvement was observed in 122 patients (77.2%) and included true cysts (91.1%), serous cystadenomas (12.3%), neuroendocrine tumors (12.3%), or combined lesions (11.5%).

Pancreatic pseudocysts arise in association with inflammatory conditions of the pancreas. During episodes of acute pancreatitis, focal pancreatic necrosis may result in accumulations of peri-pancreatic fluid collections. Over time, the fluid collections usually resolve spontaneously, but they may persist and form thick-walled cyst lesions.

PATHOGENESIS (see Table 74.2 and Chapter 73)

The pathogenesis of cystic neoplasms of the pancreas is poorly understood. Serous cystadenomas are strongly associated with mutations of the VHL gene, located on chromosome 3p25.[6] The VHL gene is likely to play a sentinel role in the pathogenesis of sporadic serous cystadenomas. In one study, 70% of the sporadic serous cystadenomas studied demonstrated loss of heterozygosity (LOH) at 3p25 with a VHL gene mutation in the remaining allele.[7] The mutations in the VHL gene probably affect most commonly the centro-acinar cell and result in hamartomatous proliferation of these small cuboidal cells.

Mucinous cystic neoplasms and intraductal papillary mucinous neoplasms most likely have a very different pathogenesis compared to serous cystadenomas. Mucinous cystic neoplasms frequently contain mutations of the K-ras oncogene and p53 tumor suppressor gene, and the frequency of this mutation increases with increasing degrees of dysplasia in the tumor. The frequency of K-ras mutation in mucinous cystic neoplasms is linearly related to the grades of atypia: 0% for normal epithelium, 29% for grade 1, 50% for grade 2, and 75% for grade 3.[8] However, the degree of atypia in intraductal papillary mucinous neoplasms does not seem to correlate with the presence of k-ras mutations. LOH of the p16 gene was observed with increasing degrees of histological atypia in intraductal papillary mucinous neoplasms, whereas LOH of the p53 gene was seen only in invasive carcinomas. Both intraductal papillary mucinous neoplasms and mucinous cystic neoplasms seem to arise from polyclonal epithelia and to be replaced by monoclonal neoplastic cells as they undergo dysplastic changes and K-ras mutation. The mechanisms controlling the switch from polyclonal expansion to monoclonal expansion are not well described.

Pancreatic pseudocysts have a completely different pathogenesis compared to serous and mucinous cystadenomas. Pseudocysts have no epithelium lining the focal fluid collections and the fluid originates from the leakage of fluid and debris from an inflammatory process in the adjacent pancreas. There are two basic mechanisms for the formation of pancreatic pseudocysts.[9] In the 'ductal-leakage' mechanism, localized necrosis of a pancreatic duct may allow the leakage of fluid out of the pancreas and into a space adjacent to the pancreas. Early in the formation of the fluid collection, often during acute pancreatitis, the space containing the fluid is not well defined and the fluid may accumulate between adjacent organs, such as the stomach, colon, liver, and small intestine. Over time, the fluid collection becomes better organized and walled-off by a thick, fibrotic wall. However, a communication between the ductal system and the pseudocyst cavity will often persist, resulting in a chronic pancreatic pseudocyst. A minority of pancreatic pseudocysts have no association with the pancreatic ductal system. Presumably, the origin of the fluid is not leakage, but rather from liquefaction necrosis of pancreatic tissue in severe acute pancreatitis. This type of focal fluid collection often takes place during acute pancreatitis and resolves spontaneously.

TABLE 74.2 PATHOGENESIS OF CYSTIC LESIONS

Types of cystic lesion	Genetic abnormalities
Serous	Mutations of VHL gene (3p25)
Mucinous	Mutations of K-ras, p53
Inflammatory	None

PATHOLOGY

Serous cystadenomas (Fig. 74.1)

These solitary microcystic lesions are usually round and arise from the pancreatic parenchyma without involvement of the ductal system. Serous tumors have three variants based on growth pattern: microcystic, macrocystic, and solid. Microcystic serous cystadenomas are the most common. They are composed of innumerable small cysts with a honeycomb-like appearance on cross-section. Microcystic serous cystadenomas may achieve a large diameter over the long term and the large lesions often have a fibrotic or calcified central scar. Macrocystic serous cystadenomas are composed of far fewer cysts, and the diameter of the cysts varies from microcystic to large cavities. The presence of discrete, large cystic cavities mimics the appearance of mucinous lesions. The cyst fluid from serous cystadenomas is thin, clear, and contains no mucin.

The epithelial cells of all types of serous cystadenomas are similar in appearance with a cuboidal shape, glycogen-rich, clear cytoplasm, and small, regular centrally located nuclei. The groups of epithelial cells usually surround small cysts in a single

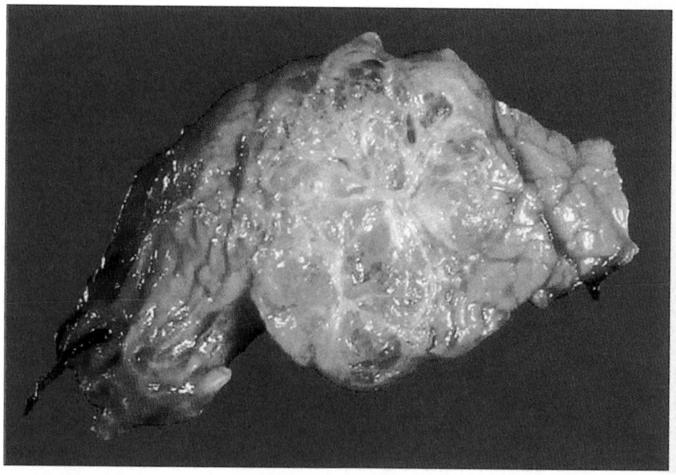

Fig. 74.1 Serous cystadenoma. Gross pathology of a serous cystadenoma.

at layer. The appearance of the surrounding stroma is variable nd ranges from highly vascular to fibrotic.

Mucinous cystic neoplasms (Fig. 74.2)

Grossly, mucinous cystic neoplasms are characteristically macrocystic with discrete individual cavities that vary in diameter. In the absence of an associated mass, malignant transformation may be suspected with focal thickening, irregularity, or ulceration of the cyst lining. Mucinous cystic neoplasms are lined by mucin-producing cells with mucin vacuoles. The World Health Organization classification divides mucinous cystic neoplasms into three types, based on the degree of epithelial dysplasia: benign, borderline, and malignant. The entire tumor is classified according to the most advanced degree of dysplasia/carcinoma present.

Mucinous cystic neoplasms of the pancreas often contain a highly cellular (so-called 'ovarian') stroma. It occurs almost exclusively in female patients, although rare cases of mucinous cystic neoplasms with ovarian stroma in male patients have been encountered. Many authorities have restricted the very definition of mucinous cystic neoplasms to include only those cystic mucinous tumors that contain ovarian stroma.

Intraductal papillary mucinous neoplasms originate in the distal main pancreatic duct in 80% of cases. As a result, they tend to cause obstructive complications such as acute pancreatitis, chronic pancreatitis, or jaundice. The presence of a papillary tumor causes dilatation of the ducts as a result of tumor growth. The degree of ductal ectasia produced varies with degree of mucin production, but duct dilatation great enough to be seen on imaging studies or gross pathologic examination is a sine qua non of the diagnosis. Mucin production may be so exuberant that extrusion from papilla of Vater is seen. The degree of dysplasia exhibited by the epithelium may range from mild to moderate to severe (carcinoma *in situ*), and the entire tumor is classified according to the greatest degree of dysplasia present.

CLINICAL PRESENTATION

Most patients with a pancreatic cystic lesion have no signs or symptoms related to the pancreatic lesion. Often the lesion is found with computed tomography (CT) or ultrasound (US) imaging performed for the evaluation of another condition such as another malignancy or liver lesions. When symptoms are present, the most common presentation is recurrent abdominal pain, nausea, and vomiting as a result of mild pancreatitis. These symptoms often reflect the presence of a lesion causing ductal obstruction or a connection with the main ductal system. Chronic abdominal pain is a rare presentation of a benign cystic lesion and suggests a malignancy or a pseudocyst. Patients with a cystic malignancy will present with symptoms and signs similar to pancreatic cancer, i.e., pain, weight loss, and jaundice. Pseudocysts may arise after an episode of acute pancreatitis or insidiously in the setting of chronic pancreatitis and are associated with chronic abdominal pain. Large pseudocysts can compress the stomach, duodenum, or bile duct, causing early satiety, vomiting, or jaundice.

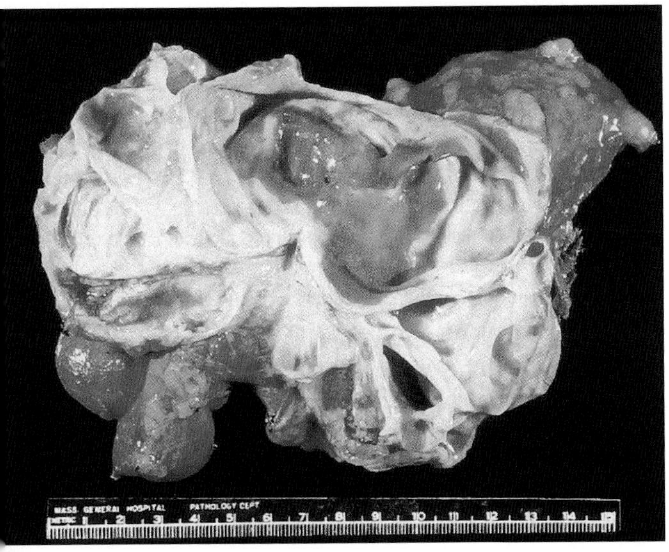

Fig. 74.2 Mucinous cystic lesion. Gross pathology of a mucinous cystic lesion.

DIFFERENTIAL DIAGNOSIS

The finding of a cystic lesion of the pancreas by imaging exams presents the clinician with a wide range of possible diagnoses. The most important differentiation is between a cystic neoplasm and a pseudocyst. Although pancreatic pseudocysts usually arise in association with pancreatitis, the acute episode of pancreatitis may not have been clinically apparent or the patient may have mild chronic pancreatitis. Evidence of inflammatory changes or calcifications in the pancreas is suggestive of a pancreatic pseudocyst. However, in the acute setting of mild pancreatitis it may be difficult to differentiate between a cystic neoplasm that has caused pancreatitis and a small pseudocyst that has formed as a result of pancreatitis.

If a pancreatic pseudocyst can be excluded on the basis of a clinical history or imaging findings, attention should be focused on the differential between the types of cystic neoplasms. The principal differentiation is between mucinous and serous lesions because the fundamental difference in management is based on the neoplastic potential of mucinous lesions. Serous lesions are often diagnosed based on the characteristic microcystic morphology that is apparent on most imaging techniques. Once a serous lesion has been confidently diagnosed and if the patient has not suffered any complications of the serous cystadenoma, the lesion may not require resection. In contrast, mucinous cystic lesions are often resected because of the propensity towards growth and malignant degeneration. Under some clinical circumstances, such as in high-risk surgical patients, differentiation between benign and malignant mucinous lesions is important. Benign mucinous lesions in high-risk patients may not require resection.

DIAGNOSTIC METHODS

CT is an excellent test for cystic lesions of the pancreas because of its widespread use and ability to detect cysts[10] (Fig. 74.3). MR imaging is used increasingly because of the lack of radiation exposure and the ability to image the pancreatic duct with MR cholangiopancreatography (MRCP). Transabdominal ultrasonography may aid in differentiating between solid and cystic lesions, but complete evaluation of the pancreas is often difficult due to overlying bowel gas.

Although seen in less than 20% of lesions, demonstration of a central scar by CT or MRI is a highly diagnostic feature of a

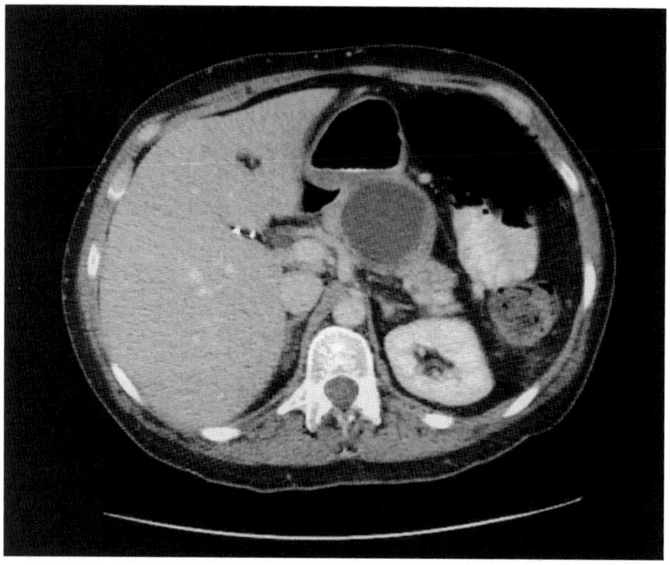

Fig. 74.3 Pseudocyst. Abdominal CT scan of a simple, thick-walled pseudocyst.

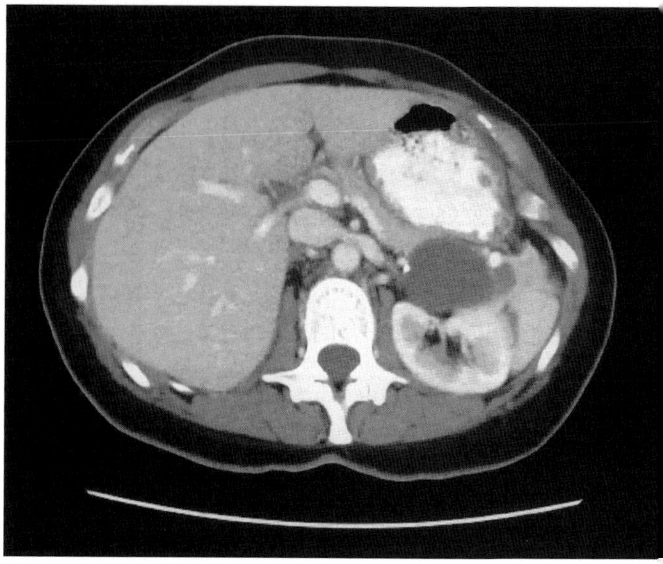

Fig. 74.4 Unilocular mucinous cystic neoplasm. Abdominal CT scan of a thin-walled, unilocular mucinous cystic neoplasm. It may be difficult to differentiate mucinous lesions from pseudocysts.

serous cystadenoma. The honeycombed or microcystic appearance of the lesion is commonly used to provide a diagnosis. However, macrocystic serous cystadenomas are difficult to diagnose with cross-sectional imaging because of the morphologic similarities with mucinous lesions. Mucinous cystic neoplasms, in contrast, are commonly diagnosed with CT based on the unilocular or macrocystic characteristics. Although not frequently seen, the finding of peripheral calcification by CT is specific for a mucinous cystic neoplasm. Intraductal papillary mucinous neoplasms may involve the main pancreatic duct exclusively, a side branch, or both. MRCP can demonstrate the diagnostic findings of pancreatic duct dilation, mural nodules, and ductal connection.

Despite these imaging features, the ability to diagnose a specific cystic lesion accurately and to determine whether malignancy is present using CT and MRI remains uncertain (Fig. 74.4). The diagnosis of a pancreatic pseudocyst is more dependent upon the clinical history and the associated findings of chronic pancreatitis. Pancreatic pseudocysts appear as unilocular fluid-filled cavities associated with parenchymal changes such as calcifications and atrophy. A pseudocyst complicated by infection or bleeding may have high-density lesions seen within the fluid.

Recently, endoscopy and endoscopic ultrasound (EUS) have been used to diagnose cystic lesions of the pancreas and guide fine needle aspiration (FNA).[11] Using the high-resolution imaging of endoscopic ultrasound, the morphologic features of various cystadenomas have recently been defined. However, the detailed imaging features of cystic neoplasms by EUS do not appear to be sufficiently accurate to differentiate between benign and malignant cystadenomas unless there is evidence of a solid mass or invasive tumor (Fig. 74.5). Fine needle aspiration under EUS guidance can be performed on small lesions within the pancreas.

Cyst fluid, aspirated using EUS guidance, can be analyzed through the use of cytology and a variety of tumor markers.[12] However, the low cellular content of cyst fluid has hampered the use of the cytologic analysis of cyst fluid. Small, cuboidal cells in cytologic specimens are diagnostic of serous cystadenomas (Table 74.3). In contrast, mucinous cystadenoma ma[y] have epithelial cells with evidence of mucin secretion or atypia. Only inflammatory cells should be present in the flui[d] aspirated from pseudocysts.

A variety of cyst fluid tumor markers have been studied t[o] help differentiate between the major types of cystic neoplasms. Several studies suggest that carcinoembryonic antigen (CEA

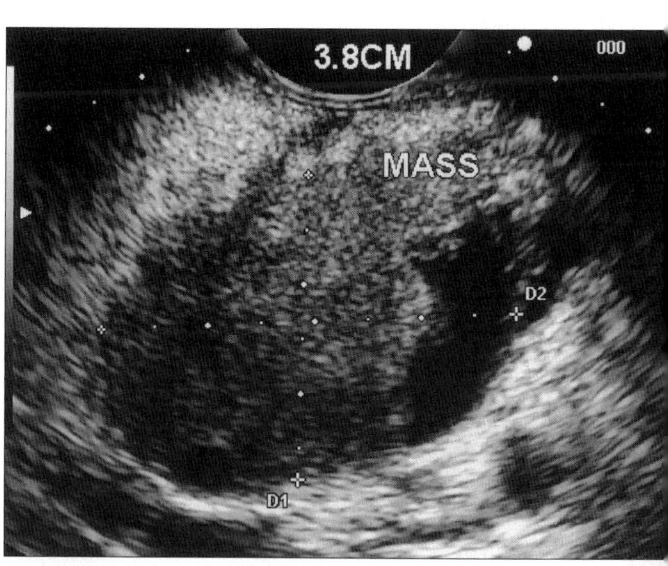

Fig. 74.5 Mucinous lesion. Endoscopic ultrasound of a malignant mucinous lesion with a mass filling the cystic space.

TABLE 74.3 DIAGNOSIS OF CYSTIC LESIONS

	Fluid	CEA	Cytology
Serous	Thin	Low	Cuboidal
Mucinous	Viscous	High	Mucinous
Pseudocyst	Thin	Low	Macrophages

or CA 72-4 are useful for identifying mucinous lesions.[13] These carbohydrate antigens are secreted by the epithelium lining mucinous lesions and are present in high concentrations. Cyst fluid concentrations of CEA and CA 72-4 are very low in serous cystadenomas. Unfortunately, there is considerable overlap in cyst fluid concentration of CEA in benign and malignant mucinous cystic lesions and pseudocysts. Cyst fluid amylase is used to differentiate between cystadenomas and pseudocysts.

Intraductal papillary mucinous neoplasms can be imaged with endoscopic retrograde cholangiopancreatography (ERCP) or EUS. The endoscopic appearance of mucin extrusion from a widely patent ampulla is diagnostic of an intraductal papillary mucinous neoplasm. Contrast retrograde pancreatography will demonstrate the characteristic findings of mucinous filling defects within the duct, diffuse ductal dilation, and cystic dilation of side branches. EUS may assist in the detection of malignancy arising from intraductal papillary mucinous neoplasms by demonstrating wall invasion and guiding fine needle aspiration.

TREATMENT AND PREVENTION

Cystic neoplasms

Surgical resection is the treatment of choice for premalignant cystic neoplasms. The decision to resect a lesion, however, is based on the presence or absence of symptoms, the risk of malignancy, and the surgical risk of the patient. High-risk patients with low-grade cystic neoplasms may be monitored with periodic CT/MRI scanning or EUS-FNA.

The increasing safety of surgical resection has prompted the use of surgery for a wider range of lesions.[14] Since most mucinous cystic neoplasms are located in the tail of the pancreas, a distal pancreatectomy is sufficient for these premalignant lesions. Unless invasive carcinoma is suspected or discovered at surgery, the spleen can often be preserved. Serous cystadenomas are resected by removing the involved portion of the pancreas: tail (tail resection), head (Whipple), or body (middle pancreatectomy). Since intraductal papillary mucinous neoplasms invade the pancreas along ductal structures, it is important that frozen section histology be used during surgery to ensure negative margins.[15] High-risk intraductal papillary mucinous neoplasms involving the entire pancreas will require total pancreatectomy. These surgical approaches often require that the patients be managed in centers with considerable experience in cystic tumors of the pancreas.

Pancreatic pseudocysts

Small pseudocysts (less than 4 cm in diameter) often resolve spontaneously and are rarely associated with clinical symptoms. Only 40% of pseudocysts less than 6 cm in diameter will require drainage because of complications or persistence. Small pseudocysts located in the tail of the pancreas and arising from acute biliary pancreatitis have a very high rate of spontaneous drainage. Prior to drainage, it is critical to confirm the diagnosis of a pseudocyst using fluid analysis and cytology. Mistakenly diagnosed pseudocysts that are drained with percutaneous drainage often do not resolve and may harbor occult malignancy.

Drainage of pseudocysts (Table 74.4)

Pancreatic pseudocysts may be drained using a variety of approaches. External drainage using CT/US guidance is the most common approach and involves the percutaneous placement of a small drainage catheter.[16] Fluid is drained into an external collection system carried by the patient. The short-term success rate for this relatively simple technique is very high, more than 90%. Patients with communicating pseudocysts, however, should not have percutaneous drainage because of the high risk of prolonged drained and fistula formation.

TABLE 74.4 DRAINAGE PROCEDURES FOR PSEUDOCYST

Type	Procedure
Surgical	Cyst-gastrostomy
Radiologic	Percutaneous cyst drainage
Endoscopic	Transgastric cyst-gastrostomy stenting

Surgical drainage of pseudocysts is performed by providing a large anastomosis between the pseudocyst wall and the stomach or small bowel. The anastomosis should be located in the most dependent portion of the cystic cavity in order to maximize drainage. Surgical drainage is probably the best approach when the pseudocyst is complicated by areas of necrosis, infection, or involves adjacent organs such as the spleen. However, maturation of a pseudocyst wall over 4–6 weeks will allow the formation of a thick wall that will provide a more secure anastomosis. Cyst-gastrostomy is the easiest approach and requires less operating time than cyst-jejunostomy. However, the risk of bleeding is greater with cyst-gastrostomy. Recent series report overall success rates for surgical drainage of 90% with major complication rates of 9% and recurrence rates of 3%.

Endoscopic drainage of pseudocysts is an alternative to surgical or radiologic drainage.[17] This type of drainage is used most commonly for uncomplicated, unilocular pseudocysts. Pseudocyst drainage is accomplished with either a transpapillary approach with ERCP or direct endoscopic stent placement across the stomach or duodenal wall. A transpapillary approach with drainage is used when the pseudocyst communicates with the main pancreatic duct, usually in the head of the pancreas. A transgastric or duodenal approach is used when the pseudocyst is directly adjacent to the gastroduodenal wall. Endoscopic ultrasound is often used to determine the size, location, and thickness of the pseudocyst wall and may reduce the rate of complications.[18] A wall thickness of more than 1 cm or the presence of large intervening vessels or varices as made evident by the EUS exam will preclude the possibility of endoscopic drainage. With the presence of a visible bulge in the wall of the stomach or the duodenum, endoscopic drainage is performed by the placement of transmural catheters or stents. If a bulge is not visible, EUS is required to provide localization of the pseudocyst. One-step EUS-directed drainage has recently been made possible with the use of pseudocyst drainage catheters that can be used in therapeutic echoendoscopes. Overall, the complication rate of elective endoscopic drainage is about 13% with success rates of more than 90% and recurrence rates of 10–20%.

COMPLICATIONS AND THEIR MANAGEMENT

Complications of cystic neoplasms are rare and consist of malignant invasion of local structures, such as the bile duct.

Endoscopic stenting is the treatment of choice unless the lesion is surgically resectable. Bleeding and infection are the most common complications of pancreatic pseudocysts. Arterial pseudoaneurysms are the most common cause of bleeding and should be managed with angiography. The treatment of choice for infected pseudocysts is external drainage.

PROGNOSIS WITH AND WITHOUT TREATMENT

The prognosis for resected cystic tumors of the pancreas is excellent.[19] There have been only rare reports of tumor recurrence in cases where the lesion was completely resected and there has been no evidence of malignant tissue in the resected specimen. Even for intraductal papillary mucinous neoplasms containing carcinoma (which comprises almost 60% of resected tumors) the 5-year survival is over 50%.[20] The worst prognosis is for advanced, transmural adenocarcinomas arising from mucinous lesions; the 5-year survival is only 30% for resected lesions

CURRENT CONTROVERSIES

With the widespread use of CT/MRI and EUS-FNA, an increasing number of cystic lesions are being identified at an early stage. Without a firm understanding of the natural history of mucinous cystadenomas, it is difficult to know when and if surgical resection should be performed. Noninvasive therapies such as chemical ablation would offer alternatives to surgical therapy.

SOURCES OF INFORMATION FOR PATIENTS AND DOCTORS

http://www.pancreasfoundation.org/

REFERENCES

1. Brugge WR, Lauwers GY, Sahani D, Fernandez-del Castillo C, Warshaw AL. Cystic neoplasms of the pancreas. N Engl J Med 2004; 351:1218–1226.
2. Kimura W, Nagai H, Kuroda A, Muto T, Esaki Y. Analysis of small cystic lesions of the pancreas. Int J Pancreatol 1995; 18:197–206.
3. Zhang XM, Mitchell DG, Dohke M, Holland GA, Parker L. Pancreatic cysts: depiction on single-shot fast spin-echo MR images. Radiology 2002; 223:547–253.
4. Compton CC. Serous cystic tumors of the pancreas. Semin Diagn Pathol 2000; 17:43–55.
5. Hammel PR, Vilgrain V, Terris B et al. Pancreatic involvement in von Hippel-Lindau disease. The Groupe Francophone d'Etude de la Maladie de von Hippel-Lindau. Gastroenterology 2000; 119:1087–1095.
6. Moore PS, Zamboni G, Brighenti A et al. Molecular characterization of pancreatic serous microcystic adenomas: evidence for a tumor suppressor gene on chromosome 10q. Am J Pathol 2001; 158:317–321.
7. Vortmeyer AO, Lubensky IA, Fogt F et al. Allelic deletion and mutation of the von Hippel-Lindau (VHL) tumor suppressor gene in pancreatic microcystic adenomas. Am J Pathol 1997; 151:951–956.
8. Yoshizawa K, Nagai H, Sakurai S et al. Clonality and K-ras mutation analyses of epithelia in intraductal papillary mucinous tumor and mucinous cystic tumor of the pancreas. Virchows Arch 2002; 441:437–443.
9. Byrne MF, Mitchell RM, Baillie J. Pancreatic pseudocysts. Curr Treat Options Gastroenterol 2002; 5:331–338.
10. Curry CA, Eng J, Horton KM et al. CT of primary cystic pancreatic neoplasms: can CT be used for patient triage and treatment? Am J Roentgenol 2000; 175:99–103.
11. Brugge WR. Role of endoscopic ultrasound in the diagnosis of cystic lesions of the pancreas. Pancreatology 2001; 1:637–640.
12. Brugge WR, Lewandrowski K, Lee-Lewandrowski E, et al. Diagnosis of pancreatic cystic neoplasms: a report of the cooperative pancreatic cyst study. Gastroenterology 2004; 126:1330–1336.
13. Frossard JL, Amouyal P, Amouyal G et al. Performance of endosonography-guided fine needle aspiration and biopsy in the diagnosis of pancreatic cystic lesions. Am J Gastroenterol 2003; 98:1516–1524.
14. Fernandez del Castillo CF, Targarona J, Thayer SP et al. Incidental pancreatic cysts: clinicopathologic characteristics and comparison with symptomatic patients. Arch Surg 2003; 138:427–434.
15. Chari ST, Yadav D, Smyrk TC et al. Study of recurrence after surgical resection of intraductal papillary mucinous neoplasm of the pancreas. Gastroenterology 2002; 123:1500–1507.
16. Andersson R, Cwikiel W. Percutaneous cystogastrostomy in patients with pancreatic pseudocysts. Eur J Surg 2002; 168:345–348.
17. De Palma GD, Galloro G, Puzziello A, Masone S, Persico G. Endoscopic drainage of pancreatic pseudocysts: a long-term follow-up study of 49 patients. Hepatogastroenterology 2002; 49:1113–1115.
18. Sanchez Cortes E, Maalak A, Le Moine O et al. Endoscopic cystenterostomy of nonbulging pancreatic fluid collections. Gastrointest Endosc 2002; 56:380–386.
19. Harper AE, Eckhauser FE, Mulholland MW. Resectional therapy for cystic neoplasms of the pancreas. Am Surg 2002; 68:353–357; discussion 357–358.
20. Kanazumi N, Nakao A, Kaneko T et al. Surgical treatment of intraductal papillary-mucinous tumors of the pancreas. Hepatogastroenterology 2001; 48:967–971.

Chapter 75

Development and miscellaneous abnormalities

Bommayya Narayanaswamy and Mark Davenport

KEY POINTS

- Developmental abnormalities of the pancreas may manifest from infancy to adulthood
- The most common presentations are as duodenal obstruction (annular pancreas), exocrine pancreatic insufficiency (hypoplasia), and recurrent pancreatitis (pancreas divisum, congential strictures, common pancreatobiliary channel)

DEVELOPMENT

The pancreas develops from the foregut between the 5th and 8th weeks of intrauterine life from multiple sources. The acinar exocrine cells, the epithelium of its duct system, and the endocrine islet cells are derived from endoderm. The blood and lymphatic vessels and stromal connective tissue develop from mesoderm and its innervation arises from neural crest ectoderm. Pancreatic endocrine cells are initially located in the walls of the ducts. Proliferation and later migration into mesenchyme occurs to form the islets of Langerhans. Islet maturation occurs with polyhormonal cells evolving into monohormonal ones arranged to form a core of insulin-producing cells surrounded by the other cell types.

Pancreatic endoderm originates as ventral and dorsal buds from the caudal part of the foregut (Fig. 75.1A,D). The dorsal bud appears initially and grows between the leaves of the dorsal mesentery. The smaller ventral bud arises adjacent to the origin of the hepatic diverticulum and slightly caudal to the dorsal bud. The caudal foregut representing the developing duodenum elongates and bows ventrally to form a loop (Fig. 75.1B). It then rotates to the right and comes to lie against the dorsal body wall creating its characteristic C-shape (Fig. 75.1E–G). The dorsal bud element now lies to the left of the duodenum and the ventral one to the right. Differential growth of the duodenal wall causes the growing ventral bud and developing bile duct to migrate dorsally with fusion of the two primordial elements. Thus, in the developed pancreas the entire body and tail, and the anterior part of the head are derived from the dorsal bud leaving the posterior part derived from the ventral bud. The uncinate process is derived from both pancreatic elements.

Initially, there are two independent embryological duct systems, one for each of the primordia. A variable amount of fusion then occurs such that the original dorsal duct territory (tail and body) drains via the proximal ventral duct (of Wirsung). The original smaller proximal dorsal duct opening persists as the accessory duct (of Santorini) and in most adults drains a small portion of the head. Duct fusion is believed to occur in the 7th week of gestation. Failure of or incomplete duct fusion is termed 'pancreas divisum'.

Functional maturation of the pancreas is first evident in the third month of intrauterine life with the appearance of secretory acini at the end of ducts. Formation of trypsin occurs around 22 weeks' gestation but full exocrine function is only achieved by the second year of life.

AGENESIS AND HYPOPLASIA

Agenesis of the entire pancreas is a very rare abnormality characterized by intrauterine growth retardation, severe metabolic acidosis, hyperglycemia, and meconium ileus and is usually fatal. Recently, some cases have been associated with point mutations in the IPF (insulin promotor factor) 1 gene, a transcription factor believed to be important in early pancreas development.[1, 2]

Partial agenesis may involve either the dorsal or ventral anlage. Dorsal agenesis is the more common and may, in some cases, be hereditary.[3] Diabetes mellitus may be associated but presentation is most often with recurrent acute pancreatitis in the ventral moiety and subsequent exocrine pancreatic insufficiency. Imaging shows absence of the body and tail of the pancreas. Partial agenesis must be distinguished from atrophy or degeneration secondary to disease.

Pancreatic hypoplasia refers to paucity or underdevelopment of the pancreas. Typically, this affects the acini with preservation of ducts and may be part of the autosomal recessive Shwachman-Diamond syndrome characterized by exocrine pancreatic insufficiency and bone marrow dysfunction.[4]

Congenital absence of the pancreatic islets is very rare and associated with intrauterine growth retardation and neonatal death. It may be inherited in an X-linked manner.[5]

ECTOPIC (SYN. HETEROTOPIC) PANCREATIC TISSUE

Pancreatic tissue may be present outside the confines of the gland itself. Most reported examples have been foregut related (i.e., stomach, duodenum, and biliary tree), although other reported sites include small bowel, Meckel's diverticulum, and colon. Ectopic pancreatic tissue may contain both exocrine and endocrine elements. Although most cases are asymptomatic and otherwise incidental findings, symptoms may result from extrinsic compression (e.g., causing obstructive jaundice or gastric outlet obstruction), peptic ulceration (causing gastrointestinal bleeding), intussusception or, rarely, malignant change. Symptomatic ectopic pancreas is treated by surgical resection.

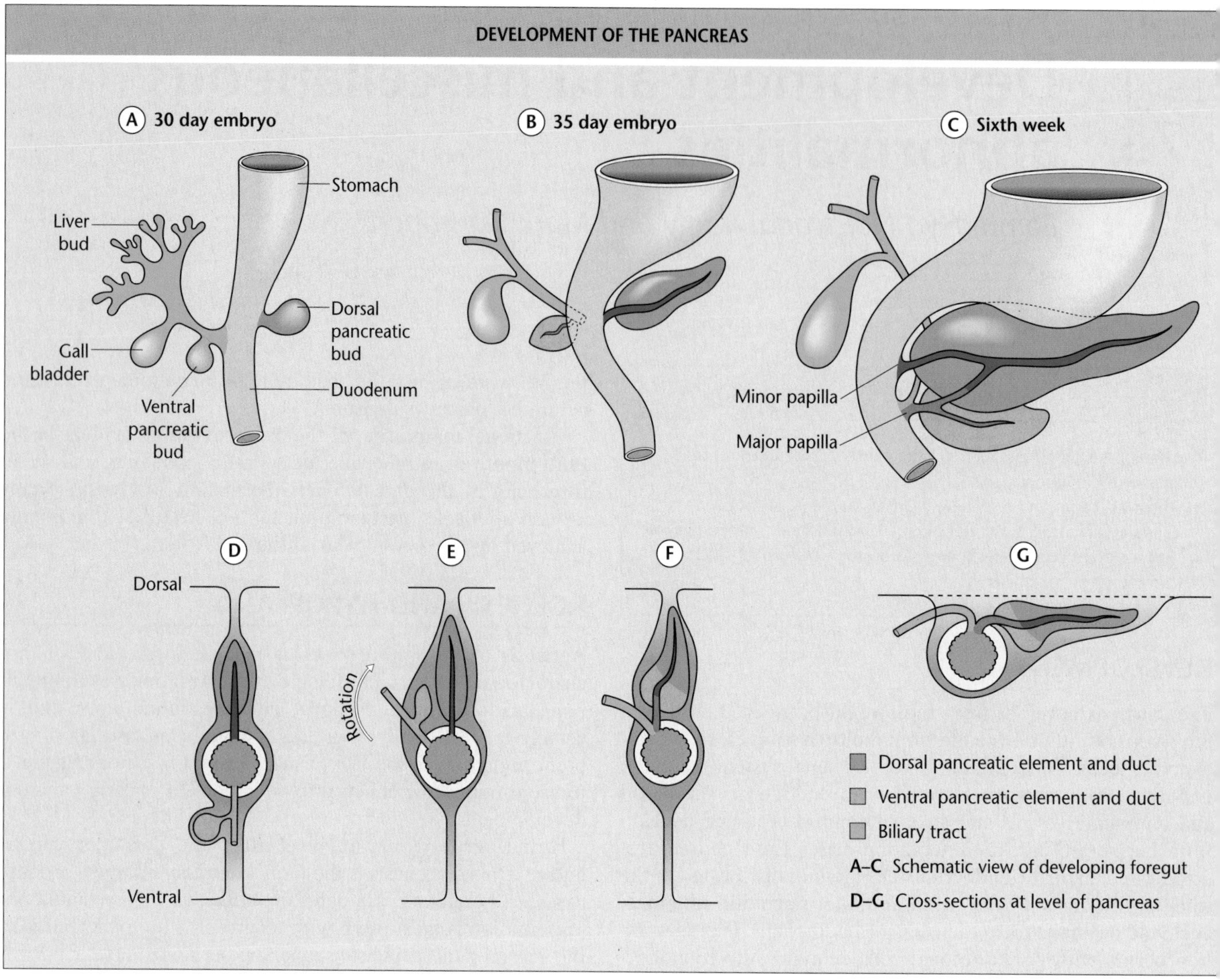

Fig. 75.1 Development of the pancreas. A–D, schematic view of developing foregut. **D–G,** cross-sections at level of pancreas.

ANNULAR PANCREAS

The second part of the duodenum may be encircled by a band of pancreatic tissue and is termed an annular pancreas. This may be due to fixation of the ventral pancreatic bud prior to its rotation or, alternatively, splitting of the ventral bud with failure of involution of the left ventral element. Certainly, the annulus has been shown immunohistochemically to be of ventral bud origin.[6]

The relationship of the annulus to the duodenum varies from juxtaposition to intramural 'invasion.' A large duct has been reported to run dorsally within the annulus, draining into the duct of Wirsung in about two-thirds of cases. Other anomalies such as duodenal atresia or stenosis and intestinal malrotation are often present in those that present during the neonatal period, while those presenting later are typically isolated. Down's syndrome is not uncommon because of its relationship with duodenal atresia and a few familial cases have been described. The true incidence is not known, as many remain asymptomatic.

Clinical presentation: Although most cases of annular pancreas are probably clinically silent, a proportion will present with the underlying duodenal obstruction, typically within the first week of life with bile vomiting. A minority will present much later in life and many cases are reported with the first symptoms only occurring in adulthood.[7] There is usually vomiting and abdominal pain due to intermittent duodenal obstruction. Acute pancreatitis, peptic ulcer disease and, rarely, biliary tract obstruction have all been associated with annular pancreas.

Diagnosis: The radiological feature of duodenal obstruction in infants is that of a 'double bubble' appearance on a plain abdominal X-ray and, given this, little more is needed prior to a laparotomy. In older children and adults, further investigations may include an upper gastrointestinal contrast series to define the nature of the duodenal obstruction and endoscopic cholangiopancreatography (ERCP) or magnetic resonance cholangiopancreatography (MRCP) to visualize pancreatic ductal arrangement. CT imaging and, most recently, endoscopic ultrasound may allow visualization of the annulus itself.

Treatment: This depends on the nature of the presentation. Duodenal obstruction is relieved by duodeno-duodenostomy performed anterior to the annulus. No attempt should be made to divide the annulus itself as this carries a high risk of istula formation. In the older child or adult presenting with pancreatitis, pancreatic duct arrangement needs to be investigated endoscopically and, in some cases, duct drainage procedures may be useful.

ANNULAR PANCREAS

- Descending duodenum encircled by ring of pancreatic tissue
- Incidence: unknown
- Often associated with duodenal atresia/stenosis
- Presentation: may be clinically silent, duodenal obstruction, pancreatitis
- Diagnosis: 'double bubble' on plain abdominal film, upper GI contrast study, CT, endoscopic US, ERCP, MRCP (not infants)
- Treatment: duodeno-duodenostomy, ? pancreatic duct drainage procedures

PANCREAS DIVISUM

Originally, the term pancreas divisum was confined to complete failure of fusion of the ventral and dorsal duct systems; however this has been expanded to encompass variants due to abnormal fusion of the two duct systems. Figure 75.2 illustrates some varieties of pancreas divisum. In most, the key observation is that the dorsal duct drains most of the gland via the accessory Santorini papilla rather than the main ampulla of Vater.

Pancreas divisum is a relatively common anatomical observation although there is discrepancy between the reported incidence at endoscopy (~5%) and that observed at autopsy (~10%). For this reason its relationship to pancreatic pathology has been questioned, at least in adults.[8] It is probable that it is not simply that the accessory duct drains most pancreatic exocrine secretions, but that there is also a relative accessory duct stenosis causing a raised ductal pressure. The term 'dominant dorsal duct syndrome' has been coined to reflect this.[9]

Clinical presentation has included recurrent abdominal pain, recurrent acute pancreatitis, and chronic pancreatitis, and in this setting usually affects the dorsal pancreas. Rarely, the ventral element drains exclusively by fine ducts into the dorsal duct, resulting in so-called ventral-segment pancreatitis.

Diagnosis: Pancreas divisum can only be definitively diagnosed by ERCP (Fig. 75.3), although a range of supportive investigations may be used to establish its relationship to clinical

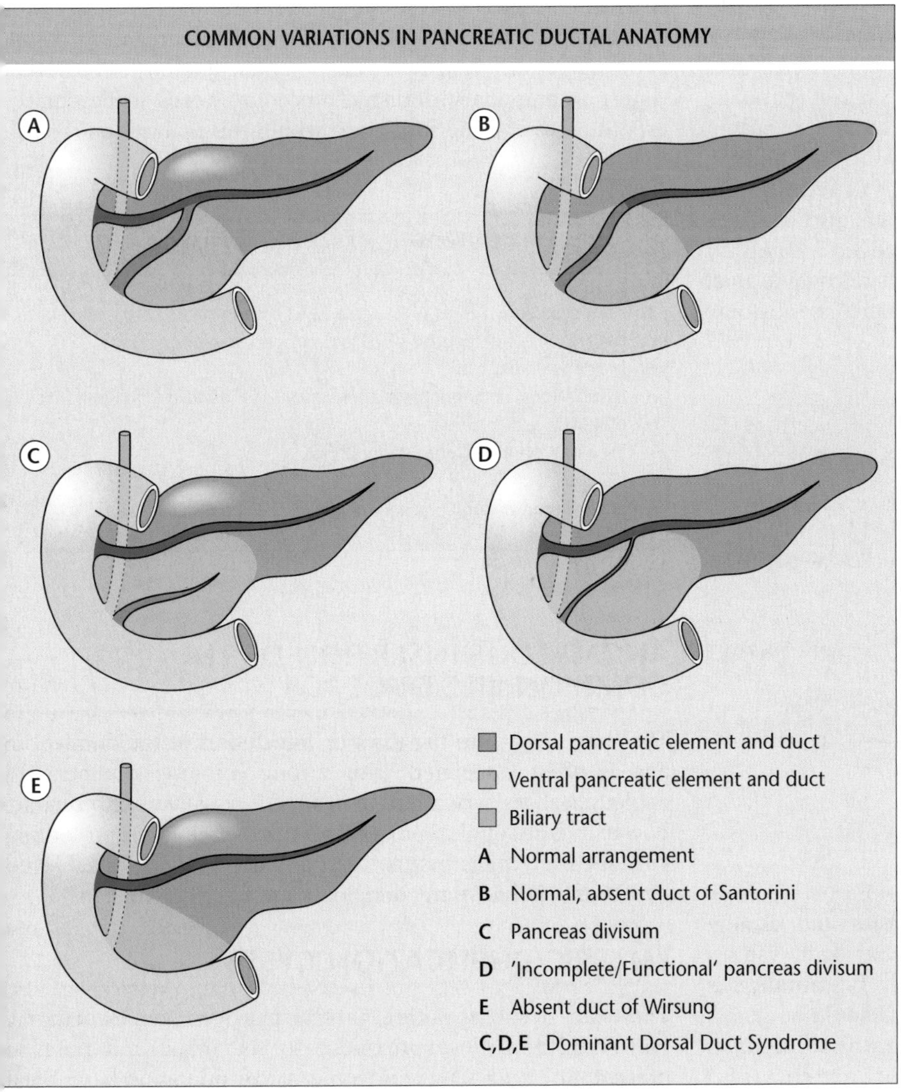

Fig. 75.2 Variations and abnormalities of pancreatic ductal anatomy. A, normal arrangement; **B,** absent accessory duct; **C,** pancreas divisum; **D,** incomplete (functional) pancreas divisum; **E,** absent duct of Wirsung. Modified from Warshaw et al.[9]

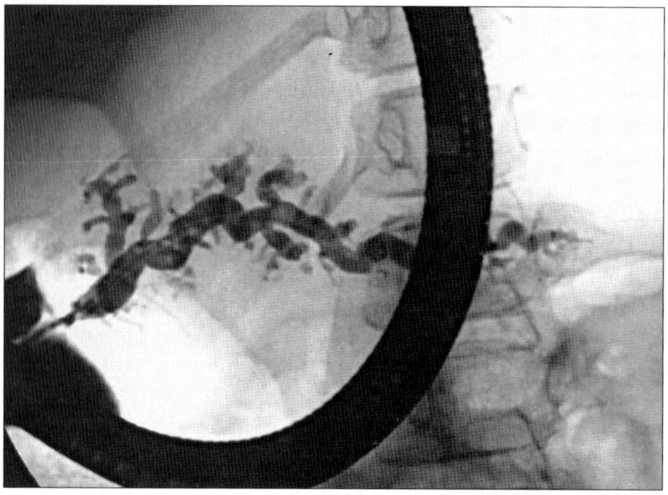

Fig. 75.3 ERCP in a 6-year-old child with recurrent pancreatitis. The main pancreatic duct is filled by cannulating the minor papilla and is dilated consistent with chronic obstruction. Symptoms relieved by longitudinal pancreaticojejunostomy.

symptoms. Thus, intravenous secretin stimulation with detection of consequent dorsal duct dilatation by ultrasonography or MR pancreatography has been described.[8]

Treatment: The aim of most intervention is to improve pancreatic duct drainage and a number of options are available. A suitable initial approach would be endoscopic dorsal duct stenting and/or sphincterotomy. Adult series suggest that most benefit is seen if the presenting symptoms have been recurrent pancreatitis rather than chronic pancreatic pain.[10] In children, if there has been symptomatic relief in terms of reduction in episode frequency then open surgical pancreatic duct drainage should be considered. This can be achieved either by transduodenal accessory ductoplasty or by a retrograde duct drainage procedure (e.g., longitudinal pancreaticojejunostomy – Puestow procedure).

PANCREAS DIVISUM

- Failure of fusion of embryonic dorsal and ventral duct systems
- Incidence: 5–10% (ERCP, autopsies)
- Presentation: may be clinically silent, recurrent pancreatitis, recurrent abdominal pain
- Diagnosis: ERCP
- Treatment (when symptomatic):
  endoscopic – dorsal duct stenting/sphincterotomy
  open surgery – dorsal duct sphincteroplasty, Puestow procedure

CONGENITAL PANCREATIC DUCT STRICTURES

This has been reported in ~3% of autopsies and usually involves the junction of the ventral and dorsal duct systems with consequent distal dorsal duct dilatation. Presentation is usually with recurrent acute pancreatitis and should be investigated with ERCP. Retrograde duct drainage will decompress the distal ducts satisfactorily.[11]

COMMON PANCREATICOBILIARY CHANNEL

The terminal parts of the common bile duct and the ventral pancreatic duct often unite outside of the medial wall of the duodenum to form a short common channel. The length of this varies from ~3 mm in infants to ~5 mm in children and adolescents. It is clearly pathological if it is long (>10 mm) and lies outside the sphincter complex (of Oddi). A common channel is a normal stage in pancreatic duct development and absorption of this into the wall of the duodenum occurs towards the end of gestation.

It is a frequent observation in choledochal malformations (~80%) and biliary atresia (~20%), and has a higher than expected incidence in gallbladder carcinoma. There is some evidence that because the common channel allows free intermixing of bile and pancreatic juices it may actually be etiological by exposing biliary epithelium to activated proteolytic enzyme attack.[12] Conversely, acute pancreatitis may also occur and is due to the abnormal presence of bile within the pancreatic duct triggering premature activation of secreted pancreatic enzymes.

ERCP or, occasionally, percutaneous transhepatic cholangiography, is diagnostic. Particularly when associated with pancreatitis, the common channel may be dilated and found to contain debris or occasionally calculi (Fig. 75.4). The aim of surgical therapy is to separate pancreatic and biliary secretions and this is achieved by excision of the bile duct malformation, cholecystectomy, and Roux-en-Y hepaticojejunostomy. Sometimes, an ampullary drainage procedure needs to be considered if there is stone formation within the channel.

COMMON PANCREATICOBILIARY CHANNEL

- Abnormal early fusion of pancreas and common bile ducts, allowing pathological intermixing of biliary and pancreatic secretions
- Incidence: unknown
- Associations: choledochal malformations, biliary atresia, gallbladder dysplasia and malignancy
- Presentation: recurrent pancreatitis
- Diagnosis: ERCP or PTC
- Management: surgical biliary diversion

ANOMALOUS INSERTION OF THE COMMON BILE DUCT

This may occur into the third or fourth part of the duodenum and is often associated with a long common channel and choledochal malformation. In itself, it is usually asymptomatic; however, Doty et al. reported two cases of children presenting with recurrent pancreatitis.[13] Symptomatic relief was achieved by hepaticojejunostomy and complete biliary diversion.

ENTERIC DUPLICATION CYSTS

These are, strictly speaking, not true pancreatic malformations. However, their close proximity to the gland and possible presentation with pancreatitis merits consideration here. Such

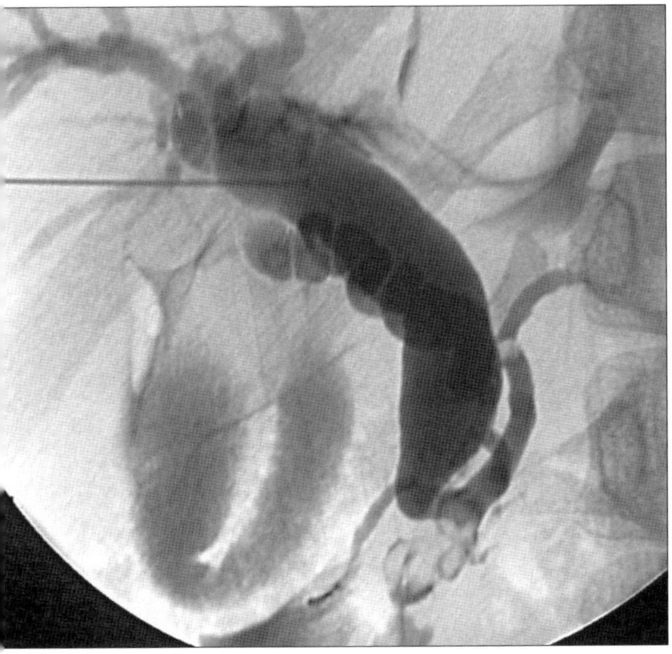

Fig. 75.4 Percutaneous transheptic cholangiogram (PTC) in a 12-year-old girl with recurrent pancreatitis and intermittent jaundice. There is a fusiform choledochal dilatation, a dilated common channel containing radiolucent debris, and a dilated main pancreatic duct. Symptoms relieved by excision of choledochal malformation, hepaticojejunostomy-en-Roux, and a transduodenal sphincteroplasty.

duplications may be entirely within the pancreatic head and may present with pancreatitis due to duct obstruction and occasionally gastritis due to hypergastrinemia.[14] A variety of imaging modalities have been suggested including ultrasonography, ERCP, CT, and intraoperative ultrasound. Incision of the overlying pancreas with complete cyst excision should be performed.

Gastric duplications abutting on the head of the pancreas may present with pancreatitis secondary to erosion or perforation of a posterior peptic ulcer into the gland. Such cysts may also directly communicate with the pancreatic duct system causing pancreatitis by blockage of the ducts with mucus and debris (Fig. 75.5).

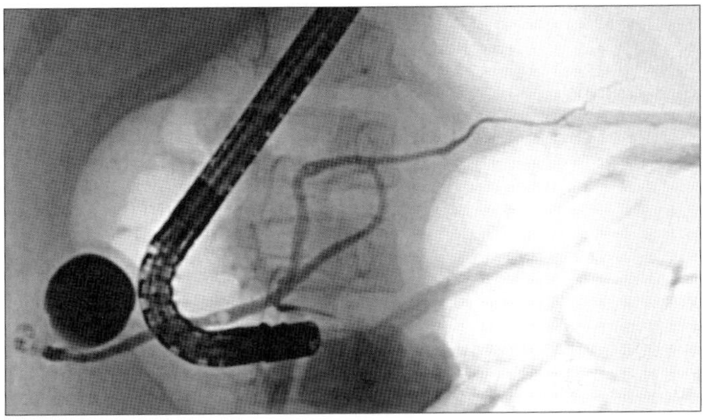

Fig. 75.5 ERCP in a 7-year-old girl with recurrent pancreatitis. There is a cyst anatomically adjacent to the gastric antrum that communicates by an accessory duct with the main pancreatic duct. Resection of the cyst showed this to be a foregut duplication cyst containing predominantly gastric mucosa.

REFERENCES

1. Stoffers DA, Zinkin NT, Stanojevic V et al. Pancreatic agenesis attributable to a single nucleotide deletion in the human IPF1 gene coding sequence. Nat Genet 1997; 15:106–110.
2. Schwitzgebel VM, Mamin A, Brun T et al. Agenesis of human pancreas due to decreased half-life of Insulin Promoter Factor 1. J Clin Endocrinol Metab 2003; 88:4398–4406.
3. Stingl H, Schnedl WJ, Krssak M et al. Reduction in hepatic glycogen synthesis and breakdown in patients with agenesis of the dorsal pancreas. J Clin Endocrinol Metab 2002; 87:4678–4685.
4. Rothbaum R, Perault J, Vlachos A et al. Shwachman-Diamond syndrome: report from an international conference. J Pediatr 2002; 141:266–270.
5. Dodge JA, Laurence KM. Congenital absence of the islets of Langerhans. Arch Dis Child 1977; 52:411–413.
6. Suda K. Immunohistochemical and gross dissection studies of annular pancreas. Acta Pathol Jpn 1990; 40:505–508.
7. England RE, Newcomer MK, Leung JW, Cotton PB. Case report: annular pancreas divisum – a report of two cases and review of the literature. Br J Radiol 1995; 68:324–328.
8. Quest L, Lombard M. Pancreas divisum: opinio divisa. Gut 2000; 47:317–319.
9. Warshaw AL, Simeone JF, Schapiro RH, Flavin-Warshaw B. Evaluation and treatment of the dominant dorsal duct syndrome (pancreas divisum redefined). Am J Surg 1990; 159:59–64.
10. Heyries L, Barthet M, Delvasto C et al. Long-term results of endoscopic management of pancreas divisum with recurrent acute pancreatitis. Gastrointest Endosc 2002; 55:376–381.
11. Tagge EP, Smith SD, Raschbaum GR et al. Pancreatic ductal abnormalities in children. Surgery 1991; 110:709–717.
12. Stringer MD, Dhawan A, Davenport M et al. Choledochal cysts: lessons from a 20 year experience. Arch Dis Child 1995; 73:528–531.
13. Doty J, Hassal E, Fonkalsrud EW. Anomalous drainage of the common bile duct into the fourth part of the duodenum. Arch Surg 1985; 120:1077–1079.
14. Siddiqui AM, Shamberger RC, Filler RM et al. Enteric duplications of the pancreatic head: definitive management by local resection. J Pediatr Surg 1998; 33:1117–1120.

Chapter 76

Cholelithiasis, choledocholithiasis, and cholecystitis

Franz Ludwig Dumoulin and Tilman Sauerbruch

KEY POINTS

- Prevalence: 10–15% in Western societies
- Risk factors: older age, female, obesity, weight loss, pregnancy, terminal ileal disease, drugs, genetic predisposition
- Formed from biliary sludge: 80% cholesterol stones, < 20% pigment stones
- Gallbladder stones: only 1/3 symptomatic (pain from obstruction of the cystic duct).
- Bile duct stones: most become symptomatic
- Clinical: biliary colic, cholecystitis, ascending cholangitis, pancreatitis
- Rarely: cystic duct obstruction (Mirizzi syndrome), cholecysto-enteric fistulae, gallstone ileus, or gallbladder cancer
- Diagnosis: transabdominal ultrasound reliable, ERCP most accurate for bile duct stones plus therapeutic intervention, MRCP for patients with low suspicion of CBD stones
- Treatment: cholecystectomy (laparoscopic) if symptomatic or CBD stones (endoscopic sphincterotomy and stone extraction or surgical common bile duct exploration). Acute cholecystitis: early cholecystectomy. Ascending cholangitis: urgent endoscopic drainage.

NTRODUCTION AND DEFINITION

allstones (concretions formed from mainly cholesterol rystals) are common in Western societies with an estimated 5% of the US population having gallstones. They are formed om biliary sludge (microlithiasis), a mixture of particulate atter and bile that occurs when solutes in bile precipitate. he most frequent symptom caused by sludge or gallstones is iliary colic, which refers to a pain attack in the right upper quadrant and epigastrium. The majority of patients with gallbladder stones (cholecystolithiasis), however, are asymptomatic. In contrast, bile duct stones (choledocholithiasis) more often induce biliary pain, jaundice, acute biliary pancreatitis, and/or ascending cholangitis. An inflammatory reaction of the gallbladder wall (cholecystitis) is usually initiated when a stone or sludge becomes impacted in the gallbladder neck or the cystic duct. Acalculous cholecystitis may occur as a consequence of an impaired microcirculation and/or infection in the absence of gallstones.

EPIDEMIOLOGY

Gallstone prevalence ranges from 10% to 15% in the Western world with considerable variation between different ethnic groups. Gallstones are more frequent with increasing age and in young women. Thus, the highest known prevalence of gallstones is more than 70% in female Pima Indians at age 25. A higher than average prevalence has also been reported from Chile, Alaska, Canada, and Bolivia. In contrast, African Americans and Asians have a lower than average risk and in sub-Saharan Africa, gallstones are rare.[1] The importance of genetic factors is further emphasized by the fact that first-degree relatives of index persons are 4.5 times more likely to develop gallstones and that several single gene defects associated with cholelithiasis have been identified (Table 76.1).[2,3] In the majority of patients, however, a complex genetic predisposition, rather than single genes, promotes gallstone formation. A variety of susceptibility loci have been mapped in the mouse and will help the future characterization of candidate genes in man.[4,5]

TABLE 76.1 GENE DEFECTS ASSOCIATED WITH GALLSTONE FORMATION

Gene	Protein/function	Proposed mechanism of gallstone formation
ABCB4	Multidrug resistance-3 p-glycoprotein (MDR3)/phosphatidylcholine flippase	Biliary phospholipid secretion ↓
CCKA-R	Cholecystokinine A receptor/receptor	Gallbladder hypomotility
ABCC7	Cystic fibrosis transmembrane regulator (CFTR)/chloride channel	bile pH↓, Bilirubin secretion ↑, fecal bile acid excretion↑
SLC10A2	Ileal bile acid transporter (IBAT)/carrier for Na^+-dependent bile acid uptake	Biliary bile acid concentration ↓
CPY7A1	Cholesterol 7 alpha hydroxylase/first and rate-limiting enzyme of bile acid synthesis	Biliary bile acid synthesis ↓

CAUSES, RISK FACTORS, DISEASE ASSOCIATIONS

Pregnancy and childbirth are important risk factors. Thus, sludge and/or gallstones develop in up to a third and 1–3% of all pregnancies, respectively. After pregnancy, sludge resolves in 60–70% and gallstones disappear in 20–30% of the patients.[6] Other risk factors are age, obesity, rapid weight loss, or weight fluctuations, while physical activity is associated with a lower risk for gallstone formation.[7] Thus, up to 25% of patients with rapid weight loss and up to 50% of the patients following gastric bypass develop sludge or gallstones. Moreover, the risk for gallstones increases with serum triglyceride levels and there is an inverse correlation to high-density lipoprotein (HDL) cholesterol in serum, but no firm correlation exists with total or low-density lipoprotein (LDL) cholesterol. Clinical conditions associated with gallstone formation are parenteral nutrition, diseases of the terminal ileum, in particular Crohn's disease (see Chapter 54), pancreatic insufficiency including cystic fibrosis, and spinal cord injury. Black pigment stones, resulting from an increase in bilirubin output are more frequently observed in chronic hemolysis and in up to 30% of patients with liver cirrhosis. A variety of drugs are known to increase the risk of gallstone or sludge formation including ceftriaxone, octreotide, estrogens, and lipid-lowering drugs such as clofibrate. Finally, bacterial cholangitis, which promotes bilirubin deconjugation, can contribute to the formation of brown pigment stones.

Over 90% of cases of cholecystitis are due to gallbladder stones or sludge. In contrast, acalculous cholecystitis is predominantly seen in critically ill patients (multiple trauma, burns, sepsis, major surgery, shock, acute renal failure, mechanical ventilation >72 h) and/or in patients with vascular disorders (atherosclerosis, vasculitis) but may also result from primary microbial infection of the gallbladder, both in immunocompetent (e.g., typhoid fever, *Campylobacter jejuni*, leptospirosis) and in immunocompromised patients (e.g., *Salmonella enteritidis*, *Candida*, cytomegalovirus (CMV), *Cryptosporidium*).[8]

CAUSES AND RISK FACTORS

RISK FACTOR	PROPOSED MECHANISM OF STONE FORMATION
GENERAL FACTORS	
Age	Biliary cholesterol secretion increases with age, bile acid secretion decreases
Female	? Pregnancy and childbirth, effect of estrogens
Genetic factors	High in Pima Indians, very low in sub-Saharan Africa
Pregnancy/ Childbearing	Biliary cholesterol secretion increased (estrogens) Gallbladder hypomotility (progesterone)
NUTRITIONAL/METABOLIC FACTORS	
Obesity	Biliary cholesterol secretion increased (HMG-CoA reductase activity increased)
Weight loss/surgery for obesity	Biliary cholesterol secretion increased Mucin secretion increased (nucleation) Gallbladder hypomotility
Parenteral nutrition	Gallbladder hypomotility
Hypertriglyceridemia/ low HDL cholesterol	HMG CoA reductase activity increased: increased biliary cholesterol secretion
DISEASE ASSOCIATIONS	
Terminal ileal disease (e.g., Crohn's)	Impaired entero-hepatic circulation/ depletion of bile acid pool
Spinal cord injury	Gallbladder hypomotility (neuronal)
Pancreatic insufficiency	Gallbladder hypomotility (decreased cholecystokinin production)
Cystic fibrosis	Altered bile composition (see above)
Cholangitis	Deconjugation of bilirubin by bacterial enzymes
Hemolysis/liver cirrhosis	Increased bilirubin load
DRUGS	
Ceftriaxone	Biliary secretion of drug/precipitation
Octreotide	Biliary cholesterol secretion increased; gallbladder hypomotility
Clofibrate	Biliary cholesterol secretion increased
Estrogens	Biliary cholesterol secretion increased
ANATOMIC ABNORMALITIES	
Biliary strictures, duodenal diverticulum	Ascending cholangitis, intraductal brown pigment stones

PATHOGENESIS

Gallstone formation

Gallstones are classified as cholesterol and pigment stones (Fig. 76.1). They form from biliary sludge by continuing aggregate precipitation. Cholesterol stones consist of >50% cholesterol monohydrate crystals, bound in a matrix of glycoproteins often with a core of calcium bilirubinate. They account for up to 80% of the stones in the Western world. Three principal mechanisms contribute to their formation: secretion of bile supersaturated with cholesterol, accelerated nucleation of cholesterol crystals, and gallbladder hypomotility.[9] In bile, cholesterol is kept in aqueous solution by the detergent action of bile acids and phospholipids. An increase in cholesterol saturation results in the formation of unilamellar and finally unstable multilamellar vesicles. Accelerated nucleation time may be due to an excess of pronucleating factors (e.g., mucin glycoproteins) or a deficiency of antinucleating factors. Finally, gallbladder hypomotility has been found in many patients with gallstones.[5]

Black pigment stones are predominantly found in patients with chronic hemolysis, liver cirrhosis, cystic fibrosis, or diseases of the terminal ileum.[10] They are composed of calcium bilirubinates and develop as a consequence of bilirubin supersatu ration of bile along with biliary proteins and mucins serving a a nidus for crystallization.

Brown pigment stones are mostly formed within the bil ducts as a consequence of bacterial infection and hydrolysis o glucuronic acid from bilirubin by bacterial beta-glucuronidase This results in a decreased solubility of deconjugated bilirubi ultimately leading to the formation of stones consisting o calcium salts of unconjugated bilirubin, deconjugated bil acids, and varying amounts of cholesterol and saturated long chain fatty acids.

Cholecystitis

Over 90% of patients with calculous cholecystitis have a obstruction of the cystic duct by the impaction of sludge or gallstone in the gallbladder neck. The increased intralumina pressure together with aggressive bile trigger an inflammator

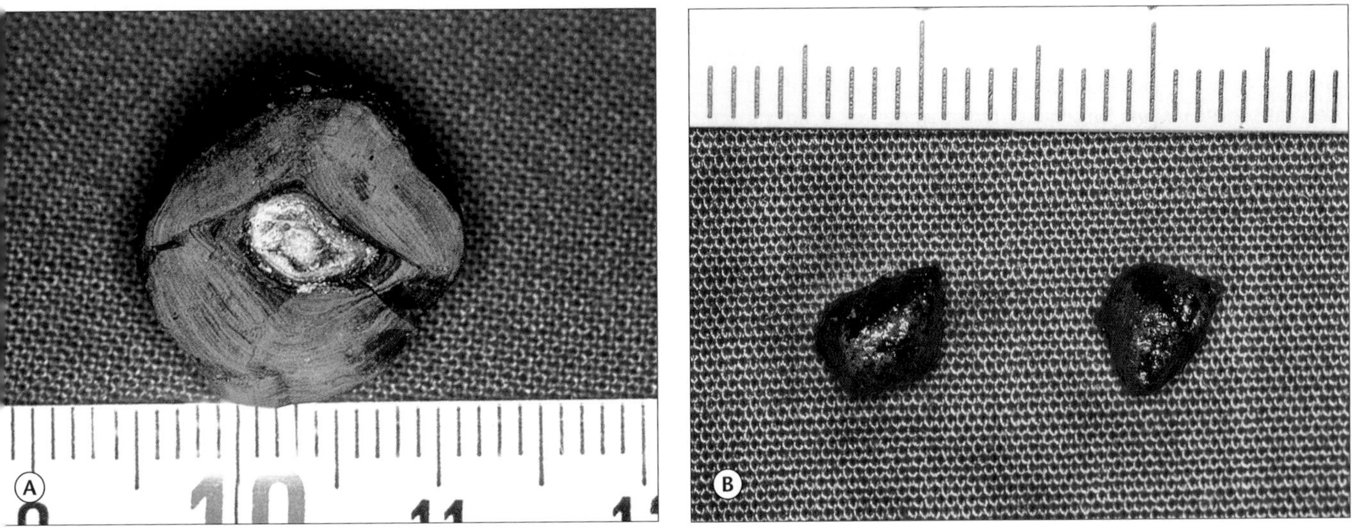

ig. 76.1 Gallbladder stones. A. Endoscopically extracted mixed bile duct stone with a typical cholesterol core that had moved from the allbladder and served as a nidus for the formation of a brown pigment shell in the common bile duct; **B.** black pigment gallbladder stones. cale bar = 1 cm.

eaction within the gallbladder wall. In about 20–50% of cases, secondary bacterial infection (most commonly by *Escherichia oli*, *Klebsiella*, and enterococci) is observed.[8] In contrast, calculous cholecystitis develops in the absence of gallstones s a result of ischemia and gallbladder stasis.[11] Acalculous holecystitis is seen with an incidence of 0.2–3% in critically l patients and/or in patients with vascular disorders (atherolerosis, vasculitis) and may also result from primary microial infection of the gallbladder.[8]

ATHOLOGY

n acute cholecystitis, the gallbladder is usually distended and, esides bile, contains stones, sludge, and an inflammatory exuate (Fig. 76.2A). Histological changes comprise an inflammaory infiltrate of polymorphous nuclear granulocytes with edema r, in advanced stages, necrosis (Fig. 76.2B). In chronic cholecystitis, the inflammatory infiltrate is replaced by lymphocytes nd plasma cells eventually resulting in mucosal atrophy and ibrous thickening of the gallbladder wall. Signs of vasculitis with ischemia and endothelial damage may dominate the histological picture in acute acalculous cholecystitis.

CLINICAL PRESENTATION

Cholelithiasis and choledocholithiasis

Biliary sludge results in stone formation in 12–80% of the patients with an incidence of complications ranging from 3% to 13%.[6] Cholecystolithiasis is asymptomatic in 60–80% of the patients. In two prospective studies on asymptomatic patients, biliary pain developed at a rate of 2% per year during the first 5 years; the overall incidence was 15–26% at 10 years. By that time, complications (cholecystitis, biliary obstruction, ascending cholangitis, pancreatitis) had developed in 3% of the patients and gallbladder carcinoma had been diagnosed in 1/161 patients.[1] Biliary pain due to intermittent obstruction of the cystic duct by a gallstone is localized in the mid-epigastrium or the right upper abdomen and may irradiate to the back or to the right shoulder. It is colicky but waves of pain are of long duration, typically lasting from 15 min to several hours. They may be

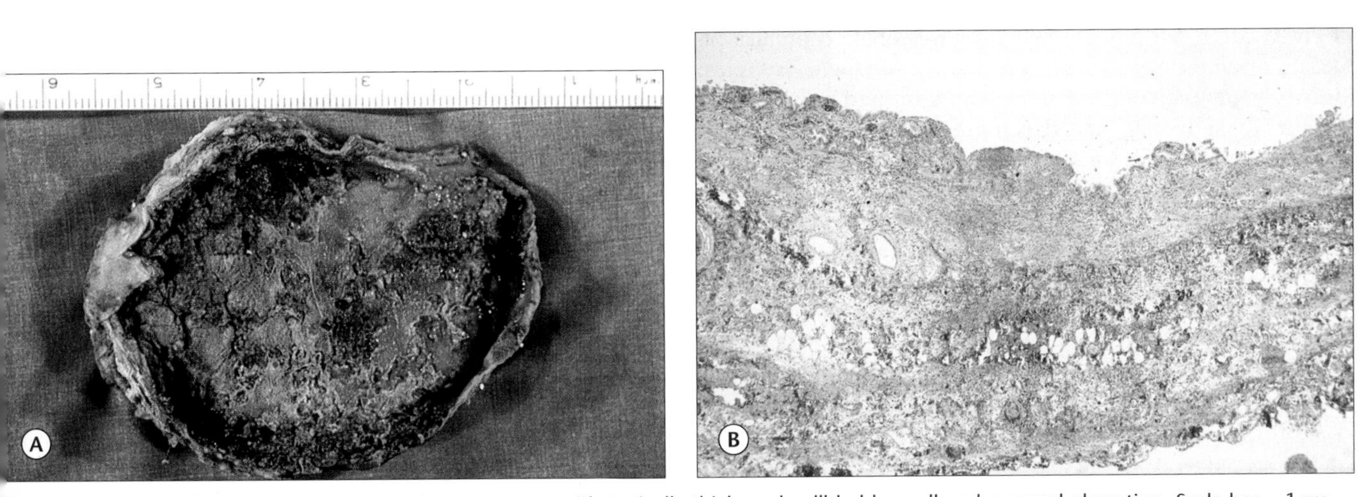

ig. 76.2 Acute cholecystitis. A. Macroscopic appearance with typically thickened gallbladder wall and mucosal ulceration. Scale bar = 1 cm. **.** Dense inflammatory infiltrate on histopathology.

accompanied by nausea and/or vomiting. Once an episode of biliary pain has occurred, the risk of repeated attacks or complications ranges from 58% to 72%; more than 90% of the complications are preceded by episodes of biliary pain.[1] Abdominal discomfort following fatty meals may have a similar predictive value.[12]

Cholecystitis

Cholecystitis typically causes worsening pain lasting longer than 5h. It is located in the right upper quadrant and accompanied by signs of inflammation such as fever, chills, and, in severe cases, signs of sepsis. Jaundice may be present in patients with sepsis or as a consequence of Mirizzi syndrome (see below). On examination, there is tenderness in the right hypochondrium with or without a palpable mass. Pain and an arrest in inspiration upon deep palpation underneath the right costal margin (Murphy's sign) may be present and has a sensitivity and specificity of 65% and 87%, respectively.[12]

The natural history of cholangiolithiasis is less well defined, but symptoms are more likely and complications are more severe than in cholecystolithiasis.[1]

CLINICAL PRESENTATION OF CHOLELITHIASIS
• Asymptomatic cholecystolithiasis • Symptomatic cholecystolithiasis with biliary pain • Complication of cholelithiasis: Cholecystitis Bile duct obstruction with jaundice/ascending cholangitis Acute biliary pancreatitis Perforation/cholecysto-enteric fistula Gallstone ileus Mirizzi syndrome Gallbladder or bile duct carcinoma

Cholangitis

Ascending cholangitis is usually due to bile duct obstruction with subsequent infection by Gram-negative enteric bacteria or enterococci. It is a potentially life-threatening complication presenting with fever, chills, and often posthepatic jaundice, and necessitates emergency treatment with fluid resuscitation, parenteral antibiotics, and decompression of the bile ducts, preferably by endoscopic means such as stone extraction or nasobiliary drainage. Concomitant cholecystitis or biliary pancreatitis should be ruled out. Long-term complications can be stricture formation, recurrent cholangitis with intrahepatic stone formation, and secondary biliary cirrhosis.

Other presentations

There are other well recognized but rare presentations. A stone impacted in the cystic duct may produce intermittent obstruction of the ductus hepatocholedochus (Mirizzi syndrome). Gallstones can erode the gallbladder wall resulting in cholecysto-enteric fistula with or without subsequent duodenal obstruction (Bouveret syndrome) or gallstone ileus.[13]

DIFFERENTIAL DIAGNOSIS

Cholecystolithiasis and choledocholithiasis

The differential diagnosis of recurrent abdominal pain comprise a great number of possible diseases. In addition to the biliar tract, abdominal pain may originate from the chest, stomac small intestine, colon, pancreas, kidneys, uterus, and ovarie Moreover, ischemic, neurogenic (e.g., from herpes zoster) c musculosketetal pain as well as pain of metabolic or toxi origin should be considered.[14] Jaundice and pain sugge choledocholithiasis, while painless jaundice favors liver diseas or malignant biliary obstruction. In patients with addition signs of inflammation, cholangitis and cholecystitis (see below must be included in the list of possible differential diagnoses

Cholecystitis

Fever, chills, and/or persistent pain localized in the right uppe quadrant lasting longer than 12h are suggestive of cholecystiti and/or cholangitis. The major differentials to be considered i a patient with persistent upper abdominal pain and signs o inflammatory reaction are acute appendicitis, acute pancreatiti pyelonephritis or stones of the right kidney, peptic ulcer disease alcohol hepatitis, hepatic abscess or tumor, and basal pneumoni with pleurisy. The differential diagnosis may be particular challenging, since patients may indeed have more than on diagnosis (e.g., cholangitis and pancreatitis). Diagnosis o acalculous cholecystitis in mechanically ventilated critically il patients is notoriously difficult. A high grade of suspicion o cholecystitis as a possible focus in critically ill patients, wit sepsis of unknown cause, is required.[15]

DIFFERENTIAL DIAGNOSIS OF BILIARY PAIN
COMMON • Symptomatic cholecystolithiasis/cholecystitis • Cholangiolithiasis/cholangitis • Acute appendicitis • Acute pancreatitis • Right kidney disease: pyelonephritis, stone • Peptic ulcer disease UNCOMMON • Liver disease (alcohol hepatitis/hepatic abscess) • Basal pneumonia with pleurisy/pulmonary embolism

DIAGNOSTIC METHODS

Cholecystolithiasis and choledocholithiasis

Physical examination during an episode of biliary pain may reveal right upper quadrant tenderness but usually is norma between the attacks. Blood chemistry will be normal in th majority of patients but may show increases in serum bilirubin alkaline phosphatase, gamma glutamyl transpeptidase an transaminases, particularly with cholangitis, or amylase in th case of biliary obstruction or pancreatitis. In cholangitis, sign of inflammation (fever, leukocytosis with left-shift, elevate C-reactive protein) may be seen and blood cultures ma become positive.

Transabdominal ultrasound is the best single test for th diagnosis of gallbladder stones (Fig. 76.3). Common bile duc

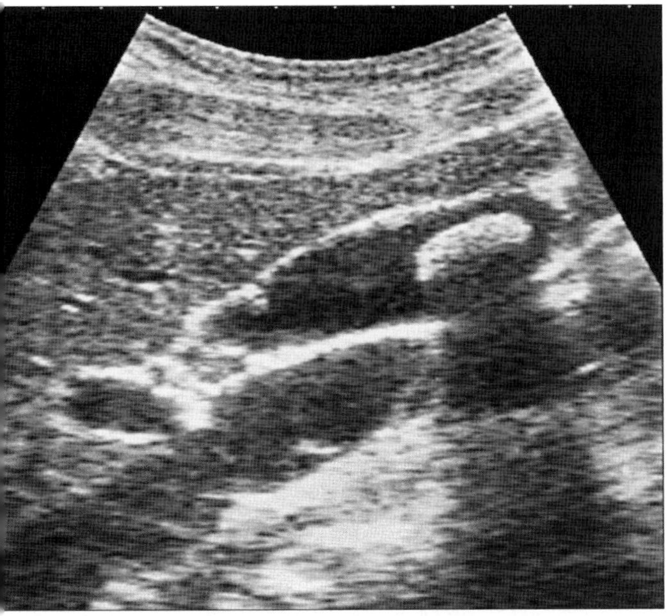

Fig. 76.3 Abdominal ultrasound of a gallbladder stone. This is easily recognized by the hyperechoic signal with dorsal acoustic shadowing.

stones may be visualized by ultrasound (Fig. 76.4) but in the majority of patients only indirect evidence, such as the presence of dilated bile ducts together with gallbladder stones, can be obtained.[16] Endoscopic retrograde cholangiography (ERCP) and, in case of inaccessibility of the papilla or technical failure, percutaneous transhepatic cholangiography (PTC) remain the gold standard for the imaging of bile duct stones (Fig 76.5). ERCP is the preferred diagnostic method in patients with a high suspicion for cholangiolithiasis since it allows subsequent therapeutic intervention. Endoscopic ultrasound has a similar diagnostic accuracy for the detection of common bile duct stones, but its precise role remains to be defined.[17,18] Magnetic resonance cholangiography (MRC) has a sensitivity and specificity of 90–95% for the detection of common bile duct stones (Fig. 76.6) and is well suited to rule out bile duct stones in patients with low or intermediate clinical suspicion. In addition, it is the imaging method of choice if the biliary tract is inaccessible to endoscopy.[19] Axial computed tomography (CT) has its role in the work-up of abdominal pain or acute abdomen and is useful in ruling out of calcified stones in patients who are evaluated for oral litholysis. Finally, intraoperative cholangiography can be performed in patients with an intermediate probability of cholangiolithiasis who undergo cholecystectomy.

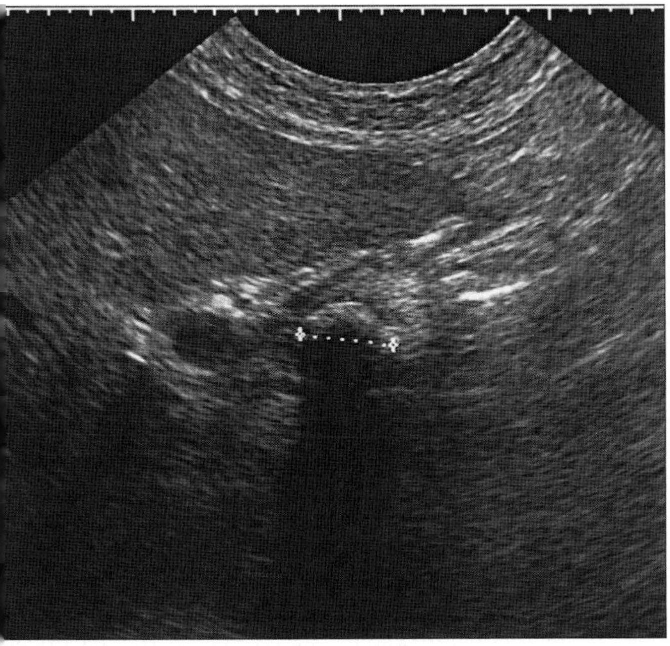

Fig. 76.4 Ultrasound of a common bile duct stone. Ultrasound of a common bile duct stone presenting as a typical hyperechoic structure with acoustic shadowing. Ultrasound can only confirm the diagnosis, but cannot rule out the presence of cholangiolithiasis, since diagnostic accuracy is limited due to interference of air from the adjacent duodenum.

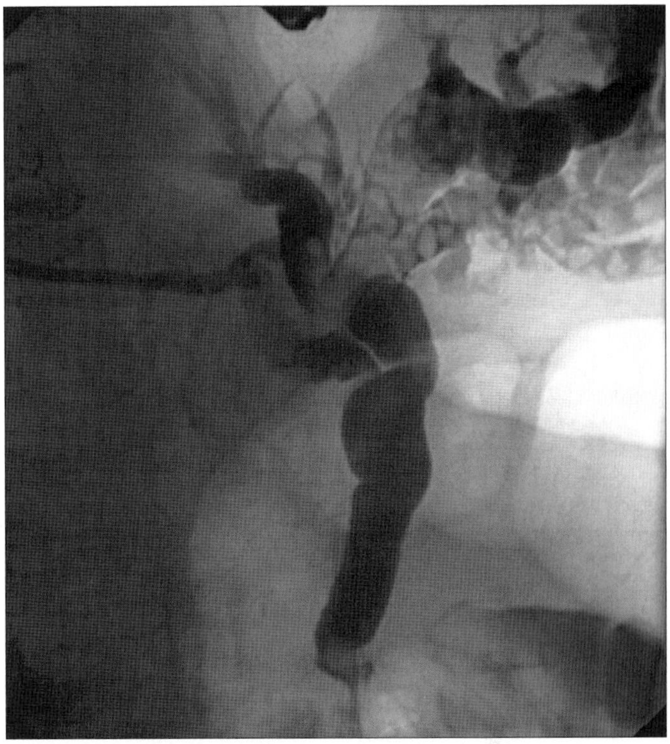

Fig. 76.5 Endoscopic retrograde cholangiography. Endoscopic retrograde cholangiography showing multiple intrahepatic stones. The 80-year-old patient had been cholecystectomized 20 years earlier. Note the dilated left-sided bile duct system with multiple filling defects.

Cholecystitis

Blood chemistry will show signs of inflammation and possibly of cholestasis; aerobe and anaerobe blood cultures may become positive.[11] Transabdominal ultrasound is the single most useful diagnostic tool with a sensitivity and specificity of >90% and >80%, respectively. Typical findings are thickening of the gallbladder wall, which, however, may also be present in patients with ascites or hypoalbuminemia, a positive sonographic Murphy's sign, emphysematous cholecystitis with gas bubbles in the gallbladder wall (so-called champagne sign), or signs of perforation or abscess formation (Fig. 76.7). Abdominal CT is useful, particularly if the initial diagnosis of abdominal pain is obscure. Ultrasound is a less reliable diagnostic tool in critically ill patients but the presence of sludge together with the above signs are useful hints. Murphy's sign, however, is rarely observed and CT scans should be performed in the critically ill with a high suspicion of cholecystitis.[15]

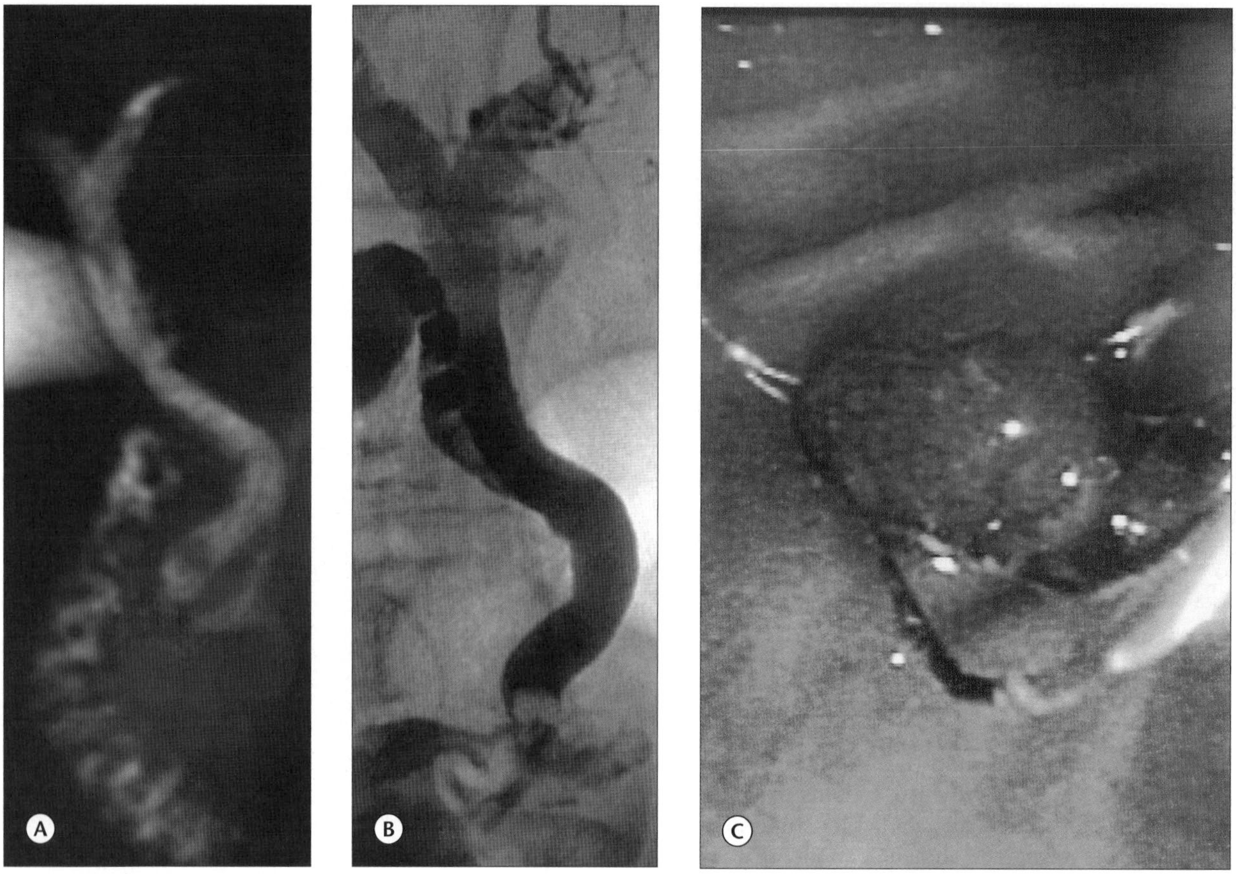

Fig. 76.6 Prepapillary common bile duct stone. Magnetic resonance cholangiography (MRC), endoscopic retrograde cholangiography (ERC), and endoscopic view of a common bile duct stone. The intraductal stone can be clearly visualized by both MRC **(A)** and ERC **(B)**. The stone was removed after sphincterotomy using a Dormia basket **(C)**. MRC courtesy of Professor Schild, Department of Radiology, University of Bonn.

DIAGNOSTIC METHODS
DIAGNOSTIC METHODS FOR CHOLELITHIASIS/CHOLECYSTITIS • Routine blood tests including blood cultures • Transabdominal ultrasound • Axial computed tomography **DIAGNOSTIC METHODS FOR BILE DUCT STONES/CHOLANGITIS** • Routine blood tests including blood cultures • Transabdominal ultrasound • ERCP (PTC) in patients with high suspicion of bile duct stones • MRCP in patients with low suspicion of bile duct stones or inaccessibility of bile ducts • Endoscopic ultrasound • Axial computed tomography

TREATMENT AND PREVENTION

Cholecystolithiasis and choledocholithiasis

Preventive measures

Prevention of stone formation is possible in high-risk situations with ursodeoxycholic acid (UDCA), 600 mg/day p.o., as adjunctive therapy to weight reduction or with cholecystokinin octapeptide (CCK-8), 50 ng/kg body weight i.v., in patients receiving long-term total parenteral nutrition.[6]

Asymptomatic cholecystolithiasis

Asymptomatic cholecystolithiasis is not an indication for cholecystectomy since the risk of complications from surgery outweighs the advantage of preventing possible complications from asymptomatic gallbladder stones including gallbladder cancer. However, some patient populations have an increased risk for the development of cholelithiasis and/or can be prone to more severe complications but do not have a significantly increased complication rate for cholecystectomy. These include patients undergoing surgery for morbid obesity (e.g., gastric bypass) or receiving solid organ transplantation other than cardiac transplant surgery.[20] Similarly, the prevention of gallbladder cancer may be an indication for cholecystectomy in male patients with gallbladder stones >3 cm (up to 10-fold increased risk for gallbladder cancer), in those with polyps >10 mm, or in those with a calcified gallbladder (cancer risk of 3–6% or up to 20%, respectively).

Symptomatic cholecystolithiasis

Emergency treatment of biliary colic is accomplished by spasmolytics (e.g., N-butyl-scopolamin 40 mg i.v.) and nonsteroidal anti-inflammatory drugs (e.g., metamizol 1 g i.v., diclofenac 75 mg i.m.). Cholecystectomy, preferably by laparoscopic approach, should be performed to avoid the 50–70% rate of recurrence as well as the 1–2% risk of complications from gallstone disease. In selected patients who do not wish to undergo an operation and have solitary, noncalcified stones

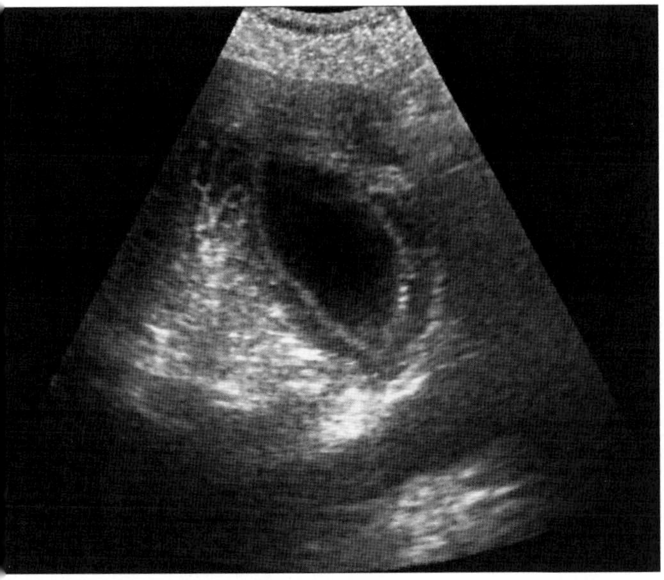

ig. 76.7 **Ultrasound appearance of cholecystitis.** In this patient, calculous cholecystitis was diagnosed during mechanical ventilation or severe pneumonia. Note the hypoechoic thickening of the gallbladder wall and the pericholecystic fluid collection. The diagnosis of acalculous cholecystitis was confirmed histologically after open holecystectomy.

vith a diameter of less than 20 mm and a well-contracting gall-bladder, an attempt of extracorporeal shock wave lithotripsy ESWL) and oral litholysis with UDCA (10–15 mg/kg body weight/day) for 6–12 months is justified.[21] Patients with tiny loating stones may profit from prolonged UDCA treatment alone.

Choledocholithiasis

Choledocholithiasis is a definite indication for treatment, even n asymptomatic patients, since complications occur more often and are more severe than in cholecystolithiasis. In the majority of patients, cholecysto- and cholangiolithiasis coexist and three options are available: (1) strict surgical treatment with (laparoscopic) cholecystectomy and bile duct exploration;[22] (2) strict therapeutic splitting with endoscopic removal of bile duct stones followed by (laparoscopic) cholecystectomy; or (3) flexible splitting.[23] While a surgical approach has the advantage of subjecting the patient to just one procedure, laparoscopic duct exploration is technically demanding and ime consuming. On the other hand, endoscopic methods for bile duct clearance with standard equipment (Dormia basket and balloon) are successful in over 90% of the patients Fig. 76.8). Treatment options for difficult stones include mechanical lithotripsy, extracorporeal shock wave lithotripsy Fig. 76.9), and electrohydraulic or laser lithotripsy.[24] Alternatively, surgical bile duct exploration remains a valuable option, n particular for large impacted stones and in patients with an ndication of cholecystectomy. Under certain circumstances e.g., elderly patients unfit for surgery with difficult-to-treat bile duct stones) endoscopic sphincterotomy and stenting are accepted alternatives. If ascending cholangitis complicates cholangiolithiasis, emergency endoscopic placement of naso-biliary drainage along with antibiotic therapy and supportive measures are warranted.

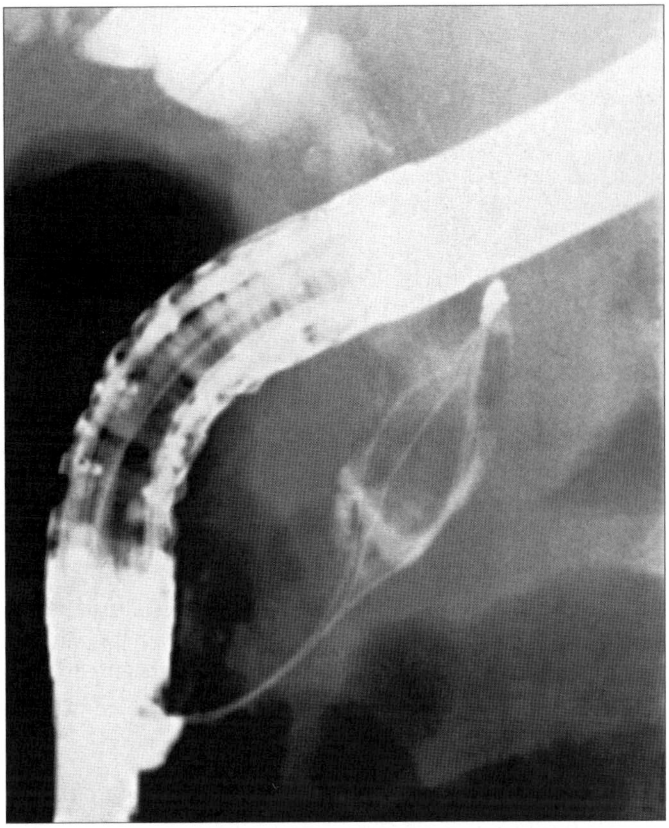

Fig. 76.8 Clearance of a common bile duct stone using a Dormia basket. The stone has already been captured inside the basket. Lithotripsy may be required prior to the extraction of larger stones.

Cholecystitis

Medical treatment

Emergency treatment consists of fasting, fluid resuscitation, spasmolytics, and analgesia, preferably with NSAIDs. In addition, intravenous antibiotic therapy covering Gram-negative enteric microorganisms (e.g., broad spectrum acyl-ureido-penicillins/third generation cephalosporins/chinolones) should be started.

Surgery

Most patients respond to initial conservative medical treatment. However, up to 20% develop signs of advanced cholecystitis (fever >38 °C, serum bilirubin >10 mg/dL or 170 μmol/L) and need emergency surgery to avoid complications such as gangrene, perforation, peritonitis, or sepsis.[8] The timing of surgery in the remaining 80% of patients is still under debate. Early laparoscopic surgery (within 48 h of the onset of symptoms) is preferred, since these patients have lower conversion and complication rates and shorter hospital stays than those undergoing delayed (>5 days after the onset of symptoms) or interval (>6 weeks after the acute episode) laparoscopic surgery. The overall complication rates of the laparoscopic approach range from 9.0% to 15.0%, with bile duct injuries between 0.7% and 1.3%, which is comparable to complications for open cholecystectomy in these patients.[25–27]

Percutaneous cholecystostomy

Percutaneous (ultrasound or CT-guided) drainage of the gallbladder is an alternative temporary treatment in patients unfit

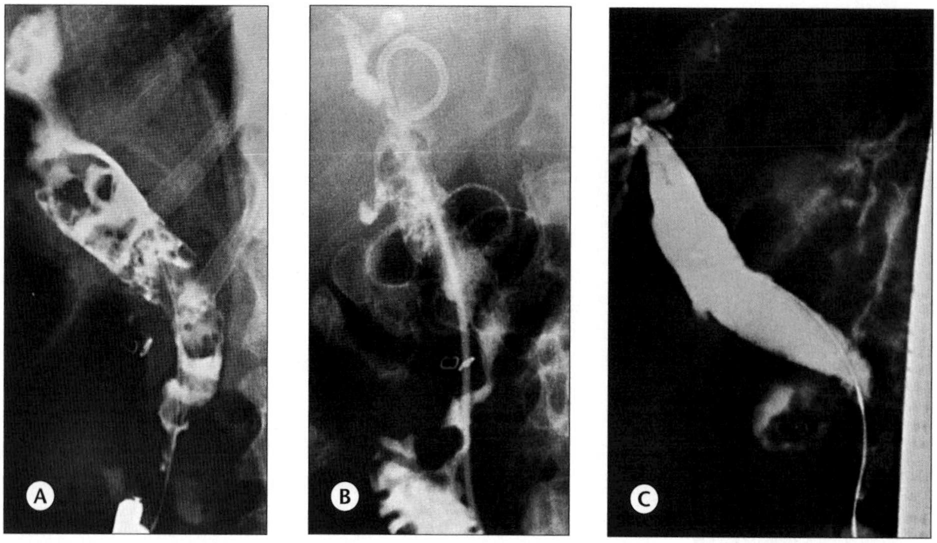

Fig. 76.9 Efficacy of extracorporeal shock wave lithotripsy (ESWL). A. Multiple filling defects due to multiple common bile duct stones. **B.** A nasobiliary drainage is inserted to facilitate visualization of stones for planned ESWL. **C.** Complete duct clearance after two ESWL treatments and subsequent ERC with extraction of stone fragments by Dormia basket and balloon.

for surgery. The possibility of a bedside procedure renders this technique a valuable treatment option in critically ill patients. Cholecystostomy without subsequent cholecystectomy can be a definite treatment for acalculous cholecystitis.

Treatment fallacies

Complications of gallstone disease may occur in combination, e.g., pancreatitis and cholangitis or ascending cholangitis with cholecystis. In these patients, concomitant complications must not be overlooked and should be treated promptly. Moreover, the acuity of cholecystitis, particularly acalculous cholecystitis, may be underestimated. Particularly in critically ill patients, a frequent interdisciplinary re-evaluation is warranted to proceed to emergency cholecystectomy (or cholecystotomy) if necessary.

COMPLICATIONS AND THEIR MANAGEMENT

Cholecystolithiasis and choledocholithiasis

The single most frequent complication of gallstone disease is cholecystitis, which has been discussed above. Other complications are mostly due to migrating or impacted stones, which may result in a variety of complications such as ascending cholangitis, acute biliary pancreatitis (discussed in Chapter 71), Mirrizi syndrome, gallstones ileus (including Bouveret's syndrome), choledocho- or cholecysto-enteric fistulae, and gallbladder cancer.

Cholecystitis may become gangrenous (2–30%) or lead to gallbladder perforation (10%) with a mortality of 30%, as well as cholecysto-enteric fistulae and gallstone ileus (see above) and/or sepsis.[8] Early diagnosis of local complications by ultrasound and/or contrast-enhanced CT is important. Treatment consists of supportive measures and emergency cholecystectomy.

Rare complications

Mirizzi syndrome (Fig. 76.10) and cholecystocholedochal fistula are two manifestations of the same process beginning with impaction of gallstone(s) in the gallbladder neck and subsequent obstruction of the hepatocholedochal duct and/or erosion with fistula formation. Presenting symptoms are pain, jaun-

TREATMENT AND PREVENTION

PREVENTION
- During weight reduction: UDCA 600 mg/day
- During prolonged parenteral nutrition: CCK-8 50 ng/kg body weight/day

SYMPTOMATIC CHOLECYSTOLITHIASIS
- NSAIDs, spasmolytics (opioids)
- (Laparoscopic) cholecystectomy

SIMULTANEOUS CHOLANGIOLITHIASIS/CHOLECYSTOLITHIASIS
- (Laparoscopic) cholecystectomy and concurrent surgical duct exploration or prior
- endoscopic duct clearance
- Palliative stenting in patients unfit for surgery

CHOLANGITIS
- Endoscopic (nasobiliary) drainage, antibiotics, supportive treatment

CHOLECYSTITIS
- Emergency therapy with fasting, fluids, analgesics, antibiotics
- Early (laparoscopic) cholecystectomy within 48 h
- Percutaneous or transpapillary drainage in critically ill patients

COMPLICATIONS OF CHOLELITHIASIS AND THEIR MANAGEMENT (PEARLS)

Cholecystitis	Supportive therapy with antibiotics Early cholecystectomy within 48–72 h (open or laparoscopic)
Biliary pancreatitis	Early endoscopic sphincterotomy in patients with obstructive jaundice or severe biliary pancreatitis Supportive therapy including prophylactic antibiotics in severe pancreatitis (see Chapter 71)
Ascending cholangitis	Supportive therapy with antibiotics and endoscopic (or percutaneous) biliary drainage
Mirizzi syndrome	Cholecystectomy (open); occasional patients unfit for surgery might be treated endoscopically with sphincterotomy/lithotripsy
Fistulae	Surgical treatment only if symptomatic

ice, and fever. It is important to make an accurate diagnosis usually by ERC). Surgical treatment is usually required, with laparoscopic procedures carrying a higher risk of complications. ERC with sphincterotomy, lithotripsy, and stone extraction may be helpful, in particular for poor surgical candidates. Fistula formation is usually identified at cholangiography. Management may be expectant (e.g., for an asymptomatic choledocho-duodenal fistula) or surgical (e.g., at the time of cholecystectomy). Treatment of gallstone ileus comprises supportive measures and emergency surgery.[13]

PROGNOSIS WITH AND WITHOUT TREATMENT

Prognosis with treatment

The prognosis of cholecystolithiasis is good. Likewise, calculous cholecystitis usually follows a benign course. The overall mortality rate after surgical treatment is less than 0.1%. However, after cholecystectomy up to 10% of the patients complain of recurrent or persistent pain, which is referred to as 'post cholecystectomy syndrome.' In some cases, this may represent continuation of preoperative nongallstone pain that was misattributed to coincidental gallstones. Acalculous cholecystitis in critically ill patients carries a poor prognosis, which depends on coexisting medical conditions and the mortality may be higher than 50%.

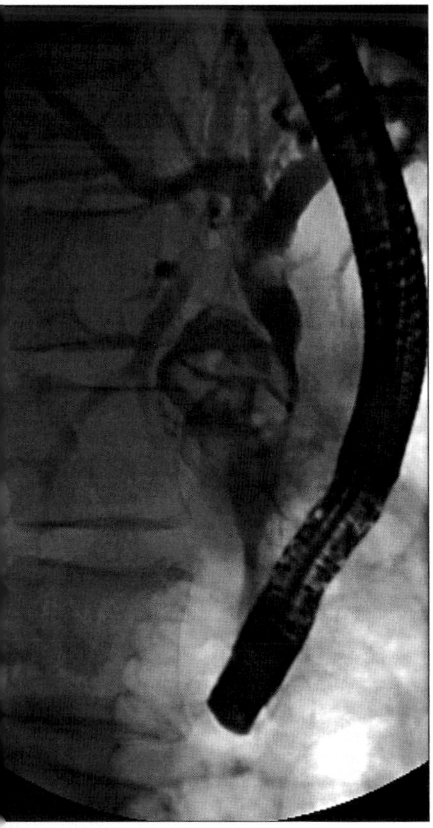

Fig. 76.10 Endoscopic retrograde cholangiography (ERC) appearance of Mirizzi's syndrome. Note the eccentric stenosis of the common hepatic duct in close vicinity to the cystic duct and the presence of multiple stones both in the gallbladder and the bile ducts. The patient underwent open cholecystectomy and a large defect in the wall of the common hepatic duct was diagnosed intraoperatively.

Prognosis without treatment

The natural history of asymptomatic gallstones has been described. Acute cholecystitis resolves spontaneously in half of the patients within 7–10 days; however, the rate of gangrenous cholecystitis with gallbladder perforation may be as high as 10%. If cholecystitis is treated without cholecystectomy, the recurrence rate is about 60% within 6 years. Ascending bacterial cholangitis has a high mortality rate if left untreated (e.g., when unrecognized). Acalculous cholecystitis carries a high mortality rate, even with appropriate treatment.

Harmful consequences of treatment

The risk of interventional endoscopy is determined by a variety of factors, including patient characteristics and comorbidity as well as the techniques used and the skills of the endoscopist. Endoscopic sphincterotomy probably carries the highest risk with pancreatitis as the most important complication (4.2–9.8%); mortality rates range between 0% and 0.4%.[24,28] The major complications of laparoscopic cholecystectomy are bile duct injuries. They occur at a rate of 0.4–0.5%, which is two to three times the rate reported for open cholecystectomy. Bile duct injuries comprise small biliary leaks closing spontaneously, biliary strictures (Fig. 76.11), which may be managed by endoscopic stent insertion, and large leaks or complete biliary obstruction usually requiring surgical repair. Other complications, e.g., injury to vessels, are less frequent. Important factors influencing the complication rate are the experience of the laparoscopic surgeon and the patient selection. Thus, patients with cholecystitis have a higher than average rate of bile duct injury and conversion to open surgery should be performed liberally.[29]

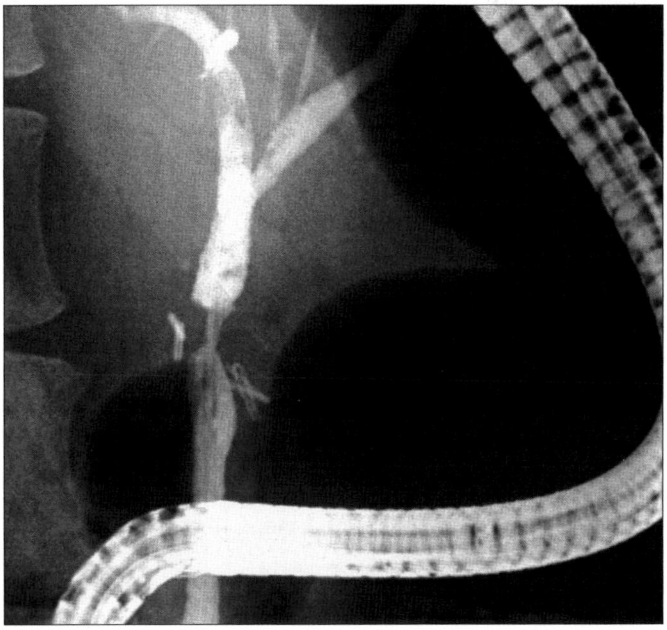

Fig. 76.11 Endoscopic retrograde cholangiography showing a bile duct stricture after laparoscopic cholecystectomy. Note the clip material after previous surgery. Longstanding cholangiolithiasis may lead to secondary biliary cirrhosis and bile duct carcinoma.

WHAT TO TELL PATIENTS

If gallstones are detected incidentally and if they are not producing any symptoms, most patients can be told not to worry about them. However, once gallstones have become symptomatic, the risk of repeated pain episodes and/or complications outweighs the risks of cholecystectomy. Surgery should be carried out by an experienced laparoscopic surgeon. The following may help to avoid developing gallstones: physical activity, moderate weight loss, or if a patient is planning to drastically reduce their body weight, they should consult their physician for prophylactic treatment with UDCA.

SOURCES OF INFORMATION FOR PATIENTS AND DOCTORS

A variety of useful websites from distinguished societies are recommended:

American Gastroenterological Association (AGA) at http://www.gastro.org
American College of Gastroenterology (ACG) at http://www.acg.gi.org
digestive.niddk.nih.gov/ddiseases/pubs/gallstones
www.gastro.org/clinicalRes/brochures/gallstones.html
www.patient.co.uk/showdoc.asp?doc=23068740
www.digestivedisorders.org.uk/leaflets/gallston.htm
http://www.hopkins-gi.org/pages/latin/templates/index.cfm?pg=disease1&organ=3&disease=33&lang_id=1
http://patients.uptodate.com/topic.asp?file=livr_dis/5577
http://www.gesa.org.au/consumer/publications/gallstones
http://cchs-dl.slis.ua.edu/patientinfo/gastroenterology/hepatic gallbladder/cholelithiasis.htm

CURRENT CONTROVERSIES AND THEIR FUTURE RESOLUTION

Major advances of our understanding of the pathogenesis of gallstone formation at the molecular level are expected and the identification of genes involved in cholesterol gallstone formation will have an impact on preventive measures. In addition clinical issues concerning the most efficient diagnostic and treatment algorithm remain to be fully investigated, including the precise diagnostic role of ERC vs MRC vs EUS or the controversy about endoscopic vs surgical bile duct clearance.

CONTROVERSIES, FALLACIES, AND PREDICTED FUTURE DEVELOPMENTS

- Identification of genetic factors involved in the pathogenesis of gallstone formation
- Definition of the relative contribution and the rational use of ERC/PTC, MRC, and EUS in the diagnosis of common bile duct stones
- Treatment of duct stones by interventional endoscopists or laparoscopic surgeons?

REFERENCES

1. Ko CW, Lee SP. Epidemiology and natural history of common bile duct stones and prediction of disease. Gastrointest Endosc 2002; 56 (Suppl 6):S165–S169.
2. Trauner M, Boyer JL. Bile salt transporters: molecular characterization, function, and regulation. Physiol Rev 2003; 83:633–671.
3. Pullinger CR, Eng C, Saleng G et al. Human cholesterol 7 alpha-hydroxylase (CYP7A1) deficiency has a hypercholesterolemic phenotype. J Clin Invest 2002; 110:109–117.
4. Lammert F, Carey MC, Paigen B. Chromosomal organization of candidate genes involved in cholesterol gallstone formation: a murine gallstone map. Gastroenterology 2001; 120: 221–238.
5. Kosters A, Jirsa M, Groen AK. Genetic background of cholesterol gallstone disease. Biochim Biophys Acta 2003; 1637:1–19.
6. Ko CW, Sekijima JH, Lee SP. Biliary sludge. Ann Intern Med 1999; 130(4 Pt 1):301–311.
7. Carey MC, Paigen B. Epidemiology of the American Indians' burden and its likely genetic origins. Hepatology 2002; 36(4 Pt 1):781–791.
8. Indar AA, Beckingham IJ. Acute cholecystitis. BMJ 2002; 325:639–643.
9. Zanlungo S, Nervi F. The molecular and metabolic basis of biliary cholesterol secretion and gallstone disease. Front Biosci 2003; 8:S1166–S1174.
10. Vitek L, Carey MC. Enterohepatic cycling of bilirubin as a cause of 'black' pigment gallstones in adult life. Eur J Clin Invest 2003; 33:799–810.
11. Barie PS, Eachempati SR. Acute acalculous cholecystitis. Curr Gastroenterol Rep 2003; 5:302–309.
12. Trowbridge RL, Rutkowski NK, Shojania KG. Does this patient have acute cholecystitis? JAMA 2003; 289:80–86.
13. Abou-Saif A, Al-Kawas FH. Complications of gallstone disease: Mirizzi syndrome, cholecystocholedochal fistula, and gallstone ileus. Am J Gastroenterol 2002; 97:249–254.
14. Kallo AN. Overview of differential diagnosis of abdominal pain. Gastrointest Endosc 2002; 56 (Suppl 6):255–257.
15. Ko CW, Lee SP. Gastrointestinal disorders of the critically ill. Biliary sludge and cholecystitis. Best Pract Res Clin Gastroenterol 2003; 17:383–396.
16. Gandolfi L, Torresan F, Solmi L, Puccetti A. The role of ultrasound in biliary and pancreatic diseases. Eur J Ultrasound 2003; 16:141–159.
17. Schwartz DA, Wiersema MJ. The role of endoscopic ultrasound in hepatobiliary disease. Curr Gastroenterol Rep 2002; 4:72–78.
18. Sivak MV Jr. EUS for bile duct stones: how does it compare with ERCP? Gastrointest Endosc 2002; 56 (Suppl 6):S175–S177.
19. Fulcher AS. MRCP and ERCP in the diagnosis of common bile duct stones. Gastrointest Endosc 2002; 56 (Suppl 6):S178–S182.
20. Kao LS, Kuhr CS, Flum DR. Should cholecystectomy be performed for asymptomatic cholelithiasis in transplant patients? J Am Coll Surg 2003; 197:302–312.
21. Howard DE, Fromm H. Nonsurgical management of gallstone disease. Gastroenterol Clin North Am 1999; 28:133–144.
22. Fielding GA. The case for laparoscopic common bile duct exploration. J Hepatobiliary Pancreat Surg 2002; 9:723–728.
23. Binmoeller KF, Schafer TW. Endoscopic management of bile duct stones. J Clin Gastroenterol 2001; 32:106–118.
24. Carr-Locke DL. Therapeutic role of ERCP in the management of suspected common bile duct stones. Gastrointest Endosc 2002; 56 (Suppl 6):S170–174.
25. Madan AK, Aliabadi-Wahle S, Tesi D, Flint LM, Steinberg SM. How early is early laparoscopic treatment of acute cholecystitis? Am J Surg 2002;183:232–236.
26. Liu TH, Consorti ET, Mercer DW. Laparoscopic cholecystectomy for acute cholecystitis: technical considerations and outcome. Semin Laparosc Surg 2002; 9:24–31.
27. Kitano S, Matsumoto T, Aramaki M, Kawano K. Laparoscopic cholecystectomy for acute cholecystitis. J Hepatobiliary Pancreat Surg 2002; 9:534–537.
28. Cotton PB, Geenen JE, Sherman S et al. Endoscopic sphincterotomy for stones by experts is safe, even in younger patients with normal ducts. Ann Surg 1998; 227:201–204.
29. Hashizume M, Sugimachi K, MacFadyen BV. The clinical management and results of surgery for acute cholecystitis. Semin Laparosc Surg 1998; 5:69–80.

Chapter 77

Sphincter of Oddi dysfunction

Evan L Fogel and Stuart Sherman

KEY POINTS

- Sphincter of Oddi dysfunction is an abnormality of sphincter of Oddi contractility
- Sphincter of Oddi dysfunction is a benign, noncalculus obstruction to flow of bile or pancreatic juice
- Manifested clinically by chronic upper abdominal pain, pancreatitis, abnormal liver function tests, or pancreatic enzymes
- In manometry testing, both the pancreatic duct and CBD should be assessed

NTRODUCTION

phincter of Oddi dysfunction (SOD) refers to an abnormal ontractility of the sphincter of Oddi (SO). It is a benign, nonalculus obstruction to flow of bile or pancreatic juice through he pancreaticobiliary junction. SOD may be manifested clinially by 'pancreaticobiliary' pain, pancreatitis, abnormal liver unction tests (LFTs), or abnormal pancreatic enzymes. Postholecystectomy pain resembling the patient's preoperative iliary colic occurs in at least 10–20% of patients. Once other otential etiologies (e.g., common duct stones, tumors, stricures near the cholecystectomy site, etc.) are ruled out, the esidual group of patients has a high frequency of SOD. Biliary and pancreatic classification systems have been developed for patients with suspected SOD (Tables 77.1 and 77.2) based on clinical history, laboratory results, and endoscopic retrograde cholangiopancreatography (ERCP) findings.

EPIDEMIOLOGY

SOD may occur in patients of any age; however, patients with SOD are typically middle-aged females. Although SOD most commonly occurs after cholecystectomy, it may be present with the gallbladder *in situ*. The frequency of diagnosing SOD in reported series varies considerably with the patient selection criteria, the definition of SOD, and whether one or both sphincters are studied by manometry. Eversman and colleagues performed manometry of the biliary and pancreatic sphincter segments in 360 patients with pancreatobiliary pain and intact sphincters.[1] In this large series, 19% had abnormal pancreatic basal sphincter pressure alone, 11% had abnormal biliary basal sphincter pressure alone, and in 31%, the basal sphincter pressure was abnormal in both segments (overall frequency of sphincter dysfunction was 61%). Among the 214 patients labeled type III by a modified Hogan-Geenen SOD classification system, the overall frequency of SOD was 59%. In the 123 type II patients, SOD was diagnosed in 65%. Similar findings were reported by Aymerich and colleagues in a series of 73 patients.[2] These two studies clearly suggest that both the bile duct and

TABLE 77.1 HOGAN-GEENEN BILIARY SPHINCTER OF ODDI CLASSIFICATION SYSTEM (POSTCHOLECYSTECTOMY) RELATED TO THE FREQUENCY OF ABNORMAL SPHINCTER OF ODDI MANOMETRY AND PAIN RELIEF BY BILIARY SPHINCTEROTOMY

Patient group classifications	Approximate frequency of abnormal sphincter manometry	Probability of pain relief by sphincterotomy		Manometry before sphincter ablation if manometry:
		Abnormal	*Normal*	
BILIARY TYPE I				
Patients with biliary-type pain, abnormal SGOT or alkaline phosphatase >2 times normal documented on two or more occasions, delayed drainage of ERCP contrast from the biliary tree >45 min, and dilated CBD >12 mm diameter	75–95%	90–95%	90–95%	Unnecessary
BILIARY TYPE II				
Patients with biliary-type pain and only one or two of the above criteria	55–65%	85%	35%	Highly recommended
BILIARY TYPE III				
Patients with only biliary-type pain and none of the three criteria	25–60%	55–65%	<10%	Mandatory

TABLE 77.2 PANCREATIC SPHINCTER OF ODDI CLASSIFICATION SYSTEM
PANCREATIC TYPE I Patients with pancreatic-type pain, abnormal amylase or lipase 1.5 times normal on any occasion, delayed drainage of ERCP contrast from the pancreatic duct (PD) >9 min, and dilated PD >6 mm diameter in the head or 5 mm in the body
PANCREATIC TYPE II Patients with pancreatic-type pain but only one or two of the above criteria
PANCREATIC TYPE III Patients with only pancreatic-type pain and no other abnormalities

pancreatic duct must be evaluated when assessing the sphincter by manometry (SOM).

Dysfunction may occur in the pancreatic duct portion of the SO and cause recurrent pancreatitis. Manometrically documented SOD has been reported in 15–72% of patients with recurrent pancreatitis, previously labeled as idiopathic.

PATHOGENESIS AND PATHOLOGY

The SO is a small complex of smooth muscles surrounding the terminal common bile duct, ventral pancreatic duct, and the common channel (ampulla of Vater), when present (Fig. 77.1). Its role is to regulate bile and pancreatic exocrine juice flow and to prevent duodenum-to-duct reflux. The SO possesses both a variable basal pressure and phasic contractile activity. The basal pressure appears to be the predominant mechanism regulating outflow of pancreaticobiliary secretion into the intestine, while phasic contractions maintain a sterile intraductal milieu. Sphincter regulation is under both neural and hormonal control. Phasic wave activity of the sphincter is closely tied to the migrating motor complex of the duodenum. Innervation of the bile duct does not appear to be essential as sphincter function is preserved following liver transplantation. Cholecystokinin (CCK) and secretin appear to be most important in causing sphincter relaxation, while vasoactive intestinal peptide and nitric oxide play a lesser role. While cholecystectomy may suppress the inhibitory effect of CCK on the sphincter, the mechanism of this effect is unknown and needs further study.

Wedge specimens of the SO obtained at surgical sphincteroplasty from SOD patients show evidence of inflammation, muscular hypertrophy, fibrosis, or adenomyosis within the papillary zone in approximately 60% of patients.[3] In the remaining 40% with normal histology, a motor disorder is suggested. Less commonly, infections (cytomegalovirus, *Cryptosporidium*, *Strongyloides*) have caused SOD.

How does SOD cause pain? From a theoretical point of view, abnormalities of SO pressure can give rise to pain by: (1) impeding the flow of bile and pancreatic juice resulting in ductal hypertension; (2) inducing ischemia arising from spastic contractions; and (3) resulting in 'hypersensitivity' of the papilla. Although unproven, these mechanisms may act alone or in concert to explain the genesis of pain.

THE SPHINCTER OF ODDI

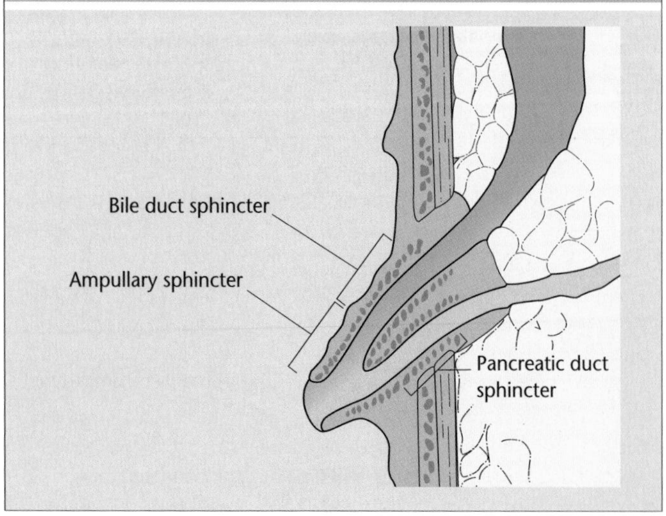

Fig. 77.1 The sphincter of Oddi.

CLINICAL PRESENTATION

Abdominal pain is the most common presenting symptom of patients with SOD. The pain is usually epigastric or right upper quadrant and lasts for 30 min to hours. It may be continuous with episodic exacerbations. It may radiate to the back or shoulder and be accompanied by nausea and vomiting, precipitated by food or narcotics. The pain may begin several years after cholecystectomy and is often similar in character to the pain leading to the cholecystectomy. Alternatively, patients may have continued pain that was not relieved by cholecystectomy. Jaundice, fever, or chills are rarely observed. Physical examination is typically characterized only by mild abdominal tenderness. The pain is not relieved by trial medications for acid peptic disease or irritable bowel syndrome. Laboratory abnormalities consisting of transient elevation of LFTs, typically during episodes of pain, are present in less than 50% of patients. Patients with SOD may present with typical pancreatic pain (epigastric or left upper quadrant radiating to the back) with or without pancreatic enzyme elevation and recurrent pancreatitis.

SOD may exist in the presence of an intact gallbladder. As the symptoms of SOD or gallbladder dysfunction cannot be reliably separated, the diagnosis of SOD is commonly made after cholecystectomy or less frequently after gallbladder abnormalities have been excluded.

CLINICAL PRESENTATION

- Most common symptom is upper abdominal pain
- Pain lasts for 30 min to hours
- May be accompanied by nausea and vomiting
- Jaundice, fever, chills are rarely seen
- Physical examination is typically remarkable only for abdominal tenderness
- May be associated with elevated LFTs, pancreatic enzymes
- May present as unexplained pancreatitis
- Most commonly diagnosed postcholecystectomy, with recurrence of pain similar to precholecystectomy
- May exist with gallbladder intact

IFFERENTIAL DIAGNOSIS

ıe diagnostic approach to suspected SOD may be influenced the presence of key clinical features. However, the clinical anifestations of functional abnormalities of the SO may not ways be easily distinguishable from those caused by organic ıes (e.g., common bile duct stones, chronic pancreatitis) or her functional nonpancreaticobiliary disorders. Standard evaltion and treatment of other more common gastrointestinal nditions, such as peptic ulcer disease, irritable bowel synome, and gastroesophageal reflux should be done simultanesly. In the absence of mass lesions, stones, or response to edical therapy trials, the suspicion for sphincter disease is creased.

DIFFERENTIAL DIAGNOSIS
Peptic ulcer disease
Reflux esophagitis
Irritable bowel syndrome/functional abdominal pain
Choledocholithiasis
Chronic pancreatitis
Ampullary tumor
Musculoskeletal pain syndromes/radiculopathy
Coronary artery disease/angina pectoris
Mesenteric ischemia
Renal colic

IAGNOSTIC METHODS

valuation of patients with suspected SOD should be initiated ith LFTs, serum amylase and/or lipase, and abdominal imaging ltrasound or computed tomography). The serum enzyme udies should be drawn during bouts of pain, if possible. Mild evations (<2 times upper limits of normal) are frequent in OD whereas greater abnormalities are more suggestive of ones, tumors, and liver parenchymal disease. Computed mography (CT) scans and abdominal ultrasounds are usually ormal but occasionally a dilated bile duct or pancreatic duct ay be found (particularly in patients with type I SOD). Because hincter of Oddi manometry (SOM) is technically demandg, invasive, not widely available, and associated with complition rates (pancreatitis in particular) reported as high as 30%, veral noninvasive and provocative tests have been designed an attempt to identify patients with SOD. The morphineostigmin provocative test (Nardi test) and radiographic assessent of the extrahepatic bile duct and pancreatic duct diameter ter secretory stimulation (by transcutaneous or endoscopic trasound or MRCP) are limited by their modest correlation ith SOM and outcome after sphincter ablation. Quantitative patobiliary scintigraphy (HBS), with or without morphine ovocation,[4] may predict an abnormal SOM and response to iary sphincterotomy. However, abnormal results may be und in asymptomatic controls, and HBS does not address the ncreatic sphincter, which may be dysfunctional and a cause r the patients' symptoms. Use of HBS and other noninvasive ethods should be reserved for situations where more finitive testing (manometry) is unsuccessful or unavailable. OM is considered by most authorities to be the gold standard for diagnosing SOD. However, because of the associated risks, this should be reserved for patients with clinically significant or disabling symptoms. In general, invasive assessment of patients for SOD is not recommended unless definitive therapy (sphincter ablation) is planned if abnormal sphincter function is found.

DIAGNOSTIC METHODS
• History and physical examination
• Liver function tests, amylase, lipase
• Abdominal ultrasound, computed tomography scan
• Esophagogastroduodenoscopy ± small bowel X-ray
• Noninvasive evaluation: endoscopic ultrasonography, MRCP, ± hepatobiliary scintigraphy
• Invasive evaluation: ERCP with sphincter of Oddi manometry

TREATMENT AND PREVENTION

The therapeutic approach in patients with SOD is aimed at reducing the resistance to the flow of bile and/or pancreatic juice caused by the sphincter of Oddi. Historically, emphasis has been placed on definitive intervention, i.e., surgical sphincteroplasty or endoscopic sphincterotomy. However, given the high complication rate in patients with suspected SOD, medical therapy with nonspecific antispasmodics or smooth muscle relaxants should be considered in all type III and less severely symptomatic type II SOD patients before considering more aggressive sphincter ablation.

Once the decision is made to evaluate the highly symptomatic patient, endoscopic sphincterotomy remains the standard therapy for patients with SOD. Most data on endoscopic therapy relates to biliary sphincter ablation alone. Clinical improvement following therapy has been reported to occur in 55–95% of patients if manometry is abnormal (Table 77.1). These variable outcomes reflect the different criteria used to document SOD, the degree of obstruction (type I biliary patients appear to have a better outcome than type II and III), the methods of data collection (retrospective versus prospective), and the techniques used to determine benefit. Although most of the studies reporting efficacy of endoscopic therapy in SOD have been retrospective, three notable randomized trials have demonstrated that in type II biliary SOD patients, SOM predicts the outcome from sphincterotomy, biliary sphincterotomy offers a long-term benefit in the majority of patients with biliary SOD, and type II patients may be more likely to respond to sphincter ablation than type III patients[5–7] (Tables 77.3 and 77.4). Performance of SOM is not necessary in type I patients, highly recommended in type II patients, and mandatory in type III patients (Table 77.1).

Evidence is now accumulating that the addition of a pancreatic sphincterotomy to an endoscopic biliary sphincterotomy in patients with pancreatic sphincter disease may improve the outcome. In patients with chronic abdominal pain and initial pancreatic sphincter hypertension (with or without biliary sphincter hypertension), performance of an initial dual pancreatobiliary sphincterotomy was associated with a lower reintervention rate (70/285, 24.6%) than biliary sphincterotomy alone (31/95, 33%; $P<0.05$).[8] Furthermore, in patients with

TABLE 77.3 CHANGE IN MEAN PAIN SCORE

Therapy	Follow-up (years)	Mean pain score		Hospital days/month		% Patients improved
		Pre-Rx	*Post-Rx*	*Pre-Rx*	*Post-Rx*	
ES (*n*=19)	3.3	9.2	3.9[a]	0.85	0.23[b]	68[c]
S-ES (*n*=17)	2.2	9.4	7.2	0.87	0.89	24
SSp±CCx (*n*=16)	3.4	9.4	3.3[a]	0.94	0.27[b]	69[c]

Change in the mean pain score (using a 0=none to 10=most severe linear pain scale), number of hospital days per month required for pain and the percentage improved in patients with manometrically documented sphincter of Oddi dysfunction randomized to endoscopic sphincterotomy (ES), sham sphincterotomy (S-ES), and surgical sphincteroplasty with or without cholecystectomy (SSp±CCx).
Data from Toouli J et al. Manometry based randomised trial of endoscopic sphincterotomy for sphincter of Oddi dysfunction. Gut 2000; 46:98–102, with permission from the BMJ Publishing Group.
[a] $P<0.04$; [b] P=0.002; [c] P=0.009; ES and SSp±CCx vs S-ES.

TABLE 77.4 CLINICAL BENEFIT CORRELATED WITH SPHINCTER OF ODDI DYSFUNCTION (SOD) TYPE

SOD type[a]	Patients improved/total no. patients		
	ES	*S-ES*	*SSp± CCx*
Type II	5/6 (83%)[b]	1/7 (14%)	8/10 (80%)[b]
Type III	8/13 (62%)	3/10 (30%)	3/6 (50%)

[a] SOD type based on Hogan-Geenen SOD classification system.
[b] $P<0.02$; ES and SSp±CCx vs S-ES.

idiopathic recurrent pancreatitis and pancreatic SOD, pancreatic sphincter ablation appears to be associated with a better long-term outcome than biliary sphincterotomy alone.[9,10]

In an attempt to be less invasive and possibly preserve long-term sphincter function, trials evaluating balloon dilation, stenting, and injection of *Botulinum* toxin (Botox) into the sphincter have been performed. Balloon dilation has been associated with unacceptably high pancreatitis rates and cannot be recommended. Similarly, trials of biliary stenting have demonstrated high pancreatitis rates, and this practice is discouraged. Botox injection into the SO may result in a reduction in the basal biliary sphincter pressure and improved bile flow; this reduction in pressure may be accompanied by symptom improvement in some patients. Although further study is warranted, Botox may serve as a therapeutic trial for SOD with responders undergoing permanent sphincter ablation.

Historically, surgery was the traditional therapy of SOD. The most common surgical approach is a transduodenal biliary sphincteroplasty with a transampullary septoplasty (pancreatic septoplasty). Early studies demonstrated a 60–70% benefit from this therapy during a 1- to 10-year follow-up. The surgical approach for SOD has largely been replaced by endoscopic therapy. Patient tolerance, cost of care, morbidity, mortality, and cosmetic results are some of the factors that favor an initial endoscopic approach. At present, surgical therapy is reserved for patients with re-stenosis following endoscopic sphincterotomy and when endoscopic evaluation or therapy is not available or technically feasible (e.g., Roux-en-Y gastrojejunostomy).

TREATMENT AND PREVENTION

- Medical therapy is indicated in all type III and mildly symptomatic type II SOD patients
- Performance of SOM is not necessary in type I patients, highly recommended in type II, and mandatory in type III patients if considering sphincterotomy
- Sphincterotomy is the endoscopic therapy of choice in appropriate patients (Table 77.1)
- Pancreatic sphincterotomy, in addition to biliary sphincterotomy, may improve outcome in patients with pancreatic sphincter dysfunction
- Balloon dilation of the sphincter and biliary stent (as opposed to sphincterotomy) should not be performed, due to high complication rates (i.e., pancreatitis)
- Use of *Botulinum* toxin sphincter injection remains experimental and its use should be confined to clinical trials
- Surgical sphincteroplasty is reserved for patients with sphincter re-stenosis following endoscopic sphincterotomy, or when endoscopic evaluation or therapy is not available or technically feasible

COMPLICATIONS AND THEIR MANAGEMEN

Most studies indicate that patients undergoing endoscop sphincterotomy for SOD have complication rates 2–5 tim higher than patients undergoing endoscopic sphincteroton for ductal stones. Pancreatitis is the most common comp cation occurring in up to 30% of patients in some series. prospective, multicenter study examining risk factors for pos ERCP pancreatitis identified suspected SOD as an indepen ent factor by multivariate analysis.[11] Endoscopic techniqu are being developed (e.g., pancreatic duct stenting) to lim such complications.[12,13,14]

A variety of methods to decrease the incidence of pos manometry pancreatitis have been proposed. These includ (1) use of an aspiration catheter; (2) gravity drainage of tl pancreatic duct after manometry; (3) a reduction of tl perfusion rate to 0.05–0.1 mL/lumen/min; (4) limitation of tl pancreatic duct manometry time to less than 2 min (or avo pancreatic manometry); (5) use of the microtransducer (no perfused) system; and (6) placement of a pancreatic stent aft ıanometry and/or sphincterotomy. The reduction in pancreatitis rates with the use of the aspirating catheter in the pancreatic duct[15] and the very low incidence of pancreatitis after ile duct manometry lend support to the notion that increased ancreatic duct hydrostatic pressure is a major cause of this omplication. Thus, when the pancreatic duct sphincter is studied by SOM, aspiration of pancreatic juice and the perfusate is strongly recommended.

While progress is being made in both patient outcomes and prevention of complications (i.e., pancreatitis), a thorough review of the risk-benefit ratio with individual patients remains mandatory prior to performance of ERCP and SOM.

REFERENCES

1. Eversman D, Fogel EL, Rusche M, Sherman S, Lehman GA. Frequency of abnormal pancreatic and biliary sphincter manometry compared with clinical suspicion of sphincter of Oddi dysfunction. Gastrointest Endosc 1999; 50:637–641.
2. Aymerich RR, Prakash C, Aliperti G. Sphincter of Oddi manometry: is it necessary to measure both biliary and pancreatic sphincter pressure? Gastrointest Endosc 2000; 52:183–186.
3. Anderson TM, Pitt HA, Longmire WP Jr. Experience with sphincteroplasty and sphincterotomy in pancreatobiliary surgery. Ann Surg 1985; 201:399–406.
4. Thomas PD, Turner JG, Dobbs BR, Burt MJ, Chapman BA. Use of 99m Tc-DISIDA biliary scanning with morphine provocation in the detection of elevated sphincter of Oddi basal pressure. Gut 2000; 46:838–841.
5. Geenen JE, Hogan WJ, Dodds WJ, Toouli J, Venu RP. The efficacy of endoscopic sphincterotomy after cholecystectomy in patients with sphincter of Oddi dysfunction. N Engl J Med 1989; 320:82–87.
6. Toouli J, Roberts-Thomson IC, Kellow J et al. Manometry based randomized trial of endoscopic sphincterotomy for sphincter of Oddi dysfunction. Gut 2000; 46:98–102.
7. Sherman S, Lehman GA, Jamidar P et al. Efficacy of endoscopic sphincterotomy and surgical sphincteroplasty for patients with sphincter of Oddi dysfunction (SOD): randomized, controlled study. Gastrointest Endosc 1994; 40:A125.
8. Park SH, Watkins JL, Fogel EL et al. Long-term outcome of endoscopic dual pancreatobiliary sphincterotomy in patients with manometry-documented sphincter of Oddi dysfunction and normal pancreatogram. Gastrointest Endosc 2003; 57:483–491.
9. Kaw M, Brodmerkel GJ. ERCP, biliary crystal analysis, and sphincter of Oddi manometry in idiopathic pancreatitis. Gastrointest Endosc 2002; 55:157–162.
10. Okolo PI 3rd, Pasricha PJ, Kalloo AN. What are the long-term results of endoscopic pancreatic sphincterotomy? Gastrointest Endosc 2000; 52:15–19.
11. Freeman ML, Nelson DB, Sherman S et al. Complications of endoscopic biliary sphincterotomy: a prospective, multicenter study. N Engl J Med 1996; 335:909–918.
12. Tarnasky PR, Palesch YY, Cunningham JT et al. Pancreatic stenting prevents pancreatitis after biliary sphincterotomy in patients with sphincter of Oddi dysfunction. Gastroenterology 1998; 115:1518–1524.
13. Fogel EL, Eversman D, Jamidar P, Sherman S, Lehman GA. Sphincter of Oddi dysfunction: Pancreatobiliary sphincterotomy with pancreatic stent placement has a lower rate of pancreatitis than biliary sphincterotomy alone. Endoscopy 2002; 34:280–285.
14. Fogel EL, Varadarajulu S, Sherman S et al. Prophylactic pancreatic duct stenting in patients with suspected sphincter of Oddi dysfunction but normal sphincter of Oddi manometry. Gastrointest Endosc 2003; 57:88.
15. Sherman S, Troiano FP, Hawes RH, Lehman GA. Sphincter of Oddi manometry: decreased risk of clinical pancreatitis with the use of a modified aspirating catheter. Gastrointest Endosc 1990; 36:462–466.

Chapter 78

Primary sclerosing cholangitis

Flavia D Mendes and Keith D Lindor

KEY POINTS

- Inflammatory and fibrosing condition of the bile ducts that leads to cholestasis and cirrhosis
- Uncommon disease, but relatively common indication for liver transplantation
- Strong association with inflammatory bowel disease
- Unclear etiology
- No available medical treatment
- Increased risk of cholangiocarcinoma

INTRODUCTION

Primary sclerosing cholangitis (PSC) is a chronic cholestatic liver disease characterized by slowly progressive inflammation and fibrosis of the intra- and extrahepatic biliary trees, culminating with the development of biliary cirrhosis.

The etiology of this condition is poorly understood, though it is accepted that several immune and nonimmune mediated mechanisms, as well as genetic predisposition, play a significant role in disease causation. It has a strong association with inflammatory bowel disease (IBD), especially ulcerative colitis. Initially regarded as a rare disease entity, it currently is one of the more common causes of liver transplantation in the US.

EPIDEMIOLOGY

The true prevalence of PSC is unknown. There is a paucity of population-based studies in PSC. In one study performed in Norway, the reported incidence and point prevalence was 1.3 and 8.5 per 100 000 people, respectively.[1] However studies from other countries report much lower rates.

In the US, the estimated prevalence based on studies of inflammatory bowel disease is 6.3 per 100 000. A recently published population-based study from Olmsted County, Minnesota found the age-adjusted incidence to be 1.25 per 100 000 person-years in men and 0.54 per 100 000 person-years in women. The prevalence in men and women was 20.9 and 6.3 per 100 000, respectively.[2] These findings suggest that the prevalence of PSC in the US is higher than initially estimated.

The condition is predominant in males; 70% of affected patients are men. The mean age at diagnosis is 40 years, but it can occur at any age.[1]

Inflammatory bowel disease (especially ulcerative colitis) has a strong association with PSC, being present in up to 80% of these patients.[3]

CAUSES, RISK FACTORS, DISEASE ASSOCIATIONS

The etiology of PSC is yet to be determined. Several immune and nonimmune mechanisms have been proposed, in the setting of genetic predisposition, which will be discussed in more detail in the pathogenesis section.

The typical PSC patient is a middle-aged man with IBD, but disease may affect both genders, occur at any age, and be present in patients without a history of IBD. Patients with a new diagnosis of PSC should be evaluated for the presence of IBD, even if no symptoms are elicited in the history. As previously mentioned, IBD is strongly associated with PSC, being present in up to 80% of these patients. On the other hand, in patients with IBD, only 2.5–7.5% have PSC.[4] Despite the close association, the courses of the two conditions run independently. The presence of PSC in patients with IBD increases substantially the risk of developing colorectal cancer; therefore, close surveillance with annual colonoscopy is advised, even in patients with quiescent IBD.[3]

No other risk factors for PSC have been clearly identified. As with ulcerative colitis, it seems that cigarette smoking has a protective effect for the development of PSC. Other conditions reportedly associated with PSC include several autoimmune disorders, such as systemic lupus erythematosus, Sjögren's syndrome, celiac sprue, and rheumatoid arthritis, as well as systemic fibrosing conditions.

CAUSES AND RISK FACTORS

- Male predominance
- Mean age at diagnosis is 40 years
- Inflammatory bowel disease
- Smoking may be a protective factor
- Autoimmune disorders
- Systemic fibrosing conditions

PATHOGENESIS

The pathogenesis of PSC is likely multifactorial. Currently, the most accepted explanation for the development of PSC is that of a genetic susceptibility, resulting in dysregulation of the immune system, which would be responsible for the inflammatory response and fibrosis that affect the intra- and extrahepatic biliary trees. Genetic predisposition is supported by reports of familial occurrence, human leukocyte antigen (HLA) associations, and more recently polymorphisms of the tumor necrosis factor gene.[3]

The role of an immune-related process is evidenced by observations of multiple cellular and humoral immunologic abnormalities, including elevated serum levels of immunoglobulins, the presence of nonspecific autoantibodies, elevated circulating immune complexes, and complement activation. The majority of patients with PSC are positive for three or more autoantibodies; however, there is no evidence that these antibodies have a pathogenic role in the disease.[5]

Other proposed mechanisms are toxic and infectious injuries, possibly related to intestinal transmigration of bacteria and toxic substances in patients with IBD. Several viral and bacterial agents have been sought as causative factors in PSC, but no evidence supports this hypothesis. Ischemic injury has also been considered, given the similar cholangiographic appearance between PSC and chemotherapy-induced strictures.

Further work is still required in order to shed light on the complex mechanisms involved in the etiology of PSC.

PATHOLOGY

Ludwig et al. have described a histological grading system for PSC. It is composed of four stages, based on which area is involved in the inflammatory and fibrotic changes: stage 1, portal; stage 2, periportal; stage 3, septal; and stage 4, cirrhosis. The classic finding of onion skin fibrosis as shown in Fig. 78.1 is seen in less than 10% of patients.[4]

CLINICAL PRESENTATION

A large number of patients are asymptomatic at the time of diagnosis, and come to medical attention because of abnormal liver enzymes. The presence of symptoms does not correlate well with disease severity. There are reports of worse survival experience in symptomatic patients compared to asymptomatic, but asymptomatic PSC patients have decreased survival compared to healthy controls.[1]

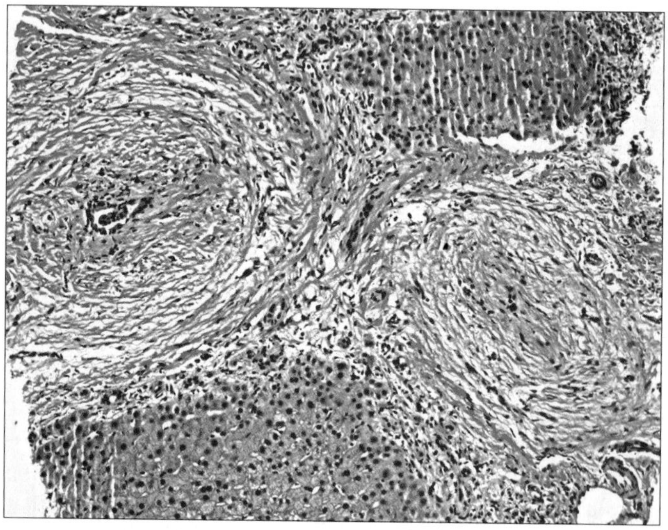

Fig. 78.1 Typical onion skin lesion that can be seen in PSC. The duct on the left is damaged and is partly surrounded by fibrous tissue. On the right, there is a fibrous scar where the duct used to be. Courtesy of Dr Thomas Smyrk.

Fatigue and pruritus are the most common complaints, and can be debilitating. Jaundice, abdominal pain, and weight loss are usually present in later stages of the disease; new onset of these symptoms in patients that were previously stable should prompt evaluation for complications such as cholangiocarcinoma. Fever and chills are concerning for ascending bacterial cholangitis.

Physical examination may be unremarkable, or may reveal hepatomegaly, splenomegaly, jaundice, and other signs of chronic liver disease.

In patients with IBD and PSC, the IBD tends to be quiescent. In fact, the two diseases tend to have completely independent courses.

CLINICAL PRESENTATION

- Asymptomatic
- Fatigue
- Pruritus
- Jaundice
- Abdominal pain
- Hepatomegaly
- Splenomegaly

CLINICAL TIPS (PEARLS)

- Suspect PSC in young to middle-aged males with IBD and cholestatic pattern of liver enzymes
- Look for IBD, even without suggestive symptoms
- Increased risk of colorectal cancer, close surveillance required
- Perform MRCP as the initial diagnostic method; if indeterminate ERCP is required to make the diagnosis
- Not all patients need liver biopsy
- No therapy available, except for liver transplantation for later disease stages
- Cholangiocarcinoma is a well-recognized complication

DIFFERENTIAL DIAGNOSIS

Several disorders may mimic the clinical picture or the cholangiographic findings characteristic of PSC. Cholelithiasis and biliary neoplasms can present in a similar way to PSC, but they could also be a complication of the disease; therefore, their presence does not exclude the diagnosis of PSC. Differentiating cholangiocarcinoma from benign dominant strictures in the setting of PSC can be particularly challenging, as they can look identical on endoscopic retrograde cholangiopancreatography (ERCP), and bile duct biopsies and cytologic brushings have a low sensitivity.[3]

Bile duct disorders, such as surgical strictures, medication, or ischemic induced bile duct injury, and acquired immune deficiency syndrome cholangiopathy all can have radiological changes very similar to PSC.

Other chronic liver diseases such as primary biliary cirrhosis, autoimmune hepatitis, viral hepatitis, drug-induced hepatitis, and metabolic liver diseases should be excluded during e initial evaluation of patients that present with abnormal ver enzymes. These diseases are readily differentiated from SC by the lack of the typical cholangiographic findings, and their own characteristic laboratory features.

DIFFERENTIAL DIAGNOSIS
• Choledocholithiasis • Biliary neoplasms • Surgical biliary strictures • Chronic bacterial cholangitis • Medication-induced biliary damage • Ischemic induced biliary injury • Acquired immune deficiency syndrome cholangiopathy • Other causes of chronic liver disease and cirrhosis (primary biliary cirrhosis, viral hepatitis, autoimmune hepatitis, hemochromatosis, Wilson's disease, alpha-1 antitrypsin deficiency, alcoholic liver disease)

DIAGNOSTIC METHODS

ndoscopic retrograde cholangiopancreatography is still onsidered the 'gold standard' for diagnosing PSC. The finding f multifocal strictures and dilatations, with beaded appearance, and occasional diverticular formation, involving the intraepatic and/or the extrahepatic biliary trees characterizes the disease (Fig. 78.2).[5] More recently, magnetic resonance cholangiography (MRC) has been increasingly used, because of reports showing good diagnostic accuracy and the advantage of not being invasive.[6] Liver biopsy is not considered necessary for diagnosis in the setting of convincing cholangiographic features. Also, its prognostic role is limited, because of the high degree of sample variability.[7]

Commonly, these patients will have abnormal liver enzymes, with alkaline phosphatase 3–5 times the upper limit of normal, and only a mild degree of elevation in the transaminases (cholestatic pattern). Development of significant hyperbilirubinemia should prompt investigation of potential complications such as dominant strictures, biliary stones, bacterial cholangitis, cholangiocarcinoma, or it may indicate disease progression. Autoantibodies are frequently present in these patients, with detection of autoantibodies in over 80% of patients; however, they are neither sensitive nor specific for the diagnosis.

DIAGNOSTIC METHODS
CHOLANGIOGRAPHIC FINDINGS • Endoscopic retrograde cholangiopancreatography ('gold standard') • Magnetic resonance cholangiography **LIVER BIOPSY** • Classic onion skin lesion only present in 10% of cases **LABORATORY DATA** • Cholestatic pattern of abnormal liver enzymes • Presence of autoantibodies

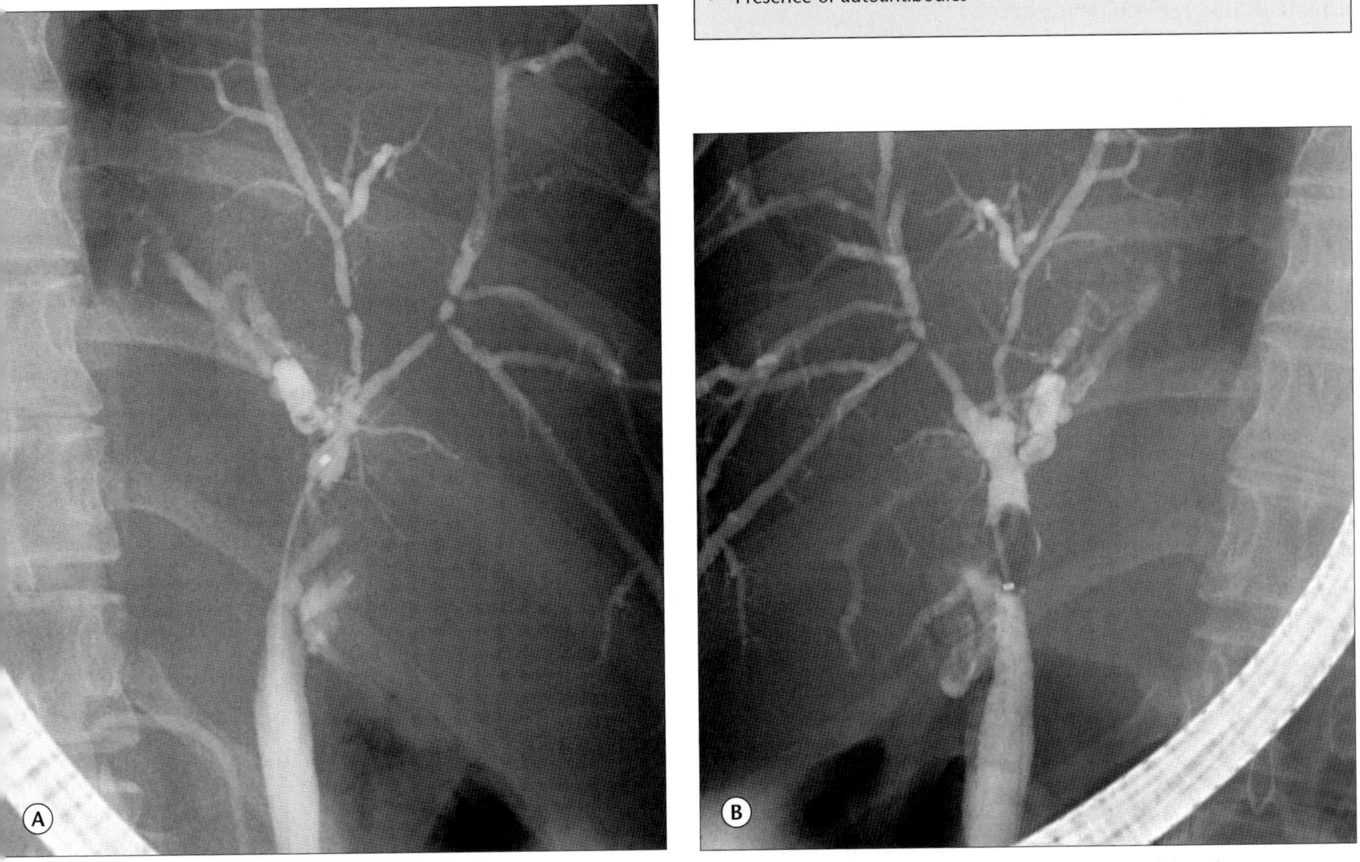

Fig. 78.2 ERCP demonstrating typical changes of PSC, involving the intrahepatic region. A. A dominant stricture involving the common hepatic duct, which was dilated and stented. **B.** Three months later, ERCP with balloon occlusion shows resolution of the endoscopically treated stricture at the common hepatic duct. Courtesy of Dr Todd H. Baron.

TREATMENT AND PREVENTION

Several treatment options have been studied for PSC, including pharmacological, endoscopic, and surgical modalities. Unfortunately, liver transplantation remains the only therapy that improves survival in these patients.

Pharmacological approaches

Ursodeoxycholic acid (UDCA) has been the drug most extensively investigated for the treatment of PSC. Despite initial promising results from uncontrolled trials, Lindor et al. in a large multicenter placebo controlled trial, found only biochemical improvement, but no benefits with regards to histological findings or time to treatment failure.[8] Current studies are evaluating the use of high-dose UDCA. The results from some studies suggest that the use of UDCA decreases the risk of colorectal cancer in patients with PSC and ulcerative colitis.

Several immunosuppressive and antifibrotic agents, including corticosteroids, methotrexate, tacrolimus, cladibrine, pentoxifylline, colchicine, penicillamine, and pirfenidone, as well as combination therapy have been evaluated in open label and placebo-controlled trials; however, none have been proven to significantly alter disease progression.[9] Nicotine use was also studied, based on the reported association of PSC and nonsmoking status, but again no beneficial effect was reported.[9]

Treatment of pruritus in these patients is another important aspect of their management, as this is a common symptom that can be disabling to some patients. Cholestyramine, a bile acid-binding resin, is a good initial choice. Rifampin, naloxone, and ondansetron are potential options for patients who do not respond to bile acid-binding resin.[10]

Endoscopic therapy

The main role of endoscopic therapy is for the treatment of dominant strictures. Some reports suggest that survival free of liver transplantation may be higher in patients who undergo endoscopic treatment of dominant strictures. These patients usually undergo balloon dilatation with or without stent placement. There is some evidence that dilatation alone is as effective as stenting, and associated with less complications.[3]

Surgical treatment

Another option for the treatment of dominant biliary strictures is surgical resection with choledochojejunostomy or hepaticojejunostomy. Ahrendt et al. reported an improved 1-, 3-, and 5-year survival and survival free of liver transplantation in selected noncirrhotic patients who underwent surgical resection, compared to endoscopic therapy.[11] These patients should be carefully selected, because surgery may have a negative impact on liver transplantation outcomes.

Liver transplantation

Orthotopic liver transplantation (OLT) continues to be the only life-extending therapy for PSC patients. Excellent outcome has been reported, with 5-year survival rates ranging from 73% to 100%.[12] It is not clear what the optimal timing for OLT is. Some advocate early OLT, because it may prevent the development of hepatobiliary malignancies, which we know have a higher incidence in these patients. Strong arguments against the early approach are the increased risk of death from colorectal cancer after OLT, as well as the possibility of recurrent PSC in 4% o patients per year after OLT.[3,11]

COMPLICATIONS AND THEIR MANAGEMEN

The complications observed in PSC are related to chroni cholestasis, mechanical bile duct obstruction, and chronic live disease.

Chronic cholestasis

Steatorrhea and vitamin deficiency (mainly A, D, and E secondary to fat malabsorption, may occur during the lat stages of the disease. This is more often seen in jaundice patients; therefore, they should be screened for fat-solubl vitamin deficiency and treated accordingly.[1] Osteoporosis i another common problem in patients with cholestatic live disease, but the exact mechanism is unclear. Currently, th recommendation is to treat patients with calcium and vitami D supplementation, as there are no published data on th efficacy of bisphosphonates for bone disease related to PSC.[1]

Mechanical biliary obstruction

Patients with PSC have an increased risk of developing recur rent bacterial cholangitis and pigmented biliary stones. Domi nant biliary strictures of the extrahepatic bile duct may occu in 7–20% of patients with PSC. These strictures are mos commonly treated with endoscopic balloon dilatation, with o without stenting. Surgical resection with choledochojejunos tomy is another approach for noncirrhotic patients; however this may be associated with adverse outcome in cases wher the patient requires future liver transplantation.[1]

Cholangiocarcinoma

Cholangiocarcinoma is a worrisome complication that may occur in 10–30% of PSC patients. Diagnosis can be extremely challenging. Endoscopic brushings and biopsies have poo sensitivity. Tumor markers (CA 19-9, CEA), imaging studies (MRI, CT, PET scan), and endoscopic sampling in combination may aid the diagnosis of a suspect lesion; however, their role for screening purposes has not been established.[3]

Chronic liver disease

Similar to all other end-stage liver diseases, patients with PSC that progress to cirrhosis may develop complications of portal hypertension, such as ascites, esophageal varices, and portosystemic encephalopathy. Management is the same for all patients with advanced liver disease, and will not be discussed further in this chapter.

PROGNOSIS WITH AND WITHOUT TREATMENT

Data from natural history studies demonstrate a median survival without liver transplantation of approximately 12 years. Several prognostic models to predict survival have been developed, using multivariate analysis. The most recent model by Kim et al. uses age, serum bilirubin, albumin, and aspartate aminotransferase, and history of variceal bleeding to estimate survival probability.[13] An advantage of this model is that it does not include liver biopsy for prognostic determination. As mentioned before, no medical therapy has been shown to rolong survival or the need for liver transplantation. Patients ith PSC have excellent outcome after OLT.

VHAT TO TELL PATIENTS

Iost patients have never heard about PSC before diagnosis. Iaving an uncommon disease may be a source of anxiety. One f the most important roles of the physician is to provide ducation about the condition. Patients appreciate knowing nat this disease progresses slowly, and they may remain symp-om free for many years. No specific lifestyle or dietary modi-cations need to be implemented. Close monitoring is recom-nended, as symptoms and complications may develop, and reatment is usually available. There is still a lot to learn about his condition. Its cause is unknown and there is no medical reatment proven to stop its progression; active investigation of effective therapies is ongoing. Referral to specialized centers should be considered, especially if the patient is interested in participating in clinical trials.

CONTROVERSIES, FALLACIES, PREDICTED FUTURE DEVELOPMENTS

- Pathogenesis still unknown
- No effective treatment
- Optimal timing for liver transplantation unclear
- Surveillance, preventive and therapeutic strategies for cholangiocarcinoma are lacking

SOURCES OF INFORMATION FOR PATIENTS AND DOCTORS

http://www.liverfoundation.org/db/articles/1015/
nddic@info.niddk.nih.gov
http://www.patient.co.uk/showdoc/513/

CURRENT CONTROVERSIES AND THEIR FUTURE RESOLUTION

Many areas in PSC require further studies. Pathogenesis of the disease needs to be better understood, in order to help target therapeutic interventions. Ongoing clinical trials with high-dose UDCA and immunosuppressive agents may bring some promising results, and studies on potential infectious agents may alter therapeutic options. Tools to identify which patients are more likely to have an aggressive course and optimal timing for liver transplantation are still not well defined. Surveillance strategies for cholangiocarcinoma are lacking, as are preventive strategies and effective therapy. Liver transplantation with preoperative chemoradiation is emerging as a promising option for highly selected patients.

REFERENCES

1. Lee YM, Kaplan MM. Management of primary sclerosing cholangitis. Am J Gastroenterol 2002; 97:528–534.
2. Bambha K, Kim WR, Talwalkar J et al. Incidence, clinical spectrum, and outcomes of primary sclerosing cholangitis in a United States community. Gastroenterology 2003; 125:1364–1369.
3. Mendes FD, Lindor KD. Primary sclerosing cholangitis. Clin Liver Dis 2004; 8:195–211.
4. Lee YM, Kaplan MM. Primary sclerosing cholangitis. N Engl J Med 1995; 332: 924–933.
5. Angulo P, Lindor KD. Primary sclerosing cholangitis. Hepatology 1999; 30:325–332.
6. Angulo P, Pearce DH, Johnson CD et al. Magnetic resonance cholangiography in patients with biliary disease: its role in primary sclerosing cholangitis. J Hepatol 2000; 33:520–527.
7. Burak KW, Angulo P, Lindor KD. Is there a role for liver biopsy in primary sclerosing cholangitis? Am J Gastroenterol 2003; 98: 1155–1158.
8. Lindor KD. Ursodiol for primary sclerosing cholangitis. Mayo Primary Sclerosing Cholangitis-Ursodeoxycholic Acid Study Group. N Engl J Med 1997; 336:691–695.
9. Chapman RW. The management of primary sclerosing cholangitis. Curr Gastroenterol Rep 2003; 5:9–17.
10. Levy C, Lindor KD. Current management of primary biliary cirrhosis and primary sclerosing cholangitis. J Hepatol 2003; 38:S24–S37.
11. Ahrendt SA, Pitt HA, Kalloo AN et al. Primary sclerosing cholangitis: resect, dilate, or transplant? Ann Surg 1998; 227:412–423.
12. Sekido H, Takeda K, Morioka D et al. Liver transplantation for primary sclerosing cholangitis. J Hepatobil Pancreat Surg 1999; 6:373–376.
13. Kim WR, Therneau TM, Wiesner RH et al. A revised natural history model for primary sclerosing cholangitis. Mayo Clin Proc 2000; 75:688–694.

Chapter 79

Cholangiocarcinoma

Konstantinos N Lazaridis and Gregory J Gores

KEY POINTS

- Cholangiocarcinoma accounts for 10–15% of all hepatobiliary malignancies. Chronic inflammation of the biliary tree and/or persistent cholestasis are predisposing factors
- Cholangiocarcinoma can be intrahepatic (30%) or extrahepatic (70%). The most common extrahepatic location is the hilar region
- Extrahepatic cholangiocarcinoma presents as progressive cholestasis, while intrahepatic cholangiocarcinoma presents with symptoms of a liver mass. Surgery is the only curative therapy, but 5-year survival is only 20–40%

INTRODUCTION

Cholangiocarcinoma is a malignant tumor of the biliary ductal system that accounts for 10–15% of all hepatobiliary malignancies.[1] Cholangiocarcinoma arises from malignant transformation of the cholangiocyte, the epithelial cell that lines both the intra- and extrahepatic bile ducts.[1] In spite of progress in better understanding the biology of cholangiocarcinoma, patients diagnosed with this tumor have a grave prognosis[2] and therapies are limited.

EPIDEMIOLOGY

Independent epidemiological studies from around the world have shown an increasing incidence of cholangiocarcinoma.[3–5] The incidence of cholangiocarcinoma in the US is approximately 7 cases per million.[6] Cholangiocarcinoma affects males and females almost equally.

RISK FACTORS, DISEASE ASSOCIATIONS

A number of established risk factors have been associated with the development of cholangiocarcinoma including primary sclerosing cholangitis (PSC), Caroli's disease, congenital choledochal cyst, chronic hepatolithiasis, liver flukes such as *Clonorchis sinensis* and *Opisthorchis viverrini*, and exposure to Thorotrast®. Nevertheless, most patients diagnosed with cholangiocarcinoma do not have history of a known predisposing factor associated with the disease. The risk for developing cholangiocarcinoma in a patient with PSC is approximately 1.5% per year after diagnosis of the cholestatic biliary disease.[7] An association between biliary-enteric drainage surgical procedures and development of cholangiocarcinoma has been reported.[8] A common feature of the risk factors in cholangiocarcinogenesis is chronic inflammation in the biliary tree and/or persistent cholestasis.

PATHOGENESIS

Chronic inflammation of the bile ducts is probably a predisposing factor of malignant transformation of cholangiocytes, which leads to the development of cholangiocarcinoma. A number of genetic and somatic alterations could lead to cholangiocarcinoma. These mechanisms include pathways to: (1) develop apoptosis resistance and divert immune surveillance of cholangiocytes; (2) acquire telomerase activity resulting in immortalization and malignant propagation of bile ducts; and (3) alter the expression of oncogenes and tumor suppressor genes leading to lack of cholangiocyte-cycle control. An inflammatory milieu within the bile ducts could cause cholangiocarcinogenesis via dysregulation or constitutive expression of growth factors, pro-inflammatory cytokines and their receptors. Pro-inflammatory cytokines can advance expression of inducible nitric oxide (NO) synthetase and thus produce NO locally, which may cause DNA damage, inhibit DNA repair and apoptosis, promote angiogenesis for tumor growth, and induce the expression of cyclooxygenase (COX)-2 that in turn restrains apoptosis, aids cell growth, and angiogenesis.

PATHOLOGY

Cholangiocarcinoma is a relatively slow-growing, locally destructive tumor of the intra- and extrahepatic bile ducts. Histologically, cholangiocarcinoma is a well- to poorly differentiated tubular adenocarcinoma arising from malignant transformation of cholangiocytes. The tumor forms glands with a prominent, dense, desmoplastic stroma. Other variants of cholangiocarcinoma include papillary adenocarcinoma, signet-ring carcinoma, squamous cell or mucoepidermoid carcinoma, and a lymphoepithelioma-like form.

Extra- vs intrahepatic cholangiocarcinoma: Macroscopically, cholangiocarcinoma is classified into the extra- and intrahepatic types. Extrahepatic cholangiocarcinoma represents two-thirds of all cholangiocarcinomas and is subdivided into: (1) hilar or upper-third; (2) middle third; and (3) distal third tumors. Hilar cholangiocarcinoma or Klatskin tumor represents ~60% of all extrahepatic biliary adenocarcinomas. On the basis of gross appearance, extrahepatic cholangiocarcinoma is grouped into sclerosing, nodular, and papillary. Sclerosing cholangiocarcinoma is the most common and develops annular thickening of the bile ducts with infiltration and fibrosis of the periductal tissues. Intrahepatic cholangiocarcinoma grows as a mass lesion, accounts for about a third of bile duct adenocarcinomas, and can be confused with hepatocellular carcinoma. Intrahepatic cholangiocarcinoma may be solitary or multinodular; it may also be well demarcated as a mass lesion or present as a diffuse, infiltrating neoplasm growing along the intrahepatic bile ducts.

The distinction of cholangiocarcinoma into extra- and intrahepatic origin is relevant not only in clinical practice, but most importantly to growing evidence that these two types of cholangiocarcinoma may be caused by different pathogenetic mechanisms including discrete genetic and/or environmental triggers.

CLINICAL PRESENTATION AND STAGING

Clinical presentation and diagnosis

Extrahepatic cholangiocarcinoma is characterized by symptoms, signs, and biochemical profile of cholestasis. Patients often present with jaundice, dark urine, pale stools, pruritus, malaise, and weight loss. The laboratory tests reveal an increased alkaline phosphatase and bilirubin. Serum CA19-9 is usually elevated. Imaging studies demonstrate dilatation of the biliary tree and often localize the level of obstruction. Unilobular bile duct obstruction is usually associated with atrophy of the affected lobe coupled with hypertrophy of the nonaffected liver lobe (i.e., the atrophy–hypertrophy complex).[9] An atrophied lobe may suggest vasculature encasement by the tumor in the affected lobe.

Endoscopic retrograde cholangiopancreatography (ERCP) is used often to define the topography of cholangiocarcinoma along the bile ducts. In addition, endoscopic biopsies and brush cytology of the bile ducts can be obtained during ERCP for pathological diagnosis of the obstructive lesion. An ERCP of a patient with a hilar cholangiocarcinoma is shown in Fig. 79.1. Nevertheless, the pathological diagnosis could be demanding, given the fact that cholangiocarcinoma is a highly desmoplastic tumor that consists mainly of fibrous tissue with few aggregations of malignant cells. This desmoplastic reaction that surrounds the bile ducts and extends into the submucosal space explains why only 30% of cholangiocarcinomas have positive findings on brush cytology.[2] Combined brush cytology and endoscopic biopsy increase the yield of positive findings to 40–70% of cholangiocarcinomas.[2] However, novel approaches including single-cell techniques such as digitized image analysis (DIA) and fluorescence *in situ* hybridization (FISH) offer promising tools to evaluate cellular aneuploidy and to assess the chromosomal duplication of cholangiocarcinoma.[10] In a recent study, DIA and FISH doubled the diagnostic yield of cholangiocarcinoma compared with the standard brush cytology.[11,12] In clinical practice, however, it is not uncommon to make the diagnosis of cholangiocarcinoma based on clinical, laboratory and imaging findings in the absence of tissue-proven diagnosis.

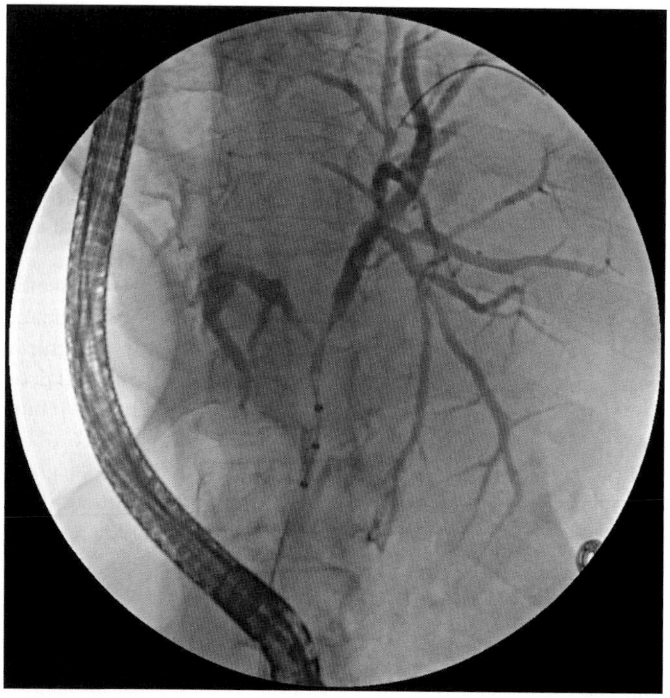

Fig. 79.1 ERCP of a hilar cholangiocarcinoma.

Patients with primary sclerosing cholangitis (PSC): Here diagnosis is challenging. In this clinical scenario, the patient may have a dominant benign biliary stricture that may be difficult to differentiate from cholangiocarcinoma (Fig. 79.2). In this situation, sudden and unexpected clinical deterioration associated with progressive elevation of alkaline phosphatase and serum CA19-9 values greater than 100 U/mL, in the absence of bacterial cholangitis, strongly suggest the development of cholangiocarcinoma complicating PSC.

The intrahepatic cholangiocarcinoma presents with nonspecific symptoms of a liver mass including symptoms of abdominal pain, anorexia, weight loss, malaise, and night sweats. An abdominal mass on exam or imaging study may be the only presentation in asymptomatic patients. Usually, the alkaline phosphatase is elevated with a normal bilirubin. Serum tumor markers such as CA19-9 and CEA are increased.[2] The diagnosis of intrahepatic cholangiocarcinoma is made by the exclusion of other primary or metastatic liver masses that could mimic its clinical and imaging features. At times, biopsy of the liver lesion is the only approach to make the correct diagnosis.

Staging (Tables 79.1, 79.2, and 79.3)

The aim of staging is to identify potential candidates for surgical resection. The value of tumor node metastasis (TNM) classification for extrahepatic cholangiocarcinoma is limited. During the clinical staging of extrahepatic cholangiocarcinoma, it is important to first define the proximal and distal boundaries of the tumor. This goal can be achieved by ERCP or percutaneous transhepatic cholangiography (PTC). Alternatively, the extent of disease can be delineated by magnetic resonance cholangiography (MRC). Second, it is important to exclude vascular encasement by the tumor of the contralateral lobe prior to partial hepatectomy as well as vascular patency of the portal vein and hepatic artery (Table 79.3). Third, regional metastases should be excluded. It appears that endoscopic ultrasound (EUS) is better than conventional abdominal imaging (i.e., CT, MRI) to assess for metastatic disease, particularly for regional lymph nodes, which can also be biopsied during EUS. In fact, 15–20% of patients with normal conventional abdominal imaging were found to have metastatic lymph node involvement by EUS.[10]

TREATMENT

The best treatment for intra- and extrahepatic cholangiocarcinoma is surgical excision. To date, chemotherapy and/or radiation therapy for cholangiocarcinoma have not been evaluated in randomized, controlled trials. Thus, their efficacy

TABLE 79.1 CLASSIFICATION OF EXTRAHEPATIC CHOLANGIOCARCINOMA

TUMOR NODE METASTASIS (TNM) PATHOLOGICAL CLASSIFICATION OF EXTRAHEPATIC CHOLANGIOCARCINOMA

Stage	Tumor	Node	Metastasis
0	T_{is}	N_0	M_0
I	T_1	N_0	M_0
II	T_2	N_0	M_0
III	T_1–T_2	N_1–N_2	M_0
IV A	T_3	Any N	M_0
IV B	Any T	Any N	M_1

T_{is}: carcinoma *in situ*. T_1: tumor invades subepithelial connective tissue (T_{1a}) or fibromuscular layer (T_{1b}). T_2: tumor invades perifibromuscular connective tissue. T_3: tumor invades adjacent structures, i.e., liver, pancreas, duodenum, stomach, gallbladder, colon. N_0: no regional lymph node metastases. N_1: cystic duct, pericholedochal, hilar lymph node metastases. N_2: peripancreatic (head only), periduodenal, periportal, celiac, superior mesenteric, posterior pancreaticoduodenal lymph node metastases. M_0: no distant metastases. M_1: distant metastases.

TABLE 79.2 CLASSIFICATION OF INTRAHEPATIC CHOLANGIOCARCINOMA

TUMOR NODE METASTASIS (TNM) PATHOLOGICAL CLASSIFICATION OF INTRAHEPATIC CHOLANGIOCARCINOMA

Stage	Tumor	Node	Metastasis
I	T_1	N_0	M_0
II	T_2	N_0	M_0
III A	T_3	N_0	M_0
III B	T_1–T_3	N_1	M_0
IV A	T_4	Any N	M_0
IV B	Any T	Any N	M_1

T_1: solitary, 2 cm or less, without vascular invasion. T_2: solitary, 2 cm or less, with vascular invasion; multiple, one lobe, 2 cm or less, without vascular invasion; solitary, greater than 2 cm, without vascular invasion. T_3: solitary, greater than 2 cm, with vascular invasion; multiple, one lobe, 2 cm or less, with vascular invasion; multiple, one lobe, with vascular invasion; multiple, one lobe, 2 cm or less, with vascular invasion; multiple, one lobe, greater than 2 cm, with or without vascular invasion. T_4: multiple, more than one lobe; invasion of major branch of portal or hepatic veins; invasion of adjacent organs other than gallbladder; perforation of visceral peritoneum. N_0: no regional lymph node metastases. N_1: regional lymph node metastases. M_0: no distant metastases. M_1: distant metastases.

in this malignancy remains unknown.[2] Overall, palliative therapies provide symptom relief without affecting survival. An overview algorithm for the treatment of cholangiocarcinoma is shown in Fig. 79.3.

Surgical therapy

For extrahepatic cholangiocarcinoma, surgery should only be carried out with the intent to cure. To have tumor-free margins, partial hepatic resection(s) are required. In fact, patients with positive surgical margins have survival comparable to patients receiving palliative care.[13] In patients with tumor-free margins, the 5-year survival is only 20–40% with an operative mortality of about 10%.[13] Following surgical resection, the main

TABLE 79.3 PROPOSED PREOPERATIVE T-STAGE CRITERIA FOR HILAR CHOLANGIOCARCINOMA

Stage	Criteria
T1	Tumor involving biliary confluence +/– unilateral extension to second-order biliary radicles
T2	Tumor involving biliary confluence +/– unilateral extension to second-order biliary radicles and ipsilateral portal vein involvement +/– ipsilateral hepatic lobar atrophy
T3	Tumor involving biliary confluence + bilateral extension to second-order biliary radicles; unilateral extension to second-order biliary radicles with contralateral portal vein involvement; unilateral extension to second-order biliary radicles with contralateral hepatic lobar atrophy; or main bilateral portal vein involvement

morbidity is infection. For intrahepatic cholangiocarcinoma, surgical resection provides the best outcome with a 3-year survival of between 40% and 60%.[13] Prognostic factors of unfavorable outcome following surgical resection of intrahepatic cholangiocarcinoma are shown in Table 79.4.

Patients with PSC: For these patients, the contribution of tumor surgical resection with the intention to cure remains questionable. First, such patients usually have end-stage liver disease and thus cannot tolerate loss of liver parenchyma. Second, cholangiocarcinoma in PSC is also associated with bile duct dysplasia[14] posing a risk for recurrent *de novo* cholangiocarcinoma development even following successful initial surgical resection. It is not surprising that the 5-year survival of patients with cholangiocarcinoma complicating PSC is less than 10%.[15] Therefore, in PSC patients with early stage cholangiocarcinoma, orthotopic liver transplantation (OLT) is the best available therapeutic approach.

Cholangiocarcinoma in the absence of PSC can be an indication for orthotopic liver transplantation in selected liver transplantation centers that have established protocols. In such medical centers, patients undergo preoperative chemotherapy and radiation therapy as well as an exploratory laparotomy to exclude metastatic disease before receiving a liver transplant. At the Mayo Clinic, Rochester, MN, the 5-year survival post-liver transplantation for patients with TNM stage I and II cholangiocarcinoma is about 80%.[16]

TABLE 79.4 INTRAHEPATIC CHOLANGIOCARCINOMA: UNFAVORABLE PROGNOSTIC FACTORS

- Preoperative CA19-9 levels >1000 U/mL
- Multifocal disease
- Liver capsule invasion
- Lack of cancer-free surgical margins
- Lymph node involvement
- Mass-forming or periductal-infiltrating type cholangiocarcinoma growth
- Expression of MUC1 by cholangiocarcinoma cells

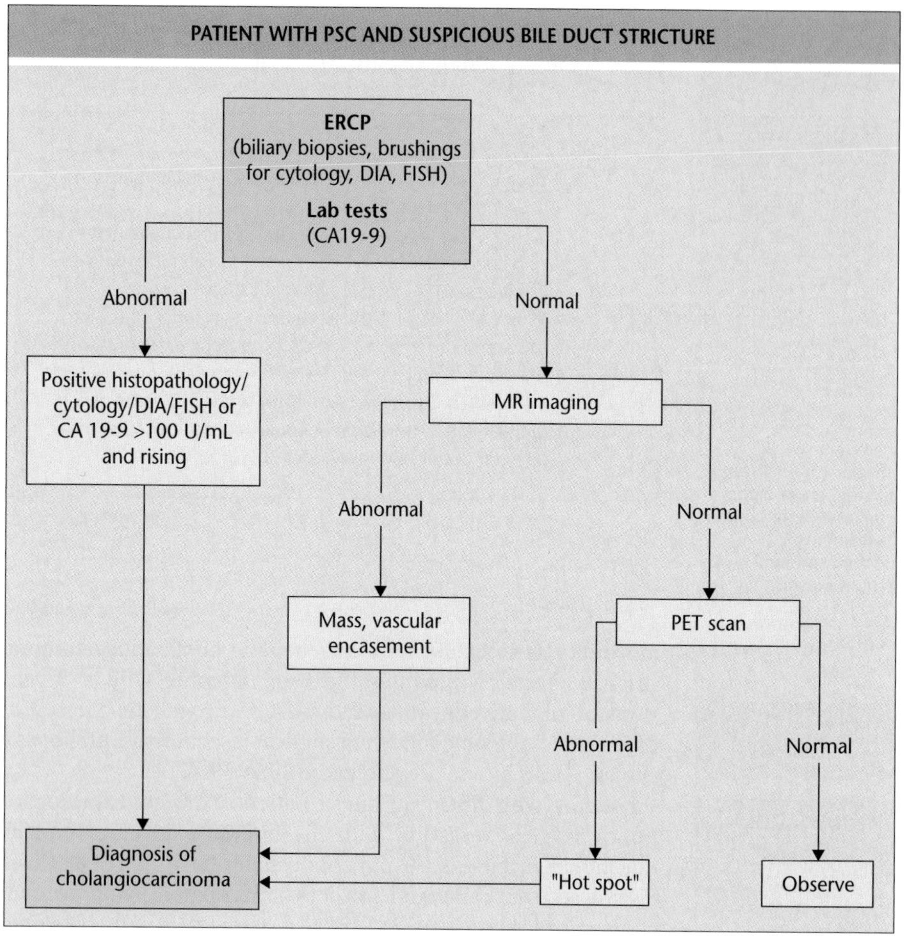

Fig. 79.2 PSC patient with suspicious bile duct stricture.

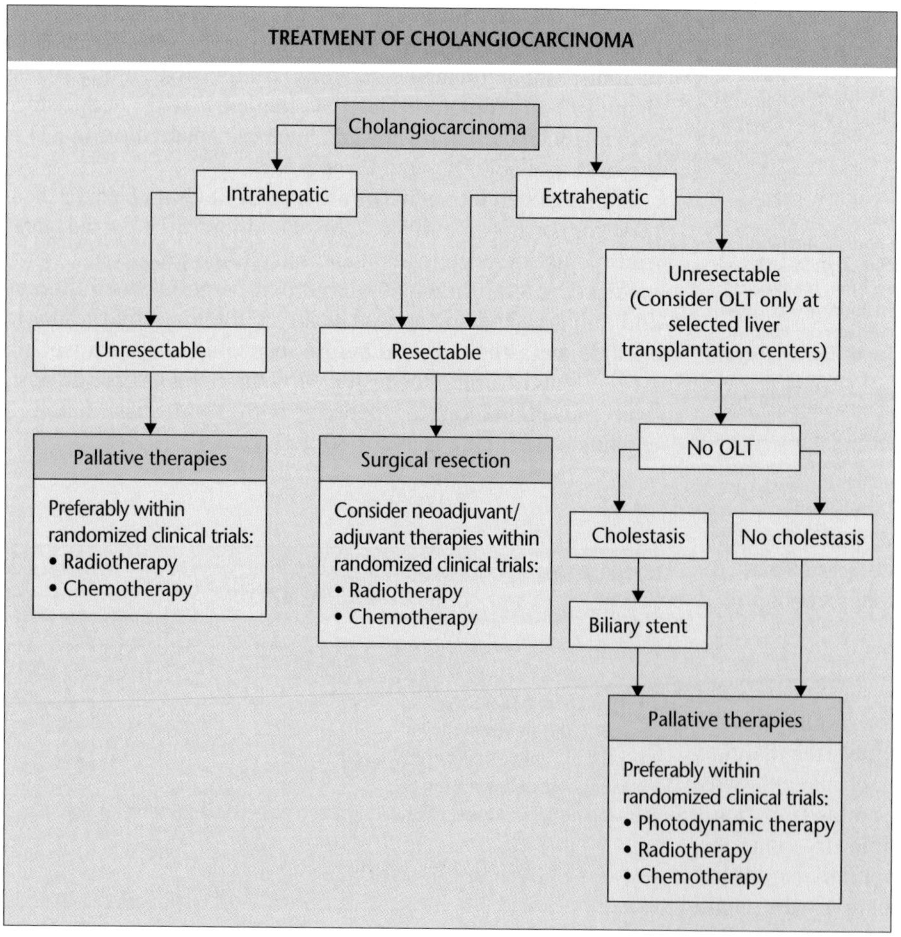

Fig. 79.3 Treatment algorithm of cholangiocarcinoma. OLT, orthotopic liver transplantation.

Palliative therapeutic approaches

Biliary stents

Endoscopic or percutaneous placement of biliary stents prevents obstructions of the biliary tree and restores near normal bile flow.[2] Biliary stents improve symptoms of fatigue, anorexia, and pruritus but not survival.[2] A preplacement MRC may be helpful to define the biliary anatomy in complex hilar tumors. The choice between a plastic vs metallic stent depends on many aspects including expected survival and availability of stent exchange. A course of antibiotics, usually ciprofloxacin, is recommended after stent placement to prevent the development of bacterial cholangitis.

Photodynamic therapy (PDT)

This therapy involves the systemic preadministration of a nontoxic, photosensitizer, such as sodium porfimer, that accumulates mainly within the malignant cholangiocarcinoma cells. Subsequently, the patient undergoes ERCP or PTC, during which laser light of 630 nm is used and energy is transferred from the photosensitizer to molecular oxygen causing cholangiocarcinoma cell apoptosis. This therapy has now been shown in a randomized, prospective controlled trial to improve patient survival and quality of life when used in conjunction with biliary stenting.[17] Patients that may benefit from PDT are those with no improvement of cholestasis following stent placement alone.

Future therapeutic directions

At present, no survival benefit has been attained in cholangiocarcinoma patients treated with chemotherapy and/or radiation therapy.[2] Randomized, controlled clinical trials are needed to address and test the usefulness of novel chemotherapeutic agents and/or radiation therapy.

As we begin to have a better understanding of the biology of cholangiocarcinoma, pharmacological inhibitors of highly expressed receptors in these tumors (i.e., cyclooxygenase-2, epidermal growth factor) should be used in future trials with or without chemotherapeutic drugs.

SOURCES OF INFORMATION FOR PATIENTS AND DOCTORS

http://www.clevelandclinic.org/gastro/endoscopy/patient/stone.htm

http://www.patient.co.uk/showdoc/27000742/

REFERENCES

1. Gores GJ. Cholangiocarcinoma: current concepts and insights. Hepatology 2003; 37:961–969.
2. Khan SA, Davidson BR, Goldin R et al. Guidelines for the diagnosis and treatment of cholangiocarcinoma: consensus document. Gut 2002; 51 (Suppl 6):VI1–9.
3. Khan SA, Taylor-Robinson SD, Toledano MB et al. Changing international trends in mortality rates for liver, biliary and pancreatic tumours. J Hepatol 2002; 37:806–813.
4. Patel T. Worldwide trends in mortality from biliary tract malignancies. BMC Cancer 2002; 2:10.
5. Taylor-Robinson SD, Toledano MB, Arora S et al. Increase in mortality rates from intrahepatic cholangiocarcinoma in England and Wales 1968-1998. Gut 2001; 48:816–820.
6. Patel T. Increasing incidence and mortality of primary intrahepatic cholangiocarcinoma in the United States. Hepatology 2001; 33: 1353–1357.
7. Bergquist A, Broome U. Hepatobiliary and extra-hepatic malignancies in primary sclerosing cholangitis. Best Pract Res Clin Gastroenterol 2001; 15:643–656.
8. Tocchi A, Mazzoni G, Liotta G et al. Late development of bile duct cancer in patients who had biliary-enteric drainage for benign disease: a follow-up study of more than 1,000 patients. Ann Surg 2001; 234:210–214.
9. Hadjis NS, Adam A, Gibson R, Blenkharn JI, Benjamin IS, Blumgart LH. Nonoperative approach to hilar cancer determined by the atrophy-hypertrophy complex. Am J Surg 1989; 157:395–399.
10. Gores GJ. Early detection and treatment of cholangiocarcinoma. Liver Transplant 2000; 6 (Suppl 2):S30–S34
11. Baron TH, Harewood A, Rumalla A et al. A prospective comparison of digital image analysis and routine cytology for the identification of malignancy in biliary tract strictures. J Clin Gastroenterol Hepatol 2004; 2:214–219.
12. Rumalla A, Baron TH, Leontovich O et al. Improved diagnostic yield of endoscopic biliary brush cytology by digital image analysis. Mayo Clinic Proc 2001; 76:29–33.
13. Jarnagin WR, Fong Y, DeMatteo RP et al. Staging, resectability, and outcome in 225 patients with hilar cholangiocarcinoma. Ann Surg 2001; 234:507–517; discussion 517–519.
14. Fleming KA, Boberg KM, Glaumann H et al. Biliary dysplasia as a marker of cholangiocarcinoma in primary sclerosing cholangitis. J Hepatol 2001; 34:360–365.
15. Boberg KM, Bergquist A, Mitchell S et al. Cholangiocarcinoma in primary sclerosing cholangitis: risk factors and clinical presentation. Scand J Gastroenterology 2002; 37: 1205–1211.
16. De Vreede I, Steers JL, Burch PA et al. Prolonged disease-free survival after orthotopic liver transplantation plus adjuvant chemoirradiation for cholangiocarcinoma. Liver Transplant 2000; 6:309–316.
17. Ortner M, Caca K, Berr F et al. Successful photodynamic therapy for nonresectable cholangiocarcinoma: a randomized prospective study. Gastroenterology 2003; 125:1355–1363.

Chapter 80

Congenital abnormalities of the biliary tract

Daniel Dhumeaux, Elie Serge Zafrani, Daniel Cherqui, and Alain Luciani

KEY POINTS

- Can affect both the intra- and extrahepatic bile ducts and can be cystic or noncystic
- Congenital cystic diseases of the intrahepatic biliary tract:
  - Von Meyenburg complexes
  - Congenital hepatic fibrosis
  - Caroli's syndrome
  - Simple cyst
  - Polycystic liver disease (with or without polycystic kidney disease)
- Congenital cystic diseases of the extrahepatic biliary tract:
  - Choledochal cyst
- Congenital noncystic diseases of the biliary tract are probably not the result of a malformation process, but rather the result of gradual destruction of bile ducts during fetal life:
  - Paucity of interlobular bile ducts (syndromic and nonsyndromic)
  - Atresia of extrahepatic bile ducts

INTRODUCTION

Congenital abnormalities of the biliary tract can affect both the intra- and the extrahepatic bile ducts. They are either inherited or not inherited, and can be divided into two main groups: cystic and noncystic. It is now widely agreed that congenital cystic diseases of bile ducts belong to a family of bile duct malformations that are mostly related to abnormal remodeling of the embryonic ductal plate ('ductal plate malformation'). Although they are congenital, all of them can be diagnosed at any age of life. Contrary to congenital cystic diseases of bile ducts, congenital noncystic diseases of bile ducts are probably not linked to a malformation process, but are rather the result of gradual destruction of bile ducts during fetal life. They are mainly diagnosed in children.

Only those congenital abnormalities of the biliary tract present in adults will be reviewed in this chapter.

CONGENITAL CYSTIC DISEASES OF INTRAHEPATIC BILE DUCTS

Introduction

This category includes entities that differ in their prevalence, manifestations, and severity, but share at least three characteristics: (1) the basic lesion of the liver consists of cysts that are either macroscopic, and therefore easily recognized by imaging techniques, or microscopic, i.e., only found at histological examination of the liver; (2) a ductal plate malformation can account for these disorders; and (3) the liver disease is frequently associated with a variety of renal disorders that are related to congenital malformations of renal tubular segments.

KEY POINTS

CONGENITAL CYSTIC DISEASES OF THE INTRAHEPATIC BILIARY TRACT

- Family of bile duct malformations that are mostly related to abnormal remodeling of the embryonic ductal plate ('ductal plate malformation')
- The basic lesion consists of cysts that are either macroscopic or microscopic
- Since ductal plate malformation can occur simultaneously at different levels of the intrahepatic biliary tree, coexistence of several cystic disorders is common
- The liver disease is frequently associated with a variety of renal disorders that are related to congenital malformations of renal tubular segments

Pathogenesis

Embryonic anomalies lead to congenital cystic diseases of the intrahepatic bile ducts. In normal embryos, at around the 8th week of gestation, a layer of cells originating from liver precursor cells, with the characteristics of biliary cells, surrounds each mesenchymal area containing the largest branches of the portal vein. This layer of cells, which is later duplicated by a second layer of the same cells, is referred to as the ductal plate. In the following weeks, ductal plates also appear more distally around smaller portal vein branches. After 12 weeks of gestation, the ductal plates are progressively remodeled around the larger portal veins near the hilum. This remodeling leads to: (1) dilatation of short segments of the double-layered ductal plate to form tubular structures; (2) subsequent incorporation of these structures as individualized bile ducts into the mesenchyme surrounding portal vein branches; and (3) disappearance of most nontubular portions of the ductal plate (Fig. 80.1).[1]

Remodeling defects, which likely cause congenital cystic diseases of intrahepatic bile ducts, result in the persistence of an excess of embryonic bile duct structures, a phenomenon referred to as 'ductal plate malformation.' When the remodeling defect is complete, ductal plate malformation appears as a circular lumen containing a fibrovascular axis (Fig. 80.2A). When it is incomplete, it may give rise either to a nearly circular lumen with an apparent polypoid projection of mesenchymal tissue (Fig. 80.2B) or to an interrupted circle of dilated bile ducts around the fibrovascular axis (Fig. 80.2C).[1]

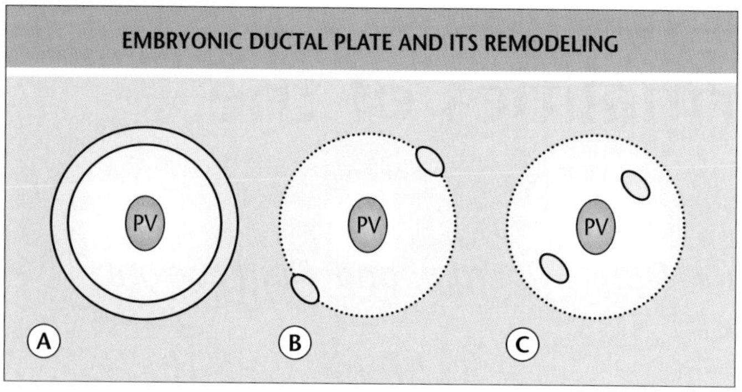

Fig. 80.1 Schematic representation of the embryonic ductal plate and of its remodeling. A. Initial ductal plate with the typical double layer of biliary cells. **B.** Remodeling of the ductal plate, with tubular dilatation in some segments and disappearance of most of the ductal plate. **C.** Incorporation of the tubular segments within the portal mesenchyme. Note the presence of a portal vein (PV) branch at the center of the embryonic portal space.

When discussing ductal plate malformation as the basic component of congenital cystic diseases of the intrahepatic bile ducts, it is important to bear in mind that: (1) the different segments of the intrahepatic biliary tree develop during successive periods of fetal life; (2) ductal plate malformation can be observed in segmental (Caroli's syndrome), interlobular (congenital hepatic fibrosis), or more peripheral bile ducts (von Meyenburg complexes, polycystic liver disease); and (3) ductal plate malformation occurring simultaneously at different levels of the intrahepatic biliary tree may explain the observed coexistence of these disorders.

Von Meyenburg complexes[1–3]

These are usually asymptomatic and are diagnosed incidentally at histological examination. They are often multiple and may occur in an otherwise normal liver or can be associated with congenital hepatic fibrosis, Caroli's syndrome, or polycystic liver disease. Von Meyenburg complexes consist of groups of more or less dilated bile ducts containing bile and embedded in fibrous tissue (Fig. 80.3). They are located within or at the periphery of the portal tracts. Von Meyenburg complexes may be secondary to a ductal-plate remodeling defect in the later phases of bile duct development, thus affecting the smallest branches of the intrahepatic biliary tree.

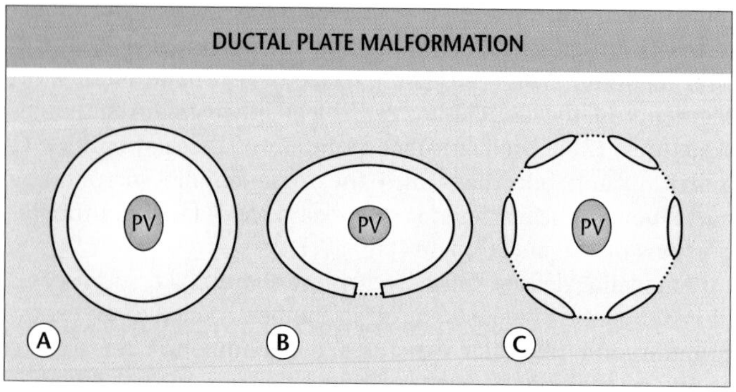

Fig. 80.2 Schematic representation of the ductal plate malformation. A. Complete lack of remodeling of the ductal plate, which appears as a continuous circular dilated duct. **B,C.** Incomplete remodeling of the ductal plate, which appears as a dilated bile duct with a polypoid projection of mesenchymal tissue **(B)** or as an interrupted circle of dilated bile ducts **(C)**. Note the presence of a portal vein (PV) branch at the center of the ductal plate malformation.

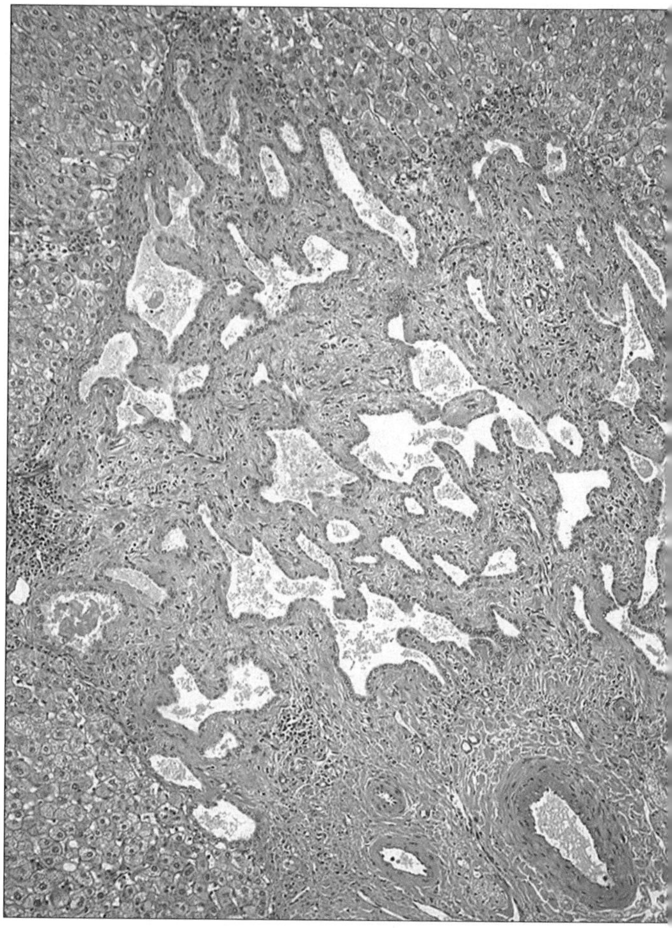

Fig. 80.3 Von Meyenburg complexes. Multiple biliary channels are lined by a cuboidal epithelium and are embedded in dense fibrous tissue. Note the irregular outline of the ducts, with polypoid projections into dilated lumens, as seen in ductal plate malformation.

KEY POINTS
VON MEYENBURG COMPLEXES
• Consist of groups of variably dilated bile ducts containing bile, embedded in fibrous tissue, mostly at the periphery of the portal tracts • Asymptomatic • Commonly diagnosed incidentally at histological examination • No therapy necessary

Congenital hepatic fibrosis[1–5]

Histologically, congenital hepatic fibrosis consists of enlargement of portal spaces by an abundant fibrous tissue containing numerous, more or less ectatic bile ducts. Some bile ducts contain bile, indicating communication with the rest of the biliary tree. Bile ducts can be so dilated that they form cysts that are nonetheless ot macroscopically visible, at least in congenital hepatic fibrosis ot associated with Caroli's syndrome. Portal veins appear to be ypoplastic. The disease can be sporadic or familial. It is inherited nd transmitted as an autosomal recessive trait. The mutant gene not clearly identified. Due to a possible association between ongenital hepatic fibrosis and recessive polycystic kidney disease, e gene *PKHD1* involved in the renal disease could be a candidate. However, several cases of congenital hepatic fibrosis ssociated with protein-losing enteropathy have recently been nked to a congenital phosphomannose isomerase deficiency.[6] n this disorder, protein hypoglycosylation secondary to the nzyme deficiency has been suggested to play a role in the defective embryonic development of intrahepatic bile ducts, but the echanism by which protein hypoglycosylation leads to ductal late malformation remains to be elucidated.

The prevalence of congenital hepatic fibrosis is about 1:100000. he main consequence of the disease is portal hypertension, ue to fibrous compression and/or hypoplasia of portal vein ranches. The first bleeding episode secondary to ruptured astroesophageal varices usually occurs between the ages of and 20 years, sometimes later. Liver failure being absent, ariceal bleeding is generally well tolerated. On clinical examiation, the liver is often enlarged, and splenomegaly is found n most of the patients. Liver biochemical tests are generally ormal, although a moderate increase in serum alkaline phoshatase and gammaglutamyltranspeptidase activities can be oted. Congenital hepatic fibrosis is occasionally complicated y recurrent, potentially life-threatening bacterial cholangitis, ven in the absence of Caroli's syndrome. Both hepatocellular nd cholangiocellular carcinomas may also complicate congenital epatic fibrosis.

The diagnostic value of imaging procedures in congenital epatic fibrosis is limited. Most frequently, reported features are iver dystrophy and indirect signs of portal hypertension. The iagnosis of congenital hepatic fibrosis is made by liver biopsy. Iowever, the diagnosis of the disease may be missed on a small iver specimen since the malformation is not always diffuse. Aagnetic resonance cholangiography is generally normal, as only mall bile ducts are dilated, at least in the absence of associated Caroli's syndrome. Congenital hepatic fibrosis is frequently assoiated with a renal malformation consisting of ectatic collecting ubules. This malformation is generally silent. It can be demontrated by intravenous pyelography or by multidetector computed omography.[7] It is found in about two-thirds of patients, and ssists with the diagnosis of congenital hepatic fibrosis. In some ases, the ectatic segments lose their communication with the urinary tract and transform into large renal cysts, referred to as autosomal recessive polycystic kidney disease.[8]

Recurrent variceal bleeding can be prevented with betablockers and/or endoscopic variceal ligation, although these treatments have not been specifically evaluated in this setting. If they fail, transjugular intrahepatic portosystemic shunt can be considered, and the risk of hepatic encephalopathy could be lower than in patients with cirrhosis, given the absence of liver failure. Surgical procedures on the biliary tree, and invasive investigations such as endoscopic retrograde cholangiography carry a risk of bacterial cholangitis and must be avoided. Liver transplantation can be offered to selected patients.

KEY POINTS

CONGENITAL HEPATIC FIBROSIS

- Characterized by enlargement of portal spaces by abundant fibrous tissue containing numerous ectatic bile ducts
- Inherited and transmitted as an autosomal recessive trait with a prevalence of about 1:100000
- The main consequence of the disease is portal hypertension, due to fibrous compression and/or hypoplasia of portal vein branches
- Variceal hemorrhage first occurs between the ages of 5 and 20 years
- It is occasionally complicated by recurrent, bacterial cholangitis, even in the absence of Caroli's syndrome
- Hepatocellular and cholangiocellular carcinomas may be a complication
- Treatment: prevention and treatment of variceal bleeding; liver transplantation

Caroli's syndrome[1–5,9]

Caroli's syndrome is a congenital disorder characterized by cystic dilatations of large, segmental intrahepatic bile ducts. The cystic dilatations may be diffuse, affecting the whole intrahepatic biliary tree (Fig. 80.4), or confined to a lobe, often the left lobe,[10] or to a segment of the liver (Fig. 80.5). Congenital dilatation of segmental bile ducts is not a single entity, and the term Caroli's syndrome is thus more appropriate than that of Caroli's disease.

Caroli's syndrome is usually associated with congenital hepatic fibrosis. In such patients, cystic dilatations are diffuse and, like congenital hepatic fibrosis, the malformation is transmitted as an autosomal recessive trait, and it may be associated with ectatic renal collecting tubules (Table 80.1). When Caroli's syndrome

TABLE 80.1 CHARACTERISTICS OF CAROLI'S SYNDROME WHETHER OR NOT ASSOCIATED WITH CONGENITAL HEPATIC FIBROSIS

	Caroli's syndrome with congenital hepatic fibrosis	Caroli's syndrome without congenital hepatic fibrosis
Hereditary transmission	Autosomal recessive	Absent
Hepatic cyst distribution	Diffuse	Diffuse or localized to one lobe or one segment
Cholangitis	Frequent	Possible
Portal hypertension	Frequent	Absent
Renal abnormalities	Ectatic collecting tubules and/or autosomal recessive polycystic kidney disease	Absent

Reproduced from Benhamou JP, Menu Y. Non-parasitic cystic diseases of the liver and intrahepatic biliary tree. In: Bircher J et al., eds. Oxford textbook of clinical hepatology. Oxford: Oxford University Press; 1999:817–823.)

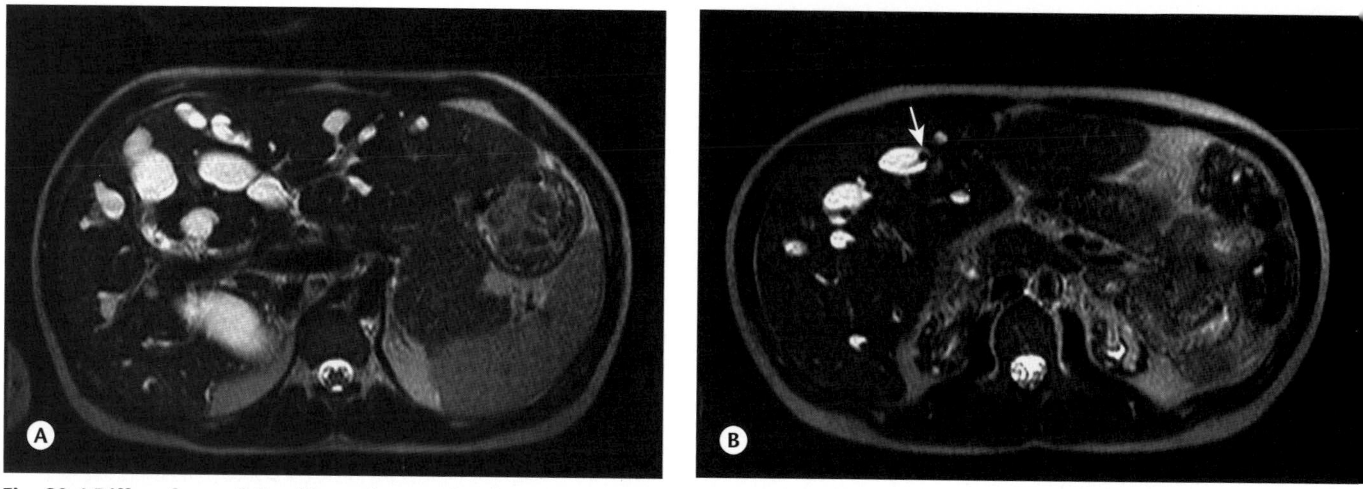

Fig. 80.4 Diffuse form of Caroli's syndrome. Heavily T2-weighted sequence of magnetic resonance imaging showing numerous cystic dilatations of the biliary tree. **A.** Note that the cysts appear to communicate with the remaining biliary tree. **B.** Hypointense dots, which probably correspond to portal vein branches, in the center of the cysts (arrow).

is not associated with congenital hepatic fibrosis, cystic dilatations are often confined to one part of the liver, the malformation is congenital but not inherited, and the disorder is not associated with renal malformations (Table 80.1).

Caroli's syndrome, which is usually present at birth, can remain asymptomatic for a long period of time, at least for the first 5–20 years of life. The main clinical manifestation is recurrent cholangitis, the prevalence of which markedly varies from one patient to another. The prognosis is bad in patients with frequent bouts of cholangitis, who are at risk of death from uncontrolled bacterial infection. Cholangitis may be complicated by liver abscesses and secondary amyloidosis. In contrast to cholangitis due to common bile duct stones, in which fever is usually associated with pain and/or jaundice, the main and often the only symptom of cholangitis in Caroli's syndrome is fever, which can be difficult to relate to cholangitis, at least in initial episodes. Jaundice and pain may occur if pigment or cholesterol stones that form in dilated bile ducts migrate to the extrahepatic biliary tree. Manifestations of portal hypertension are usually present in patients with associated congenital hepatic fibrosis. Intracystic cholangiocarcinoma occurs in approximately 7% of either diffuse or localized Caroli's syndrome.

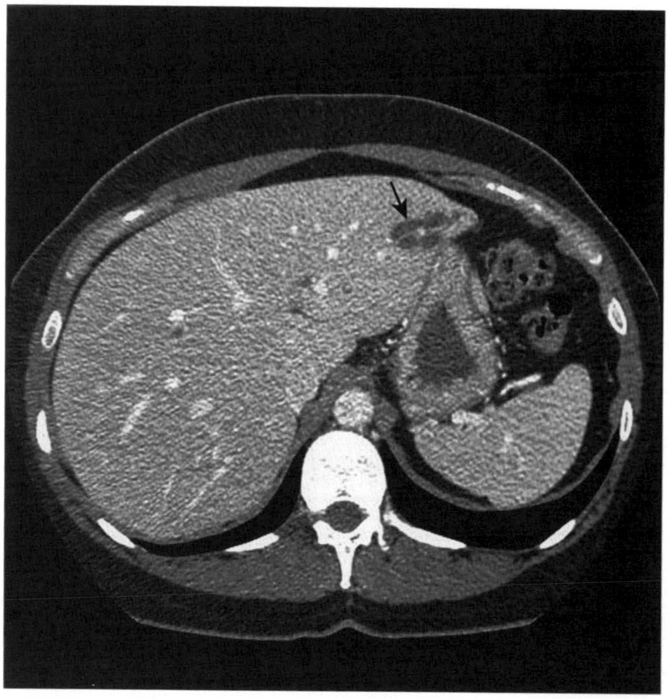

Fig. 80.5 Caroli's syndrome. Caroli's syndrome localized in segment III of the left lobe of the liver. Portal-venous-phase contrast-enhanced computed tomography shows a saccular dilatation of the biliary tree with enhanced central portal vein branch ('central dot' sign) (arrow).

Physical examination usually shows an enlarged liver. There are no signs of liver failure. Liver biochemical tests are normal, except for moderate increases in serum alkaline phosphatase and gammaglutamyl transpeptidase activities. The diagnosis of Caroli's syndrome can be suggested on imaging techniques, i.e., ultrasonography, computed tomography (CT), and magnetic resonance imaging (MRI) (Fig. 80.4 and Fig. 80.5). Computed tomography or MRI can reveal the 'central dot' sign after contrast medium injection[11] (Fig. 80.5), which may correspond to the ductal plate malformation illustrated in Fig. 80.2B. In addition to cystic dilatations, magnetic resonance cholangiography may inconstantly show communications with the biliary tree, which would be diagnostic of Caroli's syndrome. Communications can also be documented by CT or MRI after intravenous injection of biliary contrast medium. Moreover, ultrasonography, CT, and MRI can show the presence of stones within the cystic dilatations.[11] As for congenital hepatic fibrosis, invasive investigations of the biliary tree (i.e., endoscopic retrograde cholangiography or percutaneous transhepatic cholangiography) must be avoided.

Treatment consists of appropriate antibiotic therapy for patients with bacterial cholangitis. Ursodeoxycholic acid may be effective in preventing or treating intracystic stones, and should be given to all patients with Caroli's syndrome. In the localized form of Caroli's syndrome, partial hepatectomy is indicated. This treats cholangitis and prevents the development of cholangiocarcinoma. Liver transplantation may be considered for patients with the diffuse form complicated by severe recurrent cholangitis. Surgical bilioenteric anastomosis can increase the prevalence and severity of cholangitis, and is therefore not recommended.

> **KEY POINTS**
>
> **CAROLI'S SYNDROME**
>
> - Characterized by cystic dilatations of large, segmental intrahepatic bile ducts that may be diffuse or confined to a lobe or a segment of the liver
> - Usually associated with congenital hepatic fibrosis
> - Is usually asymptomatic for the first 5–20 years of life until it presents with recurrent cholangitis; unlike other types of cholangitis, the main and often the only symptom is fever (in the absence of abdominal pain)
> - Invasive investigations of the biliary tree must be avoided
> - Treatment consists of antibiotic therapy for cholangitis and ursodeoxycholic acid to prevent or treat intracystic stones
> - In the localized form of Caroli's syndrome, partial hepatectomy is indicated
> - Liver transplantation may be considered for patients with the diffuse form complicated by severe recurrent cholangitis

Simple cyst of the liver[2–5]

Simple cyst of the liver is regarded as a congenital malformation consisting of an aberrant dilated bile duct without communication with the biliary tree. It is spherical or ovoid. Its diameter increases with age, ranging from a few millimeters to more than 20 cm. There is no septation and the cystic fluid is generally clear. Small cysts are surrounded by normal liver, whereas large cysts may be responsible for atrophy of adjacent hepatic tissue. The cyst is solitary in about 50% of cases, while other patients have two or more cysts.

The prevalence of simple cysts of the liver is about 3% in the adult population. The lesions are generally sporadic, although a small number of familial cases have been observed. Simple cysts of the liver predominate in females and are generally asymptomatic. Some large cysts produce abdominal pain or discomfort. Complications include intracystic hemorrhage or infection and cyst rupture. In most patients, the lesion is discovered fortuitously at liver ultrasonography, which shows a circular or oval, well-limited and totally anechoic area, with strong posterior wall echoes. Simple cyst of the liver is not associated with renal malformations, although the association with one or two simple renal cysts, which are also very common in adults, is possible.

Asymptomatic simple cysts do not require any treatment. When large cysts produce abdominal pain or are complicated, cyst resection or, more often, cyst fenestration (i.e., partial excision of the external part of the cyst) can be performed by open surgery or preferably by laparoscopy. Injection of alcohol or of other sclerosing agents into cysts has also been attempted.

> **KEY POINTS**
>
> **SIMPLE CYST OF THE LIVER**
>
> - Aberrant dilated bile duct without communication with the biliary tree; the cyst is not septated and its fluid is clear
> - Its diameter increases with age, ranging from a few millimeters to more than 20 cm
> - The cyst is solitary in about 50% of cases
> - The prevalence of simple cysts of the liver is about 3% in the adult population. The lesion predominates in females
> - Generally asymptomatic
> - When large cysts produce abdominal pain or are complicated, cyst resection or, more often, cyst fenestration, is the therapy of choice

Polycystic liver disease

Polycystic liver disease may or may not be associated with polycystic kidney disease.

Autosomal dominant polycystic liver disease associated with polycystic kidney disease[1–3,5,12,13]

The prevalence of autosomal dominant polycystic kidney disease is observed in about 1:1000 of the general population, and related mutations of at least two genes have been described. The *PKD1* gene is located on chromosome 16 and encodes for a protein called polycystin-1.[12,13] Its mutations are found in 85–90% of patients. The *PKD2* gene is located on chromosome 4 and encodes for a protein called polycystin-2[12,13] (Table 80.2). Mutations of this gene are found in 10–15% of the patients. Some rare patients with autosomal dominant polycystic kidney disease have no *PKD1* or *PKD2* mutations, suggesting a third implicated gene (*PKD3*) which has, however, not been identified.[12] Polycystins are mainly involved in cell-to-cell or

TABLE 80.2 CHARACTERISTICS OF POLYCYSTIC LIVER DISEASE WHETHER OR NOT ASSOCIATED WITH POLYCYSTIC KIDNEY DISEASE

	Mechanism of inheritance	Aberrant gene	Chromosomal location	Protein encoded	Prevalence in the general population
Polycystic liver disease with polycystic kidney disease	Autosomal dominant	PKD_1 (85-90%) PKD_2 (10–15%) PKD_3 (<1%)	16 4 (?)	Polycystin-1 Polycystin-2 (?)	1: 1000 1: 10000 1: 100000 (?)
Polycystic liver disease without polycystic kidney disease	Autosomal dominant	*PRKCSH*	19	Hepatocystin	1:1000 (?)
	or Not inherited	-		--	(?)

From Wilson PD. Polycystic kidney disease. N Engl J Med 2004; 350:151–164, Qian Q, Li A, King BF et al. Clinical profile of autosomal dominant polycystic liver disease. Hepatology 2003; 37:164–171, and Everson GT, Taylor MRG, Doctor RB. Polycystic disease of the liver. Hepatology 2004; 40:774–782.

cell-to-matrix interactions, and loss of these functions, due to mutations, could contribute to cyst formation. It has recently been recognized that cilia can be present on various epithelial cells, such as biliary and renal epithelial cells, and that polycystins are expressed on cilia. A role of impaired cilia function in the pathogenesis of autosomal dominant polycystic kidney disease has been proposed,[12] but the mechanism of induction of the malformation remains to be determined.

The prevalence of hepatic cysts in autosomal dominant polycystic kidney disease is age-related, ranging from about 0% at 20 years to 80% at 60 years. Hepatic cysts always appear after kidney cysts. Their prevalence is higher in females than in males, pointing to the possible role of estrogens in the development of hepatic cysts. Indeed, the prevalence and the size of cysts increase with the number of pregnancies, and also in postmenopausal women receiving estrogens.[14] The cysts range from 2 mm to 20 cm in diameter. They contain a clear fluid and do not communicate with the biliary tree. Von Meyenburg complexes are thought to be the initial lesion in polycystic liver disease. Cysts could be formed over years by gradual dilatation of von Meyenburg complexes, because of stricturing of bile ducts by fibrosis surrounding them. The dilated ducts, which originally communicate with the biliary tree, might become noncommunicating when fibrosis completely obstructs the biliary flow.

The liver is enlarged and generally contains a great number of cysts. These, along with renal cysts, are readily identified by imaging procedures, such as ultrasonography, CT, and MRI. Occasionally, only one lobe, usually the left one, is affected. Liver tests are generally normal. Polycystic liver disease is often asymptomatic. Symptoms most often develop during the 4th or 5th decade of life. They are due to the mass effect of the cysts or to complications, such as intracystic hemorrhage or infection and cyst rupture. Cholangiocarcinoma has been reported as a possible complication of associated von Meyenburg complexes. In most cases, the prognosis is not related to the liver disease but rather to progressive renal failure, and kidney graft recipients can survive for many years despite marked development of hepatic cysts. The disorder is frequently associated with vascular lesions, such as intracranial aneurysms, which are observed in approximately 10% of the cases. Mitral valve abnormalities have also been described.

Patients with asymptomatic liver cysts do not require treatment. Fenestration of one or several of the largest cysts can be performed, either by open surgery or by laparoscopy (preferred) in case of marked discomfort. The efficacy of this procedure is, however, far from being of proven efficacy. When cysts predominate in one lobe and are responsible for severe discomfort, partial hepatectomy can be proposed. A small number of patients may qualify for liver transplantation, possibly combined with renal transplantation.[15]

Autosomal dominant polycystic liver disease without polycystic kidney disease[13,16,17]

Autosomal dominant polycystic liver disease without kidney cysts seems to be about as frequent as the form associated with polycystic kidney disease. The mutant gene (*PRKCSH*) is different from *PKD1* and *PKD2* genes, and is usually located on chromosome 19 and encodes for a protein called hepatocystin.[13,16] Pathogenesis, manifestations, and management of the disease are similar to those of autosomal dominant polycystic liver disease associated with polycystic kidney disease.

Nonfamilial liver polycystic disease

Rare cases of sporadic, nonfamilial liver polycystic disease have been described.

KEY POINTS
POLYCYSTIC LIVER DISEASE
• Polycystic liver disease may or may not be associated with polycystic kidney disease • Autosomal dominant polycystic kidney disease is observed in about 1:1000 of the general population, and related mutations of at least two genes have been described • The prevalence of hepatic cysts in autosomal dominant polycystic kidney disease is age-related, ranging from about 0% at 20 years to 80% at 60 years; hepatic cysts always appear after kidney cysts • The cysts range from 2 mm to 20 cm in diameter; they contain a clear fluid and do not communicate with the biliary tree • Polycystic liver disease is often asymptomatic; when present, symptoms are generally due to the mass effect of the cysts • In markedly symptomatic cysts, fenestration of one or several of the largest cysts can be performed

CONGENITAL CYSTIC DISEASES OF EXTRAHEPATIC BILE DUCTS: THE CHOLEDOCHAL CYST[2,3,5]

This congenital dilatation of the common bile duct occurs in 1 per 100 000 to 1 per 150 000 births. It is more prevalent in Far Eastern countries, especially Japan. Four types have been recognized (Fig. 80.6). Type 1, which is by far the commonest (80%), consists of segmental or diffuse, generally fusiform dilatation of the extrahepatic bile duct. Type 2 consists of saccular dilatation that forms a diverticulum of the extrahepatic bile duct. Type 3 is a choledochocele of the distal common bile duct, mostly within the duodenal wall. Type 4 associates type 1 with cystic dilatations of the intrahepatic bile ducts that are generally close to the hilum. Choledochal cyst is frequently associated with abnormal pancreato-biliary ductal anatomy with a long common segment that could favor biliary reflux of pancreatic fluid.

Choledochal cyst, which is congenital, is mainly observed in children, but can also be diagnosed in adults. Eighty per cent of patients are female. The size of choledochal cysts varies greatly from one patient to another, and the cyst may contain from some milliliters to several liters of bile. In children, the main symptom is an abdominal mass, whereas cholangitis, with or without jaundice, is the most frequent sign in adults. The cyst may also be asymptomatic, being detected incidentally during abdominal ultrasonography. Carcinoma may be associated with choledochal cyst. It can develop within the cyst or outside (namely within the liver). The prevalence of carcinoma markedly increases with age, and reaches 15% in adults. Choledochal cyst is readily diagnosed by ultrasonography and other imaging procedures, namely magnetic resonance cholangiography. The best treatment is excision of the cyst, followed by choledocho-jejunostomy. Simple anastomosis between the cyst and intestinal tract should be avoided, as it favors cholangitis and does not prevent the development of adenocarcinoma.

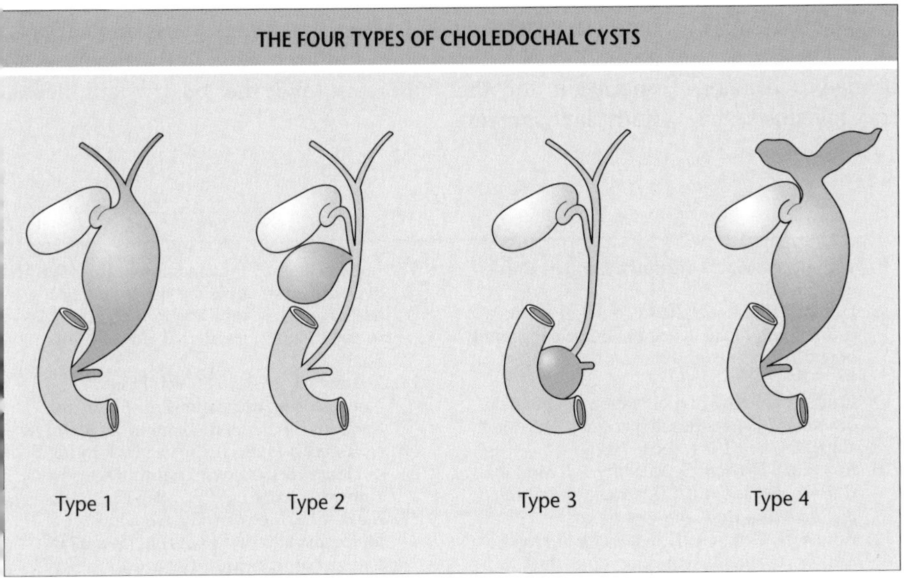

Fig. 80.6 Choledochal cysts. The four types of choledochal cysts.

KEY POINTS
CHOLEDOCHAL CYST

- Congenital dilatation of the common bile duct following four patterns, the most common being a diffuse fusiform dilatation of the common bile duct
- It occurs in 1 per 100 000 to 1 per 150 000 births, being more prevalent in Far Eastern countries, especially Japan
- Mainly diagnosed in children, but can also be diagnosed in adults; 80% of patients are female
- In children, the main symptom is an abdominal mass, whereas cholangitis, with or without jaundice, is the most frequent sign in adults
- Associated with adenocarcinoma, the prevalence of which markedly increases with age, reaching 15% in adults
- The treatment of choice is excision of the cyst, followed by choledochojejunostomy

CONGENITAL NONCYSTIC DISEASES OF BILE DUCTS

Paucity of interlobular bile ducts[1,5,18]

In children, two types of paucity of interlobular bile ducts (i.e., ductopenia) can be distinguished. The syndromic paucity, also called Alagille's syndrome, is an autosomal dominant disorder characterized by mutations of the *JAGGED1* gene located on chromosome 20. Numerous extrahepatic malformations are present. Cholestasis is generally moderate, and evolution toward cirrhosis is rare. The nonsyndromic paucity is not associated with a known genetic factor, although a high rate of consanguinity is noted in some patients. There are no extrahepatic manifestations. Cholestasis is usually severe and biliary cirrhosis occurs rapidly.

In adults, ductopenia is usually the result of progressive inflammatory destruction of interlobular bile ducts and is observed in various conditions, such as primary biliary cirrhosis, primary sclerosing cholangitis, liver allograft rejection, graft-versus-host disease, and drug-induced chronic cholestatic liver disease. Idiopathic ductopenia has also been reported in adulthood,[19–23] and might be related to an unidentified (e.g., toxic, viral, or metabolic) agent. A congenital origin, at least in some cases, is supported by: (1) reports of familial forms,[19,22,23] with possible autosomal dominant transmission[23]; and (2) clinical similarity with the nonsyndromic paucity of interlobular bile ducts observed in children, suggesting that adult disease might be a late-onset form of the childhood process.[19,20] Idiopathic ductopenia in adults is always associated with cholestasis, with or without jaundice. Its severity varies greatly from one patient to another, with a spectrum that ranges from an absence of clinical symptoms[21] to biliary cirrhosis. Ursodeoxycholic acid may improve liver biochemical tests,[19,21–23] but its impact on the disease progression is unknown. Liver transplantation is required in severe cases.[19,22]

KEY POINTS
PAUCITY OF INTERLOBULAR BILE DUCTS

- In children, there are two forms of paucity of interlobular liver ducts: the syndromic paucity (Alagille's syndrome) and the nonsyndromic paucity
- In adults, paucity of interlobular bile ducts can have several causes. Idiopathic form might be a late onset form of the nonsyndromic paucity observed in children. Treatment is ursodeoxycholic acid. Transplantation may be required in severe cases.

Atresia of extrahepatic bile ducts

Like idiopathic paucity of interlobular bile ducts, extrahepatic bile duct atresia is probably not a malformation, but rather the result of gradual destruction of the bile ducts by a necroinflammatory process of unknown etiology.[18] It is diagnosed in children and not in adults and will not, therefore, be dealt with in this chapter.

Other congenital abnormalities of extrahepatic bile ducts

Absence of gallbladder, double gallbladder, left-sided gallbladder, folded gallbladder, floating gallbladder, accessory bile ducts, and other malformations have been described.[3] These anomalies are generally not symptomatic, but awareness of their existence is important for the radiologist and the biliary and hepatic transplant surgeon.

REFERENCES

1. Desmet VJ. Congenital diseases of intrahepatic bile ducts: variations on the theme "ductal plate malformation." Hepatology 1992; 16:1069–1083.
2. Summerfield JA, Nagafuchi Y, Sherlock S et al. Hepatobiliary fibropolycystic diseases. A clinical and histological review of 51 patients. J Hepatol 1986; 2:141–156.
3. Sherlock S, Dooley J. Diseases of the liver and biliary system, 9th edn. Oxford: Blackwell Scientific Publications; 1993:548–561.
4. Benhamou JP, Menu Y. Non-parasitic cystic diseases of the liver and intrahepatic biliary tree. In: Bircher J, Benhamou JP, McIntyre N, Rizzetto M, Rodés J, eds. Oxford textbook of clinical hepatology. Oxford: Oxford University Press; 1999:817–823.
5. Ishak KG, Sharp HL. Developmental abnormalities and liver disease in childhood. In: MacSween RNM, Burt AD, Portmann BC et al, eds. Pathology of the liver, 4th edn. London: Churchill Livingston; 2002:107–154.
6. De Koning TJ, Dorland L, van Berge Henegouwen GP. Phosphomannose isomerase deficiency as a cause of congenital hepatic fibrosis and protein-losing enteropathy. J Hepatol 1999; 31:557–560.
7. Lang EK, Macchia RJ, Thomas R et al. Improved detection of renal pathologic features on multiphasic helical CT compared with IVU in patients presenting with microscopic hematuria. Urology 2003; 61:528–532.
8. Dupond JL, Miguet JP, Carbillet JP et al. Kidney polycystic disease in adult congenital hepatic fibrosis. Ann Intern Med 1978; 88:514–515.
9. Caroli J, Corcos V. La dilatation congénitale des voies biliaires intrahépatiques. Rev Med Chir Mal Foie 1964; 39:1–70.
10. Boyle MJ, Doyle GD, McNulty JG. Monobar Caroli's disease. Am J Gastroenterol 1989; 84:1437–1444.
11. Krausé D, Cercueil JP, Dranssart M et al. MRI for evaluating congenital bile duct abnormalities. J Comput Assist Tomogr 2002; 26:541–552.
12. Wilson PD. Polycystic kidney disease. N Engl J Med 2004; 350:151–164.
13. Everson GT, Taylor MRG, Doctor RB. Polycystic disease of the liver. Hepatology 2004; 40:774–782.
14. Sherstha R, McKinley C, Russ P et al. Postmenopausal estrogen therapy selectively stimulates hepatic enlargement in women with autosomal dominant polycystic kidney disease. Hepatology 1997; 26:1282–1286.
15. Swenson K, Seu P, Kinkhabwala M et al. Liver transplantation for adult polycystic liver disease. Hepatology 1998; 28:412–415.
16. Qian Q, Li A, King BF et al. Clinical profile of autosomal dominant polycystic liver disease. Hepatology 2003; 37:164–171.
17. Tahvanainen P, Tahvanainen E, Reijonen H et al. Polycystic liver disease is genetically heterogeneous: clinical and linkage studies in eight Finnish families. J Hepatol 2003; 38:39–43.
18. Desmet VJ, Roskams T, Van Eyken P. Non-cystic malformations of the biliary tract. In: Bircher J, Benhamou JP, McIntyre N, Rizzetto M, Rodés J, eds. Oxford textbook of clinical hepatology. Oxford: Oxford University Press; 1999:779–815.
19. Zafrani ES, Métreau JM, Douvin C et al. Idiopathic biliary ductopenia in adults: a report of five cases. Gastroenterology 1990; 99:1823–1828.
20. Brugera M, Llach J, Rodés J. Nonsyndromic paucity of intrahepatic bile ducts in infancy and idiopathic ductopenia in adulthood: the same syndrome? Hepatology 1992; 15:830–834.
21. Moreno A, Carreno V, Cano A et al. Idiopathic biliary ductopenia in adults without symptoms of liver disease. N Eng J Med 1997; 336:835–838.
22. Ludwig J. Idiopathic adulthood ductopenia: an update. Mayo Clin Proc 1998; 73:285–291.
23. Burak KW, Pearson DC, Swain MG et al. Familial idiopathic adulthood ductopenia: a report of five cases in three generations. J Hepatol 2000; 32:159–163.

Chapter 81

Acute viral hepatitis

Robert Thimme, Hans Christian Spangenberg, and Hubert E Blum

KEY POINTS

Virus	HAV	HBV	HCV	HDV	HEV
Viral genome	RNA(+)	DNA	RNA(+)	RNA(+)	RNA(–)
Screening test	Anti-HAV IgM	HBsAg or anti-HBc	Anti-HCV	Anti-HDV	Anti-HEV
Main transmission	Enteral	Parenteral	Parenteral	Parenteral	Enteral
Incubation period (days)	15–49	25–160	21–84	60–110	10–56
Acute hepatitis	Yes	Yes	Yes	Yes	Yes
Chronic hepatitis	No	Yes	Yes	Yes	No
Antiviral therapy during acute hepatitis	No	No	Yes	No	No
Immune prophylaxis					
Passive	+	+	–	–	–
Active	+	+	–	–	–

INTRODUCTION

Research in the last several decades has led to an enormous increase in our knowledge about the immunobiology and pathogenesis of viruses that cause acute liver disease in man. Five viruses have been identified that primarily manifest clinically as acute hepatitis: hepatitis A virus (HAV), hepatitis B virus (HBV), hepatitis C virus (HCV), hepatitis D virus (HDV), and hepatitis E virus (HEV). It is very difficult to accurately estimate the incidence of acute viral hepatitis because these infections are often asymptomatic and thus do not come to clinical attention. The Center for Disease Control and Prevention has undertaken mathematical modeling studies to estimate the past incidence of acute viral hepatitis worldwide. Based on these studies, acute hepatitis A makes up 47–49%, acute hepatitis B 33–35%, and acute hepatitis C 5–15%. Hepatitis D only occurs in association with hepatitis B. Hepatitis E is so rare that the true incidence is very difficult to estimate.[1]

HAV and HEV infections are often associated with acute icteric hepatitis and do not lead to chronic infection. By contrast, HBV, HCV, and HDV infections can lead to viral persistence that may lead to chronic hepatitis, cirrhosis, and hepatocellular carcinoma (HCC).

All five viruses have been extensively studied at the biological, molecular, and immunological level. This chapter reviews the structure, virology, and pathogenesis as well as the clinical manifestations, diagnosis, treatment, and prevention of all five hepatitis viruses. Since the pathology caused by all hepatitis viruses is very similar this will be described initially.

PATHOLOGY

Histologic examination of liver biopsies from patients with acute viral hepatitis reveals characteristic signs of acute hepatitis, such as hepatocyte ballooning, acidophilic (apoptotic) degeneration, and acidophilic (Councilman-like) body formation, readily identifiable by its oval or round shape and its hyaline and eosinophilic waxy cast. These histologic changes are most prominent near the terminal hepatic venule and are usually accompanied by lymphocytic inflammation within the lobule and portal and periportal areas. The infiltrate consists mainly of monocytic and lymphocytic cells. Hepatocyte regeneration may begin during the acute phase of infection and is recognized by thickening of the hepatocyte plates, the presence of mitotic figures, many binucleated cells, and hepatocyte rosette formation. Cholestasis is more often found in acute HAV compared to acute HBV or HCV infection. All histological changes disappear completely after resolution of acute infection. It is important to note, however, that histologic examination of the liver is rarely needed in patients with acute viral hepatitis.

ACUTE HEPATITIS A

Epidemiology

HAV has a worldwide distribution and is considered the most common cause of viral hepatitis.[2] The prevalence of HAV infection depends on the quality of water supply, level of sanitation, and age of population. In the US, the reported incidence of HAV infection is 9.1 per 100000 population per year.[1] Rates in men are consistently higher than in women.

Causes, risk factors, disease associations

The major route of transmission is person-to-person via the fecal–oral route. HAV is shed into the stool in high titers, and because it is relatively resistant to degradation by environmental conditions, the virus is spread easily within a population. Indeed, 70–90% of those exposed become infected. In the Viral Hepatitis Surveillance Study, the most common risk factor for HAV acquisition was personal contact with an HAV-infected individual (26%). Other risk factors were employment or attendance at a daycare facility (14%), intravenous drug use (11%), a history of recent travel (4%), and association with a suspected food or water-borne outbreak (3%). In 42% of cases, no known source of infection was reported.

RISK FACTORS FOR HEPATITIS A IN THE US	
Unknown	42%
Exposure by personal contact	26%
Daycare associated	14%
Intravenous drug use	11%
International travel	4%
Association with suspected outbreak	3%

Pathogenesis

HAV is a nonenveloped, positive-strand RNA virus that has been assigned to a separate genus (Hepatovirus) within the Picorna virus family.[3] The HAV RNA genome serves as messenger RNA for translation into a single polyprotein that is cleaved into 11 proteins with structural and nonstructural functions (Fig. 81.1). The structural proteins VP1–VP4 are responsible for the stability of the virus.

HAV is shed into the feces as early as 2 weeks after infection and peaks 1–2 weeks before the onset of symptoms.

There are at least four different genotypes that have a genetic heterogeneity of 15–20% with no significant differences in biologic or antigenic properties. Only one serotype exists, so that infection with one strain confers immunity to the other strains. Most evidence indicates that, as holds true for all hepatitis viruses, hepatocyte injury is secondary to the host immune response.

Clinical presentation

Between 70% and 80% of acutely HAV infected adults will develop symptoms of acute viral hepatitis. By contrast, more than 90% of children younger than 5 years remain asymptomatic during acute HAV infection. The onset of symptomatic hepatitis A is abrupt with prodromal symptoms such as fatigue, weakness, anorexia, nausea, abdominal pain, and vomiting. Jaundice develops in 90% of patients within 1–2 weeks after the onset of prodromal symptoms, typically shortly after darkening of urine occurs. The appearance of jaundice may be associated with pruritus and extrahepatic manifestations such as an evanescent rash, arthralgias, and, less commonly, leukocytoclastic vasculitis, glomerulonephritis, transient renal failure, or transient sensory neuropathy. With the exception of anorexia, prodromal symptoms resolve with the onset of jaundice. The duration of jaundice is less than 2 weeks in the majority of patients. Physical examination may reveal scleral jaundice and mild enlargement of the liver. Complete clinical and biochemical recovery is seen in 60% of patients within 2 months and in nearly 100% of patients within 6 months. After resolution of acute HAV infection, patients have a lifelong immunity against HAV infection that is mediated by IgG anti-HAV (Fig. 81.2).

Atypical course of acute HAV infection: Two have been described: cholestatic and relapsing hepatitis A. The course of cholestatic HAV infection is prolonged and characterized by jaundice that lasts 2–8 months. Cholestatic hepatitis is associated with symptoms of pruritus, fatigue, weight loss, loose stools and is often associated with extrahepatic manifestations. However, spontaneous recovery occurs. Relapsing hepatitis A has been described in 6–12% of cases in children and adults. An initial phase of acute infection with remission (lasting 4–15 weeks) is followed by a relapse. The pathogenesis of relapsing hepatitis is unknown. The prognosis is excellent.

Diagnostic methods

The detection of IgM anti-HAV during the acute phase of symptomatic or asymptomatic hepatitis and for 3–6 months thereafter is diagnostic of acute HAV infection. IgG anti-HAV may also be present early in the acute phase of infection; however, the presence of IgG anti-HAV without IgM anti-HAV

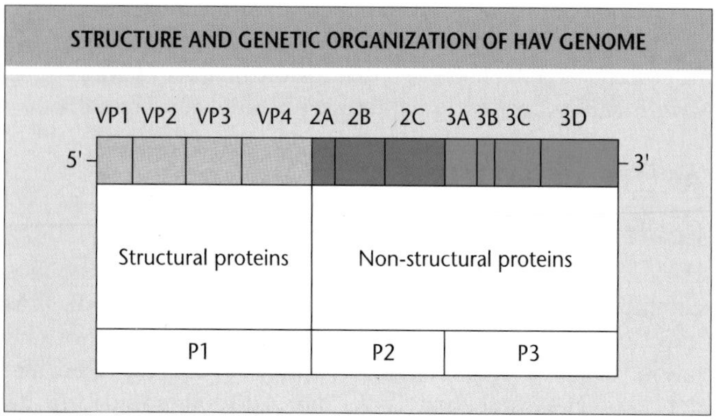

Fig. 81.1 Structure and genetic organization of HAV genome.

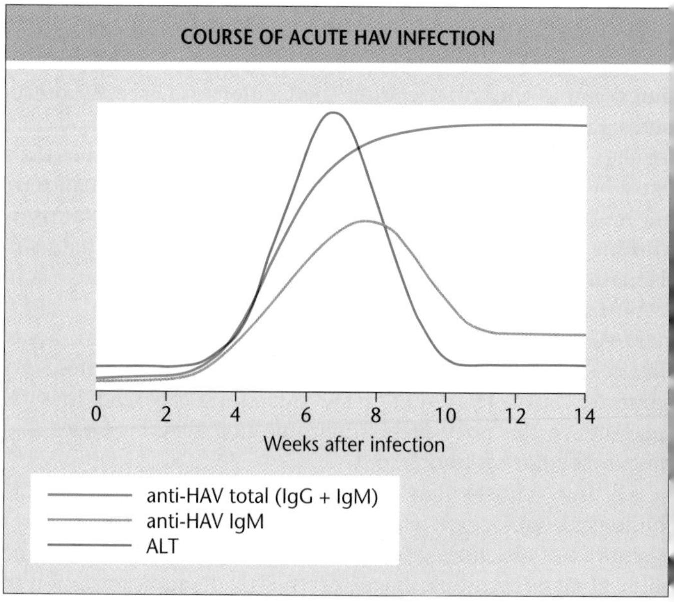

Fig. 81.2 Clinical, biochemical, and serological course of acute HAV infection.

CLINICAL PRESENTATION AND SYMPTOMS OF ACUTE HEPATITIS A
Children: 90% asymptomatic
Adults: 70–80% symptomatic
• Dark urine (94%)
• Lassitude (91%)
• Anorexia (90%)
• Jaundice (90%)
• Nausea (87%)
• Weakness (77%)
• Fever (76%)
• Vomiting (71%)
• Headache (70%)
• Abdominal pain (65%)

trongly suggests other causes of hepatitis. Serum IgM anti-IAV levels peak during the acute or early convalescent phase of infection and decline to undetectable levels after 3–4 months. gG anti-HAV remains detectable for decades and is responsible for the lifelong immunity following clinical recovery. The letection of HAV RNA in blood or stool is not necessary for he diagnosis of acute HAV infection.

Treatment and prevention

Supportive measures are the only treatment for acute HAV nfection. Isolation of infected persons is not necessary because shedding of virus into the feces has already declined prior to he onset of symptoms. Hospitalization is only recommended or patients with severe anorexia or vomiting or for patients who develop acute liver failure. Cholestatic hepatitis may be reated by a short course of prednisolone (30 mg/day with tapering over 1–2 weeks). Liver transplantation should be considered early in cases of acute liver failure.

Prevention of HAV infection requires maintenance of high hygienic standards and appropriate use of immunoprophylaxis. Travelers to endemic regions should be advised to avoid drinking water or ice of uncertain origin and eating uncooked food. Immunoprophylaxis can be achieved by passive transfer of anti-HAV immunoglobulins or by active immunization. The major current use of immunoglobulin is for postexposure prophylaxis of household contacts of infected individuals and for travelers to endemic regions. Administration of immunoglobulin before exposure will prevent infection in 85–95% of exposed persons, administration within 1–2 weeks after exposure will prevent or attenuate infection, and administration more than 2 weeks after exposure is ineffective.

Active immunization: Two licensed HAV vaccines are currently available (Havrix®, Glaxo Smith Kline, and VAQTA®, Merck Sharp and Dohme). These vaccines are highly immunogenic, leading to a seroconversion rate of up to 95% after a single injection and 100% after three injections. Therefore, postvaccination testing for a serologic response is not recommended. It is anticipated that protective antibody levels last for more than 20 years. Seroconversion results in protection against HAV infection. Active immunization is recommended, e.g., for travelers to endemic areas, medical staff in pediatric clinics, persons in childcare facilities, and intravenous drug users.

Prognosis with and without treatment

Hepatitis A is typically a benign, self-limited infection. Most patients recover completely within 2 months after the onset of disease. Underlying chronic liver disease and an age above 40 years are associated with increased severity and a higher risk of acute liver failure. Fulminant hepatitis A is rare and chronic HAV infection does not occur. [2]

ACUTE HEPATITIS B

Epidemiology

Hepatitis B virus (HBV), the prototype member of the Hepadnaviridae family, is a noncytopathic, hepatotropic virus with more than 350 million infected individuals worldwide.[4] The prevalence of HBV infection varies in different geographic regions of the world ranging from 0.1% in the Western world up to 15% in Asian and African countries. The incidence of HBV infection in high-prevalence countries is hard to estimate. It is well documented, however, that the implementation of HBV vaccination programs has led to a substantial decrease of HBV infection and its most common complications, such as chronic hepatitis, cirrhosis, and HCC. In the US, the incidence of acute HBV infection has decreased from 70 cases per 100 000 persons in 1985 to 40 cases per 100 000 persons in 1991. Men are more commonly infected than women and peak prevalence is between 10 and 29 years of age.[5]

Causes, risk factors, disease associations

HBV is parenterally transmitted via blood or blood products or by sexual or perinatal exposure. HBV infection occurs in regions with high prevalence mostly in early childhood via horizontal transmission, but also in rare cases by vertical transmission. HBV persistence is much greater in infants (90%) than in adults (<5%). In regions with low prevalence, spread of infection occurs predominantly horizontally and adolescents and adults are at a greater risk of acquiring HBV infection. High-risk groups in the Western world include intravenous drug users, homosexuals, household contacts and sexual contacts with HBV-infected individuals, patients with multiple sexual contacts, healthcare workers, and patients requiring hemodialysis.

Pathogenesis

The infectious virion is an enveloped nucleocapsid containing the viral polymerase bound to an open circular DNA genome, which consists of a full-length 3.2 kbp minus strand and an incomplete plus strand (Fig. 81.3). After infection, the viral genome is released into the nucleus where DNA repair enzymes process and join the viral minus and plus strands, yielding the 3.2 kbp covalently closed circular DNA that serves as template for viral transcription. The viral genome is organized into four open reading frames (ORFs) controlled by four independent promoters and a single common polyadenylation signal, yielding four overlapping viral RNA species of 3.5, 2.4, 2.1, and 0.7 kb length. The 3.5 kb transcript encodes polymerase, core, and precore proteins and serves as pregenomic RNA that is reverse transcribed into minus strand DNA as the first step in viral replication. The 2.4 and 2.1 kb transcripts encode the large, middle, and small hepatitis B surface antigens (HBsAgs) that make up the viral envelope. The small HBsAg defines the HBV subtypes by the determinant a. Furthermore, the major

STRUCTURE AND GENETIC ORGANIZATION OF HBV GENOME

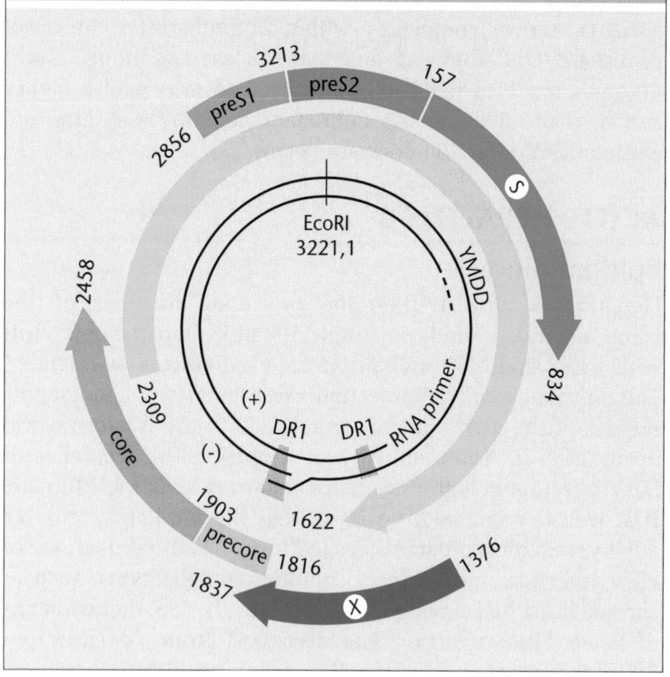

Fig. 81.3 Structure and genetic organization of HBV genome.

humoral immune response is directed against this antigen. The 0.7 kb transcript encodes the X-protein, which has transcriptional trans-activating potential and may be involved through its interaction with p53 in HCC development.

While HBV can be divided into eight genotypes A–H there is remarkably little genomic variability in this virus. Besides this classification system, the identification of the common determinant a and two pairs of allelic variations, a/y and w/r, has led to the definition of the four major subtypes of HBsAg: adw, adr, ayw, and ayr. HBV variants with mutations in the precore, surface, X gene, and the core promoter regions have been identified (Table 81.1). HBV mutants may accumulate because of a survival advantage – by evading the host immune response or by enhanced viral replication. The G1896A (precore/core) mutant was first reported in patients with fulminant hepatitis or chronic active hepatitis. The basis of the selectio of this mutant was thought to be related to the escape fro immune recognition by anti-HBe; molecular studies showe that stability and replicative capacity were enhanced. How ever, in clinical studies in patients with this mutation the leve of HBV DNA were not increased. Mutations in the S gene hav been reported in infants born to carrier mothers who deve oped HBV infection despite vaccination and in liver transplai recipients who developed HBV reinfection despite prophylax with hepatitis B immunoglobulin.[6]

TABLE 81.1 HEPATITIS B VARIANTS

Gene	Molecular effect	Clinical relevance
Pre-S/S	Change of subtype determinant d/y, w/r	?
	Loss of group-specific determinant a	Diagnosis escape Vaccine escape Immune escape
Precore/core	Loss of HBeAg ? change in T cell recognition ? direct cytopathic effect	HBeAg negative Severe clinical course of infection Fulminant hepatitis
X	?	?
Polymerase	Dysfunction of polymerase	? HBV latency, persistence

HBV is noncytopathic for the infected hepatocytes. Since th disease spectrum associated with HBV infection is very var able, the host response to HBV infection must play a critic role in disease pathogenesis. Indeed, based on studies of HB pathogenesis in man and animal models, it is clearly estal lished that hepatitis is initiated by an antigen-specific antivir cellular immune response. Indeed, several studies have show that viral clearance during acute HBV infection is associate with the induction of a vigorous and polyclonal T cell respons Both HBV-specific CD4 and CD8+ T cell responses are detectabl in acutely infected individuals. The CD8+ T cells, howeve seem to play the major role with respect to the clearance c the virus and liver disease.[7] The CD8+ T cells do not only pe form cytopathic effector functions but also contribute to vir clearance by the secretion of inflammatory cytokines such a interferon gamma (IFNγ) and tumor necrosis factor alpha (TNFα These cytokines are capable of acting noncytopathically throug two distinct pathways that result in HBV nucleocapsid co elimination and destabilization of viral DNA.

Clinical presentation

Acute HBV infection varies from an asymptomatic infectio to cholestatic hepatitis and acute liver failure. After an incu bation period of about 75 days (26–160 days) HBV infectio may cause clinical symptoms with cholestatic hepatitis an jaundice. This is generally accompanied by fatigue and genera discomfort. However, acute HBV infection may also be asymp tomatic. Interestingly, these patients have a higher risk o chronic HBV infection. Usually, acute HBV infection is sel limiting and lasts at most for 4 months. Rarely, acute HB infection can be fulminant (about 1%) and may lead to acut liver failure.

Extrahepatic disease manifestations are common in acut HBV infection and include a variety of manifestations. Mos manifestations can be explained by HBsAg-containing immun complexes that are responsible for arthralgias and rashes, bu also for the severe serum sickness-like syndrome. This syn drome includes fever, symmetric arthralgias of the small joints urticaria, and, especially in children, acrodermatitis papulosa Furthermore, hematological manifestations may range fron isolated lymphopenia or thrombocytopenia to agranulocytosi or aplastic anemia. In addition, cardiac (bradycardia, hyper tension, myocarditis) and respiratory manifestations (pleura effusion, infection), vasculitis, arteritis of medium-sized arter ies, glomerulonephritis, polymyalgia rheumatica, type II mixe essential cryoglobulinemia, and neurological and psychiatri pathologies (apathy, depression, sleeplessness, headache, poly neuropathy, and Guillain-Barré syndrome) can be associate with acute HBV infection. In general, the extrahepatic manifes tations resolve spontaneously. In severe cases, plasmapheresi may be indicated.

Diagnostic methods

Virological markers (HBsAg, HBeAg) and markers of viral replication (HBV DNA by hybridization assays) become detectable usually within the first 6 weeks after HBV infection. This is long before the onset of clinical symptoms or biochemical abnormalities. These markers remain positive throughout the prodromal phase and the early phase of illness. Coinciding with the onset of biochemical abnormalities, IgM anti-HBc becomes detectable and may persist for many months before IgG anti-HBc develops. Anti-HBs becomes positive last and indicates that HBV infection has resolved.

Biochemical markers of acute HBV infection are elevated serum alanine aminotransferase (ALT) and serum aspartate aminotransferase (AST) levels that are usually 500U/L or higher. Bilirubin levels usually do not exceed 10mg/dL.

In summary, the combination of clinical symptoms, biochemical abnormalities, and typical serological findings, as summarized in Fig. 81.4, allow a clear differentiation of acute resolving HBV infection from acute HBV infection followed by chronic infection.

Treatment and prevention

In adults, there is no need for a specific treatment of acute HBV infection because it resolves in most symptomatic patients. Therefore, treatment is limited to supportive measures. Acute HBV infection can be prevented by three strategies: behavior modification to prevent disease transmission, passive immunoprophylaxis, and active immunoprophylaxis. Behavior modifications, such as changes in sexual practices and needle exchange programs for intravenous drug users, have reduced HBV transmission. Passive immunoprophylaxis with hepatitis B immune globulin is used in neonates born to HBsAg-positive mothers, after needle stick exposure, after sexual exposure, and after liver transplantation of HBV-infected patients. Active immunization is highly effective and leads to anti-HBs in more than 95% of healthy vaccine recipients. There are currently two hepatitis B vaccines available in the US (Engerix-B®, Recombivax®). HBV protective levels of antibody persist in the majority of vaccine recipients (68% at 4years). Even though antibody levels can decline to the point at which anti-HBs is no longer detectable, protection is not necessarily lost. Therefore, routine testing of antibodies and routine booster vaccination are not recommended. Only persons with high risk of HBV infection should be revaccinated.[8]

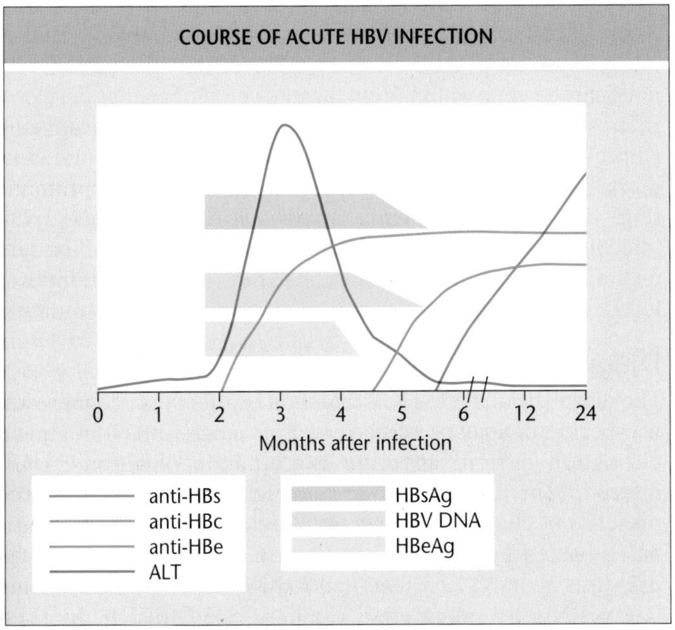

Fig. 81.4 Clinical, biochemical, and serological course of acute HBV infection.

Prognosis with and without treatment

The overall prognosis of acute HBV infection is very good. Specific treatment of acute HBV infection is not recommended; prevention of HBV infection is most important.

ACUTE HEPATITIS C

Epidemiology

Acute HCV infection is the third most common cause of acute viral hepatitis (5–15%). The annual incidence of acute HCV infection in the US decreased from an average of 230000 new cases per year in the 1980s to 38000 cases per year in the 1990s. This decline is primarily due to the institution of HCV screening of blood donors in 1989 and the establishment of safer needle-using practices among intravenous drug users.[9]

Causes, risk factors, disease associations

HCV is transmitted by percutaneous (e.g., blood transfusion, needle stick inoculation) or nonpercutaneous (e.g., sexual contact or perinatal) exposure to infectious blood or blood-derived body fluids. The factor most strongly associated with acute HCV infection is intravenous drug use, which is responsible for about 68% of HCV cases. Additional risk factors include sex with HCV-infected partners, high-risk sexual behavior (together about 18% of cases), occupational exposure to blood (primarily contaminated needle sticks), and, very rarely, healthcare related procedures. In up to 10% of cases, the source of HCV infection remains unknown (Table 81.2).

Pathogenesis

HCV is a small, enveloped, single-stranded RNA virus that belongs to the family of flaviviruses. The HCV genome is approximately 9600 nucleotides long and contains a single ORF that encodes a large viral polypeptide precursor of 3010–3033 amino acids. The cleavage of the protein by viral and cellular proteases results in the structural and nonstructural viral proteins (Fig. 81.5). Viral replication is very rapid and it is estimated that 10^{10}–10^{12} virions are produced per day. The lack of a proofreading function of the viral polymerase in part accounts for the fact that the HCV RNA genome mutates

TABLE 81.2 MODES OF HEPATITIS C TRANSMISSION

- Intravenous drug use
- Cocaine snorting
- Accidental occupational exposure (i.e., needlestick)
- Exposure to contaminated medical equipment
- Tatooing or body piercing
- Sexual
- Mother–infant
- Blood transfusion (currently uncommon)

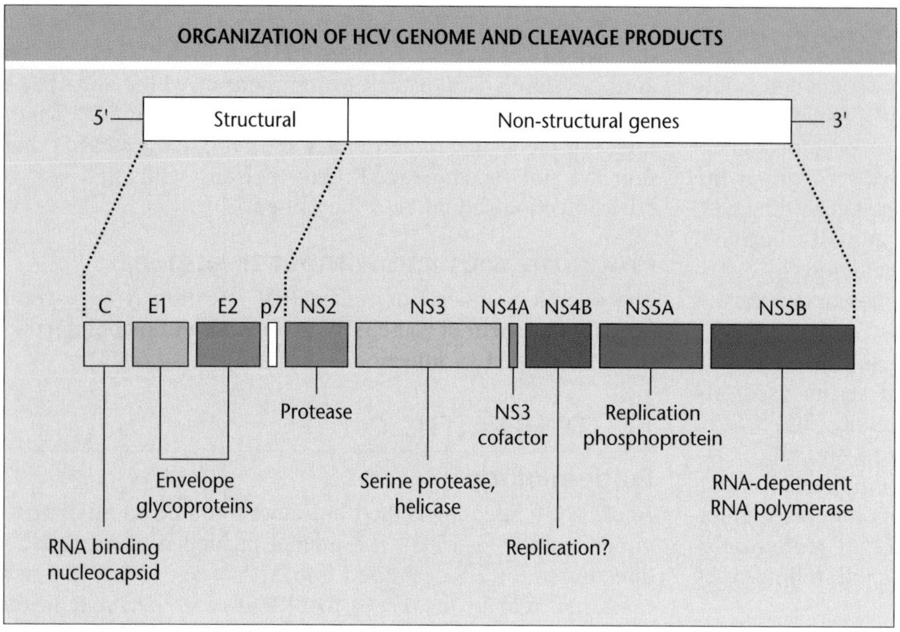

Fig. 81.5 Organization of HCV genome. Structure and genetic organization of HCV genome and polyprotein cleavage products.

frequently. As a result, HCV circulates as a population of quasispecies with individual viral genomes differing by 1–5% in nucleotide sequence, presenting a major challenge to the immune-mediated control of HCV infection. Phylogenetic analysis has revealed six major genotypes with further subtypes. In the US and Western Europe, genotypes 1a and 1b are most common, followed by genotypes 2 and 3. The virus has the propensity to persist in the majority of acutely infected patients (55–85%).[10]

The immunological and virological mechanisms that determine the outcome of infection are still not completely understood although it is generally accepted that the control of HCV is mediated primarily by virus-specific T cells. Indeed, viral clearance is associated with multispecific and vigorous HCV-specific CD4+ and CD8+ T cell responses that accumulate in the liver and exert cytotoxic (e.g., killing of infected hepatocytes) and noncytotoxic (e.g., secretion of antiviral cytokines such as IFNγ) effector functions. By contrast, viral persistence develops in acutely infected patients with no or only weak and dysfunctional HCV-specific T cell responses.[11] In addition, the development of viral mutations that escape the immune response may also be an important mechanism of viral persistence. The role of circulating anti-HCV antibodies during acute HCV infection remains unknown. Several studies have shown that neutralizing antibodies are produced during natural infection despite the high rate of viral persistence. The most likely explanation for the ineffectiveness of the antibody response may be the rapid occurrence of viral escape mutations.

Multiple episodes of acute hepatitis C have been observed in polytransfused thalassemic children and reinfection of chimpanzees after HCV recovery from the infection has been described indicating that no sterilizing immunity exists in HCV infection. A recent study in intravenous drug users showed, however, that a group of individuals who had recovered from HCV infection had only a 50% risk of being reinfected compared to previously uninfected persons. Similar results have been obtained in chimpanzees. Rechallenge of animals after recovery from HCV infection with homologous or heterologous virus resulted in fast and efficient control of infection. These results suggest that sterilizing immunity to HCV infection does not exist but that acquired immunity can develop that protects against viral persistence. Depletion studies in chimpanzees have demonstrated that CD8+ T cells mediate this protective immunity.

Clinical presentation

Acute HCV infection is usually asymptomatic and therefore it is rarely recognized clinically. Jaundice may develop in 25% of acutely infected patients, whereas 10–20% may present with nonspecific symptoms such as fatigue, nausea, myalgias, low-grade fever, and vomiting. The clinical symptoms occur 2–12 weeks (average 7 weeks) after infection and last 3–12 weeks. HCV RNA appears in blood within 2 weeks of infection and is followed by an elevation of serum ALT/AST. HCV antibodies are first detectable at the time of liver disease (Figs 81.6 and 81.7). Acute HCV infection can be severe and prolonged but it is rarely fulminant. Approximately 85% of infected patients do not clear the virus within 6 months, and chronic hepatitis develops. Interestingly, the small number of patients who develop clinically symptomatic acute hepatitis C seem to clear the virus more frequently than those who are clinically asymptomatic (Fig. 81.8).[12] Extrahepatic manifestations of acute HCV infection are less often seen than during chronic infection and include fever, arthralgias, urticaria, mixed cryoglobulinemia, leucocytoclastic vasculitis, and bone marrow suppression.

Diagnostic methods

The diagnosis of acute HCV infection is difficult since there are no specific diagnostic tests to identify acute infection and to distinguish it from an acute exacerbation of chronic HCV infection. The diagnosis of acute infection is suggested by the presence of clinical or biochemical evidence of acute hepatitis accompanied by anti-HCV and/or HCV RNA in serum. Thus, diagnosis requires serologic (anti-HCV) and virologic testing (HCV RNA by polymerase chain reaction (PCR)). In most cases, however, the diagnosis can be made based upon anti-HCV testing alone.

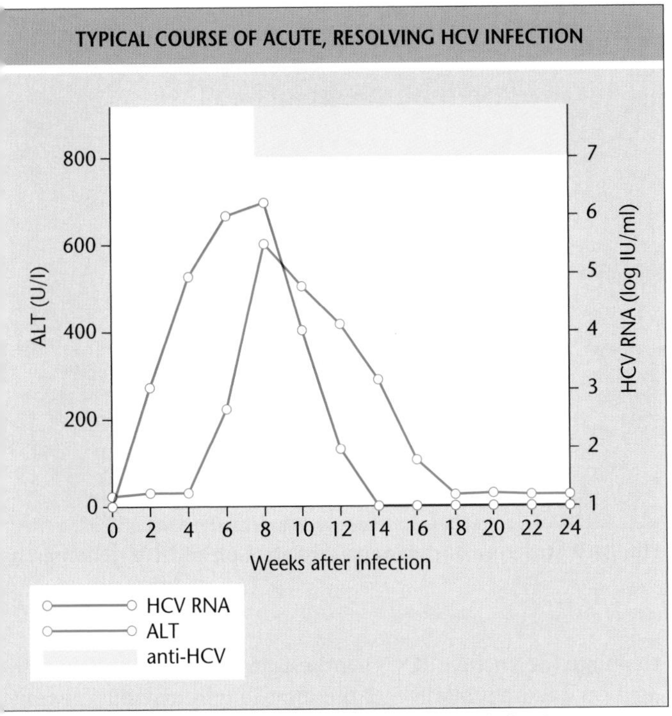

Fig. 81.6 Typical course of acute, resolving HCV infection.

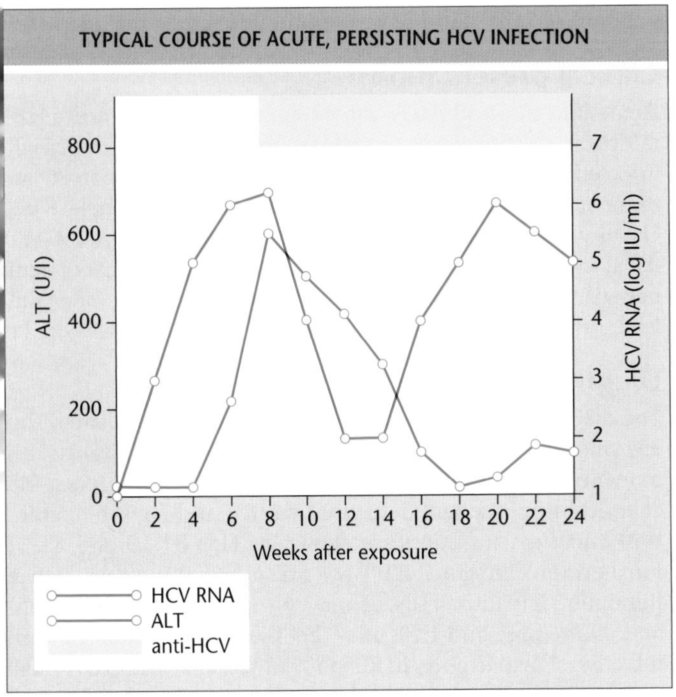

Fig. 81.7 Typical course of acute, persisting HCV infection.

Treatment and prevention

The high propensity of acute HCV infection to become chronic has provided the rationale for treating patients with acute HCV infection to prevent chronicity. Even though most studies on therapy of acute HCV have been small, uncontrolled, and heterogeneous with respect to patient characteristics, treatment regimens, and follow-up evaluations, the currently available data support treatment of patients with acute HCV infection. However, the available data are insufficient to draw firm

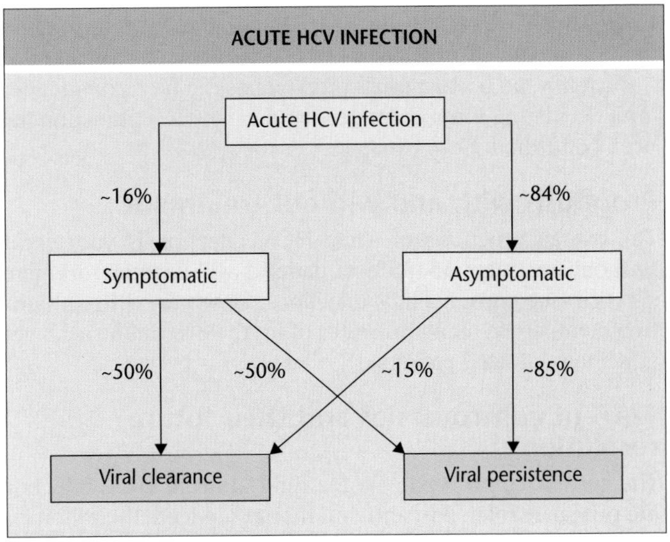

Fig. 81.8 Acute HCV infection.

conclusions as to which patient should be treated, when therapy should be started, and what regimen should be used. In a German multicenter study, 44 patients (most of them with acute symptomatic HCV infection) were treated with alpha interferon daily for 4 weeks then 3 times weekly for an additional 20 weeks. Importantly, all but one patient (98%) had a sustained virological response with normal ALT levels and no detectable HCV RNA 6 months after cessation of therapy.[13] Although this study has clearly shown that early antiviral therapy with alpha interferon may prevent the progression to chronicity, uncertainties remain with respect to the therapeutic regimen (alpha interferon monotherapy versus combination therapy with alpha interferon and ribavirin) and the time for initiation of therapy, particularly considering that up to 50% of symptomatic patients show spontaneous viral clearance and would be treated unnecessarily.

A recent study that accounted for a high spontaneous viral clearance rate in symptomatic patients (52% in this study), showed that a delay of therapy with alpha interferon with or without ribavirin in patients who had not cleared the virus by 3 months was still successful in 80%. Overall, this strategy led to a viral clearance (spontaneous or treatment-induced) in 91% of patients.[14] By contrast, asymptomatic patients were unable to clear the virus spontaneously and should therefore be treated as early as possible. In view of these data, antiviral therapy should be considered early; however, delaying therapy by 2–4 months after the onset of symptoms may be a reasonable therapeutic strategy. Since this recommendation is not based on large controlled trials and since the actual standard therapy with pegylated interferon and ribavirin has not been tested, inclusion of patients with acute HCV infection in controlled clinical trials is recommended.

Prevention of HCV infection has been achieved by screening and testing of blood donors and virus inactivation of plasma derived products. However, further strategies for reducing or eliminating the potential risk for HCV transmission from high-risk behaviors such as risk reduction counseling and services, need to be more widely implemented. Primary prevention of intravenous drug use will eliminate the greatest risk factor for HCV infection. There is no effective vaccine and no effective postexposure prophylaxis against HCV infection available.

However, the development of HCV vaccines is a very active field of research.

Currently, no postexposure prophylaxis can be recommended until circulating virus is detected and acute HCV infection has been confirmed.

Prognosis with and without treatment

The overall prognosis of acute HCV infection is very good. Without treatment 55–85% of patients will develop viral persistence (see chronic HCV infection). However, with antiviral treatment, viral elimination rates of up to 98% can be achieved in acutely infected patients.

Current controversies and their future resolution

The current controversies in the field of acute HCV infection are primarily related to antiviral therapy. Indeed, the following key questions need to be addressed: (1) who should be treated; (2) when should therapy be started; and (3) what treatment regimen should be used? Further therapeutic studies of acute HCV infection through prospective randomized controlled trials of adequate size and design should be performed.

ACUTE HEPATITIS D

Epidemiology

HDV was first discovered by Rizetto and coworkers in 1977.[15] These investigators estimated that 15 million individuals are infected with HDV. This was based on the assumption that approximately 5% of HBsAg carriers are infected with HDV. Although HBV is required for HDV replication, the geographic distribution of HDV does not match that of HBV. Areas of high HDV prevalence include Italy, regions in Eastern Europe, Colombia, Venezuela, Western Asia, and some Pacific islands. For the US it has been estimated that 7500 acute HDV infections occur annually.

Causes, risk factors, disease associations

As HBV infection is a prerequisite for HDV infection, modes of HDV transmission are similar to those of HBV infection. In Western countries, the major mode of transmission is intravenous drug use. Sexual transmission of HDV has been reported but is quite low compared to HBV. Since the geographic distribution of HDV is not identical to that of HBV, other factors may determine the prevalence of HDV infection.

Extrahepatic manifestations do not differ from those of acute HBV infection. However, antibodies against liver kidney microsomes (LKM) can be found in about 20% of patients.

Pathogenesis

HDV is a 36-nm particle containing the viral RNA genome and the delta antigen. HDV RNA encodes for only one protein, which is produced in two forms – a large (LHDAg) and a small (SHDAg) protein (Fig. 81.9).[16] The short form promotes viral replication whereas the long form inhibits it. The circular RNA genome is of negative polarity and is transcribed into a linear anti-genomic transcript and mRNA for HDAg. The replication process requires the host RNA-dependent RNA polymerase. The genomic, positive-strand circular HDV RNA becomes the template for successive rounds of minus strand synthesis. Thereafter, the multimeric, linear, minus strand RNA serves as

STRUCTURE AND GENETIC ORGANIZATION OF HDV GENOME

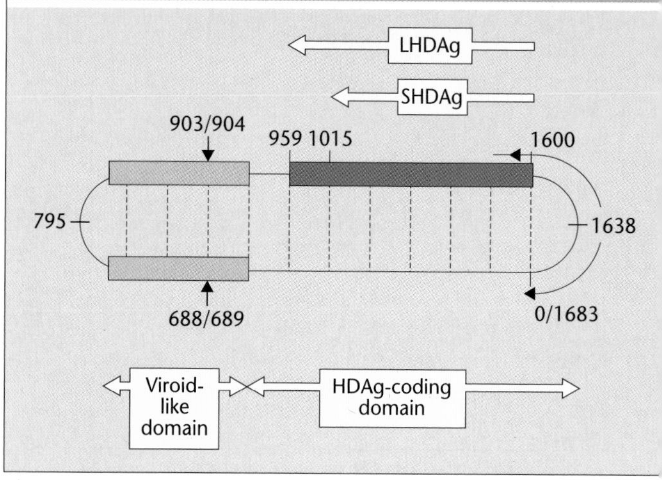

Fig. 81.9 Structure and genetic organization of HDV genome.

template for positive RNA synthesis, followed by cleaving and ligation leading finally to the unit-length circular genome. Together with the HDAg, which is translated from a cytoplasmic, polyadenylated antigenomic mRNA, HDV particles are enveloped by HBsAg. Therefore, HDV replication is independent of HBV, but HBV is required for viral spread.[17]

Clinical presentation

Acute infection with HDV can be simultaneous with acute HBV infection (coinfection) or can occur in patients chronically infected with HBV (superinfection). The clinical course and outcome of both infections are quite different (Table 81.3). Usually after an incubation period of about 70 days (60–110 days) most patients develop clinical symptoms typical of acute hepatitis with jaundice, fatigue, nausea, myalgias, low-grade fever, and vomiting.

Diagnostic methods

The diagnosis of acute HDV infection is based on elevated liver enzymes (ALT, AST) and bilirubin, HBsAg positivity, and detection of anti-HDV. The typical course of symptoms, biochemical findings, and detection of HBV and HDV in coinfection and superinfection are shown in Figs 81.10 and 81.11. Furthermore, in the 2–20% of HDV infections that lead to fulminant hepatitis, HBsAg may be transiently undetectable and, therefore, anti-HBc may be the only marker of HBV infection. Furthermore, in 20–30% of patients with HBV/HDV coinfection, a second peak of ALT elevations can be observed. These patients, for unknown reasons, are at higher risk of

TABLE 81.3 CLINICAL COURSE OF HDV COINFECTION AND SUPERINFECTION

	Coinfection (%)	Superinfection (%)
Spontaneous resolution	90–95	5–10
Fulminant hepatitis	2–20	10–20
Chronic hepatitis	2–7	70–95

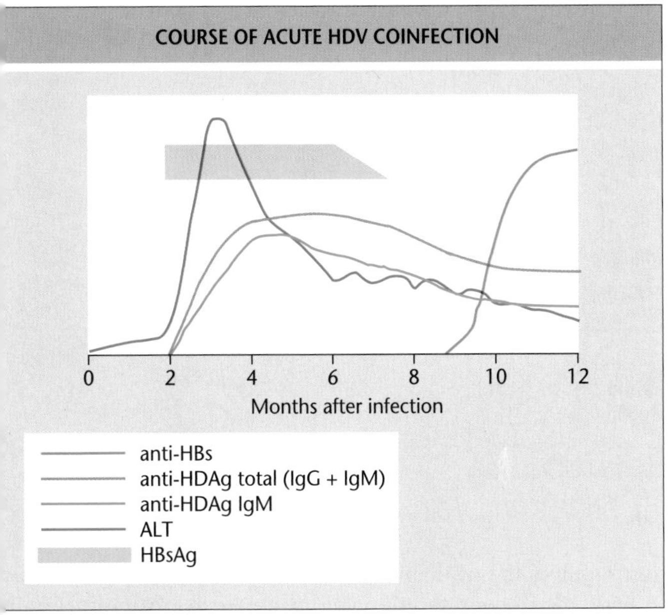

ig. 81.10 Clinical, biochemical, and serological course of acute IDV coinfection.

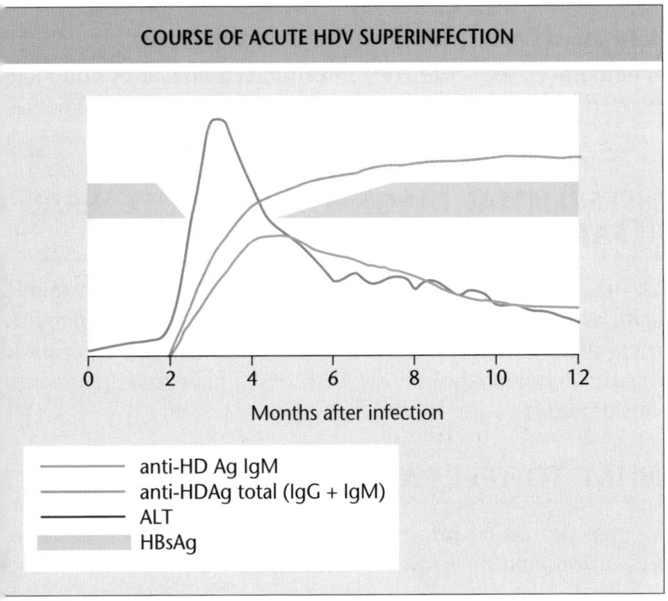

ig. 81.11 Clinical, biochemical, and serological course of acute IDV superinfection.

leveloping fulminant hepatitis. However, in general, patients with HBV/HDV superinfection are at a greater risk of developing subfulminant or fulminant hepatitis (10–20%). The most important diagnostic tool is the detection of anti-HDV.[18]

Treatment and prevention

There is no specific treatment for acute HDV infection neither in the case of coinfection nor in the case of superinfection. Since HDV is transmitted parenterally and dependent on HBV infection, the prevention strategies for HDV are identical to those for HBV.

Unfortunately, to date, there is no specific active or passive vaccine for HDV available.[19]

Prognosis with and without treatment

The overall prognosis of acute HDV infection depends on whether HDV presents as a coinfection or as a superinfection with HBV (Table 81.3). Treatment of acute HDV infection is not recommended.

ACUTE HEPATITIS E

Epidemiology

Worldwide, two geographic patterns of HEV infection can be observed: areas of high HEV prevalence with major outbreaks and substantial numbers of sporadic cases; and nonendemic regions, in which HEV infection accounts for only a few cases. In endemic areas, outbreaks have a periodicity of 5–10 years. In nonendemic countries, such as the US and Western Europe, cases of acute HEV infection are uncommon and occur primarily in travelers returning from endemic areas.

Causes, risk factors, disease associations

Fecal–oral spread, mainly by contaminated drinking water, is the predominant mode of HEV transmission in endemic regions. Percutaneous and blood-borne modes of transmission may also contribute to the spread of HEV. The secondary attack rates in households of HEV-infected patients range from 0.2% to 2.2%. This is in dramatic contrast to the high transmission rates in households of HAV infected persons that range from 50% to 75%. This difference between both viruses may be explained by the instability of HEV in the environment, lower viral titers of HEV in the stool, differences in infectious dose needed to produce infection or a higher frequency of subclinical disease.

Pathogenesis

HEV is a nonenveloped, positive-strand RNA virus. It has been classified as a member of the Caliciviridae. Unlike other RNA viruses, HEV has an RNA genome that encodes structural and nonstructural proteins through the use of discontinuous and partially overlapping ORFs (Fig. 81.12). ORF1 encodes nonstructural proteins, ORF2 encodes structural proteins, and the function of the ORF3-encoded protein is currently unknown.

After intravenous inoculation of primates, elevated serum ALT levels have been observed after 10–19 days. The shedding of virus into feces starts before symptoms develop. The titer of virus in stool during acute HEV infection is much lower compared to acute HAV infection.

Geographically distinct isolates of HEV have been identified and are classified into four different genotypes.

The pathogenesis of acute HEV infection is not known. It is believed, however, that early ALT elevations are caused by direct cytopathic effects while later ALT rises may be immune-mediated. The pathogenesis of the severe hepatitis E observed in pregnant women in the third trimester is also unknown.

Clinical presentation

Clinical signs and symptoms of hepatitis E are very similar to acute hepatitis A. The incubation period is about 40 days. The prodromal phase is characterized by fever (23–97%) and malaise (95–100%) while the icteric phase is characterized by jaundice, dark urine, anorexia, abdominal pain, and vomiting. Less common symptoms include diarrhea, pruritus, arthralgias, and urticarial rash.

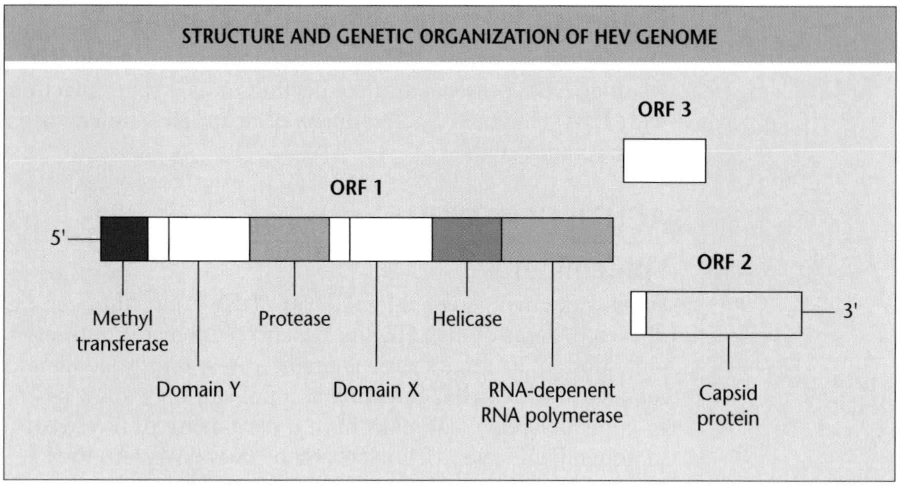

Fig. 81.12 Structure and genetic organization of HEV genome. ORF, open reading frame.

As in acute HAV infection, cholestatic acute HEV infection may occur and has a good prognosis. Generally, acute HEV infection is mild and symptoms resolve within 6 weeks. Fulminant hepatitis E has been seen in 10–20% of pregnant women, especially if the infection is acquired in the third trimester.

COMMON CLINICAL FEATURES OF ICTERIC HEPATITIS E

- Malaise (95–100%)
- Anorexia (66–100%)
- Abdominal pain (37–82%)
- Nausea, vomiting (29–100%)
- Fever (23–97%)
- Pruritus (14–59%)

Diagnostic methods

Serologic testing for evidence of acute HEV infection includes assays for both IgM and IgG anti-HEV. In clinical practice, the diagnosis of acute HEV infection is usually made by exclusion since many laboratories do not have diagnostic tests for HEV. Testing for anti-HEV should be considered in patients with typical signs of acute HAV infection who are IgM anti-HAV negative.[20]

Treatment and prevention

As in hepatitis A, management of acute HEV infection is largely symptomatic and supportive. Prevention of HEV infection requires the availability of clean water supplies. Travelers to endemic regions should avoid water or ice from uncertain origin and uncooked food. Immunoglobulins or monoclonal antibody preparations for passive immunoprophylaxis are not available for hepatitis E. Active immunization strategies are currently being developed.

Prognosis with and without treatment

In nonfatal cases, acute HEV infection is followed by complete recovery without the development of viral persistence. Whether protection from reinfection is life long is unclear.

DIFFERENTIAL DIAGNOSIS OF ACUTE VIRAL HEPATITIS

All other pathogens that can cause acute hepatitis can mimic acute viral hepatitis. Furthermore, as some acute viral infections present with jaundice, other reasons for cholestatic hepatitis (choledocholithiasis, PBC, PSC) have to be taken into consideration.

WHAT TO TELL PATIENTS

Patients should be informed about the nature of the disease, prevention, and postexposure strategies.

SOURCES OF INFORMATION FOR PATIENTS AND DOCTORS

http://www.gastro.org/clinicalRes/brochures/cvh.html

EFERENCES

1. Alter MJ, Mast EE. The epidemiology of viral hepatitis in the United States. Gastroenterol Clin North Am 1994; 23:437–455.
2. Melnick JL. History and epidemiology of hepatitis A virus. J Infect Dis 1995; 171 (Suppl 1): S2–8.
3. Feinstone SM, Kapikian AZ, Purcell RH. Hepatitis A: detection by immune electron microscopy of a viruslike antigen associated with acute illness. Science 1973; 182:1026–1028.
4. Ganem D, Prince AM. Hepatitis B virus infection: natural history and clinical consequences. N Engl J Med 2004; 350:1118–1129.
5. Alter MJ. Epidemiology and prevention of hepatitis B. Semin Liver Dis 2003; 23:39–46.
6. Chisari FV. Rous-Whipple Award Lecture. Viruses, immunity, and cancer: lessons from hepatitis B. Am J Pathol 2000; 156:1117–1132.
7. Thimme R, Wieland S, Steiger C et al. CD8(+) T cells mediate viral clearance and disease pathogenesis during acute hepatitis B virus infection. J Virol 2003; 77: 68–76.
8. Lok AS, Heathcote EJ, Hoofnagle JH. Management of hepatitis B: 2000 – summary of a workshop. Gastroenterology 2001; 120:1828–1853.
9. Lauer GM, Walker BD. Hepatitis C virus infection. N Engl J Med 2001; 345:41–52.
10. Reed KE, Rice CM. Overview of hepatitis C virus genome structure, polyprotein processing, and protein properties. Curr Top Microbiol Immunol 2000; 242:55–84.
11. Thimme R, Oldach D, Chang KM et al. Determinants of viral clearance and persistence during acute hepatitis C virus infection. J Exp Med 2001; 194:1395–1406.
12. Orland JR, Wright TL, Cooper S. Acute hepatitis C. Hepatology 2001; 33:321–327.
13. Jaeckel E, Cornberg M, Wedemeyer H et al. Treatment of acute hepatitis C with interferon alfa-2b. N Engl J Med 2001; 345:1452–1457.
14. Gerlach JT, Diepolder HM, Zachoval R et al. Acute hepatitis C: high rate of both spontaneous and treatment-induced viral clearance. Gastroenterology 2003; 125:80–88.
15. Rizzetto M, Canese MG, Arico S et al. Immunofluorescence detection of new antigen-antibody system (delta/anti-delta) associated to hepatitis B virus in liver and in serum of HBsAg carriers. Gut 1977; 18:997–1003.
16. Branch AD, Benenfeld BJ, Baroudy BM et al. An ultraviolet-sensitive RNA structural element in a viroid-like domain of the hepatitis delta virus. Science 1989; 243:649–652.
17. Lai MM. The molecular biology of hepatitis delta virus. Annu Rev Biochem 1995; 64: 259–286.
18. Negro F, Rizzetto M. Diagnosis of hepatitis delta virus infection. J Hepatol 1995; 22: 136–139.
19. Taylor JM. Hepatitis delta virus. Intervirology 1999; 42:173–178.
20. Mast EE, Krawczynski K. Hepatitis E: an overview. Annu Rev Med 1996; 47:257–266.

Chapter 82A

Chronic hepatitis B

Patrick Marcellin, Tarik Asselah, and Nathalie Boyer

KEY POINTS

- Therapy is aimed at reducing HVB replication and necroinflammatory activity, inducing HBeAg seroconversion and clearance of HBsAg
- Results of interferon-α and PEG-interferons are not optimal. Applicability is limited by side-effects
- Lamivudine is highly effective and safe, but limited by development of resistance. Adefovir dipivoxil is as effective and safe as lamivudine, but does not induce resistance
- Interferon-α + lamivudine is not superior to monotherapy

TABLE 82A.1 NUCLEOSIDE AND NUCLEOTIDE ANALOGS FOR THE TREATMENT OF CHRONIC HEPATITIS B

Drug	Status
Lamivudine	Approved
Adefovir dipivoxil	Approved
Entecavir	Phase III trial
Emtricitabine (FTC)	Phase III trial
Telbivudine (L-dT)	Phase III trial
Clevudine (L-FMAU)	Phase II trial
L-dC, L-dA	Phase I trial

FTC, fluorothiacytidine; L-dT; L-deoxythymidine; L-FMAU, 2-fluoro-5-methyl-β-L-arabinofuranosyluracil; L-dC, L-deoxycytidine; L-dA, L-deoxyadenosine.

NTRODUCTION

'he epidemiology, risk factors, and diagnosis of hepatitis B are escribed in Chapter 81; therefore, this chapter focuses mainly n the treatment of chronic hepatitis B.

Three agents are currently approved for the treatment of hronic hepatitis B: interferon-α (IFN-α), lamivudine, and defovir. Each agent has inherent limitations for use in the reatment of chronic hepatitis B.[1–3] Interferon is effective in a ninority of patients and has frequent side effects that limit its olerability.[4,5] The efficacy of lamivudine is limited by the emergence of drug-resistant hepatitis B virus (HBV) mutants, restricting its utility as a long-term therapy for chronic hepatitis B. defovir, which has been registered recently, induces an nhibition of viral replication, is well tolerated, and is associated vith a low incidence of resistance.

Lamivudine and adefovir have the advantages of oral administration and excellent safety profiles. However, they induce sustained response after withdrawal of therapy in only a ninority of patients and therefore the treatment needs to be dministered indefinitely in the majority of patients. As a esult, more effective therapy with more potent drugs used lone or in combination is needed and the treatment of hepatitis 3 remains an open issue.

After a brief summary of the natural history of chronic hepatitis B (including serologic diagnosis at each of the different hases), this review first summarizes the results obtained vith currently available treatments, IFN-α, lamivudine, and defovir. The second part of the review summarizes recent esults obtained with pegylated interferon, the combination f pegylated interferon with lamivudine, the combination of amivudine with adefovir, and newer antiviral agents such as ntecavir, emtricitabine, telbivudine and clevudine. Entecavir nd emtricitabine just achieved phase III clinical trials. The ther drugs are in early phase III or still in phase II clinical studies, and so the information available is limited (Table 82A.1).

NATURAL HISTORY OF CHRONIC HEPATITIS B

Chronic hepatitis can induce liver cirrhosis and hepatocellular carcinoma (HCC).[1–3] Chronic HBV infection is a dynamic process with an early replicative phase and active liver disease, and a late low or nonreplicative phase with remission of liver disease. Perinatally acquired HBV infection is characterized by a prolonged ‘immunotolerant’ phase with hepatitis B e antigen (HBeAg) positivity, high levels of serum HBV-DNA, normal levels of aminotransferases, minimal liver damage, and very low rates of spontaneous HBeAg clearance. Patients with childhood or adult acquired infection and chronic hepatitis B usually present in the ‘immunoactive’ phase with raised levels of aminotransferases and liver necroinflammation at histologic examination (HBeAg-positive chronic hepatitis). The rate of spontaneous HBeAg seroconversion may vary in relation to the degree of activity of the liver disease. Seroconversion from HBeAg to antibody to HBeAg (anti-HBe) marks the transition from chronic hepatitis to an inactive hepatitis B surface antigen (HBsAg) carrier state with low or undectable serum HBV-DNA and normal levels of aminotransferases, and confers a favourable long-term outcome with a very low risk of cirrhosis or HCC in the majority of patients. HBsAg clearance may occur at the rate of around 1% per year in chronically HBV-infected adults (resolved hepatitis B).

HBV-DNA persistence: However, about 20–30% of patients followed prospectively continue to have or redevelop high levels of HBV-DNA and active hepatitis despite HBeAg seroconversion. These patients usually have HBV variants unable

PHASES IN THE NATURAL HISTORY OF CHRONIC HEPATITIS B
• **Immunotolerant phase (in perinatally acquired hepatitis B)** Very high HBV-DNA, HBeAg positive, normal ALT level, minimal liver damage Low rate of spontaneous HBeAg clearance
• **Immunoactive phase** High HBV-DNA, HBeAg positive, raised ALT level, liver necroinflammation Variable rate of spontaneous HBeAg clearance
• **Inactive carrier state** Low or undetectable HBV-DNA, HBeAg negative, anti-HBe positive, normal ALT level May evolve to HBeAg-negative chronic hepatitis or to resolution of hepatitis B
• **HBeAg-negative chronic hepatitis** High HBV-DNA, HBeAg negative, anti-HBe positive, raised ALT level, liver necroinflammation Low rate of spontaneous disease remission
• **Resolved hepatitis B** Clearance of HBsAg

to express HBeAg (HBeAg-negative chronic hepatitis). HBeAg-negative chronic hepatitis represents a late phase in the natural history of chronic HBV infection and is associated with a low rate of spontaneous disease remission.

Cirrhosis: Longitudinal studies of patients with chronic hepatitis B indicate that, after diagnosis, the 5-year cumulative incidence of developing cirrhosis ranges from 8% to 20%. Morbidity and mortality rates in chronic hepatitis B are linked to the evolution to cirrhosis or HCC. The 5-year probability of survival is approximately 80–86% in patients with compensated cirrhosis. The 5-year cumulative incidence of cirrhosis decompensation is approximately 20%. Patients with decompensated cirrhosis have a poor prognosis (14–35% probability of survival at 5 years).

HCC: The incidence of HCC has increased worldwide and today it constitutes the fifth most common cancer, representing about 5% of all cancers worldwide.[1–3] The incidence of HCC appears to vary geographically and correlates with the underlying stage of liver disease. The risk of HCC is highest for patients with cirrhosis and usually arises in the setting of a compensated cirrhosis that may be clinically silent. The annual incidence in HBV carriers ranges between 0.2% and 0.6%, but reaches 2% once cirrhosis is established. The oncogenic mechanism leading to liver cancer involves different pathways that have not been fully elucidated. Prevention through universal vaccination has effectively decreased the incidence of liver cancer, and new therapeutic agents may delay or avoid the establishment of cirrhosis. The only chance for long-term survival after HCC diagnosis is to achieve early detection through regular surveillance by ultrasonography and alfa-fetoprotein (AFP) determination, which will allow effective therapy, such as surgical resection, liver transplantation, or percutaneous ablation, to be undertaken.

OBJECTIVES OF TREATMENT

The objective of treatment is to decrease HBV replication in order to decrease liver necroinflammation, thereby preventing the progression of fibrosis and the development of cirrhosis and its complications, including HCC, and thereby improving survival.

The response to treatment can be classified in three phases. Th first phase is characterized by a decrease in HBV replicatio reflected by a reduction in serum HBV-DNA levels; liver necroi flammation diminishes and fibrosis is stabilized or may eve regress, but the risk of reactivation persists. If the antiviral effe is sufficient (fewer than 100 000 copies of HBV-DNA per milliliter sustained, and accompanied by an effective immune respons with clearance of infected hepatocytes, loss of serum HBeAg wit appearance of anti-HBe antibodies (HBe seroconversion) ma occur, which marks a second phase, with a low risk of reactiva tion. If HBV replication is abolished (as reflected by the absenc of detectable HBV-DNA in the serum by sensitive assays), wit stable HBe seroconversion, a third phase characterized by los of detectable HBsAg (with or without the appearance of ant HBs) may occur, associated with complete disappearance o liver necroinflammation and no risk of reactivation.

PHASES IN THE RESPONSE TO THERAPY
• Decreased HBV replication
• HBeAg seroconversion (HBeAg negative, anti-HBe positive)
• Clearance of HBsAg (with or without appearance of anti-HBs)

CURRENT TREATMENTS

Interferon-α

IFN-α has been used in the treatment of chronic hepatitis B fo many years. It exerts an antiviral effect on infection with HB by two mechanisms. First, IFN-α has a direct antiviral effect b inhibiting synthesis of viral DNA and by activating antivira enzymes. Second, IFN-α exaggerates the cellular immune respons against hepatocytes infected with HBV by increasing the expres sion of class I histocompatibility antigens and by stimulating th activity of helper T lymphocytes and natural killer lymphocytes Thus, IFN-α induces an early decrease of HBV replicatio (reflected by a decrease in HBV-DNA serum levels) and a lat (about 2 months later) increase in aminotransferase levels.

Many controlled studies of IFN-α in patients with chroni hepatitis B have been reported, using various schedules. Th percentage of treated patients who achieve HBe seroconversio ranges from 11% to 79%. This discrepancy could be due, i part, to the different therapeutic schedules, but is mostly th result of the population of patients included in these trials. A number of factors are predictive of response to IFN-α. Lo serum HBV-DNA levels and high serum alanine aminotrans ferase (ALT) levels are the best predictors of response. Alsc the occurrence of infection with HBV at birth or early in th patient's life (as is often the case in countries where HB infection is hyperendemic, such as southeast Asia) is a facto associated with poor response to IFN-α. In white caucasia patients infected with HBV as adults, IFN-α induces HBe sero conversion in about one-third of cases. A dosage of 5 MU dail or 10 MU three times a week for 4–6 months, allows goo efficacy with a satisfactory tolerance.[3]

Lamivudine

Lamivudine, a nucleoside analog, directly inhibits HBV-DNA polymerase. Lamivudine was first developed as a revers

TREATMENT AND PREVENTION

AGENTS USED IN THE TREATMENT OF HEPATITIS B

APPROVED

- Interferon-α
  Sustained response in a low percentage of patients (seroconversion occurs in about a third of Caucasians who acquired infection as adults)
  Frequent side effects limit its tolerability
- Lamivudine
  Rarely leads to a sustained response, requiring indefinite treatment
  Well tolerated
  Efficacy of lamivudine is limited by the frequent emergence of drug-resistant HBV mutants, restricting its utility as a long-term therapy
- Adefovir
  Rarely leads to a sustained response, requiring indefinite treatment
  Well tolerated
  Associated with a low incidence of resistance

UNDER INVESTIGATION

- Pegylated interferon
  Seems to be more effective than standard interferon
- Combination of pegylated interferon and lamivudine
  Does not appear to be superior to pegylated interferon monotherapy
- Combination of lamivudine and adefovir
- Newer antiviral agents
  Entecavir
  Emtricitabine
  Telbivudine
  Clevudine

ranscriptase inhibitor for use in human immunodeficiency irus (HIV) infection. It also has activity against HBV at lower oncentrations. Randomized controlled trials have shown the fficacy of lamivudine in the treatment of patients with HBeAg-positive and HBeAg-negative chronic hepatitis B.

amivudine in HBeAg-positive chronic hepatitis B

One randomized placebo-controlled trial[6] showed that almost ll treated patients (98%) had a reduction of serum HBV-DNA evels. Serum HBV-DNA levels became undetectable (<0.7 mEq/ nL) in 44% of patients on lamivudine, compared with 16% of hose on placebo. At 1 year of treatment, HBe seroconversion ates were 17% versus 6%; normalization of serum ALT concentration was observed in 41% versus 7%, and histologic mprovement (decrease of at least two points in the Knodell core) occurred in 52% versus 23% of patients on lamivudine versus placebo, respectively. The rates of virologic, biochemical, and histologic response observed in three other randomized controlled trials showed similar results, with HBeAg seroconversion rates ranging from 17% to 21%.[6–9] The tolerability and safety of lamivudine are excellent; with an incidence of adverse events similar to that of placebo. Lamivudine therapy seems to be well tolerated for up to 5 years.

Resistance: The major drawback of lamivudine is the high ncidence of viral resistance related to mutations in the YMDD notif. Indeed, even when the HBeAg seroconversion rate is ncreased by continuing treatment, the frequency of resistance ncreases with time from 24% at 1 year to 38% at 2 years, 50% at 3 years, and 67% at 4 years.[1,3,10]

The emergence of lamivudine resistance is usually associated with moderate increases of HBV-DNA in the serum, and ALT levels that may remain lower than baseline for several months.[11] However, severe cases have been reported in patients with cirrhosis. In patients who develop lamivudine-resistant mutants, adefovir is effective and should be initiated rapidly if an increase in ALT levels is observed, especially in patients with cirrhosis who have a risk of hepatic decompensation. In order to diagnose the emergence of resistance earlier (before the appearance of detectable serum HBV-DNA by standard assays and before the increase in ALT concentration ensues), monitoring of serum HBV-DNA by a sensitive quantitative assay is useful. Indeed, an increase of serum HBV-DNA of 1 log generally reflects the appearance of a resistant mutant, and this allows a switch to adefovir several months before the increase of ALT levels.

In cases of HBe seroconversion, it is usually recommended that treatment be prolonged for 3–6 further months to decrease the risk of reactivation.[2,3] In the absence of HBe seroconversion, the usual recommendation is to continue treatment as long as HBV replication is suppressed and serum ALT levels remain normal, and until the appearance of viral resistance.

HBeAg-negative chronic hepatitis B

In patients with HBeAg-negative chronic hepatitis B, a randomized controlled study[12] showed an efficacy similar to that observed in patients with HBeAg-positive chronic hepatitis B with the same rate of resistance. HBV-DNA was undetectable (non-PCR-based assays) after 12 months of therapy in 90% of patients (70% with PCR-based assays). Serum ALT levels normalized in 75% of patients. A fall in HBV-DNA and normalization of ALT occurred in only 5% of patients on placebo. A histologic response was observed in 60% of treated patients. Predictors of response to lamivudine have not been established in this population. In patients with a virologic response at the end of a 12-month course of lamivudine, the sustained response rate 6 months after treatment was less than 5%.

The rate of resistance observed in patients with HBeAg-negative chronic hepatitis was similar to that observed in those with HBeAg-positive chronic hepatitis. Lamivudine-resistant mutants appeared in 10–40% of patients after 1 year of therapy, and in 50–60% of those treated continuously for 3 years.[13] As occurs in HBeAg-positive patients, the emergence of lamivudine-resistant mutant HBV was accompanied by an increase in HBV-DNA and, after a few months, by raised ALT levels. Flares occurred in 30% of patients, and were symptomatic or severe in some. As for HBeAg-positive patients, treatment with adefovir is generally effective in patients who develop lamivudine resistance.

Adefovir

Adefovir dipivoxil, the oral prodrug of adefovir, has been recently approved for the treatment of chronic hepatitis B. Adefovir is a nucleotide analog of adenosine monophosphate. In vivo, adefovir dipivoxil is converted to the parent compound, adefovir, and via two phosphorylation reactions to adefovir diphosphate, the active intracellular metabolite that interacts with HBV polymerase. Adefovir diphosphate acts as a competitive inhibitor and chain terminator of viral replication.

Two large randomized controlled trials have demonstrated that adefovir dipivoxil is effective in patients with HBeAg-positive or HBeAg-negative chronic hepatitis B. Also, it effectively suppresses lamivudine-resistant HBV in patients with chronic hepatitis B post-liver transplantation, in patients with compensated or decompensated liver disease, and in those patients coinfected with HIV.

HBeAg-positive chronic hepatitis B

A large randomized placebo-controlled study enrolled 515 patients randomized to receive adefovir dipivoxil 10 mg daily ($n=172$), adefovir 30 mg daily ($n=173$), or placebo ($n=170$) for 48 weeks.[14] The placebo and adefovir groups were similar at baseline. The antiviral activity of adefovir dipivoxil was demonstrated by a significant decrease in serum HBV-DNA levels, measured using a sensitive PCR assay. There was a rapid decrease in the median serum HBV-DNA level in patients treated with adefovir dipivoxil, and at week 48 the median change from baseline in serum HBV-DNA was significantly greater for adefovir 10 mg ($-3.5\log_{10}$) than for placebo ($-0.5\log_{10}$ copies/mL). Also, significantly more patients taking adefovir had undetectable serum HBV-DNA levels (<400 copies/mL) (21% versus 0%; $p<0.001$). After 48 weeks of treatment, HBeAg seroconversion was observed in 12% versus 6% ($p<0.05$), ALT normalization was achieved in 48% versus 16% ($p<0.001$), and histologic improvement (at least 2 points of the Knodell score) occurred in 53% versus 25% ($p<0.001$) of patients receiving adefovir 10 mg versus placebo, respectively.[15]

Histology: Results of the blinded ranked assessment of baseline and week 48 biopsies demonstrated that patients treated with adefovir 10 mg had a greater improvement in necroinflammatory activity ($p<0.001$) and fibrosis ($p<0.001$). Using the Ishak fibrosis score, fibrosis improved in 34% versus 19%, and fibrosis progressed in 11% versus 21%.[16]

The **tolerability and safety profile** of adefovir at a dose of 10 mg was similar to that of placebo. Adefovir at a dose of 30 mg was associated with an increased creatinine level in some patients. This increase was moderate, occurred after 24 weeks of treatment, and resolved in all cases after withdrawal of the drug. However, this observation led to the choosing and approval of the 10-mg dose as that with the best risk : benefit ratio.

Maintenance: The durability of the response after withdrawal of treatment is not well known because treatment was maintained according to the design of the trial. However, cessation of therapy in some patients without HBe seroconversion was associated with relapse. Therefore, maintenance therapy is recommended. Preliminary results suggest that the antiviral effect is maintained and that the rate of virologic response with HBe seroconversion increases with the duration of therapy.[14] However, a longer follow-up is planned (up to 5 years) in order to answer the questions of durability and of the possible increased efficacy of long-term treatment.

An extensive genotyping study has been carried out in all patients with detectable HBV-DNA (by PCR assay). Systematic sequencing did not show any cases of emergence of adefovir-resistant mutant HBV after 48 weeks of treatment with adefovir.[17]

HBeAg-negative chronic hepatitis B

A large randomized placebo-controlled study of adefovir dipivoxil has been performed in patients with HBeAg-negative chronic hepatitis B.[18] Patients were randomized in a 2 : 1 ratio to receiv either adefovir dipivoxil 10 mg ($n=123$) or placebo ($n=62$) fo 48 weeks. Adefovir 10 mg once daily resulted in a significa reduction in serum HBV-DNA levels at week 48 compare with placebo, with a median decrease of $3.9\log_{10}$ copies/m versus $1.3\log_{10}$ copies/mL ($p<0.001$). Some 51% of patien treated with adefovir dipivoxil had no detectable HBV-DNA a measured by PCR, compared with none in the placebo grou ($p<0.001$). ALT normalization was achieved in 72% versu 29% ($p<0.001$).

Histology: Significantly more patients in the adefovir grou had histologic improvement from baseline to week 48 compare with the placebo group (64% versus 33%; $p<0.001$). Blinde ranked assessment of baseline and week 48 biopsies showe significant differences between the adefovir and placebo group 80% versus 42% for necroinflammation ($p<0.001$), 48% versu 25% for fibrosis ($p<0.001$); fewer patients had worsening c fibrosis (4% versus 38%).

At 144 weeks of therapy with 10 mg adefovir daily, th antiviral effect was maintained with an excellent tolerabilit and without the occurrence of nephrotoxicity.[19] The incidence c resistance was very low (around 16%). It seems that the HB strains resistant to adefovir are sensitive to lamivudine.

NEW TREATMENTS

Pegylated interferon

More recently, the efficacy of interferon has improved with th replacement of standard interferon by interferon conjugate with polyethylene glycol (PEG-IFN). This new form of inter feron reduces elimination by the kidneys, thus significantl increasing the half-life and resulting in more stable plasm concentrations that last for 1 week. Moreover, pegylation reduce the immunogenicity of the protein (reduction of the produc tion of anti-IFN antibodies). Finally the number of injection has been reduced from thrice to once weekly, thanks to improve pharmacokinetics, which is obviously more comfortable fo the patient.

Two PEG-IFNs that differ in the quality and quantity o conjugated PEG to IFN have been produced: 12 kD of linea PEG for IFN-α2b and 40 kD ramified PEG for IFN-α2a. In both cases PEG-IFNs have been shown to be twice as effective overall than the corresponding nonpegylated interferons in chronic hepatitis C. Therefore, the efficacy of PEG-IFNs has been recently assessed in the treatment of chronic hepatitis B

The first randomized controlled study of PEG-IFN-α2a has been performed in patients with HBeAg-positive chronic hepa titis B.[20] Treatment duration and follow-up were each 24 weeks At the end of follow-up, loss of HBeAg was observed in 29–37% of patients receiving PEG-IFN-α2a (at a dose of 90 180, or 270 µg per week) versus 25% of patients who receivec standard IFN-α2a. Dose modification for adverse avents or laboratory abnormalities occurred in 22–30% of patients receiving PEG-IFN-α2a. This study strongly suggests that PEG IFN-α2a is at least as effective as standard IFN-α2a for the treatment of chronic hepatitis B. This study does not prove any superiority of PEG-IFN-α2a over standard IFN-α2a, because the dose of IFN-α2a used was relatively low (4.5 million unit three times a week) and the differences observed between the three PEG-IFN-α2a treatment groups and the standard IFN α2a were not significant. However, a retrospective analysi showed that the rates of response were higher with PEG-IFN among the most difficult to treat patients (with high HBV DNA level or low ALT levels). Side effects associated with PEG-IFN were comparable to those observed with standard interferon.

Combination of pegylated interferon with lamivudine

HBeAg-positive chronic hepatitis

In a large randomized controlled study, 307 patients with HBeAg-positive chronic hepatitis B received either the combination of PEG-IFN-α2b 100 μg per week with lamivudine 100 mg per day or PEG-IFN-α2b with placebo.[21] Treatment was given for 52 weeks. According to the protocol, the dose of PEG-IFN-α2b was reduced to 50 μg at week 32. About 80% of the patients completed the therapy on full dose. Approximately 10% of patients prematurely discontinued PEG-IFN, mainly between week 0 and week 32. Preliminary results showed a response rate (HBeAg loss) of 40% at the end of treatment, sustained at the end of follow-up. There was no difference in response rates between the two treatment groups. Major predictors of response were HBV genotype and pretreatment ALT level. The response rate was 60% for genotype A versus 42% for genotype B, 32% for genotype C, and 28% for genotype D. Response was 34% for those with ALT levels under three times the upper limit of normal and 50% for those with ALT levels more than five times the upper limit of normal. This study suggests that in patients with HBeAg-positive chronic hepatitis B, the combination of PEG-IFN-α2b with lamivudine (with the simultaneous regimen used) is not superior to PEG-IFN-α2b used as monotherapy.

HBeAg-negative chronic hepatitis

A phase III, partially double-blind, study has evaluated the efficacy and the safety of PEG-IFN-α2a alone or in combination with lamivudine versus lamivudine in patients with HBeAg-negative chronic hepatitis B.[22] Patients were randomized to one of the following treatments: (a) PEG-IFN-α2a 180 μg once weekly plus oral placebo once daily for 48 weeks; (b) PEG-IFN-α2a 180 μg once weekly plus lamivudine 100 mg once daily for 48 weeks; or (c) lamivudine 100 mg once daily for 48 weeks.

In total, 552 patients were enrolled in the study. At the end of the 24 weeks post-treatment follow-up, the two PEG-IFN treatment arms (with or without lamivudine) showed the same efficacy, which was superior to that observed in the lamivudine-alone treatment arm. Normal serum ALT levels were observed in 59%, 60%, and 44% of the patients respectively, and virologic response (serum HBV-DNA level less than 20 000 copies/mL) in 43%, 44%, and 29%. This study suggests that in patients with HbeAg-negative chronic hepatitis B the combination of PEG-IFN-α2a with lamivudine (with the simultaneous regimen used) is not superior to PEG-IFN-α2a used in monotherapy.

Combination of adefovir with lamivudine

The concept of improving the efficacy by combining two analogs is based on the hypothesis that the combination will maximize viral suppression and decrease the occurrence of viral resistance.

One randomized study evaluated the efficacy of the combination of adefovir with lamivudine, compared with lamivudine alone or adefovir alone in patients with lamivudine-resistant HBV.[15] There was no significant difference in serum HBV-DNA reduction or in the rate of ALT normalization between the adefovir–lamivudine combination group and the adefovir monotherapy group. Of note, serum HBV-DNA levels remained stable during the study in patients who remained on lamivudine monotherapy. Therefore, the clinical benefit of continuing lamivudine therapy once resistance has developed appears to be questionable.

Another study compared the efficacy of the combination of adefovir with lamivudine versus lamivudine alone in the treatment of naive patients.[16] There was no significant difference in response rates at the end of 1 year. However, there was a lower incidence of lamivudine resistance (2% versus 20%).

These two studies do not answer the question of the benefit of long-term treatment with the combination of adefovir and lamivudine in comparison to adefovir monotherapy. Large randomized controlled trials are needed to address this issue.

NEW ANTIVIRAL AGENTS

Entecavir

Entecavir, a cyclopentyl guanosine analog, is a potent inhibitor of HBV DNA polymerase, inhibiting both the priming and elongation steps of viral DNA replication. Entecavir is phosporylated to its triphosphate (the active compound) by cellular kinases. It is a selective inhibitor of HBV-DNA and is also effective against lamivudine-resistant mutants, but less effective than against wild-type HBV.

In a 24-week double-blind randomized trial, the safety and efficacy of entecavir in three different doses (0.01, 0.1, and 0.5 mg/day) was compared to that of lamivudine (100 mg daily). One hundred and sixty-nine patients were included.[23] Both the 0.1 and 0.5 mg/day doses of entecavir were superior to lamivudine in viral load reduction, as measured by PCR. A clear dose–response relationship was observed. Of patients treated with entecavir 0.5 mg, 84% had an HBV-DNA level below the lower limit of detection of the assay (0.7 mEq/mL) compared with 57% of patients treated with lamivudine and 62% of those treated with 0.1 mg entecavir. Entecavir was well tolerated at all doses; most adverse events were mild to moderate and transient, with no significant differences observed between the different doses of entecavir and lamivudine. This study indicates that the 0.5-mg dose of entecavir could be optimal. Phase III studies are currently evaluating the efficacy in comparison with lamivudine, and the safety of entecavir given for 48 weeks in HbeAg-positive and HbeAg-negative patients and in those with lamivudine-resistant HBV.

Emtricitabine

Emtricitabine (FTC; fluorothiacytidine) is a cytosine nucleoside analog with antiviral activity against both HBV and HIV. In a randomized double-blind study, 94 Asian patients (77 HBeAg-positive and 21 HBeAg-negative) were randomized to receive 25, 100, or 200 mg emtricitabine daily.[24] The median decreases in viral load were 2.6, 3.1, and 2.9 $\log_{10}$ copies/mL for the three doses, respectively. The proportions of patients with undetectable HBV-DNA at week 48 were 38%, 42%, and 61% for the three doses. At week 48, HBeAg loss was observed in 40% of the HBeAg-positive patients (ranging from 32% to 50% depending on the dose). The results of this study suggest that the optimal dose of emtricitabine is 200 mg once daily. Genotypic analysis performed at week 48 showed that 12% of patients treated with 100 mg emtricitabine and 6% of those treated with 200 mg developed drug-resistant HBV.

Phase III clinical trials are under way to determine the long-term safety and efficacy of emtricitabine. However, the role of emtricitabine as a monotherapy may be limited by its structural similarity to lamivudine, with the risk of development of drug resistance.

OTHER NUCLEOSIDE AND NUCLEOTIDE ANALOGS

Phase II studies assessed the safety and efficacy of several nucleoside or nucleotide analogs. Among them, tenofovir, a nucleotide analog, telbuvidine (L-dT; L-deoxythymidine), and clevudine are promising drugs whose preliminary studies indicated a potent antiviral effect on HBV and a satisfactory safety profile that need to be confirmed by phase III studies.[25]

SUMMARY

In recent years marked progress has been made in the treatment of chronic viral hepatitis. Preliminary results suggest that PEG-IFNs are at least as effective as standard interferon in the treatment of chronic hepatitis B. So far, the combination of PEG-IFN with lamivudine, used simultaneously, is disappointing in terms of short-term efficacy. However, long-term efficacy needs to be addressed and different schedules of combination (e.g., sequential) need to be evaluated.

A number of nucleoside analogs with favorable toxicity profiles and a promise of increased effectiveness against HBV are in various stages of clinical development. Results of phase III trials confirmed the efficacy of entecavir and emtricitabine, which will probably be approved in the near future for the treatment of chronic hepatitis B.

The future of chronic hepatitis B therapy seems to be in the combination of different drugs. Ideally, the optimal drugs to combine would meet the following criteria: they should have a potent antiviral effect and an excellent safety profile, and the duration of therapy should be limited. Indeed, the concept of combination therapy has been developed recently in order to increase efficacy and decrease the occurrence of viral resistance. However, so far there are few data available and no combination therapy has demonstrated a benefit compared with monotherapy. More potent drugs and new combinations together with the understanding of the mechanisms of resistance to therapy are challenges to improve the efficacy of treatment and decrease in the future the global burden related to chronic hepatitis B.

SOURCES OF INFORMATION FOR PATIENTS AND DOCTORS

http://www.gastro.org/clinicalRes/brochures/cvh.html

REFERENCES

1. Lok AS, Heathiste EJ, Hoofnagle JH. Management of hepatitis B: summary of a workshop. Gastroenterology 2001; 120:1828–1853.
2. Conjeevaram HS, Lok AS. Management of chronic hepatitis B. J Hepatol 2003; 38(Suppl 1):S90–S103.
3. EASL International Consensus Conference on Hepatitis B. Consensus statement. J Hepatol 2003; 38:533–540.
4. Hoofnagle JH, Di Bisceglie AM. The treatment of chronic viral hepatitis. N Engl J Med 1997; 226:347–356.
5. Wong DKH, Cheung AM, O'Rourke K, Naylor CD, Detsky AS, Heathcote J. Effect of alpha-interferon treatment in patients with hepatitis B e antigen-positive chronic hepatitis B. Ann Intern Med 1993; 119:312–323.
6. Dienstag JL, Schiff E, Wright T et al. for the US Lamivudine Investigator Group. Lamivudine as initial treatment for chronic hepatitis B in the United States. N Engl J Med 1999; 341:1256–1263.
7. Lai CL, Chien RW, Leung NWY et al. and the Asia Hepatitis Lamivudine Study Group. A one year trial of lamivudine for chronic hepatitis B. N Engl J Med 1998; 339:61–68.
8. Schalm SW, Heathcote J, Cianciara J et al. International Lamivudine Study Group. Lamivudine and alpha interferon combination treatment of patients with chronic hepatitis B infection: a randomised trial. Gut 2000; 46:562–568.
9. Schiff E, Karayalcin S, Grimm I et al. and the International Lamivudine Investigator Group. A placebo controlled study of lamivudine and interferon alpha 2b in patients with chronic hepatitis B who previously failed interferon therapy. Hepatology 1998; 28(Suppl):388 (Abstract).
10. Liaw YF, Leung NW, Chang TT et al. Effects of extended lamivudine therapy in Asian patients with chronic hepatitis B. Gastroenterology 2000; 119:172–180.
11. Zoulim F, Trépo C. Drug therapy for chronic hepatitis B: antiviral efficacy and influence of hepatitis B virus polymerase mutations on the outcome of therapy. J Hepatol 1998; 29:151–168.
12. Tassopoulos N, Volpes R, Pastore G et al. and the Lamivudine Precore Mutant Study Group. Efficacy of lamivudine in patients with hepatitis B e antigen-negative/hepatitis B virus DNA-positive (precore mutant) chronic hepatitis B. Hepatology 1999; 29:889–896.
13. Lau DT, Khokhar MF, Doo E et al. Long-term therapy of chronic hepatitis B with lamivudine. Hepatology 2000; 32:828–834.
14. Marcellin P, Chang TT, Lim SG et al. for the Adefovir Dipivoxil 437 Study Group. Adefovir dipivoxil for the treatment of hepatitis B e antigen-positive chronic hepatitis B. N Engl J Med 2003; 348:808–816.
15. Peters MG, Hann HW, Martin P et al. Adefovir dipivoxil alone and in combination with lamivudine in patients with lamivudine-resistant chronic hepatitis B. Gastroenterology 2004; 126:91–101.
16. Sung JJY, Lai JY, Zeuzme S et al. A randomised double-blind phase II study of lamivudine (LAM) compared to lamivudine plus adefovir dipivoxil (ADV) for treatment naïve patients with chronic hepatitis B (CHB): week 52 analysis. J Hepatol 2003; 38(Suppl 2): 69.
17. Yang H, Westland CE, Delaney WE et al. Resistance surveillance in chronic hepatitis B patients treated with adefovir dipivoxil for up to 60 weeks. Hepatology 2002; 36:464–473.
18. Hadziyannis SJ, Tassopoulos NC, Heathcote EJ et al. for the Adefovir Dipivoxil 438 Study Group. Adefovir dipivoxil for the treatment of hepatitis Be antigen-hepatitis B. N Engl J Med 2003; 348:800–807.
19. Hadziyannis S, Tassopoulos N, Chang TT. Three year study of adefovir dipiroxide (ADV) demonstrates sustained efficacy in presumed precore mutant chronic hepatitis B (CHB) patients in a long term safety and efficacy study (LTSES). J Hepatol 2004; 40: S17.
20. Cooksley G, Piratvisuth T, Lee SD et al. Peginterferon alpha 2a (40KD): an advance in the treatment of hepatitis B e antigen-positive chronic hepatitis B. J Viral Hepatol 2003; 10:298–305.
21. Janssen HLA, Sentruk H, Zeuzem S et al. Peginterferon alfa 2b and lamivudine combination therapy compared with peginterferon alfa 2b for chronic HbeAg-positive hepatitis B: a randomized controlled trial in 307 patients. Hepatology 2003; 38:1323.
22. Marcellin M, Lau G, Bonino F et al. for the Peginterferon alfa-2a HBeAg-negative Chronic Hepatitis B Study Group. N Engl J Med 2004; 351:1206-1207. N Engl J Med 2004; 351:1206–1207.
23. Lai CL, Rosmawati M, Lao J et al. Entecavir is superior to lamivudine in reducing HBV DNA in patients with chronic hepatitis B infection. Gastroenterology 2002; 123:1831–1838.
24. Leung N, Gish RG, Wang C et al. A randomized double-blind comparison of 3 doses of emtricitabine in patients with chronic hepatitis B given 48 weeks of treatment. Hepatology 2001; 34:349 (Abstract).
25. Marcellin P, Mommeja-Marin H, Sacks SL et al. A phase II dose-escalating trial of clavudine in patients with chronic hepatitis B. Hepatology 2004; 40:140–148.

Chapter 82B

Chronic viral hepatitis C

Xavier Forns and Jose M Sánchez-Tapias

KEY POINTS

- Hepatitis C virus (HCV) is an RNA virus of the Flaviviridae family that causes a persistent infection in around 3% of the world's population
- Diagnosis of HCV infection is based on the detection of antibodies against several HCV proteins (anti-HCV); in most cases, the presence of anti-HCV indicates active HCV replication, which is established by the detection of HCV RNA
- Chronic hepatitis caused by HCV has a very protracted course; after decades of infection some individuals will develop cirrhosis and hepatocellular carcinoma
- Acquisition of HCV infection at an older age, HIV, coinfection, and alcohol abuse are some of the factors associated with rapid disease progression
- Liver biopsy is the gold standard to establish the degree of liver damage caused by chronic HCV infection; although not essential, it is a useful element in treatment decisions

INTRODUCTION

The hepatitis C virus (HCV), a positive-strand RNA virus of the Flaviviridae family, is a major cause of chronic liver disease (CLD) worldwide. About 170 million people (3%) are chronically infected with HCV. The majority of persistently infected individuals develop chronic hepatitis and a significant proportion will develop liver cirrhosis or hepatocellular carcinoma (HCC). In the US, HCV is the main etiological agent of CLD, and HCV-related CLD causes about 10 000 deaths per year and is the leading cause of liver transplantation.

The viral genome encodes a polyprotein of approximately 3000 amino acids; the structural proteins (core, two glycoproteins (E1, E2)) constitute the amino-terminal third of the polyprotein whereas the nonstructural proteins constitute the carboxy-terminal part of the polyprotein (Fig. 82B.1). HCV exhibits extensive genetic heterogeneity and has been classified into six major genotypes and over 100 subtypes. In each infected individual, HCV circulates as a quasispecies, which is a mixture of closely related but distinct genomes. The viral genomes within a quasispecies typically differ by 1–2%. As in other RNA viruses, the lack of proofreading activity of the HCV-RNA-dependent RNA polymerase introduces errors during the replication process and explains the high genetic heterogeneity of HCV.

EPIDEMIOLOGY

The prevalence of HCV infection varies greatly throughout the world, from <0.5% of the population in the Scandinavian countries to >20% in Egypt. About three million people (1%) are infected in the US.

RISK FACTORS

Risk factors depend on HCV transmission mechanisms. Transmission through transfused contaminated blood or blood derivatives was an important mechanism for the spread of HCV. However, following screening with highly sensitive anti-HCV EIA tests, the risk of transfusion-related HCV transmission fell to about 1/100 000 donations. Recently, HCV-RNA determination in blood pools has reduced this risk to even lower rates (1/500 000 to 1/1 000 000 donations).

Intravenous illicit drugs: Their use remains an important mechanism of HCV transmission. Infection occurs mostly during the first year of drug abuse and 40–80% of addicts are chronically infected. Nasal inhalation of cocaine may also be an important risk factor, probably related to cannulae sharing.

Sexual transmission is uncommon but possible. Transmission may occur when genital ulcers, hematuria, or menstrual flux are present. Sexual promiscuity, either homo- or heterosexual, is associated with an increased prevalence of HCV infection. Preventive measures are recommended in the situations mentioned above, but not in individuals with stable partners.

Vertical or perinatal transmission occurs in about 5% of children born to infected mothers. Transmission correlates with the level of viremia and is higher (around 20%) when mothers are coinfected with the human immunodeficiency virus (HIV).

The mechanism of transmission is uncertain in a high proportion of infected individuals (10–50%, depending on the geographic area). This may be the case in individuals subjected to invasive medical procedures, surgery, or who have received therapeutic injections or vaccinations with inadequately sterilized material. The use of nondisposable material in the past and the less stringent medical practices may explain the higher prevalence of HCV infection of unknown origin in individuals over 60 years of age.

Hemodialysis: HCV transmission related to medical procedures (nosocomial transmission) was a great concern in hemodialysis units, but very strict adherence to universal precaution measures has virtually eradicated *de novo* HCV infection in this setting. Epidemics have also been described in conventional hospital wards for hematological patients and in patients undergoing endoscopic or other (even minimally) invasive procedures. Lack of observance of the universal rules or inadequate sterilization of instruments has consistently been related to HCV transmission in these circumstances. Transmission of HCV to healthcare workers through accidental needlesticks is uncommon,

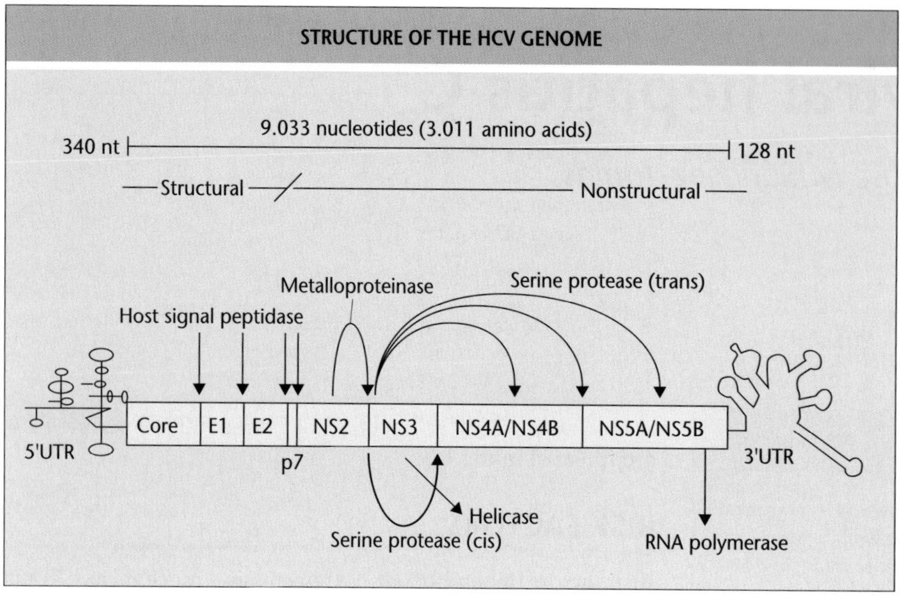

Fig. 82B.1 Structure of the HCV genome. Schematic representation of the structure and function of the HCV genome. UTR, untranslated region.

while transmission to a patient from an infected physician or nurse seems to be extremely rare.

RISK FACTORS

- Transmission of HCV trough blood products has been practically eliminated since the implementation of anti-HCV screening
- Intravenous drug abuse is the main mechanism of HCV transmission in the Western world
- Sexual transmission of HCV is uncommon in individuals with stable partners, but the risk increases with sexual promiscuity
- Perinatal transmission of HCV occurs mainly in cases of mothers with high HCV viral load or HIV coinfection
- Nosocomial HCV transmission should be considered in individuals with acute hepatitis C without other risk factors for HCV acquisition, who have undergone a healthcare-related procedure within the previous 3 months

PATHOGENESIS

The ability to cause chronic infection is a remarkable feature of HCV. Pathogenesis is largely unknown, but includes viral factors (genetic variability) and host factors (immune response). There is a strong and multispecific cellular immune response against HCV antigens in patients capable of clearing HCV, whereas cellular immunity against HCV appears to be weak in individuals who develop chronic infection.

The presence of replicative virions inside hepatocytes is the leading cause of liver damage, which possibly results from a combined immune-mediated attack against infected liver cells and a cytopathic effect of HCV itself.

PATHOLOGY

Liver biopsy findings vary from minimal portal inflammation with little or no fibrosis to significant necroinflammatory changes with expanding fibrosis and distorted hepatic architecture. Despite its morbidity and sampling error, liver biopsy still remains the gold standard to assess the degree of liver damage in chronic hepatitis C. Scoring systems aimed to evaluate separately the intensity of necroinflammatory changes (grading) and the extension of fibrosis (staging) in the liver have been described. Currently, there is an increasing interest in the development of noninvasive procedures to assess liver inflammation and fibrosis using biochemical markers and imaging techniques.

CLINICAL PRESENTATION

HCV infection ranges from asymptomatic hepatitis to severe forms of CLD, such as decompensated cirrhosis and HCC. HCV infection can also cause extrahepatic disorders, mostly through autoimmune mechanisms.

Acute hepatitis C

A silent course and a marked tendency to become chronic are prominent features of acute hepatitis C. In post-transfusional cases, the incubation period ranges from 2 to 26 weeks. In symptomatic patients, who represent about 25% of the cases, the clinical manifestations are usually mild and include fatigue, nonspecific digestive complaints, and, in some cases, jaundice. Severe forms of acute hepatitis are rare and HCV possibly does not cause fulminant hepatitis. In acute hepatitis C, the elevation of transaminases is usually less prominent than in hepatitis caused by other viruses.

Acute hepatitis C resolves spontaneously in 10–40% of cases. It must not be considered resolved until normal transaminase values and persistently negative HCV-RNA are documented for several months, as these markers often fluctuate during the acute phase. Chronic infection, as indicated by persistence of HCV-RNA in serum, may occur in some subjects with persistently normal ALT serum levels.

Chronic hepatitis and cirrhosis

Chronic hepatitis C is characterized by the persistence of elevated aminotransferase values and by the presence of HCV-RNA in serum. However, in some patients serum transaminases remain normal for long periods of time. These patients usually have mild hepatic disease.

Most patients are asymptomatic, but some of them complain ˈ nonspecific symptoms, such as an increased tendency to ɛcome fatigued or abdominal discomfort. Besides increased ninotransferases, other abnormalities may be seen, such elevated gamma-glutamyltranspeptidase, serum ferritin gammaglobulin, or a decreased platelet count. In general, .ese abnormalities are associated with more advanced sease.

Progression to cirrhosis is usually silent and is suspected the presence of a decreasing platelet count or inversion the aspartate aminotransferase/alanine aminotransferase ᴧST/ALT) ratio. In addition, ultrasonography abnormalities ıch as distortion of liver architecture, portal vein enlarge-ent, and splenomegaly should also suggest the presence cirrhosis. Patients with cirrhosis usually remain compen-ted for many years: after a 5-year follow-up time, hepatic ɛcompensation occurs in less than 20% and HCC develops around 7% of the patients. Coinfection with HIV or cohol consumption can accelerate the appearance of com-ications.

epatocellular carcinoma

ıe relationship between chronic HCV infection and HCC is ell established. The strength of this association in different ırts of the world is variable, probably due to differences in evalence of other carcinogenic factors. Pre-existing cirrhosis almost a *sine qua non* condition for the development of CC in chronic hepatitis C. The annual rate of appearance of CC in European patients with compensated cirrhosis is 3%, hich is lower than in Japanese patients. Male gender, age ver 55 years, and high alpha-fetoprotein (AFP) values are osely related to the appearance of HCC. Biannual abdominal trasonography and AFP are the preferred methods to screen ıtients with cirrhosis for early detection of HCC.

xtrahepatic manifestations

ɛveral extrahepatic disorders have been related to HCV fection (Table 82B.1). The association between HCV infec-on and mixed cryoglobulinemia is particularly evident, as dicated by the 90% prevalence of anti-HCV in patients with ixed cryoglobulinemia, the identification of HCV-RNA in the yoprecipitate and the good response, at least initially, to terferon (IFN) therapy. Cryoglobulins are detected in about)% of patients with chronic hepatitis C, but symptoms related cryoglobulinemia are relatively rare.

IAGNOSTIC METHODS

he diagnosis of hepatitis C is based on the detection of specific ıtibodies and on the detection of the viral genome.

nti-HCV testing

ighly sensitive and specific enzyme immunoassays (EIA) are vailable for the identification of antibodies against HCV ıtigens. Anti-HCV can be detected by EIA as soon as 3–6 eeks after infection and is useful in the diagnosis of acute ɛpatitis. Strongly positive reactions are found in patients with ıronic infection. False-negative results can occur in immuno-ıppressed patients (HIV infection, patients on hemodialysis), hereas false-positive results are rare (less than 5% in low-risk ɔpulations such as volunteer blood donors).

TABLE 82B.1 EXTRAHEPATIC MANIFESTATIONS OF HCV INFECTION

DOCUMENTED ASSOCIATION
- Cryoglobulinemia
- Membrane proliferative glomerulonephritis
- Serum autoantibodies
- Non-Hodgkin's lymphoma
- Porphyria cutanea tarda
- Lichen planus

PROBABLE OR COINCIDENTAL ASSOCIATION

Hematological
- Monoclonal gammopathies
- Idiopathic thrombocytopenia

Dermatological
- Erythema nodosum
- Erythema multiforme
- Urticaria
- Pruritus

Endocrine
- Autoimmune thyroiditis, thyroid autoantibodies
- Diabetes mellitus

Ocular and salivar
- Sjögren's syndrome
- Corneal ulcer, uveitis

Miscellaneous
- Idiopathic pulmonary fibrosis
- Systemic lupus erythematosus
- Guillain-Barré syndrome

HCV RNA detection

The presence of HCV RNA can be tested in serum, liver tissue, peripheral blood lymphocytes, or other specimens by molecular biology techniques. In clinical practice, the qualitative or quantitative determination of serum HCV-RNA is widely used.

For diagnostic purposes, the region amplified belongs to the well-conserved 5′ noncoding region of the viral genome. Commercial PCR kits are available for the qualitative and quantitative determination of HCV RNA using semiautomatic analyzers. These kits are reproducible and offer excellent sensitivity (around 100 IU/mL of HCV RNA). HCV-RNA viral load can be determined using fully automated competitive quantitative PCR-based assays, which have an acceptable linear range (10^2–10^7 IU/mL). Serum HCV RNA can also be quantified by signal-amplification through hybridization of amplified HCV-cDNA to branched DNA probes.

Qualitative determination of serum HCV RNA is required in different situations: anti-HCV-positive patients with normal ALT levels, patients with more than one potential cause of liver disease (i.e., hemochromatosis), CLD with autoimmune features, immunosuppressed individuals, or to evaluate the response to therapy. HCV-RNA quantification is useful (along with genotype determination) to define treatment schedules (see below) and to evaluate response to therapy.

HCV genotype

Direct sequencing of specific genomic regions is the gold standard for HCV genotyping. However, more simple techniques, such as hybridization of amplified HCV-cDNA on immobilized genotype-specific DNA probes, are reliable for clinical or epidemiological studies.

TREATMENT

The current treatment of hepatitis C is based on IFN-alfa and ribavirin, a nucleoside analog. According to the type of response, patients are classified as: sustained virological responders (SVR, normalization of ALT and clearance of HCV RNA that persists 6 months after treatment withdrawal); transient responders or relapsers (normalization of ALT and clearance of HCV RNA during treatment, followed by the reappearance of viral RNA and increase in ALT after treatment); and nonresponders (lack of normalization of ALT and persistence of HCV RNA during treatment).

Acute hepatitis

Since acute hepatitis C is a relatively rare disease, studies aimed to evaluate potential therapies have not been performed. As spontaneous resolution will occur in up to 40% of patients, the decision to offer therapy or not may be difficult. However, complete resolution was recently observed in 90% of patients treated with IFN monotherapy. The optimal treatment in terms of duration, dosing of IFN, and association with ribavirin is not well established. The administration of IFN-alfa (3 MU t.i.w. for 24 weeks), with or without ribavirin, starting 4–6 months after onset, is probably adequate. Presumably, treatment with pegylated IFN will be at least equally effective.

Chronic hepatitis

Treatment of chronic hepatitis C is an important health problem that has not been solved satisfactorily. The mid- and long-term prognosis of hepatitis C is not necessarily unfavorable and the current available therapies have numerous side effects and are very expensive. For these reasons, the decision to treat or not to treat may be difficult and must be taken on an individual basis. In general, therapy may be deferred in patients with mild chronic hepatitis and low probability of response. In contrast, treatment is indicated in patients with more advanced disease.

IFN and ribavirin

Two large trials including more than 1500 patients demonstrated the increased efficacy of the combination of IFN and ribavirin compared to IFN monotherapy. Using a treatment schedule of IFN-alfa (3 MU 3 times a week) associated with ribavirin (1000–1200 mg/day), the overall SVR rate was 41%, as compared with 16% in those treated with IFN-alfa monotherapy. Infection with genotype non-1, low viral load, young age, mild hepatic fibrosis, and female gender were associated with a more favorable response. Fig. 82B.2 shows the response rate observed in different subgroups of patients according to virological features at baseline.

Pegylated IFN (PEG-IFN) is a new pharmaceutical form of IFN, obtained through the binding of IFN-alfa to one or multiple polyethyleneglycol molecules, thereby delaying its clearance and increasing its efficacy. PEG-IFN administered once a week achieves a slow decline of IFN plasma levels, avoiding the extreme fluctuations that occur with the thrice weekly administration of non-pegylated IFN.

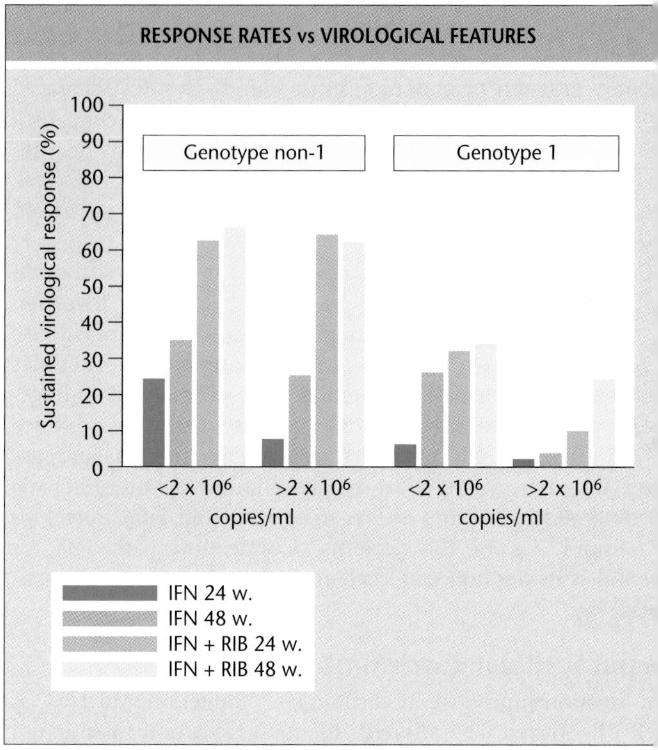

Fig. 82B.2 Response rates vs virological features. Sustained virological response rate observed in two large pivotal trials comparing IFN monotherapy and IFN plus ribavirin combination therapy, according to HCV genotype and viral load.[7,10]

Two large clinical trials have demonstrated that pegylate IFN monotherapy leads to a significantly greater SVR tha standard IFN monotherapy. Two large international multicente clinical trials have recently shown that PEG-IFN (either alfa 2 or alfa 2b) plus ribavirin increases the rate of SVR compare to standard IFN plus ribavirin (Tables 82B.2 and 82B.3). There fore, the standard treatment for chronic hepatitis C is current pegylated IFN plus ribavirin. SVR in patients infected wit HCV genotype 2 or 3 is greater than in those infected wit HCV genotype 1 or 4. Recently, another large controlled tri has shown that 48 weeks of combined therapy are necessar for optimal results in HVC-genotype 1 infected patients wherea 24 weeks of treatment with a reduced ribavirin dose is suff cient for optimal results in patients infected with HCV-genotyp 2 or 3 (Fig. 82B.3).

Side effects

IFN frequently causes unpleasant side effects (Table 82B.4 Young patients generally tolerate treatment better than olde individuals, although there is a marked individual variabilit of the incidence, type, and intensity of side effects. Severe sid effects are very uncommon, but they may be serious c irreversible.

The most significant side effect of ribavirin is hemolyti anemia, which is reversible and of variable severity but occu in the majority of patients. Dose reduction is often necessar because of significant anemia but ribavirin withdrawal is rarel needed. Ribavirin-induced hemolysis may be a concern whe planning therapy in patients with chronic anemia, such as thos on hemodialysis, or in patients with heart disease. Ribavirin i teratogenic and contraception is recommended to both me and women undergoing therapy.

TABLE 82B.2 RESPONSE RATE IN PEG-IFN vs STANDARD IFN THERAPY

herapy	Weeks on therapy	Number of cases	Virological response (%)		
			Overall	Genotype 1	Genotype 2 or 3
N α-2b (3 MU t.i.w.)	48				
bavirin (1–1.2 g/day)	48	505	47	34	79
EG-IFN α-2b					
1.5 µg/kg/week	4				
0.5 mg/kg/week	44				
bavirin (1–1.2 g/day)	48	514	47	33	80
EG-IFN α-2b	48				
.5 µg/kg/week)					
bavirin (0.8 g/day)	48	511	54	42	82

stained virological response rate observed in a large multicenter trial of interferon-ribavirin combination chronic hepatitis C. Standard α-2b interferon vs pegylated α-2b interferon were compared.[6]

TABLE 82B.3 RESPONSE RATE IN PEG-IFN vs STANDARD IFN THERAPY

herapy	Weeks on therapy	Number of cases	Virological response (%)		
			Overall	Genotype 1	Genotype 2 or 3
N α-2b (3 MU, t.i.w.)	48				
bavirin (1–1.2 g/day)	48	444	44	36	61
EG-IFN α-2a	48				
(180 µg/w)					
acebo	48	224	29	21	45
EG-IFN α-2a	48				
(180 µg/week)					
bavirin (1–1.2 g/day)	48	453	56	46	76

stained virological response rate observed in a large multicenter trial aimed to evaluate pegylated α-2a terferon as monotherapy or in combination with ribavirin in comparison with standard α-2b interferon us ribavirin combination therapy.[3]

TABLE 82B.4 SIDE EFFECTS OF THERAPY IN PATIENTS WITH CHRONIC HEPATITIS C

ELATED TO INTERFERON

ommon but usually mild

Flu-like symptoms: fever, headache, rigors, joint pain, muscle ache
Constitutional: tiredness, poor appetite, loss of weight, impotence
Neuropsychiatric: insomnia, mild depression, impaired concentration, irritability, bad mood
Digestive: nausea, diarrhea
Cutaneous: exanthema, loss of hair, reaction at injection site
Hematological: neutropenia, thrombocytopenia
Biochemical: hypertriglyceridemia

ncommon or rare but serious

Neuropsychiatric: major depression, suicidal ideation, psychosis, delirium, confusion, convulsions, ataxia, extrapiramidal alterations
Immunological: thyroid disease, psoriasis, sarcoidosis, interstitial pneumonitis, hemolytic anemia, exacerbation of other autoimmune disorders
Miscellaneous: retinopathy, bone marrow aplasia, diabetes mellitus

ELATED TO RIBAVIRIN

Hemolytic anemia, cough, digestive intolerance, hyperuricemia, potential teratogenicity

Treatment of patients relapsing or nonresponding to previous IFN monotherapy

In relapsers to IFN monotherapy, combination therapy for 24 weeks induces SVR in nearly one half of the patients. Response rate ranges from 100% among previous relapsers infected with non-1 HCV genotype and low viral load, to 25% among those infected with HCV genotype 1 and a high viral load. Presumably, relapsers to IFN and a less favorable virological profile may benefit from PEG-IFN plus ribavirin combination administered for 48 weeks, but large confirmatory studies have not been performed.

In IFN monotherapy nonresponders, the probability of responding to combination therapy is low, although those with a favorable virological profile may benefit from this combination. More aggressive therapeutic approaches are under evaluation.

Treatment of chronic hepatitis C in special situations

The indication of therapy in patients with persistently normal aminotransferases is unclear, since the risk of disease progression appears to be low in these cases. Response rates, however, are comparable to those achieved in patients with elevated aminotransferases.

RESPONSE RATES vs LENGTH OF THERAPY AND DOSING SCHEDULE

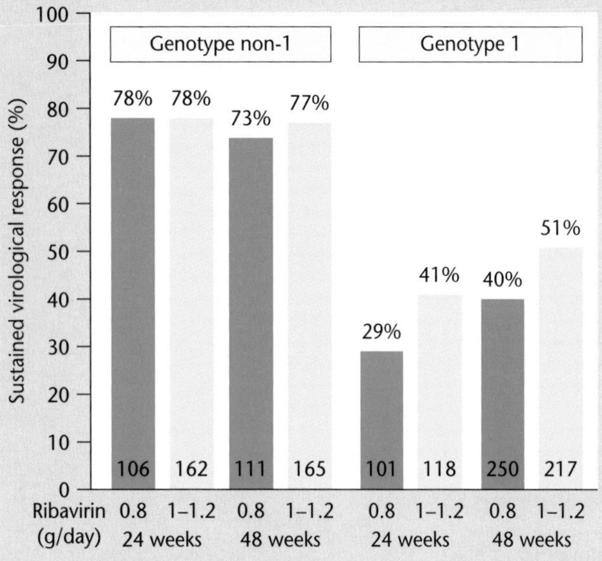

Fig. 82B.3 Sustained virological response rate to a weekly fixed dose of 180 μg of PEG-IFN α-2a in combination with variable doses of ribavirin, according to the length of therapy and HCV-genotype.[5] Number of patients in each treatment group is shown.

Treatment with PEG-IFN plus ribavirin achieves a sustained response in approximately one-third of the patients with compensated cirrhosis, but the rate of response is higher in patients infected with genotypes 2 and 3. Ongoing studies are aimed to assess the effects of long-term therapy on the outcome of cirrhosis.

Chronic hepatitis C follows an accelerated course in HIV-infected patients. An increase in mortality and morbidity from HCV-related liver disease is being recognized among coinfected patients, in whom HIV infection is under control following antiretroviral therapy. Treatment of hepatitis C in coinfected individuals can be administered following the same criteria established for HIV-negative patients. However, current data suggest that the efficacy of therapy appears to be lower and side effects are more frequent in coinfected individuals. In addition, drug toxicity requires close monitoring, particularly in individuals on antiretroviral therapy.

PROGNOSIS WITHOUT TREATMENT

Data on the natural history of HCV chronic infection are somewhat contradictory. Studies following patients from the onset of the infection suggested that HCV infection is a relatively benign disease. After 20 years of follow-up most patients

TREATMENT

- Acute hepatitis C resolves spontaneously in around 30–50% of infected individuals; treatment of the remaining individuals with interferon achieves more than 80% of sustained virological response
- In chronic hepatitis C, the best treatment regimen in patients infected with genotypes 2 and 3 is pegylated interferon plus ribaviri for 6 months (more than 80% of sustained viral clearance)
- In chronic hepatitis C, the best treatment regimen in patients infected with genotypes 1 and 4 is pegylated interferon plus ribaviri for 12 months (around 50% of sustained virological response)
- Patients with compensated cirrhosis can be treated with similar therapeutic regimens, but sustained virological response rates are slightly lower than those previously stated
- Analysis of large cohorts of patients treated with combination therap (interferon and ribavirin) indicates that sustained virological respons is associated with a significant improvement of necroinflammatory activity and liver fibrosis

remain asymptomatic and the incidence of clinically releva events (cirrhosis, hepatic decompensation, HCC) appears be low. In contrast, studies evaluating the long-term outcor of patients with already diagnosed chronic hepatitis sugg that after two decades of follow-up, a significant proportion patients (20–30%) develop cirrhosis. Most likely, these studi indicate that progression to cirrhosis is a late event, whi probably requires three, four, or more decades of persiste infection.

Fibrosis progression is not uniform in all patients, and f progressors (cirrhosis could develop in less than 20 years aft infection), intermediate progressors (cirrhosis could appe between 20–50 years after infection), and slow or minimal pr gressors (cirrhosis development could take more than 50 yea or could never occur) have been recognized. Factors that appe to be associated with fast progression of fibrosis are male gend older age at time of the infection, and alcohol consumpti (even in relatively small amounts).

WHAT TO TELL PATIENTS

Different sources of information for patients with chror hepatitis C are available. Websites from patient associatio and booklets edited by official organizations offer detail information on clinical aspects of the disease, life-style reco mendations, and treatment options.

SOURCES OF INFORMATION FOR PATIENTS AND DOCTORS

http://www.gastro.org/clinicalRes/brochures/cvh.html

EFERENCES

. Forns X, Purcell RH, Bukh J. Quasispecies in viral persistence and pathogenesis of hepatitis C virus. Trends Microbiol 1999; 7:402–410.
. Forns X, Bukh J. The molecular biology of hepatitis C virus. Genotypes and quasispecies. Clin Liver Dis 1999; 3:693–716, vii.
. Fried MW, Shiffman M, Reddy KR et al. Peginterferon alfa-2a plus ribavirin for chronic hepatitis C virus infection. N Engl J Med 2002; 347:975–382.
. Hoofnagle JH. Hepatitis C: the clinical spectrum of disease. Hepatology 1997; 26:15S–20S.
. Hadziyannis SJ, Sette H Jr, Morgan TR et al. PEGASYS International Study Group. Peginterferon-alpha2a and ribavirin combination therapy in chronic hepatitis C: a randomized study of treatment duration and ribavirin dose. Ann Intern Med 2004; 140:346–355.
. Manns MP, McHutchison JG, Gordon SC et al. Peginterferon alfa-2b plus ribavirin compared with interferon alfa-2b plus ribavirin for initial treatment of chronic hepatitis C: a randomised trial. Lancet 2001; 358:958–965.
7. McHutchison JG, Gordon SC, Schiff ER et al. Interferon alfa-2b alone or in combination with ribavirin as initial treatment for chronic hepatitis C. Hepatitis Interventional Therapy Group. N Engl J Med 1998; 339:1485–1492.
8. NIH Consensus Statement on Management of Hepatitis C:2002. Hepatology 2002; 5 (Suppl).
9. Pawlotsky JM. Molecular diagnosis of viral hepatitis. Gastroenterology 2002; 122: 1554–1568.
10. Poynard T, Marcellin P, Lee SS et al. Randomised trial of interferon alpha2b plus ribavirin for 48 weeks or for 24 weeks versus interferon alpha2b plus placebo for 48 weeks for treatment of chronic infection with hepatitis C virus. International Hepatitis Interventional Therapy Group (IHIT). Lancet 1998; 352: 1426–1432.
11. Seeff LB. Natural history of hepatitis C. Hepatology 1997; 26:21S–28S.

Further reading

McHutchison JG, Poynard T. Combination therapy with interferon plus ribavirin as initial treatment of chronic hepatitis C. Semin Liver Dis 1999; 19 (Suppl 1):57–66.

Chapter 82C

Chronic viral hepatitis D

Patrizia Farci and Maria Eliana Lai

KEY POINTS

- HDV is a unique defective virus that requires the obligatory helper function of HBV for its assembly and transmission
- HDV can be acquired by simultaneous coinfection with HBV or by superinfection of a chronic HBsAg carrier
- HDV is transmitted through the same routes as HBV; it has a worldwide distribution, although a significant decline in HDV prevalence has occurred in developed countries over the past decade
- HDV is a highly pathogenic virus that causes acute and chronic liver disease
- Chronic hepatitis D is the least common but most severe and rapidly progressive form of chronic viral hepatitis, leading to cirrhosis in 80% of cases within 5–10 years
- The clinical symptoms, the biochemical tests, and the histopathologic features of chronic hepatitis D are indistinguishable from those seen in the other forms of chronic viral hepatitis
- Definitive diagnosis of chronic hepatitis D is based on serological and virological testing specific for HDV
- Interferon-alfa is the only licensed drug of proven benefit for the treatment of chronic hepatitis D, although more than 50% of patients do not respond and side effects are common
- High doses of interferon-alfa for at least 1 year should be offered to all patients with well compensated chronic hepatitis D; liver transplantation is the only option for end-stage liver disease

INTRODUCTION

Chronic hepatitis D is a disease caused by persistent infection over 6 months) with hepatitis D virus (HDV),[1] a unique defective RNA virus that requires the obligatory helper function of hepatitis B virus (HBV) for its assembly and transmission. HDV is the smallest animal virus (1700 nucleotides) and the only one to possess a circular RNA genome and a single structural protein, hepatitis delta antigen (HDAg), that are encapsidated by the hepatitis B surface antigen (HBsAg).[2] Because of the obligatory link with HBV, infection with HDV occurs only in persons who simultaneously harbor HBV. There are essentially two modes of HDV infection: simultaneous coinfection with HBV or superinfection of an HBsAg carrier. Anti-HBs-positive individuals, being immune to HBV, are not susceptible to HDV. HDV is a highly pathogenic virus that causes acute and chronic liver disease. Chronic hepatitis D is the least common, but most severe form of viral hepatitis.

EPIDEMIOLOGY

Transmission

The routes of HDV transmission are the same as for HBV, i.e., primarily by parenteral exposure to blood or blood products, through the inapparent parenteral route involving nonsexual interpersonal contacts, as well as through the sexual route.

Geographic distribution

Infection with HDV has a worldwide distribution, although there is considerable geographic variation.[3] It has been estimated that 5% of HBsAg carriers are also coinfected with HDV, leading to a total of 15 million persons infected with HDV in the world. The prevalence is higher in South America, South Pacific islands, West Africa, the Mediterranean basin, the Middle East and Central Asia than in Northern Europe and North America, where the infection is mainly confined to intravenous drug users.

Over the past decade, there has been a significant decline in the prevalence of HDV in the Mediterranean area,[4] most likely due to implementation of universal HBV vaccination, together with improved socioeconomic and hygienic conditions, as well as universal precautions for the control of acquired immune deficiency syndrome. In parallel with this decline, however, new foci of HDV infection have emerged in other regions, including southeastern Russia, the Okinawa island, Northern India, and Albania.[2]

Three major genotypes have been identified, which differ in their global distribution. Genotype I is the most prevalent worldwide; genotype II is found predominantly in Eastern Asia, whereas genotype III has been identified only in South America.[3]

CAUSES, RISK FACTORS, DISEASE ASSOCIATIONS

The risk of HDV transmission in developed countries remains high mainly among intravenous drug users, whereas it has virtually disappeared among polytransfused subjects and hemophiliacs as a result of blood screening for HBV, use of viral inactivation procedures, and HBV vaccination campaigns. Molecular epidemiological studies have confirmed that promiscuous sexual activity, as well as nonsexual interpersonal contact, particularly among household contacts of chronically infected persons, represents other important risk factors especially in endemic areas.[2]

PATHOGENESIS AND PATHOLOGY

The mechanism whereby HDV infection induces liver damage remains poorly understood. There is controversy as to the relative roles played by direct pathogenic effects of HDV versus immune-mediated mechanisms.[2] Differences in pathogenicity could be related to biological differences among HDV genotypes. Genotype III was linked with outbreaks of fulminant hepatitis in South America, suggesting higher pathogenicity. However, genotype I is associated with a wide spectrum of disease severity,[2] including fulminant hepatitis, which argues against this hypothesis.

There are no histopathologic features that can differentiate chronic hepatitis D from the other types of chronic viral hepatitis, except that the former exibits more severe necroinflammatory lesions. The most characteristic feature is a marked intralobular infiltration and an eosinophilic degeneration of the hepatocytes.

CLINICAL PRESENTATION

Natural history

Since the HBsAg carrier state permits continuous replication of HDV, over 90% of HDV superinfected carriers develop acute hepatitis D that progresses to chronicity. Chronic hepatitis D is the most severe and rapidly progressive form of chronic viral hepatitis, leading to cirrhosis in about 80% of cases (in 15% within 1–2 years from the onset of acute hepatitis). Once established, HDV-associated cirrhosis may be a stable disease for many years, although the risk of mortality is twice and the risk of hepatocellular carcinoma three times that observed in patients with compensated HBV-associated cirrhosis alone.[5] The association of HDV with severe liver disease has been confirmed at all ages. However, the clinical spectrum of chronic hepatitis D varies widely.[6] In open populations in endemic areas, such as the Greek island of Rhodes, American Samoa, and the small Japanese island of Miyako, a high proportion of anti-HD positive individuals showed no signs of liver disease. Differences in disease outcome could be related to viral, host, or still undefined environmental factors. Studies of viral interaction have provided controversial data: whereas some reports suggested that in triple infection HDV inhibits both HBV and hepatitis C virus (HCV), others showed a dominant role of HCV. Coinfection with human immune deficiency virus does not seem to influence the natural history of chronic hepatitis D.

As a consequence of the dramatic decline in the incidence of HDV infection, the current clinical scenario of HDV-associated disease is changing. Occurrence of new, florid forms of hepatitis D is rare and advanced liver cirrhosis has become the dominant form. A paradigm example is the increasing prevalence of cirrhosis over the past two decades among patients with chronic hepatitis D in Italy.[7]

Clinical features

The clinical presentation of chronic hepatitis D is variable. It may be asymptomatic and discovered incidentally, or it may present with general symptoms such as fatigue, malaise, anorexia, right upper quadrant discomfort, or with complications of cirrhosis.[6] There are no specific clinical features, although half the patients report a previous episode of acute hepatitis, which likely represents the time of superinfection with HDV, and many exhibit splenomegaly.[2] Most patients are anti-HBe positive and, because HDV inhibits HBV replication, have no eviden or low levels of HBV DNA detected by polymerase chain rea tion (PCR). Chronic hepatitis D is associated with autoimmu manifestations, including in 13% of cases the presence of live kidney antibody microsomal type 3, directed against uridin diphosphate-glucuronyl-transferases.

DIFFERENTIAL DIAGNOSIS

The clinical symptoms, the biochemical markers, and the hist pathologic changes of chronic hepatitis D are indistinguishab from those observed in other forms of chronic viral hepatiti except for their tendency to be more severe. Thus, diagnosis chronic hepatitis D is based on serological and virological testin

DIAGNOSTIC METHODS

Diagnosis of chronic HDV infection is usually based on the find ing of HDAg in the liver and high titers of antibodies to HDA (anti-HD) in the serum. The direct detection of HDAg in th serum by conventional immunoassay during the chronic pha of infection is hampered by antigen sequestration in immur complexes with high-titered circulating antibodies. Chronic HD infection is associated with continuing synthesis of IgM ant HD, which provides prognostic information on the course of th infection: its persistence is associated with chronic active diseas whereas its disappearance predicts impending resolution.[2]

The introduction of PCR for the detection of HDV RNA ha provided the most sensitive tool for the diagnosis of HD infection and for monitoring the efficacy of antiviral agents.[6]

SURVIVAL UNTIL TRANSPLANTATION OR DEATH IN PATIENTS TREATED WITH INTERFERON

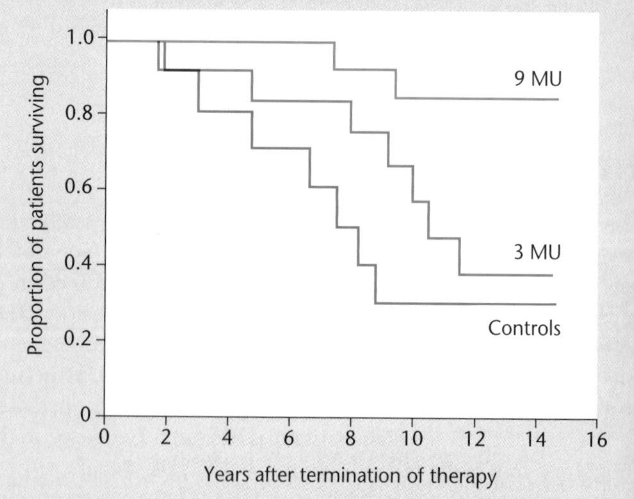

Fig. 82C.1 Survival until liver transplantation or death in interferon-treated patients. Cumulative survival until liver transplantation or death among patients treated with 9 MU of interferon or 3 MU and in untreated controls. Survival was significantly longer in the high-dose group than in controls (*P*=0.0027) or in the low-dose group (*P*=0.0190). Survival did not differ significantly between the low-dose group and the controls (*P*=0.3280) Reproduced with permission from Farci P et al. Long-term benefit of interferon alpha therapy of chronic hepatitis D: regression of advanced hepatic fibrosis. Gastroenterology 2004; 126(7):1740–1749.

REATMENT AND PREVENTION

eatment of chronic hepatitis D is not yet satisfactory. Several tiviral agents, such as acyclovir, famciclovir, ribavirin, and nivudine have been tried, but only interferon-alfa (IFN-alfa) s been shown to be beneficial.[8] Experience with combination erapy with lamivudine and IFN is limited, although prelimi-ry data are not promising. Results from trials using pegyl-ed IFN are not yet available.

IFN-alfa is the only licensed drug for the treatment of chronic patitis D. Its efficacy is related to the dose and duration of erapy. In one controlled trial, high doses of IFN (9 MU three nes weekly for 48 weeks) induced ALT normalization in % of patients at the end of treatment and in 50% after nonths of follow-up.[8] The biochemical response correlated th histologic improvement, whereas the effects on HDV NA were limited. The results of several studies confirmed that earance of HDV RNA occurs in less than 10% of treated patients, although individuals who clear HDV RNA may ultimately lose HBsAg as well.[9] In these studies, however, the efficacy of IFN was usually evaluated on the basis of the short-term biochemical and virological response.

The **long-term effects of IFN** in the natural history of chronic hepatitis D have only been investigated recently. High doses of IFN (9 MU three times weekly for 48 weeks) were found to significantly improve the long-term clinical outcome and survival of patients with chronic hepatitis D (Fig. 82C.1).[10] Remarkably, half the patients had a sustained biochemical response for up to 15 years of follow-up, which was associated with a significant improvement in hepatic function, loss of IgM anti-HD and sustained decrease in the levels of HDV replication, with subsequent clearance of HDV RNA and in some cases of HBV. The most dramatic finding was the absence of fibrosis in some patients with long-term biochemical response and an initial diagnosis of active cirrhosis (Fig. 82C.2).

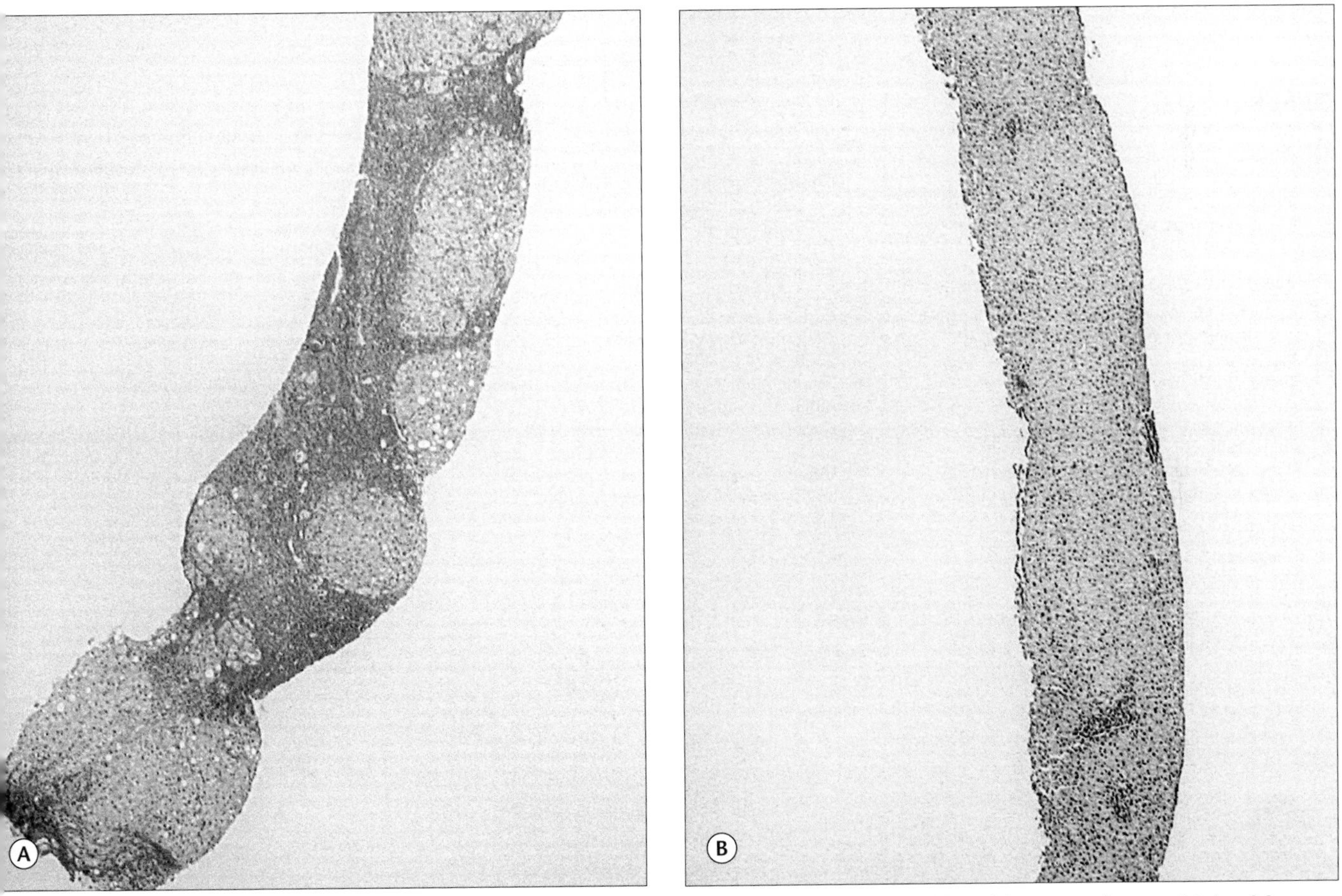

g. 82C.2 Liver biopsy specimens from a patient with chronic hepatitis D. Photomicrographs of liver biopsy specimens obtained from a atient with chronic hepatitis D before and 12.8 years after the completion of treatment with 9 MU of interferon alfa-2a. A. A specimen otained before treatment. An active micronodular cirrhosis with small nodules surrounded by wide fibrous septa is seen (picrosirius stain, x25). A specimen obtained from the same patient 12.8 years after the completion of therapy. Grade of activity and stage of fibrosis were established cording to the scoring system of Knodell. The intensity of the necroinflammatory lesions was measured by grade of activity, which comprised e sum of three scores, including interface hepatitis +/– bridging necrosis (0–10), lobular necrosis and inflammation (0–4), and portal flammation (0–4). Fibrosis was scored on a scale of 0–4, with 0 indicating absence of fibrosis, 1 fibrous portal expansion, 3 bridging fibrosis, nd 4 cirrhosis. Inflammatory activity and fibrosis can no longer be identified in the needle biopsy (picrosirius stain, x25). Serum HDV RNA, as easured by nested PCR, became undetectable 13 months prior to the last liver biopsy, and HBsAg 14 months after the last liver biopsy; all the ver enzymes were normal and the hepatic function was dramatically improved. At the time of the last liver biopsy there were no clinical atures of portal hypertension: there was no evidence of esophageal or gastric varices at endoscopy, the diameter of the portal vein and of the pleen were normal by ultrasound, and the platelet count was normal. Reproduced with permission from Farci P et al. Long-term benefit of terferon alpha therapy of chronic hepatitis D: regression of advanced hepatic fibrosis. Gastroenterology 2004; 126(7): 1740–1749.

Current recommendations

Based on data currently available, the best regimen for the treatment of chronic hepatitis D appears to be high doses of IFN-alfa (e.g., 9 MU three times weekly or 5 MU daily) taken for at least 1 year. In responders, therapy should be continued as long as possible, until HDV RNA and HBsAg are lost, based on individualized regimens in which the dose is titered according to serum ALT levels and tolerance. Therapy should be offered to all patients with well-compensated HDV liver disease. However, because side effects are common, medical monitoring is critical for the early detection and management of medical and psychiatric complications. Patients with end-stage HDV-liver disease should be considered for liver transplantation.[9] The risk of HDV reinfection of the graft is lower than that of ordinary HBV reinfection and can be prevented by the continuous administration of anti-HBs immunoglobulins.

Although IFN remains the only drug of proven benefit for chronic hepatitis D, about 50% of the patients do not respond. IFN seems to be ineffective in children. These limitations emphasize the need for improving the efficacy of IFN treatment, as well as for identifying innovative approaches and new, effective antivirals. Using a novel mouse model capable of suppo ing HDV replication, prenylation inhibitors were shown to highly effective in clearing HDV viremia, thereby opening n perspectives for the treatment of chronic hepatitis D.[11]

Prevention

Prevention of HDV infection can be achieved by active imm nization against HBV. However, there are currently no mea such as a specific HDV vaccine, of protecting over 300 milli global HBsAg carriers from HDV superinfection. Despite gre advances in understanding the molecular biology of HD much remains to be unraveled in order to devise more effe tive therapies and vaccines for the control of this unique vir which still represents a major challenge to both clinicians a virologists.

SOURCES OF INFORMATION FOR PATIENTS AND DOCTORS

http://www.gastro.org/clinicalRes/brochures/cvh.html

REFERENCES

1. Rizzetto M, Canese MG, Arico S et al. Immunofluorescence detection of new antigen-antibody system (delta/anti-delta) associated to hepatitis B virus in liver and in serum of HBsAg carriers. Gut 1977; 18:997–1003.
2. Rizzetto M, Smedile A. Hepatitis D. In: Schiff E, Sorrell M, Maddrey W, eds. Diseases of the liver. Lippincott Williams and Wilkins; 2002: 863–875.
3. Casey JL, Brown TL, Colan EJ et al. A genotype of hepatitis D virus that occurs in northern South America. Proc Natl Acad Sci USA 1993; 90:9016–9020. [First identification of the three major HDV genotypes and association of genotype III with a severe form of acute hepatitis in South America.]
4. Gaeta GB, Stroffolini T, Chiaramonte M et al. Chronic hepatitis D: a vanishing disease? An Italian multicenter study. Hepatology 2000; 32:824–827.
5. Fattovich G, Giustina G, Christensen E et al. Influence of hepatitis delta virus infection on morbidity and mortality in compensated cirrhosis type B. The European Concerted Action on Viral Hepatitis (Eurohep). Gut 2000; 46:420–426.
6. Farci P. Delta hepatitis: an update. J Hepatol 2003; 39 (Suppl 1):S212–S219. [A recent comprehensive review of hepatitis D.]
7. Rosina F, Conoscitore P, Cuppone R et al. Changing pattern of chronic hepatitis D in Southern Europe. Gastroenterology 1999; 117:161–166.
8. Farci P, Mandas A, Coiana A et al. Treatmen of chronic hepatitis D with interferon alfa-2 N Engl J Med 1994; 330:88–94.
9. Rizzetto M, Rosina F. Treatment of hepatitis D. In: Zuckerman AJ, Thomas HC, eds. Viral hepatitis. 2nd edn. Edinburgh: Churchill Livingstone; 1997: 387–393.
10. Farci P, Roskams T, Chessa L et al. Long-ter benefit of interferon alpha therapy of chron hepatitis D: regression of advanced hepatic fibrosis. Gastroenterology 2004; 126(7): 1740–1749.
11. Bordier BB, Ohkanda J, Liu P et al. In vivo antiviral efficacy of prenylation inhibitors against hepatitis delta virus. J Clin Invest 2003; 112:407–414.

Chapter 83

Liver parasites

The editors

KEY POINTS
• Infection by liver flukes predisposes to cholangiocarcinoma • Schistosomiasis and kala azar are associated with granuloma liver disease • The gastrointestinal tract is the principal site of nematode infection • Hydatid cysts cause a spectrum of effects, from asymptomatic to fatal anaphylaxis due to rupture • Amebiasis is a cause of bloody diarrhea • The liver is commonly involved in malaria infection, but liver failure is rare

The liver may be parasitized by helminths or protozoa, some of which also infest the gut (see Chapter 52).

TREMATODES

Amongst helminths, trematodes (flukes) are a major cause of specific liver disease (Table 83.1). Granulomatous reaction to eggs in the liver causes fibrosis with two schistosomal species, *Schistosoma hematobium* and *S. japonica*. In the case of liver flukes (*Fasciola*, *Chlonorchis*, and *Opisthorchis*; Table 83.1), liver infection is via the biliary system where inflammatory responses cause acute febrile illnesses with jaundice; long-term infection is a major cause of cholangiocarcinoma. The liver can also be involved during infection with the lung fluke *Paragonimus*.

NEMATODES

The gut is the principal site of nematode infection, although infection may occur via the skin and is usually established by

TABLE 83.1 TREMATODES (FLUKES) AFFECTING THE LIVER

	Blood flukes *Schistosoma*	*Fasciola hepatica*	**Liver flukes** *Chlonorchis siniensis*	*Opisthorchis*
Definitive host	Human	Sheep (humans)	Humans	Humans, cats, dogs
Intermediate host	Snail	Snail	Freshwater fish	Freshwater fish
Geography	*S. mansoniae:* Africa, Middle East *S. japonica:* Far East	Worldwide	China, Japan, Korea, Vietnam	Poland, Russia (*O. felineus*) Thailand (*O. viverrini*)
Mode of acquisition	Water: skin	Eating contaminated plants (e.g., watercress)	Eating raw or pickled fish	Eating raw or pickled fish
Site infestation	Mesenteric veins	Biliary radicals	Biliary system	Biliary system
Liver pathology	Granulomatous reaction to eggs in portal radicals	Inflammatory response to biliary worms	Inflammatory or fibrotic response to biliary worms	Inflammatory or fibrotic response to biliary worms
Liver: clinical	Chronic: fibrosis causing portal hypertension Hepatoma, especially with hepatitis B co-infection	Acute: fever, hepatomegaly, eosinophilia ± jaundice	Acute: fever, hepatomegaly, eosinophilia, jaundice Cholangitis Cholangiocarcinoma	Acute: fever, hepatomegaly, eosinophilia, jaundice Cholangitis Cholangiocarcinoma (*O. viverrini*)
Diagnosis	Fecal eggs CIEP, ELISA	CIEP, ELISA	Fecal eggs ELISA	Fecal eggs ELISA
Treatment	Praziquantel Oxamniquine	Bithionol Dehydroemetine Not praziquantel	Praziquantel	Praziquantel
Additional comments	*S. haematobium* (Africa, South America, Caribbean): urinary schistosomiasis			

CIEP, counter-current immunoelectrophoresis; ELISA, enzyme-linked immunosorbent assay.

a complex process of migration (Table 83.2). Nematodes may migrate secondarily into the biliary tree, causing jaundice or hepatomegaly.

CESTODE INFECTION – ECHINOCOCCOSIS

Ingestion of foods contaminated with dog feces containing granular cysts can result in the development of hydatid cysts in the liver (70%), lungs, or other sites (Table 83.3). Cysts are often asymptomatic or cause pressure symptoms; rupture may lead to severe anaphylactic shock and death. Treatment is with albendazole and surgery may be necessary.

PROTOZOAL INFESTATIONS

Kala azar is a chronic granulomatous infection of the liver cause by *Leishmania donovani* (Table 83.4). It is characterized b progress hepatosplenomegaly and treated by pentavalent ant monial agents. *Entamoeba histolytica* causes human amoebiasi most commonly characterized by diarrhea, which may be blood The liver can be involved with an amebic abscess. Metronidazol (or tinidazole) is the drug of choice for amebic abscess, bu diloxanide furoate should also be given to clear enteric infectio

Malaria is an acute multisystem disorder – jaundice and/c liver involvement is frequent. Amongst the consequences c

TABLE 83.2 NEMATODES AFFECTING THE LIVER

	Ascaris lumbricoides	*Toxocara canis and cati*	*Strongyloides stercoralis*
Definitive host	Humans	Dogs and cats	Humans
Intermediate host	None	None	Larvae develop in soil
Geography	Worldwide	Worldwide	(Sub)tropics, south-east Europe, USA
Mode of acquisition	Eating contaminated vegetables	Contamination from definitive host	Skin penetration
Site infestation	Intestine → liver → lungs → intestine → feces	Intestine, then liver, brain, and eye by migration	Skin → lungs → intestine → feces
Liver pathology	May migrate into biliary tree	Invasion provokes hemorrhage, necrosis, granuloma and eosinophilia	Immunosuppressed patients → hyperinfestation → multiple organs including liver
Liver: clinical	Obstructive jaundice, cholangitis, abscess	Tender hepatomegaly	Jaundice
Other clinical features	Acute-phase reaction, cough, wheeze, dyspnea, intestinal obstruction	Acute-phase reaction, larva migrans, visual disturbance, encephalitis, convulsions	Itch, low-grade fever, cough, wheeze, diarrhea, eosinophilia
Diagnosis	Eggs in feces Ultrasonography: bile duct worms	Larvae in tissues (liver biopsy) ELISA	Larvae in feces, intestinal aspirate or biosy CIEP, ELISA
Treatment	Mebendazole Pyrantel pamoate Levamisole	Diethylcarbamazine Thiabendazole Albendazole	Albendazole

CIEP, counter-current immunoelectrophoresis; ELISA, enzyme-linked immunosorbent assay.

TABLE 83.3 CESTODES: *ECHINOCOCCUS*

Organism	*Echinococcus granulosus* (tapeworm)
Reservoir	Dog (definitive host), sheep, pigs, etc. (intermediate hosts)
Vector	Feco-oral (dogs to humans)
Geography	South America, southern Africa, Australasia, Mediterranean, Iceland, Alaska, northern Europe
Mode of acquisition	Human = accidental intermediate host (contaminated dog feces)
Site infestation	Liver, lung, brain
Liver pathology	Compression IVC, HPV, hepatic veins, insidious liver dysfunction, cholangitis
Other clinical features	Small cyst leaks: flushing, urticaria; major rupture: anaphylaxis
Diagnosis	US, CT liver, CXR, ELISA.
Treatment	Albendazole, mebendazole

ELISA, enzyme-linked immunosorbent assay.

TABLE 83.4 PROTOZOA INVOLVING THE LIVER

	Kala azar	Amebic abscess	Malaria
Organism	*Leishmania donovani*	*Entamoeba histolytica*	*Plasmodium falciparum, P. vivax, P. ovale, P. malariae*
Reservoir	Small mammals, dogs (humans)	Humans	Humans
Vector	Sandfly	Feco-oral	Mosquitos
Geography	Mediterranean, north-east Africa, Indian subcontinent, China	Worldwide, especially (sub)tropics	(Sub)tropics
Mode of acquisition	Sandfly bite	Feco-oral	Mosquito bite
Site infestation	Mononuclear phagocytes	Colon	→ Hepatocytes → red cells → hepatoctes (*P. vivax* and *P. ovale*)
Liver pathology	Parasitized Kupffer cells proliferate, form granulomas. Extracellular PAS-positive material	Nonpurulent abscess	Mononuclear infiltrate, Kupffer cell hyperplasia, sinusoidal dilatation
Liver: clinical	Progressive hepatosplenomegaly Hepatocellular jaundice if severe	Mass, fever, rupture	Hemolysis → jaundice; tender liver; cholestasis; blackwater fever; hypoglycemia; liver failure rare
Other clinical features	Acute fever, black skin Pancytopenia	Bloody diarrhea	Fever, headache, coma, pulmonary edema, diarrhea, hypoglycemia, lactic acidosis, dysrhythmias
Diagnosis	IFAT, ELISA, DNA probes, skin test. Giemsa stain of spleen smears or liver biopsy sample	CIEP, ultrasonography, computed tomography	Thin- and thick-film blood microscopy
Treatment	Pentavalent antimonials ± interferon-γ or allopurinol Pentamidine, amphotericin, paromomycin	Metronidazole or tinidazole (or (dehydro)emetine), followed by diloxanide furoate	*P. malariae:* chloroquine *P. vivax* and *P. ovale:* chloroquine, then primaquine *P. falciparum:* quinine, Malarone or Riamet, then Fansidar or doxycycline
Additional comments		Some add chloroquine to metronidazole Aspirate abscess if imminent rupture or no response	Malarone contains proguanil + atovaquone Riamet contains artemether + lumefantrine (parenteral artemether and atesunate are also available on a named patient basis in the UK) Fansidar contains pyrimethamine + sulfadoxine

CIEP, counter-current immunoelectrophoresis; ELISA, enzyme-linked immunosorbent assay; IFAT, immunofluorescent antibody technique; PAS, periodic acid–Schiff (stain).

liver involvement is the development of hypoglycemia. Treatment and prophylaxis are complicated, and dependent upon the species involved and local patterns of resistance. The main drugs for treatment are shown in Table 83.4. Most countries maintain up-to-date advice services for travelers on optimal prophylaxis.

SOURCES OF INFORMATION FOR PATIENTS AND DOCTORS

http://cchs-dl.slis.ua.edu/patientinfo/infectious/byorganism/parasitic/schistosomiasis.htm

Chapter 84

Bacterial and fungal infections of the liver

Alexander Gimson

KEY POINTS
Liver dysfunction may arise due to direct infection or inflammatory mediators The liver plays a major role in the host's response to infection The predominant histologic abnormality is canalicular cholestasis and/or focal hepatocyte fat droplets in periportal cell infiltrates • TNF-alpha, IL-1, IL-6, bacterial lipopolysaccharides, and endotoxin inhibit bile sort export protein • Investigation includes ultrasound and appropriate cultures

NTRODUCTION

. wide range of bacterial, protozoal, and fungal infections ay cause liver dysfunction. This dysfunction may be effected directly, consequent on production during the septic process f various mediators and cytokines, or by direct parenchymal r biliary invasion. This chapter will not consider further other arasitic infections (see Chapter 52), bacterial abscesses within e liver (see Chapter 117), or spontaneous bacterial peritonitis cirrhosis (see Chapter 98).

The liver plays a major role in modulating the host's response) sepsis, and for this reason prior impairment of liver meta-olic function due to chronic liver disease, alcohol use, or drugs ltering splanchnic hemodynamics may alter the adequacy of is response and the body's ability to respond successfully) a septic challenge. The liver constitutes a major component f the host's innate immune system elaborating complement, oluble and membrane-bound recognition receptors, cells of e monocyte/macrophage lineage of which Kupffer cells con-titute a large majority, and various cytokines (tumor necrosis actor-α (TNF), interleukin 1 (IL1), IL6, IL12, and IL18). The roducts of the initial contact between host immune effector ells and an invading organism also release various active medi-tors that modulate hepatocellular intermediary metabolism.

HEPATIC DYSFUNCTION DURING SEPSIS

Epidemiology

Abnormal liver blood tests have been described in a wide range of septic scenarios, ranging from isolated intra-abdominal bscess to lobar pneumonia or bacteremia (Table 84.1). It may ccur in up to 10% of cases with community acquired pneu-nonia, 35% of those with positive blood cultures,[1] and is a niversal finding in some series with septicemic shock. It is robably more common in neonates and infants less than 1 year of age who have a low bile salt independent bile flow, than in adults, but does not otherwise relate to age, gender, organism isolated, nutritional state, or site of sepsis.

TABLE 84.1 CLINICAL SYNDROMES OF SEPSIS ASSOCIATED WITH LIVER DYSFUNCTION

Lobar pneumonia
Bacteremia
Multiple organ failure syndrome (even in absence of sepsis)
Related to specific organisms
Toxic shock syndrome

Pathogenesis

The predominant histological abnormality in all these cases is a canalicular cholestasis, occasionally with focal hepatocyte fat droplets and periportal cell infiltrates. In most series, there is a disproportionately high bilirubin compared to minor changes in aminotransferases and alkaline phosphatase. These changes are consequent on release of a range of inflammatory mediators during the septic process. TNF-α, IL1, IL8, and activated complement (C5a) may all induce leukostasis within sinusoids and enhanced adherence to hepatic endothelial lining cells. Subsequent transmigration and adherence to parenchymal hepatic cells can result in cytotoxicity. Endothelin-1 can activate both Kupffer and Ito cells with myofibroblast transformation, sinusoidal constriction, and heterogeneity of liver blood flow, effects which nitric oxide attempts to reverse. Most importantly, TNF-α, IL1, and IL6 as well as bacterial lipopolysaccharide and endotoxin result in inhibition of specific bile salt export protein on the canalicular membrane and the sodium-dependent Na taurocholate co-transporting polypeptide on the basolateral membrane.[2] Organic anion transport is also impaired, resulting in impaired bile salt and bilirubin uptake from sinusoids and clearance into a canaliculus.

Clinical presentation

In a minority of cases, jaundice is the initial presenting feature along with fever, rigors, and confusion. More commonly abnormal liver blood tests appear after 24–48h. The source of the sepsis may be clinically apparent or only revealed after specific cultures are obtained. A wide range of organisms has been associated with abnormal liver blood tests, both Gram-positive and Gram-negative (Table 84.2). The presence of abnormal liver blood tests is not an independent adverse risk factor for survival (Table 84.3)

TABLE 84.2 BACTEREMIC MICROORGANISMS ASSOCIATED WITH JAUNDICE OF SEPSIS

Escherichia coli
Klebsiella
Pseudomonas aeruginosa
Salmonella
Bacteroides
Clostridium perfringens
Staphylococcus aureus
Streptococcus pneumoniae

TABLE 84.3 DIFFERENTIAL DIAGNOSIS OF ABNORMAL LIVER BLOOD TEST

Cholestasis of sepsis, lobar pneumonia, bacteremia
Adult respiratory distress syndrome; multiple organ failure syndrome
Related to infection by specific microbiological organisms (see Table 84.4)
Drug hepatotoxicity or parenteral nutrition-induced changes
Biliary obstruction
Postcardiopulmonary bypass (postpump jaundice)
Ischemic hepatopathy following shock/splanchnic hypoperfusion
Hepatosplenic candidiasis
De novo acute liver disease
Exacerbations of chronic liver disease

Investigation and treatment

Liver blood test abnormalities occurring in the scenarios shown in Table 84.1 should initially be investigated with an abdominal ultrasound scan. This may reveal evidence of prior chronic liver disease and portal hypertension, biliary obstruction, or focal septic fluid collections. Sets of blood cultures as well as sputum, urine, and, where appropriate, stool cultures are crucial. Where sepsis is suspected early treatment with broad spectrum antibiotics are indicated, even before culture results are available, as early therapy is important.

Prognosis

During lobar pneumonia and bacteremia the presence of jaundice or abnormal liver blood tests is not associated with an adverse prognosis.[1] In the adult, respiratory distress syndrome abnormal liver blood tests constitute one organ failure and the total number of organ failures accurately predicts mortality. Hepatic dysfunction is a component of scoring systems that predict mortality (APACHE II, SOFA).

DIRECT HEPATIC INVOLVEMENT WITH SPECIFIC MICROORGANISMS

A range of bacteria may directly infect the liver. Hepatic involvement is common with these organisms (Table 84.4), although the extent of the resulting dysfunction is highly variable depending on the host response. Mechanisms of liver dysfunction may occur through both indirect mechanisms (often cytokine-mediated changes) as well as by direct infection of parenchymal or Kuppfer cells.[3] Some patients may rarely progress to larger abscess formation; this is dealt with in Chapter 117. Hepatic dysfunction may also occur with bo *Coxiella burnetti* and *Rickettsia rickettsii* (Rocky Mount spotted fever) infection, both Gram-negative obligate int cellular organisms. *Coxiella* causes a granulomatous hepati and *Rickettsia* a portal tract lymphocytic infiltration.

MYCOBACTERIAL INFECTIONS WITHIN THE LIVER

Epidemiology

The prevalence of mycobacterial infection is on the increase a consequence of the spread of acquired immune deficien syndrome (AIDS) and increased global travel, which dissen nates the organism from endemic zones. *Mycobacterium tube culosis, M. bovis, M. kansasii, M. gordonae,* and *M. aviu intracellulare* may cause hepatic infection. Risk factors for t development of a mycobacterial infection include HIV carriag intravenous drug use, alcoholism, diabetes mellitus, renal failu and current drug-induced or disease-related immunosuppre sion. Reactivation of prior mycobacterial infection may occ years after the primary infection. Disseminated or milia tuberculosis occurs in approximately 10% of cases, in whi liver involvement is universal.

Pathology

The most common pattern is of a granulomatous liver disea predominantly of lobular distribution, with epithelioid ar chronic inflammatory cells, and occasional giant cells. Th granulomas do not have diagnostic features and central caseatic may occur in up to 50%. In patients who are severely debi tated, an associated microvesicular steatosis, reactive hepatit and peliosis hepatis have also been reported. The host respon dictates the extent of granuloma formation. In immunosu pressed HIV cases, the granulomas are loose aggregates of cel with abundant acid-alcohol-fast bacilli on Ziehl-Nielson stai ing, whereas in the more immunocompetent with florid gran lomas the bacteria are often difficult to detect.

Clinical features

There is no characteristic clinical presentation of hepatic tube culosis, which can be notoriously protean and mimic mar other diseases. Hepatomegaly with mild elevations of alkalir phosphatase and γ-glutamyl transpeptidase is most commo but rarely an acute liver failure syndrome may be present wi encephalopathy and hypoglycemia. Weight loss is often prese or features of other organ involvement including pulmonar pleural spaces, genitourinary, gastrointestinal tracts, and region lymphadenopathy. During miliary tuberculosis, liver involve ment is inevitable and tuberculous peritonitis may accompar any hepatic involvement. Fever is variable but a pyrexia c unknown origin may point to the diagnosis.

Investigations and differential diagnosis

There is a wide differential, which depends on the clinic context, and tuberculosis should be considered in any patie from an endemic zone or in one of the high-risk categori mentioned above. In HIV cases, antiretroviral drug hepato toxicity, viral hepatitis (hepatitis B and C), cytomegaloviru and parvovirus infection need to be excluded. In others pre senting with a granulomatous hepatitis, the differential include other bacterial or metazoal causes of granulomas (*Brucell*

TABLE 84.4 HEPATIC INVOLVEMENT WITH SPECIFIC MICROORGANISMS

Organism	Epidemiology	Pathology	Clinical features	Underlying disease associations, risk factors	Investigations and diagnosis	Treatment
Listeria monocytogenes	Declining prevalence from maximum of 1 case / 970 births. Found in milk, coleslaw, paté, soft cheeses	α,β listeriolysin may mediate pathogenesis; microabscesses in liver, granuloma, cholestatic hepatitis	Mild influenza-like illness; fever; meningitis in 50%; stillbirth, premature delivery, rarely widespread infection of other organs[4]	Those with liver involvement often have underlying cirrhosis; hematological malignancy, steroids, immunosuppression, organ transplantation	Elevated transaminases Neutrophilia Leucocytosis, low glucose, elevated protein in CSF Differential includes viral hepatitis, leptospirosis, bacteremia	Ampicillin ± aminoglycoside
Brucella mellitensis, abortus, suis	*B. mellitensis* from goats and cattle in Mediterranean basin; *B. abortus* from cattle and *B. suis* from pigs in North America	Granulomas, extent dependent on host immune response in early disease; portal tract infiltration and fibrosis	Acute phase with fever, rigors , arthralgia, hepatosplenomegaly Chronic phase with recurring pyrexia over 2-week period; fatigue malaise, with late hepatosplenomegaly a rare presentation	–	Elevated transaminases, alkaline phosphatase in 30%. Blood cultures (Castaneda techniques) and rising titer agglutinating antibodies	Doxycycline
Legionella pneumophila	Males >females; over age 40 years; contaminated water cooling systems, water supplies	Widespread dissemination to many organs; mild portal infiltrate with neutrophils in sinusoids	Features of chest infection, jaundice less common[5]	Smokers, alcoholics, chronic lung disease	Elevated aminotransferases and alkaline phosphatase in 50%. Jaundice in 10%. Serological confirmation of diagnosis	Erythromycin, clarithromycin
Burckholderia pseudomallei Melioidosis	Endemic in South East Asia. In soil, water entry via wounds in skin; inhalation	Exotoxin/protease mediates inflammation and necrosis. Epithelioid and giant cell granulomas	Fever, rigors, cough, chest infection, meningitis; hepatosplenomegaly[6]	Chronic liver disease, diabetes mellitus, renal failure, and other immunosuppressed states	Jaundice 40% Diagnosis from blood cultures or aspirated pus from abcesses	Ceftazidine
Francisella tularensis Tularemia	N. America, Europe, Russia. From tick and deer flies. Reservoir in squirrels, hares, musk rats. Common in summer in hunters	Coagulative necrosis with surrounding inflammatory cell infiltrate; may form abcess	Different syndromes. Most common: fever, rash, ulcer at site of bite, regional lymphadenopathy; also lung, oropharynx, eye involvement	Elderly, chronic disease	Abnormal liver blood tests in 10% with high aminotransferases Gram –ve rod from blood culture or on serology	Streptomycin, gentamycin tetracyclines

TABLE 84.4 HEPATIC INVOLVEMENT WITH SPECIFIC MICROORGANISMS—Cont'd

Organism	Epidemiology	Pathology	Clinical features	Underlying disease associations, risk factors	Investigations and diagnosis	Treatment
Treponema pallidum	Up to 10% have liver involvement but liver blood test abnormal in up to 40% of those with secondary syphilis. Often confused with associated viral hepatitis	Unknown; possible portal lymph node involvement with biliary obstruction, autoantibody mediated or portal pyemia. Granulomas, patchy necrosis	During secondary syphilis, weight loss, jaundice, maculopapular rash[7]	Other associated infections; hepatitis B, hepatitis C, HIV	White cell count normal; LFTs variable but alkaline phosphatase > aminotransferase TPHA+ve, FTA-ABS +ve. US may show focal hypoechoic lesion in liver, nonenhancing on CT scan	Procaine benzylpenicillin (procaine penicillin)
Neisseria gonococcus	Fitz-Hugh-Curtis syndrome of perihepatitis. Predominantly found in women; 1% of those with cervical infection	Direct spread from Fallopian tubes to peritonitis and perihepatitis	Right upper quadrant pain, tenderness, fever	–	White cell count elevated. Laparoscopy reveals violin string adhesions[8] Culture organism from peritoneal washings	

LFTs, liver funtion tests.

Coxiella, Treponema, Francisella, Listeria, melioidosis, schistosomiasis (see Chapter 83)), sarcoidosis, Hodgkin's lymphoma, and drug hepatotoxicity (see Chapter 104).

The mainstay of diagnosis is histological staining of acid-fast bacilli by the Ziehl-Nielsen method. Culture of the organism from a biopsy specimen is slow (up to 6 weeks) and more rapid automated culture tests are being developed. Molecular diagnosis is rapidly expanding and *M. tuberculosis* nucleic acid amplification tests now have an 80% positive predictive rate and a 90% negative predictive rate. Despite that, culture will remain important for drug sensitivity testing.

Treatment

The strain and drug sensitivity are critical to eradication of tuberculosis. Initial intensive therapy with isoniazid, rifampicin, pyrazinamide, and ethambutol for 8 weeks is followed by isoniazid and rifampicin for 16 weeks. Directly observed therapy strategy (DOTS) is promoted in developing countries. Drug toxicity is an important side effect[9] and hepatotoxicity occurs in up to 5–10% of cases (see Chapter 92). Monitoring of liver blood tests during the first month is recommended. Isoniazid, rifampicin, pyrazinamide, and ethambutol are all implicated in hepatotoxicity, but it is most common with isoniazid, which causes hepatitis. Coexisting chronic liver disease, alcoholism, slow acetylation phenotype, and coadministration with rifampicin all increase the risk. Rifampicin more commonly causes a cholestatic picture.

LEPTOSPIROSIS

Definition and serovars

Leptospirosis is caused by two species of *Leptospira*: pathogenic *Leptospira interogans* and the saprophytic *L. biflexa*. *Leptospira interogans* has 19 subspecies and 170 serovariants, which include the well-known *L. icterohaemorrhagiae*, *L. hebdomadis*, *L. canicola*, among others. The host in European countries is predominantly the rat, but *Leptospira* may occur widely in dogs, hedgehogs, and raccoons. Transmission to humans occurs most commonly in summer and autumn from water contaminated by urine, into which the spirochete has been shed, entering through breaches in skin or mucosal surfaces. Asymptomatic seroconversion is common especially in high-risk occupations such as sewerage and water workers. Recreational exposure to contaminated water during sailing and canoeing is increasing.

Pathology

The pathogenesis of both the histological changes in liver and kidney, which are often not dramatic, and the development of end-organ dysfunction, which may be severe, is poorly understood. The incubation phase is between 7 and 13 days followed by a septicemic phase for 2–3 days with a localized phase where end-organ damage to kidney, liver, myocardium, muscles, and skin may predominate.

In the liver, jaundice is due to both conjugated hyperbilirubinemia with cholestasis and hepatocyte ballooning as well an unconjugated fraction due to hemolysis from disseminated intravascular coagulation.

Clinical features

An anicteric illness starts during the septicemic phase with fever >39 °C, chills, rigors, headaches with meningism, conjunctival suffusion, and muscle aches/pain. There is a marked neutrophil leucocytosis and high creatine kinase, but only minor elevations in aminotransferases and alkaline phosphatase. Leptospires are detectable in blood cultures. The subsequent phase of immune localization occurs 1–3 days later when the organism may be found in urine. It is associated with a lower fever but more evidence of end-organ damage. The majority of infections follow such an anicteric course.

An icteric form (Weil's disease) may occur with any serovar, but may be more common with *L. icterohaemorrhagiae*, and represents a more severe illness with renal dysfunction[10] and frank jaundice. Bilirubin may rise to levels higher than 800 mmol/L with only minor elevation in aminotransferases or alkaline phosphatase. Prothrombin time if prolonged is a reflection of intravascular coagulation as is thrombocytopenia.

Differential diagnosis

In any patient presenting with acute jaundice and renal impairment Weil's disease must be considered. Alcoholic hepatitis with hepatorenal syndrome may also present with leucocytosis but any fever is usually milder. Wilson's disease may also have an acute presentation with renal failure, and severe viral hepatitis (hepatitis A, B/D, cytomegalovirus (CMV), Epstein-Barr virus (EBV), parvovirus) will need to be excluded.

TREATMENT

Mild infections may be treated with doxycycline, but severe disease needs penicillin. A Jarisch Herxheimer reaction may occur but should not deter treatment. In Weil's disease, intensive care may be needed with maintenance of oxygen delivery and arterial perfusion, intermittent positive pressure ventilation, as well as dialysis when renal failure develops.

FUNGAL INFECTIONS AND THE LIVER

Hepatosplenic candidiasis

Candidemia and disseminated candidiasis including hepatosplenic invasion is becoming increasingly recognized in patients following cancer therapy, organ transplantation, and in the critically ill in intensive care units. Risk factors for hepatosplenic candidiasis are given in Table 84.5. In some cases, liver invasion is preceded by documented candidemia but in 50% there may be no prior positive blood cultures.

TABLE 84.5 FACTORS PREDISPOSING TO INVASIVE *CANDIDA* INFECTIONS
• Neutropenia: primary or secondary to malignancy or anticancer therapy
• T-lymphocyte; impaired function or depletion: primary or secondary to disease or immunosuppressant drugs
• Complement deficiency
• Diabetes mellitus
• Prior antibiotic therapy
• Gastrointestinal mucosal defect
• Intravenous catheters; central venous lines

Clinical features

Candidemia may be detected in a critically ill patient who is pyrexial and commonly neutropenic. Hepatosplenic involvement is suggested by an elevated alkaline phosphatase and occasional right upper pain.[11] Fever may have been resistant to broad-spectrum antibiotics. Imaging techniques including ultrasonography and computed tomography (CT) scanning may show focal lesions but these are often only seen when the white cell count has rebounded.

Differential diagnosis

The clinical context is usually of a critically ill patient with abnormal liver blood tests (Table 84.3) and/or pyrexia of unknown origin. Diagnosis is often difficult. Liver biopsy may be inappropriate in such ill patients and scanning has a low predictive value. Empirical therapy is often suggested, as the consequences of delayed diagnosis are serious.

Treatment

There is clear evidence from randomized controlled trials that prophylaxis with azoles (fluconazole) in high-risk cases can prevent significant mucosal colonization and invasive candidiasis. Where possible, treatment should always be accompanied by attempts to reverse the predisposing factors leading to *Candida* invasion, which should be dictated by fungal sensitivity testing but this is often slow. Treatment starts with amphotericin B in a liposomal preparation when renal function is at risk. Newer antifungals including voriconazole and caspofungin have shown early promise but experience of these is still limited.[12]

REFERENCES

1. Franson TR, Hierholzer WJ Jr, LaBrecque DR. Frequency and characteristics of hyperbilirubinemia associated with bacteremia. Rev Infect Dis 1985; 7:1–9.
2. Bolder U, Ton-Nu HT, Schteingart CD, Frick E, Hofmann AF. Hepatocyte transport of bile acids and organic anions in endotoxemic rats: impaired uptake and secretion. Gastroenterology 1997; 112:214–225.
3. Cunha BA. Systemic infections affecting the liver. Some cause jaundice, some do not. Postgrad Med 1988; 84:148–158, 161–163, 166–168.
4. Samra Y, Hertz M, Altmann G. Adult listeriosis – a review of 18 cases. Postgrad Med J 1984; 60:267–269.
5. La Scola B, Michel G, Raoult D. Isolation of *Legionella pneumophila* by centrifugation of shell vial cell cultures from multiple liver and lung abscesses. J Clin Microbiol 1999; 37: 785–787.
6. Piggott JA, Hochholzer L. Human melioidosis. A histopathologic study of acute and chronic melioidosis. Arch Pathol 1970; 90:101–111.
7. Schlossberg D. Syphilitic hepatitis: a case report and review of the literature. Am J Gastroenterol 1987; 82:552–553.
8. Cano A, Fernandez C, Scapa M, Boixeda D, Plaza G. Gonococcal perihepatitis: diagnostic and therapeutic value of laparoscopy. Am J Gastroenterol 1984; 79:280–282.
9. Mitchell I, Wendon J, Fitt S, Williams R. Anti-tuberculous therapy and acute liver failure. Lancet 1995; 345:555–556.
10. Covic A, Goldsmith DJ, Gusbeth-Tatomir P, Seica A, Covic M. A retrospective 5-year study in Moldova of acute renal failure due to leptospirosis: 58 cases and a review of the literature. Nephrol Dial Transplant 2003; 18: 1128–1134.
11. Kontoyiannis DP, Luna MA, Samuels BI, Bodey GP. Hepatosplenic candidiasis. A manifestation of chronic disseminated candidiasis. Infect Dis Clin North Am 2000; 14:721–739.
12. Tiraboschi IN, Bennett JE, Kauffman CA et al. Deep Candida infections in the neutropenic and non-neutropenic host: an ISHAM symposium. Med Mycol 2000; 38 (Suppl 1):199–204.

Chapter 85

Primary biliary cirrhosis

James Neuberger

KEY POINTS

- Progressive immune-mediated destruction of the intrahepatic bile ducts
- Affects predominantly middle-aged women (90%)
- Associated with other autoimmune diseases
- Characterized by itching and lethargy
- The antimitochondrial antibody is diagnostic
- Ursodeoxycholic acid may retard progression

INTRODUCTION

Primary biliary cirrhosis (PBC) is a chronic progressive cholestatic disease of unknown cause, characterized by a granulomatous destruction of the middle sized intrahepatic bile ducts. The condition affects primarily middle-aged women, although the disease in males runs a similar course. The condition has not been described in children. There is a widespread disturbance of both the humoral and cellular immune system. The hallmark of PBC is the antimitochondrial antibody (AMA), which is virtually diagnostic of the condition. Other disease-specific autoantibodies include antibodies to the nuclear pore complex (such as gp210 and Sp100). The main clinical symptoms of PBC are lethargy and pruritus. There is an association with other autoimmune diseases, especially sicca syndrome and thyroid disease. There is no curative treatment but ursodeoxycholic acid may delay progression. Liver transplantation is the treatment for patients with end-stage disease but the condition recurs in some patients.

Since the first description by Addison and Gull in 1857, it is clear that the spectrum of disease varies greatly, from the asymptomatic patient in whom progression is very slow and the effect on survival is minimal, to those who present with decompensated liver disease.

EPIDEMIOLOGY

Studies on the epidemiology of PBC have been limited by a variety of factors, including differences in methodology. Changes in reported incidence and prevalence may reflect differences in disease awareness rather than real differences. Nonetheless, there is evidence of spatial clustering and there is worldwide variation in the epidemiology.

The reported incidence of PBC varies from 2 to 50 per million per year. The reported prevalence ranges from 15 to 400 per million.

PBC is most common in Europe and North America and very rare in Africa and the Indian subcontinent. Australia and Japan have intermediate rates reported. Migrants from high to low incidence areas (or vice versa) tend to acquire the incidence of the host country.

CAUSES, RISK FACTORS, DISEASE ASSOCIATIONS

Causes

The cause of PBC is unknown and several hypotheses have been proposed but none has been accepted:

Autoimmune: The association with other autoimmune diseases, the HLA association, and the disturbance of the immune system has led to the concept that PBC is an autoimmune disease. However, there is no response to immunosuppression and, unlike most autoimmune diseases, there is no childhood counterpart.

Infectious: The similarity between the antigen recognized by the AMA and some bacterial proteins has led some to suggest that PBC is triggered by bacteria, including *Escherichia coli* and *Novospingobium arotmaticivorans*.[1] Others have suggested that mycobacteria or retroviruses may trigger PBC.[2]

Xenobiotic: Some have suggested that a xenobiotic may trigger PBC but, again, no proof exists at this time.

Risk factors

PBC is most commonly seen in women and in middle age and in association with other autoimmune diseases. There is also a geographic variation suggesting that a variety of factors, both host and environmental, are important.

There is an increased risk in first-degree relatives: the sibling relative risk (λ_s) for PBC is 10.5[3] which is similar to that of rheumatoid arthritis (8) and ulcerative colitis, but slightly below that of Crohn's disease (20) or multiple sclerosis (20).

Several studies have addressed the HLA associations in PBC but have not always distinguished those HLA types that are associated with disease susceptibility from those that are associated with disease progression. However, there appears to be an association with the haplotype DRB1*08. Other haplotypes that have been associated with PBC include the CTLA4*G and IL1RN-IL1B haplotypes and the C4B2 haplotype.

Disease associations

There are many disease associations with PBC. The more common associations are with sicca syndrome and thyroid disease.

CAUSES AND RISK FACTORS
CAUSES • Unknown • Suggested Autoimmune Infection (bacterial or viral) Xenobiotic **RISK FACTORS** • Female gender • Middle age • Positive family history • Other autoimmune disease • HLA DRB1*08

Rheumatological:
- Sjögren's syndrome: the association between PBC and sicca syndrome varies but some studies suggest that up to 90% of patients with PBC have sicca syndrome
- Raynaud's syndrome
- Arthritis – usually affects the small joints of the hands and feet
- Sclerodactyly
- Calcinosis
- CREST (calcinosis, Raynaud's syndrome, esophageal involvement and telangiectasia) syndrome

Autoimmune disease:
- Thyroid disease (usually hypothyroidism in up to 20%)
- Celiac syndrome (note the presence of anti-endomysial and anti-tissue transglutaminase antibodies is not always associated with subtotal villous atrophy)
- Diabetes mellitus
- Pernicious anemia
- Addison's disease
- Systemic lupus erythematosis

Renal disease:
- Glomerulonephritis
- Urinary tract infection (especially *E. coli*)

Bone disease:
- Osteopenia
- Osteomalacia

Respiratory problems:
- Sarcoidosis
- Pulmonary fibrosis

Skin diseases:
- Pemphigus pemphigoid
- Scleroderma
- Lichen planus

Lipids:
- Hyperlipidemia: elevated serum cholesterol is common, especially in early disease
- Xanthoma
- Xanthelasma (Fig. 85.1)
- Neuropathy
- There appears to be no increased risk of morbidity or mortality from cerebrovascular or cardiovascular disease

Malignancy:
- Increased risk of hepatocellular carcinoma, especially in men with PBC

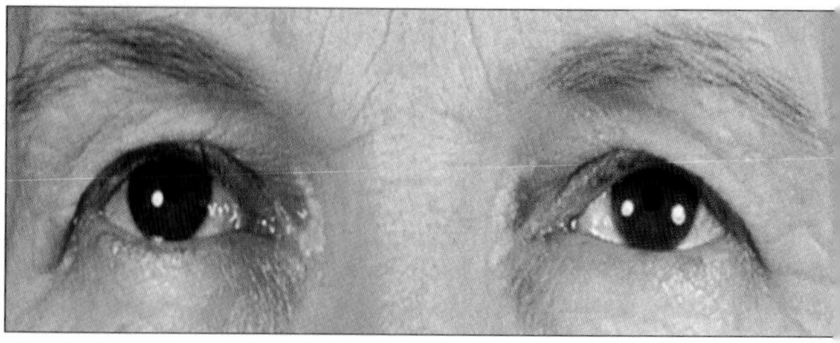

Fig. 85.1 Xanthelasmata in a patient with primary biliary cirrhosis.

- There is controversy whether there is an increased incidence of extrahepatic malignancies, but most studies suggest not

Gastrointestinal disease:
- Pancreatitis
- Gallstones
- Ulcerative colitis
- Crohn's disease

PATHOGENESIS

The pathogenesis of the disease is unknown (see causes above).

The pathogenesis of the other complications of PBC is that of portal hypertension and liver disease in general and will not be covered here. The cause of fatigue in patients with PBC is unknown but is of central origin. Altered central neurotransmission with emphasis on the central role of corticotropin releasing hormone has been suggested but conclusive information is lacking.

The cause of pruritus is uncertain (see Chapter 17). The rapid response to bile diversion and to transplantation suggests that there is some factor(s) in bile that causes the itching. The severity of itch does not correlate with the stage or rate of progression of disease. Initially, the itching was attributed to bile acids, which are elevated in PBC and bile acid sequestrants relieve the itching. However, neither tissue nor plasma levels of bile acid correlate with the degree of itch. Similarly, histamines are elevated in patients with PBC but antihistamines are relatively ineffective in treating itch. More recently, attention has focused on the role of opioid substances that accumulate in PBC and are potent pruritogens. Furthermore, opioid receptor antagonists can induce a withdrawal-like syndrome in patients with PBC and opioid receptor antagonists can help alleviate the itching.

PATHOLOGY

Scoring systems: Several have been proposed for the histological classification of PBC; these broadly agree with each other but there are some subtle differences. The commonly used systems (e.g., those of Ludwig, Sheuer, and Popper) recognize four stages with stage 4 representing cirrhosis, stage 1 bile duct damage, and stages 2 and 3 intermediate degrees of fibrosis. These systems are not widely used in clinical practice since the clinical correlation with disease stage and progression is poor and sampling variation causes difficulties in studying disease progression.

In the early stages of disease, there is an inflammatory infiltration, located primarily in the portal and periportal areas with associated bile duct damage and loss. The portal inflammatory cells are predominantly lymphocytes but eosinophils asma cells, histiocytes, and neutrophils are also present. Bile ıct injury is confined to the interlobular ducts of diameter –80 μm. Inflammatory infiltration of the bile duct epithelium associated with disruption of the epithelium and granulo-atous destruction. In the early stages, the disease process is tchy. There is apoptosis of the bile duct cells.

As the disease progresses, there is progressive bile duct loss ıd portal lymphoid aggregates develop. Bile ductular prolifer-ion occurs.

In the early stages, the parenchymal damage is scant but with sease progression, there is some inflammatory infiltration ıd interface hepatitis may be seen.

Fibrosis develops in three phases: there is an initial fibrous ortal expansion, which leads to portal–portal linkages, which ventually develops into a true cirrhosis. Ductular prolifera-on and cholate stasis will develop.

LINICAL PRESENTATION

ıere are several ways in which patients with PBC can esent. With increasing recognition of PBC and greater access laboratory diagnostics, more patients are being diagnosed at early stage, before the onset of symptoms. Classification is help as it carries prognostic information.

Presymptomatic patients are found to have evidence of PBC ısually the anti-mitochondrial antibody) but no clinical, iochemical, or even histologic features of disease.

Asymptomatic patients have biochemical and histologic atures of PBC but not the characteristic symptoms. PBC may e detected while investigating for other conditions such as cca syndrome. Symptomatic patients complain of lethargy nd itching. Itching occurs in up to 70% of patients with PBC; is not related to the stage or severity of disease and may be eneralized or localized. There is often a cyclical pattern and ıe itching is worse in winter and at night. Pregnancy may xacerbate the itching. Lethargy occurs in up to 90% of atients with PBC and, like pruritus, does not correlate with isease stage. Abdominal pain is relatively common.

Liver decompensation: patients present with symptoms or gns of decompensated disease, such as jaundice, ascites, ariceal bleeding, or hepatic encephalopathy.

CLINICAL PRESENTATION

ASYMPTOMATIC
- Patients found to have PBC during investigations for other conditions

SYMPTOMATIC
- Pruritus
- Lethargy
- Abdominal pain
- Jaundice
- Ascites
- Variceal bleeding

IFFERENTIAL DIAGNOSIS

he list for differential diagnosis of PBC is not long. Recently, here has been much controversy about the overlap of yndromes.[4] The variants associated with PBC are:

Autoimmune cholangitis (AIC): In AIC, patients have all the clinical, biochemical, and histologic features of PBC but AMA are not present. The natural history of AIC and response to treatment is identical to that of PBC. Some of these patients will develop AMA and others have AMA detected by other techniques, such as immunoblotting or ELISA. Hence, these patients should be treated as for PBC and most consider them to be a variant of PBC.

PBC/Autoimmune hepatitis (AIH) overlap: Some patients have high titers of antinuclear antibodies, high levels of serum transaminases, and significant interface hepatitis on liver histology. Indeed, some may meet the criteria for the diagnosis of AIH. Whether these patients represent a true overlap between PBC and AIH or just one end of the spectrum of PBC is controversial. While treatment with corticosteroids, as for AIH, is associated with a reduction of transaminases and the severity of interface hepatitis, the natural history resembles that of PBC rather than AIH. There are occasional reports of patients having a transition from PBC to AIH.

PBC/primary sclerosing cholangitis (PSC) overlap: There are a few reports of an overlap between PBC and PSC. The clinical and pathogenetic implications are uncertain.

DIFFERENTIAL DIAGNOSIS

- Primary sclerosing cholangitis
- Autoimmune hepatitis
- Sarcoidosis
- Drug reaction
- Gallstones

OVERLAP SYNDROMES AND VARIANTS
- Autoimmune cholangitis
- PBC/AIH
- PBC/PSC
- Sequential PBC and AIH

DIAGNOSTIC METHODS

AMA

The diagnostic hallmark of PBC is the AMA: although there are several AMAs seen in normal and disease states, the AMA that reacts with the E2 component of pyruvate dehydrogenase is virtually diagnostic of PBC. In Europe, most laboratories still use indirect immunofluorescence on composite tissue sections to define the autoantibodies. AMA may be masked by other autoantibodies; especially in older people, low titer AMA (up to 1:40) may be found. The specificity of the AMA for PBC with PDC-E2 can be confirmed by commercially available ELISA or by immunoblotting.

Other autoantibodies

A variety of antinuclear antibodies are associated with PBC, with different staining patterns. Of these, those that react with the nuclear pore complex, Sp100 and gp210, are also diagnostic of PBC but are seen less frequently.

Immunoglobulins

As with other causes of liver disease, immunoglobulins are usually increased polyclonally but PBC is associated with a rise in IgM, seen in over 90% of patients.

Biochemistry

The liver tests show a cholestatic pattern and are nonspecific. There is an early rise in serum alkaline phosphatase and GGT, which is not of prognostic significance. As the disease progresses, the serum bilirubin rises and the serum albumin falls.

Imaging the liver

This is rarely helpful in making the diagnosis but the liver is usually enlarged.

Liver histology

The histological features of PBC are described above. In cases of classical PBC (i.e., a middle-aged woman with itching and cholestatic liver tests, elevated serum IgM, and high titer AMA) there is usually no need to do a liver biopsy to make the diagnosis of PBC, although histology may help with management to look for the presence or absence of cirrhosis.

DIAGNOSTIC METHODS

SEROLOGY
- Biochemical:
  - may be normal
  - usually cholestatic
- Immunological:
  - elevated serum immunoglobulins (esp. IgM)
  - autoantibodies:
    - antimitochondrial
    - antinuclear

HISTOLOGY
- Granulomatous cholangitis
- Vanishing bile duct syndrome

IMAGING
- Rarely helpful in diagnosis
- May exclude other conditions

TREATMENT AND PREVENTION

At present, there is no effective prevention of PBC.

Treatment

Specific

Without a clear pathogenesis, it is difficult to design a logical strategy for treatment. Undertaking clinical trials for drug effectiveness in PBC is difficult because of the long natural history; the increasing use of liver transplantation for those with end-stage disease makes the use of death as an end-point unrealistic and there are no validated surrogate end-points. Therefore, interpretation of the clinical trials must be viewed in light of these observations. Most studies have been underpowered with either too few patients being studied or followed up or are too short so that there is a possibility that significant benefits may not be detected.

Ursodeoxycholic acid (UDCA) is currently the only dru that is licensed for use in PBC. The mode of action uncertain but the drug has many effects in PBC: (1) prote tion of cell membranes against the detergent effects hydrophobic bile acids; (2) immunomodulatory effec including reduction of MHC class I and II expression o hepatocytes and biliary epithelial cells and reduction in titer AMA and in the eosinophilia; (3) stimulation of biliar excretion of endogenous bile acids; and (4) anti-apoptot effects.

In patients with PBC, UDCA at a dose of 10–15 mg/kg/da is safe and well tolerated. There is an improvement in the live tests, a reduction in the rate of fibrosis, and development varices. There is no consistent effect on symptoms. There also a reduction in the development of colonic polyps an of colonic cancer.[5] Although two meta-analyses have show no effect of UDCA on patient survival, several studies hav shown that use of UDCA does improve outcome and dela time to transplantation.[6–9] Since there are very few advers side effects (mainly gastrointestinal disturbance), most clin cians recommend its use.

Other drugs have been assessed in PBC. There is som evidence that ciclosporin and azathioprine are effective prednisolone and budesonide may also have a benefici effect, although there are concerns about the risks c developing osteoporosis and in those with cirrhosi budesonide may precipitate portal vein thrombosis. There is n strong evidence base for a beneficial effect of methotrexate, d penicillamine, bezafibrate, colchicine, rifampicin, silymarin sulindac, or thalidomide. A recent study has suggested that th anti-estrogen tamoxifen may be of benefit. Other agents unde evaluation include HMGcoA reductase inhibitors an mycophenolate.

Liver transplantation

Liver transplantation is indicated for those with intractabl symptoms that make life intolerable (such as intractable itch o recurrent encephalopathy) or those with an anticipated surviva of less than 1 year. Most centers now report 5-year survival i excess of 80%. PBC does recur in the allograft in up to 40% by 10 years but this is of little clinical impact.

Pruritus

The mainstay for the treatment of itching is cholestyramine. I is effective in 80% of cases provided the dose and duration o therapy is adequate. The main side effect is gastrointestina upset. Since the sequestrant binds other drugs, caution mus be used when patients are taking multiple therapies. The dru is most effective when taken before and after breakfast, wit other doses throughout the day. It usually takes several week for the treatment to be effective; then the dose can be reduce to 4 g daily or twice daily.

For those who are intolerant of cholestyramine or in whon it is ineffective, rifampicin 300 mg/day should be tried. Thi drug is effective but may be hepatotoxic so liver tests need t be monitored. The drug is also a potent enzyme inducer. There after, naltrexone, an opioid receptor antagonist should b tried. The starting dose is 25 mg/day and this can be increase to 250 mg/day. The drug may induce a withdrawal-like state, i which case the drug should be introduced at a very low dos and gradually increased.

A small number of patients respond to a low dose of corti-)steroids. Antihistamines are usually ineffective. Other treat- ent options that may help include plasmaphoresis and MARS nolecular adsorbent recirculation systems).

ethargy

here is no effective treatment for the symptom of lethargy. ometimes anti-depressants are effective. Antioxidant therapy ineffective. Ondansetron 30 mg twice daily has been assessed; is associated with constipation and is relatively ineffective.

TREATMENT AND PREVENTION

SPECIFIC
- Licenced – ursodeoxycholic acid 10–15 mg/kg/day
- Possibly effective
  Corticosteroids
  Cyclosporin
  Azathioprine
  Tamoxifen

LIVER TRANSPLANTATION
- For end-stage disease or intractable symptoms
- PBC recurs in about 40% at 10 years

PRURITUS
- First line: bile acid sequestrants such as cholestyramine (up to 28 g/day)
- Second line: rifampicin 300 mg/day
- Third line: naltrexone starting at 25 mg/day
- Other: plasmaphoresis, bile duct diversion; molecular adsorbent recirculating system (MARS) dialysis
- Transplantation

HYPERLIPIDEMIA
- Statins
- Fibrates

OSTEOPENIA
- Life style advice
- Vitamin D and calcium
- Alendronate
- Raloxifene

Iyperlipidemia

'atients with PBC have high serum cholesterol levels but the erum HDL and LDL are usually increased in the early stages f the disease, although they fall with disease progression. The ole of drug treatment is not well described: statins and ezafibrate seem well tolerated but a clear benefit has not een documented.

)steopenia

'here is an increased risk of osteopenia, associated with female ender, menopause, and cholestasis. There have been several tudies on drug treatment but these are usually small and under- owered. All patients should get life style advice (avoid excess lcohol, stop smoking, increase weight-bearing exercise). It is ensible to give calcium (1.5 g/day) and vitamin D (800 units/day) o all. Where there is bone density loss, biphosphonates, ormone therapy, and vitamin K may be helpful. There is urrently no good data to recommend any one of these options n PBC.

Malabsorption

Prolonged cholestasis and use of bile acid sequestrants may be associated with malabsorption of the fat-soluble vitamins A, D, E, and K. Appropriate supplementation should be offered.

PROGNOSIS

The prognosis of PBC will vary. The serum bilirubin remains the best guide in identifying those with advancing disease: a serum bilirubin of 150 µmol/L implies a prognosis of survival for less than 18 months. A number of prognostic models have been developed: these are useful for identifying prognostic markers and for population studies but are less useful when applied to individual patients. The Mayo risk score is most widely used; the MELD (model for end-stage liver disease) score is used for those with end-stage disease. The major risk factors for death are serum bilirubin, age, serum albumin, and the development of ascites or peripheral edema. Older patients tend to have a slow progression of disease. Cirrhosis correlates weakly with survival.

As described above, there is controversy whether UDCA alters the survival; most reports suggest that the time to transplantation or death is increased by 5–10 years.

Presymptomatic

Survival is probably similar to an aged and sex matched population.

Asymptomatic

Symptoms develop on average within 5–10 years of diagnosis.

Symptomatic

In the absence of transplantation, decompensated disease develops within 10 years.

End-stage disease

Serum bilirubin is the best prognostic marker.

WHAT TO TELL PATIENTS

Patients should be fully informed as to the nature and natural history of the disease.

The patients should be informed that:
- the disease is progressive;
- there is an increased risk of disease in first-degree members;
- patients are not infectious;
- complications and associated diseases should be screened for;
- pruritus can usually be treated;
- lethargy cannot usually be treated;
- transplantation offers a good but not perfect safety net.

SOURCES OF INFORMATION FOR PATIENTS AND DOCTORS

The following patient support groups are available to give help and information:

American Liver Foundation at http://www.liverfoundation.org
PBC Foundation at http://www.pbcfoundation.org.uk
PBCers at http://www.pbcers.org
British Liver Trust at http://www.britishlivertrust.org.uk
Canadian Liver Foundation at http://www.liver.ca

http://www.liverfoundation.org/db/articles/1014
http://www.patient.co.uk/showdoc/26739247/
http://www.patient.co.uk/showdoc/511/

CONTROVERSIES, FALLACIES
ETIOLOGY • What is the etiology? • What is the role of host and environment? • Why female? • What is the role of AMA? • Do viruses or bacteria trigger the disease? **TREATMENT** • Role of UDCA? • What is the role of other treatments?

CURRENT CONTROVERSIES AND THEIR FUTURE RESOLUTION

The greatest controversy remains the effectiveness UDCA but given its widespread use and difficulties in runni clinical trials in PBC, it is unlikely that this argument w be resolved. Combinations of UDCA with other drugs ha not been shown to add efficacy. Novel approaches at prese include trials of oral tolerance (so far ineffective) ar antiretroviral therapy (preliminary data, but potential toxic).

The enigma of the close association between PBC ar AMA is still to be unraveled: the antigens have bee identified and cloned but a pathogenetic relationship is st uncertain.

In short, all we need is a cause and a cure.

REFERENCES

1. Selmi C, Balkwill DL, Invernizzi P et al. Patients with primary biliary cirrhosis react against a ubiquitous xenobiotics-metabolizing bacterium. Hepatology 2003; 38:1250–1257.
2. Xu L, Shen Z, Guo L et al. Does a beta retrovirus infection trigger primary biliary cirrhosis? Proc Natl Acad Sci 2003; 100:8454–8459.
3. Jones DE, Watt FE, Metcalf JV et al. Familial primary biliary cirrhosis reassessed: a geographically based population study. J Hepatol 1999; 30:402–407.
4. Woodward J, Neuberger J. Autoimmune overlap syndromes. Hepatology 2001; 33:994–1002.
5. Serfaty L, De Leusse A, Rosmorduc O et al. Ursodeoxycholic acid therapy and the risk of colorectal adenoma in patients with primary biliary cirrhosis: an observational study. Hepatology 2003; 38:203–209.
6. Goulis J, Leandro G, Burroughs AK. Randomised controlled trials of ursodeoxycholic acid therapy for primary biliary cirrhosis: a meta analysis. Lancet 1999; 354:1053–1060.
7. Gluud C, Christensen E. Ursodeoxycholic ac for primary biliary cirrhosis. Cochrane Database Syst Rev 2002; 1:CD000551.
8. Poupon RE, Lindor KD, Pares A et al. Combined analysis of the effect of treatment with ursodeoxycholic acid on histologic progression in primary biliary cirrhosis. J Hepatol 2003; 39:12–16.
9. Paumgartner G. Ursodeoxycholic acid for primary biliary cirrhosis: treat early to slow progression. J Hepatol 2003; 39:112–114.

Chapter 86

Autoimmune hepatitis and overlap syndromes

H Bantel, C P Strassburg, and M P Manns

KEY POINTS

- AIH is characterized by female predominance, hypergammaglobulinemia, circulating autoantibodies and a good response to immunosuppressive treatment
- There are three types of AIH
- Type 1 represents the most common form and is characterized by the presence of antinuclear antibodies (ANA) and/or anti-smooth muscle antibodies (SMA)
- Type 2 is characterized by the presence of liver kidney microsomal antibodies (LKM-1)
- AIH type 3 is characterized by autoantibodies against soluble liver antigen (SLA/LP)
- 'Overlap syndrome' describes a disease condition in which clinical, biochemical, and serological features of AIH coexist with those of another autoimmune liver disease (primary biliary cirrhosis, primary sclerosing cholangitis)
- AIH and overlap syndromes are often associated with extrahepatic immune-mediated syndromes including autoimmune thyroiditis, rheumatoid arthritis, and diabetes mellitus

INTRODUCTION

In 1950 Waldenström described a chronic inflammatory liver disease in a young woman; this condition is now termed autoimmune hepatitis (AIH) and represents a chronic, mainly periportal hepatitis characterized by female predominance, hypergammaglobulinemia, circulating autoantibodies, and a good response to immunosuppressive treatment.[1] Serologic detection of autoantibodies is one of the distinguishing features that has led to the subclassification of autoimmune hepatitis into three groups (Table 86.1). AIH type I represents the most common form of AIH and is characterized by the presence of antinuclear antibodies (ANA) and/or anti-smooth muscle antibodies (SMA). The target autoantigen of type 1 autoimmune hepatitis is unknown. Characteristic antibodies of AIH type 2 are liver kidney microsomal antibodies (LKM-1) directed against cytochrome P450 (CYP)2D6 and, with lower frequency, against UDP-glucuronyltransferases (UGT). The complex associations of autoantibodies directed against microsomal antigens are summarized in Fig. 86.1.[2,3] AIH type 3 is characterized by autoantibodies against soluble liver antigen (SLA/LP) directed towards the UGA-suppressor transfer RNA (tRNA)-associated protein.[4]

The term 'overlap syndrome' describes a disease condition in which clinical, biochemical, and serological features of autoimmune hepatitis coexist with those of another autoimmune liver disease, most frequently with primary biliary cirrhosis (PBC) but also with primary sclerosing cholangitis (PSC), and depending on the definition, also with hepatitis C. In adult patients an overlap of PBC and AIH is the most common occurrence although it remains unclear whether this is a true coexistence of both diseases or an immunoserological overlap characterized by the presence of antinuclear (ANA) and antimitochondrial (AMA) antibodies. Many ANA-positive patients do not show immunoreactivity against AMA despite a cholestatic liver enzyme profile. This phenomenon has been termed autoimmune cholangiopathy (AIC) or AMA-negative PBC. The coexistence of AIH and PSC has only been conclusively shown in pediatric patients but its existence has been suggested in the adult AIH population. Apart from coexisting, autoimmune liver diseases can also develop into each other (sequential manifestation).[5]

EPIDEMIOLOGY

Originally described in Caucasian Northern Europeans and North Americans, autoimmune hepatitis has a worldwide distribution. This disease affects 100000–200000 persons in the United States[6] and accounts for 4% of transplant recipients in Europe[7] and 5.9% in the US.[8] In Northern Europe, the prevalence is estimated at 170 cases per 1 million. Reliable data on the prevalence of autoimmune overlap syndromes is not available. The overlap of AIH and PBC or of AIH and PSC both appear to be present in about 8% of AIH patients.[9,10] In contrast, AIH features can be present in about 9% of PBC patients.[11] In about 24% of autoimmune diseases of the liver a syndrome of autoimmune cholangiopathy is present.[12] Figure 86.2 summarizes overlapping features of AIH type 1 and PBC.

CAUSES, RISK FACTORS, DISEASE ASSOCIATIONS

AIH and overlap syndromes are often associated with extrahepatic immune-mediated syndromes including autoimmune thyroiditis, rheumatoid arthritis, and diabetes mellitus (Table 86.2).

Most of these autoimmune diseases appear to be inheritable because they are clustered in families. This inherited susceptibility is complex and is likely to rely on a combination of numerous different genes, which most notably include immunogenetic markers (HLA-genes) and cytokine genes. However, the lack of concordance of most autoimmune diseases in identical twin pairs implicates that other environmental and host factors, such as bacterial or viral infections, dysregulated apoptosis, or cytokine profile, may be relevant for development of autoimmune diseases.

TABLE 86.1 CLINICAL CHARACTERISTICS AND DISTINGUISHING FEATURES OF THE THREE SUBCLASSES OF AIH

Clinical features	AIH type 1	AIH type 2	AIH type 3
Diagnostic autoantibodies	ANA/SMA	LKM-1	SLA/LP
Target antigen	Nuclear antigens Smooth muscle actin unknown (??)	Cytochrome P450 (CYP)2D6 UDP-glucuronosyltransferase UGTIA	UGA-suppressor (tRNA)-associated protein
Prevalence of all AIH types (%)	80%	20% in Europe 4% in the US	<20%
Common age at presentation	Bimodal (16–30 and >50 years)	Pediatric (2–14 years)	20–40 years
Extrahepatic associated diseases (%)	41	34	58
HLA association	B8, DR3, DR4	B14, DR3, C4AQO	Unknown
Progression to cirrhosis (%)	45	82	75

PATHOGENESIS

Autoimmunity is characterized by T-cell-dependent immunopathological responses to auto/neo-antigens leading to inflammatory tissue injury. An autoimmune response can be triggered by the HLA class II-dependent presentation of specific antigenic peptides to T cells via antigen-presenting cells (APCs). As a response to cytokines, exposed T cells become activated and differentiate into Th1 or Th2 cells. Pro-inflammatory cytokines are believed to play an important role in the initiation of the autoimmune response.[13] Owing to cytokine activation autoimmune diseases are often observed in associated viral or bacterial infections. Another mechanism is called 'molecular mimicry As an example, a major B cell epitope of cytochrome P450 which is targeted by LKM-1 autoantibodies in AIH-2, share sequence homology with the herpes simplex virus antigen II 175 (Fig. 86.3).[2]

The immune response is normally tightly regulated. T- and B cell homeostasis and the removal of autoreactive T cells ar regulated by apoptosis. The failure of control by apoptosis may therefore contribute to the initiation and perpetuation of autoimmune hepatitis and autoimmune overlap syndromes.[14] Thi could be explained by the inability to kill autoreactive cells, o

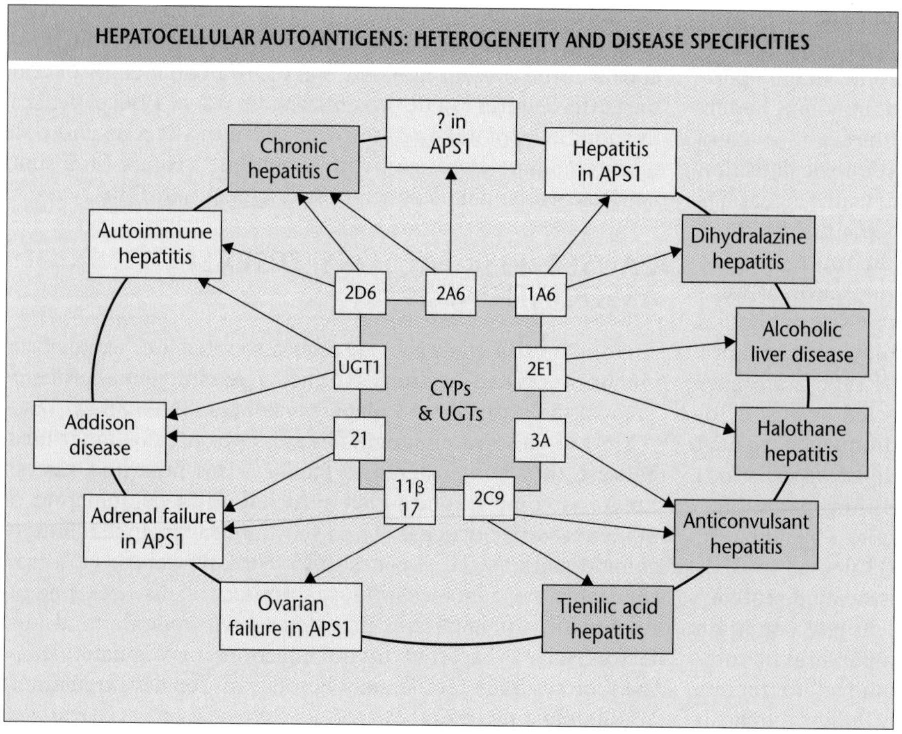

Fig. 86.1 Hepatocellular autoantigens. The heterogeneity of hepatocellular autoantigens and their disease specificities.

SEROLOGICAL PROFILES OF OVERLAPPING SYNDROME BETWEEN AIH AND PBC

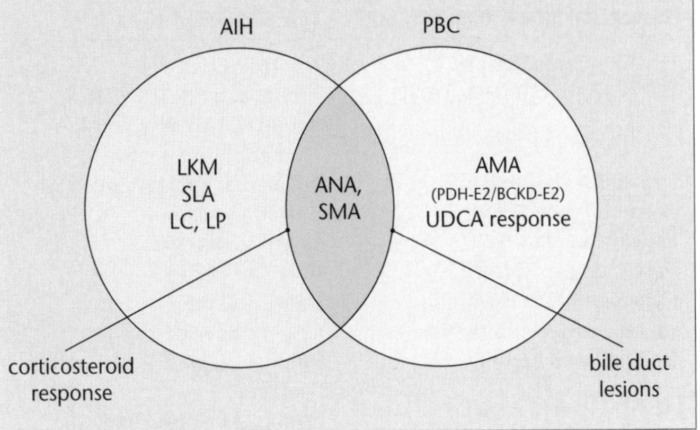

Fig. 86.2 Overlapping syndrome. Serological profiles of an overlapping syndrome between autoimmune hepatitis and primary biliary cirrhosis.

LKM-1 AUTOEPITOPES WITH HERPES VIRUS PROTEINS: VIRAL MIMICRY

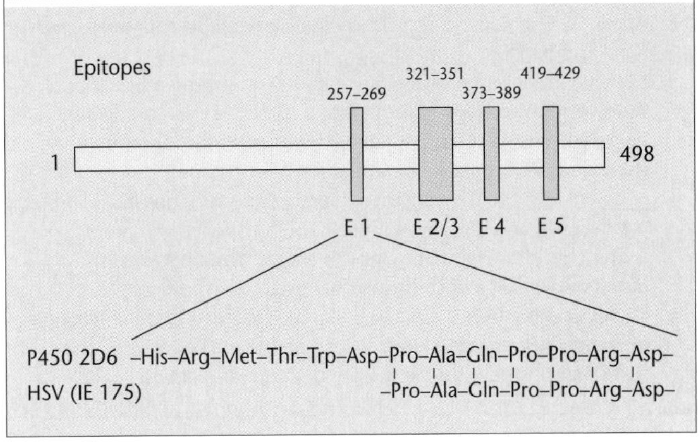

Fig. 86.3 Sequence homologies. Sequence homologies of LKM-1 autoepitopes with herpes virus proteins. Evidence of viral mimicry.

by inducing autoimmunity against cellular constituents modified by apoptosis.

Genetic factors have been implicated in the susceptibility to autoimmune hepatitis. In particular, polymorphisms of genes influencing lymphocyte homeostasis, such as the TNF-alpha promoter gene (TNF-α), the complement factor C4 gene, and the CTLA-4 gene contribute to increased susceptibility to AIH.[15] One hypothesis suggests that inheritance of specific HLA class II alleles modified at critical sites, provides one of the crucial steps for the development of AIH. The relevance of genetic alterations for AIH is further underlined by the observation that chronic hepatitis occurs in 10–18% of patients with the autoimmune polyendocrine syndrome type 1 (APS1), an autosomal recessive disorder caused by mutations in a single gene (AIRE). APS-1 is characterized by various autoimmune diseases mainly affecting endocrine glands.[16]

There has been no report of a genetic predisposition for overlap syndromes.

TABLE 86.2 EXTRAHEPATIC AUTOIMMUNOLOGIC DISEASE ASSOCIATIONS OF AIH

Hematologic diseases	Autoimmune hemolytic anemia
	Thrombocytopenic purpura
	Pernicious anemia
	Eosinophilia
Gastrointestinal diseases	Inflammatory bowel disease[a]
	Celiac disease
Rheumatologic diseases	Synovitis[a]
	Rheumatoid arthritis
	CREST syndrome
	Systemic sclerosis
	Sjögren's syndrome
Endocrinologic diseases	Diabetes mellitus
	Autoimmune thyroid disease[a]
Others	Proliferative glomerulonephritis
	Lichen planus
	Vitiligo
	Nail dystrophy
	Alopecia
	Uveitis
	Erythema nodosum

[a] Most frequently observed.

AUTOIMMUNE HEPATITIS

Pathology

AIH is characterized by periportal hepatitis with lymphocytic infiltrates, plasma cells, and piecemeal necrosis. A lobular hepatitis can be observed, but is only indicative of AIH in the absence of copper deposits or biliary inflammation. The presence of granulomas and iron deposits also argue against AIH.

Clinical presentation

About 25% of patients show an acute onset of AIH and rare cases of fulminant progression of AIH leading to acute liver failure have also been reported.[17] Commonly, the clinical presentation of AIH resembles that of other forms of chronic hepatitis. AIH is therefore characterized by nonspecific features, such as fatigue, right upper quadrant pain, jaundice, mild pruritus, arthralgias, and, when frank cirrhosis has developed, frequently also by spider angiomas and palmar erythema. In later stages, signs of portal hypertension including ascites, bleeding esophageal varices, and encephalopathy dominate this chronic progressive liver disease.

Both patients who present acutely and those who present with chronic hepatitis often show histologic evidence of cirrhosis at the onset of symptoms implicating that subclinical disease is the diagnostic challenge because it often precedes the onset of disease symptoms. As many as 25% of patients initially show signs of decompensated liver cirrhosis.[18] In particular, autoimmune hepatitis (especially type 2) is associated with a wide variety of other disorders, most of which are of immunological origin (Table 86.2).

Differential diagnosis

The clinical presentation of AIH is indistinguishable from other causes of acute or chronic hepatitis including liver cirrhosis. The clinical picture of AIH can therefore resemble those of viral

CLINICAL PRESENTATION

- About 25% of patients present with acute hepatitis and, rarely, with fulminant hepatitis
- More commonly, the clinical presentation of AIH resembles that of other forms of chronic hepatitis and is therefore characterized by nonspecific features such as fatigue, right upper quadrant pain, jaundice, mild pruritus, and arthralgias
- Histologically, there is periportal hepatitis with lymphocytic infiltrates, plasma cells, and piecemeal necrosis. Both patients who present acutely and those who present with chronic hepatitis often show histologic evidence of cirrhosis at the onset of symptoms
- The diagnosis of AIH is established by the exclusion of other etiologies of chronic hepatitis and can be aided by the use of a revised numeric score that describes the probability of having the disease

hepatitis, drug-, or alcohol-induced hepatitis. Other entities in the differential diagnosis of AIH include nonalcoholic steatohepatitis (NASH), genetic hemochromatosis, and alpha-1 antitrypsin deficiency. Cryptogenic hepatitis, an etiologically undefined chronic hepatitis, should also be included in the differential diagnosis of AIH. Patients with cryptogenic hepatitis are negative for viral as well as for autoantibody markers. It remains unknown how many of these patients suffer from AIH without detectable autoantibodies. In about 13% of patients who were initially negatively tested for ANA, SMA, and LKM, detection of SLA autoantibodies contributed to their clarification. These patients clinically resemble those of AIH type I with respect to age and sex distribution, HLA antigen profile, inflammatory activity, and response to therapy. If cholestatic signs and immunoserological markers of AIH are present, overlap syndromes have to be included in the differential diagnosis.

Diagnostic methods

The diagnosis of AIH is established by the exclusion of other etiologies of chronic hepatitis (Table 86.3). The diagnosis can be aided by the use of a revised numeric score that describes the probability of having the disease (Table 86.4). The sensitivity of the scoring system to establish definite or probable AIH is 89.9%. However, the specificity of the initial version of this score for discriminating AIH from overlapping syndromes such as AIH/PBC or AIH/PSC was low. In the revised AIH score, patients with histologic and cholangiographic evidence of PBC or PSC should be viewed as having variants of cholestatic diseases and not AIH. Specifically, well-defined granulomas, typical bile duct pathology of PSC, and PBC and substantial marginal bile duct proliferation with cholangiolitis and copper accumulation exclude AIH. Cholangiography is recommended for all patients who score as definite or probable AIH but do not respond to steroid treatment. Liver biopsy is generally recommended for grading and staging of the disease and for decision making regarding treatment of AIH, although a disease-specific histological feature does not exist for AIH and therefore limits its usefulness in the diagnosis of AIH.

Treatment and prevention

The standard initial treatment of AIH is either prednisone monotherapy (50 mg/day and tapering regimen) or combination therapy with prednisone (30 mg/day) and azathioprine (1–2 mg/kg/day). Both are equally effective, although combination therapy is generally preferred because it allows for the reduction of prednisone, frequently to a dose lower than 10 mg, thereby reducing the steroid-associated unwanted side effects. Remission is achieved in 87% of patients within 3 years of treatment. However, a sustained response is only observed in 17% of patients after stopping treatment after an initial treatment period of at least 2 years. To prevent relapse episodes, treatment should not be terminated without histological evidence of a complete remission and drug withdrawal should proceed gradually over a 3- to 6-month period. Azathioprine monotherapy (2 mg/kg/body weight) after prednisone withdrawal is a therapeutic option for the steroid-free maintenance of remission. The induction of remission by azathioprine monotherapy is not effective.

TABLE 86.3 AUTOIMMUNE HEPATITIS: A DIAGNOSIS OF EXCLUSION

Suspected differential diagnosis	Test performed to exclude
Hepatitis C infection (HCV)	Anti HCV (HCV RNA)
Hepatitis B and D (HBV, HDV)	HBsAg, anti HBc (HBV DNA) Anti-HDV, HDV RNA only when HBsAg positive
Hepatitis A virus (HAV)	Antibodies, serology: IgG, IgM
Hepatitis E virus (HEV)	Only if suspected
Epstein-Barr virus (EBV)	Only if suspected
Herpes simplex virus (HSV)	Only if suspected
Cytomegalovirus (CMV)	Only if suspected
Varicella zoster virus (VZV)	Only if suspected
Drug-induced hepatitis	History, if applicable withdrawal of drug LKM-2, LM autoantibody in selected cases
Primary biliary cirrhosis (PBC)	Anti mitochondrial antibodies (AMA) Specification of reactivity: PDH-E2, BCKD-E2 Liver histology: copper deposition in bile ducts Unresponsive to steroids
Primary sclerosing cholangitis (PSC)	Cholangiography
Wilson's disease	Ceruloplasmin, urine copper, eye examination, quantitative copper in liver biopsy
Hemochromatosis	Serum ferritin, serum iron, transferrin saturation, HFE gene test (C282Y, H63D?) Liver histology: iron staining, quantitative iron in biopsy
Alpha-1-antitrypsin deficiency	Serum alpha-1-antitrypsin (if abnormal isoelectric focusing: PiZZ/PiSS/PiMZ/PiSZ genotype ?)

Complications and their management

Treatment failure is marked by deterioration during therapy and occurs in 13% of patients. This situation justifies the termination of conventional therapy and the institution of high-dose regimens or use of alternative drugs. High-dose prednisone

TREATMENT AND PREVENTION

- The standard initial treatment of AIH consists of prednisone monotherapy (50 mg/day and tapering regimen) or combination therapy with prednisone (30 mg/day) and azathioprine (1–2 mg/kg/day)
- Combination therapy is generally preferred because it allows for the reduction of prednisone, frequently to a dose lower than 10 mg
- Remission is achieved in 87% of patients within 3 years of treatment. However, a sustained response is only observed in 17% of patients
- To prevent relapse episodes, treatment should not be terminated without histological evidence of a complete remission and drug withdrawal should proceed gradually over a 3- to 6-month period
- In cases of treatment failure (~13% of the cases), higher doses of prednisone and azathioprine can be considered or the use of alternative drugs (e.g., cyclosporine A, cyclophosphamide, tacrolimus)

lone (60 mg/day) or a lower dose (30 mg/day) in combination vith azathioprine (150 mg/day) induces biochemical remission n more than 60% of patients within 2 years. In cases of incomplete response, immunosuppression should be changed to alterative drugs. Drug-related adverse effects can be improved vith dose reduction, and a 50% decrease in dose is the first ourse of action. Alternatively, in the maintenance of remission rednisone can be substituted for azathioprine monotherapy. hus, side effects of steroids such as psychosis, diabetic decomensation, severe weight gain, and symptomatic osteopenia an be prevented by increasing the azathioprine dose or by zathioprine monotherapy. In order to maintain remission vithout or with little steroid side effects, topical steroids like udesonide are under investigation.

If standard therapy fails, alternative drugs such as cyclosporine A, cyclophosphamide, mycophenolate mofetil, or tacrolimus an be considered. However, since these strategies have not een evaluated in randomized trials, they should only be dministered after consultation with specialized hepatological enters. Liver transplantation remains as a therapeutic option or patients with treatment failure who do not reach remission espite therapy for years and who progress to cirrhosis with igns of decompensation.[19] This procedure also may be used to escue patients who present with fulminant hepatic failure econdary to autoimmune hepatitis. The long-term outlook fter liver transplantation is excellent, with 5-year survival ates of 92%. The recurrence of AIH after liver transplantation s independent of persistent autoantibodies and ranges between 1% and 35%.[20] Individual adjustments of immunosuppresive therapy after transplantation in patients with AIH may be ecessary to prevent or control the recurrence of AIH.

OVERLAP SYNDROMES

Pathology

n addition to lymphocytic interface hepatitis, a characteristic eature of AIH, florid lesions of middle-sized bile ducts with ortal inflammation and formation of granulomas can be bserved in AIH/PBC overlap syndrome. The AIH/PSC overlap

TABLE 86.4 INTERNATIONAL DIAGNOSTIC CRITERIA FOR AIH

Parameter	Score
GENDER	
Female	+2
Male	0
SERUM BIOCHEMISTRY	
Ratio of elevation of serum alkaline phosphatase vs aminotransferase	
>3.0	−2
1.5–3	0
<1.5	+2
TOTAL SERUM GLOBULIN, γ-GLOBULIN, OR IGG	
Times upper normal limit	
>2.0	+3
1.5–2.0	+2
1.0–1.5	+1
<1.0	0
AUTOANTIBODIES (TITERS BY IMMUNOFLUORESCENCE ON RODENT TISSUES) (ADULTS)	
ANA, SMA or LKM-1	
>1:80	+3
1:80	+2
1:40	+1
<1:40	0
ANTIMITOCHONDRIAL ANTIBODY	
Positive	−4
Negative	0
HEPATITIS VIRAL MARKERS	
Negative	+3
Positive	−3
OTHER ETIOLOGIC FACTORS	
History of drug usage	
Yes	−4
No	+1
Alcohol (average consumption)	
<25 g/day	+2
>60 g/day	−2
Genetic factors: HLA DR3 or DR4	+1
Other autoimmune diseases	+2
Response to therapy	+2
Complete	+3
Relapse	+3
LIVER HISTOLOGY	
Interface hepatitis	+1
Predominant lymphoplasmacytic infiltrate	+1
Rosetting of liver cells	−5
None of the above	−3
Biliary changes	−3
Other changes	+2
Seropositivity for other defined autoantibodies	

For details refer to International Autoimmune Hepatitis Group Report. Review of criteria for diagnosis of autoimmune hepatitis. J Hepatol 1999; 31:929–938. Interpretation of aggregate scores: definite AIH, greater than 15 before treatment and greater than 17 after treatment; probable AIH 10–15 before treatment and 12–17 after treatment.

syndrome is characterized by lymphocytic interface hepatitis and fibrous obliterative cholangitis, the histologic hallmark of PSC.

Clinical presentation

In an overlap syndrome, the classical appearance of the individual disease component is mixed with features of another autoimmune liver disease. Thus, in addition to the above-discussed nonspecific symptoms such as chronic fatigue associated with AIH, clinical signs of cholestasis including pruritus and jaundice can occur with overlap syndromes.

Differential diagnosis

Depending on the leading symptoms, the differential diagnosis includes all forms of cholestatic and noncholestatic liver diseases such as PBC, PSC, AIC, AIH, viral hepatitis, Wilson's disease, hemochromatosis, and alpha-1 antitrypsin deficiency.

Diagnostic methods

The diagnosis of an overlap syndrome relies on the biochemical profile (either cholestatic with elevated alkaline phosphatase, gamma glutamyltransferase, and bilirubin levels, or hepatocellular with elevated aspartate aminotransferase and alanine aminotransferase levels in addition to elevated gammaglobulins), the histology showing portal inflammation with or without the involvement of bile ducts, and the autoantibody profile showing AMA directed against antigens of the oxoacid dehydrogenase complex (PDH-E2, BCKD-E2, OADC-E2 (PBC)) or pANCA (PSC), and autoantibodies associated primarily with AIH such as liver kidney microsomal antibodies (LKM), soluble liver antigen antibodies (SLA/LP), or ANA. In cholestatic cases cholangiography detects sclerosing cholangitis. Immunglobulins are elevated in all autoimmune liver diseases; in PBC the elevation of immunoglobulin M is more pronounced.

Treatment and prevention

As a general rule, the leading disease component is treated. In an overlap syndrome presenting as hepatitis, immunosuppression with prednisone (or combination therapy with azathioprine) is initiated. In cholestatic disease ursodeoxycholic acid (13–15 mg/kg body weight/day) is administered. Both treatments can be combined when biochemistry and histology suggest a relevant additional disease component.[5]

Complications and their management

It has been suggested that corticosteroid-resistant patients with AIH/PBC overlap syndrome benefit from cyclosporine A therapy. However, validated therapeutic guidelines for overlap syndromes and their complications are not yet available because of their low prevalence. As discussed above, liver transplantation is the treatment of choice in end-stage autoimmune liver diseases irrespective of etiology once the presence of advanced cirrhosis has been ensured.[5]

PROGNOSIS WITH AND WITHOUT TREATMENT

The natural history and prognosis of AIH are largely define by the inflammatory activity present at diagnosis and mor importantly by the presence or development of cirrhosis Patients with periportal hepatitis develop cirrhosis in 17% within 5 years. However, when bridging necrosis or necrosis o multiple lobules is present, cirrhosis develops in 82%. Th presence of cirrhosis indicates a mortality of 58% in 5 year However, the presence of cirrhosis at the beginning of trea ment does not influence response or short-term outcome. Th course of AIH is also significantly influenced by the HLA antigen profile of the affected individual. In this way HLA B antigen profile is associated with severe inflammation at preser tation and a higher likelihood of relapse after treatment. Patient with HLA DR3 have a lower probability of reaching remissio show a higher relapse rate, and require transplantation mor often. HLA DR4-positive individuals have a higher age of onse (or diagnosis) and a more benign outcome. In overlap syndrome with dominating features of PSC an increased risk (~20%) o developing cholangiocarcinoma exists. In PBC-dominating over lap syndromes the prognosis depends on the stage of cirrhosi according to the Child-Pugh criteria.

WHAT TO TELL PATIENTS

Autoimmune hepatitis and overlap syndromes are chronic non infectious diseases that require long-term treatment. If therap is adequate, the prognosis of both autoimmune hepatitis an overlap syndromes is excellent. Compared to other chroni liver diseases, autoimmune hepatitis under remission is les frequently associated with the development of liver cirrhosis During pregnancy close monitoring of disease activity in hepatological center is recommended. If liver transplantatio is required, the results are excellent.

ADVICE

Treatment should not be terminated without histological evi dence of complete remission and erratic modifications of th therapeutic regimen should not be performed during therapy In case of pregnancy or planned pregnancy a hepatologica center should be contacted to plan an efficient therapeutic an monitoring strategy.

SOURCES OF INFORMATION FOR PATIENTS AND DOCTORS

http://www.liverfoundation.org/db/articles/1011
http://www.patient.co.uk/showdoc/23068926/

REFERENCES

1. International Autoimmune Hepatitis Group Report. Review of criteria for diagnosis of autoimmune hepatitis. J Hepatol 1999; 31:929–938.
2. Manns MP, Griffin KJ, Sullivan KF, Johnson EF. LKM-1 autoantibodies recognize a short linear sequence in P450IID6, a cytochrome P-450 monooxygenase. J Clin Invest 1991; 88:1370–1378.
3. Strassburg CP, Alex B, Zindy F et al. Identification of cyclin A as a molecular target of antinuclear antibodies (ANA) in hepatic and non-hepatic autoimmune diseases. J Hepatol 1996; 25:859–866.
4. Manns MP, Gerken G, Kyriatsoulis A, Staritz M, Meyer zum Büschenfelde KH. Characterization of a new subgroup of autoimmune chronic hepatitis by autoantibodies against a soluble liver antigen. Lancet 1987; 1:292–294.
5. Vogel A, Wedemeyer H, Manns MP, Strassburg CP. Autoimmune hepatitis and overlap syndromes. J Gastroenterol Hepatol 2002; 17 (Suppl 3):S389–S398.
6. Jacobson DL, Gange SJ, Rose NR, Graham NMH. Epidemiology and estimated population burden of selected autoimmune diseases in the United States. Clin Immunol Immunopathol 1997; 84:223–243.
7. European Liver Transplant Registry 2001. www.ELTR.com
8. Wiesner RH, Demetris AJ, Belle SH et al. Acute hepatic allograft rejection: incidence, risk factors, and impact on outcome. Hepatology 1998; 28:638–645.
9. Czaja AJ. The variant forms of autoimmune hepatitis. Ann Intern Med 1996; 125: 588–598.
10. Van Buuren HR, van Hoogstraten HJE, Terkivatan T, Schalm SW, Vleggaar FP. High prevalence of autoimmune hepatitis among patients with primary sclerosing cholangitis. J Hepatol 2000; 33:543–548.
11. Chazouilleres O, Wendum D, Serfaty L, Montembault S, Rosmorduc O, Poupon R. Primary biliary cirrhosis-autoimmune hepatitis overlap syndrome: Clinical features and response to therapy. Hepatology 1998; 28:296–301.
12. Czaja AJ, Carpenter HA. Autoimmune hepatitis with identical histologic features of bile duct injury. Hepatology 2001; 34:659–665.
13. Vergani D, Mieli-Vergani G 2000. The role of T cells in autoimmune hepatitis. In: Manns MP, Paumgartner G, Leuschner U, eds. Immunology and liver. Dordrecht: Kluwer Academic Publishers; 2000:133–136.
14. Chervonsky AV. Apoptotic and effector pathways in autoimmunity. Curr Opin Immunol 1999; 11:684–688.
15. Agarwal K, Czaja AJ, Jones DE, Donaldson PT. Cytotoxic T lymphocyte antigen-4 (CTLA-4) gene polymorphisms and susceptibility to autoimmune hepatitis. Hepatology 2000; 31:49–53.
16. Obermayer-Straub P, Strassburg CP, Manns MP. Autoimmune polyglandular syndrome type 1. Clin Rev Allergy Immunol 2000; 18:167–183.
17. Nikias GA, Batts KP, Czaja AJ. The nature and prognostic implications of autoimmune hepatitis with acute presentation. J Hepatol 1994; 19:225–232.
18. Roberts SK, Therneau TM, Czaja AJ. Prognosis of histological cirrhosis in type 1 autoimmune hepatitis. Gastroenterology 1996; 110:848–857.
19. Tillmann HL, Jackel E, Manns MP. Liver transplantation in autoimmune liver disease: selection of patients. Hepatogastroenterology 1999; 46:3053–3059.
20. Manns MP, Bahr MJ. Recurrent autoimmune hepatitis after liver transplantation: when non-self becomes self. Hepatology 2000; 32:868–870.

Chapter 87

Alcoholic liver diseases

Rajeshwar P Mookerjee and Rajiv Jalan

KEY POINTS

- ALD is responsible for 44% of all cirrhosis-related mortality in the UK
- The total number of alcohol-related deaths is increasing with the greatest rise noted in women
- A threshold of alcohol is believed to be important in developing ALD: 40–80 g/day in males and 20–40 g/day in females
- Despite apparent thresholds, there is not a particular amount of alcohol that will predictably cause ALD
- Amongst alcohol abusers, the majority (>60%) develop fatty liver disease, which is largely reversible following abstinence
- 8–20% of alcohol abusers will present as alcoholic hepatitis, which may be superimposed on cirrhosis
- The pathogenesis of alcoholic hepatitis is not fully understood and the mortality remains high (>40% in some series)

INTRODUCTION

The word 'alcohol' dates back to 1543 (a Latin derivative of the term 'al-kuhl') when it was used by Arabic chemists to refer to substances such as essences that were obtained by distillation. Ethyl alcohol is metabolized at the rate of about 7 g (0.3 oz)/h in a healthy human (a little less than the amount in an average 'drink') and larger quantities or drinking faster leads to an accumulation of alcohol for the liver to process. Alcoholism refers to a subgroup of heavy drinkers (8% of men and 3% of women in the UK) who are dependent on and have a tolerance to alcohol and are unable to control their drinking behavior and craving. These individuals are at risk of alcoholic liver disease (ALD), which accounts for greater than 50% of presentations of UK liver disease and is responsible for 44% of all cirrhosis-related mortality, with the resultant economic burden that this entails.[1]

Alcoholic cirrhosis was the primary indication for liver transplantation in the UK between 1996 and 2000. However, the pathophysiology of severe ALD, as seen in alcoholic hepatitis, is poorly understood with treatment modalities being largely supportive and lack of consensus on more specific interventions.

EPIDEMIOLOGY

There is a marked heterogeneity in the severity of presentation of clinical disease and in the susceptibility of individuals to ALD. There is believed to be a 'threshold' daily amount and length of time of alcohol intake that has to be exceeded in order for ALD to develop. This has been proposed as being a daily intake of alcohol over 10–12 years of doses in excess of 40–80 g/day for males (equating to 3–6 12-oz cans of beer) and 20–40 g/day for females (Fig. 87.1).[2] The lower thresholds are now widely accepted, especially with the increased recognition of high alcohol intake amongst younger drinkers, especially young women. In a report compiled by the UK Department of National Statistics, the total number of alcohol-related deaths has increased every year since 1979, with the number of deaths (5543) almost doubling in number by the year 2000. Within the last 3 decades, there has been a fourfold increase in mortality from liver cirrhosis in 45–54-year-old men and an eightfold cirrhosis mortality increase in 35–44-year-old men, largely attributable to ALD. Whilst death rates for males remain higher than those for females, in the younger age groups the rates for women are now approaching those for men (Figs 87.2 and 87.3).

Despite the need for a threshold with respect to dose and length of time for the development of ALD, there is not a

RISK ESTIMATES FOR ALCOHOLIC CIRRHOSIS

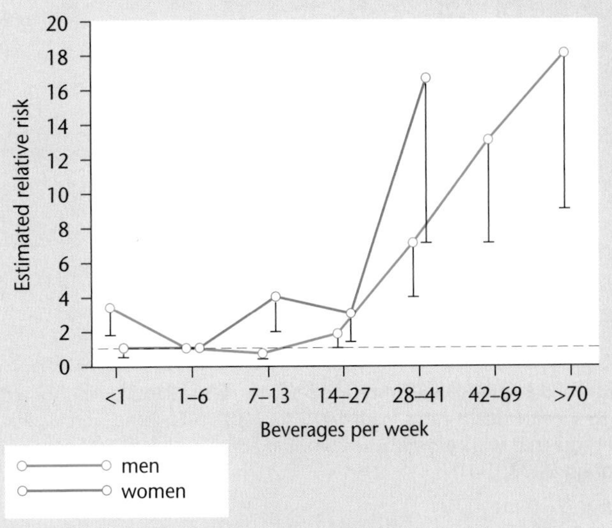

Fig. 87.1 Relative risk estimates for development of alcohol-induced cirrhosis. Alcohol intake classified as <1 beverage (<12 g); 1–6 beverages (12–72 g); 7–13 beverages (84–156 g); 14–27 beverages (168–324 g); 28–41 beverages (336–492 g); 42–69 beverages (504–828 g); 70 beverages (840 g). The group with an alcohol intake of 1–6 beverages (12–72 g) per week is the reference group (relative risk = 1). The vertical lines are estimated lower 95% confidence limits. Reproduced with permission from Becker et al. Hepatology 1996; 23:1027.

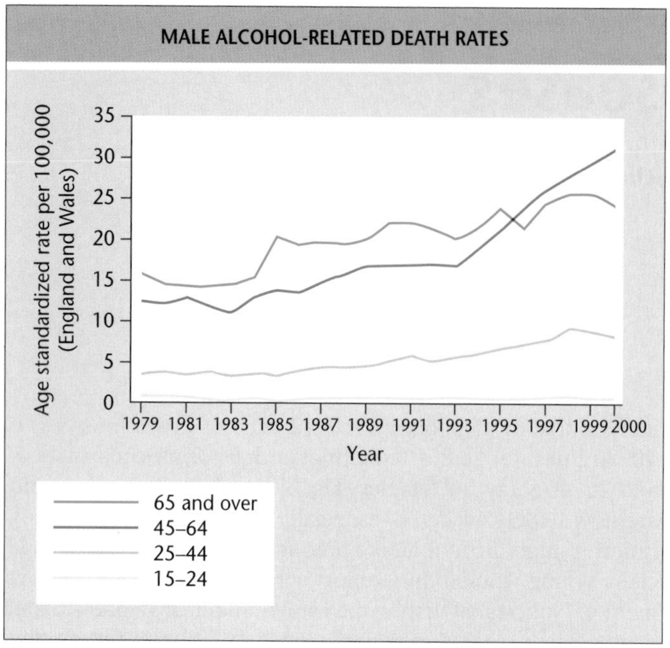

Fig. 87.2 Male alcohol-related death rates. Male alcohol-related age-specific death rates from 1979 to 2000 in England and Wales. Reproduced with permission from Barker et al. Health Stat Quart Spring 2003;1-10.

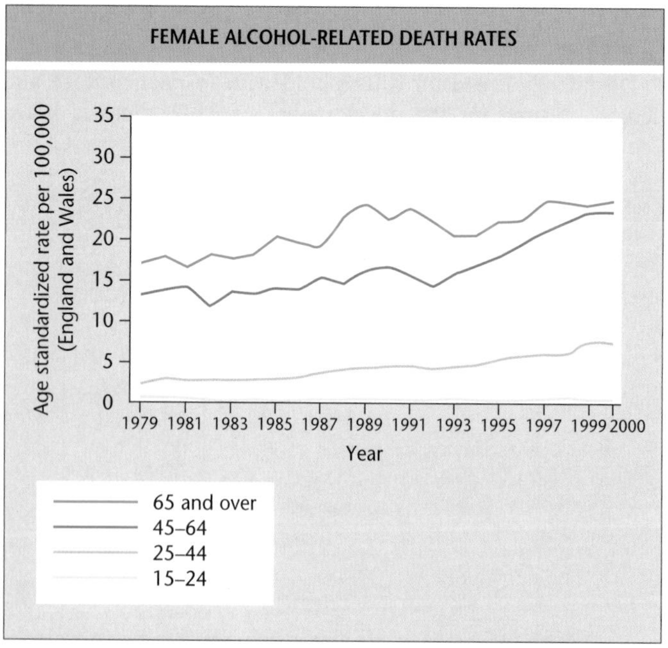

Fig. 87.3 Female alcohol-related death rates. Female alcohol-related age-specific death rates from 1979 to 2000 in England and Wales. Reproduced with permission from Barker et al. Health Stat Quart Spring 2003; 1-10.

particular amount of alcohol that will predictably cause ALD. Among long-term alcohol abusers, the majority will develop fatty liver but only 10–35% develop alcoholic hepatitis and 8–20% will get alcoholic cirrhosis, albeit these two histological forms of the disease often coexist on a biopsy. It remains controversial whether alcoholic hepatitis is a prerequisite for the development of cirrhosis.

RISK FACTORS

Quantity of alcohol consumed

Longitudinal studies such as The Dionysos Study, performed in two Northern Italian towns,[3] has suggested that the risk of developing ALD increases with increasing daily intake above a threshold of 30g ethanol/day in both sexes. This is consistent with observations of decreased ALD during the times of ‘Prohibition’ and World War rationing. Drinking alcohol outside meal times and drinking multiple different alcoholic beverages also increases the risk of ALD. This may explain geographic differences in prevalence of ALD in countries where a ‘pub culture’ exists as opposed to countries in which alcohol is often consumed during meals in the form of wine.

Gender

Women appear to have a greater risk of developing ALD than men, even when factors such as body weight and amount of alcohol ingested are taken into consideration. Human data to explain the gender differences is lacking but alcohol-fed animal models illustrate some potential mechanisms. Firstly, alcohol-fed female rats have greater hepatic steatosis, inflammation and necrosis compared to males.[4] Moreover, there is increased sensitivity to endotoxin in estrogen-treated rats with increased production of the pro-inflammatory cytokine tumor necrosis factor α (TNFα) and the endotoxin receptor CD14, which is likely to compound liver injury. Estrogens also increase the expression of alcohol dehydrogenase (ADH) with resultant higher levels of production of the metabolite acetaldehyde which may account for increased reactive oxygen species generation in female rats fed alcohol.

Obesity

Lipid metabolism is significantly deranged in ALD and, accordingly, a diet rich in fat is likely to increase pro-oxidant damage in alcoholic patients. Recent studies have shown worse histopathological changes in obese alcoholics than in lean patients and demonstrated that the body mass index is an independent risk factor for fibrosis in ALD, which may have therapeutic implications.[5] Obese alcoholics have been shown to have reduced insulin secretion and insulin is an inhibitor of the P450 enzyme, CYP2E1, a possible explanation for the increased oxidant damage in obese alcoholics. Moreover, a diet rich in polyunsaturated fats can induce CYP2E1, which generates peroxidative damage.

Concomitant viral infection

There is a high prevalence of hepatitis C viral (HCV) infection in chronic alcoholics, with 15–50% of this screened population with liver disease having a positive HCV-RNA. The combination of HCV plus alcohol leads to more severe histological features with a relative risk for developing cirrhosis estimated at 8.7, compared to ALD patients without HCV infection.[6] The presence of HCV is a major risk factor for the development of hepatocellular cancer in patients with alcoholic cirrhosis, the 10-year absolute cumulative risk being 81% in anti-HCV-positive alcoholic cirrhotics compared with 19% in anti-HCV-negative patients. The synergistic effects of HCV and alcohol relates to the effects on the immune system and on hepatocellular responses to injury.

Genetics

Even taking into account the above risk factors, some individuals still develop ALD despite consuming lower levels of alcohol, which suggests that in addition to environmental factors, genetic factors are likely to increase the risk of developing ALD. Genetic polymorphisms have been described for the metabolizing enzyme systems ADH and CYP2E1, which may account for the increased sensitivity to alcohol in Asian populations. Furthermore, polymorphisms have also been identified to pro-inflammatory cytokines such as TNFα that may increase the susceptibility to hepatic injury.[7]

Thus, alcohol probably works as a 'potential hepatotoxin,' with the development of liver disease depending on the balance of host attributes and coexisting external factors, such as gender, polymorphism of alcohol-metabolizing enzymes, immunological factors, exposure to other substances/drugs, hepatic viral infections, nutritional deficiencies, and obesity.

CAUSES AND RISK FACTORS

- Quantity of alcohol consumed and drinking outside of meal times
- Women are at higher risk secondary to unfavorable metabolic and pro-inflammatory effects of estrogen
- Obesity and diets rich in polyunsaturated fats – increased oxidative stress
- Concomitant hepatitis C infection
- Genetic polymorphisms such as alcohol metabolizing enzymes and inflammatory mediators such as TNFα

PATHOGENESIS

Consequences of alcohol metabolism

Ethanol is metabolized by two major pathways: (1) oxidation to acetaldehyde by cytosolic ADH and subsequent oxidation to acetate by mitochondrial aldehyde dehydrogenase (ALDH) coupled to the reduction of NAD to NADH; and (2) metabolism by CYP2E1, which also generates acetaldehyde, in addition to numerous free radicals. Acetaldehyde is thought to have a direct toxic effect on cells by the formation of protein adducts by binding to cysteine residues. These modified proteins may then evoke an immune response and the production of autoantibodies perpetuating an inflammatory response.[8] The change in redox state (increased NADH formation) impairs normal carbohydrate and lipid metabolism, whilst decreasing the supply of ATP to cells. Gluconeogenesis is impaired, leading to the diversion of generated acetyl CoA to ketogenesis and synthesis of free fatty acids. The inhibition of mitochondrial β-oxidation coupled with the additional inhibitory effect on lipolysis by acetate leads to hepatic steatosis and the generation of reactive oxidant species through lipid peroxidation.[9] The loss of normal mitochondrial function, together with modified cellular proteins through adduct formation, leads to derangements in apoptotic signaling pathways. Thus, following an initial pathological derangement such as steatosis, there follows a number of potentially injurious responses, such as promotion of endotoxin mediated necro-inflammation, known as the 'second-hit hypothesis (Fig. 87.4).

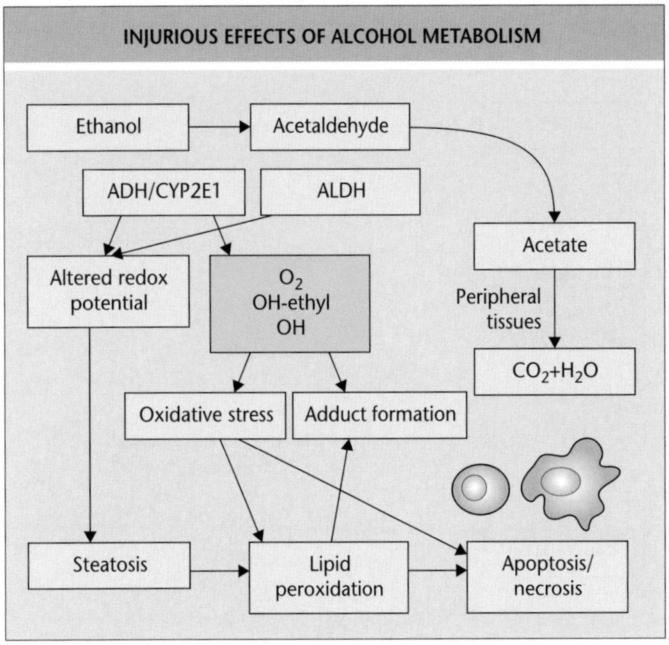

Fig. 87.4 Injurious effects of alcohol metabolism. Schematic representation of the injurious effects of alcohol metabolism. Reproduced with permission from Stewart et al. Trends Mol Med 2001; 7:409.

The role of endotoxin and pro-inflammatory cytokines

Alcohol promotes gut permeability to bacterial translocation and bacterial overgrowth. Bacterial lipopolysaccharide (LPS) binds to Kupffer cells through inducible receptors such as CD14 and Toll-like receptor-4 causing Kupffer cell activation, resulting in the production of pro-inflammatory cytokines such as TNFα and the neutrophil-attracting chemokine, IL-8. The liver inflammation that ensues is perpetuated by the further generation of neutrophil oxidative burst and protease production, and the continued pro-apoptotic drive through increased mitochondrial permeability transition, promoted by TNFα.[10] Immune responses to alcohol are illustrated in Fig. 87.5. Furthermore, alcohol appears to 'prime' peripheral blood mononuclear cells to increase cytokine generation in response to LPS stimulation, and sensitizes hepatocytes to the inflammatory and pro-apoptotic effects of cytokines.[9] The concept of priming and sensitization, following an initial primary hit injury response, implies a series of sequential events in the progression of liver injury following alcohol exposure. Thus, reducing gut bacterial load or modulation of pro-inflammatory cytokines may prevent further injury driven by a 'second hit' response.

CLINICAL PRESENTATION

Physical examination reveals variable clinical features that reflect the underlying severity of the disease. Often, the examination will not distinguish ALD from non-ALD causes (see Chapter 19), without accompanying history and supportive laboratory data. Patients with steatosis are usually asymptomatic, though they may present with hepatomegaly. Patients who progress to steatohepatitis may also be asymptomatic, but more commonly present with hepatomegaly, or the full-blown picture of alcoholic hepatitis (10–70%) with tender hepatomegaly, jaundice, fever,

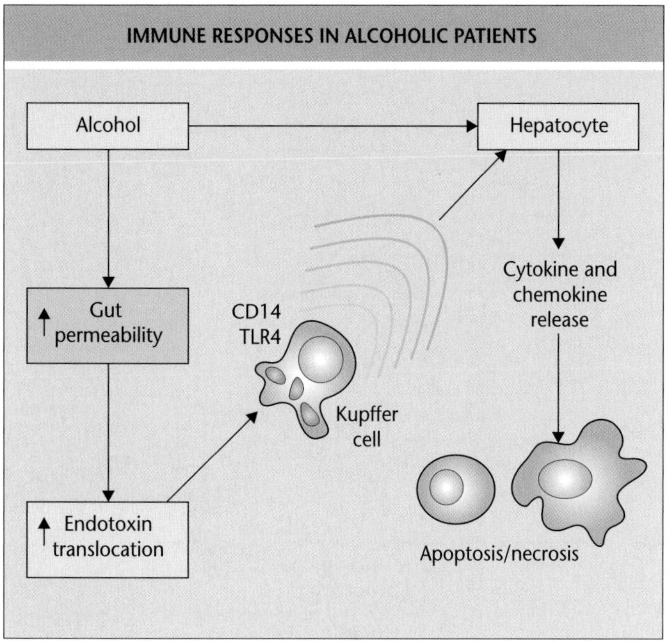

Fig. 87.5 Immune responses in alcoholic patients. Reproduced with permission from Stewart et al. Trends Mol Med 2001; 7:409.

ascites, hepatic encephalopathy, anorexia, malaise, or even hepatorenal syndrome. Portal hypertension may be a feature, with ascites, splenomegaly, and abdominal wall collaterals, even in the absence of cirrhosis (see Chapter 96). Cutaneous manifestations of alcohol excess include Dupuytren's contracture and rosacea (Fig. 87.6), where alcohol causes flushing, as well as manifestations of cirrhosis such as telangiectases and palmar erythema (Fig. 87.7). Peripheral neuropathy or cerebellar ataxia may be present. The cutaneous manifestations were described most aptly in a rhyme by the late Dame Sheila Sherlock 'An older miss muffet sat on a tuffet drinking her whisky and gin, red hands and a spider developed outside her, such are the wages of sin'. Patients may also show signs of feminization with hypogonadism and gynecomastia and hypoalbuminemia (leukonychia) (see Chapter 19). Patients with well-compensated alcohol-induced cirrhosis may have very few symptoms or signs of liver disease. However, as the disease advances, most patients will have features of portal hypertension and hepatocellular dysfunction (cachexia and jaundice). The liver often decreases in size, the left hepatic lobe becoming more prominent, whilst the entire liver adopts a hard and nodular consistency. The probability of one or more of these clinical manifestations of liver disease developing is 25–30% per decade. Mortality tends to increase in parallel with the severity of portal hypertension and hepatic dysfunction. It is important to note that none of the physical signs and symptoms is pathognomonic for ALD.

Wernicke's encephalopathy (WE) (see Chapter 100): This is an important clinical presentation which is often overlooked. Patients may present with confusion, ataxia, and varying levels of impaired consciousness, which may be confused with drunkenness or the effect of associated head injury. Ophthalmoplegia and nystagmus occurs in only 30% of cases and signs of accompanying malnutrition should alert one to the possibility of WE. If the diagnosis is missed, a significant proportion of patients (84%) will go on to develop Korsakoff's psychosis with short-term memory loss and long-term morbidity.[11]

DIFFERENTIAL DIAGNOSIS

No single physical examination finding or constellation of findings is specific for ALD. Thus, the differential diagnosis can be wide. The presence of clinical signs of feminization and palmar erythema are highly suggestive in a cirrhotic patient who admits drinking alcohol. Furthermore, other liver disorders may contribute to or compound pre-existing alcoholic liver disease despite abstinence, such as nonalcoholic fatty liver disease and hepatitis C. Histologically, nonalcoholic steato-

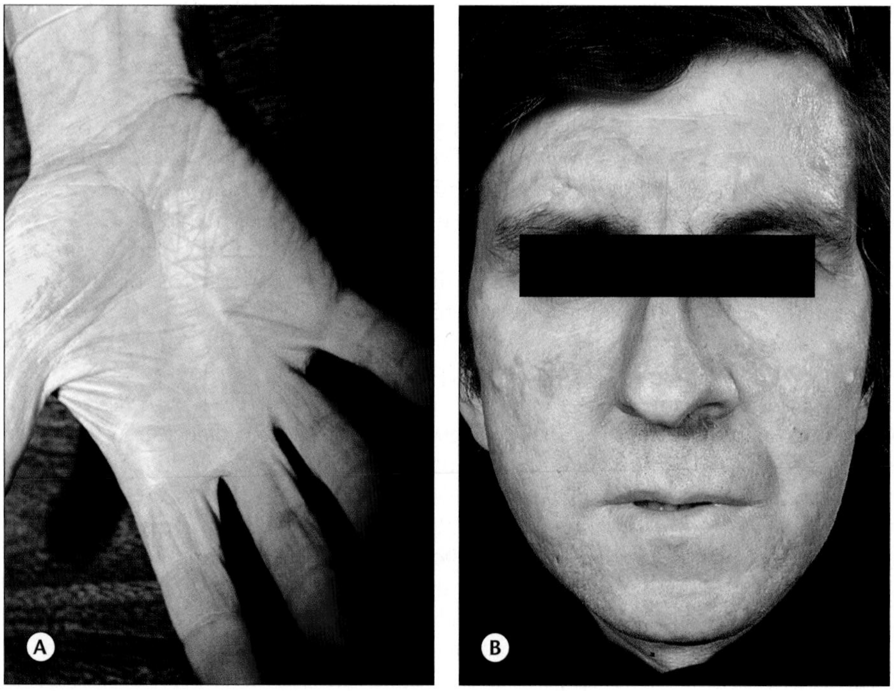

Fig. 87.6 Signs associated with alcohol excess. A. Dupuytren's contracture (see also Fig. 19.5). **B.** Rosacea associated with excess consumption of alcohol, which causes flushing.

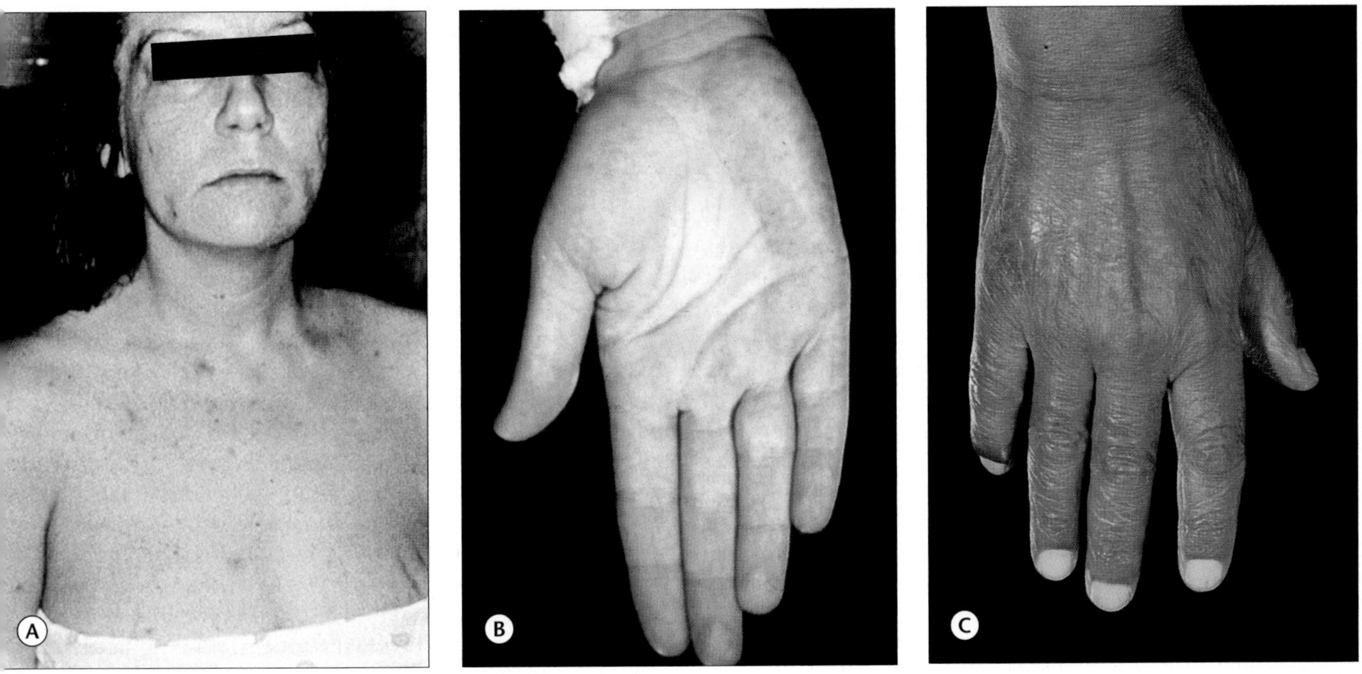

Fig. 87.7 **Manifestations of cirrhosis in alcoholic liver disease. A.** Multiple spider nevi. **B.** Palmar erythema. **C.** Leukonychia.

hepatitis can be indistinguishable from alcoholic hepatitis, albeit the patients would be unlikely to have the same degree of severity of presentation of their cirrhosis (see Chapter 88).

DIAGNOSTIC METHODS

Historical features

A screening tool for alcohol abuse is the CAGE questionnaire (Table 87.1). A CAGE score cut-off of 2 or more positive answers is indicative of alcohol dependency, with a specificity of >91% and a sensitivity of 70–96%.[5] A potential criticism of this screening method is that it may fail to identify individuals who do not incur social or psychological consequences from alcohol ingestion.

Laboratory test abnormalities

Serum aminotransferases are often elevated in ALD but the degree of enzyme elevation provides no indication of the severity of liver injury. A pattern most commonly seen in ALD is a serum aspartate aminotransferase (AST) level two to three times greater than the alanine aminotransferase (ALT) level, with neither elevated more than seven times the upper limit of normal. Elevation of gamma glutamyl transferase (GGT) is more sensitive (70%) than AST or ALT with a reduced specificity of 65–80% for excessive alcohol consumption. A high serum bilirubin may be present but this is often in a patient with alcoholic steatohepatitis, unless there is concomitant bile duct obstruction. Abnormalities of synthetic function (albumin and prothrombin time) manifest as liver disease progresses or in the acute presentation of alcoholic hepatitis. A commonly used prognostic index in alcoholic hepatitis is the 'Maddrey's discriminant function', which is calculated using the equation: $4.6 \times$ (PT patient − PT control) + total bilirubin (mg/dL). If this value exceeds 32, the in-hospital mortality is in excess of 50%.[12]

Lipids: Chronic alcohol consumption is often associated with hypertriglyceridemia, hyperuricemia, hypokalemia, and hypomagnesemia, as well as elevated mean corpuscular erythrocyte volume (MCV). The metabolic abnormalities normalize with abstinence and/or adequate replacement. The elevation in MCV is often found in persons ingesting more than 50 g alcohol/day, with a sensitivity of 27–52% and specificity of 85–90%.[7] Carbohydrate deficient transferrin (CDT) is a more sensitive test (58–69%) for current or recent alcohol use and is 82–92% specific. With alcohol intakes >10 g/day there is a positive correlation between CDT and alcohol intake. CDT is superior to GGT or MCV in detecting alcohol abuse. Leukocytosis and thrombocytopenia are also common in alcoholic hepatitis. Occasionally, patients have leukemoid reactions with counts of 100 000 white blood cells (WBC)/mm^3 in the absence of infection. These may improve if the acute inflammatory state resolves. There is also evidence that serum concentrations of tumor necrosis factor-α (TNF-α), interleukin-6 (IL-6), and interleukin-8 (IL-8) correlate with mortality in patients with alcoholic hepatitis, but measurements of these cytokines are not routinely available in clinical practice.[13]

TABLE 87.1 CAGE QUESTIONNAIRE
*C*utting down on drinking
*A*nnoyance at others' concerns about drinking
*G*uilty feelings about drinking
*E*ye opener: requirement of alcohol early in the morning
2 or more positive answers = alcohol dependency

Imaging

Sonography, computerized tomography, and magnetic resonance imaging are useful in suggesting steatosis, but they can neither define its cause nor exclude associated alcoholic hepatitis. Furthermore, these imaging modalities can detect evidence of portal hypertension (collateral vessels, ascites, and splenomegaly) before it becomes clinically apparent and exclude the presence of biliary obstruction.

Liver biopsy

Histological assessment provides a sensitive method of evaluating the severity of liver cell injury and the degree of fibrosis, which can be used to define prognosis and treatment options. It is the only reliable way of detecting alcoholic steatohepatitis and fibrosis in individuals with minimal or atypical symptoms. Histology also helps clarify the predominant condition in patients with coexisting liver diseases such as viral hepatitis. For accurate histological interpretation in ALD, the samples should contain more than six portal tracts.

Steatohepatitis: Most 'heavy' drinkers will have histological evidence of steatosis, with fat deposition in the centrilobular or perivenular regions. Subjects who have severe mixed micro/macrovesicular pattern, and/or giant mitochondria are more likely to develop fibrosis and evolve to cirrhosis.[14] In patients with alcoholic hepatitis (AH), there is characteristic ballooning degeneration of hepatocytes with polymorphonuclear cell infiltration, moderate to severe fatty infiltration, and Mallory bodies (intracellular eosinophilic inclusions which represent masses of intermediate filaments). The presence of Mallory bodies suggests a more serious disease. It is thought that immunological reactions directed against these cellular components may contribute to the pathogenesis of ALD. Other features of AH histology includes pericellular fibrosis and sclerosing hyaline necrosis. It is also common for features of cirrhosis to be noted in patients with AH (Fig. 87.8).

DIAGNOSTIC METHODS

- History: CAGE questionnaire (reliable predictor of dependency)
- Laboratory tests: no single definitive test; AST 2 or more times greater than ALT, elevated γGT and MCV and high carbohydrate-deficient transferrin may all be suggestive
- Imaging: sonography/CT/MRI may help to define steatosis and evidence of portal hypertension
- Histology: defines severity, guides treatment if alcoholic hepatitis present, and clarifies predominant condition if viral disease coexists

TREATMENT AND PREVENTION

Treatment for ALD can be subdivided into (1) long-term management of ALD, (2) acute management of AH, and (3) management of the complications of cirrhosis resultant from ALD.

Long-term management

Abstinence from alcohol is vital in order to prevent further liver injury, fibrosis, and possibly hepatocellular carcinoma. There are limited, retrospective studies evaluating the effect of abstinence on the progression of ALD. There is a suggestion of resolution of steatosis from total abstinence and that decompensated patients with jaundice or ascites benefit from abstinence.[15] Abstinence can be achieved by psychological support and/or pharmacological interventions. The former is cost effective and requires only minimal training to implement, with some evidence of benefit. Table 87.2 gives indications for detoxification. Pharmacological agents that have been shown to generate abstinence, such as naltrexone and acamprosate, have efficacy in some chronic alcoholics but there are no large studies evaluating these drugs in patients with ALD.[16] Patients who are smokers or obese should undergo lifestyle modifications to reduce the increase in oxidative stress generated by these additional factors, which may contribute to progression of disease.

Nutrition

Protein calorie malnutrition is common in ALD and indicative of a poor prognosis, with increased risk of infection, ascites and encephalopathy. Studies suggests that supplementation of a regular diet in decompensated alcoholic cirrhotic patients can reduce hospitalizations for infections.[17] Changes in dietary feeding patterns is also required as cirrhotics obtain >70% of their nonprotein calories from fat, after an overnight fast compared with 40% in normal volunteers. Thus, ALD patients with cirrhosis should have frequent interval feeding with importance being attributed to a night-time snack and breakfast, to improve nitrogen balance. These patients are also likely to require a diet higher in protein (>1.5 g/kg) and energy (>40 kcal/kg), especially during episodes of decompensation or infection.

Pharmacological therapies

To date there has been no consistent survival benefit with adjunctive pharmacotherapy. However, some agents have shown beneficial effects and await randomized controlled trials.

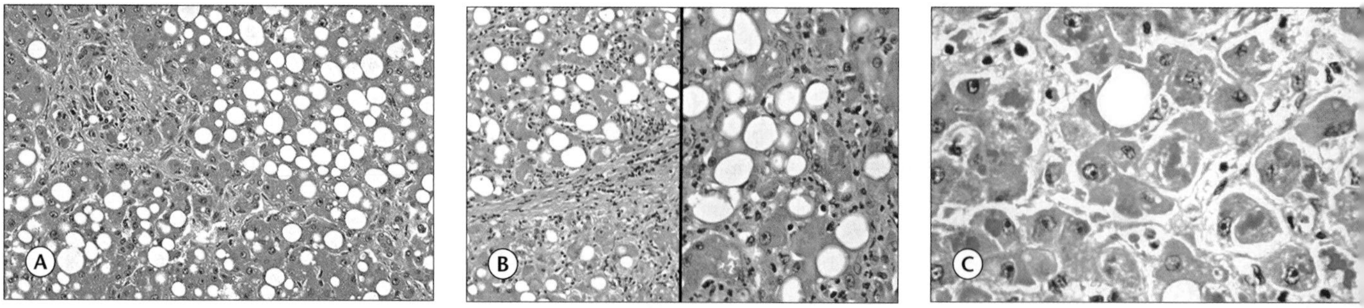

Fig. 87.8 Histology. A. Histologic appearance of hepatic fatty change with high alcohol intake. Lipid accumulation in hepatocytes is seen as clear vacuoles with H&E staining. **B.** Histological section of alcoholic hepatitis; Mallory's hyaline, neutrophils, hepatocyte necrosis, collagen deposition, and fatty change are noted. **C.** Mallory's hyaline; at high magnification, globular red hyaline material is seen within hepatocytes.

TABLE 87.2 INDICATIONS FOR DETOXIFICATION

Hospital detoxification is advised if the patient:
- Has confusion or hallucinations
- Has a history of previous complicated withdrawals
- Is known to have epilepsy or a history of fits
- Is malnourished
- Has severe diarrhea or vomiting
- Has suicidal intent or a history of psychiatric illness
- Has previously failed home-assisted withdrawal
- Has multiple substance abuse
- Community detoxification
- For patients with mild to moderate withdrawal symptoms

Propylthiouracil (PTU) is believed to reduce the hypermetabolic state and the relative hypoxic damage to centrolobular areas. There has been one randomized controlled trial, which demonstrated a 2-year improved mortality in those who continue drinking.[18]

Colchicine is suggested as a treatment for ALD because of its antifibrotic effects. It has many potential therapeutic mechanisms of action including inhibition of collagen production, enhancement of collagenase activity, and anti-inflammatory functions. A recent meta-analysis of 14 randomized controlled trials found no benefit of colchicine treatment.[19]

Silymarin, an active component of the herb 'milk thistle,' has antioxidant activities, protects against lipid peroxidation, and has anti-inflammatory and antifibrotic effects. Two large trials to date have demonstrated conflicting results on survival benefit.

S-Adenosylmethionine (SAMe) is a precursor for the synthesis of glutathione, with consequent antioxidant properties. It also acts as a methyl donor for a number of molecular pathways, whilst also converting methionine to cysteine, a pathway with reduced activity in ALD patients. SAMe downregulates production of TNFα in animal models of liver injury. One large trial to date has shown a significant reduction in mortality and/or liver transplantation requirement in patients with Child A and B cirrhosis.[20]

Dilinoleoylphosphatidylcholine (a form of lecithin/soybean extract) has antioxidant, anti-fibrotic, and anticytokine activity in experimental rat models of ALD. A large Veterans Affairs (VA) cooperative study has failed to show any significant benefit in human ALD.

Vitamin E deficiency in ALD is established and supplementation is thought to have potential benefits including membrane stabilization, reduced NFkB activation, and TNFα production. The one large published randomized supplementation study with 500 IU vitamin E has failed to show any significant benefit to date. The dosage used is half that used in smaller studies applied to alcoholic hepatitis.

Table 87.3 gives a list of the pharmacological therapies tried to date and the evidence supporting their usage.

The role of transplantation

ALD is one of the commonest indications for liver transplantation. However, liver transplantation for advanced ALD remains a controversial issue in the light of increasing donor shortages and concerns over the risk of post-transplant recidivism. Current data suggests patients transplanted for ALD do as well as patients transplanted for other clinical indications.[21] However, the majority of patients with ALD are not listed for liver transplantation for multiple reasons including continued alcohol consumption, improvement of liver function with abstinence, and deterioration with multiorgan failure where the patient is deemed 'too sick' for transplantation.

TABLE 87.3 PHARMACOLOGICAL THERAPIES IN ALD

Therapeutic agent	No. of trials	No. of patients	No. of trials favoring therapy	
			Significant	Trend
LONG-TERM THERAPY IN ALCOHOLIC LIVER DISEASE				
PTU	1	310	1	0
Colchicine	1	45	1	0
SHORT-TERM THERAPY IN ALCOHOLIC HEPATITIS				
Corticosteroids	12	749	5	
Amino acid supplements	8	291	2	4
Insulin/glucagon (intravenous)	4 (+ 1 abstract)	307	1	2
PTU	2	105	0	1
Anabolic steroids				
Testosterone	2	140	0	0
Oxandrolone	2	173	1	1
Colchicine	1	72	0	0

Reproduced with permission from McCullough and O'Connor. Am J Gastroenterol 1998; 93:11 2022–2036.

Management of alcoholic hepatitis

Most trials on AH are restricted to patients with a discriminant function (DF) >32 and have assessed short-term mortality (inpatient stay or 28-day mortality). Management of patients with less severe presentations of AH, who have a better prognosis, and in those who have survived after their initial severe presentation, is focused on achieving abstinence. Specific therapies for severe AH are targeted on our current understanding of disease mechanisms, including the importance of inflammatory cytokine pathways and oxidative stress.

Corticosteroids

The rationale for steroid use is to decrease the immune response and proinflammatory cytokine drive, in part by modulation of NFκB transcriptional activity. There have been 12 randomized trials to date with 5 demonstrating a reduction in 28-day mortality, whilst 7 showed no reduction. The trials varied in their inclusion and exclusion criteria, including severity of AH, and only two had histological confirmation of AH. This is needed to differentiate patients with acute AH from those with cirrhosis alone who decompensate after continued drinking. Most trials also differ in the dosing and duration of treatment, and most trials excluded patients with active GI bleeding, active infection, and renal failure. Six meta-analyses have followed, the most recent being nonconventional, by pooling the results from the three largest studies; this showed a benefit in steroid-treated patients (Fig. 87.9). However, in view of the continued risks

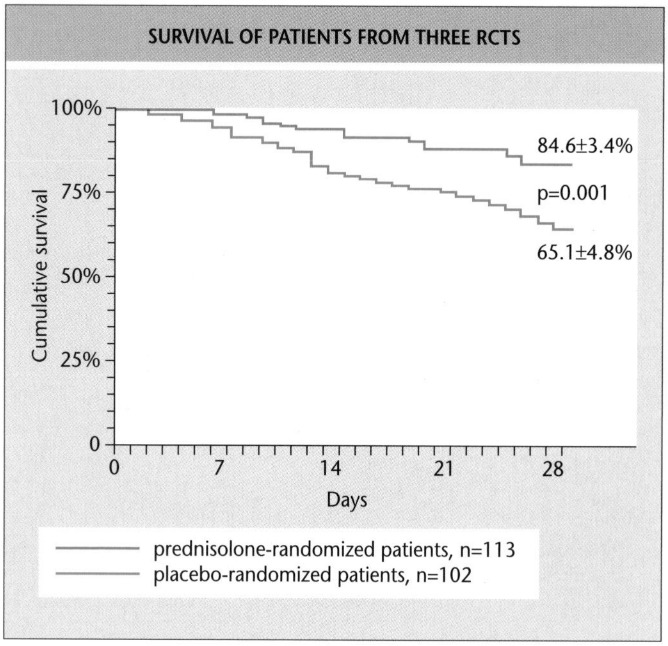

Fig. 87.9 Survival of patients from three RCTs. Twenty-eight-day survival of patients with DF=32 from three RCTs. Reproduced with permission from Mathurin et al. J Hepatol 2002; 36:480-487.

from infection in steroid-treated patients and the lack of conclusive benefit from treatment, the debate over steroid usage persists. There is likely to be a benefit in a subgroup of patients, with severe AH and/or hepatic encephalopathy, in the absence of infection or recent GI bleeding, albeit, this clearly limits the application of this treatment.

Pentoxifylline (PTX)

Pentoxifylline is a nonselective phosphodiesterase inhibitor that has also been shown to reduce TNFα gene transcription. A large, randomized trial of PTX [22] showed a significant reduction in mortality compared with placebo, largely from a reduction in deaths from hepatorenal syndrome.

Anti-TNF strategies

Infliximab, a chimeric monoclonal antibody to TNFα, has been reported in two small, nonrandomized studies, with improvements in inflammatory indices, biochemistry, and apparent short-term mortality. Short-term improvement in histological severity is depicted in Fig. 87.10. Treatment with infliximab has also been shown to result in an acute reduction in hepatic venous pressure gradient (HVPG) of >38% within 24h of treatment (Fig. 87.11).[23] This decrease in HVPG persists up until the time of discharge and may account for the apparent improvement in early mortality in previous studies.

Other anti-TNF treatments, such as the TNFα antagonist etanercept, are under evaluation.

Enteral nutrition

AH is a catabolic state and there is a correlation between severity of malnutrition and mortality in patients with AH. Early indications of benefit from trials of enteral nutrition have been confirmed by a recent study comparing enteral nutrition with steroid therapy,[24] which showed no difference in 28-day mortality but a lower 1-year mortality in enterally fed patients.

Artificial liver support

The molecular adsorbents system (MARS) has been applied to patients with severe AH and the development of organ failure, to bridge patients to transplantation or recovery. A small study reported significant improvements in bilirubin, renal function, and decreased encephalopathy.[25] Larger trials are still awaited.

Antioxidant therapies

There have been three trials on the use of antioxidants in AH, either compared to placebo or steroid therapy. None of the trials conferred any survival benefit with the use of *N*-acetylcysteine, selenium, vitamins A, C, and E, and allopurinol.

Complications of AH

Hepatorenal syndrome

In patients with AH, the development of renal failure is associated with a survival of less than 10%, even with intensive

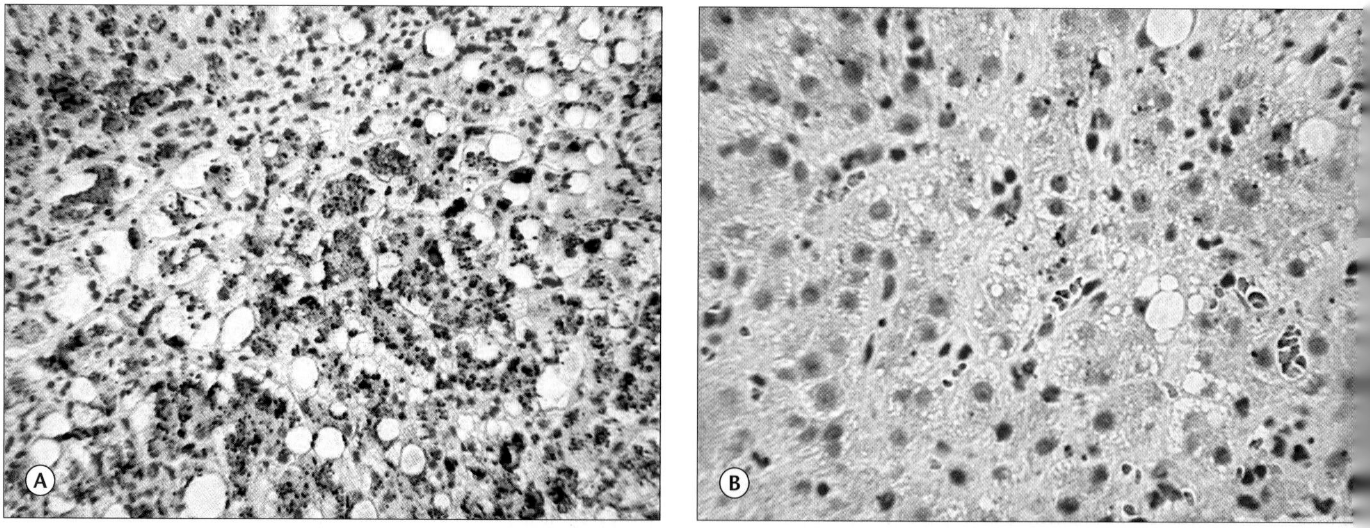

Fig. 87.10 TNF immunohistochemistry before **(A)** and after **(B)** infliximab therapy. Reproduced with permission from Tilg et al. J Hepatol. 2003

HVPG CHANGES WITH INFLIXIMAB

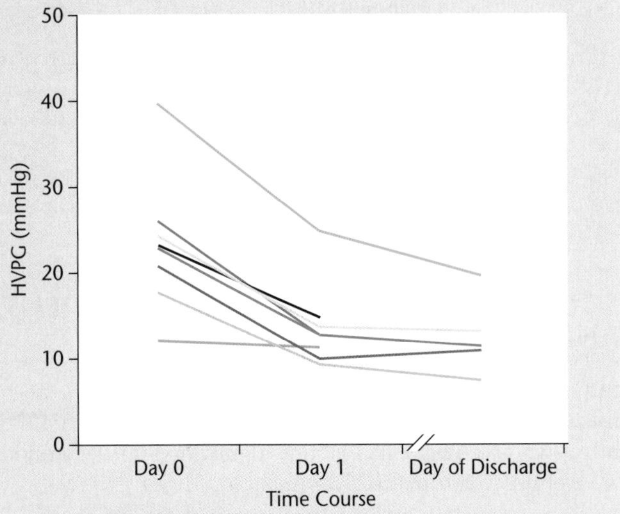

ig. 87.11 Changes in HVPG in patients treated with infliximab. eproduced with permission from Mookerjee et al. Gut 2003; 2:1182-1187.

nanagement and renal support. However, recent data suggest hat a combination of albumin infusions and use of the splanchic vasoconstrictor agent, terlipressin, can lead to a significant mprovement in creatinine, mean arterial pressure, and supression of the renin–angiotensin system, with a consequent mprovement in mortality.[26] Randomized controlled trials of his treatment in AH are awaited.

nfection

atients with AH have significant derangements in both adapive and innate immune responses. Furthermore, an increase in ut permeability increases the risk of bacterial translocation nd subsequent sepsis. Infection is a common complication nd a reason for decompensation in AH. The risk of infection s further compounded by therapies such as corticosteroids nd infliximab. An early screen for infection using cultures of lood, ascitic fluid, urine, a screening chest X-ray, and seroogical markers such as C-reactive protein are an important art of the management. Further screens for infection must e undertaken if steroid therapy is instituted, and appropriate ntimicrobials commenced if infection is confirmed.

Osteopenia and osteoporotic fracture

 recent study has demonstrated a high incidence of osteopenia nd fractures in patients with ALD cirrhosis, alcohol having a lirect inhibitory effect on osteoblast function coupled with nalnutrition in these patients.[27]

ROGNOSIS

lcoholic steatosis

This is considered a nonprogressive lesion that reverses after essation of alcohol. In some individuals, fibrosis of terminal epatic venules develops, which may herald the development f cirrhosis or there is a mixture of macro/microvesicular fat, which may progress to steatohepatitis and/or cirrhosis.

TREATMENT AND PREVENTION

LONG-TERM MANAGEMENT
- Abstinence through detoxification programs
- Nutrition: frequent interval meals including breakfast and night-time snack to improve nitrogen balance
- Pharmacological adjuvants: no consistent survival benefit demonstrated for any agent
- Liver transplantation: data suggests ALD patients benefit as much as other causes of cirrhosis but controversies over post-transplant recidivism and donor shortages limit numbers performed

MANAGEMENT OF ALCOHOLIC HEPATITIS
- Corticosteroids: benefits shown in selected patients especially those with hepatic encephalopathy but without renal failure, sepsis, or acute GI bleeding; controversy over survival benefit data continues
- Pentoxifylline: survival benefit shown amongst patients who also develop hepatorenal syndrome
- Infliximab: two small studies to date have shown improved survival at 28 days and one has demonstrated a significant improvement in HVPG and regional blood flow
- Nutrition: severe malnutrition correlates with mortality in AH – a study with enteral nutrition showed lower 1-year mortality compared to prednisolone treatment
- Artificial liver support: MARS may have a role in organ failure
- Antioxidant therapies: no proven benefit to date

Alcoholic hepatitis

The presence of hepatic inflammation is probably the most important histological prognostic indicator. The mortality from AH in some series has been noted to be as high as 50% in patients with severe disease (DF >32). TNFα has been shown to correlate with mortality. However, cytokine assays are not routinely available. Other risk factors for worse outcome include female gender and additional liver injury from viral infections or drug toxicity.

Alcoholic cirrhosis

The outcome of patients with cirrhosis is dictated by the development of complications of portal hypertension (such as variceal bleeding and ascites), onset of hepatic encephalopathy, and hepatocellular carcinoma. Alcohol consumption continues to influence prognosis even after the development of cirrhosis. Patients with decompensated cirrhosis who remain abstinent have a 5-year survival of 60% versus only 30% if they continue to drink alcohol.[28]

CURRENT CONTROVERSIES

Many aspects of ALD continue to promote controversy, from agreement on pathogenetic mechanisms, to accepted 'safe' limits of drinking or a consensus on the treatment of alcoholic hepatitis. Despite apparent improvements in mortality and clinical state with anti-TNFα therapy, it has been difficult to show any discernible change in TNFα levels, following treatment. This may reflect the importance of TNFα interacting with its receptors (TNF receptor I and II) to evoke a clinical effect. Receptor concentration may be more useful in gauging prognosis and treatment response than measurement of TNFα.[29] Improved understanding of genetic polymorphisms, including those for alcohol dehydrogenase and TNFα promoters and the effects of estrogen on alcohol-induced liver injury, has helped to validate more conservative 'safe' limits for drinking and may explain the lack of correlation between intake and liver injury. Data on steroid treatment in AH remains controversial, despite recent data suggesting that early changes in bilirubin might predict those likely to respond to therapy.[30] Further studies assessing anti-TNF agents are awaited and human studies on anti-apoptotic agents and antifibrotics are likely to reveal new therapies to tackle the ever-increasing burden of ALD.

Liver transplantation remains the most effective treatment for end-stage ALD but also evokes the greatest controversy relating to moral and ethical issues. At present, most centers offer transplantation to patients with severe disease (Child C cirrhosis) if they have demonstrated a period of abstinence (traditionally, 6 months) since there is evidence that these patients have the best outcome. Future developments in the field of hepatocyte transplantation may offer new hope for patients with AH.

CONTROVERSIES

- Alcohol thresholds: there are no data to suggest that a given alcohol intake will definitely cause ALD
- TNFα is believed to be important in the pathogenesis of ALD but shows no discernible change after anti-TNF therapy, despite clinical benefit; should we be measuring TNF receptors?
- Steroid therapy: debate on survival benefit persists
- Liver transplantation: requirement for 6 months' abstinence despite proven benefit in patients with Child disease; moral and ethical issues

SOURCES OF INFORMATION FOR PATIENTS AND DOCTORS

http://www.patient.co.uk/showdoc/23068925/
http://patients.uptodate.com/topic.asp?file=gen_hlth/4978
http://www.prodigy.nhs.uk/clinicalguidance/releasedguidance/webBrowser/pils/PL253.htm

REFERENCES

1. Alcohol Related Liver Disease Working Party. http://www.britishlivertrust.org.uk
2. Becker U, Deis A, Sorensen TI et al. Prediction of risk of liver disease by alcohol intake, sex, and age: a prospective population study. Hepatology 1996; 23:1025–1029.
3. Bellentani S, Saccoccio G, Costa G et al. Drinking habits as cofactors of risk for alcohol induced liver damage. The Dionysos Study Group. Gut 1997; 41:845–850.
4. Moshage H. Alcoholic liver disease: a matter of hormones? J Hepatol 2001; 35:130–133.
5. Raynard B, Balian A, Fallik D et al. Risk factors of fibrosis in alcohol-induced liver disease. Hepatology 2002; 35:635–638.
6. McCullough AJ, O'Connor JF. Alcoholic liver disease: proposed recommendations for the American College of Gastroenterology. Am J Gastroenterol 1998; 93:2022–2036.
7. Arteel G, Marsano L, Mendez C, Bentley F, McClain CJ. Advances in alcoholic liver disease. Best Pract Res Clin Gastroenterol 2003; 17: 625–647.
8. Albano E. Free radical mechanisms in immune reactions associated with alcoholic liver disease. Free Radic Biol Med 2002; 32:110–114.
9. Stewart S, Jones D, Day CP. Alcoholic liver disease: new insights into mechanisms and preventative strategies. Trends Mol Med 2001; 7:408–413.
10. Purohit V, Russo D. Cellular and molecular mechanisms of alcoholic hepatitis: introduction and summary of the symposium. Alcohol 2002; 27:3–6.
11. Thomson AD, Cook CC, Touquet R, Henry JA. The Royal College of Physicians report on alcohol: guidelines for managing Wernicke's encephalopathy in the accident and emergency department. Alcohol Alcohol 2002; 37:513–521.
12. Maddrey WC, Boitnott JK, Bedine MS et al. Corticosteroid therapy of alcoholic hepatitis. Gastroenterology 1978; 75:193–199.
13. McClain CJ, Barve S, Deaciuc I, Kugelmas M, Hill D. Cytokines in alcoholic liver disease. Semin Liver Dis 1999; 19:205–219.
14. Teli MR, Day CP, Burt AD, Bennett MK, James OF. Determinants of progression to cirrhosis or fibrosis in pure alcoholic fatty liver. Lancet 1995; 346:987–990.
15. Morgan MY. The prognosis and outcome of alcoholic liver disease. Alcohol Alcohol (Suppl) 1994; 2:335–343.
16. Palmer AJ, Neeser K, Weiss C, Brandt A, Comte S, Fox M. The long-term cost-effectiveness of improving alcohol abstinence with adjuvant acamprosate. Alcohol Alcohol 2000; 35:478–492.
17. Hirsch S, Bunout D, de la Maza P et al. Controlled trial on nutrition supplementation in outpatients with symptomatic alcoholic cirrhosis. J Parenter Enteral Nutr 1993; 17: 119–124.
18. Orrego H, Blake JE, Blendis LM, Compton KV, Israel Y. Long-term treatment of alcoholic liver disease with propylthiouracil. N Engl J Med 1987; 317:1421–1427.
19. Rambaldi A, Gluud C. Colchicine for alcoholic and non-alcoholic liver fibrosis and cirrhosis. Cochrane Database Syst Rev 2001:CD002148.
20. Mato JM, Camara J, Fernandez de Paz J et al. S-adenosylmethionine in alcoholic liver cirrhosis: a randomized, placebo-controlled, double-blind, multicenter clinical trial. J Hepatol 1999; 30:1081–1089.
21. Stewart SF, Day CP. The management of alcoholic liver disease. J Hepatol 2003; 38 (Suppl 1):S2–S13.
22. Akriviadis E, Botla R, Briggs W et al. Pentoxifylline improves short-term survival in severe acute alcoholic hepatitis: a double-blind, placebo-controlled trial. Gastroenterology 2000; 119:1637–1648.
23. Mookerjee RP, Sen S, Davies NA et al. TNF an important mediator of portal and systemic haemodynamic derangements in alcoholic hepatitis. Gut 2003; 52:1182–1187.
24. Cabre E, Rodriguez-Iglesias P, Caballeria J et al. Short- and long-term outcome of severe alcohol-induced hepatitis treated with steroids or enteral nutrition: a multicenter randomized trial. Hepatology 2000; 32:36–42.
25. Jalan R, Sen S, Steiner C et al. Extracorporeal liver support with molecular adsorbents recirculating system in patients with severe acute alcoholic hepatitis. J Hepatol 2003; 38:24–31.
26. Ortega R, Gines P, Uriz J et al. Terlipressin therapy with and without albumin for patients with hepatorenal syndrome: results of a prospective, nonrandomized study. Hepatology 2002; 36:941–948.
27. Carey EJ, Balan V, Kremers WK, Hay JE. Osteopenia and osteoporosis in patients with end-stage liver disease caused by hepatitis C and alcoholic liver disease: not just a cholestatic problem. Liver Transpl 2003; 9:1166–1173.
28. Diehl AM. Liver disease in alcohol abusers: clinical perspective. Alcohol 2002; 27:7–11.
29. Naveau S, Emilie D, Balian A et al. Plasma levels of soluble tumor necrosis factor receptors p55 and p75 in patients with alcoholic liver disease of increasing severity. J Hepatol 1998; 28:778–784.
30. Mathurin P, Abdelnour M, Ramond MJ et al. Early change in bilirubin levels is an important prognostic factor in severe alcoholic hepatitis treated with prednisolone. Hepatology 2003; 38:1363–1369.

Chapter 88

Nonalcoholic fatty liver disease

Arthur J McCullough

KEY POINTS

- Non-alcoholic fatty liver disease (NAFLD) is emerging as the most frequent liver disease in developed countries
- The diagnosis of NASH implies steatosis associated with lobular inflammation plus ballooning degeneration or fibrosis
- The most important risk factors for NASH are obesity, diabetes, age over 45, hypertension, hypertriglyceridemia and increased ALT
- NASH may progress to cirrhosis and liver failure
- Insulin resistance and cytokine activation are thought to play a key role in the pathophysiology of NASH
- There is currently no specific treatment for NASH. Therapy is mainly directed to correct nutritional habits and comorbidities

INTRODUCTION, INCLUDING DEFINITION

Nonalcoholic steatohepatitis (NASH) is one form of a larger spectrum of nonalcoholic fatty liver disease (NAFLD), with histologic findings ranging from fat alone, to fat plus inflammation, to fat plus hepatocyte injury (ballooning degeneration), to fat with fibrosis. Only fat plus hepatocyte injury and fibrosis should be considered to be NASH (Table 88.1). The significance of these histologic categories rests on the fact that both the prevalence and clinical outcome vary by histologic category.[1]

Examples of the histological appearance of the two most clinically relevant types of NAFLD – fat alone and NASH – are shown in Figure 88.1.

TABLE 88.1 TYPES OF NAFLD RELATED TO CLINICAL OUTCOME

Category	Pathology	Clinicopathologic correlation
Type 1	Simple steatosis	Known to be nonprogressive
Type 2	Steatosis plus lobular inflammation	Probably benign (not regarded as NASH)
Type 3	Steatosis, lobular inflammation, and ballooning degeneration	NASH without fibrosis may progress to cirrhosis
Type 4	Steatosis, ballooning degeneration, and Mallory bodies, and/or fibrosis	NASH with fibrosis – may progress to cirrhosis and liver failure

Only types 3 and 4 are considered to be NASH.

EPIDEMIOLOGY

The incidence of NAFLD/NASH is unknown and, as shown in Table 88.2, estimates of the prevalence vary depending on the methodology used to make the diagnosis.

Prevalence: Because of the imprecision of the diagnostic modalities available, the prevalence of NAFLD can be, at best, an estimate. An example of this difficulty is displayed in Table 88.3, which provides three different prevalence rates based on three different analyses of the National Health and Nutritional Examination Survey (NHANES III), which was performed between 1988 and 1994 in more than 12 000 adults from the general US population. NAFLD was diagnosed based on increased serum levels of liver enzymes – alanine aminotransferase (ALT), aspartate aminotransferase (AST), and γ-glutamyltransferase (GGT) – in the absence of other causes. The prevalence ranged between 2.8% and 23%. This wide discordance was due to differences in inclusion criteria. However, the essence of the uncertainty in the prevalence rates resides in the problem of defining NAFLD in epidemiologic studies based on noninvasive tests without a liver biopsy.[2]

The 23% prevalence rate is likely the most accurate because it is consistent with the ultrasonographic screening studies shown in Table 88.2. Based on the best performed general population screening studies, the prevalence of NAFLD is between 16% and 20% in lean patients, and 19–76% in obese patients. Using these rates and assuming that 23% of the population is obese; the overall prevalence of NAFLD is between 17% and 33%. In the population studies, the ratio of NASH to NAFLD was one-third to half. Therefore, the prevalence of NASH would rest between 5.7% (conservative estimate) and 16.5% (liberal estimate). Although these current prevalence rates are already high, they are expected to increase in industrialized countries in concert with the rapidly increasing prevalence of obesity and type 2 diabetes.

CAUSES, RISK FACTORS, DISEASE ASSOCIATIONS

Insulin resistance

As insulin resistance is the essential underling pathophysiologic factor associated with fatty liver, NAFLD/NASH is now considered to be the hepatic component of the insulin resistance syndrome, which has been defined in different ways.

The World Health Organization (WHO) classification is based on the presence of at least one of two essential conditions plus two other criteria. This classification can be applied to diabetic populations, but is not useful in a general setting.

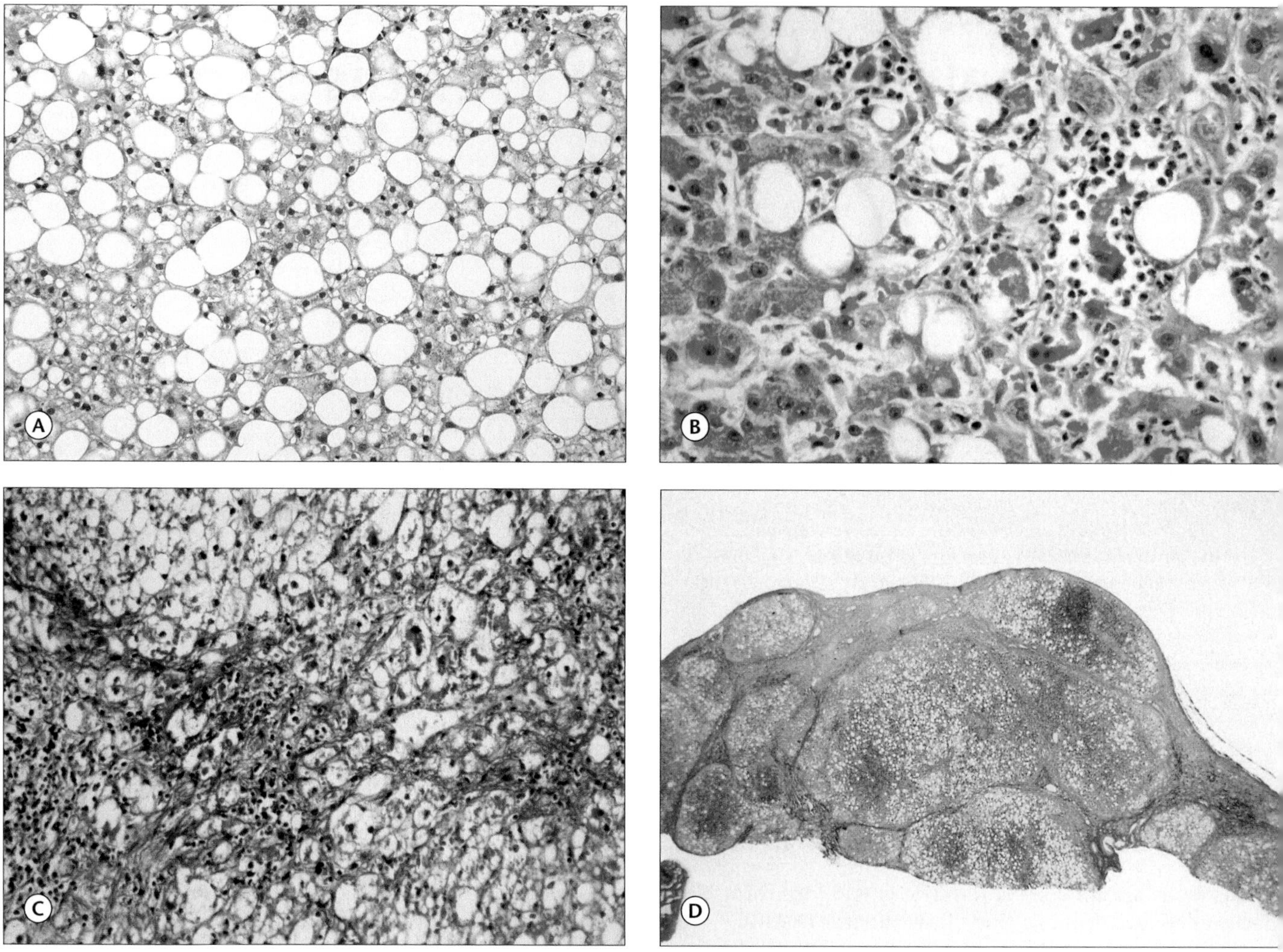

Fig. 88.1 Histologic findings in NASH. A. Hepatic steatosis. **B.** Ballooning and Mallory hyaline. **C.** Sinusoidal/pericellular fibrosis. **D.** NASH cirrhosis.

The Third Report of the National Cholesterol Education Program's Expert Panel on Detection, Evaluation, and Treatment of High Blood Cholesterol in Adults (Adult Treatment Panel III; ATPIII)[3] defines the metabolic syndrome as the pres ence of any three categorical and discrete risk factors that ca be measured easily.

The risk of hepatic steatosis increases exponentially with eac additional component of the metabolic syndrome. In addition the presence of the metabolic syndrome makes it more likel that a patient will have NASH rather than steatosis.[4]

TABLE 88.2 PREVALENCE OF NAFLD AND NASH

Type of study	Prevalence (%)
General population screening	
Ultrasonography	16–23 (76)
Liver enzymes	3–23
Selected populations	
Surgical patients	
Adult living liver donors	20
Bariatric surgery	56–86 [14–29]
Post-mortem analysis	
Hospitalized patients	3(19)
Random deaths	16–24 [2.1]
Patients undergoing liver biopsy	15–84 [1.2–48]

Numbers in parentheses indicate the prevalence of NAFLD in obese patients. Numbers in square brackets indicate the prevalence of NASH in studies in which liver biopsies were performed.

Obesity

A number of studies have established obesity as a risk facto not only for hepatic steatosis, but also for the presence of an progression to cirrhosis.

The distribution of fat may be more important than the tota fat mass. Compared with total fat mass, visceral fat is a stronge predictor of hepatic steatosis, as well as hyperinsulinemia decreased hepatic insulin extraction, and peripheral insuli resistance. Decreasing visceral fat has been shown to decreas hepatic insulin resistance. Lean patients with NASH may hav central adiposity. This may explain NAFLD in the subgroup o nonobese patients who are frequently of Asian origin.

Diabetes

Diabetes is an independent predictor for cirrhosis and live related deaths in patients with NAFLD.[5] The reason for this i unclear, but may be due to additional oxidative stress in diabetics

TABLE 88.3 PREVALENCE OF NAFLD IN THE NATIONAL HEALTH AND NUTRITIONAL EXAMINATION SURVEY (NHANES III)

	Analysis 1	Analysis 2	Analysis 3
Prevalence (%)	23	2.8	7.9
Liver enzymes (units/L)	AST, ALT, GGT (>30)	ALT (>43)	AST, ALT Women: >31, >31 Men: >37, >40
Exclusions	Appropriate	Diabetics	Appropriate

ALT, alanine aminotransferase; AST, aspartate aminotransferase; GGT, γ-glutamyltransferase.

DIAGNOSTIC METHODS

COMPARISON OF DIAGNOSTIC CRITERIA FOR METABOLIC SYNDROME

World Health Organization proposal	Adult Treatment Protocol III proposal[a]
Altered glucose regulation or insulin resistance *plus* two of the following:	Any three of the following:
Obesity: BMI >30 kg/m² *or* WHR >.0 (M) or >0.9 (F)	Waist girth: >102 cm (M) or >88 cm (F)
High triglycerides: >150 mg/dL *or* Low HDL cholesterol: <35 mg/dl (M) or <39 mg/dL (F)	Arterial pressure: ≥130/85 mmHg
Hypertension (≥150/90 mmHg	Triglycerides: ≥150 mg/dL
Microalbuminuria: ≥20 μg/ml	HDL cholesterol: <40 mg/dL (M) or <50 mg/dL (F) Glucose: ≥110 mg/dL

[a] Classification proposed by the Third Report of the National Cholesterol Education Expert Panel on detection, evaluation and treatment of high blood cholesterol in adults.[3]
BMI, body mass index; F, female; HDL, high density lipoprotein; M, male; WHR, waist:hip ratio.

Risk factors

In addition to histology (the presence or absence of NASH), certain risk factors predict the development of progressive fibrosis and cirrhosis; the most important of these are obesity, diabetes, age, hypertension, AST:ALT ratio, triglycerides, raised ALT, iron, the extent of steatosis, and inflammation.[5,6]

Table 88.4 displays the strongest predictive factors along with their acronyms, which may be helpful in deciding whether a liver biopsy is indicated in patients with NAFLD.

Data from the BARD acronym, for example, would predict that a patient with fatty liver on ultrasonography who is less than 45 years old, with neither obesity nor diabetes, and an AST:ALT ratio of less than 0.8 has only a minimal risk of significant fibrosis. In contrast, a 50-year-old patient with diabetes and an AST:ALT ratio greater than 1 would have a 66% chance of having fibrosis.

TABLE 88.4 PREDICTION ACRONYMS FOR ADVANCED FIBROSIS IN NAFLD

	BARD	BAAT	HAIR
BMI	3	3	
Age	3	3	
AST:ALT	3		
ALT		3	3
Diabetes	3		
Triglycerides		3	
Hypertension			3
Insulin resistance index			3

BARD: BMI ≥30; age ≥45 years; ratio of AST:ALT ≥1; diabetes.
BAAT: BMI ≥28; age ≥50 years; ALT ≥twice normal value; triglycerides ≥1.7 mmol/L.
HAIR: hypertension; ALT ≥40 units/L; insulin resistance ≥5.0 (defined by the Quicki equation).

PATHOGENESIS

An overall schematic for the pathogenesis of NAFLD/NASH is provided in Figures 88.2 and 88.3. Epidemiologic and migration studies link obesity to societal lifestyle changes, decreased physical activity, and an alteration in the dietary patterns that has occurred in industrialized countries over the past 50 years.

Once obesity has developed, the expanded fat mass functions as an endocrine organ that secretes increased amounts of tumor necrosis factor α, resistin, leptin, angiotensinogen, and cortisol, as well as decreased amounts of adiponectin. All of these hormones are known to have a definite or potential role in the development of either fat alone or NASH.[7]

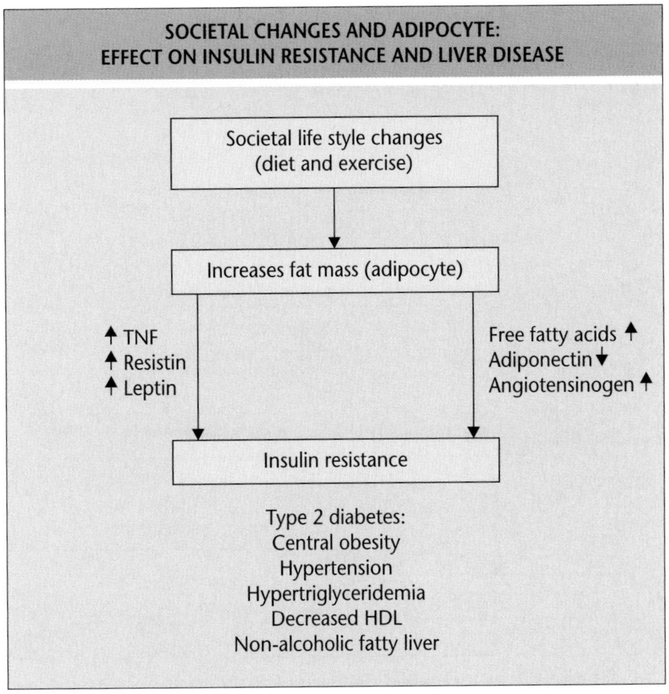

Fig. 88.2 Societal changes and adipocytes: the effect on insulin resistance and liver disease. The cascade effect of societal life changes on the development of insulin resistance and nonalcoholic fatty liver disease is shown.

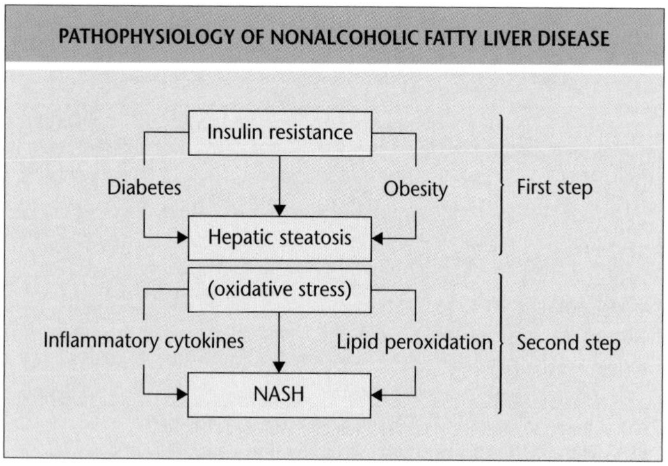

Fig. 88.3 Pathophysiology of nonalcoholic fatty liver disease. The two-step hypothesis in the development of NASH is shown. Insulin resistance is the first step that leads to hepatic steatosis, which, once developed, may advance to NASH (the second step) as a result of inflammatory cytokines and lipid peroxidation.

Insulin resistance is the essential first step in the pathophysiology of NAFLD and may be present prior to the development of obesity and/or type 2 diabetes B (Fig. 88.3). As shown in Figure 88.4, the influx of fatty acids to the liver (due to peripheral insulin resistance) combined with alteration in their hepatic metabolism (increased lipid synthesis and decreased triglyceride export) results in hepatic steatosis, which itself accelerates hepatic insulin resistance. Once developed, the hepatic steatosis may take two different paths with different clinical outcomes.[8,9] It may remain as steatosis or may progress to NASH.

Hepatic steatosis

Patients with steatosis alone have a benign clinical course without histologic clinical progression when followed for up to 19 years.[10] However, this 'benign' steatosis is not quiescer Up to 3–5% of these patients may progress to cirrhosis. The is activation of hepatic stellate cells, stimulation of apoptot proteins, and upregulation of mitochondrial uncoupling protei Despite these abnormalities (which have the potential to cau cell injury), hepatic histology (other than steatosis) and functic are normal.

NASH

It is unclear why only a subgroup of patients with NAFL develop NASH. However, lipid-laden hepatocytes may act as reservoir of hepatotoxic agents and are susceptible to 'secor hit' injury by compounds such as endotoxin, cytokines, an environmental toxins.[11]

Oxidative stress: NASH is associated with lipid peroxidatic caused by oxidative stress resulting from either lysosomal proces ing or increased oxidation of fatty acids by mitochondria, pe oxisomes, or cytokines.[12] These oxidative processes produce fr electrons, hydrogen peroxide, and reactive oxygen species whi depleting the potent antioxidants (glutathione and vitamin E Oxidative stress also stimulates insulin resistance and the sy thesis of several cytokines through both the upregulation of tra scription by nuclear translocation of nuclear factor-κB (NF-κI and the byproducts of lipid peroxidation – malondialdehyd (MDA) and 4-hydroxynonenal (HNE).[12–14] The combination these events causes hepatocyte injury through lipid peroxid tion and the stimulation of cytokine production (Fig. 88.5).

Bacterial toxin: The other proposed pathophysiologic mec anism for the development of NASH may involve increase delivery of portal-derived hepatotoxins to a sensitized fatt liver as a result of small intestinal bacterial overgrowth. Hov ever, even if this mechanism were operative, the resultant live injury would likely be mediated through cytokine-induce oxidative stress.[12]

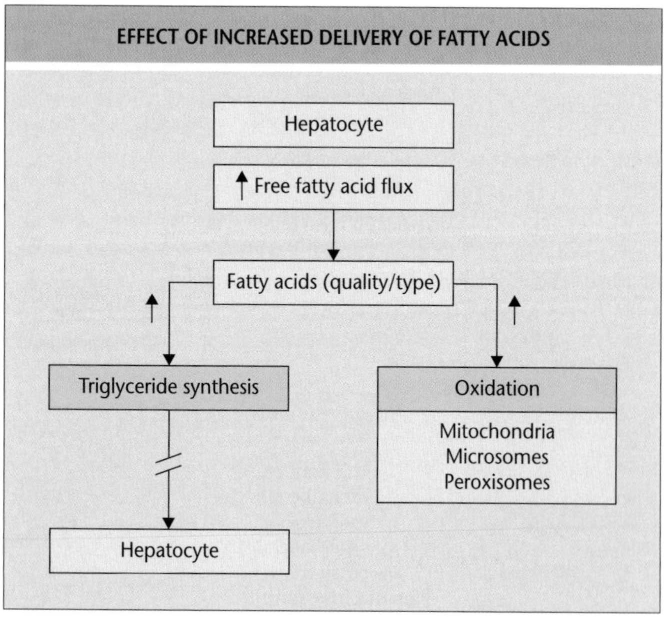

Fig. 88.4 Effect of increased delivery of fatty acids. Increased delivery of fatty acids results in hepatic steatosis due to increased lipid synthesis and decreased export of very low density lipoprotein (VLDL) triglycerides. Oxidation of fatty acids is increased due to increased PPAR(peroxisome proliferator activated receptors)-α.

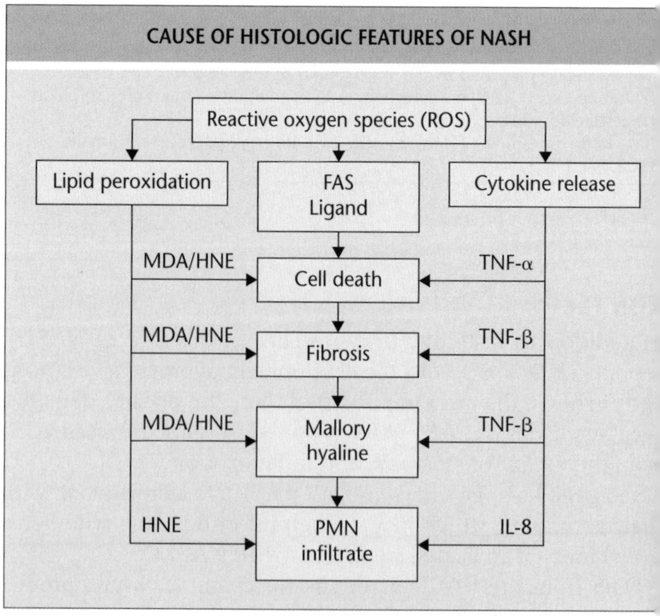

Fig. 88.5 Causes of the histologic features of NASH. Both lipid peroxidation and inflammatory cytokines can cause many or all of the histologic features of NASH: cell death (apoptosis), fibrosis, Mallory hyaline, and inflammatory infiltrates. IL, interleukin; TGF, transforming growth factor; TNF, tumor necrosis factor; MDA/HNE, malondialdehyde and 4-hydroxynonenal.

ATHOLOGY

onsensus regarding histologic nomenclature and categorization f this disease is only now emerging. Portal-based scoring systems uch as Ishak or Metavir) are not appropriate for NAFLD, which as more abnormalities in the central area of the hepatic lobule.

The histologic features of NAFLD fall into four general cateories. A promising new scoring system is a modification of the runt system[15] and has been proposed by a National Institutes f Health-funded NASH Clinical Research Network (CRN), nd shown in Table 88.5. The necessary histologic components diagnose NASH are: steatosis (macrovesicular greater than icrovesicular, accentuated in zone 3); mixed, mild lobular flammation; scattered polymorphonuclear leukocytes as well s mononuclear cells; and hepatocellular ballooning, most pparent near steatotic liver cells, typically most prominent in one 3. Other histologic features that are usually present, but not ecessary for the diagnosis of NASH, include: zone 3 perisinuoidal fibrosis, lipogranulomas, occasional acidophilic bodies, igmental Kupffer cells, and contiguous glycogenated nuclei. ess commonly present are Mallory hyaline, megamitochondria, nd positive iron staining.

TABLE 88.5 HISTOLOGIC SCORING SYSTEM FOR NAFLD

Feature	Score
1. STEATOSIS	
A. Grade	
Absent (< 5%)	0
5–33%	1
33–66%	2
>66%	3
B. Location	
Zone 3	0
Zone 1	1
Azonal	2
Panacinar	3
C. Microvesicular steatosis	
Absent	0
Present	1
2. INFLAMMATION	
A. Lobular inflammation (no. foci per 200× field)	
None	0
<2	1
2–4	2
>4	3
B. Portal inflammation	
None to minimal	0
Greater than minimal	1
C. Large lipogranulomas	
Absent	0
Present	1

TABLE 88.5 HISTOLOGIC SCORING SYSTEM FOR NAFLD—cont'd

Feature	Score
D. Microgranulomas	
Absent	0
Present	1
3. LIVER CELL INJURY	
A. Ballooning degenerations	
None	0
Few balloon cells	1
Many cells or prominent ballooning	2
B. Acidophilic bodies	
None to rare	0
Many	1
C. Mallory bodies	
None to rare	0
Many	1
D. Pigmented macrophages	
None to rare	0
Many	1
4. FIBROSIS STAGE	
0 (none)	0
1a (mild, zone 3, perisinusoidal)	1
1b (moderate, zone 3, perisinusoidal)	1
1c (portal/periportal)	2
2 (perisinusoidal and portal/periportal)	1
3 (bridging fibrosis)	3
4 (cirrhosis)	4

Although current highly detailed scoring systems are of little practical use, the importance of relating the natural history to histological findings has been emphasized by a system that involves four types of broad histologic classification, briefly described in Table 88.1 and Figure 88.6.

CLINICAL PRESENTATION

Patient demographics

Table 88.6 provides patient demographics from a number of studies. Most cases of NAFLD occur in the fifth and sixth decades of life, but may also occur in children. The condition is more frequent in females and in those with a high prevalence of type 2 diabetes mellitus, obesity, and hypertriglyceridemia. Three studies indicate that the typical clinical profile needs to be expanded to include male patients with normal weight and with no abnormalities of either glucose or lipid metabolism.

NAFLD has been reported in all ethnic groups, with preliminary data suggesting an overrepresentation in Hispanics and underrepresentation in African Americans.

Symptoms

A large proportion of patients with NAFLD are asymptomatic. Fatigue, malaise, and vague right upper quadrant abdominal

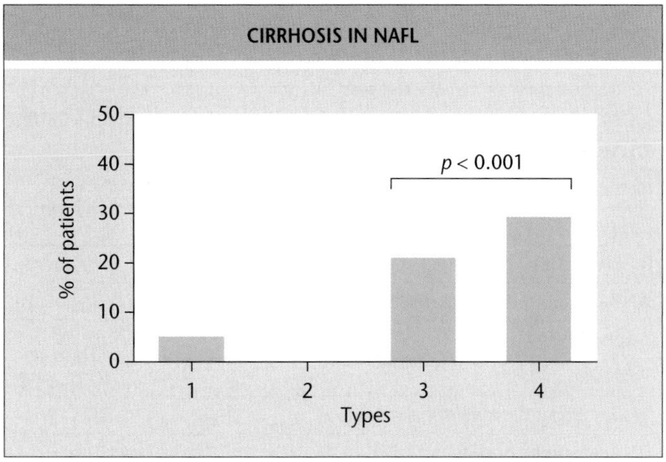

Fig. 88.6 Cirrhosis in nonalcoholic fatty liver disease. Cirrhosis occurs most prominently in NAFLD types 3 and 4 (NASH). There is only minimal risk for the development of cirrhosis in patients with types 1 and 2.

discomfort bring some patients with NASH to medical attention. Typically, patients with NAFLD present with other conditions and are found only incidentally to have abnormal liver function or hepatomegaly, the latter occurring in up to 75% of patients.

Fatigue correlates poorly with histologic stage. Although right upper quadrant pain (thought to be caused by distention of Glisson's capsule) is usually mild and nonspecific, it may be mistaken for gallstone disease. If diabetes is present, complications from visceral (bowel dysmotility and small bowel bacterial overgrowth) and peripheral neuropathy (pain and orthostatic hypotension) may also be present.

Physical examination

These patients usually have unremarkable findings on physical examination.[16] Most are obese with an increased waist circumference, and those who do not usually have increased visceral adiposity. Hypertension occurs in 15–70% of patients. Stigmata of chronic liver disease (muscle wasting, spider telangiectasis, gynecomastia, palmar erythema) are rarely seen on initial presentation, but when present suggest advanced fibrotic diseas Fluid retention (peripheral edema and ascites) and hepat encephalopathy may occur when cirrhosis is present. Abno malities in fat distribution should be sought to diagnose lip dystrophies. Females may exhibit hirsutism and acne, whic suggest polycystic ovary syndrome. Acanthosis nigrica (especially in children) with its associated hyperpigmente velvety plaques found in body folds is a feature of insul resistance. Finally intermittent disconjugate gaze (thought t be part of a generalized mitochondrial dysfunction) may occ in 15–20% of patients.

DIFFERENTIAL DIAGNOSIS

Exclusion of other disease

It is important to exclude other diseases associated with increase fat. These 'secondary' causes of hepatic steatosis (listed in Tab 88.7) are not typically associated with insulin resistance.[17] It particularly important to exclude alcohol and hepatitis C vir (HCV)-associated disease.

By definition, excessive alcohol consumption excludes th diagnosis of NAFLD. A wide range of alcohol consumption ha been used to define NAFLD, from complete abstinence to 14 and 210 g weekly for females and males respectively. Therefo there is no consensus regarding the definition of 'nonalcoholi As it is difficult objectively to confirm the daily use of 10–20 alcohol (currently the limit usually used to exclude NAFLD females and males respectively), clinicians need to be dilige in quantitating alcohol consumption.

It is also important to exclude HCV, which often is associate with hepatic steatosis, with appropriate serologic testing. patients with biochemical evidence of iron overload, genet testing (*HFE* gene) or liver biopsy for iron quantification ma be necessary.

DIAGNOSTIC METHODS

Liver biopsy

Liver biopsy is considered the gold standard for diagnosis an is the only method for differentiating NASH from steatos

TABLE 88.6 PATIENT DEMOGRAPHICS

Study	*n*	Age (years)	Female (%)	Diabetes (%)	Obesity (%)	Hyperlipidemia (%)	Symptomatic (%)	Advanced fibrosis (%)
Ludwig[25]	20	54	65	25	90	67	NA	15
Diehl[26]	39	52	81	55	71	20	23	39
Lee[27]	49	53	78	51	69	4	0	34
Powell[28]	42	49	83	36	93	81	52	50
Bacon[29]	33	47	42	21	39	21	36	39
Pinto[30]	32	48	75	34	47	28	6	55
Laurin[31]	40	48	73	28	70	40	NA	NA
Matteoni[10]	132	53	53	33	70	92	NA	15
Angulo[32]	144	51	67	28	60	27	NA	NA
Willner[33]	90	51	51	46	87	61	12	28
Chitturi[34]	66	47	41	39	57	82	(most)	33
Marchesini[4]	304	42	17	7	25	3	NA	21

NA, data not available.

TABLE 88.7 PROPOSED CLASSIFICATION FOR NAFL[a]

PRIMARY

Conditions associated with:

- Metabolic syndrome
- Diabetes mellitus (type II)
- Obesity
- Hyperlipidemia

SECONDARY

Drugs

- Corticosteroids
- Synthetic estrogens
- Amiodarone
- Perhexiline
- Calcium channel blockers

Surgical procedures

- Gastroplexy
- Jejunoileal bypass
- Extensive small bowel resection
- Biliopancreatic diversion

Miscellaneous

- Abeta/hypobeta-lipoproteinemia
- Weber-Christian disease
- Total parenteral nutrition with glucose
- Environmental toxins
- Small bowel diverticulosis
- Lipodystrophy
- Human immunodeficiency virus
- Malnutrition (both marasmus and kwashiorkor)

[a] This classification refers to conditions and diseases associated only with macro/microvesicular steatosis. Conditions associated with predominantly microvesicular steatosis are excluded.

with or without inflammation.[15] Disagreements exist, however, regarding the necessity for performing liver biopsy in patients with NAFLD. A liver biopsy in these patients can be used to exclude other liver diseases, distinguish steatosis from NASH, estimate prognosis, and determine the progression of fibrosis over time. The arguments against performing a liver biopsy include: a generally good prognosis, lack of effective therapy, and the associated risk and cost. Therefore, radiologic and serum chemistries have been investigated as alternative noninvasive methods for the diagnosis of NAFLD and its different histologic subtypes.

Radiology

Ultrasonography, computed tomography, magnetic resonance imaging, and proton magnetic resonance spectroscopy (^{1}H-MRS), the latter being more sensitive when fat involves less than 30% of the liver volume, have been used to diagnose NAFLD.[18] However, differences between NASH and steatosis are not apparent with any of the radiologic modalities. Although ultrasonography has limitations, practicality and cost issues have made it the most common imaging modality used for evaluating hepatic steatosis.[12]

Serum chemistry

Increased aminotransferase activities are the most common abnormality in NAFLD; levels are usually raised only modestly, in the range of a 2–5-fold increase. Alkaline phosphatase concentration is increased 2–3-fold in less than half of patients. Serum albumin and bilirubin levels are rarely abnormal unless cirrhosis has developed. Raised serum levels of ferritin are reported in approximately 50% of patients with NAFLD, usually with no evidence of hepatic iron overload.

The AST:ALT ratio is usually less than 1. When the ratio is greater than 1, this suggests an advanced fibrotic form of NAFLD. Hematologic measurements are usually normal, unless cirrhosis has led to hypersplenism. Several small selected case studies have reported antinuclear antibodies in 10–46% of patients with NAFLD. The significance of this observation is unclear.

Although liver function test results may be raised in NAFLD, values can be normal and the degree of abnormality does not correlate with the degree of steatosis or fibrosis.

TREATMENT AND PREVENTION

A management and treatment algorithm is proposed in Figure 88.7 and has been reviewed recently.[19–21]

Histologic confirmation

Although the role of liver biopsy in NAFLD remains uncertain, many clinicians believe that patients with unexplained abnormal liver function test results or a fatty liver on radiological examination should undergo liver biopsy, especially if they are high risk for having NASH (obesity, diabetes, age above 45 years, or warning signs of fibrotic disease). This approach identifies those patients with NAFLD about whom the clinician should be most concerned.

Treatment of co-morbid diseases

Treatment of the co-morbid conditions usually associated with NAFLD (type 2 diabetes, obesity, and/or hypertriglyceridemia)

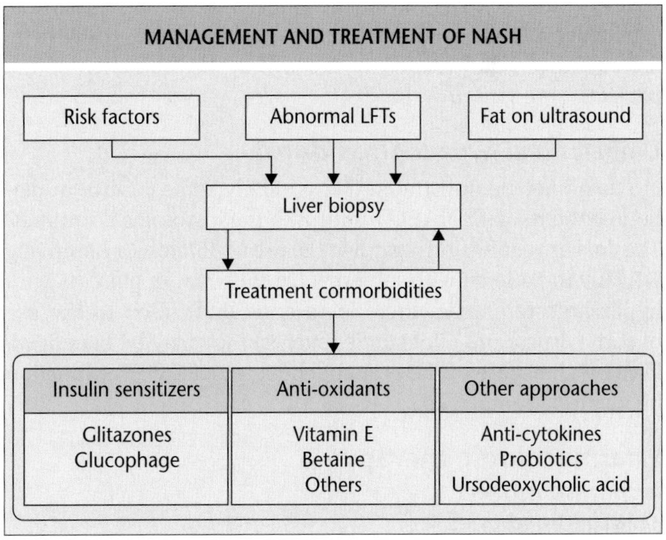

Fig. 88.7 Management and treatment of NASH. A management and treatment algorithm is proposed. If fat is found on a radiologic test or there is unexplained abnormal liver function (especially in the setting of risk factors suggestive of advanced fibrosis), a liver biopsy is indicated either before or after the treatment of co-morbidities. If there is improvement in liver function and/or steatosis on ultrasonography, liver biopsy may not be necessary. All the therapies below the broken line have not yet been shown to be clinically effective in NAFLD and are not recommended for routine clinical use at present.

is essential in these patients.[14] This approach is consistent with overall good clinical care; however, the benefits of this strategy have been inconsistent. Clinicians disagree regarding whether treatment of co-morbidities should be initiated before or after a liver biopsy has been performed.

Weight loss

Serum transaminase levels almost always improve with weight loss (with as little as 5–10% decrease in bodyweight), but they are poor predictors of histological appearance, which does not always improve and may in fact worsen if weight loss occurs too rapidly. Gradual weight loss (1–2 lb per week) with an overall goal of 10% weight loss over 6 months is recommended as a safe and effective clinical strategy, especially in patients who are 30% overweight.

With success, further weight loss can be attempted, if indicated. Multiple interventions and strategies, including diet modifications, physical activity, behavioral therapy, and pharmacotherapy with orlistat, or a combination of these treatment modalities is recommended. The particular treatment modality should be individualized, taking into consideration the body mass index (BMI) and presence of concomitant risk factors and other diseases. Given the lack of clinical trials in this area, these overall recommendations are a useful and safe first step for obese patients with NAFLD.

The only prospective study using restrictive bariatric surgery in patients with NAFLD was very effective in diminishing hepatic injury.[22]

Type of diet

A number of different diets have been suggested, including: the American Heart Association's healthy heart diet, the Diabetic Diet as recommended by the American Diabetes Association, a low glycemic diet, and diets enriched with omega-3 polyunsaturated fatty acids. However, the effect of these diets in NAFLD is unproven. Diets used to produce weight loss must always be individualized and related to the overall health status of the patient.

Diabetes and hypertriglyceridemia

No data have demonstrated that good glycemic control in diabetic patients with NAFLD improves the histological findings. The data are conflicting regarding the use of fibrates for improving NAFLD in patients with hypertriglyceridemia. In patients with hypercholesterolemia, there is no contraindication to the use of statin drugs, and pilot studies suggest they may be beneficial. However, because of the potential hepatotoxicity, liver function needs to be monitored.

Pharmacologic therapy

Insulin sensitizers

Thiazolidinediones

Pilot trials have been performed using thiazolidinediones (troglitazone, rosiglitazone, and pioglitazone), a relatively new class of antidiabetic drugs that act as PPAR-γ agonists and increase insulin sensitivity in fat tissue. Each of these drugs improved serum levels of transaminases, with some improvement in steatosis and fibrosis. However, they all have the potential for hepatotoxicity. Therefore, the nascent but promising results of these pilot studies need to be evaluated in well controlled studies prior to general clinical use.

Glucophage

Glucophage improves insulin sensitivity by decreasing hepati lipid production, which in turn increases hepatic sensitivity t insulin and thereby suppresses hepatic glucose production. Tw studies (of which only one was controlled) have demonstrate that glucophage decreases liver function, but histologi findings have not been shown to improve.

Antioxidants

Although two initial trials suggested that vitamin E improve NAFLD, the only controlled trial showed no benefit of vitami E (combined with vitamin C) over placebo. Betaine has improve liver function, with some improvement in histologic findings i uncontrolled small pilot studies. Although *N*-acetylcysteine, mil thistle, *S*-adenosylmethionine (SAMe), and antioxidant cocktail have been used in preliminary studies, there are insufficient dat to discuss any of the results in detail. Three trials have bee performed with phlebotomy to remove iron (hypothesized t be a pro-oxidant in NAFLD). All showed improvement in live function, but none was controlled and no histologic exami nation was undertaken.

Others

Although there is a rationale for the use of ursodeoxycholi acid, probiotics, anticytokines, and nonabsorbable antibiotics insufficient data exist to employ such therapy at the presen time.

Prevention

No studies have directly evaluated preventive therapies.

Preventing disease

Extracting information from studies in patients with obesit and diabetes, weight loss and exercise are reasonable strategie as well as being good for general health. Although man specific therapeutic interventions have been implemented i NAFLD, epidemiologic data suggest that a change in behavio that would affect energy balance by as little 420 kJ/day woul prevent weight gain and arrest the epidemics of both obesit and NAFLD.

Preventing complications

Vaccination for viral hepatitis

Although no data are available for this strategy in NAFLD vaccinating for hepatitis A and B may be worthwhile and i employed by many clinicians.

Screening for hepatocellular carcinoma

Hepatocellular carcinoma (HCC) is now recognized to develo in cirrhosis secondary to NAFLD/NASH. Therefore, man clinicians employ interval assessments with screening ultra sonography and/or α-fetoprotein, even without existing cost effectiveness studies.

COMPLICATIONS AND THEIR MANAGEMENT

The only complications that occur in NAFLD are those asso ciated with the adverse clinical outcomes (cirrhosis, acute live failure, and HCC) that are part of its natural history. The man agement of these outcomes are standard treatment for thes complications of cirrhosis in general.

ROGNOSIS WITH AND WITHOUT REATMENT

Vithout treatment

.s shown in Figures 88.6 and 88.8, cirrhosis develops in 5–25% of patients with NASH. Once developed, 40% of these atients may succumb to liver-related death over a 10-year eriod,[9] the mortality rate being similar to or worse than that f cirrhosis associated with hepatitis C. NASH is also now onsidered the major cause of cryptogenic cirrhosis. NASH-ssociated cirrhosis may also decompensate into subacute liver ilure, progress to HCC, and recur after transplantation. In ontrast, steatosis alone is reported to have a more benign inical course, although progression of fibrosis in cirrhosis has ccurred in 3% of these patients with steatosis alone.[9]

Vith treatment

o specific therapy has been shown to be effective in NAFLD/ ASH. However, of those therapies being considered, only ustained weight loss with or without bariatric surgery has the otential to alter the natural history of NAFLD.

VHAT TO TELL PATIENTS

atients need to partner with their physicians in the management of NAFLD in a number of important ways and become ctively involved in their own care.

Diet

n general, patients should follow a well balanced diet. One such iet is recommended by the National Cholesterol Education Program (http://www.nhlbi.nih.gov/about/ncep). This diet makes specific recommendations regarding total calorie intake, as well as the amount and type of fat and carbohydrate for patients who do not have to lose weight. If the patient has diabetes, specific recommendations have been made by the American Diabetes Association.[23]

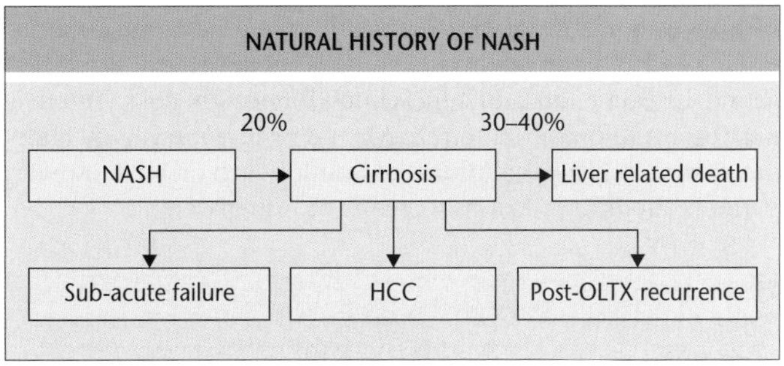

Fig. 88.8 Natural history of NASH. HCC, hepatocellular carcinoma; OLTX, orthotopic liver transplantation.

Dietary supplements

Many patients seek advice regarding the efficacy and safety of vitamins, herbs, or other nutritional supplements. Unfortunately, there is insufficient information in this area to make sound recommendations, although general recommendations can be made.

Weight loss

Overweight patients (BMI $>25\,kg/m^2$) should be given a diet with a goal of losing and sustaining an initial weight loss of 10%

TREATMENT AND PREVENTION

USE OF NUTRITIONAL SUPPLEMENTS AND MEDICATIONS IN NAFLD

Possibly harmful		Possibly helpful	
Supplements	**Medications**	**Supplements**	**Medications**
St John's wort	Acetaminophen[d]	Vitamin E[h]	Betaine[k]
Ephedrine-containing compounds	Tamoxifen[e]	MVI[i]	Ursodeoxycholic acid[k]
Excessive vitamin A[a]	Amiodarone[e]	SAMe[j,k]	Metformin[k,l]
Glucosamine[b]	Iron[f]	Milk thistle[k]	Statins[k,m]
Others[c]	Estrogen[g]		Thiazolidinediones[k,l]

[a] Vitamin A should not be used in excess of that contained in a daily multivitamin (MVI), which is 5000 IU.
[b] As hexosamines in general cause insulin resistance, glucosamine should be used with some caution.
[c] All other herbs should be considered as possible causes of injury and should be avoided.
[d] Acetaminophen should be restricted to less than 2–3 g daily. Repeated or ongoing use of acetaminophen or longer than 3 days with daily doses above 1.5 g should be discouraged. Many over-the-counter (OTC) nedications contain acetaminophen; therefore the amount of acetaminophen in OTC medications should be sought carefully.
[e] This drug may cause hepatic injury that histologically looks similar to NAFLD/NASH. Therefore, the benefit risk of using these drugs in NAFLD/NASH should be considered carefully.
[f] As iron may cause oxidative stress in the liver, iron supplements should be used only as per standard nanagement for anemia. Transferrin saturation should not exceed 50%.
[g] Estrogens used as oral contraceptive pills or hormonal replacement therapy do not have to be discontinued.
[h] Vitamin E should not be used at doses greater than 800 IU daily.
[i] A daily multivitamin (MVI) with iron content <20 mg should be used.
[j] SAMe, *S*-adenosylmethionine.
[k] The use of this supplement or medication should not be encouraged. However, there are uncontrolled studies suggesting their benefit in NAFLD.
[l] This agent is approved for use in patients with type II diabetes.
[m] The use of the statins used as cholesterol-lowering agents is not contraindicated (and may be beneficial) n NAFLD. However, baseline and interval measurements of liver function should be performed.

of bodyweight. The weight loss should be gradual and should not exceed 2 lb per week, as per the National Heart, Lung and Blood Institute (NHLBI) guidelines for weight loss. There is insufficient information to recommend or discourage any alternative diet (such as the Atkins' or South Beach diets). However, patients should not fast as a means of losing weight.

TREATMENT AND PREVENTION

WEIGHT LOSS DIET[a]

Nutrient	Recommended intake
Calories[b]	Approximately 500–1000 kcal/day reduction from usual state
Total fat[c]	30% or less of total calories
Saturated fatty acids[d]	8–10% of total calories
Monounsaturated fatty acids	Up to 15% of total calories
Polyunsaturated fatty acids	Up to 10% of total calories
Cholesterol[d]	<300 mg/day
Protein[e]	Approximately 15% of total calories
Carbohydrate[f]	55% or more of total calories
Sodium chloride	No more than 100 mmol/day (approximately 2.4 g sodium or 6 g sodium chloride)
Calcium[g]	1000–1500 mg/day
Fiber[f]	20–30 g/day

[a] This table provides guidelines for Step I weight loss as suggested in a monograph provided by the National Heart, Lung and Blood Institute (2000) entitled "The practice guide. Identification, evaluation and treatment of obesity in adults."

[b] A reduction in calories of 500–1000 kcal/day will help achieve a weight loss of 1–2 lb/week. Alcohol provides unneeded calories and displaces more nutritious foods. Alcohol consumption not only increases the number of calories in a diet but has been associated with obesity in epidemiologic as well as experimental studies. The impact of alcohol calories on a person's overall caloric intake needs to be assessed and approximately controlled.

[c] Fat-modified foods may provide a helpful strategy for lowering total fat intake but will be effective only if they are also low in calories and there is no compensation by calories from other foods.

[d] Patients with high blood cholesterol levels may need to use the Step II diet to achieve further reductions in low density lipoprotein cholesterol levels; in the Step II diet, saturated fats are reduced to less than 7% of total calories, and cholesterol levels to less than 200 mg/day. All of the other nutrients are the same as in Step I.

[e] Protein should be derived from plant sources and lean sources of animal protein.

[f] Complex carbohydrates from different vegetables, fruits, and whole grains are good sources of vitamins, minerals, and fiber. A diet rich in soluble fiber, including oat bran, legumes, barley, and most fruits and vegetables, may be effective in reducing blood cholesterol levels. A diet high in all types of fiber may also aid in weight management by promoting satiety at lower levels of calories and fat intake. Some authorities recommend 20–30 g fiber daily, with an upper limit of 35 g.

[g] During weight loss, attention should be given to maintaining an adequate intake of vitamins and minerals. Maintenance of the recommended calcium intake of 1000–1500 mg/day is especially important for women who may be at risk of osteoporosis.

Exercise

Regular exercise is a useful adjunct to weight loss and improves the success of weight loss. The Institute of Medicine recommends that regular physical activity of at least 1 h per day should be performed.

Alcohol and cigarette use

Alcohol should not be used at all, or restricted to no more than minimal ceremonial use. Cigarette use has now been recognized as a risk factor for fibrosis in other forms of liver disea[se] and should therefore be strongly discouraged.

Physician management of co-morbid diseases

The recognized co-morbidities and diseases associated wi[th] NAFLD, along with specific management recommendation[s] are shown in the box.

TREATMENT AND PREVENTION

MANAGEMENT OF CO-MORBIDITIES IN NAFLD

Co-morbidity	Management goals/issues
Type 2 diabetes	HgbA1c <7% should be sought Insulin sensitizing agents rather than insulin or sulfonylureas are preferred
Hypercholesterolemia	Referral to PCP or specialist for cholesterol levels >130 mg/dL in nondiabetics and >100 mg/dL in diabetics
Hypertriglyceridemia	Referral to PCP or specialist for fasting triglycerides >200 mg/dL
Hypertension	Referral to PCP or specialist for repeated systolic blood pressure (BP) >140 mmHg and/or diastolic BP >90 mmHg in diabetics. In diabetics, referral for systolic BP >130 mmHg and/or a diastolic BP >85 mmHg
Angina	Symptoms of coronary heart disease should be sought and referred to PCP or specialist as needed
Obstructive sleep apnea (OSA)	Symptoms of OSA (snoring, disruptive sleep, etc.) should be sought. If present, referral to a specialist should be obtained for possible sleep study and therapy
Polycystic ovary syndrome (PCOS)	Women with hirsutism and nonmenopausal menstrual irregularity (>9 menstrual cycles yearly) should be referred to PCP or gynecologist for possible PCOS
Occupational hepatotoxin	A history of ongoing exposure to volatile hydrocarbons should be sought and suggestions for changing workplace conditions made

PCP, primary care provider

Sources of information for patients and doctor[s]

Although the above recommendations regarding diet and exe[r]cise should be strongly encouraged, these recommendations a[re] often difficult to achieve. Therefore, continual encourageme[nt] should be utilized even if the absolute goals are not achieve[d]. Patients can obtain additional information on NAFLD from th[e] American Liver Foundation (http://www.liverfoundation.or[g]) and the National Digestive Diseases Information Clearinghous[e] (http://digestive.niddk.nih.gov) and the Institute of Medicin[e] (http://www.iom.edu).

Other websites:

http://www.patient.co.uk/showdoc/23068929/
http://www.patient.co.uk/showdoc/40024505/
http://patients.uptodate.com/topic.asp?file=livr_dis/5305
http://www.liverfoundation.org/db-select/article[s/]CatNonAlcy/1/1/ascend/Validated

CURRENT CONTROVERSIES AND FUTURE RESOLUTION

A number of important controversies and questions remain relevant to NAFLD and NASH:[24]

- What are the histologic criteria that differentiate NASH from NAFLD?
- What minimal amount of alcohol use separates alcoholic from nonalcoholic fatty liver disease?
- Why does only a subset of patients with NAFLD develop NASH?
- Are there noninvasive methods other than liver biopsy that distinguish NAFLD from NASH?
- What is the interaction between genetic and environmental factors in the development of NAFLD?
- Is our current knowledge of the natural history and pathophysiology of NAFLD sufficient to recommend management algorithms or treatments that are cost-effective and safe?
- As the normal limits for ALT in population studies have been revised downward, with values individualized by sex and obesity, what should be considered an abnormal ALT value?

Unfortunately, these questions remain unanswered at the present time. However, the pathologists from the NASH Clinical Research Network in the United States have published in preliminary form a histologic scoring system for NASH. It will be published in 2005 and is likely to be widely accepted. In addition, a number of therapeutic trials are being initiated that will test the efficacy of insulin sensitizers (glucophage and thiazolidinediones), antioxidants (vitamin E, betaine, and SAMe), ursodeoxycholic acid, and probiotics. These studies should be completed within the next 3 years. Until such time, clinicians and patients with NAFLD will need to implement the general therapeutic strategies outlined above.

REFERENCES

1. Youssef WI, McCullough AJ. Steatohepatitis in obese individuals. Best Pract Res Clin Gastroenterol 2002; 16:737–747.
2. Yu AS, Keefe EB. Elevated AST or ALT to nonalcoholic fatty liver disease: accurate predictor of disease prevalence? Am J Gastroenterol 2003; 98:955–956.
3. Executive Summary of the Third Report of the National Cholesterol Education Program (NCEP) Expert Panel on detection, evaluation, and treatment of high blood cholesterol in adults (Adult Treatment Panel III). JAMA 2001; 285:2486–2497.
4. Marchesini G, Bugianesi E, Forlani G et al. Non-alcoholic fatty liver, steatohepatitis and the metabolic syndrome. Hepatology 2003; 37:917–923.
5. Younossi ZM, Gramlich T, Matteoni CA, Bopari N, McCullough AJ. Non-alcoholic fatty liver disease in patients with type 2 diabetes. Clin Gastroenterol Hepatol 2004; 2:262–265.
6. Angulo P. Non-alcoholic fatty liver disease. N Engl J Med 2002; 346:1221–1231.
7. Tilg H, Diehl AM. Cytokines in alcoholic and nonalcoholic steatohepatitis. N Engl J Med 2000; 343:1467–1476.
8. Marchesini G, Brizi M, Bianchi G et al. Nonalcoholic fatty liver disease: a feature of the metabolic syndrome. Diabetes 2001; 50:1844–1850.
9. Kim JK, Fillmore JJ, Chen U et al. Tissue specific over expression of lipoprotein lipase causes tissue specific insulin resistance. Proc Natl Acad Sci USA 2001; 98:7522–7527.
10. Matteoni CA, Younossi ZM, Gramlich T et al. Nonalcoholic fatty liver disease: a spectrum of clinical and pathological severity. Gastroenterology 1999; 116:1413–1419.
11. Day CP, James OFW. Steatohepatitis: A tale of two "hits"? Gastroenterology 1998; 114:842–845.
12. Chitturi S, Farrell GC. Etiopathogenesis of nonalcoholic steatohepatitis. Semin Liv Dis 2001; 21:27–41.
13. Day CP. Pathogenesis of steatohepatitis. Best Pract Clin Gastroenterol 2002; 16:663–678.
14. Youseff WI, McCullough AJ. Diabetes mellitus, obesity and hepatic steatosis. Semin Gastrointestinal Dis 2002; 13:17–30.
15. Brunt EM. Nonalcoholic steatohepatitis: definition and pathology. Semin Liv Dis 2001; 21:3–16.
16. AGA Technical Review on Nonalcoholic Fatty Liver Disease. Gastroenterology 2002; 123:1705–1725.
17. Falck-Ytter, Younossi ZM, Marchesini G, McCullough AJ. Clinical features and natural history of non-alcoholic steatosis syndromes. Semin Liv Dis 2001; 21:17–26.
18. Siegelman ES, Rosen MA. Imaging of hepatic steatosis. Semin Liv Dis 2001; 21:71–80.
19. Harrison SA, Kadakia S, Lang KA, Schenker S. Nonalcoholic steatohepatitis. What we know in the new millennium. Am J Gastroenterol 2002; 97:2714–2724.
20. Agarwal S, Bonkovsky HL. Management of nonalcoholic steatohepatitis. J Clin Gastroenterol 2002; 35:253–261.
21. Alba LM, Lindor K. Nonalcoholic fatty liver disease. Aliment Pharmacol Ther 2003; 17:977–986.
22. Dixon JA, Bhathal PS, Hughs NR, O'Brien PE. Nonalcoholic fatty liver disease: improvement in liver histological analysis with weight loss. Hepatology 2004; 39:1647–1654.
23. Franz MJ, Bantle JP, Beebe JD et al. for the American Diabetes Association. Nutrition principles and recommendations in diabetes. Diabetes Care 2004; 27:S36–S46.
24. Younossi ZM, Diehl AM, Ong JP. Nonalcoholic fatty liver disease: an agenda for clinical research. Hepatology 2002; 35:746–752.
25. Ludwig J, Viaggiano TR, McGill DB, Ott BJ. Nonalcoholic steatohepatitis. Mayo Clinic experiences with a hitherto unnamed disease. Mayo Clin Proc 1980; 55:434–438.
26. Diehl AM, Goodman Z, Ishak KG. Alcohollike liver disease in nonalcoholics. A clinical and histologic comparison with alcohol-induced liver injury. Gastroenterology 1988; 95:1056–1062.
27. Lee RG. Nonalcoholic steatohepatitis: a study of 49 patients. Hum Pathol 1989; 20:594–598. Review.
28. Powell EE, Cooksley WG, Hanson R, et al. The natural history of nonalcoholic steatohepatitis: a follow-up study of forty-two patients for up to 21 years. Hepatology 1990; 11:74–80.
29. Bacon BR, Farahvash MJ, Janney CG, Neuschwander-Tetri BA. Nonalcoholic steatohepatitis: an expanded clinical entity. Gastroenterology 1994; 107:1103–1109.
30. Pinto HC, Baptista A, Camilo ME, et al. Nonalcoholic steatohepatitis. Clinicopathological comparison with alcoholic hepatitis in ambulatory and hospitalized patients. Dig Dis Sci 1996; 41:172–179.
31. Laurin J, Lindor KD, Crippin JS, Gossard A, et al. Ursodeoxycholic acid or clofibrate in the treatment of non-alcohol-induced steatohepatitis: a pilot study. Hepatology 1996; 23:1464–1467.
32. Angulo P, Keach JC, Batts KP, Lindor KD. Independent predictors of liver fibrosis in patients with nonalcoholic steatohepatitis. Hepatology 1999; 30:1356–1362.
33. Willner IR, Waters B, Patil SR, et al. Ninety patients with nonalcoholic steatohepatitis: insulin resistance, familial tendency, and severity of disease. Am J Gastroenterol 2001; 96:2957–2961.
34. Chitturi S, Abeygunasekera S, Farrell GC, et al. NASH and insulin resistance: insulin hypersecretion and specific association with the insulin resistance syndrome. Hepatology 2002; 35:373–379.

Chapter 89

Hemochromatosis

John M Kauffman and Norman D Grace

KEY POINTS

- Most common genetic disorder in Caucasians, especially of Celtic ancestry
- Autosomal recessive mutation of the HFE gene
- C282Y/C282Y homozygous mutation responsible for at least 85% of cases of HH
- C282Y/H63D compound heterozygous mutations may also cause a milder HH
- Extrahepatic manifestations may include congestive heart failure, diabetes, arthropathy, pituitary insufficiency, and skin hyperpigmentation

NTRODUCTION

ı its fullest phenotypic expression, hemochromatosis is a rogressive, multiorgan disease of excessive iron deposition. he excess iron is a result of increased intestinal iron absorp- on, inappropriate to the level of total body iron stores. The rincipal organs affected include the liver, heart, pancreas, and kin, with involvement of these last two organs giving rise ɔ the archaic term 'bronze diabetes.' Whereas the initial case eport of the disease was described in a clinic lecture on glycos- ria in 1865,[1] it was not until 1889 that von Recklinghausen uggested the term 'hemochromatosis,'[2] and recognized that ron deposition was responsible for the hyperpigmentation. he authoritative text on hemochromatosis was published by heldon in 1935,[1] and systematically detailed the accepted 311 eported cases of the disease to that date. In these patients, 7% presented with the triad of diabetes, skin hyperpigmen- ation, and hepatomegaly. The diagnosis was commonly made nly on autopsy and was felt to be a rare disease. The high ercentage of alcoholics in these early descriptions of iron verload clouded the recognition that hemochromatosis is not disease of alcoholism.

Nearly 40 years passed before the autosomal recessive nature of hereditary hemochromatosis (HH) was established.[3] The ene associated with HH was sequenced in 1996[4] and subse- quently labeled *HFE*. Two different single point mutations in his gene, located on the short arm of chromosome 6, appear o be responsible for the large majority of cases of HH. The principal mutation (C282Y) results in the substitution of yrosine for cysteine at the 282 position of the HFE gene product. A secondary mutation of less importance (H63D) results in the substitution of aspartate for histadine at the 63 amino acid position.

EPIDEMIOLOGY

Although representing the most common genetic disorder in Caucasians, HH demonstrates great prevalence variability worldwide. The highest frequency occurs in European populations, specifically in Ireland and the Basque region,[5] whereas it is rare in the African and Asian populations. Epidemiological data suggest that the original mutation occurred either in the Celtic or the Viking populations.[6] Clinically, the most significant mutation is the C282Y gene defect. In the homozygous state, the C282Y gene mutation appears to be responsible for 85–90% of HH, whereas the H63D mutation seems to result in iron overload only in the compound heterozygous state with C282Y. On a worldwide basis, the gene frequency of C282Y is 1.9%, but the gene frequency in a group of Caucasian patients attending a health appraisal clinic in the US was 6.3%. The H63D mutation is more common (15.2%). In the Basque region, the H63D mutation has been found in up to 30.4% of chromosomes.[5] The C282Y/C282Y homozygous state approaches 5 in 1000, or 0.5% of the population in the US, Australia, and northern Europe.[5,7]

Although rare and not an important epidemiological cause of HH, genetically transmitted hemochromatosis occurs in some families without defects in the *HFE* gene. In southern Europe, particularly Italy, there are reports of non-*HFE* iron overload syndromes indistinguishable from the classical HH occurring in a large family. The defect appears to be a missense mutation in the ferroportin gene, resulting in an autosomal dominant form of hemochromatosis.[8]

The penetrance of the homozygous C282Y gene mutation remains unclear. In an Australian population-based study of 3011 white adults, 16 (0.5%) were homozygous for the C282Y gene.[7] Of these, half had symptoms consistent with HH, including hepatomegaly, skin pigmentation, and arthritis. The serum ferritin was elevated in 7 of the 12 homozygotes who had no previous diagnosis of HH. After a follow-up of 4 years, the serum ferritin of four homozygotes remained within the normal range. In a large study of 41038 patients attending a health appraisal clinic in the US, 152 C282Y homozygotes were identified.[9] Evidence of iron overload in homozygous men, as assessed by elevated serum ferritin levels and elevated transferrin saturations, was present in 76% and 77%, respectively, when frequent blood donors were excluded. The symptoms commonly associated with HH, including general poor health, diabetes, arthralgias, arrhythmias, impotence, and skin hyperpigmentation, however, were not significantly different from the large control population. As no tissue biopsies were obtained, the degree of abnormal iron deposition and liver fibrosis was not assessed.

The heterozygous C282Y state and the compound heterozygous C282Y/H63D state may have served a vital role in early human evolution, preventing iron deficiency through increased hemoglobin and mean erythrocyte volume levels. Hepatic complications of iron overload in heterozygotes appear to be extremely rare. However, the heterozygous state may play a significant, synergistic role in other liver diseases, such as NASH, viral hepatitis, and alcoholic liver disease.

CAUSES, RISK FACTORS, DISEASE ASSOCIATIONS

The homozygous C282Y/C282Y mutation confers an increased risk for iron overload. This occurs through increased intestinal iron absorption. There is no mechanism for the intestine to increase iron excretion, which is typically 1 mg of iron daily. Therefore, increased absorption leads to a net increase in the iron balance, resulting in progressive accumulation. Patients with HH can absorb up to 4 mg of iron daily. Generally, the disease is not manifested early in life, as a total of 10–20 g of iron is necessary prior to the development of tissue injury.[10] A hepatic iron concentration threshold of 283 µmol/g liver is associated with an increased risk of cirrhosis. Women are relatively protected earlier in life because of the iron loss associated with menstruation. When compared to age-matched men, women show a decreased ferritin level (911 µg/L compared to 1911 µg/L) and less iron removed by venesection (5.5 g compared to 8.6 g). Moreover, women had a reduced risk for development of cirrhosis (25.6% compared to 13.8%).[11] Hepatic iron concentrations and hepatic iron indices, however, were similar in men and women.

Extrahepatic manifestations of HH include diabetes, bronze discoloration of the skin, arthralgias, impotence, and cardiac involvement. Iron deposition in the respective tissues is responsible for these complications. Progressive accumulation of iron in the myocardium can result in a dilated cardiomyopathy, conduction defects, and congestive heart failure in advanced cases.

Disease interactions: Several liver diseases are known to be potentiated by the concomitant consumption of excessive alcohol. Progression of fibrosis to cirrhosis was nine times more likely in HH patients who consumed more than 60 g alcohol per day,[12] with similar results seen with a cut-off value of 40 g. Serum ferritin and transferrin saturation were both statistically higher in those that consumed more that 60 g per day. Moreover, the incidence of hepatocellular carcinoma was greater in this group. Similar results have been reported in a French study, where serum ferritin, serum iron, transferrin saturation, and alanine and aspartate aminotransferases were all significantly elevated in the HH population with excessive alcohol consumption.

Hepatitis C (HCV) is a common cause of chronic viral hepatitis in Western Europe and the US. Given the frequency of HH, it is not uncommon for patients to present with combined HH and HCV. The progression to advanced fibrosis and cirrhosis occurs at a younger age and at a lower hepatic iron concentration in patients with both disease processes, compared to patients with HH alone. This supports a potentiating effect of HCV and HH on fibrogenesis. The presence of a single C282Y allele in patients with HCV appears to influence progression to advanced liver fibrosis. Increased hepatic iron staining and an increased hepatic iron concentration[13] were found in patients with HCV and the heterozygous presence of the C282Y allele. Overall, progression of fibrosis in the presence of the single allele appears to be accelerated only in a minority of cases.

CAUSES AND RISK FACTORS

- Prevalence of C282Y/C282Y homozygous state may be 0.5% in populations of Northern European extraction
- C282Y mutation of *HFE* results in an inappropriate increase in iron absorption
- Body iron loss is unregulated, and stable around 1 mg daily
- Patients with HH can absorb up to 4 mg of iron daily
- Liver injury in HH is accelerated by excessive alcohol consumption
- Fibrosis in HH may be accelerated by concomitant infection with hepatitis C or NASH

PATHOGENESIS

Iron homeostasis is predominantly regulated by the liver. The liver serves as a reservoir for iron storage, largely incorporated with ferritin. The normal *HFE* gene encodes a protein that is expressed in multiple organs, including the liver, and throughout the gastrointestinal tract. In the proximal small intestine, the site of iron absorption, the HFE protein localizes deep within the crypt enterocytes. The normal HFE protein appears to bind to β_2-microglobulin. This complex associates with the transferrin receptor 1 in the duodenal crypt enterocyte, and regulates iron uptake from serum transferrin into the crypt cells, thus providing the intestinal enterocytes with a sensing mechanism for the body's iron stores. Crypt enterocytes ultimately migrate and differentiate into villus enterocytes. Iron absorption is maximal in the villus enterocytes of the duodenum, and these cells are primed for their level of iron absorption based on the iron stores sensed within the crypts. The intestinal iron sensing mechanism provided by the HFE complex thus permits a mechanism for regulation of intestinal iron absorption. In the presence of reduced circulating transferrin iron, decreased iron uptake occurs within the crypt enterocytes. This leads to increased iron absorption at the apical membrane in the mature villus enterocytes.

Figure 89.1 displays the uptake of iron from the intestinal lumen and transfer through the enterocyte, with ultimate transport across the basolateral membrane into the blood.[14] Ferric iron is reduced to the ferrous state through the brush border membrane enzyme Dcytb (duodenal cytochrome b).[15] The apical membrane protein DMT-1 (divalent metal transporter-1) transports iron into the enterocyte from the gut lumen. On the basolateral membrane, iron is transported out of the enterocyte by ferroportin 1, a membrane-bound protein. Derangement of any of these iron transport mechanisms or enzymes can result in perturbations of iron metabolism.

In classical HH, the C282Y mutation of the HFE protein prevents binding with β_2-microglobulin at the basolateral membrane. The result is an inappropriately low measurement of plasma iron, leading to increased villus enterocyte iron absorption. In mice studies with deletions of the HFE gene, profound iron accumulation within the liver was noted.[16] Subsequent knockout studies support the role of the HFE protein in the regulation of duodenal uptake of transferrin-bound iron from

UPTAKE AND TRANSPORT OF IRON INTO THE BLOOD

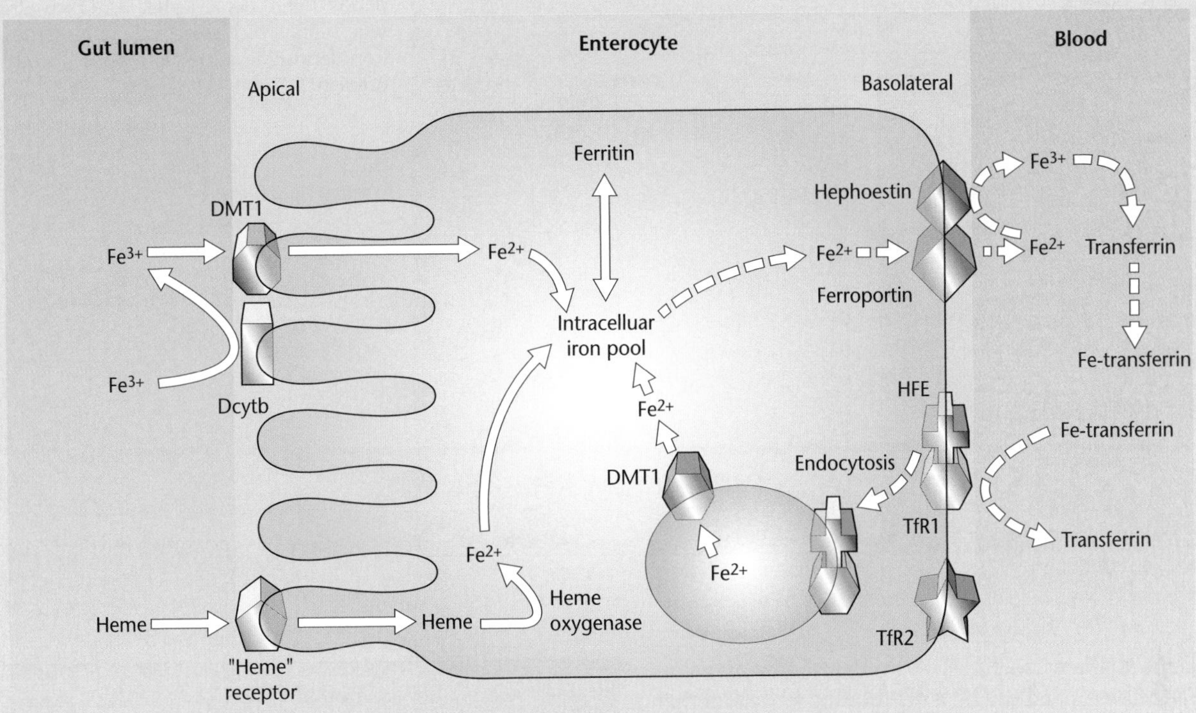

g. 89.1 **Uptake and transport of iron.** Dietary ferric iron is reduced to ferrous iron by the membrane-bound protein called Dcytb. rrous iron is transported into the cell by DMT1. Iron is transported across the basolateral surface by ferroportin 1. Uptake of serum nsferrin-bound iron into the enterocyte occurs at the basolateral surface. This process is mediated by TfR1 (transferrin receptor 1). is receptor, in turn, is regulated by the hemochromatosis protein (HFE) and β2-microglobulin. HFE appears to reduce the affinity of TfR1 r transferrin. The role of a second transferrin receptor, TfR2, in iron absorption is unknown.[14]

asma. The precise mechanism whereby HFE affects iron omeostasis remains unknown, but recently hepcidin, a protein nthesized in the liver, has been proposed to play a pathonic role.[17] Hepcidin levels are reduced in patients with assical HH.

ATHOLOGY

gure 89.2 shows the typical findings associated with epatic iron overload. Perls' Prussian blue stain shows iron eposition within the hepatocytes. Iron is preferentially calized to the periportal regions of the lobule, with a zonal radation. Other processes that may lead to more mild cases of on overload commonly result in iron deposition first in the upffer cells with no preferential localization to the periportal egions.

LINICAL PRESENTATION

opulation screening with iron saturation and ferritin frequently etects asymptomatic patients with phenotypic expression of H. Additionally, many patients present to their physicians ith a family history of HH. In a fortunate majority of these ases, the disease is diagnosed in the premorbid phase when o symptoms or significant liver fibrosis have developed. In ther cases, HH develops insidiously. Patients usually have no ymptoms during iron accumulation in the early stages of HH prior to end organ injury. Typically, iron accumulation is minimal before 20 years of age, by which time less than 5 g of iron have accumulated. Progressive iron accumulation between ages 20 and 40 years results in an asymptomatic state of iron overload (usually less than 20 g of iron). With iron accumulation beyond 20 g, organ dysfunction may result. With ever more iron deposition in the hepatocytes, liver fibrosis can develop and evolve into cirrhosis. Even in the early cirrhotic phase, symptoms can be minimal or nonspecific. The presence of cirrhosis, however, places patients at an increased risk for the development of hepatocellular carcinoma.

Liver-related symptoms: Many symptoms of HH are secondary to the underlying liver dysfunction. These symptoms, therefore, may be present in other causes of liver injury. These include the nonspecific complaints of fatigue or lethargy. Common symptoms of advanced liver disease of any etiology include spider angiomata, palmar erythema, testicular atrophy, hypogonadism, and weight loss. The development of portal hypertension may result in hypersplenism, encephalopathy, and gastric and esophageal varices.

Non liver-related symptoms: When present, skin hyperpigmentation is an important sign that calls for testing for HH, as few other liver diseases result in this finding. This presentation is secondary to increased melanin, not iron, and is secondary to pituitary insufficiency. Adult onset diabetes is common in Western countries. Iron accumulation in the pancreas may result in pancreatic endocrine dysfunction and adult-onset but

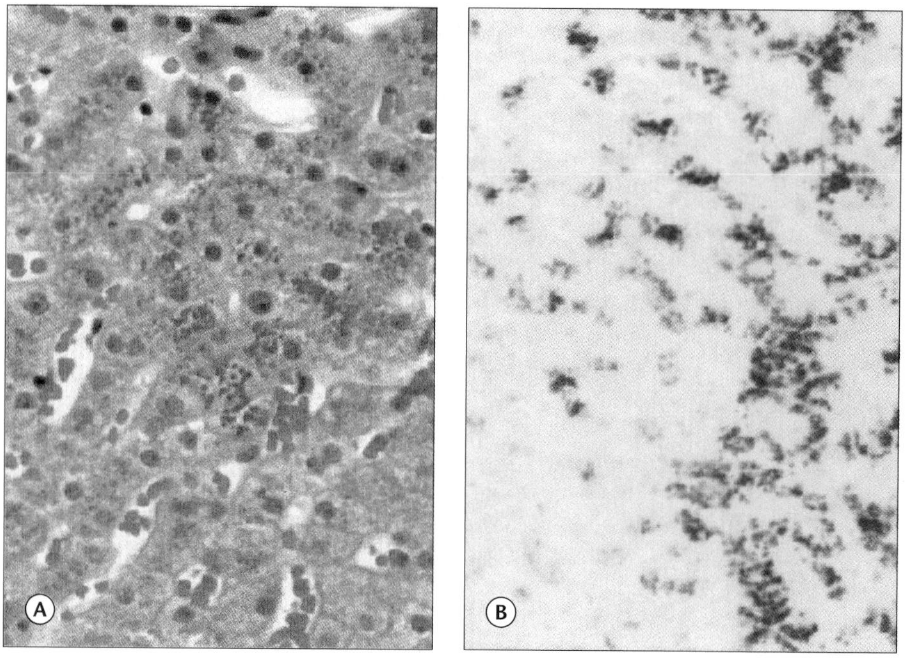

Fig. 89.2 Typical findings associated with hepatic iron overload. A. A hematoxylin ar eosin stain revealing cytoplasmic pigment deposition in hepatocytes. **B.** A Perls' Prussia blue stain, which selectively stains ferric iron Iron deposition occurs in a portal to central gradient.

insulin-deficient diabetes mellitus. Arthralgias may develop prior to hepatic fibrosis and can be a debilitating symptom that does not usually improve with phlebotomy therapy. Cardiac dysfunction from iron overload may result in arrhythmias, dilated cardiomyopathy, and congestive heart failure.

CLINICAL PRESENTATION

- HH typically does not become symptomatic prior to 40 years of age, when iron stores surpass the threshold for liver injury
- Liver iron overload can lead to advanced fibrosis without significant transaminase elevation
- Upon liver iron saturation, extrahepatic iron accumulation may develop with the following potential complications:
  - skin hyperpigmentation
  - adult onset, insulin-dependent diabetes mellitus
  - arthralgias/arthritis
  - congestive heart failure, dilated cardiomyopathy, and cardiac arrythmias
- Patients with HH and cirrhosis are at an increased risk for hepatocellular carcinoma

DIFFERENTIAL DIAGNOSIS

The two *HFE* gene mutations most associated with HH are the C282Y/C282Y (>85%) and C282Y/H63D (>5%) mutations. The presence of excess hepatic iron, however, can occur secondary to non-HFE-related conditions. Secondary iron overload from blood transfusions, ineffective erythropoiesis, or chronic hemolytic conditions can result in hepatocytic iron overload. Thus, sideroblastic anemia, aplastic anemia, or severe thalassemias may result in a parenchymal iron overload indistinguishable from HH. In extreme cases, dietary iron overload or iron injections can contribute.

CLINICAL PEARLS

- The treatment of HH prior to the development of cirrhosis is associated with a normal life expectancy
- Population screening should focus on the phenotypic expression of iron overload, not the genotype
- Family screening should focus on the genotype
- Patients with homozygous C282Y who are age <40 and normal liver tests have a low prevalence of hepatic fibrosis, making liver biopsy unnecessary

Genetic causes of iron overload not related to the *HFE* gen may result in massive iron overload. These include juvenil hemochromatosis, which is an autosomal recessive diseas that presents in the 2nd and 3rd decades of life and is linke to chromosome 1q. The gene is now called *HFE 2*. Iro overload appears in a similar pattern to HH, but at a muc earlier age. Mutations in the transferrin receptor 2 (TFR2) gen on 7q, called *HFE 3*, can result in a rare, recessive disorde similar to HH.[18] The function of TFR2, and its role in iro overload, remain to be elucidated. Ferroportin gene mutation have been reported to cause a hereditary iron overloa condition indistinguishable from HH in 15 related individual in Italy.[8]

Several common chronic liver diseases may predispose t excess iron deposition. These conditions include alcoholic live disease, chronic hepatitis B and C, and nonalcoholic fatty live disease. In these cases, however, the degree of iron overload i less than HH, as manifested by the fewer number of phle botomies before anemia develops.

DIAGNOSTIC METHODS

Initial laboratory testing typically includes serum iron, tota iron binding capacity (TIBC), and ferritin. Elevated transferri

DIFFERENTIAL DIAGNOSIS
Multiple blood transfusions secondary to: – aplastic anemia – sideroblastic anemia – thalassemia – chronic hemolytic anemia Chronic hepatitis B and C Alcoholic liver disease Nonalcoholic fatty liver disease Aceruloplasminemia Juvenile hemochromatosis (*HFE 2*) Transferrin receptor 2 mutations (*HFE 3*) Ferroportin 1 mutations (*HFE 4*) Exogenous iron supplementation

turation above 45% and elevated serum ferritin are sugges- ve of iron overload. Higher transferrin saturations are more ecific for HH. Ferritin, however, is an acute phase reactant d is commonly elevated in inflammatory conditions, cases of alignancy, and in non-iron-related causes of liver disease, cluding hepatitis C, alcoholic liver disease, and nonalcoholic tty liver disease. The presence of tissue iron overload defini- vely provides the diagnosis of hemochromatosis. The hepatic on index (HII) quantifies hepatic iron and corrects for the ogressive iron accumulation seen in older subjects. It is cal- ılated by dividing the hepatic iron content in micromoles by e patient's age in years. A value of >1.9 correlated highly ith the diagnosis of HH.

A **liver biopsy** is commonly recommended during the initial valuation and diagnosis of patients presenting with symptoms nd laboratory testing suggestive of HH. This helps confirm the iagnosis in some cases, but more importantly permits meas- rement of the degree of liver fibrosis. In select cases, how- ver, a biopsy may not be necessary. Whereas the presence of dvanced fibrosis cannot be determined with great accuracy sing serological markers, the absence of advanced fibrosis can e accurately predicted in most patients lacking high-risk dicators.[19] These indicators include a ferritin >1000, absence f hepatomegaly, abnormal serum aminotransferases, and an ge >40 years. Therefore, current recommendations are to efer biopsy if these indicators are absent.

DIAGNOSTIC METHODS
• Serum tests: – serum iron, total iron binding capacity, and ferritin – transferrin saturation >45% suggests iron overload – elevated ferritin suggests iron overload, but may also be elevated as an acute phase reactant – HFE genotype • Liver biopsy: – provides direct measurement of hepatic iron and degree of fibrosis – hepatic iron index corrects for progressive iron accumulation with age – not necessary if ferritin <1000, age <40, and transaminases are normal

TREATMENT AND PREVENTION

Once the diagnosis of HH has been made, hemochromatosis is easily and successfully treated by phlebotomy therapy. The venesection of 400–500 mL is equivalent to approximately 200–250 mg of iron. Excess total body iron can exceed 20–30 g, commonly resulting in the need for weekly phlebotomy for months until evidence of iron depletion results in a failure of the hematocrit to rebound after phlebotomy. Once normalization of iron stores is accomplished, phlebotomy frequency may be reduced to once every 1–6 months, depending on the response of the hematocrit to phlebotomy. Once iron stores are depleted, ferritin levels typically fall below 50 ng/mL. A reasonable target for the transferrin saturation is below 25%. Dietary changes are not necessary, but patients should be advised to avoid iron-containing vitamin preparations. Vitamin C promotes iron absorption and, for this reason, supplements of this vitamin should be avoided as well.

Although the genetic predisposition to iron overload cannot be prevented, all first-degree relatives of patients with known HH should be screened at an age not earlier than 25 years. Initial screening can be performed either with HFE genotype testing, or with measurement of the fasting transferrin saturation and serum ferritin.[20]

As alcohol greatly accentuates the expression of HH, including the risk for development of cirrhosis and symptomatic development of hemochromatosis (including skin hyperpigmentation) all patients with HH should be advised to abstain from alcohol, or to consume with extreme restraint.

TREATMENT AND PREVENTION
• Phlebotomy to remove excess iron is the treatment of choice • 400–500 mL of blood is equivalent to 200–250 mg of iron • Weekly phlebotomy may be necessary for months to deplete excess iron stores • After iron depletion, periodic phlebotomy every 3–6 months • Goal is to maintain ferritin levels between 25 and 50 ng/mL • Avoidance of vitamin C, which promotes iron absorption • Avoidance of alcohol, which accelerates the progression of fibrosis

COMPLICATIONS AND THEIR MANAGEMENT
• Diagnosis after cirrhosis predisposes to hepatocellular carcinoma (HCC) • Extrahepatic manifestations may include congestive heart failure, diabetes, and arthropathy; these typically do not improve with phlebotomy therapy • Phlebotomy therapy results in improvement in liver function tests, decreases the risk for HCC, decreases cardiac arrhythmias, and skin hyperpigmentation • Possible progression to end-stage liver disease and need for transplantation

PROGNOSIS WITH AND WITHOUT TREATMENT

The prognosis of patients treated with phlebotomy therapy prior to the onset of cirrhosis or diabetes is excellent. A study of patients with clinical, biochemical, and histological evidence of HH but no cirrhosis followed for 14.1 years revealed identical survival rates in a matched normal population.[21] However, cumulative survival in patients with HH and cirrhosis was significantly reduced when compared to noncirrhotic patients with HH. The development of diabetes as a complication of HH also affects survival. In patients with cirrhosis and HH, 71.8% had diabetes, in contrast to 16.5% in noncirrhotic HH patients.[21] Moreover, survival is significantly reduced in patients with diabetes, but without cirrhosis. Untreated HH predisposes to the usual complications of cirrhosis, including liver cancer and liver failure. The development of liver cancer in the setting of cirrhosis secondary to HH appears to have an increased frequency when compared to cirrhosis secondary to causes other than HH.

End-stage liver disease or hepatocellular carcinoma secondary to HH is frequently treated by orthotopic liver transplantation. Excess iron has the potential to cause extrahepatic organ dysfunction, including cardiac and pancreatic dysfunction. Therefore, survival after liver transplantation might be expected to be reduced when compared to non-iron-loaded patients. The 5-year survival of patients transplanted with a hepatic iron index greater than 1.9 was found to be 48%, compared to matched controls with a 77% 5-year survival.[22] The reduced survival was mainly attributable to increased bacterial a particularly fungal infections.

WHAT TO TELL PATIENTS

An important message to relay to patients with HH is that disease is curable and that survival is no different from t of controls if the disease is treated prior to the developm of complications, particularly cirrhosis. Treatment is hig effective, relatively easy, and devoid of significant side effe The FDA has approved the use of HH patients' blood as do blood. Therefore, with certain restrictions, phlebotomi units may be used for blood donation. Substantial changes lifestyle are not necessary. Dietary changes are not usua necessary, although avoidance of vitamin C supplementat is reasonable.

SOURCES OF INFORMATION FOR PATIENTS AND DOCTORS

The National Institute of Diabetes and Digestive and Kidn Diseases (NIDDK) has a website with additional informati on hemochromatosis that may be informative for patie (http://digestive.niddk.nih.gov/ddiseases/pubs/hemochroma sis/index.htm).

http://patients.uptodate.com/topic.asp?file=livr_dis/2974&titl Hemochromatosis

http://www.liverfoundation.org/db/articles/1013

REFERENCES

1. Sheldon JH. Haemochromatosis. London: Oxford University Press; 1935.
2. von Recklinghausen FD. Über Hamochromatose. Tagebl Versamml Natur Artze Heidelberg 1889; 62:324.
3. Simon M, Bourel M, Genetet B et al. Idiopathic hemochromatosis. Demonstration of recessive transmission and early detection by family HLA typing. N Engl J Med 1977; 297:1017–1021.
4. Feder JN, Gnirke A, Thomas W et al. A novel MHC class I-like gene is mutated in patients with hereditary haemochromatosis. Nat Genet 1996; 13:399–408.
5. Merryweather-Clarke AT, Pointon JJ, Shearman JD et al. Global prevalence of putative haemochromatosis mutations. J Med Genet 1997; 34:275–278.
6. Smith BN, Kantrowitz W, Grace ND et al. Prevalence of hereditary hemochromatosis in a Massachusetts corporation: is Celtic origin a risk factor? Hepatology 1997; 25:1439–1446.
7. Olynyk JK, Cullen DJ, Aquilia S et al. A population-based study of the clinical expression of the hemochromatosis gene. N Engl J Med 1999; 341:718–724.
8. Montosi G, Donovan A, Totaro A et al. Autosomal-dominant hemochromatosis is associated with a mutation in the ferroportin (SLC11A3) gene. J Clin Invest 2001; 108: 619–623.
9. Beutler E, Felitti VJ, Koziol JA et al. Penetrance of 845G→A (C282Y) HFE hereditary haemochromatosis mutation in the USA. Lancet 2002; 359:211–218.
10. Bassett ML, Halliday JW, Powell LW. Value of hepatic iron measurements in early hemochromatosis and determination of the critical iron level associated with fibrosis. Hepatology 1986; 6:24–29.
11. Moirand R, Adams PC, Bicheler V et al. Clinical features of genetic hemochromatosis in women compared with men. Ann Intern Med 1997; 127:105–110.
12. Fletcher LM, Dixon JL, Purdie DM et al. Excess alcohol greatly increases the prevalence of cirrhosis in hereditary hemochromatosis. Gastroenterology 2002; 122:281–289.
13. Tung BY, Emond MJ, Bronner MP et al. Hepatitis C, iron status, and disease severity: relationship with HFE mutations. Gastroenterology 2003; 124:318–326.
14. Trinder D, Fox C, Vautier G et al. Molecular pathogenesis of iron overload. Gut 2002; 51:290–295.
15. McKie AT, Barrow D, Latunde-Dada GO et al. An iron-regulated ferric reductase associated with the absorption of dietary iron. Science 2001; 291:1755–1789.
16. Zhou XY, Tomatsu S, Fleming RE et al. HFE gene knockout produces mouse model of hereditary hemochromatosis. Proc Natl Aca Sci USA 1998; 95:2492–2497.
17. Petrangelo A. Hereditary hemochromatosis. A new look at an old disease. N Engl J Me 2004; 350:2383–2397.
18. Camaschella C, Roetto A, Cali A et al. The gene TFR2 is mutated in a new type of haemochromatosis mapping to 7q22. Nat Ger 2000; 25:14–15.
19. Guyader D, Jacquelinet C, Moirand R et al. Noninvasive prediction of fibrosis in C282Y homozygous hemochromatosis. Gastroenterolo 1998; 115:929–936.
20. Tavill AS. Diagnosis and management of hemochromatosis. Hepatology 2001; 33:1321–1328.
21. Niederau C, Fischer R, Purschel A et al. Long-term survival in patients with hereditary hemochromatosis. Gastroenterology 1996; 110:1107–1119.
22. Brandhagen DJ, Alvarez W, Therneau TM et al. Iron overload in cirrhosis-HFE genotype and outcome after liver transplantation. Hepatology 2000; 31:456–460.

Chapter 90

Alpha$_1$-antitrypsin deficiency

Giorgina Mieli-Vergani and Nedim Hadžić

KEY POINTS

- The commonest genetic indication for liver transplantation in children
- Autosomal codominant inheritance
- Only PiZZ A1ATD associated with liver disease
- Presence of PAS-positive, diastase-negative deposits in the liver biopsy is suggestive of PiZZ A1ATD
- Pathogenesis of liver disease is incompletely understood
- Wide range of clinical severity of liver disease
- Majority of PiZZ individuals are asymptomatic

NTRODUCTION

lpha$_1$-antitrypsin deficiency is the commonest metabolic cause f chronic liver disease (CLD) in Caucasians and the leading enetic indication for liver transplantation in children.[1] In ddition, smokers with alpha$_1$-antitrypsin deficiency are at risk f developing chronic obstructive lung disease in adulthood. ther complications such as vasculitis, glomerulonephritis, and anniculitis have also been described.

Alpha$_1$-antitrypsin is a highly polymorphic 55-kD glycorotein, which belongs to the serine protease inhibitor (serpin) perfamily[2] and is the product of the Pi gene, which resides n chromosome location 14q31-32.1. Alpha$_1$-antitrypsin is roduced at a rate of 34 mg/kg/day, primarily by hepatocytes, ut also by alveolar macrophages and intestinal endothelial ells.[2,3] Alpha$_1$-antitrypsin undergoes a structural change when s reactive center is exposed to the attached target protease uring activation. This conformational change has the role of activating the protease at the end of the acute phase response.[2] he alpha$_1$-antitrypsin variants other than the wild-type (PiMM) ppear to be less stable, leading to an increased incidence of pontaneous opening of the main sheet of the molecule and, onsequently, abnormal folding, augmented polymerization, nd retention within the hepatocytes. This has been well ocumented for the PiZZ alpha$_1$-antitrypsin variant.[4,5]

PIDEMIOLOGY

lpha$_1$-antitrypsin deficiency is a condition affecting mainly aucasians, although individuals with different variants have een anecdotally reported from other ethnicities.[6] Normal serum evels of the alpha$_1$-antitrypsin protein are associated with the iMM phenotypes, while alpha$_1$-antitrypsin deficiency is characerized by absent or significantly reduced serum alpha$_1$-ntitrypsin levels and phenotypic profiles PiNull, PiZ, and PiS on serum isoelectric focusing. Almost one hundred genetic alpha$_1$-antitrypsin variants have been described to date.[7] PiZ and PiS deficiency are related to 342 Glu→Lys and 264 Glu→Val point mutations, respectively.[7] Alpha$_1$-antitrypsin deficiency is inherited in an autosomal codominant fashion. The prevalence of PiZ and PiS alleles in nonconsanguineous populations of European descent is estimated to be between 0.5% and 2% and 1% and 9%, respectively.[7]

CAUSES, RISK FACTORS, DISEASE ASSOCIATIONS

PiZZ alpha$_1$-antitrypsin deficiency leads to CLD in 10–20% of affected children.[8] Liver disease has also been described with rare Pi S_{iiyama} and M_{malton} variants of alpha$_1$-antitrypsin. Possible genetic modifiers leading to the development of CLD in only a minority of the affected individuals with the PiZZ phenotype are yet to be identified. There is a wide range of the severity of liver disease in the symptomatic PiZZ children. Of those, approximately one-quarter progress to end-stage CLD and require liver replacement during childhood.[1,8] Presence of fibrosis in the liver biopsies and jaundice after 6 months of age are associated with the highest risk of developing end-stage CLD in childhood.[1]

Chronic obstructive lung disease can develop in PiNull, PiZ, and PiS alpha$_1$-antitrypsin deficiency, albeit only in a small proportion of patients and in strong association with smoking. There is no information as yet on whether symptomatic children with liver disease are at risk of developing lung disease later in life.

PATHOGENESIS AND PATHOLOGY

The mechanisms of liver and lung disease in alpha$_1$-antitrypsin deficiency are different. Adults appear to develop chronic obstructive lung disease as a direct consequence of low serum levels of the alpha$_1$-antitrypsin protein, resulting in decreased protease inhibitory activity during inflammatory processes in the lungs.

The pathogenesis of liver disease is less clear. It has been suggested that conformational changes of the unstable alpha$_1$-antitrypsin variants lead to retention of polymers of abnormally folded alpha$_1$-antitrypsin in the hepatocyte endoplasmic reticulum (Fig. 90.1).[4,5] Their presence can be demonstrated by immunoperoxidase staining in the fetal livers as early as 19 weeks postconception (Fig. 90.2),[9] when exposure to triggers of acute phase response is minimal. Some early studies have suggested an increased prevalence of light-for-gestational age infants

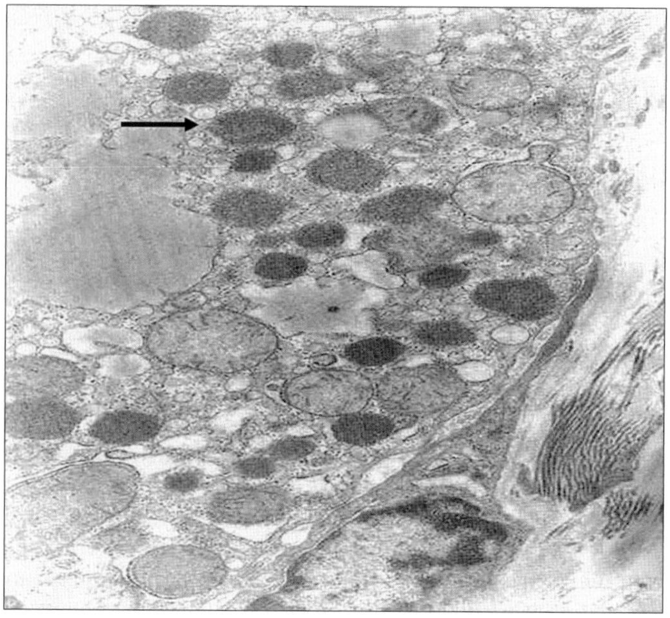

Fig. 90.1 A1AT deposits. Amorphous material representing deposits of A1AT in the endoplasmic reticulum of hepatocytes of a patient with PiZZ A1ATD (arrow) (electromicroscopy, x6500).

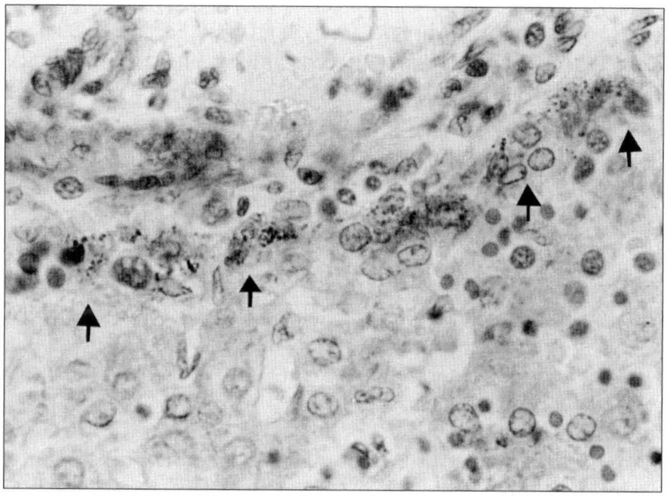

Fig. 90.2 A1ATD deposits. Postmortem liver specimen from a fetus with PiZZ A1ATD, aborted at 19 weeks of gestation, demonstrating granular deposits of A1ATD (arrows) (immunoperoxidase, x300). From Malone et al. Pediatric Pathology 1989; 9:623–631.

amongst PiZZ children who later require liver transplantation.[10] Whether liver injury could be related to accumulation of Z alpha$_1$-antitrypsin polymers is unknown. However, these polymers are present also in the 80–85% of PiZZ alpha$_1$-antitrypsin-deficient individuals who do not develop clinically overt liver disease and therefore are unlikely to be major effectors of damage *per se*.

Liver histology in infancy demonstrates non-specific portal and lobular hepatitis with variable cholestasis, mild biliary features, and fibrosis (Fig. 90.3). The appearances can sometimes mimic biliary atresia. Presence of periportal macrovesicular fat may represent an important diagnostic clue (Fig. 90.4 and Fig. 90.5). The demonstration of magenta-colored alpha$_1$-antitrypsin deposits on periacid Schiff (PAS) stain is usually not possible within the first 3–6 months of life. Presence of PAS-positive,

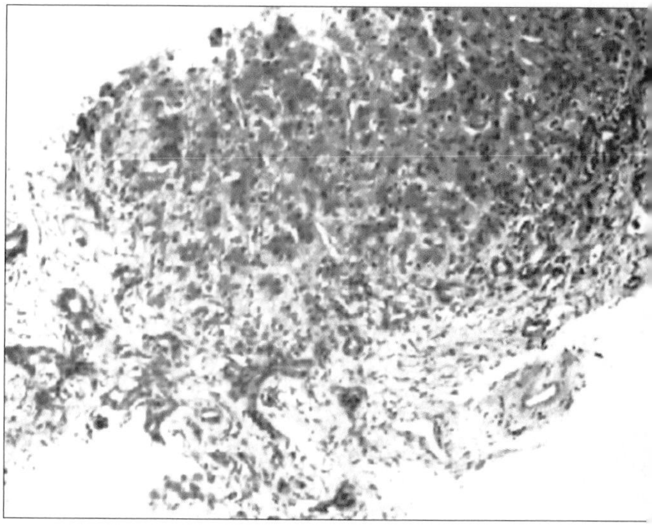

Fig. 90.3 Liver histology in infant with PiZZ A1ATD. Expansion of the portal tracts, bile duct reduplication, and portal inflammation similar to histological features of large bile duct obstruction are seen (hematoxilin & eosin, x150).

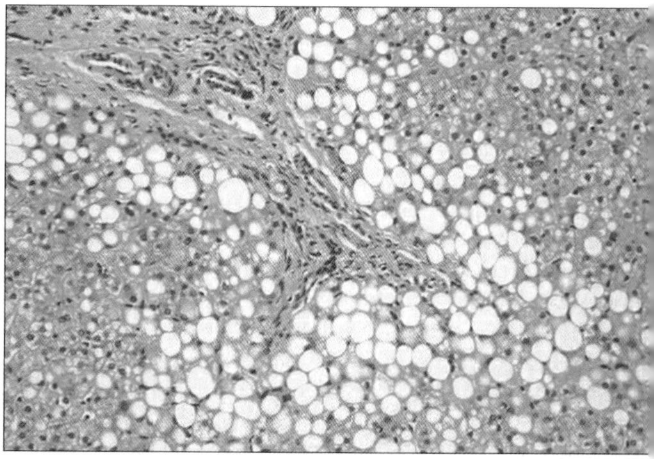

Fig. 90.4 Macrovesicular fatty deposition. Macrovesicular fatty deposition in the periportal regions and incipient fibrosis in an infant with PiZZ A1ATD (hematoxilin & eosin, x180).

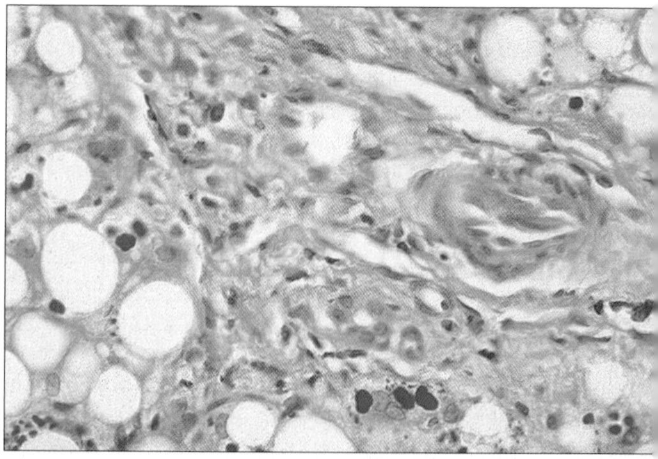

Fig. 90.5 Macrovesicular fatty change and globules of A1ATD (PAS, x250).

astase-resistant granules and globules in the periportal hepa-cytes of older children is highly suggestive of alpha$_1$-antitrypsin ·ficiency (Fig. 90.6), but conventional phenotyping or geno-ping is still required for the diagnosis, since these granules e seen in PiZ heterozygotes and, at times, in hepatocellular ırcinoma or alcoholic hepatitis in adult patients with PiMM ıenotype. Children with alpha$_1$-antitrypsin deficiency-related ·er disease who present later during childhood usually have active fibrosis or frank cirrhosis.

LINICAL PRESENTATION

lpha$_1$-antitrypsin deficiency may present at any stage of life.

CLINICAL PRESENTATION
Prolonged neonatal jaundice
Pale stools and dark urine
Signs of chronic liver disease later in childhood (much less common)

leonatal

lpha$_1$-antitrypsin deficiency most commonly presents in the eonatal period with:

- prolonged neonatal jaundice;
- pale stools;
- dark urine;
- elevated liver enzymes; and
- (less frequently) vitamin K-responsive coagulopathy.[10]

Childhood

pproximately 15% of the symptomatic PiZZ children present ter during childhood with the signs of established CLD, includ-ıg hepatosplenomegaly, impaired liver synthetic function, and/or omplications of portal hypertension. Standard biochemical ıdices of liver function tests are deranged, but with no clear attern. One study has suggested that presence of cholestasis t 6 months of age indicates a poor prognosis.[1]

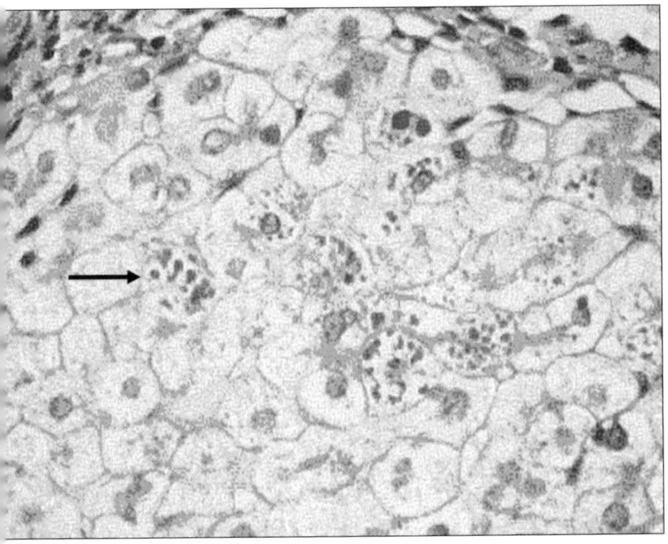

ig. 90.6 **Cytoplasmic granules and globules.** Cytoplasmic granules nd globules representing deposits of A1AT in a patient with PiZZ 1ATD (arrow) (PAS, x150).

Abdominal ultrasound scan (USS) is usually unremarkable at presentation in infancy. Later, nonspecific abnormal appearances of the liver parenchyma, abnormal portal flow, splenomegaly or mild ascites, suggestive of CLD, can be observed.

Screening

Asymptomatic individuals with CLD can be detected on family screening, instituted when the diagnosis is made in the proband.

Adults

Homozygous and heterozygous forms of PiZZ alpha$_1$-antitrypsin deficiency are increasingly recognized in adults with cryptogenic cirrhosis or CLD associated with alcoholism, iron overload, autoimmunity, or chronic hepatitis B and C.[11,12] It is conceivable that possession of a PiZ allele may represent a comorbidity element in the 'multiple hit' theory of pathogenesis of the liver injury. The liver disease can remain clinically silent for many years since there are anecdotal reports of abnormal biochemical liver indices associated with precocious emphysema as well as incidental findings of cirrhosis at postmortem in asymptomatic PiZZ adults.

Malignancy

Individuals with PiZZ alpha$_1$-antitrypsin deficiency are at an increased long-term risk of developing hepatocellular carcinoma or cholangiocarcinoma.[11] Interestingly, some of the patients with these malignancies have been noncirrhotic and inconsistently alpha-fetoprotein positive.

Incidental detection

PiSS alpha$_1$-antitrypsin deficiency has been detected incidentally in children with various forms of liver disorders, in keeping with the estimated high PiS allele prevalence of 4–10% in Southern and Western Europe.[7] Abnormal polymerization of alpha$_1$-antitrypsin in PiSS individuals has been demonstrated *in vitro*,[2] but does not appear to lead to its retention in the hepatocytes and consecutive liver damage in children.

Differential diagnosis

At presentation in early infancy alpha$_1$-antitrypsin deficiency must be distinguished from biliary atresia, neonatal sclerosing cholangitis, cystic fibrosis and Alagille syndrome. Diagnosis should be made by determining the specific alpha$_1$-antitrypsin phenotype, and if necessary genotype, since blood levels of alpha$_1$-antitrypsin, an acute phase reactant, are often within the normal range in deficient infants with inflammatory conditions. In the less common postinfantile presentation, the diagnosis is often suggested by the presence of PAS-positive, diastase-resistant material on liver histology (Fig. 90.6). Clinically, other causes of CLD in childhood such as autoimmune liver disease, Wilson disease, and storage disorders need to be ruled out.

DIFFERENTIAL DIAGNOSIS
• Biliary atresia
• Neonatal nonspecific giant cell hepatitis
• Cystic fibrosis
• Perinatal sclerosing cholangitis
• Alagille syndrome
• Bile salt export pump (BSEP) deficiency

DIAGNOSTIC METHODS

The diagnosis of alpha$_1$-antitrypsin deficiency may be suspected on low serum levels of the protein or absent alpha$_1$ bands on the agarose gel serum protein electrophoresis, particularly in older children, but the abnormal phenotype should be confirmed by isoelectric focusing on polyacrylamide gel, which is based on the different mobility of the alpha$_1$-antitrypsin variants (Fig. 90.7). Occasionally, in the jaundiced infants differentiation between Z and S band may be difficult on isoelectric phenotyping. Genotyping by allele specific oligonucleotide probe hybridization should be undertaken in selected cases, such as antenatal diagnosis, presence of severe jaundice, or history of very recent blood transfusions. Parental testing to document their heterozygosity is mandatory for confirmation of the diagnosis.

TREATMENT AND PREVENTION

There is no effective way of modifying the natural history of CLD in PiZZ alpha$_1$-antitrypsin deficiency. The only proven treatment for PiZZ alpha$_1$-antitrypsin deficiency-related CL is liver transplantation. There are reports that transplante patients with alpha$_1$-antitrypsin deficiency may be more pror to develop hypertension in the immediate postoperative perio due to subclinical renal involvement.[3] Overall survival rat in alpha$_1$-antitrypsin deficiency are similar to other indic tions for elective liver transplantation.[1,13] With a successf transplant the phenotype is changed to that of the donor. It still unclear whether alpha$_1$-antitrypsin recipients have a increased risk of developing calcineurin inhibitor-relate nephrotoxicity and whether they are protected from lun complications in adult life.

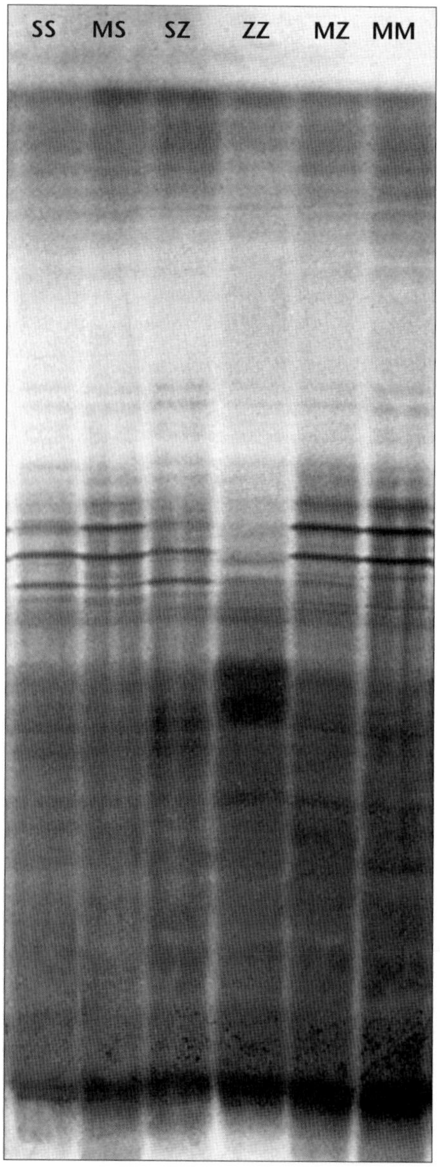

Fig. 90.7 Isoelectric phenotyping. Isoelectric phenotyping demonstrating alpha-1-antitrypsin deficiency PiSS (lane 1), PiSZ (lane 3), and PiZZ (lane 4), heterozygous states PiMS (lane 2) and PiMZ (lane 5), and normal phenotype PiMM (lane 6).

DIAGNOSTIC METHODS
• Measurement of the serum levels of A1AT (nonspecific) • Phenotyping using isoelectric focusing • Genotyping using allele specific oligonucleotide probe hybridization

Avoidance of additional risk factors such as active and pas sive smoking or heavy drinking is advisable in individuals wit the PiZ allele, though there is no clear evidence that this preven liver and lung disease.

Genetic counseling is difficult because of the varying clinic severity and difficulty in predicting the prognosis. Early serie have reported up to 75% concordance in severity of liver diseas among siblings,[10] though this should be confirmed in large studies. Prenatal diagnosis can be made from genetic analys after chorionic villi sampling at 8–10 weeks' gestation.

A better understanding of the pathogenesis of liver injury i alpha$_1$-antitrypsin, in particular the role of the abnormal fold ing of the PiZ variant and the assisted export of the abnorma protein from the hepatocytes, will hopefully lead to effectiv treatment and/or prevention of liver damage.

TREATMENT AND PREVENTION
• No proven modifiers or preventative measures for liver disease at present • Standard medical support and management of complications of chronic liver disease • Liver transplantation only effective treatment for severe liver disease

COMPLICATIONS AND THEIR MANAGEMENT

Children with severe CLD related to alpha$_1$-antitrypsin deficiency can develop complications such as portal hypertension hypoalbuminemia, and ascites at any time during childhood Liver decompensation is more common in infancy and early puberty. Standard treatment of CLD complications, such a banding or sclerotherapy of bleeding varices, albumin supplementation, and diuretics may help temporarily, but the appearance or reappearance of jaundice, hypoalbuminemia, and prolonged prothrombin time usually heralds a rapid evolution to liver failure and indicates the need for urgent consideration to transplant.

PROGNOSIS WITH AND WITHOUT TREATMENT

The prognosis of liver disease in alpha$_1$-antitrypsin deficiency is related to the degree of biochemical dysfunction at presentation and severity of the histological changes, in particular to the presence of fibrosis.[1] About 5% of PiZZ infants undergo rapid decompensation requiring transplantation in the first years of life, but in 95% the hepatitis settles and the quality of life is good. Of these, 25% show no further evidence of liver disease, 25% develop cirrhosis requiring transplantation before the second decade of life, and the remainder continue to exhibit biochemical and/or clinical evidence of liver disease, which may decompensate in adult life.[10] The long-term susceptibility of children presenting with liver disease in infancy for developing chronic obstructive lung disease is still unknown. PiZZ individuals, including noncirrhotic ones, have slightly increased lifelong risk of developing hepatocellular carcinoma.

SOURCES OF INFORMATION FOR PATIENTS AND DOCTORS

http://www.alpha1.org/

REFERENCES

1. Francavilla R, Castellaneta SP, Hadzic N et al. Prognosis of alpha-1-antitrypsin deficiency-related liver disease in the era of paediatric liver transplantation. J Hepatol 2000; 32:986–992.
2. Carrell R, Lomas DA. Mechanisms of disease: Alpha-1-antitrypsin deficiency – a model for conformational diseases. N Engl J Med 2002; 346:45–53.
3. Primhak RA, Tanner MS. Alpha-1 antitrypsin deficiency. Arch Dis Child 2001; 85:2–5.
4. Sifers RN, Finegold MJ, Woo SLC. Molecular biology and genetics of alpha-1-antitrypsin deficiency. Sem Liver Dis 1992; 12:301–310.
5. Lomas DA, Evans DL, Finch JT, Carrell RW. The mechanism of Z alpha$_1$-antitrypsin accumulation in the liver. Nature 1992; 357:605–607.
6. de Serres FJ. Worldwide racial and ethnic distribution of alpha-1-antitrypsin deficiency. Chest 2002; 122:1818–1829.
7. Miravittles M. Alpha$_1$-antitrypsin deficiency: epidemiology and prevalence. Resp Med 2000; 94:S12–S15.
8. Sveger T. Liver disease in alpha-1-antitrypsin deficiency detected by screening of 200,000 infants. N Engl J Med 1976; 294:1316–1321.
9. Malone M, Mieli-Vergani G, Mowat AP, Portmann B. The fetal liver in PiZZ alpha-1-antitrypsin deficiency: a report of five cases. Pediatr Pathol 1989; 9:623–631.
10. Psacharopoulos HT, Mowat AP, Cook PJ et al. Outcome of liver disease associated with alpha 1 antitrypsin deficiency (PiZ). Implications for genetic counselling and antenatal diagnosis. Arch Dis Child 1983; 58:882–887.
11. Zhou H, Fischer HP. Liver carcinoma in PiZ alpha-1-antitrypsin deficiency. Am J Surg Path 1998; 22:742–748.
12. Propst T, Propst A, Dietze O, Judmaier G, Braunsteiner H, Vogel W. High prevalence of viral infections in adults with homozygous and heterozygous α_1-antitrypsin deficiency and chronic liver disease. Ann Intern Med 1992; 117:641–645.
13. Filipponi F, Soubrane O, Labrousse F et al. Liver transplantation for end-stage liver disease associated with alpha-1-antitrypsin deficiency in children: pretransplant natural history, timing and results of transplantation. J Hepatol 1994; 20:72–78.

Chapter 91

Wilson's disease

Peter Ferenci

KEY POINTS

- Wilson's disease involves mutation of *ATB7B*, a P-type ATPase responsible for copper transport
- More than 200 distinct mutations are known, affecting the gene on chromosome 13
- Copper accumulation occurs in liver and brain
- Presents at any age, but most commonly in children and young adults, with liver disease and/or neuropsychiatric disease
- Diagnosis requires a panel of tests including slit-lamp examination for Kayser-Fleischer rings, serum ceruloplasmin and copper balance studies
- Treatment is by copper chelation, interference with absorption, and liver transplantation. Treatment markedly improves outlook in a disease that was previously universally fatal

NTRODUCTION, INCLUDING DEFINITION

'ilson's disease is an inherited disorder in which defective biliary ccretion of copper leads to its accumulation, particularly in the ver (Fig. 91.1), brain (Fig. 91.2), and cornea (Kayser-Fleischer ngs;[1,2] see Fig. 91.3). Wilson's disease is due to a mutation in gene on chromosome 13 that encodes for a P-type ATPase that lays a central role in copper extrusion.[3–5] Clinical presentaon can vary, but the key features of Wilson's disease are liver isease and cirrhosis developing early in childhood or young dult life, neuropsychiatric disturbances, muddy brown Kayserleischer rings around the cornea, and acute episodes of emolysis.

AUSES AND EPIDEMIOLOGY

/ilson's disease is a genetic disorder that is found worldwide. Iore than 200 distinct mutations have been described in the Vilson gene.[6] The importance of individual mutations varies om country to country. Most commonly in northern, central, nd eastern European populations[7–9] there is an H1069Q misense mutation (43.5%), or mutations of exon 8 (6.8%), 3400 elC (3%), and P969Q (1.6%).[10,11] Elsewhere different mutaons are more common: A1003T and P969Q in Turkey and .778L in the Far East.[12]

ATHOGENESIS

Vilson's disease is recognized to be more common than preiously thought, with a gene frequency of 1 in 90–150 and an incidence (based on adults presenting with neurologic symptoms) of at least 1 in 30 000–50 000.[13] Normal dietary consumption and absorption of copper exceeds need, and homeostasis is maintained exclusively by biliary excretion of copper. The Wilson gene, localized to chromosome 13, encodes a copper-transporting P-type APTase (*ATP7B*). This protein resides in the trans-Golgi network and is responsible for transporting copper from intracellular chaperone proteins into the secretory pathway, both for excretion into bile and for incorporation into apo-ceruloplasmin for the synthesis of functional ceruloplasmin.[3–5]

The development of Wilson's disease is due to the accumulation of copper in affected tissues. The electron structure of copper readily facilitates the synthesis of reactive oxygen species, affecting mitochondrial respiration and causing a decrease in cytochrome C activity. This is an early event in liver damage and is accompanied by lipid peroxidation. In the brain there is preferential deposition of copper in basal ganglia, for reasons that are uncertain, and pathogenic mechanisms are also less clear than in the liver.

PATHOLOGY

In most patients there is a greater than 5-fold increase in copper in the liver. This is associated with nonspecific liver biopsy findings including fatty intracellular accumulations, marked steatosis, portal and periportal lymphocyte infiltration, necrosis, and fibrosis. Rhodamine staining reveals focal copper stores in about 10% of patients. Ultrastructurally there is progressive mitochondrial and peroxisome damage.

Changes in the brain

In the brain there is a ubiquitous excess of copper associated with neuronal cavitation and death. This leads to a characteristic 'giant panda' appearance on MRI (see Chapter 127)[14]. Excess copper distribution is also seen in the kidney, where copper has functional effects in a minority of patients.

CLINICAL PRESENTATION

The most common presentations are with liver disease or neuropsychiatric disturbance.[15–17] Clinically evident liver disease may precede neurologic manifestations by as much as 10 years and most patients have some degree of liver disease at presentation.

Acute hepatitis

Wilson's disease enters into the differential diagnosis of any young patient presenting with acute hepatitis. Its clinical presentation may be indistinguishable from that of viral hepatitis, with jaundice

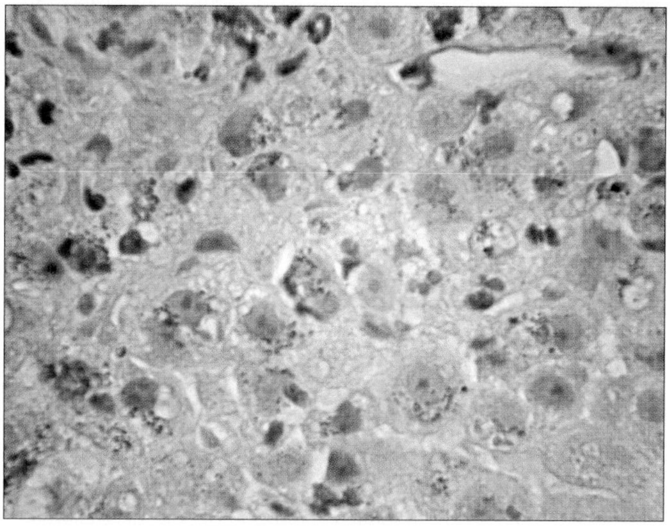

Fig. 91.1 Accumulation of copper in the liver. Rhodanin staining.

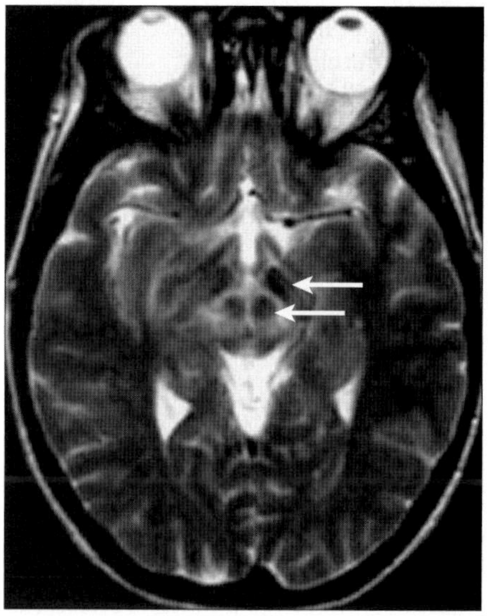

Fig. 91.2 Characteristic changes of Wilson's disease on MRI. Abnormal high intensity signal in the mid-brain tegmentum, possibly due to edema, accentuates the difference with low intensity signals from red nuclei, substantia nigra and superior colliculus resulting in ears (top arrow) and eyes (bottom arrow) of the panda. From Jacobs et al.[14]

and abdominal discomfort. Rapid deterioration can occur with fulminant liver failure. Wilson's disease accounts for 6–12% of all patients with fulminant hepatic failure who are referred for emergency transplantation.[18,19] Prominent hepatic failure may lead to large amounts of stored copper, which induce a severe hemolytic anemia.

Chronic hepatitis and cirrhosis

Wilson's disease may present with cirrhosis at a young age. Histologically there is chronic hepatitis and/or advanced cirrhosis. The presentation may be indistinguishable from other forms of chronic active hepatitis, with symptoms including jaundice, malaise, and vague abdominal complaints.

Neuropsychiatric disease

This commonly occurs in the mid-teens or twenties, although later presentation is possible. Subtle motor disorders such as tremor, speech, and writing problems progress to juvenile parkinsonism characterized by tremor and rigidity, with dysarthria, dysphagia, and sometimes apraxia.[16] Wilson disease may present as reduced performance in school, bu there are other psychiatric presentations including moo lability, depression, exhibitionism, and psychosis that accou for about one-third of presentations.

Patients may present with liver disease alone, neuropsy chiatric disease alone, or both, although liver disease is usuall present when a neuropsychiatric presentation occurs.

Other clinical manifestations

Less common presentations include hypercalciuria and nephr calcinosis, cardiac manifestations (arrhythmias, myopathy and chondrocalcinosis and osteoarthritis, similar to that see with hemochromatosis.

Physical signs

The hallmark of Wilson's disease is the Kayser-Fleischer rin (Fig. 91.3), which is present in 95% of patients with neurologi symptoms and somewhat over half of those without.

Kayser-Fleischer rings are more evident when the cornea i examined under a slit lamp; this should be done if a ring is nc obvious. Neurologic signs include tremor and extrapyramid rigidity. Signs of liver disease are nonspecific. Diagnosti vigilance is important because Kayser-Fleischer rings may b absent in up to 50% of patients with Wilson's disease affectin the liver.

DIFFERENTIAL DIAGNOSIS

Acute hepatitis with Wilson's disease presents similarly t other acute cases of hepatitis, whether viral, toxic, or drug induced. Similarly, Wilson's disease should enter into the diag nosis of all patients with chronic hepatitis and cirrhosis, a routine histologic changes are nonspecific. When Wilson' disease presents neurologically, it may be misdiagnosed as behavioral problem because initial symptoms may be subtl and presentation is during adolescence. More advanced move ment disorders in a young person should provoke considera tion of Wilson's disease, but the diagnosis may be overlooke where the presentation suggests a primarily psychologic o psychiatric disorder. Whether a diagnosis of Wilson's diseas is pursued may depend upon a Kayser-Fleischer ring bein noticed. Where the diagnosis is entertained on clinical grounds it is easy to confirm.

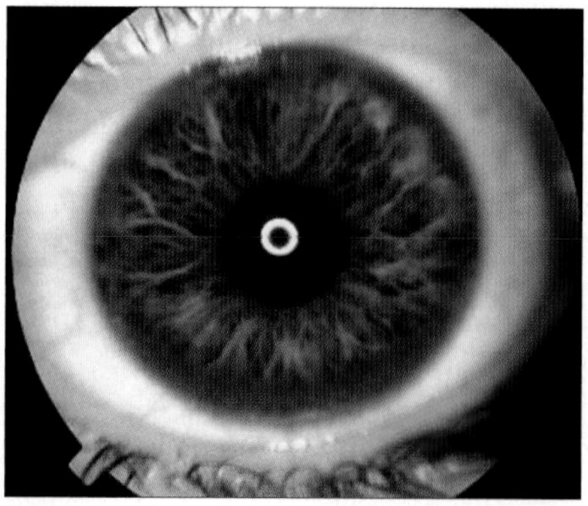

Fig. 91.3 Kayser-Fleischer rings in the cornea.

IAGNOSTIC METHODS

ypically, the presence of Kayser-Fleischer rings and/or a low rum ceruloplasmin level is sufficient to establish a diagnosis. /here Kayser-Fleischer rings are not present (as is common in ver disease), ceruloplasmin levels are not always reliable because ey may be low for reasons other than Wilson's disease (e.g., utoimmune hepatitis, familial aceruloplasminemia),[20] hereas inflammation in the liver or elsewhere may cause the ruloplasmin concentration to rise to normal levels, reflecting s identity as an acute-phase protein. Thus, for many patients combination of tests of copper content or excretion may be eeded. Although all the tests show a strong correlation with /ilson's disease, none is completely specific and a range of sts may often be needed (Table 91.1).

Molecular genetic testing for Wilson's disease is cumbersome and, therefore, not yet routine because there are so many potential mutations. A likely development is a multiplex polymerase chain reaction for the most frequent mutations seen in a particular geographic region.[7,8,12]

FAMILY SCREENING

It is very important to screen the family of patients presenting with Wilson's disease because the chance of a sibling being a homozygote – and therefore developing clinical disease – is 25%. Amongst offspring the chance is 0.5%.[21] There is difficulty in diagnosing heterozygote carriers with certainty, but family members can be screened by mutational analysis for the specific mutation found in the index case.

DIAGNOSTIC METHODS

ROUTINE TESTS FOR DIAGNOSIS OF WILSON'S DISEASE

Test	Typical finding	Proportion abnormal	Comments
Kayser-Fleischer rings by slit lamp	Present	95% neurologic; 50% liver	
Serum ceruloplasmin	Decreased	>50%	Ceruloplasmin level raised with inflammation (acute phase). Overestimated by immunologic assay. Other causes of deficiency include ceruloplasmin anemia
24-h copper	>100 mg/day	88%	May increase with hepatic necrosis
Serum-free copper	>10 mg/dL	Most	May increase with hepatic necrosis
Hepatic copper	>250 mg/g dry weight	82%	May be increased with other cholestasis

TABLE 91.1 SCORING SYSTEM DEVELOPED AT THE EIGHTH INTERNATIONAL MEETING ON WILSON'S DISEASE, LEIPZIG, 2001

Typical clinical symptoms and signs		Other tests	
Kayser-Flesicher rings		**Liver copper (in absence of cholestasis)**	
Present	2	>5× ULN (>250 µg/g)	2
Absent	0	50–250 µg/g	1
Neurologic symptoms		Normal (<50 µg/g)	–1
Severe	2	Rhodamine-positive granules[a]	1
Mild	1	**Urinary copper (in absence of acute hepatitis)**	
Absent	0	Normal	0
Serum ceruloplasmin		1–2× ULN	1
Normal (>0.2 g/L)	0	>2× ULN	2
0.1–0.2 g/L	1	Normal, but >5× ULN after D-penicillamine	2
<0.1 g/L	2	**Mutation analysis**	
Coombs-negative hemolytic anemia		Two chromosome mutations	4
		One chromosome mutation	1
Present	1	No mutations detected	0
Absent	0		
TOTAL SCORE	**Evaluation:**		
≥4	Diagnosis established		
3	Diagnosis possible, more tests needed		
≤2	Diagnosis very unlikely		

[a]If no quantitative liver copper analysis available. ULN, upper limit of normal.

TREATMENT

A number of drugs are available for the definitive treatment of Wilson's disease, including penicillamine, trientine, zinc, tetrathiomolybdate, and, of course, dimercaprol. The American Association for the Study of Liver Disease has recommended that all symptomatic patients with Wilson's disease should receive a chelating agent (penicillamine or trientine).[22,23] Once the diagnosis has been made, treatment needs to be lifelong.

Penicillamine

This chelating agent mobilizes copper from proteins, allowing it to be excreted in the urine.[22] The usual dose is 1–1.5 g per day, and a response is generally seen within months, when the dose may be reduced to 0.5–1 g daily. Compliance and effectiveness can be monitored by repeated measurements of 24-h urinary copper levels, which may ultimately settle at a level of more than 500 mg/day.

Adverse events are common with penicillamine, so that 20% or more of patients may need to be switched to other treatments. Penicillamine induces pyridoxine deficiency in a dose-dependent fashion, and interferes with collagen and elastin formation so that some patients develop cutis laxa and elastosis perforans serpiginosa. All patients should receive pyridoxine 50 mg per week to avoid deficiency. Penicillamine also commonly causes immune-mediated adverse effects; these include systemic lupus erythematosus, immune complex nephritis, leukopenia and thrombocytopenia, optic neuritis, myasthenia gravis, Goodpasture's syndrome, and pemphigus. The onset of these symptoms is an indication to stop the drug immediately.

Trientine

This copper-chelating agent, which leads to enhanced urinary copper excretion, is at least as potent as penicillamine with far fewer side effects.[24,25] It may become the treatment of first choice, but at present this is not the case because of a lack of direct comparisons with penicillamine.

Ammonium tetrathiomolybdate

Ammonium tetrathiomolybdate complexes with copper in the intestinal tract to prevent absorption and in the circulation where it renders copper unavailable for cellular uptake.[26] As yet, experience with this drug is limited, although it is effective at removing copper from the liver; however, sufficiently effective but continuous use may cause copper deficiency.

Zinc

Zinc interferes with copper absorption, firstly by competir for a common carrier for absorption and secondly by inducir metallothionin in enterocytes, allowing copper absorbed int them to be excreted by desquamation.[27] A further advantag of zinc is that induction of metallothionin in liver protec hepatocytes against copper toxicity.

Most data on zinc come from uncontrolled studies of dosage ranging from 75 to 250 mg per day.[28] Zinc is probably les effective than chelating agents in the treatment of establishe Wilson's disease, although data are limited and uncontrolled Its greatest use is in presymptomatic patients. Whether a com bination therapy with chelators has advantages is not yet know

Liver transplantation

Transplantation is frequently necessary for patients presentin with fulminant hepatitis or decompensated cirrhosis due t Wilson's disease.[18,19] Because the biochemical defect in Wilson disease is in the liver, transplantation corrects the underlyin problem. In the past, the median survival was about 2.5 year and better for patients having a transplant for chronic advance liver disease than for those with fulminant hepatic failure Survival is improving; the longest survival recorded is 20 years Limited observation suggests that the neurologic symptoms c patients who need liver transplantation may also improve as result.

PREGNANCY

Successful treatment means that some women with Wilson' disease become pregnant.[29–31] Counseling should indicate tha the likelihood of finding a homozygote amongst children i 0.5%; haplotype analysis of the partner is justified. The patient' copper status should be optimized prior to therapy. Althoug there is some concern over the teratogenicity of penicillamine the risks of withdrawing treatment outweigh those o continuing it.

PROGNOSIS

Untreated Wilson's disease is universally fatal, with mos patients dying from liver disease and a minority from progres sive neurologic disease. With chelation treatment and live transplantation, prolonged survival has become the norm although mortality has not been assessed prospectively. I

TABLE 91.2 PROGNOSTIC INDEX IN ACUTE WILSON'S DISEASE

	Score 0	Score 1	Score 2	Score 3	Score 4
Serum bilirubin (μmol/L)	<100	100–150	151–200	201–300	>301
AST (× ULN)	<2.5	2.6–3.5	3.6–5	5.1–7.5	>7.5
PTT (no. of seconds more than control)	<4	4–8	9–12	13–20	>21

A score of 7 is associated with a high probability of death.
AST, aspartate aminotransferase; PTT, partial thromboplastin time; ULN, upper limit of normal.
Modified from Nazer et al.[32]

eneral, prognosis depends on the severity of liver disease. iver function becomes normal over 1–2 years in most patients ith no or compensated cirrhosis at presentation, and then emains stable without progressive liver disease. At the other nd of the spectrum, medical therapy is rarely effective in patients resenting with fulminant Wilson's disease. A prognostic index as been developed, although not validated prospectively Table 91.2). A score of greater than 7 is always associated with eath. Patients presenting with neurologic symptoms fare better, specially if liver disease is limited. Neurologic symptoms ppear to be partly reversible with treatment, sometimes after n initial worsening. In patients undergoing autotopic liver transplantation, survival may be slightly reduced early on, but appears normal (for transplant population) thereafter.

SOURCES OF INFORMATION FOR PATIENTS AND DOCTORS

http://www.wilsonsdisease.org/
http://digestive.niddk.nih.gov/ddiseases/pubs/wilson/
http://www.wemove.org/wil/
http://www.acsu.buffalo.edu/~drstall/wilsons.html
http://www.eurowilson.org/

REFERENCES

1. Scheinberg IH, Sternlieb I. Wilson's disease. Major problems in internal medicine, Vol 23. Philadelphia: Saunders; 1984.
2. Gitlin JD. Wilson disease. Gastroenterology 2003; 125:1868–1877.
3. Robertson WM. Wilson's disease. Arch Neurol 2000; 57:276–277.
4. Tao YT, Gitlin JD. Hepatic copper metabolism: insights from genetic disease. Hepatology 2003; 37:1241–1247.
5. Lutsenko S, Petris MJ. Function and regulation of the mammalian copper-transporting ATPases: insights from biochemical and cell biological approaches. J Membr Biol 2003; 191:1–12.
6. Cox DW. Molecular advances in Wilson disease. In: Boyer JL, Ockner RK. Progress in liver disease. Vol X. Philadelphia: WB Saunders; 1996: 245–264.
7. Maier-Dobersberger T, Ferenci P, Polli C et al.The His1069Gln mutation in Wilson´s disease: detection by a rapid PCR-test, clinical course and liver biopsy findings. Ann Intern Med 1997; 127:21–26.
8. Caca K, Ferenci P, Kuhn HJ, et al. High prevalence of the H1069Q mutation in East German patients with Wilson disease: rapid detection of mutations by limited sequencing and phenotype–genotype analysis. J Hepatol 2001; 35:575–581.
9. Firneisz G, Lakatos PL, Szalay F, Polli C, Glant TT, Ferenci P. Common mutations of *ATP7B* in Wilson disease patients from Hungary. Am J Med Genet 2002; 108:23–28.
10. Garcia-Villareal L, Daniels S, Shaw SH, et al. High prevalence of the very rare Wilson disease gene mutation Leu708Pro in the Island of Gran Canaria (Canary Islands, Spain): a genetic and clinical study. Hepatology 2000; 32:1329–1336.
11. Loudianos G, Dessi V, Lovicu M, et al. Mutation analysis in patients of Mediterranean descent with Wilson disease: identification of 19 novel mutations. J Med Genet 1999; 36:833–836.
12. Shimizu N, Nakazono H, Takeshita Y, et al. Molecular analysis and diagnosis in Japanese patients with Wilson's disease. Pediatr Int 1999; 41:409–413.
13. Ferenci P, Steindl-Munda P, Vogel W et al. Diagnostic value of quantitative hepatic copper determination in patients with Wilson disease. (in press).
14. Jacobs DA, Markowitz CE, Liebeskind DS, Galetta SL. The "double panda sign" in Wilson's disease. Neurology 2003; 61:969.
15. Ferenci P, Caca K, Loudianos G et al. Diagnosis and phenotypic classification of Wilson disease. Final report of the Proceedings of the Working Party at the 8th International Meeting on Wilson disease and Menkes disease, Leipzig, Germany, 2001. Liver Int 2003; 23:139–142.
16. Oder W, Grimm G, Kollegger H, Ferenci P, Schneider B, Deecke L. Neurological and neuropsychiatric spectrum of Wilson's disease. A prospective study in 45 cases. J Neurol 1991; 238:281–287.
17. Schilsky ML, Scheinberg IH, Sternlieb I. Prognosis of Wilsonian chronic active hepatitis. Gastroenterology 1991; 100:762–767.
18. Schilsky ML, Scheinberg IH, Sternlieb I. Liver transplantation for Wilson's disease: indications and outcome. Hepatology 1994; 19:583–587.
19. Khanna A, Jain A, Eghtesad B, Rakela J. Liver transplantation for metabolic liver diseases. Surg Clin North Am 1999; 79:153–162, ix.
20. Cauza E, Maier-Dobersberger T, Ferenci P. Plasma ceruloplasmin as screening test for Wilson's disease. J Hepatol 1997; 27:358–362.
21. Ferenci P. Diagnosis and current therapy of Wilson's disease. Aliment Pharmacol Ther 2004; 19:157–165
22. Roberts EA, Schilsky ML. AASLD practice guidelines: a practice guideline on Wilson disease. Hepatology 2003; 37:1475–1492.
23. Walshe JM, Yealland M. Chelation treatment of neurological Wilson's disease. Q J Med 1993; 86:197–204.
24. Scheinberg IH, Jaffe ME, Sternlieb I. The use of trientine in preventing the effects of interrupting penicillamine therapy in Wilson's disease. N Engl J Med 1987; 317:209–213.
25. Walshe JM. The management of pregnancy in Wilson's disease treated with trientine. Q J Med 1986; 58:81–87.
26. Brewer GJ, Dick RD, Johnson V et al. Treatment of Wilson's disease with ammonium tetrathiomolybdate: I. Initial therapy in 17 neurologically affected patients. Arch Neurol 1994; 51:545–554.
27. Hoogenraad TU. Zinc treatment of Wilson's disease. J Lab Clin Med 1998; 132:240–241.
28. Ferenci P. Zinc treatment of Wilson's disease. In: Kruse-Jarres JD, Schölmerich J (eds). Zinc and diseases of the digestive tract. Lancaster: Kluwer Academic Publishers; 1997:117–124.
29. Scheinberg IH, Sternlieb I. Pregnancy in penicillamine-treated patients with Wilson's disease. N Engl J Med 1975; 293:1300–1302.
30. Stremmel W, Meyerrose KW, Niederau C, Hefter H, Kreuzpaintner G, Strohmeyer G. Wilson's disease: clinical presentation, treatment, and survival. Ann Intern Med 1991; 115:720–726.
31. Brewer GJ, Johnson VD, Dick RD, Hedera P, Fink JK, Kluin KJ. Treatment of Wilson's disease with zinc XVII: treatment during pregnancy. Hepatology 2000; 31:364–370.
32. Nazer H, Ede RJ, Mowat AP, Williams R. Wilson's disease: clinical presentation and use of prognostic index. Gut 1986; 27:1377–1381.

Chapter 92

Drug-induced and toxic liver disease

Stefan Russmann and Jürg Reichen

KEY POINTS

- Drugs have become the leading cause of acute liver failure in Western countries
- The clinical and histologic picture of drug-induced liver disease may resemble liver disease of any other origin
- Individual susceptibility to idiosyncratic hepatotoxicity is determined by a combination of predisposing genetic and/or environmental factors
- Diagnosis is based on (a) exclusion of other causes; (b) a detailed drug history including phytotherapeutics, illicit drugs, and environmental hepatotoxins; (c) temporal relationship of exposure and symptoms and signs of liver disease; and (d) extrinsic evidence
- Hepatotoxicity by individual drugs may have a typical latency time and a typical clinical and laboratory presentation, which may assist in identifying the causative agent in patients taking several drugs
- When severe hepatotoxicity is suspected, potential causative drugs must be stopped immediately
- Presumed liver disease after acetaminophen overdose must be treated immediately with *N*-acetylcysteine. There is no evidence-based treatment for other hepatotoxins

INTRODUCTION, INCLUDING DEFINITION

The liver is functionally interposed between the site of resorption and the systemic circulation; it is also the major organ for metabolism of foreign substances. These conditions render the liver not only the most important organ for detoxification of foreign substances but also a major target of their toxicity. Indeed, hepatotoxicity is the most frequent cause of drug-induced mortality and consequently of safety-related drug withdrawal from the market. Toxicity may be mainly dose dependent and predictable – referred to as *intrinsic hepatotoxicity*. Many environmental hepatotoxins, including halogenated molecules and toxic mushrooms, share these features. The discovery of intrinsic hepatotoxicity of active substances in preclinical or early clinical studies usually denotes the end of the substance's further development. Except for acetaminophen (paracetamol), which induces intrinsic hepatotoxicity, most cases of drug-induced liver disease are *idiosyncratic*, i.e., they are rare and unpredictable adverse reactions to a drug where the dose plays no or only a minor role. Therefore, these reactions are usually identified during the post-marketing period. Every prescribing physician should be vigilant in patients with liver disease of unknown origin and report suspicious cases, particularly when newly marketed drugs are involved. Examples of drugs that had to be withdrawn recently due to hepatotoxicity are bromfenac, troglitazone, trovafloxacin, and benzbromarone, and in many countries kava-containing phytotherapeutics.

EPIDEMIOLOGY

More than 1000 drugs have been associated with idiosyncratic hepatotoxicity[1] and, together with cases of intrinsic acetaminophen toxicity after intentional and nonintentional overdose, result in a considerable absolute number of cases. Two European studies have estimated a population-based annual risk of hepatic adverse reactions of about 8 per 100 000 inhabitants.[2,3] This risk includes mildly increased levels of transaminases without clinical signs of liver disease. The risk of drug-induced acute liver failure is more significant. Whereas in Eastern countries viral hepatitis is still the main cause of acute liver failure, drug-induced hepatotoxicity is now the leading cause of acute liver failure and transplantation in Western countries. In the USA, acute liver failure affects about 2000 persons per year. In a recent study about 40% of cases were found to be due to acetaminophen and 13% were caused by idiosyncratic drug reactions. The overall mortality rate was 33%, being lower for acetaminophen and higher in idiosyncratic drug-induced liver failure. A further 23% of patients survived only after liver transplantation.[4] In the UK, more than 70% of all cases of acute liver failure follow acetaminophen overdosage. Importantly, most patients had been in good health and the median age was less than 40 years.

The incidence of hepatotoxicity for a specific drug is difficult to determine because very large epidemiologic studies would be required. For most idiosyncratic hepatotoxins, the frequency of hepatotoxicity may range from 1 in 10 000 to 1 in 100 000 first-time users, but amoxicillin–clavulanic acid and cimetidine may have a higher incidence.[5] However, if a given number of well documented reports of severe drug-induced liver disease are identified through spontaneous post-marketing reporting systems, a risk–benefit assessment may be urgently required. An estimate of risk may be obtained from the number of reports (as a surrogate for real incident cases) and the sales data (as a surrogate for exposure). The estimate may be corrected for underreporting (generally, fewer than 10% of severe adverse drug reactions are reported) and other factors. However, this method always provides a rather crude estimation of the real incidence and is subject to bias. Pharmacoepidemiological studies based on large automated patient databases can provide much more reliable estimates if they are well-designed, but availability of such studies is still limited. The risk–benefit assessment of recently introduced potentially hepatotoxic drugs is therefore a difficult challenge for regulatory authorities, manufacturers, and prescribing physicians.

MECHANISMS AND RISK FACTORS

Mechanisms

Hepatocytes, cholangiocytes, and stellate and sinusoidal endothelial cells can all be involved in drug-induced liver disease. In hepatocytes many different intracellular organelles and their function may be primary targets of hepatotoxicity.[6–8] Mitochondrial dysfunction is a major mechanism of hepatotoxicity.[9] Recently, hepatic drug transport proteins such as organic anion transporting polypeptides, multidrug resistance(-associated) protein, and the bile salt export pump, as well as nuclear receptor-mediated regulation of drug metabolism and transport, have also been shown to play an important role in hepatotoxicity.[10,11] Eventually, more or less specific inactivation of vital cellular functions, activation of the apoptosis cascade, or activation of cytotoxic immune mechanisms lead to dysfunction and possibly cell death. Whereas the hepatotoxic mechanisms of many intrinsic hepatotoxins have been investigated in animal and in vitro models, the mechanisms and modulating factors that are involved in idiosyncratic hepatotoxicity tend to be more complex and difficult to identify and reproduce. Only the presence of risk factors and the interaction of several mechanisms may lead to overt liver disease. Further, taken in different dosages and by different patients, a single drug may cause liver disease via multiple mechanisms and with different clinical presentations. The major mechanisms of drug-induced liver disease are presented in Figure 92.1.

Risk factors

The large number of different mechanisms and processes involved in hepatotoxicity constitute multiple targets for its modulation. Risk factors can be divided in two major categories: genetic and environmental. Because toxicity is exerted mostly through a metabolite rather than the parent drug, factors that affect metabolite formation may be considered particularly important. Accordingly genetic polymorphisms and environmental induction or inhibition of drug-metabolizing enzymes are particularly relevant.

With regard to genetic factors, an interesting observation is that three-quarters of patients with drug-induced liver failure are female.[4] A person's sex may affect both the use and the susceptibility to hepatotoxins. Predisposing metabolic or immunologic risk factors may explain the rare occurrence of idiosyncratic hepatotoxicity. For a given drug, both factors may play a role. For example, in halothane hepatotoxicity the risk is increased when a toxifying metabolic pathway is activated and a previous exposure has additionally resulted in the formation of specific antibodies. In addition, the toxicity of intrinsic hepatotoxins is subject to modification, as discussed below for acetaminophen.

Pre-existing liver disease is generally believed to play a relatively minor role as a risk factor for hepatotoxicity, but there are some well documented exceptions. Hepatotoxicity caused by isoniazid is more common in patients with viral hepatitis and/or human immunodeficiency virus (HIV) infection,[12] and patients undergoing antiretroviral treatment for HIV infection have a higher risk of severe hepatotoxicity when co-infected with the hepatitis B or C viruses, particularly if the regimen contains protease inhibitors.[13] HIV infection also increases the

CAUSES AND RISK FACTORS

- Toxic potential of drug
- Genetic factors that affect metabolism, detoxification, and hepatic transport proteins
- Female sex
- Age
- Enzyme induction or inhibition
- Alcohol and other drugs
- Underlying disease

risk of liver toxicity from cotrimoxazole. Irrespective of the role of pre-existing liver disease as a risk factor for hepatotoxicity, the development of hepatotoxicity in this setting will further impair liver function. Modulating factors of hepatotoxicity are summarized in Table 92.1.

PATHOLOGY

Drug-induced liver disease may mimic virtually any liver pathology. It may present as necrosis, cholestasis, steatohepatitis, granulomatous hepatitis, autoimmune hepatitis, veno-occlusive disease, fibrosis, cirrhosis, or benign and malignant liver tumors. Therefore the histologic picture must usually be classified as compatible rather than specific for a particular drug. Nevertheless some histologic features may be recognized as typical for certain drugs, drug classes, or hepatotoxic mechanisms. Necrosis limited to zone 3 may indicate the involvement of metabolism by CYP450 enzymes, as they are more abundant in the centrilobular region, as is typical for acetaminophen toxicity. In contrast, immune-mediated inflammatory reactions with lymphocellular infiltrates and eosinophilia may primarily affect portal areas and are typical for hypersensitivity reactions with aromatic antiepileptics. Figure 92.2 summarizes some important histologic features.

SPECIFIC HEPATOTOXICITY

Acetaminophen (paracetamol)

When given in recommended doses acetaminophen is a fairly safe drug, but its intrinsic toxicity at higher doses makes it the single most important cause of acute liver failure in Western countries. It is metabolized predominantly by conjugation reactions with sulfate and glucuronide. Only a small fraction is metabolized by cytochrome P450 2E1 (CYP2E1) to form the highly reactive and hepatotoxic metabolite *N*-acetyl-benzoquinone imide (NAPQI). NAPQI is normally rapidly detoxified by binding to intracellular glutathione (GSH), but if the daily dose of acetaminophen exceeds 10–15 g the conjugating capacity of the liver is overwhelmed and NAPQI formation increases, leading to cytolysis accompanied by extremely high plasma transaminase levels (Fig. 92.3). Because cytochrome P450 enzymes are located predominantly in hepatocytes near the central vein, the typical histologic picture is centrilobular necrosis (see Fig. 92.2A). In the presence of risk factors such as alcohol abuse or malnutrition that increase NAPQI formation and/or deplete GSH stores even therapeutic doses may cause severe liver injury. Whereas the acute ingestion of alcohol competitively inhibits the formation of NAPQI, chronic alcohol abuse induces CYP2E1 and additionally decreases glutathione production.[8] If treatment with the

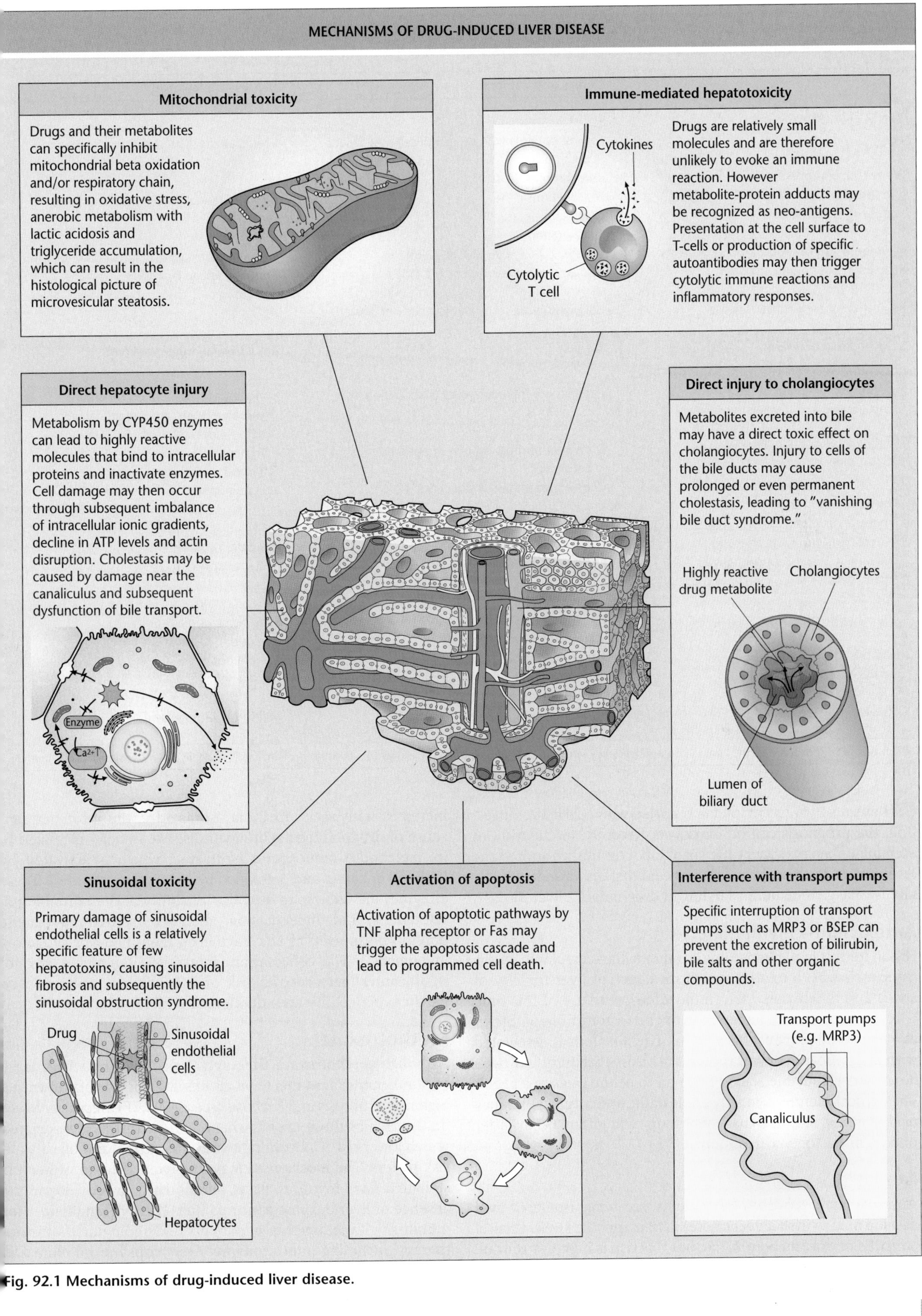

MECHANISMS OF DRUG-INDUCED LIVER DISEASE
Mitochondrial toxicity
Drugs and their metabolites can specifically inhibit mitochondrial beta oxidation and/or respiratory chain, resulting in oxidative stress, anerobic metabolism with lactic acidosis and triglyceride accumulation, which can result in the histological picture of microvesicular steatosis.
Immune-mediated hepatotoxicity
Cytokines
Cytolytic T cell
Drugs are relatively small molecules and are therefore unlikely to evoke an immune reaction. However metabolite-protein adducts may be recognized as neo-antigens. Presentation at the cell surface to T-cells or production of specific autoantibodies may then trigger cytolytic immune reactions and inflammatory responses.
Direct hepatocyte injury
Metabolism by CYP450 enzymes can lead to highly reactive molecules that bind to intracellular proteins and inactivate enzymes. Cell damage may then occur through subsequent imbalance of intracellular ionic gradients, decline in ATP levels and actin disruption. Cholestasis may be caused by damage near the canaliculus and subsequent dysfunction of bile transport.
Enzyme
Ca2+
Direct injury to cholangiocytes
Metabolites excreted into bile may have a direct toxic effect on cholangiocytes. Injury to cells of the bile ducts may cause prolonged or even permanent cholestasis, leading to "vanishing bile duct syndrome."
Highly reactive drug metabolite
Cholangiocytes
Lumen of biliary duct
Sinusoidal toxicity
Primary damage of sinusoidal endothelial cells is a relatively specific feature of few hepatotoxins, causing sinusoidal fibrosis and subsequently the sinusoidal obstruction syndrome.
Drug
Sinusoidal endothelial cells
Hepatocytes
Activation of apoptosis
Activation of apoptotic pathways by TNF alpha receptor or Fas may trigger the apoptosis cascade and lead to programmed cell death.
Interference with transport pumps
Specific interruption of transport pumps such as MRP3 or BSEP can prevent the excretion of bilirubin, bile salts and other organic compounds.
Transport pumps (e.g. MRP3)
Canaliculus

Fig. 92.1 Mechanisms of drug-induced liver disease.

TABLE 92.1 MODULATING FACTORS OF HEPATOTOXICITY

	Details and comments	Representative drugs
GENETIC FACTORS		
Sex	75% of patients with drug-induced liver failure are female	Seems to affect most drugs
Polymorphisms of enzymes or regulators of drug metabolism (toxifying and detoxifying reactions)	Cytochromes P450 *N*-acetyltransferase GSH *S*-transferase Sulfoxidation	 Isoniazid (controversially discussed)
Polymorphisms of drug transport proteins	See text (OATP, BSEP, MDR, MRP)	Bosentan, estrogens, anabolic steroids
Regulation of immune response	Human leukocyte antigens (HLA)	Aromatic antiepileptics Sulfa drugs
Regulation of antioxidant defense mechanisms	GSH synthetase (clinical relevance not proven)	?
Mitochondrial disorders	See text	Antiretroviral drugs, valproate
ACQUIRED AND ENVIRONMENTAL FACTORS		
Induction or inhibition of drug metabolism and hepatic transporters	Cytochrome P450 enzymes transcription factor SXR	Isoniazid, acetaminophen (rifampin, carbamazepine, phenobarbital, and alcohol act as inducers)
Previous drug exposure (for immune reactions)	Formation of drug–protein or autoimmune antibodies	Halothane Ticrynafen
Activation or inhibition of xenobiotic receptors and transcription factors that regulate drug metabolism	Constitutive androstane receptor (CAR)	Acetaminophen
Pre-existing liver disease affecting metabolic activity, functional liver cell mass, defense mechanisms, or capacity for regeneration	Chronic viral hepatitis Alcoholic cirrhosis	Isoniazid, ritonavir Acetaminophen
Concomitant diseases	HIV	Sulfamethoxazole, isoniazid
Age	Risk increases with age	Isoniazid
Malnourishment	Anorexia nervosa, cachexia	Acetaminophen
Obesity	Also association between obesity and overall incident liver disorders	Halothane
Concomitant exposure to other liver toxins	Alcohol	Methotrexate, isoniazid

BSEP, bile salt export pump; HIV, human immunodeficiency virus; MDR, MRP, multidrug resistance(-associated) protein; OATP, organic anion transporting polypeptide.

GSH precursor *N*-acetylcysteine is started within 24 h after ingestion, the prognosis can be improved. Recently, modulation of acetaminophen toxicity by the xenobiotic constitutive androstane receptor has been proposed,[14] a concept that may also be important for the general understanding of drug-induced liver disease.

Amoxicillin–clavulanic acid

For an idiosyncratic hepatotoxin, amoxicillin–clavulanic acid is associated with a relatively high incidence of liver toxicity of about 1 in 5000 users.[5] Given the widespread use of this drug combination, it is not uncommon to encounter this hepatotoxicity in general practice. Because amoxicillin alone is associated with a significantly lower risk and no cross-reactivity has been described, clavulanic acid is assumed to be the causative agent. The clinical picture is mostly cholestatic, and a typical latency of 1–2 weeks implies that symptoms will often occur after treatment has been discontinued.

Isoniazid

Approximately 10–20% of patients receiving isoniazid will develop mild to moderate increases in transaminase levels. Clinical hepatitis occurs in about 0.1%, but this risk is higher if routine transaminase monitoring is not performed. The incidence also increases with age.[12] In India, isoniazid is the most frequent cause of drug-induced acute liver disease. Toxicity is related to its metabolite monoacetyl hydrazine, which is activated by CYP450 enzymes and detoxified by *N*-acetyltransferase-2. These enzymes are subject to genetic variability and environmental alterations, and, indeed, slow acetylator status and genetic polymorphism of CYP2E1 have been identified as risk factors in humans.[15] The concomitant intake of rifampin or alcohol significantly increases the risk of liver disease, which can be partly explained by an induction of CYP450 enzymes.[12]

Methotrexate

Although methotrexate therapy for psoriasis in which large (several grams) amounts have accumulated is associated with a high risk of fibrosis and cirrhosis (see Fig. 92.2F), the use of lower doses, such as those used in rheumatoid arthritis, is associated with a lower risk. Concomitant intake of alcohol and obesity are risk factors. The mechanism may involve activation of hepatic stellate cells to myofibroblasts, and fibrosis may develop in the absence of liver enzyme abnormalities. There are guidelines for monitoring liver function in patients undergoing methotrexate therapy, including indications for liver biopsy at baseline and during treatment; however, these are controversial.[16]

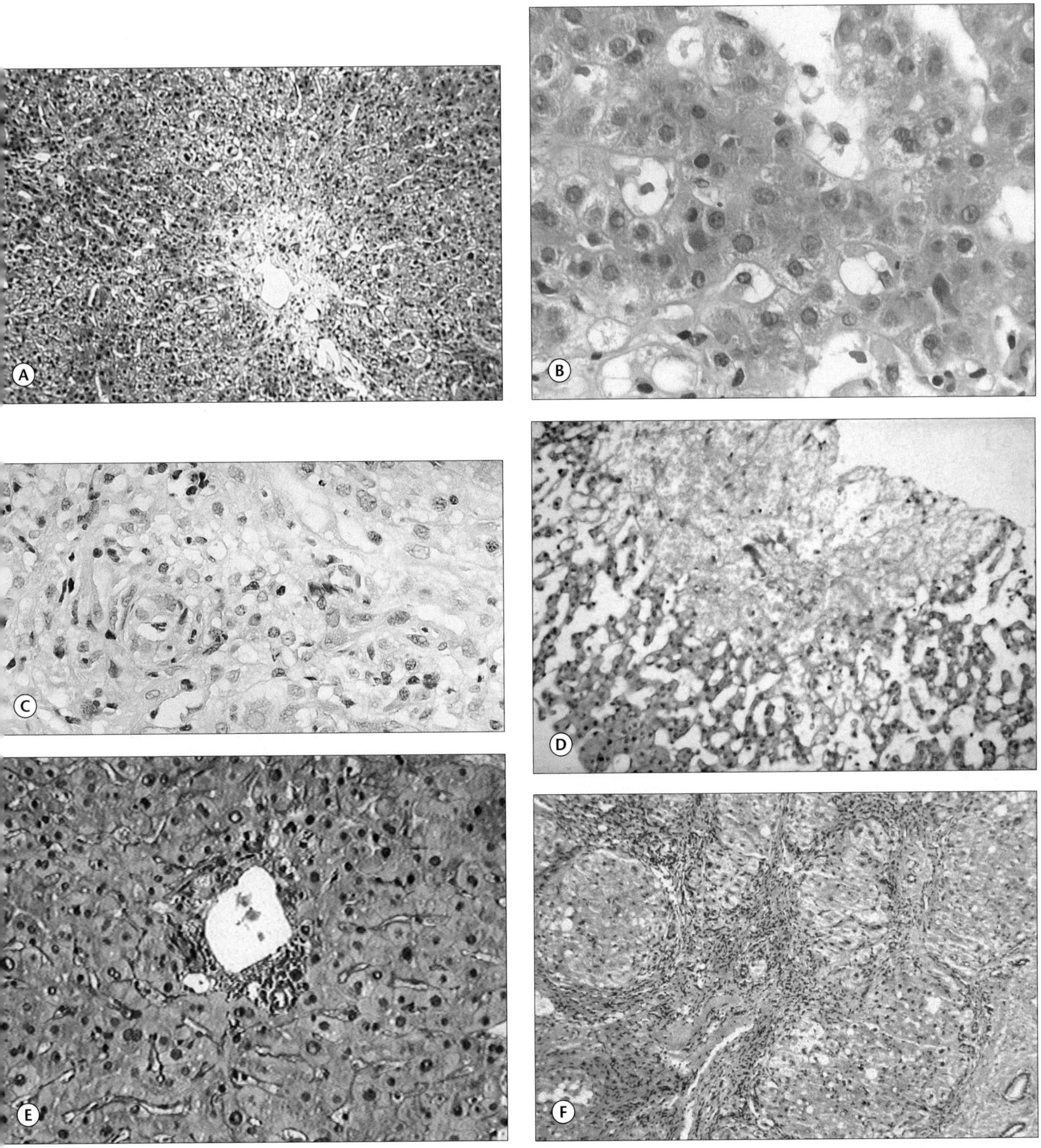

Fig. 92.2 **Histologic manifestations of drug-induced liver disease.** **A,** Hepatotoxicity after acetaminophen overdose with predominant centrilobular necrosis. **B,** Cholestatic liver injury typically caused by amoxicillin–clavulanic acid. **C,** Kava-induced hepatitis showing an inflamed portal field. The mixed cellular infiltrate is dominated by lymphocytes, but also shows eosinophils and activated macrophages. (From Russmann et al. Ann Intern Med 2001; 135:68–69.) **D,** Sinusoidal obstruction syndrome with marked sinusoidal dilatation after chemotherapy with cyclophosphamide. **E,** Ductopenia as a rare long-term complication of cholestatic drug-induced liver injury. **F,** Methotrexate-induced liver cirrhosis.

Bosentan

This recently introduced endothelin receptor antagonist is a good example of a drug that causes liver damage by inhibiting hepatic transport proteins. In clinical trials, bosentan caused dose-dependent reversible liver injury in 2–18% of patients. Subsequent in vitro studies were able to demonstrate inhibition of the bile salt export pump for bosentan and its metabolite, a presumed mechanism of cholestatic liver injury in patients.[17]

TABLE 92.2 SELECTION OF IMPORTANT HEPATOTOXINS

Substance or drug	Comment
REGISTERED DRUGS	
Acetaminophen	
Amiodarone	Mitochondrial toxicity leading to microvesicular steatosis
	i.v. form contains potentially hepatotoxic solvent
Antiretrovitral drugs (e.g., ritonavir)	Mitochondrial toxicity, strong indication in HIV makes clinical decision to stop treatment difficult
Aromatic antiepileptics (e.g., carbamazepine, phenytoin)	Liver involvement in approx. 50% of hypersensitivity reactions
Amoxicillin–clavulanic acid	
Azathioprine	Sinusoidal toxicity, cirrhosis
Bosentan	Inhibitor of bile salt export pump
Cyclophosphamide	Sinusoidal toxicity
Inhalational anesthetics	
Isoniazid	
Methotrexate	
NSAIDs (e.g., diclofenac)	Widespread use results in a considerable absolute number of cases
Phenprocoumon	Long latency time (3–12 months)
Sulfamethoxazole	Presumed cause of cotrimoxazole-induced toxicity
	HIV infection is a risk factor
PHYTOTHERAPEUTICS	
Kava (*Piper methysticum*)	Withdrawn from the market in many countries due to several recent cases of related fulminant liver failure
Chaparral leaf	Several case reports of acute and cholestatic hepatitis related to chaparral-containing dietary supplements
Germander	Withdrawn from the market in France due to several related cases of acute hepatitis; toxicity mediated by metabolites of Furan-containing diterpenoids
RECREATIONAL OR ILLICIT DRUGS	
Anabolic steroids	Frequently abused in bodybuilding community; easily available via the internet
Cocaine	Dose-dependent toxicity that may be enhanced by concomitant alcohol intake; other toxic manifestations are myocardial infarction, rhabdomyolysis and shock
Ecstasy (MDMA)	Several cases of acute liver disease and even liver failure; associated hyperthermia may also play a causal role for its hepatotoxicity
NATURAL AND ENVIRONMENTAL HEPATOTOXINS	
Aflatoxins	Produced by *Aspergillus flavus*, which grows on humid grains and nuts; may be an important cause of hepatocellular carcinoma in tropical countries
Bacillus cereus toxin	Mitochondrial toxicity; food contamination possible
Halogenated molecules	Strong intrinsic toxicity; classic experimental hepatotoxins (e.g., carbon tetrachloride)
Phosphorus	Strong intrinsic toxicity; classic experimental hepatotoxin
Pyrrolizidine alkaloids (occur in several plant families; e.g., *Senecio*, *Crotalaria*, and *Heliotropium* spp)	Intrinsic sinusoidal toxicity leading to SOS
Toxic mushrooms (*Amanita phalloides*, *Lepiota helveola*, and *Gyromitra* spp)	Intrinsic toxicity
Vitamin A	Acute hepatotoxicity has occurred after ingestion of bear liver; chronic overdose may cause fibrosis

HIV, human immunodeficiency virus; MDMA, methylenedioxymetamphetamine; NSAID, nonsteroidal anti-inflammatory drug; SOS, sinusoidal obstruction syndrome.

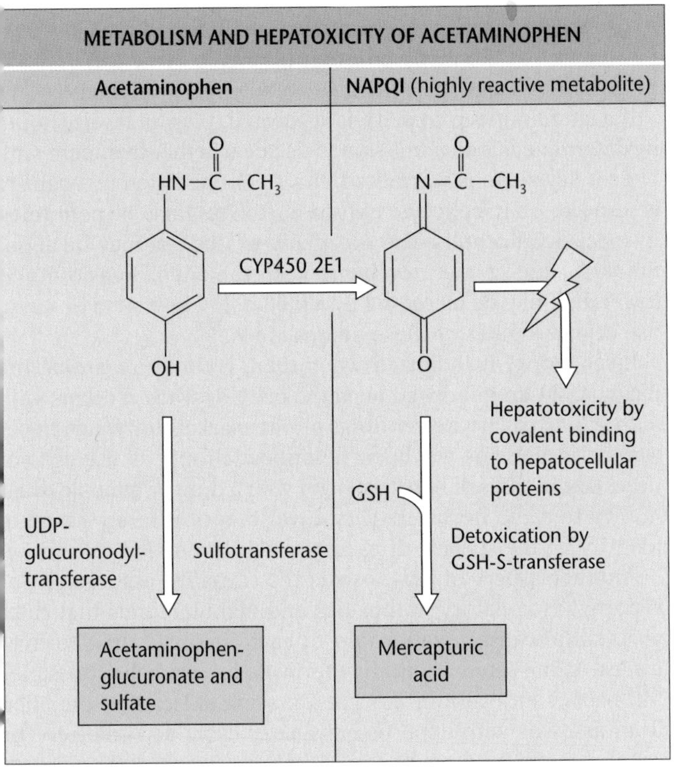

Fig. 92.3 Metabolism and hepatotoxicity of acetaminophen.

Sinusoidal obstruction syndrome (veno-occlusive disease)

In this condition sinusoidal endothelial cells, rather than hepatocytes, are the primary target of toxicity. Chemotherapy with cyclophosphamide, pyrrolizidine alkaloids that are constitutively expressed by several plants, and azathioprine are typical drugs. It is presumed that these substances or their reactive metabolites cause a profound intracellular depletion of GSH in sinusoidal endothelial cells, leading to cell injury with subsequent fibrosis of the hepatic sinusoids, resulting in a specific histologic picture (see Fig. 92.2D). The clinical presentation is typically acute with sudden onset of severe abdominal pain, hepatomegaly, and ascites.[18]

Inhalational anesthetics

Although the use of halothane in anesthesia has essentially been abandoned, the unraveling of its mechanism of hepatotoxicity has made a major contribution to the understanding of immune-mediated toxic liver damage. Whereas toxicity after the first exposure is very rare, after frequent exposures antibodies against CYP2E1-mediated trifluoroacetylated (TFA) metabolite–protein adducts can lead to severe immune-mediated liver injury. Modern inhalational anesthetics – enflurane, isoflurane, sevoflurane, and desflurane – are chemically related to halothane but are metabolized to a much lesser extent; therefore fewer TFA proteins are formed and the incidence of hepatotoxicity is much lower.[19]

Liver disease from herbal remedies

The therapeutic benefit of herbal remedies in liver disease lacks convincing scientific evidence, but an increased use of alternative agents in Western countries has resulted in a rising number of liver disease actually caused by them.[20] In addition to cases in which herbal remedies are identified as the cause of liver disease, idiosyncratic herbal hepatotoxicity may also be responsible for a high proportion of fulminant hepatic failure of an unidentified cause.[21] Products derived from kava (piper methysticum) were recently withdrawn from the market in many countries after several well documented cases of acute liver failure had been reported. There is also concern about extraction methods that do not remove pyrrolizidine alkaloids from plants that are used for herbal remedies, and products of uncontrolled quality that may contain unknown hepatotoxins.

Environmental hepatotoxicity

A large number of substances may cause intrinsic hepatotoxicity through environmental exposure. In industrial settings, halogenated molecules have a high hepatotoxic potential. Fortunately accidental exposure has dramatically decreased during the past 50 years, once the problem of environmental toxicity had been recognized and corresponding protective measures introduced. Today these substances play a role mainly in experimental hepatotoxicity, but they must still be considered in the differential diagnosis of liver diseases of unknown origin, particularly in nonindustrialized countries and if occurrence is epidemic. Accidental ingestion of toxic mushrooms or plants that contain pyrrolizidine alkaloids with consequent liver injury has been described worldwide. For a comprehensive discussion of environmental hepatotoxicity the reader is referred to detailed literature on this topic.[22]

CLINICAL PRESENTATION

Given the wide spectrum of hepatotoxic mechanisms and resulting pathologies, the clinical presentation of drug-induced liver disease ranges from mild clinical symptoms of liver disease, such as nausea, loss of appetite, abdominal discomfort, and mild alterations in laboratory test results, to pronounced cytolytic or cholestatic patterns of liver enzyme abnormalities with jaundice, or even acute liver failure with hepatic coma and multiorgan failure. Systemic immune-mediated hypersensitivity reactions with liver involvement may additionally present with fever, rash, lymphadenopathy, and eosinophilia.

Although clinical presentation is generally nonspecific for a given drug, some typical features can help in the differential diagnosis; for example:

- Extremely high transaminase levels in acetaminophen overdose
- Acute onset with ascites and abdominal pain in sinusoidal obstruction syndrome
- Hypersensitivity syndrome in aromatic epileptic hepatotoxicity.

As presented in Table 92.3, the pattern of liver enzyme alterations can also be typical for certain drugs and has been used to differentiate primarily cytolytic or cholestatic hepatic reactions.[23] However, the enzyme pattern may change during the course of the liver injury, and liver disease should be named according to histologic findings, if possible.

The temporal relationship between liver disease and initiation and discontinuation of the suspected drug is an important aspect, because latency times typical for certain drugs can be useful in the differential diagnosis and may provide some evidence about the mechanism involved. Onset of hepatotoxicity by intrinsic hepatotoxins such as acetaminophen or toxic mushrooms occurs

TABLE 92.3 DEFINITION OF DRUG-INDUCED LIVER INJURY ON THE BASIS OF ENZYMATIC PRESENTATION

Cytolytic liver injury	Cholestatic liver injury	Mixed liver injury
Isolated increase of ALT >2× N *or* R >5	Isolated increase of AP >2× N *or* R <2	ALT and AP increase >2× N *and* 2<R<5

'Liver injury,' as defined by enzyme levels, is present if alanine aminotransferase (ALT) or conjugated bilirubin levels are raised more than 2-fold, or if there is a combined increase in aspartate aminotransferase (AST), alkaline phosphatase (AP), and conjugated bilirubin levels (at least one parameter raised more than 2-fold). Further subclassification is shown in the table body. N, upper limit of normal; R, ALT/AP, where enzyme activities are expressed as multiples of N.

within 48 h of ingestion, whereas T cell-mediated immunologic reactions may have a latency time of several weeks or even months, but shorter in case of a rechallenge. Amoxicillin–clavulanate-induced cholestasis typically occurs 1–2 weeks after exposure, and therefore often occurs after the drug has been discontinued. Phenprocoumon tends to have an unusually long latency time of 3–12 months. In both instances, long latency times may mistakenly exclude causal drugs in the etiology of liver disease.

CLINICAL PRESENTATION

- The clinical and pathologic presentation of drug-induced liver injury may mimic liver disease of any other cause.
- Individual hepatotoxins tend to have a typical pattern of clinical, laboratory, and histologic presentation.

DIFFERENTIAL DIAGNOSIS

Drug-induced liver disease is usually a diagnosis of exclusion.

DIFFERENTIAL DIAGNOSIS

- Viral serology (hepatitis A, B, C, cytomegalovirus, Epstein-Barr virus)
- Exclusion of obstructive biliary disease
- Autoimmune hepatitis
- Exclusion of metabolic liver disease

DIAGNOSTIC METHODS

Causality assessment of drug-induced liver disease can be based on the following criteria:

- Detailed drug history including phytotherapeutics, illicit drugs, and environmental hepatotoxins
- Temporal relationship between exposure and onset of symptoms and signs of liver disease
- Information on discontinuation of drug and possibly after rechallenge
- Presence of known risk factors
- Exclusion of other causes
- Information about hepatotoxic potential and typical features of the involved drugs (extrinsic evidence)
- Specific diagnostic evidence (usually not available)

If acetaminophen toxicity is suspected, plasma levels should be determined upon admission to decide whether treatment with *N*-acetylcysteine is warranted. If a T cell-mediated mechanism is suspected, a lymphocyte transformation test may be performed in specialized centers. The specificity of this test may be about 80–90%, but it has not been well validated. Sensitivity is lower and may be increased by a metabolizing system or direct use of metabolites, if these are available.[24]

Liver biopsy is indicated when there is doubt regarding the diagnosis of drug-induced hepatotoxicity or when it occurs with a drug (particulary newer drugs on the market) for which hepatotoxicity has not yet been described. Biopsy is usually not necessary in cases of hepatotoxicity with a drug or multiple drugs known to cause hepatotoxicity. Liver biopsy is rarely useful in identifying the specific drug responsible for toxicity.

Another aspect of diagnosis is the causality assessment for reports to regulatory authorities and manufacturers that categorizes the causal relationship of each involved drug to liver disease using semiquantitative terms (e.g., 'unlikely,' 'possible,' 'probable,' and 'certain'). A good assessment can be obtained if an assessor with expertise evaluates cases according to the criteria mentioned above, and different weights are given to extrinsic criteria and types of reaction. Standardized scales that formally assess causality have been developed mainly for regulatory purposes.[25] Although these scales certainly help to generate structured reports and ensure that the most important critical parameters of causality assessment are addressed, they also have important disadvantages. First, in clinical practice their use is difficult and may contribute little to the management of individual patients. Second, typical features of hepatotoxicity related to a specific drug may not be considered, and standardization can therefore introduce systematic bias; for example, the onset of liver disease after discontinuation of amoxicillin–clavulanic acid therapy can lead to an underestimation of its causal role. Another frequently encountered and relevant example is the intake of acetaminophen after the first symptoms of drug-induced liver disease, possibly combined with a 'positive' history of alcohol use, which in fact may be minimal. In this situation lack of high serum levels of transaminases and lack of zone 3 necrosis on histologic examination can virtually rule out acetaminophen as the cause, but this may not be considered in a standardized assessment. These limitations can lead to poor interassessor reproducibility, and in the worst case may be systematically abused by an assessor who is not free of a conflict of interest, resulting in a pseudo-objective underassessment of the associated risk. Unfortunately this is not just a theoretical consideration. Limitations of standardized scales therefore have to be considered carefully, and it must be realized that they can only support but not replace specialized expertise.

CLINICAL TIPS

- Always consider hepatotoxicity in liver disease of unclear origin.
- Drug history must be chronologically exact and should include phytotherapeutics and exposure to environmental hepatotoxins.
- Stop suspicious drugs without a vital indication immediately.

DIAGNOSTIC METHODS

- Exclude other pathologies by imaging, viral serology, and autoimmune markers.
- A comprehensive drug history and careful differential diagnosis are the keys to the diagnosis of drug-induced liver disease, which mostly is a diagnosis of exclusion.
- Improvement after dechallenge of suspected drugs has an important diagnostic value. Rechallenge is the only proof of the causal role of a drug, but can be life-threatening and is therefore usually contraindicated. If the causal role is unclear and the drug has a vital indication, a reintroduction under close monitoring may be considered. If several drugs are involved this should be done sequentially.
- Specific immunologic in vitro testing is possible but not validated, and usually not available in routine clinical practice.

TREATMENT AND PREVENTION

With the exception of *N*-acetylcysteine for acetaminophen toxicity, there is no evidence-based specific treatment for drug-induced liver disease. If an immunologic mechanism is suspected, it seems plausible to attempt treatment with steroids, although the benefit has never been proven because numbers are too small for controlled clinical trials. Therefore, if severe liver injury with clinical symptoms is suspected, the most important action is to discontinue all drugs except low-suspicion drugs with a vital indication. A special problem is the mild to moderate, and sometimes only transient, drug-induced increase in transaminase levels. If there are no clinical symptoms of liver disease and no therapeutic alternative (e.g., tuberculostatic chemotherapy), therapy may be continued with close monitoring of liver enzymes and clinical symptoms. The success of primary preventive monitoring depends on compliance, incidence, and kinetics of the development of severe liver disease. Whereas for isoniazid and methotrexate intensive monitoring clearly reduces the risk of severe liver disease, for most idiosyncratic hepatotoxins a benefit is possible, but has never been formally proven. Sometimes an isolated increase of γ-glutamyl transferase may be interpreted as a sign of drug-induced liver injury, but it may just reflect an induction of CYP450 enzymes and is not a specific sign of liver injury.

Furthermore, the understanding and identification of risk factors has important preventive implications. Avoidance of known environmental risk factors, including drug interactions, decreases the incidence of hepatotoxicity, and recent advances in genetics allow the identification of previously unknown genetic risk factors. Ideally individual genetic patient screening before prescription would decrease the number of adverse drug reactions. However, for most idiosyncratic hepatotoxins the complexity of involved post-transcriptional and environmental factors may prevent this approach from ever having a major impact.

TREATMENT AND PREVENTION

- Administer *N*-acetylcysteine as soon as possible for acetaminophen-induced toxicity.
- There is no established treatment for other causative drugs. Steroids may be tried if an immune-mediated mechanism is suspected.

PROGNOSIS

The prognosis is generally good if the drug is stopped at the first symptom or sign of liver disease. In contrast – particularly when injury is caused by idiosyncratic hepatotoxins and when exposure is continued – irreversible fulminant liver failure may occur with a high mortality rate. Rechallenge in case of allergic reactions poses a high risk and should therefore be avoided. A typical feature of cholestatic drug-induced liver disease is a prolonged recovery of several weeks or even months after discontinuation of causal drug. Despite this protracted course, the prognosis is usually good, although vanishing bile duct syndrome may rarely develop with a poor prognosis.

WHAT TO TELL PATIENTS

Patients at risk of developing drug-induced liver disease should be told to contact a physician immediately if symptoms of liver disease occur (i.e., jaundice, itching, nausea and vomiting, loss of appetite, abdominal discomfort, or discoloration of stools and urine). If risk factors are present, patients must be advised to avoid them. For patients with a previous history of drug-induced liver disease, re-exposure with the causative drug and related substances must be avoided. Ideally patients should carry an allergy card that contains information about the manifestation and the causative drugs, including substance name and trade names of all products that contain the causative substances.

CURRENT CONTROVERSIES AND THEIR FUTURE RESOLUTION

Recent developments in genetics, immunology, cell biology, pharmacology, and toxicology have provided new insights into drug hepatotoxicity. Whereas the main mechanisms are mostly understood, the complex interactions of potential hepatotoxins with genetic and environmental risk factors, and the regulation of hepatic susceptibility and secondary responses, are still unclear. Severe drug-induced liver disease therefore remains unpredictable for most drugs. A better understanding of pathogenesis, particularly of idiosyncratic hepatotoxicity, has the potential of identifying previously unknown genetic and environmental risk factors and new therapeutic targets, and of increasing the sensitivity and specificity of screening for potentially hepatotoxic substances during drug development. New therapeutic approaches may include specific pharmacologic alteration of apoptotic pathways and immune responses, and may thus prevent further damage after a hepatotoxin's initial strike. Although preventive genetic screening for drug-induced liver disease is in the pipeline, the sole identification of risk factors is unlikely to reliably predict and prevent rare idiosyncratic hepatotoxicity, if the complex interaction of the involved processes is not well understood. The chances of prediction may be better for drugs with a higher incidence of hepatotoxicity, but if therapeutic alternatives are available these drugs may be withdrawn from the market before the mechanism has been investigated and the efficacy of screening proven. Therefore vigilant prescribers who report incident cases, sensitive pharmacovigilance systems, and epidemiological post-marketing studies continue to be important measures for the rapid identification and estimation of incidence and related patient risk of hepatotoxicity. In the absence of reliable incidence data and predictability, the evaluation of a drug's risk–benefit ratio will continue to be subject to controversial discussions. Phytotherapeutics are equally concerning, and for some preparations, such as dietary supplements, less strict regulatory requirements for proof of efficacy, safety, and patient information may be insufficient to protect the consumer. Professional networks that collect comprehensive information on incident cases of hepatotoxicity, including material for genetic testing, may be an important step to improve evaluation and research of drug-induced liver disease.[26]

COMPLICATIONS AND CONTROVERSIES

- The mechanisms of idiosyncratic hepatotoxicity of most drugs are unknown.
- The complex interaction of several risk factors is poorly understood.
- Whether genotyping or phenotyping prior to therapy will ever be able to reduce morbidity and mortality related to drug-induced liver disease is as yet undetermined.
- Methods to determine and report causality assessment in individual cases and the risk–benefit ratio of potentially hepatotoxic drugs are still controversial.

REFERENCES

1. Biour M, Poupon R, Grange JD, Chazouilleres O. Hépatotoxicité des médicaments. 13e mise à jour du fichier bibliographique des atteintes hépatiques et des médicaments responsables. Gastroenterol Clin Biol 2000; 24:1052–1091.
2. Ibanez L, Perez E, Vidal X, Laporte JR. Prospective surveillance of acute serious liver disease unrelated to infectious, obstructive, or metabolic diseases: epidemiological and clinical features, and exposure to drugs. J Hepatol 2002; 37:592–600.
3. Sgro C, Clinard F, Ouazir K et al. Incidence of drug-induced hepatic injuries: a French population-based study. Hepatology 2002; 36:451–455.
4. Ostapowicz G, Fontana RJ, Schiodt FV et al. Results of a prospective study of acute liver failure at 17 tertiary care centers in the United States. Ann Intern Med 2002; 137:947–954.
5. Garcia Rodriguez LA, Ruigomez A, Jick H. A review of epidemiologic research on drug-induced acute liver injury using the general practice research data base in the United Kingdom. Pharmacotherapy 1997; 17:721–728.
6. Kaplowitz N. Biochemical and cellular mechanisms of toxic liver injury. Semin Liver Dis 2002; 22:137–144.
7. Pessayre D, Haouzi D, Fau D, Robin MA, Mansouri A, Berson A. Withdrawal of life support, altruistic suicide, fratricidal killing and euthanasia by lymphocytes: different forms of drug-induced hepatic apoptosis. J Hepatol 1999; 31:760–770.
8. Lee WM. Drug-induced hepatotoxicity. N Engl J Med 2003; 349:474–485.
9. Pessayre D, Fromenty B, Mansouri A, Berson A. Hepatotoxicity due to mitochondrial injury. In: Kaplowitz N, DeLeve L, eds. Drug-induced liver disease. New York: Marcel Dekker; 2003:55–83.
10. Bohan A, Boyer JL. Mechanisms of hepatic transport of drugs: implications for cholestatic drug reactions. Semin Liver Dis 2002; 22:123–136.
11. Liddle C, Goodwin B. Regulation of hepatic drug metabolism: role of the nuclear receptors PXR and CAR. Semin Liver Dis 2002; 22:115–122.
12. Garg PK, Tandon RK. Antituberculous agents-induced liver injury. In: Kaplowitz N, DeLeve L, eds. Drug-induced liver disease. New York: Marcel Dekker; 2003:505–517.
13. Sulkowski MS. Hepatotoxicity associated with antiretroviral therapy containing HIV-1 protease inhibitors. Semin Liver Dis 2003; 23:183–194.
14. Zhang J, Huang W, Chua SS, Wei P, Moore DD. Modulation of acetaminophen-induced hepatotoxicity by the xenobiotic receptor CAR. Science 2002; 298:422–424.
15. Huang YS, Chern HD, Su WJ et al. Cytochrome P450 2E1 genotype and the susceptibility to antituberculosis drug-induced hepatitis. Hepatology 2003; 37:924–930.
16. Reuben A. Methotrexate controversies. In: Kaplowitz N, DeLeve L, eds. Drug-induced liver disease. New York: Marcel Dekker; 2003:653–675.
17. Fattinger K, Funk C, Pantze M et al. The endothelin antagonist bosentan inhibits the canalicular bile salt export pump: a potential mechanism for hepatic adverse reactions. Clin Pharmacol Ther 2001; 69:223–231.
18. DeLeve LD, Shulman HM, McDonald GB. Toxic injury to hepatic sinusoids: sinusoidal obstruction syndrome (veno-occlusive disease). Semin Liver Dis 2002; 22:27–42.
19. Kenna JG. Mechanism, pathology and clinical presentation of hepatotoxicity of anesthetic agents. In: Kaplowitz N, DeLeve L, eds. Drug-induced liver disease. New York: Marcel Dekker; 2003:405–424.
20. Stedman C. Herbal hepatotoxicity. Semin Liver Dis 2002; 22:195–206.
21. Estes JD, Stolpman D, Olyaei A et al. High prevalence of potentially hepatotoxic herbal supplement use in patients with fulminant hepatic failure. Arch Surg 2003; 138:852–858.
22. Zimmerman HJ. Environmental hepatotoxicity. In: Zimmerman HJ, ed. Hepatotoxicity, 2nd edn. Philadelphia: Lippincott Williams & Wilkins; 1999:201–426.
23. Benichou C. Criteria of drug-induced liver disorders. Report of an international consensus meeting. J Hepatol 1990; 11:272–276.
24. Maria VA, Victorino RM. Diagnostic value of specific T cell reactivity to drugs in 95 cases of drug induced liver injury. Gut 1997; 41:534–540.
25. Lucena MI, Camargo R, Andrade RJ, Perez-Sanchez CJ, Sanchez De La Cuesta F. Comparison of two clinical scales for causality assessment in hepatotoxicity. Hepatology 2001; 33:123–130.
26. Hepatotoxicity clinical research network. Hepatology 2002; 36:277.

Chapter 93

Genetic and metabolic liver diseases in childhood

Giorgina Mieli-Vergani and Richard Thompson

KEY POINTS

- Several genetic syndromes may present in childhood with jaundice or other features of liver dysfunction
- Many have dysmorphia of the face or internal organs
- Alagille syndrome associated with mutations of the JAG-1 gene has typical facial features
- Level of γ-glutamyl transferase can be used to distinguish different causes of cholestasis
- Genetic causes of liver disease in childhood may require transplantation

INTRODUCTION

Nearly all liver diseases have at least a partly genetic cause – even viral hepatitis has genetic determinants of outcome. Some conditions have a more obvious genetic origin, either by familial recurrence, or by frequently occurring in consanguineous families. Furthermore most liver diseases present with features of metabolic disturbance. Of these, many fit into the typical definition of metabolic diseases (Fig. 93.1). Preceding chapters have covered several such disorders. The conditions covered in this chapter are those that are most likely to be seen by clinicians presenting with a 'liver phenotype,' often cholestatic. Table 93.1 depicts such conditions; the most common are described in detail.

ALAGILLE SYNDROME

Epidemiology and pathogenesis

Alagille syndrome is reported to have an incidence of 1 per 70 000 population and a worldwide distribution. This is likely to be an underestimate. There is a strong association with heterozygous mutations in the *JAG1* gene.[1,2] Mutations are, however, not fully penetrant, with some parents having the same mutations with few or no features. In addition nearly all mutations are family specific. This severely limits the use of genetics for diagnostic purposes.

Clinical presentation and pathology

The cardinal feature of Alagille syndrome is the presence of *intrahepatic cholestasis with a biliary hypoplasia*, evident as a relative paucity of bile duct on liver biopsy. Clinically the syndrome presents with:

- Persistent cholestasis
- Intense pruritus
- Hepatomegaly
- Congenital heart defects – peripheral pulmonary stenosis, tetralogy of Fallot
- Notched or butterfly dorsal vertebrae
- Eye defects – most frequently posterior embryotoxon
- Characteristic facial features – broad forehead, pointed chin resulting in triangular face (Fig. 93.2).

In the neonatal period the liver biopsy findings may be inconclusive and the facial features less obvious. The cholesta-

TABLE 93.1 CONDITIONS PRESENTING WITH A "LIVER PHENOTYPE" – FEATURES AND GENETIC CAUSE

Condition	Features	Gene	Protein	Reference
Alagille syndrome	IC, heart, bone, eye, kidney abnormalities	*JAG1*	JAG1	1, 2
BSEP deficiency	Low GGT IC	*ABCB11*	BSEP	3
FIC1 deficiency	Low GGT IC, extrahepatic features	*ATP8B1*	FIC1	4, 5
ARC syndrome	Arthrogryposis, renal dysfunction, cholestasis, low GGT IC	*VPS33B*	VPS33B	6
Aagenaes syndrome	Low GGT IC, lymphedema	*Ch 15*	Unknown	7
Bile acid synthesis defects	Most low GGT IC, neurologic abnormalities in some	Various	Various	8
MDR3 deficiency	Low GGT IC, gallstones, ICP	*ABCB4*	MDR3	9
North American Indian childhood cirrhosis	High GGT IC	*CIRH1A*	Cirhin	10
Neonatal sclerosing cholangitis	High GGT IC	Unknown		11
Dubin-Johnson syndrome	Conjugated jaundice	*ABCC2*	MRP2	12
Crigler-Najjar syndrome	Unconjugated jaundice	*UGT1A1*	UGT1A1	13

ARC, arthrogryposis; BSEP, bile salt export pump; GGT, γ-glutamyl transferase; IC, intrahepatic cholestasis; ICP, intrahepatic cholestasis of pregnancy; MDR3, multidrug resistance protein-3.

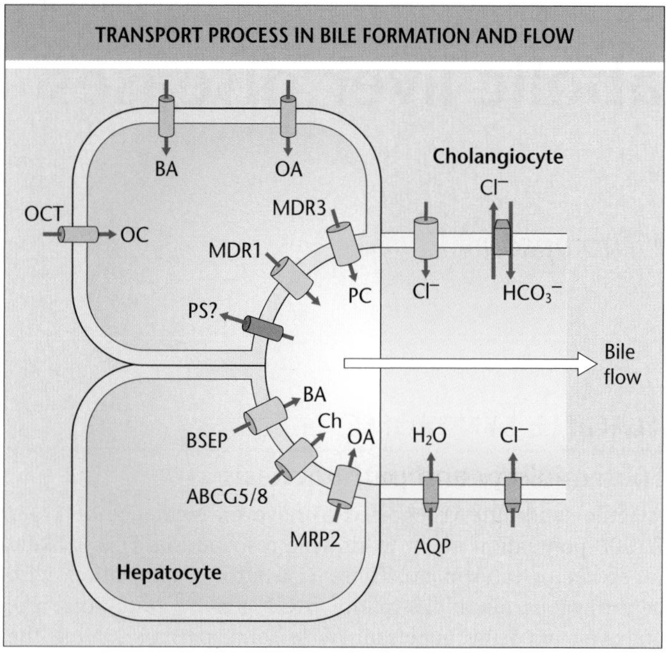

Fig. 93.1 Major transport processes in bile formation and flow. In particular, the classes of uptake transporter in the hepatocyte basolateral membrane are indicated, as are the apical transporters of the cholangiocyte membrane. The individual transporters of the canalicular membrane are shown, as featured in the text. OCT, organic action transporters; OATP, organic anion transporting polypeptides; NTCP, sodium taurocholate co-transporting polypeptide; MDR, multidrug resistance protein; FIC1, familial intrahepatic cholestasis protein-1; BSEP, bile salt export pump; ABCG5/8, cholesterol-transporting heterodimer; MRP2, multidrug resistance-associated protein-2; CFTR, cystic fibrosis transmembrane conductance regulator; AQP, aquaporins; AE, anion exchanger, OC, organic cations; OA, organic anions; BA, bile acids; PC, phosphatidylcholine; PS, phosphatidylserine; Ch, cholesterol.

ALAGILLE SYNDROME ASSOCIATED WITH MUTATIONS OF THE *JAG1* GENE

- Characterized by intrahepatic cholestasis and biliary hypoplasia
- Typical facial features and xanthomata
- May require liver transplantation
- Congenital heart defects (pulmonary stenosis, tetralogy of Fallot) may cause greater health limitation

sis is often characterized by markedly increased serum level of cholesterol, with development of xanthomata (Fig. 93.3 Growth failure is a major feature in most cases.

Management

The cholestasis of Alagille syndrome may be severe enough t justify liver transplantation. However, it does frequently improv after the first decade. The overall prognosis is largely determine by the severity of the heart disease. Peripheral pulmonar stenosis is often asymptomatic, but may require dilatation an stenting before liver transplantation. Most of the extrahepati features are clearly not corrected by liver transplantation.

FAMILIAL INTRAHEPATIC CHOLESTASIS

Whilst most cholestatic liver diseases are marked by raised serur levels of γ-glutamyl transferase (GGT), a number of condition are characterized by normal levels. In most cases when a live disease is associated with normal levels of GGT there is a accompanying failure of bile salt excretion. This may be primar or secondary. Secondary failure of secretion of bile acids ma be seen in severe liver disease, and is not uncommon in acut liver failure. Primary failure of bile acid secretion may be du

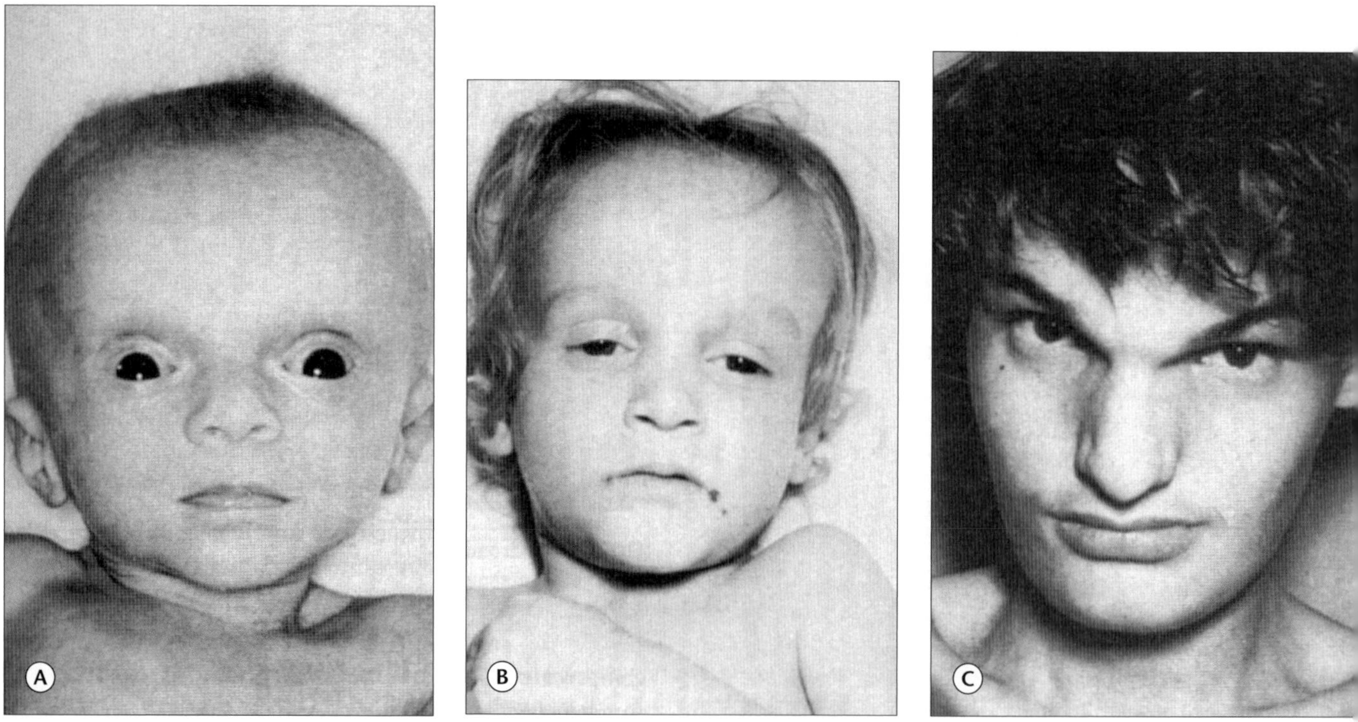

Fig. 93.2A–C Alagille syndrome at various ages. From Alagille D, Estrada A, Hadchouel M et al. Syndromic paucity of interlobular bile ducts (Alagille syndrome or arteriohepatic dysplasia): review of 80 cases. J Pediatr. 1987; 110:195–200. Reproduced with permission from Elsevier.

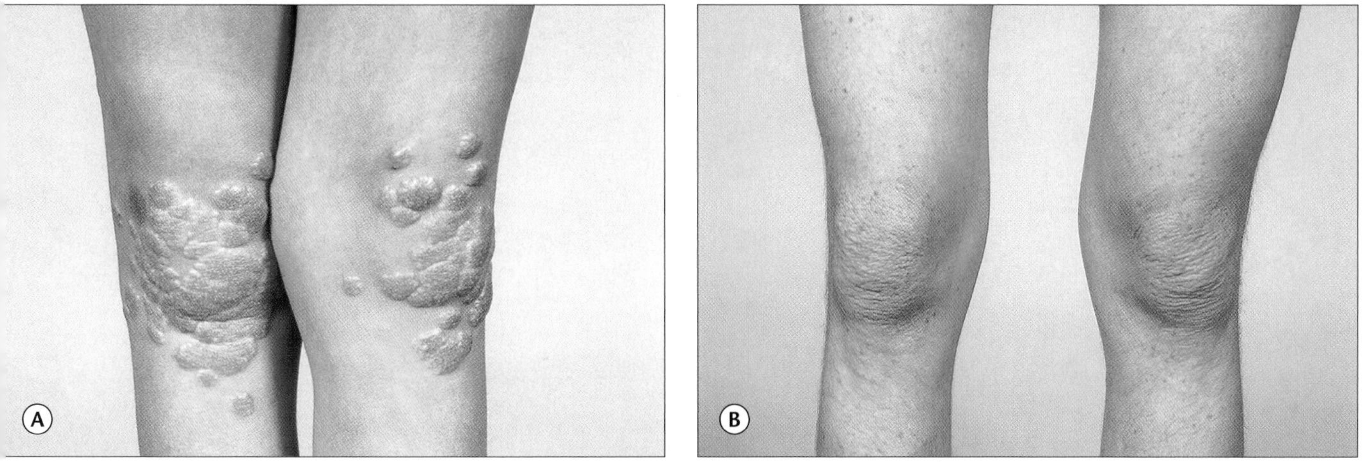

Fig. 93.3 Alagille syndrome: xanthomata. Lobulated tumors occur over the elbows and knees (A), or along the course of the tendons, when they may be known as xanthoma tendinosum. B. This child with Alagille syndrome was treated successfully with a liver transplant. Reproduced from Du Vivier A. Atlas of clinical dermatology, 3rd edn. London: Churchill Livingstone, 2002, with permission from Elsevier.

to failure of bile salt synthesis[8] or transport. Although bile acid synthesis defects are relatively rare, they are usually treatable with oral bile acid therapy. For this reason it is essential to screen the urine for abnormal metabolites.

Progressive familial intrahepatic cholestasis with low GGT

Pathogenesis and epidemiology

Most cases of progressive familial intrahepatic cholestasis (PFIC) are of the low, or normal, GGT type. Two causes of low GGT PFIC have been identified so far:

- *Bile salt export pump (BSEP) deficiency* – due to mutations in the gene encoding the BSEP of the canalicular membrane (*ABCB11*)[3]
- *Familial intrahepatic cholestasis-1 (FIC1) deficiency* – caused by mutations in *ATP8B1*.[4,5] The function of the FIC1 protein is unknown, although it may be an aminophospholipid flipase.

ABCB11 is expressed only in the liver; *ATP8B1* is, however, widely expressed. Collectively these two conditions have an incidence of approximately 1 in 50 000. Although originally thought of as occurring only in isolated populations, approximately one-third of patients with FIC1 are compound heterozygotes, rising to two-thirds for BSEP deficiency.

Clinical presentation

BSEP deficiency usually presents in the first 3 months with a giant cell hepatitis and continues to a progressive cholestasis, with jaundice and itching.

FIC1 deficiency is usually milder in onset, may have a fluctuating course, and is accompanied by nonspecific features of cholestasis on light microscopy. As well as progressive cholestasis, with jaundice and itching, FIC1 deficiency results in a number of extrahepatic features, especially diarrhea and malabsorption, in excess of what would be expected from the cholestasis.

A significant minority also has:

- Sensorineural deafness
- Pancreatitis
- Pancreatic insufficiency
- Abnormal sweat electrolytes.

Pathology

Immunohistochemical staining for BSEP is becoming available as a discriminatory diagnostic tool (Fig. 93.4). FIC1 staining is not yet available. A number of other canalicular proteins do, however, appear to be absent in patients with FIC1 deficiency, most notably GGT and CD26; this can be used to aid diagnosis. Transmission electron microscopy can be diagnostic in FIC1 deficiency, showing coarsely granular bile in the canalicular space – Byler bile (Fig. 93.5).

Management

Both BSEP and FIC1 deficiencies have largely been managed conservatively, or by liver transplantation. Both require aggressive nutritional management, such as medium-chain triglyceride supplements. Some patients require parenteral dosing to maintain adequate fat-soluble vitamin levels. Pruritus can be very difficult to treat. Rifampin, with or without ursodeoxycholic acid (in modest doses), is probably the best treatment, although far from ideal.

Surgical interventions, such as partial external biliary diversion and ileal exclusion, have been attempted. There is very little information on the latter, but the former works in some patients. In FIC1 deficiency success cannot so far be predicted. For BSEP deficiency, however, it appears that patients with 'milder' mutations (with some retention of function) do much better. Liver transplantation is an excellent treatment for BSEP deficiency. For FIC1 deficiency, although transplantation greatly improves the cholestasis, the extrahepatic features remain. The malabsorption can be particularly difficult after transplantation. Several patients with BSEP deficiency have developed either hepatocellular carcinoma or cholangiocarcinoma; neither has been reported in FIC1 deficiency.

Progressive familial intrahepatic cholestasis with high GGT

Three types of recessive cholestatic liver disease with raised levels of serum GGT have so far been identified. Overall there are fewer data available than for low GGT disease, reflecting the fact that these conditions seem to be rarer.

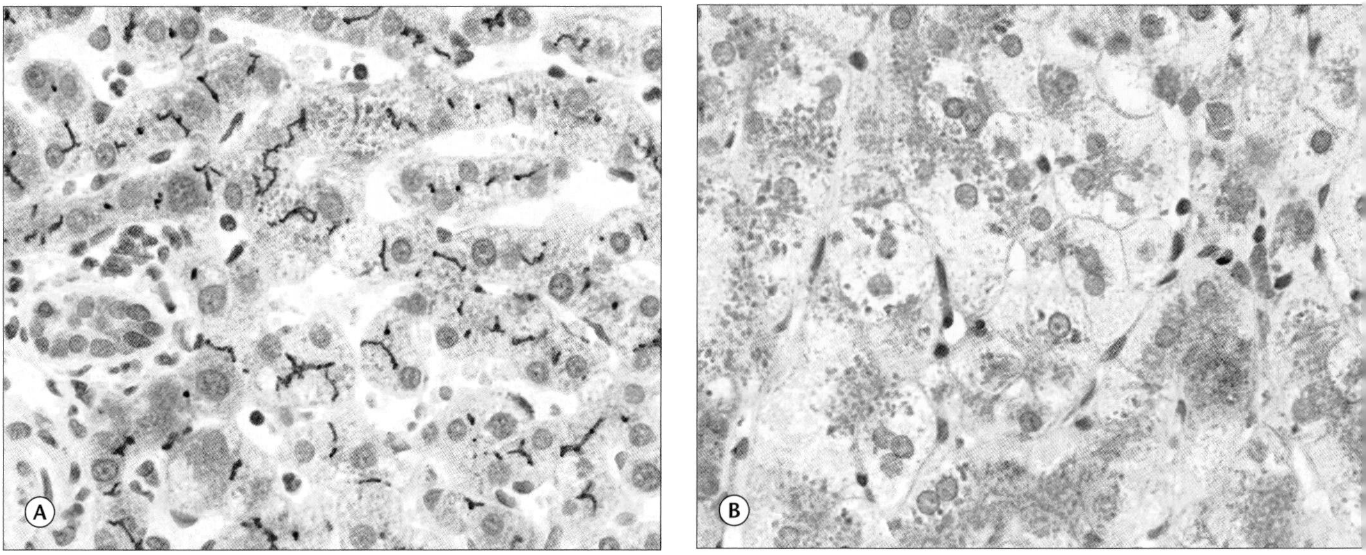

Fig. 93.4 Bile salt export pump deficiency. A. Normal liver. **B.** BSEP deficiency. Rabbit polyclonal antibody against human BSEP/hematoxylin counterstain. Original magnification ×400. Courtesy of Dr Y Meier and Dr B Steiger, University of Zurich.

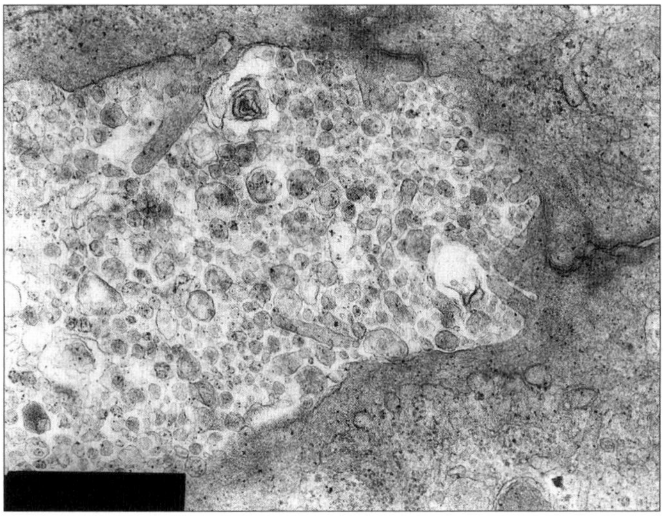

Fig. 93.5 Byler bile. Osmium tetroxide–uranyl acetate–lead citrate. Original magnification ×40 000. (Patient materials courtesy of Dr L Szönyi.) Kindly provided by A S Knisely.

PROGRESSIVE FAMILIAL INTRAHEPATIC CHOLESTASIS WITH LOW GGT

MAIN CAUSES
- Bile salt export pump (BSEP) deficiency (mutation of *ABCB11* gene)
- Familial intrahepatic cholestasis-1 (FIC1) deficiency (mutations in *80P8B1* gene)

BSEP DEFICIENCY
- Giant cell hepatitis and progressive cholestasis
- Requires nutritional management with medium-chain triglycerides
- Liver transplantation helpful

FIC1 DEFICIENCY
- Cholestasis with Byler bile (coarsely granular bile)
- Extrahepatic manifestations
- Liver transplantation treats only hepatic problem

North American Indian childhood cirrhosis

This condition is uniquely found in Ojibway-Cree children from northwestern Quebec, Canada. It is a recessive condition due to a missense mutation (R565W) in the protein cirhin. The phenotype is very similar to that of extrahepatic biliary atresia, with transient neonatal jaundice, followed by progression to biliary cirrhosis and portal hypertension. This will make the function of cirhin all the more interesting, once it has been elucidated.

Neonatal sclerosing cholangitis

This is a recessive condition that mimics biliary atresia. The genetics and pathogenesis have not yet been fully defined; however, there does seem to be a spectrum, ranging from patients who require liver transplantation in the first year of life to those who are controlled for many years on ursodeoxycholic acid.

Multidrug resistance protein-3 (MDR3) deficiency

Pathology and clinical presentation

This is the best characterized form of intrahepatic cholestasis, with high levels of serum GGT. MDR3 is an ATP-binding cassette-type protein that resembles the multidrug resistance P-glycoprotein and is expressed in the canalicular membrane of hepatocytes, where it is involved in the transport of phospatidylcholine to bile.

A complete lack of MDR3 function is associated with a complete lack of phosphatidylcholine in bile. This is the main phospholipid in bile; without it, bile acids cannot form mixed micelles and instead the bile consists of highly detergent, free bile acids. This causes major damage to both hepatocytes and cholangiocytes, as is reflected on histologic inspection (Fig. 93.6).

There is a wide spectrum of severity in MDR3 deficiency. Although most patients so far described present in the first few months of life, there is a range of phenotypes that present later. As phospholipids, along with bile acids, are essential in maintaining cholesterol in solution, some patients present with intrahepatic cholelithiasis. There are also patients with late-onset cholestatic disease, presenting in the second or even third decade. Furthermore, heterozygotes for severe mutations, for

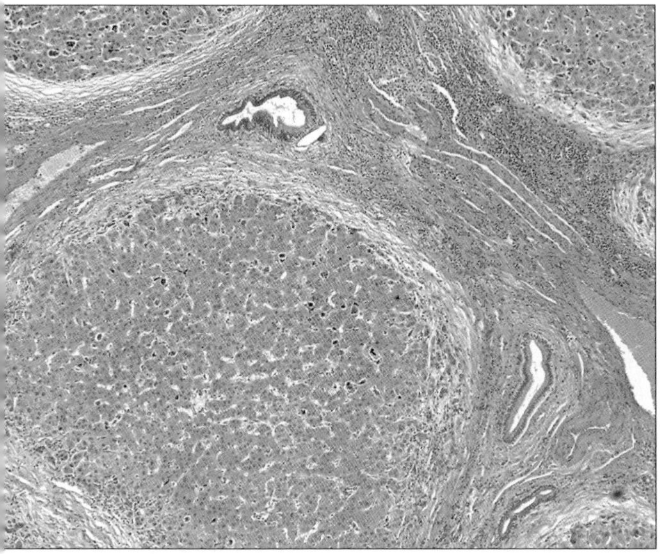

ig. 93.6 **MDR3 deficiency.** Hematoxylin and eosin stain. Original ıagnification ×4. Photo kindly provided by Alex S Knisely.

xample mothers of patients with severe disease, can suffer rom cholestasis of pregnancy.

Management

Most patients with early-onset MDR3 deficiency will come to ver transplantation, although some respond to ursodeoxy-holic acid treatment. This is understandable, as anything that educes the hydrophobicity of the bile should help. However, there are no phospholipids at all, even ursodeoxycholic acid annot help. The mouse model of MDR3 deficiency (*mdr2* eficiency) indicates that this condition may be an excellent andidate for hepatocyte transplantation, which has not yet een tried in humans.

PROGRESSIVE FAMILIAL INTRAHEPATIC CHOLESTASIS WITH HIGH GGT

NORTH AMERICAN CHILDHOOD CIRRHOSIS

- *R565W* gene mutation (protein product cirhin)
- Transient neonatal jaundice and later cirrhosis

NEONATAL SCLEROSING CHOLANGITIS

- Mimics biliary atresia
- Treatment ranges from ursodeoxycholic acid to liver transplantation

MULTIDRUG RESISTANCE PROTEIN-3 (MDR3) DEFICIENCY DEFICIENCY

- Mutation in MDR P-like glycoprotein involved transport of phosphatidylcholine
- Highly detergent, free bile acids damage hepatocytes and cholangiocytes
- Treatment ranges from ursodeoxycholic acid to liver transplantation

SUPPORT FOR PATIENTS AND PARENTS

Many of the intrahepatic cholestases are very distressing and ifficult to treat. The majority of treatments are supportive. Unfortunately even liver transplantation does not cure Alagille syndrome or FIC1 deficiency. Patients with Alagille syndrome benefit from skilled input from cardiologists and endocrinologists, as well as from those who care for the liver disease. For all patients with cholestasis, the liver disease requires multidisciplinary input if the secondary consequences are to be minimized. The recessive conditions discussed can all be tested for in subsequent pregnancies, should the parents so wish. The complex genetics of Alagille syndrome make testing very difficult, as there is not a one to one relationship between mutations and phenotype.

The multidisciplinary team caring for these patients needs to include nurse specialists and dietitians capable of helping the parents look after their child. In addition the following organizations seek to help the families of children with liver disease in various ways:

UK: Children's Liver Disease Foundation. http://www.childliverdisease.org/
USA: Children's Liver Association for Support Services. http://www.classkids.org/
Australia: Children's Liver Alliance. http://www.liverkids.org.au/
South Africa: Children's Liver Disease Foundation, South Africa. http://www.realcom.co.uk/cldfsa/

REFERENCES

1. Oda T, Elkahloun AG, Pike BL et al. Mutations in the human *Jagged1* gene are responsible for Alagille syndrome. Nat Genet 1997; 16:235–242.
2. Li L, Krantz ID, Deng Y et al. Alagille syndrome is caused by mutations in human *Jagged1*, which encodes a ligand for Notch1. Nat Genet 1997; 16:243–251.
3. Strautnieks SS, Bull LN, Knisely AS et al. A gene encoding a liver-specific ABC transporter is mutated in progressive familial intrahepatic cholestasis. Nat Genet 1998; 20:233–238.
4. Klomp LW, Vargas JC, van Mil SW et al. Characterization of mutations in *ATP8B1* associated with hereditary cholestasis. Hepatology 2004; 40:27–38.
5. Bull LN, van Eijk MJ, Pawlikowska L et al. A gene encoding a P-type ATPase mutated in two forms of hereditary cholestasis. Nat Genet 1998; 18:219–224.
6. Gissen P, Johnson CA, Morgan NV et al. Mutations in *VPS33B*, encoding a regulator of SNARE-dependent membrane fusion, cause arthrogryposis–renal dysfunction–cholestasis (ARC) syndrome. Nat Genet 2004; 36: 400–404.
7. Bull LN, Roche E, Song EJ et al. Mapping of the locus for cholestasis–lymphedema syndrome (Aagenaes syndrome) to a 6.6-cM interval on chromosome 15q. Am J Hum Genet 2000; 67:994–999.
8. Bove KE, Daugherty CC, Tyson W et al. Bile acid synthetic defects and liver disease. Pediatr Dev Pathol 2000; 3:1–16.
9. de Vree JM, Jacquemin E, Sturm E et al. Mutations in the *MDR3* gene cause progressive familial intrahepatic cholestasis. Proc Natl Acad Sci USA 1998; 95:282–287.
10. Chagnon P, Michaud J, Mitchell G et al. A missense mutation (R565W) in cirhin (*FLJ14728*) in North American Indian childhood cirrhosis. Am J Hum Genet 2002; 71:1443–1449.
11. Mieli-Vergani G, Vergani D. Sclerosing cholangitis in the paediatric patient. Best Pract Res Clin Gastroenterol 2001; 15:681–690.
12. Paulusma CC, Kool M, Bosma PJ et al. A mutation in the human canalicular multispecific organic anion transporter gene causes the Dubin-Johnson syndrome. Hepatology 1997; 25:1539–1542.
13. Bosma PJ. Inherited disorders of bilirubin metabolism. J Hepatol 2003; 38:107–117.

Chapter 94

Disturbances of bilirubin metabolism

Dean Cekic, Igino Rigato, and Claudio Tiribelli

KEY POINTS

- Hereditary syndromes in which hyperbilirubinemia is related to a genetic disorder of bilirubin transport and metabolism
- Divided in those leading to unconjugated hyperbilirubinemia and those related to conjugated hyperbilirubinemia
- Unconjugated hyperbilirubinemia syndromes are caused by anomalies in bilirubin-conjugating capacity:
  - Gilbert
  - Crigler-Najjar (types I and II)
- Conjugated hyperbilirubinemia syndromes are caused by impaired extrusion of bilirubin into the bile canaliculus:
  - Dubin-Johnson
  - Rotor

INTRODUCTION

Bilirubin is the terminal product of heme present in hemoglobin, myoglobin, and some enzymes. An adult healthy person produces 250–300 mg of bilirubin per day: 80% derives from hemoglobin (breakdown of senescent erythrocytes), 15–20% derives from the turnover of myoglobin, cytochromes and other hemoproteins, and less than 3% derives from destruction of immature red blood cells in the bone marrow. This fraction is greatly increased in cases of ineffective erythropoiesis such as hemoglobinopathies, megaloblastic anemia, and lead intoxication.

Heme degradation is performed by the reticuloendothelial enzyme heme oxygenase, which is particularly abundant in spleen and liver Kupffer cells, the principal sites of red cell breakdown. This enzyme opens the heme ring, freeing the iron ion and forming a tetrapyrrolic chain with the final formation of biliverdin and carbon monoxide. The reaction requires oxygen and NADPH. The conversion of biliverdin to bilirubin is catalyzed by the cytosolic enzyme biliverdin reductase, which reduces biliverdin using NADH or NADPH[1] (Fig. 94.1).

Once released in the blood and due to its very poor water solubility, practically all (more than 99.9%) of the bilirubin binds to serum albumin, the main bilirubin carrier protein in blood; less than 0.1% of the pigment is unbound to albumin (free bilirubin). This fraction, however, can increase in the presence of some drugs, for example sulfonamides, nonsteroidal anti-inflammatory drugs, and some radiological contrast agents, which inhibit the binding of bilirubin to albumin.

Free bilirubin present in Disse's space is internalized by hepatocytes. The mechanism(s) of bilirubin uptake is not yet fully clarified. Although it is known that bilirubin uptake is saturable, indicating the presence of membrane transporters, the carrier molecule responsible for this transport is still undetermined. Once internalized by the hepatocyte, bilirubin is metabolized by the enzyme uridinediphosphoglucuronosyltransferase (UGT), located in the endoplasmic reticulum, which conjugates bilirubin with one or two molecules of glucuronic acid rendering it hydrosoluble. Bilirubin glucuronides are then extruded into the bile canaliculus by the membrane transporter 'multidrug resistance protein 2' (MRP2 or ABCC2) and eventually secreted into the duodenum[1] (Fig. 94.2.)

Any abnormality causing slowing or blockage of this rather complicated metabolic pathway will lead to disturbances of bilirubin metabolism.

Definition

The **inherited disorders of bilirubin metabolism** or 'familial nonhemolytic hyperbilirubinemias' are defined as hereditary syndromes where the cause of hyperbilirubinemia is related to a genetic disorder of bilirubin transport and metabolism. They may be divided in unconjugated and conjugated hyperbilirubinemias, the first being the Gilbert syndrome and the Crigler-Najjar syndrome types I and II, and the second the Dubin-Johnson and Rotor syndromes. Gilbert syndrome and the Crigler-Najjar syndrome are caused by anomalies mostly in bilirubin conjugating capacity, while the Dubin-Johnson syndrome is caused by impaired extrusion of bilirubin into the bile canaliculus.

Gilbert syndrome is defined as a mild, benign, unconjugated hyperbilirubinemia without signs of increased hemolysis and with normal routine liver function tests and hepatic histology. Crigler-Najjar syndrome II is defined as moderate/severe, familial, unconjugated hyperbilirubinemia sensitive to phenobarbital treatment, while Crigler-Najjar syndrome I is a severe unconjugated hyperbilirubinemia unresponsive to phenobarbital administration. Dubin-Johnson and Rotor syndromes are each defined as a chronic, benign, intermittent jaundice with conjugated hyperbilirubinemia and bilirubinuria.

EPIDEMIOLOGY

The Gilbert syndrome is the most common familial hyperbilirubinemia, and the most frequent cause of increased plasma bilirubin levels in man. It is estimated that it occurs in 3–10% of the total population. However, this prevalence could be an underestimate due to the naturally occurring fluctuations of bilirubinemia in these subjects. The male/female ratio in Gilbert syndrome is 8:1; this is probably due to a greater heme loading originating from muscle myoglobin metabolism or hormonal

BILIRUBIN METABOLISM

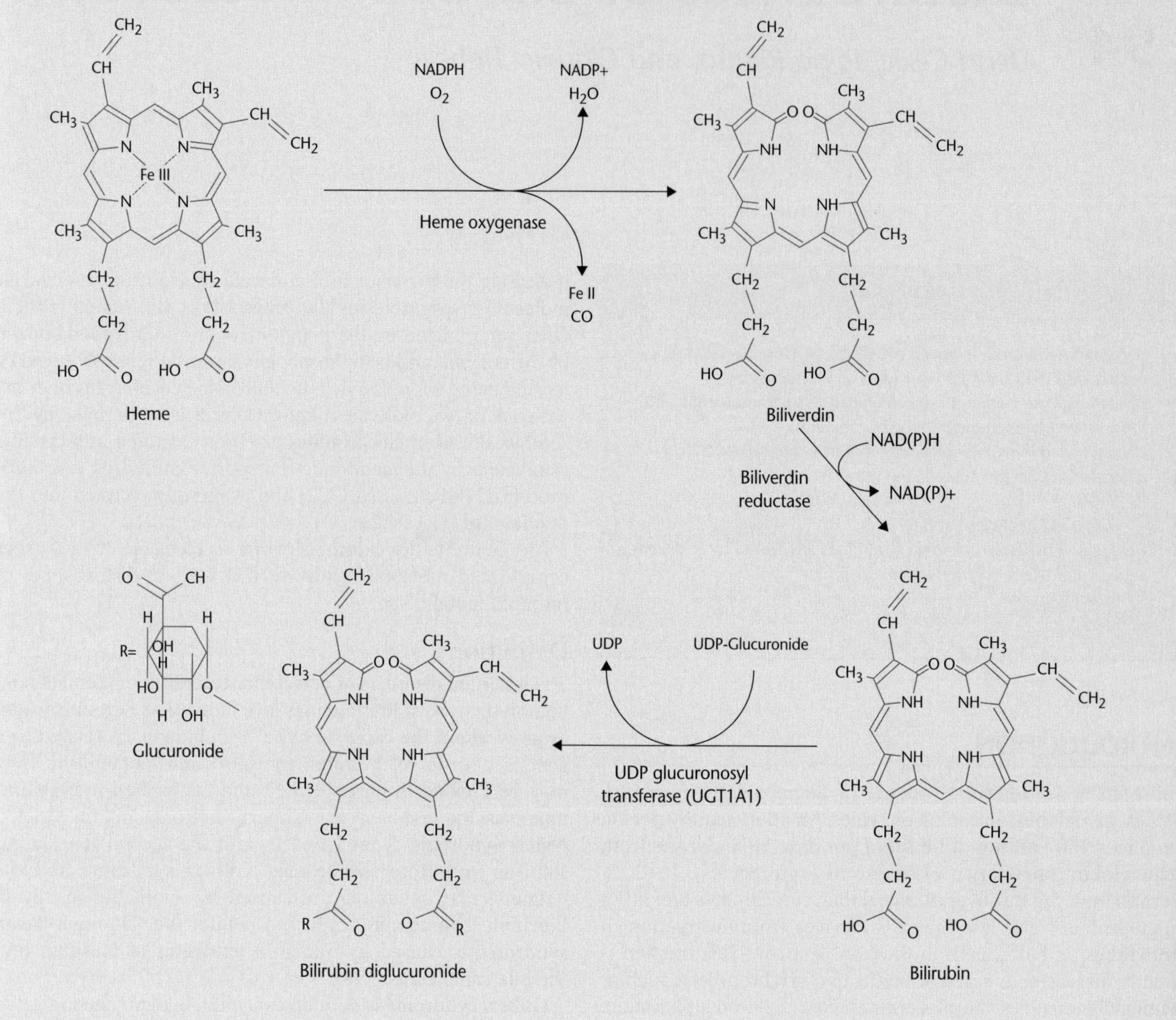

Fig. 94.1 Bilirubin metabolism. Bilirubin derives from heme metabolism by heme-oxygenase and biliverdin reductase. UGT1A1 conjugates bilirubin with glucuronic acid forming bilirubin mono- or diglucuronides.

differences. The discovery of TATA box mutation at the A1 exon of UGT as a major cause of Gilbert syndrome opened the way to genetic population studies. The mutation is extremely frequent: 34–40% of Caucasians contribute one mutated allele, while 12–16% are homozygote.[2] Based on these data (12–16% homozygote, 3–10% affected), it is apparent that other factors are needed for the clinical expression of Gilbert syndrome.

In contrast to the Gilbert syndrome, both Crigler-Najjar I and II syndromes are very rare, affecting one in 1×10^6 newborns.

The Dubin-Johnson syndrome and Rotor's syndrome are also extremely rare, although the former is more prevalent in Sephardic Jews.

CAUSES AND PATHOGENESIS

The UGT gene

The UGT gene is a complex of 100 kb located on the q37 region of chromosome 2. It consists of four common exons named 2–5 that encode the carboxy-terminal portion of the enzyme, and 13 variable exons named A1–A13, codifying the amino-terminal part of each isoform. All exons are preceded by a 5′ flanking regulatory region that controls transcription and splicing as an effect of specific signals. During transcription, the transcript of each single variable exon is found with the transcripts of common exons, forming nine different mRNA that encode different UGT isoforms. Exons 12 and 13 do not contain regulatory regions, while mutations in exons 11 and 1

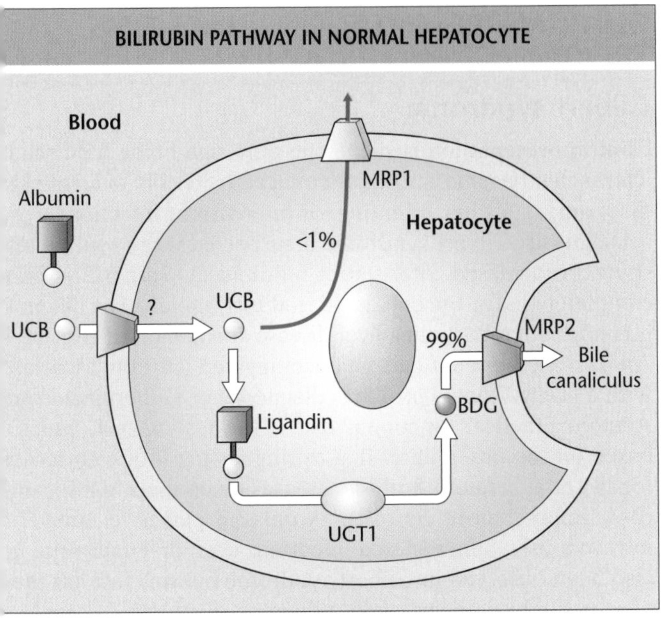

ig. 94.2 Bilirubin pathway in normal hepatocyte. Bilirubin irculates in blood tightly bound to albumin. The free portion of nconjugated bilirubin (UCB) enters the hepatocyte through an nknown carrier system. Inside the hepatocyte, UCB is bound to gandin, transformed into bilirubin diconjugate (BDG) by eticuloendothelial enzyme UGT1 and secreted into bile canaliculus y multidrug resistance protein 2 (MRP2). Less than 1% of bilirubin secreted in unconjugated form in the blood, most probably by ultidrug resistance protein 1 (MRP1).

revent transcription. The carboxy-terminal part of the enzyme odified by common exons is responsible for glucuronidation, while the amino-terminal portion codified by each of the variable exons determines the substrate specificity of the isoform. The isoform containing exon A1 (UGT1A1) is responsible for bilirubin glucuronidation (Fig. 94.3).[3]

Gilbert syndrome

The main cause of Gilbert syndrome is a mutation in the 5′ flanking region of the A1 exon where the 'TATA box' promoter hat binds the transcription factor is located. The sequence of this promoter is normally $A(TA)_6TAA$. In subjects with Gilbert syndrome the sequence is mutated in both alleles of the A1 exon by the insertion of two nucleotides TA changing the sequence to $A(TA)_7TAA$. This causes a reduction of 70% in the A1 exon transcription activity and therefore in conjugation capacity.[4]

Strong evidence suggests that the abnormalities observed in Gilbert syndrome are more complex than those that can be deduced from genetic analysis of UGT. This is in line with the discrepancy between the genetic (TATA7) and phenotypic (increased plasma levels of unconjugated bilirubin) expression of the syndrome (see above). Experimental evidence suggests that in addition to reduced conjugating activity, Gilbert subjects have an impaired uptake of bilirubin and other related organic anions. Studies using bromosulfophtalein (BSP), a molecule that simulates bilirubin, show a significantly reduced hepatic uptake in patients with Gilbert syndrome compared to normal subjects, suggesting that the still undefined membrane transporter(s) may have a reduced affinity for the substrate, probably because of underlying mutations.

KEY POINTS

GILBERT SYNDROME

- Most common inherited disorder of bilirubin metabolism, affecting 3–10% of the general population
- Defined as a mild, benign, unconjugated hyperbilirubinemia without signs of increased hemolysis and with normal routine liver function tests and hepatic histology
- Main cause is a mutation at the A1 exon of the uridinediphosphoglucuronosyltransferase (UGT) gene
- Clinically silent except for mild unconjugated hyperbilirubinemia (1–5 mg/dL) that becomes more pronounced and clinically apparent with fasting, vomiting, or intercurrent infections
- Diagnosis is established with a fasting test that shows a 2–4-fold increase in serum bilirubin after a 400 calorie/day diet for 24 h
- Since Gilbert syndrome is associated with a reduced liver uptake of other organic anions, an impaired metabolism of some drugs may occur (e.g., irinotecan, indinavir) in these patients

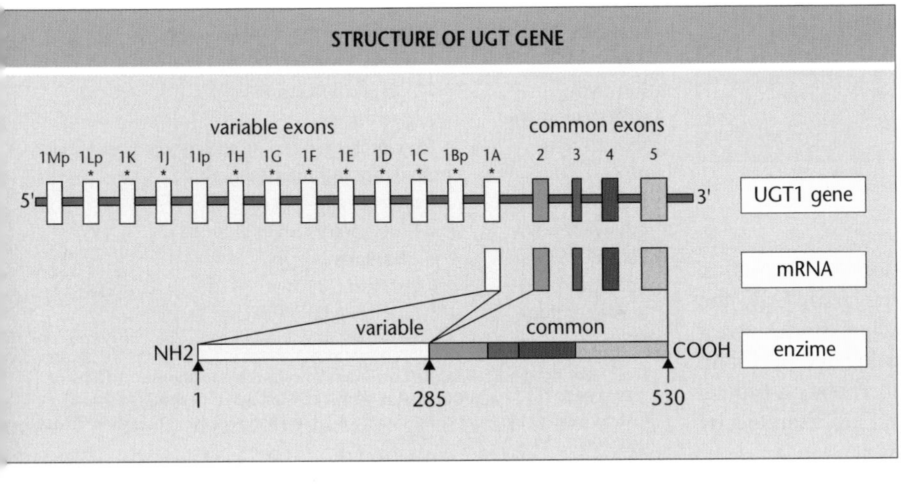

Fig. 94.3 Structure of the UGT gene. The human UGT gene contains 13 unique exons (1A-M) and four common exons (2–5). p, pseudoexon;* TATA box.

Crigler-Najjar syndrome types I and II

The mutations present in Crigler-Najjar syndrome I involve the coding regions of the UGT gene. The type of mutation is mainly nonsense or frameshift, leading to truncated and/or nonfunctional UGT or preventing its transcription, thereby completely abolishing bilirubin conjugating activity. The mutations are found in all exons, both variable and common. In mutations affecting variable exon A1 only bilirubin conjugation is impaired, while common exon (2–5) mutations impair conjugation in general, affecting the metabolism of several other molecules besides bilirubin. Crigler-Najjar type I is a disease of autosomal recessive inheritance.

Unlike Crigler-Najjar type I where bilirubin conjugation is totally abolished, some conjugating activity is still present in type II syndrome. Although the enzyme is synthesized at lower than normal levels and is less functional, its expression/function can be increased by the administration of phenobarbital. The mutations described are of missense type, altering the enzyme conformation but not abolishing its transcription. This greatly diminishes bilirubin conjugation by lowering it to less than 5%. As for type I, the inheritance is autosomal recessive. Beside missense mutation homozygosity, one relatively frequent combination is a nonsense mutation of one allele and a mutated 'TATA' box mutation on the other.[4]

KEY POINTS

CRIGLER-NAJJAR SYNDROME

- Crigler-Najjar syndrome is very rare, affecting one in 1×10^6 newborns; it is of autosomal recessive inheritance
- Main cause is a mutation that involves the coding regions of the UGT gene; unlike Crigler-Najjar syndrome type I where bilirubin conjugation is totally abolished, some conjugating activity is still present in type II
- Type I is characterized by the presence, at birth, of severe unconjugated hyperbilirubinemia (20–30 mg/dL), which may lead to severe neurological complications (kernicterus) and is unresponsive to phenobarbital; type II is characterized by lower levels of unconjugated hyperbilirubinemia (8–12 mg/dL) and is sensitive to phenobarbital
- The diagnosis is made by demonstrating the absence of UGT 1A1 activity on a liver biopsy specimen and confirmed by genotyping UGT1A1 alleles
- Early detection of kernicterus (lethargy and hypotonia) is key in type I Crigler-Najjar syndrome in order to prevent irreversible neurological damage; treatment should be initiated promptly with phototherapy to reduce hyperbilirubinemia
- Avoiding factors that may exacerbate jaundice (e.g., infections) is a crucial aspect in the management of this condition
- OLT is the only permanent cure for these patients

Dubin-Johnson syndrome

The cause of Dubin-Johnson syndrome is a nonsense mutation of the coding region of the gene for MRP2 (ABCC2), the canalicular membrane transporter that normally extrudes a vast number of metabolites into bile, including conjugated bilirubin. Bilirubin glucuronides reflux back into blood creating a typical pattern of conjugated hyperbilirubinemia and are excreted by the kidneys causing bilirubinuria.

CLINICAL PRESENTATION, DIAGNOSIS, TREATMENT, AND PROGNOSIS

Gilbert syndrome

Clinical presentation is silent, the only sign being mild scler icterus that becomes more pronounced (clinically evident jau dice) during fasting, vomiting, or intercurrent infections.

Diagnosis: Gilbert syndrome is suspected when routine tes show an increased total serum bilirubin (1–5 mg/mL), almo completely in the unconjugated (indirect) moiety. The diagnos is confirmed by excluding liver disease and hemolysis (Fig. 94.4 An increased level of plasma unconjugated bilirubin associate with a (TATA7) gene profile is diagnostic of Gilbert syndrom A more practical functional test is the fasting test, which based on the observation that during fasting (400 calories/da for 24 h) the serum bilirubin increases much more significant (2–4 times) than in controls.[5] A delayed plasma clearance intravenously administered nicotinic acid or rifampicin ha also been observed in Gilbert syndrome but this test has mo of a pathophysiological than a diagnostic value.[5]

Why is establishing the diagnosis of Gilbert syndrome usefu For one, it is important to reassure the subject that life expe tancy and morbidity will not be influenced by this disord and that jaundice will be lifelong and may increase wit coexisting illnesses. Also, since Gilbert syndrome is associate with a reduced liver uptake of other organic anions, an impaire metabolism of some drugs may occur.[6] These drugs includ irinotecan and TAS-103 (both inhibitors of the topoisomeras I), as well as indinavir that can lead to pronounced hype bilirubinemia due to both impaired conjugation and increase hemolysis.[6] Several other drugs (Table 94.1) have been reporte to be potentially toxic in Gilbert syndrome because of th decrease in glucuronidation and/or hepatic elimination.[7]

Treatment: Although phenobarbital has been proposed t decrease serum bilirubin levels in Gilbert syndrome, its us should be recommended only for cosmetic purposes.

Crigler-Najjar I and II

Clinical features: Type I is characterized by the presence, a birth, of severe unconjugated hyperbilirubinemia (20–30 mg/dL

TABLE 94.1 DRUGS THAT HAVE MODIFIED METABOLISM IN PATIENTS WITH GILBERT SYNDROME AND TYPE OF EXPERIMENTAL EVIDENCE

Drug	Experimental evidence
Menthol	↓ Glucuronidation *in vivo*
Tolbutamine	↓ Glucuronidation *in vivo*
Rifamycin	↓ Glucuronidation *in vivo*
Acetaminophen	↓ Clearance *in vivo*
Irinotecan	Toxicity in case report and retrospective study
TAS	Dose-limiting toxicity in phase I study
Indinavir	↑ Adverse effect *in vivo*
Ethinylestradiol	↓ Glucuronidation *in vitro*
Lorazepam	↓ Clearance *in vivo*
Rifampicin-SV	↓ Clearance *in vivo*
Buprenorphine	↓ Glucuronidation *in vivo*

Data from Bosma PJ. Inherited disorders of bilirubin metabolism. J Hepatol 2003; 38:107–117 and Burchell B, Soars M, Monaghan G et al. Drug-mediated toxicity caused by genetic deficiency of UDP-glucuronosyltransferases. Toxicol Lett 2000; 112–113:333–340.

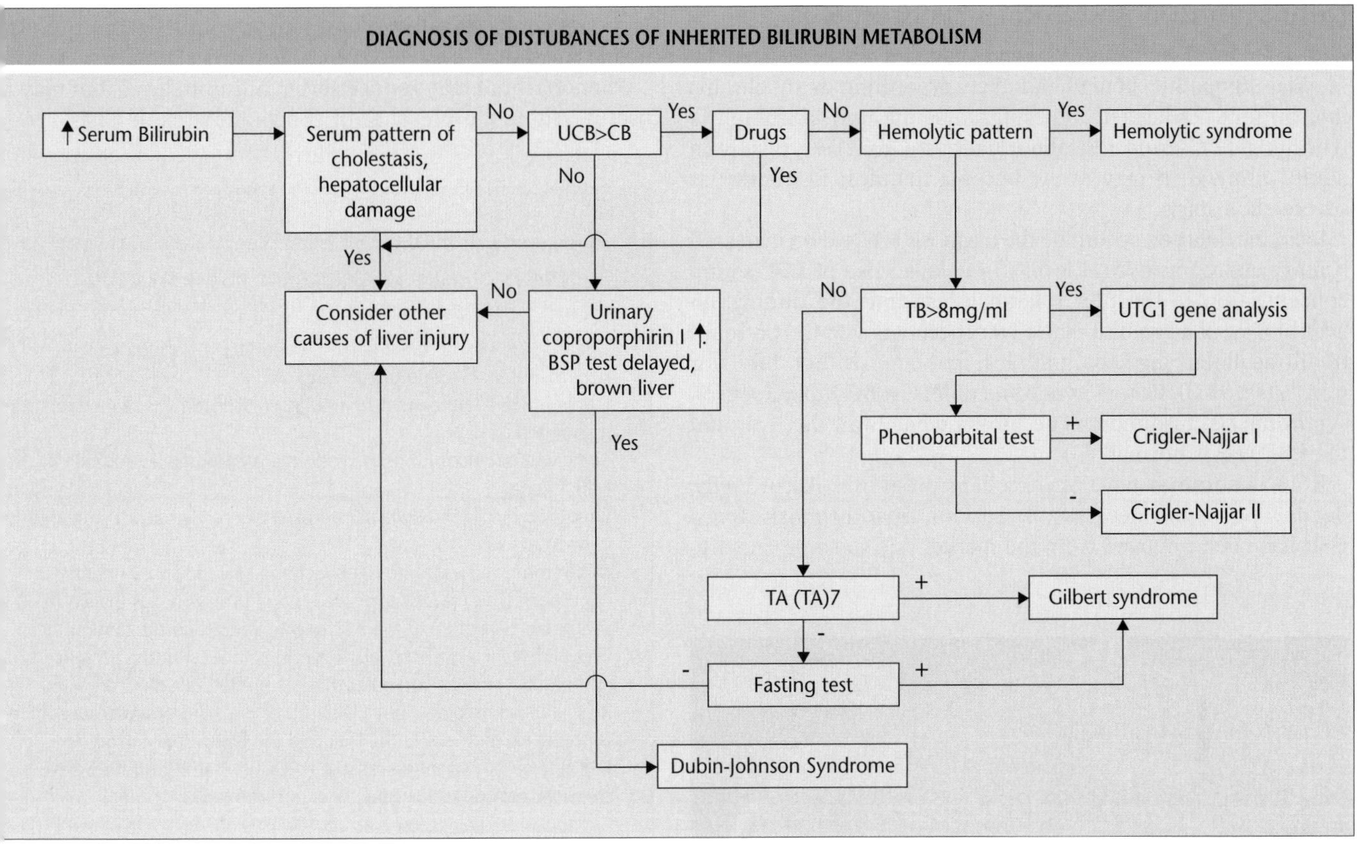

Fig. 94.4 Algorithm for the diagnosis of disturbances of inherited bilirubin metabolism. UCB, unconjugated bilirubin; CB, conjugated bilirubin; TB, total bilirubin; BSP, bromosulfophthalein; $TA(TA)_7$, see text.

without other signs or symptoms. Patients are otherwise healthy; however, if hyperbilirubinemia remains untreated, it will lead to severe neurological complications, the so-called bilirubin-induced neurodysfunction (BIND), which may proceed to the irreversible and much more serious picture of kernicterus. Type II is characterized by lower levels of unconjugated hyperbilirubinemia, ranging between 8 and 12 mg/dL. In this case the only clinical manifestation is jaundice.[8]

Diagnosis: The differential diagnosis between Crigler-Najjar syndrome types I and II is based on serum bilirubin levels (almost double in those with type I) and the different response to phenobarbital. In Crigler-Najjar syndrome type I patients there is no response to treatment with phenobarbital while in type II a reduction of about 50% in serum bilirubin is commonly observed after phenobarbital. The diagnosis is made by demonstrating the absence of UGT 1A1 activity on a liver biopsy specimen and confirmed by genotyping UGT1A1 alleles.[9]

Treatment: At present, the only permanent cure is orthotopic liver transplantation (OLT), which permanently corrects the metabolic defect. The optimal timing for OLT is before school age and definitely before adolescence.[10]

Kernicterus is the most important and severe complication of Crigler-Najjar syndrome and is of prognostic significance. Early detection is key in order to prevent irreversible neurological damage. Its clinical presentation is often characterized by lethargy and hypotonia. If hyperbilirubinemia is not treated, the patient will become hypertonic and may develop fever and a high-pitched cry. Cerebellar symptoms are rarely reported in children while they are prominent in adolescents.

Phototherapy: In order to reduce the probability of kernicterus, neonates with Crigler-Najjar syndrome must be immediately treated with phototherapy to reduce hyperbilirubinemia and their survival will be dependent on the indefinite continuation of this therapy. With age, however, the efficacy of phototherapy is reduced unless the number of treatment hours is increased (from 10–12 to 16–18 h/day) due to increased skin thickness and unfavorable body surface/weight ratio. Treatment with protoporphyrin IX, a potent heme oxygenase inhibitor, has been suggested as an adjuvant to phototherapy as it appears to increase its effect. Since infections or other concomitant illnesses can potentially exacerbate jaundice and lead to kernicterus, avoiding factors that may exacerbate jaundice is a crucial aspect in the management of this condition. In case of acute bilirubin encephalopathy due to the exacerbation of jaundice, the duration of phototherapy must be increased. Oral calcium supplementation, through sequestration of fecal bilirubin, makes phototherapy more efficient. Albumin infusion and plasmapheresis must be considered when the effect of other therapies is insufficient. In any case, OLT is the only permanent cure for these patients.[9]

Before phototherapy was introduced in 1968, most children with Crigler-Najjar syndrome type I died in early infancy or developed kernicterus in adolescence or early adulthood. The progresses in phototherapy technology allow patients affected by Crigler-Najjar syndrome I to reach adolescence and even adulthood but the risk of developing kernicterus is still pending. Great hope is placed in the development of gene therapy, which is not actually feasible or available at the present time.

Dubin-Johnson and Rotor's syndrome

Dubin-Johnson and Rotor's syndrome are characterized by familial idiopathic benign jaundice presenting with chronic intermittent conjugated hyperbilirubinemia and bilirubinuria without other serum test abnormalities. Onset is typically in adults although it may rarely become manifest in infancy as severe cholestasis.

In Dubin-Johnson syndrome the diagnosis is based on increased urinary coproporphyrin I levels,[9] a delayed rise of BSP serum concentration in the BSP tolerance test, and the finding, on liver biopsy, of a greenish-black liver specimen with the presence of intracellular pigment granules that are neither bile nor iron[11] (Fig. 94.5). Rotor's syndrome differs from Dubin-Johnson syndrome because there is no brown pigment in the liver and the BSP test is normal.[12]

Both syndromes have an excellent prognosis. Accordingly, liver biopsy is not necessary to reach a final diagnosis. Since BSP has been removed from the market due to some anaphylactic reactions, this test is not longer considered in the diag nostic work-up.

Phenobarbital may reduce serum bilirubin levels but may b useful only in the presence of concomitant cholestasis.

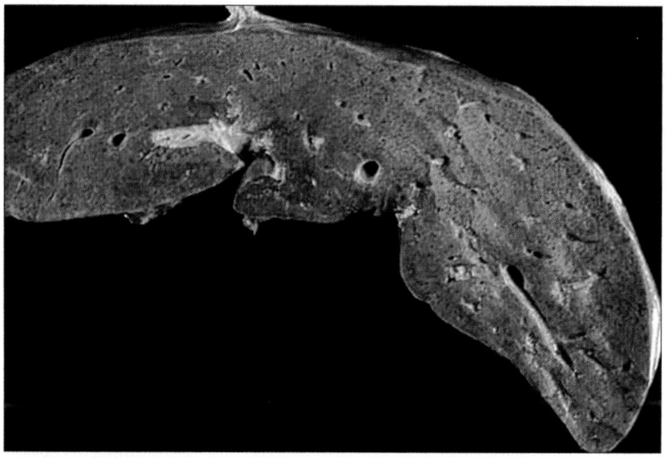

Fig. 94.5 Dubin-Johnson syndrome. Liver of patient with Dubin-Johnson syndrome showing the distinctive blackish-brown color.

KEY POINTS

DUBIN-JOHNSON SYNDROME AND ROTOR SYNDROME

- Characterized by chronic, benign, intermittent conjugated hyperbilirubinemia and bilirubinuria
- Extremely rare, although Dubin-Johnson syndrome is more common in Sephardic Jews
- The cause of Dubin-Johnson syndrome is a nonsense mutation of the MRP2 gene
- Onset is typically in adults although it may rarely become manifest in infancy as severe cholestasis
- Dubin-Johnson syndrome is characterized by increased urinary coproporphyrin I levels, a delayed rise of bromosulfophthalein (BSP) serum concentration in the BSP tolerance test and the finding, on liver biopsy, of a greenish-black liver specimen with the presence of intracellular pigment granules that are neither bile nor iron
- Rotor syndrome differs from Dubin-Johnson syndrome because there is no brown pigment in the liver and the BSP test is normal
- BSP test is not currently available and since both syndromes have an excellent prognosis, liver biopsy is not warranted

SOURCES OF INFORMATION FOR PATIENTS AND DOCTORS

Gilbert's syndrome:
http://www.patient.co.uk/showdoc/316/
Crigler-Najjar:
http://www.patient.co.uk/showdoc/40001363/
Dubin-Johnson:
http://www.patient.co.uk/showdoc/40001223/

REFERENCES

1. Ostrow JD, ed. Bile pigments and jaundice: molecular, metabolic and medical aspects. New York: Marcel Dekker; 1986.
2. Bosma PJ, Chowdhury JR, Bakker C et al. The genetic basis of the reduced expression of bilirubin UDP-glucuronosyltransferase 1 in Gilbert's syndrome. N Engl J Med 1995; 333:1171–1175.
3. Gong QH, Cho JW, Huang T et al. Thirteen UDP glucuronosyltransferase genes are encoded at the human UGT1 gene complex locus. Pharmacogenetics 2001; 11:357–368.
4. Kadakol A, Ghosh SS, Sappal BS, Sharma G, Chowdhury JR, Chowdhury NR. Genetic lesions of bilirubin uridine-diphosphoglucuronate glucuronosyltransferase (UGT1A1) causing Crigler-Najjar and Gilbert syndromes: correlation of genotype to phenotype. Hum Mutat 2000; 16:297–306.
5. Gentile S, Orzes N, Persico M, Marmo R, Bronzino P, Tiribelli C. Comparison of nicotinic acid- and caloric restriction-induced hyperbilirubinaemia in the diagnosis of Gilbert's syndrome. J Hepatol 1985; 1:537–543.
6. Bosma PJ. Inherited disorders of bilirubin metabolism. J Hepatol 2003; 38:107–117.
7. Burchell B, Soars M, Monaghan G et al. Drug-mediated toxicity caused by genetic deficiency of UDP-glucuronosyltransferases. Toxicol Lett 2000; 112-113:333–340.
8. Crigler JF Jr, Najjar VA. Congenital familial nonhemolytic jaundice with kernicterus. Pediatrics 1952; 10:169–180.
9. Jansen PL. Diagnosis and management of Crigler-Najjar syndrome. Eur J Pediatr 1999; 158 (Suppl 2):S89–S94.
10. Gridelli B, Lucianetti A, Gatti S et al. Orthotopic liver transplantation for Crigler-Najjar type I syndrome. Transplant Proc 1997; 29:440–441.
11. Dubin IN, Johnson FB. Chronic idiopathic jaundice with unidentified pigment in liver cells; a new clinicopathologic entity with a report of 12 cases. Medicine (Baltimore) 1954; 33:155–197.
12. Schiff L, Billing BH, Oikawa Y. Familial nonhemolytic jaundice with conjugated bilirubin in the serum; a case study. N Engl J Med 1959; 260:1315–1318.

Chapter 95

Cirrhosis of the liver

Gennaro D'Amico and Giuseppe Malizia

KEY POINTS
• Cirrhosis is a frequent disease worldwide – the main causes are hepatitis C and B virus infection and alcohol abuse • Prognosis of cirrhosis is dictated by development of portal hypertension-related complications, liver failure and systemic infections • The only curative treatment for decompensated cirrhosis is liver transplantation

NTRODUCTION AND DEFINITION

irrhosis is a 'diffuse process characterized by fibrosis and ıe conversion of normal liver architecture into structurally ɔnormal nodules'.[1] It represents the end stage of chronic liver amage resulting from several different causes and leading to ltered hepatic function and portal hypertension.

PIDEMIOLOGY AND CAUSES

he estimated prevalence of cirrhosis around the world is 100 ?.5–400) per 100 000 subjects.[2] In 2001, 796 000 people died om cirrhosis, according to the 2002 World Health Organiation report. In Europe, a decline in mortality in the first half f the 1980s was related to a decrease in per capita alcohol ɔnsumption.[3] However, younger generations of northern and astern Europe have shown an increased risk of death from rrhosis, possibly owing to use of alcohol at younger age, viral epatitis, and changed dietary habits.[3] In the UK, almost 3000 eaths from cirrhosis or chronic liver disease are reported very year (about 40% due to alcohol-related disease), with a end towards an increase in the mortality rate.

In Italy in 1992 almost 15 000 patients died from cirrhosis ılmost 28 deaths per 100 000 population), with a trend towards decrease in the subsequent years. The most frequent cause was epatitis C virus (HCV) infection (alone 47.7%, associated with ther factors 72.7%), followed by alcohol (alone 8.7%, associated ith other factors 32.9%) and HBV infection (alone 3.4%, ssociated with other factors 13.8%). In the USA in 1998 more ıan 5.5 million prevalent cases of chronic liver disease or cirıosis were estimated, with a rate of 2030 cases per 100 000 opulation. The mortality rate was approximately 25 000 deaths).3 deaths per 100 000) annually. In two sentinel counties in the SA the most common etiology of chronic liver disease was HCV 57%), followed by alcohol (24%), nonalcoholic fatty liver isease (9.1%), and hepatitis B (4.4%).[4] A comprehensive list f etiologic factors of cirrhosis is given in Table 95.1.

TABLE 95.1 MAIN ETIOLOGIC FACTORS IN CIRRHOSIS
• Hepatitis C virus
• Hepatitis B or B/D virus
• Alcohol
• Autoimmune hepatitis
• Metabolic disorders
Hemochromatosis
Wilson's disease
α_1-Antitrypsin deficiency
Nonalcoholic steatohepatitis
Diabetes
Glycogen storage diseases
Abetalipoproteinemia
Porphyria
• Biliary diseases
Primary biliary cirrhosis
Primary sclerosing cholangitis
Intrahepatic or extrahepatic biliary obstruction
• Venous outflow obstruction
Budd-Chiari syndrome
Veno-occlusive disease
Cardiac failure
• Drugs (amiodarone, methotrexate) and toxins
• Intestinal bypass
• Obesity
• Indian childhood cirrhosis
• Cryptogenic cirrhosis

CAUSES AND RISK FACTORS
MAIN CAUSES OF CIRRHOSIS
• In the Western World the most common etiology of cirrhosis by far is infection with hepatitis C virus, followed by alcohol abuse. • Other important factors are hepatitis B infection (decreasing as a result of large-scale vaccination) and nonalcoholic steatohepatitis (probably imcreasing as a result of increasing obesity). • Autoimmune, metabolic, biliary, and genetic disorders account for the largest remaining proportion of cirrhosis. • The relative proportion of patients with 'cryptogenic' cirrhosis is decreasing progressively.

PATHOGENESIS

Cirrhosis is characterized by the progressive accumulation of collagen types I and III in the liver parenchyma, including the space of Disse with the consequent 'collagenization of sinusoids.' This results in the alteration of both the exchange between hepatocytes and plasma and the regulation of intrahepatic resistance to blood flow. In cirrhosis of different etiologies, active fibrogenesis has been related to the increased expression of transforming growth factor-β (TGF-β) and platelet-derived growth factor (PDGF), which stimulate the activation and proliferation of hepatic stellate cells, the main source of extracellular matrix in the fibrotic liver. A significant correlation between growth factor expression, fibrogenesis, and necroinflammatory activity has been also shown. However, active fibrogenesis may be present in conditions with minimal inflammation and marked ductular proliferation (i.e., biliary atresia). A role in fibrogenesis has therefore been proposed for ductular proliferation, associated with periductular fibrosis, neutrophil infiltration, and increased expression of fibrogenic growth factors.[5] (See Chapters 102, 103, 105, and 106 for the pathophysiology of the main complications of cirrhosis.)

PATHOLOGY

The morphologic classification, based on the size of the nodules, identifies three types of cirrhosis:

- **Micronodular** – characterized by nodules mostly less than 3 mm in diameter, surrounded by fibrous tissue, and generally lacking terminal veins and portal tracts. Found mostly in alcoholic cirrhosis, hemochromatosis, and bile duct obstruction.
- **Macronodular** – characterized by nodules of variable size, from more than 3 mm to a few centimeters, so that it may be difficult to recognize the nodular structure. In this type, nodules contain both portal tracts and terminal veins. Common in chronic viral hepatitis and autoimmune hepatitis.
- **Mixed** – composed of both micronodules and macronodules.

The morphologic classification has a limited diagnostic value because macronodular forms may represent the late evolution of micronodular forms.

Histologically, cirrhosis is characterized by nodular regeneration, scarring with formation of diffuse fibrous septa, and a variable degree of parenchymal necrosis.

CLINICAL PRESENTATION

Clinically, cirrhosis can be divided in compensated and decompensated stages, each with different diagnostic, therapeutic, and prognostic implications.

Compensated cirrhosis

Cirrhosis may be totally asymptomatic and diagnosed fortuitously during routine biochemical testing or clinical or ultrasonographic abdominal examination. It may also become evident during abdominal surgery or at autopsy (in older reports accounting for 30–40% of all cases). Nonspecific asthenia, malaise, right upper quadrant abdominal discomfort, or sleep disturbances may be the only complaints.

Physical examination (Table 95.2): Spider angiomas may be found, mostly on the trunk, face, and upper limbs (Fig. 95.1) (see also Chapter 19). Their number and size correlate with disease severity. Palmar erythema (Fig. 95.2), involving the thenar and hypothenar eminences, is the expression of a dense network of arteriovenous anastomoses. White nails may also appear (Fig. 95.3). Common in male patients is hair loss on the chest and abdomen. Gynecomastia and loss of libido may also occur. Petechiae and ecchymoses may be present as a result of thrombocytopenia

CLINICAL PRESENTATION

COMPENSATED CIRRHOSIS

- Asthenia, malaise, right upper quadrant abdominal discomfort, or sleep disturbances may be the only complaints.
- Physical signs secondary to alterations of estrogen metabolism – palmar erythema and spider angiomata – are common.
- Hepatomegaly is very common, although liver size can be normal or reduced. However, liver consistency is invariably increased.
- Splenomegaly and collateral circulation on the abdominal wall may be present as a consequence of portal hypertension.

DECOMPENSATED CIRRHOSIS

- Ascites, gastrointestinal hemorrhage, jaundice, and portosystemic encephalopathy (flapping tremor, bradylalia, and mental state alterations) are the main signs of decompensation.
- Malnutrition and muscle wasting may be present, particularly in alcoholic cirrhosis.
- Hypotension and tachycardia due to hyperdynamic circulation secondary to portal hypertension may also occur.

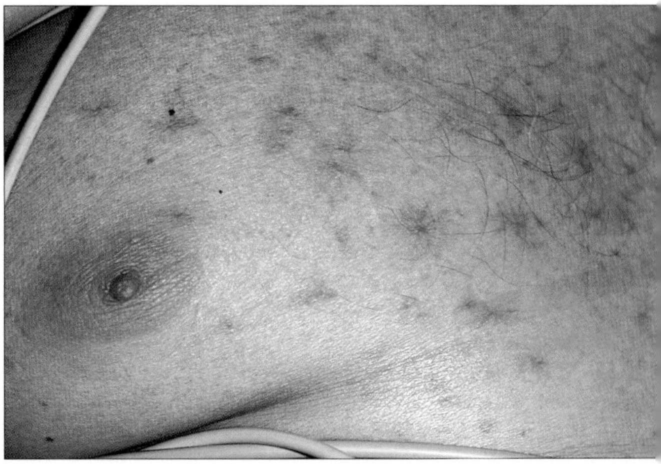

Fig. 95.1 Spider nevi seen on upper truncal region.

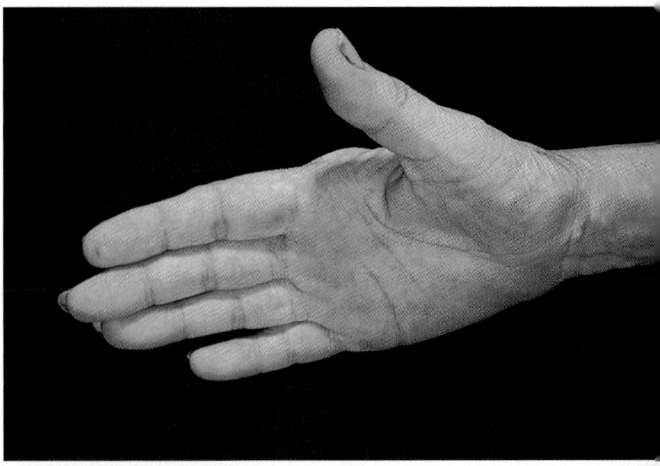

Fig. 95.2 Palmar erythema.

TABLE 95.2 DIAGNOSIS OF CIRRHOSIS

CLINICAL FINDINGS
- Asthenia
- Malaise
- Right upper quadrant abdominal discomfort
- Loss of libido
- Sleep disturbances
- Palmar erythema
- Dupuytren's contracture
- Spider nevi
- White nails
- Gynecomastia
- Hair loss (chest and abdomen)
- Hepatomegaly
- Splenomegaly
- Abdominal wall collaterals
- General deterioration, muscle wasting
- Jaundice
- Ascites
- Ankle edema
- Flapping tremor
- Bradylalia
- Mental state alteration (coma)
- Fetor hepaticus
- Gastrointestinal hemorrhage (hematemesis, melena)
- Hypotension, tachycardia
- Dyspnea, cyanosis

LABORATORY FINDINGS
- AST:ALT ratio >1
- Low platelet count
- Hypoalbuminemia
- Hypergammaglobulinemia
- Prolonged prothrombin time
- Hyperbilirubinemia

ULTRASONOGRAPHIC FINDINGS
- Liver nodular surface
- Reduced portal flow velocity
- Portal vein diameter >13 mm
- Lack (or reduction <30%) of respiratory variations of splenic and superior mesenteric veins

ENDOSCOPIC FINDINGS
- Esophageal varices
- Gastric varices
- Congestive gastropathy

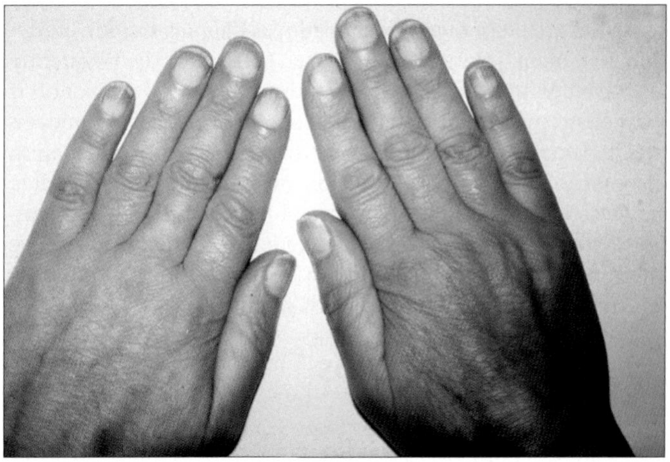

Fig. 95.3 Leukonychia (white nails) occur in cirrhosis but also in other situations.

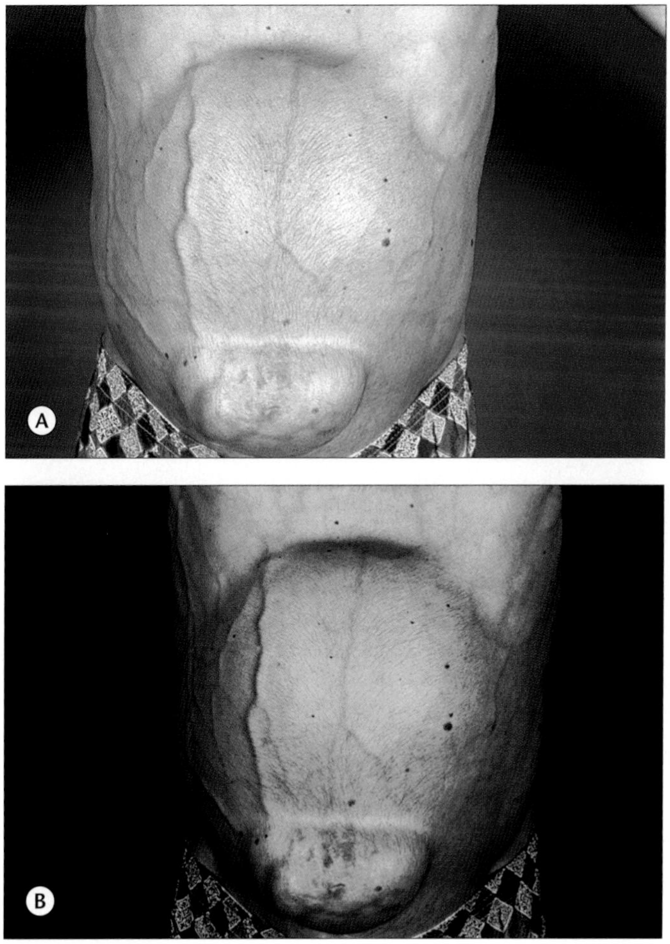

Fig. 95.4 Prominent abdominal veins (and a paraumbilical hernia) in a patient with cirrhosis and ascites. A. Under normal light. **B.** Under infra-red light. Blood flow is away from the umbilicus.

nd/or prolonged prothrombin time. Dupuytren's contracture, volving the palmar fascia, is particularly common in alcoholic atients. Hepatomegaly is very common, but liver size may also e normal or reduced. However, the consistency of the liver is variably harder than normal. Splenomegaly is frequent and dicates the presence of portal hypertension. Collateral circulation on the abdominal wall may develop as a consequence of ortal hypertension (Fig. 95.4).

ecompensated cirrhosis

gns of decompensation – ascites, variceal hemorrhage, jaundice, and/or portosystemic encephalopathy – are found at esentation in a proportion of patients, varying between 20% d 63%. Ascites is by far the most frequent sign of decompensation, being present in 80% of patients with decompensated cirrhosis (see Chapters 19 and 103).

Physical examination (Table 95.2): Patients with advanced cirrhosis often present with malnutrition and muscle wasting, particularly in alcoholic cirrhosis. In decompensated cirrhosis, jaundice and/or ascites may appear as manifestations of liver dysfunction and portal hypertension. Other signs of decompensation are those of encephalopathy, as flapping tremor, bradylalia, and mental state alterations (see Chapter 101). Frequently associated with encephalopathy and severe liver dysfunction is a sweetish smell of the breath, called fetor hepaticus. Moreover, hypotension and tachycardia due to hyperdynamic circulation secondary to portal hypertension may be present. Dyspnea may also occur due to the presence of large ascites, pleural effusions, and/or alterations of the pulmonary circulation (hepatopulmonary syndrome, pulmonary hypertension, pulmonary arteriovenous anastomoses) (see Chapter 99).

DIAGNOSTIC METHODS

In clinical practice, liver biopsy (see Chapter 134) still remains the gold standard for assessing liver fibrosis and cirrhosis, despite the limitations of sampling error and interobserver variability. However, even though 'definitive' tests such as histologic diagnosis are important for patients and for the quantitative evaluation of treatment outcomes in clinical studies, noninvasive tests to estimate disease probability are necessary. The accuracy of these probabilistic tests is strictly dependent on disease spectrum and patient selection.

Compensated cirrhosis

The clinical history is helpful, particularly in determining the cause of cirrhosis. Exposure to viral hepatitis, workplace hazards, a history of transfusions or surgery, drug addiction, alcohol abuse, and a family history of cirrhosis may change the pre-test probability of the disease and suggest a cause.

The presence of a firm liver has been shown to be the most accurate sign of cirrhosis, with a diagnostic accuracy of 83%, followed by the presence of collateral circulation (accuracy 76%).[6]

DIAGNOSTIC METHODS

DIAGNOSTIC APPROACH TO CIRRHOSIS: KEY POINTS

- Liver biopsy is the gold standard for the diagnosis of cirrhosis, but potential limitations are sample variation, observer variability, and complications for the patient.
- Compensated cirrhosis can be diagnosed with an accuracy of about 90% by a combination of clinical (firm liver, other), biochemical (AST:ALT ratio >1, platelet count below 140×10^9/L, prolonged prothrombin time, other), ultrasonographic (liver nodular surface, reduced portal flow velocity, portal vein diameter >13 mm, and lack or reduction to less than 30% of respiratory variations of splenic and superior mesenteric veins) and endoscopic (esophageal and/or gastric varices, congestive gastropathy) findings.
- When a precise definition of stage of fibrosis or grading of inflammation is required, liver biopsy is needed.
- The detection of signs of decompensation, such as ascites, variceal bleeding, and encephalopathy, in patients with virologic, serologic, and biochemical markers of liver disease rules in the diagnosis of cirrhosis.

Routine laboratory tests: A value ≥1 for the ratio of aspartate aminotransferase to alanine aminotransferase (AST/ALT ratio, or AAR) has been proposed as a simple low-cost predictor of cirrhosis in viral cirrhosis.[7] A reduced platelet count (≤150 to ≤130×10^9/L) can also indicate the presence of cirrhosis. In several studies a prolonged prothrombin time also correlated with the presence of cirrhosis. Recently, serum hyaluronate measurement has been shown to have an accuracy of about 90%, being particularly useful for excluding the presence of cirrhosis. Further noninvasive indices based only on a combination of laboratory test results have been proposed for the prediction of cirrhosis, but there is still a need for external validation.[8]

Ultrasonography is a useful tool for diagnosis as it may detect nodularity of the liver surface, portal hypertension, splenomegaly, and ascites. The sensitivity of ultrasonography in detecting portal hypertension has been shown to be 80%, with a specificity of 100% when assessing the lack (or reduction to less than 30%) of respiratory variations of splenic and superior mesenteric veins.[9] More recently, ultrasonographic detection of liver nodular surface and reduction of mean portal velocity showed 79% sensitivity and 80% specificity.[10]

Upper digestive endoscopy has a definite role in the diagnostic work-up as it may identify the presence of esophageal or gastric varices and congestive gastropathy. In compensated patients, the presence of esophageal varices has a sensitivity of 40% and a specificity of 99%.[11]

In a series of 277 patients with abnormal liver function selected prospectively for liver biopsy, the presence of a firm liver was found to be an independent predictor of cirrhosis, together with a platelet count ≤140×10^9/L and portal vein diameter ≥13 mm at ultrasonography in the absence of respiratory variations of splenic or mesenteric veins.[11]

In conclusion, a combination of clinical, biochemical, ultrasonographic, and endoscopic data can establish the diagnosis of cirrhosis without liver biopsy with an accuracy of about 90% (Table 95.3). However, when a precise determination of stage of fibrosis and degree of inflammation is required, liver biopsy is necessary (see Chapter 134).

Decompensated cirrhosis

The detection of signs of decompensation, such as ascites, variceal bleeding, and encephalopathy, in patients with virologic, serologic, and biochemical markers of liver disease basically rule in the diagnosis of cirrhosis. Abdominal ultrasonography and upper digestive endoscopy are required to evaluate the need for prophylaxis of variceal hemorrhage (see Chapter 101) and to exclude the presence of hepatocellular carcinoma (see Chapter 102), respectively.

TREATMENT AND PREVENTION

For the treatment of clinical manifestations and complication of decompensated cirrhosis, see Chapters 96–103, 106, and 107

The treatment of compensated cirrhosis is essentially base on careful avoidance of alcohol and hepatotoxic drugs, an on the early detection of initial signs of decompensation. A adequate nutritional regimen should include 1.0–1.2 g protei per kg bodyweight.

Theoretically the treatment of cirrhosis, particularly in th compensated phase of the disease, should be aimed at th interruption of fibrogenesis and the resorption of fibrosis. How ever, so far no drugs have been approved as antifibrotic agen in humans and the most effective way to eliminate or reduc hepatic fibrosis is to treat the underlying liver disease. A redu tion in fibrosis has been reported in some patients with chron infection with HCV treated with interferon-α and ribaviri

TABLE 95.3 OPERATING CHARACTERISTICS OF SIGNS AND TESTS IN THE DIAGNOSIS OF CIRRHOSIS

;ign/Test	Sensitivity %	Specificity %	LR+	LR–
'irm liver	89	47	1.67	0.23
'latelet count <140.000/mmc	59	85	4.0	0.48
ST/ALT ratio>1*	53 (44–78)	96 (90–100)	11.7 (7.3–53)	0.48 (0.25–0.59)
Jltrasonography:				
Lack (or reduction to <30%) of respiratory variations of splenic and mesenteric veins	80	100	∞	0.20
Liver nodular surface/reduced portal flow velocity	79	80	3.9	0.26
ndoscopy: esophageal varices	40	99	40	0.60
iver biopsy	80	100	∞	0.20

R+, likelihood ratio for a positive result; LR–, likelihood ratio of a negative result.
Median (range) from seven studies.

/hether this effect may be reproduced also in cirrhotic patients under investigation.

No treatment has yet been shown to be effective in prevent-g the development or progression of esophageal varices.

OMPLICATIONS AND THEIR MANAGEMENT

ariceal bleeding, ascites, encephalopathy, and jaundice are the ajor clinical manifestations of liver cirrhosis. The appearance these complications marks the transition from the *compen-ted* phase to the *decompensated* phase of cirrhosis.

leeding from esophageal varices

ne incidence of variceal bleeding is approximately 2% per ar in patients without varices at diagnosis, 5% in those with nall varices, and 15% in those with medium or large varices. Independent of variceal size, major indicators of the risk of eeding are Child-Pugh class, ascites, and red wheal marks ewly formed vessels on the variceal wall). These risk indica-rs have been combined in the North Italian Endoscopic Club IEC) index[12] which, identifying patients with a predicted year bleeding risk ranging from 6% to 76%, is the best avail-le system for predicting the first variceal bleeding, although accuracy is far from satisfactory.

Portal pressure: Esophageal varices do not bleed below a reshold portal pressure level (as determined by the hepatic nous pressure gradient; HVPG) of 12 mmHg;[13,14] this risk is gnificantly reduced if the HVPG is reduced by 20% or more om baseline.[15] Variceal pressure is significantly related to riceal size, red signs, and severity of liver dysfunction, as ell as with the risk of bleeding and death.[16] The relationship tween variceal pressure and the risk of bleeding is mediated rough the variceal wall tension, which is inversely related to e wall thickness.

Ruptured esophageal varices cause 60–70% of all upper strointestinal bleeding episodes in cirrhosis[17] (Fig. 95.5). ariceal bleeding is diagnosed on endoscopy, either by blood urting from a varix or white nipple or clot adherent on a varix, by varices without other potential sources of bleeding. ebleeding is distinguished from the initial bleeding episode a bleed-free period of at least 24 h. Variceal bleeding ceases ontaneously in 40–50% of patients, and treatment achieves ntrol of bleeding within 24 h from admission in nearly 75%.[17] Active bleeding on endoscopy, bacterial infection, and HVPG >20 mmHg are predictors of failure to control bleeding. The immediate mortality rate from uncontrolled bleeding is approximately 5%, and 6-week rebleeding occurs in 20%. Active bleeding at emergency endoscopy, gastric varices, low albumin level, high blood urea nitrogen level, and HVPG above 20 mmHg have been reported as predictive of early rebleeding risk.

Prognosis: The 6-week mortality rate after variceal bleeding is 20%, with nearly half of the deaths caused by bleeding or early rebleeding and a quarter occurring in the first 5 days. Albumin, bilirubin, creatinine, encephalopathy, hepatocellular carcinoma, the number of blood units transfused, bacterial infection, and HVPG above 20 mmHg are predictors of 6-week mortality.

After a first episode of variceal bleeding there is a 63% rebleeding risk and 33% risk of death within 1 year. Reduction of HVPG to less than 12 mmHg totally prevents recurrent bleeding.[14,15]

Development of ascites and encephalopathy

Ascites develops after HVPG has increased to more than 12 mmHg, when the associated vasodilatation causes under-

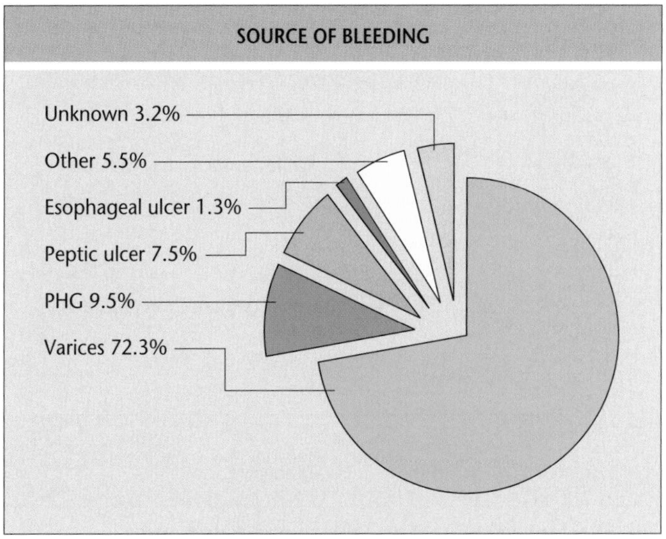

Fig. 95.5 Sources of bleeding. Source of bleeding in a series of 465 consecutive patients with cirrhosis.[20] PHG, portal hypertensive gastropathy.

filling of the vascular capacity, fall in the glomerular filtration rate, and renal sodium retention. At diagnosis, the prevalence of ascites ranges from 20% to 60%, according to referral pattern.[18,19] The incidence of ascites is about 5% per year and, together with variceal bleeding, is the most frequent mode of transition from compensated to decompensated cirrhosis.

Less frequent is the development of encephalopathy, with an incidence of approximately 2–3% per year.[18,19] The incidence of encephalopathy in the absence of ascites or previous bleeding is, however, even lower. Jaundice follows the same pattern as encephalopathy, with a low incidence in the range of 2–3% per year, and almost always occurs in patients with other severe manifestations of advanced cirrhosis. Therefore, the most important indicators of decompensated cirrhosis are variceal bleeding and ascites, whereas encephalopathy and jaundice indicate a very advanced stage of the disease.

PROGNOSIS

The outcome of cirrhosis is determined by three major factors: (1) survival time within the compensated phase; (2) the intensity of transition from the compensated to the decompensated phase; and (3) survival while in the decompensated phase.

Compensated cirrhosis

The natural history of compensated cirrhosis is still poorly defined, because patients are almost invariably free of symptoms and the diagnosis is usually prompted by a casual discovery of abnormal liver function. Patients with compensated cirrhosis die after transitioning into decompensation. The 10-year survival rate for compensated patients is nearly 90%, while the median survival after decompensation is about 2 years (Fig. 95.6). The progression to decompensation parallels the development and progression of portal hypertension. The 10-year transition rate to decompensation is 50% (Fig. 95.7).

In patients with compensated cirrhosis the development and enlargement of esophageal varices mark the progression of the disease towards a more advanced stage.

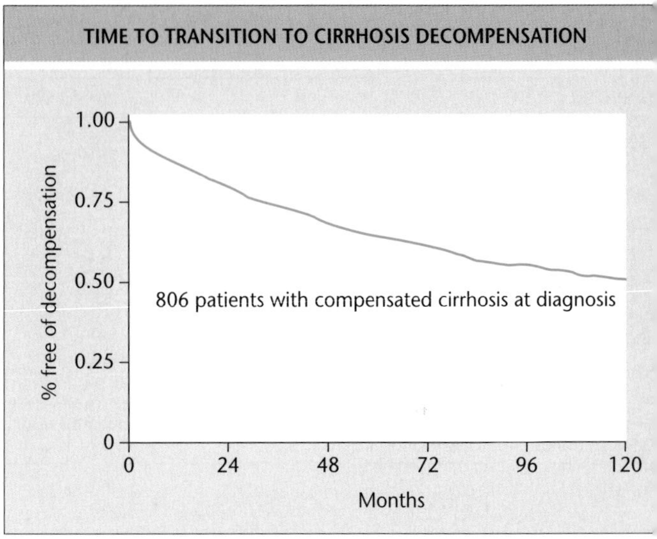

Fig. 95.7 Time to transition to cirrhosis decompensation. Transition to cirrhosis decompensation (variceal bleeding, ascites, encephalopathy, jaundice) in a cohort of 806 patients with compensated cirrhosis at diagnosis.

When cirrhosis is diagnosed, the prevalence of varices rang from 20% in compensated patients to 60% in those presentin with ascites. Two recent large cohort studies showed that th incidence of esophageal varices in patients with newly diag nosed cirrhosis is nearly 5% per year (Fig. 95.8).

Varices do not develop below a threshold HVPG 10–12 mmHg.[13] Above this threshold, the median time to th development of varices and/or bleeding or other complicatio of portal hypertension is about 4 years. Worsening liver functio and continued exposure to alcohol are associated with an increa of HVPG and an increasing risk of developing varices.[20]

Once varices have developed, they increase in size fro small to large before they eventually rupture and bleed. Lar prospective studies show a median progression probabili from small to large varices of 0.07 per year. Improvement

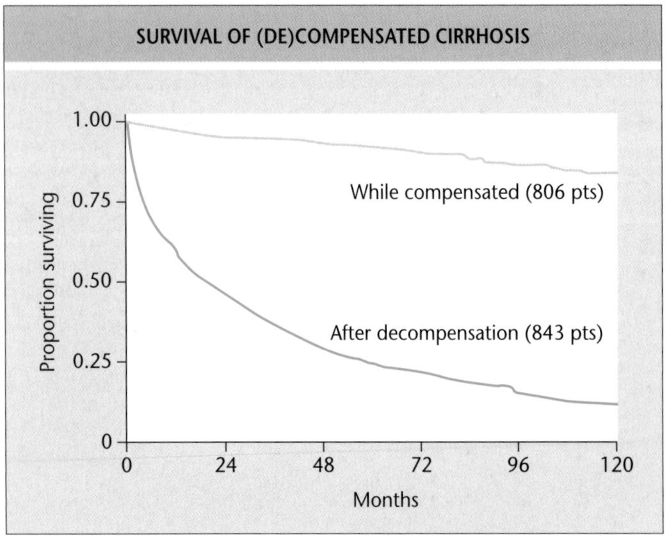

Fig. 95.6 Survival of patients with compensated and decompensated cirrhosis. Data from two large prospective studies of the natural history of cirrhosis. Survival time of compensated patients was censored when they developed decompensation.

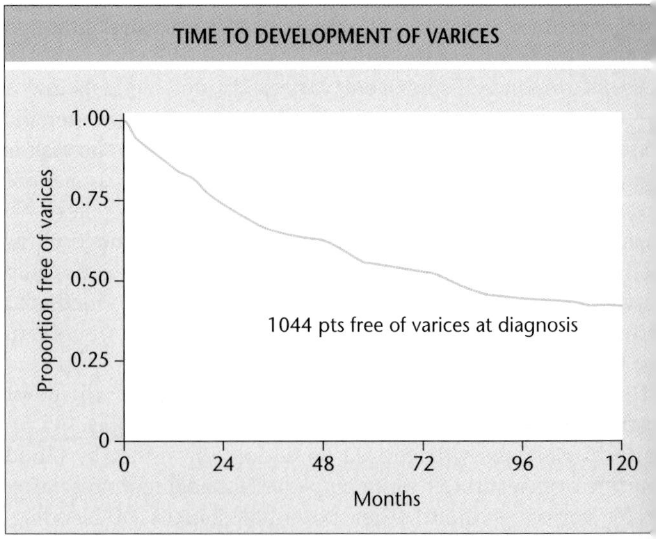

Fig. 95.8 Time to development of varices. Data for a series of 104 patients free of varices at diagnosis from two large prospective studi on the natural history of cirrhosis.

er function and abstinence from alcohol may result in a crease or even disappearance of varices,[20] probably through lecrease in HVPG, as occurs for spontaneous or treatment-luced HVPG reductions.[14] Thus, HVPG plays a key role in th the development and the progression of varices.

ncreasing size of esophageal varices is associated with increas- ; bleeding risk (4-fold from absent to small varices, and old from small to large varices). A similar increase in risk s been shown for the development of ascites and mortality. n clinical practice, the size of varices is the most widely ed indicator of risk of first variceal bleeding, because this k is significantly reduced by prophylactic therapy in patients th medium to large varices. As noninvasive tests (particu-ly platelet count and abdominal ultrasonography) have not en proven accurate enough to avoid endoscopy in patients io are negative for the test, all patients with cirrhosis should endoscopically screened for the presence of esophageal rices at the diagnosis of cirrhosis.[15] Endoscopy should be peated every 2–3 years in patients without varices. In patients th compensated cirrhosis and small varices, endoscopy should repeated every 1–2 years to detect the progression from small large varices.[15] In decompensated patients without varices with small varices, endoscopy should be repeated yearly.

ırvival of decompensated cirrhosis

e median survival after first variceal hemorrhage is about ear (2 years if time zero is day 30 after the onset of bleed-;), and after the development of ascites it is 2 years.[18,19] icephalopathy and jaundice usually appear after bleeding ascites, and the median survival after the first episode of cephalopathy or after the appearance of jaundice is there-e shorter than that for bleeding or ascites. The most frequent uses of death are bleeding, liver failure with hepatic coma, psis, and hepatorenal syndrome.

utcome of cirrhosis as related to clinical stage

combining individual patient data from two large prospec-e studies of the natural history of cirrhosis,[18,19] four stages the progression of the disease can be identified (Fig. 95.9):

- *age 0* – absence of esophageal varices and ascites. Mortality rate is as low as 1% per year. Patients exit this stage when they develop varices (7% per year) and/or ascites (4.4% per year).
- *age 1* – varices without ascites and without bleeding. Mortality rate is 3.4% per year, significantly higher than at stage 0. Patients leave this stage when they develop ascites (6.6% per year) and/or bleeding (4% per year).
- *age 2* – ascites with or without esophageal varices that have not bled. Mortality rate at this stage is 20% per year, significantly higher than in the two former stages. Besides death, patients leave this stage by developing bleeding at a rate of 7.6% per year.
- *age 3* – variceal bleeding with or without ascites. Mortality rate is 57% per year (about half of these deaths occur within 6 weeks of the bleeding episode).

rognostic scores

ie Child-Pugh score[21] is the most widely used system (see iapter 150). Although it was empirically set without any statis-al basis, it is highly reliable in identifying prognostically ferent subgroups of patients (classes A, B, and C) in particular clinical situations occurring in the course of cirrhosis. For this reason, it has been widely used to stratify patients included in clinical trials for cirrhosis, particularly in portal hypertension, and has been, until recently, included among the most important criteria used by the United Network for Organ Sharing (UNOS) for liver allocation. The UNOS has now replaced the

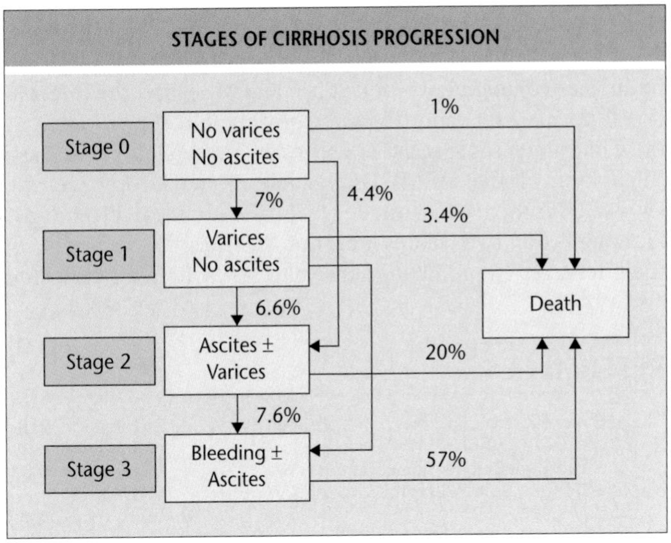

Fig. 95.9 Stages in the progression of cirrhosis. Different stages of progression of cirrhosis according to the development of esophageal varices, ascites, and bleeding. Transition rates from one stage to the next are drawn from the cumulative analysis of two prospective studies on the natural history of cirrhosis.

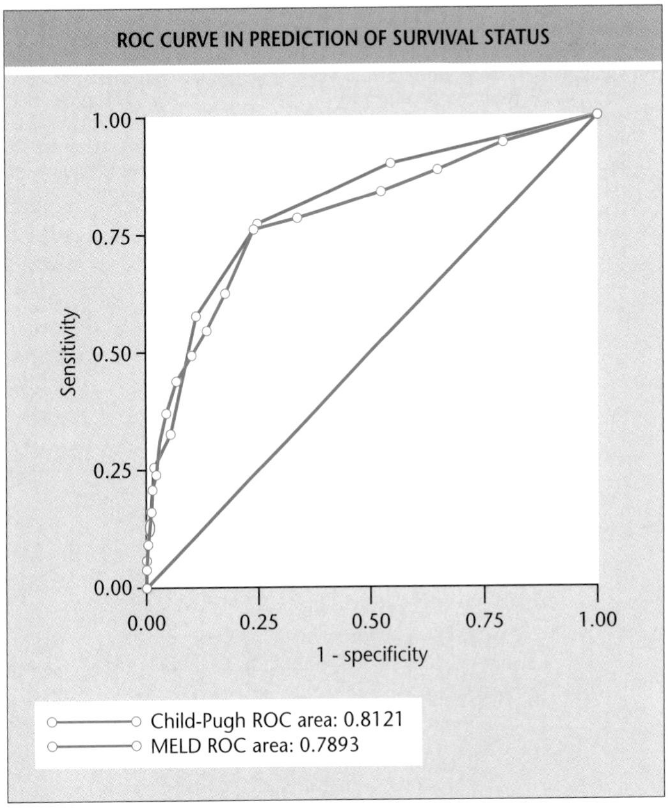

Fig. 95.10 Receiver–operator characteristic (ROC) curves in prediction of survival status. ROC curves for Child-Pugh score and MELD in the prediction of 6-month survival status in a cohort of 494 cirrhotic patients.

Child-Pugh score with the Model for End-stage Liver Disease (MELD);[22] MELD is based on objective variables not affected by subjective judgment – bilirubin, creatinine, and the international normalized ratio (INR) for prothombin time – whereas the Child-Pugh score includes ascites and encephalopathy. Easy calculation of the MELD is available at the UNOS website (www.UNOS.org/resources/meldPeldCalculator.asp). Although the two scores are not significantly different in their accuracy in predicting survival (Fig. 95.10), it is expected that the interobserver agreement for classifying cirrh patients in prognostically different subgroups will be hig with MELD.

SOURCES OF INFORMATION FOR PATIENTS AND DOCTORS

http://www.gastro.org/clinicalRes/brochures/cirrhosis.html

REFERENCES

1. Anthony PP, Ishak KG, Nayak NC, Poulsen HE, Scheuer PJ, Sobin LH. The morphology of cirrhosis: definition, nomenclature and classification. Bull Wld Health Organ 1977; 55:521–540.
2. La Vecchia C, Levi F, Lucchini F Franceschi S, Negri E. Worldwide patterns and trends in mortality from liver cirrhosis, 1955 to 1990. Ann Epidemiol 1994; 4:480–486.
3. Corrao G, Ferrari P, Zambon A, Torchio P, Aricò S, Decarli A. Trends of liver cirrhosis mortality in Europe, 1970–1989: age–period–cohort analysis and changing alcohol consumption. Int J Epidemiol 1997; 26:100–109.
4. Kim WR, Brown RS, Terrault NA, El-Serag H. Burden of liver disease in the United States: summary of a workshop. Hepatology 2002; 36:227–242.
5. Malizia G, Brunt EM, Peters MG, Rizzo A, Broekelmann TJ, McDonald JA. Growth factor and procollagen type I gene expression in human liver disease. Gastroenterology 1995; 108:145–156.
6. Oberti F, Valsesia E, Pilette C et al. Noninvasive diagnosis of hepatic fibrosis or cirrhosis. Gastroenterology 1997; 113:1609–1616.
7. Giannini E, Risso D, Botta F et al. Validity and clinical utility of the aspartate aminotransferase–alanino aminotransferase ratio in assessing disease severity and prognosis in patients with hepatitis C virus-related chronic liver disease. Arch Intern Med 2003; 163:218–224.
8. Imbert-Bismut F, Ratziu V, Pieroni L, Charlotte F, Benhamou Y, Poynard T. Biochemical markers of liver fibrosis in patients with hepatitis C virus infection: a prospective study. Lancet 2001; 357: 1069–1075.
9. Bolondi L, Gandolfi L, Arienti V, Caletti GC, Corcioni E, Gasbarrini G. Ultrasonography in the diagnosis of portal hypertension: diminished response of portal vessels to respiration. Radiology 1982; 142:167–172.
10. Gaiani S, Gramantieri L, Venturoli N et al. What is the criterion for differentiating chronic hepatitis from compensated cirrhosis? A prospective study comparing ultrasonography and percutaneous liver biopsy. J Hepatol 1997; 27:979–985.
11. Tinè F, Caltagirone M, Cammà C et al. Clinical indicants of compensated cirrhosis: a prospective study. In: Dianzani MU, Gentilini P, eds. Chronic liver damage. Amsterdam: Elsevier; 1990:187–198.
12. North Italian Endoscopic Club. Prediction of the first variceal hemorrhage in patients with cirrhosis of the liver and esophageal varices. A prospective multicenter study. N Engl J Med 1988; 319:983–989.
13. Garcia-Tsao G, Groszmann RJ, Fisher RL, Conn HO, Atterbury CE, Glickman M. Portal pressure, presence of gastroesophageal varices and variceal bleeding. Hepatology 1985; 5:419–424.
14. Groszmann RJ, Bosch J, Grace N et al. Hemodynamic events in a prospective randomized trial of propranolol vs placebo in the prevention of the first variceal hemorrhage. Gastroenterology 1990; 99: 1401–1407.
15. Bosch J, Abraldes JC, Groszmann R. Curr management of portal hypertension. J Hep 2003; 38:S54–S68.
16. Rigau J, Bosch J, Bordas JM et al. Endosc measurement of variceal pressure in cirrho correlation with portal pressure and varic hemorrhage. Gastroenterology 1989; 96: 873–880.
17. D'Amico G, De Franchis R. Upper digesti bleeding in cirrhosis. Post-therapeutic outc and prognostic indicators. Hepatology 20 38:599–612.
18. D'Amico G, Morabito A, Pagliaro L, Maru E. Survival and prognostic indicators in compensated and decompensated cirrhosis Dig Dis Sci 1986; 31:468–475.
19. Pagliaro L, D'Amico G, Pasta L et al. Port hypertension in cirrhosis: natural history. In: Bosch J, Groszmann R, eds. Portal hypertension: pathophysiology and treatm Cambridge, MA: Blackwell Scientific; 199 72–92.
20. Vorobioff J, Groszmann RJ, Picabea E et a Prognostic value of hepatic venous pressu gradient measurements in alcoholic cirrho a 10-year prospective study. Gastroenterol 1996; 111:701–709.
21. Pugh RN, Murray-Lyon IM, Dawson JL, Pietroni MC, Williams R. Transection of th esophagus for bleeding oesophageal varic Br J Surg 1973; 60:646–649.
22. Kamath PS, Wiesner RH, Malinchoc M et a A model to predict survival in patients wi end-stage liver disease. Hepatology 2001; 33:464–470.

Chapter 96

Portal hypertension

Juan Carlos García-Pagán, Roberto J Groszmann, and Jaime Bosch

KEY POINTS

- Portal hypertension is defined by an increase in the portal pressure gradient (PPG: the difference between portal and inferior vena cava pressure); portal hypertension becomes clinically significant when the PPG is >10 mmHg (normal <5 mmHg)
- PPG is determined by the product of blood flow and vascular resistance within the portal venous system; portal hypertension is initiated by an increased resistance to portal blood flow and aggravated by an increased portal venous inflow
- The site of increased resistance to portal blood flow is the basis for the classification of portal hypertension: prehepatic (e.g., portal vein thrombosis), intrahepatic (e.g., cirrhosis), and posthepatic (e.g., hepatic vein thrombosis, heart disease)
- PPG is most commonly assessed clinically by measuring the hepatic venous pressure gradient (or HVPG, the difference between wedged and free hepatic vein pressures) at hepatic vein catheterization; HVPG accurately reflects portal pressure both in alcoholic and viral cirrhosis, but not in prehepatic portal hypertension (see Chapter 133)
- Bleeding from ruptured esophageal or gastric varices is the main complication of portal hypertension, and a major cause of death and of liver transplantation in patients with cirrhosis
- The risk of bleeding increases with increasing pressure and size of the varices and decreased thickness of the variceal wall (reflected by the presence of red color signs)
- Patients with large varices (5 mm diameter) who have never bled should be treated to prevent first bleeding; continued drug therapy with propranolol or nadolol is highly effective; in patients with contraindications to beta-blockers, endoscopic band ligation may be considered
- In acute variceal hemorrhage, vasoactive drug therapy (mainly terlipressin or somatostatin since evidence for octreotide is weak) has been shown to be as effective and safer than emergency endoscopic therapy; the combination of early vasoactive drug administration plus endoscopic treatment increases the efficacy of either treatment alone and is the recommended approach
- Failures of medical treatment to control bleeding should be managed aggressively by using emergency TIPS or shunt surgery
- Patients surviving an episode of variceal bleeding are at a high risk of rebleeding; medical therapies, using beta-blockers +/– nitrates or endoscopic band ligation, are the recommended first-line treatments; failures of medical therapy may be treated by associating drug therapy and endoscopic treatment, or by means of TIPS or surgical portal-systemic shunts; liver transplantation should be considered for patients with a Child-Pugh score over 9 points

INTRODUCTION

Portal hypertension is a frequent clinical syndrome, defined as a pathological increase in the portal venous pressure. The pressure gradient between the portal vein and the inferior vena cava (portal perfusion pressure of the liver or portal pressure gradient) increases above normal levels (1–5 mmHg.) When the portal pressure gradient rises above 10–12 mmHg, complications of portal hypertension can arise and this level is defined as clinically significant portal hypertension.

CAUSES AND CLASSIFICATION

Portal hypertension can be caused by any disease interfering with blood flow at any level within the portal venous system. According to its anatomical location, the diseases causing portal hypertension are classified as prehepatic (diseases involving the splenic, mesenteric, or portal veins), intrahepatic (acute and chronic liver diseases), or posthepatic (diseases interfering with the venous outflow of the liver) (Table 96.1).[1] Cirrhosis of the liver is by far the most common cause of portal hypertension in the world, followed by hepatic schistosomiasis. All other causes account for less than 10% of the cases, which explains why these are sometimes referred to as 'noncirrhotic portal hypertension.'

PATHOPHYSIOLOGY

The portal pressure gradient is the result of the interaction between portal blood flow and the vascular resistance that opposes that flow. This relationship is defined by Ohm's law in the equation:

$$\Delta P = Q \times R$$

in which ΔP is the portal pressure gradient (PPG), Q is blood flow within the entire portal venous system (which in portal hypertension also includes portal-systemic collaterals), and R is the vascular resistance of the entire portal venous system. It follows that portal pressure may increase because of an increase in portal blood flow, an increase in resistance, or a combination of both (Fig. 96.1).[1]

Increased resistance to portal blood flow is the primary factor in the etiology of portal hypertension and may occur at any site within the portal venous system. In cirrhosis, increased intrahepatic resistance is the consequence of anatomical and functional alterations. The first is due to the distortion of the liver vascular architecture caused by fibrosis, scarring, and nodule formation. Also, pathological analyses suggest that thrombosis of medium and small portal and hepatic veins contributes to the anatomical increase in resistance.[2] Functional increase in resistance is due to active contraction of different liver cell types, in response to several agonists. These cells include

TABLE 96.1 PORTAL HYPERTENSION: ETIOLOGY

PREHEPATIC
- Splenic vein thrombosis
- Portal vein thrombosis
- Congenital stenosis of the portal vein
- Extrinsic compression of the portal vein
- Arteriovenous fistulae (splenic, aortomesenteric, aortoportal, and hepatic artery–portal vein)[a]

INTRAHEPATIC
- Partial nodular transformation
- Nodular regenerative hyperplasia
- Congenital hepatic fibrosis
- Peliosis hepatis
- Polycystic disease
- Idiopathic portal hypertension
- Hypervitaminosis A
- Arsenic, copper sulfate, and vinyl chloride monomer poisoning
- Sarcoidosis
- Tuberculosis
- Primary biliary cirrhosis
- Schistosomiasis
- Amyloidosis
- Mastocytosis
- Rendu-Osler disease
- Liver infiltration in hematologic diseases
- Acute fatty liver of pregnancy
- Severe acute viral hepatitis
- Chronic active hepatitis
- Hepatocellular carcinoma
- Hemochromatosis
- Wilson's disease
- Hepatic porphyrias
- Alpha-1 antitrypsin deficiency
- Cyanamid toxicity
- Chronic biliary obstruction
- Cirrhosis due to hepatitis B and C virus infection
- Alcoholic cirrhosis
- Alcoholic hepatitis
- Veno-occlusive disease

POSTHEPATIC
- Budd-Chiari syndrome
- Congenital malformations and thrombosis of the inferior vena cava
- Constrictive pericarditis
- Tricuspid valve diseases

[a] This is the only instance where portal hypertension is not initiated by an increased resistance to portal blood flow.

vascular smooth muscle cells of the intrahepatic vasculature (i.e., small portal venules in portal tracts), activated hepatic stellate cells (HSCs) (pericyte cells located in the perisinusoidal space of Disse with extensions that wrap around the sinusoids and reduces its caliber after contraction), and the abundant myofibroblasts located in fibrous septa that may compress regenerating nodules and venous channels within fibrous septa.[1] This dynamic, reversible component may represent up to 40% of the increased intrahepatic resistance in cirrhosis. The increased vascular tone is due to an imbalance between an increased production of vasoconstrictors, such as endothelin, norepinephrine (noradrenaline), angiotensin II, vasopressin, leukotrienes, and thromboxane A2 (associated with an exaggerated response of the hepatic vascular bed to vasoconstrictors), and an in ficient release of hepatic vasodilators (nitric oxide and v dilating prostaglandins) (Fig. 96.1).[3,4]

Portal venous inflow: In addition, an increased portal ve inflow is characteristically observed in advanced stages of p hypertension, which results from marked arteriolar vasodila of splanchnic organs draining into the portal vein. This incre blood flow maintains and aggravates the portal hyperten syndrome (Fig. 96.1).[1] Splanchnic vasodilation is likely t multifactorial and involves neurogenic, humoral, and l mediators. Many candidate substances have been propo Among them, the more important are the paracrine vasoac factors produced by the vascular endothelium, such as n oxide, but also prostacyclin and carbon monoxide. Moreo endocannabinoids and glucagon have also been shown to a role in the pathogenesis of the circulatory abnormal associated with portal hypertension (Fig. 96.1).[1]

Vasoactive mediators: It is remarkable that the hemodyna disturbances observed in the mesenteric and the hepatic vasc bed are completely divergent. Indeed, while the mesent vascular bed exhibits vasodilation, hyporesponse to vaso strictors, and increased response to endothelium-depen vasodilators, the liver circulation exhibits vasoconstrict increased response to vasoconstrictors, and decreased resp to endothelium-dependent vasodilators. The vasoactive media involved in these alterations are similar, but work in opp directions. A decreased production of NO in the hepatic vasc bed, contributing to increase hepatic vascular resistance associated with an overproduction of NO in the splanc territory, contributing to increase portal blood flow.[5]

Collaterals: Development of portal-collateral circula (including gastroesophageal varices) is another important c sequence of portal hypertension. Development of collatera triggered by an increased portal pressure, and involves dilation of pre-existing vascular channels connecting the po and systemic circulation, as well as angiogenesis by vasc endothelial growth factor (VEGF) and probably other fact Portal-collateral circulation itself may modulate portal press In advanced cirrhosis, over 90% of portal blood may be shu through collaterals. In these circumstances, collateral resista will markedly influence the overall resistance to portal bl flow and, therefore, portal pressure.

Complications: Variceal hemorrhage is the main complica of portal hypertension. The so-called explosion theory is most accepted hypothesis to explain variceal rupture. This the suggests that the main event leading to bleeding is an exces hydrostatic intravariceal pressure, determined by an increa portal pressure (Fig. 96.2). In support of this hypothesis, m studies have shown that variceal bleeding does not occur if hepatic venous pressure gradient (HVPG) does not reac threshold value of 12 mmHg. The risk of bleeding increase parallel with the size of the varices and presence of red color si

Variceal pressure, variceal size, and wall thickness determ variceal wall tension (the inwardly directed force exerted the variceal wall opposing the expansion due to increa variceal pressure) (Fig. 96.2). Variceal bleeding occurs w the tension exerted by the thin wall of the varices goes bey a critical value determined by the elastic limit of the ves According to Frank's modification of Laplace's law, vari wall tension (WT) can be defined by the equation:

$$WT = (P_i - P_e) \times r/w$$

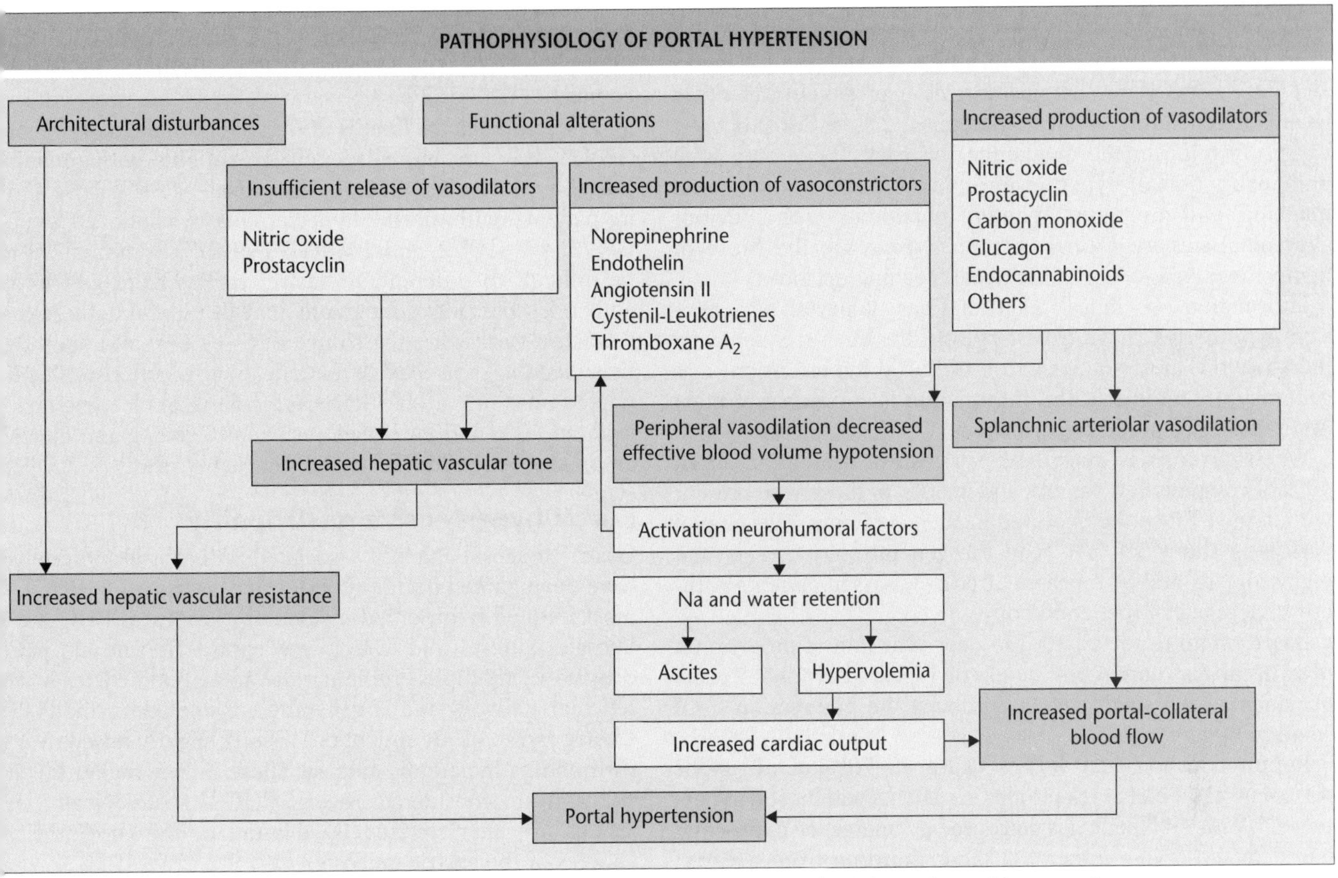

. 96.1 **Pathophysiology of portal hypertension.** Mechanisms involved in the pathophysiology of portal hypertension.

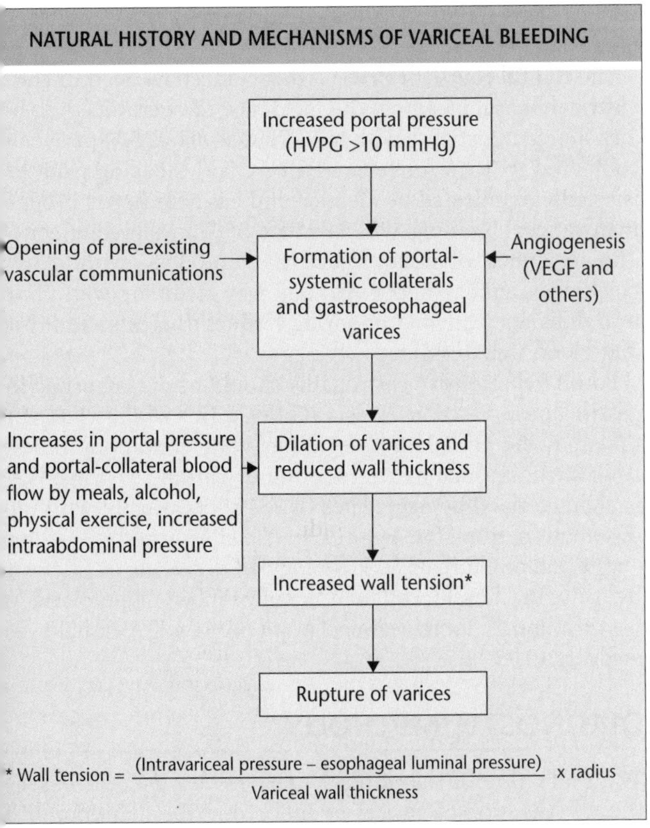

. **96.2 Natural history of gastroesophageal varices and echanisms of bleeding.**

where P_i is the intravariceal pressure, P_e the pressure in the esophageal lumen, r is the radius of the varix, and w the thickness of its wall.

This equation indicates that a large variceal size multiplies the deleterious effects of a high intravariceal pressure increasing the tension exerted on the wall of the varices; a big varix with thin walls will reach a high wall tension (and risk of bleeding) at much lower variceal pressures than a small varix with thick walls. This equation explains the prognostic value of the red color signs (which reflect areas where the wall of the varices is especially thin), of variceal size, and of increased portal pressure.[6]

CLINICAL PRESENTATION AND NATURAL HISTORY

The importance of portal hypertension is defined by the frequency and severity of its complications: massive upper gastrointestinal bleeding from ruptured gastroesophageal varices and portal hypertensive gastropathy, ascites, renal dysfunction, hepatic encephalopathy, arterial hypoxemia, disorders in the metabolism of drugs or endogenous substances that are normally eliminated by the liver, bacteremia, and hypersplenism. This chapter focuses on portal hypertension-related gastrointestinal bleeding.

Gastroesophageal varices

These are the most clinically relevant collaterals, since their rupture is a major cause of death in cirrhosis. Gastroesophageal collaterals and varices develop from connections between the short gastric and coronary veins and the esophageal, azygos, and intercostal veins. Ectopic varices may develop at other locations depending on local anatomical factors. Most ectopic varices develop in the duodenum (primarily associated with prehepatic portal hypertension), in the colon and small intestine, and are more frequent in patients with previous abdominal surgery. Overall, ectopic varices are the cause of hemorrhage in 1–5% of all variceal bleeding episodes.

Information on clinical manifestations of portal hypertension is primarily drawn from cirrhosis, the most frequent and therefore the most studied cause of portal hypertension. It is generally accepted that this information is applicable to most other causes of portal hypertension.

When cirrhosis is diagnosed, varices are present in about 40% of compensated patients and in 60% of those who present with ascites. Since the expected incidence of newly developed varices is about 5% per year, the general consensus is that endoscopy should be repeated after 2–3 years in patients without varices at the first endoscopy.

Based on an expected 10–15% per year rate of progression of variceal size, endoscopy should be repeated every 1–2 years in patients with small varices to detect the progression from small to large varices.

Ruptured esophageal varices cause 60–70% of all upper gastrointestinal bleeding episodes in patients with portal hypertension. Variceal bleeding is diagnosed at emergency endoscopy based on observing either: (1) blood spurting from a varix; (2) white nipple or clot adherent to a varix; and (3) varices without other potential sources of bleeding. Active bleeding at endoscopy, bacterial infection, advanced liver failure,[7] and HVPG >20 mmHg[8] are significant prognostic indicators of failure to control bleeding.

Early rebleeding: The incidence ranges between 30% and 40% in the first 6 weeks and therefore its prevention should be a primary objective in the management of variceal bleeding. The rebleeding risk peaks in the first 5 days with 40% of all rebleeding episodes occurring in this period, remaining high during the first 2 weeks and declining slowly in the next 4 weeks. Six weeks after the index episode, the risk of bleeding essentially returns to baseline.

Six-week mortality after variceal bleeding is about 30%. Almost 60% of deaths are caused by uncontrolled bleeding, either during the initial episode or after early rebleeding.[9] The most consistently reported predictors of death are Child-Pugh classification (see Chapter 95), blood urea nitrogen (BUN) or creatinine, age, active alcohol abuse, active bleeding at endoscopy, and HVPG. Early rebleeding is the most important and most consistently reported late prognostic indicator of 6-week mortality.

Patients surviving a first episode of variceal bleeding have a very high risk of rebleeding and death. Median rebleeding incidence within 1–2 years is 63%.[9] The corresponding mortality figure is 33%. Because of these high risks, all patients surviving a variceal bleeding should be treated for prevention of rebleeding independently of other risk indicators.[10]

Gastric varices

The natural history of gastric varices is far less known than that of esophageal varices. Gastric varices are classified as those that are a continuation of esophageal varices (GOV), either along the lesser curve of the stomach (GOV1) or i the fundus (GOV2), and those that are isolated (IGV) (i.e., connected with esophageal varices), which are more rare, a may be located in the fundus (IGV1) or elsewhere in the stom (IGV2). IGV are more frequent in patients with prehep portal hypertension. Overall, the prevalence of gastric vari in patients with portal hypertension is about 20% (1 GOV1, 4% GOV2, and 2% IGV 1 or 2).[11] Sometimes it m be difficult to differentiate gastric varices from gastric fo and endoscopic ultrasonography may be helpful in these cas

Gastric varices are the source of 5–10% of all upper dig tive bleeding episodes in patients with cirrhosis. Bleedi related mortality after a first gastric variceal bleeding episo is about 20% and long-term recurrent bleeding and morta are in the same order as for esophageal varices.

Portal hypertensive gastropathy

Gastric mucosal changes associated with portal hypertens have been named portal hypertensive gastropathy (PHG). T most frequently observed elementary lesions of PHG are 'mosaic pattern' and 'cherry red spots.' The mosaic patt consists of multiple erythematous areas outlined by a wh reticular network and is generally considered as 'mild' PH Cherry red spots are round, red lesions, slightly raised over surrounding hyperemic mucosa. These carry a higher bleed risk and are considered 'severe' PHG.[12] Histologically, th lesions are characterized by dilation of the capillaries a venules of the gastric mucosa.

At the time of diagnosis of cirrhosis, the prevalence of P is about 30% and its incidence is about 12% per year. patients with advanced cirrhosis these figures may be as h as 70% and 30%, respectively. Endoscopic therapy of esophag varices (especially injection sclerotherapy) is a possible r factor for PHG.

The **clinical course of PHG** is characterized by overt or chro gastric mucosal bleeding. The incidence of overt bleeding fr any source in patients with mild PHG is about 5% per year, compared to 15% for severe PHG. Overt bleeding from PH is usually manifested by melena, and has a far better progno than variceal bleeding, with less than 5% mortality per episo The incidence of minor mucosal blood loss, without ov bleeding, is about 8% per year and may result in severe chro iron deficiency anemia requiring frequent hospital admissi and blood transfusions.

Portal hypertensive gastropathy should be distinguished fr gastric antral vascular ectasia (GAVE). This is a distinct ent that may be found in association with conditions differ from cirrhosis such as scleroderma or chronic gastritis. GA is characterized by aggregates of red spots usually with rad distribution from the pylorus to the antrum of the stoma ('watermelon stomach'). Histology of GAVE is characteriz by smooth muscle cell and myofibroblast hyperplasia a fibrohyalinosis. From a clinical point of view, GAVE behaves a severe PHG.

DIAGNOSTIC METHODS

The evaluation of the portal hypertensive patient is based the visualization of varices at endoscopy, the definition of porto-collateral anatomy by ultrasonography, and/or angiog phy, and the measurement of portal pressure.

CLINICAL PRESENTATION

- When cirrhosis is diagnosed, varices are present in about 50% of patients; patients without varices develop varices at a rate of 6% per year, and should be screened endoscopically for development of varices every 2–3 years; patients with small varices should be re-endoscoped every 1–2 years for enlargement
- Variceal bleeding episodes present with massive hematemesis and melena from ruptured esophageal varices in 60–70%, gastric varices in 5–10%, and ectopic varices in 1–5% of cases
- Variceal bleeding is diagnosed at emergency endoscopy based on observing either: (1) blood spurting or oozing from a varix; (2) white nipple or clot adherent on a varix; (3) varices without other potential sources of bleeding
- Severity of liver failure, active bleeding at diagnostic endoscopy, and degree of portal pressure elevation correlate with failure to control bleeding
- Six-week mortality after variceal bleeding is about 20%; death risk indicators are Child-Pugh, creatinine, active bleeding, HVPG, and associated conditions (infections, hepatocellular carcinoma)
- Gastric mucosal changes associated with portal hypertension (portal hypertensive gastropathy, PHG) are frequently observed as the 'mosaic pattern' (mild PHG) and 'cherry red spots' (severe PHG)
- Overt bleeding from PHG is usually manifested by melena, with less than 5% mortality; incidence of occult blood loss is about 8% per year in patients with mild PHG and up to 25% in those with severe PHG, in whom severe chronic iron deficiency anemia may result; rebleeding from PHG is prevented with nonselective beta-blockers (40–50% efficacy)

Imaging techniques are very useful in the initial evaluation the portal hypertensive patient. Frequently, portal hyper-nsion is first detected by the finding on ultrasonography a dilated portal vein, portosystemic collaterals, ascites, or lenomegaly. Patency of the portal vein or the presence of ortal vein thrombosis should be investigated in every portal ypertensive patient. Portal venography obtained at the venous hase of splenic and mesenteric angiography has been replaced y noninvasive methods such as Doppler ultrasonography with cho enhancement, helical computed tomography (CT) scans, nd magnetic resonance imaging (MRI). Retrograde wedged epatic venography, using CO_2 as contrast media during hepatic ein catheterization, is a safe technique that allows an adequate sualization of the portal vein in over 70% of patients with rrhosis.[13] Ultrasonography, CT scans, and MRI are as accurate angiography in detecting portal vein thrombosis. Ultra-onography is the preferred initial investigation because of its w cost and high accuracy.

ndoscopy

t endoscopy it is important to assess semi-quantitatively the ppearance and size of any esophageal varix, as well as the resence of red color signs (Fig. 96.3). Endoscopy should clude a careful evaluation for the presence of gastric varices, hich in some cases may require endosonography, and the resence, extent, and severity of portal hypertensive gastro-athy (Fig. 96.4).

Measurement of portal pressure

lease refer to Chapter 133 for details of measurement of ortal pressure.

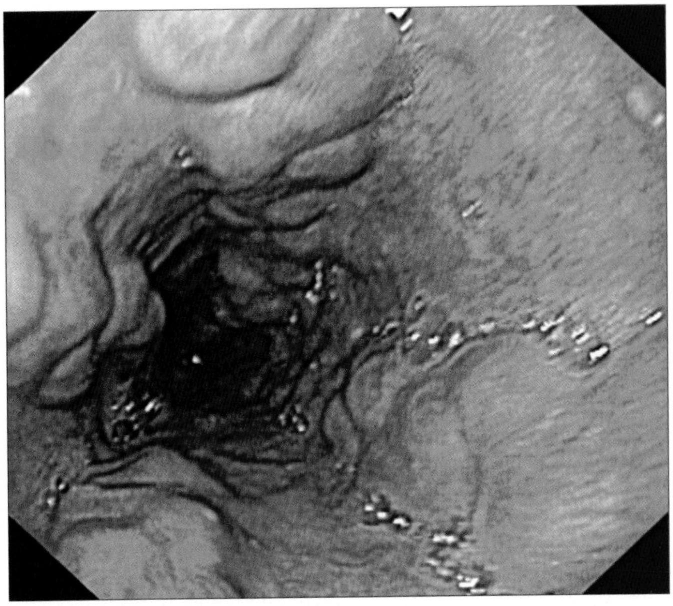

Fig. 96.3 Esophageal varices. (Courtesy of Dr F. Mondelo and Dr J. Llach.)

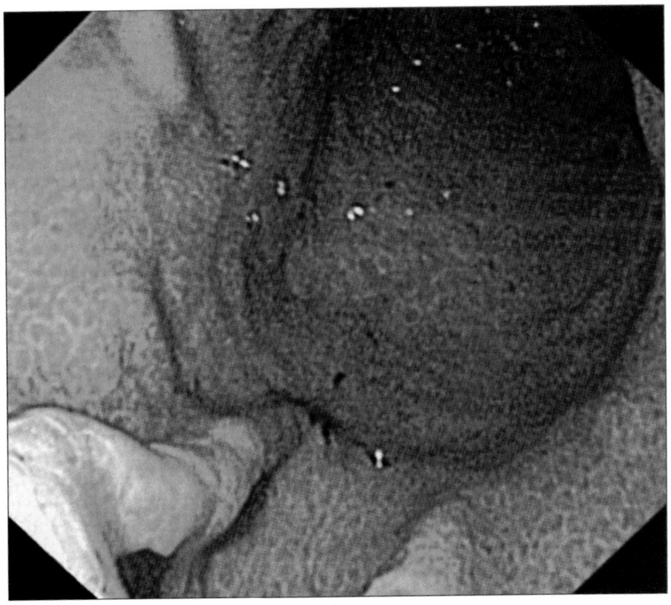

Fig. 96.4 Portal hypertensive gastropathy. (Courtesy of Dr J. M. Bordas and Dr J. Llach.)

Measurement of variceal pressure

Esophageal variceal pressure can be measured at endoscopy by either direct puncture or by using endoscopic pressure-sensitive gauges. The latter technique allows the measurement of variceal pressure without puncturing the varices, and therefore without the risk of precipitating variceal hemorrhage. Endoscopic pressure measurements can be difficult, especially in small varices. Variceal pressure has been shown to correlate with the risk of bleeding and pharmacological reduction of variceal pressure has been associated with a low actuarial probability of variceal bleeding.[14]

Endosonography

Endosonography is used for the diagnosis of gastric fundal varices when endoscopy offers doubtful results and to estimate the risk of variceal recurrence after varices have been eradicated by endoscopic therapy. In this later situation, the finding of grossly dilated periesophageal veins or of patent perforating veins below the gastroesophageal junction carries a high risk of variceal recurrence.

DIAGNOSTIC METHODS

- The evaluation of the portal hypertensive patient is based on visualization of varices at endoscopy, definition of the porto-collateral anatomy by ultrasonography and/or angiography, and measurement of portal pressure
- Angiographic techniques are being replaced by noninvasive methods such as Doppler ultrasonography with echo enhancement, helical CT scans, and MRI; ultrasonography is the preferred initial investigation; the presence of portal vein thrombosis should always be investigated
- Frequently, portal hypertension is first detected by the presence of a dilated portal vein, portosystemic collaterals, ascites or splenomegaly
- Endoscopy should assess the presence and size of esophageal varices, as well as the presence of red signs, and should include a careful evaluation for the presence of gastric varices
- Endosonography may be useful in the diagnosis of gastric fundal varices when endoscopy is equivocal
- Hepatic vein catheterization with measurement of HVPG is the preferred method to determine portal pressure, and provides strong prognostic information

TREATMENT AND PREVENTION

Prevention of the first bleed from esophageal varices

Pharmacological treatment

Nonselective beta-blockers reduce portal pressure through a reduction in portal and collateral blood flow. This is achieved through the reduction in cardiac output caused by beta-1 adrenergic blockade, and by splanchnic vasoconstriction due to the blockade of beta-2 adrenoceptors in the splanchnic arteries. Several meta-analyses have consistently shown a significant reduction of the bleeding risk, from 25% with nonactive treatment to 15% with beta-blockers[9] over a median follow-up of about 2 years. This beneficial effect was found in patients either with or without ascites, and with good or poor liver function. In addition, nonselective beta-blockers are associated with an almost significant reduction in mortality, and with a significant reduction in bleeding-related deaths. These beneficial effects are restricted to patients with relatively big varices (>5 mm diameter). Results in patients with small varices are heterogeneous.

About 15% of patients have contraindications to the use of beta-blockers. The most frequent include active pulmonary obstructive disease, aortic valve disease, and other diseases such as atrioventricular heart block, and peripheral arterial insufficiency, which may be worsened by beta-blockers. Sinus bradycardia and insulin-dependent diabetes are relative contraindications. The incidence of side effects among treated patients is in the order of 15%. The most frequent are fatigue, dyspnea, bronchospasm, and reduction of sexual activity. About 5% of side effects require treatment discontinuation, while others are managed by decreasing the dose; however, this may lead to a decreased efficacy.

Propranolol and nadolol are the nonselective beta-block most widely used in the pharmacological treatment of por hypertension. Propranolol should be prescribed initially 20–40 mg b.i.d. and titrated on a bi-weekly basis, up to a ma mum of 160 mg b.i.d. Similar concepts apply to nadolol, wh should be prescribed initially at 20 mg a day, in a single da dose, and titrated every 2–3 days up to a maximum of 160 m Patients should be instructed not to discontinue treatment a told that they will be treated on a life-long basis, since bleedi risk increases sharply after discontinuation of beta-blockers

Other treatments: Administration of short-acting (nytroglycer NTG) or long-acting (isosorbide di-nitrate, ISDN, or isosorbic 5-mono-nitrate, IMN) nitrates decreases portal pressure.[1] Or IMN has been evaluated in clinical trials for the prevention variceal bleeding, failing to show any benefit in the preventi of first bleeding.[16]

The association of a vasoconstrictor (such as propranolol nadolol) with a vasodilator (such as IMN) achieves a fall portal pressure greater than that caused by either drug alone The combination of IMN with beta-blockers has been compar with beta-blockers alone in three RCTs.[9] The combined resu of these three studies do not support the use of combinati therapy for the prevention of first variceal bleeding.

Spironolactone lowers HVPG in patients with cirrhosis. association with nadolol has been compared with nadolol alo for the prevention of first variceal bleeding and again no benefit the association was observed in reducing first variceal bleeding.

Endoscopic therapy

Published prophylactic clinical trials using sclerotherapy clear indicate that sclerotherapy should not be used for the preve tion of first variceal bleeding because the risks outweigh t benefits.[12] Endoscopic banding ligation (EBL) has greater ef cacy and lower side effects than sclerotherapy. EBL has bee compared to beta-blockers in the prevention of first bleedin No significant differences either for bleeding or death we observed between both treatments, but EBL had a higher cos Thus, there is no evidence to support the use of EBL as firs line prophylactic therapy. However, it may be considered f patients with high-risk varices and contraindications to bet blockers (Fig. 96.5).

Treatment of acute bleeding from esophageal varices

General management

Variceal bleeding is a medical emergency and its manageme should be undertaken in an intensive care setting by a team experienced medical staff, including a clinical hepatologis endoscopist, and surgeon. It is essential to have well-traine nurses. Therapy is greatly facilitated if decision-making follow a written protocol (Fig. 96.6). The initial therapy is aimed correcting hypovolemic shock, preventing complications ass ciated with gastrointestinal bleeding, and achieving hemostas at the bleeding site.

Blood volume replacement should be initiated as soon possible to avoid complications from hypovolemic shock an decreased perfusion of vital organs. Overtransfusion should b avoided, not only because of the risks inherent with bloo transfusion, but also because it increases portal pressure wit a consequent risk of continued bleeding or rebleeding. Curre consensus (Baveno III) is to transfuse packed red blood cel

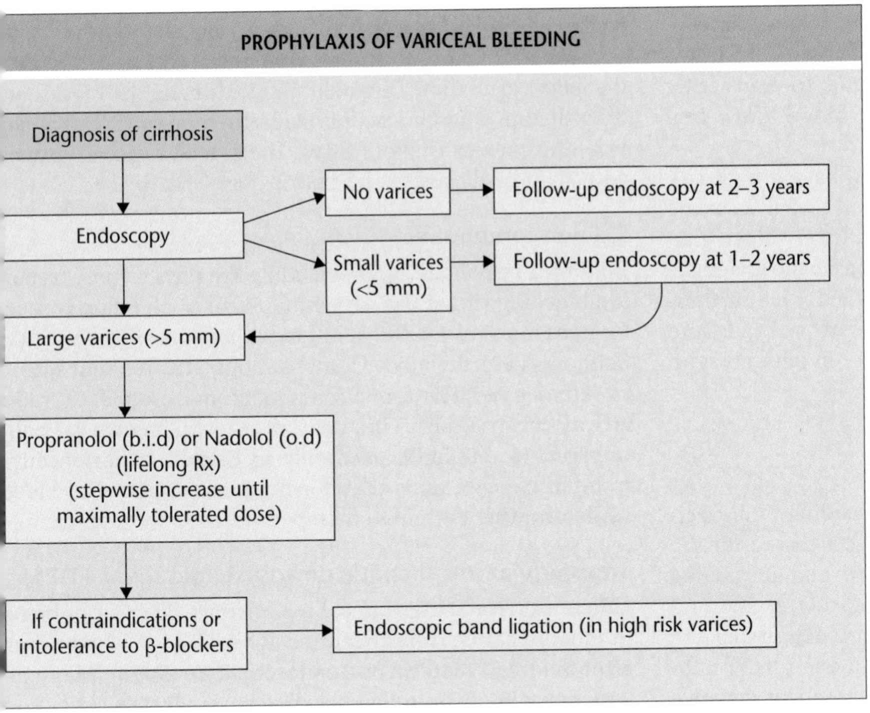

Fig. 96.5 Prevention of first variceal bleeding. Therapeutic algorithm.

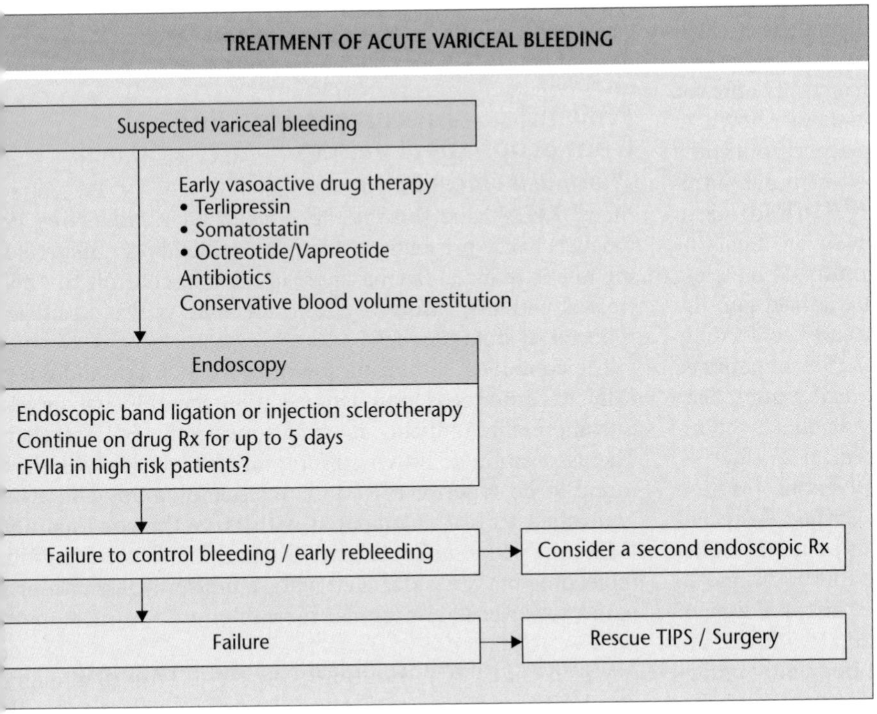

Fig. 96.6 Acute variceal bleeding. Therapeutic algorithm.

the hematocrit is below 25%, with a target hematocrit of -30%. Plasma (or expanders) should be given to maintain a tolic blood pressure over 80 mmHg and a heart rate <120 bpm. **Aspiration** of blood or gastric secretions is especially frequent patients with impaired consciousness due to shock or hepatic cephalopathy. Suspected or proven aspiration should be treated mediately with antibiotics. Its prevention is based on close pervision by a well-trained nurse, orotracheal intubation in matose patients, and aspiration of the gastric contents through indwelling nasogastric tube. The latter is not universally used; wever, it allows the enteral administration of drugs in comatose patients and is a useful method for monitoring the activity of bleeding. In addition, removal of blood from the upper gastrointestinal tract may help to prevent and correct hepatic encephalopathy, which is a frequent complication of variceal hemorrhage.

Renal function should be supported by maintaining the systemic circulation. Saline infusions should be avoided. It is crucial to avoid the administration of nephrotoxic drugs, especially aminoglycosides and nonsteroidal anti-inflammatory agents. The use of terlipressin to arrest the bleeding may have the additional advantage of protecting from hepatorenal syndrome.

Massive or tense ascites should be treated by paracentesis, preferably with albumin replacement. This has been shown to improve the hemodynamic conditions and to transiently decrease portal pressure, portal-collateral blood flow, and variceal pressure.

Antibiotics: Patients with variceal bleeding have a high risk of bacterial infections (near 50% as compared to 5–7% in the general population). A recent meta-analysis[19] has shown that antibiotic prophylaxis using quinolones decreases the incidence of bacterial infections and increases the survival rate. Furthermore, bacterial infections significantly increase the risk of failure to control bleeding and the hospital mortality in patients with cirrhosis and gastrointestinal bleeding.

Specific treatment

Pharmacological treatment

This should be started as soon as variceal bleeding is suspected, even prior to diagnostic endoscopy. Drugs assessed for the treatment of acute bleeding are vasopressin and its analog terlipressin, and somatostatin and its analogs octreotide and vapreotide. Vasopressin and terlipressin have been associated with nitroglycerin (NTG) in some trials. Meta-analysis of published RCTs clearly shows that either terlipressin or somatostatin are the best therapeutic options. Octreotide improves the efficacy of emergency sclerotherapy in controlling bleeding, but there is no evidence supporting its use as single therapy. If vasopressin is used, it should be associated with nitroglycerin because this reduces the side effects and enhances its efficacy.

Terlipressin is the only treatment that has been shown to improve prognosis of variceal bleeding in placebo-controlled RCTs and meta-analyses. Terlipressin is used in bolus intravenous (IV) injections at doses of 2mg every 4–6h for up to 48h. It should not be used in patients with severe heart or vascular disease. After achieving an initial control of bleeding (a 24-h bleeding free period) the dose can be halved and the treatment maintained for 5days to prevent early rebleeding. Side effects of terlipressin may occur in nearly 25% of patients, the more frequent being relatively mild: abdominal cramps, diarrhea, bradycardia, and hypertension. Severe side effects requiring discontinuation of the drug are in the order of 2–4%.[20]

Somatostatin is used by continuous intravenous infusion of 250μg/h following an initial bolus of 250μg. A recent study suggested that high-risk patients (with active bleeding at endoscopy) should receive a greater dose (500μg/h and to associate repeat 250μg boluses during the initial hours of therapy).[21] Treatment may be maintained for up to 5days. Side effects of somatostatin are usually mild, most frequently bradycardia, hyperglycemia, diarrhea, and abdominal cramps. '5-day success' (control of bleeding, no further bleeding, no death) is achieved in about 70% of patients using either terlipressin or somatostatin.

Endoscopic therapy

Endoscopic therapy using either injection sclerotherapy or banding ligation is recommended as soon as an experienced endoscopist is available. Emergency endoscopic injection sclerotherapy of esophageal varices stops bleeding in about 80–90% of patients. However, it requires a skilled endoscopist and is associated with serious complications in 10–20% of patients, with an overall mortality of 2%.[9] RCTs indicate that emergency sclerotherapy is not superior to pharmacological therapy in achieving 5-day success. EBL may be slightly better t sclerotherapy. Recent studies and meta-analysis suggest the best results are obtained by combining early vasoac drug therapy and endoscopic sclerotherapy or EBL (Fig. 96 Five-day success is about 80%. The use of variceal obtura with tissue adhesives is no better than EBL.

Balloon tamponade

Balloon tamponade stops bleeding by direct compressio the bleeding site at the varices. Control of bleeding is succ ful in as much as 80–90%, but most patients will rebleed w balloon(s) are deflated. Complications are frequent and be lethal in 6–20% (aspiration pneumonia, esophageal rupt airway obstruction). Because of these drawbacks ball tamponade should be used only by skilled, experienced s in intensive care units only for temporary control of bleec while awaiting definitive therapy.

Transjugular intrahepatic portosystemic shunt (TIPS)

When used for acute variceal hemorrhage, TIPS stops bleec in most patients. It has been mostly used as a salvage ther after failure of medical and endoscopic treatment. Many of patients with uncontrolled bleeding have advanced liver fail which probably accounts for the high 6-week mortality, ra ing from 27% to 55%. Shunt surgery using interposition me caval graft shunts or traditional portacaval shunts may be alternative to TIPS in Child A patients (Fig. 96.6).

Prevention of recurrent bleeding from esophageal varices

Pharmacological treatment

Many RCTs have proved the efficacy of nonselective be blockers in the prevention of variceal rebleeding.[12] The reble ing rate is reduced from a mean of 63% in controls to 42% treated patients.[9] Mortality from bleeding is also significar reduced by beta-blockers.

The combined administration of propranolol or nadolol p IMN was introduced after demonstrating that IMN enhanced portal pressure reducing effect of nonselective beta-blocker The association of IMN with propranolol or nadolol has be found to be superior to endoscopic sclerotherapy and at le equivalent to EBL. Compared with TIPS, the combination IMN and propranolol is less effective for the prevention rebleeding but it is associated with significantly less encepha pathy, lower cost, and similar mortality.

Monitoring pharmacological treatment response

The HVPG response to continued therapy with beta-block correlates with its clinical efficacy. The risk of rebleeding almost nil when HVPG falls <12mmHg, and is dramatic reduced (to 18%) in patients decreasing HVPG >20% of ba line, even when the 12mmHg target is not reached. It is s unclear whether patients with an insufficient hemodyna response to pharmacological therapy will benefit from alt native treatments. These patients probably benefit from add EBL to drug therapy.

Endoscopic treatment

Endoscopic injection sclerotherapy of esophageal varices s nificantly reduces both the rebleeding and death risk.[22] Rec rence of varices occurs in nearly 40% of patients within 1 y from eradication, requiring further sessions. Serious side effects are dysphagia, esophageal stenosis, and bleeding from esophageal ulcers, which may account for 14% of all rebleeding episodes. EBL has proven to be superior to sclerotherapy and has less frequent and severe complications.[12] However, EBL does not improve survival compared with sclerotherapy and it is associated with higher recurrence of varices.[22]

Combined endoscopic and pharmacological treatment

The combination of injection sclerotherapy and beta-blockers has been associated with a significant reduction in rebleeding compared to either treatment used alone, but with no differences in mortality. The limited information on the combination of EBL plus beta-blockers suggests that it is more effective than EBL alone.[23] Therefore, the combination of EBL with a nonselective beta-blocker is particularly recommended in patients who have bled under either treatment alone. In these patients, the substitution of the failing treatment with another treatment should not be preferred to their combination. This combination may also be considered in HVPG nonresponders to drug therapy.

TIPS and surgery

TIPS and shunt surgery are very useful in the prevention of recurrent bleeding. Patients with severe or repeat rebleeding episodes while on beta-blockers (+/– ISMN) in combination with endoscopic therapy should be considered for 'rescue' therapy with TIPS or shunt surgery (Fig. 96.7).

Treatment of gastric varices

Results of pharmacological therapy in the prevention of first bleeding in patients with esophageal varices can most probably be extended to patients with gastric varices.

The optimal treatment of acute gastric variceal bleeding is not known. The usual initial treatment is a vasoactive drug(s). Balloon tamponade, with the Linton-Nachlas tube, is preferred over the Sengstaken tube, as a temporary treatment. The tissue adhesive isobutyl-2-cyanoacrylate (bucrylate), mixed with lipiodol has been found to be efficacious and superior to ethanolamine in nonrandomized studies, achieving hemostasis in 90% of patients. In a recent RCT, endoscopic obturation using cyanoacrylate proved more effective and safer than band ligation in the management of bleeding gastric varices.[24] However, cerebral embolism has been reported with tissue adhesives. Thrombin has provided good hemostasis in some studies. Since the rebleeding rate after endoscopic treatment is high, it is recommended that an early decision should be made for TIPS or surgery in patients rebleeding from gastric varices. Salvage TIPS is very effective, with more than 90% success rate for initial hemostasis and an early rebleeding rate below 20%, often from nonvariceal sources, e.g., sclerosis ulcers. In clinical practice, nonselective beta-blockers are used as first-line therapy for the prevention of recurrent bleeding. TIPS, shunt surgery, or variceal obturation are recommended in failures of pharmacological treatment.

Treatment of portal hypertensive gastropathy (PHG) and gastric antral vascular ectasia (GAVE)

There is no indication for the primary prophylaxis of bleeding from PHG.

Acute bleeding from PHG should first be treated with the same vasoactive drugs as for variceal bleeding, although there are no RCTs specifically designed for PHG. Prevention of recurrent bleeding from PHG should be based on nonselective

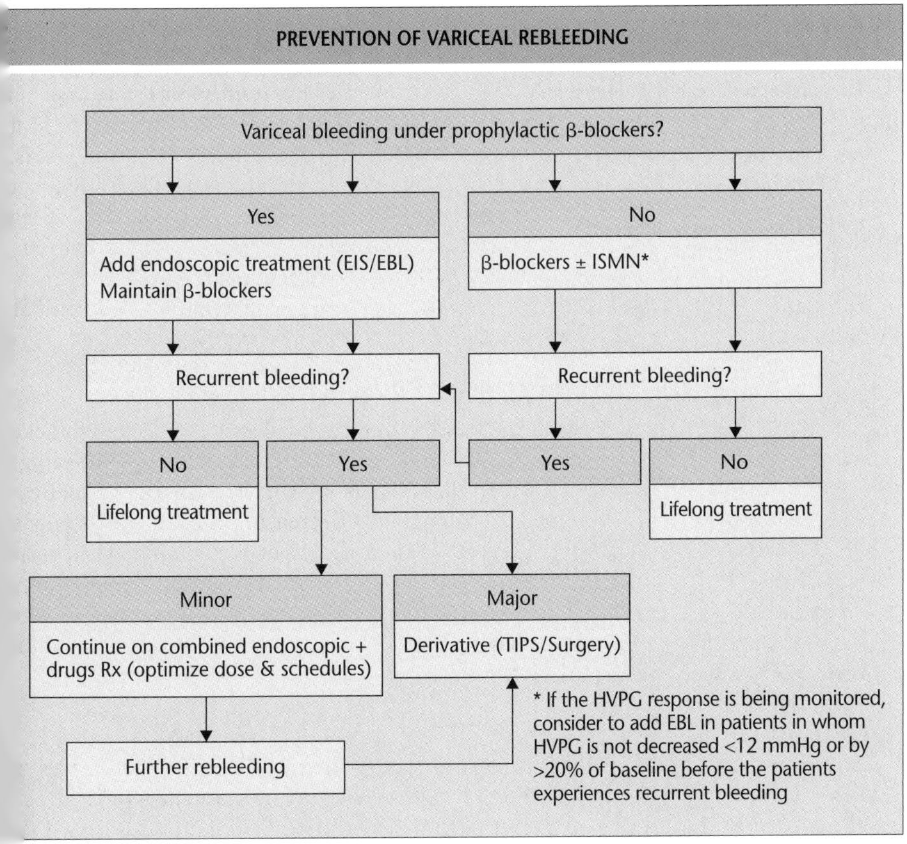

Fig. 96.7 Prevention of recurrent variceal bleeding. EIS, endoscopic injection sclerotherapy; EBL, endoscopic band ligation.

beta-blockers.[10,25] Adequate iron supplementation may be useful to prevent or correct chronic iron-deficiency anemia in patients with severe PHG. TIPS may be considered as an alternative therapy for the rare patient that has repeated severe bleeding from PHG despite pharmacological therapy. Argon plasma coagulation or neodymium:yttrium-aluminum-garnet (Nd:YAG) laser may also be useful.

Patients bleeding from GAVE may benefit from endoscopic ablation, either by argon plasma coagulation, Nd:YAG laser, or heater probe. TIPS and beta-blockers are not effective for the prevention of recurrent bleeding from GAVE. Selected patients with severe recurrent bleeding or uncontrollable acute bleeding from GAVE may benefit from antrectomy with Billroth I anastomosis.

REFERENCES

1. Bosch J, Garcia-Pagan JC. Complications of cirrhosis. I. Portal hypertension. J Hepatol 2000; 32 (Suppl 1):141–156.
2. Wanless IR, Wong F, Blendis LM et al. Hepatic and portal vein thrombosis in cirrhosis: possible role in development of parenchymal extinction and portal hypertension. Hepatology 1995; 21:1238–1247.
3. Gupta TK, Toruner M, Chung MK, Groszmann RJ. Endothelial dysfunction and decreased production of nitric oxide in the intrahepatic microcirculation of cirrhotic rats. Hepatology 1998; 28:926–931.
4. Graupera M, Garcia-Pagan JC, Pares M et al. Cyclooxygenase-1 inhibition corrects endothelial dysfunction in cirrhotic rat livers. J Hepatol 2003; 39:521.
5. Wiest R, Groszmann RJ. The paradox of nitric oxide in cirrhosis and portal hypertension: too much, not enough. Hepatology 2002; 35: 478–491.
6. NIEC. Prediction of the first variceal hemorrhage in patients with cirrhosis of the liver and esophageal varices. A prospective multicenter study. The North Italian Endoscopic Club for the Study and Treatment of Esophageal Varices [see comments]. N Engl J Med 1988; 319: 983–989.
7. D'Amico G, de Franchis R. Upper digestive bleeding in cirrhosis. Post-therapeutic outcome and prognostic indicators. Hepatology 2003; 38:599–612.
8. Moitinho E, Escorsell A, Bandi JC et al. Prognostic value of early measurements of portal pressure in acute variceal bleeding. Gastroenterology 1999; 117:626–631.
9. D'Amico G, Pagliaro L, Bosch J. Pharmacological treatment of portal hypertension: an evidence-based approach. Semin Liver Dis 1999; 19:475–505.
10. Grace ND, Groszmann RJ, Garcia-Tsao G et al. Portal hypertension and variceal bleeding: an AASLD single topic symposium. Hepatology 1998; 28:868–880.
11. Spina GP, Arcidiacono R, Bosch J et al. Gastric endoscopic features in portal hypertension: final report of a consensus conference, Milan, Italy, September 19, 1992. J Hepatol 1994; 21:461–467.
12. de Franchis R. Updating consensus in portal hypertension: report of the Baveno III Consensus Workshop on definitions, methodology and therapeutic strategies in portal hypertension. J Hepatol 2000; 33:846–852.
13. Debernardi-Venon W, Bandi JC, Garcia-Pagan JC et al. CO(2) wedged hepatic venography in the evaluation of portal hypertension. Gut 2000; 46:856–860.
14. Escorsell A, Bordas JM, Castaneda B et al. Predictive value of the variceal pressure response to continued pharmacological therapy in patients with cirrhosis and portal hypertension. Hepatology 2000; 31:1061–1067.
15. Abraczinskas DR, Ookubo R, Grace ND et al. Propranolol for the prevention of first esophageal variceal hemorrhage: a lifetime commitment? Hepatology 2001; 34:1096–1102.
16. Garcia-Pagan JC, Villanueva C, Vila MC et al. Isosorbide mononitrate in the prevention of first variceal bleed in patients who cannot receive beta-blockers. Gastroenterology 2001; 121:908–914.
17. Garcia-Pagan JC, Feu F, Bosch J, Rodes J. Propranolol compared with propranolol plus isosorbide-5-mononitrate for portal hypertension in cirrhosis. A randomized controlled study. Ann Intern Med 1991; 114:869–873.
18. Abecasis R, Kravetz D, Fassio E et al. Nadolol plus spironolactone in the prophylaxis of first variceal bleed in nonascitic cirrhotic patients: A preliminary study. Hepatology 2003; 37: 359–365.
19. Bernard B, Grange JD, Khac EN et al. Antibiotic prophylaxis for the prevention of bacterial infections in cirrhotic patients with gastrointestinal bleeding: a meta-analysis. Hepatology 1999; 29:1655–1661.
20. Escorsell A, Ruiz DA, Planas R et al. Multicenter randomized controlled trial of terlipressin versus sclerotherapy in the treatment of acute variceal bleeding: the TEST study. Hepatology 2000; 32:471–476.
21. Moitinho E, Planas R, Bañares R et al. Multicenter randomized controlled trial comparing different schedules of somatostatin in the treatment of acute variceal bleeding. J Hepatol 2001; 35:712–718.
22. de Franchis R, Primignani M. Endoscopic treatments for portal hypertension. Semin Liver Dis 1999; 19:439–455.
23. Lo GH, Lai KH, Cheng JS et al. Endoscopic variceal ligation plus nadolol and sucralfate compared with ligation alone for the prevention of variceal rebleeding: a prospective, randomized trial. Hepatology 2000; 32:461–465.
24. Lo GH, Lai KH, Cheng JS, Chen MH, Chiang HT. A prospective, randomized trial of butyl cyanoacrylate injection versus band ligation in the management of bleeding gastric varices. Hepatology 2001; 33:1060–1064.
25. Perez-Ayuso RM, Pique JM, Bosch J et al. Propranolol in prevention of recurrent bleeding from severe portal hypertensive gastropathy in cirrhosis. Lancet 1991; 337:1431–1434.

Chapter 97

Ascites and hepatorenal syndrome

Andrés Cárdenas, Pere Ginès, and Vicente Arroyo

KEY POINTS

- Ascites and renal dysfunction in patients with cirrhosis are the consequence of the homeostatic activation of vasoconstrictor and sodium-retaining systems triggered by a decrease in effective arterial blood volume due to a marked arterial vasodilation located in the splanchnic circulation
- While patients with moderate ascites are best managed with the combination of sodium restriction and diuretics, large-volume paracentesis plus volume replacement is the best treatment option for patients with large ascites
- Ascites refractory to diuretic therapy can be successfully managed by either repeated large-volume paracentesis or transjugular intrahepatic portosystemic shunts; however, repeated paracentesis with concomitant albumin administration is safer and has fewer side effects and is the recommended initial therapy for refractory ascites
- The development of dilutional hyponatremia also carries a poor prognosis in cirrhosis; newer agents aimed at counteracting the effects of the antidiuretic hormone are promising but are not yet available for use in clinical practice
- HRS continues to be a major cause of mortality in patients with cirrhosis and ascites, but effective therapeutic methods have been introduced recently, including the administration of vasoconstrictor drugs or transjugular intrahepatic portosystemic shunts; these methods may increase survival and help patients reach liver transplantation

NTRODUCTION

scites is the pathological accumulation of free fluid in the eritoneal cavity. This term derives from the Greek root 'askos,' neaning bag. Although ancient Egyptians and Greeks acknowl-dged a possible link between liver disease and ascites, Erasitratus f Cappadoccia, circa 300 BC,[1] described the 'hardness of the ver' as a risk factor for ascites formation. One of the most elebrated figures with ascites and cirrhosis was Ludwig van eethoven who was treated with serial large-volume paracen-esis and died of hepatic failure in 1827.[2]

PIDEMIOLOGY

n the natural history of cirrhosis, patients may develop signifi-ant complications of renal function manifested by sodium etention, water retention, and renal vasoconstriction. These re responsible for fluid accumulation in the form of ascites, ilutional hyponatremia, and hepatorenal syndrome, respec-vely. Ascites is the most common complication of cirrhosis esulting in poor quality of life, increased risk for infections, renal failure, and high mortality rates. Nearly 60% of patients with compensated cirrhosis develop ascites within 10 years of the disease.[3] The development of ascites in cirrhosis is a poor prognostic feature because it has been estimated that approximately 50% of these patients will die in approximately 3 years without liver transplantation.[4] Therefore, the presence of ascites in a cirrhotic patient is an indication for liver transplantation. Dilutional hyponatremia and hepatorenal syndrome are later events that carry an even worse prognosis.

CAUSES

The causes of ascites and its differential diagnosis are specified in Chapter 20. Cirrhosis is by far the most frequent cause of ascites. This chapter will therefore focus on the pathophysiology, clinical features, diagnostic methods and current therapy of ascites, dilutional hyponatremia, and hepatorenal syndrome in cirrhosis.

PATHOPHYSIOLOGY OF ASCITES AND RENAL FUNCTION ABNORMALITIES IN CIRRHOSIS

In cirrhosis, the presence of bridging fibrosis and nodule formation distorts the normal architecture of the hepatic sinusoids thereby causing an increased resistance to flow from the portal vein into the liver. This event causes significant effects in the portal venous system with development of sinusoidal portal hypertension and collateral vein formation with shunting of blood from the portal to the systemic circulation. In the splanchnic arterial bed, development of vasodilation contributes to portal hypertension by increasing flow and inducing changes in the microcirculation that predispose to increased filtration of plasma. Several vasodilator factors, in particular nitric oxide, are responsible for this vasodilatory effect.[5] Aside from changes in splanchnic hemodynamics, patients with ascites develop a hyperdynamic state characterized by reduced systemic vascular resistance and arterial pressure, increased cardiac output, and activation of vasoconstrictor and antinatriuretic systems (renin-angiotensin and sympathetic nervous systems and antidiuretic hormone).[6] Splanchnic vasodilation by decreasing effective arterial blood volume leads to stimulation of central baroreceptors thereby triggering the activation of vasoconstrictor systems, which interact with the kidney leading to the development of sodium and water retention, as well as renal vasoconstriction (Fig. 97.1). Inability to excrete sodium is the earliest renal alteration and occurs before water retention and renal vasoconstriction (see Fig. 97.2).[7] The major clinical consequence of water retention is dilutional hyponatremia, which

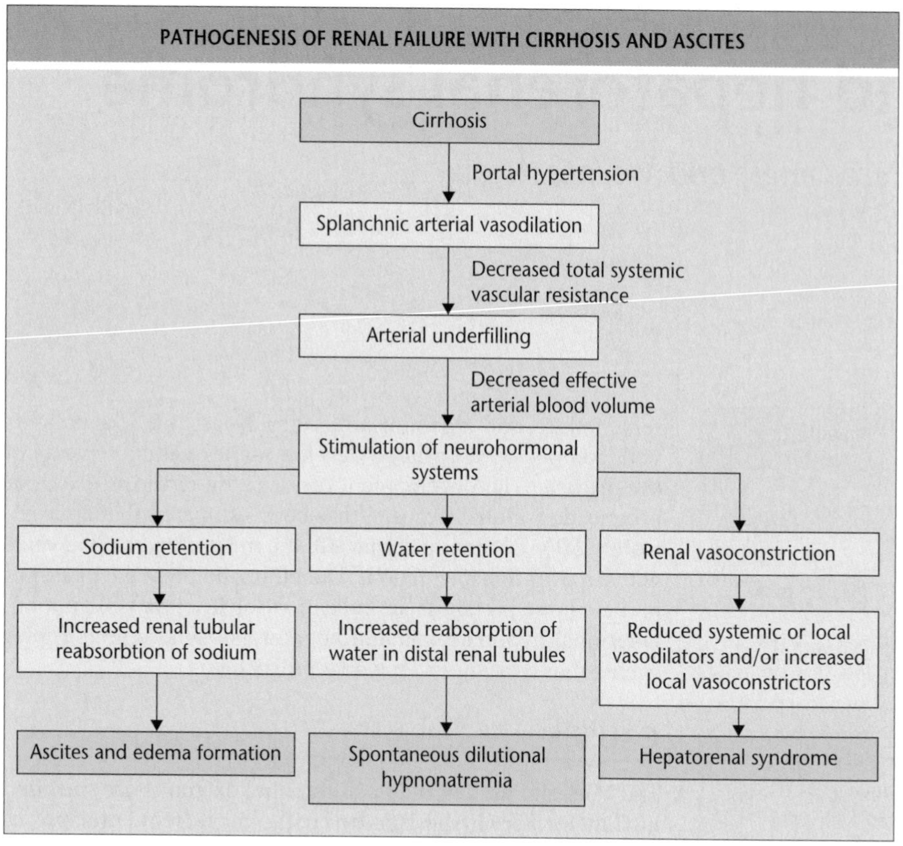

Fig. 97.1 Pathogenesis of functional renal failure in patients with cirrhosis and ascite The neurohumoral effects of the renin-angiotensin-aldosterone system (RAAS), the sympathetic nervous system (SNS), and arginine vasopressin (AVP) on systemic circulation and renal function in cirrhosis wit ascites are responsible for sodium and water retention as well as the hepatorenal syndrom The levels of these vasoconstrictors are highe in patients with hepatorenal syndrome.

occurs despite significant sodium retention because water is retained in excess of sodium.[8] Renal vasoconstriction develops late in the disease and manifests as hepatorenal syndrome (HRS).[9,10] The degree of renal failure may range from a modest renal impairment (serum creatinine levels between 1.2 and 1.4 mg/dL) to severe renal failure (serum creatinine above 1.5 mg/dL and oliguria/anuria).[11]

CLINICAL PRESENTATION

The clinical features of patients presenting with ascites are described in detail in Chapter 20.

TREATMENT

The first and most important aspect in the management of patients with cirrhosis and ascites is the evaluation for liver transplantation.[12] Early referral is advocated due to the short survival once patients develop this complication. Education of patients regarding a sodium-restricted diet (70–90 mmol/day) is one of the mainstays of management in all patients with cirrhotic ascites.[13] A more stringent restriction is generally not well tolerated and patients become noncompliant. Although in a low proportion of patients ascites may decrease with this measure alone, it is essential when diuretics are added. Finally, in patients with alcoholic cirrhosis, alcohol abstention is one of the most important steps in the management of ascites.

Nonrefractory ascites

Patients with mild to moderate ascites respond well to diuretics. The best initial regimen for minimizing ascites is spironolactone 100 mg/day with or without furosemide (20–40 mg/day).[1] If there is no response, compliance with diet and medication should be confirmed, and diuretics may then be increased in stepwise fashion every 5–7 days by doubling doses to a maxi mal dose of spironolactone of 400 mg/day and a maximal dos of furosemide of 160 mg/day. The goal is to achieve an averag weight loss of 300–500 g per day in patients without edem and 800–1000 g per day in those with peripheral edema.[15] A greater degree of weight loss may induce volume depletion an renal failure. After minimizing ascites, sodium restriction shoul be maintained while the dose of diuretics may be reduced a needed.

Tense ascites: These patients are probably best managed b therapeutic paracentesis. A detailed description of this tech nique can be found in Chapter 149. Complete removal of ascite in one tap or repeated taps of 4–6 L/day in combination wit intravenous albumin (6–8 g per liter tapped) has been show to be quick, effective, and associated with a lower number o complications than conventional diuretic therapy.[16] After therapeutic tap, postparacentesis circulatory dysfunction ma develop; this is a circulatory derangement with marked activa tion of the renin-angiotensin system that occurs 24–48 h afte the procedure.[17] This disorder is clinically silent, not sponta neously reversible, and associated with hyponatremia, rena impairment, decreased survival, and may be prevented wit the administration of plasma expanders.[18] Albumin has prove superior to dextran-70, polygeline, and saline following para centesis of more than 5 L.[19] Patients with a known history o cirrhosis and without any complications can be managed a outpatients. However, patients in whom tense ascites is th first manifestation of cirrhosis or those with associated hepat ephalopathy, gastrointestinal bleeding, or bacterial infections uire hospitalization. Most of these patients have marked lium retention and need to be started or continued on rela-ly high doses of diuretics after paracentesis together with w sodium diet.

EATMENT STRATEGY FOR PATIENTS WITH NONREFRACTORY ASCITES

LD TO MODERATE ASCITES

w-sodium diet (70–90 mmol/day) and spironolactone (100 mg/day as gle dose). Monitor body weight daily and urine sodium weekly. Ideal ight loss should be between 300 and 500 g/day in patients without ripheral edema and 800–1000 g/day in patients with peripheral ema. Furosemide 20–40 mg/day may be used in combination with ironolactone to increase the natriuretic effect[a]

NSE ASCITES

erapeutic paracentesis plus intravenous albumin (6–8 g/liter of ascites moved)[b]

there is no response, check compliance with treatment and low-sodium t. Increase the dose of diuretics in stepwise fashion every 5–7 days up to 0 mg/day of spironolactone and 160 mg/day of furosemide.

fter the tap; if the patient was not on diuretics begin with spironolactone 00–200 mg/day) and furosemide (20–40 mg/day) to maintain the patient th mild or no ascites. If the patient was on diuretics before begin with a dose gher than previously.

fractory ascites

proximately 10% of patients with ascites are refractory to atment with diuretics.[20] In refractory ascites, sodium excre-n cannot be achieved either because patients do not respond high doses of diuretics (spironolactone 400 mg/day and osemide 160 mg/day) or because they develop side effects t preclude their use.[20] Current treatment strategies include eated therapeutic paracentesis plus intravenous albumin, and nsjugular intrahepatic portosystemic shunts (TIPS). Perito-ovenous shunts, although very effective, were abandoned due significant complications when compared to paracentesis.[21] erapeutic paracentesis is the most accepted initial therapy refractory ascites. Patients, on average, require a tap every 4 weeks and the majority may be treated as outpatients, king this option easy to perform and cost effective.[22] TIPS, on-surgical method of portal decompression, acts as a side-side portocaval shunt that reduces sinusoidal and portal pres-e and decreases ascites and diuretic requirements in these tients.[23] The main disadvantage with TIPS is frequent obstruc-n of the prosthesis, which precipitates rapid reaccumulation ascites in some patients.[23] Major side effects include hepatic cephalopathy and impairment in liver function.[22,24]

Four randomized controlled studies comparing TIPS with eated paracentesis showed that TIPS is associated with a ver rate of ascites recurrence.[22,25–27] However, hepatic cephalopathy was seen in 30–50% of patients treated with PS. The studies reported discrepant findings with respect to rvival: one showed improved survival with paracentesis,[25] other a survival benefit with TIPS,[26] and two demonstrated difference.[22,27] Finally, the cost of treating patients with ractory ascites with TIPS was higher than the cost of repeat-paracentesis plus albumin.[22] In view of these contradic-ns, it is difficult to advocate TIPS as the initial treatment for refractory ascites. TIPS placement should be evaluated on a case-by-case basis and probably reserved for patients with preserved liver function, without hepatic encephalopathy, with loculated fluid, or those unwilling to undergo repeated taps.

TREATMENT STRATEGY FOR PATIENTS WITH REFRACTORY ASCITES

INITIAL THERAPY

- Total paracentesis plus intravenous albumin (6–8 g/liter of ascites removed)

MAINTENANCE THERAPY

- Maintain a low-sodium diet (70–90 mmol/day) constantly
- In patients taking the highest doses of diuretics, check urinary sodium; if less than 30 mEq/day, stop diuretic therapy
- Total paracentesis plus intravenous albumin when necessary (approximately every 2–3 weeks)
- Consider use of TIPS in patients with preserved hepatic function, no hepatic encephalopathy, either with loculated fluid, or unwilling to have repeated paracentesis

Dilutional hyponatremia

Impairment of solute-free water excretion is common in advanced cirrhosis and occurs months after the onset of sodium retention (Fig. 97.2). The major clinical consequence of this disorder is the development of dilutional hyponatremia, which is defined as a serum sodium concentration less than 130 mEq/Lt in the presence of ascites or edema.[8] The pathogenesis of impairment of solute-free water excretion in cirrhosis is complex and involves a reduced delivery of filtrate to the ascending limb of the loop of Henle, reduced renal synthesis of prostaglandins, and most importantly, increased nonosmotic secretion of antidiuretic hormone.

In most patients, dilutional hyponatremia is asymptomatic, but in some it may be associated with symptoms such as anorexia,

RENAL FUNCTION ABNORMALITIES VS DEGREE OF LIVER DISEASE

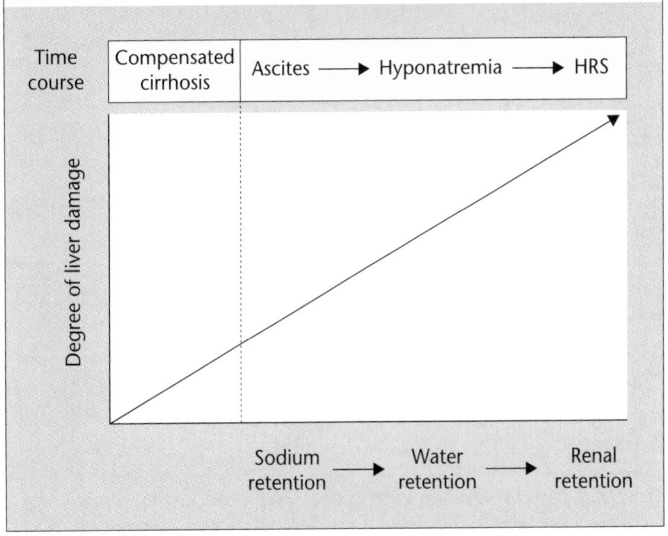

Fig. 97.2 Renal function abnormalities vs degree of liver disease. Time course of renal functional abnormalities and their relationship to the underlying degree of liver disease in patients with cirrhosis. HRS, hepatorenal syndrome.

poor concentration, lethargy, nausea, vomiting, and occasionally seizures. Water restriction of approximately 1 L/day prevents the progressive decrease in serum sodium concentration but does not correct hyponatremia. The administration of hypertonic saline solutions is not recommended because it invariably leads to further expansion of extracellular fluid volume and accumulation of ascites and edema. Preliminary phase II studies show that antagonists of the V2 receptor of antidiuretic hormone increase solute-free water excretion and improve serum sodium concentration in hyponatremic patients with cirrhosis and ascites.[28,29] These drugs selectively antagonize the water-retaining effect of antidiuretic hormone in the cortical collecting duct. Several phase II–III studies are being conducted in order to learn more about the efficacy and safety of these drugs. These compounds, when available for use in clinical practice, would offer a novel therapeutic approach for the treatment of dilutional hyponatremia in cirrhotic patients with ascites.

Hepatorenal syndrome

One of the ultimate and most serious complications of cirrhotic ascites is HRS, a unique form of functional renal failure without identifiable renal pathology that occurs in approximately 10% of patients with advanced cirrhosis or acute liver failure.[9] HRS may develop acutely or subacutely. Type 1 HRS is an acute and rapidly progressive form of renal failure with an expected survival of 2 weeks, while in type 2 HRS, renal failure is usually less severe and shows little or no progression compared to that of type 1 HRS (Fig. 97.3).[9] The latter patients usually have refractory ascites and a better prognosis compared to those with type 1. In the majority of patients, HRS develops in the setting of advanced liver disease and in others, in the setting of acute liver failure. In either case these patients, particularly those with type 1 HRS are unstable and require hospitalization, preferrably in an intensive care unit.

PATIENT SURVIVAL WITH TYPE 1 AND 2 HRS

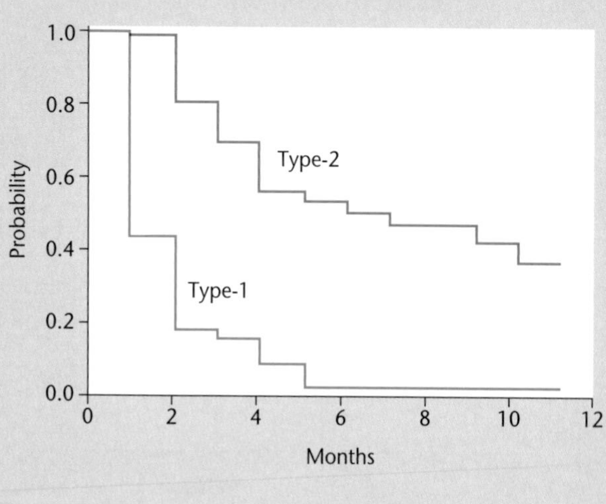

Fig. 97.3 Patient survival with type 1 and type 2 HRS. On average, patients with type 1 HRS have a median survival of 2 weeks whereas patients with type 2 HRS have a longer median survival time of approximately 6 months. Reproduced from Gines et al. Hepatorenal syndrome. The Lancet 2003; 362:1819-1827 with permission from Elsevier.

DIAGNOSTIC CRITERIA OF HEPATORENAL SYNDROME

MAJOR CRITERIA

- Low glomerular filtration rate, as indicated by serum creatinine greater than 1.5 mg/dL or 24-h creatinine clearance lower than 40 mL/min
- Absence of shock, ongoing bacterial infection, fluid losses, and current treatment with nephrotoxic drugs
- No sustained improvement in renal function (decrease in serum creatinine to 1.5 mg/dL or less or increase in creatinine clearance to 40 mL/min or more) following diuretic withdrawal and plasma volume expansion
- Proteinuria lower than 500 mg/day and no ultrasonographic eviden of obstructive uropathy or parenchymal renal disease

ADDITIONAL CRITERIA

- Urine volume lower than 500 mL/day
- Urine sodium lower than 10 mEq/L
- Urine osmolality greater than plasma osmolality
- Urine red blood cells less than 50 per high-power field
- Serum sodium concentration lower than 130 mEq/L

Accepted therapies for HRS include liver transplantati vasoconstrictors, and portosystemic shunts. Liver transplan tion is the best treatment for suitable candidates with HRS it offers a cure for both the diseased liver and the renal failu The presence of HRS is associated with increased morbid and early mortality after transplantation.

Although the use of renal vasodilator drugs such as dopam and prostaglandin analogs to treat HRS was adopted by ma physicians in the past, this practice has been progressiv abandoned during the last decade due to lack of data confir ing adequate benefit.[30] Other treatments such as endothe blockers (BQ123) and *N*-acetylcysteine have been reported, studies with larger numbers of patients are needed to confi their role in HRS.[31,32] Currently, the use of systemic vasoc strictors such as vasopressin analogs or alpha-adrenergic agoni in association with octreotide and human albumin seems to the most promising approach given that several uncontroll studies have confirmed their benefit in HRS.[9]

The most studied vasoconstrictor in HRS is terlipressin. Int venous terlipressin along with albumin as a plasma expan is associated with a significant improvement of renal functi and normalization of serum creatinine in approximately tw thirds of patients.[33–36] Administration of midodrine, an alp adrenergic agonist in association with octreotide, a glucag inhibitor, and albumin has also proved efficacious in HRS Nonetheless, octreotide alone does not improve HRS.[38] Fina norepinephrine (noradrenaline) in combination with albun expansion also improves renal function in HRS.[39] After st ping therapy, which typically lasts between 5 and 15 da recurrence is uncommon. Due to limited information and t possibility of ischemic side effects, treatment with vasoc strictors should probably be restricted to patients with type HRS. The main end-point of therapy is a reduction of ser creatinine below 1.5 mg/dL so that suitable transplant can dates can undergo transplantation without renal failure, whi may decrease morbidity and improve survival.[40] Nontra plant candidates may also benefit by reducing readmissio morbidity, and mortality, but this has not been proved. Final

TIPS may improve renal function in type 1 HRS.[41,42] However, the effects on renal function and the clinical course of patients after TIPS is variable; some have a delayed response whereas others do not respond at all. Although uncontrolled studies suggest that TIPS improves prognosis in type 1 and 2 HRS,[42] the impact on survival remains to be assessed. Hemodialysis is not routinely recommended in HRS; however, it may be reasonable to use in suitable liver transplant candidates as a bridge to transplantation when there is no response to vasoconstrictors or TIPS or patients develop severe volume overload, metabolic acidosis, or refractory hyperkalemia.

RECOMMENDATIONS FOR USING VASOCONSTRICTORS IN HEPATORENAL SYNDROME

- Total duration of treatment: 5–15 days
- Vasoconstrictors:
  - Terlipressin 0.5 mg intravenously every 4 h with an increase of the dose in a stepwise fashion (i.e., every 2–3 days) to 1 mg/4 h and then up to 2 mg/4 h in cases showing no response to therapy
  - Midodrine 7.5 mg orally three times daily with an increase to 12.5 mg three times daily if needed and octreotide 100 μg subcutaneously three times daily with an increase to 200 μg three times daily if needed
  - Norepinephrine (noradrenaline) 0.5–3 mg/h continuous intravenous infusion
- Intravenous albumin 1 g/kg on day 1, followed by 20–40 g/day

[a] Only major criteria are necessary for the diagnosis of hepatorenal syndrome.

PROGNOSIS

Although there are no established prognostic models for patients with cirrhosis and ascites there are some predictive factors related to renal and circulatory function that are useful in identifying candidates for liver transplantation. These factors include dilutional hyponatremia, marked hypotension, serum creatinine >1.2 mg/dL, and avid sodium retention (urine sodium less than 10 mEq/day).[43] However, the best and quickest way of identifying patients in need of liver transplantation is to recognize those with severe renal functional abnormalities such as refractory ascites or HRS. Interestingly, in patients with ascites, parameters of renal function and systemic hemodynamics are better predictors of prognosis than liver tests, such as albumin, bilirubin, and prothrombin time.

REFERENCES

1. Dawson A. Historical notes on ascites. Gastroenterology 1960; 39:790–791.
2. Reuben A. Out came copious water. Hepatology 2002; 36:261–264.
3. Ginès P, Quintero E, Arroyo V et al. Compensated cirrhosis: natural history and prognostic factors. Hepatology 1987; 7:122–128.
4. Ginès P, Fernández-Esparrach G. Prognosis of ascites. In: Arroyo V, Ginès P, Rodés J, Schrier RW, eds. Ascites and renal dysfunction in liver disease. Malden: Blackwell Science; 1999:431–441.
5. Martin PY, Ginès P, Schrier RW. Nitric oxide as a mediator of hemodynamic abnormalities and sodium and water retention in cirrhosis. N Engl J Med 1998; 339:533–541.
6. Cárdenas A, Bataller R, Arroyo V. Mechanisms of ascites formation. Clin Liver Dis 2000; 4: 447–465.
7. Jiménez W, Martínez-Pardo A, Arroyo V et al. Temporal relationship between hyperaldosteronism, sodium retention and ascites formation in rats with experimental cirrhosis. Hepatology 1985; 5:245–250.
8. Cárdenas A, Ginès P. Pathogenesis and treatment of dilutional hyponatremia in cirrhosis. In: Arroyo V, Forns X, Garcia-Pagan JC, Rodes J, eds. Progress in the treatment of liver diseases. Barcelona: Ars Medica; 2003:31–42.
9. Ginès P, Guevara M, Arroyo V, Rodés J. Hepatorenal syndrome: diagnosis and management. The Lancet 2003; 362:1819–1827.
10. Cárdenas A, Uriz J, Ginès P, Arroyo V. Hepatorenal syndrome. Liver Transpl 2000; 4 (Suppl 1):S63–71.
11. Ginès P, Cárdenas A, Schrier R. Liver disease and the kidney. In: Schrier R, ed. Diseases of the kidney and urinary tract, 7th edn. Philadelphia: Lippincott Williams & Wilkins; 2001:2167–2203.
12. Carithers RL, Jr. Liver transplantation. American Association for the Study of Liver Diseases. Liver Transpl 2000; 6:122–135.
13. Sherlock S, Dooley J. Ascites. In: Sherlock S, Dooley J, eds. Diseases of the liver and biliary system. Blackwell Science; 2002:127–146.
14. Moore KP, Wong F, Gines P et al. The management of ascites in cirrhosis: report on the consensus conference of the International Ascites Club. Hepatology 2003; 38:258–266.
15. Shear L, Ching S, Gabuzda GJ . Compartmentalization of ascites and edema in patients with hepatic cirrhosis. N Engl J Med 1970; 282: 1391–1396.
16. Ginès P, Arroyo V, Quintero E et al. Comparison of paracentesis and diuretics in the treatment of cirrhotics with tense ascites. Results of a randomized study. Gastroenterology 1987; 93:234–241.
17. Ruiz-del-Arbol L, Monescillo A, Jiménez W, Garcia-Plaza A, Arroyo V, Rodés J. Paracentesis-induced circulatory dysfunction: mechanism and effect on hepatic hemodynamics in cirrhosis. Gastroenterology 1997; 113:579–586.
18. Ginès P, Tito L, Arroyo V et al. Randomized comparative study of therapeutic paracentesis with and without intravenous albumin in cirrhosis. Gastroenterology 1988; 94:1493–1502.
19. Ginès A, Fernandez-Esparrach G, Monescillo A et al. Randomized trial comparing albumin, dextran 70, and polygeline in cirrhotic patients with ascites treated by paracentesis. Gastroenterology 1996; 111:1002–1010.
20. Arroyo V, Ginès P, Gerbes AL et al. Definition and diagnostic criteria of refractory ascites and hepatorenal syndrome in cirrhosis. International Ascites Club. Hepatology 1996; 23: 164–176.
21. Ginès P, Arroyo V, Vargas V et al. Paracentesis with intravenous infusion of albumin as compared with peritoneovenous shunting in cirrhosis with refractory ascites. N Engl J Med 1991; 325:829–835.
22. Ginès P, Uriz J, Calahorra B et al. Transjugular intrahepatic portosystemic shunting versus paracentesis plus albumin for refractory ascites in cirrhosis. Gastroenterology 2002; 123: 1839–1847.
23. Shiffman ML, Jeffers L, Hoofnagle JH, Tralka TS. The role of transjugular intrahepatic portosystemic shunt for treatment of portal hypertension and its complications: a conference sponsored by the National Digestive Diseases Advisory Board. Hepatology 1995; 22:1591–1597.
24. Casado M, Bosch J, Garcia-Pagan JC et al. Clinical events after transjugular intrahepatic portosystemic shunt: correlation with hemodynamic findings. Gastroenterology 1998; 114: 1296–1303.
25. Lebrec D, Giuily N, Hadengue A et al. Transjugular intrahepatic portosystemic shunts: comparison with paracentesis in patients with cirrhosis and refractory ascites: a randomized trial. J Hepatol 1996; 25:135–144.
26. Rossle M, Ochs A, Gulberg V et al. A comparison of paracentesis and transjugular intrahepatic portosystemic shunting in patients with ascites. N Engl J Med 2000; 342:1701–1707.
27. Sanyal A, Genning C, Reddy RK et al. The North American Study for Treatment of Refractory Ascites. Gastroenterology 2003; 124:634–641.
28. Wong F, Blei AT, Blendis LM, Thuluvath PJ. A vasopressin receptor antagonist (VPA-985) improves serum sodium concentration in patients with hyponatremia: a multicenter, randomized, placebo-controlled trial. Hepatology 2003; 37:182–191.
29. Gerbes AL, Gulberg V, Ginès P et al. VPA Study Group. Therapy of hyponatremia in cirrhosis with a vasopressin receptor antagonist: a randomized double-blind multicenter trial. Gastroenterology 2003; 124:933–939.
30. Arroyo V, Bataller R, Guevara M. Treatment of hepatorenal syndrome in cirrhosis. In: Arroyo V, Ginès P, Rodés J, Schrier RW, eds. Ascites and renal dysfunction in liver disease. Malden: Blackwell Science; 1999:492–510.

31. Soper CP, Latif AB, Bending MR. Amelioration of hepatorenal syndrome with selective endothelin-A antagonist. Lancet 1996; 347: 1842–1843.
32. Holt S, Goodier D, Marley R. Improvement in renal function in hepatorenal syndrome with N-acetylcysteine. Lancet 1999; 353:294–295.
33. Uriz J, Ginès P, Cardenas A et al. Terlipressin plus albumin infusion: an effective and safe therapy of hepatorenal syndrome. J Hepatol 2000; 33:43–48.
34. Moreau R, Durand F, Poynard T et al. Terlipressin in patients with cirrhosis and type 1 hepatorenal syndrome: a retrospective multicenter study. Gastroenterology 2002; 122: 923–930.
35. Solanki P, Chawla A, Garg R. Beneficial effects of terlipressin in hepatorenal syndrome: a prospective, randomized placebo-controlled clinical trial. J Gastroenterol Hepatol 2003; 18:152–156.
36. Halimi C, Bonnard P, Bernard B. Effect of terlipressin (Glypressin) on hepatorenal syndrome in cirrhotic patients: results of a multicentre pilot study. Eur J Gastroenterol Hepatol 2002; 14:153–158.
37. Angeli P, Volpin R, Gerunda G et al. Reversal of type 1 hepatorenal syndrome with the administration of midodrine and octreotide. Hepatology 1999; 29:1690–1697.
38. Pomier-Layrargues G, Paquin SC, Hassoun Z et al. Octreotide in hepatorenal syndrome: a randomized, double-blind, placebo-controlled, crossover study. Hepatology 2003; 38:238–243.
39. Duvoux C, Zanditenas D, Hezode C et al. Effects of noradrenalin and albumin in patients with type I hepatorenal syndrome: a pilot study. Hepatology 2002; 36:374–380.
40. Restuccia T, Ortega R, Guevara M et al. Treatment of hepatorenal syndrome before transplantation. Effect on posttransplantation outcome. J Hepatol 2004; 40:140–146.
41. Guevara M, Ginès P, Bandi JC et al. Transjugular intrahepatic portosystemic shunt in hepatorenal syndrome: effects on renal function and vasoactive systems. Hepatology 1998; 28:416–422.
42. Brensing KA, Textor J, Perz J et al. Long term outcome after transjugular intrahepatic portosystemic stent-shunt in non-transplant cirrhotics with hepatorenal syndrome: a phase II study. Gut 2000; 47:288–295.
43. Llach J, Ginès P, Arroyo V et al. Prognostic value of arterial pressure, endogenous vasoactive systems, and renal function in cirrhotic patients admitted to the hospital for the treatment of ascites. Gastroenterology 1988; 94:482–487.

Chapter 98

Spontaneous bacterial peritonitis

Guadalupe Garcia-Tsao

KEY POINTS

- Cirrhotic patients develop bacterial infections at a higher rate than hospitalized patients at large (~30% vs 6%) and the most common is spontaneous bacterial peritonitis (SBP)
- SBP is an infection of ascites in the absence of a contiguous source of infection (e.g., intestinal perforation, abscess)
- The most common bacteria responsible for SBP are aerobic Gram-negative organisms, with *E. coli* being the predominant organism
- Patients with a poor liver function are particularly susceptible to develop SBP (and other bacterial infections); a low ascites protein content (<1.0 g/dL) is an independent predictor of SBP development
- Hepatic hydrothorax results from passage of ascites into the pleural space; this fluid can also become infected (spontaneous bacterial empyema); an entity that has identical implications as SBP and that can occur in the absence of SBP or ascites
- Early detection, prompt antibiotic therapy and, in selected cases, volume expansion with albumin, have been key factors in reducing SBP-related mortality
- Patients who recover from an episode of SBP are at a high risk of developing recurrence of SBP (70% at 1 year)
- Median survival in patients who develop SBP is ~9 months and therefore these patients require prompt liver transplant evaluation

INTRODUCTION

Spontaneous bacterial peritonitis (SBP) is an infection of ascites characteristic of the cirrhotic patient that occurs in the absence of hollow viscus perforation and in the absence of an intra-abdominal inflammatory focus such as an abscess, acute pancreatitis, or cholecystitis. The term SBP is restricted to the primary peritonitis that develops in a cirrhotic patient. The entity was first recognized in the early 1900s; however, it was not fully characterized until 1971, when the term SBP was first coined.[1] Although an infecting organism can be isolated from ascitic fluid in over half the patients, a percentage of cirrhotic patients with SBP have evidence of peritoneal inflammation (elevated ascites polymorphonuclear cell count) but an organism cannot be isolated from ascites fluid. Since culture-negative SBP has the same implications as culture-positive SBP, in the following discussion the term SBP encompasses both entities.

EPIDEMIOLOGY

Recent large prospective series report bacterial infection rates in cirrhotic patients (either at the time of admission or during hospitalization) of 32–34%.[2] These figures contrast with a 5–7% infection rate reported in hospitalized patients at large. SBP is the most common type of infection, accounting for about 25% of all infections in hospitalized cirrhotic patients (37% of infections in those with ascites). More than half of the episodes of SBP are detected at the time of admission to the hospital while the rest develop during hospitalization. The prevalence of SBP appears to be lower in the outpatient setting where a 3.5% rate of SBP was reported in a retrospective study of patients subjected to serial therapeutic paracenteses.[3] In prospective studies, the 12-month incidence of first episode of SBP in cirrhotic patients with ascites ranges between 11%[4] and 29%.[5] Incidence is highly dependent on ascites total protein content (0% in patients with an ascites protein >1 g/dL vs 20% in patients with an ascites protein <1 g/dL).[4]

CAUSES, RISK FACTORS, DISEASE ASSOCIATIONS

Two factors are predictive of the development of bacterial infections in hospitalized cirrhotic patients: the severity of the liver disease and admission for gastrointestinal (GI) hemorrhage.

Studies uniformly show that patients who develop SBP have a greater impairment in liver function than patients with ascites who do not develop this complication. Liver synthetic function tests correlate with serum and ascites complement levels that in turn correlate with opsonic activity, a critical element in bacterial phagocytosis. Therefore, with more severe liver dysfunction there is a greater impairment in antibacterial defense mechanisms. Ascites protein has been shown to correlate very closely with ascites complement levels and with ascites opsonic activity,[6] accounting for the importance of ascites protein levels as predictive of the development of SBP.

In addition to a low ascites protein, two other parameters have been related to a higher risk of developing SBP, a high serum bilirubin (>3.2 mg/dL) and a low platelet count (<98 000/mm^3),[7] both of which are indicative of a more severe liver disease.[8] High-risk patients defined using these parameters have a high (55%) 1-year probability of developing a first episode of SBP.

SBP is monomicrobial in over 90% of cases. Aerobic Gram-negative organisms are responsible for the great majority (72–80%) of cases, *Escherichia coli* being the most frequently isolated organism. The next most frequent microorganisms isolated in SBP are Gram-positive cocci, mainly *Streptococcus* sp. (20%) with enterococci accounting for 5% of cases. Blood cultures are positive in roughly half the cases of SBP.

PATHOGENESIS

Given the predominance of enteric organisms isolated from ascites, bacterial translocation (passage of viable microorganisms from the intestinal lumen to mesenteric lymph nodes and other extraintestinal sites) has been postulated as the initial mechanism in the pathogenesis of SBP.[9] Experimental studies demonstrate that translocation to mesenteric lymph nodes occurs only in cirrhotic animals with ascites (which have a more impaired liver function) and is always present in those with infected ascites.[9] The decreased incidence of SBP by the use of orally administered nonabsorbable antibiotics (selective intestinal decontamination) is compatible with a causal relationship between bacterial translocation and development of bacterial infections in cirrhosis.[10–12]

The presence of bacteremia in half the cases of SBP and the occurrence of isolated bacteremia in cirrhotic patients without an obvious primary focus of infection (spontaneous bacteremia), suggest that bacteria gain access to the systemic circulation prior to infecting the peritoneal fluid.

Cirrhotics have an acquired deficiency in antibacterial activity and this explains their increased susceptibility to develop bacterial translocation and bacteremia, even when bacteria are arising from sources other than the gut (Fig. 98.1). The reticuloendothelial system (RES) is the main defensive system against bacteremia and is located in the liver where Kupffer cells (tissue macrophages) are its major components. In cirrhosis, the phagocytic activity of the RES is altered because of portosystemic shunting and because of a decreased bactericidal activity of Kupffer cells. Additionally, low serum complement levels lead to decreased peripheral bactericidal activity. This decreased antibacterial activity would explain how a transient bacteremia (arising from the gut or other sources) would become persistent (Fig. 98.1). In the patient with ascites, bacteria present in the systemic circulation will reach ascites and, once microorganisms colonize ascites, the development of SBP will depend on the defensive capacity of the fluid. Low ascites complement lead to decreased ascites bactericidal activity and to a greater risk for SBP (Fig. 98.1).[6]

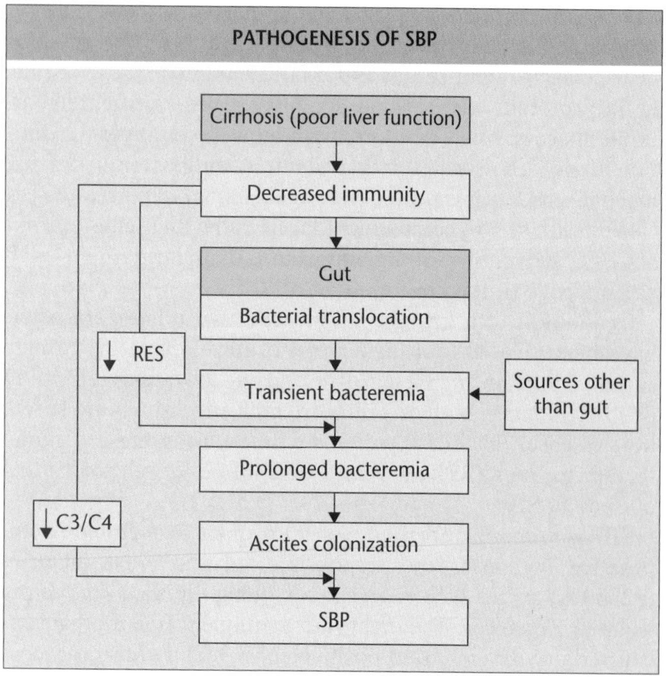

Fig. 98.1 Pathogenesis of SBP. RES, reticuloendothelial system; C3/C4, complement (fractions 3 and 4) levels.

CLINICAL PRESENTATION

SBP usually presents in a patient with overt ascites; however, it has been described in patients with ascites detectable only by ultrasound.

The typical features of SBP consist of symptoms and signs of a generalized peritonitis, that is, diffuse abdominal pain, fever, abdominal tenderness with rebound tenderness, and decreased bowel sounds. However, patients rarely present with the complete picture and single elements of the typical presentation occur more frequently, with isolated fever or abdominal pain being the most frequent presenting manifestations. Patients may present with other less typical signs and symptoms such as hypothermia, hypotension, and diarrhea. The presence of unexplained encephalopathy and/or deterioration in renal function in a patient with ascites should always raise the suspicion of SBP. Similarly, peripheral leukocytosis with a shift to the left, even in the absence of symptoms/signs of SBP should also raise the suspicion of SBP.

CLINICAL PRESENTATION

- SBP generally presents in a cirrhotic patient with overt ascites
- Typical symptoms/signs are those of generalized peritoneal inflammation, i.e., abdominal pain, fever, decreased or absent abdominal sounds, and rebound tenderness
- Patients with SBP may, however, be entirely asymptomatic or will present with unexplained encephalopathy and/or deterioration in renal function
- Renal dysfunction is the main complication of SBP

DIFFERENTIAL DIAGNOSIS

The majority of cirrhotic patients with ascites and peritoneal infection have SBP. However, a small group of patients have a peritonitis that is secondary to hollow viscus perforation, a contiguous abscess (e.g., perinephric), or an intra-abdominal inflammatory process (e.g., acute pancreatitis or cholecystitis). With the exception of peritonitis secondary to the latter condition, in which the precise nature of peritoneal infection can be more or less easily established, the differential diagnosis between SBP and secondary peritonitis is difficult. The differentiation is important because secondary peritonitis usually requires surgical intervention and the decision to undertake surgery has to be a careful one as surgery can lead to further deterioration of an already decompensated cirrhotic patient. The presence of secondary bacterial peritonitis should be suspected primarily when a suspected SBP fails to respond to antibiotic therapy, that is, lack of a significant decrease (or even an increase) in ascites PMN in the follow-up paracentesis performed 2 days after initiating therapy. Secondary peritonitis can be suspected earlier when more than one organism is isolated from ascites (particularly when anaerobic bacteria and/or fungi are isolated). It has been postulated that patients o have two of the following ascites findings, glucose <50 mg/dL, otein >1.0 g/dL, or LDH >normal serum levels, have a higher obability of having secondary peritonitis[13] and that ascites cinoembryonic antigen and alkaline phosphatase levels may markers of intestinal perforation; however, the usefulness these tests has not been validated.

Another condition that should be distinguished from SBP is acterascites,' that is, a positive ascites bacteriological culture the absence of an inflammatory reaction in the peritoneal id (i.e., normal PMN count). This most likely represents the ase of ascites colonization (Fig. 98.1) and could evolve to P or resolve spontaneously. Once the diagnosis of bacterascites made (usually 2–4 days after the paracentesis, when the micro-ological results are available), it is recommended to repeat paracentesis for PMN count and culture. If the patient has idence of infection (fever, leukocytosis) at this time, if the IN count is now compatible with SBP, or if the culture con-ues to be positive, initiation of antibiotic therapy is warranted.

DIFFERENTIAL DIAGNOSIS

- The main entity to be considered in the differential diagnosis of SBP is secondary bacterial peritonitis, i.e., a peritoneal infection secondary to a local source of infection, such as an abscess or intestinal perforation, which usually requires surgical intervention
- Secondary bacterial peritonitis should be suspected when a suspected SBP fails to respond to antibiotic therapy
- Secondary bacterial peritonitis should also be suspected upon finding multiple organisms on culture, particularly if anaerobes or fungi are among the infecting organisms
- Upon suspecting secondary bacterial peritonitis, work-up should be continued with imaging studies (abdominal computed tomography)
- A positive ascites culture in the absence of an elevated ascites PMN count (bacterascites) is not equivalent to SBP and should lead to repeat diagnostic paracentesis to confirm the finding

IAGNOSTIC METHODS

s outlined recently,[14] a diagnostic paracentesis should be per-rmed in: (1) any patient with cirrhosis and ascites admitted the hospital; (2) any cirrhotic patient that develops symp-ms or signs compatible with SBP; and (3) any cirrhotic patient ith worsening renal function and/or hepatic encephalopathy. patients with hepatic hydrothorax in whom an infection is ispected and in whom SBP has been ruled out, a diagnostic oracentesis should be performed to rule out spontaneous acterial empyema, an entity akin to SBP that may occur in e absence of ascites or SBP.[15] In patients with clinically ndetectable ascites in whom SBP is suspected, an abdominal trasound should be obtained to determine whether fluid can e obtained for analysis.

Although isolation of an infecting organism is definitive in stablishing the diagnosis of SBP, ascites cultures are negative up to 60% of patients with clinical manifestations com-atible with SBP and increased ascites polymorphonuclear cell PMN) counts despite the use of sensitive culture methods. herefore, the diagnosis of SBP is established when objective vidence of a peritoneal inflammatory reaction is present, i.e., n elevated ascites PMN count. The highest diagnostic accuracy is obtained with a cutoff at 250/mm^3 and therefore the diagnosis of SBP is currently defined as an ascites PMN count >250/mm^3. This count is performed manually in most laboratories and may not be available in all hospitals after hours. An alternative to manual PMN counting is the use of reactive strips for leukocyte esterase that has been reported as having a 98% positive predictive value;[16] however, local validation may be necessary.

Bacteriological cultures of ascites (10 mL inoculated into blood culture bottles) and blood cultures should be obtained prior to the initiation of therapy.

If and when secondary bacterial peritonitis is suspected, imaging studies should be performed, mainly abdominal computed tomography.

DIAGNOSTIC METHODS

- SBP should be suspected and a diagnostic paracentesis should be performed in any cirrhotic patient with ascites: (1) at admission; (2) in the presence of any symptom or sign suggestive of SBP (pain, tenderness, fever, ileus); and (3) in the presence of renal dysfunction and/or hepatic encephalopathy
- The diagnosis of SBP is based on the ascites polymorphonuclear cell count; a cell count of >250/mm^3 is diagnostic of SBP
- Ascites (in blood culture bottles) and blood cultures should be performed upon the suspicion of SBP to maximize the possibilities of isolating an infecting organism
- Reactive strip agents appear to be reasonable alternatives to cell count when manual cell count is not immediately available

TREATMENT AND PREVENTION

Treatment: Management recommendations in these areas are based on evidence in the literature and the results of a consensus conference on the diagnosis and management of SBP sponsored by the International Ascites Club.[14] Once an ascitic (or pleural) fluid PMN count >250/mm^3 is detected, antibiotic therapy needs to be started (Table 98.1) before obtaining bacteriological culture results. The most effective, safe, and overall accepted drug is cefotaxime (or other third generation cephalosporin) administered intravenously (at a minimum dose of 2 g every 12 h) with which the overall resolution of SBP occurs in approximately 80–90% of the patients (Table 98.1).[17] The combination of amoxicillin and clavulanic acid administered intravenously has been shown to be as effective and safe as cefotaxime.[18] In patients with community-acquired SBP, no encephalopathy, and a normal renal function, oral ofloxacin is an acceptable alternative,[19] provided that the local prevalence of quinolone-resistant organisms is low. Cirrhotic patients are particularly prone to develop nephrotoxicity from aminoglycosides and therefore their use should be avoided.[20] Treatment should be administered for a minimum of 5 days, although the median time to resolution of SBP is 8 days in prospective trials and this is probably a 'safer' length of time (Table 98.1). A control paracentesis performed 48 h after starting therapy is recommended to assess the response to therapy and the need to modify antibiotic therapy (depending on the isolation of a causative organism) and/or to initiate investigations to rule out secondary peritonitis. Failure of initial therapy occurs in up to 23%

TABLE 98.1 ANTIBIOTIC TREATMENT FOR SPONTANEOUS BACTERIAL PERITONITIS

First Author	Year published	SBP episodes	Initial antibiotic	Overall SBP resolution[a]	Failure of initial antibiotic[b]	Cases resolved after modifying initial antibiotic	Days to resolution	In-hospital mortality
Felisart[23]	1985	22	Cefotaxime (2g/4h)	19 (86%)	5/33 (15%)	9%	NR	NR
Runyon[24]	1991	47	Cefotaxime (2g/8h/10days)	41 (87%)	6 (13%)	4%	–	20 (42%)
		43	Cefotaxime (2g/8h/5days)	40 (93%)	3 (7%)	5%	–	14 (33%)
Gomez-Jimenez[25]	1993	30	Cefonicid (2g/12h)	26 (87%)	6 (20%)	0	8.4	11 (37%)
		30	Ceftriaxone (2g/24h)	28 (93%)	2 (7%)	–	9.1	9 (30%)
Rimola[26]	1995	66	Cefotaxime (2g/6h)	53 (80%)	15 (23%)	3%	9.0	22/71 (31%
		70	Cefotaxime (2g/12h)	60 (86%)	15 (21%)	7%	8.8	15/72 (21%
Ricart[27]	2000	24	Cefotaxime (1g/6h)	20 (83%)$^{+}$	5 (21%)	12.5%	8.0	5 (21%)
		24	Amoxicillin/ clavulanate	21 (88%)$^{+}$	5 (21%)	17%	8.1	3 (12%)
Navasa[28]	1996	64[c]	Cefotaxime	54 (92%)	9 (17%)	6%	7.0	11 (17%)
		59[c]	Ofloxacin	61 (95%)	10 (17%)	12%	8.0	12 (20%)
Sort[36]	2000	63[c]	Cefotaxime	59 (94%)	10 (16%)	10%	6.0	18 (29%)
		63[c]	Cefotaxime[d] albumin	62 (98%)	6 (10%)	8%	5.0	6 (10%)

Results are from randomized clinical trials in which antibiotic schedules resulted in SBP resolution rates ≥80% (reproduced with permission from Garcia-Tsao G. Treatment of spontaneous bacterial peritonitis. In: Arroyo et al., Therapy in hepatology. Barcelona: Ars Medica).
NR, not reported for SBP.
[a] Includes resolution after modification of initial antibiotic therapy.
[b] Failure defined by one or more of the following: clinical symptoms and signs not improving or worsening, nonsignificant reduction in ascites on repeat paracentesis 2–3 days later, isolation of a nonsusceptible pathogen, superinfection (new, nonsusceptible pathogen), severe side effect, or death during therapy. Failure would lead to modification in antibiotic unless cause is death.
[c] Uncomplicated SBP.
[d] Only response to initial antibiotic is reported.

of cases (Table 98.1). In the presence of an obvious clinical improvement, this control paracentesis may not be necessary. Intravenous antibiotics can be safely switched to oral antibiotics after 2 days of therapy and once a response to therapy is demonstrated by a decrease in ascites PMN.

Prevention of SBP is currently based on selective intestinal decontamination with nonabsorbable or poorly absorbable antibiotics against Gram-negative organisms. Cost issues aside, the complications of long-term unrestricted antibiotic prophylaxis are well known and include the emergence of resistant bacterial strains and the change in the spectrum of bacteria causing SBP (and other infections). There are two subsets of cirrhotic patients who are at a high risk of developing SBP and in whom antibiotic prophylaxis has been shown to be effective. These are patients who have recovered from an episode of SBP and patients admitted with gastrointestinal (GI) hemorrhage.

Prophylaxis: Cirrhotic patients who have recovered from an episode of SBP obviously possess the necessary risk factors for its development and therefore their probability of developing a second episode is elevated, around 70% over the next year.[21] In patients with previous SBP, prophylaxis has been shown decrease the recurrence of SBP to 20%, a striking benefici effect. Based on this study, one can justify the use of proph lactic antibiotics in this subset of patients, even though there no data on patient survival. The antibiotic used is norfloxacin a dose of 400 mg orally every day. The use of weekly quinolon has been shown to be less effective in preventing SBP recu rence and is therefore not recommended. Prophylaxis shou be continuous until disappearance of ascites (i.e., patients wi alcoholic hepatitis), death, or transplant.

Cirrhotic patients with GI hemorrhage develop infections (SB and other) during hospitalization at high rates ranging betwee 35% and 66%. Short-term (7 days) antibiotic prophylaxis in the patients has been uniformly found to be effective not only preventing bacterial infections but also in reducing in-hospit mortality.[22] Based on these results, antibiotic prophylaxis this subset of patients should be routinely used. The preferre antibiotic is norfloxacin at a dose of 400 mg orally twice a da for 7 days (or less if patient is to be discharged from the hospital

Currently, there are insufficient data to support the use of lon term antibiotic prophylaxis in cirrhotic patients with ascit ho are not bleeding and who have not had a previous episode f SBP, independent of its protein content.

TREATMENT AND PREVENTION

- The recommended empirical antibiotics for SBP are third generation cephalosporins or the combination of a beta-lactam/beta-lactamase
- Aminoglycosides should be avoided in cirrhotic patients as they are prone to develop nephrotoxicity
- Duration of antibiotic therapy should be for a minimum of 5 days, but a prudent length is probably 8 days
- The use of albumin infusion (to increase effective arterial volume) has been shown to decrease development of renal dysfunction and to improve survival in SBP
- At least one repeat paracentesis should be performed 2 days after starting antibiotics; a decrease in PMN <25% from baseline and/or deterioration in clinical condition define treatment failure
- Long-term antibiotic prophylaxis with norfloxacin is warranted in patients who have recovered from an episode of SBP
- Short-term antibiotic prophylaxis with norfloxacin is warranted in patients admitted with gastrointestinal hemorrhage
- There is not enough evidence to support the use of antibiotics for primary prophylaxis of SBP, particularly given the rise in quinolone- and bactrim-resistant organisms in chronic norfloxacin users

OMPLICATIONS AND THEIR MANAGEMENT

ne of the most serious complications and the most important redictor of death in patients with SBP is the development of enal impairment, which occurs in about a third of the patients. t has been considered that renal impairment occurs as a result f a decrease in effective arterial blood volume. With the bjective of determining whether plasma volume expansion an prevent renal impairment, a randomized study comparing efotaxime + albumin vs cefotaxime alone was performed in atients with SBP.[23] While the rate of infection resolution was he same in both groups, patients that received albumin had ignificantly lower rates of renal dysfunction (10% vs 33%), n-hospital mortality (10% vs 29%), and 3-month mortality 22% vs 41%) compared to patients who did not receive lbumin. The inpatient mortality rate of 10% is the lowest lescribed so far for SBP (Table 98.1). The dose of albumin used was arbitrary, 1.5 g/kg of body weight during the first 6 h, followed by 1 g/kg on day 3. The group of patients that appeared to be more likely to benefit from the addition of albumin was characterized by having a serum bilirubin >4 mg/dL and evidence of renal impairment at baseline (blood urea nitrogen (BUN) >30 mg/dL and/or creatinine >1.0 mg/dL), and this is the population of patients in whom albumin should be currently recommended.

The development of infections by quinolone-resistant organisms is the main complication of long-term norfloxacin prophylaxis. A recent study performed in a large number of cirrhotic patients hospitalized with an infection demonstrated that Gram-negative bacteria isolated from patients on long-term quinolone prophylaxis were significantly more likely to be not only quinolone-resistant but also trimethoprim/sulfamethoxazole-resistant compared to patients not on prophylaxis. Patients who develop SBP on prophylactic quinolones have been shown to respond as well to cefotaxime as patients not on prophylaxis. Experimental studies using nonantibiotic maneuvers such as probiotics (*Lactobacillus*) have been shown to be ineffective in reducing bacterial translocation but others using cisapride[24] and conjugated bile acids[25] seem hopeful.

PROGNOSIS WITH AND WITHOUT TREATMENT

In initial series published in the 1970s, the mortality associated with an episode of SBP exceeded 80%. In prospective studies from the last decade, with well-defined criteria for the diagnosis of SBP, the mortality rate has been reported as being around 20–30% (Table 98.1). This decrease in mortality is the result of an increased awareness and early detection of the entity with prompt initiation of antibiotic therapy.

Lower mortalities have been observed in series that included patients with 'uncomplicated' SBP defined as those without GI hemorrhage, severe encephalopathy, ileus, or septic shock and a creatinine at diagnosis <3 mg/dL (Table 98.1). Notably, a 100% cure and survival with antibiotic therapy alone is reported in patients with uncomplicated SBP who additionally have community-acquired SBP, no encephalopathy, and a BUN at diagnosis <25 mg/dL.[19]

Median survival in patients who develop SBP is ~9 months and it is uncertain whether it is affected by prophylaxis or albumin. Therefore, patients who have developed an episode of SBP require prompt liver transplant evaluation.

REFERENCES

1. Conn HO, Fessel JM. Spontaneous bacterial peritonitis in cirrhosis: variations on a theme. Medicine 1971; 50:161–197.
2. Fernandez J, Navasa M, Gomez J et al. Bacterial infections in cirrhosis: epidemiological changes with invasive procedures and norfloxacin prophylaxis. Hepatology 2002; 35: 140–148.
3. Evans LT, Kim WR, Poterucha JJ, Kamath PS. Spontaneous bacterial peritonitis in asymptomatic outpatients with cirrhotic ascites. Hepatology 2003; 37:897–901.
4. Llach J, Rimola A, Navasa M et al. Incidence and predictive factors of first episode of spontaneous bacterial peritonitis in cirrhosis with ascites: relevance of ascitic fluid protein concentration. Hepatology 1992; 16:724–727.
5. Andreu M, Sola R, Sitges-Serra A et al. Risk factors for spontaneous bacterial peritonitis in cirrhotic patients with ascites. Gastroenterology 1993; 104:1133–1138.
6. Runyon BA, Morrissey RL, Hoefs JC, Wyle FA. Opsonic activity of human ascitic fluid: a potentially important protective mechanism against spontaneous bacterial peritonitis. Hepatology 1985; 5:634–637.
7. Guarner C, Sola R, Soriano G et al. Risk of a first community-acquired spontaneous bacterial peritonitis in cirrhotics with low ascitic fluid protein levels. Gastroenterology 1999; 117: 414–419.
8. Garcia-Tsao G. Identifying new risk factors for spontaneous bacterial peritonitis: how important is it? Gastroenterology 1999; 117: 495–499.
9. Garcia-Tsao G, Lee FY, Barden GE et al. Bacterial translocation to mesenteric lymph nodes is increased in cirrhotic rats with ascites. Gastroenterology 1995; 108:1835–1841.
10. Soriano G, Guarner C, Tomas A et al. Norfloxacin prevents bacterial infection in cirrhotics with gastrointestinal hemorrhage. Gastroenterology 1992; 103:1267–1272.
11. Gines P, Rimola A, Planas R et al. Norfloxacin prevents spontaneous bacterial peritonitis recurrence in cirrhosis: results of a double-blind,

placebo-controlled trial. Hepatology 1990; 12:716–724.
12. Grange JD, Roulot D, Pelletier G et al. Norfloxacin primary prophylaxis of bacterial infections in cirrhotic patients with ascites – A double-blind randomized trial. J Hepatol 1998; 29:430–436.
13. Akriviadis EA, Runyon BA. Utility of an algorithm in differentiating spontaneous from secondary bacterial peritonitis. Gastroenterology 1990; 98:127–133.
14. Rimola A, Garcia-Tsao G, Navasa M et al. Diagnosis, treatment and prophylaxis of spontaneous bacterial peritonitis: a consensus document. J Hepatol 2000; 32:142–153.
15. Xiol X, Castellvi JM, Guardiola J et al. Spontaneous bacterial empyema in cirrhotic patients: a prospective study. Hepatology 1996; 23: 719–723.
16. Castellote J, Lopez C, Gornals J et al. Rapid diagnosis of spontaneous bacterial peritonitis by use of reagent strips. Hepatology 2003; 37:893–896.
17. Runyon BA, McHutchison JG, Antillon MR et al. Short-course versus long-course antibiotic treatment of spontaneous bacterial peritonitis. Gastroenterology 1991; 100:1737–1742.
18. Ricart E, Soriano G, Novella M et al. Amoxicillin-clavulanic acid versus cefotaxime in the therapy of bacterial infections in cirrhotic patients. J Hepatol 2000; 32:596–602.
19. Navasa M, Follo A, Llovet JM et al. Randomized, comparative study of oral ofloxacin versus intravenous cefotaxime in spontaneous bacterial peritonitis. Gastroenterology 1996; 111:1011–1017.
20. Garcia-Tsao G. Further evidence against the use of aminoglycosides in cirrhotic patients. Gastroenterology 1998; 114:612–613.
21. Tito L, Rimola A, Gines P et al. Recurrence of spontaneous bacterial peritonitis in cirrhosis: frequency and predictive factors. Hepatology 1988; 8:27–31.
22. Bernard B, Grange JD, Khac EN et al. Antibiotic prophylaxis for the prevention of bacterial infections in cirrhotic patients with gastrointestinal bleeding: a meta-analysis. Hepatology 1999; 29:1655–1661.
23. Sort P, Navasa M, Arroyo V et al. Effect of intravenous albumin on renal impairment and mortality in patients with cirrhosis and spontaneous bacterial peritonitis. N Engl J Med 1999; 341:403–409.
24. Pardo A, Bartoli R, Lorenzo-Zuniga V et al. Effect of cisapride on intestinal bacterial overgrowth and bacterial translocation in cirrhosis. Hepatology 2000; 31:858–863.
25. Lorenzo-Zuniga V, Bartoli R, Planas R et al. Oral bile acids reduce bacterial overgrowth, bacterial translocation, and endotoxemia in cirrhotic rats. Hepatology 2003; 37:551–557

Chapter 99

Hepatopulmonary syndrome and portopulmonary hypertension

Miguel R Arguedas and Michael B Fallon

KEY POINTS

Hepatopulmonary syndrome
- Intrapulmonary vasodilatation
- Develops with hepatic synthetic dysfunction and/or portal hypertension
- Present in 8–20% of patients with cirrhosis
- Liver transplantation generally curative

Portopulmonary hypertension
- Intrapulmonary vasoconstriction and arterial remodeling
- Develops in the setting of portal hypertension
- Present in 3–12% of patients with advanced liver disease
- Liver transplantation generally contraindicated

INTRODUCTION

Pulmonary dysfunction in liver disease has been noted for more than 100 years. Two distinct pulmonary vascular disorders have emerged over the last 15 years as important complications in patients with hepatic dysfunction or portal hypertension. The hepatopulmonary syndrome (HPS) occurs when intrapulmonary vasodilatation causes a widened age-corrected alveolar–arterial oxygen gradient with or without hypoxemia.[1] Portopulmonary hypertension (POPH) results when pulmonary arterial constriction and remodeling lead to increased pulmonary arterial pressure.[2] The presence of HPS and POPH increase morbidity and mortality in patients with liver disease. Liver transplantation is effective in HPS whereas it is currently contraindicated in patients with moderate or severe POPH.

EPIDEMIOLOGY

HPS is more common than POPH. As many as 40–50% of patients with cirrhosis have evidence of intrapulmonary vasodilatation using contrast echocardiography and 8–20% will have sufficient vasodilatation to cause hypoxemia and fulfill criteria for HPS.[1] POPH appears to occur in 1–2% of patients with portal hypertension, although in patients evaluated for liver transplantation, the prevalence may be higher (3–12%).

CAUSES, RISK FACTORS, DISEASE ASSOCIATIONS

HPS and POPH are found most commonly in the setting of cirrhosis and portal hypertension. Recently, the spectrum of abnormalities associated with the development of HPS has broadened to include portal hypertension without cirrhosis (hepatic venous outflow obstruction, prehepatic portal hypertension) and hepatic dysfunction in the absence of established portal hypertension (acute and chronic hepatitis). The presence and severity of POPH does not appear to correlate with the degree of hepatic dysfunction or portal hypertension. Controversy exists regarding whether HPS is more common or severe in patients with advanced cirrhosis.

PATHOGENESIS AND PATHOLOGY

The pathogenesis of HPS and POPH are incompletely understood. Since either disorder can develop in the setting of cirrhosis and portal hypertension, they may share pathogenetic mechanisms. Potential mechanisms common to both disorders include effects mediated by shear stress, cytokine and endothelin-1 alterations occurring in liver disease (Fig. 99.1). In human HPS, nitric oxide overproduction appears to contribute to intrapulmonary vasodilatation.[3] In experimental HPS, both endothelin-1-induced endothelial nitric oxide synthase activation and intravascular macrophage accumulation and production of nitric oxide and carbon monoxide trigger vasodilatation.[4–6] Less is known about the underlying mechanisms for POPH and no experimental models have been developed. However, shear stress, vasoactive mediator, genetic and inflammatory effects leading to endothelial dysfunction, and smooth muscle cell proliferation have been postulated based on studies in primary pulmonary hypertension.[2] One emerging hypothesis is that the pulmonary endothelial response to liver disease and portal hypertension (nitric oxide overproduction in HPS versus dysfunction and injury in POPH) is important in determining whether HPS or POPH develops.

CLINICAL PRESENTATION

Dyspnea is the most common complaint in patients with either HPS or POPH. However, moderate to severe HPS or POPH may be present in the absence of dyspnea. Patients with HPS typically complain of the insidious onset of exertional dyspnea, which progresses. Platypnea (an increase in dyspnea when standing), spider angiomata, cyanosis, and clubbing are often found in moderate to severe HPS and may increase the clinical suspicion for the diagnosis.[7] Clubbing appears to be a relatively specific finding in HPS (Fig. 99.2). POPH appears to be more commonly asymptomatic, is infrequently associated with cyanosis or marked hypoxemia, and is not associated with platypnea. Chest discomfort and syncope are features of advanced POPH. An elevated jugular venous pressure, an accentuated P2 component or a tricuspid regurgitation murmur may be found on examination in POPH. Lower extremity edema out of proportion to ascites may be observed as POPH progresses.

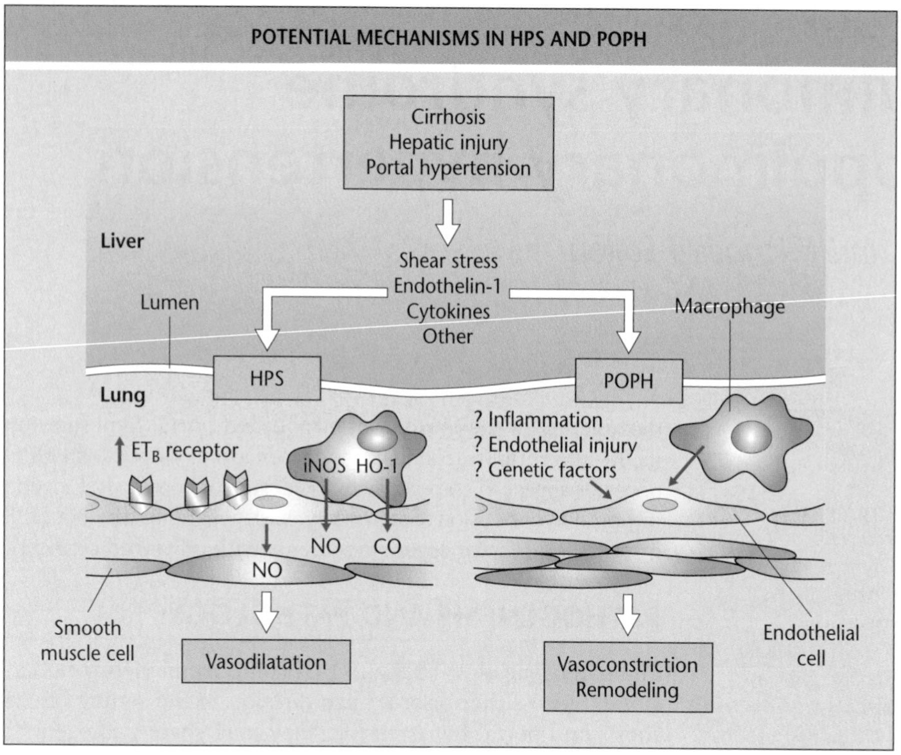

Fig. 99.1 Potential mechanisms in HPS and POPH. Liver injury and/or portal hypertension trigger alterations that influence the production and release of vasoactive mediators and cytokines and modulate vascular shear stress. In experimental HPS, hepatic endothelin-1 release stimulates pulmonary vascular endothelial nitric oxide synthase derived nitric oxide (NO) production through an increased number of endothelin B receptors (ET_B receptor) leading to vasodilatation. Macrophages also accumulate in the vascular lumen and produce NO from inducible nitric oxide synthase (iNOS) and carbon monoxide (CO) from heme oxygenase-1 (HO-1) contributing to vasodilatation. In POPH, similar events possibly modified by genetic factors and the inflammatory response may result in endothelial injury and smooth muscle proliferation with vascular remodeling.

DIFFERENTIAL DIAGNOSIS

Dyspnea is a common symptom in cirrhosis and has multiple causes. For clinical purposes, these causes may be grouped into those arising due to the presence of liver disease and those independent of the presence of liver disease. Specifically, decompensated liver disease may be associated with deconditioning, muscle wasting, tense ascites, and/or hepatic hydrothorax and certain specific causes of cirrhosis may be associated with lung injury. The most common causes of intrinsic cardiopulmonary disease are chronic obstructive pulmonary disease and congestive heart failure. It is important to recognize that both HPS and POPH may coexist with these other causes of dyspnea and hypoxemia.[8]

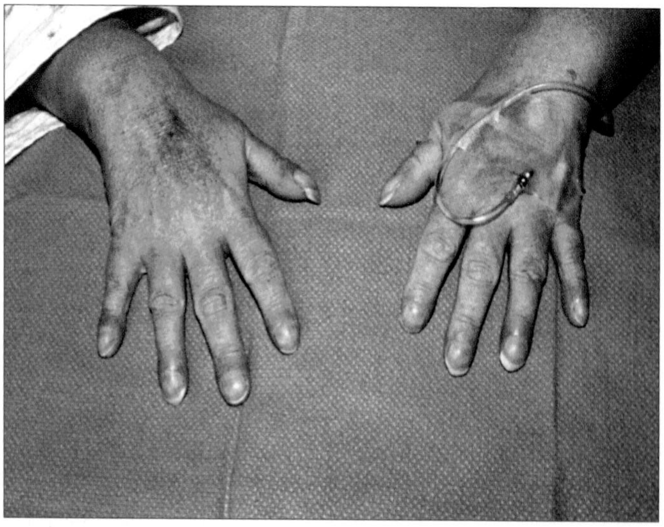

Fig. 99.2 Digital clubbing in a patient with HPS. Clubbing appears to be a relatively specific clinical marker for the presence of HPS.

CLINICAL PRESENTATION

Hepatopulmonary syndrome	Portopulmonary hypertension
Often asymptomatic but symptoms include:	Often asymptomatic but symptoms include:
Dyspnea (most common)	Dyspnea (most common)
Platypnea	Chest pain
	Syncope
Signs:	Signs:
Spider angiomata	Jugular distention
Digital clubbing	Accentuated P2
Cyanosis	Tricuspid regurgitation murmur
	Anasarca
Symptoms/signs may correlate with severity of underlying cirrhosis	Symptoms/signs do not correlate with severity of underlying cirrhosis
Hypoxemia common	Hypoxemia uncommon

DIAGNOSTIC METHODS

In patients where dyspnea and/or physical examination findings raise the possibility of HPS or POPH, diagnostic screening is appropriate. As both conditions may be asymptomatic, screening is also appropriate in patients undergoing evaluation for liver transplantation, since the presence of HPS or POPH may influence candidacy for and timing of liver transplantation. An algorithm for screening is outlined in Fig. 99.3.

Hepatopulmonary syndrome

The diagnosis of HPS rests on documenting the presence of pulmonary gas exchange abnormalities due to intrapulmonary vasodilatation. When other causes for arterial blood gas abnormalities coexist with intrapulmonary vasodilatation it may be

CAUSES OF DYSPNEA AND HYPOXEMIA IN CHRONIC LIVER DISEASE

INTRINSIC CARDIOPULMONARY DISEASE INDEPENDENT OF CIRRHOSIS
- Chronic obstructive pulmonary disease
- Congestive heart failure
- Other: pneumonia, atelectasis, asthma, restrictive lung disease

CONDITIONS ASSOCIATED WITH LIVER DISEASE

General Complications
- Deconditioning and muscular wasting
- Ascites
- Hepatic hydrothorax

Pulmonary Vascular Disorders
- Hepatopulmonary syndrome
- Portopulmonary hypertension

Specific Lung–Liver Disease Associations
- Primary biliary cirrhosis: pulmonary hemorrhage, fibrosing alveolitis, pulmonary granulomas
- Alpha-1 antitrypsin deficiency: panacinar emphysema

difficult to define if HPS is contributing to gas exchange abnormalities. The most sensitive technique for detecting gas exchange abnormalities is measurement of the arterial blood gas and calculation of the alveolar–arterial oxygen gradient with age correction (abnormal >20 mmHg, Fig. 99.1). This test can detect mild abnormalities prior to the development of hypoxemia. Pulse oximetry is an alternative noninvasive modality that indirectly measures oxygen saturation and screens for hypoxemia. In cirrhosis, pulse oximetry may overestimate arterial oxyhemoglobin saturation. A threshold value of <97% is needed to reliably detect hypoxemia.[9] The most commonly employed screening technique to detect HPS is contrast echocardiography. A positive test occurs when there is delayed visualization (after the 3rd heartbeat after injection) of intravenously administered microbubbles in the left cardiac chambers. Radionuclide lung perfusion scanning, which quantifies intrapulmonary shunting, is useful to define whether HPS is contributing to hypoxemia in patients with concomitant intrinsic lung disease.[10] Radionuclide lung perfusion scanning is less sensitive as a screening test than contrast echocardiography.

Portopulmonary hypertension

The diagnosis of POPH is established by documenting an elevated mean pulmonary arterial pressure in the absence of volume overload or intrinsic cardiopulmonary disease. Doppler echocardiography is used to screen for POPH.[2] This study allows measurement of the tricuspid regurgitant jet and permits estimation of the pulmonary artery pressure. Combining Doppler echocardiography with contrast injection provides screening for both POPH and HPS. An estimated systolic pulmonary arterial pressure of >40 mmHg is used to define the need for direct measurement of pulmonary pressures by right heart catheterization. A mean pulmonary artery pressure of >25 mmHg with a pulmonary capillary wedge pressure <15 mmHg, confirms the diagnosis of pulmonary arterial hypertension. An elevated transpulmonary gradient (mean pulmonary artery pressure – pulmonary capillary wedge pressure >10 mmHg) and pulmonary vascular resistance (>120 dyn/s/cm^{-5}) are additional measurements used to distinguish POPH from pulmonary venous hypertension.

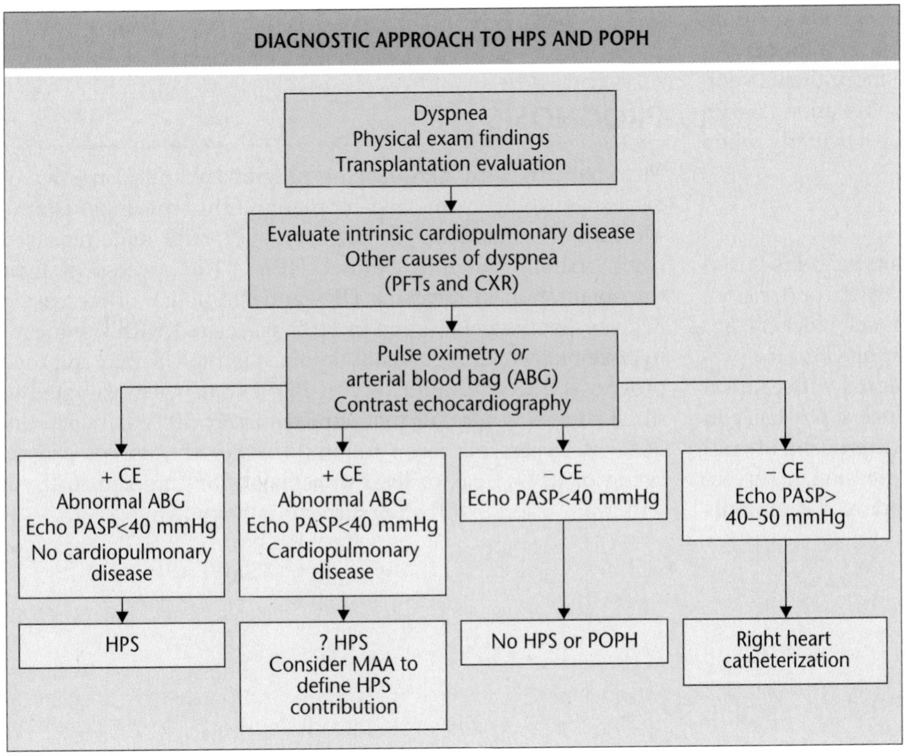

Fig. 99.3 Diagnostic Approach to HPS and POPH. In patients where symptoms or examination findings suggest cardiopulmonary dysfunction or in those being considered for liver transplantation, screening for HPS and POPH is appropriate. Other causes for cardiopulmonary disease are evaluated using chest radiography (CXR) and pulmonary function testing (PFTs). Pulse oximetry or arterial blood gases (ABGs) are used to detect gas exchange abnormalities. Standard simplified formulae may be used to calculate the alveolar–arterial oxygen gradient and correct values for age. Contrast echocardiography with Doppler (CE) is performed. If CE is positive for intrapulmonary shunting and gas exchange abnormalities are present without intrinsic cardiopulmonary disease then HPS is present. If similar findings are found in a patient with intrinsic cardiopulmonary disease then radionuclide lung perfusion scanning using technetium-labeled macroaggregated albumin particles (MAA) may define if HPS is contributing to ABG abnormalities. If CE is negative and Doppler calculation of pulmonary arterial systolic pressure (PASP) is low then HPS and POPH are unlikely. If CE is negative and estimated PASP is high, then right heart catheterization is indicated to confirm the presence of POPH.

TREATMENT AND PREVENTION

There are no clearly effective medical therapies to reverse HPS or POPH. However, prospective randomized studies have not been performed to date and most of the data has arisen from case reports and retrospective series.

TREATMENT AND PREVENTION	
Hepatopulmonary syndrome	**Portopulmonary hypertension**
No effective medical therapies	Medical therapies improve symptoms
Appropriate interventions: Oxygen therapy (if PaO_2 <60 mmHg) Referral to specialized center Liver transplantation evaluation	Appropriate interventions: Referral to specialized center Epoprostenol infusion
Liver transplantation only effective treatment modality	Liver transplantation generally contraindicated
No specific prevention available	No specific prevention available

Hepatopulmonary syndrome

From a practical standpoint, patients with HPS who are hypoxemic should be considered for long-term oxygen therapy to improve symptoms and assessed for candidacy for liver transplantation. In patients where specialized evaluation and liver transplantation are not options, selective intestinal decontamination and garlic preparations could be considered.[1] Transjugular intrahepatic portosystemic shunt (TIPS) has been attempted in a small number of cases, but convincing evidence for sustained improvement is lacking. Liver transplantation is the only proven therapy for HPS based upon resolution or significant improvement in gas exchange postoperatively in more than 80% of reported patients.[1] The length of time for resolution after transplantation varies and may be more than 1 year. In addition, mortality is increased after transplantation in HPS patients compared to subjects without HPS particularly when hypoxemia is severe.[11]

Portopulmonary hypertension

Medical treatment for portopulmonary hypertension is based largely on experience in primary pulmonary hypertension. However, anticoagulation and calcium channel blockers are not recommended. The use of beta-adrenergic blockers for prevention of variceal bleeding should be considered with caution given the potential for cardiac depression. Chronic prostacyclin (epoprostenol) infusion results in clinical improvement and increased survival in primary pulmonary hypertension. In several series of POPH, epoprostenol infusion[12,13] improved symptoms and lowered pulmonary artery pressures but has not been shown to prolong survival. Whether epoprostenol improves transplant candidacy has not been studied. In addition, there are reports of worsening ascites, splenomegaly, and hypersplenism associated with long-term epoprostenol use. Preliminary studies with subcutaneous and inhaled prostacyclin analogs have shown promising results. Endothelin receptor antagonists are effective in primary pulmonary hypertension, but cases of hepatotoxicity raise concern over their use in advanced liver disease. POPH is not considered an indication for liver transplantation. Retrospective data and clinical experience support the theory that moderate to severe POPH (mean pulmonary artery pressure >35 and PVR >250 $dyn/s/cm^{-5}$ or mean pulmonary artery pressure >50 mmHg) is a contraindication to transplantation due to a perioperative mortality of approximately 50% and lack of reversibility of pulmonary hypertension. Patients with mild portopulmonary hypertension (mean pulmonary artery pressure <35 mmHg) appear to have no increase in cardiopulmonary mortality after liver transplantation.[14] The outcome after liver transplantation in intermediate severity portopulmonary hypertension and in patients who have improvement on long-term medical therapy is less well defined and requires further evaluation.

COMPLICATIONS

The presence of HPS appears to significantly decrease survival in patients with cirrhosis through an increase in liver-related complications.[15] This observation has led to the hypothesis that hypoxemia may worsen hepatic function in HPS. In addition, a number of unique postoperative complications after liver transplantation have been observed in patients with HPS including pulmonary hypertension, cerebral vascular accidents, sepsis/respiratory failure, cardiac arrhythmias, and postoperative deterioration in oxygenation.[1] The major complication in patients with POPH is progressive right heart failure and cor pulmonale.

PROGNOSIS

Most patients with HPS develop progressive and worsening of gas exchange over time and spontaneous improvement is rare. Mortality is significant in patients with HPS and increased over cirrhotic patients without HPS.[15] The success of liver transplantation in reversing HPS and the policy of increasing priority for transplantation in HPS associated with significant hypoxemia, which is currently in place in the US, may improve prognosis. The natural history of POPH has been evaluated in small studies. A mortality of approximately 50% at 1 year and 70% at 5 years has been found. Whether the use of prostacyclin or its analogs or liver transplantation targeted to those with mild disease will alter survival is unknown.

EFERENCES

1. Fallon M, Abrams G. Pulmonary dysfunction in chronic liver disease. Hepatology 2000; 32: 859–865.
2. Budhiraja R, Hassoun PM. Portopulmonary hypertension: a tale of two circulations. Chest 2003; 123:562–576.
3. Rolla G, Brussino L, Colagrande P. Exhaled nitric oxide and impaired oxygenation in cirrhotic patients before and after liver transplantation. Ann Intern Med 1998; 129:375–378.
4. Luo B, Liu L, Tang L et al. Increased pulmonary vascular endothelin B receptor expression and responsiveness to endothelin-1 in cirrhotic and portal hypertensive rats: a potential mechanism in experimental hepatopulmonary syndrome. J Hepatol 2003; 38:556–563.
5. Rabiller A, Nunes H, Lebrec D et al. Prevention of gram-negative translocation reduces the severity of hepatopulmonary syndrome. Am J Resp Crit Care Med 2002; 166:514–527.
6. Zhang J, Ling Y, Luo B et al. Analysis of pulmonary heme oxygenase-1 and nitric oxide synthase alterations in experimental hepatopulmonary syndrome. Gastroenterology 2003; 125:1441–1451.
7. Martinez GP, Barbera JA, Visa J et al. Hepatopulmonary syndrome in candidates for liver transplantation. J Hepatol 2001;34(5):651–657.
8. Martinez G, Barbera J, Navasa M et al. Hepatopulmonary syndrome associated with cardiorespiratory disease. J Hepatol 1999; 30:882–889.
9. Abrams GA, Sanders MK, Fallon MB. Utility of pulse oximetry in the detection of arterial hypoxemia in liver transplant candidates. Liver Transpl 2002; 8:391–396.
10. Abrams G, Nanda N, Dubovsky E, Krowka M, Fallon M. Use of macroaggregated albumin lung perfusion scan to diagnose hepatopulmonary syndrome: a new approach. Gastroenterology 1998; 114:305–310.
11. Arguedas M, Abrams GA, Krowka MJ, Fallon MB. Prospective evaluation of outcomes and predictors of mortality in patients with hepatopulmonary syndrome undergoing liver transplantation. Hepatology 2003;37:192–197.
12. Kuo P, Johnson L, Plotkin J et al. Continuous intravenous epoprostenol for the treatment of portopulmonary hypertension. Transplantation 1997; 63:604–606.
13. Krowka M, Frantz R, McGoon M et al. Improvement in pulmonary hemodynamics during intravenous epoprostenol (prostacyclin): a study of 15 patients with moderate to severe portopulmonary hypertension. Hepatology 1999; 30:641–648.
14. Krowka M, Plevak D, Findlay J et al. Pulmonary hemodynamics and perioperative cardiopulmonary-related mortality in patients with portopulmonary hypertension undergoing liver transplantation. Liver Transpl 2000; 6: 443–450.
15. Schenk P, Schoniger-Hekele M, Fuhrmann V et al. Prognostic significance of the hepatopulmonary syndrome in patients with cirrhosis. Gastroenterology 2003; 125:1042–1052.

Chapter 100

Hepatic encephalopathy

Andres T Blei

KEY POINTS
• Hepatic encephalopathy (HE) reflects the spectrum of neurologic abnormalities seen in liver failure • HE occurs in the presence of hepatocellular dysfunction and/or portal–systemic shunting • There are three types of HE: Type A – associated with acute liver failure Type B – associated with portal–systemic bypass Type C – associated with cirrhosis

INTRODUCTION AND DEFINITION

Behavioral abnormalities in patients with liver disease have been recognized since antiquity. Hippocrates had noted that 'those who are mad on account of phlegm are quiet, but those on account of bile are vociferous, vicious and do not keep quiet' (quoted in reference 1). Nowadays, hepatic encephalopathy (HE) can be defined in broad terms as *neurologic abnormalities seen in liver failure*, encompassing a wide range of neuropsychiatric signs and symptoms seen in patients with acute liver failure (ALF) and cirrhosis. A recent consensus has been reached, where HE type A refers to patients with encephalopathy associated with *A*LF, type B reflects encephalopathy associated with portal–systemic *b*ypass, and type C corresponds to HE in subjects with *c*irrhosis.[2] The term portal–systemic encephalopathy has also been used synonymously with HE, although the consensus statement argued against its use in view of its more restricted focus.

EPIDEMIOLOGY

The appearance of encephalopathy is a serious development in the course of ALF. In some patients the course is very rapid, with encephalopathy developing shortly after the appearance of jaundice. In others, the interval between jaundice and the development of HE may be weeks or even months (see Chapter 101). Estimates of the prevalence of ALF in the USA suggest an annual incidence of approximately 2000 cases per year.[3] Neurologic complications may be the cause of death in patients with ALF, in contrast to the encephalopathy associated with other forms of HE in cirrhosis, where seldom is the neurologic picture the cause of death.

Portal–systemic bypass refers to a direct communication between the portal and the systemic circulation. It may be the result of surgical or radiologic decompression of portal hypertension, best exemplified by transjugular intrahepatic portal–systemic shunting (TIPS) (see Chapter 147). It may also occur as part of a congenital venous anomaly, with no evidence of liver disease.[4] In such patients, a direct communication between the portal and hepatic veins can be detected (Fig. 100.1). This is an extremely rare condition, but one that allows an independent assessment of the role of portal–systemic shunting in the pathogenesis of HE.

In cirrhosis, the most common disease in which HE is identified, abnormalities of mental state are generally seen in patients with more advanced liver failure. In the Child-Pugh classification, alterations of mental state correspond to classes B and C. More subtle forms of encephalopathy, also termed minimal encephalopathy, may be observed in a considerably wider population of subjects with cirrhosis.

CAUSES AND RISK FACTORS

Cirrhosis

HE in cirrhosis occurs in three major settings.

CAUSES AND RISK FACTORS
CAUSES AND RISK FACTORS OF HEPATIC ENCEPHALOPATHY IN CIRRHOSIS
• **Most common precipitating factors that result in an episode of HE** Gastrointestinal bleeding Uremia (dehydration) Infection • **Less common precipitating factors** Use of sedatives Constipation Dietary indiscretion Hypokalemia • **Portal–systemic shunting and chronic HE** Disease related – large splenorenal collateral Radiologically induced – post-TIPS • **Liver failure** Associated with chronic HE Acute-on-chronic liver failure involves severe HE

Precipitating factors

Most patients with cirrhosis develop HE as a result of a precipitating event that results in an acute increase in a toxin load to the brain. Of these, gastrointestinal bleeding, uremia, and infection are the most common precipitants. Other factors include a high-protein diet, hypokalemia, constipation, and

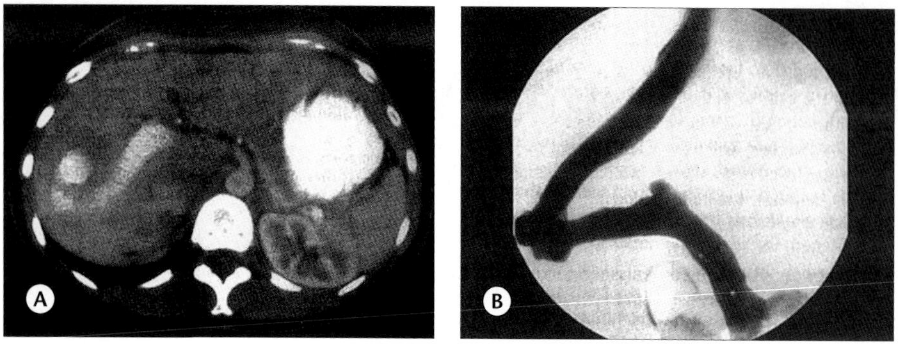

Fig. 100.1 Communication between portal and hepatic veins. A. Spiral abdominal computed tomogram demonstrating a massively enlarged portal vein running towards the hepatic vein. **B.** Portal venous system injection performed from the right transjugular approach. Portal venogram showing a direct connection from the portal vein to the hepatic vein in a patient with congenital portal–systemic shunt. From Crespin et al. Intrahepatic portal-hepatic venous anastomosis: a portal-systemic shunt with neurological repercussions. American Journal of Gastroenterology 2000; 95:1568–1572, with permission from Blackwell Publishing.

the use of sedatives and/or psychotropic drugs. Dehydration and discontinuation of antiencephalopathy medication also needs to be considered. The identification and removal of the precipitating factor is a key diagnostic and therapeutic strategy in the management of these patients.

Portal–systemic shunting

Development of a portal–systemic collateral circulation is a classic feature of cirrhosis once a critical value of portal pressure is reached. The anatomic features of this circulation are described in Chapter 96. In some patients with cirrhosis, a large spontaneous portal–systemic collateral develops, mostly as a splenorenal connection. These patients may develop HE in the absence of a precipitating event. Nowadays, it is more common to find this type of encephalopathy after placement of a transjugular intrahepatic stent. In patients with cirrhosis and long-standing portal–systemic shunting, acquired hepatolenticular degeneration can develop, also termed hepatocerebral degeneration.

Liver failure

Patients may present with chronic encephalopathy, with frequent acute episodes, or with a low-grade persistent abnormality. In addition, the term 'acute-on-chronic' liver failure has been coined to describe patients with cirrhosis and clinical decompensation, who present with HE in combination with renal failure and hemodynamic instability.[5] The increasing prevalence of cirrhosis in the West, as a result of hepatitis C and obesity, has resulted in a larger number of patients with this picture, which can be summarized as encephalopathy + deep jaundice + severe coagulopathy. Clinically, the alteration in mental state is quite severe and does not respond readily to removal of the precipitating factor.

Acute liver failure

In ALF, encephalopathy can also occur as the result of the same precipitating factors as in cirrhosis. However, liver failure is the main consideration, and evolution of encephalopathy to a deeper alteration of the sensorium is associated with the development of brain edema and intracranial hypertension.[6]

PATHOGENESIS

Elucidation of the cause of encephalopathy needs to take account of the presence of liver failure and portal–systemic shunting, the anatomic substrates of encephalopathy. For many years, research has focused on the nature of putative toxins that escape liver uptake and enter the systemic circulation. This substance would have to be generated in the intestine, exhibit a high concentration in the portal vein, be avidly eliminated by the liver on first pass, and exert neurotoxic effects. It may be related to dietary protein ('meat intoxication' is a classic clinical association) or to bacterial metabolism in the colon, as poorly absorbable antibiotics, such as neomycin, improve mental state in patients with encephalopathy.

Ammonia fits all of these requirements. It is a nitrogenous product of bacterial metabolism in the colon, with a concentration in the portal vein that is approximately 10-fold higher than that in the systemic circulation, and is taken up very efficiently by the liver (close to 85% on first pass), where it is utilized mainly for the synthesis of urea. Ammonia is also used for the synthesis of glutamine in perivenous hepatocytes, a process that in normal conditions closely controls the levels of ammonia entering the systemic circulation. An interorgan traffic of ammonia exists: muscle and brain use ammonia for amidation of glutamate in order to generate glutamine. Glutamine in the circulation is utilized by the kidney and small bowel, and deamination of this amino acid results in the generation of ammonia (Fig. 100.2).

Neurological changes: At pathologic concentrations, ammonia produces alterations in brain function. The main element affected is the cortical astrocyte, the only cell in the brain that contains glutamine synthetase, which is required for glutamine synthesis. An excess of intracellular glutamine is associated with astrocyte swelling, which impairs intercellular communications with neurons and endothelial cells. As a result, abnormalities arise in diverse neurotransmitter systems, such as the glutamate and gamma-aminobutyric acid (GABA) systems (Fig. 100.3). The protean manifestations of the syndrome can be traced to the variable degree of astrocyte alteration and the resultant abnormalities in intercellular communications in different parts of the brain.[7]

Other factors exert effects that are synergistic with those of ammonia. Clinically, infection is a common precipitating factor and its association with changes in mental state is the product of multiple mechanisms by which cytokines, generated as a result of bacterial infection, affect brain function.[8] Traditionally, other products of bacterial metabolism in the colon, such as short-chain fatty acids, phenols, and mercaptans, are thought to exert synergistic effects with ammonia. A role for circulating GABA and endogenous benzodiazepines – prominent hypotheses in the 1980s and 1990s – has been discredited with the results of experimental and clinical studies.

Biochemical changes: Accumulation of manganese in basal ganglia may play a role in the frequent finding of extrapyramidal

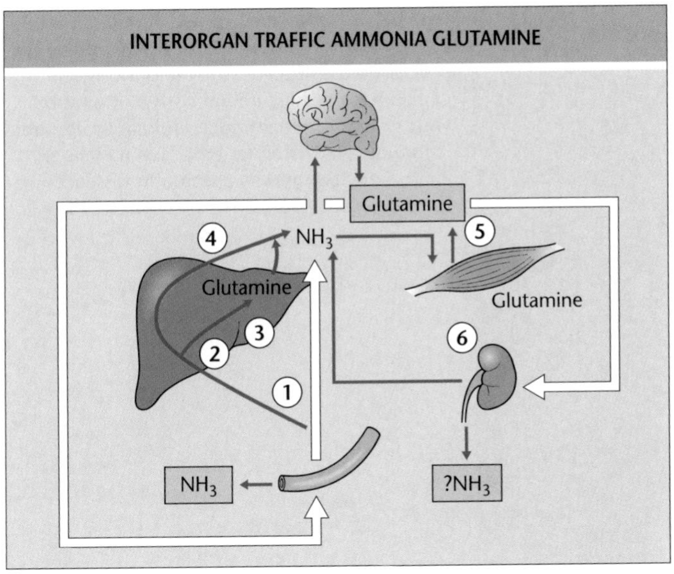

Fig. 100.2 Interorgan traffic of ammonia and glutamine. Ammonia (NH_3), generated in the small bowel mucosa and via the action of colonic bacteria, is normally converted into urea (2) and glutamine (3) in the liver. Extrahepatic (1) and intrahepatic (4) shunts result in increased ammonia levels in the periphery, where it is taken up by muscle (5) and brain. Amidation of glutamate to glutamine occurs, and glutamine is released into the circulation. Glutamine is taken up by kidney (6) and small bowel, where it is used for metabolic needs. Ammonia is generated in these organs via the action of glutaminase. Elimination of ammonia can occur via the fecal route, with a recent study suggesting that the kidneys are able to eliminate ammonia.

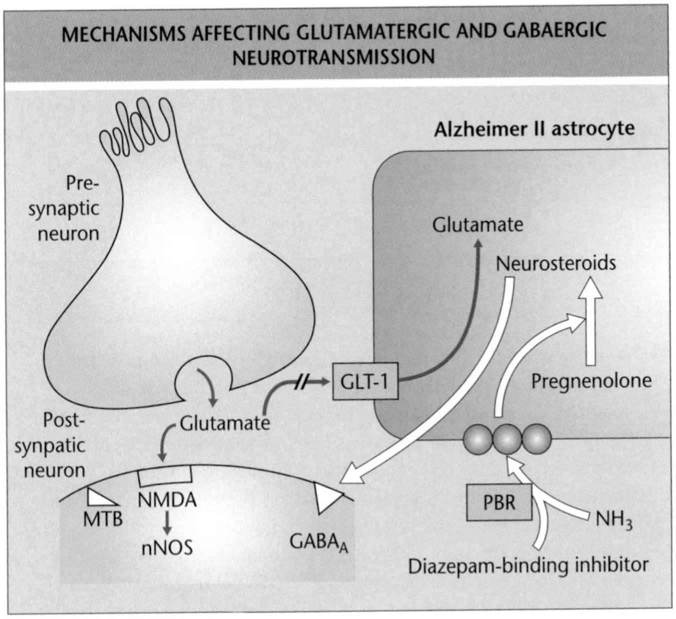

Fig. 100.3 Mechanisms affecting glutamatergic and GABAergic neurotransmission. Under normal circumstances, avid reuptake of presynaptically released glutamate into astrocytes occurs via transporters, of which GLT-1 is prominent. In HE, swollen astrocytes (Alzheimer type II) have decreased activity of GLT-1, resulting in an increased concentration of glutamate to bind at the postsynaptic neuron to either metabotropic (MTB) or *N*-methyl-D-aspartate (NMDA) receptors. Binding to the latter results in activation of neuronal nitric oxide synthase (nNOS) with production of nitric oxide. Ammonia, through peripheral benzodiazepine receptors (PBRs) in the mitochondria of astrocytes, can increase the synthesis of neurosteroids, which are powerful agonists of the gamma-aminobutyric acid type A ($GABA_A$) receptor in neurons.

symptomatology in patients with advanced cirrhosis, the result of altered dopaminergic neurotransmission. Portal–systemic shunting and decreased biliary excretion result in an increased availability of systemic manganese.[9] Tryptophan is an amino acid whose entry into the brain is favored as a result of exchange with the increased intracerebral glutamine. Tryptophan is a precursor of serotonin, and altered serotoninergic neurotransmission may underlie some of the classic descriptions of altered sleep–wake cycles seen in early stages of encephalopathy.

PATHOLOGY

Autopsy studies of patients with cirrhosis who die in hepatic coma are striking for the lack of gross anatomic changes. At microscopy, a constant feature is the presence of glial changes, the so-called Alzheimer type II astrocyte. Seen on immersion fixation, the enlarged nucleus of the astrocyte – its defining feature – corresponds to the same swollen cell seen on perfusion fixation of the brain (Fig. 100.4). Astrocyte swelling is a key element in our current understanding of the mechanisms responsible for HE.

In patients with ALF, the degree of astrocyte swelling may be maximal, associated with an increase in total brain water content. Brain edema can be detected in vivo, and at autopsy swelling of the cerebral cortex with loss of sulci, together with a heavier brain, can be detected. Transtentorial brain herniation as a result of intracranial hypertension is a major cause of death in ALF. In cirrhosis, radiologic studies also suggest an increase in brain water content.[10] However, progression to intracranial hypertension is not a feature.

Hepatocerebral degeneration is associated with anatomic changes in basal ganglia, especially in the lenticular nucleus and globus pallidus. Microcavitations may be detected. This pathology resembles changes seen in Wilson's disease, and hence the term 'acquired hepatolenticular degeneration' has been coined.[11]

CLINICAL PRESENTATION

Symptoms and signs

Changes in mental state

Patients may present with minor changes in behavior, more often detected by a family member. These include somnolence, confusion, and difficulty with simple mathematic calculations. Inversion of the sleep–wake cycle may be present, with patients having difficulty with falling asleep during the night and sleeping through the day (stage I). As encephalopathy progresses, lethargy is more prominent (stage II). In stage III, patients may be incoherent and unable to communicate effectively with their surrounding; stupor may also be present. In stage IV, patients are in coma, with varying degree of response to painful stimuli. Clinical symptoms are for the most part reversible, and in the case of overt encephalopathy will improve within a 72-h interval.

Neuromuscular abnormalities

The presence of asterixis is a classic and useful physical sign of encephalopathy. The 'liver flap' is elicited by asking the patient to extend both upper extremities, open the fingers, and retroflex the wrists. The inability to maintain the position defines the presence of asterixis. The mechanisms responsible for this physical sign have not been elucidated, but the presence of asterixis

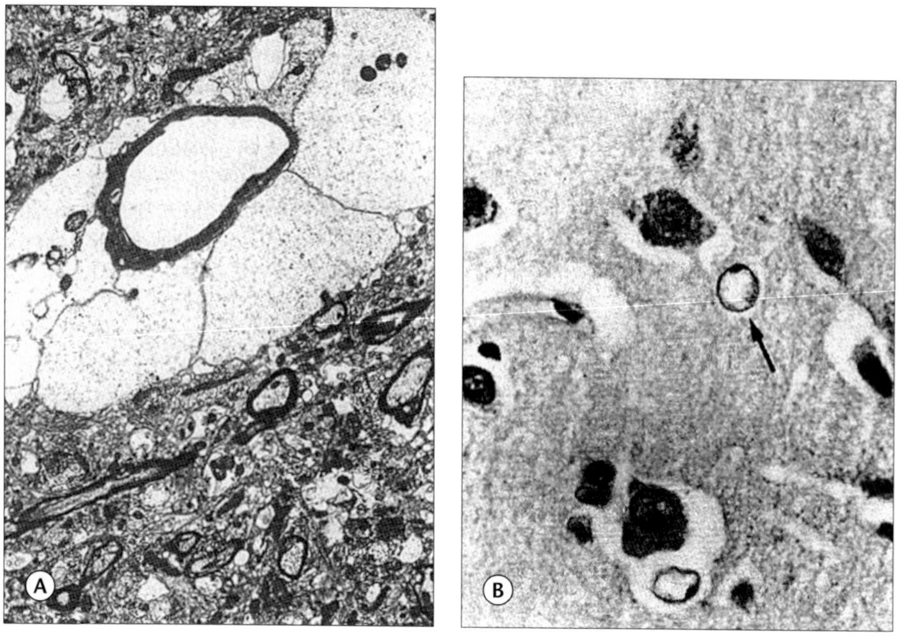

Fig. 100.4 Alterations of astrocytic morphology in liver failure. A. Hydropic foot-processes of astrocytes surround a cerebral capillary from the cerebral cortex of a rabbit with galactosamine-induced fulminant hepatic failure. **B.** An Alzheimer type II astrocyte, with a large nucleus and its chromatin displaced to the side. With courtesy of RF Butterworth.

in other metabolic encephalopathies, such as uremia and carbon dioxide narcosis, suggests a common nonspecific mechanism.

Long tract signs

Patients in deeper stages of coma may exhibit a transient Babinski reflex and clonus, which are important to differentiate from the repercussions of a cerebrovascular accident. Recent magnetic resonance imaging (MRI) studies have noted the presence of changes in the pyramidal tract consistent with edema.[12]

Brain edema

Swelling of the brain may be undetected, and intracranial pressure may rise to 60 mmHg (normal to 15 mmHg) with no clinical signs. Once displacement of brain tissue has occurred, papillary abnormalities and decerebrate posturing may be seen. The presence of a fixed, dilated pupil denotes the presence of brain herniation.

Extrapyramidal symptomatology

In patients with advanced liver disease it is common to detect mutism, associated on occasions with rigidity and tremor. These are classic parkinsonian symptoms.[13] Subjects with hepatocerebral degeneration may have particular difficulties with gait and ataxia; dementia may also be present.

Respiratory findings

Patients hyperventilate with deep encephalopathy, most likely as a result of glutamate-induced stimulation of the respiratory center. Respiratory alkalosis is common. Mercaptans have been associated with a particular pungent breath odor present in subjects with liver failure – fetor hepaticus. The odor has received florid descriptions, including one of roasted almonds, reflecting difficulties in its description.

DIFFERENTIAL DIAGNOSIS

Two are the settings in which it is important to consider a differential diagnosis. In the first, when the patient is not known to have liver disease, the presence of an altered mental state requires careful consideration of other causes of neurologic impairment, including structural diseases of the brain. Imaging of the brain and lumbar puncture may be required to exclude cerebrovascular accidents, tumors, cerebral hemorrhage, or meningitis. Abnormal physical findings suggestive of liver disease, together with general laboratory tests and an elevated level of ammonia, lead to the correct diagnosis.

CLINICAL PRESENTATION

ACUTE PRESENTATION (EPISODIC HE)
- Precipitant-induced
- Spontaneous
- Recurrent

CHRONIC PRESENTATION (PERSISTENT HE)
- Mild
- Severe
- Treatment dependent

MINIMAL HE
- Neurocognitive disturbance

CLINICAL TIPS

- A family member may be the best source for the patient's history.
- Asterixis (short, repetitive movements reflecting the inability to maintain the position) can also be elicited by asking the patient to squeeze the healthcare provider's hand or to stick out the tongue.
- The search for a precipitating factor may include a diagnostic paracentesis if ascites is present, as well as passage of a nasogastric tube to exclude gastrointestinal bleeding.
- Determination of ammonia levels is useful once, to determine the presence of a biochemical abnormality. It is not useful for follow-up.
- Recurrent HE in the absence of liver failure suggests the presence of a large spontaneous portal–systemic collateral.

DIFFERENTIAL DIAGNOSIS
DIFFERENTIAL DIAGNOSIS OF ABNORMAL MENTAL STATE IN CIRRHOSIS

- In all subjects – exclude presence of psychoactive drugs
- With fever and leukocytosis – lumbar puncture to exclude meningitis
- In active alcoholism – rule out subarachnoid hemorrhage
- Alcoholism and confusion – consider Wernicke's encephalopathy
- Asterixis – uremia, hypercapnia, hypomagnesemia
- Decerebrate posturing – rule out brainstem lesions; liver patients have normal neuroopthalmologic findings
- Psychosis – in liver patients, short duration and acute onset; agitation is a feature of acute liver failure rather than cirrhosis
- Dementia – seen in long-standing portal–systemic shunting; exclude vitamin B_{12} deficiency, hypothyroidism, lues

More complex is the exclusion of other causes of an abnormal mental state when the patient is already known to have liver disease. Patients with alcoholism may develop Wernicke's encephalopathy as a result of thiamine deficiency, with paralysis of conjugated gaze. Cryptococcal meningitis may occur in patients with advanced liver failure and may present with chronic symptomatology. Asterixis can be present in other conditions, as stated above, but may also be a manifestation of phenytoin toxicity. Dementia is a feature of established acquired hepatocerebral degeneration and requires exclusion of other usual causes.

DIAGNOSTIC METHODS

Staging

The Glasgow Coma Scale assists in the differentiation of patients in stage 4 encephalopathy (Table 100.1).

TABLE 100.1 GLASGOW COMA SCALE

Feature	Score
EYES OPEN	
Spontaneously	4
To command	3
To pain	2
No response	1
BEST MOTOR RESPONSE	
Obeys verbal orders	6
Painful stimulus, localizes pain	5
Painful stimulus, flexion response	3
Painful stimulus, extension	2
No response	1
BEST VERBAL RESPONSE	
Oriented and conversant	5
Disoriented and conversant	4
Inappropriate words	3
Incomprehensible sounds	2
No response	1

Total score from zero (worst) to 15 (best).

Measurement of ammonia

The main value of this measurement lies in defining the presence of severe liver disease and the likelihood that changes in sensorium are due to HE. Although the serum levels correlate with stages of encephalopathy,[14] there is substantial overlap between values so that staging is not helped with these measurements. Decisions are made by following the mental state.

The only exception may be ALF. An elevated ammonia level, above 200 mg/dL, appears to be predictive of the development of brain edema and cerebral herniation.[15] In addition, arterial values are preferable to venous samples, because there is an arteriovenous difference in the concentration of ammonia, more marked in patients with ALF. The samples should be kept in a cold environment and assayed promptly to avoid in situ generation of ammonia.

Neuropsychologic testing

Patients with cirrhosis may exhibit cognitive defects in the absence of overt neurologic findings. The term minimal encephalopathy describes this situation, in which neuropsychologic tests uncover abnormalities, focused mainly on the area of attention. Patients with Child's class B or C disease, and who have esophageal varices, are more likely to exhibit such abnormalities. A psychometric hepatic encephalopathy score (PHES) can be used to quantify this disturbance.[16] It combines the results of the Reitan Trail test A and B, the block design test, and the digit symbol test.

Brain imaging

A hyperresonant globus pallidus is often seen in MRI studies of patients with chronic liver disease (Fig. 100.5). It is not associated with encephalopathy, and most likely reflects the deposition of manganese in this area. Magnetic resonance spectroscopy can detect the increase in brain glutamine, as well as the reduction in myoinositol, another organic osmolyte, whose decrease can be viewed as a compensation for the altered intracerebral osmolarity caused by glutamine (Fig. 100.6).[17]

DIAGNOSTIC METHODS

- **Neurologic examination**
  West Haven criteria (reviewed in reference 2)
  Glasgow Coma Scale (see Table 100.1)
- **Laboratory tests**
  Ammonia levels, only at diagnosis
- **Brain imaging**
  Magnetic resonance imaging excludes other pathology
  Computed tomography can show brain atrophy, a nonspecific finding
  Magnetic resonance spectroscopy is a research tool
- **Neuropsychologic testing**
  Psychometric hepatic encephalopathy score (PHES)[17] – Reitan trail tests A and B, digit symbol test, block design test, line tracing test

TREATMENT AND PREVENTION

There are strategies to follow when a patient presents with cirrhosis and overt HE. The reader is referred to Chapter 101 for details.

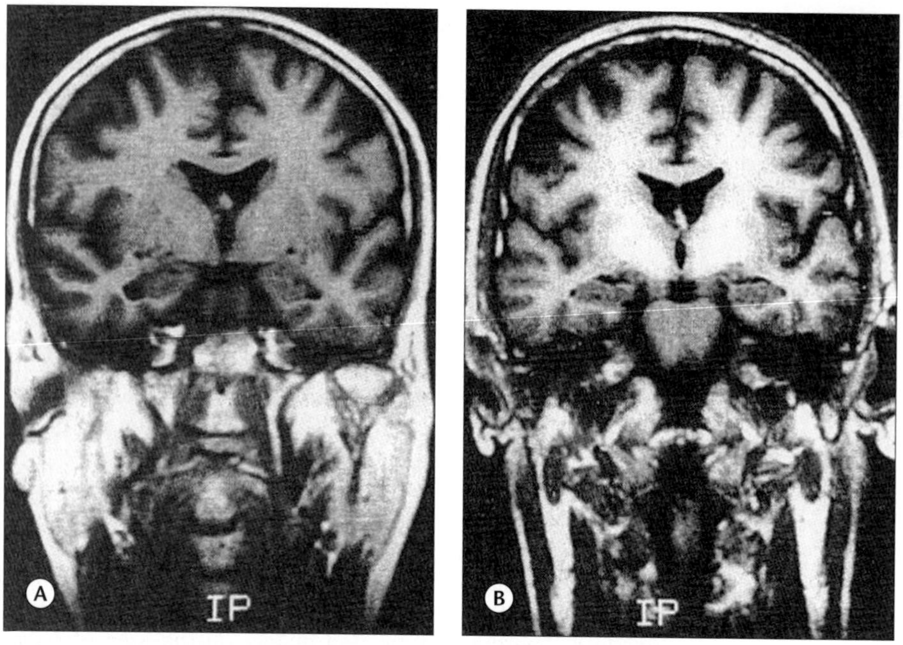

Fig. 100.5 Radiologic alterations in cirrhosi Magnetic resonance image of a normal contr (left) compared to that of a cirrhotic individu (right), with conspicuous changes in the area of the basal ganglia. A hyperresonant globus pallidus can be seen. From Oxford Textbook of Clinical Hepatology (2nd edn), with permission.

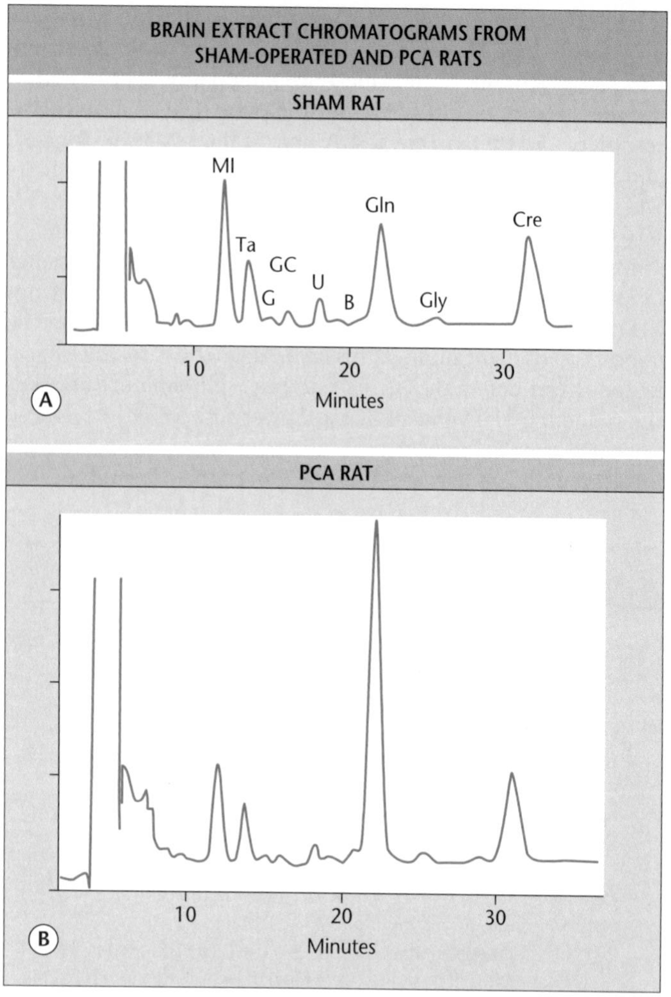

Fig. 100.6 Brain extract chromatograms from rats with a sham operation and portacaval anastomosis (PCA). High-performance liquid chromatograms of brain extracts from a sham-operated rat (A) and a rat that underwent PCA (B), 6 weeks after surgery. MI, myoinositol; Ta, taurine; G, glycerophosphoroethanolamine; GC, glycerophosphocholine; U, urea; B, betaine; Gln, glutamine; Gly, glycine; Cre, creatine. A marked increase in glutamine is offset by a reduction in myoinositol and taurine. Reproduced from Cordoba et al, Hepatology 1996; 24:919–923. © John Wiley & Sons Limited. Reproduced with permission.

General supportive measures

Dehydration as a result of diuretic therapy is a common com plication and fluid should be replaced intravenously. Correc tion of metabolic disturbances, especially hypokalemia, i important. Hypoxemia, common in subjects with cirrhosis may also aggravate the neurologic picture. Recent studies poin to the deleterious effects of hyponatremia on brain function,[1] and efforts should be made to normalize serum sodium levels Patients with deeper stages of encephalopathy are at risk o aspiration and may require intubation for airway protection.

Catharsis should be assured, although this is usually provid ed by the administration of nonabsorbable disaccharides (see below). Protein restriction may initally be necessary in a severely encephalopathic individual, but such measures should be avoidec in the long run. Patients with cirrhosis are hypercatabolic anc may require up to 1.5 g/kg protein per day.[19] Vegetable anc dairy-based protein are preferred over animal protein as the dietary source. Branched-chain amino acids may be used ir patients who are intolerant of dietary protein.

TREATMENT AND PREVENTION

- **General supportive measures**
  Correction of dehydration and electrolyte disturbances, hypokalemia, hyponatremia
  Supplementary oxygen
  Catharsis
  Dietary protein restriction can be deleterious; switch to vegetable and dairy-based protein sources
- **Removal and treatment of precipitating factor**
- **Specific therapy**
  Focus on the gut – decrease ammonia production:
  a. Nonabsorbable disaccharides
  b. Antibiotics (neomycin, metronidazole)
  Focus on the liver – increase conversion of ammonia to urea:
  a. Zinc supplementation with zinc deficiency
  Focus on the brain – antagonize abnormal neurotransmission:
  a. Flumazenil if concern over benzodiazepine ingestion
  b. Bromocriptine for parkinsonian features

Identify and treat the precipitating factor

A careful history should be obtained, including the use of hypnotics and sedatives – a common problem in these patients. General laboratory tests should be performed, and the possibility of gastrointestinal bleeding considered, even without overt signs of hemorrhage. In patients with ascites, a diagnostic paracentesis is required to exclude spontaneous bacterial peritonitis, as such patients may present with encephalopathy as the sole clinical manifestation. Infection should be excluded in other territories, and blood and urine samples should be obtained.

Provide specific therapy

The armamentarium for the treatment of HE is not wide. Furthermore, the use of medications for HE is not supported by large, well designed clinical trials. Still, a rationale for their use and clinical experience has resulted in the wide adoption of such therapies by the practicing community.

Reduce generation of toxins from the gastrointestinal tract

Most therapies for HE target the gastrointestinal tract and attempt to reduce the generation of ammonia by the colon.[20]

Nonabsorbable disaccharides

Nonabsorbable disaccharides, such as lactulose and lactitol, can be administered orally or via enema; the latter is useful in patients with deep HE in whom a quicker arousal is sought. The section on drugs (see Chapter 136) describes the mode of action of these compounds. Oral administration can be started with 15–30 ml every 12 h. The goal is to obtain three soft bowel movements per day. Chronic use is hampered by poor compliance, as the sweet taste is not palatable for some, and flatulence and abdominal cramping can be quite bothersome. Excessive diarrhea will result in hypernatremia, a factor that can independently alter the mental state by causing hyperosmolarity.

Antibiotics

Poorly absorbed oral neomycin can be administered at a dose of 2–6 g/day, although little evidence is available to support such an indication. If neomycin is provided in such a setting, renal and auditory testing should be provided, as there is some absorption of this aminoglycoside. A malabsorption syndrome has also been described with chronic use. Metronidazole is another antibiotic that may be effective in HE. The bacterial flora affected by this antibiotic is quite different from that affected by neomycin, suggesting other effects, probably on the generation of ammonia in the small bowel. The dose of metronidazole in liver disease has to be lowered, because the hepatic clearance of the drug is reduced in liver failure; 250 mg twice daily should be the starting dose.

Improve hepatic elimination of ammonia

Zinc is a co-factor in all reactions of the urea cycle. Patients with cirrhosis and zinc deficiency will improve their ability to synthesize urea after the provision of zinc. Long-term zinc supplementation may be useful for patients with mild chronic forms of encephalopathy.[21] The role of other approaches to improve the capacity of the liver to detoxify ammonia, such as sodium benzoate and ornithine-aspartate, is still under investigation.

Improve neurotransmission

Flumazenil, a benzodiazepine receptor antagonist, has been used to reverse quickly the sedative effects of benzodiazepine on the brain. In HE, studies using 1 mg intravenously have indicated an improvement in mental function when compared to placebo.[22] However, the effects were not striking and the improvement was transient. The lack of an oral formulation has precluded further research with this drug.

Bromocriptine, a dopamine agonist, may improve mental state in patients with chronic encephalopathy who exhibit extrapyramidal symptomatology. It is not commonly used and requires neurologic consultation.

PROGNOSIS

The presence of HE is a serious prognostic development in liver disease. In ALF, it defines the disease and spontaneous survival is limited once deeper stages of encephalopathy have been reached. In cirrhosis, the 1-year survival rate after any episode of encephalopathy is only 40%[23] (Fig. 100.7), although causes of death are related to other complications of chronic liver disease. Even the presence of minimal hepatic encephalopathy is associated with a reduced survival.[24] In appropriate candidates, the presence of encephalopathy signals the need to consider liver transplantation. In the United States, the MELD (Model for End-stage Liver Disease) score, used to assign priority for transplantation, does not take the presence of encephalopathy into account. As a result, many institutions have patients with recurrent encephalopathy who require multiple hospital admissions before a donated liver becomes available.

The impact of therapy for HE in cirrhosis on survival has not been evaluated. One of the difficulties of such a study would

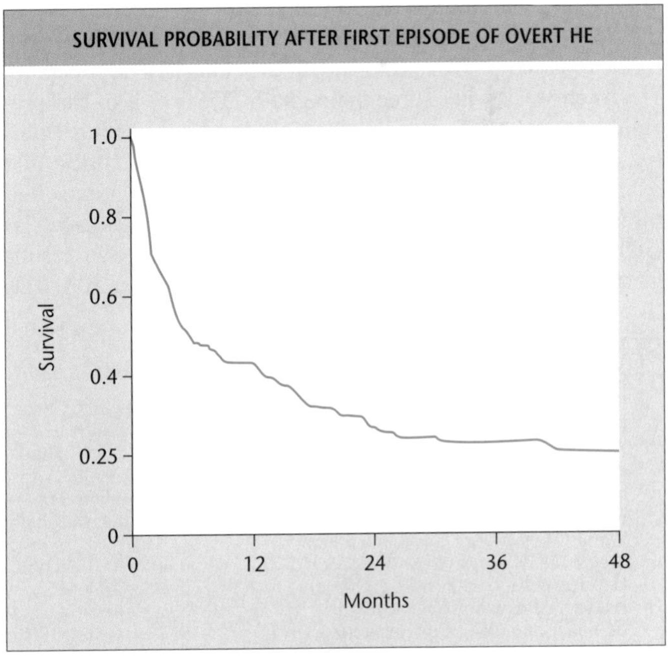

Fig. 100.7 Survival after first episode of overt HE. Survival probability of 111 cirrhotic patients presenting with a first episode of overt HE. Time zero of the curve corresponds to the time of diagnosis of HE. Note that the survival rate at 1 year is 40%. Reprinted from Bustamante J et al, Journal of Hepatology 1999; 30:891 with permission from The European Association for the Study of the Liver. Reproduced with permission from Elsevier.

be the ability for patients to be treated for a prolonged period with currently available medications. Studies have also examined brain function after liver transplantation. Cognitive deficits can be detected 1–2 years after the procedure.[25] The possibility arises that some deficits associated with HE are not totally reversible; however, these patients have undergone a major surgical procedure and are on a wide range of immunosuppressive drugs. Better controlled studies are required to examine this question.

WHAT TO TELL PATIENTS

Hepatic encephalopathy is the medical term used to describe changes of brain function that result from liver disease. The liver normally clears the blood of substances that can hurt the brain. When the liver is chronically injured, both the function of the liver cells as well as the blood circulating through the organ are altered. This combination favors the appearance of excessive levels of such substances in the general circulation. These toxins can now enter the brain.

Ammonia is a leading cause of HE, as it normally originates in the intestine, especially by the metabolism of bacteria in the colon. Ammonia is not the sole toxin, and many other candidates have been examined over the years. Ammonia is still the main player, and though its increased levels can be measured in the bloodstream, serial measurements do not help in deciding the best treatment for the condition. Rather, it is the evaluation of mental state that dictates the clinical approach.

The mental state can evolve from mild confusion to disorientation, lethargy, and somnolence. Coma may occur at deeper stages. Almost all episodes of encephalopathy are reversible. A precipitating event, such as gastrointestinal bleeding or an infection, is brought under control and, together with treatment of HE, an improvement in mental state occurs. Most of the time, such improvement will occur over a 48–72-h period.

Most patients with HE need to be admitted to hospital. Treatment of HE has three main goals: (1) control of the precipitating event; (2) general measures (e.g., intravenous fluids for dehydration, correction of electrolyte abnormalities, and oxygen supplementation); (3) provision of medications that target the intestine, including nonabsorbable sugars, such as lactulose and lactitol, whose metabolism by bacteria results in ammonia being trapped in the intestine. The goal of this therapy is to induce three soft bowel movements a day. The medication may cause excessive diarrhea, flatulence, and abdominal cramping. An alternative is to use a poorly absorbable antibiotic, neomycin, reducing the bacterial count in the colon. Chronic use of neomycin requires medical supervision, as there may be deleterious effects on renal and auditory function.

CURRENT CONTROVERSIES AND THEIR FUTURE RESOLUTION

Three major developments are expected in this area:

1. Better understanding of the neurologic mechanisms responsible for the development of HE.[26] Studies in animal models and in isolated astrocytes will provide deeper insights into the neurochemical abnormalities seen in HE. Included in this area is the study of the mechanisms responsible for brain edema,[27] as an increase in brain water content is seen throughout the spectrum of chronic liver disease. Such studies should translate into improved therapeutic measures in the future.
2. Testing of new approaches to improve HE. Several products are being evaluated for their clinical efficacy. They are focused on changing the nature of the colonic flora. Probiotics are currently being evaluated with this rationale in mind.[28] Another nonabsorbable antibiotic, rifaximin, may be efficacious in this condition.[29]
3. Minimal encephalopathy. For many years, the presence of minimal encephalopathy was viewed as a curiosity, not worthy of specific treatment. Recent studies indicate an impact of minimal encephalopathy on daily activities and quality of life,[30] as well as in the ability to drive a vehicle.[31] An improvement of these parameters with treatment of HE would widen the therapeutic options for caregivers of patients with chronic liver disease.

Unraveling the pathogenesis of HE is important for the treatment of patients with liver failure. It is also a window to many other neurologic conditions in which reversibility is not readily attainable. The sum of experimental data is that hepatic coma (a neuronal condition) arises primarily from an astrocyte-related pathology. Such a paradigm provides novel insights into the nature of consciousness.[32]

REFERENCES

1. Reuben A. There's nothin' like a dame. Hepatology 2002; 35:983–985.
2. Ferenci P, Lockwood A, Mullen K et al. Hepatic encephalopathy – definition, nomenclature, diagnosis, and quantification: final report of the working party at the 11th World Congresses of Gastroenterology, Vienna, 1998. Hepatology 2002; 35:716–721.
3. Hoofnagle JH, Carithers RL Jr, Shapiro C, Ascher N. Fulminant hepatic failure: summary of a workshop. Hepatology 1995; 21:240–252.
4. Watanabe A. Portal–systemic encephalopathy in non-cirrhotic patients: classification of clinical types, diagnosis and treatment. J Gastroenterol Hepatol 2000; 15:969–979.
5. Sen S, Williams R, Jalan R. The pathophysiological basis of acute-on-chronic liver failure. Liver 2002; 22(Suppl):5–13.
6. Vaquero J, Chung C, Cahill ME, Blei AT. Pathogenesis of hepatic encephalopathy in acute liver failure. Semin Liv Dis 2003; 23:259–269.
7. Norenberg MD. Astroglial dysfunction in hepatic encephalopathy. Metab Brain Dis 1998; 13:319–335.
8. Blei AT. Infection, inflammation and hepatic encephalopathy, synergism redefined. J Hepatol 2004; 40:327–330.
9. Layrargues GP, Rose C, Spahr L et al. Role of manganese in the pathogenesis of portal–systemic encephalopathy. Metab Brain Dis 1998; 13:311–317.
10. Cordoba J, Alonso J, Rovira A et al. The development of low-grade cerebral edema in cirrhosis is supported by the evaluation of (1)H-magnetic resonance abnormalities after liver transplantation. J Hepatol 2001; 35: 598–604.
11. Wijdicks EF, Wiesner RH. Acquired (non-Wilsonian) hepatocerebral degeneration: complex management decisions. Liver Transpl 2003; 9:993–994.
12. Cordoba J, Raguer N, Flavia M et al. T2 hyperintensity along the cortico-spinal tract in cirrhosis relates to functional abnormalities. Hepatology 2003; 38:1026–1033.
13. Burkhard PR, Delavelle J, Du Pasquier R, Spahr L. Chronic parkinsonism associated with cirrhosis: a distinct subset of acquired hepatocerebral degeneration. Arch Neurol 2003; 60:521–528.
14. Kramer L, Tribl B, Gendo A et al. Partial pressure of ammonia versus ammonia in hepatic encephalopathy. Hepatology 2000; 31:30–34.
15. Clemmensen JO, Larsen FS, Kondrup J et al. Cerebral herniation in patients with acute liver failure is correlated with arterial ammonia concentration. Hepatology 1999; 29:648–653.

16. Weissenborn K, Ennen JC, Schomerus H et al. Neuropsychological characterization of hepatic encephalopathy. J Hepatol 2001; 34:768–773.
17. Laubenberger J, Haussinger D, Bayer S et al. Proton magnetic resonance spectroscopy of the brain in symptomatic and asymptomatic patients with liver cirrhosis. Gastroenterology 1997; 112:1610–1616.
18. Restuccia T, Gomez-Anson B, Guevara M et al. Effects of dilutional hyponatremia on brain organic osmolytes and water content in patients with cirrhosis. Hepatology 2004; 39:1613–1622.
19. Marchesini G, Bianchi G, Rossi B et al. Nutritional treatment with branched-chain amino acids in advanced liver cirrhosis. J Gastroenterol 2000; 35(Suppl):7–12.
20. Blei AY. Diagnosis and treatment of hepatic encephalopathy. Baillières Best Pract Res Clin Gastroenterol 2000; 14:959–974.
21. Marchesini G, Fabbri A, Bianchi G et al. Zinc supplementation and amino acid-nitrogen metabolism in patients with advanced cirrhosis. Hepatology 1996; 23:1084–1092.
22. Goulenok C, Bernard B, Cadranel JF et al. Flumazenil vs. placebo in hepatic encephalopathy in patients with cirrhosis: a meta-analysis. Aliment Pharmacol Ther 2002; 16:361–372.
23. Bustamante J, Rimola A, Ventura PJ et al. Prognostic significance of hepatic encephalopathy in patients with cirrhosis. J Hepatol 1999; 30:890–895.
24. Kamath PS, Weisner RH, Malinchoc M et al. A model to predict survival in patients with end-stage liver disease. Hepatology 2001; 33: 464–470.
25. Mechtcheriakov S, Gzaziadei IW, Mattedi M et al. Incomplete improvement of visuo-motor deficits in patients with minimal hepatic encephalopathy after liver transplantation. Liver Transpl 2004; 10:77–83.
26. Butterworth RF. Pathogenesis of hepatic encephalopathy: new insights from neuroimaging and molecular studies. J Hepatol 2003; 39:278–285.
27. Blei AT. Pathogenesis of brain edema in acute liver failure. Neurochem Int 2004; in press.
28. Qing L, Zhong PD, Da Hang H et al. Synbiotic modulation of gut flora: effect on minimal hepatic encephalopathy in patients with cirrhosis. Hepatology 2004; 39:1441–1449.
29. Mas A, Rodes J, Sunyer L et al. Comparison of rifaximin and lactitol in the treatment of acute hepatic encephalopathy: a result of a randomized, double-blind, double-dummy, controlled clinical trial. J Hepatol 2003; 38:51–58.
30. Groeneweg M, Quero JC, De Bruijn I et al. Subclinical hepatic encephalopathy impairs daily functioning. Hepatology 1998; 28:45–49.
31. Wein C, Koch H, Popp B et al. Minimal hepatic encephalopathy impairs fitness to drive. Hepatology 2004; 39:739–745.
32. Fields RD, Stevens-Graham B. New insights into neuron–glial communication. Science 2002; 298:556–562.
33. Olde Damink SW, Jalan R, Redhead DN et al. Interorgan ammonia and amino acid metabolism in metabolically stable patients with cirrhosis and a TIPSS. Hepatology 2002; 36: 1163–1171.

Chapter 101

Acute liver failure

John G O'Grady and Julia Wendon

KEY POINTS

- Acute liver failure is a complex multisystemic illness that evolves after catastrophic liver damage, manifest by the development of coagulopathy and encephalopathy within days or weeks
- Hepatitis viruses and drugs (toxic and idiosyncratic reactions) account for the majority of cases
- The natural history is very variable, depending among other things on age, etiology, grade of encephalopathy, and complications
- Liver transplantation is the best therapy for severe cases. About half of patients will require it. Thus, early referral to specialist centers, appropriate monitoring and therapy of emerging complications, and listing for urgent transplantation are key elements in patient management
- Encephalopathy is constant but of varying severity. It can be complicated by cerebral edema, which may cause brain death. Measurement of intracranial pressure (ICP) should be considered. ICP should be maintained below 25 mmHg
- Cardiovascular support, mechanical ventilation, and correction of renal failure are frequently required
- Prevention and treatment of sepsis, metabolic monitoring, and adequate enteral feeding, together with active surveillance of coagulopathy, are other important aspects of management
- The potential to develop 'bridges to transplantation' with extracorporeal liver support devices has yet to be determined

INTRODUCTION

Acute liver failure (ALF) is a complex multisystemic illness that evolves after a catastrophic insult to the liver. The liver damage is manifest by the development of a coagulopathy and encephalopathy within days or weeks of the liver injury. ALF is a heterogenous condition incorporating a range of clinical syndromes. The dominant factors that give rise to this heterogeneity include the underlying etiology, the age of the patient, and the duration of time over which the disease evolves. Three classifications of ALF are currently used and are outlined in Table 101.1.

The natural history of the condition is very variable within this spectrum and survival rates without transplantation range from 10% to 90% for different cohorts. The key components of the management strategy are:

- assessment of the severity of the disease and the associated prognosis;
- prevention or treatment of complications;
- liver transplantation when spontaneous survival is considered unlikely; and
- possible utilization of liver support devices.

Integrated multidisciplinary protocols are now achieving considerably improved survival rates in the range from 40% to 90% depending on the underlying etiology.

ETIOLOGY AND EPIDEMIOLOGY

There is considerable geographic variation in the etiology of ALF (Table 101.2). Viruses and drugs account for the majority of cases. However, a significant number of patients with no definable cause are classified as seronegative or being of indeterminate etiology. The overall incidence of ALF complicating acute hepatitis in the US is 0.9% and this equates to about 2000 deaths annually. Most of the drug-induced cases are rare idiosyncratic reactions, but some like acetaminophen are dose-related toxic events.

Viral

ALF is an uncommon complication of viral hepatitis, occurring in 0.2–4% of cases depending on the underlying etiology. The risk is lowest with hepatitis A, but is increasing with delayed

TABLE 101.1 DEFINITIONS OF ALF IN CURRENT USE

	US	FRANCE	UK
Trigger event	First symptom	Jaundice	Jaundice
Term	Fulminant hepatic failure	Fulminant hepatic failure	Hyperacute liver failure
Time to encephalopathy	8 weeks	2 weeks	<7 days
Term	Late-onset liver failure	Subfulminant hepatic failure	ALF
Time to encephalopathy	9–26 weeks	3–12 weeks	8–28 days
Term			Subacute liver failure
Time to encephalopathy			29–84 days

TABLE 101.2 GEOGRAPHIC VARIATION IN THE ETIOLOGY OF ALF

	UK	US	France	India	Japan
Acetaminophen	54%	40%	2%	–	–
Drug reactions	7%	12%	15%	5%	–
Seronegative	17%	17%	18%	24%	45%
Hepatitis A or B	14%	12%	49%	33%	55%
Hepatitis E	–	–	–	38%	–
Other causes	8%	19%	16%	–	–

exposure from childhood to adulthood. This trend may be modified by the appropriate targeting of populations at risk for vaccination against hepatitis A. Hepatitis B can cause ALF through a number of scenarios (Table 101.3). The incidence of the delta virus appears to be decreasing, while vaccination and antiviral drugs should have some impact on the other mechanisms. Hepatitis C is rarely recognized as the sole cause of ALF.

Hepatitis E is common in parts of Asia and Africa and the risk of developing ALF increases to over 20% in pregnant women, being particularly high during the third trimester. Hepatitis E is also encountered in Europe and the US and may account for up to 8% of cases that would previously have been described as seronegative hepatitis. Unusual causes of viral ALF include herpes simplex 1 and 2, herpesvirus-6, varicella zoster, Epstein-Barr virus and cytomegalovirus.

Seronegative hepatitis is the commonest presumed viral cause in some parts of the Western world. In the UK, it accounts for 56% of such cases. Middle-aged females are most frequently affected and it occurs sporadically. The diagnosis is one of exclusion. There is considerable uncertainty whether much, or all, of this category is due to a viral infection.

Drugs

Acetaminophen overdose accounts for about 40% of cases of ALF in the UK and US.[1] It is usually taken with suicidal or parasuicidal intent, but up to 8–30% cases follow the therapeutic use of acetaminophen. Factors increasing susceptibility to acetaminophen toxicity include regular alcohol consumption, antiepileptic therapy (enzyme induction), and malnutrition. ALF develops in only 2–5% of those taking overdoses, and the mortality is highest at doses exceeding 48g.

Idiosyncratic drug reactions usually develop during the first exposure to the drug. Some of the offending agents are listed in Table 101.4. The diagnosis is largely made on the basis of a temporal relationship between exposure to the drug and the development of ALF. Estimates of the risk of developing ALF as a result of an idiosyncratic reaction range from 0.001% for nonsteroidal antiinflammatory drugs to 1% for the isoniazid/rifampicin combination. Ecstasy (methylenedioxymethamphetamine – a synthetic amphetamine) has been associated with a number of clinical syndromes ranging from rapidly progressive ALF associated with malignant hyperpyrexia to subacute liver failure.

Other etiologies

ALF associated with pregnancy tends to occur during the third trimester. There are three recognized patterns, although a considerable degree of overlap exists:

- acute fatty liver of pregnancy – primagravids carrying a male fetus are most at risk;
- HELLP syndrome (hemolysis, elevated liver enzymes, low platelets); and
- ALF complicating preeclampsia or eclampsia.

In addition, there is a range of unusual causes of ALF:

- Wilson's disease may present as ALF, usually during the second decade of life. It is characterized clinically by a Coomb's negative hemolytic anemia and demonstrable Kayser-Fleischer rings in the majority of cases.
- Poisoning with the mushroom *Amanita phalloides* is most commonly seen in central Europe, South Africa, and the West coast of the US. Severe diarrhea, often with vomiting, is a typical feature and commences five or more hours after ingestion of the mushrooms. Liver failure develops 4–5 days later.
- Autoimmune chronic hepatitis may present as ALF but it is usually no longer responsive to corticosteroid therapy.
- The Budd-Chiari syndrome may present with ALF and the diagnosis is suggested by hepatomegaly and ascites and confirmed by the demonstration of hepatic vein thrombosis.
- Malignant infiltration, especially with lymphoma, is typically associated with hepatomegaly.
- Ischemic hepatitis is being increasingly recognized as a cause of ALF, especially in older patients.
- Pediatric causes include neonatal hemochromatosis, mitochondrial disorders, tyrosinemia, galactosemia, and fructose intolerance.

DIFFERENTIAL DIAGNOSIS

The etiology of ALF must be accurately identified. The contribution of histology to the assessment of ALF is controversial. Histologic features may suggest specific diagnoses including sodium valproate toxicity (microvascular steatosis), malignant

TABLE 101.3 ALF ASSOCIATED WITH HEPATITIS B

	HBsAg	IgM anti-core	HBeAg	HBeAb	HBV DNA	Comment
Acute infection	Variable	Positive	Variable	Variable	Usually negative	Hyperactive immune response
Seroconversion	Positive	Negative	Negative	Positive	Negative	Immune-mediated
Replication surge	Positive	Negative	Variable	Variable	High	Spontaneous or after immunosuppression
Delta superinfection	Positive	Negative	Variable	Variable	Low	New positive serology for delta virus

TABLE 101.4 DRUGS CAUSING ALF

CATEGORY 1: COMMONER CAUSES
- Acetaminophen
- Halothane
- Isoniazid/rifampicin
- Nonsteroidal anti-inflammatory drugs (NSAIDs)
- Sulphonamides
- Flutamide
- Sodium valproate
- Carbamazepine
- Ecstasy

CATEGORY 2: RARER CAUSES
- Benoxyprofen
- Phenytoin
- Isoflurane
- Enflurane
- Tetracycline
- Allopurinol
- Ketoconazole
- Monoamine oxidase inhibitors (MAOIs)
- Disulphiram
- Methyldopa
- Amiodarone
- Tricyclic antidepressants
- Propylthiouracil
- Gold
- 2,3-Dideoxyinosine (ddI)

infiltration, Wilson's disease (cirrhosis), pregnancy-related syndromes and the Budd-Chiari syndrome. Confluent necrosis is the commonest histological finding and its severity has been used to assess prognosis. However, nodules of regeneration may occur randomly, particularly in subacute liver failure, and a biopsy from such a site will underestimate the gravity of the condition.

PROGNOSIS

Numerous variables correlate with prognosis in ALF. The underlying etiology is a powerful determinant of prognosis. The grade of encephalopathy also correlates strongly with outcome (both the grade at presentation and the maximum grade attained). The prognosis deteriorates further when grade 4 encephalopathy is complicated by cerebral edema, and even further when the latter coexists with renal failure. Reliance on the development of these clinical complications to determine prognosis is not helpful when defining the scope and application of liver transplantation. Furthermore, subsets of patients have very poor prognoses without the development of cerebral or renal failure. The use of transplantation mandates the need for early indicators of prognosis so that those in need can be identified at the earliest possible opportunity.

Determination of prognosis drives two fundamental management issues, i.e., the need for referral to specialist centers and the indications for transplantation. Indications for referral to specialist units have been suggested for acetaminophen and other etiologies of ALF (Tables 101.5 and 101.6). Separate criteria have been identified for use within specialist centers to identify the cohort most in need of liver transplantation.

The King's College criteria, which are early indicators of prognosis, often pre-empt advanced encephalopathy and can be applied quickly and easily.[2] In nonacetaminophen cases, etiology, the age of the patient, and the interval between the onset of jaundice and the development of encephalopathy are the static variables used to assess prognosis. These are combined with two commonly used dynamic parameters, serum bilirubin and prothrombin time, to complete the model (Table 101.7). In acetaminophen cases, the pH of arterial blood has the strongest predictive value, and a pH <7.30 suggests a very poor prognosis. In patients who did not develop an acidosis, the coexistence of a prothrombin time >100 s (international normalized ratio (INR) 6.7), serum creatinine $>300\,\mu$mol/L, and grade 3 encephalopathy was necessary to be reasonably certain

DIAGNOSIS/DIFFERENTIAL DIAGNOSIS

Etiology	Investigation	Comment
Hepatitis A (HAV)	IgM anti-HAV	95% positive initially – 100% on repeat testing
Hepatitis B and D (HBV, HDV)	Full profile	See Table 101.3 for interpretation
Hepatitis E (BEV)	Anti-HEV	IgM antibody test not routinely available
Seronegative hepatitis	All tests	Diagnosis of exclusion
Acetaminophen	Drug levels in blood	May be negative on third or subsequent days after overdose
Idiosyncratic drug reactions	Eosinophil count	Most diagnoses based on temporal relationship
Ecstasy	Blood, urine, hair analysis	Medium-term exposure can be mapped from analysis of hair
Autoimmune	Autoantibodies, IgGs	High titers or anti-KLM suggest diagnosis
Pregnancy-related syndromes		
– fatty liver	Ultrasound, uric acid, histology	First pregnancy
– HELLP syndrome	Platelet count	Disseminated intravascular coagulation a prominent feature
– toxemia	Serum transaminases	Very high transaminases, appropriate obstetric history
Wilson's disease	Urinary copper, ceruloplasmin	Deeply jaundiced, anemic, second decade of life
Amanita phalloides	–	History of ingestion of mushrooms, diarrhea
Budd-Chiari syndrome	Ultrasound or venography	Ascites, prominent caudate lobe on imaging
Malignancy	Imaging and histology	Imaging may be interpreted as normal
Ischemic hepatitis	Transaminases	Transaminases very high
Heatstroke	Myoglobinuria	Rhabdomyolysis a prominent feature

TABLE 101.5 REFERRAL FOLLOWING ACETAMINOPHEN INGESTION

Day 2	Day 3	Day 4
Arterial pH <7.30 INR >3.0 or PT >50 s Oliguria Creatinine >200 µmol/L Hypoglycemia	Arterial pH <7.30 INR >4.5 or PT >75 s Oliguria Creatinine >200 µmol/L Encephalopathy Severe thrombocytopenia	INR >6 or PT >100 s Progressive rise in PT to any level Oliguria Creatinine >300 µmol/L Encephalopathy Severe thrombocytopenia

The presence of any of the above criteria should prompt referral.
INR, international normalized ratio; PT, prothrombin time.

TABLE 101.6 REFERRAL IN NON-ACETAMINOPHEN ETIOLOGIES

Hyperacute	Acute	Subacute
Encephalopathy Hypoglycemia PT >30 s INR >2.0 Renal failure Hyperpyrexia	Encephalopathy Hypoglycemia PT >30 s INR >2.0 Renal failure	Encephalopathy Hypoglycemia (less common) PT >20 s INR >1.5 Renal failure Serum sodium <130 µmol/L Shrinking liver volume

The presence of any of the above criteria should prompt referral.
INR, international normalized ratio; PT, prothrombin time.

TABLE 101.7 POOR PROGNOSIS INDICATORS IN NON-ACETAMINOPHEN ETIOLOGIES

Parameter	Sensitivity	Specificity	Positive predictive accuracy
Prothrombin time >100 s or INR >6.7	34%	100%	46%
Any three of the following: unfavorable etiology (seronegative hepatitis or drug reaction), age <10 or >40 years, acute or subacute categories, serum bilirubin >300 µmol/L	93%	90%	92%

of a poor prognosis (Table 101.8). Despite the prompt identification of patients with a poor prognosis after an acetaminophen overdose, liver transplantation can only be achieved in a minority of cases because of very rapid progression of the disease. Serum lactate levels have been found to complement the acetaminophen criteria.[3] The criteria were not validated in a number of rare etiologies particularly pregnancy-related syndromes, Wilson's disease, and *Amanita phalloides* poisoning. In France, the factor V levels are used in preference to either the prothrombin time or INR. Factor V levels <20% in patients under the age of 30 years and <30% in older patients are indicative of a poor prognosis once encephalopathy develops.

A small liver on clinical or radiologic assessment, or more particularly a liver that is found to be shrinking rapidly, is a poor prognostic indicator. This feature is especially useful in subacute liver failure when the degree of encephalopathy and the severity of the derangement of coagulation may not be particularly marked. In Japan, CT scanning has been used to assess both the size of the liver and the functional reserve and this was useful in determining prognosis. The limitations of histologic assessment have been previously addressed.

TREATMENT

Overall strategy

Each patient with ALF needs an overall management plan that starts with identification of etiology and an initial assessment of prognosis. There are a few drugs with defined roles in specific etiologies of ALF. Appropriate patients should be referred to specialist centers offering liver transplantation. Patients are monitored for complications, which are treated as they emerge to the point of recovery, death, or transplantation. Patients not initially considered for transplantation may change status on the basis of prognostic indicators or the pattern of clinical complications that emerges. Likewise, patients listed for transplantation may develop complications that preclude this intervention or occasionally may show unexpected signs of recovery before a donor organ becomes available. The final decision on transplantation is made when an organ is available and should involve the multidisciplinary team. The potential to develop 'bridges to transplantation' with extracorporeal liver support devices has yet to be determined.

TABLE 101.8 POOR PROGNOSIS INDICATORS IN ACETAMINOPHEN-INDUCED ALF

Parameter	Sensitivity	Specificity	Positive predictive
Arterial pH <7.30	49%	99%	81%
All three of the following concomitantly: prothrombin time >100 s or INR >6.5, creatinine >300 µmol/L and grade 3–4 encephalopathy	45%	94%	67%

TREATMENT		
Etiology	**Drug**	**Comment**
Acetaminophen	*N*-Acetylcysteine	(a) Antidote role depending on blood levels within 16h (Fig. 101.1) (b) Disease modifying effect with later use
Hepatitis B	Lamivudine, adefovir	Most effective in cases with high levels of viral replication
Amanita phalloides	Penicillin	Early administration required
Autoimmune hepatitis	Steroids	Response not predictable and risk of infection problematic

Encephalopathy

Pathophysiology: Hepatic encephalopathy encompasses a wide spectrum of neuropsychiatric disturbances associated with both acute and chronic liver dysfunction. The diagnosis of encephalopathy is essentially a clinical diagnosis and is graded from 1 to 4 depending on clinical severity (Table 101.9). The development of encephalopathy is essential for the diagnosis of ALF. Deep levels of encephalopathy (grades 3/4) are associated with the development of cerebral edema and the potential risk of cerebral herniation. Patients with acute and hyperacute liver failure are at greater risk of developing grade IV coma and cerebral edema.

The etiological factors in the development of encephalopathy remain unclear but it is believed that there is a build up of putative toxins (including ammonia, mercaptans, gamma-aminobutyric acid, endogenous benzodiazepines and serotonin/tryptophan) resulting in neurological dysfunction with abnormality of cerebral astrocytic and neuronal function.[5] The development of cerebral edema in patients with ALF is thought to relate, amongst other things, to the speed of onset. In patients with CLD there is control of intracellular osmolarity but in ALF time does not allow such adaptation and cellular edema may result.[6] The pathogenesis of cerebral edema in ALF incorporates both vasogenic and cytotoxic mechanisms. There is marked variability of cerebral blood flow in patients with ALF with hyperemia being seen with increased prevalence in patients with cerebral edema.[5] This hyperemia occurs predominantly in the posterior circulation, an area that in animal studies demonstrates predominant vasogenic edema. By contrast cytogenic edema is seen predominantly in the anterior brain.

Cerebral ammonia uptake is thought to be of importance in the accumulation of glutamate and astrocyte swelling. The relationship between arterial ammonia and cerebral uptake is not clear although increased levels have been observed in patients who died from cerebral death compared to those who survive or succumb to a noncerebral cause. Inflammatory mediators are also of importance in the development of deeper levels of coma. A correlation between increasing components of the systemic inflammatory response syndrome (SIRS) and progressive coma has been observed.[7] This effect appears to be related to 'inflammation' *per se* as compared to culture-positive sepsis and may reflect the effects of cytokines and other pro-inflammatory substances on the blood–brain barrier.

Management: The clinical management of the cerebral complications of ALF has been developed predominantly in a pragmatic manner and by the extrapolation of data from the neurosurgical literature rather than from the results of large randomized controlled clinical trials. Patients whose conscious level deteriorates to grade 3/4 coma are best managed with control of the airway and elective intubation, sedation, and ventilation. Sedation may be undertaken with a variety of compounds but the standard would be to utilize an opiate and a sedative, e.g., propofol and/ or a benzodiazepine. Both agents have anticonvulsant activity and propofol has been suggested to be of benefit in the treatment of surges in intracranial pressure (ICP).

The maintenance of a cerebral perfusion pressure of greater than 55 mmHg has been suggested as optimal. It is of note, however, that patients with ALF do not autoregulate to pressure and as such increases in blood pressure may be associated with increased cerebral blood flow and potentially increased intracranial pressure. The relationship between cerebral blood flow and arterial CO_2 is maintained and in most patients normocapnia is ideal. Short periods of hypocapnia may be considered in patients with significant elevations of ICP if cerebral hyperemia is thought to be contributing to the cerebral hypertension. It is essential to ensure that cerebral hypoxia does not develop. Optimal management of such patients requires the institution of multi-modality monitoring, including the placement of a reverse jugular line. This will allow a degree of assessment of cerebral blood flow, with an aim to have jugular venous saturations within the normal range 55–80%. The measurement of cerebral blood flow may also be estimated at the bedside utilizing Doppler velocity assessment of the middle cerebral artery.

Measurement of intracranial pressure should be considered in patients who have progressed to grade 3/4 coma. The decision to place an intracranial monitor must be driven by a balance of risk and benefit for any given individual patient. The procedure carries risk of bleeding and this varies with the placement site (epidural, subdural, or parenchymal).[8] The risk of bleeding may be modified by coagulation support at the time of placement and technical expertise. There are little data

TABLE 101.9 PARSONS-SMITH SCALE OF HEPATIC ENCEPHALOPATHY

Grade	Clinical features	Neurological signs	Glasgow coma scale
0/subclinical	Normal	Only seen on neuropsychometric testing	15
1	Trivial lack of awareness, shortened attention span	Tremor, apraxia, incoordination	15
2	Lethargy, disorientation, personality change	Asterixis, ataxia, dysarthria	11–15
3	Confusion, somnolence to semi-stupor, responsive to stimuli	Asterixis, ataxia	8–11
4	Coma	± Decerebration	<8

on the advantages of ICP bolt placement although one study, whilst not showing mortality benefit, did demonstrate an increased time span during which therapeutic interventions may be undertaken.[9] It is our policy to place an ICP bolt in patients who are 'deemed to be at risk.' This may relate to jugular venous saturations outside the normal range, requirement for vasopressors, pupillary abnormalities, and/or systolic hypertension.

Treatment of patients with cerebral edema requires information as to the relationship between cerebral blood flow and intracranial pressure along with systemic blood pressure. The normal treatment targets would be to maintain jugular venous saturations greater than 55 mmHg and ICP <25 mmHg with normal pupillary responses. Patients whose ICP rises are sustained beyond 25 mmHg will require treatment. The normal first line treatment is still mannitol, 0.5 g/kg given as a bolus with an appropriate subsequent diuresis. It is essential that serum osmolarity is maintained at less than 320 mOsmol to avoid damage to the blood–brain barrier and worsening of vasogenic edema.

Some patients remain resistant to treatment and in these cases other therapies may be considered. Hypothermia resulted in a decrease in cerebral blood flow, decreased ICP, and decreased cerebral ammonia uptake in one small study.[10] Indomethacin (0.5 mg/kg) has also been reported in a small number of cases to be of benefit. A recent small controlled study has also suggested that maintaining serum sodium levels in the normal range may be of benefit in decreasing incidence of elevated intracranial hypertension.[11]

In some patients, hypotension may result in decreased cerebral perfusion pressure and vasopressor therapy may be required. This is normally achieved with an agent such as norepinephrine but increasingly vasopressin agonists are being utilized. This agent should be used with care in patients with ALF given a recent study demonstrating an increase in cerebral blood flow and ICP over and above that expected from the increase in blood pressure.[12]

Cardiovascular

Patients with ALF develop a hyperdynamic circulation with peripheral vasodilation and central volume depletion. Hypotension is common and may initially respond to volume repletion. Assessment of volume reponsiveness in the clinical setting may be difficult and pressure measurements are a poor indicator of volume status. Hypotension that does not respond to volume requires invasive hemodynamic monitoring and frequently institution of pressor agents. Increasingly it is recognized that volume responsiveness should be determined by dynamic rather than static variables.

The requirement for pressor agents should raise the possibility of adrenal dysfunction, a frequent occurrence in patients with sepsis and hypotension. Patients with ALF have been demonstrated to have impaired response to adrenocorticotropic hormone (ACTH).[13] The response at 30 and 60 min in terms of cortisol should be examined following 250 µg ACTH in all patients with ALF who are requiring pressor agents. A subnormal response should result in consideration of hydrocortisone replacement therapy, normally given for a period of 10 days.

Respiratory

Ventilatory support is frequently required in patients with ALF, though this normally pertains to decreased conscious level rather than hypoxia in the initial stages of disease. Common respiratory complications are pleural effusions, atelectasis, and intrapulmonary shunts. The development of pulmonary sepsis may or may not proceed to adult respiratory distress syndrome (ARDS). Similarly, ARDS may be precipitated by extrapulmonary sepsis or inflammation.

Pulmonary sepsis should be aggressively sought and treated. In ventilator-dependent patients this will normally require bronchoalveolar lavage to acquire the appropriate specimens.

Ventilatory strategies are influenced by the respiratory component of the disease as well as the multiorgan involvement that is characteristic of ALF. Thus, patients with deep levels of coma and at risk of cerebral edema will require close attention to CO_2 levels and tailored sedation regimens. Hypercapnia may have to be tolerated in patients progressing to ARDS. Pleural effusions may require drainage if they are impeding ventilation. Weaning may be facilitated by undertaking tracheostomy during the recovery period of ALF.

Renal

Renal failure is common in the setting of ALF and may have an incidence as high as 50%. This is particularly so with acetaminophen-induced liver failure where the drug may also exert a direct toxic effect on the renal tubule. The etiology of renal dysfunction is frequently multifactorial with hepatorenal failure being a rare occurrence whilst acute tubular necrosis and prerenal renal failure are more common precipitants. Volume therapy and maintenance of intrathoracic blood volume is essential in the management of such patients as is the avoidance of nephrotoxins. Urinary electrolytes may add further information as to the etiology of the renal failure and the presence of significant proteinuria should trigger screening for other forms of renal disease. Intra-abdominal hypertension may reduce renal perfusion pressure and the measurement of intra-abdominal pressure should be considered a valuable component of monitoring.

Management: Established renal failure requires the institution of renal replacement therapy (RRT). It is clear that it is inappropriate to delay initiation of RRT until standard renal criteria for dialysis are established. Early consideration should be given to control of fluid balance, acid-base disturbances, and avoidance of rapid changes in osmolarity. The hemodynamic instability and associated cerebral complications of this patient group have resulted in the application of continuous modes of RRT rather than intermittent hemodialysis.[14] Inability of the liver to metabolize and utilize lactate or acetate buffer solutions means that bicarbonate buffers are preferred in this setting as these provide more effective control of acid-base status. Extrapolation from data in critically ill patients with acute renal failure suggests the optimal filtration rate is 35 mL/kg/h.

Anticoagulation may also be problematic in a setting of coagulopathy. A balance needs to be achieved between risk of bleeding and platelet protection across an extracorporeal filter. A prostaglandin such as epoprostenol may be advantageous in terms of decreased bleeding and prolonging filter life. Alternatively, circuits may be run without anticoagulation, with regional heparinization or utilizing citrate. In patients with thrombocytopenia, consideration should be given to the diagnosis of heparin-induced thrombocytopenia and if confirmed heparin should be withdrawn and anticoagulation achieved with an alternative agent, e.g., lepirudin.

Sepsis

Both culture-positive and culture-negative systemic inflammatory response syndromes are common in patients with ALF who are functionally immunosuppressed with impaired cell-mediated immunity, complement levels, and phagocytosis. Therefore, scrupulous attention with regard to washing of hands and line care needs to be applied to decrease risk of nosocomial infection. Regular culture screens are required and antimicrobials are indicated in patients with any clinical suggestion of sepsis. Prophylactic antifungals should be considered, especially in those listed for transplantation. The choice of antimicrobial agent should be driven by local resistance patterns. Antimicrobial therapy should be reviewed in the light of culture results on a daily basis.

Metabolic and feeding

Enteral nutrition should commence within 12 h of admission assuming there are no contraindications. In patients with large aspirates (>200 mL/4 h), a prokinetic agent should be commenced and erythromycin (250 mg i.v. every 6 h) appears to be more effective than metoclopramide. Endoscopic placement of a postpyloric feeding tube should be considered in refractory cases. The optimal nature of enteral feed used has not been investigated but metabolic data on these patients demonstrate increased calorific requirements. Patients with ALF demonstrate both peripheral and hepatic insulin resistance. Tight glycemic control results in improved outcome and less cholestasis in a general intensive care unit population and it would seem reasonable to extrapolate this management to patients with ALF.

Metabolic acidosis is a relatively frequent occurrence that may relate to lactic acidosis, hyperchloremic acidosis, or renal failure. The hyperlactatemia may be resultant upon volume depletion and resolve with appropriate fluid loading and/or may reflect the inability of the liver to metabolize the lactate produced. A failure for blood lactate to normalize following volume loading is associated with a poor prognosis.

Coagulopathy

The correction of coagulopathy should not be undertaken routinely as it may complicate the determination of prognosis. However, repletion of coagulation factors is necessary for clinical bleeding and prophylactically before major invasive procedures. Thrombocytopenia is common and may be associated with disseminated intravascular coagulation (DIC) and these patients are at particular risk of hemorrhage.

Liver transplantation

The impact of liver transplantation on the management of ALF is considered revolutionary. ALF now accounts for 5–12% of all liver transplant activity. Donor organ allocation systems prioritize patients with acute liver and 45–50% of patients undergo transplantation. Up to 25% of patients are deemed to have contraindications to transplantation and the remainder deteriorate before an organ is allocated.

Patient selection

The development of encephalopathy in association with a progressive coagulopathy is a commonly used selection criterion. However, survival rates of 39–67% are being achieved with medical management in some etiologies, risking unnecessary transplants using this approach. The King's College Hospital criteria (Tables 101.7 and 101.8) indicating a poor prognosis have been used as a method of selecting patients for liver transplantation. This model is considered to: (1) be sensitive to the urgency with which patients with a poor prognosis need to be identified; (2) be easily and widely applicable; (3) not be reliant on the development of advanced disease; and (4) maximize the time available to obtain a suitable donor organ.

Another pragmatic approach is to list all patients with ALF for transplantation and make the decision to proceed when an organ becomes available. This approach may maximize the delivery of transplantation to this patient population, but increases the risk of unnecessary transplantation.

The removal of patients from the waiting list when the clinical condition deteriorates to the extent that transplantation is futile is both emotive and difficult. No definite role has yet been confirmed for ICP monitoring or cerebral metabolic rates for oxygen in deciding the vexed question of when potentially irreversible brain damage should preclude the use of liver transplantation. Accelerating inotrope requirements, uncontrolled sepsis, and severe respiratory failure are other imprecise contraindications to transplantation. These contraindications are age sensitive as younger patients are more resilient and more likely to reverse these complications after liver transplantation.

Transplant operation

The repletion of coagulation factors, and platelets where necessary, prior to surgery adequately reverses the clinical coagulopathy in most cases, and intraoperative blood losses are remarkably low. This reflects both the poor correlation between studies of coagulation factors and the risk of surgical bleeding, and the absence of portal hypertension. Cerebral edema may be problematic during the dissection phase and the period immediately after reperfusion. In contrast, it often improves dramatically during the anhepatic phase of the transplant operation. Cerebral autoregulation is restored within 48 h of successful transplantation and monitoring of intracerebral pressure and cerebral perfusion pressure should continue during this period in patients susceptible to cerebral edema.

Auxiliary liver transplantation has been pioneered for patients with the potential to recover normal liver function and morphology. In theory, it combines the advantages of transplantation with the ability to withdraw immunosuppression when regeneration has been demonstrated in the native liver. In practice, the prediction of regenerative capacity to normal morphology has not been easy. The neurologic and hemodynamic benefits derived from the removal of the diseased liver are reduced with this approach, and in unstable patients standard orthotopic transplantation is preferred. Functional studies using radionuclide scans and liver histology are used to assess the degree of regeneration in the native liver. When the native liver returns to normal morphology and function, the auxiliary transplant is sacrificed either passively by withdrawing immunosuppression or actively with surgical resection.

The profile of sepsis, including fungal infection, seen in ALF extends into the post-transplant period and is further aggravated by the necessary immunosuppressive therapy. Patients transplanted for ALF are routinely included in antimicrobial prophylactic regimens targeted at high-risk patients. Renal function may improve dramatically in the immediate postoperative period but more often renal support may be necessary for many weeks after successful transplantation. The potent immunosuppressive agents and some antimicrobial drugs commonly used are potentially nephrotoxic and the use of these agents should be modified to promote the return of renal function.

Results

Registry data indicate that the overall survival rates are in the region of 60–65%, but individual centers have reported higher survival in the 75–90% range. Patients receiving liver transplants for ALF (median age 28 years) are younger than those undergoing elective transplantation (median age 44 years). The age of the patient influences selection for liver transplantation in ALF more than in elective transplantation.

Prognostic factors: The factors that influence outcome after liver transplantation are multiple. The etiology of the underlying disease correlated with outcome in some centers. The best results were achieved for transplantation for Wilson's disease and the worst for idiosyncratic drug reactions. In acetaminophen-induced liver failure, survival was best when transplant was performed within 4 days of the overdose. This reflects the role of sepsis in the continued deterioration in these patients and the inability of liver transplantation to reverse this complication. Survival rate decreases with progression of encephalopathy at the time of transplantation; in one series, the figures were 90% for grade 1, 77% for grade 2, 79% for grade 3, and 54% for grade 4. As with liver transplantation in general, renal function correlated with outcome and serum creatinine levels above 200 μmol/L or 1.5 mg/dL were associated with a poorer outcome. Acidosis and Apache III score at the time of transplantation were good indicators of the severity of the illness and correlated with outcome. However, none of these parameters were sufficiently discriminatory to use as criteria to disqualify individual cases from transplantation.

Liver support

A variety of liver support systems have been described and assessed aiming to improve outcome, provide an environment for regeneration and possible spontaneous recovery, or support the patient until liver transplantation is an option. Such therapies may be applied to patients with ALF, acute or chronic decompensation of liver disease, and those with graft dysfunction following liver transplant. It is important to note that the requirements of these groups are different and should not be confused when assessing the efficacy of these therapeutic strategies.

Available systems: The systems available at the present time to support the failing liver are bioartificial livers utilizing cell-based therapies or extracorporeal liver perfusion (using human or porcine livers), and dialysis-based methods or plasmapheresis. A recent systematic review of the literature examined 198 patients who had been exposed to extracorporeal liver perfusion.[15] Long-term survival was 28% and was similar to that of standard of care. Independent predictors of positive outcome appeared to be age <20 years, level of encephalopathy grade 3 or 4, a perfusion time of >10 h, and use of human or baboon livers. Such systems must, however, be recognized as being very expensive, both in resource and time.

Charcoal hemoperfusion: The initial enthusiasm for this system emanated from an uncontrolled study of 75 patients in which a significant survival benefit in the treated patients as compared with historical controls was found (65% vs 15%).[16] A subsequent controlled study failed to demonstrate a survival benefit in the active limb.[17]

Hybrid systems have utilized a mixture of charcoal and cellular mechanisms. The Berlin extracorporeal liver support system utilizes a very elegant three-dimensional capillary structure containing hepatocytes. Provisional work with this system suggests it is safe and provides hemodynamic stability but controlled trials are lacking. Another bioartificial liver device utilized 50 g of hepatocytes on collagen-coated microcarriers. It was incorporated into an extracorporeal circuit where the patient's plasma is separated before being run over charcoal columns and then exposed to the porcine hepatocytes. This system was applied for 6–7 h and in original studies was shown to provide significant improvement in Glasgow coma score with a significant fall in ICP and improvement in cerebral perfusion pressure.[18] This system also demonstrated significant falls in blood ammonia, bilirubin, and creatinine. However, a randomized controlled trial involving 147 patients with ALF and 27 patients with primary graft nonfunction found no overall difference in 30-day survival rates, when reported in abstract form.[19] However, there did appear to be a significant benefit in terms of survival for acetaminophen-induced ALF and those patients who developed encephalopathy within 2 weeks of jaundice.

The **ELAD system** incorporates hepatocytes in the form of hepatoblastoma cells (C_3A cell line) that are grown to confluence in the extracapillary compartment of a hollow fiber filter. Initial studies incorporated veno-venous access with no oxygenator and the system was shown to be biocompatible but to have little effect on measured clinical parameters.[20] A more sophisticated ELAD circuit incorporated plasma separation and an oxygenator system prior to the patient's plasma being exposed to the hepatocytes; clinical trials with this have not yet progressed beyond the phase 2 stage.

Other systems: Liver support systems that do not utilize biological components include albumin dialysis (molecular adsorbent recirculating system: MARS) and plasmapheresis. Albumin dialysis has been advocated for the removal of both water-soluble and albumin-bound toxins providing the albumin dialysis is incorporated with standard dialysis or hemofiltration. The controlled trials assessing this modality have examined patients with acute or chronic liver failure only. Case series have been reported in patients with ALF demonstrating improved biochemistry and amino acid profiles, hemodynamic stability, and neurological improvement. Plasmapheresis protocols have utilized membrane filtration with a pore size of 0.65 mm and exchanged 15% of body weight on up to three consecutive occasions.[21] Improvement in encephalopathy, cerebral blood flow, and cerebral perfusion pressure has been documented without any deleterious change in ICP. Mean arterial pressure improved significantly with an improvement in systemic vascular resistance. As with MARS therapy there is as yet a lack of controlled clinical data.

EFERENCES

Bernal B. Changing patterns of causation and the use of transplantation in the United Kingdom. Semin Liver Dis 2003; 23:227–237.

O'Grady JG, Alexander GJ, Hallyar KM, Williams R. Early indicators of prognosis in fulminant hepatic failure. Gastroenterology 1989; 97:439–445.

Bernal W, Donaldson N, Wyncoll D, Wendon J. Blood lactate as an early indicator of outcome in paracetamol-induced acute liver failure. Lancet 2002; 359:558–563.

Bernuau J, Goudeau A, Poynard T et al. Multivariate analysis of prognostic factors in fulminant hepatitis B. Hepatology 1986; 6:648–651.

Strauss GI, Knudsen GM, Kondrup J, Moller K, Larsen FS. Cerebral metabolism of ammonia and amino acids in patients with fulminant hepatic failure. Gastroenterology 2001; 121: 1109–1119.

Cordoba J, Gottstein J, Blei AT. Glutamine, myo-inositol and organic brain osmolytes after portocaval anastomosis in the rat: implications for ammonia induced brain edema. Hepatology 2000; 24:919–923.

Rolando N, Wade J, Davalos M et al. The systemic inflammatory response syndrome in acute liver failure. Hepatology 2000; 32:734–739.

8. Blei AT, Olafsson S, Webster S, Levy R. Complications of intracranial pressure monitoring in fulminant hepatic failure. Lancet 1993; 341:157–158.
9. Keays RT, Alexander GJ, Williams R. The safety and value of extradural intracranial pressure monitors in fulminant hepatic failure. J Hepatol 1993; 18:205–209.
10. Jalan R, Damink SW, Deutz NE, Lee A, Hayes PC. Moderate hypothermia for uncontrolled intracranial hypertension in acute liver failure. Lancet 1992; 354:1164–1168.
11. Murphy N, Auzinger G, Bernel W, Wendon J. The effect of hypertonic sodium chloride on intracranial pressure in patients with acute liver failure. Hepatology 2004; 39:464–470.
12. Shawcross DL, Davies NA, Mookerjee RP et al. Worsening of cerebral hyperemia by the administration of terlipressin in acute liver failure with severe encephalopathy. Hepatology 2004; 39:471–475.
13. Harry R, Auzinger G, Wendon J. The clinical importance of adrenal insufficiency in acute hepatic dysfunction. Hepatology 2002; 36: 395–402.
14. Davenport A. The management of renal failure in patients at risk of cerebral edema/hypoxia. New Horiz 1995; 3:717–724.
15. Pascher A, Sauer IM, Hammer C, Gerlach JC, Neuhaus P. Extracorporeal liver perfusion as hepatic assist in acute liver failure: a review of world experience. Xenotransplantation 2002; 9:309.
16. Gimson AE, Braude S, Mellon PJ, Canalese J, Williams R. Earlier charcoal haemoperfusion in fulminant hepatic failure. Lancet 1982; 2:681–683.
17. O'Grady JG, Gimson AE, O'Brien CJ et al. Controlled trials of charcoal hemoperfusion and prognostic factors in fulminant hepatic failure. Gastroenterology 1988; 94:1186–1192.
18. Chen SC, Mullon C, Kahaku E et al. Treatment of severe liver failure with a bioartificial liver. Ann N Y Acad Sci 1997; 831:350–360.
19. Stephens et al (abst) AASLD 2001.
20. Ellis AJ, Hughes RD, Wendon JA et al. Pilot-controlled trial of the extracorporeal liver assist device in acute liver failure. Hepatology 1996; 24:1446–1451.
21. Clemmesen JO, Larsen FS, Ejlersen E, Schiodt FV, Ott P, Hansen BA. Haemodynamic changes after high-volume plasmapheresis in patients with chronic and acute liver failure. Eur J Gastroenterol Hepatol 1997; 9:55–60.

Chapter 102

Tumors of the liver

María Varela, Natascha Celli, Margarita Sala, and Jordi Bruix

KEY POINTS

- Defined as focal solid or liquid lesions
- With the common and widespread use of imaging techniques, incidental liver tumors are increasingly being diagnosed. They range widely in epidemiology, risk factors, clinical characteristics, diagnosis, treatment, and prognosis
- Can be divided in two major categories: cystic and solid lesions

Cystic lesions:
- Simple cyst
- Hydatid cyst
- Hepatic abscess (pyogenic or amebic)

Solid lesions:
- Hemangioma
- Focal nodular hyperplasia
- Hepatocellular adenoma
- Hepatic metastasis
- Hepatocellular carcinoma
- Fibrolamellar carcinoma
- Intrahepatic cholangiocarcinoma
- Angiosarcoma
- Hepatic epithelioid hemangioendothelioma
- Biliary cystadenoma and cystadenocarcinoma

ITRODUCTION

mors of the liver are defined as focal solid or liquid lesions at can be differentiated from the normal anatomy of the liver imaging techniques. They range from benign asymptomatic ions to malignant aggressive neoplasms. The clinical prevance of focal hepatic lesions has increased due to recent vances in imaging techniques and their widespread use.[1]

The diagnosis of a focal liver lesion is based on clinical findgs, imaging techniques, and, most commonly, on histopathogic analysis.[1–3] An incidental lesion in an asymptomatic patient th no history of liver disease or known neoplasia is usually nign. The most prevalent benign lesions are simple cysts, mangiomas, and focal nodular hyperplasia (FNH).[4] In a patient th a known cancer of any origin, liver metastases will be the ost probable diagnosis. Finally, a liver lesion in a cirrhotic tient is most likely a hepatocellular carcinoma (HCC). The st medical history may also suggest a diagnosis. Thereby, a ghly vascularized nodule in a healthy young woman on oral ntraceptives should raise the suspicion of hepatocellular enoma, and a liver tumor in a patient with sclerosing cholantis should suggest the presence of cholangiocarcinoma. milarly, biochemical data including viral and tumor markers ay be helpful clinically.

Radiologic techniques indicate whether the tumor has a liquid (cysts, abscesses) or solid (benign or malignant tumors) content. The vascularization profile may also suggest its possible nature.[4] However, both benign (FNH or hepatocellular adenoma) and malignant (HCC, carcinoid) tumors may show arterial hypervascularization. Doppler ultrasonography (US), contrast-enhanced US, dynamic computed tomography (CT), and dynamic magnetic resonance imaging (MRI) define the vascular pattern and, together with analysis of the nodule characteristics, may strongly suggest the diagnosis. Nevertheless, in the majority of cases the final diagnosis will be established solely by biopsy.

Given the wide spectrum of liver tumors, the following sections will separately review the epidemiology, pathology, clinical presentation, diagnosis, and treatment of the most common cystic and solid hepatic lesions.

CYSTIC LESIONS

Simple cyst

Some 2–7% of the general population is affected by a simple cyst.[5–8] Cysts contain serous liquid, are covered by cuboidal epithelium, and do not communicate with the biliary ducts.[5–7] In most cases they are solitary, and, if multiple, should prompt the suspicion of hepatic and/or renal polycystic disease. Symptoms are absent until their size is larger than 10 cm in diameter; anecdotally, they may cause jaundice, hemorrhage, or infection.[6–7] Diagnosis is easily established by US demonstrating a simple liquid lesion with well defined, thin walls, associated with strong posterior wall echoes.[7–8] CT scan (Fig. 102.1) depicts a hypointense lesion with no changes through all the phases of the dynamic study. Treatment, if any, should be symptomatic. Only complicated cysts may benefit from percutaneous drainage or surgical resection.[7]

Hydatid cyst (see Chapter 83)

Echinococcosis is a zoonosis caused by cestodes belonging to the genus *Echinococcus* (family Taeniidae). It can affect the liver, lung, central nervous system, and others.[9] Hepatic cysts rupture into the peritoneum, pleural space, or biliary tract in one-third of cases. Thicker walls with potential calcification, septa, and split walls with floating membranes differentiate hydatid from simple cysts.[9] Distinction from biliary cystadenoma or cystadenocarcinoma may require biopsy. Serology is positive in 70% of cases. Treatment should be based on the administration of mebendazole or albendazole, even in surgical cases.[10]

Hepatic abscess

Pyogenic hepatic abscesses are usually produced by bacteria from the gastrointestinal tract. In 40% of cases they complicate

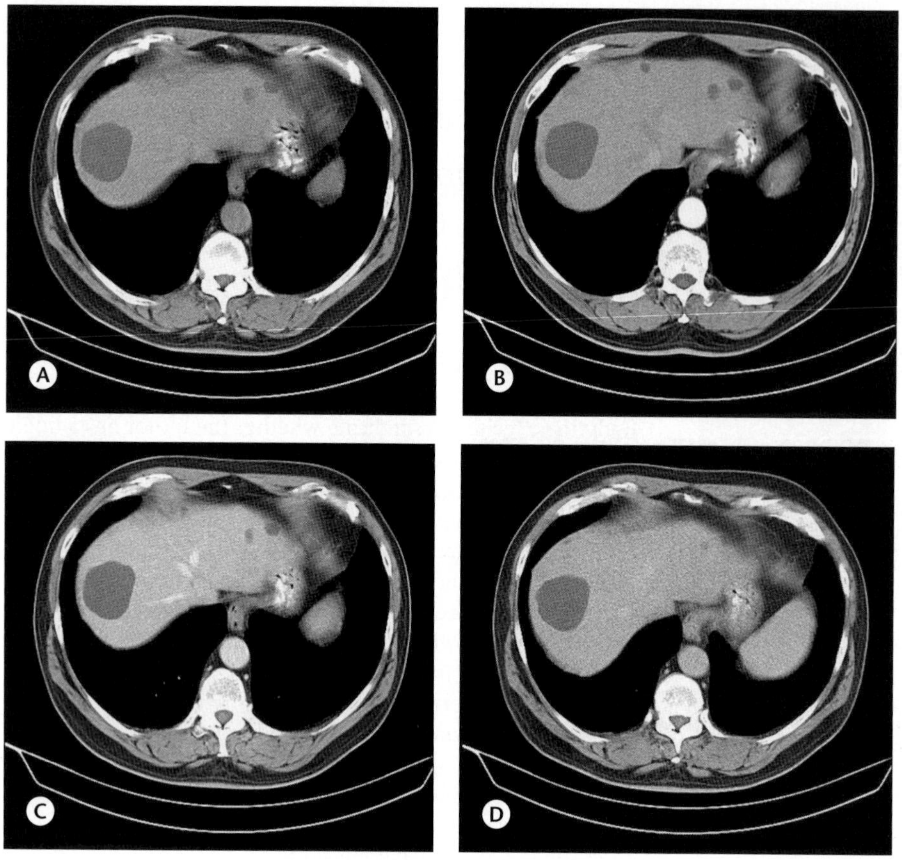

Fig. 102.1 Simple liver cysts. CT scan with contrast enhancement shows a big simple c within the right lobe (arrow) and multiple small simple cysts within the left lobe (arrov **A.** Basal phase. **B.** Arterial phase. **C.** Portal phase. **D.** Equilibrium phase.

cholangitis, and the remainder result from portal bacteremia secondary to gastrointestinal infections such as diverticulitis or appendicitis.[2,11] The clinical suspicion is based on the presence of malaise, fever, anorexia, right upper quadrant pain, and leukocytosis. CT confirms the diagnosis by demonstrating one or more cystic lesions with internal bubbles and ill-defined margins.[2,11] Blood cultures are positive in 60% of cases.[11] Treatment includes antibiotics and percutaneous or surgical drainage.[11]

Pyogenic abscess must be distinguished from amebic hepatic abscess. This is uncommon in developed countries, but may occur in travelers to endemic areas. Clinical manifestations and imaging techniques do not allow distinction from pyogenic abscess. Ameba serology is positive in more than 90% of cases. The best treatment is metronidazole, frequently associated with percutaneous drainage.

SOLID LESIONS

Hepatic hemangioma

Hemangioma is the most frequent tumor of the liver, with a prevalence of 0.4–7.4%.[2,5,12] It is composed of large vascular channels lined by mature, flattened, endothelial cells, enclosed in a fibroblastic stroma.[2,5,6] Hemangiomas are usually solitary and small, but can reach 20 cm in diameter.[12] Even then, most patients are asymptomatic and diagnosis is incidental. Their course is benign, although they may grow slightly during pregnancy or estrogen treatment. Bleeding is extremely infrequent and should suggest another diagnosis. Giant hemangiomas may become symptomatic in the event of infarction or thrombosis. Exceptionally a hemangioma can lead to thrombocytopenia, localized coagulopathy, and microangiopathic hemoly anemia (Kasabach-Merritt syndrome).

US shows a well defined hyperechogenic lesion. MRI is best technique to establish the diagnosis (100% sensitivity, 9 specificity) (Fig. 102.2) upon finding a typical globular peri eral enhancement with progressive hyperintense filling T2-weighted images.[13,14] Treatment should be symptomatic

Focal nodular hyperplasia

FNH is a benign tumor with a prevalence of 0.01% in general population. In most cases it is solitary and smaller th 5 cm (Fig. 102.3), but it may be larger and multiple in 20% cases. It is considered a regenerative cell response to an ab rant dystrophic artery.[1,2,5–7] Normal hepatocytes form plates c or two cells thick, and in the margins of the nodule promin bile ductular reaction with positive staining for orcein can observed, a characteristic that is used to distinguish FNH fr hepatic adenoma. The presence of a central fibrotic scar c taining the feeding artery is a characteristic finding and is us to establish the CT or MRI diagnosis in the absence of biop (Fig. 102.4).[15–17] MRI evidences this central scar as an i intense nodule in T1-wedged images, and as isointense mildly hyperintense in T2-weighted images.

FNH is more common in young women[2,6] and usually rep sents an incidental finding in asymptomatic subjects. The clini evolution is uneventful with no potentially severe compli tions. Thus, no treatment is recommended.[1,2,7]

Hepatocellular adenoma

Hepatocellular adenoma is a very uncommon tumor (prevaler 0.001%) that is found more frequently in young women.[2,6,7

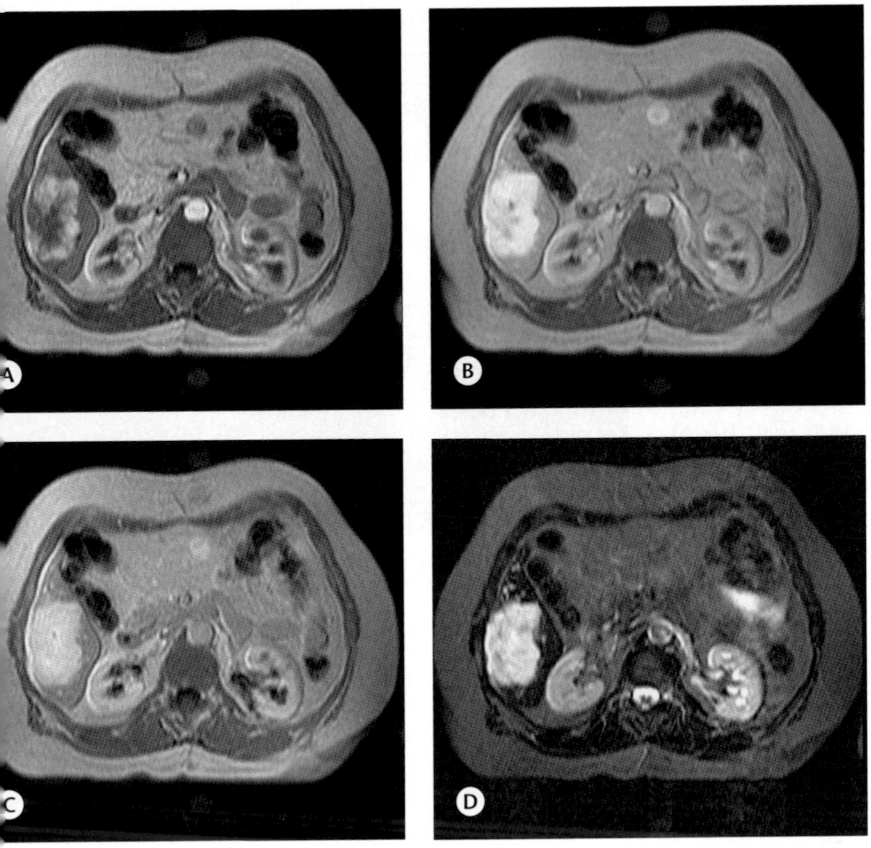

Fig. 102.2 Small hepatic hemangioma. Contrast-enhanced MRI shows this small hepatic hemangioma as a hyperintense nodule on T2-wedged images. **A.** Arterial phase. **B.** Portal phase. **C.** Equilibrium phase. **D.** T2 wedged image.

ssociated with oral contraceptive or anabolic treatment, and h glycogen storage disease type Ia (von Gierke disease).[2,5–7] most instances it is a solitary lesion, but in up to 10–20% of es more than one adenoma can be detected. In these patients patic adenomatosis due to a genetic abnormality has to be nsidered.[2,5,7,16] Hepatic adenoma is composed of normal patocytes without atypia, arranged in plates separated by ated sinusoids. It lacks portal spaces or biliary ducts.[2,6]

Most patients with hepatic adenoma report mild abdominal n. The most frequent complication is necrosis and bleeding. is can prompt severe hemoperitoneum from subcapsular enomas.[15,16] Malignant transformation has been demonstrated a minority of patients, and justifies treatment – resection or rcutaneous ablation.[1,5,7]

Distinction between hepatic adenoma and FNH may be difficult, en with the most sensitive imaging techniques and pathologic amination.[7] MRI depicts a hyperintense signal on T2-wedged ages, an iso-signal intensity on T1-wedged images, and rapid wash-in and wash-out of gadolinium (enhancement of hepatic adenoma in the arterial phase, whereas in parenchymal phases the tumor is isointense with respect to the liver tissue).[2,6,7,17]

Hepatic metastasis

Most malignant liver tumors are metastases from cancers that originate in other organs,[2,18] the most frequent being lung, colon,

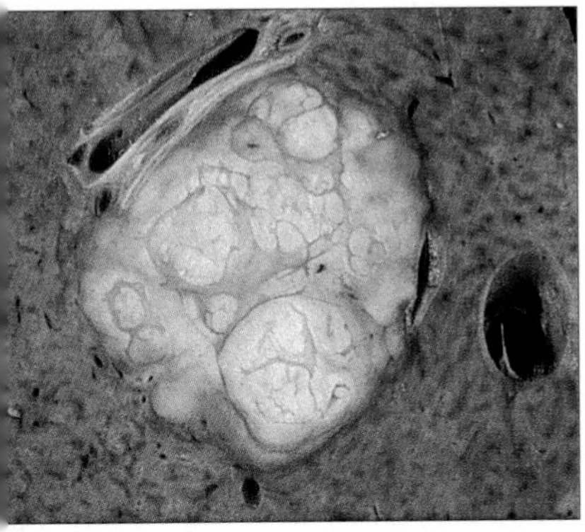

Fig. 102.3 Focal nodular hyperplasia. The section of the liver segment containing the tumor shows a mass smaller than 3 cm in diameter, with a typical central fibrotic scar.

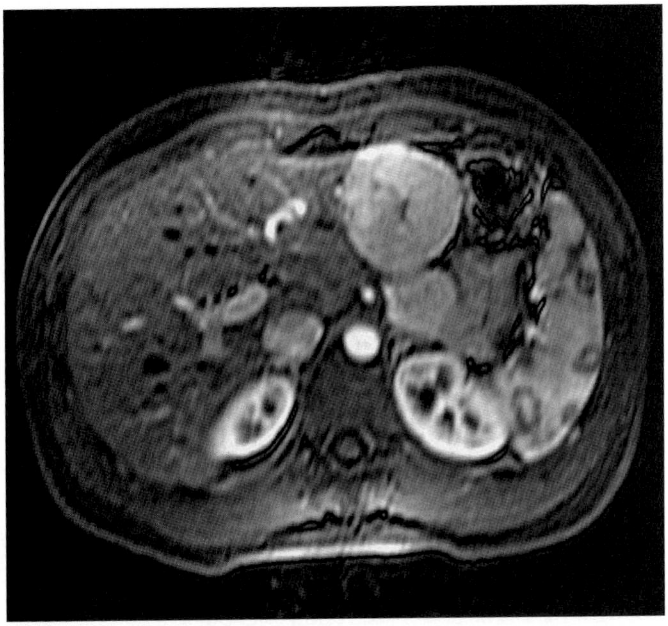

Fig. 102.4 Focal nodular hyperplasia. With contrast enhanced dynamic MRI it is possible to identify a mass in the left hepatic lobe with a central fibrotic scar, which confirms the diagnosis of focal nodular hyperplasia.

stomach, pancreas, gallbladder, breast, and ovaries. Metastatic involvement of the liver implies a poor prognosis, except in patients with colorectal or neuroendocrine metastases that can be treated surgically (Fig. 102.5).

Searching for the primary tumor and biopsy confirmation is justified if the patient may benefit from therapy such as surgery or systemic chemotherapy.[18] Fine-needle aspiration biopsy has an 85% diagnostic sensitivity with more than 95% specificity. Tumor markers can also be useful. Serum carcinoembryonic antigen levels are increased in 90% of colorectal cancer (CRC) metastases, CA125 can rise in pancreatic and ovarian cancer, and prostate-specific antigen is specific for prostate tumors. On CT, liver metastases are hypovascular lesions that in some neoplasms may have a specific pattern (Fig. 102.6). Contrast uptake in the arterial phase on CT or MRI suggests carcinoid tumor, melanoma, sarcoma, hypernephroma, or thyroid neoplasia.[2,6,17] Isotopic studies using labeled somatostatin analogs can identify neuroendocrine tumors.

Surgical resection of liver metastases may prolong survival in patients with CRC, neuroendocrine tumors, and some renal carcinomas, but for other neoplasms the indication of surgery is still controversial. Patients with up to four CRC metastases who can be successfully resected may achieve a 40% survival rate at 5 years. Neadjuvant chemotherapy may also improve outcome.[19] In neuroendocrine tumors, resection may be curative when associated with resection of the primary tumor.[20,21]

Hepatocellular carcinoma

HCC is the fifth most common neoplasm in the world, and the third most common cause of cancer-related death, with more than half a million new cases diagnosed yearly.[22] It usually develops in the setting of chronic liver disease, and cirrhosis represents the strongest predisposing factor.

Epidemiology: There are significant geographic differences in HCC incidence (age-adjusted incidence rate is 8.7×10^5 in developed countries and 14.7×10^5 in developing countries),

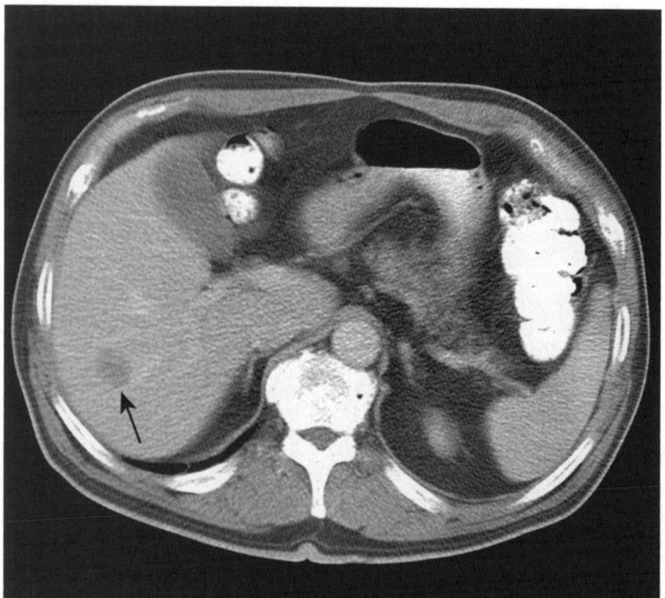

Fig. 102.5 **Metastases from colorectal carcinoma.** On contrast-enhanced CT, CRC metastases are depicted as hypovascular lesions with peripheral contrast uptake (arrow).

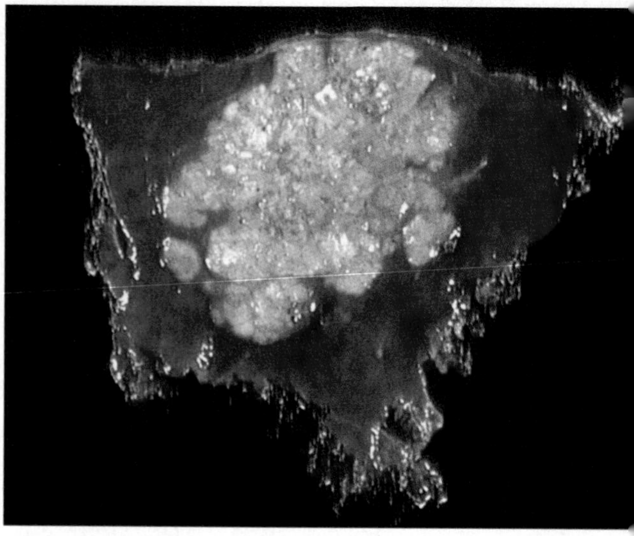

Fig. 102.6 **Colorectal metastasis.** This section of the liver reveals heterogeneous multilocular mass with ill-defined margins.

reflecting the heterogeneous distribution of its main etiol factors (Table 102.1).[23] In Asia and Africa, hepatitis B v infection is the predominant risk factor, and the risk is increa by ingestion of aflatoxin B1-contaminated food that is associa with a specific mutation in the *p53* tumor suppressor gene these areas, HCC may develop early in life, mostly in a non rhotic liver. By contrast, in developed countries, HCC aff older patients with hepatitis C virus (HCV) or alcohol-rela cirrhosis.[23] The incidence of HCC has increased in the p decade as a consequence of higher rates of HCV infection improvements in the management and survival of cirrh patients. In these patients surveillance with US and measu ment of α-fetoprotein levels every 6 months is recommen to detect the tumor in early phases, while still amenable curative therapies.[24]

Diagnosis: In patients without underlying liver disease, diagnosis of HCC should be based on cytohistologic crite By contrast, in cirrhotic patients the diagnosis can be establis by noninvasive criteria (Fig. 102.7).[24] Thereby, HCC can be c fidently diagnosed if a focal lesion more than 2 cm in diame with arterial hypervascularization is identified by two imag techniques (four techniques considered: US, spiral CT, MRI, angiography) or by one imaging technique (tumor >2 cm w arterial hypervascularization) together with an α-fetoprot level >400 mg/mL. HCC is usually seen as a hypoechogenic heterogeneous nodule with marked enhancement in the a rial phase after contrast administration on US, CT, and M (Figs 102.8–102.10). MRI angiography has the highest diagno accuracy for HCC >1 cm.[25] Thus, MRI angiography is con ered the optimal test for staging early HCC (Fig. 102.11).

In cirrhotic patients it is important to distinguish early sm HCC from macroregenerative nodules and dysplastic nodu as well as from atypical hemangiomas and metastases. Nodu of between 1 and 2 cm require a diagnostic biopsy (Fig. 102. A negative biopsy does not rule out malignancy, and so repe ed biopsies may be necessary. Establishing a diagnosis of H in nodules <1 cm is difficult and the recommendation is follow them by US every 3 months to detect tumor growth

Transplantation and outcome: Prognosis depends on tur stage, degree of liver failure, general condition, and treatment.[2

BLE 102.1 ANNUAL INCIDENCE OF HCC IN CHRONIC LIVER DISEASE OF VARIOUS ETIOLOGIES

	Incidence
V carrier without cirrhosis	0.4–0.6%*
V-related cirrhosis	2–6% per year
V-related cirrhosis	3–8%
rhosis from genetic hemochromatosis	5%
ary primary cirrhosis	Low risk
rhosis from autoimmune hepatitis or primary sclerosing cholangitis	Very low risk

sk increased if infection is acquired in childhood.
/, hepatitis B virus; HCV, hepatitis C virus.

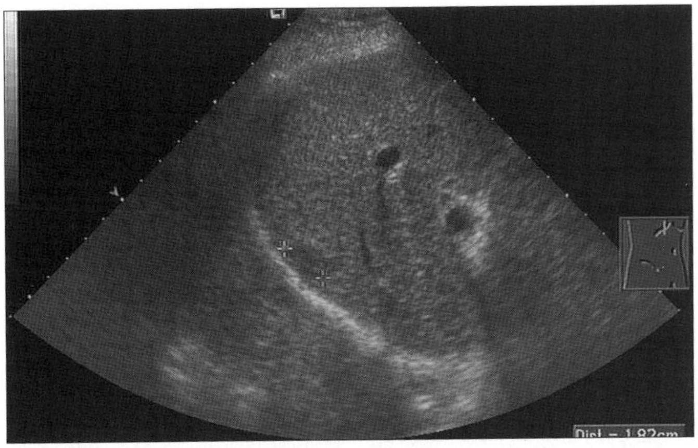

Fig. 102.8 Small hepatocellular carcinoma. HCC (diameter <2 cm) seen as a hypoechoic focal lesion on regular US.

ently, the Barcelona Clinic Liver Cancer Group has proposed stratification of patients with HCC into four major cate- es, each with a different treatment (Fig. 102.13).[26] Stage 0 situ HCC) corresponds to patients with very early tumors cm, differentiated, and without the ability to disseminate. h curative therapies, the 5-year survival rate is 80%.[26] Stage umors are slightly more advanced, although still at an early e (single nodules, or fewer than three nodules <3 cm), and suitable for resection, orthotopic liver transplantation (OLT), percutaneous ablation. The 5-year survival rate is 50–70% patients in whom the optimal treatment is selected. ection is therefore of benefit only in patients with solitary C in whom the underlying cirrhosis has not led to signifi- t portal hypertension or hyperbilirubinemia. Transplantation he preferred approach for patients with decompensated hosis and a single tumor (Fig. 102.14) and for those with to three nodules <3 cm.

)ther treatments: Percutaneous ablation by ethanol injection radiofrequency should be considered in patients at stage 0

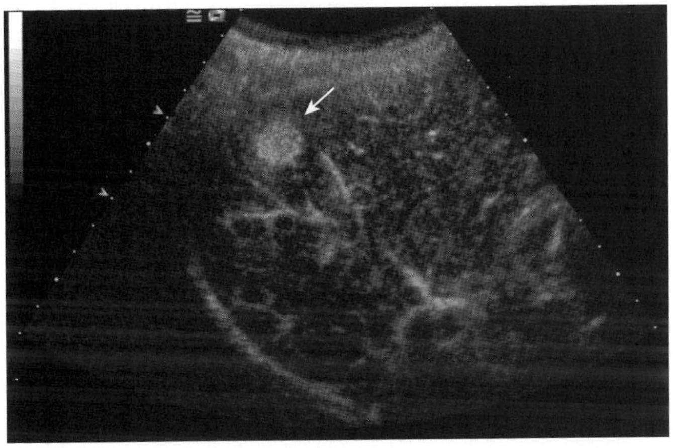

Fig. 102.9 Small hepatocellular carcinoma. HCC (arrow) depicted as a hypervascular lesion on the arterial phase of contrast-enhanced US. The vessels feeding the tumor can be identified.

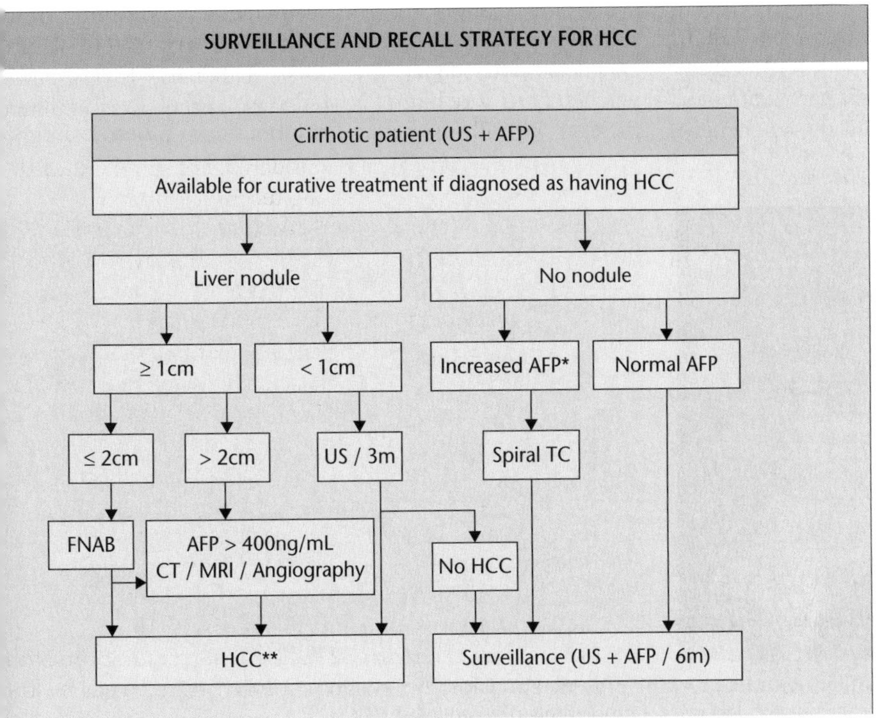

Fig. 102.7 Surveillance and recall strategy for HCC. AFP, α-fetoprotein; CT, computed tomography; HCC, hepatocellular carcinoma; MRI, magnetic resonance imaging; US, ultrasonography; *AFP levels to be defined. **Pathological confirmation or noninvasive criteria. From Bruix et al.,[24] with permission.

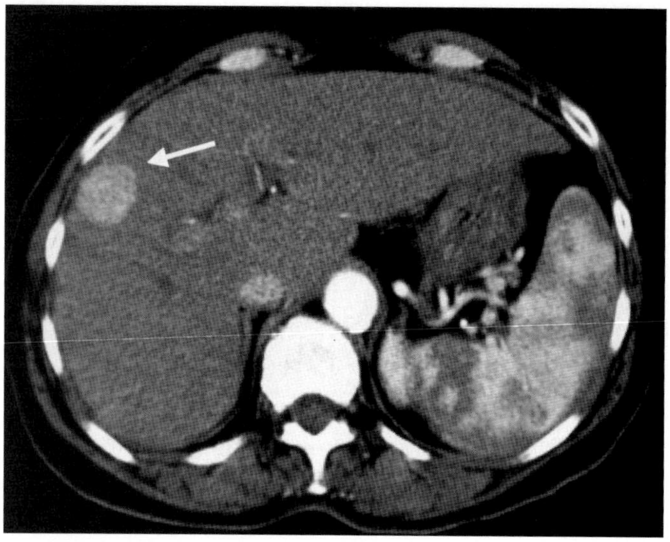

Fig. 102.10 Hepatocellular carcinoma. Contrast-enhanced CT shows a 3.5-cm HCC located in the right hepatic lobe (arrow), depicted as a hypervascular lesion in the arterial phase of the study.

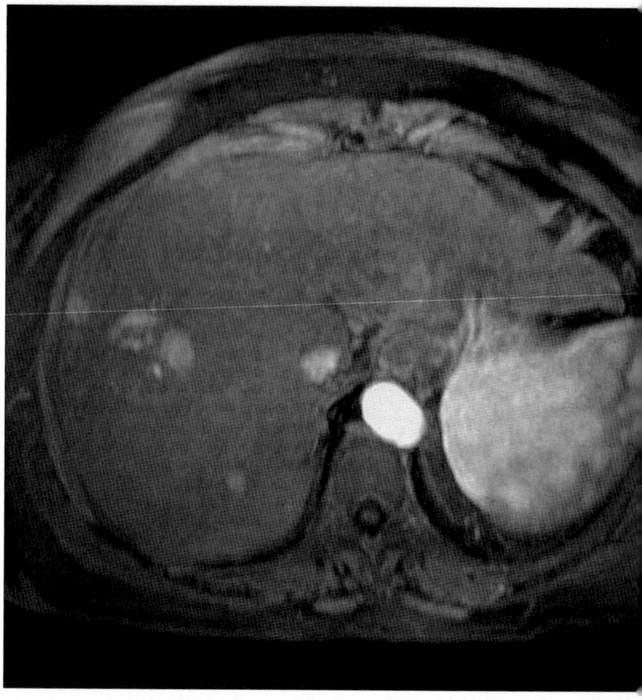

Fig. 102.11 Hepatocellular carcinoma. Contrast-enhanced MRI of 4-cm HCC located in the right hepatic lobe, depicted as a hypervascu lesion in the arterial phase.

or A who are not eligible for surgery.[26–28] Patients with stage B disease are still asymptomatic with large or multifocal HCC without vascular invasion or extrahepatic spread, and are optimal candidates for chemoembolization.[29] This requires selective catheterization of the hepatic artery feeding the tumor, with injection of a chemotherapeutic agent followed by the injection of gelfoam or polyvinyl alcohol to prevent backflow. The procedure is well tolerated and achieves tumor necrosis in more than 50% of the patients, who thereafter achieve an improved survival rate exceeding 50% at 3 years. Stage C denotes patients with advanced tumors and vascular involvement, extrahepatic spread, or physical impairment who do not benefit from any available therapy and, thus, should be assessed for new antitumoral agents in randomized controlled trials. Finally, patients with stage D tumors have a very poor physical status and/or major tumor burden (Okuda stage 3), and should receive symptomatic treatment. Their median survival is less than 6 months. Patients with Child-Pugh grade C HCC at any stage who are not candidates for liver transplantation belong to this group and do not benefit from antitumoral treatment as outcome is poor due to liv failure.

Fibrolamellar carcinoma

Fibrolamellar carcinoma is an uncommon variant of HC (1–9%), frequent in Western countries, and most prevalent young patients without chronic liver disease. Therefore, it m be differentiated from benign liver lesions. Usually it consi of a large, single, nonencapsulated intrahepatic mass with fibrotic calcified central scar. The diagnosis is usually late, w symptoms related to mass and malignant syndrome. The fetoprotein level is normal in more than 90% of patien Diagnosis and staging are based on spiral CT and/or MI percutaneous core biopsy is needed in cases of atypical imagi Patients with fibrolamellar carcinoma have a better progno

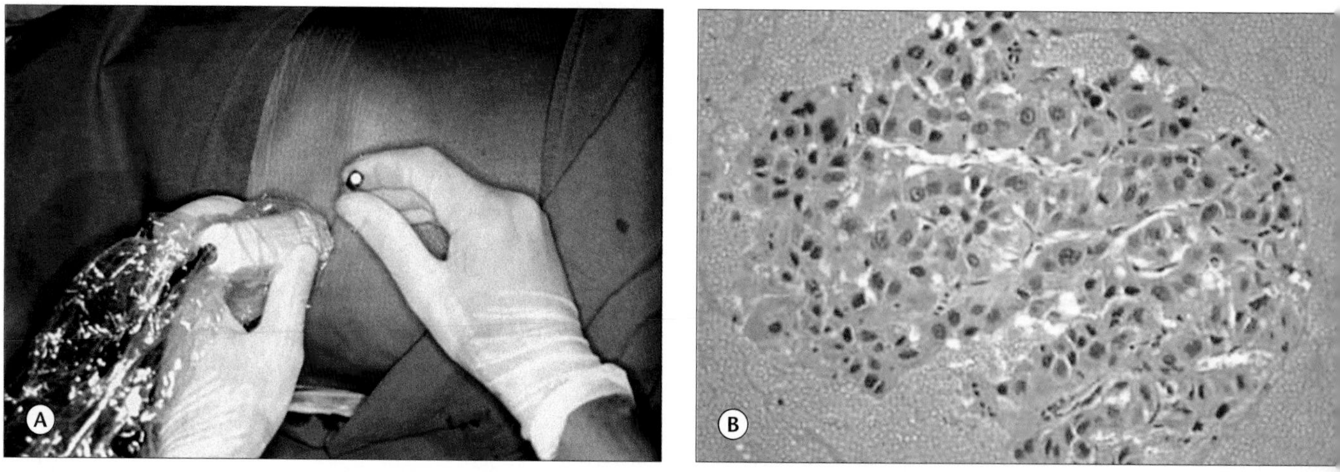

Fig. 102.12 Fine-needle aspiration biopsy in a patient with HCC. A. The procedure is guided by US using the free-hand technique. **B.** Ligh microscopy using conventional hematoxylin and eosin staining indicates a moderately differentiated HCC.

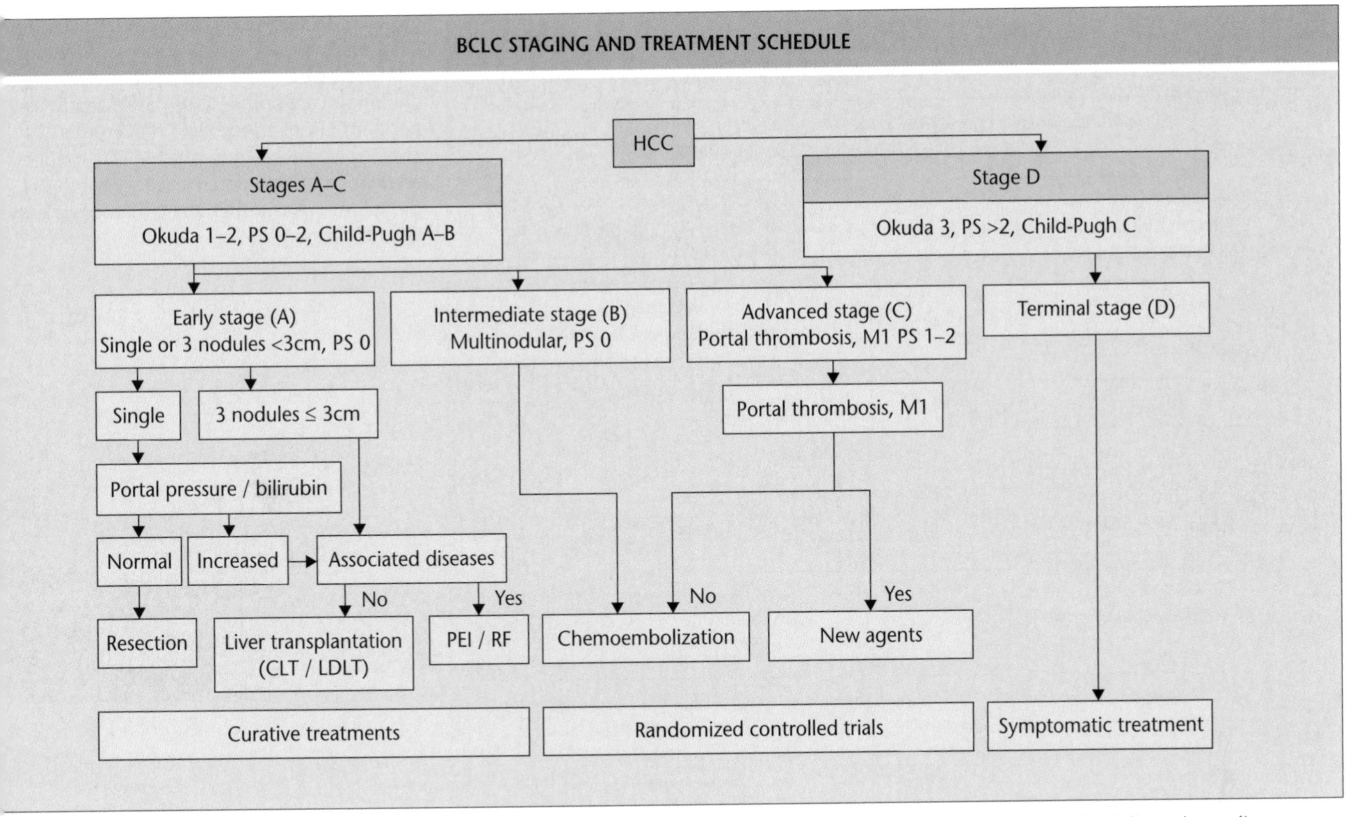

ɟ. 102.13 **Barcelona Clinic Liver Cancer staging and treatment schedule.** CLT, cadaveric liver transplantation; LDLT, liver donor liver ınsplant; PEI; percutaneous ethanol injection; PS, performance status; RF, radiofrequency. Reprinted with permission from Elsevier he Lancet, 2003; 362:1907–1917).

an those with classic HCC, and aggressive surgical resection liver transplantation is feasible in around 80%, with a 5-year rvival rate of 67%.[30]

ıtrahepatic cholangiocarcinoma

trahepatic cholangiocarcinoma is less common than extra-patic ductal cholangiocarcinoma, and appears as a focal mass sion.[31] It is an adenocarcinoma that originates from intra-patic biliary epithelial cells (Fig. 102.15). Although sclerosing olangitis, recurrent pyogenic cholangitis by *Chlonorchis nensis*, and choledocal cysts are predisposing factors for ductal olangiocarcinoma,[2,31,32] their relationship with intrahepatic olangiocarcinoma is not clear. CT shows a basal hypodense lesion with a hypovascular pattern,[31] associated with portal-phase peripheral enhancement. The tumor becomes symptomatic upon reaching a large size, and the sole therapeutic option is surgical resection, which is an option in only a minority of patients who may then have a 3-year survival rate of 40–60% (Fig. 102.16).[31,32] Liver transplantation has poor results and is not recommended.

Angiosarcoma

This is the most common mesenchymal malignant tumor of the liver.[33] It originates from the endothelial cells of the sinu-

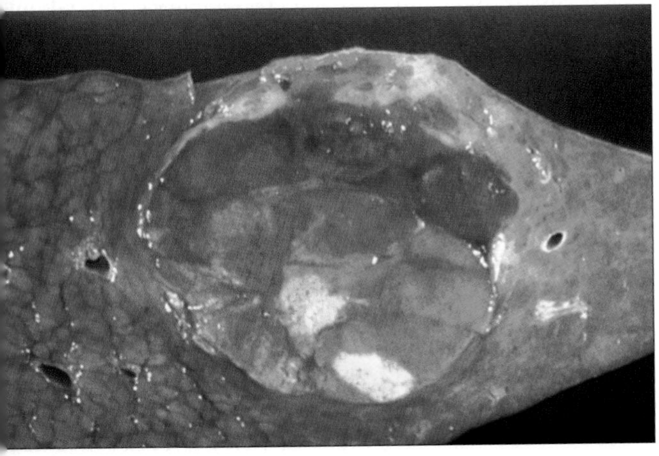

g. 102.14 **Large HCC replacing part of the right lobe.** The green pearance reflects bile production.

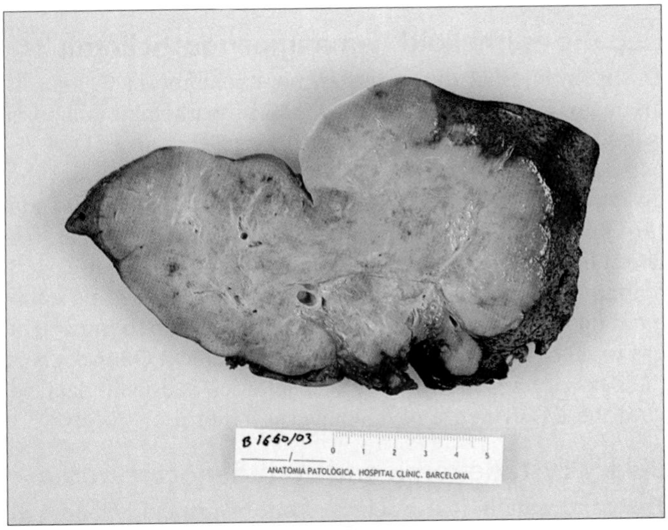

Fig. 102.15 Intrahepatic cholangiocarcinoma. The large tumor has an irregular infiltrative margin; the central area is fibrotic.

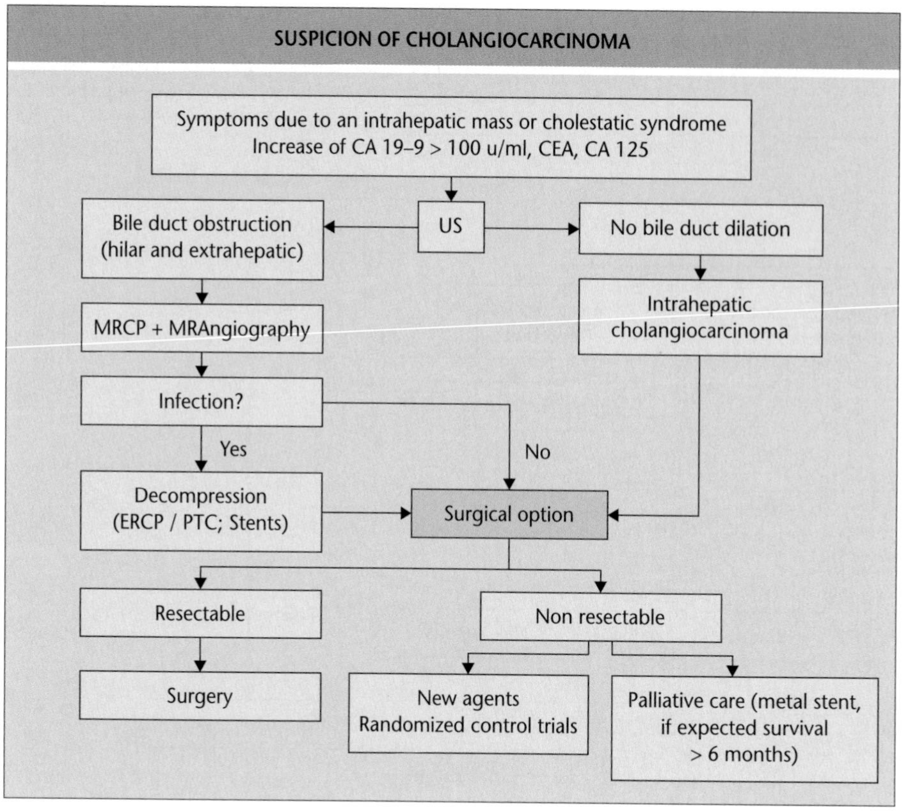

Fig. 102.16 Suspicion of cholangiocarcinor Diagnostic algorithm for patients in whom cholangiocarcinoma is suspected. CC, cholangiocarcinoma; CEA, carcinoembryoni antigen; ERCP, endoscopic retrograde cholangiopancreatography; MRCP, magneti resonance cholangiopancreatography; PTC, percutaneous transhepatic cholangiography US, ultrasonography.

soidal lining, and generally appears in adults (male:female ratio 3:1). The tumor cells infiltrate the sinusoids, hepatic and portal veins, and finally substitute the hepatic parenchyma. Angiosarcoma has been associated with thorotrast and vinyl chloride exposure.[33] Symptoms may mimic those of chronic liver disease, but in 15% of patients angiosarcoma is diagnosed because of acute hemoperitoneum due to tumor rupture. Liver biopsy establishes the diagnosis.[33] Dynamic CT shows gradual contrast enhancement and homogeneity in the late phase. MRI shows that the tumor is homogeneously hypointense on T1-weighted imaging and hyperintense on T2-weighted imaging.[33] Diagnosis is usually made at an advanced stage when surgery is not feasible, and prognosis is dismal.[34]

Hepatic epithelioid hemangioendothelioma

This is an unusual tumor that is more common in women. It originates from endothelial cells, and histopathologic diagnosis is based on staining for vascular markers CD31 and CD34. Its pathogenesis is unknown; symptoms are nonspecific and the evolution is unpredictable. It can remain stable for years and then progress in a very aggressive way. On imaging studies, the lesion has a solid appearance and mimics metastatic disease.[33] Solitary tumors may be resected, but, if multiple, the sole treatment option is liver transplantation. The decision to transplant has to take into account the frequently indolent course versus the risks of transplantation. Transplantation is usually delayed until there is evidence of unequivocal tumor progression.[35]

Biliary cystadenoma and cystadenocarcinoma

These are tumors that originate from biliary epithelium and mainly affect women. They are detected as multiloculated lesions. The sole treatment option is surgical resection.

DIFFERENTIAL DIAGNOSIS

Four different clinical situations can be considered for tl categorization of liver tumors (Fig. 102.17):[1,4]

- Cystic lesion
- Solid lesion in a healthy patient
- Solid lesion in a patient with chronic liver disease
- Solid lesion in a patient with known or suspected neoplasi

Cystic lesion

US is sufficient to establish the liquid content of a focal lesi in the liver. Clinical characteristics, hydatidic and amebic serolog and CT or MRI will make the differential diagnosis betwe simple cyst, hepatic and/or renal polycystic disease, hydat cyst, pyogenic abscess, and amebic abscess. The differentiati with cystoadenoma and cystoadenocarcinoma is difficult an if suspected, usually requires image-guided biopsy or histolog analysis of the resected lesion. It should be noted that meta tases from ovaries, pancreas, or neuroendocrine tumors ma sometimes have a cystic aspect.

Solid lesion in a healthy patient

The most prevalent lesion is hemangioma, which can be easi diagnosed by US and MRI. If the patient is a young wom with a background of oral contraceptive use, it will be nece sary to rule out FNH and hepatic adenoma. FNH is much mo frequent and indolent. Although MRI can differentiate bo entities in two-thirds of the cases,[7,16] biopsy will be required doubtful cases and will establish the malignant nature of tl nodules in asymptomatic patients and in those with atypic and unexpected tumors. If the nature of the lesion is st equivocal, surgical resection is recommended.

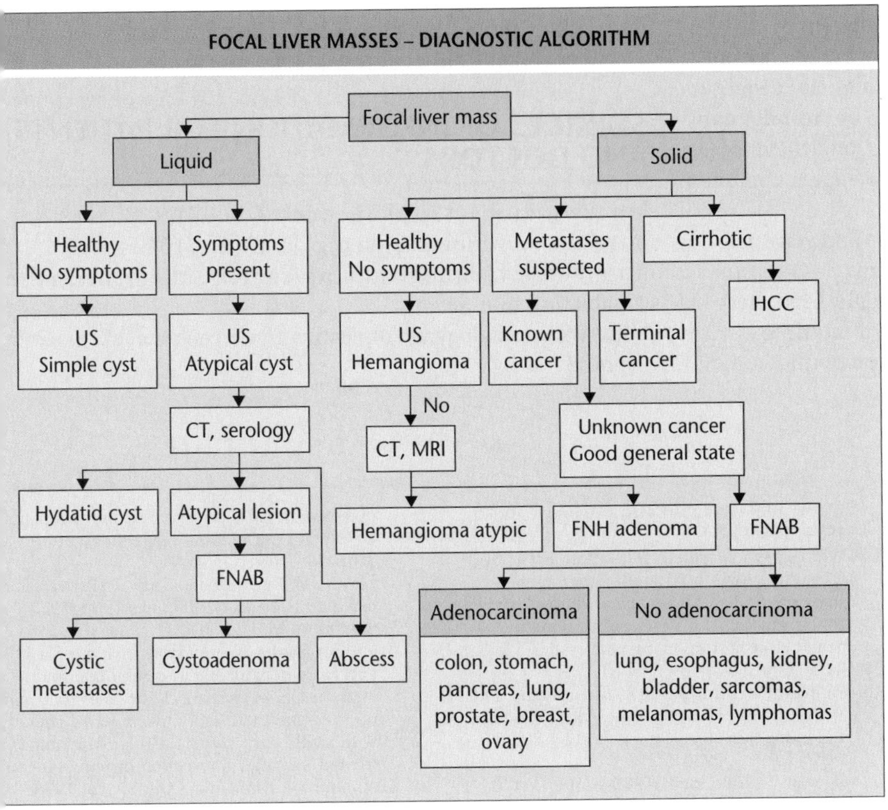

Fig. 102.17 Diagnostic algorithm for a focal hepatic lesion. CT, computed tomography; FNAB, fine-needle aspiration biopsy; FNH, focal nodular hyperplasia; HCC, hepatocellular carcinoma; MRI, magnetic resonance imaging; US, ultrasonography.

olid lesion in a patient with chronic liver isease

he diagnostic strategy in these patients has been established y the panel of experts set up by the European Association for e Study of the Liver.[24] Lesions greater than 2 cm in cirrhotic atients can be confidently diagnosed by imaging techniques; e diagnosis of lesions between 1 and 2 cm should be based n biopsy. Finally, lesions smaller than 1 cm must be followed very 3 months with US because currently available imaging chniques are unable clearly to distinguish regenerative nodules om dysplastic foci or early HCC.

olid lesion in a patient with neoplasia

hree different settings can be considered:[18]

. Patients with a known primary neoplasm who are found to have liver metastases during staging or after treatment of the primary tumor. In these cases, histologic analysis is necessary only if there are doubts regarding the etiology of the focal lesion.
. Patients with a good general condition and an unknown primary tumor. The search for the primary tumor is based on biopsy of the lesion. Adenocarcinomas and poorly differentiated malignancies are the most common histologic patterns.
  a. Adenocarcinoma (well or moderately differentiated) – CRC must be ruled out if the biopsy discloses a potentially gastrointestinal origin, especially in patients older than 50 years and/or with a carcinoembryonic antigen level above 5 ng/mL. Gastric and pancreatic cancer should be excluded in jaundiced patients with high CA19.9 or high CA125 levels. If a nondigestive origin is suspected, it is necessary to exclude lung and prostate cancer, specially in patients with a prostate-specific antigen level above 4 ng/mL, rising acid phosphatase concentration, or osteoblastic bone metastases. Breast and ovarian cancer should be ruled out in women.
  b. Poorly differentiated malignancy – immunohistochemical techniques for cytokeratins are useful in this setting.

TABLE 102.2 IMMUNOPEROXIDASE STAINING OF LIVER BIOPSY

Tumor type	Immunoperoxidase marker
Carcinoma	Cytokeratin (CK20 in gastrointestinal adenocarcinomas, CK7 in respiratory or gynecologic malignancies), EMA
Lymphoma	CLA, EMA (±)
Sarcoma	Vimentin, desmin, factor VIII antigen
Melanoma	S-100, HMB-45, vimentin, NSE, CD68
Neuroendocrine	Chromogranin, synaptophysin, cytokeratin, EMA, NSE
Germ cell	Cytokeratin, EMA, HCG, AFP
Prostate cancer	PSA, cytokeratin 5, 14, 18, EMA
Breast cancer	Cytokeratin 5/6, 8/18/19, EMA, ER, PR
Thyroid cancer	Thyroglobulin, cytokeratin 19, EMA, calcitonin

EMA, epithelial membrane antigen; CLA, common leucocyte antigen; NSE, neuron-specific enolase; HCG, human chorionic gonadotropin; AFP, α-fetoprotein; PSA, prostate-specific antigen; ER, estrogen receptor; PR, progesterone receptor.

They may help to distinguish carcinomas (lung, breast, prostate, pancreas, kidney, and urinary bladder) from other tumors. Neuroendocrine tumors may be diagnosed by staining for neuron-specific enolase or cromogranin. Identification of lymphomas, sarcomas, and melanomas also require specific staining and molecular techniques (Table 102.2).

3. Patients with an unknown primary tumor and seriously impaired general status (performance status 3–4) with constitutional syndrome (wasting and weight loss), liver failure, severe biochemical alterations, and multiple metastatic sites. Given the lack of any therapeutic benefit, workup should be minimized in these patients and management directed towards comfort care.

SOURCES OF INFORMATION FOR PATIENTS AND DOCTORS

http://www.patient.co.uk/showdoc/27000742/
http://www.liverfoundation.org/db/articles/1040
http://www.radiologyinfo.org/content/interventional/r ablation.htm
http://www.radiologyinfo.org/content/interventional/chemoemb htm

REFERENCES

1. Reddy KR, Schiff E. Approach to a liver mass. Sem Liver Dis 1993; 13:423–435.
2. Rubin RA, Mitchell DG. Evaluation of the solid hepatic mass. Med Clin North Am 1996; 80:907–928.
3. Ishak KG, Goodman ZD, Stocker JT. Tumors of the liver and intrahepatic bile ducts. In: Rosai J, Sobin LH, eds. Atlas of tumor pathology. Washington, DC: Armed Forces Institute of Pathology; 2001.
4. Ros PR, Davis GL. The incidental focal liver lesion: photon, proton, or needle? Hepatology 1998; 27:1183–1190.
5. Horton KM, Bluemke DA, Hruban RH et al. CT and MR imaging of benign hepatic and biliary tumors. Radiographics 1999; 19: 431–451.
6. Fulcher AS, Sterling RK. Hepatic neoplasms. J Clin Gastroenterol 2002; 34:463–471.
7. Benhamou JP, Menu Y. Non-parasitic cystic diseases of the liver and intrahepatic biliary tree. In: Bircher J, Benhamou JP, McIntyre N, Rizzeto M, Rodes J, eds. Oxford textbook of clinical hepatology, 2nd edn. Oxford: Oxford Medical Publications; 1999:817–823.
8. Kew MC. Hepatic tumors and cysts. In: Feldman M, Friedman LS, Sleisenger MH, eds. Sleisenger & Fordtran's gastrointestinal and liver disease, 7th edn. Philadelphia: Saunders; 2002:1577–1602.
9. Bresson-Hadni S, Miguet JP, Vuitton DA. Echinococcosis of the liver. In: Bircher J, Benhamou JP, McIntyre N, Rizzeto M, Rodes J, eds. Oxford textbook of clinical hepatology, 2nd edn. Oxford: Oxford Medical Publications; 1999:1066–1076.
10. Khuroo MS, Wani NA, Javid G et al. Percutaneous drainage compared with surgery for hepatic hydatid cysts. N Engl J Med 1997; 337:881–887.
11. Kibbler CC, Sánchez-Tapias JM. Bacterial infection and the liver. In: Bircher J, Benhamou JP, McIntyre N, Rizzeto M, Rodes J, eds. Oxford textbook of clinical hepatology, 2nd edn. Oxford: Oxford Medical Publications; 1999:989–993.
12. Gandolfi L, Leo P, Solmi L et al. Natural history of hepatic haemangiomas: clinical and ultrasound study. Gut 1991; 32:677–680.
13. Mitchell DG, Saini S, Weinreb J et al. Hepatic metastases and cavernous hemangiomas: distinction with standard and triple-dose gadoteridol-enhanced MR imaging. Radiology 1994; 193:49–57.
14. Whitney WS, Herfkens RJ, Jeffrey RB et al. Dynamic breath-hold multiplanar spoiled gradient-recalled MR imaging with gadolinium enhancement for differentiating hepatic hemangiomas from malignancies at 1.5 T. Radiology 1993; 189:863–870.
15. Weimann A, Burckhardt R, Klempnauer J et al. Benign liver tumors: differential diagnosis and indications for surgery. World J Surg 1997; 21:983–991.
16. Cherqui D, Rahmouni A, Charlotte F et al. Management of focal nodular hyperplasia and hepatocellular adenoma in young women: a series of 41 patients with clinical, radiological and pathological correlations. Hepatology 1995; 22:1764–1781.
17. Hussain SM, Zondervan PE, Ifzermans JNM et al. Benign versus malignant hepatic nodules: MR findings with pathologic correlation. Radiographics 2002; 22:1023–1039.
18. Pavlidis N, Briasoulis E, Hainsworth J, Greco FA. Diagnostic and therapeutic management of cancer of an unknown primary. Eur J Cancer 2003; 39:1999–2005.
19. Kemeny MM, Goldberg D, Beatty JD et al. Results of a prospective randomized trial of continuous regional chemotherapy and hepatic resection as treatment of hepatic metastases from colorectal primaries. Cancer 1986; 57:492–498.
20. Kulke MH, Mayer RJ. Medical progress: carcinoid tumors. N Engl J Med 1999; 340:858–868.
21. Fenwick SW, Wyatt JI, Toogood GJ et al. Hepatic resection and transplantation for primary carcinoid tumors of the liver. Ann Surg 2004; 239:210–219.
22. Parkin DM, Bray F, Ferlay J, Pisani P. Estimating the world cancer burden: GLOBOCAN 2000. Int J Cancer 2001; 94:153–156.
23. Bosch X, Ribes J, Borras J. Epidemiology of primary liver cancer. Semin Liver Dis 1999; 112: 463–472.
24. Bruix J, Sherman M, Llovet JM et al. Clinical management of hepatocellular carcinoma. Conclusions of the Barcelona-2000 EASL Conference. J Hepatol 2001; 35:421–430.
25. Burrell M, Llovet JM, Ayuso MC et al. MRI angiography is superior to helical CT for detection of HCC prior to liver transplantatio an explant correlation. Hepatology 2003; 38:1034–1042.
26. Llovet JM, Burroughs A, Bruix J. Hepatocellul carcinoma. Lancet 2003; 362:1907–1917
27. Sakamoto M, Hirohashi S. Natural history and prognosis of adenomatous hyperplasia and early hepatocellular carcinoma: multi-institutional analysis of 53 nodules followed up for more than 6 months and 141 patients with single early hepatocellular carcinoma treated by surgical resection or percutaneou ethanol injection. Jpn J Clin Oncol 1998; 28:604–608.
28. Arii S, Yamaoka Y, Futagawa S et al. Results of surgical and nonsurgical treatment for small-sized hepatocellular carcinomas: a retrospective and nationwide survey in Japa Hepatology 2000; 32:1224–1229.
29. Llovet JM, Bruix J. Systematic review of randomized trials for unresectable hepatocellular carcinoma: chemoembolizatio improves survival. Hepatology 2003; 37:429–442.
30. Pinna AD, Iwatsuki S, Lee RG et al. Treatmer of fibrolamellar hepatoma with subtotal hepatectomy or transplantation. Hepatology 1997; 26:877–883.
31. Gores GJ. Cholangiocarcinoma: current concepts and insights. Hepatology 2003; 37:961–969.
32. Khan SA, Davidson BR, Goldin R et al. Guidelines for the diagnosis and treatment of cholangiocarcinoma: consensus document Gut 2002; 51(Suppl VI):vi1–9.
33. Bruguera M, Rodés J. Malignant mesenchym tumours of the liver. In: Bircher J, Benhamo JP, McIntyre N, Rizzeto M, Rodes J, eds. Oxford textbook of clinical hepatology, 2nd edn. Oxford: Oxford Medical Publications; 1999:1545–1550.
34. Kitami M, Yamada T, Sato A et al. Diffuse hepatic angiosarcoma with a portal venous supply mimicking hemangiomatosis. J Comput Assist Tomogr 2003; 27:626–629.
35. Madariaga JR, Marino IR, Karavias DD et al Long-term results after liver transplantation for primary hepatic epithelioid hemangioendothelioma. Ann Surg Oncol 1995; 2:483–487.

Chapter 103

Vascular disorders of the liver

Dominique-Charles Valla

NTRODUCTION

lterations of hepatic vasculature have different consequences epending on the type of vessels primarily involved, that is, large r small arteries, large or small portal veins, large or small hepatic eins, or hepatic sinusoids. These primary vascular disorders that ay result in liver or biliary damage should be distinguished from ascular changes secondary to liver or biliary disease. Although ese secondary vascular changes may in turn aggravate biliary or arenchymal damage, they will not be considered in this chapter.

IEPATIC ARTERY DISORDERS

KEY POINTS
HEPATIC ARTERY DISORDERS
• Hepatic artery dissection and aneurysms are usually iatrogenic in origin and remain silent in the majority of cases • Obstruction of large hepatic arteries is generally without consequence, except for the obstruction that occurs in the liver transplant patient • Injury to the peribiliary plexus causes ischemic cholangiopathy • Arteriovenous fistulae are produced by the rupture of an arterial aneurysm into a portal vein branch, resulting in clinically significant portal hypertension when associated with chronic liver disease • Hereditary hemorrhagic telangiectasia causes multiple arteriovenous shunts, which can induce cardiac failure, ischemic cholangiopathy, or portal hypertension

pidemiology and etiology

Iepatic artery lesions include dissection,[1] aneurysms,[2] arterio-enous fistulae,[3,4] and thrombosis. They are increasingly diag-osed with current imaging modalities. They remain, however, xtremely rare in the general population. In many cases, these rterial lesions share similar causes and are therefore present n the same patient. Iatrogenic injury during interventional adiologic procedures[1] or during surgery constitute the main auses, and include transplant-related arterial injury. These atrogenic causes are followed by blunt or penetrating trauma, ystemic disorders (polyarteritis nodosa, Wegener's granulo-natosis, Behçet's disease, and systemic lupus erythematosus), onnective tissue disorders (Marfan's disease, Ehler-Danlos yndrome, fibromuscular dysplasia), and systemic infections bacterial endocarditis, tuberculosis, syphilis). Atheroma of the epatic artery is rare. Hepatic involvement in hereditary hemor-hagic telangiectasia is relatively uncommon.[4]

Dissection and aneurysms

A distinction should be made between a true aneurysm, in which the dilatation involves all three layers of the arterial wall, and a false aneurysm, where the dilatation results from rupture of the intima and the media with preservation of the adventitia. Most traumatic and infectious aneurysms are false aneurysms. Hepatic arterial dissection and aneurysms may rupture into the peritoneal cavity, the liver, the bile ducts (causing hemobilia), or the intrahepatic or extrahepatic portal vein. The risk of rupture increases with the size and number of aneurysms.[2] A diameter of less than 2 cm has a low risk of rupture. Fibromuscular dysplasia and polyarteritis nodosa are also associated with an increased risk of rupture. Pregnancy may precipitate the rupture of pre-existing aneurysms. Large extrahepatic aneurysms may cause obstructive jaundice or portal vein thrombosis. Doppler ultrasonography (US) and computed tomography (CT) or magnetic resonance imaging (MRI) vascular reconstruction are the key diagnostic investigations. The use of percutaneous angiography is limited to therapeutic evaluation. Expectant management is appropriate in patients with silent aneurysms less than 2 cm in diameter. Percutaneous transarterial embolization or stenting has become the preferred therapy for large or symptomatic lesions. A ruptured aneurysm is best managed using emergency embolization therapy after appropriate resuscitation. Surgery can be used where interventional radiology fails or is unsuitable.

Arterioportal fistula

In most cases, arterioportal fistulae are produced by the rupture of a false aneurysm of the hepatic artery into a neighboring portal vein branch. There is a moderate increase in portal pressure, although usually not to a clinically significant level. In patients in whom an arterioportal fistula is associated with clinically significant portal hypertension, the presence of a concomitant chronic liver disease should be considered. Such an association may not be fortuitous as traumatic injury is more common in alcoholics or drug users. Large fistulae can induce mesenteric to hepatic arterial stealing, resulting in intestinal ischemia.[3] A solitary arterioportal fistula can be managed with embolization using a transarterial or transhepatic portal approach.[3] However, spreading or dislodgment of the embolized material can lead to portal or mesenteric vein thrombosis. In asymptomatic patients with a small intrahepatic arterioportal fistula, expectant management is recommended.

Hereditary hemorrhagic telangiectasia

Most cases of hepatic arteriovenous fistula are related to hereditary hemorrhagic telangiectasia.[4] Randomly and widely distributed telangiectases are surrounded by various degree of fibrous tissue. Nodular hyperplasia and sinusoidal fibrosis are common. The diagnosis can be made at Doppler US on the basis of a marked enlargement of the hepatic arteries with increased blood flow velocity, together with the extrahepatic cardinal features of the disease. Rarely patients with this condition have liver involvement without extrahepatic features. Massive shunting from the hepatic arterial bed to the hepatic venous bed may cause high-output cardiac failure in the absence of any apparent consequences on liver function or portal hemodynamics. Ischemic cholangiopathy may occur due to blood stealing away from the peribiliary plexus (see below). When present, portal hypertension is related either to the association of nodular regenerative hyperplasia and perisinusoidal fibrosis, or to arterioportal shunting. In patients with portal hypertension, ill-explained ascites may occur. Embolization of the hepatic artery has been associated with encouraging short-term results and with severe – sometimes fatal – ischemic damage to the liver or bile ducts. The outcome after liver transplantation appears to be excellent. When the main complication is cardiac dysfunction, transplantation should be considered before severe heart failure occurs.

Thrombosis

Thrombosis usually develops in the setting of a pre-existing anomaly of a hepatic artery (dissection, stenosis, or aneurysm). A hepatic artery may be blocked without consequences as long as the accompanying portal vein remains patent and the peribiliary plexus is unaffected. This is due to the rapid development (within hours) of extensive collaterals from large intrahepatic or extrahepatic arteries, and also from the peribiliary capillary plexus. Damage to the peribiliary plexus, however, leads to bile duct ischemia. Such damage has been reported in the following settings: after transcatheter embolization small-sized particles (less than 120 mm in diameter); after intrahepatic arterial infusion of toxic substances (fluoxidine or alcohol); and in association with systemic disorders characterized by microcirculatory impairment. Clinically significant ischemic cholangiopathy consists of bile duct necrosis (producing bilomas), or stenosis predominating at the midportion of the common bile duct or at the hepatic duct confluence. Concurrent obstruction of portal vein and hepatic artery causes parenchymal infarction in the doubly obstructed territory. Outside the transplant setting, obstruction of the large hepatic arteries does not require intervention. There is no established therapy to recanalize a damaged peribiliary plexus.

PORTAL VEIN DISORDERS

These disorders include aneurysm, fistula, and obstruction. The so-called portal vein cavernoma corresponds to the network of hepatopetal collaterals that develops following permanent obstruction of the portal vein, of its main radicles, or of its main branches.

Portal aneurysm

Aneurysm is usually defined as an increase in portal vein diameter that acquires a fusiform or saccular aspect. It is an extremely uncommon condition of unknown cause that may be congenital. Aneurysms may rupture or thrombose. Most cases of portal aneurysm are recognized fortuitously by abdominal imaging. Expectant management is reasonable.

KEY POINTS

PORTAL VEIN DISORDERS

- Portal vein thrombosis is related to prothrombotic disorders and/or local factors
- Decompensated cirrhosis may precipitate portal vein thrombosis
- Complications of portal vein thrombosis include intestinal ischemia, portal hypertension, and compression of the bile ducts by a cavernoma
- Early anticoagulation allows repermeation in 75% of patients with recent thrombosis
- At the late stage of cavernoma, anticoagulation therapy should be decided on a case by case basis
- Obliterative intrahepatic portal venopathy produces portal hypertension The main cause worldwide is schistosomiasis. In some patients, a prothrombotic disorder is present and is presumably its cause

Acute thrombosis of a previously normal portal vein can b associated with a marked but transient enlargement of th thrombosed portion that may lead to an erroneous diagnos of a thrombosed pre-existing portal aneurysm.

Spontaneous portacaval fistulae

Spontaneous fistulae are characterized by large-sized commu nications between the portal vein and either the hepatic arter (arterioportal fistula, described above) or the inferior ven cava (portacaval fistula) in the absence of chronic liver diseas Spontaneous portacaval fistulae of unknown pathogenesis hav been described in two entities, each with a different locatio In the first entity – congenital absence of the portal vein – th extrahepatic portal vein cannot be visualized by mesenteric c celiac angiography, and there is a fistula between a mesenteri vein and the inferior vena cava. In the second entity, one c several intrahepatic fistulae are visualized. Both entities ar identified in neonates screened for congenital galactosemi (portosystemic shunting induces hypergalactosemia), and fror their association with other developmental anomalies. As simila intrahepatic shunts can develop in patients with acquired chroni liver disease, it has been suggested that intrauterine blockag of the intrahepatic circulation may lead to the developmer of congenital portacaval fistulae. In most cases, there is n evidence for a familial transmission.

Enlargement of the hepatic arteries suggests compensator arterialization. Morphometry may show paucity of intrahepati portal veins. Macroregenerative nodules (resembling focal nodula hyperplasia) or nodular regenerative hyperplasia may develop probably as a result of an imbalance between an increase arterial perfusion and a reduced portal inflow. There are anec dotal reports of adenoma, hepatoblastoma, and hepatocarcinoma Although liver function is well maintained, patients may develo portal– systemic encephalopathy, usually after the age of 50 years Diagnosis is made using duplex Doppler US or vascular recon struction at MRI or CT. Most patients do not require any treatmen In patients with debilitating portal–systemic encephalopathy percutaneous transhepatic embolization of the shunt shoul probably be attempted first, retaining liver transplantation as a final option. Correct characterization of the macronodule may require limited surgical resection. Extensive hepatectomy should be avoided because there is concern that regeneratio may be impaired given the lack of portal inflow.

ortal vein obstruction

xtrahepatic portal vein thrombosis

ne portal vein can become obstructed by malignant tumors as result of invasion or compression. Primary tumors of the ver, pancreas, or bile ducts are most commonly implicated. Vhen not related to a tumor, portal vein obstruction is due to rombosis.[5]

Causes of portal vein thrombosis (PVT) can be systemic and ocal.[5,6] The cause is usually not apparent at the time of pres-ntation. Therefore, workup must be systematic. All known ereditary or acquired thrombogenic factors have been impli-ated in the genesis of PVT, with primary myeloproliferative isorders and protein S deficiency as leading causes.[6,7] Com-on local factors include portal vein injury (cannulation, section, gation, anastomosis, splenectomy); portal venous stasis (due cirrhosis, obliterative portal venopathy, or hepatic venous utflow block); and inflammatory conditions in the splanchnic rea (appendicitis, diverticulitis, inflammatory bowel disease, ancreatitis, cholangitis, liver abscesses). Systemic and local auses are frequently combined. Surgery for portal hyperten-on has been a major cause of PVT in the past. Despite exten-ve workup, a number of cases of PVT remain unexplained.

Liver impairment: In the particular setting of cirrhosis without epatocellular carcinoma, the risk of extrahepatic PVT is related the severity of liver disease, occurring in less than 1% of atients with Child-Pugh class A, and in up to 15% of candi-ates for liver transplantation or portosystemic shunting. ntrahepatic PVT is even more common in the explanted liver about 50%). There is evidence that extrahepatic PVT in a hild-Pugh class A patient is often precipitated by an underlying ommon thrombophilic state.

Upstream from the portal vein thrombus, preserved mesen-eric venous arches prevent ischemic damage to the gut, whereas nvolvement of these arches induces intestinal ischemia. Down-tream from the thrombus, the liver is protected from clinically ignificant damage due to increased arterial blood flow (the uffer response), and to the rapid development of hepatopetal ollaterals (the cavernoma). The cavernoma, however, does not ompletely relieve the extrahepatic block, so that portal hyper-ension ensues.

Upon obstruction of a major branch of the portal vein, with atency of remaining branches, the hepatic parenchyma under-oes atrophy due to apoptosis; if the obstruction is sudden and omplete, it undergoes necrosis. In the unobstructed territory, owever, the hepatic parenchyma undergoes hypertrophy related o hepatocellular proliferation. The mechanisms signaling this daptation are not yet understood.

Owing to the development of noninvasive imaging, extra-epatic PVT is now often diagnosed at an early acute stage acute pyelophlebitis) in patients with abdominal pain, often ssociated with fever. When diagnosis and therapy are delayed, rolonged ischemia may induce intestinal necrosis, peritonitis, nd multiorgan failure. When thrombosis is precipitated by an bscess in the splanchnic area, spiking fever, chills, and positive lood cultures indicate the presence of septic pyelophlebitis. Vhen the initial episode goes unnoticed, the condition is recog-ized at a late, cavernomatous stage, usually as a fortuitous iscovery of portal hypertension. Bleeding from gastro-sophageal varices has become an uncommon presentation of VT. However, recurrent gastrointestinal bleeding is the major omplication of longstanding PVT. The second major complication is recurrent thrombosis, usually in the portal venous territory and less commonly in other venous beds. Bile duct compression by portal collaterals is emerging as an important source of morbidity including bacterial cholangitis, cholecystitis, and chronic cholestasis.

CT and Doppler US are the key diagnostic procedures. The main diagnostic challenge is to identify a possible cause. Local factors are investigated mainly by abdominal imaging modalities. Underlying prothrombotic disorders require systematic hematologic workup.

The **treatment of PVT** depends on its stage (acute or cavernomatous) at the time of diagnosis.[6] While spontaneous recanalization is rare, recanalization of a recently thrombosed portal vein can be expected to occur in more than 75% of patients treated promptly with anticoagulation. Failure of treatment should be declared only after an anticoagulation period of at least 6 months. When re-permeation has been achieved, current data support continued anticoagulation in patients with an underlying prothrombotic disorder. In patients with portal cavernoma, pharmacologic or endoscopic therapy for primary or secondary prevention of variceal hemorrhage appear useful. Evidence suggests that anticoagulation in these patients may decrease the risk of recurrent thrombosis without increasing the risk or the severity of gastrointestinal bleeding. Therefore, anticoagulation can be proposed to patients with portal cavernoma, particularly those with an underlying thrombogenic condition and when no treatable local factor has been documented.

In patients so treated, the outcome is excellent and death occurs largely from unrelated diseases at an old age. The prognostic factors for bleeding include the size of esophageal varices and a past history of bleeding. The main prognostic factor for recurrent thrombosis is the presence of an underlying prothrombotic condition. The likelihood of biliary complications increases with time.

Obstruction of intrahepatic portal veins

The major cause of intrahepatic portal vein obstruction worldwide is schistosomiasis (see Chapter 83). The entity termed portal obstructive venopathy is distinct from, although frequently complicated by, extrahepatic PVT. It is characterized by the obstruction of small intrahepatic portal veins.[8] This entity has been reported under numerous denominations, including noncirrhotic intrahepatic portal hypertension in clinical reports, and hepatoportal sclerosis or noncirrhotic portal fibrosis in pathologic studies. In Western countries, exposure to arsenicals, vinyl chloride monomer, and thorium sulfate had been recognized as a cause of obliterative portal venopathy. Recent studies indicate that underlying thrombogenic conditions are frequently found in these patients. However, in a proportion the cause remains unknown.

Pathologically, portal tracts are devoid of normal veins.[8] The small intrahepatic portal veins are absent, thrombosed, or replaced by a fibrous scar. Characteristically, multiple small vascular channels (microscopic equivalent to the cavernoma) are found within the portal tracts, at their periphery, or at random within the lobule. Fibrous enlargement of the portal tracts, nodularity of the parenchyma, patchy sinusoidal dilatation, and sinusoidal fibrosis are common. Atrophy of the parenchyma is reflected by the approximation of portal tracts and central veins.

Clinical presentation is almost always with portal hypertension. Liver failure is rare or occurs after a course of several decades. The prognosis is better than that of cirrhotic portal hypertension, and is mostly related to accompanying diseases. Superimposed extrahepatic PVT is seen in half the patients. There is no specific therapy. Anticoagulation can be proposed when an underlying thrombogenic condition is present. Portal hypertension can be managed as recommended for cirrhotic patients.

HEPATIC VEIN DISORDERS

KEY POINTS
HEPATIC VEIN DISORDERS
• The Budd-Chiari syndrome is related to prothrombotic disorders, among which myeloproliferative disorders are the most frequent • Clinical manifestations result from an increased sinusoidal pressure and ischemic injury. An acute presentation is commonly associated with evidence of longstanding hepatic outflow obstruction • Obstruction of the intrahepatic or extrahepatic portal vein aggravates the disease • Therapy includes anticoagulation and interventions aimed at restoring hepatic venous outflow (angioplasty, TIPS or surgical portacaval shunts, or transplantation)

Definition

In addition to arteriohepatic or portohepatic fistulae (see above), hepatic veins can also become obstructed. The Budd-Chiari syndrome is characterized by an obstruction of the hepatic venous outflow tract at the level of small hepatic veins, large hepatic veins, or suprahepatic segment of the inferior vena cava.[9] Although secondary Budd-Chiari syndrome is related to invasion or compression of the veins by an extravenous lesion, the primary condition is related to primary phlebitis or thrombosis. Veno-occlusive disease is currently not considered a primary disorder of the hepatic veins and is discussed below as a sinusoidal disorder.

Epidemiology, causes, risk factors, associated disorders

Budd-Chiari syndrome is a rare condition. Causes of secondary Budd-Chiari syndrome include malignancies that invade the hepatic venous outflow tract (liver, kidney, or adrenal tumors) or that develop in the vicinity of the terminal portion of the inferior vena cava (leiomyosarcoma, myxoma).[9–11] Alveolar hydatid disease behaves like a malignant tumor of the liver (see Chapter 102). Focal nodular hyperplasia or liver cysts, when large and located near the junction of the hepatic veins and the inferior vena cava, can block these veins. Causes of primary Budd-Chiari syndrome include systemic thrombogenic disorders (primary myeloproliferative disorder, protein C deficiency, factor V Leiden mutation and antiphospholipid syndrome, paroxysmal nocturnal hemoglobinuria), inflammatory disorders (granulomatous venulitis, inflammatory bowel disease, amebic abscess), and some other risk factors (estroprogestative agents, pregnancy).[7] A combination of causes is common. Usually, the underlying condition is not apparent at presentation, which justifies a systematic workup for a thrombogenic disorder. Generally, the local factor triggering thrombosis at this uncommon locatic remains unknown.

Pathogenesis

Hepatic vein or inferior vena cava thrombosis can be dia nosed at three different stages: a fresh thrombus, a localize fibrous stenosis, or complete obliteration of the vein. In the F East a membranous obstruction of the terminal inferior ve cava is the predominant form of Budd-Chiari syndrome, whereas in the West a fresh thrombus or localized stenosis the hepatic veins appears to be more frequent.[10] Figure 103 illustrates the typical course of Budd-Chiari syndrome.

Obstruction of the hepatic venous outflow tract has du consequences.[10] First, sinusoidal pressure rises, leading congestion, portal hypertension, increased lymph productio (resulting in the formation of protein-rich ascitic fluid), and th development of collaterals that bypass the obstructed portio of the hepatic veins. Second, the sudden interruption in hepat venous blood outflow may lead to ischemic necrosis and resu in liver insufficiency. Hepatic perfusion is restored by an increas in arterial blood flow, an increase in portal pressure, and th development of intrahepatic and extrahepatic venous collatera (which should be distinguished from portosystemic collaterals Fibrosis develops is the areas of ischemic necrosis.

At advanced stages of the disease, irregularly distributed, thron bosed, intrahepatic portal veins are found. Extrahepatic portal ve thrombosis occurs in about 20% of cases. The areas where bot portal veins and hepatic veins are thrombosed undergo infarctio or parenchymal extinction (i.e., transformation into a fibro area devoid of parenchymal cells). By contrast, the areas wit thrombosed portal veins, but patent hepatic veins, undergo hype trophy (nodular regenerative hyperplasia), sometimes in an ex berant form (regenerative macronodules). At imaging, these art rialized macronodules closely mimic hepatocellular carcinom

Clinical manifestations

Hepatic vein thrombosis can run a long asymptomatic cours and be discovered incidentally. There is little clinicopathologi correlation, an acute presentation frequently being associate with histopathologic features of chronic damage with supe imposed features of recent injury.[9–11] The acute presentatio includes upper abdominal pain, liver enlargement, ascites c recent onset, increased serum levels of transaminases, decrease levels of coagulation factors, and impaired renal function. Th chronic presentation, in the form of decompensated liver diseas is the most common. The course is unpredictable. In some patient complete spontaneous remission occurs with or without recurre manifestations, whereas in others there is an unremittin aggravation of liver insufficiency and portal hypertension.

Diagnosis

Diagnosis should be considered whenever a patient with known prothrombotic disorder develops liver disease; whe ever a patient with acute and severe liver disease has an enlarge painful liver and massive ascites; in patients with ascitic flui protein content greater than 3.0 g/dL; and in all patients pre senting with chronic liver disease that remains unexplaine once all common viral, autoimmune, and metabolic causes hav been ruled out.[9–11]

Diagnosis is made on the basis of the findings at duple Doppler US and MRI.[9,10] The most specific and sensitive sig

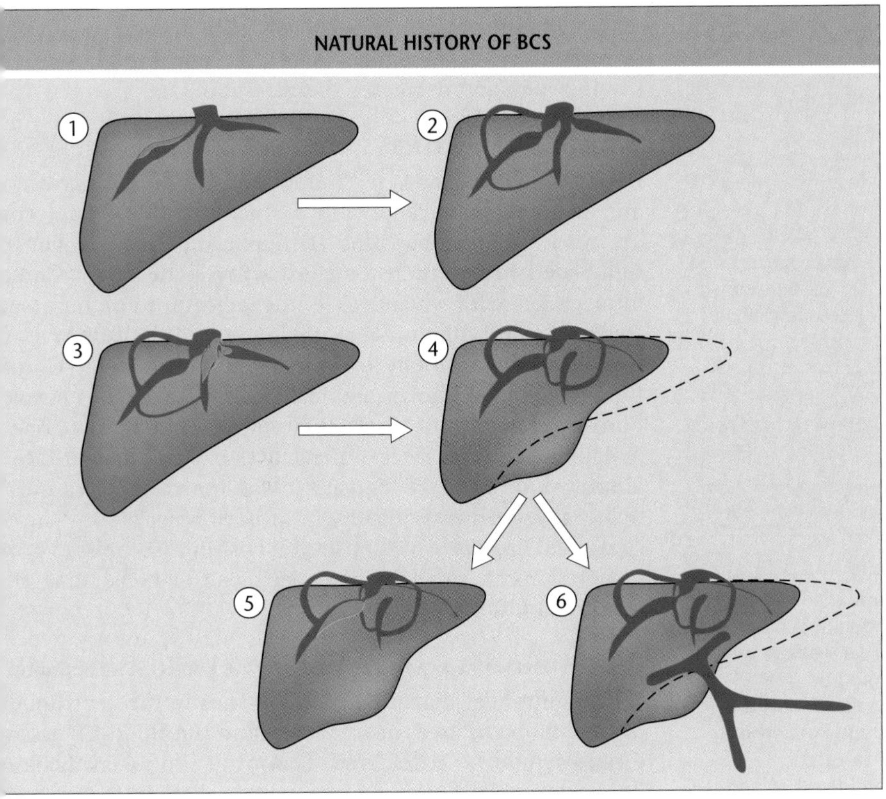

Fig. 103.1 Natural history of Budd-Chiari syndrome. (1) Initially, there is rapid or progressive formation of a thrombus, usually in a major hepatic vein, close to its ostium in the inferior vena cava. (2) This is followed by the formation of a short-length stenosis (as depicted) or by complete obliteration of the vein (not shown). Collaterals develop connecting obstructed territories with patent hepatic or extrahepatic veins in the vicinity. (3) In a subsequent stage, there is rapid or progressive development of a thrombus in another major hepatic vein. (4) Short-length or diffuse stenosis again develops, together with collaterals. There may be atrophy of the parenchyma in the obstructed territory, with compensatory hypertrophy of the preserved territories (most commonly the caudate lobe). (5) A thrombus can then develop in a vein that had remained partially (as depicted) or completely (not shown) patent. (6) Or a thrombus can develop in the portal vein. Depending on the velocity of the obstructive process, steps 1–4 can take place without notice. Symptoms would develop only when obstruction was rapid, or when most of the venous outflow tract was obstructed. Steps 5 and 6 are probably always associated with symptoms. A scenario in which complete thrombosis of all three major hepatic veins occurs simultaneously appears to be rare.

e altered flow pattern within the hepatic veins, hepatic venous llateral circulation, and patchy alterations in the parenchy-al perfusion pattern. Hepatic venography, which is not required r diagnosis, still remains an irreplaceable tool for delineating e venous lesion and for planning intervention therapy.

reatment

ıerapy for hepatic vein thrombosis has not been well eval-ıted.[10] An algorithm for management is presented in Figure)3.2. Anticoagulant therapy is rational and has likely improved e outcome of the disease over the past two decades. Ascites ıd portal hypertensive bleeding can be treated as recom-ended for patients with cirrhosis. In symptomatic patients ith short-length stenosis on the hepatic veins or inferior vena ıva, percutaneous angioplasty (with or without stenting, and ith or without thrombolysis) can be attempted first. When ıgioplasty fails or is unfeasible, transjugular intrahepatic ortosystemic shunting (TIPS) appears promising because of a w procedure-related mortality rate. However, the incidence ıd consequences of secondary TIPS dysfunction await further valuation. Surgical portacaval shunts have had a small impact ı survival, probably because of a high operative mortality te and a high incidence of late shunt stenosis. Based on trospective cohort studies, liver transplantation may increase ırvival in the most severe cases.

rognosis

ne natural history of Budd-Chiari syndrome is poorly known. recent series (which included patients diagnosed in a 10–25-ear period receiving various forms of therapy), half of the atients had 10-year survival rate above 90%, and the other alf had a 50% 10-year mortality rate.[9,10] Most fatalities occur the first 12 or 18 months after presentation. Age and Child-Pugh score are well established independent predictors of a poor outcome. Acute exacerbation of a longstanding disease and extrahepatic portal vein thrombosis are associated with a particularly poor outcome.

HEPATIC SINUSOIDAL DISORDERS

Disorders that exclusively or predominantly affect the sinusoids are rare. The most typical, formerly known as veno-occlusive disease, was recently renamed sinusoidal obstruction syndrome.[12] It is related to acute toxic injury of the sinusoidal endothelial cells. Other sinusoidal disorders are characterized by one of the three following sinusoidal lesions:

KEY POINTS
HEPATIC SINUSOIDAL DISORDERS
• Sinusoidal obstruction syndrome, a toxic injury to sinusoidal endothelium, is encountered mainly following myeloablative therapy • Other sinusoidal disorders include perisinusoidal fibrosis, sinusoidal dilatation and peliosis, fibrin deposition, and infiltration with various types of benign or malignant cell

- Fibrosis, likely due to enhanced matrix deposition in the perisinusoidal space
- Deposition of abnormal substances within the perisinusoidal space
- Cellular infiltration of the sinusoids.

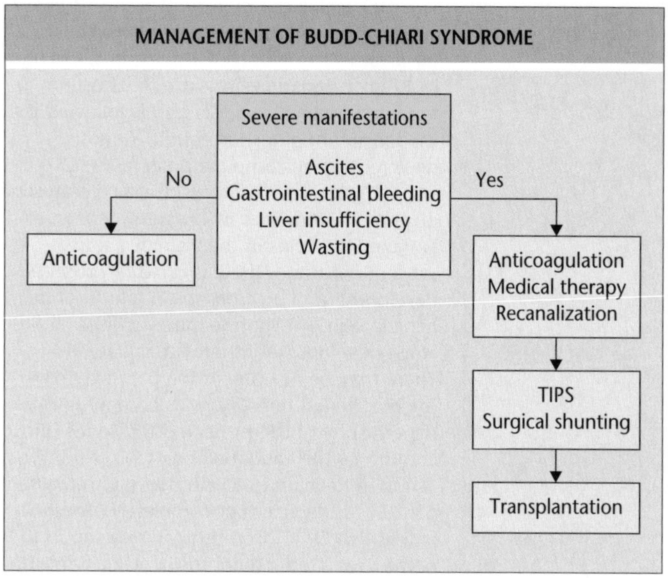

Fig. 103.2 Management of Budd-Chiari syndrome. Patients with absent or mild manifestations are treated with lifelong anticoagulation and, if possible, correction of the underlying disorder. Patients with manifestations of decompensated liver disease should be treated medically and, if feasible, with percutaneous recanalization of the obstructed veins. In patients with failed recanalization, and whose symptoms are not well controlled, transjugular intrahepatic portosystemic shunt (TIPS) insertion should be considered. When TIPS insertion fails, surgical portosystemic shunting can be considered in patients with a good liver function and uncontrolled portal hypertension. Transplantation should be considered in patients with severe liver insufficiency or failed shunts. Preservation of portal vein patency is of the utmost importance.

Sinusoidal obstruction syndrome

Sinusoidal obstruction syndrome characterized by an initially acute endothelial cell damage, followed by detachment and embolization to the central area of the lobule producing post-sinusoidal outflow block.[12] Histologically, the subendothelial space of central and subendothelial veins is widened and occupied by cellular debris. There is congestion and necrosis within the centrilobular area, followed by subendothelial deposition of fibrous tissue in central and sublobular veins, and in the sinusoids. Causes include exposure to certain toxic substances (pyrrolizidine alkaloids, azathioprine, various chemotherapeutic agents), hepatic irradiation, or the combination of irradiation and chemotherapy (as currently used in myeloablative therapy). Clinical manifestations mimic Budd-Chiari syndrome: tender hepatomegaly, ascites, and raised serum bilirubin levels. In the context of myeloablative therapy, these manifestations begin 10–30 days after initiation of therapy. The severity is variable, ranging from silent forms to fulminant hepatic failure. The incidence and severity of sinusoidal obstruction syndrome are influenced by the particular myeloablative protocol, as well as previous infection with the hepatitis C virus. Some patients recover completely, whereas others develop fatal forms, usually associated with multiorgan failure. The diagnosis is made once other possible causes of liver disease have been ruled out (particularly severe sepsis and hyperacute graft versus host disease). When the presence of other liver diseases is possible, transvenous liver biopsy coupled with hepatic venous pressure gradient measurement is useful. A poor prognosis is correlated with high serum transaminase levels, high hepatic venous pre sure gradient, development of portal vein thrombosis, re insufficiency, and decreased oxygen saturation.

Sinusoidal fibrosis

Pure sinusoidal fibrosis with predominance in the periveno area is usually associated with venous scarring.[13] Main caus are resolved steatohepatitis (alcoholic or nonalcoholic) a right-sided heart failure or constrictive pericarditis. Chro intoxication with vitamin A is the prototype for pure sin soidal fibrosis without zonal predominance. A distinctive fe ture is the hypertrophy of lipid-laden stellate cells. Chro therapy with methotrexate has been related to sinusoi fibrosis, although the distinction with coexistent alcoholic metabolic liver disease is difficult. Mastocytosis may lead to almost pure form of perisinusoidal fibrosis. All causes obliterative portal venopathy have been associated with pu sinusoidal fibrosis, which raises the possibility of missed por vein lesions in small biopsy specimens demonstrating pu sinusoidal fibrosis.

Pure sinusoidal dilatation and peliosis hepatis

When sinusoidal dilatation predominates in the centrilobul or mediolobular area, heart failure and the Budd-Chiari sy drome should be considered. Periportal sinusoidal dilatati has been reported in association with oral contraceptive use patients with concomitant inflammatory conditions such Crohn's disease. Sinusoidal dilatation without zonal predom nance can be found in patients with various granulomato disorders, in those on azathioprine or anabolic steroids, or patients with antiphospholipid syndrome.[14] Peliosis hepa differs from pure sinusoidal dilatation by the presence of blo lakes that lack endothelium. Chronic debilitating conditio including infection and cancer, have been incriminated in t past, but patients had frequently been treated with anabo steroids. Infection of immunodeficient patients with *Bartone henselae* causes a treatable form of peliosis.

Manifestations of sinusoidal dilatation range from asym tomatic mild abnormalities in serum liver tests, to painful liv enlargement and portal hypertension with marked cholesta features. Prognosis is determined largely by the underlyi disorder, with possible resolution when the disorder is tre able. In many patients, sinusoidal dilatation has been ass ciated with, or followed, by nodular regenerative hyperplas which suggests a link between these two pathologic entities.

Infiltration of the sinusoids

Various substances, including immune globulin light cha (myeloma), various amyloid substances (AL type in myelom AA type in chronic inflammatory disorders), or immu globulin A (alcoholics), can be deposited in the perisinusoid space. Liver enlargement and cholestatic liver tests are t main manifestations of these lesions.

The sinusoidal lumen may be the site of fibrin deposition conditions where intravascular activation of coagulation occu such as pre-eclampsia (see Chapter 32), the hemolytic–urem syndrome, and thrombotic thrombocytopenic purpura. Liv hematoma and intraperitoneal rupture may occur, albeit rare Upper abdominal pain occurring in the setting of the HELI syndrome heralds the development of intrahepatic or extr hepatic bleeding.

In sickle cell anemia, falciform cells within the sinusoids use painful liver enlargement and abnormal liver enzymes. Diffuse infiltration of the sinusoids with abnormal cells may :cur in patients with breast carcinoma, undifferentiated carci- ma, lymphomas and leukemias, mastocytosis, and the hemophagocytic syndrome. In rare instances, the disorder presents with apparently pure liver involvement. Liver enlargement is constant. Ascites and acute liver failure are frequent. Prognosis is poor.

EFERENCES

. Yoon DY, Park JH, Chung JW, Han JK, Han MC. Iatrogenic dissection of the celiac artery and its branches during transcatheter arterial embolization for hepatocellular carcinoma: outcome in 40 patients. Cardiovasc Intervent Radiol 1995; 18:16–19.

. Abbas MA, Fowl RJ, Stone WM et al. Hepatic artery aneurysm: factors that predict complication. J Vasc Surg 2003; 38:41–45.

. Vauthey JN, Tomczak RJ, Helmberger T et al. The arterioportal fistula syndrome: clinicopathologic features, diagnosis, and therapy. Gastroenterology 1997; 113:1390–1401.

. Garcia-Tsao G, Korzenik JR, Young L et al. Liver disease in patients with hereditary hemorrhagic telangiectasia. N Engl J Med 2000; 343:931–936.

. Sarin SK, Agrawal SR. Extrahepatic portal vein obstruction. Semin Liver Dis 2002; 22:43–58.

6. Condat B, Pessione F, Hillaire S et al. Current outcome of portal vein thrombosis in adults: risk and benefit of anticoagulant therapy. Gastroenterology 2001; 120:490–497.
7. Janssen HL, Meinardi JR, Vleggaar FP et al. Factor V Leiden mutation, prothrombin gene mutation, and deficiencies in coagulation inhibitors associated with Budd-Chiari syndrome and portal vein thrombosis: results of a case–control study. Blood 2000; 96: 2364–2368.
8. Hillaire S, Bonte E, Denninger MH et al. Idiopathic non-cirrhotic intrahepatic portal hypertension in the West: a re-evaluation in 28 patients. Gut 2002; 51:275–280.
9. Janssen HL, Garcia-Pagan JC, Elias E, Mentha G, Hadengue A, Valla DC. Budd-Chiari syndrome: a review by an expert panel. J Hepatol 2003; 38:364–371.
10. Valla DC. The diagnosis and management of the Budd-Chiari syndrome: consensus and controversies. Hepatology 2003; 38:793–803.
11. Okuda K. Inferior vena cava thrombosis at its hepatic portion (obliterative hepatocavopathy). Semin Liver Dis 2002; 22:15–26.
12. DeLeve LD, Shulman HM, McDonald GB. Toxic injury to hepatic sinusoids: sinusoidal obstruction syndrome (veno-occlusive disease). Semin Liver Dis 2002; 22:27–42.
13. Okudaira M, Ohbu M, Okuda K. Idiopathic portal hypertension and its pathology. Semin Liver Dis 2002; 22:59–72.
14. Bruguerra M, Aranguibel F, Ros E, Rodes J. Incidence and clinical significance of sinusoidal dilatation in liver biopsies. Gastroenterology 1978; 75:474–478.

Chapter 104

Granulomas of the liver

Miquel Bruguera Cortada

KEY POINTS

- Liver granulomas are focal accumulations of chronic inflammatory cells, including macrophages, easily demarcated from the surrounding tissue, which develop as a reaction to foreign agents
- There are multiple causes of hepatic granulomas, the most frequent being sarcoidosis and tuberculosis
- The clinical manifestations, treatment, and prognosis are those of the underlying etiology, although in some cases liver granulomas per se can lead to hepatomegaly and elevations in alkaline phosphatase
- The differential diagnosis can be made histologically by searching for the etiologic agent within the granuloma and/or by analyzing the location and morphological characteristics of the granuloma
- The clinical history, including a drug history, is of the essence in establishing the cause for liver granulomas

ɴTRODUCTION

. granuloma is a focal accumulation of chronic inflammatory ells, including macrophages, easily demarcated from the sur-ɔunding tissue, which develops as a reaction to foreign agents. he causes of hepatic granulomas are numerous (Table 104.1), nd identifying an etiology is often difficult.

PIDEMIOLOGY

ranulomas are found in 2–10% of liver biopsies in large series. he frequency of detection depends on the population studied, e prevalence of risk factors for granulomas in different geo-raphic area, and the frequency with which liver biopsies are erformed in the evaluation of febrile disorders of unknown rigin. Examination of multiple sections of liver biopsies icreases the diagnostic yield.

Sarcoidosis and tuberculosis are the two most common causes f hepatic granulomas in most series. In developed countries, arcoidosis is the main cause, followed by tuberculosis; in nderdeveloped countries, tuberculosis is the main cause.

ATHOGENESIS AND PATHOLOGY

athology

here are several types of granulomas depending on the type nd arrangement of cells.

. **Epithelioid granulomas:** These are the most common and are composed of epithelioid cells surrounded by lymphocytes.

TABLE 104.1 CAUSES OF HEPATIC GRANULOMAS

INFECTIONS

Bacterial
- Tuberculosis
- Atypical mycobacteria (especially in AIDS)
- Leprosy
- Brucellosis
- (Salmonellosis, tularemia, melioidosis, listeriosis, yersiniosis, Whipple's disease)

Mycotic
- Histoplasmosis
- Coccidioidomycosis
- (Blastomycosis, candidiasis, cryptococcosis, actinomycosis, toxoplasmosis, aspergillosis, nocardiosis)

Parasitic
- Schistosomiasis
- Toxocariasis
- (Ascaridiasis, fascioliasis, tongueworm)

Rickettsial
- Q fever
- Boutonneuse fever

Spirochetal
- Secondary syphilis

Viral
- (CMV infection, mononucleosis, psittacosis)

CHEMICALS
- Therapeutic drugs
- Beryllium
- Silica
- Talc

LIVER DISEASES
- Primary biliary cirrhosis
- Primary sclerosing cholangitis
- Fatty liver
- (Chronic hepatitis C, hepatitis A, hepatocellular carcinoma)

SYSTEMIC DISEASES
- Sarcoidosis
- Crohn's disease
- Hodgkin's disease
- Wegener granulomatosis
- Temporal arteritis
- Hypogammaglobulinemia
- Polymyalgia rheumatica

Epithelioid cells are activated macrophages that have lost their phagocytic properties and have developed synthetic and secretory activity with production of large amounts of cytokines. Giant cells formed by the fusion of the membranes of epithelioid cells can be seen within the granulomas. The giant cells contain from 6 to over 50 nuclei arranged either in a compact cluster (foreign body type) or along the periphery of the cell (Langhan's type) (Fig. 104.1). The foreign body granulomas may contain inclusions of particulate material, such as talc, silicone, starch, or droplets of mineral oil, usually within cytoplasmic vacuoles. Specific stains may reveal the presence of fungi, ova, or bacteria within the epithelioid granuloma. Necrosis of macrophages in the center of the granuloma is not uncommon. In late stages, granulomas may contain variable amounts of collagen. Fibrous tissue may undergo hyalinization and, after a long time, calcification. Granulomas may be found in the portal tracts, in the acinar parenchyma, or in both sites. Coalescence of single granulomas may occur.

2. **Lymphohistiocytic granulomas** are focal but poorly delimited clusters of lymphocytes and macrophages, without epithelioid cells. They are generally a nonspecific finding, resulting from clean-up of necrotic hepatocytes by Kupffer cells.
3. **Lipogranulomas** are a collection of lymphocytes and macrophages localized around extracellular fat, originating from fat-laden hepatocytes that have undergone necrosis. Mineral oil granulomas are similar reactions to ingested oil, which is present in the form of multiple vacuoles within macrophages. They are commonly located near the terminal venules.
4. **Fibrin-ring granulomas** have characteristically a central fat vacuole, surrounded by macrophages, lymphocytes, and neutrophils, as well as by strands of fibrin at the periphery forming a ring (Fig. 104.2).

Pathogenesis

Granulomas are the result of a cell-mediated immune reaction of the hepatic mononuclear phagocytic system to a foreign substance or antigen. The foreign material or the infecting agent may be present within the granuloma but is often no identifiable.

The process of transformation of macrophages into epithe lioid cells depends on the secretion of gamma-interferon an tumor necrosis factor beta (TNFβ) by activated T helper lym phocytes responding to the presence of a persistently retaine antigen.

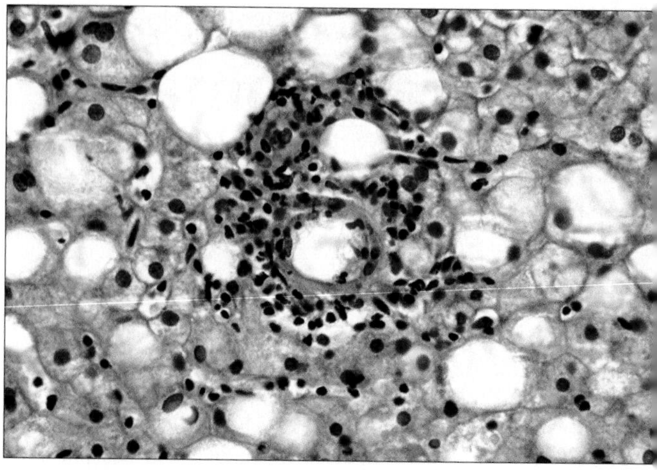

Fig. 104.2 Q fever. A central clear space surrounded by macrophag lymphocytes, and neutrophils also contains a peripheral fibrosis ring HE stain, x415.

CAUSES

Sarcoidosis

Sarcoidosis is a systemic granulomatous disease of unknow etiology that involves several organs. It is characterized clinicall by fever, pulmonary infiltrates, lymphadenopathy, and uveiti There are no specific diagnostic tests. Noncaseating epithelioi granulomas with multinucleated giant cells are present in affect ed organs, usually in high number (Fig. 104.3). With healing granulomas are usually replaced by collagen and later underg hyalinization. In the liver, they may be located anywhere withi the lobules, but they are more numerous in the portal tract and periportal zones (Table 104.2).

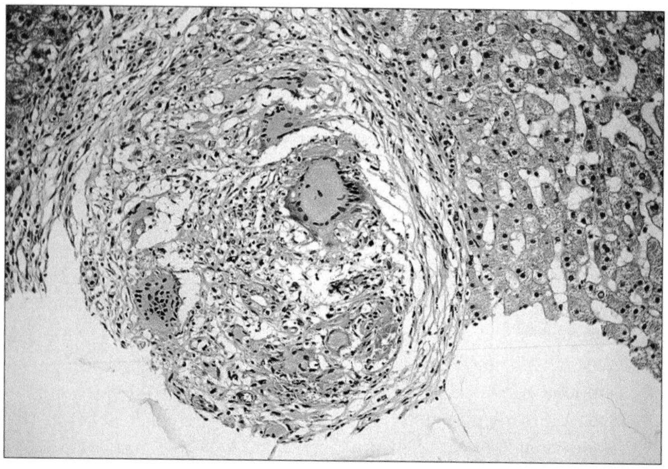

Fig. 104.1 Tuberculosis. An epithelioid granuloma with a multinucleated cell (Langhan's type). Hematoxylin-eosin (HE) stain, x210.

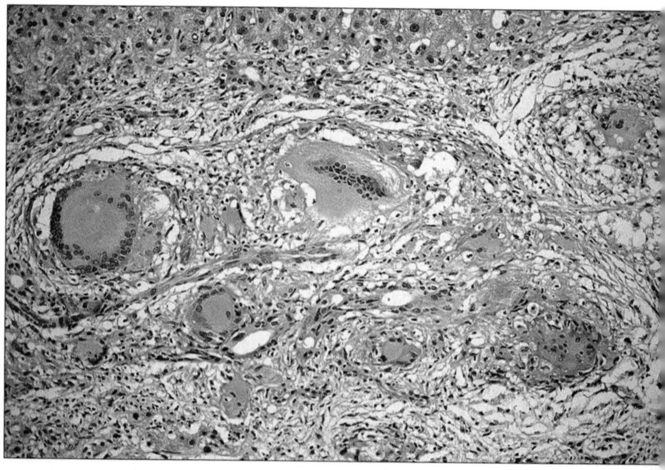

Fig. 104.3 Sarcoidosis. Confluent granulomas containing giant multinucleated cells. HE stain, x2103

TABLE 104.2 MANIFESTATIONS OF SARCOIDOSIS IN THE LIVER
Asymptomatic hepatic and splenic enlargement (30–50% of cases)
Nonnecrotizing epithelioid granulomas (>90%)
Elevated serum alkaline phosphatase levels (nearly 100%)
Elevated angiotensin converting enzyme levels (50–80%)
Intrahepatic cholestasis due to vanishing bile duct syndrome (rare)
Extrahepatic cholestasis due to lymph node enlargement at porta hepatis (rare)
Portal hypertension (rare)

Hepatic and spleen enlargement occurs in 30–50% of patients as the result of the presence of granulomas in both organs. Laboratory examination reveals mild-to-moderate elevation of serum alkaline phosphatase activity. Serum aminotransferases are normal or only slightly elevated. Serum angiotensin converting enzyme levels are increased in 50–80% of patients. Liver biopsy specimens contain epithelioid granulomas in nearly all patients with sarcoidosis. Thus, a liver biopsy is the recommended procedure to confirm a presumptive diagnosis of sarcoidosis

Hepatic involvement by sarcoidosis is usually asymptomatic and is not affected by treatment with corticosteroids. In a few patients, hepatic disease presents as chronic cholestasis or as portal hypertension. Cholestasis is due to the progressive destruction of the interlobular bile ducts by granulomas. The portal tracts lacking bile ducts are fibrotic and contain proliferating cholangioles. These changes may be confused with those of primary biliary cirrhosis, but sarcoidosis is not associated with serum antimitochondrial antibodies. Chronic cholestasis in sarcoidosis may also be caused by enlarged lymph nodes in the hilar region.

The **syndrome of intrahepatic cholestasis** associated with sarcoidosis presents with jaundice, pruritus, and fever. Most cases have been described in young African American men. The course of the syndrome is protracted, lasting several decades, despite treatment with ursodeoxycholic acid or corticosteroids, before reaching an end-stage liver disease. Liver transplantation has been performed in patients with advanced liver disease.

Portal hypertension develops as a consequence of granulomatous destruction and obliteration of portal vein branches at the level of the portal tracts. It seems to be an uncommon manifestation of sarcoidosis. It may lead to variceal hemorrhage, which should be treated by the administration of propranolol or by endoscopic sclerotherapy of esophageal varices.

Tuberculosis

Hepatic granulomas are found in more than 90% of patients with disseminated tuberculosis, but only in 25% of patients with tuberculosis confined to the lung. Diagnosis of tuberculosis is easy when caseating granulomas are found, particularly if the Ziehl-Neelsen stain reveals acid-fast bacilli. Acid-fast bacilli are rarely found in patients with only lung involvement, but very often in patients with disseminated disease. Polymerase chain reaction (PCR) has a high sensitivity and specificity to detect *Mycobacterium tuberculosis* DNA in tissues, and should be done when tuberculosis is suspected.

Mycobacteria of the *M. avium* complex are relatively common in AIDS patients. Liver involvement by this agent causes clusters of macrophages containing a high number of bacilli, rather then well-formed granulomas.

Leprosy

Hepatic granulomas are common in patients who have lepromatous leprosy (up to 75%), but much less frequently in patients who have tuberculoid leprosy. The lepromatous granulomas are composed of histiocytes with clear-to-foamy cytoplasm that contain a high number of acid-fast bacilli (*M. leprae*) (Fig. 104.4). The granulomas of tuberculoid leprosy are composed of epithelioid cells and rarely contain bacilli.

Q fever

Infection with *Coxiella burnetti* may present as a febrile disease with severe headache and pneumonia or as a febrile hepatitis. Hepatic involvement is characterized by fibrin-ring granulomas associated with macrovesicular steatosis. Diagnosis is based on serology.

Brucellosis

Granulomas are the most frequent histological change in brucellosis. Recent infection with *Brucella* species is accompanied by hepatic granulomas in 50% of cases. Most granulomas are of the lymphohistiocytic type. Epithelioid granulomas are seen less frequently, particularly in chronic brucellosis.

Whipple's disease

In rare cases, hepatic granulomas with PAS-positive macrophages have been reported in Whipple's disease.

Hodgkin's disease

In Hodgkin's disease, granulomas are usually epithelioid and are seen in both portal tracts and lobules. There is some evidence that prognosis is better in patients with granulomas in the liver than in those without granulomas. Granulomas are probably the result of a response to a tumor antigen.

Drug-induced granulomas

Granulomas can be associated with a number of drugs (Table 104.3). Granulomas may be found within portal tracts and in the parenchyma. Upon withdrawal of the causative drug they quickly resolve without fibrosis. In the absence of a test that

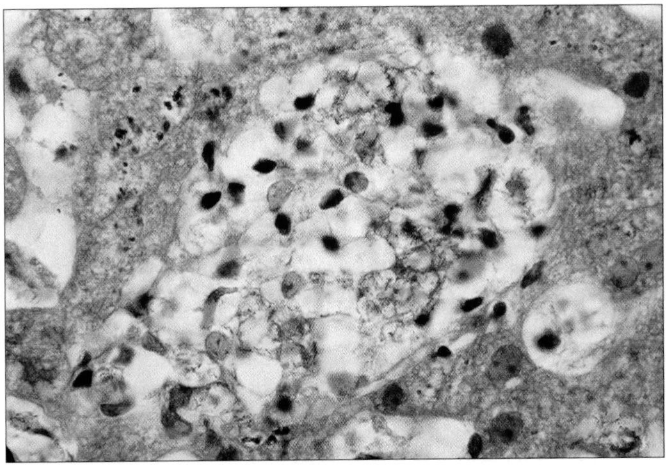

Fig. 104.4 Leprosy. Aggregates of foamy histiocytes that contain acid-alcohol bacilli. Ziehl-Neelsen stain, x415.

TABLE 104.3 THERAPEUTIC DRUGS ASSOCIATED WITH HEPATIC GRANULOMAS

Allopurinol	Nitrofurantoin
Amoxicillin-clavulanic acid	Phenylbutazone
Carbamazepine	Phenytoin
Diltiazem	Procainamide
Hydralazine	Quinidine
Mebendazole	Sulfonamides
Methyldopa	Tocainide

allows the diagnosis of drug hepatotoxicity, a reaction to a drug can only be suspected when the granulomas contain a high number of eosinophils.

Liver diseases

Granulomas are found in approximately 25% of patients with primary biliary cirrhosis, typically in portal tracts, surrounding damaged bile ducts, particularly in early stages of the disease. They have been seen in some patients with chronic hepatitis C, treated and not treated with interferon. Granulomas developing in treated patients are probably related to interferon-induced sarcoidosis.

CLINICAL PRESENTATION

Most patients present with systemic manifestations of the causative disorder, such as fever, malaise, weight loss, and anorexia, rather than symptoms related to the liver involvement. The presence of granulomas in the liver may be suspected by liver enlargement and a raised serum alkaline phosphatase. Pain in the right upper quadrant can be seen in some cases.

Granulomas are often an unexpected finding in a liver biopsy carried out for the work-up of asymptomatic abnormalities of liver tests.

Imaging studies may show no abnormalities, or there may be a diffuse nonhomogeneous appearance. Focal lesions may be detected by computed tomography (CT) scanning or ultrasound imaging when there is coalescence of many granulomas. Calcifications can be seen on plain radiographic films.

DIAGNOSIS/DIFFERENTIAL DIAGNOSIS

The diagnostic approach to hepatic granulomas requires a systematic histological evaluation of the granulomas themselves, of their topographic location, and of any associated changes in the surrounding liver tissue. The following stains should be done when the hematoxylin-eosin-stained section does not provide clues as to the cause of the granulomas: Ziehl-Neelsen for acid-fast bacilli and silver impregnation stain for fungi.

Evaluation of a patient in whom hepatic granulomas are found must include information on occupation, travel history, residence in foreign countries, and exposure to therapeutic drugs or industrial agents. The pathologist should attempt a systematic microscopic examination of the specimen containing the granulomas.

The first thing the pathologist must do is search for the presence of the etiologic agent within the granuloma, such as ova of *Schistosoma* (Fig. 104.5), mycobacteria or fungi (identified with special stains), or talc or silica identified under a polarizing microscope. In many cases, the pathologist cannot find the etiologic agent, but may suggest several possible causes based on the location of the granulomas or on some other morphological features:

1. Coalescence of granulomas, absence of necrosis, partial hyaline fibrosis, and location in portal and periportal areas suggest sarcoidosis.
2. Portal tract granulomas surrounding a damaged bile duct suggest primary biliary cirrhosis.
3. Two types of cytoplasmic inclusions, Schaumann's bodies (basophil structures with concentric proteinaceous calcified laminations) and asteroid bodies (star-like radiating structures within a clear space), are found in approximately half of the sarcoid granulomas, and very infrequently in granulomas of other etiologies.
4. Necrotizing granulomas suggest the presence of tuberculosis or fungal infections.
5. A relatively high number of eosinophils among the cellular population of the granuloma suggests a drug reaction or a parasitic disease.
6. The most common cause of fibrin-ring granulomas is Q fever, but they have been reported in rare instances associated with allopurinol treatment, leishmaniasis, mononucleosis, hepatitis A, CMV infection, and Hodgkin's disease.
7. Central purulent necrosis with presence of leucocytes suggests *Yersinia* infection or cat-scratch disease.
8. The presence of granuloma in the vicinity of an artery in a portal tract suggests the presence of granulomatous arteritis, either drug-induced or associated with systemic vasculitis.

When a clinical diagnosis of a granulomatous disease, such as primary biliary cirrhosis, sarcoidosis, or vasculitis, has been established based on clinical features, the etiology of granulomas found in the liver may be firmly suspected, even in the absence of any histological characteristic specific for this diagnosis.

The treatment and prognosis of hepatic granulomas depend on their cause.

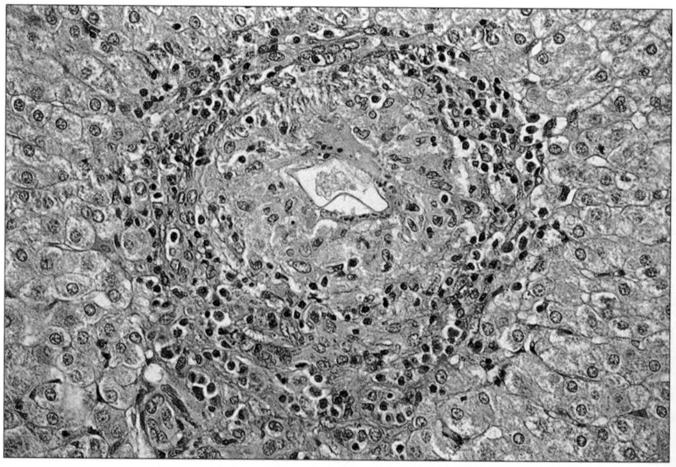

Fig. 104.5 Schistosomiasis. An epithelioid granuloma with remains of an ova of *Schistosoma*. HE stain, x210.

:EFERENCES

Alcantara-Payawal DE, Matsumura M, Shiratori Y et al. Direct detection of Mycobacterium tuberculosis using polymerase chain reaction assay among patients with hepatic granuloma. J Hepatol 1997; 27:620–627.

Harada K, Minato H, Hiramatsu K, Nakanuma Y. Epithelioid cell granulomas in chronic hepatitis C: immunohistochemical character and histological marker of favourable response to interferon-α therapy. Histopathology 1998; 33:216–221.

3. Ishak KG. Sarcoidosis of the liver and bile ducts. Mayo Clin Proc 1998; 73:467–472.
4. Lefkowitch JH. Hepatic granulomas. J Hepatol 1999; 30:40–45.
5. Mueller S, Boehme MW, Hofmann WJ et al. Extrapulmonary sarcoidosis primarily diagnosed in the liver. Scand J Gastroenterol 2000; 35:1003–1008.
6. Ryan BM, McDonald GS, Pilkington R. The development of hepatic granulomas following interferon-α2b therapy for chronic hepatitis C infection. Eur J Gastroenterol Hepatol 1998; 10:349–351.
7. Valla DC, Benhamou JP. Hepatic granulomas and hepatic sarcoidosis. Clin Liver Dis 2000; 4:269–285.
8. Denk H, Scheuer PJ, Baptista A et al. Guidelines for the diagnosis and interpretation of hepatic granulomas. Histopathology 1994; 25: 209–218.
9. Ferrell LD. Hepatic granulomas: a morphologic approach to diagnosis. Surg Pathol 1990; 3:87–106.

Chapter 105

Liver diseases and pregnancy

J Eileen Hay

KEY POINTS

- Hepatic dysfunction occurs in 3–5% of pregnant women. This may be related to hyperemesis gravidarum (0.3–2% in the first trimester of pregnancy), intrahepatic cholestasis of pregnancy (~ 0.1%), severe pre-eclampsia (1–2%); HELLP syndrome (Hemolysis, Elevated Liver tests, Low Platelets) (0.1–0.6%), and acute fatty liver of pregnancy (0.005%)

INTRODUCTION

Most pregnant women remain healthy during the physiologic adaptations to pregnancy but pathophysiologic changes may occur, including five unique liver diseases seen only in the pregnant or postpartum period.[1,2] Hyperemesis gravidarum is intractable nausea and vomiting in the first trimester;[3] intrahepatic cholestasis of pregnancy (ICP) is pruritus and liver dysfunction in second half of pregnancy.[4,5] Severe pre-eclampsia may cause hepatic dysfunction;[6] some cases are complicated further by hemolysis (H), elevated liver tests (EL), and low platelets (LP) – the HELLP syndrome.[7] In acute fatty liver of pregnancy (AFLP), microvesicular fatty infiltration of hepatocytes in the third trimester results in acute liver failure (Fig. 105.1).[8]

Any liver disease in a young woman of childbearing age may occur coincidentally during pregnancy and often resolves with few effects on the pregnancy. Similarly, patients with early, well compensated chronic liver disease may have successful pregnancies but, in the rare pregnant patient with cirrhosis and/or portal hypertension, complications frequently occur.

CAUSES AND INCIDENCE OF LIVER DISEASE IN PREGNANCY

Liver diseases in pregnancy fall into three main categories:

- liver diseases unique to pregnancy
- liver diseases occurring coincidentally in the pregnant patient
- pre-existing chronic liver disease.

Liver diseases unique to pregnancy all have characteristic timing in relation to the pregnancy (Fig. 105.2). Although jaundice is uncommon (0.1%), hepatic dysfunction occurs in 3–5% of pregnant women with most cases due to liver diseases unique to pregnancy.[9] Severe pre-eclampsia is the commonest cause of liver dysfunction in pregnancy (1–2% of all deliveries); 2–12% of cases of severe preeclampsia (0.1–0.6% of all deliveries) are complicated further by the HELLP syndrome.[7] ICP occurs worldwide with striking geographic variations. In the USA it occurs in 0.1% pregnancies, with jaundice in 20% of cases, and is the second most common cause of jaundice in pregnancy after viral hepatitis. Hyperemesis gravidarum occurs in 0.3–2.0% of pregnancies. AFLP is generally considered to be the least common of the pregnancy-associated liver diseases (0.005% of pregnancies), although recent studies have suggested its incidence may be considerably higher.

Viral hepatitis has the same incidence and clinical features in the pregnant population as in the nonpregnant, and is the commonest cause of jaundice in pregnancy.[10] Apart from hepatitis E (rare in the USA), the hepatitis viruses and pregnancy have little or no effect on one another; the prevention of perinatal transmission of hepatitis B virus is very important. Herpes simplex hepatitis is a rare but treatable cause of fulminant hepatitis in the third trimester (Fig. 105.3A). Although gallstones are common, especially in multiparous patients, symptomatic cholelithiasis is infrequent – usually biliary colic, less commonly pancreatitis or cholecystitis. The Budd-Chiari syndrome is rare and usually occurs in the postpartum period, often associated with antiphospholipid syndrome, thrombotic thrombocytopenic purpura (TTP), pre-eclampsia, and septic abortion. Sepsis associated with pyelonephritis or abortion is a cause of jaundice in early pregnancy.

Chronic hepatitis B is present in 0.5–1.5% of pregnancies, and chronic hepatitis C in 2.3% of some indigent populations. An uncomplicated pregnancy with no disease flare is expected in mild disease. Patients with treated autoimmune or Wilson disease may have successful pregnancies, but must be adequately managed before and during pregnancy. Most patients with advanced cirrhosis and/or portal hypertension are infertile but, if pregnancy occurs, increased maternal complications occur including variceal hemorrhage (20–25%), hepatic failure, encephalopathy, and rupture of splenic artery aneurysms.[2]

CLINICAL PRESENTATION

DIAGNOSTIC APPROACH TO LIVER DISEASE IN PREGNANCY

- Are there any features of chronic liver disease (including liver transplantation)?
- Is the presentation compatible with acute viral hepatitis?
- Are there features to suggest biliary disease?
- Is there any history of drugs or toxins?
- Are there features of Budd-Chiari syndrome?
- Is there any evidence or risk factors for sepsis?
- Is the presentation compatible with one of the liver diseases unique to pregnancy?

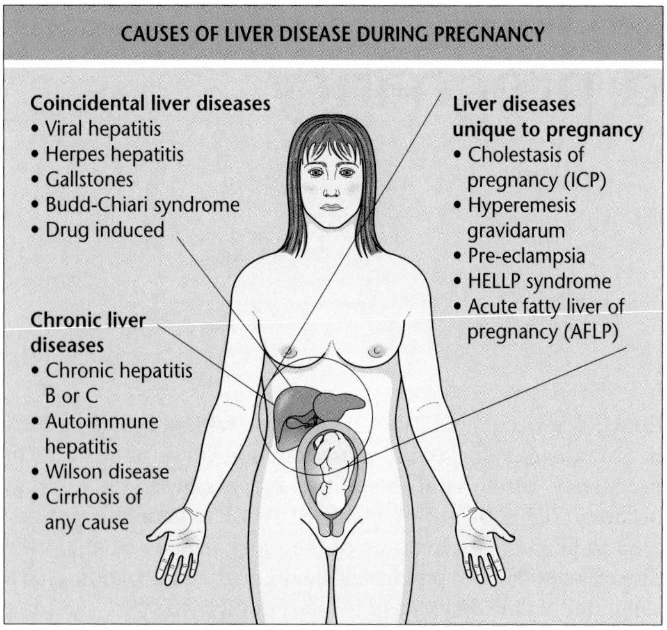

Fig. 105.1 Causes of liver disease during pregnancy.

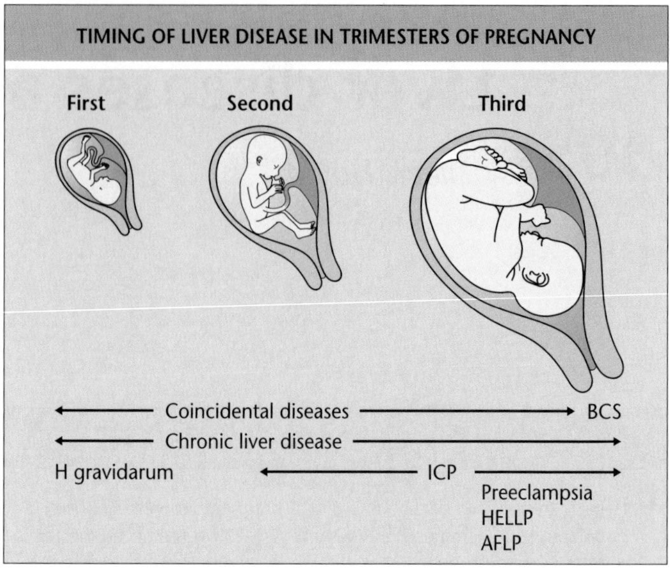

Fig. 105.2 Timing of liver disease in the trimesters of pregnancy. AFLP, acute fatty liver of pregnancy; BCS, Budd-Chiari syndrome; HELLP, hemolysis (H), elevated liver tests (EL), and low platelets (LP) syndrome; H gravidarum, hyperemesis gravidarum; ICP, intrahepatic cholestasis of pregnancy.

ETIOLOGY OF PREGNANCY-ASSOCIATED LIVER DISEASES

The etiologies of the liver diseases unique to pregnancy remain obscure, with overlap among pre-eclampsia, HELLP, and AFLP. Hyperemesis gravidarum and ICP are not associated with pre-eclampsia. Hyperemesis gravidarum is an enigmatic, multifactorial, neurohormonal disorder of pregnancy in which hormonal (raised estrogen and chorionic gonadotropin levels, transient hyperthyroidism) and immunologic abnormalities are found.[3]

The etiology of ICP is probably multifactorial.[5,11] An exogenous influence is suggested by the seasonal and geographic variability, the potential role of dietary factors (selenium deficiency), the proven role of exogenous progestogen therapy, and the recurrence rate of only 45–70% in multiparous patients. The pathogenesis is clearly related in some way to female sex hormones (genetic and/or exogenous), perhaps involving a genetically abnormal or exaggerated hepatic metabolic response to the physiologic increase in estrogen levels during pregnancy. Abnormalities in progesterone metabolism are also seen, with impaired sulfation in some patients.[12] The familial cases and ethnic clustering strongly suggest a genetic predisposition to ICP. Mothers with ICP have been identified who are heterozygous, with homozygous babies, for genetic abnormalities in canalicular transport proteins, the same abnormalities being responsible for the rare group of diseases known as the

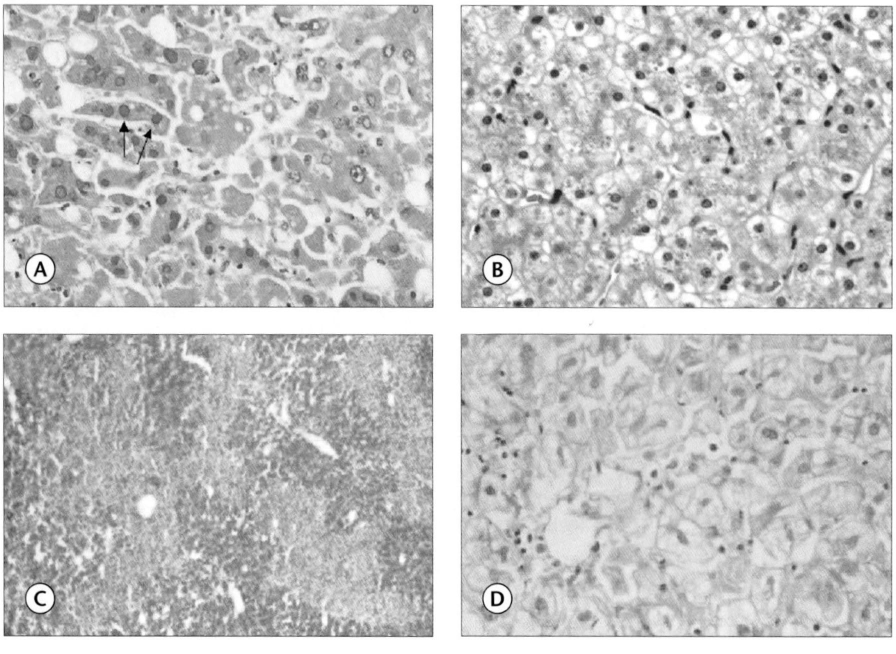

Fig. 105.3 Histologic appearance of the liver during pregnancy. A. Hematoxylin and eosin stain of herpes hepatitis in the third trimester shows typical acidophilic intranuclear inclusions (arrows). **B.** Hematoxylin and eosin stain of intrahepatic cholestasis of pregnancy shows bland cholestasis without inflammation or necrosis. **C.** Sudan stain (low power) of acute fatty liver of pregnancy shows the zonal distribution of diffuse fatty infiltration (red staining) predominantly in zone 3. **D.** Hematoxylin and eosin stain (high power) of same patient shows hepatocytes stuffed with microvesicular fat and centrally located nuclei. **C, D** Reproduced from the Mayo Clinic Gastroenterology and Hepatology Board Review, with permission from the Mayo Foundation.

PATHOGENIC MECHANISMS OF INTRAHEPATIC CHOLESTASIS OF PREGNANCY

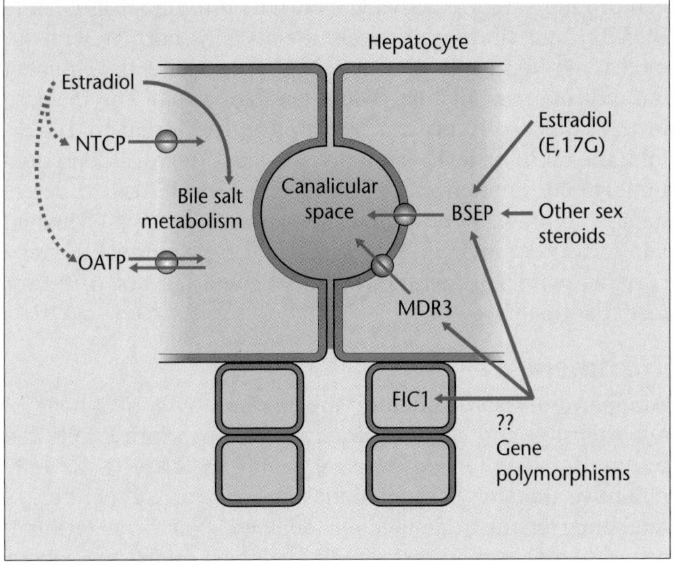

Fig. 105.4 Pathogenic mechanisms of intrahepatic cholestasis of pregnancy. Potential sites of inhibition of normal biliary excretion mechanisms on the hepatocyte and cholangiocyte in intrahepatic cholestasis in pregnancy. BSEP, bile salt export pump; $E_2$17G, estradiol 17β-D-glucuronide; FIC1, product of the familial intrahepatic cholestasis gene; MDR3, multidrug resistance protein 3; NTCP, sodium taurocholate co-transporting polypeptide; OATP, organic anion transporting polypeptide.

progressive familial intrahepatic cholestasis (PFIC) syndromes (Fig. 105.4).[13] Abnormalities in placental bile acid transport systems and/or the high circulating bile acid levels may contribute to fetal loss due to asphyxia from vasospasm of the placental vessels.

The **etiology of pre-eclampsia** appears to involve defective placentation leading to generalized endothelial dysfunction. Liver dysfunction may result from vasoconstriction of the hepatic vascular bed. In the HELLP syndrome, microangiopathic hemolytic anemia causes periportal hemorrhage, necrosis, and fibrin deposition in the liver; as this increases in severity, the hemorrhage dissects from zone 1 to affect the whole lobule, extending the area of necrosis and leading to large hematomas, capsular tears, and hepatic rupture.

In AFLP, microvesicular fatty infiltration of hepatocytes leads to acute liver failure; its etiology may involve abnormalities in intramitochondrial fatty acid oxidation (FAO).[14,15] Some babies of mothers with AFLP are homozygous for enzymes essential for normal FAO, the best characterized being LCHAD (long-chain 3-hydroxacyl-coenzyme A dehydrogenase) deficiency.[15] This suggests that maternal heterozygosity, with fetal homozygosity, for deficiency of an enzyme responsible for normal FAO may overwhelm the increased metabolic demands on fatty acid metabolism of later pregnancy, perhaps exacerbated by external factors, and result in AFLP.

HYPEREMESIS GRAVIDARUM

Hyperemesis gravidarum is intractable vomiting of such severity as to necessitate intravenous hydration.[3] It occurs in the first trimester of pregnancy, typically between 4 and 10 weeks of gestation, and is complicated by high transaminase levels (up to 20-fold above the normal range) in 50% of patients and occasional jaundice. The diagnosis is made on clinical features of intractable, dehydrating vomiting in the first trimester. When the levels of transaminases are high, viral hepatitis must be excluded. In the rare patient who requires a liver biopsy to exclude more serious disease, the hepatic histologic appearance is generally normal with no inflammation or necrosis; occasionally cholestasis with rare cell dropout will be seen. Hospitalization is necessary for hydration and parenteral nutrition, and therapy is generally symptomatic.

INTRAHEPATIC CHOLESTASIS OF PREGNANCY

Clinical features

ICP is characterized by severe pruritus, mild jaundice, and biochemical cholestasis appearing in the second half of pregnancy and disappearing after delivery, typically to recur in subsequent pregnancies.[4] Pruritus, starting around 25–32 weeks of gestation, in a patient with no other signs of liver disease is strongly suggestive of ICP, especially if ICP occurred in previous pregnancies. The pruritus affects all parts of the body, is worse at night, and may be so severe that the patient is suicidal. Occasionally the cholestasis is complicated by diarrhea or steatorrhea. Jaundice occurs in 10–25% of patients and usually follows the pruritus by 2–4 weeks. Jaundice without pruritus is rare. A mild to 10–20-fold increase in transaminase levels is seen; bilirubin concentration is usually less than 5 mg/dL.

Diagnosis

Diagnosis in the first pregnancy is generally made on typical clinical features, confirmed by rapid postpartum disappearance of the pruritus. Serum bile acid levels are always increased; they may be 100 times above normal and may correlate with fetal risk. Liver biopsy is needed only to diagnose a more serious liver disease; in ICP the liver has a near-normal appearance with mild cholestasis and minimal or no hepatocellular necrosis (see Fig. 105.3B). The differential diagnosis of cholestasis in pregnancy includes coincidental cholestatic diseases (drugs, cholestatic viral hepatitis, sepsis, gallstones) and pre-existing chronic biliary disease.

DIFFERENTIAL DIAGNOSIS

CAUSES OF CHOLESTASIS IN PREGNANCY

- **Coincidental liver diseases**
  Gallstones
  Viral hepatitis
  Drugs
  Sepsis
- **Chronic liver disease**
  Primary biliary cirrhosis
  Primary sclerosing cholangitis, etc.
- **Liver diseases unique to pregnancy**
  Intrahepatic cholestasis of pregnancy

Treatment and prevention

With ICP the main risk is to the fetus (premature delivery and perinatal death), and fetal monitoring for chronic placental insufficiency is essential. Unfortunately this will not prevent all fetal deaths; acute anoxic injury can be prevented only by delivery as soon as the fetal lungs are mature.

Maternal management is symptomatic to relieve pruritus. Exogenous progesterone therapy should be discontinued and may result in remission of the pruritus. Several small trials of ursodeoxycholic acid (UDCA) 0.6–1 g daily have consistently shown clinical and biochemical improvement; the fetal outcome was improved, with less prematurity and no adverse fetal or maternal effects. High-dose UDCA (1.5–2.0 g/day) has recently been shown to relieve pruritus in most cases, to reduce abnormal maternal bile acid levels, and to be completely safe for the fetus; in addition, the babies born to these mothers had almost normal bile acid levels in comparison to babies of untreated mothers.[16,17] Cholestyramine can sometimes give relief of pruritus in 1–2 weeks, but biochemical parameters, maternal malabsorption, and fetal prognosis are not improved. Dexamethasone (12 mg daily for 7 days), by suppressing feto-placental estrogen production, improves symptoms, liver function, and fetal lung maturity in some patients with ICP and no adverse effects. Other agents have generally been ineffective.

PRE-ECLAMPSIA

Pre-eclampsia is a disease of the third trimester; liver involvement occurs in only a minority of patients with severe disease with right upper abdominal pain, jaundice, and a tender, normal-size liver. Transaminase levels range from mild to 10–20-fold increases; bilirubin concentration is usually less than 5 mg/dL.

No specific therapy is needed for the hepatic involvement of pre-eclampsia, and its only significance is as an indicator of severe disease with need for immediate delivery to avoid eclampsia, hepatic rupture, or necrosis. HELLP and AFLP may complicate pre-eclampsia.

THE HELLP SYNDROME

Clinical features

Severe pre-eclampsia is complicated in 2–12% of cases by the HELLP syndrome. Most patients with HELLP present with epigastric or right upper quadrant pain (65–90%), nausea and vomiting (35–50%), a 'flu-like illness (90%), or headache (30%). They usually have edema and weight gain (60%), right upper quadrant tenderness (80%), and hypertension (80%). Jaundice is uncommon (5%). Some patients have no obvious pre-eclampsia. Most patients (71%) present between 27 and 36 weeks' gestation, but pre-eclampsia may occur earlier or up to 48 h after delivery. HELLP is commoner in multiparous and older patients.

Diagnosis

The diagnosis of HELLP must be quickly established due to maternal and fetal risk, and requires the presence of all three criteria:

1. Hemolysis with an abnormal blood smear, raised LDH concentration (>600 U/L), and increase in indirect bilirubin
2. Aspartate aminotransferase (AST) level above 70 U/L
3. Platelet count of less than 100×10^9/L, and in severe cases less than 50×10^9/L.

Prothrombin time, activated partial thromboplastin time (APTT), and fibrinogen levels are usually normal with no increase in fibrin split products, but occasionally disseminated intravascular coagulation (DIC) may be present. The increase in transaminase levels can be variable, from mild to 10–20-fold; the bilirubin level is usually less than 5 mg/dL. Computed tomography (limited views) is indicated in HELLP to detect hepatic rupture, subcapsular hematomas, intraparenchymal hemorrhage, or infarction (Fig. 105.5); these abnormalities may correlate with a reduction in platelet count but not with liver test abnormalities.

Treatment

Antepartum stabilization of the mother with treatment of hypertension and seizure prophylaxis is a priority, followed by transfer to a tertiary referral center. Delivery is the only definitive therapy; if the patient is near term and/or there is fetal lung maturity, immediate delivery should be effected, probably by cesarean section although well established labour should be allowed to proceed in the absence of obstetric complications or DIC. Many (40–50%) will require Cesarean section, especially primigravidae remote from term. Blood or blood products are given to correct hypovolemia, anemia, or coagulopathy. Management remote from term is controversial, and sometimes in milder cases at less than 34 weeks a more conservative approach with high-dose glucocorticoids is taken in an attempt to prolong the pregnancy and improve fetal lung maturity; this therapy may also help to aid maternal stability during the transfer time to a tertiary referral center. Once delivered, most babies do very well.

Most patients have rapid early resolution of HELLP after delivery with normalization of the platelet count by 5 days. The persistence of thrombocytopenia, hemolysis, progressive increases in bilirubin and creatinine levels for more than 72 h, and the development of complications are usually taken as indications for plasmapheresis, although no clinical trials have

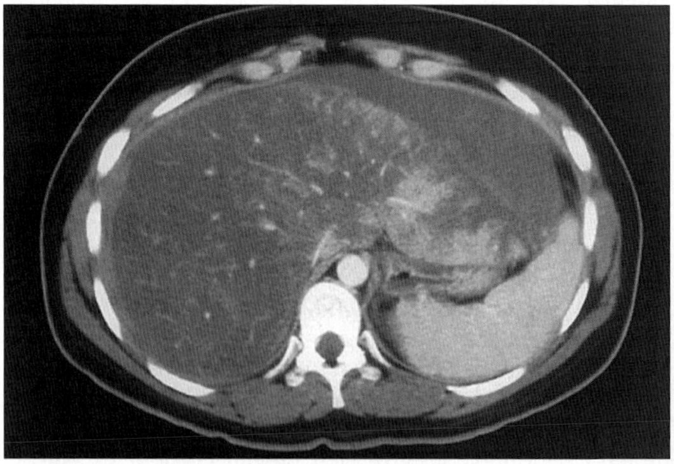

Fig. 105.5 Computed tomogram of the abdomen in severe HELLP. A large subcapsular hematoma can be seen extending over the left lobe, as well as the heterogeneous, hypodense appearance of the right lobe due to extensive necrosis with 'sparing' of a small area of the left lobe (compare perfusion to that of normal spleen). Reproduced from the Mayo Clinic Gastroenterology and Hepatology Board Review, with permission from the Mayo Foundation.

established the efficacy of this treatment. Serious maternal complications are common – DIC (20%), abruptio placentae (16%), acute renal failure (8%), pulmonary edema (8%), adult respiratory distress syndrome (1%), severe ascites (8%), and hepatic failure (2%) – and maternal mortality rates range from 1% to 25%. Worsening liver failure after the first 3–5 days following delivery necessitates consideration of liver transplantation in the rare case.

Hepatic hemorrhage without rupture is generally managed conservatively in stable patients with close hemodynamic monitoring in an intensive care unit, correction of coagulopathy, immediate availability of large-volume transfusion of blood and blood products, immediate intervention for rupture, and follow-up diagnostic computed tomography as needed. Exogenous trauma must be avoided – abdominal palpation, convulsions, emesis, and unnecessary transportation.

Liver rupture, with hemorrhage into the peritoneum, is a rare life-threatening complication of HELLP, usually preceded by intraparenchymal hemorrhage and a contained subcapsular hematoma in the right lobe. Survival depends on aggressive hemodynamic support and immediate surgery, although the best surgical management is still controversial. The maternal mortality rate from hepatic rupture is 50%, with high perinatal mortality from placental rupture, intrauterine asphyxia, or prematurity.

ACUTE FATTY LIVER OF PREGNANCY

Clinical features

AFLP occurs almost exclusively in the third trimester from 28 to 40 weeks, most commonly at 36 weeks; 50% of patients are nulliparous, with an increased incidence in twin pregnancies. The presentation is variable, from asymptomatic to fulminant liver failure. The typical patient has 1–2 weeks of anorexia, nausea, vomiting, and right upper quadrant pain, and is ill-looking with jaundice, hypertension, edema, ascites, a small liver, hepatic encephalopathy, and pre-eclampsia (50%). Intrauterine death may occur.

Transaminase levels vary from near-normal to more than 1000 mg/dL, usually about 300 mg/dL; bilirubin concentration is usually less than 5 mg/dL, but is higher in patients with severe or complicated disease. Other typical abnormalities are normochromic, normocytic anemia, high white blood cell count, normal to low platelet count, abnormal prothrombin time, APTT, and fibrinogen levels, with or without DIC, metabolic acidosis, renal dysfunction or oliguric renal failure, hypoglycemia, high ammonia, and often biochemical pancreatitis.

Diagnosis

The differential diagnoses of the severely ill patient with liver failure in the third trimester are AFLP, HELLP, thrombotic thrombocytopenic purpura, hemolytic–uremic syndrome, and fulminant viral hepatitis. The diagnosis is generally made on clinical and biochemical features. Computed tomography is more sensitive than ultrasonography in the detection of AFLP. Liver biopsy is rarely indicated for management, but is essential for a definitive diagnosis of AFLP. Microvesicular, and infrequently macrovesicular, fatty infiltration is most prominent in zone 3; this fat consists of free fatty acids. There is lobular disarray with pleomorphism of hepatocytes and mild portal inflammation with cholestasis (see Fig. 105.3C and D).

DIAGNOSTIC METHODS

DIAGNOSTIC DIFFERENCES BETWEEN ACUTE FATTY LIVER OF PREGNANCY (AFLP) AND THE HELLP SYNDROME

	AFLP	HELLP
Parity	Nulliparous, twins	Multiparous, older
Jaundice	Common	Uncommon
Encephalopathy	Present	Absent
Platelet count	Low to normal	Low
Prothrombin time	Prolonged	Normal
APTT	Prolonged	Normal
Fibrinogen	Low	Normal or increased
Glucose	Low	Normal
Creatinine	High	High
Ammonia	High	Normal
Computed tomography	Fatty infiltration	Hemorrhage

APTT, activated partial thromboplastin time.

Treatment

In AFLP, early diagnosis, immediate fetal delivery, and intensive supportive care are essential for both maternal and fetal survival. Delivery is usually effected by cesarean section (epidural anesthesia will allow better ongoing assessment of coma grade), but rapid controlled vaginal delivery with fetal monitoring is probably safer if the cervix is favorable. Correction of coagulopathy and thrombocytopenia, and prophylactic antibiotics are recommended. There is no proven effective therapy for AFLP apart from termination of the pregnancy.

By 2–3 days after delivery, liver function and encephalopathy will improve, but intensive supportive care for acute liver failure is needed until the recovery of liver function occurs, sometimes over days but occasionally delayed for weeks or months. The maternal mortality rate is now 10–18%, with a fetal mortality rate of 9–23%. Infectious and bleeding complications remain the most life threatening. Patients who are critically ill at the time of presentation, who develop complications (encephalopathy, hypoglycemia, coagulopathy, bleeding), or who continue to deteriorate despite emergency delivery, should ideally be transferred to a liver center. Liver transplantation is rarely indicated because of the great potential for recovery with delivery, but should be considered in patients whose clinical course continues to deteriorate with advancing fulminant hepatic failure after the first 1–2 days' postpartum without signs of hepatic regeneration.

PROGNOSIS FOR FUTURE PREGNANCIES

In ICP, pruritus and liver dysfunction resolve immediately after delivery with no maternal mortality, recurring in 45–70% of subsequent pregnancies and occasionally with oral contraceptives. Patients with ICP may develop more gallstones and gallbladder disease. Some rare familial cases of apparent ICP have persisted postpartum, with progression to subsequent fibrosis and cirrhosis.

The risk of recurrence of HELLP in subsequent pregnancies is poorly defined (up to 25%), but subsequent pregnancies carry an increased risk of pre-eclampsia, preterm delivery, intrauterine growth retardation, and abruptio placentae. Many patients do not become pregnant again after AFLP, either by choice because of the devastating effect of the illness or by necessity as a result of hysterectomy to control postpartum bleeding. However, AFLP does not tend to recur in subsequent pregnancies, although rare cases have been reported. Because LCHAD (long-chain 3-hydroxyacyl-coenzyme dehydrogenase) deficiency is present in many of these infants, later neonatal problems may occur.[14,15]

REFERENCES

1. Wolf JL. Liver disease in pregnancy. Med Clin North Am 1996; 80:1167–1187.
2. Sandhu BS, Sanyal AJ. Pregnancy and liver disease. Gastroenterol Clin North Am 2003; 32:407–436.
3. Koch KL, Frissora CL. Nausea and vomiting during pregnancy. Gastroenterol Clin North Am 2003; 32:201–234.
4. Bacq Y, Sapey T, Brechot M et al. Intrahepatic cholestasis of pregnancy: a French prospective study. Hepatology 1997; 26:358–364.
5. Germain AM, Carvajal JA, Glasinovic JC et al. Intrahepatic cholestasis of pregnancy: an intriguing pregnancy-specific disorder. J Soc Gynecol 2002; 9:10–14.
6. Norwitz ER, Hsu C-D, Repke JT. Acute complications of preeclampsia. Clin Obstet Gynecol 2002; 45:308–329.
7. Sibai BM, Ramadan MK, Usta I et al. Maternal morbidity and mortality in 442 pregnancies with hemolysis, elevated liver enzymes and low platelets (HELLP syndrome). Am J Obstet Gynecol 1993; 169:1000–1006.
8. Mabie WC. Acute fatty liver of pregnancy. Gastroenterol Clin North Am 1992; 21:951–959.
9. Ch'ng CL, Morgan M, Hainsworth I et al. Prospective study of liver dysfunction in pregnancy in southwest Wales. Gut 2002; 51:876–880.
10. Hay JE. Viral hepatitis in pregnancy. Viral Hepatitis Rev 2000; 6:205–215.
11. Lammert F, Marschall H-U, Glantz A et al. Intrahepatic cholestasis of pregnancy: molecular pathogenesis, diagnosis and management. J Hepatol 2000; 33:1012–1021.
12. Meng L-J, Reyes H, Axelson M et al. Progesterone metabolites and bile acids in serum of patients with intrahepatic cholestasis of pregnancy: effect of ursodeoxycholic acid therapy. Hepatology 2997; 26:1573–1579.
13. Yang Z, Shao Y, Bennett MJ et al. Fetal genotypes and pregnancy outcomes in 35 families with mitochondrial trifunctional protein mutations. Am J Obstet Gynecol 2002; 187:715–720.
14. Rakheja D, Bennett MJ, Rogers BB. Longchain L-3-hydroxyacyl-coenzyme A dehydrogenase deficiency: a molecular and biochemical review. Lab Invest 2002; 82:815–824.
15. Strauss AW, Bennett MJ, Rinaldo P et al. Inherited long-chain 3-hydroxyacyl-CoA dehydrogenase deficiency and a fetal–maternal interaction cause maternal liver disease and other pregnancy complications. Sem Perinatol 1999; 23:100–112.
16. Serrano MA, Brites D, Larena MG et al. Beneficial effect of ursodeoxycholic acid on alterations induced by cholestasis of pregnancy in bile acid transport across the human placenta. J Hepatol 1998; 28:829–839.
17. Mazzella G, Nicola R, Francesco A et al. Ursodeoxycholic acid administration in patients with cholestasis of pregnancy: effects on primary bile acids in babies and mothers. Hepatology 2001; 33:504–508.

Chapter 106

Liver transplantation: indications and selection of candidates and immediate complications

Patrick S Kamath and John J Poterucha

KEY POINTS

- Liver transplantation is the only established therapy for patients with end-stage liver diseases. It is also indicated in fulminant liver failure, in some biliary malformations, and in some hepatocellular carcinomas
- Survival after liver transplantation is approximately 80% at 3 years. Donor organ shortage is a major limitation in adult liver transplant and is responsible for significant mortality while on the waiting list. Strategies to increase the number of donor organs include the use of marginal livers, split liver, and living donors

INTRODUCTION

Liver transplantation is now an established treatment to improve quality of life and prolong survival in patients with end-stage liver disease. Liver transplantation is currently associated with a 1-year patient survival above 90% in most liver diseases, and a 3-year survival of approximately 80%.

Surgical techniques used in liver transplantation are summarized in Fig. 106.1.

INDICATIONS FOR LIVER TRANSPLANTATION

The indications for liver transplantation in adults are fulminant liver failure, end-stage liver disease, hepatocellular carcinoma, and metabolic liver disease. In children, the most common indication for liver transplantation is biliary atresia followed by alpha-1-antitrypsin deficiency. The most common indication for adult liver transplantation is end-stage liver disease. Indications for liver transplantation in this group are general and disease specific.

General indications

These indications for liver transplantation are the complications of liver disease that are associated with poor survival. These include spontaneous bacterial peritonitis, refractory ascites and hepatorenal syndrome, hepatic encephalopathy that is refractory to treatment, and superimposed hepatocellular carcinoma. In many patients, impaired quality of life related to fatigue and malnutrition is an additional consideration.

In general, patients with end-stage liver disease with a Child-Pugh score ≥7 should be considered for liver transplantation. In patients with cholestatic liver disease such as primary biliary cirrhosis and primary sclerosing cholangitis, a rising bilirubin is an indicator of poor outcome. Intractable pruritus or osteopenic bone disease and, in patients with primary sclerosing cholangitis, recurrent bacterial cholangitis, are again indications for liver transplantation.

Disease-specific considerations for liver transplantation and evaluation

Hepatitis C and hepatitis B

Currently, the most frequent indication for liver transplantation in many countries is cirrhosis secondary to chronic hepatitis C. Recurrence of hepatitis C post liver transplantation is invariable. Moreover, in patients who have recurrent hepatitis C, the course is accelerated with approximately 20% of patients developing cirrhosis within 5 years. Recurrence of hepatitis C is more likely in patients with pretransplant viral loads $>1\times10^6$ copies/mL. Therefore, in patients who can tolerate treatment, efforts should be made to reduce viral loads pretransplantation.

A positive hepatitis B e antigen and/or high hepatitis B viral DNA pretransplantation is associated with recurrence of hepatitis B in the graft. A combination of lamivudine or adefovir with hepatitis B immunoglobulin (to maintain anti-HBs levels >100 IU/mL) is recommended for all patients with hepatitis B undergoing liver transplantation.

Alcoholic liver disease

Survival post liver transplantation in patients with alcoholic liver disease is no different from that in patients with other etiologies of liver disease. Typically, an abstinence period of approximately 6 months, adequate rehabilitation, and a stable social support system are required for liver transplantation. It is important that patients continue to remain in an alcohol rehabilitation program following liver transplantation because of a rate of recidivism of approximately 15%. Recidivism is associated with lower compliance with immunosuppression and, therefore, a risk of graft loss.

Primary biliary cirrhosis and primary sclerosing cholangitis

Risk scores for primary biliary cirrhosis and primary sclerosing cholangitis have been of invaluable help in the decision-making regarding liver transplantation. Patients should be referred for liver transplantation when their chance of 1-year survival based on the Mayo risk scores is <90%.

Autoimmune hepatitis

Recurrence of autoimmune hepatitis post liver transplantation occurs in about 20% of patients. Given the risk of recurrence, we recommend that steroids are not tapered away completely in these patients post liver transplantation.

Budd-Chiari syndrome

Patients with a fulminant presentation, i.e., those with hepatic encephalopathy within 8 weeks of symptoms, are best

DECEASED DONOR LIVER TRANSPLANTATION

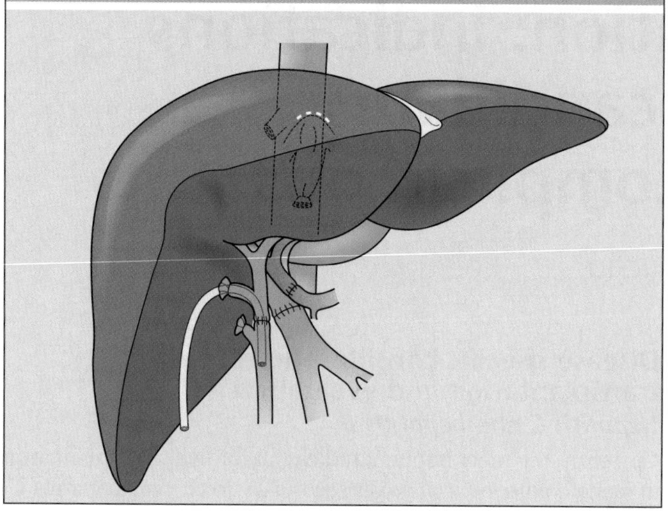

Fig. 106.1 Deceased donor liver transplantation. Donor inferior vena cava to recipient hepatic vein confluence 'piggy-back' anastomosis, choledochocholedochostomy, biliary tube in donor cystic duct. Reproduced from Rosen CR. Liver diseases necessitating transplantation. In: Kelly KA et al., eds. Mayo Clinic in Gastrointestinal Surgery, with permission from Mayo Foundation for Medical Education and Research.

managed by liver transplantation. Patients with Budd-Chiari syndrome and cirrhosis, those with acute Budd-Chiari syndrome who fail a transjugular intrahepatic portosystemic shunt (TIPS) procedure, and patients with subacute Budd-Chiari syndrome who fail shunt surgery should be considered for liver transplantation. Liver transplantation reverses the underlying thrombotic disorder in patients with protein C, protein S, and anti-thrombin III deficiency. However, multiple thrombophilic disorders can occur in the same patient; therefore, we recommend long-term anticoagulation post liver transplantation (in the absence of contraindications).

Hepatic malignancies

Hepatocellular carcinoma is the most common tumor for which liver transplantation is carried out. The Milan criteria (a single tumor <5 cm in diameter, or three tumor lesions or less, the largest being no greater than 3 cm) are used to select patients for liver transplantation. There should be no evidence of metastatic disease. In patients meeting these criteria, the long-term survival rate is similar to survival in patients being transplanted for decompensated cirrhosis.

Evaluation of patients with hepatocellular carcinoma includes an extensive search for extrahepatic metastases (Table 106.1). After confirming that the hepatocellular cancer is localized to the liver, then transarterial chemoembolization of the tumor is recommended and repeated every 2 months as required.

The **cholangiocarcinoma protocol** includes preoperative radiation (both brachytherapy as well as external beam radiation) and chemotherapy. Following this, an operative staging is carried out and, if it is confirmed that the tumor is localized to the liver, the patient may then undergo liver transplantation.

Neuroendocrine tumors: Liver transplantation may be carried out for such patients and those with metastases localized to the liver. The primary tumor in such patients requires resection

TABLE 106.1 PROTOCOLS FOR EVALUATION OF PATIENTS WITH MALIGNANT TUMORS
HEPATOCELLULAR CARCINOMA PROTOCOL – INITIAL EVALUATION
CT chest
CT abdomen and pelvis (repeated with CT chest every 3 months until transplantation)
CT head
Bone scan (entire skeleton)
CHOLANGIOCARCINOMA PROTOCOL
CT chest
CT abdomen
Bone scan (entire skeleton)
Endoscopic ultrasound of biliary tree
NEUROENDOCRINE TUMOR PROTOCOL
CT chest
CT abdomen/pelvis (repeated every 4–6 months until transplantation)
Bone scan
Octreotide scan
Echocardiogram

before liver transplantation. Rectal carcinoid is an exclusion criterion because of the aggressive nature of the tumor.

CONTRAINDICATIONS TO LIVER TRANSPLANTATION

Absolute contraindications

In general, the more experienced a liver transplantation center, the fewer the absolute contraindications for liver transplantation.

INDICATIONS FOR LIVER TRANSPLANTATION: FULMINANT HEPATIC FAILURE[a]
VIRAL HEPATITIS
Viral
Types A, B, C (rare), D, and E
Herpes simplex
Drug
Acetaminophen
Isoniazid
Nonsteroidals
Halothane
Valproic acid
TOXINS
Amanita phalloides
Yellow phosphorus
VASCULAR
Budd-Chiari syndrome
Ischemic hepatitis
Heat stroke
METABOLIC
Wilson's disease
Reye's syndrome
Acute fatty liver of pregnancy
Hereditary tyrosinemia

[a] List is not all-inclusive; only most common conditions are presented.

INDICATIONS FOR LIVER TRANSPLANTATION
Cirrhosis due to: • Viral hepatitis: hepatitis B, hepatitis C • Alcoholic liver disease • Autoimmune liver disease • Nonalcoholic steatohepatitis • Cryptogenic liver disease • Primary biliary cirrhosis • Primary sclerosing cholangitis Polycystic liver disease Malignancy: • Hepatocellular carcinoma • Cholangiocarcinoma • Metastatic neuroendocrine tumors Metabolic liver disease: • α-1 antitrypsin deficiency • Hereditary hemochromatosis • Wilson's disease • Glycogen storage disorders • Primary oxalosis • Familial amyloidosis

Advanced, irreversible neurological deficit and cardiopulmonary disease are absolute contraindications to liver transplantation. Portopulmonary hypertension is not a contraindication if the mean pulmonary arterial pressure is <35 mmHg, or can be reduced to <35 mmHg with epoprostenol; if the mean pulmonary arterial pressure is between 35 and 50 mmHg with a pulmonary vascular resistance <250 dyn/s/cm^{-5}, liver transplantation can still be carried out. When the mean pulmonary arterial pressure is greater than 50 mmHg, mortality post liver transplantation is greater than 50%, ruling out liver transplantation as a viable option.

Hepatopulmonary syndrome is not a contraindication, but when associated with a PaO_2 of <50 mmHg and a pulmonary arterial shunt of >30% it generally has a poor outcome.

Patients with coronary artery disease, including those who have undergone coronary artery bypass grafting, have a higher post-transplant mortality and morbidity. In view of the systemic vasodilatation in patients with cirrhosis, cardiac function may deteriorate after transplantation because of increased afterload. Patients with cardiomyopathy and those with lethal cardiac arrhythmias should be excluded from liver transplantation.

Uncontrolled infection, either intrahepatic, such as related to cholangitis or liver abscesses, or extrahepatic, is a contraindication to liver transplantation.

Previous extrahepatic malignancy is not a contraindication, provided the treatment carried out, the grade of malignancy, and the clinical picture suggest a low likelihood of metastatic spread. For most malignancies, a 2-year disease-free period immediately prior to liver transplantation is required. However, the disease-free interval should be longer for high-grade malignancies such as malignant melanoma.

Relative contraindications

Selected patients over the age of 65 who are in otherwise 'pristine' health should be considered for liver transplantation. With the advent of highly active antiretroviral treatment, excellent post-transplant survival is seen in patients with HIV infection and a CD4 count >400 mm^{-3}.

Patients with morbid obesity do not have significantly higher post liver transplantation mortality or morbidity than less obese patients.

CONTRAINDICATIONS TO LIVER TRANSPLANTATION
Absolute • Extrahepatic malignancy • Uncontrolled sepsis • Irreversible/advanced neurological disease • Irreversible/advanced cardiovascular disease • Irreversible/advanced pulmonary disease • Active substance abuse • Uncontrolled major psychosis • Fibrosing cholestatic hepatitis C[a]
Relative contraindications • Age >65 years • Cholangiocarcinoma • HIV infection • Pulmonary hypertension • Paroxysmal nocturnal hemoglobinuria • Extensive portal vein thrombosis

[a] In most centers.

SELECTION OF CANDIDATES FOR LIVER TRANSPLANTATION

Following input from the liver transplantation team, patients accepted for transplantation are placed on a waiting list and undergo further investigations outlined in Table 106.2. Patients who have a history of substance abuse are evaluated by a substance counselor. A carotid ultrasound is carried out in patients >50 years of age. A dobutamine stress echocardiogram is carried out in patients at risk for coronary artery disease. This includes patients over the age of 50 years, a family history of coronary artery disease, or a personal history of diabetes mellitus, hyperlipidemia, or chest pain.

In the US and in regions of Europe and South America, once a patient with end-stage liver disease is activated for liver transplantation, priority for cadaveric organ allocation is based on the MELD system (model for end-stage liver disease). Prior to February 2002 in the US, prioritization for liver transplantation in patients with chronic liver disease was heavily weighted in favor of waiting time. Because of the perceived unfairness of heavily weighting transplantation in favor of waiting time rather than on severity of illness, the United Network of Organ Sharing (UNOS) moved its prioritization scheme to the MELD system. The MELD score is a mathematical score based on serum creatinine, international normalized ratio (INR) for prothrombin time, and serum bilirubin. Complications of liver disease like spontaneous bacterial peritonitis, hepatic encephalopathy, and variceal bleeding do not influence the accuracy of the model.

Patients who meet criteria for fulminant hepatic failure (Table 106.3), post-transplant primary graft nonfunction, and hepatic artery thrombosis are given highest priority for organ allocation. For patients with cirrhosis, the patient with the

TABLE 106.2 LIVER TRANSPLANT EVALUATION

LIVER TRANSPLANT STEP 1 EVALUATION		LIVER TRANSPLANT STEP 2 EVALUATION
ABO/Rh/RBC Ab	Ceruloplasmin	EBV and varicella-zoster virus serologies
Complete blood counts	Protein electrophoresis	Urine cultures: CMV, bacteria, fungi
Iron studies	Smooth muscle antibody	Tuberculin skin test
Ferritin	Antimitochondrial antibody	Sinus X-ray
Vitamins A, D, E, B_{12}, folate	Alpha-1-antitrypsin phenotype	Standard renal clearance
Prothrombin time	Antinuclear antibody	
Sodium	Hepatitis serology	Mammogram (females >40 years)
Potassium	HCV-PCR	Echocardiogram
Calcium	Hemochromatosis gene	Dobutamine stress echocardiogram (>50 years)
Phosphorus		Carotid ultrasound (>50 years)
Glucose	Lipid profile	Dental X-rays and examination
Alkaline phosphatase	Testosterone	CT Abdomen (to screen for HCC) if creatinine ≤ 1.4 mg/dL
Total bilirubin	sTSH	Vaccines: 1. Pneumovax
Direct bilirubin	Parathormone	2. Hepatitis A
Creatinine		3. Hepatitis B
Albumin		4. Tetanus booster
Chloride		5. Influenza
Alpha fetoprotein	HIV	Evaluation by: 1. Transplant surgeon
CA 19-9	HTLV-1	2. Pulmonologist
PSA (males >40)	Serology RPR	3. Infectious diseases
CMV serology		4. Psychiatry
Arterial blood gas		**Additional tests (if required)**
Urinalysis		ERCP (if dominant biliary stricture)
24-h urine Na^+		Colon cancer screen
Drug abuse urine survey		
Ultrasound: hepatobiliary and pelvis (if female)		**LIVER TRANSPLANT STEP 3**
Upper gastrointestinal endoscopy		Dietitian
Electrocardiogram		Physical therapy
Bone Densitometry Spine		Anesthesia
Evaluation by: 1. Hepatologist		Preoperative surgical class
2. Social Services		Tours of intensive care area and transplant inpatient area
3. Transplant Coordinator		Nurse coordinator
4. Substance abuse team (if necessary)		

TABLE 106.3 CRITERIA FOR LIVER TRANSPLANTATION IN FULMINANT HEPATIC FAILURE

CRITERIA OF KING'S COLLEGE, LONDON:

Acetaminophen patients:

Arterial pH <7.3 or INR >6.5 and serum creatinine >3.4 mg/dL

Non-acetaminophen patients:

INR >6.5 or any three of the following variables:

- age <10 years or >40 years
- etiology: non-A, non-B hepatitis; halothane hepatitis; idiosyncratic drug reaction
- duration of jaundice before encephalopathy >7 days
- INR >3.5

CRITERIA OF HOPITAL PAUL-BROUSSE, VILLEJUIF:

Hepatic encephalopathy and factor V level <20% in patients <30 years, or factor V level <30% in patients ≥30 years

INR, international normalized ratio. From Keefe EB. Liver transplantation: current status and novel approaches to liver replacement. Gastroenterology 2001; 120:749–762, with permission from American Gastroenterological Association.

highest MELD score within a particular UNOS region an blood group receives priority for liver transplantation. Th advantage of MELD-based allocation is that the sickes patients are more likely to receive liver transplantation. Lowe socioeconomic groups and minorities, who were disadvan taged by a system based on waiting time, are no longe disadvantaged. Contrary to initial fears, post liver transplan mortality has not increased; moreover, mortality on th waiting list has decreased after implementation of the MELI system.

EXPANDING THE DONOR POOL

The major limitation of liver transplantation is the worldwid shortage of donor organs, which leads to an increased numbe of deaths while awaiting transplantation. Increasing the number of donor organs requires use of marginal livers, split livers, an live donors.

ʌarginal livers

ivers from deceased donors are considered marginal if there an increased risk of initial poor function, primary nonfunc-on, delayed graft, or patient survival. Marginal livers are robably best used for stable patients disadvantaged by the urrent MELD-based allocation system. Marginal livers include: vers from donors older than 70 years, livers with steatosis, on-heart-beating donors, and livers from donors with hepa-tis virus infection. Older donors also have an increased risk f previously undiagnosed malignancy. Transplantation of donor vers with less than 30% steatosis gives similar results to trans-lantation of nonsteatotic livers. Transplantation of livers with reater than 60% steatosis is not advised given the high inci-ence of initial poor function or delayed graft function. Trans-lantation of livers with 30–60% steatosis should only be con-idered when there are no other risk factors for poor function.

Non-heart-beating donors are from individuals who have evere neurologic damage but who do not meet criteria for rain death; therefore, organs cannot be procured until cessa-on of cardiopulmonary function. Controlled non-heart-beating onors are taken off life support in an operating room with the rocurement team in place. Uncontrolled non-heart beating onors have an unplanned cessation of cardiopulmonary unction, often before arriving at the hospital. Ischemic times re therefore longer than seen in controlled non-heart-beating onors. Allograft survival from an uncontrolled non-heart-eating donor is low and such livers should only be used when ocumented warm ischemic time is short.

Livers from donors who are hepatitis B surface antigen HBsAg)-negative but anti-HBc-positive transmit hepatitis B to he recipient in 33–78% of cases. Recipients of anti-HBs (without nti-HBc) livers are only rarely infected. Livers from anti-HBc-ositive donors are considered mainly for recipients with hepatitis , who are going to receive postoperative therapy regardless of he hepatitis B status of the donor.

Hepatitis C-positive donors should only be used for hepatitis -positive recipients and only if there is no histological evi-ence of liver disease. Graft and patient survival of liver trans-plants in hepatitis C-positive recipients is the same whether they receive a hepatitis C-positive or hepatitis C-negative liver.

Split grafts

Split liver transplantation is the use of a liver from a single donor for two recipients. The recipients need to be relatively small and often either one or both recipients are children. Splitting of the liver can either be performed *in vivo* at liver procurement or *ex vivo* prior to implantation. Graft function is generally good although there is a higher risk of biliary and vascular complications compared with the use of whole-organ grafts.

Living donors

Living donor liver transplantation is used for patients who are not able to receive a cadaver liver in a timely fashion but have no contraindications to cadaver liver transplantation. Rapid regeneration of the liver both in donor and recipient helps prevent delayed graft function. About 90% of regeneration occurs within 4 weeks of transplantation.

Living donor liver transplantation (LDLT) for pediatric recipients involves removing either the left lateral liver or left lobe from a parent. The small size of the left lobe does not provide enough liver mass for adults. Donation of the right lobe provides enough mass for many adults, although the operation is more challenging than deceased donor liver transplantation (see Fig. 106.2A,B).

Evaluation of the potential donor (Fig. 106.3) is kept separate from evaluation of the recipient to avoid donor coercion. Evaluation is often spread out over 2–4 weeks to ensure that the potential donor has adequate time to contemplate the risks of living liver donation. After initiation of the first visit with the transplant center, about 60–70% of potential donors will go on to donate a liver.

Mortality in donors is about 0.5%. About 5% of donors will have a complication necessitating hospitalization, reoperation, or transfusion. Overall, recipient outcomes are similar to historical rates of deceased donor transplantation. Hepatic artery thrombosis is seen in 2–6% of recipients, portal vein throm-

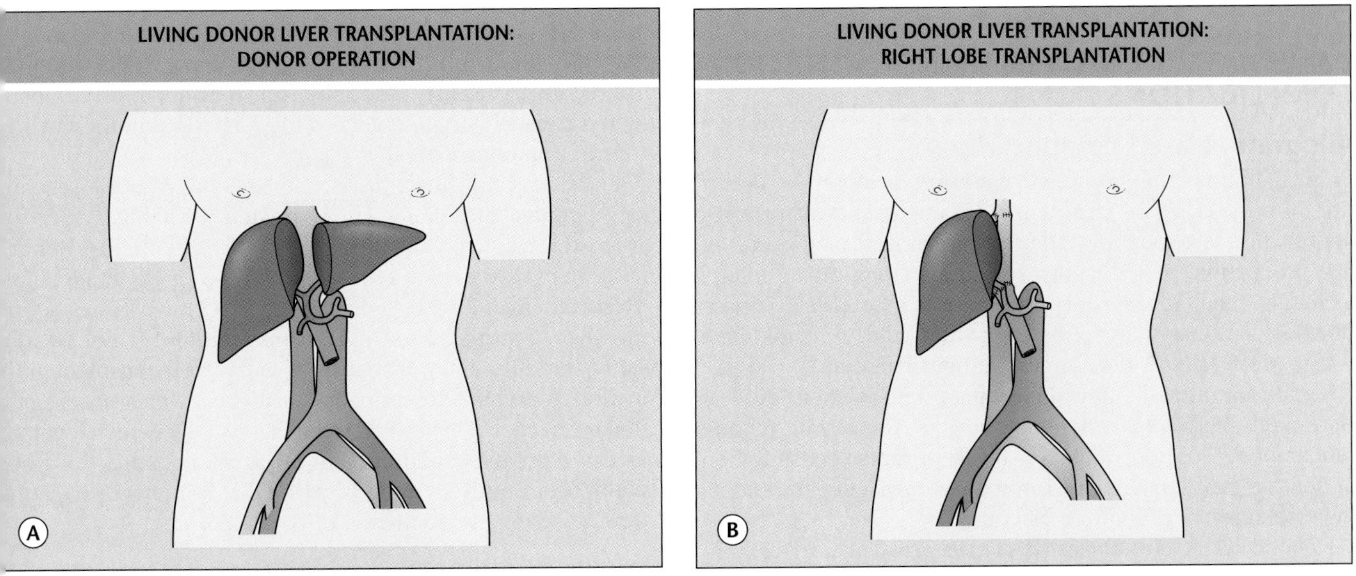

ig. 106.2 Living donor liver transplantation. A. Donor operation. **B.** Right lobe implantation. Reproduced from Rosen CR. Liver diseases ecessitating transplantation. In: Kelly KA et al., eds. Mayo Clinic in Gastrointestinal Surgery, with permission from Mayo Foundation for ʌedical Education and Research.

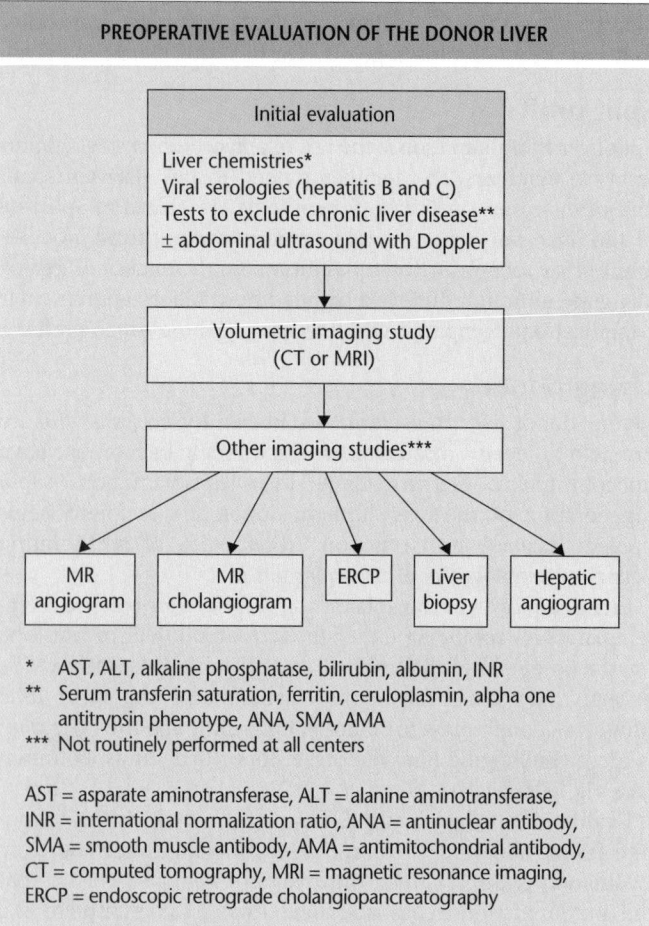

PREOPERATIVE EVALUATION OF THE DONOR LIVER

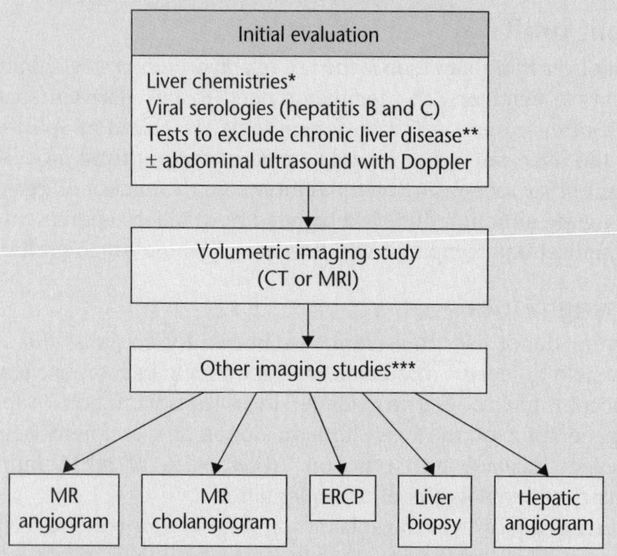

* AST, ALT, alkaline phosphatase, bilirubin, albumin, INR
** Serum transferin saturation, ferritin, ceruloplasmin, alpha one antitrypsin phenotype, ANA, SMA, AMA
*** Not routinely performed at all centers

AST = asparate aminotransferase, ALT = alanine aminotransferase, INR = international normalization ratio, ANA = antinuclear antibody, SMA = smooth muscle antibody, AMA = antimitochondrial antibody, CT = computed tomography, MRI = magnetic resonance imaging, ERCP = endoscopic retrograde cholangiopancreatography

Fig. 106.3 Preoperative diagnostic algorithm for evaluation of the donor liver. Reproduced from Rosen CR. Liver diseases necessitating transplantation. In: Kelly KA et al., eds. Mayo Clinic in Gastrointestinal Surgery, with permission from Mayo Foundation for Medical Education and Research.

bosis in 2.5–6%, hepatic venous outflow obstruction in about 10%, and biliary complications in 30%.

IMMEDIATE POST LIVER TRANSPLANTATION COMPLICATIONS

Allograft-related complications

Primary nonfunction is a relatively rare phenomenon, occurring in only 1–2% of transplants. Characteristics of primary nonfunction are portosystemic encephalopathy, absence of bile production, coagulopathy, and multisystem organ failure, including renal insufficiency. Risk factors for primary nonfunction are marginal donor livers and cold ischemia time >18h. Most patients need urgent retransplantation.

Significant intra-abdominal bleeding occurs in about 20% of transplant recipients and about half of these will require reoperation. Coagulopathy as a result of factor consumption or delayed graft function and thrombocytopenia due to residual hypersplenism contribute to bleeding.

Hepatic artery thrombosis (HAT) is a dreaded early complication of liver transplantation, and occurs in 2–12% of transplant recipients. Predictors of HAT are pediatric transplantation, complex arterial anastomoses, and tobacco use by donors. Our center performs a Doppler ultrasound of the hepatic arter and portal vein on the first and seventh postoperative day. Impending HAT may be heralded by the ultrasonographi findings of a resistive index <0.5, systolic acceleration, c increased focal peak velocity. If HAT is diagnosed earl operative repair is usually advised. If diagnosed later, retrans plant may be necessary because of late complications includin diffuse ('ischemic-type') biliary strictures or liver abscesses.

Hepatic venous outflow obstruction due to stenosis at th inferior vena caval anastomosis occurs in 1–2% of transplant. Use of the 'piggyback' technique (preservation of the recipier inferior vena cava with anastomosis of the donor inferior ven cava to the recipient hepatic vein confluence) (Fig. 106.1) ma carry a slightly higher risk of hepatic venous outflow obstruc tion. Hepatic venous outflow obstruction is often successfull treated by transvenous dilation with or without stenting. Porta vein stenosis or thrombosis is rare after liver transplantatio but may lead to portal hypertension.

Biliary complications occur in about 8–15% of liver trans plant recipients. Bile leaks tend to occur early, within 1 mont after liver transplantation, while strictures generally occur late The development of biliary complications mandates a carefu search for HAT. At our center, nearly all patients will have biliary tube using a ureteral catheter placed via the dono cystic duct at the time of surgery. This allows monitoring c graft bile output and access for cholangiography. Our policy i to carry out routine cholangiography on the fifth and twenty first postoperative days. Leaks from choledochojejunostom usually require reoperation while those from choledochochole dochostomy can usually be observed or treated with sphinc terotomy or temporary transpapillary biliary stenting.

Biliary strictures can be anastomotic or nonanastomotic Anastomotic strictures in patients with choledochocholedo chostomy are usually managed endoscopically. Choledocho jejunostomy anastomotic strictures are usually managed wit percutaneous stenting. Diffuse strictures may be a complica tion of hepatic artery thrombosis or recurrence of primar sclerosing cholangitis and are initially managed with percuta neous stenting.

Cellular rejection occurs in 30–50% of liver transplant recip ients. Rejection typically occurs early, usually within 1 mont after transplantation. Late cellular rejection can be confuse with recurrent disease, especially recurrent hepatitis C. Docu mented late cellular rejection is often related to subtherapeuti levels of immunosuppressive agents.

Our center performs a protocol liver biopsy on the sevent post-operative day. Rejection is treated with high doses o corticosteroids, which is effective in 90% of patients. Refrac tory patients are treated either with OKT-3 or thymoglobulin

Recurrent liver disease generally occurs >1 month after ortho topic liver transplantation (OLT) and therefore is not usuall part of the differential diagnosis of early post-transplant graf function. A notable exception is hepatitis C, which may mimi cellular rejection. Hepatitis C viremia is usually detected withi 2 weeks of transplantation. Clinical acute hepatitis does no usually occur until 1–6 months post-OLT. Features of hepatiti C and rejection are compared in Table 106.4.

Miscellaneous early complications

Pulmonary complications of liver transplantation include atelec tasis and pneumonia. Pleural effusions, especially right-sided

TABLE 106.4 DIFFERENTIATING POST-TRANSPLANT ACUTE RECURRENT HEPATITIS C AND REJECTION

	Acute hepatitis C	Rejection
Time after liver transplantation	1–6 months	1–4 weeks
Jaundice	Common	Uncommon
HCV RNA level	Steep increase	Variable
Histology	Lobular hepatitis with hepatocyte swelling and acidophil bodies	Portal hepatitis, endotheliitis, lymphocytic cholangitis

occur in nearly all patients but may be particularly troublesome in patients with hepatic hydrothorax prior to transplantation. Pre-existing hepatopulmonary syndrome usually resolves although complete resolution may take months.

A **hyperdynamic circulation** persists for a few weeks after transplantation. Rarely, patients develop a dilated cardiomyopathy without a clear cause. Supportive medical management is often necessary and myocardial function generally returns to normal within a few weeks.

Neurologic symptoms occur in 12–20% of patients. Most common are mental status changes that are probably multifactorial although often attributed to immunosuppression. More serious central nervous system complications are seizures due to calcineurin inhibitors such as cyclosporine and tacrolimus, intracranial hemorrhage due to hypertension and coagulopathy, and central pontine myelinosis due to changes in serum osmolality and sodium.

Abnormalities of renal function are an important clinical problem because of the current priority given to patients with pretransplant renal dysfunction. Patients with hepatorenal syndrome have delayed return to function and many probably have an element of acute tubular necrosis that leads to residual renal dysfunction. Calcineurin inhibitors may also lead to impaired renal function after transplantation, especially if drug levels are high.

Infection: Improvements in prophylaxis have led to a decreased incidence in serious infections after liver transplantation. In the first 2 weeks, most infections are bacterial and originate in the biliary tree, peritoneal cavity, wound, urinary tract, and lungs. Fungal infections, especially due to *Candida* species, can also occur early. Viral infections, in particular those due to cytomegalovirus, occur a little later, usually 3–8 weeks after transplant.

Gastrointestinal bleeding is usually due to ulcers, viral infections of the gut, or from the jejunojejunostomy in patients with choledochojejunostomy. Diarrhea is very common after transplantation and is probably due to medications. Use of antibiotics may also lead to pseudomembranous colitis, although this complication is uncommon in our practice, perhaps due to oral selective bowel decontamination.

REFERENCES

1. Adam R, McMaster P, O'Grady JG et al. Evolution of liver transplantation in Europe: report of the European liver transplant registry. Liver Transpl 2003; 9:1231–1243.
2. Brandhagen D, Fidler J, Rosen C. Evaluation of the donor liver for living donor liver transplantation. Liver Transpl 2003; 9:S16–S28.
3. Brown RS, Russo MW, Lai M et al. A survey of liver transplantation from living adult donors in the United States. N Engl J Med 2003; 348: 818–825.
4. Busuttil RW, Goss JA. Split liver transplantation. Ann Surg 1999; 229:313–321.
5. Busuttil RW, Tanaka K. The utility of marginal donors in liver transplantation. Liver Transpl 2003; 9:651–663.
6. Forman LM, Lewis JD, Birlin JA, Feldman HI, Lucey MR. The association between hepatitis C infection and survival after orthotopic liver transplantation. Gastroenterology 2002; 22: 889–896.
7. Gores GJ. A spotlight on cholangiocarcinoma. Gastroenterology 2003; 125:1536–1538.
8. Halpern SD, Ubel PA, Caplan AL. Solid-organ transplantation in HIV-infected patients. N Engl J Med 2002; 347:284–287.
9. Kamath PS, Wiesner RH, Malinchoc M et al. A model to predict survival in patients with end-stage liver disease. Hepatology 2001; 33: 464–470.
10. Keeffe EB. Liver transplantation: current status and novel approaches to liver replacement. Gastroenterology 2001; 120:749–762.
11. Kim WR, Dickson ER. Timing of liver transplantation. Semin Liver Dis 2000; 20:451–464.
12. Krowka MJ, Mandell S, Ramsay MA et al. Hepatopulmonary syndrome and portopulmonary hypertension: a report of the multicenter liver transplant database. Liver Transpl 2004; 10:174–182.
13. Llovet JM, Fuster J, Bruix J. The Barcelona approach: diagnosis, staging and treatment of hepatocellular carcinoma. Liver Transpl 2004; 10:S115–120.
14. Mazariegos GV, Molment EP, Kramer DJ. Early complications after orthotopic liver transplantation. Surg Clin North Am 1999; 79:109–129.
15. Menon KVN, Shah VH, Kamath PS. The Budd-Chiari syndrome. N Engl J Med 2004; 350: 578–585.
16. Rosado B, Kamath PS. Transjugular intrahepatic portosystemic shunts: an update. Liver Transpl 2003; 9:207–217.
17. Rosen CB. Liver diseases necessitating liver transplantation. In: Kelly KA, Sarr MG, Hinder RA, eds. Mayo Clinic Gastrointestinal Surgery. Philadelphia: W.B. Saunders; 2004:209–223.
18. Wiesner RH, Edwards E, Freeman R et al. Model for end-stage liver disease (MELD) and allocation of donor livers. Gastroenterology 2003; 124:91–96.
19. Wiesner RH, Rakela J, Ishitani MB et al. Recent advances in liver transplantation. Mayo Clinic Proceedings 2003; 78:197–210.

Chapter 107

Long-term management and recurrence of primary liver disease

Marina Berenguer and Teresa L Wright

KEY POINTS

- Recurrence of hepatitis B virus infection occurs in 75–90% of cases if no prophylaxis is done. Antiviral therapy with nucleoside/nucleotide analogs prior to transplantation diminishes the risk of recurrence
- Recurrent HVC infection is universal, and leads to cirrhosis in ~ 30% of cases at 5 years. Pre-transplant antiviral therapy may reduce recurrence but applicability is limited. Results of post-transplantation therapy are not optimal, except in genotype-2
- PBC and sclerosing cholangitis recur in 20% of cases at 5 years

INTRODUCTION

Liver transplantation has become the definitive therapy for a wide range of acute and chronic liver diseases, giving excellent survival rates of 90–95% and 65–80% after 1 and 5 years of follow-up respectively. Among several circumstances that may pose a threat to long-term survival, the greatest is probably recurrence of the original liver disease, a complication that may occur for most diseases requiring liver transplantation.[1]

RECURRENT HEPATITIS B VIRUS INFECTION

In the absence of prophylactic therapy, hepatitis B virus (HBV) recurs in 75–90% of cases. The presence of HBV-DNA prior to transplantation is the best predictor of disease recurrence, with the highest rates of recurrence (75% at 2 years) reported in hepatitis B surface antigen (HBsAg)-positive cirrhotic patients with evidence of active viral replication (HBV-DNA and/or hepatitis B e antigen [HBeAg] positive). Lower recurrence rates are observed in patients without detectable HBeAg or HBV-DNA (2-year actuarial risk: 67%), in fulminant hepatitis (17%), or in those coinfected with the delta virus (32%). With long-term hepatitis B imunoglubulin (HBIg) prophylaxis, the recurrence rate decreases in patients without active HBV replication (17–38%), but remains unchanged (70–96%) in those with positive HBV-DNA.[1–3]

Natural history of HBV recurrence

Recurrence is more aggressive than that observed in the immune-competent population. Less than 5% maintain a normal graft in the medium to long term. Typically, patients develop acute hepatitis after detection of HBsAg in serum, with progression to chronic hepatitis and cirrhosis within 2 years of transplantation. One particular entity called fibrosing cholestatic hepatitis develops in a small subset of patients. It is characterized histologically by the presence of periportal and perisinusoidal fibrosis, ballooned hepatocytes with cell loss, pronounced cholestasis, and a paucity of inflammatory activity. Immunohistochemical stains show marked cytoplasmic expression of viral antigens, which in conjunction with the lack of inflammatory infiltrate suggests a direct cytopathic effect of the virus. The clinical course is rapidly progressive with severe cholestasis, hypoprothrombinemia, and liver failure within weeks of onset. Early death is common after liver retransplantation. Patients who survive the postoperative period develop an even more aggressive recurrent disease. Fibrosing cholestatic hepatitis develops predominantly in patients with high levels of viremia before transplantation and in those infected with precore mutants.[1–3]

Prevention of HBV graft reinfection (Fig. 107.1)

Lifelong passive immunization with high-dose HBIg

Lifelong passive immunization with high-dose HBIg (polyclonal antibodies directed against the viral envelope) was until recently the 'standard of care.' Its use is followed by an overall reduction in the rate of recurrence to 27%, 35%, 40%, and 42% at 1, 2, 5, and 10 years respectively, with substantial differences observed between patients who are HBV-DNA-positive before transplantation and those who are HBV-DNA-negative (5-year actuarial recurrence rate 77% and 33% respectively). Almost no new cases of recurrence are observed after 5 years following liver transplantation.[1–3] The adverse prognosis of patients with active viral replication before transplantation may be overcome with more aggressive use of HBIg or by the use of HBIg in combination with lamivudine. Indeed, recurrence in these patients may be reduced to approximately 16–35% by maintaining anti-HBs titers above 500 IU/L through aggressive HBIg use, at least during the first 6 months. This aggressive regimen has also been shown to improve outcome in patients retransplanted for fibrosing cholestatic hepatitis.[1–3]

Treatment regimens mostly include the administration of 10 000 IU HBIg intravenously during the anhepatic phase and 10 000 IU HBIg daily for the first week post-transplantation. Subsequent dosing is either given on a fixed schedule (generally on a monthly basis) or based on anti-HBs titers (readministration when antiHBs dosage is less than 100 IU/L). Given the great individual variability in the pharmacokinetic profile of immunoglobulins, the best approach is to individualize immunoprophylaxis by adjusting the dose of HBIg to obtain an anti-HBs titer above 500 IU/L during the first week after transplantation, above 250 IU/L from day 8 to day 90, and above 100 IU/L thereafter.

Limitations: Despite its clear efficacy, HBIg has limitations, including high cost, limited availability, and efficacy. Causes of breakthrough are probably multifactorial and include inadequate

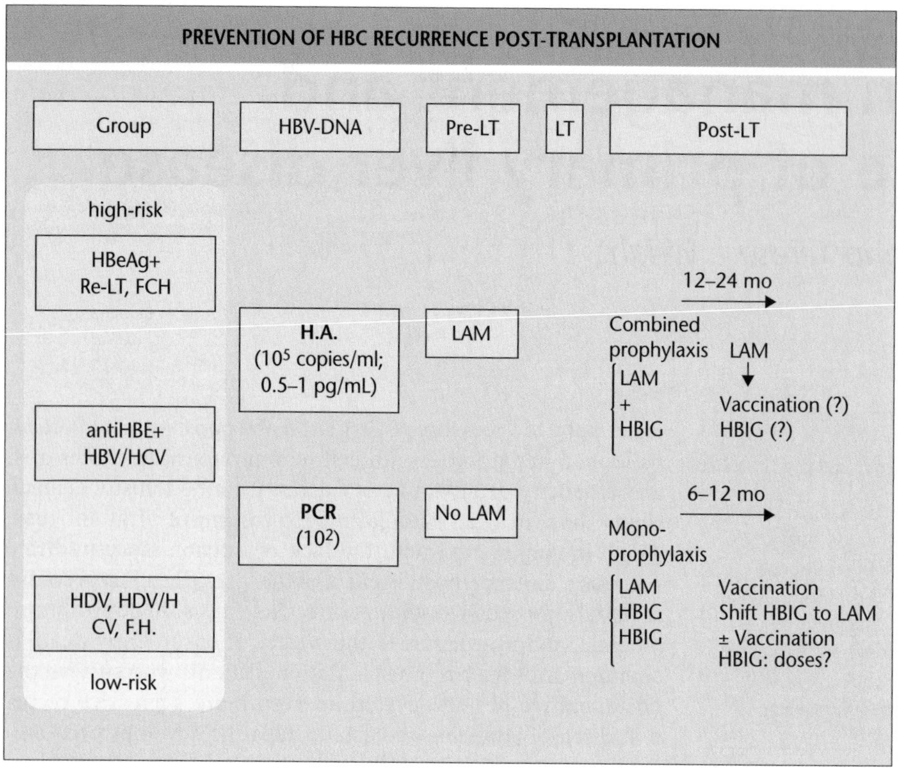

Fig. 107.1 Prevention of HBV recurrence following liver transplantation. Algorithm based on risk of recurrence. LT, liver transplantation; LAM, lamivudine; HBIg, hepatitis B immunoglobulins; HBV, hepatitis B virus; HDV, hepatitis delta virus; HCV, hepatitis C virus; FH, fulminant hepatitis; FCH, fibrosing cholestatic hepatitis; Re-LT, retransplantation; HA, hybridization assays; PCR, polymerase chain reaction.

anti-HBs titers following transplantation, HBV overproduction from extrahepatic sites, and/or mutations in the region of the surface gene of the HBV genome encoding the 'a' determinant region (the putative region for antibody binding) due to immune pressure selection. In addition, discontinuing HBIg, even after a long time, may lead to recurrence. Indeed, HBV-DNA has been detected by highly sensitive molecular techniques in the serum, liver, and peripheral blood monocyte cells (PBMCs) in 50% of HBsAg-negative patients on HBIg prophylaxis, suggesting that indefinite treatment is required.[2,3]

In order to overcome the limitations of HBIg, several alternatives are being evaluated, as described below.

Antiviral treatment prior to transplantation to inhibit viral replication (Table 107.1)

Nucleoside analogs are well tolerated, are orally administered, and have a potent antiviral effect inducing a rapid clearance of HBV-DNA from serum. Recent experience with these drugs, particularly lamivudine, in cirrhotic patients awaiting transplantation is encouraging. Lamivudine decreases HBV replication

TABLE 107.1 PRE-LIVER TRANSPLANTATION ANTIVIRAL THERAPY IN PATIENTS WITH HBV CIRRHOSIS

Reference	No. of patients	HBeAg-positive (%)	Mean follow-up pre-LT (months)	Decreased Child-Pugh score[a] (%)	Lamivudine resistance (%)
Villeneuve et at.[14] (2000)	35	57	19	66	13 (25% at 2 years)
Kapoor et al.[15] (2000)	18	55	17.9	50	17
Sponseller et al.[16] (2000)	5	100	–	60	–
Yao & Bass[17] (2000)	23	74	13	61	9
Marzano et al.[18] (2001)	33	27	5.6	33	3
Fontana et al.[19] (2002)	154	64	5.7	–	27

[a] Decrease in Child-Pugh score of more than 2 points.

to undetectable levels, allowing the transplant to be performed in conditions with a low risk of recurrence.[3] The major drawback is the development of 'resistance' to lamivudine with HBV-DNA reappearance, which is especially frequent after 6 months of therapy. Although most patients with resistant mutants have low serum HBV-DNA levels, flares of liver disease have been reported with the development of lamivudine-resistant mutants. In addition, development of resistant mutants while on the waiting list may lead to reluctance to perform liver transplantation. Lamivudine should therefore be initiated based on the expected waiting time for a transplant. On the other hand, it should also be considered that some patients with decompensated cirrhosis may improve on lamivudine therapy.[3]

Adefovir dipivoxil has also been used as pre-emptive therapy, but the data are limited. Adefovir has the advantage of being active against lamivudine-resistant strains. Recent data from 40 patients with decompensated cirrhosis and breakthrough associated with the development of lamivudine-resistant mutants showed that adefovir at doses of 10 mg daily was safe and significantly inhibited serum HBV-DNA levels.[3] The major concern with this drug is the potential for renal toxicity, which may be significant in patients with hepatic decompensation. The dose should be adjusted to creatinine clearance, and renal function should be monitored carefully. In addition, the reduction in viral replication occurs less rapidly with adefovir than with lamivudine. The best posttransplantation prophylaxis in patients with lamivudine-resistant mutants is still uncertain, but probably should be based on triple therapy (lamivudine, adefovir, high-dose HBIg).

Antiviral treatment after liver transplantation

Once transplantation has been performed there are several alternatives to prevent recurrence (Fig. 107.1):[2,3]

- *Continue the pre-emptive therapy with lamivudine initiated before transplantation.* Although this approach is initially effective, therapy is limited by the emergence of HBV mutants; this occurs in 40% and 60% at 1 and 3 years respectively.
- *Combination therapy with HBIg and nucleoside analogs.* In addition to a synergistic effect that lowers recurrence rates to less than 10%, combination therapy has the potential advantages of allowing the administration of lower doses of HBIg (400–2000 IU), resulting in a significant cost reduction, as well as a reduction in the development of resistant mutants, a frequent occurrence when each of the agents is administered separately) (Table 107.2).

At present, the main unanswered question relates to *long-term prophylaxis*. There is a need to define the optimal dose and duration of HBIg (indefinitely versus limited periods of time). Two approaches have been investigated:[4]

1. A*ctive HBsAg vaccination* aimed at inducing active immunity against HBV, without the need for additional antiviral treatment. Results from preliminary studies are disparate: good results were obtained in some studies, but the response to HBV vaccination was poor in others. Larger trials using different vaccination protocols over a longer observation period are needed to determine the real efficacy of this approach.
2. *Substituting HBIg with lamivudine in the long term.* Successful results using this alternative have already been reported by some authors in low-risk patients. More data are needed to define the efficacy of this approach in high-risk individuals.

An individualized multistep prophylactic regimen to prevent HBV recurrence is summarized in Figure 107.1.

Treatment of HBV disease of the graft

There are three different categories of patients who are potential candidates for HBV therapy after liver transplantation and who require different therapeutic schedules:

- Those who underwent liver transplantation in the pre-HBIg/lamivudine era
- Those who underwent liver transplantation in the post-HBIg/lamivudine era and who have broken through treatment
- Those with apparently de novo acquisition of HBV.

Nucleoside analogs are the cornerstone of therapy in the transplant population due to their potent antiviral effect and lack of side effects. Resistance remains the main limitation. Lamivudine 100 mg daily (adjusted for renal function) leads to biochemical improvement with rapid loss of HBV-DNA in serum, not only in patients with chronic hepatitis B but also in the setting of

TABLE 107.2 COMBINED PROPHYLAXIS WITH LAMIVUDINE + HBIG

	No. of patients	HBV-DNA + pre-LT	Pre-LT lamivudine (%)	HBIg (IU × 10^3)		HBV recurrence (%)	Follow-up (months)
				1st month	Monthly		
Markowitz et at.[20] (1998)	14	4	70	80 i.v.	10 i.v.	0	13
Yao et al.[21] (1999)	10	2	90	10–80 i.v.	1.48 i.m.	10	15.6
Yoshida et al.[22] (1999)	6	4	60	43.4 i.m.	4–6.8 i.m.	0	18
McCaughan et al.[23] (1999)	9	8	NA	3.2 i.m. total NA	0.4 i.m.	0	15.6
Han et al.[24] (2000)	59	NA	100	80 i.v	10 i.v.	0	15
Angus et al.[25] (2000)	32	16	100	0.4–0.8 i.m.	0.4–0.8 i.m.	3	18.5
Rosenau et al.[26] (2001)	21	13	90	40 i.v. total NA	2 i.v. total NA	10	20
Marzano et al.[18] (2001)	25	25	100	46.5 i.v.	5 i.v.	4	31

NA, data not available.

TREATMENT AND PREVENTION

ANTIVIRAL THERAPY FOR HEPATITIS B IN LIVER TRANSPLANT RECIPIENTS

Timing of infection	Antiviral therapy
LT in the pre-HBIg and/or lamivudine era	Nucleoside/nucleotide analogs (lamivudine, adefovir, entecavir)
LT in the post-HBIg/lamivudine era (potentially resistant mutants)	Antivirals active against resistant mutants (adefovir, entecavir)
De novo HBV infection	Nucleoside/nucleotide analogs (lamivudine, adefovir, entecavir)

TREATMENT AND PREVENTION

STRATEGIES TO PREVENT DE NOVO HBV INFECTION

HBc/HBs donor	HBc/HBs recipient	Risk	Therapy
+/+	–/–	High (>50%)	Lamivudine/combination
or	+/–	0–13%	Lamivudine/monitoring
+/–	+/+	Low (<5%)	Monitoring/lamivudine
–/+	Any	Very low	No prophylaxis
IgMHBc	Any	High	Lamivudine/combination
HBsAg	Any	High	Lamivudine/combination
HBV-DNA	Any	High	Combination

Adapted from Munoz SJ Liver Transpl 2002; 8(Suppl 1):S82–S87.

acute hepatitis B and in the most severe cases of fibrosing cholestatic hepatitis. Therapy also achieves histologic improvement in the inflammatory grade. HBV-DNA negativization is obtained in 68–100% of patients treated for periods of 12–36 months. Continuous treatment is required because relapse is the rule once the drug is discontinued. Unfortunately, prolonged therapy is associated with the development of breakthrough (more than 50%), with a rise in serum HBV-DNA and alanine aminotransferase levels. Molecular analysis of mutations has shown changes in the DNA polymerase gene. Although drug-resistant mutants are not consistently associated with hepatic disease progression, severe and fatal hepatitis B infection can occur.

New hepatitis B antiviral agents such as adefovir allow successful treatment of lamivudine-resistant variants. It is not yet known whether patients who are treated for lamivudine resistance with adefovir need to continue on lamivudine. Given the potential for progressive liver disease upon recurrence, it seems prudent to continue therapy with both drugs. Experience with adefovir (at a dose of 10 mg daily) indicates effective suppression of viral replication. Treatment may be limited by renal toxicity. Experience with entecavir is limited.

Prevention and treatment of de novo HBV infection

The prevalence of de novo HBV hepatitis ranges from 2% to 8%, and is generally related to transmission from an HbsAg-negative anti-HBc-positive donor. The most significant factor associated with transmission is the serologic status of the receptor, the risk being almost zero in patients who are anti-HBs-positive, minor (about 10%) in those who are anti-HBs-negative but anti-HBc-positive, and high (50–70%) in those with no markers of previous exposure to HBV. Although there have been reports of severe progression, the natural history of de novo hepatitis B is generally more benign than that described for recurrent hepatitis B. To avoid de novo HBV infection, two complementary approaches may be undertaken:

- **HBV vaccination prior to liver transplantation** – Results of accelerated vaccination regimen (double doses of 40 μg at 0, 1, and 2 months with a follow-up vaccine at 6 months) have been disappointing, with low response rates (40%).
- **Anti-HBc testing of the donor** – limiting the use of organs from anti-HBc-positive donors to recipients already infected with HBV and using them only in special circumstances in those not infected.

Retransplantation

Retransplantation for recurrent HBV disease is currently rare. If necessary, outcomes can be improved by avoiding late retransplantation when hepatic failure is too advanced and renal insufficiency has developed, by using antiviral therapy to clear the virus prior to retransplantation, and by using an aggressive prophylactic regimen to prevent reinfection.[1]

RECURRENT HEPATITIS C VIRUS INFECTION

Natural history of recurrent hepatitis C (Fig. 107.2)

Recurrent infection, defined as the presence of hepatitis V virus (HCV) in serum, is universal.[5,6] In these circumstances a rapid and sharp decline in viral load occurs immediately after removal of the infected liver followed by a progressive increase in serum HCV-RNA, reaching pretransplantation levels as soon as day 4 and up to 10–20-fold higher at 1 month.[6] Recurrence of infection is associated with histologic evidence of liver injury in the majority of patients. Progression to cirrhosis occurs in a proportion that varies between 6% and 23% at a median of 3–4 years after transplantation, the cumulative risk at 5–7 years ranging from 10% to 44%.[5,7] Liver enzymes do not correlate with viremia or with histologic disease severity, and protocol liver biopsies are generally needed to identify progression to severe forms of chronic hepatitis. Importantly, delayed severe liver damage is not infrequent (30%) among recipients with an initially 'benign' recurrence of HCV.[5,7] The presence of some degree of fibrosis at baseline appears to predict this severe form of recurrent hepatitis C. In a small proportion of patients (<10%), an accelerated course of liver injury leading to liver failure has been observed, reminiscent of that described in HBV-infected recipients with fibrosing cholestatic hepatitis.

The course of hepatitis C is more aggressive in immunocompromised than in immunocompetent patients, with significantly higher rates of fibrosis progression (0.3 fibrosis units per year [0.004–2.19 units] versus 0.2 fibrosis units per year [0.09–0.8 units], $p<0.0001$) and consequently a shorter time to the development of cirrhosis (9–12 versus 20–30 years). These differences are also present once cirrhosis is established, with a higher risk of clinical decompensation in immunocompromised patients (42% versus 5–10% in 1 year).[5,7,8]

Recent data suggest that disease progression, and thus the risk of developing *severe* HCV-hepatitis posttransplantation, has been increasing in recent years.

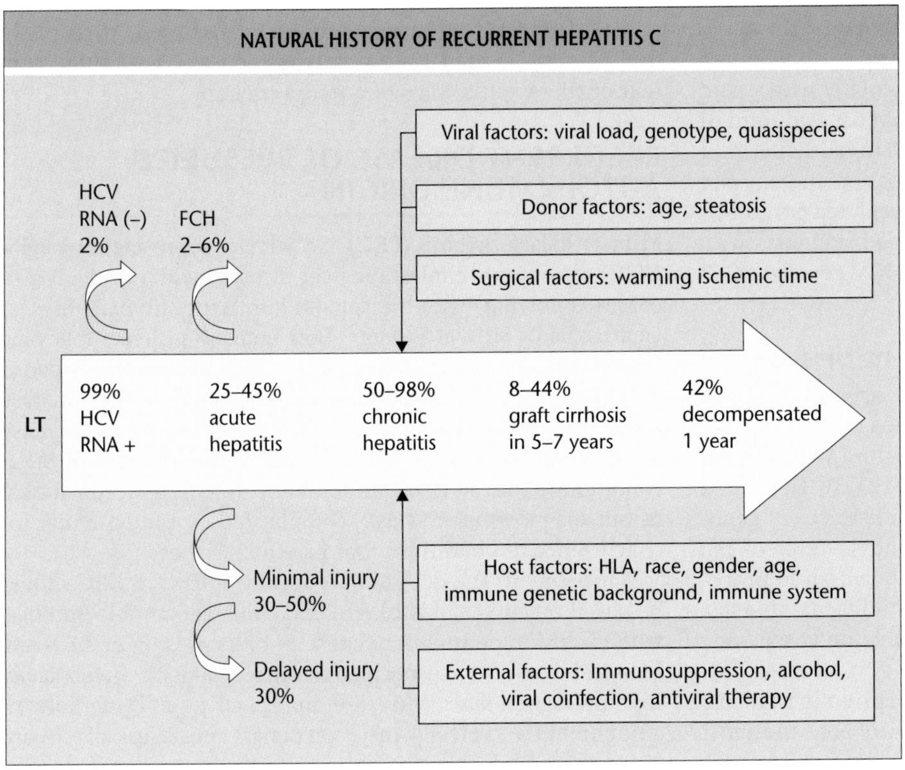

Fig. 107.2 Natural history of recurrent hepatitis C. Patterns of recurrence and factors associated with fibrosis progression. FCH, fibrosing cholestatic hepatitis; HCV, hepatitis C virus; HLA, human leukocyte antigen; LT, liver transplantation.

The negative clinical impact of HCV infection is demonstrated by two recent studies showing that HCV infection significantly impairs patient and allograft survival (60–70% versus 76–77% in non-HCV controls at 5 years).[5,7]

Prognostic factors

One-third of patients with recurrent HCV progress to cirrhosis, whereas another third remains stable.

Immune status: The major determinant of accelerated progression is immunosuppression.[7–9] Patients who are more severely immunosuppressed, such as those receiving high doses of steroids or antilymphocyte globulin, are at higher risk of progressing to cirrhosis than those less immunosuppressed. The worse outcome of recurrent hepatitis C noted recently may be partly due to the introduction of more potent immunosuppressive agents.[5,8,9] Given the negative effect of intense immune suppression, steroid boluses should be minimized and antilymphocyte globulin avoided. When doubt exists between rejection and hepatitis C, serial biopsies should be performed to clarify the clinical picture rather than adding immunosuppression blindly.

The level of viremia before transplantation or early posttransplantation correlates with the severity of recurrent hepatitis C.[6] In contrast, the influence of HCV genotype is unclear. Patients who develop cytomegalovirus viremia are at increased risk of severe HCV recurrence. Coinfection with HBV may influence histologic disease severity, but results are conflicting.[8]

Other factors: The age of the donor has been found to be independently associated with disease severity, disease progression, and survival. The increasing donor age may partly explain the worse outcome seen in recent years. The degree of necroinflammatory activity and fibrosis staging observed on the initial liver biopsy, as well as some histologic findings such as steatosis, ballooning degeneration, cholestasis, and confluent necrosis, may help to predict subsequent progression to severe disease. Prolonged rewarming time during allograft implantation and non-caucasian race have also been associated with severe recurrent disease. Although the use of living donors could theoretically lead to better outcomes by avoiding some of the known negative factors (age of the donor, rewarming time, steatosis, levels of viremia), preliminary data suggests that the results are, in fact, worse than those observed with cadaveric organs.[5,7,8]

Prevention of infection and/or HCV-related disease

In contrast to HBV, there are no universally effective measures to prevent recurrence of HCV. Antiviral therapy may be attempted before and/or early after transplantation to prevent disease recurrence or diminish the risk of aggressive progression.[10,11]

Post-transplantation pre-emptive treatment

Treatment with interferon initiated during the first 3 weeks after transplantation does not appear to modify disease progression. Combination with ribavirin may produce better results, particularly in those infected with non-1 genotypes. Sustained virologic and biochemical responses are achieved in 20% of patients infected with HCV genotype 1, but in 80–100% of those with genotype 2. Applicability of posttransplantation interferon plus ribavirin is low due to side effects and the low proportion of patients meeting entry criteria, particularly with regard to anemia, neutropenia, and thrombocytopenia.

Pretransplantation therapy

Before transplantation, interferon therapy is poorly tolerated and can lead to further deterioration of hepatic function. In addition, patients with advanced cirrhosis are at increased risk for bone marrow suppression during combination therapy and can suffer severe, even life-threatening, infections. Stepwise increases of antiviral agents may improve tolerability. The applicability of pretransplantation antiviral therapy is also limited because few patients meet entry criteria, particularly with regard to thrombocytopenia and leukopenia, and almost one-third of patients need to discontinue therapy owing to side effects. If tolerated, sustained responses with combination therapy are similar to those obtained in patients with compensated cirrhosis.[10] This is potentially a good option in selected patients (with relatively good liver function infected with HCV genotype 2–3 or with genotype 1 and low viral load).

Treatment of HCV-related recurrent disease

Results with interferon or ribavirin as single agents have been disappointing. The efficacy is improved when both drugs are administered in combination for 6–12 months, with overall sustained response rates of 9–33% (Table 107.3). The broad range of response probably relates to the differences in genotype distribution, timing of intervention, and severity of the underlying hepatitis C. Most studies have shown an improvement in liver histology among those responding to therapy. Tolerability of interferon and ribavirin is variable, and frequently leads to dose reduction or discontinuation.[11]

In conclusion, and given the limitations of currently available drugs, treatment of established disease is probably the most cost-effective option. Although limited by a relatively low efficacy, tolerance appears to be better and treatment is offered only to patients who develop progressive disease. Serial protocol liver biopsies may identify early histologic changes that herald an aggressive course. This allows antiviral therapy to be started at an earlier stage, when a response appears to occur more frequently.

Retransplantation

Outcome is generally poor, but may be improved if performed prior to the development of significant renal impairment and hepatic failure. If retransplantation is considered, attempts to do it should be made in a timely fashion and within the context of therapeutic trials of antiviral therapy.[12]

RECURRENT DISEASE OF PRESUMED AUTOIMMUNE ORIGIN

Primary biliary cirrhosis (PBC) and **primary sclerosing cholangitis (PSC)** are chronic cholestatic liver diseases with excellent outcomes following liver transplantation, with survival rates of approximately 80% at 5 years.[13] Both entities may recur following transplantation, with overall rates of 20% at 5 years. The diagnosis is suggested by increased bilirubin and alkaline phosphatase levels, the development of pruritus, reappearance or increase of antimitochondrial antibody titers, or development of other conditions believed to be autoimmune in nature. Confirmation of this diagnosis is, however, complicated by the potential for concurrence of conditions that may mimic these diseases.[13]

Management: The definition of recurrent PBC or PSC should be based on clinical, histologic, and cholangiographic findings, with exclusion of any other cause of biliary lesion or stricture. In most instances of suspected recurrence, patients are clinically asymptomatic, liver tests are nonspecific, and markers of autoimmunity typically recur or persist regardless of disease recurrence. The selection of a specific immunosuppressive regimen is still unclear. It has been suggested that cyclosporin-based regimens with slow steroid tapering are preferable to tacrolimus in patients with PBC. Therapeutic strategies for the prevention or treatment of recurrent PBC remain to be defined. In patients with PSC, therapeutic options for nonanastomotic strictures include radiologic or surgical therapies. Retransplantation may be considered in those with failing grafts. Both intermediate graft and patient survival rates are excellent and unaffected by recurrent disease.

TABLE 107.3 COMBINATION THERAPY WITH INTERFERON-α AND RIBAVIRIN IN PATIENTS WITH RECURRENT HEPATITIS C

Reference	No. of patients	Treatment regimen	Biochemical response/virologic response (%)	Sustained biochemical response/ sustained virologic response (%)[a]	Histological improvement	Discontinued
Bizollon et al.[27] (1997)	21	6 mo IFN+Rbv+6 mo RbV	100/48	86/24	Yes	14
Alberti et al.[28] (2001)	18	12 mo IFN+Rbv+ long-term RbV	83/44	78/33	Yes	22
Ahmad et al.[29] (2001)	60	6 mo IFN (n=40) vs 12 mo combination (n=20)	20 vs 25/15 vs 40	NA vs NA/2.5 vs 20	No	25
De Vera et a.[30] (2001)	32	IFN+Rbv≥12 mo	77/9	71/9	No	40
Gopal et al.[31]	12	IFN+Rbv indefinitely	NA/50	NA/8	NA	0
Narayanan et al.[32] (2002)	26	12 mo IFN+Rbv	42/35	NA	Yes	50
Lavezzo et al.[33] (2002)	57	12 mo IFN–Rbv (n=30) vs 6 mo IFN-Rbv (n=27)	66 vs 53/23 vs 33	37 vs 30/17 vs 22	Yes	5
Samuel et al.[34] (2003)	52	IFN+Rbv (n=28) vs placebo (n=24)	NA/32	18/21	No	43

[a] A sustained virologic response was significantly higher in patients with HCV genotypes 2, 3, 4 and than in those with HCV genotype 1.
IFN, interferon; Rbv, ribavirin; NA, data not available.

DIFFERENTIAL DIAGNOSIS		
CONDITIONS MIMICKING THE RECURRENCE OF THE ORIGINAL DISEASE		
Primary biliary cirrhosis	**Primary sclerosing cholangitis**	**Autoimmune**
• Viral hepatitis • Biliary obstruction • Chronic rejection • Acute hepatitis • Drug toxicity • Graft versus host disease	• Ischemic strictures (hepatic thrombosis, preservation injury) • Strictures secondary to ascending cholangitis following choledochojejunostomy • Chronic rejection • ABO incompatibility • Viral infection cytomegalovirus	• Viral hepatitis • Acute rejection • Biliary obstruction • Drug toxicity

Autoimmune hepatitis: Survival in these patients undergoing transplantation is excellent. Recurrent disease may, however, become an issue with prolonged follow-up, with an incidence ranging from 8% at 1 year to 60% after 5 years. Recurrence has not been linked to a specific immunosuppressive regimen. However, most studies have emphasized the hazards of discontinuing immunosuppression, particularly steroids, as its reintroduction is frequently accompanied by an improvement in liver function tests. Such biochemical response is, however, not always associated with histologic resolution. Thus, a slow and careful tapering of immunosuppressive drugs, particularly prednisone, is recommended. The definition of recurrent autoimmune hepatitis should be based not only on histologic findings but also on biochemical, serologic, and clinical criteria. Recurrence should be strongly suspected in recipients with a sustained increase in transaminase levels, consistent histopathology, positive autoimmune markers (antinuclear antibodies, smooth muscle antibodies, anti-liver–kidney–microsomal antibodies) with or without raised IgG or gamma-globulin levels and a history of steroid dependency. Other causes of graft hepatitis should be excluded. A small proportion of these patients develop serious disease requiring retransplantation (approximately 4%), but most respond to increases in immunosuppression. Graft and patient survival rates do not appear to be affected in the midterm.

REFERENCES

1. Rosen HR. Hepatitis B and C in the liver transplant recipient: current understanding and treatment. Liver Transpl 2001; 7(Suppl 2):S87–S98.
2. Shouval D, Samuel D. Hepatitis B immune globulin to prevent hepatitis B virus graft reinfection following liver transplantation: a concise review. Hepatology 2000; 32:1189–1195.
3. Villamil FG. Prophylaxis with anti-HBs immune globulins and nucleoside analogues after liver transplantation for HBV infection. J Hepatol 2003; 39:466–474.
4. Berenguer M, Wright TL. Treatment of recurrence of hepatitis B in transplant patients. J Hepatol 2003; 39(Suppl 1):S190–S193.
5. Berenguer M, Lopez-Labrador FX, Wright TL. Hepatitis C and liver transplantation. J Hepatol 2001; 35:666–678.
6. Charlton M. Liver biopsy, viral kinetics, and the impact of viremia on severity of hepatitis C virus recurrence. Liver Transpl 2003; 9(Suppl 3):S58–S62.
7. Gane E. The natural history and outcome of liver transplantation in hepatitis C virus-infected recipients. Liver Transpl 2003; 9(Suppl 3):S28–S34.
8. Berenguer M. Host and donor pre- and post-liver transplant risk factors impacting on HCV recurrence. Liver Transpl 2003; 9(Suppl 3):S44–S47.
9. McCaughan GW, Zekry A. Impact of immunosuppression on immunopathogenesis of liver damage in hepatitis C virus-infected recipients following liver transplantation. Liver Transpl 2003; 9(Suppl 3):S21–S27.
10. Everson GT. Treatment of patients with hepatitis C virus on the waiting list. Liver Transpl 2003; 9(Suppl 3):S90–S94.
11. Berenguer M, Wright TL. Treatment strategies for hepatitis C: intervention prior to liver transplant, pre-emptively or after established disease. Clin Liver Dis 2003; 7:631–650.
12. Rosen H, Prieto M, Casanovas-Taltavull T et al. Validation and refinement of survival models for liver retransplantation. Hepatology 2003; 38:460–469.
13. Faust TW. Recurrent primary biliary cirrhosis, primary sclerosing cholangitis, and autoimmune hepatitis after transplantation. Liver Transpl 2001; 7(Suppl):S99–S108.
14. Villeneuve J, Condreay LD, Willems B et al. Lamivudine treatment for decompensated cirrhosis resulting from chronic hepatitis B. Hepatology 2000; 31:207–210.
15. Kapoor D, Gutpan RC, Wakil S et al. Beneficial effects of lamivudine in hepatitis B virus related decompensated cirrhosis. J Hepatol 2000; 33:308–312.
16. Sponseller 2000, Bacon DR, Di Bisceglie AM. Clinical improvement in patients with decompensated liver disease caused by hepatitis B after treatment with lamivudine. Liver Transpl 2000; 6:715–720.
17. Yao FY, Bass NM. Lamivudine treatment in patients with severely decompensated cirrhosis due to replicating hepatitis B infection. J Hepatol 2000; 33:301–307.
18. Marzano A, Salizzoni M, Debernardi-Venon W et al. Prevention of hepatitis B virus recurrence after liver transplantation in cirrhotic patients treated with lamivudine and passive immunoprophylaxis. J Hepatol 2001; 34:903–910.
19. Fontana RJ, Keeffe EB, Carey W et al. Effect of lamivudine treatment on survival of 309 North American patients awaiting liver transplantation for chronic hepatitis B. Liver Transpl 2002; 8:433–439.
20. Markowitz JS, Martin P, Conrad AJ et al. Prophylaxis against hepatitis B recurrence following liver transplantation using combination lamivudine and hepatitis B immune globulin. Hepatology 1998; 28:585–589.
21. Yao FY, Osorio RW, Roberts JP et al. Intramuscular hepatitis B immune globulin combined with lamivudine for prophylaxis against hepatitis B recurrence after liver transplantation. Liver Transpl Surg 1999; 5:491–496.
22. Yoshida EM, Erb SR, Partovi N et al. Liver transplantation for chronic hepatitis B infection with the use of combination lamivudine and low-dose hepatitis B immune globulin. Liver Transpl Surg 1999; 5:520–525.
23. McCaughan GW, Spencer J, Koorey D et al. Lamivudine therapy in patients undergoing liver transplantation for hepatitis B virus precore mutant-associated infection: high resistance rates in treatment of recurrence but universal prevention if used as prophylaxis with very low-dose hepatitis B immune globulin. Liver Transpl Surg 1999; 6:512–519.
24. Han SH, Ofman J, Holt C et al. An efficacy and cost-effectiveness analysis of combination hepatitis B immune globulin and lamivudine to prevent recurrent hepatitis B after orthotopic liver transplantation compared with hepatitis B immune globulin monotherapy. Liver Transpl 2001; 6:741–748.
25. Angus PW, McCaughan GW, Gane EJ et al. Combination low-dose hepatitis B immune globulin and lamivudine therapy provides effective prophylaxis against posttransplantation hepatitis B. Liver Transpl 2000; 6:429–433.

26. Rosenau J, Bahr MJ, Tillman HL et al. Lamivudine and low-dose hepatitis B immune globulin for prophylaxis of hepatitis B reinfection after liver transplantation: possible role of mutations in the YMDD motif prior to transplantation as a risk factor for reinfection. J Hepatol 2001; 34:895–902.
27. Bizollon T, Palazzo U, Ducerf C et al. Pilot study of the combination of interferon alfa and ribavirin as therapy of recurrent hepatitis C after liver transplantation. Hepatology 1997; 26:500–504.
28. Alberti AB, Belli LS, Airoldi A et al. Combined therapy with interferon and low-dose ribavirin in posttransplantation recurrent hepatitis C: a pragmatic study. Liver Transpl 2001; 7:870–876.
29. Ahmad J, Dodson SF, Demetris AJ, Fung JJ, Shakil AO. Recurrent hepatitis C after liver transplantation: a nonrandomized trial of interferon alfa alone versus interferon alfa and ribavirin. Liver Transpl 2001; 7:863–869.
30. De Vera ME, Smallwood GA, Rosado K et al. Interferon-alpha and ribavirin for the treatment of recurrent hepatitis C after liver transplantation. Transplantation 2001; 71:678–686.
31. Gopal DV, Rabkin JM, Berk BS et al. Treatment of progressive hepatitis C recurrence after liver transplantation with combination interferon plus ribavirin. Liver Transpl 2001; 7:181–190.
32. Narayanan M, Poterucha JJ, El-Amin OM et al. Treatment of posttransplantation recurrence of hepatitis C wih interferon and ribavirin: lessons on tolerability and efficacy. Liver Transpl 2002; 8:623–629.
33. Lavezzo B, Franchello A, Smedile A et al. Treatment of recurrent hepatitis C in liver transplants: efficacy of a six versus twelve month course of interferon alfa 2b with ribavirin. J Hepatol 2002; 37:247–252.
34. Samuel D, Bizollon T, Feray C et al. Interferon-alpha 2b plus ribavirin in patients with chronic hepatitis C after liver transplantation: a randomized study. Gastroenterology 2003; 124:642–650.

Chapter 108

Gastrointestinal tract in systemic disease

Ulf Müller-Ladner and Jürgen Schölmerich

KEY POINTS

- Vasculitis affecting the gut is often occult
- Signs of systemic inflammation and continuous abdominal pain are important clues
- Immunosuppression is usually required
- Biologic therapies show promise for the future
- Vascular involvement in antiphospholipid syndrome carries a high mortality
- Gastrointestinal tract involvement is common (and under diagnosed) in systemic sclerosis
- Sjögren's syndrome is a multi system disease; the more proximal the gastrointestinal tract, the more common the involvement

NTRODUCTION

.lthough the gastrointestinal (GI) tract is not generally regard-
l as one of the primary organ systems affected by systemic auto-
nmune or inflammatory rheumatic diseases, numerous mech-
nisms for these diseases are operative in or around the various
ructures and compartments of the GI tract. Vasculitis or intra-
ascular phenomena associated with immunologic symptoms,
ıch as mesenteric or portal vein thrombosis in catastrophic anti-
hospholipid syndrome, may cause ischemic dysfunction. Altera-
ons of matrix metabolism can also affect the functional integrity
f the GI tract, as in systemic sclerosis. Immune processes can
estroy essential exocrine functions, as in Sjögren's syndrome.
ı this chapter, these immunologic, mesenchymal, intravascular,
nd perivascular matrix-related and glandular alterations, and
ıeir impact on the morbidity of patients, are described.

.PIDEMIOLOGY

ystemic autoimmune diseases can affect the GI tract at any age;
ı some patients, especially those with vasculitides or systemic
clerosis, GI symptoms may precede the underlying systemic
isease and facilitate (or delay) its diagnosis. As well as the
pecific GI phenomena of the individual diseases as described
ı detail below, the epidemiology of GI involvement follows the
haracteristics of the respective systemic disease. In general, sex
nd age do not influence the occurrence or severity of the GI
ıanifestations. As an example, Table 108.1 shows the frequency
f intestinal involvement in different vasculitides. Of note, due
ı the systemic character of autoimmune rheumatic diseases, post-
ıortem examinations reveal that occult or subclinical involve-
ıent of the GI tract, although not causing any clinical problems,
ıay be observed in a substantial proportion of patients.

There are many similarities in the factors driving both immunologic and inflammatory diseases within and around the GI tract. A classic example – of the similarities found in rheumatoid arthritis and inflammatory bowel diseases – is shown in Table 108.2.

VASCULITIDES AND THE ANTIPHOSPHOLIPID SYNDROME

Pathology

Vasculitides are diseases characterized by inflammation within or around the vessel wall usually followed by alteration of the vascular blood flow and integrity of the vessel and secondary damage to the dependent organ. In the antiphospholipid syndrome, vascular obstruction is caused by aggregation of antiphospholipid antibodies with the lipid surfaces of platelets and vessels. Figure 108.1 illustrates the histopathology of the development of intestinal infarction following occlusion of the respective vessel.

Clinical presentation

Owing to their multifaceted appearance, clinical symptoms of vasculitides can be overt (e.g., when cutaneous or mucosal vasculitis appears) or occult (when restricted to a limited number of organs, including the intestine). Vasculitis involving the GI tract is often occult. Patients with vasculitides involving the GI tract most commonly present with abdominal pain, GI bleeding, ileus, intestinal ischemia, and necrosis or hematochezia. Figure 108.2 illustrates the endoscopic view of severe colonic ischemia. Most vascular disease is due to arteriosclerosis (see Chapter 67) and less than 10% is caused by vasculitides, so a

TABLE 108.1 FREQUENCY OF INTESTINAL INVOLVEMENT IN PRIMARY AND SECONDARY VASCULITIDES

Frequency of intestinal involvement	Type of vasculitis
Up to 90%	Schönlein-Henoch purpura
Up to 50%	Panarteritis nodosa, Churg-Strauss syndrome, vasculitis in systemic lupus erythematosus
Up to 30%	Behçet's syndrome
5–15%	Takayasu's arteritis, Wegener's granulomatosis, vasculitis in rheumatoid arthritis
Less than 5%	Lymphomatoid granulomatosis, giant cell arteritis, thromboangiitis obliterans

TABLE 108.2 SIMILARITIES IN PATHOPHYSIOLOGY AND RESPONSE TO TREATMENT IN RHEUMATOID ARTHRITIS AND INFLAMMATORY BOWEL DISEASES

Parameter	Inflammatory bowel disease (UC and CD)	Systemic disease (rheumatoid arthritis)
STIMULI		
Genetic factors	HLA DR2 (UC) HLA DQB1*0402, DRB1*1502 (CD) HLA B27	HLA DR4
Micro-organisms	Bacteria	Unclassified (retro)viruses, bacterial peptidoglycans
IMMUNE PHENOMENA		
Antibodies	Anti-*Saccharomyces cerevisiae* antibodies, anti-pancreas acini antibodies, perinuclear cytoplasmic antibodies	Rheumatoid factor, anti-citrullinated peptide antibodies
Cytokines	IL-1, IL-6, TNF-α, and various others	IL-1, IL-6, TNF-α, and various others
Inflammatory mediators	Prostaglandins, cyclo-oxygenases, chemokines, leukotrienes, nitric oxide	Prostaglandins, cyclo-oxygenases, chemokines, leukotrienes, nitric oxide
EXTRAFOCAL MANIFESTATIONS		
Skin	Erythema nodosum	Rheumatic nodules
Other organs	Reactive arthritis	Serositides
HISTOPATHOLOGY		
Cellular infiltrates	Lymphocytes, macrophages, mast cells	Lymphocytes, macrophages, dendritic cells
Vasculitis	Possible	Possible
Tissue destruction	Fistula (CD), expression of MMPs	Invading synovium, expression of MMPs and cysteine proteinases
Fibrosis	Intestinal stenosis	Secondary ankylosis
RESPONSE TO IMMUNOMODULATORS		
Steroids	+	+
Immunosuppressants	+	+
Cyclo-oxygenase inhibitors	–	+
Salicylates	+	(+) (sulfasalazine)
Biologics	+	+
Antibiotics	+ (quinolones, imidazoles)	? (minocycline)

CD, Crohn's disease; HLA, human leukocyte antigen; IL, interleukin; TNF, tumor necrosis factor; MMP, matrix metalloproteinase; UC, ulcerative colitis.

high index of suspicion is needed to differentiate these conditions from embolic, thrombotic, or arteriosclerotic ischemia in a patient suffering from severe abdominal pain. Pain starting 30–60 min postprandially favors an arteriosclerotic cause, whereas signs of systemic inflammation in combination with continuous GI symptoms should prompt consideration of vasculitis.[1,2] Mesenteric ischemia due to arteriosclerosis should be considered if a bruit is heard in the abdomen, although absence of this sign does not exclude the diagnosis (see Chapter 67). Symptomatic antiphospholipid syndrome can lead to obstruction of single major gastrointestinal veins and arteries, and also to hyperacute occlusion of the complete intestinal vasculature in catastrophic antiphospholipid syndrome.

Differential diagnosis

The overall goal is determination of the disease causing the vasculitic symptoms; therefore, patient history as well as clinical and serologic parameters are essential to allow rapid diagnosis and initiation of treatment. Identifying the cause of vasculitis from the classification criteria of the American College of Rheumatology and the Chapel Hill Consensus Conferences[1] does not identify specific diagnoses so much as distinct syndromes. Moreover, although indicators are useful, specific markers are lacking. For daily clinical practice, the differentiation between primary and secondary vasculitides is useful. In primary vasculitides the type of vasculitis is directly related to the size o the inflamed vessel, whereas secondary vasculitides can b directly associated with rheumatic or connective tissu diseases, malignant diseases, infections, toxic substances, an

DIAGNOSTIC METHODS

LABORATORY 'INDICATORS' FOR DISTINCT VASCULITIDES

Parameter	Found in
Eosinophilia	Churg-Strauss syndrome
HLA B51	Behçet's syndrome
HLA DR4	Rheumatoid arthritis
Antinuclear antibodies*	Systemic lupus erythematosus (all connective tissue diseases
Anti-double-strand DNA antibodies*	Systemic lupus erythematosus
Rheumatoid factor*	Rheumatoid arthritis
Cytoplasmic antineutrophil cytoplasmic (antiproteinase-3) antibodies	Wegener's granulomatosis
Perinuclear antineutrophil cytoplasmic (antimyeloperoxidase) antibodies	Microscopic polyangiitis

Only those parameters marked with an asterisk form part of the classification criteria of the individal disease entity.

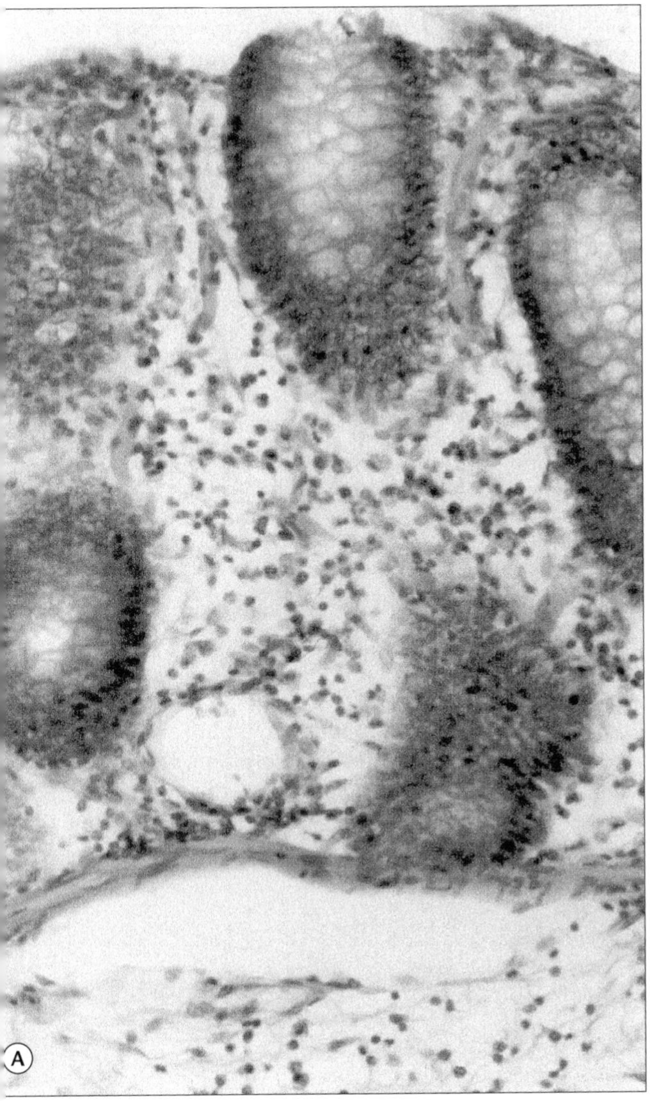

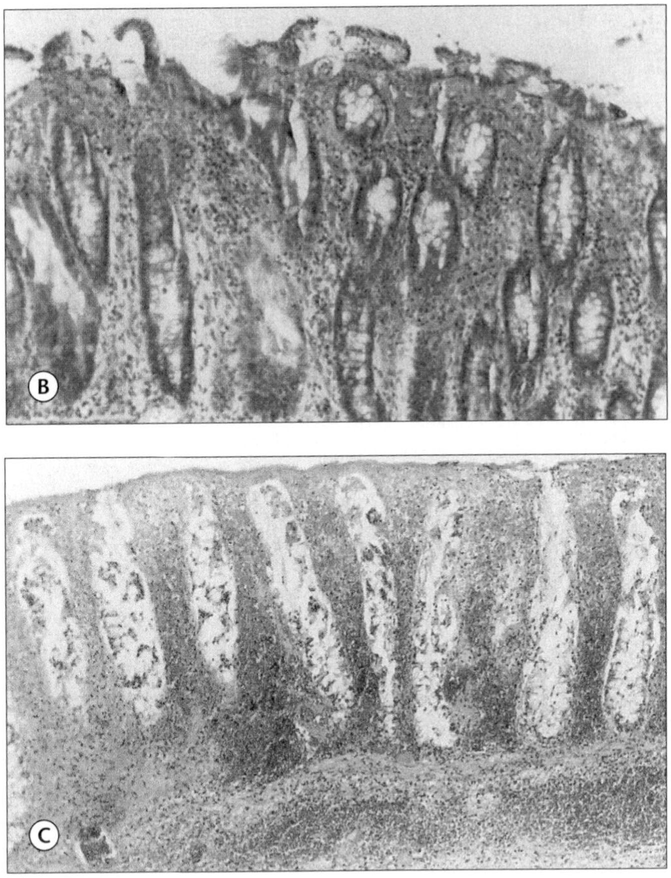

Fig. 108.1 Histologic appearance of the development of intestinal ischemia following infarction of a major vessel. A. Diffuse edema of the mucosa. **B.** Extravasation of erythrocytes into the edematous mucosa. **C.** Hemorrhagic infarction of the mucosa.

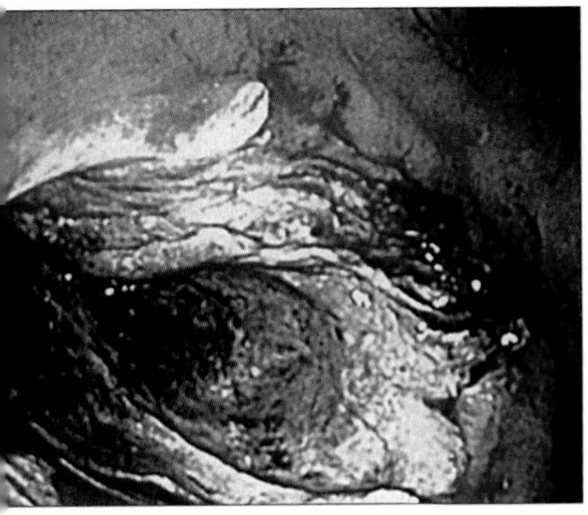

Fig. 108.2 Severe colonic ischemia. Endoscopic appearance of severe colonic ischemia with initiation of necrosis and hematochezia.

ugs. Diagnosis of antiphospholipid syndrome is usually ₁sed on the occurrence of venous or arterial thrombosis, or a story of fetal loss in combination with the respective ₁tiphospholipid antibodies.[3,4]

iagnostic methods

s well as laboratory indicators favoring specific diagnosis, it is commended that serum concentrations of lactate and coag- ation parameters be determined. All patients with suspected ischemia should have plain abdominal radiography to look for evidence of ileus, intestinal edema, and perforation. Mesenteric angiography (see Chapter 67) should be performed to identify potentially surgically correctable lesions (Fig. 108.3). Incomplete stenosis without ischemia of one of the major abdominal vessels results in typical bruits when abdominal auscultation is performed.

Treatment and prevention

The therapeutic approach is dependent on the type of vasculitis or vascular obstruction, and on the localization, intensity, and extent of the subsequent ischemia.

Intestinal ischaemia

Necrosis of the intestine requires immediate surgical intervention, and in subacute progressive mesenteric ischemia both surgical and interventional radiologic strategies including balloon dilatation, embolectomy, or bypass surgery of the affected mesenteric vessel should be performed.

Anti-inflammatory/immunosuppressive treatment

To prevent irreversible vascular obstruction during the course of prolonged inflammation, immunosuppressive therapy

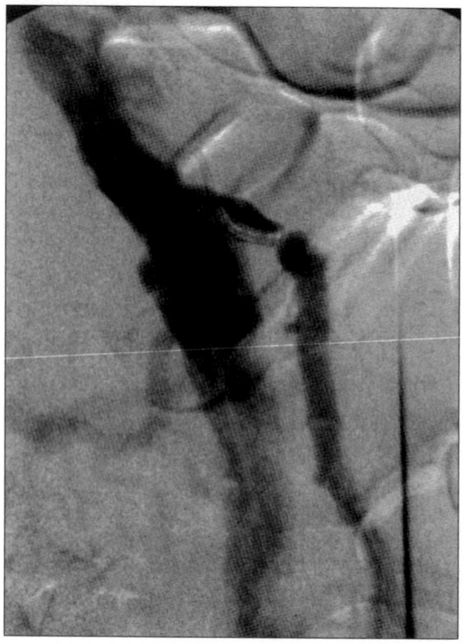

Fig. 108.3 Stenosis and occlusion of blood vessels. Angiography reveals stenosis of the superior mesenteric artery and occlusion of the inferior mesenteric artery.

should be started as soon as the diagnosis of vasculitis has been established. The box shows an overview of current medication used for treatment of active disease and maintenance of remission in vasculitis, although the evidence base is often limited.

Treatment of active disease

Administration of high-dose corticosteroids (prednisolc 100 mg/day or higher dosage in life-threatening situations), gi until GI symptoms decrease, is the treatment of choice. In so primary vasculitides, such as Wegener's granulomatosis a panarteritis nodosa, corticosteroids should be supplemented w cyclophosphamide (2 mg/kg/day). Other useful immunosuppress drugs include methotrexate, azathioprine, mycophenolate mofe tacrolimus, ciclosporin A, and leflunomide, and data incre ingly favor the use of biologic therapies including chimeric a humanized antitumor necrosis factor-α (TNF-α) antibodi soluble TNF-α receptor, and anti-CD20 antibodies (rituxima

Maintenance of remission

Corticosteroids should be tapered after improvement of syn toms and inflammation parameters, although this can ta years – especially in polymyalgia rheumatica and Takayas syndrome. To avoid severe side effects, a maintenance dc of prednisolone greater than 5–7.5 mg should be avoid Disease-modifying immunosuppressive drugs can be used help achieve this.

Specific treatments

Immunomodulation by immunoglobulins is useful especially Kawasaki's syndrome. Immunoadsorption columns can be us to reduce levels of pathogenic autoantibodies and proinfla matory molecules. In Behçet's syndrome, colchicine may

TREATMENT AND PREVENTION

THERAPEUTIC REGIMEN FOR INDUCTION OR MAINTENANCE OF REMISSION IN VASCULITIDES INVOLVING THE GI TRACT

Therapeutic options for vasculitis involving the GI tract	Goal	Regimen
Prednisolone	Induction, maintenance of remission	1–1.5 mg/kg/day p.o., up to 1000 mg/day i.v. in life-threatening situations
Cyclophosphamide	Induction, maintenance of remission	2–4 mg/kg/day p.o. (in addition to steroids), up to 1000 mg/m^2 in life-threatening situations
Methotrexate	Induction (moderate activity), maintenance of remission	7.5–30 mg/kg/week p.o./i.v. s.c. (add 5 mg folic acid p.o. 24 h later)
Azathioprine	Induction (moderate activity), maintenance of remission	2–4 mg/kg/day (adjust 6-thioguanine concentration to 150–350 pmol/0.8×10^9 erythrocytes)
Cyclosporine A	Maintenance of remission	5 mg/kg/day p.o. (adjust to serum concentration)
Leflunomide	Maintenance of remission	100 mg/day p.o. for 3 days followed by 10–20 mg/day p.o.
Sulfasalazine (Behçet's syndrome)	Maintenance of remission	2–6 mg/kg/day p.o.
Colchicine (Behçet's syndrome)	Maintenance of remission	0.5–2 mg/day p.o.
Mycophenolate mofetil	Maintenance of remission	2–3 g/day p.o.
Tacrolimus	Maintenance of remission	0.1–0.3 mg/kg/day p.o.
TNF-α inhibitors	Induction(?), maintenance of remission(?)	3–10 mg/kg i.v. every 4–8 weeks (infliximab); 20–40 mg s.c. every other week (adalimumab); 25 mg s.c. twice weekly (etanercept)

ective, and co-trimoxazole can control vasculitic symptoms d maintain remission in patients with mild to moderate ms of Wegener's granulomatosis.

Virostatic drugs, including interferon-α and ribavirin, can be ed in vasculitides triggered by hepatitis B or C, such as panar- itis nodosa and hepatitis C-associated cryoglobulinemia. sodilators such as calcium antagonists and prostaglandins useful in thromboangiitis obliterans but not in other intes- al vasculitides. In vascular thrombosis due to antiphospholipid ndrome, sufficient anticoagulation using intravenous heparin eds to be started immediately, usually replaced by long-term ostly lifelong) application of coumarin at a later date.

omplications and their management

outlined above, because of the life-threatening character of this nplication intestinal necrosis or severe obstruction of intestinal ssels requires immediate diagnostic and therapeutic action. scular obstruction due to catastrophic antiphospholipid syn- ome, however, is still associated with a mortality rate of about %, irrespective of state-of-the art immediate intensive care.

mplications of treatment

ng-term use of steroids requires continuous monitoring and erapy of side effects such as impaired glucose metabolism, reased risk of hypertension, osteoporosis, and immunosup- ession, as well as the development of cataract and glaucoma. e of immunosuppressants and biologics not only favors oical and atypical (opportunistic) infections including tuber- losis, but may also lower the threshold for the development malignancies such as lymphoma during anti-TNF-α therapy d of urinary tract carcinoma after cyclophosphamide therapy. ring immunosuppressive therapy, safe contraception is ndatory for both male and female patients (except for those ceiving steroids), and the use of azathioprine and ciclosporin ould be restricted to active patients.

ATHOGENESIS OF SYSTEMIC SCLEROSIS

athology

stemic sclerosis is characterized clinically by inflammation, scular damage, and autoimmune phenomena, resulting predominantly in progressive fibrosis of the skin, lung, and heart, as well as all parts of the GI tract. Although recent data have revealed various novel aspects in the pathogenesis of systemic sclerosis, no general pathogenetic concept has yet been accepted. As with skin sclerosis, key mechanisms hypothesized to be operating in the pathogenesis of systemic sclerosis including the GI tract[5–7] are the patient's genetic background, external stimuli, cellular and humoral activation of the immune system, inflammation, vascular damage, and upregulation of proto-oncogenes.[5,8] Figures 108.4 and 108.5 illustrate the presence of chemotactic proinflammatory molecules in the stomach and duodenum of a patient with systemic sclerosis and severe organ involvement. Finally, the cascade of events in systemic sclerosis results in fibroblast activation and overproduction of extracellular matrix (Fig. 108.6). In addition, decreased collagenase activity may also contribute to irreversible fibrosis followed by atrophy of smooth muscles and neuronal degeneration. It has also been hypothesized that in the GI tract the earliest defect in the pathogenesis of dysmotility in systemic sclerosis is located in the cholinergic nerves supplying the muscle, rather than sclerosis of the muscle itself.[9]

Clinical presentation

Esophageal dysmotility and reflux symptoms occur in up to 90% of patients; the stomach is affected in about 50%, the small bowel in up to 70%, the colon in 20–50%, and 50–70% of patients report anorectal problems. In addition, other GI organs such as the liver, gallbladder, and pancreas may be affected.[10] Of note, organ involvements of the diffuse form of systemic sclerosis tend to be more severe than those of the limited form.[8]

Differential diagnosis

In patients who show the typical cutaneous features, correct diagnosis is easy. Suggestive features include extensive skin thickening, starting with sclerodactyly (Fig. 108.7) followed by spreading cutaneous fibrosis, and resulting in digital ulcers and severe ischemia, perioral fibrosis, and impairment of articular flexibility; in combination with anti-Scl70 or anticentromere antibodies, correct diagnosis is easy to achieve. However, in

TREATMENT AND PREVENTION

RECOMMENDATIONS FOR IMMUNOSUPPRESSANTS IN VASCULITIC PATIENTS DURING PREGNANCY

rug	Problems, side effects	Recommendation
redniso(lo)ne	Blood pressure, diabetes, osteoporosis, cataract, glaucoma	+
zathioprine	Leucopenia, pancreatitis	+ in active patients
iclosporin	Hypertension, renal impairment, hypertrichosis	(+) in active patients
1ethotrexate	Teratogenic	–
eflunomide	Teratogenic, abortion	–
1ycophenolate mofetil	Teratogenic	–
yclophosphamide	Teratogenic, mutagen	–
NF-α inhibitors	Lymphoma, tuberculosis, opportunistic infections	–

NF, tumor necrosis factor.

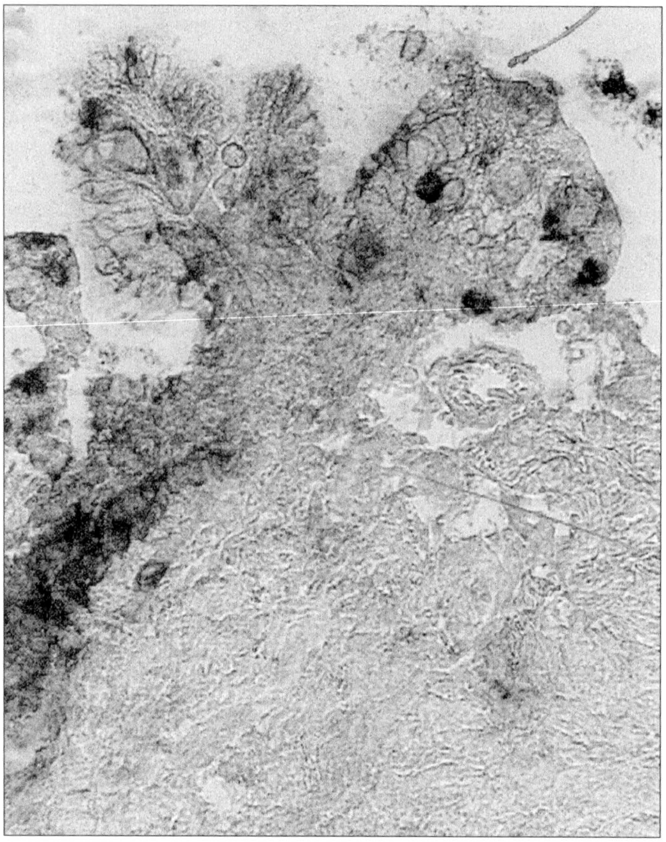

Fig. 108.4 Expression of chemokines. Strong RANTES chemokine expression (black staining) in the mucosa of the stomach of a patient with systemic sclerosis.

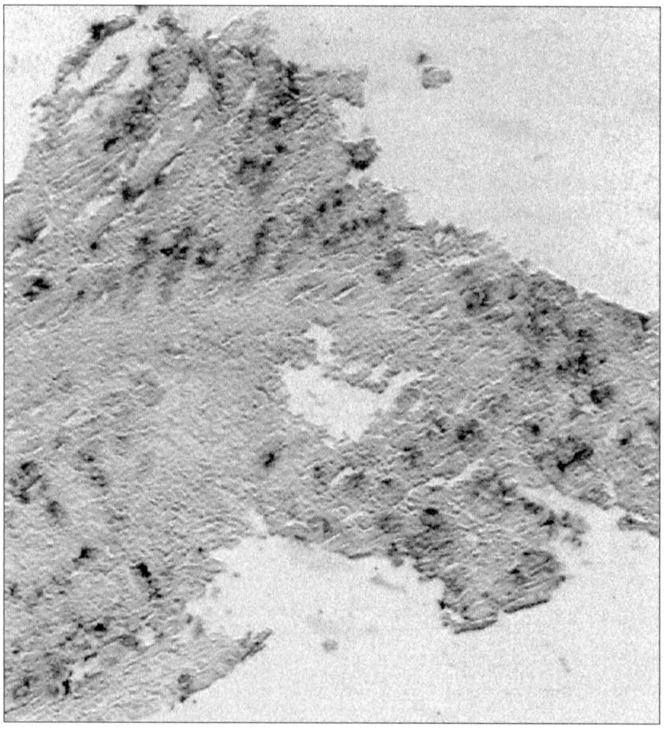

Fig. 108.5 Expression of chemokines. Macrophage chemotactic protein-3 (MCP-3) chemokine expression (black staining) in the duodenum of a patient with systemic sclerosis. Note the intensive fibrosis in deeper layers of the intestinal mucosa.

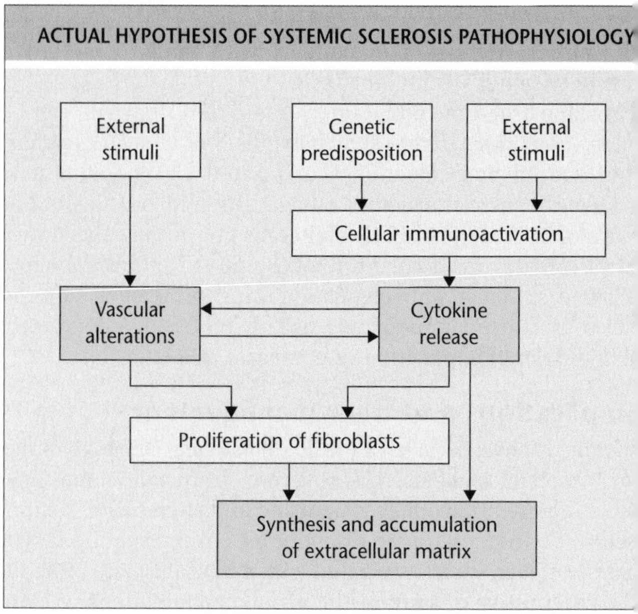

Fig. 108.6 Hypothesis for the pathophysiological development systemic sclerosis.

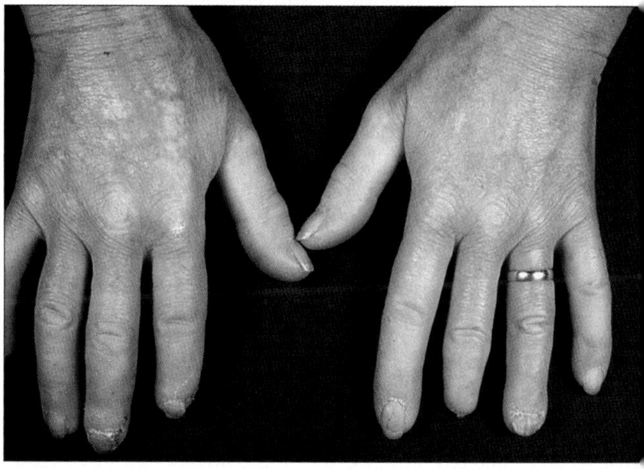

Fig. 108.7 Sclerodactyly. Note sausage-shaped fingers due to sclerodermatous thickening and digital shortening due to previous infarction.

patients with limited cutaneous involvement, lone Raynau phenomenon, and an atypical antibody pattern, the prese of occult GI tract involvement may easily be overlooked high index of suspicion is needed in patients with lo esophageal dysmotility, unclear gastroesophageal ref symptoms, malabsorption, and small bowel dysmotility.

Diagnostic methods

Scleroderma of the GI tract is underdiagnosed. Test se tion[11–13] should reflect the suspected site of disease. Esophag manometry assesses directly the motility of the esophagus a lower esophageal sphincter. Similarly, 24-h pH monitor reveals the daytime-dependent extent of gastric reflux into esophagus. Gastroscopy provides additional information structural damage of the esophagus and stomach, and allo direct histologic biopsy evaluation. Swallowing of radioact barium contrast media allows kinetic evaluation of the phagogastric movements, but is currently used less fre-ently than other techniques. Motility of the small intestine neasured by barium follow-through radiography of the small wel, especially for patients with intestinal pseudoobstruction. Kylose testing, jejunal cultures, and hydrogen glucose and tulose breath testing can help to assess malabsorption and cterial overgrowth. As the anorectum is the predominantly ected part of the large intestine, investigation of the colon is important part of the clinical evaluation. Opaque markers tz markers) can be used to measure transit times, rectal nometry evaluates the involvement and extent of rectal rosis in patients with systemic sclerosis, and sigmoidoscopy d colonoscopy reveal structural alterations of the large estine. In patients with intestinal pseudo-obstruction, nputed tomography, as illustrated in Figure 108.8, reveals ensive thickening of the intestinal mucosa.

DIAGNOSTIC METHODS

VALUATION OF INVOLVEMENT OF GI TRACT IN SYSTEMIC SCLEROSIS

lethod	Evaluation of
ophageal manometry	Esophageal dysmotility, sphincter pressure
4-h pH monitoring	Extent of gastroesophageal reflux
astroscopy	Structural gastroesophagal alterations
arium opaque meal	Gastroesophageal motility
mall-bowel barium follow-through X-ray	Intestinal motility
-Xylose test, jejunal cultures, hydrogen glucose and lactulose breath tests	Malabsorption and bacterial overgrowth
paque (Sitz) markers	Intestinal transit time, intestinal pseudo-obstruction
ectal manometry	Rectal fibrosis
igmoidoscopy/colonoscopy	Structural alterations
omputed tomography	Intestinal pseudo-obstruction

Treatment and prevention

Currently, no evidence-based disease-modifying regimen for systemic sclerosis exists. Most patients take low-dose steroids and/or D-penicillamine to inhibit overall disease activity.[5,14,15] Several therapeutic approaches for individual organs of the GI tract have proven to be effective. A (secondary) sicca syndrome requires treatment with artificial saliva, and owing to the high risk for development of caries, these patients should see a dentist every 6 months. Symptoms of gastroesophageal reflux can be treated effectively with proton pump inhibitors. However, in most of patients high doses (e.g., 20–40 mg pantoprazole or omeprazole orally, twice daily) are needed to resolve the majority of symptoms, including reflux-associated asthma-like attacks. In some patients with severe reflux, the addition of H_2 blockers at night ('sequential acid blocking') has an additional effect, although in preclinical studies this effect was found not to be significant in the majority of patients. Reduced intestinal motility has become more problematic since cisapride was taken off the market due to the risk of cardiac arrhythmia. Therefore, the effect of other prokinetic drugs such as metoclopramide, domperidone, and erythromycin needs to be evaluated for each patient separately, especially in those suffering from intestinal pseudo-obstruction (see Chapter 62). Stenoses of the GI tract, whether in the esophagus, stomach, small and large intestine, or anus, are best treated mechanically with balloon dilatation. Other treatment strategies, such as the injection of botulinum toxin, are usually much less effective than in other GI diseases.

Complications and their management

Although cutaneous fibrosis is the most obvious and impressive alteration in systemic sclerosis, the prognosis and quality of life is frequently determined by intestinal and visceral as well as pulmonary involvement. As well as the organ dysfunctions outlined above, some complications require more attention. Intestinal pseudo-obstruction with subsequent symptoms of ileus can become life-threatening. Rapid conservative nonsurgical decompression using nasogastric suction in combination with prokinetics can avoid the need for surgical intervention. Untreated reflux esophagitis can lead to acute esophageal

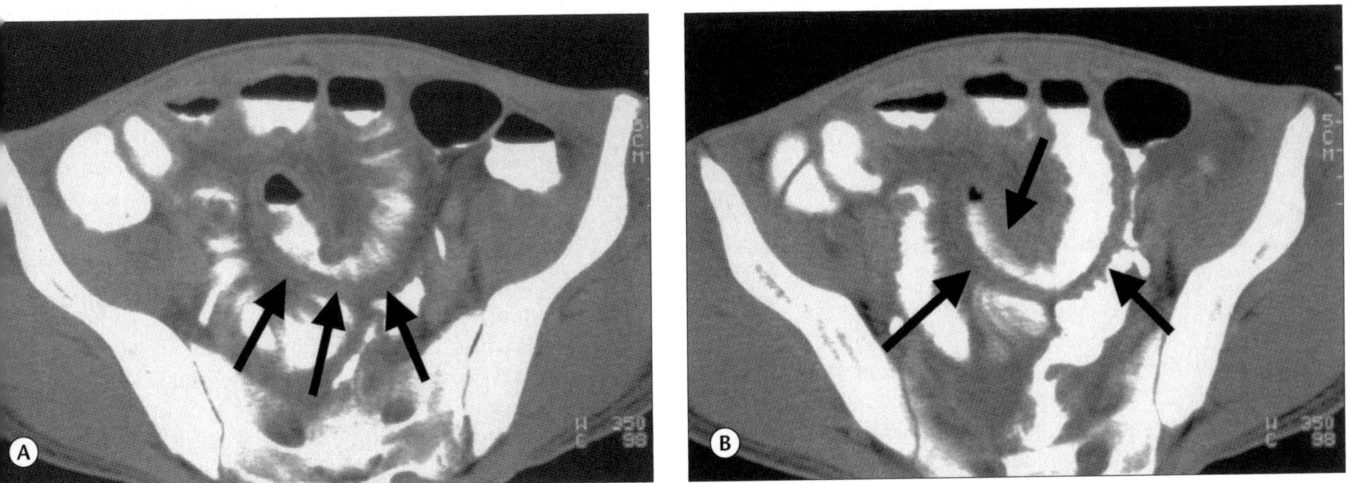

g. 108.8 **Thickening of intestinal mucosa.** Computed tomograms showing thickening (arrows) of the small and large bowel resulting from tensive fibrosis in a patient with long-term systemic sclerosis. Parts **A** and **B** both show the same segment of the bowel, which was scanned quentially by CT within a short period of time, illustrating that the thickening persists during peristaltic waves. Courtesy of Professor S uerbach, Institute for Radiology, University of Regensburg, Germany.

bleeding, and chronic esophagitis may be an early sign of Barrett's dysplasia and adenocarcinoma.

PATHOGENESIS OF SJÖGREN'S SYNDROME

Pathology

Sjögren's syndrome is a multisystemic disease of largely unknown etiology, although the inflammatory and autoimmune mechanisms can involve every organ system. Pathologic processes take place in both exocrine (salivary glands) and nonexocrine tissues, including the eye, skin, kidneys, pulmonary system, joints, muscle, and nervous system, and in the gastrointestinal tract the mucosa, pancreas, and hepatobiliary system.[16–19] The dominant histopathologic feature of Sjögren's syndrome is the presence of lymphoplasmacellular infiltrates in affected glands and organs, mostly associated with autoantibody production such as anti-Ro/SSA and anti-La/SSB antibodies.

In long-term disease after an extended period of inflammation, fibrosis replaces the original tissue accompanied by a loss of specific (exocrine) function of the respective organ or tissue, especially in the (peri)oral salivary glands. In the GI tract, the gastric mucosa appears atrophic with similar $CD4^+$ lymphocytic infiltrates as in the perioral glands. Parietal cell antibodies can also be detected. However, these intestinal alterations are not completely specific for primary Sjögren's syndrome: they may also be seen in secondary Sjögren's in patients with other autoimmune diseases.

Clinical presentation

In 1933, Hendrik Sjögren presented the first patients suffering from this syndrome, already emphasizing the systemic nature of this disease. Some 90% of patients are female, with a mean age at onset of 50 years.

CLINICAL PRESENTATION

INITIAL SYMPTOMS OF SJÖGREN'S SYNDROME

Initial symptom	Frequency (%)
Ocular symptoms	50
Xerostomia	40
Arthralgia or arthritis	30
Swollen major salivary glands	25
Raynaud's disease	20
Fever or malaise	10
Dyspareunia	5
Lung involvement	2
Renal involvement	2

Xerostomia

Xerostomia of the mouth is the predominant symptom, frequently associated with 'burning sensations,' dysgeusia, dysphagia, soreness when speaking for an extended period of time, and the rapid development of caries and periodontitis (see Chapter 1). Clinical examination reveals a dry and sticky oral mucosa, a reduction of saliva production, and atrophy of the sensory papillae of the tongue. In established Sjögren's syndrome, rhagades, severe dental lesions, and oral candidiasis can be observed. The consistency of the parotid and s mandibular glands is usually increased without being painf and in active patients these glands can be substantially enlarg Unilateral swelling may occur, but in most patients all t salivary glands are affected.

The esophagus, stomach, small intestine, and pancreas are t organs of the GI tract that are most frequently affected, in p because of exocrine gland atrophy.[16–19] In contrast, the liv and biliary system are involved more rarely, predominantly a result of autoimmune mechanisms.[17,20]

Esophagus

In some patients a reduction of esophageal motility, especia in the upper part, can be observed. In the lower parts of t esophagus, spontaneous biphasic and triphasic contractions c occur in up to 30% of patients. As well as dysfunction of t exocrine glands of the esophagus, myositis of the musculature the esophagus and antibodies against M_3 muscarinic recept have been discussed as underlying pathogenetic mechanisms

Malabsorption

There are numerous case reports of patients with Sjögre syndrome who show also signs of malabsorption, Croh disease, and celiac disease.[22,23] In a more complex setti individual patients have a combination of Sjögren's disea primary sclerosing cholangitis, and chronic pancreatitis, whi is most likely due to autoimmune reactions against an (unknow ductal antigen present in all three disease entities.

Hepatobiliary

The occurrence of an exocrine dysfunction of the pancreas Sjögren's patients is variable. Some studies show a significa alteration of pancreatic function in up to 50%, which can associated with increased serum pancreatic amylase levels a autoantibodies against pancreatic ductal structures due intrapancreatic inflammatory and autoimmune processe Hepatomegaly occurs in up to 50% of Sjögren's patients, on third also show an increase in serum levels for hepatic a biliary enzymes.

Differential diagnosis

Diagnosis of primary or secondary Sjögren's syndrome is bas on a combination of ocular and oral symptoms together wi histopathologic findings, involvement of salivary glands, a specific autoantibodies (Table 108.3). In primary Sjögren syndrome, which is easier to define because there is no ne to fulfil a second set of criteria for the underlying diseas criterion 2 is replaced by the presence of antibodies again SSA/Ro, SSB/La, antinuclear antibodies, or rheumatoid fact Using these criteria, a sensitivity of 93.5% and a specificity 94.0% for primary Sjögren' s syndrome can be achieved.

For secondary Sjögren's the sensitivity is 85.1% and th specificity 93.5% for differentiation from mixed connecti tissue diseases without secondary Sjögren's syndrome. A antimitochondrial antibodies occur in 10% of patients wi Sjögren's syndrome, the differential diagnosis should alwa include primary biliary cirrhosis.[20]

Diagnostic methods

Diagnosis can often be established on the basis of the medic history and clinical examination. Formal diagnosis is esta

TABLE 108.3 DIAGNOSIS OF SECONDARY SJÖGREN'S SYNDROME
OCULAR SYMPTOMS A positive answer to at least one of the following three questions: • Have you had daily, persistently troublesome dry eyes for more than 3 months? • Do you have a recurrent sensation of sand or gravel in the eyes? • Do you use tear substitutes more than three times a day? and/or
ORAL SYMPTOMS A positive answer to at least one of the following three questions: • Have you had a daily feeling of dry mouth for more than 3 months? • Have you had recurrent or persistently swollen salivary glands as an adult? • Do you frequently drink liquids to aid in swallowing dry foods?
EVIDENCE FOR AN UNDERLYING SYSTEMIC RHEUMATIC DISEASE OTHER THAN SJÖGREN'S SYNDROME
TWO OF THE FOLLOWING SYMPTOMS: • Positive Schirmer test or rose Bengal score • Positive histopathologic finding (lymphocytic infiltrates in the salivary glands) • Salivary gland involvement shown by sialography, scintigraphy, or reduced unstimulated salivary flow

DIFFERENTIAL DIAGNOSIS
OTHER DISEASES LEADING TO XEROSTOMIA OR KERATOCONJUNCTIVITIS SICCA
Sarcoidosis
Bacterial and viral infections
Trauma
Neurotropic keratitis
Vitamin A deficiency
Erythema multiforme
Drugs
Graft versus host disease

…shed by salivary gland biopsy and histopathologic findings of … least one 'inflammatory' focus of at least 50 lymphocytes …er 4 mm^2, but is rarely necessary, may cause complications …ch as fistulae, and is not completely specific for Sjögren's …sease. A recent study showed that up to 15% of healthy indi…duals had 'typical' lymphocytic infiltrates in salivary gland …iopsies.[24]

Sialometry is unhelpful in the diagnosis of Sjögren's syn…rome because of high interindividual variability and the vast …umber of drugs that can affect salivary production, but this …vestigation may be used to monitor therapeutic effects in …dividual patients.

Sialography can help to distinguish secondary from primary …jögren's syndrome by showing structural alterations of the …uctal system in 60–95% of those with the primary syndrome. …owever, this investigation is rather painful and not specific, as …0% of Sjögren's patients do not show such radiologic altera…ons whereas 20% of healthy individuals do.

Scintigraphy using radioactive technetium can also be used to measure saliva production by salivary glands. Typically, in Sjögren's patients only minute amounts of the radiodiagnosticum are taken up by the diseased glands, but the specificity of the method appears to be rather low.

Treatment and prevention

Treatment of the reduced or absent excretory salivary functions of the exocrine glands is most important to improve the overall clinical status of Sjögren patients.[25] In general, regular application of artificial saliva (dependent on the symptoms of the individual patient) is the therapeutic basis for the treatment of Sjögren's syndrome. Products based on methylcellulose have been shown to be the most effective. Chewing gum and sugar-free drops can provide additional effects on the remaining saliva production.

Use of disease-modifying drugs such as steroids and immunosuppressants, unfortunately, has only a limited effect on xerostomia and the symptoms of ocular sicca syndrome. Parasympathomimetics can be effective but, owing to their side effects, the evidence base for their value for long-term clinical application is still limited.[26,27] Systemic symptoms and sequelae such as arthritis and vasculitis are usually treated with therapeutic regimens that follow those of rheumatoid arthritis, primary vasculitides, and mixed connective tissue diseases. Owing to the very limited data addressing therapy of exocrine pancreas dysfunction, substitution of pancreas enzymes should be tried; when the biliary system is affected, ursodeoxycholic acid may be an option for treatment.

Complications and their management

Oral candidiasis is the most important secondary infection based on a reduced mucosal defense. As soon as diagnosis has been established by clinical inspection and microbiology, local therapy with antimycotics such as amphotericin or nystatin needs to be started. In severe cases, fluconazole given orally is the drug of primary choice. To avoid reinfection, larger mucosal defects should be treated with local adstringents and/or disinfectants. Most importantly, constant monitoring and treatment of ocular ulcers and caries should be performed all patients with Sjögren's syndrome.

PROGNOSIS WITH AND WITHOUT TREATMENT

In general, the reduction in overall health status and quality of life in systemic diseases ranges from minor temporary sequelae to acute life-threatening conditions regardless whether the individual symptoms originate from the GI tract or from other organs. Apart from severe complications, the prognosis of all systemic diseases with regard to mortality and morbidity can be good when adequate stage-dependent and long-term monitoring and treatment of the patient is applied. On the other hand, quality of life is significantly reduced in the majority of patients, as with other long-term disabling diseases.

WHAT TO TELL PATIENTS

First, it is mandatory to explain to patients the nature and course of GI symptoms in the context of the underlying systemic disease. Second, the need for a lifelong monitoring (and potentially treatment) by experts in the individual discipline should be underlined. Third, patients should be made aware that environmental factors, such as infections, may act to exacerbate the underlying disease, via immune mechanisms. Vaccination against common infectious diseases such as influenza, hepatitis B, *Haemophilus influenza*, and *Streptococcus pneumoniae* may be helpful.

SOURCES OF INFORMATION FOR PATIENTS AND DOCTORS

These include continuous online reports such as:
http://www.rheuma21st.com
http://www.jointandbone.org
http://uptodate.com
http://www.utdol.com
Sjogrens:
http://www.sjogrens.org/
Systemic sclerosis:
http://www.rheumatology.org/publications/classification/systsc asp?aud=prs

REFERENCES

1. Müller-Ladner U. Vasculitides of the gastrointestinal tract. Bailliéres Best Pract Res Clin Gastroenterol 2001; 15:59–82.
2. Dalle I, Geboes K. Vascular lesions of the gastrointestinal tract. Acta Gastroenterol Belg 2002; 64:213–219.
3. Asherson RA. Infections, antiphospholipid antibodies, and antiphospholipid syndromes. Online. Available: http://www.rheuma21st.com (Cutting Edge Reports, 22 July 2002).
4. Alarcón-Segovia D, Boffa MC, Branch W et al. Prophylaxis of the antiphospholipid syndrome: a consensus report. Lupus 2003; 12:499–503.
5. Cohen S, Laufer I, Snape WJ, Shiau Y-F, Levine GM, Jimenez S. The gastrointestinal manifestations of scleroderma. Pathogenesis and management. Gastroenterology 1980; 769:155–166.
6. Sjögren RW. Gastrointestinal disorders in scleroderma. Arthritis Rheum 1994; 37:1265–1282.
7. Rose S, Young MA, Reynolds JC. Gastrointestinal manifestations of scleroderma. Gastroenterol Clin N Am 1998; 27:563–594.
8. Steen VD, Medsger TA Jr. Severe organ involvement in systemic sclerosis with diffuse scleroderma. Arthritis Rheum 2000; 43:2437–2444.
9. Iovino P, Valentini G, Giacci C et al. Proximal stomach function in systemic sclerosis: relationship with autonomic nerve function. Dig Dis Sci 2001; 46:723–730.
10. Lock G, Holstege A, Lang B, Schölmerich J. Gastrointestinal manifestations of progressive systemic sclerosis. Am J Gastroenterol 1997; 92:763–771.
11. Clements PJ, Becvar R, Drosos AA, Ghattas L, Gabrielli A. Assessment of gastrointestinal involvement. Clin Exp Rheumatol 2003; 21(Suppl 29):S15–S18.
12. Ling TC, Johnston BT. Esophageal investigations in connective tissue disease: which tests are most appropiate. J Clin Gastroenterol 2001; 32:33–36.
13. Marie I, Levesque H, Ducrotte P et al. Gastric involvement in systemic sclerosis: a prospective study. Am J Gastroenterol 2001; 96:77–83.
14. Müller-Ladner U, Benning K, Lang B. Current therapy of systemic sclerosis (scleroderma). Clin Invest 1993; 71:257–263.
15. Steen VD. Treatment of systemic sclerosis. Am J Clin Dermatol 2001; 2:315–325.
16. Constantopoulos SH, Tsianos EV, Moutsopoulos HM. Pulmonary and gastrointestinal manifestations of Sjögren's syndrome. Rheum Dis Clin N Am 1992; 18:617–635.
17. Nishimori I, Morita M, Kino J et al. Pancreatic involvement in patients with Sjögren's syndrome and primary biliary cirrhosis. Int J Pancreatol 1995; 17;47–54.
18. Skopouli FN, Barbatis C, Moutsopoulos HM. Liver involvement in primary Sjögren's syndrome. Br J Rheumatol 1994; 33:745–748.
19. Ostuni PA, Gazzetto G, Chieco-Bianchi F et al. Pancreatic exocrine involvement in primary Sjögren's syndrome. Scand J Rheumatol 1996; 25:47–51.
20. Tsianos EV, Hoofnagle JH, Fox PC et al. Sjögren's syndrome in patients with primary biliary cirrhosis. Hepatology 1990; 11:730–734.
21. Goldblatt F, Gordon TP, Waterman SA. Antibody-mediated gastrointestinal dysmotility in scleroderma. Gastroenterolo 2002; 123:1144–1150.
22. Sobhani I, Brousse N, Vissuzaine C et al. A diffuse T lymphocytic gastrointestinal mucosal infiltration associated with Sjögren syndrome resulting in a watery diarrhea syndrome and responsive immunosuppress therapy. Am J Gastroenterol 1998; 93:2584–2586.
23. Hsieh TY, Lan JL, Chen DY. Primary Sjögren's syndrome with protein-losing gastroenteropathy: report of two cases. J Formos Med Assoc 2002; 101:519–522.
24. Radfar L, Kleiner DE, Fox PC, Pillemer SR Prevalence and clinical significance of lymphocytic foci in minor salivary glands o healthy volunteers. Arthritis Rheum 2002; 47:520–524.
25. Van der Reijden WA, Vissink A, Veerman EC Amerongen AV. Treatment of oral dryness related complaints (xerostomia) in Sjögren' syndrome. Ann Rheum Dis 1999; 58:465.
26. Vivino FB, Al-Hashimi I, Khan Z et al. Pilocarpine tablets for the treatment of dry mouth and dry eye symptoms in patients with Sjögren's syndrome: a randomized, placebo-controlled, fixed dose, multicenter trial P92-01 study group. Arch Intern Med 1999; 159:174–181.
27. Petrone D, Condemni JJ, Fife R, Gluck O, Cohen S, Dalgin P. A double-blind, randomize placebo-controlled study of cemiveline in Sjögren's syndrome patients with xerostom and keratoconjunctivitis sicca. Arthritis Rheum 2002; 46:748–754.

Chapter 109

Gut and pancreatic endocrine tumors

Fathia Gibril and Robert T Jensen

KEY POINTS

- Gastroenteropancreatic tumors (GEPs) originate from the neuroendocrine cells of the gastrointestinal tract
- They are classified by histologic staining patterns
- Associated syndromes are determined by growth factors and amines secreted
- Treatment is directed at the hormone excess state and the tumor itself
- Non functional tumors produce symptoms by direct invasion or hepatic metastasis
- Somatostatin receptor scintigraphy (SRS) is the modality of choice for localizing primary and metastatic tumors

NTRODUCTION

;astroenteropancreatic endocrine tumors (GEPs) originate ·om the diffuse neuroendocrine system of the gastrointestinal ·act, which is comprised of various amine- and peptide-roducing cells. GEP tumors were originally classified as PUDomas (amine precursor uptake and decarboxylation) as ere carcinoids, pheochromocytomas, and melanomas because ney share a number of features (Table 109.1).[1,2] The present hapter focuses on noncarcinoid GEP tumors of the gastro-ntestinal tract as carcinoid tumors are discussed in detail in :hapter 110.

'ATHOLOGY

;EPs are usually composed of a monotonous sheet of small ound cells with uniform nuclei and infrequent mitoses. GEPs re now principally recognized by their histological staining atterns due to shared cellular proteins (Table 109.1). Currently, nmunocytochemical localization of chromogranin A is most videly used (Table 109.1).

Ultrastructurally, GEPs possess electron-dense neurosecre-ory granules and frequently contain small clear vesicles that orrespond to synaptic vesicles of neurons. They synthesize umerous peptides, growth factors, and amines, which may be ecreted, giving rise to various specific clinical syndromes Table 109.2). The diagnosis of the specific syndrome requires he clinical features of the disease (Table 109.2). Pathologists annot distinguish between benign and malignant GEPs unless netastases or invasion is present.[1,2]

TABLE 109.1 GENERAL CHARACTERISTICS OF GASTROENTEROPANCREATIC (GEP) ENDOCRINE TUMORS

A. SHARED GENERAL NEUROENDOCRINE CELL MARKERS

- Chromogranins (A, B, C) are acidic monomeric soluble proteins (49 000 mol. wt) found in the large secretory granules; chromogranin A is generally used
- Neuron-specific enolase (NSE) is the gamma-gamma dimer of the enzyme enolase and is a cytosolic marker of neuroendocrine differentiation
- Synaptophysin is a membrane glycoprotein (38 000 mol. wt) found in small vesicles of neurons and GEP endocrine tumors

B. SIMILARITIES IN BIOLOGIC BEHAVIOR

- Generally slow-growing, but a proportion are aggressive
- Secrete biologically active peptides/amines, which can cause clinical symptoms
- Generally have high densities of somatostatin receptors ($sst_{2,3,11}$) which are used for both localization and in treatment

C. PATHOLOGIC SIMILARITIES

- All are APUDomas showing amine precursor uptake and decarboxylation
- Ultrastructurally they have dense-core secretory granules (>80 nm)
- Histologically they appear similar with few mitoses and uniform nuclei
  - Frequently synthesize multiple peptides/amines, which can be detected immunocytochemically but may not be secreted
  - Presence or absence of clinical syndrome or type cannot be predicted by immunocytochemical studies
  - Histological classifications do not predict biologic behavior; only invasion or metastases establishes malignancy

D. MOLECULAR SIMILARITIES

1. Common: chromosomal loss of 3p (8–47%), 3q (8–41%), 11q (21–62%), 6q (18–68%); frequent chromosomal gains at 17q (10–55%), 7q (16–68%)
2. Less common: alterations at MEN1 gene locus (11q13) and $p16^{INK4a}$ (9p21) occur in a proportion (10–30%)
3. Uncommon: alterations in common oncogenes (Ras, Jun, Fos, etc.) or in common tumor suppressor genes (p53, retinoblastoma)

CLINICAL SYNDROMES

GEPs can be classified into nine definite functional syndromes, two possible functional syndromes, and nonfunctional tumors (nonfunctional PETs) (Table 109.2). Each functional syndrome is characterized by specific symptoms due to the ectopically secreted hormone (Table 109.2). Nonfunctional PETs secrete

TABLE 109.2 GASTROENTEROPANCREATIC (GEP) ENDOCRINE TUMOR SYNDROMES

Name	Biologically active peptide(s) secreted	Tumor location	Malignant (%)	Associated with MEN1 (%)	Main symptoms/signs
I. ESTABLISHED FUNCTIONAL SYNDROMES					
Zollinger-Ellison syndrome (ZES)	Gastrin	Duodenum (70%) Pancreas (25%) Other sites (5%)	60–90	20–25	Pain (79–100%) Diarrhea (30–75%) Esophageal symptoms (31–56%)
Insulinoma	Insulin	Pancreas (>99%)	<10	4–5	Hypoglycemic symptoms (100%)
VIPoma (Verner-Morrison syndrome, pancreatic cholera, WDHA)	Vasoactive intestinal peptide	Pancreas (90%, adult) Other (10%, neural, adrenal, periganglionic)	40–70	6	Diarrhea (90–100%) Hypokalemic (80–100%) Dehydration (83%)
Glucagonoma	Glucagon	Pancreas (100%)	50–80	1–20	Rash (67–90%) Glucose intolerance (38–87%) Weight loss (66–96%)
GRFoma	Growth hormone-releasing hormone	Pancreas (30%) Lung (54%) Jejunum (7%) Other (13%)	>60	16	Acromegaly (100%)
Somatostatinoma	Somatostatin	Pancreas (55%) Duodenum/jejunum (44%)	>70	45	Diabetes mellitus (63–90%) Cholelithiases (65–90%) Diarrhea (35–90%)
ACTHoma	ACTH	Pancreas (4–16% all ectopic Cushing's)	>95	Rare	Cushing's syndrome (100%)
GEP causing carcinoid syndrome	Serotonin ? tachykinins	Pancreas (<1% all carcinoids)	60–88	Rare	Diarrhea, flushing, asthma
GEP causing hypercalcemia	PTHrP Others unknown	Pancreas (rare cause of hypercalcemia)	84	Rare	Abdominal pain due to hepatic metastases
II. POSSIBLE FUNCTIONAL SYNDROMES					
GEP secreting calcitonin	Calcitonin	Pancreas (rare cause of hypercalcitonemia)	>80	16	Diarrhea (50%)
GEP secreting renin	Renin	Pancreas	Unknown	No	Hypertension
III. NON FUNCTIONAL SYNDROMES					
PPoma/nonfunctional	None	Pancreas (100%)	>60	18–44	Weight loss (30–90%) Abdominal mass (10–30%) Pain (30–95%)

no products that cause a specific clinical syndrome. The symptoms caused by nonfunctional PETs are entirely due to the tumor *per se*.

EPIDEMIOLOGY

The prevalence of clinically significant GEPs is approximately 10 cases/million, the most common being insulinomas, gastrinomas, and nonfunctional PETs, which each have an incidence of 0.5–2 cases/million/year. VIPomas (vasoactive intestinal peptide) are 2–8 times less common, glucagonomas are 17–30 times less common, and somatostatinomas are the least common. In autopsy studies, 0.5–1.5% of all cases have a GEP which is not a carcinoid tumor, but in less than 1 in 1000 cases a functional tumor was thought to occur.

GEPs commonly show malignant behavior (Table 109.2). Except for insulinomas, <10% of which are malignant, 50–100% of GEPs in different series were found to be malignant (Table 109.2).[1–3] A number of factors have been identified that are important prognostic factors in determining survival and the aggressiveness of these tumors (Table 109.3). The presence of liver metastases is the single most important prognostic factor.

GENETIC FACTORS

In general, GEPs have not been found to have alterations in common oncogenes (Ras, Myc, Fos, Src, Jun) or common tumor suppressor genes (p53, retinoblastoma susceptibility gene (Table 109.1).[4] Recent studies on GEPs report alterations in the MEN1 gene, p16/MTS1 tumor suppressor gene, DPC 4/Smad 4 gene, amplification of the HER-2/neu proto-oncogene growth factors and their receptor expression, and deletions of unknown tumor suppressor genes as well as gains in other unknown genes (Table 109.3).[4]

DISEASE ASSSOCIATIONS

A number of diseases due to various genetic disorders are associated with an increased incidence of GEPs. The most impor-

TABLE 109.3 PROGNOSTIC FACTORS IN GASTROENTEROPANCREATIC ENDOCRINE TUMORS

I. CLINICAL/LABORATORY/TUMORAL FEATURES
- Presence of liver metastases
- Extent of liver metastases
- Presence of lymph node metastases
- Primary tumor size
- Primary tumor site
- Female gender
- MEN1 syndrome absent
- Markedly increased plasma tumor levels (increased chromogranin A in some studies; gastrinomas – increased gastrin level)

II. VARIOUS HISTOLOGIC FEATURES
- Depth of invasion
- Tumor differentiation
- High growth indices (PCNA expression, high K_i 67 index)
- High mitotic counts
- Vascular or perineural invasion
- Various cytometric features (i.e., aneuploidy)

III. MOLECULAR FEATURES
- Ha-Ras oncogene or p53 overexpression
- Increased HER2/neu expression (P=0.032)
- Loss of heterozygosity at chromosome 1q, 3p, 3q, or 6q (P=0.0004)
- EGF receptor overexpression (P=0.034)
- Gains in chromosome 7q, 17q, 17p, 20q

ant is multiple endocrine neoplasia type 1 (MEN1). MEN1 is an autosomal dominant disorder due to a defect in a 10-exon gene on chromosome 11q13, which encodes for a 610-amino-acid nuclear protein, menin. Patients with MEN1 develop:
- hyperparathyroidism (95–100%);
- GEPs (80–100%);
- pituitary adenomas (54–80%); and
- gastric carcinoids (13–30%).

MEN1 patients develop both nonfunctional PETs (80-100%) and functional GEPs (80%). Of the latter, the commonest clinical syndromes are:
- Zollinger-Ellison syndrome (54%);
- insulinomas (21%);
- glucagonomas (3%); and
- VIPomas (1%).

MEN1 accounts for 20–25% of all patients with Zollinger-Ellison syndrome and 4% of those with insulinomas and a low percentage (<5%) of the other GEPs.

Three phacomatoses are associated with GEPs:
1. von Hippel-Lindau (VHL) disease: characterized by cerebellar hemangioblastomas, renal cancer, and pheochromocytomas, with 10–17% developing a GEP (mostly nonfunctional although insulinomas and VIPomas are reported).
2. von Recklinghausen's disease (NF-1): up to 12% develop an upper gastrointestinal carcinoid, often periampullary commonly classified as somatostatinomas, but rarely associated with insulinomas or Zollinger-Ellison syndrome. Nonfunctional PETs and functional GEPs have been reported.
3. Tuberous sclerosis: nonfunctional PETs and functional GEPs have been reported in a few cases.

DIAGNOSIS AND TREATMENT OF GEP SYNDROMES

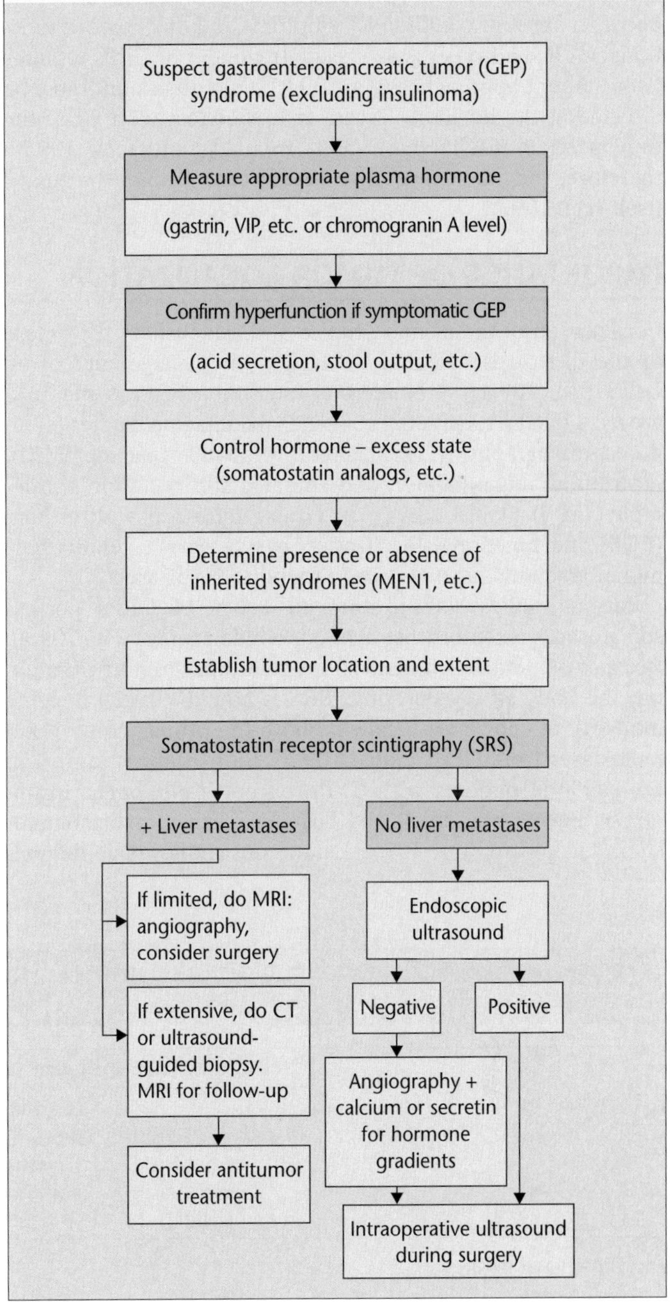

Fig. 109.1 Diagnosis and treatment of GEP syndromes. General approach to diagnosis and treatment of all GEP syndromes except insulinomas (infrequently malignant (<15%) and less frequently localized with somatostatin receptor scintigraphy (SRS) – see Fig. 109.4). For other tumors, SRS is the most sensitive localization technique and allows imaging of the entire body. Endoscopic ultrasound or angiography with venous sampling for hormonal gradients can detect primary tumors in more than 20% of patients who have normal findings at SRS. The identification of liver or distal metastases is important because it is the primary determinant of whether surgical resection should be performed as well as a determinant of prognosis (see Fig. 109.9).

APPROACH TO MANAGEMENT

Functional GEPs usually present clinically with symptoms due to the ectopically secreted hormone. It is not until late in the course of the disease that the tumor *per se* causes symptoms.

In contrast, all of the symptoms caused by nonfunctional PETs are due to the tumor *per se* (Fig. 109.1). The mean delay between onset of continuous symptoms and diagnosis of functional GEP syndromes is 4–7 years. Treatment of GEPs requires two different approaches (Fig. 109.1). First, treatment must be directed at the hormone excess state. Second, with all of the tumors except insulinomas, >50% are malignant (Table 109.2); therefore, treatment must also be directed against the tumor itself (Fig. 109.1).

IMPORTANCE OF TUMOR LOCALIZATION

Localization of the primary tumor and establishing the extent of the disease is essential to the proper management of all GEPs (Fig. 109.1).[5–9] Numerous tumor localization methods are used in GEPs including conventional imaging studies (computed tomography (CT), magnetic resonance imaging (MRI), ultrasound, angiography), and somatostatin receptor scintigraphy (SRS) (Table 109.4). In GEPs, endoscopic ultrasound (EUS) and functional localization by measuring venous hormonal gradients have also been found to be of use.

Recent studies showed that 90–100% of GEPs possess somatostatin receptors that bind octreotide analogs (Fig. 109.2). Because of its sensitivity and ability to localize tumors throughout the body at any one time, SRS is now the initial imaging modality of choice for localizing both the primary tumor and metastases from GEPs (Table 109.4). SRS localizes tumors in 56–100% of patients with GEPs, except insulinomas. Insulinomas are usually small and have low densities of somatostatin receptors (Table 109.4). Numerous studies have demonstrated that SRS has greater sensitivity than conventional imaging studies in localizing both the primary tumor and metastases (Fig. 109.3).[5,7] Occasional false-positive responses with SRS can occur (12% in one study) because numerous normal tissues as well as other diseased tissues can have high densities of somatostatin receptors, including granulomas, thyroid diseases, and activated lymphocytes.[5,10] For GEPs located in the pancreas, endoscopic ultrasound is highly sensitive, localizing 77–94% of insulinomas, which occur almost exclusively within the pancreas (Table 109.4, Fig. 109.4). SRS is also more sensitive at identifying liver metastases, as seen in Fig. 109.3 (middle panels). SRS is also more sensitive than bone scanning (Fig. 109.3, bottom panels) for localizing and assessing the extent of bone metastases from malignant GEPs. Functional localization measuring hormone gradients after intra-arterial calcium injections in insulinomas (insulin) or gastrin gradients after secretin injections in gastrinoma is a sensitive method being positive in 80–100% of patients. However, this method gives only regional localization.

GASTRINOMA (ZOLLINGER-ELLISON SYNDROME; Fig. 109.5)

Pathology and presentation

A gastrinoma is a neuroendocrine tumor secreting gastrin which results in hypergastrinemia causing gastric acid hypersecretion, leading to the Zollinger-Ellison (ZE) syndrome. The gastric acid hypersecretion causes peptic ulcer disease (PUD) which is often refractory and severe, as well as diarrhea. The most common presenting symptoms are abdominal pain

TABLE 109.4 COMPARATIVE ABILITY OF LOCALIZATION METHODS TO IDENTIFY INSULINOMAS AND GASTRINOMAS

	PANCREATIC ENDOCRINE TUMORS			
	Insulinomas	Gastrinomas		
		Sensitivity (%)		Specificity (%)
		Recent NIH studies (mean [range])	Literature (mean [range])	Literature (mean [range])
EXTRAHEPATIC LESIONS				
Ultrasound	27 [10–39]	13 [9–16][c]	23 [0–28]	92 [92–93]
CT scan	30 [0–40]	38 [31–51][c]	38 [0–59]	90 [83–100]
MR imaging	10 [0–25]	40 [30–57][c]	22 [20–25]	100 [100]
Angiography	60 [35–90]	43 [28–57][c]	68 [35–68]	89 [84–94]
SRS	25 [12–50]	69 [58–78]	72 [57–77]	86
Endoscopic ultrasound	89 [71–94]	–	60 [58–100]	95 [84–100]
METASTATIC LIVER DISEASE				
Ultrasound	–[b]	46[c]	14 [14–63]	100
CT scan	–	42[c]	54 [35–72]	99 [94–100]
MR imaging	–	71	63 [43–83]	92 [88–100]
Angiography	–	65[c]	62 [33–86]	98 [96–100]
SRS	–	92	97 [92–100]	90 [90–100]

[a] Mean data [range] are shown.
[b] Metastatic insulinomas are uncommon (<10% of all cases) and there is not sufficient data available for this analysis.
[c] $P < 0.05$ compared to SRS alone.
CT scan, computed tomographic scan; MR imaging, magnetic resonance imaging; SRS, somatostatin receptor scintigraphy.

STRUCTURE OF SOMATOSTATIN AND SYNTHETIC ANALOGS

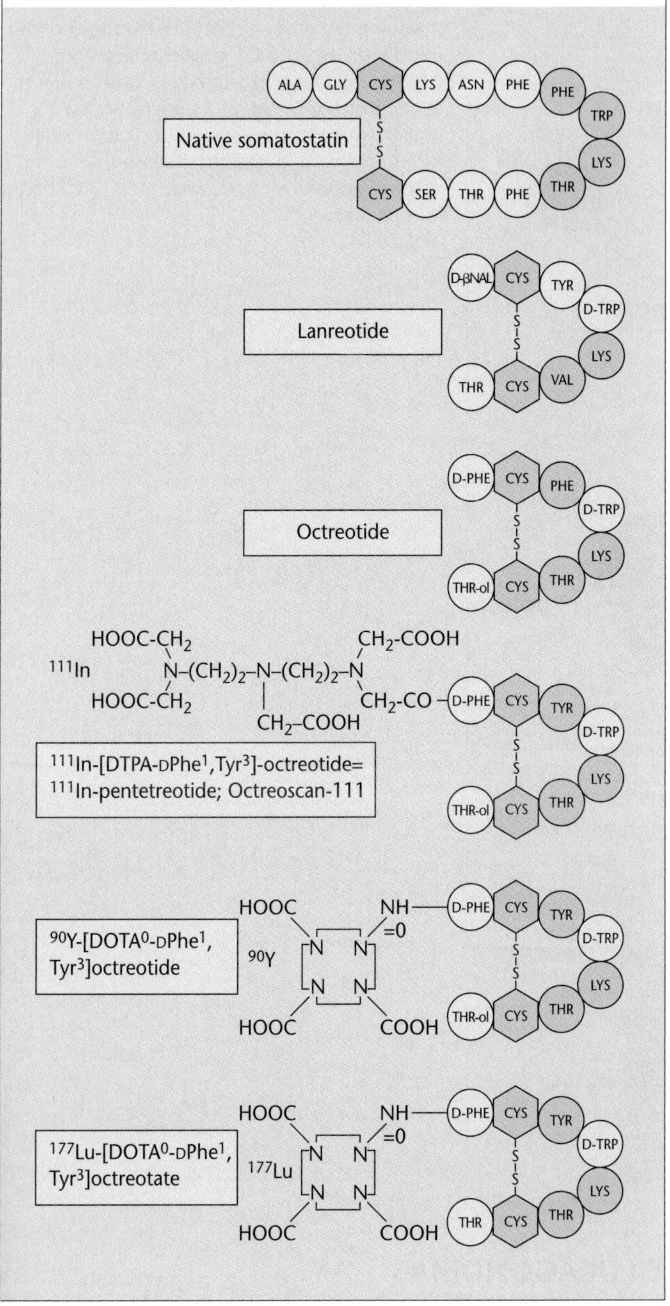

Fig. 109.2 Structure of somatostatin and synthetic analogs. Structure of somatostatin and synthetic analogs used for diagnostic or therapeutic indications.

(70–100%), diarrhea (37–73%), and gastroesophageal reflux disease (GERD) (30–35%). 10–20% have diarrhea only.[11] Most patients have a typical duodenal ulcer. It is important to consider gastrinoma in the context of peptic ulcer:

- with diarrhea;
- in the absence of *Helicobacter pylori* or NSAID use;
- unusual or multiple locations;
- persistent or refractory to treatment;
- prominent gastric folds; and
- findings suggestive of MEN1.

Gastrinomas may also present with chronic unexplained diarrhea alone.

Most gastrinomas (50–70%) are present in the duodenum, followed by the pancreas (20–40%), and other intra-abdominal sites (Fig. 109.6). Rarely, extra-abdominal primaries are found (Fig. 109.6). Sixty to ninety per cent of gastrinomas are malignant (Table 109.2) with metastatic spread to lymph nodes and liver. Distant metastases to bone occur in 12–30% of patients with liver metastases.

Diagnosis

Nearly all patients have an increased fasting plasma gastrin making this the screening test of choice if elevated resting gastric juice should be recovered. A fasting gastrin of >1000 pg/mL (10-fold increase) and resting intragastric pH <2.0 is generally diagnostic of a gastrinoma. In patients who have had a polya partial gastrectomy, the differential diagnosis of a retained antrum syndrome (retained antral mucosa at the tip of the afferent loop) may require investigation by scintigraphy.

Where the intragastric pH is <2 and the gastrin elevation less pronounced (<1000 pg/mL) the differential diagnosis includes *H. pylori* antral G cell hyperplasia/hyperfunction, gastric outlet obstruction or, rarely, renal failure. These patients require determination of basal acid output and a secretin provocative test to identify whether a gastrinoma is present (Fig. 109.5) (see Chapter 131).

Treatment

Gastric acid hypersecretion can nearly always be controlled by proton pump inhibitors once or twice daily, with dose titrated up until control is achieved. H_2-receptor antagonists are also effective but require high and more frequent doses.

More than 50% of the patients that are not cured (>60% of all patients) will die from tumor-related causes. Imaging studies are essential to localize the extent of the tumor. All patients with gastrinomas, without MEN1, should be considered for surgery by a surgeon with specialized experience. In the absence of liver metastases, 60% of such patients achieve short-term and 30% long-term cure.[13] Surgery may also be possible where hepatic metastases are limited. In patients with MEN1, long-term surgical cure is rare.

INSULINOMA (Fig. 109.4)

Pathology and presentation

An insulinoma is an endocrine tumor thought to be derived from beta cells that ectopically secrete insulin, which results in hypoglycemia. A differential diagnosis includes:

- inadvertent or surreptitious use of insulin or oral hypoglycemic agents;
- alcoholism;
- severe liver disease;
- poor nutrition; and
- other extrapancreatic tumors.

The most reliable test is a fast of up to 72 h, which will establish the diagnosis of insulinoma using the following criteria in 98% of patients by 48 h[1–3]:

- blood glucose ≤40 mg/dL;
- serum insulin >6 μU/mL; and
- ratio of insulin to glucose (in mg/dL) >0.3 (Fig. 109.4).

Measurement of pro-insulin levels, C-peptide levels, insulin antibodies, and sulfonylurea levels should enable inadvertent or surreptitious use of insulin or hypoglycemic agents to be distinguished.

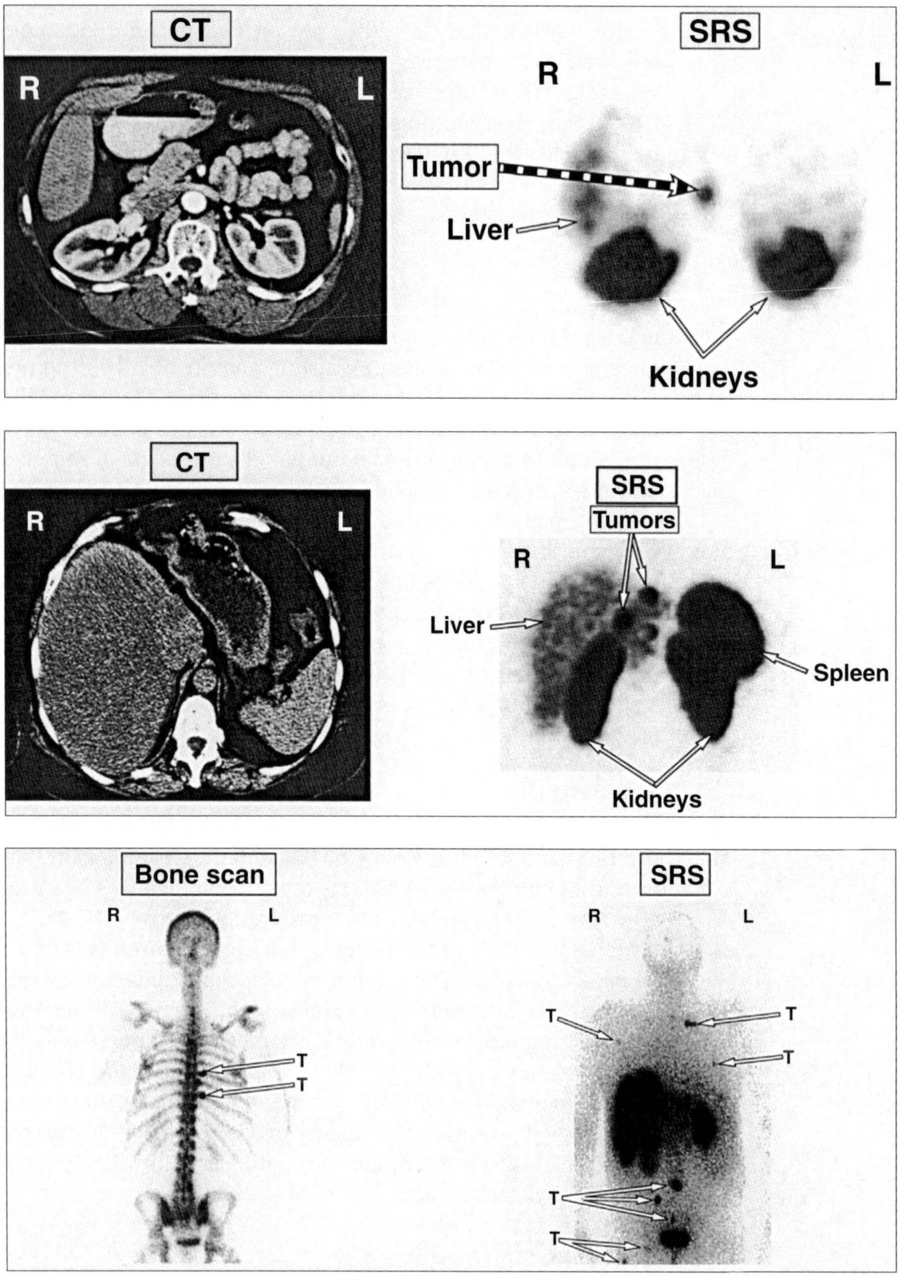

Fig. 109.3 Somatostatin receptor scintigraphy (SRS). Increased sensitivity of SRS in localizing a primary GEP (top), metastatic disease to liver (middle), or to bone (bottom). In the top and middle panels, the CT scan was negative whereas SRS localized tumor in both patients. In the bottom panel, in a patient with a malignant GEP, the SRS demonstrated much more extensive metastatic disease than bone scanning demonstrated, which led to a change in management.

Treatment

Only 5–15% of insulinomas are malignant; therefore, after appropriate imaging (discussed below), surgery should be performed (Fig. 109.4). In results from different studies, 75–95% of patients are cured by surgery. Prior to surgery the hypoglycemia can be controlled by frequent small meals and the use of diazoxide (150–800 mg/day). Approximately 50–60% of patients respond to diazoxide. Other agents that are effective in some patients in controlling the hypoglycemia include verapamil and diphenylhydantoin. Long-acting somatostatin analogs such as octreotide (Fig. 109.2) are acutely effective in 40% of patients. However, octreotide needs to be used with care because it inhibits growth hormone secretion and can alter plasma glucagon levels and therefore in some patients can worsen the hypoglycemia. For the 5–15% of patients with malignant insulinomas the above drugs or somatostatin analogs are initially used. If these are not effective, various antitumor treatments can be used.

GLUCAGONOMAS

Pathology and presentation

A glucagonoma is an endocrine tumor of the pancreas tha[t] secretes excessive amounts of glucagon that causes a distinc[t] syndrome characterized by dermatitis, glucose intolerance, o[r] diabetes and weight loss.[1,2] Glucagonomas principally occu[r] between 45 and 70 years of age. It is clinically characterized b[y] a dermatitis (migratory necrolytic erythema) (67–90%), accompanied by glucose intolerance (40–90%), weight loss (66–96%), anemia (33–85%), diarrhea (15–29%), and thromboembolism (11–24%).[14] The characteristic rash starts usually as an annula[r] erythema at intertriginous and periorificial sites, especially i[n] the groin or buttock. A characteristic laboratory finding i[s] hypoaminoacidemia, which occurs in 26–100% of patients.

Glucagonomas are generally large tumors at diagnosis wit[h] an average size of >5 cm.[14] Fifty to eighty-two per cent hav[e] evidence of metastatic spread at presentation, usually to th[e]

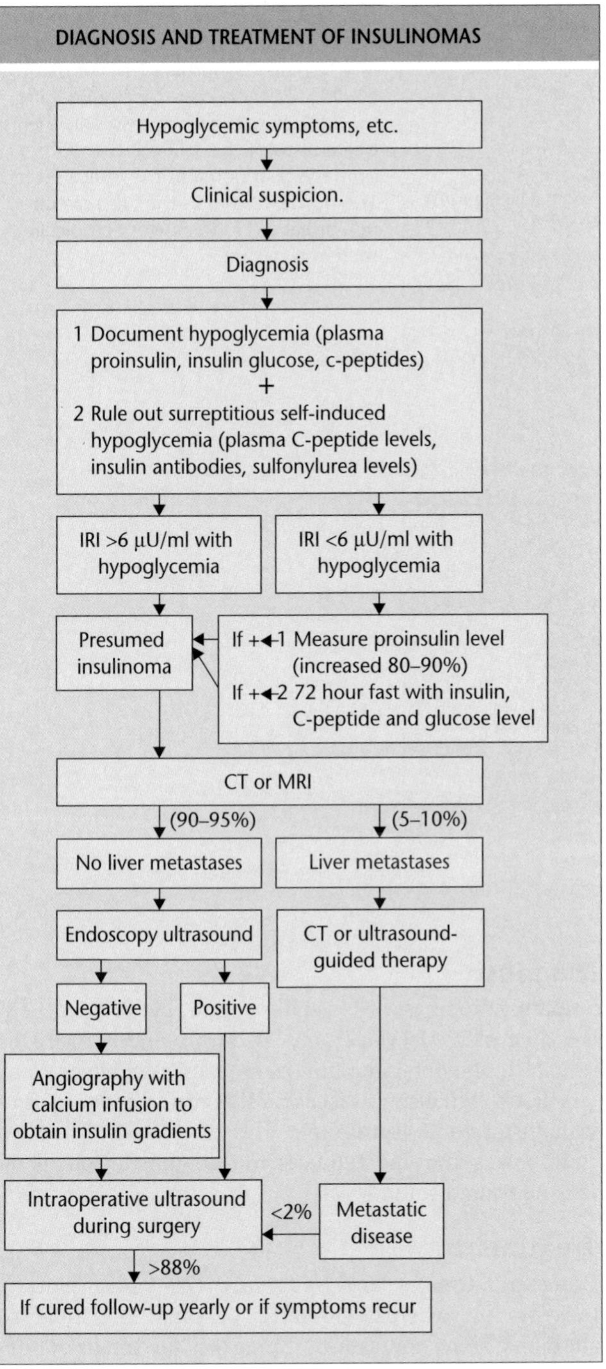

ig. 109.4 Diagnosis and treatment of a patient with insulinomas. Document the hypoglycemia, and rule out other causes (including elf-induced hypoglycemia caused by surreptitious use of insulin or ulfonylureas). The 72-h fast is most commonly used to monitor plasma insulin, glucose, and C-peptide levels. Hypoglycemia with plasma insulin-like immunoreactivity (IRI) >6 μU/mL allows presumed diagnosis of insulinoma. Hypoglycemia with IRI <6 μU/mL requires additional evaluation. Insulinomas are usually benign (90–95% of cases). Malignant cases can be detected with a CT scan or MR imaging for liver metastases. Endoscopic ultrasound (EUS) is more sensitive than other imaging studies for detection of primary insulinomas in 80–95% of cases (Table 109.4). If EUS does not localize the insulinoma, selective intra-arterial injection of calcium with sampling of hepatic veins for insulin concentrations should be performed to localize the insulinoma to the appropriate pancreatic area. Intraoperative ultrasound should be used routinely.

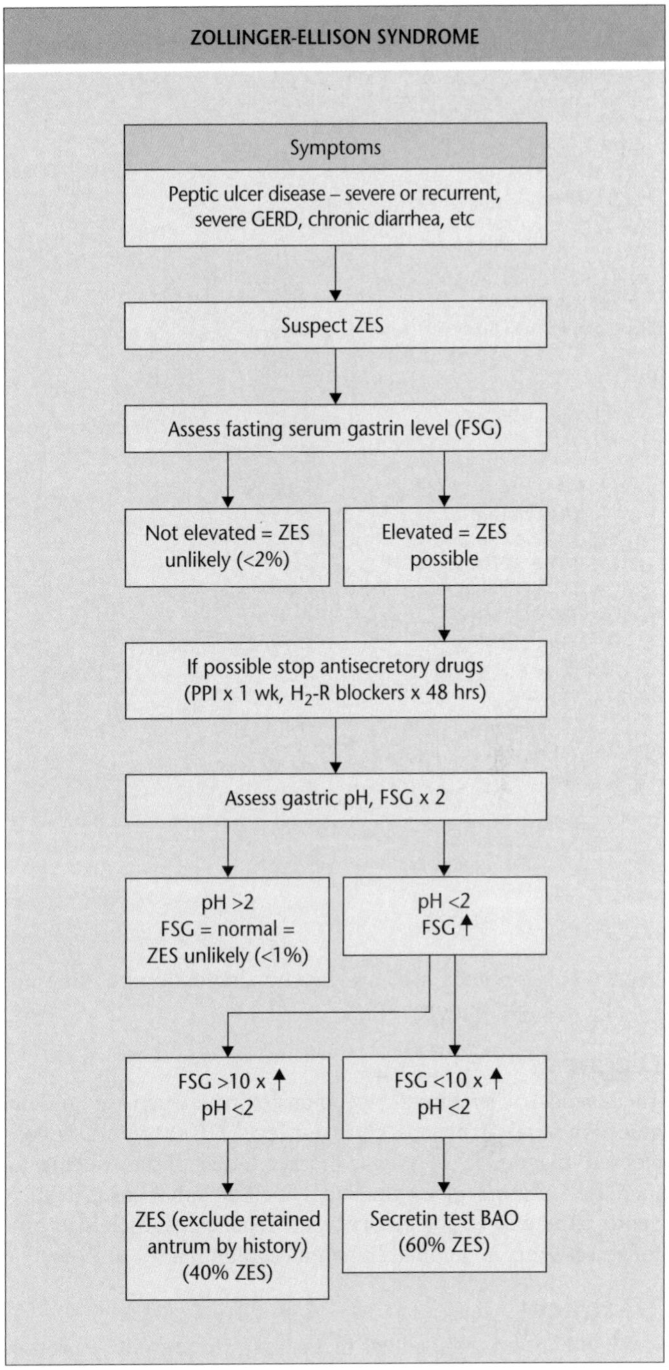

Fig. 109.5 Zollinger-Ellison syndrome (ZES). More than 98% of patients with ZES have an elevated fasting gastrin level (FSG) when first seen. Whereas FSG levels that are normal exclude >98% of ZES patients, increased FSG levels can be due to achlorhydria, to antisecretory drugs, or other causes of hypersecretion (usually <10-fold increased). If the FSG level is increased, evaluate gastric pH off antisecretory drugs (PPIs x 1 week, H_2-receptor blockers x 48 h) if it can be safely done. In a recent large series[12] all ZES patients had a fasting gastric pH <2. A secretin test and assessment of basal acid output (BAO) is necessary to distinguish numerous other conditions that can cause pH <2 and increased FSG (usually <10-fold). Secretin tests are positive in 87% (>200 pg/mL increase) of ZES patients and BAO >15 mEq/h (no gastric surgery) (>5 mEq/h) in >90% of patients.[12]

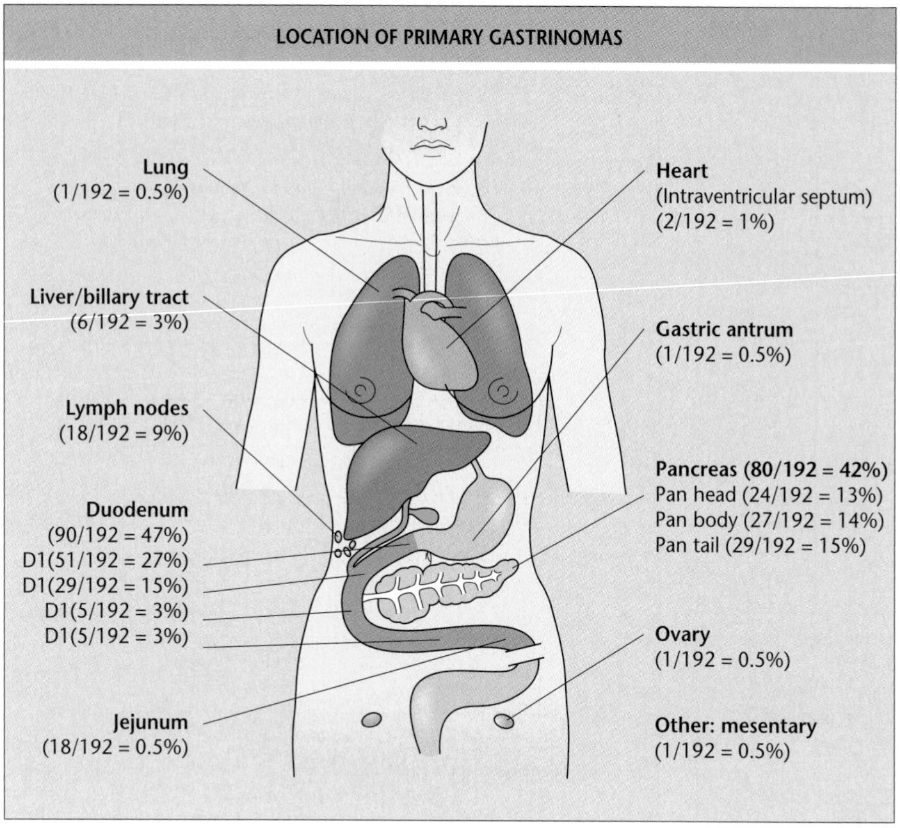

Fig. 109.6 Location of primary gastrinomas. Primary gastrinoma location was determined in 192 patients (surgery (*n*=166), autopsy (*n*=11), or endoscopy biopsy/imaging (*n*=15)). Results are expressed as the percentage of the 192 patients with a primary gastrinoma in the indicated location. The primary listed in the lung occurred in a non-small cell lung cancer ectopically secreting gastrin.

liver. Glucagonomas are rarely extrapancreatic and they are usually a single tumor.

Diagnosis

The diagnosis is confirmed by demonstrating an increased plasma glucagon level. A plasma glucagon level >1000 pg/mL is considered diagnostic of glucagonoma. Other diseases causing increased plasma glucagon levels include renal insufficiency, acute pancreatitis, hypercorticism, hepatic insufficiency, prolonged fasting, or familial hyperglucagonomia.[13]

Treatment

In 50–80% of patients, liver metastases are present at presentation so curative surgical resection is not possible. Surgical debulking in patients with advanced disease or other antitumor treatments may be beneficial. Long-acting somatostatin analogs such as octreotide or lanreotide (Fig. 109.2) improve the skin rash in 75% of patients and may improve the weight loss, pain, and diarrhea, but usually do not improve the glucose intolerance.

SOMATOSTATINOMA SYNDROME

Pathology and presentation

About two-thirds of somatostatinomas (tumors with somatostatin-like immunoreactivity) produce a clinical syndrome (somatostatinoma syndrome) due to excessive somatostatin secretion. Characteristic features are diabetes mellitus, gallbladder disease, diarrhea, and steatorrhea.[1,2]

The mean age at diagnosis is 51 years.

Diagnosis

Somatostatinomas are usually found by accident either at the time of cholecystectomy or during endoscopy. Duodenal somatostatin-containing tumors are increasingly associated with von Recklinghausen's disease. Most of these do not cause the somatostatinoma syndrome. The diagnosis of the somatostatinoma syndrome requires the demonstration of elevated plasma somatostatin levels.

Treatment

Pancreatic tumors are frequently (70–92%) metastatic at presentation whereas 30–69% of small intestinal somatostatinomas have metastases. Surgery is the treatment of choice for those without widespread hepatic metastases. Symptoms in patients with the somatostatinoma syndrome may be improved by octreotide treatment (Fig. 109.2).

VIPOMAS (Fig. 109.7)

Pathology and presentation

VIPomas are endocrine tumors that secrete excessive amounts of vasoactive intestinal peptide (VIP), which causes a syndrome characterized by large-volume diarrhea, hypokalemia, and dehydration.[1,2] This syndrome is also called Verner-Morrison syndrome, pancreatic cholera, and WDHA (watery diarrhea, hypokalemia and achlorhydria) syndrome. The mean age of patients with this syndrome is 49 years; however, it can occur in children. The principal symptoms are large-volume diarrhea (100%) severe enough to cause hypokalemia (80–100%), dehydration (83%), hypochlorhydria (54–76%), and flushing

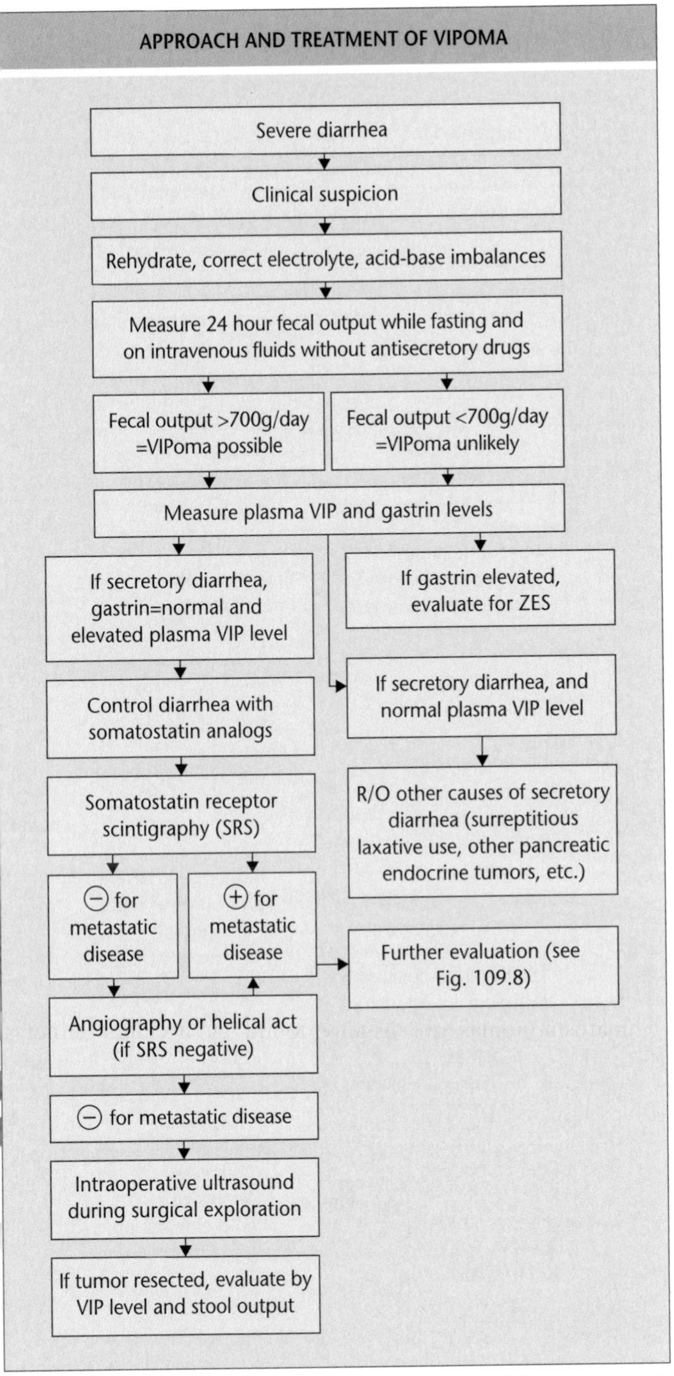

Fig. 109.7 Approach and treatment of a patient with a suspected vasoactive intestinal polypeptide-secreting tumor (VIPoma). VIPomas cause secretory diarrhea >700 g/day. Measure 24-h fecal output after correction of electrolyte or acid-base in fully rehydrated and fasted patient, who is off all antisecretory drugs (octreotide s.c. >1 week, octreotide LAR (>2 months)). Angiography is recommended if SRS is negative prior to surgery because it can detect small liver metastases not imaged by SRS. If metastatic disease is present and unresectable or if no tumor is found, postoperative treatment with long-acting somatostatin analogs (octreotide, lanreotide) should be continued. The dosage should be adjusted to control symptoms. If metastatic disease is present and there is progressive disease or symptoms are not controlled with octreotide, chemotherapy should be considered (see Fig. 109.8).

(20%). The diarrhea is secretory in nature, persisting during fasting, is almost always >1 L/day and in 70% >3 L/day (Fig. 109.7).[1,2,15]

In adults, 80–90% of VIPomas are pancreatic in location with the rest due to VIP-secreting pheochromocytomas, intestinal carcinoids, and rarely ganglioneuromas. These tumors are usually not multiple, 50–75% are in the pancreatic tail and 37–68% have hepatic metastases at diagnosis. In children <10 years old the syndrome is usually due to ganglioneuromas or ganglioblastomas. These are less malignant (10%).

Diagnosis

The diagnosis requires the demonstration of an elevated plasma VIP level and the presence of large-volume diarrhea (Fig. 109.7). A VIPoma is unlikely if stool volume is <700 mL/day. Other diseases that can give a secretory large-volume diarrhea include gastrinomas, chronic laxative abuse, carcinoid syndrome, systemic mastocytosis, rarely medullary thyroid cancer, diabetic diarrhea, and AIDS (Fig. 109.7).[15]

Treatment

The most important initial treatment in these patients is to correct their dehydration and electrolyte losses. Because 37–68% of adults with VIPomas have metastatic disease in the liver at presentation, a significant number of patients cannot be cured surgically. In these patients, long-acting somatostatin analogs such as octreotide or lanreotide (Fig. 109.2) are the drugs of choice. Octreotide will control the diarrhea in 87% of patients. In nonresponsive patients, the combination of glucocorticoids and octreotide has proved helpful in a small number of patients. Other drugs reported to be helpful in small numbers of patients include prednisone (60–100 mg/day), clonidine, indomethacin, phenothiazines, loperamide, lidamidine, lithium, propanolol, and metochlorpramide.

NONFUNCTIONAL PETS

Pathology and presentation

Nonfunctional PETs are endocrine tumors that originate in the pancreas and either secrete no products or their secreted products do not cause a specific clinical syndrome. The symptoms are due entirely to the tumor *per se*. Nonfunctional PETs almost always secrete chromogranin A (90–100%), chromogranin B (90–100%), PP (58%), and alpha-human chorionic gonadotropin (HCG) (40%).[1,2,16,17] Nonfunctional PETs usually present late in their disease course with invasive tumors and hepatic metastases (64–92%) and the tumors are usually large (72% >5 cm).[1,2,16,17] These tumors are usually solitary except in patients with MEN1 where they are multiple. The most common symptoms are abdominal pain (30–80%), jaundice (20–35%), weight loss, fatigue or bleeding, and 10–15% are found incidentally.[1,2,16,17] The average time from the beginning of symptoms to diagnosis is 5 years.[1,2,16,17]

Diagnosis

The diagnosis is only established by histologic confirmation in a patient with a PET without either clinical symptoms or elevated plasma hormone levels of one of the established syndromes (Table 109.2). Plasma pancreatic polypeptide (PP) is increased in 22–71% of patients and should strongly suggest the diagnosis in a patient with a pancreatic mass. Elevated plasma PP is not diagnostic of this tumor because it is elevated in a number of other conditions such as chronic renal failure, old age, inflammatory conditions, and diabetes.

Treatment

Unfortunately, surgical curative resection can be considered only in the minority of the patients because 64–92% present with metastatic disease. Treatment needs to be directed against the tumor *per se* as discussed in the section on advanced disease

RARER TUMORS

GRFomas are endocrine tumors that secrete excessive amounts of growth hormone-releasing factor (GRF) and are therefore an uncommon cause of acromegaly[1,2] that is indistinguishable from classical acromegaly. These are found in lung (47–54%), pancreas (29–30%), small intestine (8–10%), and other sites (12%), presenting at a mean age of 38 years. The pancreatic tumors are usually large (>6 cm) and liver metastases are present in 39%. GRFomas are an uncommon cause of acromegaly. The diagnosis is established by performing plasma assays for GRF and growth hormone. Surgery is the treatment of choice if diffuse metastases are not present. Long-acting somatostatin analogs such as octreotide or lanreotide (Fig. 109.5) are the agents of choice, with 75–100% of patients responding.

OTHER RARE GEPS

Cushing's syndrome (ACTHoma) due to a GEP occurs in 4–16% of all ectopic Cushing's syndrome cases. Paraneoplastic hypercalcemia due to a GEP releasing PTH-RP, a PTH-like material or unknown factor, is rarely reported. The tumors tend to be large and liver metastases are usually present. Most (88%) appear to be due to release of PTH-RP. PETs can occasionally cause the carcinoid syndrome (Table 109.2). PETs secreting calcitonin have recently been proposed as a specific clinical syndrome. One-half of the patients had diarrhea, which disappeared with resection of the tumor. This is classified in Table 109.2 as a possible specific disorder because so few cases have been described. Recently, a renin-producing GEP was described in a patient presenting with hypertension (Table 109.2).[18] Ghrelin is a 28-amino-acid peptide recently described with a number of metabolic effects. In a recent study, only 1 in 24 patients (4%) with a PET had elevated plasma ghrelin levels and the patient was asymptomatic, suggesting no specific syndrome is associated with release of ghrelin by a GEP.

TREATMENT OF ADVANCED (DIFFUSE METASTATIC) DISEASE (Fig. 109.8) (see Chapter 110)

Principles

The single most important prognostic factor for survival is the presence of liver metastases (Table 109.3, Fig. 109.9).[4,19] With gastrinomas the 10-year survival without liver metastases is

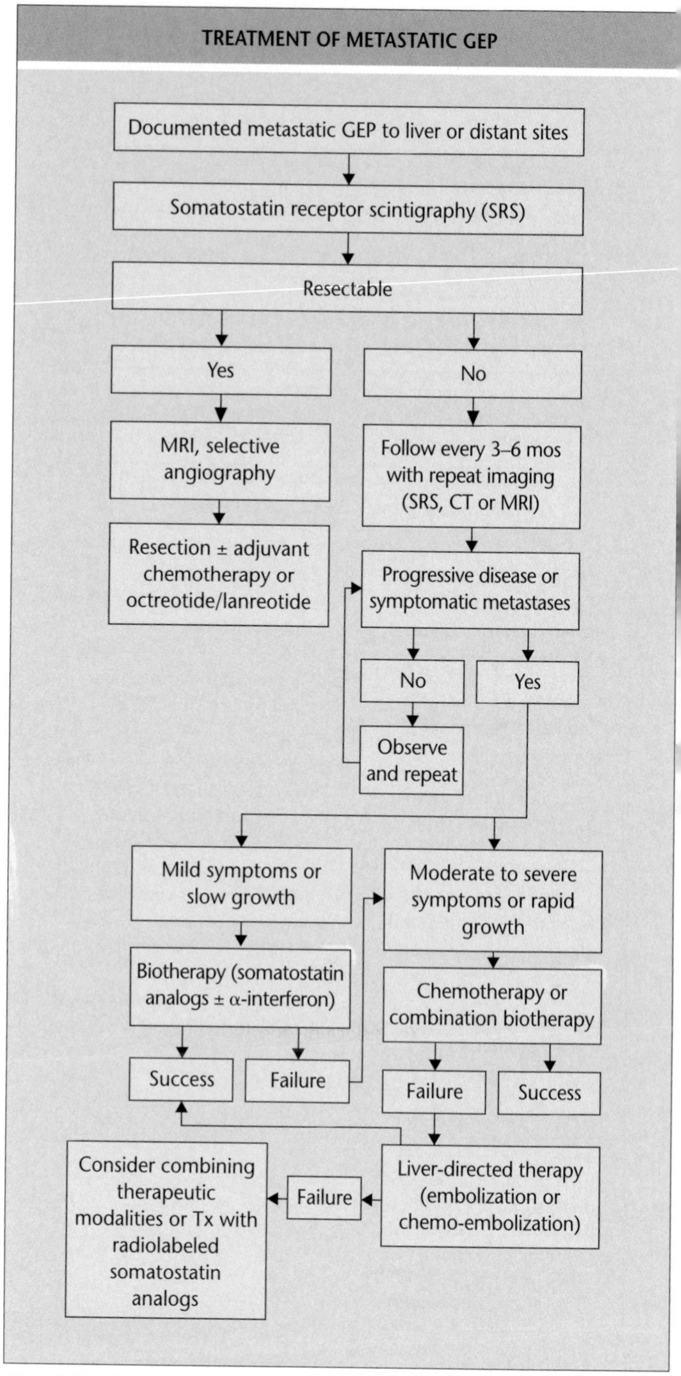

Fig. 109.8 Treatment of a patient with a metastatic GEP. For all GEPs except metastatic insulinomas, recent studies demonstrate that SRS should be the initial tumor localization method because of its greater sensitivity and ability to give a complete body scan. Consider surgical resection by a surgeon with specific expertise if likely morbidity acceptable. MR imaging and selective angiography help to locate liver metastases and detect possible small lesions not imaged on the SRS. If the tumor is not resectable, control symptoms with long-acting somatostatin analog (octreotide or lanreotide) (Fig. 109.2). If tumor growth slow, use somatostatin or alpha-interferon. If growth is rapid or symptoms are not controlled combine somatostatin analogs and alpha-interferon or use chemotherapy. If symptoms or tumor growth are still not controlled and disease is localized to the liver, consider liver-directed antitumor treatments (embolization, chemoembolization). For advanced disease, recent studies suggest treatment with ^{111}In-, ^{90}Y-, or ^{177}Lu-labeled somatostatin analogs may be beneficial.

8%; with limited metastases in one hepatic lobe it is 78%, nd with diffuse metastases, 16% (Fig. 109.9). Therefore, treatment for advanced metastatic disease is important. A number f different modalities are reported to be effective including ytoreductive surgery (removal of all visible tumor), chemotherapy, somatostatin analogs, alpha-interferon, hepatic embolization alone or with chemotherapy (chemo-embolization), radiotherapy, and liver transplantation (Fig. 109.8).

pecific antitumor treatments

Cytoreductive surgery is only possible in 9–22% of patients where there are limited hepatic metastases, though surgery may increase survival (Fig. 109.8).[1,19] Cytotoxic chemotherapy, currently with streptozotocin and doxorubicin[1,2] has been reported to cause tumor shrinkage in 30–70% of patients.

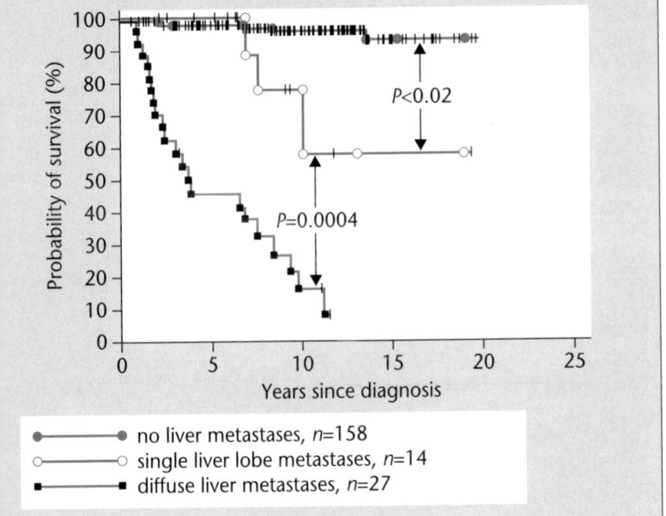

Fig. 109.9 Effect of liver metastases on survival. Survival plotted in the form of Kaplan-Meier for 1999 consecutive patients with gastrinomas followed at the National Institute of Health (NIH).

Octreotide and lanreotide (Figs 109.2 and 109.8) as well as alpha-interferon rarely decrease tumor size but are tumoristatic, stopping further growth in 26–95% of patients, though with an uncertain duration and effect on survival. Hepatic embolization and chemo-embolization (with dacarbazine, cisplatin, doxorubicin, 5-fluorouracil, or streptozotocin) have been reported to decrease tumor bulk and to help control the symptoms of the hormone-excess state.[1,2] These modalities are generally reserved for cases in which treatment with somatostatin analogs, interferon, or chemotherapy fails (Fig. 109.8).

Radiotherapy with radiolabeled somatostatin analogs (Fig. 109.2) that are internalized by the tumors is a new approach that is now being investigated. Three different radionuclides are used. High doses of [^{111}In-DTPA-DPhe^{1}]octreotide, yttrium-90 coupled by a DOTA chelating group to octreotide, or octreotate are used as well as ^{177}lutetium-coupled analogs (Fig. 109.2).[6,8,21,22] Recent studies using treatment with the ^{111}In compounds or ^{177}lutetium compounds caused tumor stabilization in 41% and 40%, respectively, and a decrease in tumor size in 30% and 38%, respectively, of patients with advanced metastatic gastrointestinal GEPs.

Liver transplantation has been abandoned as a treatment of most metastatic tumors to the liver. However, for metastatic NETs it is still a consideration. In a recent review of 103 cases of malignant NETs,[23] the 2- and 5-year survival rates were 60% and 47%, respectively. However, recurrence-free survival was low (<24%). It was concluded that for younger patients with metastatic gastrointestinal neuroendocrine tumors limited to the liver, liver transplantation may be justified.

SOURCES OF INFORMATION FOR PATIENTS AND DOCTORS

http://digestive.niddk.nih.gov/ddiseases/pubs/zollinger/
http://www.rarediseases.org/
http://www.royalfree.org.uk/patientinformation.asp?page=endocrineclinic.htm
http://www.ipsen.ltd.uk/page.php?sid=patients&tid=net&uid=infopack
German:
http://www.insulinoma.net

REFERENCES

1. Alexander RA, Jensen RT. Pancreatic endocrine tumors. In: DeVita VT, Hellman S, Rosenberg SA, eds. Cancer: principles and practice of oncology, 6th edn. Philadelphia: Lippincott Williams & Wilkins; 2001:1788–1813.
2. Metz DC, Jensen RT. Endocrine tumors of the gastrointestinal tract and pancreas. In: Rustgi AK, ed. Gastrointestinal cancers. New York: W.B. Saunders; 2003:681–720.
3. Grant CS. Insulinoma. In: Doherty GM, Skogseid B, eds. Surgical endocrinology. Philadelphia: Lippincott Williams & Wilkins; 2001:345–360.
4. Corleto VD, Delle Fave G, Jensen RT. Molecular insights into gastrointestinal neuroendocrine tumors: importance and recent advances. Dig Liver Dis 2002; 34:668–680.
5. Gibril F, Jensen RT. Diagnostic use of radiolabeled somatostatin analogues in patients with gastroenteropancreatic endocrine tumors. Dig Liver Dis 2004; 36:S106–120.
6. de Jong M, Valkema R, Jamar F et al. Somatostatin receptor-targeted radionuclide therapy of tumors: preclinical and clinical findings. Semin Nucl Med 2002; 32:133–140.
7. Kwekkeboom DJ, Krenning EP. Somatostatin receptor imaging. Semin Nucl Med 2002; 32:84–91.
8. deJong M, Kwekkeboom D, Valkema R et al. Radiolabelled peptides for tumour therapy: current status and future directions. Plenary lecture at the EANM 2002. Eur J Nucl Med Mol Imaging 2003; 30:463–469.
9. van der Lely AJ, de Herder WW, Krenning EP et al. Octreoscan radioreceptor imaging. Endocrine 2003; 20:307–311.
10. Gibril F, Reynolds JC, Chen CC et al. Specificity of somatostatin receptor scintigraphy: a prospective study and the effects of false positive localizations on management in patients with gastrinomas. J Nucl Med 1999; 40: 539–553.
11. Roy P, Venzon DJ, Shojamanesh H, et al. Zollinger-Ellison syndrome: clinical presentation in 261 patients. Medicine 2000; 79(6): 379–411.
12. Roy P, Venzon DJ, Feigenbaum KM et al. Gastric secretion in Zollinger-Ellison syndrome: correlation with clinical expression, tumor extent and role in diagnosis – A prospective NIH study of 235 patients and review of the literature in 984 cases. Medicine (Baltimore) 2001; 80:189–222.
13. Norton JA, Fraker DL, Alexander HR et al. Surgery to cure the Zollinger-Ellison syndrome. N Engl J Med 1999; 341:635–644.
14. Guillausseau PJ, Guillausseau-Scholer C. Glucagonomas: clinical presentation, diagnosis, and advances in management.

In: Mignon M, Jensen RT, eds. Endocrine tumors of the pancreas: recent advances in research and management. Frontiers in Gastrointestinal Research. Basel: S. Karger; 1995:183–193.
15. Jensen RT. Overview of chronic diarrhea caused by functional neuroendocrine neoplasms. Semin Gastrointest Dis 1999; 10:156–172.
16. Hochwald SN, Conlon KC, Brennan MF. Nonfunctional pancreatic islet cell tumors. In: Doherty GM, Skogseid B, eds. Surgical endocrinology. Philadelphia: Lippincott Williams & Wilkins; 2001:361–373.
17. Gullo L, Migliori M, Falconi M et al. Nonfunctioning pancreatic endocrine tumors: a multicenter clinical study. Am J Gastroenterol 2003; 98:2435–2439.
18. Langer P, Bartsch D, Gerdes B et al. Renin producing neuroendocrine pancreatic carcinoma – a case report and review of the literature. Exp Clin Endocrinol Diabet 2002; 110:43–49.
19. Jensen RT. Natural history of digestive endocrine tumors. In: Mignon M, Colombel JF, eds. Recent advances in pathophysiology and management of inflammatory bowel diseases and digestive endocrine tumors. Paris: John Libbey Eurotext; 1999:192–219.
20. Sarmiento JM, Que FG. Hepatic surgery for metastases from neuroendocrine tumors. Surg Oncol Clin North Am 2003; 12:231–242.
21. Valkema R, de Jong M, Bakker WH et al. Phase I study of peptide receptor radionuclide therapy with [In-DTPA]octreotide: The Rotterdam experience. Semin Nucl Med 2002; 32:110–122.
22. Kwekkeboom DJ, Bakker WH, Kam BL et al. Treatment of patients with gastro-entero-pancreatic (GEP) tumours with the novel radiolabelled somatostatin analogue [(177)Lu-DOTA(0),Tyr(3)]octreotate. Eur J Nucl Med Mol Imag 2003; 30:417–422.
23. Lehnert T. Liver transplantation for metastatic neuroendocrine carcinoma. Transplantation 1998; 66:1307–1312.

Chapter 110

The carcinoid syndrome

Eva Tiensuu Janson and Kjell Öberg

KEY POINTS

- Carcinoid syndrome is associated with carcinoid tumors that have metastasized to the liver or retroperitoneal area
- 60% have metastases at diagnosis, and 5-year survival is about 60%
- Midgut carcinoids produce deeper flushing than full gut carcinoids
- Diarrhea can be caused by excess serotonin, obstruction, or mesenteric ischemia
- Urinary 5-hydroxyindoleacetic acid is the first line screening test
- Tumor localization is by computerized tomography, magnetic resonance imaging, positron emission tomography, and scintigraphy
- Management includes surgical resection, radiofrequency ablation, chemotherapy, alpha-interferon, and somatostatin analogs

INTRODUCTION

The carcinoid syndrome was first described in 1954. Although the presence of serotonin producing midgut carcinoid tumors was recognized earlier, the association between the slowly growing tumor of the small intestine and the carcinoid syndrome including facial flushing, diarrhea, right-sided heart failure because of valvular disease, and bronchial constriction had not been made. This syndrome usually develops in patients with carcinoid tumors of the small intestine with liver metastases. Only in rare cases is the syndrome associated with a carcinoid tumor of the lung or other locations.

Hormones secreted from the tumor cells are believed to induce the symptoms. These symptoms may be severe enough to prevent the patient from carrying out daily activities. In some cases, the syndrome can become life threatening and a carcinoid crisis develops with severe flushing and diarrhea accompanied by bronchial constriction and hypotension. Since most patients can be treated successfully the recognition of the syndrome by clinicians is important. As this is a rare disease patients should be referred to specialist centers where highly competent multidisciplinary care can be given so that patients can experience long-term survival with a good quality of life.

EPIDEMIOLOGY

The overall incidence of carcinoid tumors is 1–2 cases per 100 000 people. However, in autopsy material, incidences of up to 8.4 per 100 000 people have been reported.[1] The male to female ratio is close to 1:1 and the median age at diagnosis is about 60 years.

In a large series of over 13 000 patients with carcinoid syndrome in the US between 1950 and 1999, two-thirds had their primary tumor in the gastrointestinal tract and one-fourth in the tracheobronchopulmonary area.[2] Of those with gastrointestinal tumors, 42% were in the small bowel and about half in the ileum. These statistics are compromised by the inclusion of duodenal tumors, which are usually gastrinomas rather than true carcinoids. More than 60% of the patients already had metastases at diagnosis, and the 5-year survival was 60%.

PATHOGENESIS AND PATHOLOGY

Enterochromaffin cells in the small intestine belong to the APUD (amino precursor uptake and decarboxylation) system (see Chapter 109). These cells have the ability to take up and decarboxylate amino acid precursors of biogenic amines such as serotonin and catecholamines (Fig. 110.1). It is from these cells located in the crypts of Lieberkuhn that classical midgut carcinoid tumors arise. Enterochromaffin cells can reduce silver salts, hence the tumors were previously called argentaffinomas; they are identified by Masson's staining. Today the histopathological diagnosis is based on immunohistochemistry with antibodies against chromogranin A and serotonin (Fig. 110.2).[3] Other characteristics of midgut carcinoid tumors include the presence of VMAT-1 (vesicular membrane amino acid transporter 1) and synaptophysin expressed in the tumor cells.

The histological growth patterns of midgut carcinoid tumors can be classified as insular, trabecular, glandular, undifferentiated, and mixed. The different growth patterns may represent different biological behavior but the exact implication still remains to be elucidated.

CLINICAL PRESENTATION

Most patients suffering from a carcinoid tumor present with facial flushing and diarrhea, which indicates the presence of a carcinoid syndrome (Table 110.1). The syndrome develops in patients with liver metastases as well as in patients with retroperitoneal metastases and is induced by biologically active amines and peptides produced by the tumor.[4] When metastases develop in the liver or retroperitoneal area the secretory products released from the tumor escape the liver metabolism and may appear undegraded in the circulation.

Flushing is typically restricted to the face and upper thorax, but can be even more extended in severe cases. Usually, the flush has a short duration of up to a few minutes and is most frequent in the morning. It may be induced by alcohol, physical or psychological stress, and spicy food. The flush is thought to be caused by vasoactive peptides produced by the tumor cells.[5] These peptides belong to the tachykinin family and

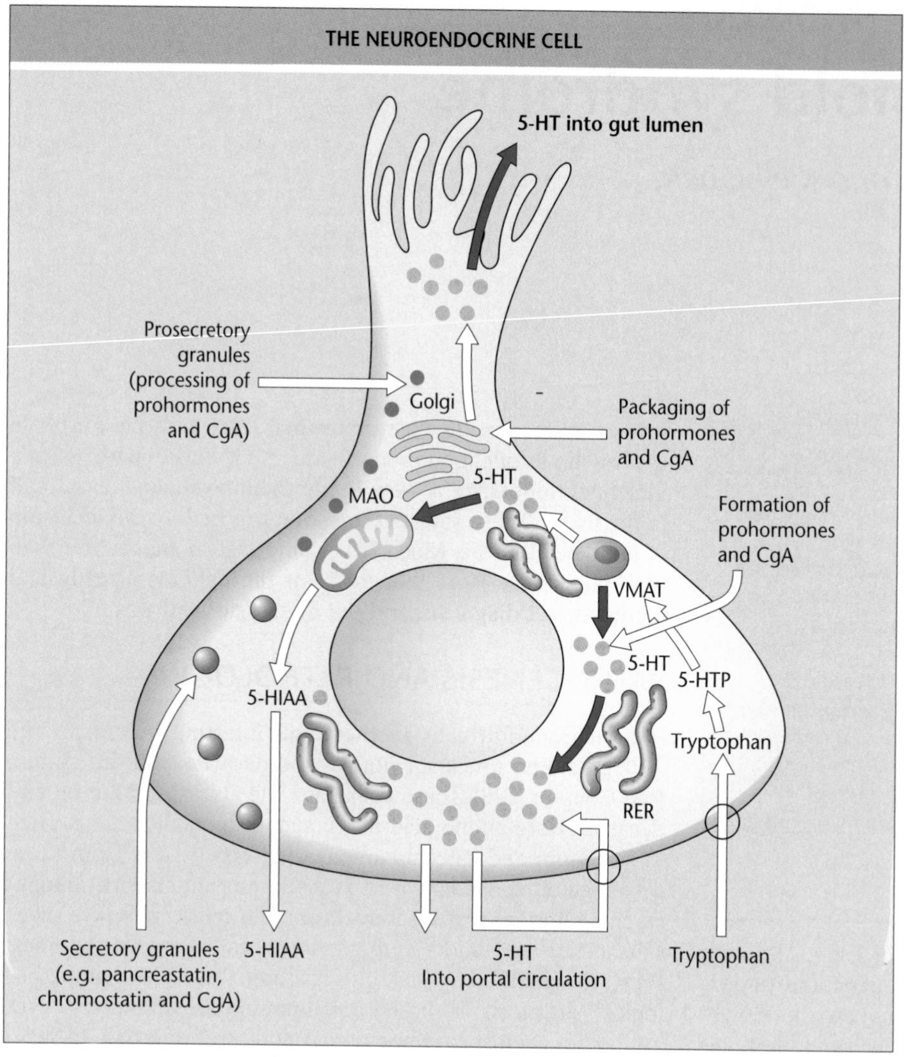

Fig. 110.1 The neuroendocrine cell. The neuroendocrine cell has the ability to take up amino acids such as tryptophan from the circulation. The amino acid precursor is processed in the cell to produce serotonin, which is stored together with chromogranin A (CgA) in the secretory granules until release back into the circulation. 5-HT, 5-hydroxytryptamine; 5-HIAA, 5-hydroxyindole acetic acid; 5-HTP, 5-hyroxytryptophan; VMAT, vesicular membrane amino acid transporter; RER, rough endoplasmic reticulum.

include substance P and neuropeptide K. The flush associated with a midgut carcinoid tumor is usually deep red as opposed to the flush that develops in patients with histamine-producing foregut carcinoid tumors. The histamine-induced flush has a bright red color. These patients also usually suffer from increased lacrimation and salivation together with a swollen face. In midgut carcinoid patients with long-standing disease, the flush may become chronic and the patient can lose the ability to recognize their flushes. Those patients can also present with facial telangiectasia caused by years of more or less constant flushing.

The diarrhea is typically most frequent in the morning. However, some patients may have diarrhea throughout the day and even during the night. This may be the most difficult symptom to handle for the patient and it is also the symptom that most frequently brings the patient to the doctor. Some patients can suffer from 10 to 15 bowel actions daily making it almost impossible to carry out daily activities. Other patients may only have noticed a slight change in the consistency of the stools. The diarrhea may be associated with loss of weight. The hormone thought to induce diarrhea is serotonin.[6]

Diarrhea in carcinoid patients may also have other causes, including tumor growth with intestinal obstruction. These patients usually have pain in association with their diarrhea. Pain and diarrhea may also be due to mesenteric ischemia due to involvement of the mesenteric artery (see below). In these patients, the diarrhea is typically worse after meals and associated with loss of weight and abdominal pain.

Symptoms of right-sided heart failure may also bring the patient to the doctor.[7] These patients usually have had their carcinoid tumor for many years. They may have suffered from flushing and diarrhea for a long period of time without seeking medical care. The valves of the right side of the heart are affected in most patients, while only a minority shows involvement of the valves in the left side of the heart. Tricuspid regurgitation is most common, often combined with tricuspid stenosis and/or pulmonary stenosis or regurgitation. The patient suffers

TABLE 110.1 THE CARCINOID SYNDROME

Symptom	Frequency	Causative agent
Flushing	85–90%	Tachykinins
Diarrhea	70%	Serotonin
Bronchial constriction	15%	Histamine
Carcinoid heart disease	30%	Unknown

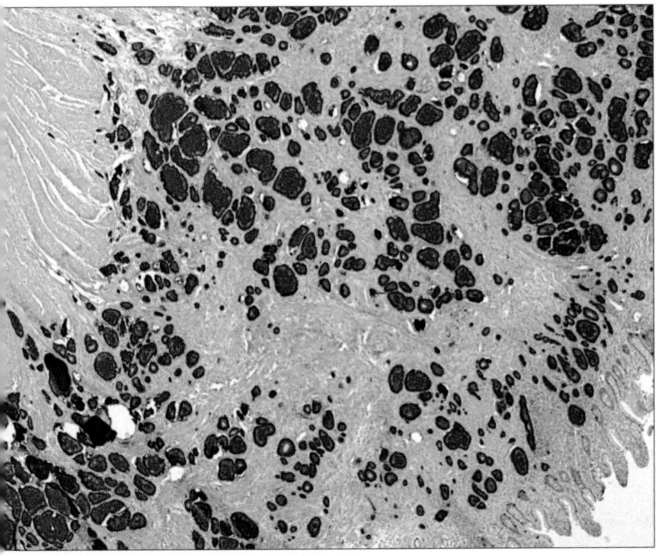

g. 110.2 **Chromogranin A staining.** A tumor specimen showing an sular growth pattern from a patient with a midgut carcinoid tumor nmunostained for chromogranin A.

om dyspnea and may present with edema as a sign of right-ded heart failure. There is a correlation between pretreatment rinary 5-hydroxyindoleacetic acid and heart disease, though is may only be an indicator of a more advanced disease. evertheless, tachykinins have been proposed to induce carci-oid heart disease, but this remains unproven.

Bronchial wheezing is observed in about 15% of patients ith midgut carcinoid tumors. If this is the most prominent ymptom the patient is often misdiagnosed as having asthma.

Abdominal pain is not a part of the carcinoid syndrome, but ay be one of the most important symptoms of a midgut arcinoid tumor. In some patients, complete or partial intes-nal obstruction may be the cause of pain and in these patients cute operation may reveal the tumor. Apart from intestinal bstruction caused by the primary tumor in the small intes-ne, ischemia may also induce severe pain in some patients. ypically, a mesenteric lymph node grows around the mesen-eric artery, strangling the blood flow. This may cause ischemia the intestine and give rise to both pain and diarrhea (see hapter 59). The pain is usually worse after meals. In some atients the ischemia is accompanied by malabsorption and eight loss. These patients should always be evaluated by a irgeon since surgery may improve the patient's status.

IFFERENTIAL DIAGNOSIS

Iany patients presenting with diarrhea as part of a carcinoid yndrome are misdiagnosed as suffering from infectious diar-nea or inflammatory bowel disease.

acial flushing

ther possible causes need to be considered including:

- Food intake and medication (see Table 110.2).
- The menopausal flushing usually involves the whole body with concomitant sweating.
- Important mediators might be calcitonin gene-related peptide (CGRP), histamine, serotonin, and tachykinins.

TABLE 110.2 FLUSHING RELATED TO DRUGS

- Bromocriptin
- Tamoxifen
- Nicotinic acid
- Opiates
- Calcium channel blockers
- Metronidazole
- Ketoconazole
- Chlorpromazine
- Cephalosporin

- Medullary carcinoma of the thyroid may cause slight facial flushing because of CGRP, calcitonin, or prostaglandins.
- High levels of vasoactive intestinal peptide produced in Verner-Morrison syndrome may cause a bluish-red whole body flush because of vasodilatation.
- Gastrin-producing tumors in Zollinger-Ellison syndrome may cause flushing.
- Mastocytosis is a rare disease of mast cell proliferation that occurs both cutaneously and systemically. The mast cell granule contains histamine, heparin, and arachidonic acid, which are metabolized to prostaglandin PGD_2.

DIFFERENTIAL DIAGNOSIS

- Menopausal flushing
- Carcinoid syndrome
- Mastocytosis
- Pheochromocytoma
- Medullary thyroid carcinoma
- Endocrine pancreatic tumors (VIP, gastrin)
- Spinal cord injury
- Emotional flushing
- Alcohol and drugs
- Food related

DIAGNOSTIC METHODS

Clinical history and a physical examination are often helpful. Measurement of the serotonin metabolite 5-hydroxyindole acetic acid (U-5HIAA) in 24-h urine is the most frequently used biochemical marker. However, levels may be normal (Table 110.3) and elevated[8] levels of plasma chromogranin A

TABLE 110.3 NUMBER OF PATIENTS WITH ELEVATED TUMOR MARKER

Tumour marker	No. elevated/No. tested	%
U-5HIAA	187/246	76
Chromogranin A	75/86	87
Neuropeptide K	69/149	46

Patients were measured at their first visit to a referral center (data from Janson ET et al. Carcinoid tumors: analysis of prognostic factors and survival in 301 patients from a referral center. Ann Oncol 1997; 8:685–690)

and, in patients with severe flushing, neuropeptide K can be helpful. The diagnosis is confirmed by chromogranin A and serotonin immunoreactivity in tumor cells on histopathology. Ki67 immunostaining, a measure of proliferation, helps to identify more aggressive tumors.

Tumor localization and spread can be evaluated by radiology, e.g., contrast enhanced computerized tomography (CT) and magnetic resonance imaging (MRI).[9] Abdominal ultrasonography is useful to guide a needle biopsy from liver metastases.

More than 95% of midgut carcinoid tumors express somatostatin receptors, which can be detected by scintigraphy using radiolabeled somatostatin analogs (Fig. 110.3). The method can guide treatments since patients expressing receptors usually respond to treatment with somatostatin analogs. Somatostatin receptor scintigraphy also helps in planning surgery by giving accurate information about distant metastasis, e.g., bone or supraclavicular lymph nodes (Fig. 110.4).[10]

Positron emission tomography (PET) is another imaging technique that can be used to characterize both metabolic and biochemical features in tumor disease (Fig. 110.5). Unlike most cancer cells, neuroendocrine tumors do not have increased glucose metabolism, so ^{18}F-fluoro-2-deoxy-D-glucose PET scanning is not useful. ^{11}C labeled 5-hydroxytryptophan (^{11}C-5-HTP) is very sensitive in localizing small primary tumors and metastases and is superior to CT.[11]

TREATMENT AND PREVENTION

Interventional treatments

Surgery

Surgical treatment should always be considered for patient with midgut carcinoid tumors. Curative surgery is seldor possible except in cases where the tumors cause complet intestinal obstruction leading to acute operation before distar metastases have occurred. However, debulking surgery shoul always be considered since reduction of tumor mass ma improve the quality of life as well as prolong survival for th patient.[12] Resection of the tumor in the small intestine shoul always be considered since many patients have or develo abdominal pain related to the primary tumor. Many patient with midgut carcinoid tumors also have a mesenteric metas tasis that grows around the mesenteric artery resulting i impairment of blood flow to the intestine. This mesenteri metastasis may give rise to severe problems with both pai and diarrhea because of intestinal ischemia, and should there fore be removed whenever possible. Resection of liver metas tases should also be considered in all patients in order t reduce tumor burden.

Liver embolization is also used to treat liver metastases Since the liver has a dual blood supply, vascular occlusion o the hepatic artery that supplies the carcinoid metastases ca induce necrosis of branch tumor cells, leaving the norma

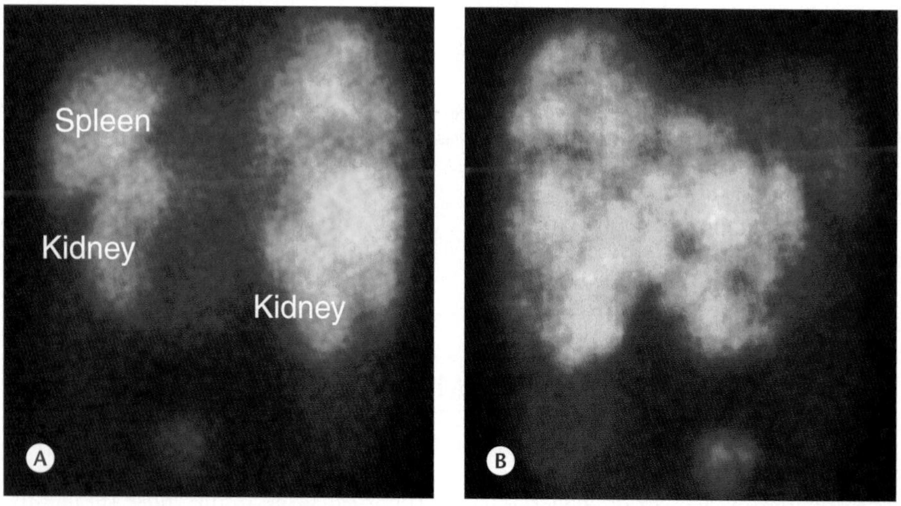

Fig. 110.3 Somatostatin receptor scintigraphy. Somatostatin receptor scintigraphy showing intense uptake of liver metastases in a patient with a midgut carcinoid tumor. **A.** Dorsal view; **B.** frontal view.

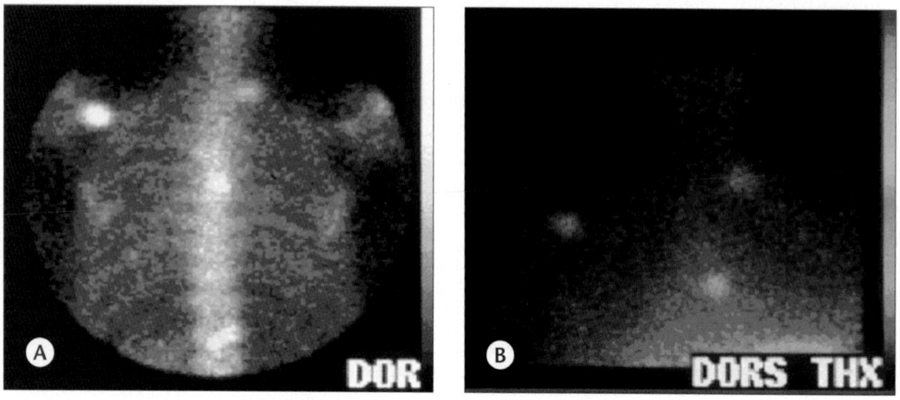

Fig. 110.4 Detection of bone metastases. **A.** A bone scintigram and **B.** somatostatin receptor scintigraphy (octreoscan) showing bone metastases in a patient with a midgut carcinoid tumor. There is a good correlation between the two methods in detecting the bone metastases.

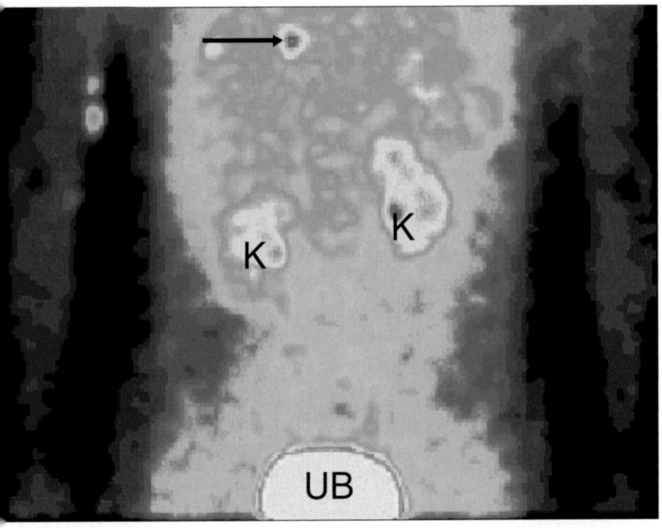

ig. 110.5 Positron emission tomography. Positron emission ›mography with ^{11}C-5-hydroxytryptophan as tracer showing the ›calization of liver metastases in a patient with a midgut carcinoid ımor. This patient had radical surgery 5 years earlier and showed ıcreasing tumor markers. Conventional radiology could not localize ıe recurrence, while the PET examination revealed the metastatic ›cation (arrow). K, kidney; UB, urinary bladder.

epatic parenchyma depending on the portal vein for blood upply with only limited damage. Most patients undergoing ver embolization develop a 'postembolization syndrome,' ıcluding abdominal pain, fever, nausea, and transient increase f liver enzymes. In some patients, the outflow of hormones rom the necrotic tumor cells may induce a carcinoid crisis and his may be prevented by continuous infusion of somatostatin nalogs in the postembolization period. To avoid development f a hepatorenal syndrome, forced diureses should be carried ut until liver enzymes fall to normal levels. Other severe omplications reported in clinical trials include ischemic ecrosis of the gallbladder and the small bowel, gastro-ıtestinal bleeding, duodenal and gastric ulcers, sepsis, hepatic bscesses, and thromboembolic complications. In clinical trials, the biochemical response rate is about 40–50% while up to 40% of patients show a significant decrease in tumor size.[13] The responses usually last for 10–12 months. After this time period, collaterals have developed. However, the procedure can be repeated although the effect may decrease with the number of embolizations performed.

Radiofrequency (RF) ablation has recently been incorporated into the treatment arsenal for patients with neuroendocrine tumors. RF induces frictional heating of the tumor resulting in coagulation and necrosis. Treatment can be performed either during surgery or percutaneously. The method is very promising but the place for this treatment modality still has to be established in clinical studies.[14]

Liver transplantation has been performed in some centers, with varying results. There are reports with long-term postoperative survival in at least a subpopulation of patients with midgut carcinoid tumors. However, it is of utmost importance to make a careful preoperative evaluation to exclude metastases outside the liver before transplantation is performed.[15]

Patients with carcinoid heart disease should be considered for heart surgery with replacement of the affected valves. The timing of heart surgery should be carefully monitored and it is recommended that the carcinoid syndrome be under control before the operation.

Drug therapy

Since most patients cannot be cured by surgery, medical treatment has to be used. Cytotoxic chemotherapy has not been shown to be very effective. There are several studies using single agents, but all of these show poor results with few biochemical and tumor size responses. Different combinations have also been utilized and the most frequently studied combination is streptozotocin and 5-fluorouracil[2] but in a randomized trial no obvious benefit was detectable in comparison to alpha-interferon.[16] Other combinations have been shown to be equally poor and chemotherapy should not be used for midgut carcinoid patients (see Table 110.4). There is a definite need for new and more effective cytotoxic agents for these patients.

TABLE 110.4 CYTOTOXIC THERAPY IN CARCINOID TUMORS

Drug	Dose, regimen	No. patients	OR (%)	Median duration (months)
SINGLE AGENTS				
Doxorubicin	60 mg/m^2 q. 3–4 w	81	21	6
5-FU	500 mg/m^2 x 5 d q. 5 w	30	17–26	3
Streptozotocin	500–1500 mg/m^2/d x 5 d q. 5 w	14	0–17	2
Dacarbacine	250 mg/m^2/d x 5 d q. 4–5 w	15	13	4.5
Cisplatin	45–90 mg/m^2 q. 3–4 w	16	6	4.5
COMBINATIONS				
Streptozotocin	500 mg/m^2/d x 5 q. 3–6 w	175	7–33	3–7
+ 5-FU	400 mg/m^2/d x 5 q. 3–6 w			
Streptozotocin	1000 mg/m^2/w for 4 w	10	40	5
+ Doxorubicin	25 mg/m^2/w then q. 2 w			
Streptozotocin	500 mg/m^2 /d q. 6 w	24	39	6.5
+ Cyclophosphamide	100 mg/m^2 once q. 3 w			
Etoposide	130 mg/m^2/d x 3 d q. 4 w	13	0	–
+ Cisplatin	45 mg/m^2/d x 2 d q. 4 w			

Alpha-interferon is used in the treatment of carcinoid tumors. It is thought to inhibit cell proliferation and induce immune cell-mediated cytotoxicity. However, the exact mechanism active in tumor treatment still remains to be elucidated. Apart from the antiproliferative effect, alpha-interferon may also have an antiangiogenic effect, which may be of importance in antitumor treatment.

The dose of alpha-interferon should be individually titrated and most patients receive 3–5 MU 3 days per week. In trials using higher doses, treatment outcome did not improve, while the side effects became intolerable.[17] The leukocyte count may be used to monitor the alpha-interferon treatment – to have a good clinical effect the leukocyte count should be below 3. If the leukocyte count falls below 2 the dose of alpha-interferon should be reduced. Since the doses that are effective are rather low, the patients can continue with treatment for many years.

In clinical trials using alpha-interferon, biochemical responses have been shown in up to 66% of the patients.[18] However, the response rate varies among studies (Table 110.5). The same is true for the radiological response rates, which may vary between 0% and 25%. In a large study including 111 patients with midgut carcinoid tumors, 42% showed a biochemical response and 16% had a significant reduction in tumor size.[19]

The most frequent adverse reactions include tiredness and depression, for which antidepressant drugs are used with good results. Another problem with alpha-interferon treatment is the development of autoimmune reactions.[20] In one study, almost 20% of patients with midgut carcinoid tumors treated with alpha-interferon developed some kind of autoimmune reaction. The most frequently affected organ is the thyroid, but severe autoimmune disorders including systemic lupus erythematosus and vasculitis may occur. In most patients the symptoms disappear when alpha-interferon treatment is interrupted. The frequencies of different autoimmune side effects are summarized in Table 110.6. Development of interferon antibodies is observed during treatment with recombinant alpha-interferon. However, only high titers of neutralizing antibodies seem to be of importance for the clinical response to interferon treatment.

Alpha-interferon also depresses bone marrow function with anemia, leukocytopenia, and thrombocytopenia. The anemia may play a role in the tiredness experienced by many patients treated with alpha-interferon. Even though there is a decrease in leukocyte count the patients are not at a higher risk than others for developing infections. Instead, most patients report fewer viral infections than the rest of the family members indicating a protective effect of alpha-interferon.

TABLE 110.6 A SUMMARY OF AUTOIMMUNE REACTIONS DURING ALPHA-INTERFERON TREATMENT

Reaction	Frequency
Binding antibodies against interferon-alpha 2a	45%
Neutralizing antibodies against interferon-alpha 2a	38%
High titers	28%
Binding antibodies against interferon-alpha 2b	51%
Neutralizing antibodies against interferon-alpha 2b	17%
High titers	4%
Development of autoantibodies during therapy	
Microsomal thyroid antigen or thyroglobulin	8%
Antinuclear antibodies	14%
Thyroid disease (autoimmune hyper/hypothyreosis)	13%
Pernicious anemia	3%
Vasculitis	1.5%
Systemic lupus erythematosus	0.7%

Somatostatin is a peptide hormone that acts on specific membrane receptors for which five different subtypes have been identified. The biological effect of somatostatin comprises inhibition of hormone secretion, inhibition of exocrine pancreatic function, and apoptotic and antiangiogenic effects among others. The expression of somatostatin receptors on tumor cells forms the target for somatostatin analog treatment.[21] The analogs available for clinical use (octreotide and lanreotide) bind with high affinity to receptor subtypes 2 and 5, which are thought to mediate inhibition of hormone secretion. Somatostatin analogs can reduce hormone release by between 27% and 75%[22] (Table 110.7) reducing symptoms and improving quality of life. Unfortunately, fewer patients (<10%) show a significant reduction in tumor size, although higher doses may be more effective. In a small trial of high dose of lanreotide tumor size was reduced in 30% of the patients.[23] Patients who fail to respond to one somatostatin analog may respond to the other. Initially, short-acting somatostatin analogs requiring 2–3 injections per day were used. The advent of long-acting compounds allowing monthly injections has been a significant advance.

Treatment with somatostatin analogs is usually well tolerated. Initial side effects include nausea and a mild abdominal pain but these symptoms usually decline with time. Since somatostatin inhibits the secretion of pancreatic juice, replacement therapy with pancreatic enzymes may be needed in order to avoid diarrhea due to steatorrhea. Other side effects include

TABLE 110.5 EFFECT OF ALPHA-INTERFERON ON MIDGUT CARCINOID TUMORS

Author (year)	No. patients	Biochemical response (%)	Subjective response (%)	Tumor volume response (%)
Moertel (1989)	27	39	65	20
Schober (1992)	16	66	85	25
Öberg (1991)	111	42	68	15
Joensuu (1992)	14	50	56	0
Bajetta (1993)	34	24	26	12
Biesma (1992)	20	60	83	11

TABLE 110.7 EFFECT OF SOMATOSTATIN ANALOGS ON MIDGUT CARCINOID TUMORS

uthor (year)	Regimen	Biochemical response (%)	Symtomatic response (%)	Radiological response (%)
CTREOTIDE				
vols (1986)	150μg x 3/d	72	88	0
berg (1991)	50μg x 2/d	27	50	9
rnold (1996)	200μg x 3/d	33	–	0
CTREOTIDE LONG-ACTING RELEASE				
arland (2003)	20 mg every 4 w	–	85	0
OMATULINE				
nthony (1993)	3000μg x 3/d	72	–	50
OMATULINE PROLONGED RELEASE				
uszniewski (1996)	30 mg every 2 w	42	55	0
ymenga (1999)	30 mg every 1–2 w	27	54	8
icci (2000)	30 mg every 2 w	42	70	8

evelopment of gallbladder stones or sludge. Bradycardia has en observed in a few patients treated with somatostatin alogs and glucose levels should be monitored since somatoatin affects the secretion of both insulin and glucagons and nsequently may affect blood glucose levels.

The combination of somatostatin analogs and alpha-interferon s been used in several clinical trials. The combination can be ed if either therapy proves to be ineffective, and may induce new biochemical and symptomatic response in more than)% of the patients. In one recent study, the effect of the mbination on tumor growth was evaluated.[24] The combinaon could induce stabilization of tumor size in about 60% of e patients even though all were in a progressive state when e study was initiated (see Table 110.8).

During the last decade, tumor targeting treatment using radiobeled somatostatin analogs has been included in the theraeutic arsenal for patients with neuroendocrine tumors. Several nall studies have been reported using octreotide labeled with fferent isotopes including ^{111}In and ^{90}Y and both biochemical d radiological responses are observed (Table 110.9).[25] Recently, other isotope, ^{177}Lu, has been introduced. New trials have to e performed in order to establish the exact role of this treatent for carcinoid patients. The isotope or combination of otopes that will induce the best results remains to be idenfied. The problem of how to select patients suitable for this nd of treatment also needs to be solved.

TABLE 110.8 EFFECT OF ALPHA-INTERFERON AND SOMATOSTAIN ANALOG COMBINED ON CARCINOID TUMORS

Author (year)	Biochemical response (%)	Symtomatic response (%)	Radiological response (%)
Janson (1993)	72	49	0
Frank (1999)	75	66	0

Symptomatic treatment for patients with carcinoid tumors are used to reduce symptoms induced by the tumor. Since one of the major features of the carcinoid syndrome is diarrhea, antidiarrheal agents such as loperamide may be of benefit for the patient. In some patients, nicotinamide supplement should be given. Bronchospasm may be treated with bronchodilators in the same way as ordinary asthmatic patients.

COMPLICATIONS AND THEIR MANAGEMENT

One of the most difficult complications that may occur in a patient with a midgut carcinoid tumor is the 'carcinoid crisis' that can develop, especially in patients undergoing surgery or other manipulations of the tumor.[26] The patient typically presents with a long-standing flush, hypotension, and tachycardia. Bronchial constriction may also be present. The best

TABLE 110.9 OVERVIEW OF SELECTED TRIALS WITH RADIOACTIVE SOMATOSTATIN ANALOGS IN CARCINOID PATIENTS

uthor (year)	Compound	No. patients	Biochemical response (%)	Radiological response (%)
renning (1996)	[^{111}In]-octreotide	1	0	0
IcCarthy (1998)	[^{111}In]-octreotide	5	–	20
anson (1999)	[^{111}In]-octreotide	3	33	0
renning (1999)	[^{111}In]-octreotide	10	–	10
Valdherr (2001)	[^{90}Y]-octreotide	8	–	12.5
wekkeboom (2003)	[^{177}Lu]-octreotide	12	–	33

treatment is continuous intravenous infusion of a somatostatin analog. It is worth mentioning that infusion of adrenaline in order to cause vasoconstriction leading to higher blood pressure might be life threatening since adrenaline may stimulate the tumor to release further hormone.

Another complication commonly found in carcinoid patients is the intestinal ischemia caused by obstruction of the mesenteric artery by a lymph node. Surgery is the treatment of choice for these patients.

TABLE 110.10 SURVIVAL IN PATIENTS WITH MIDGUT CARCINOID TUMORS

Overall from diagnosis	92 months
Overall from start of treatment	67 months
According to extent of disease:	
only lymph node metastases	108 months
<5 liver metastases	159 months
>5 liver metastases	53 months

Data from Janson ET et al. Carcinoid tumors: analysis of prognostic factors and survival in 301 patients from a referral center. Ann Oncol 1997; 8:685–690.

PROGNOSIS WITH AND WITHOUT TREATMENT

The prognosis for patients with midgut carcinoid tumors varies among different studies. There are some prognostic factors such as tumor burden and levels of hormone production. In a multivariate analysis, the plasma level of chromogranin A before treatment was initiated turned out as an independent prognostic factor.[8] For patients with a carcinoid syndrome, the median survival in nontreated patients is about 2 years according to the literature.[27] In more recent publications, the 5-year survival rate is between 50% and 90% for patients with metastases at diagnosis (Table 110.10).[8] A special feature of carcinoid tumors is the ability to develop metastases mar years after the primary tumor has been removed. Therefor patients operated radically for a midgut carcinoid tum should be followed for several years. For early detection recurrent disease, measurement of plasma levels chromogranin A is probably the best marker and when th starts to rise U-5HIAA should be collected. To localize th recurrence, PET examination with ^{11}C-5-HTP might prov helpful in early cases since these usually are difficult to fin with conventional radiology.

REFERENCES

1. Schnirer II, Yao JC, Ajani JA. Carcinoid: A comprehensive review. Acta Oncol 2003; 42:672–692.
2. Modlin IM, Lye KD, Kidd M. A 5-decade analysis of 13,715 carcinoid tumors. Cancer 2003; 97:934–959.
3. Rindi G, Capella C, Solcia E. Cell biology, clinicopathological profile, and classification of gastro-enteropancreatic endocrine tumors. J Mol Med 1998; 76:413–420.
4. Thorson Å, Biörck G, Björkman G, Waldenström J. Malignant carcinoid of the small intestine with metastases to the liver, valvular heart disease of the right side of the heart (pulmonary stenosis and tricuspid regurgitation without septal defects), peripheral vasomotor symptoms, bronchoconstriction, and an unusual type of cyanosis. Am Heart J 1954; 47:795–817.
5. Norheim I, Theodorsson E, Norheim E, Brodin E et al. Tachykinins in carcinoid tumors: Their use as a tumor marker and possible role in the carcinoid flush. J Clin Endocrinol Metab 1986; 63:605–612.
6. Feldman JM, O'Dorisio TM. Role of neuropeptides and serotonin in the diagnosis of carcinoid tumors. Am J Med 1986; 81:41–48.
7. Moller JE, Connolly HM, Rubin J et al. Factors associated with progression of carcinoid heart disease. N Engl J Med 2003; 348:1005–1015.
8. Janson ET, Holmberg L, Stridsberg M et al. Carcinoid tumors: Analysis of prognostic factors and survival in 301 patients from a referral center. Ann Oncol 1997; 8:685–690.
9. Pelage JP, Soyer P, Boudiaf M et al. Carcinoid tumors of the abdomen: CT features. Abdom Imaging 1999; 24:240–245.
10. Krenning EP, Kwekkeboom DJ, Bakker WH et al. Somatostatin receptor scintigraphy with [^{111}In-DTPA-D-Phe1]- and [^{123}I-Tyr3]-octreotide: the Rotterdam experience with more than 1000 patients. Eur J Nucl Med 1993; 20:716–731.
11. Orlefors H, Sundin A, Ahlstrom H et al. Positron emission tomography with 5-hydroxytryptophan in neuroendocrine tumors. J Clin Oncol 1998; 16:2534–2541.
12. Hellman P, Lundström T, Öhrvall U et al. Effect of surgery on the outcome of midgut carcinoid disease with lymph node and liver metastases. World J Surg 2002; 26:991–997.
13. Eriksson BK, Larsson EG, Skogseid BM et al. Liver embolization of patients with malignant neuroendocrine gastrointestinal tumors. Cancer 1998; 83:2293–2301.
14. Hellman P, Ladjevardi S, Skogseid B et al. Radiofrequency tissue ablation using cooled tip for liver metastases of endocrine tumors. World J Surg 2002; 26:1052–1056.
15. Fenwick SW, Wyatt JI, Toogood GJ et al. Hepatic resection and transplantation for primary carcinoid tumors of the liver. Ann Surg 2004; 239:210–219.
16. Oberg K, Norheim I, Alm G. Treatment of malignant carcinoid tumors: a randomized controlled study of streptozocin plus 5-FU and human leukocyte interferon. Eur J Cancer Clin Oncol 1989; 25:1475–1479.
17. Moertel CG, Rubin J, Kvols LK. Therapy of metastatic carcinoid tumor and the malignant carcinoid syndrome with recombinant leukocyte A interferon. J Clin Oncol 1989; 7:865–868.
18. Schober C, Schmoll E, Schmoll HJ et al. Antitumour effect and symptomatic control with interferon alpha 2b in patients with endocrine active tumours. Eur J Cancer 1992; 10: 1664–1666.
19. Oberg K, Eriksson B. The role of interferons in the management of carcinoid tumors. Acta Oncol 1991; 30:519–522.
20. Rönnblom LE, Alm GV, Öberg KE. Autoimmunity after alpha-interferon therap for malignant carcinoid tumors. Ann Intern Med 1991; 115:178–183.
21. Reubi JC, Kvols LK, Waser B et al. Detectio of somatostatin receptors in surgical and percutaneous needle biopsy samples of carcinoids and islet cell carcinoma. Cancer Res 1990; 50:5969–5977.
22. Kvols LK, Moertel CG, O'Connell MJ et al. Treatment of the malignant carcinoid syndrome. Evaluation of a long-acting somatostatin analogue. N Engl J Med 1986; 315:663–666.
23. Anthony L, Johnson B, Hande K et al. Somatostatin analogue phase I trial in neuroendocrine neoplasms. Acta Oncol 199 32:217–223.
24. Frank M, Klose KJ, Wied M et al. Combinatio therapy with octreotide and alpha-interfero effect on tumor growth in metastatic endocrine gastroenteropancreatic tumors. Am J Gastroenterol 1999; 94:1381–1387.
25. Jong M, Kwekkeboom D, Valkema R et al. Radiolabelled peptides for tumour therapy: current status and future directions. Eur J Nucl Med 2003; 30:463–469.
26. Marsh HM, Martin JK Jr, Kvols LK et al. Carcinoid crisis during anesthesia: successfu treatment with somatostatin analogue. Anesthesiology 1987; 66:89–91.
27. Moertel CG, Sauer WG, Dockerty MB et al. Life history of the carcinoid tumor of the small intestine. Cancer 1961; 14:901–912.

Chapter 111

AIDS and the gut

C Mel Wilcox

KEY POINTS

- Diseases of the GI tract are common in AIDS
- There are often multiple co-existent diseases
- Age related GI complications have substantially diminished in frequency since the introduction of highly active anti-retroviral therapy (HAART)
- Odynophagia suggests esophageal infection or ulceration with candida, herpes simplex virus or cytomegaly virus
- *Cryptosporidium parvum* is the most common small bowel pathogen in AIDS
- Microsporidia is identified in 10-20% of HIV infected patients with diarrhea
- Kaposi's sarcoma often involves the stomach or small bowel and is often asymptomatic but may present with abdominal pain, bleeding or obstruction
- *Mycobacterium avium* complex is the most common micro bacterial infection complicating AIDS in the USA
- *Clostridium difficile* colitis and cytomegaly virus are common in AIDS

INTRODUCTION

Since the first descriptions in 1981 of acquired immunodeficiency syndrome (AIDS), extraordinary strides have been made in our understanding of the human immunodeficiency virus (HIV) and the pathogenesis of disease. While the incidence of HIV infection in developed countries has stabilized, the epidemic continues unabated in developing countries and explosive growth within the next decade is predicted in Eastern Europe, the Soviet Union, as well as India. Although a dramatic fall in AIDS-related gastrointestinal complications has occurred since the introduction of highly active antiretroviral therapy (HAART),[1] these complications remain important because of their prevalence worldwide, morbidity, and impact on healthcare resources. Because of the many potential causes of gastrointestinal disease in these patients, this chapter will take an organ-based approach to review etiologies, manifestations, evaluation, and therapy.

GENERAL PRINCIPLES

Several important principles, many of which are unique to patients with AIDS, guide the evaluation of the HIV-infected patient with gastrointestinal complaints:

1. The rule of parsimony does not apply to patients with AIDS as multiple coexistent diseases are commonplace.
2. Opportunistic infections occur when immunodeficiency is severe. Therefore, the CD4 lymphocyte count will stratify the risk for an opportunistic process.[2]
3. Opportunistic disorders are frequently systemic. Identification of a pathogen outside of the gut (e.g., blood, bone marrow) may establish a presumptive cause of gastrointestinal symptoms.
4. Demonstration of a pathogen in tissue is the most specific means of establishing an etiologic diagnosis.
5. Recurrence is common for all opportunistic infections unless immunodeficiency is reversed.
6. Institution of HAART, when associated with immune reconstitution, is the best 'treatment' for all complications associated with HIV-related immunodeficiency.

OROPHARYNGEAL DISEASES

Diseases of the oropharynx are common in HIV infection, and oropharyngeal candidiasis (thrush) remains one of the most common index manifestations of AIDS. Oropharyngeal or hypopharyngeal pain generally reflects an ulcerative process, and aphthous ulcers are the most common cause of single or multiple well-circumscribed ulcers. Other causes of oropharyngeal ulcers in these patients include herpes simplex virus (HSV), cytomegalovirus (CMV), and, rarely, other infections. Kaposi's sarcoma appears as characteristic purple plaques or nodules (Fig. 111.1). Biopsy of oropharyngeal lesions should be performed when the appearance of the lesion is nondiagnostic, neoplasia is suspected, or empiric therapy is ineffective. With the exception of thrush where local therapies are effective, treatment for oropharyngeal diseases parallels that for the esophagus (see below).

ESOPHAGEAL DISEASES

Pathogenesis

Disorders of the esophagus are frequent in patients with AIDS, observed in up to 40% of patients who do not receive highly active antiretroviral therapy (HAART). *Candida* esophagitis is etiologic in 40–70% of patients followed by viral diseases, most commonly CMV.[3–5] Another important cause of esophageal disease is the HIV-associated aphthous or idiopathic esophageal ulcer, the pathogenesis of which remains poorly understood. Multiple coexistent esophageal disorders may be identified in 10% of patients; this complicates management.

Symptoms

Although dysphagia may be reported, odynophagia is an important and reliable clue to the presence of an esophageal infection or ulcer. When symptoms are localized to the neck or throat, hypopharyngeal rather than esophageal disease should

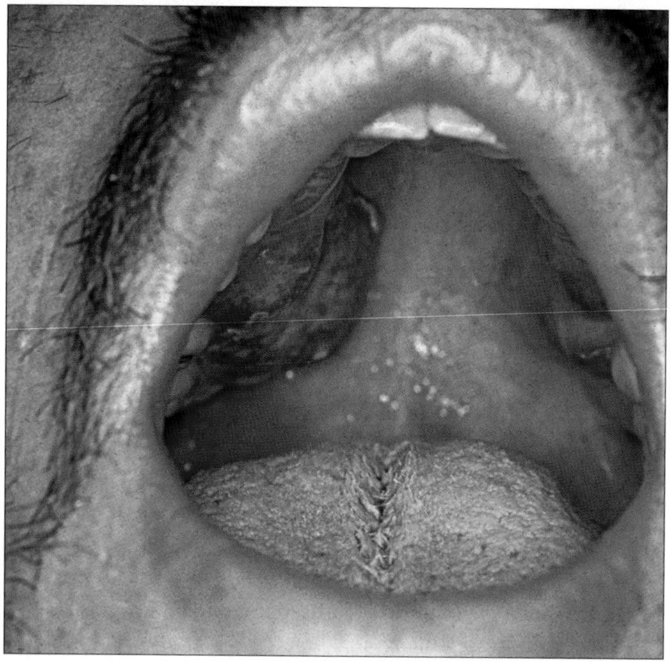

Fig. 111.1 Kaposi's sarcoma of the hard palate. Two large purple nodular lesions are seen on the hard palate of this patient with AIDS.

be suspected and evaluated accordingly. Examination of the oropharynx may provide clues to the cause of esophageal complaints. Most patients (66%) with *Candida* esophagitis have concomitant thrush. Oropharyngeal ulcerations are frequently associated with HSV esophagitis but rarely are present with CMV esophagitis and idiopathic esophageal ulcer.

Empirical management

Because of the high frequency of *Candida* esophagitis, empirical antifungal therapy with oral fluconazole (loading dose of 200mg followed by 100mg daily) is an appropriate initial management strategy for AIDS patients with the new onset of esophageal symptoms.[4] Since the clinical response of *Candida* esophagitis to therapy is very rapid, if no symptomatic response is apparent within the first 3days of initiating fluconazole, especially in the patient with severe symptoms, upper endoscopy should be performed rather than initiation of further empirical trials.

Diagnosis

Endoscopy with biopsy is the definitive diagnostic test for esophageal disease in AIDS. At the time of endoscopic evaluation, the appearance of some disorders is diagnostic, and ulcerative lesions may be biopsied (Fig. 111.2). When an ulcer is identified, multiple biopsies (at least 10) should be obtained to maximize sensitivity. Vigorous biopsy of the ulcer base essential for detecting CMV, while HSV is identified in squ mous epithelium from the ulcer edge (Fig. 111.3). Cytologic brushings and viral culture of ulcer tissue generally adds ve little over multiple biopsies alone. Immunohistochemical stai for viral pathogens improve the diagnostic yield and specifici over routine hematoxylin and eosin staining. Additional hist logical staining for other infections may be used selective based upon the clinical, endoscopic and histological finding An ulcer can be considered idiopathic when infections a excluded by appropriate histological studies and if pill-induce esophagitis and reflux disease are not suggested by the clinic presentation and endoscopic findings.

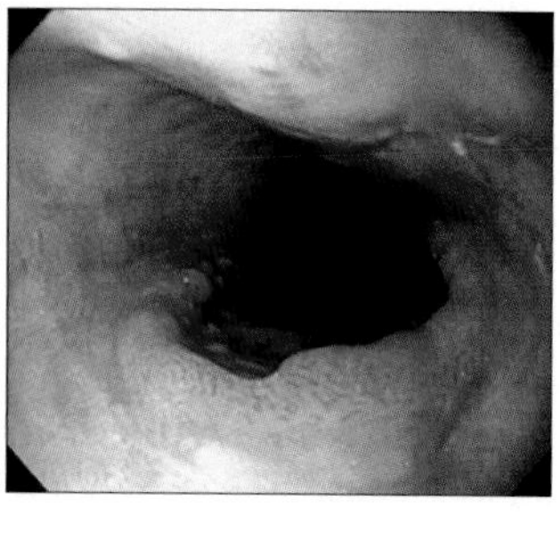

Fig. 111.2 Idiopathic esophageal ulcer. Large well-circumscribed ulcer with heaped up margins in the proximal esophagus. The endoscopic appearance may mimic CMV esophagitis.

Treatment

Therapy for esophageal diseases in patients with AIDS highly effective. Fluconazole (100mg/day) is currently the dru of choice for *Candida* esophagitis because of its exceller absorption, minimal drug interactions and side effects, an superior efficacy.[6]

Effective therapies are also available for both HSV and CM esophagitis. At most centers, intravenous ganciclovir is th drug of choice for CMV because of its relative tolerability an lower cost. Cidofovir is an attractive option for some patien given its once weekly administration. The primary side effe of ganciclovir is myelosuppression, whereas both foscarnet an cidofovir are nephrotoxic and may cause electrolyte distu bances (e.g., hypocalcemia, hypophosphatemia). Valganciclovi a new oral agent, has excellent absorption reaching serum cor centrations equivalent to ganciclovir. Although effective fo the treatment of CMV retinitis,[7] treatment of gastrointestina disease has not been well studied but may represent an optior Without HAART, the relapse rate following therapy is 40–50% similar to HSV.

For patients with idiopathic esophageal ulcers, both prednison and thalidomide are very effective. Prednisone should be adminis tered for 1month beginning with a dose of 40mg/day an tapering by 10mg each week. This regimen is well tolerate and once weekly fluconazole (100mg) will reduce any oro pharyngeal or esophageal candidiasis, which may complicat steroid use and confuse the clinical response. Thalidomide ha been successful in rare patients who fail to respond t

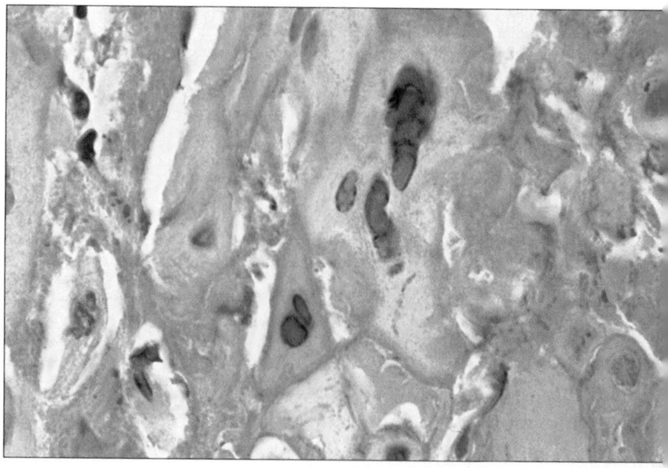

Fig. 111.3 Herpes simplex virus. High-power photomicrograph shows several cells with multinucleated inclusions characteristic of HSV

prednisone. This agent must be used cautiously and with the appropriate safeguards.

GASTRIC DISEASES

Clinically apparent gastric disorders are relatively infrequent in patients with AIDS. While a number of infections have been reported, CMV is the most frequent opportunistic infection involving the stomach in AIDS, and usually causes one or multiple ulcers. Kaposi's sarcoma often involves the stomach, but is generally asymptomatic unless the lesions are large and bulky which may then lead to abdominal pain, pyloric obstruction, or bleeding (Fig. 111.4). As with all gut symptoms, nonopportunistic causes deserve consideration regardless of the CD4 count.

Epigastric pain, nausea, and vomiting are the most common symptoms of gastric diseases, but are nonspecific. Overt gastrointestinal hemorrhage suggests ulceration. Nausea and vomiting are particularly common complaints in HIV-infected patients, and may reflect a variety of different etiologies including medications. In light of the broad differential diagnosis of upper gastrointestinal complaints in patients with AIDS, endoscopy and mucosal biopsy are generally required for definitive diagnosis. Computerized tomography (CT) may suggest the presence of gastric disease, but may also identify extraintestinal disease implicating a widely disseminated process.

SMALL BOWEL DISEASES

Intestinal disorders are among the most frequent complications in HIV-infected patients, and this high frequency may be related to altered gut immune function. A reduction in the number of CD4 lymphocytes in the lamina propria, which parallels the decrease in systemic CD4 cells, as well as decreased levels of secretory IgA in intestinal secretions in AIDS predispose to intestinal infection. In addition, the reduced number of mucosal CD4 lymphocytes may be responsible for alterations in small intestinal morphology and function (see below).

Pathogenesis

Small bowel disease in AIDS patients is usually caused by opportunistic infections.

Cryptosporidium parvum

Worldwide, *Cryptosporidium parvum*, a coccidian parasite, is the most common small bowel pathogen. While a self-limited illness in normal hosts, the incidence and severity of disease parallel the degree of immunodeficiency in HIV-infected patients. Patients with a CD4 count $>200/mm^3$ may have a self-limited illness while in those with a CD4 count $<50/mm^3$, the disease is chronic, typically severe, and associated with poor survival.[8]

While the spectrum of the disease is variable, diarrhea caused by *C. parvum* infection is characteristically secretory and can result in dehydration, electrolyte disturbances, and weight loss. The diagnosis can be established by modified acid-fast staining of fresh stool but examination of multiple stool specimens is generally required to increase yield. If stool tests are negative and the disease is suspected clinically, duodenal or ileal biopsies will usually establish the diagnosis;[9] colonic biopsies may occasionally be positive. Numerous medications have been used to treat cryptosporidiosis, generally without success. The most effective therapy is HAART, which if associated with immune reconstitution, can result in complete remission.[10]

Microsporidia

Microsporidia have emerged as one of the most common gastrointestinal opportunistic infections in AIDS, identified in 10–20% of HIV-infected patients with diarrhea worldwide.[11] Gastrointestinal disease is caused by two species, *Enterocytozoon bienusi* and *Encephalitozoon intestinalis*, with *E. bienusi* accounting for over 80% of cases of gastrointestinal disease. The clinical illness is milder than cryptosporidia, and dehydration, electrolyte disturbances, and marked weight loss suggest some other process; rarely, these pathogens may be found in an asymptomatic patient. On small bowel biopsy, the organisms appear as small round structures in the supranuclear portion of the enterocyte cytoplasm (Fig. 111.5). Colonic involvement has not been reported. Unlike *E. bienusi*, *E. intestinalis* can be identified in the lamina propria and because it is invasive, disseminated disease to other organs can be observed. These small intracellular parasites may be difficult to appreciate on hematoxylin-eosin staining, and additional staining methods such as tissue Gram stain are often required; electron microscopy has been considered the gold standard for diagnosis and permits a species-specific diagnosis. Stool tests are also available to detect the organism but the sensitivity remains low.

Therapeutic options for *E. bienusi* are limited. Despite initial promising reports, metronidazole has been shown to be largely ineffective. In contrast, *E. intestinalis* infection responds to albendazole, with some patients achieving clinical and microbiological cure;[12] *E. bienusi* responds poorly to this agent. As with cryptosporidia, HAART can result in complete remission,

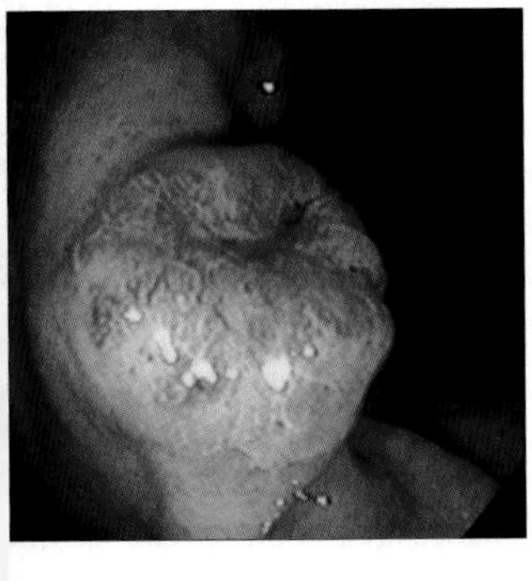

Fig. 111.4 Gastric Kaposi's sarcoma. Multiple raised lesions with central umbilication and subepithelial hemorrhage involving the gastric body.

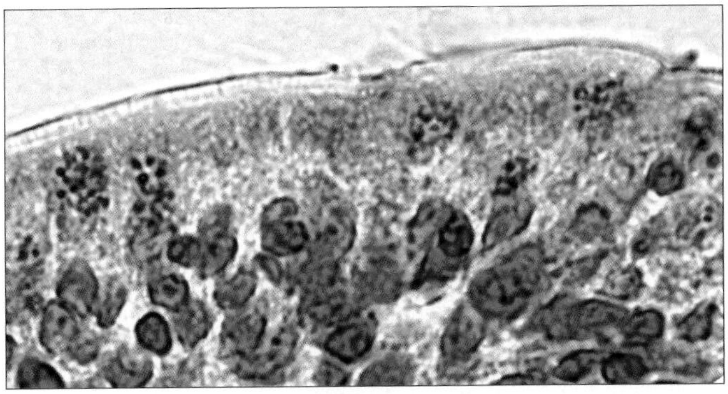

Fig. 111.5 Small bowel microsporidiosis. Tissue Gram stain of small bowel biopsy shows multiple small round Gram-positive organisms in clusters in epithelial cell.

but if immune deficiency returns, relapse occurs which underscores the interaction of immune function and these opportunistic intestinal infections.[10]

Other pathogens

Other small bowel parasitic diseases in AIDS include infection with *Isospora* and *Cyclospora*. *Isospora* has been most commonly reported as a diarrheal pathogen in developing countries. Cyclospora has recently been identified as a small bowel pathogen in both developed and developing countries. Trimethoprim-sulfamethoxazole (double-strength tablet b.i.d. for 10–14 days) is effective therapy for both pathogens, which may explain the infrequency of infection in countries where *Pneumocystis* prophylaxis is routine. There is no difference in the incidence or clinical expression of giardia and ameba in HIV-infected patients as compared with normal hosts.

Mycobacterium avium complex

Mycobacterium avium complex, a disease of late-stage AIDS, is the most common mycobacterial infection complicating AIDS in the US, while *Mycobacterium tuberculosis* (TB) is generally a disease of developing countries. Although diarrhea and abdominal pain may be observed in disseminated *Mycobacterium avium* complex, fever and wasting tend to dominate the clinical presentation.[13] Diarrhea is usually mild or moderate in severity even when small bowel infection is extensive. Acid-fast staining of stool is less sensitive than is culture for detection of *Mycobacterium avium* complex. Small bowel biopsy is the definitive diagnostic test (Fig. 111.6). Current multidrug regimens against *Mycobacterium avium* complex are effective due to the high *in vitro* efficacy of clarithromycin, azithromycin, and ethambutol.[14] Nevertheless, therapy is not considered curative and must be taken indefinitely unless HAART is instituted.

Tuberculosis

Tuberculosis (TB) may involve any portion of the gastrointestinal tract, but ileal involvement is most frequent. In contrast to *Mycobacterium avium* complex, TB may occur at any stage of immunodeficiency and can be cured with 9–12 months of multidrug therapy, provided drug resistance is not present. The recurrence rate following successful therapy, even for extrapulmonary disease, is low.

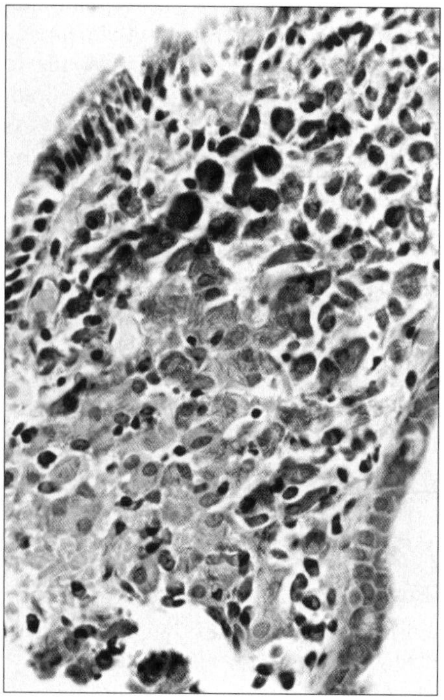

Fig. 111.6 *Mycobacterium avium* complex infection of the small bowel. AFB stain of small bowel biopsy showing multiple bacteria in macrophages causing an appearance mimicking that of Whipple's disease.

Viral diseases

Viral diseases of the small bowel are uncommon causes of chronic diarrhea in patients with AIDS. CMV intestinal disease presents as abdominal pain or bleeding due to mucosal ulceration, rather than as diarrhea. The role of HIV-1 as a direct small bowel pathogen remains controversial (see below).

Neoplasms

Neoplasms, including Kaposi's sarcoma and lymphoma, may involve the small bowel leading to abdominal pain, bleeding, obstruction, or intusussception. Endoscopy with biopsy can be used for diagnosis when the lesion is in the proximal bowel while surgical evaluation will be required for an obstructing lesion or to remove a more distal tumor.

HIV enteropathy

The term HIV enteropathy has been applied to the AIDS patient with diarrhea in which no cause can be found despite extensive evaluation. This entity is diagnosed less commonly today probably due to the rise in use of endoscopic examination for evaluation, recognition of emerging infections, and use of HAART. A variety of pathologic and functional abnormalities of the small intestine have been identified in HIV-infected patients, many of which are independent of opportunistic infections. These changes are usually observed when immunodeficiency is advanced. Chronic inflammation of both the small and large bowel, small bowel atrophy resembling celiac disease, as well as functional abnormalities of the small intestine, including reduced mucosal enzyme levels (e.g., lactase), malabsorption of sugars (D-xylose) and vitamins (B_{12}), and increased small bowel permeability have all been described. Some of these histological changes could be the result of loss of lamina propria CD4 lymphocytes, as these cells appear to have a trophic effect on the intestinal mucosa.[15]

COLONIC DISEASES

In contrast to the frequency of protozoan infections of the small intestine, bacteria and CMV are the most important colonic pathogens in patients with AIDS. The spectrum of bacterial pathogens parallels the normal host.

Clostridium difficile colitis remains common in patients with AIDS, and the clinical presentation, response to therapy, and relapse rate is no different in HIV-infected patients than in other patients. As in the normal host, bacterial colitis presents acutely with fever, abdominal pain, and watery or bloody diarrhea.

CMV colitis is one of the more common causes of chronic diarrhea in late-stage HIV disease, most patients having a CD4 count $<70/mm^3$. Although the presentation of CMV colitis is variable, the hallmarks of disease are abdominal pain and watery diarrhea.[16] Fever is inconsistent, whereas weight loss is almost universal. Gastrointestinal bleeding and perforation are infrequent complications. CMV colitis should be suspected in any AIDS patient with abdominal pain, chronic diarrhea, weight ss, and repeatedly negative stool culture and ova and parasite aminations.

In most patients with advanced immunodeficiency and colo-ctal symptoms, stool testing and endoscopic evaluation of e colon are most appropriate. While a number of other infec-ons and neoplasms may involve the colon, differentiation tween them clinically and endoscopically may be difficult. ne endoscopic findings in CMV colitis include isolated ulcera-ons, patchy subepithelial hemorrhage, or lesions resembling cerative colitis or Crohn's disease (Fig. 111.7).[17] Rarely, the sease may be limited to the right colon, and colonoscopy is cessary for diagnosis. CT may suggest the diagnosis when the lon is markedly thickened, although this finding is nonspecific. ne diagnosis of CMV colitis is best established by identification the pathognomonic viral cytopathic effect in colonic biopsy ecimens. Treatment is similar for disease elsewhere in the gut.

PPROACH TO THE AIDS PATIENT VITH DIARRHEA

iven the breadth of potential infectious causes of diarrhea nd the possibility of either small or large bowel involvement, systematic approach to diagnosis is essential (Fig. 111.8). hree important questions should be addressed when evalu-ing these patients:

. Is the diarrhea due to disease of the small bowel, colon, or some combination? The site of disease should be determined on the basis of a careful history and physical examination.
. Is the patient at risk for an opportunistic infection? The differential diagnosis should be based on the CD4 lymphocyte count. When the CD4 count is $<100/mm^3$, opportunistic processes are most likely.
. Have the appropriate stool tests been completed?

Symptoms of small bowel disease include crampy periumbil-al abdominal pain, flatulence, borborygmi, large stool volume articularly with fasting), nausea, and vomiting. Lower abdom-al pain and symptoms of proctitis point to inflammatory isease of the distal colon. Fever suggests an infectious cause f diarrhea and, when present, blood cultures should be obtained. Veight loss and severe immunodeficiency in a patient with hronic diarrhea strongly suggests an underlying opportunistic nfection. It should be recognized that drug-induced diarrhea ssociated with HAART (nelfinavir, ddI) is very frequent, is enerally mild, and use of a drug holiday may help make a resumptive diagnosis.

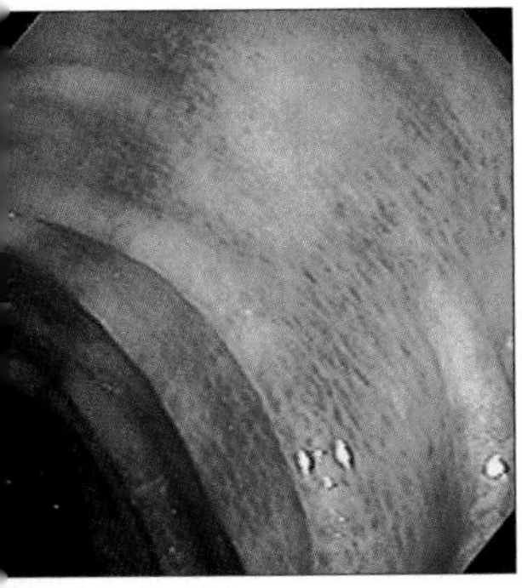

Fig. 111.7 CMV colitis. Patchy subepithelial hemorrhage in the distal colon typical for CMV. This appearance may mimic inflammatory bowel disease.

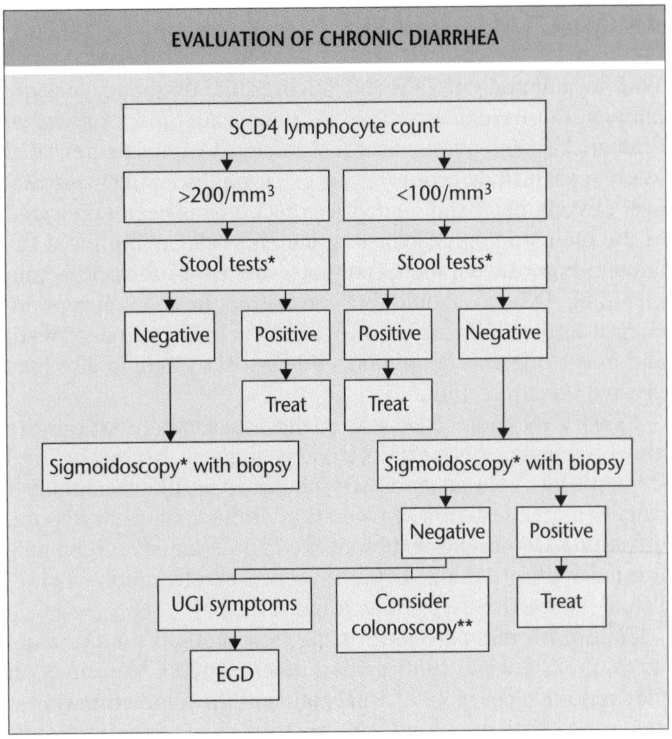

Fig. 111.8 Evaluation of chronic diarrhea. Suggested approach to the evaluation of chronic diarrhea in HIV-infected patients. *Fecal leukocytes, culture for enteric pathogens, assay for *Clostridium difficile* toxin, and examination(s) for ova and parasites. ** Colonoscopy should be considered when sigmoidoscopy is negative and colonic disease is highly suspected. UGI, upper gastrointestinal.

The presence of fecal leukocytes points to colitis and warrants evaluation for bacterial causes (e.g., *C. difficile*) and CMV colitis. If testing for *C. difficile* toxin and routine bacterial cultures of the stool are negative and symptoms of proctitis are present, sigmoidoscopy is appropriate. In the setting of severe immunodeficiency, if multiple stool tests are negative and fecal leukocytes are absent, evaluation of the distal colon or full colonoscopy with ileoscopy increase the diagnostic yield[9,16] and mucosal biopsies should be routinely taken regardless of the endoscopic appearance. The appropriate number of stool samples for bacterial culture, ova, and parasite examination, and *C. difficile* toxin necessary before proceeding to endoscopic evaluation is unknown. Most investigators suggest three samples, although up to six samples further increases the diagnostic yield.[18] In the hospitalized patient or when symptoms are severe, we proceed to endoscopic evaluation after one negative result. Colonoscopy may be required if there are concomitant right-sided abdominal complaints. Given the etiologic spectrum of infectious causes, broad-spectrum empirical antimicrobial therapies are not routinely recommended.

If no cause of diarrhea is found, symptomatic therapy is indicated. Antimotility drugs may be safely administered while obtaining additional stool studies. When diarrhea is mild, a bulking agent and antimotility drug such as loperamide are helpful. When diarrhea is more severe, tincture of opium can be very effective. Although there was initial enthusiasm for octreotide, a randomized, double-blind, placebo-controlled trial failed to document its effectiveness.[19]

ANORECTAL DISEASES

With the adoption of 'safe-sex' practices, the frequency of acute anorectal disorders, especially in homosexual men, has fallen dramatically. Infectious disorders related to unprotected anal intercourse include acute gonorrheal, syphilitic, and chlamydial proctitis. Human papilloma virus infection has been implicated as the main etiologic factor in squamous cell carcinoma of the anus in homosexual men. Traumatic disease of the anorectum including fissures should be considered in the appropriate clinical setting. Idiopathic anorectal ulcers have been described, and non-Hodgkin's lymphoma and Kaposi's sarcoma also may involve the anorectum.

As with all anorectal diseases, the usual manifestations are anorectal pain, dyschezia, bleeding, urgency, tenesmus, and frequent low-volume stools. Dyschezia (painful evacuation) is usually a manifestation of ulceration of the anal canal (fissure, infection). Careful inspection of the anorectum should be performed with attention to the presence of ulceration, fissure, fistula, hemorrhoids, or mass lesions.

Culture of perianal ulcers is the best method for the diagnosis of HSV, while confirmation of suspected CMV infection may require ulcer biopsy. Visualization of the anorectum is best performed with anoscopy and proctoscopy, or sigmoidoscopy. When dyschezia is severe, evaluation under conscious sedation or general anesthesia may be required.

PANCREATIC DISEASES

Disorders of the pancreas are uncommon in HIV-infected patients.

Acute pancreatitis, the most common manifestation in AII patients, most commonly arises from drugs, hyperlipidemi gallstones, or rarely infection.[20] Mild increases in serum amyla are frequent in AIDS patients and are clinically unimportant the asymptomatic patient. Infectious causes of pancreatitis patients with AIDS are multiple, although their diagnosis difficult because pancreatic biopsy is rarely performed. Mc cases of opportunistic pancreatic diseases are clinically sile and are diagnosed at autopsy, with pancreatic involvement bei part of a widespread disseminated infection. The role of end scopic retrograde cholangiopancreatography (ERCP) is simil to any other patient.

CONCLUSIONS

While the prevalence of gastrointestinal complications has fall due to HAART, gastrointestinal complaints remain a freque source of morbidity. Given the wide spectrum of potenti causes, the evaluation must be tailored to the history, physic examination, and routine laboratory tests including the CI lymphocyte count. Optimism should be maintained when eva uating these patients given the high diagnostic yield of current available tests as well as the efficacy of available medic therapy including HAART.

SOURCES OF INFORMATION FOR PATIENTS AND DOCTORS

http://www.fao.org/DOCREP/005/Y4168E/Y4168E00.HTM

REFERENCES

1. Monkemuller KE, Call SA, Lazenby AJ, Wilcox, CM. Declining prevalence of opportunistic gastrointestinal disease in the era of combination antiretroviral therapy. Am J Gastroenterol 2000; 95:457–462.
2. Bacellar H, Munoz A, Hoover DR et al. for the Multicenter AIDS cohort study. Incidence of clinical AIDS conditions in a cohort of homosexual men with CD4+ cell counts < 100/mm^3. J Infect Dis 1994; 170:1284–1287.
3. Bonacini M, Young T, Laine L. The causes of esophageal symptoms in human immunodeficiency virus infection: A prospective study of 110 patients. Arch Intern Med 1991; 151: 1567–1572.
4. Wilcox CM, Alexander LN, Clark WS, Thompson SE. Fluconazole compared with endoscopy for human immunodeficiency virus-infected patients with esophageal symptoms. Gastroenterology 1996; 110:1803–1809.
5. Wilcox CM, Schwartz DA, Clark WS. Causes, response to therapy, and long-term outcome of esophageal ulcer in patients with human immunodeficiency virus infection. Ann Intern Med 1995; 122:143–149.
6. Barbaro G, Barbarini G, Caladeron W et al. Fluconazole versus itraconazole for *Candida* esophagitis in acquired immunodeficiency syndrome. Gastroenterology 1996; 111:1169–1177.
7. Martin DF, Sierra-Madero J, Walmsley S et al. A controlled trial of valganciclovir as induction therapy for cytomegalovirus retinitis. N Engl J Med 2002; 346:1119–1126.
8. Manabe YC, Clark DP, Moore RD et al. Cryptosporidiosis in patients with AIDS: correlates of disease and survival. Clin Infect Dis 1998; 27:536–542.
9. Kearney DJ, Steuerwald M, Koch J, Cello JP. A prospective study of endoscopy in HIV-associated diarrhea. Am J Gastroenterol 1999; 94:556–559.
10. Carr A, Marriott D, Field A et al. Treatment of HIV-1-associated microsporidiosis and cryptosporidiosis with combination antiretroviral therapy. Lancet 1998; 351:256–261.
11. Weber R, Bryan RT, Schwartz DA, Owen RL. Human microsporidial infections. Clin Microbiol Rev 1994; 7:426–461.
12. Dore GJ, Marriott DJ, Hing MC, Harkness JL, Field AS. Disseminated microsporidiosis due to *Septata intestinalis* in nine patients infected with the human immunodeficiency virus: Response to therapy with albendazole. Clin Infect Dis 1995; 21:70–76.
13. Havlik JA, Horsburgh CR, Metchock B et al. Disseminated *Mycobacterium avium* complex infection: clinical identification and epidemiologic trends. J Infect Dis 1992; 165:577–580.
14. Shafran SD, Singer J, Zarowny DP et al. A comparision of two regimens for the treatment of *Mycobacterium avium* complex bacteremia in AIDS: Rifabutin, ethambutol, and clarithromycin versus rifampin, ethambutol, clofazimine, and ciprofloxacin. N Engl J Med 1996; 335:377–383.
15. Keating J, Bjarnason I, Somasundaram S et al. Intestinal absorptive capacity, intestina permeability and jejunal histology in HIV and their relation to diarrhoea. Gut 1995; 37:623–629.
16. Wilcox CM, Schwartz DA, Cotsonis GA, Thompson WE III. Evaluation of chronic unexplained diarrhea in human immunodeficiency virus infection: determination of the best diagnostic approach. Gastroenterology 1996; 110:30–37.
17. Wilcox CM, Chalasani N, Lazenby A, Schwartz DA. Cytomegalovirus colitis in acquired immunodeficiency syndrome: a clinical and endoscopic study. Gastrointest Endosc 1998; 48:39–43.
18. Blanshard C, Francis N, Gazzard BG. Investigation of chronic diarrhea in acquired immunodeficiency syndrome. A prospective study of 155 people. Gut 1996; 39:824–832
19. Simon DM, Cello JP, Valenzuela J et al. Multicenter trial of octreotide in patients with refractory acquired immunodeficiency syndrome-associated diarrhea. Gastroenterology 1995; 108:1753–1760.
20. Bush ZM, Kosmiski LA. Acute pancreatitis in HIV-infected patients: are etiologies changin since the introduction of protease inhibitor therapy? Pancreas 2003; 27:E1–E5.

Chapter 112

Graft-versus-host disease

George B McDonald and David J Kearney

KEY POINTS
• Graft-versus-host disease (GvHD) is caused by 'foreign' (allogeneic) immune cells • GvHD is common after hematopoietic cell transplantation, uncommon after organ transplantation, and rare after blood transfusion • It presents with fever, anorexia, diarrhea, skin rash, and jaundice • It may be rapidly fatal if not promptly recognized and treated • Two forms of GvHD exist (acute and chronic), each with different characteristics

INTRODUCTION AND DEFINITION

Graft-versus-host disease (GvHD) occurs when someone else's immune cells are introduced into a patient who cannot reject them. These allogeneic cells, and the inflammatory response they invoke, damage the gut, liver, skin, tissues such as salivary and lacrimal glands, and the immune system. GvHD is common after hematopoietic cell transplantation but rare after blood transfusions or transplantation of a solid organ harboring immune cells. Acute GvHD may be fatal unless recognized promptly and treated aggressively. Chronic GvHD, a more indolent disease in long-term survivors of transplantation, has clinical features of autoimmune disorders.

EPIDEMIOLOGY

Acute GvHD affects 50–70% of allogeneic transplant patients.[1] More severe GvHD develops when donors are mismatched for class I and II alleles, or sex mismatched or of increased parity. In some patients with cancer, acute GvHD is deliberately induced in order to kill tumor cells via donor lymphocytes (graft-versus-tumor effect). Acute GvHD occurs in approximately 10% of patients after autologous transplants (a patient's own cells are reinfused), usually affecting only the skin and upper gut. Rarely, patients who receive syngeneic cells (from an identical twin) may develop GvHD.

Chronic GvHD develops in 33% of patients who survive 150 days following matched sibling transplant, in 49% of mismatched related transplants, and in 64% of matched unrelated donor transplants.[1]

CAUSES, RISK FACTORS, DISEASE ASSOCIATIONS

GvHD is caused by hematopoietic cell transplantation or the transfusion of allogeneic cells via blood or organ transplant. GvHD can be induced deliberately by the abrupt discontinuation of prophylactic medications and by infusing donor lymphocytes.

CAUSES AND RISK FACTORS	
Acute GvHD	**Chronic GvHD**
• Donor HLA histocompatibility • HLA DRB1 allele disparity • Sex-mismatched donor • Increased parity in female donor • Increased patient age • High-dose irradiation in conditioning regimen • Inadequate GvHD prophylaxis • Cytokine gene polymorphisms	• Donor HLA histocompatibility • Increased patient age • Peripheral blood stem cells • Prior acute GvHD • Use of ciclosporin prophylaxis (rather than tacrolimus) • Cytokine gene polymorphisms

PATHOGENESIS

The pathophysiology of GvHD in humans is very complex.[1] Tissue damage caused by myeloablative regimens activates host antigen-presenting cells that stimulate donor T cells. Fatal GvHD also occurs after nonmyeloablative allografting and rarely after transfusion alone.

Tissue damage results from the generation of cytokines and cytotoxic T lymphocytes and natural killer (NK) cells, leading to damage of the skin, gut, and liver. Target cells are in the proliferative zone at the base of intestinal crypts, the parafollicular bulge and basal dermal areas of skin, and small bile ducts. Tumor necrosis factor-α (TNF-α) and interleukin-1α (IL-1α) are critical to the rapid development of GvHD, particularly in the gut. After severe damage to intestinal mucosa, skin, and liver, patients may reach a point where re-epithelialization is not sufficient to sustain life.

PATHOLOGY

The hallmark of intestinal GvHD is apoptosis of epithelial cells in crypts, recognized by clusters of nuclear and cytoplasmic debris (Fig. 112.1).[2,3] T-cell infiltration may not be present early in the course of GvHD. With progression, whole crypts may disappear, then focal areas of mucosa, followed by mucosal sloughing.

In the liver, early findings in GvHD are minimal; later, abnormalities in small bile ducts appear – dysmorphic epithelial cells, apoptosis, dropout of cells, and T-cell infiltrates in and around small bile ducts (Fig. 112.2).[4] Cholestasis is usually present,

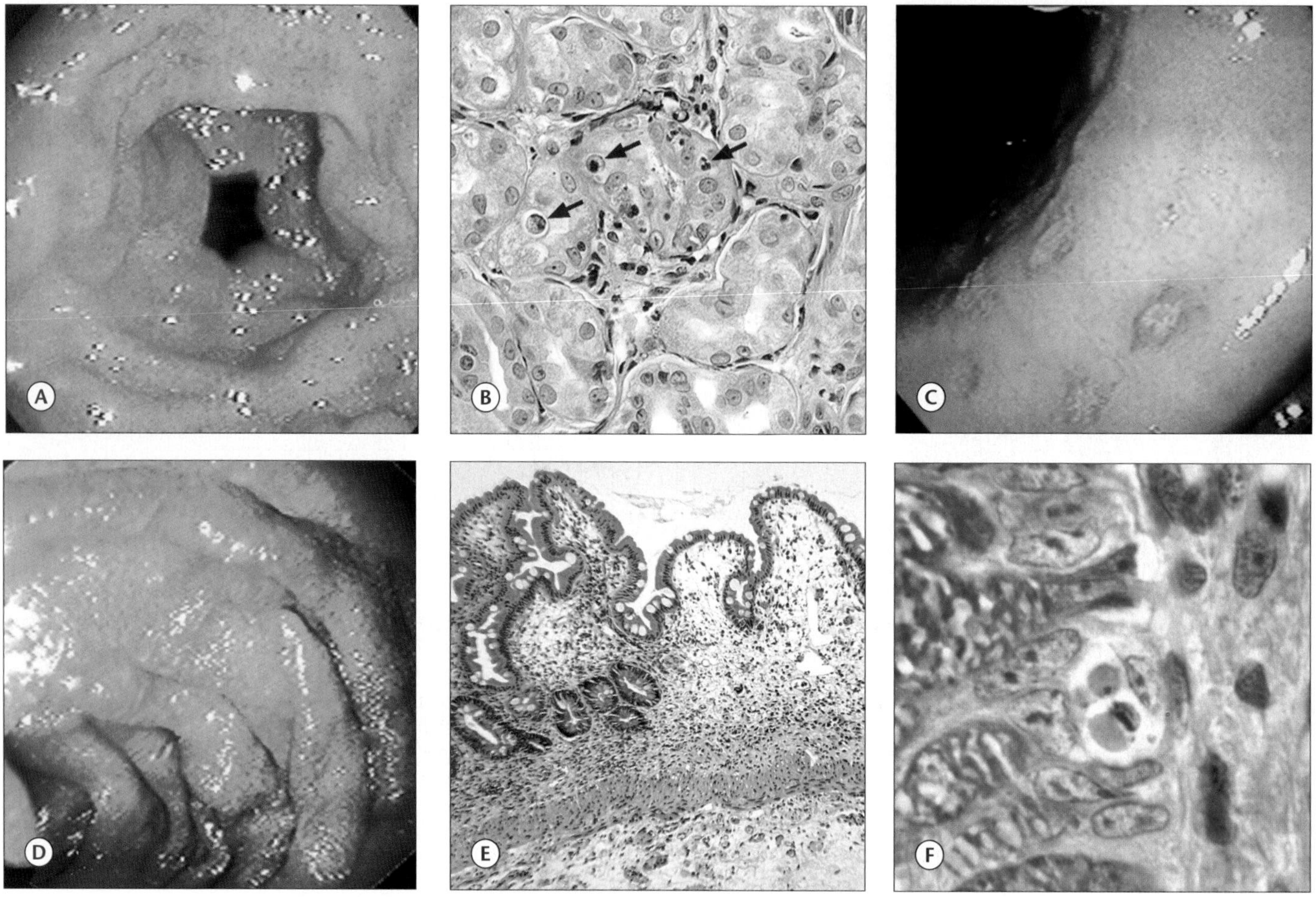

Fig. 112.1 Endoscopic and histologic features of acute GvHD involving the gastrointestinal tract. A. Mucosal edema and erythema of the gastric antrum. **B.** Photomicrograph of gastric biopsy specimen, showing apoptotic epithelial cells (arrows), crypt destruction, and small numbers of infiltrating lymphocytes. **C.** Multiple shallow ulcers on the lesser curvature of the stomach. **D.** Mucosa in the small intestine, showing erythema, edema, and multiple small erosions with hemorrhage. **E.** Photomicrograph of small intestinal mucosa, showing absence of crypt epithelium on the right. **F.** Photomicrograph of colonic mucosa biopsy specimen, showing cell fragments of an epithelial cell that has undergone apoptosis (apoptotic body), adjacent to normal crypt epithelium.

and in prolonged cholestasis bile thrombi and pericentral hepatocyte changes are evident. A hepatitic variant of GvHD can occur after immunosuppressive drugs have been withdrawn, or after donor lymphocyte infusion; biopsy shows lobular inflammation and acidophil bodies, along with typical abnormalities of small bile ducts (Fig. 112.2) – a finding absent in fulminant viral hepatitis.[5]

In chronic GvHD, histologic findings in intestinal mucosa and liver are similar to those in acute GvHD. Excessive fibrosis in the submucosal tissues of the esophagus, small intestine, and colon can be seen in severe cases.

CLINICAL PRESENTATION

Generalized symptoms of acute GvHD are a result of 'cytokine storm,' i.e., local release of TNF-α and IL-1α within gut and skin, and circulating IL-6.[1]

Anorexia, early satiety, nausea, and vomiting are common presenting symptoms, sometimes with intense abdominal pain and voluminous diarrhea. Anorexia and nausea may occur in isolation as an enigmatic illness.

Diarrhea: In mild GvHD, stool volumes are under 500 mL/day, and in severe GvHD volumes may exceed 2 L/day with persistence of diarrhea even without oral intake. The pathogenesis of early diarrhea is related to intestinal cytokine release; apoptotic crypt cells are infrequent. Later, T cell-mediated crypt damage occurs and excessive TNF-α is released throughout the gut, in some cases leading to extensive sloughing of mucosa.

Abdominal pain caused by transmural edema is a harbinger of severe GvHD. As GvHD progresses, distention from luminal fluid causes pain.

Occult gastrointestinal bleeding is very common after transplantation when platelet counts are low. GvHD is the most common cause of severe intestinal bleeding after transplantation;[6] bleeding is from oozing ulceration rather than a single artery.

Dysphagia and odynophagia are rare in acute esophageal GvHD, occurring only with extensive mucosal destruction.

Cholestatic jaundice is a feature of severe acute GvHD. With progressive disease, small bile ducts are damaged, eventually resulting in ductopenia. Extensive hepatocellular necrosis is rare in this setting.

Signs and symptoms of *chronic GvHD* occur without a previous diagnosis of acute GvHD in about 20% of cases; more commonly, acute GvHD melds into chronic GvHD (progressive onset) or resolves, only to reappear (quiescent onset). Morbidity and mortality rates are highest after a progressive onset. In its full-blown state, chronic GvHD may resemble scleroderma

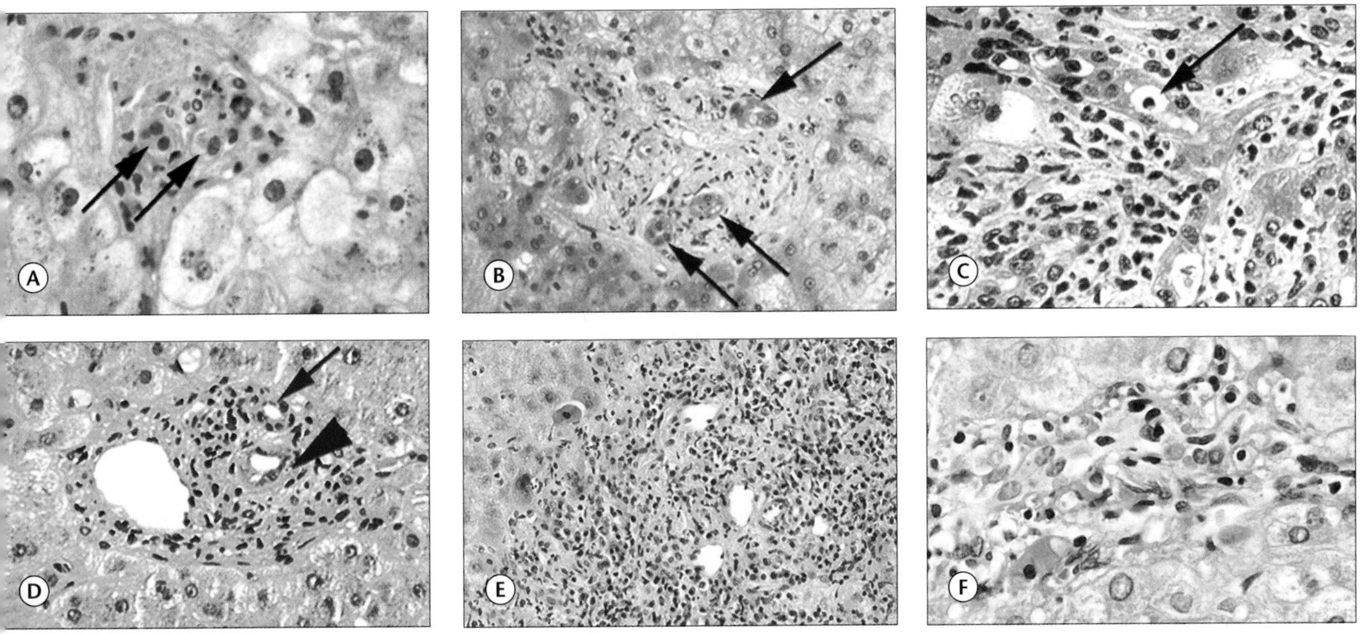

Fig. 112.2 **Histologic features of acute and chronic GvHD of the liver. A.** Portal area, with damaged small bile ducts (arrows) and surrounding bile-filled hepatocytes (28 days after transplant). **B.** Portal area with three abnormal small bile ducts, each showing epithelial cell dropout, cytoplasmic eosinophilia, and vacuolization (82 days after transplant). There are few lymphocytes in this portal area. **C.** Portal space with lymphocytic infiltrate and dysmorphic small bile ducts showing variation in shape and size and dropout (40 days after transplant). The arrow points to an apoptotic epithelial cell. **D.** Portal space with small bile ducts in chronic GvHD (465 days after transplant). The arrow points to a small bile duct with decreased numbers of epithelial cells, and the arrowhead to a bile duct remnant with no intact epithelium. **E.** Hepatitic presentation of chronic GvHD (760 days after transplant). An enlarged portal space with lymphocytes admixed with plasma cells, eosinophils, and neutrophils, obscuring small bile ducts. The limiting plate has extensive interface hepatitis with periportal acidophil bodies. **F.** Small portal space with markedly damaged small bile duct infiltrated by lymphocytes (patient with a hepatitic presentation 184 days after transplant). The bile duct has a shrunken outline, with vacuolated and eosinophilic cytoplasm and nuclear dropout.

lichen planus, Sjögren's syndrome, eosinophilic fasciitis, rheumatoid arthritis, and primary biliary cirrhosis. In some, the presentation is subtle with weight loss, weakness, or failure to thrive in children. Dysphagia is caused by extensive oral ulcerations or esophageal webs, strictures, and submucosal fibrosis. Liver involvement in chronic GvHD presents as isolated increase in alkaline phosphatase concentration or cholestatic jaundice, or as an acute hepatitis (after immunosuppressive medications have been discontinued abruptly).[5]

CLINICAL PRESENTATION

Acute GvHD	Chronic GvHD
• Fever, malaise • Skin erythema, maculopapular rash, bullae, sloughing • Anorexia, satiety, nausea, vomiting • Diarrhea • Abdominal pain • Gastrointestinal bleeding • Jaundice • Dysphagia	• Skin lesions (erythema, hyperkeratosis, desquamation, atrophy, fibrosis) • Cholestasis • Acute hepatitis • Ocular sicca syndrome • Oral atrophy, erythema, lichenoid lesions • Bronchiolitis obliterans • Esophageal webs, strictures • Diarrhea • Myositis, myasthenia gravis, contractures • Vaginitis, vaginal strictures

DIFFERENTIAL DIAGNOSIS

Anorexia, satiety, nausea, and vomiting after conditioning therapy usually wane by day 10–15 posttransplant. After day 20, upper gut symptoms are from GvHD in approximately 85% of allograft recipients.[7] The remaining 15% have medication intolerance (ciclosporin, voriconazole, trimethoprim–sulfamethoxazole, mycophenolate mofetil) or appetite suppression from high-calorie parenteral nutrition.

Diarrhea caused by conditioning is uncommon after day 10–15 posttransplant. After this time, patients with high-volume diarrhea (>1 L/day) almost always have GvHD as the cause.[8] Infection as a cause of diarrhea accounts for less than 15% of cases; the organisms responsible include *Clostridium difficile*, *C. septicum*, astrovirus, adenovirus, rotavirus, and cytomegalovirus (CMV). Parasites and bacterial enteric pathogens are rare. Oral magnesium supplements commonly cause diarrhea. Malabsorption of dietary sugars and fat, related to mucosal damage from conditioning therapy or GvHD, causes diarrhea.

Abdominal pain has a wide differential diagnosis posttransplant, but intra-abdominal catastrophes are unusual. Pseudo-obstruction is common in the first month after transplant, from opioid or anticholinergic medications. Distention is common among patients who received vincristine (an enteric neurotoxin) before transplantation. Painful hepatomegaly results from hepatic engorgement (sinusoidal obstruction syndrome). Hemorrhagic cystitis (caused by cyclophosphamide or viral infection) causes severe, crampy pain in the lower abdomen and hematuria. Passage of biliary sludge can cause upper abdominal pain,

DIFFERENTIAL DIAGNOSIS	
DIFFERENTIAL DIAGNOSIS OF GASTROINTESTINAL AND HEPATIC PROBLEMS	
Problems in patients with acute GvHD	**Differential diagnosis**
Anorexia, satiety, nausea, vomiting	• Persistent toxicity from conditioning therapy • Medication side effect • Parenteral nutrition • Infection with a herpesvirus (HSV, CMV) • Fungal or bacterial esophagitis • Brain lesion (increased intracranial pressure)
Diarrhea	• Persistent toxicity from conditioning therapy • Bacterial infection (clostridia) • Viral infection (adenovirus, astrovirus, CMV, rotavirus) • Magnesium-containing medicines (oral) • Disaccharide malabsorption • Motilin agonists (e.g., tacrolimus) • Fungal overgrowth • Parasites, enteric bacterial pathogens
Abdominal pain	• Pseudo-obstruction (usually caused by mu-opioids or anticholinergics) • Liver pain (sinusoidal obstruction syndrome) • Enteritis from the conditioning regimen • Hemorrhagic cystitis • Biliary pain (cholecystitis, biliary sludge syndrome) • Hematomas (abdominal wall, intestine) • Intestinal perforation • Acute pancreatitis • Intestinal mucosal infection • Intestinal infarction • Epstein-Barr virus lymphoproliferative disease
Gastrointestinal bleeding	• Mucosal trauma from retching • Mucosal necrosis caused by conditioning therapy • Gastric antral vascular ectasia • Ulceration of intestinal mucosa by infection • Iatrogenic (biopsy sites) • Epstein-Barr virus lymphoproliferative disease
Jaundice	• Sinusoidal obstruction syndrome • Cholangitis lenta (cholestasis of sepsis) • Medication-related liver injury • Hemolysis ± renal failure • Viral infection • Biliary obstruction • Epstein-Barr virus lymphoproliferative disease
Dysphagia and odynophagia	• Oral mucositis from the conditioning regimen • Intramural esophageal hematoma • Esophageal infection • Acid–pepsin esophagitis • Pill esophagitis

nausea, and vomiting, and may be confused with GvHD. Dissecting hematomas in either the abdominal wall or intestine rarely develop in thrombocytopenic patients. Intestinal perforation rarely occurs in patients who are not receiving corticosteroids; the sites of perforation are usually colonic diverticula and CMV ulcers. Intestinal infarction is caused by occlusion of mesenteric arteries with *Aspergillus*. Epstein-Barr virus-lymphoproliferative disease (EBV-LPD) develops only in patients being treated for GvHD.

Severe gastrointestinal bleeding is uncommon, largely due to prophylaxis of CMV and fungal infection.[6] Vascular ectasias of gastric and duodenal mucosa can lead to protracted bleeding unless ablated by laser endoscopy. In thrombocytopenic patients, duodenal biopsy sites may bleed. Rarely, a patient with an intramucosal tumor will bleed when the tumor is lysed by high-dose therapy. Gastric mucosal trauma from retching rarely causes significant bleeding. Bleeding caused by *C. septicum* (typhlitis), CMV, zygomyces, and EBV-LPD involving the gut occur sporadically.

Jaundice after transplantation has multiple causes, making a diagnosis of liver GvHD difficult.[9] Sinusoidal obstruction syndrome (formerly known as veno-occlusive disease) is a form of liver injury caused by the conditioning regimen; jaundice usully appears before day 10, often accompanied by hepatomegaly nd weight gain – features that are unusual with GvHD. Jaundice n patients with sepsis (cholangitis lenta) may be indistinguishble from hepatic GvHD. High ciclosporin levels inhibit bilirubin transport. The combination of mild cholestasis plus either emolysis (related to hemolytic uremic syndrome) or renal failure nay lead to deeper jaundice. Biliary obstruction is usually elated to passage of biliary sludge. Jaundice and serum levels f alanine and aspartate aminotransferases greater than 1000 U/L re commonly caused by sinusoidal obstruction syndrome or cute viral hepatitis (herpes simplex virus (HSV), varicellaoster virus (VZV), adenovirus, hepatitis B virus), but this resentation can also be a manifestation of chronic GvHD.

Dysphagia and odynophagia are rarely caused by acute GvHD. In severe chronic GvHD esophageal webs, rings, and trictures are more common, particularly in patients with skin, nouth, and eye involvement. Chronic fungal infection and HSV sophagitis can be seen in patients with chronic GvHD, and ome pills used after transplant may lead to esophageal damage.

DIAGNOSTIC METHODS

Acute GvHD: A clinical diagnosis of acute gastrointestinal GvHD s acceptable when the patient is at risk, all clinical hallmarks are resent, alternate conditions in the differential diagnosis are unlikely, nd a skin biopsy is positive for GvHD. The only common intestinal nfection that cannot be identified by stool culture is CMV.[8]

Endoscopy: When the diagnosis of intestinal GvHD is in loubt, endoscopy and mucosal biopsy are needed. What the ndoscopist sees carries equal weight to mucosal histological indings: mucosal edema and erythema in mild cases, friability nd erosions in moderate cases, and large areas of mucosal ecrosis, ulceration, and slough in severe cases (see Fig. 112.1).[3] The pathologist relies on lymphocyte aggregates, apoptosis of rypt cells, and crypt cell dropout to diagnose intestinal GvHD see section on Pathology), but cannot find apoptotic crypt cells n areas devoid of epithelium. The antrum is the preferred site or biopsy. Duodenal biopsies carry a higher risk of bleeding. Biopsies (six to ten in number) should be taken from both ulcerated tissue and surrounding epithelium, and serially sectioned o optimize the yield for focal findings including CMV. Biopsy naterial, placed in viral transport media, should be cultured or herpesviruses using molecular methods.

Liver biopsy: A certain diagnosis of hepatic GvHD requires iver biopsy (see Fig. 112.2), but often such a diagnosis is moot f there is biopsy-proven GvHD elsewhere. Most liver biopsies in his setting are done via a transvenous route. Liver tissue should e sent for histologic examination, immunohistology if a virus s suspected, and viral culture (adenovirus and herpesviruses).

Chronic GvHD: Diagnosis is based on clinical findings and istology of oral, skin, and gut biopsies. When patients present with dysphagia, a cine barium contrast X-ray is useful to identify pper esophageal webs and strictures. Endoscopy should be lone cautiously because of perforation risk. Liver biopsy may e required if the cause of cholestasis is in dispute or if acute epatitis develops (Fig. 112.2).

TREATMENT AND PREVENTION

Consultants in gastroenterology and hepatology play only an dvisory role in the treatment of GvHD. Initial treatment is usually with glucocorticoids: prednisone 2 mg/kg for patients with more severe symptoms and 1 mg/kg for patients with minor skin rashes or upper gut symptoms.[1] Topical oral corticosteroids are a useful adjunct to prednisone among patients with anorexia, nausea, and vomiting. Mortality in patients with grade II–IV GvHD is lowest in those who achieve a complete response to initial treatment. Incomplete responses or failure to respond trigger additional immunosuppressive therapy. Treatment of chronic GvHD is difficult; some patients stay on immunosuppressive therapy for several years. There is no universally effective salvage regimen for patients whose chronic GvHD fails to respond to initial therapy.

DIAGNOSTIC METHODS	
DIAGNOSTIC METHODS FOR GASTROINTESTINAL AND HEPATIC GVHD	
Acute GvHD	**Chronic GvHD**
• Clinical evaluation and assessment of pretest probability of GvHD • Tissue biopsy of skin • Stool culture (viruses, *C. difficile*, fungi) • Endoscopic appearance of gut mucosa • Tissue biopsy and culture of gut mucosa and liver	• Clinical evaluation • Oral examination and lip biopsy • Tissue biopsy of skin • Schirmer test (lacrimal gland function) • Endoscopic appearance and biopsy of esophageal and gut mucosa • Liver biopsy

COMPLICATIONS AND THEIR MANAGEMENT

Many complications of GvHD are caused by side effects of treatment: hypercortisolism from prednisone use, renal and neurologic damage from ciclosporin and tacrolimus, hepatic toxicity from a mélange of drugs, and infection of the lungs, sinuses, brain, gut, liver, kidneys, bladder, and bloodstream.

Intestinal infections in patients with GvHD (HSV, CMV, and *Candida* species) are infrequent because of antiviral and antifungal prophylaxis.[6] Unusual infections include necrotizing enteritis and colitis caused by adenovirus; esophagitis and gastritis caused by VZV; and mold infections of the stomach, small intestine, or colon. Each of these infections is treatable. VZV infections usually develop after acyclovir prophylaxis has been discontinued; presentation can be subtle, with abdominal distention, pain, and rising serum alanine aminotransferase levels.

Hepatobiliary infections include fungal abscesses, herpesvirus and adenovirus infections, hepatitis B and C exacerbations, and development of EBV-LPD.[9] HSV, VZV, and adenovirus hepatitis may lead to fulminant hepatic failure. Hepatitis B and C are seldom problems while patients remain on immunosuppressive drugs, but hepatitis may flare during immune recovery. Fatal hepatitis B can be prevented by prophylactic lamivudine or adefovir.

Acute pancreatitis is a common finding at autopsy among patients with refractory GvHD, but symptoms are unusual. Prednisone and ciclosporin crystals in bile have been suggested as causes. Rarely, patients with extensive chronic GvHD develop pancreatic atrophy and insufficiency.

Intestinal perforation occurs rarely, despite denudation of mucosa in severe GvHD. Perforation of colonic diverticula is

TREATMENT AND PREVENTION	
Acute GvHD	**Chronic GvHD**
PREVENTION • Donor screening for class I and II antigens • Immunosuppressive drug prophylaxis (ciclosporin or tacrolimus + methotrexate) • Antimicrobial prophylaxis • T-cell depletion • Ursodiol prophylaxis **PRIMARY TREATMENT** • Prednisone 1–2 mg/kg/day • Oral beclomethasone dipropionate 8 mg/day **SECONDARY TREATMENT OPTIONS** • Antithymocyte globulin • Additional immunosuppressive drugs (sirolimus, mycophenolate mofetil) • Anti-T-cell monoclonal antibodies • Anticytokine monoclonal antibodies • Psoralen and ultraviolet A irradiation (PUVA) • Extracorporeal photophoresis • Control of infection	**PRIMARY TREATMENT OPTIONS** • Ciclosporin or tacrolimus + prednisone • Thalidomide **SECONDARY TREATMENT OPTIONS** • Azathioprine • Thalidomide • Alternating ciclosporin and prednisone • Tacrolimus • Psoralen and ultraviolet A irradiation (PUVA) • Extracorporeal photophoresis • Control of infection • Supportive care

usually seen among patients on high-dose prednisone therapy. Perforated CMV ulcers are now rare.

Pneumatosis intestinalis and pneumoperitoneum can be caused by intestinal GvHD or CMV infection. This condition must be distinguished from mucosal necrosis caused by gas-forming organisms or infarction. The diagnosis usually comes as a radiologic surprise. Air can be seen in the peritoneal cavity and mediastinum as a relatively benign event in patients with pneumatosis intestinalis.

Aspiration and bronchiolitis are complications of esophageal strictures and webs from chronic GvHD. Untreated chronic GvHD may lead to obliteration of the esophageal lumen. Aspiration pneumonitis must be distinguished from bronchiolitis obliterans with organizing pneumonia, a form of pulmonary GvHD.

PROGNOSIS WITH AND WITHOUT TREATMENT

Acute and chronic GvHD must be treated to avoid death and chronic disability, particularly among recipients of stem cells from HLA-nonidentical donors.[1] In acute GvHD, the prognosis is poorest among patients whose GvHD had an early onset and failed to respond completely to initial therapy. Mortality in patients with chronic GvHD is related to the extent of disease, a progressive-type onset, thrombocytopenia, weight loss, and poor performance score. The adverse effects of treatment for GvHD are themselves causes of death (infections and the debilitating effects of prolonged glucocorticoid exposure).

WHAT TO TELL PATIENTS

Until patients experience GvHD, seldom do they have a clear idea of how sick they may become, and how difficult and prolonged the treatment may be. These resources are useful:

- Blood and Marrow Transplant Information Network (http://www.bmtinfonet.org) – provides electronic access to books and newsletters, and a patient–survivor link service
- BMT-Talk (http://listserv.acor.org/archives/bmt-talk.html) – home page for a mailing list that hosts communications between patients, survivors, and caregivers
- BMT Support Online (http://www.bmtsupport.org) – provides two online support groups, one for patients the other for caregivers
- National BMT link (http://www.bmtlink.org) – links transplant patients with survivors who can provide emotional support

Community physicians may find *Thomas' Hematopoietic Cell Transplantation*[1] useful.

CURRENT CONTROVERSIES AND THEIR FUTURE RESOLUTION

The dilemma facing investigators is how to achieve stable engraftment without causing GvHD, while preserving a graft-versus-tumor effect after allogeneic transplant. The solution to refractory acute and chronic GvHD will come from advances in immunogenetics, T-cell biology, and identification of antigens on epithelial stem cells that are the targets of alloimmune attack.

REFERENCES

1. Blume KG, Forman SJ, Appelbaum FR. Thomas' hematopoietic cell transplantation, 3rd edn. Oxford: Blackwell Publishing; 2004.
2. Washington K, Bentley RC, Green A, Olson J, Treem KR, Krigman HK. Gastric graft-versus-host disease: a blinded histologic study. Am J Surg Pathol 1997; 21:1037–1046.
3. Ponec RJ, Hackman RC, McDonald GB. Endoscopic and histologic diagnosis of intestinal graft-vs.-host disease after marrow transplantation. Gastrointest Endosc 1999; 49:612–621.
4. Shulman HM, Sharma P, Amos D, Fenster LF, McDonald GB. A coded histologic study of hepatic graft-versus-host disease after human marrow transplantation. Hepatology 1988; 8:463–470.
5. Strasser SI, Shulman HM, Flowers ME et al. Chronic graft-vs-host disease of the liver: presentation as an acute hepatitis. Hepatology 2000; 32:1265–1271.
6. Schwartz JM, Wolford JL, Thornquist MD et al. Severe gastrointestinal bleeding after marrow transplantation, 1987–1997: incidence, causes, and outcome. Am J Gastroenterol 2001; 96:385–393.
7. Wu D, Hockenbery DM, Brentnall TA et al. Persistent nausea and anorexia after marrow transplantation: a prospective study of 78 patients. Transplantation 1998; 66:1319–1324.
8. Cox GJ, Matsui SM, Lo RS et al. Etiology and outcome of diarrhea after marrow transplantation: a prospective study. Gastroenterology 1994; 107:1398–1407.
9. Strasser SI, McDonald GB: Hepatobiliary complications of hematopoietic stem cell transplantation. In: Schiff ER, Sorrell MF, Maddrey WC, eds. Schiff's diseases of the liver, 9th edn. Philadelphia: JB Lippincott; 2003:1636–1663

Chapter 113

Radiation and other physicochemical injury

Dermot P B McGovern

RADIATION DAMAGE TO THE GUT

KEY POINTS

- Relatively common and increasing problem
- Acute radiation enteritis and colitis are usually self limiting and occur at the time of radiation exposure
- Chronic radiation enteritis and colitis may occur any time up to 30 years after exposure
- Chronic radiation damage is due to a chronic obliterative vasculitis
- Presentation depends on part of gastrointestinal tract affected by radiation exposure
- The most commonly affected sites are the small bowel and distal colon
- Radiation damage can mimic many 'other' conditions seen in the gut
- Treatment is largely based on anecdotal reports and there is an evidence-based void on therapeutic interventions
- Prognosis is usually good but patients can suffer from intestinal failure

Introduction

Radiation enteritis and colitis (radiation enteropathy) are caused by acute or chronic injury to the gut as a result of exposure to therapeutic or supra-therapeutic levels of ionizing radiation. The damaging effect of radiation on the gut was first recognized at the end of the nineteenth century and can occur acutely (usually short lived) or up to 30 years after radiation exposure.

Epidemiology

Up to 12 000 people a year in the UK receive pelvic irradiation and many more undergo radiotherapy that may affect other parts of the gastrointestinal tract. The data on the overall prevalence of acute or chronic radiation enteritis following exposure is not consistent and studies estimate that between 2% and 20% of patients receiving radiotherapy will go on to develop chronic radiation enteritis.[1] This may occur anywhere from 6 months to 30 years after exposure (mean approximately 2 years). However, other data suggest that over 80% of patients who had received radiotherapy complained of a persistent change in their bowel habit although radiation damage is not always the cause. A further study estimated that there was a 5% chance of gastrointestinal complications at 5 years when the small intestine had been exposed to 4500–5000 centiGrays (cGy) or the large bowel to 6000–6500 cGy.

Following therapeutic radiation there are three possible gastrointestinal sequelae:

1. no clinical manifestations;
2. manifestations that affect the patient's quality of life; and
3. manifestations that may affect the patient's health (e.g., strictures, bleeding, secondary neoplasia; see 'Complications and their management').

The target of radiotherapy is usually situated in the pelvis (as gynecological and prostatic malignancies are amongst the most common malignancies treated with radiotherapy) and so the recto-sigmoid is the most commonly affected site although the small bowel is also commonly involved. The esophagus and rectum are relatively radioresistant compared to the more sensitive stomach and small bowel. This radiosensitivity is in large part due to the increased turnover of crypt epithelium within the gastric and small bowel mucosa. Within the small bowel, the duodenum, upper jejunum, and terminal ileum are the most frequently affected areas as these are relatively 'fixed' structures.

Causes, risk factors

The cause of radiation enteritis is simply an exposure to ionizing radiation that has caused acute or chronic damage to the gut. There are a number of factors known to increase the risk of developing radiation colitis including:

- concomitant chemotherapy;
- high-dose radiation therapy;
- uremia;
- diabetes mellitus;
- pelvic inflammatory disease;
- hypertension;
- thin body habitus;
- abdominal or pelvic surgery;
- accelerated fractionation regimens of delivering radiotherapy; and
- radiation intracavity implants[2]

Pathogenesis

Acute radiation enteropathy is caused by radiation-induced cell death (apoptosis) and the most vulnerable of cells are those in the G2 and M phases of the cell cycle. For this reason, stem cells located at the base of crypts are particularly vulnerable thereby leading to a dearth of differentiated cells (descendants of the stem cells) and a loss of mucosal integrity. This denuding of the gut mucosa lasts for the duration of the therapy and subsides 10–15 days after the radiotherapy has stopped. Loss of mucosal integrity increases gut permeability to bacteria and other antigens and also to loss of electrolytes and fluid, and therefore the predominant feature of acute radiation enteritis is diarrhea.

Chronic radiation enteropathy is due to a progressive, occlusive vasculitis that may affect all layers of the bowel wall. Ischemia and hypoxia is caused by arterial or venous thrombosis and hyalinization of blood vessel walls. Ischemia leads to mucosal atrophy, thickening, and ulceration and also muscularis fibrosis and serosal thickening. The transmural changes seen in chronic radiation enteropathy can present with symptoms of an inflammatory colitis, stricturing disease, or even bowel perforation.

Mechanism: There have been significant advances in the understanding of the molecular changes seen in chronic radiation enteritis. A number of pathways and key inflammatory mediators have been implicated in disease pathogenesis including:

- Production of free radicals, which causes cell death through disruption of the cell membrane and single or double-stranded DNA breaks.
- Increased apoptosis through induced levels of the tumor suppressor gene *p53*.
- Transforming growth factor β (TGFβ) is a pivotal growth factor that is involved in immune responses, extracellular matrix deposition (and hence fibrosis) and cell growth and differentiation, and is a potent pro-inflammatory and pro-fibrotic cytokine. Radiation causes a significant rise in TGFβ expression and activity and this may, in part, account for some of the micro- and macroscopic changes seen and also direct future lines of therapeutic investigation in radiation enteritis.
- In addition, other studies have implicated the following as being potentially pathogenic in radiation enteropathy: decreased mast cell response to secretagogs; increased inducible nitric oxide synthase (iNOS); suppression of Na/K ATPase pump activity leading to malabsorptive diarrhea; altered ICAM-1, tumor necrosis factor-α (TNF-α), interleukin-1, serotonin, vasoinactive polypeptide, substance P, peptide YY, motilin, and choline acetyltransferase expression.
- Animal model work has shown that radiation exposure can induce large and small bowel giant migrating contractions perhaps leading to decreased gut transit time. The same study also suggested an overall decrease in proximal small bowel contractile activity but the authors suggested that the main effect on motility is from the giant migrating contractions.[3]

Pathology

Many of the macro- and microscopic pathological findings in radiation enteritis and colitis are nonspecific and can be seen in other types of inflammatory bowel conditions. Macroscopically, there can be narrowing of the gut lumen with proximal bowel dilatation, gut wall thickening, frank ulceration, and even perforation. Microscopically, the pathologist may see an inflammatory cell infiltrate, diffuse collagen deposition, a progressive occlusive vasculitis and vascular sclerosis, and mucosal and serosal thickening (see Fig. 113.1 and Fig. 113.2).

Clinical presentation

Acute radiation gut injury is common and occurs soon after the onset of radiotherapy and is characterized by the typical colitis/enteritis symptoms of diarrhea, abdominal discomfort, tenesmus and, less frequently, overt rectal bleeding. The prognosis for acute radiation enteritis is excellent, as the mucosal damage will almost always resolve spontaneously as new cryp epithelial cells regenerate. Symptoms may start a few hour after starting treatment and will usually resolve within 2 week after therapy has ceased.

Chronic radiation-induced gut injury can present with symp toms of constipation and altered motility as well as with th symptoms seen in acute enteritis or even from the symptom of complications of radiation exposure such as adhesions, per foration, secondary cancer, or fistula formation.

The clinical presentation of radiation enteritis is largely dic tated by which anatomical section of the gastrointestinal trac has been exposed to the ionizing radiation (Table 113.1).

Differential diagnosis

Radiation-induced gut inflammation can mimic any other caus of inflammation and the key to making the diagnosis is to hav

TABLE 113.1 CLINICAL PRESENTATION OF RADIATON INJURY ACCORDING TO SITE EXPOSED

GORAL CAVITY AND PHARYNX
• Mucositis • Transient change in taste and smell (radiotherapy affects bitter and salt taste compared with chemotherapy, which largely affects the sweet and sour senses) • Doses of 60–70 Gy can lead to taste impairment for several years
ESOPHAGUS
• Esophagitis • >60 Gy can cause perforation • Decreased motility
STOMACH
• Gastritis and ulceration (radiation ulcers are usually 0.5–2 cm in diameter and situated in the antrum) • Decreased acid secretion, which can last from 6months to many years (radiation has been used as therapy for peptic ulceration) • Chronic atrophic gastritis
SMALL BOWEL (FIG. 113.1)
• Jejunitis and ileitis • Perforation • Stricture • Altered motility • Fistulae • Adhesions
COLON
• Colitis and ulceration • Stricture • Altered motility • Adhesions • Secondary cancer
ANORECTUM
• Decreased anal contractility and rectal compliance • Increased electrosensory threshold • Internal anal sphincter damage • Proctitis

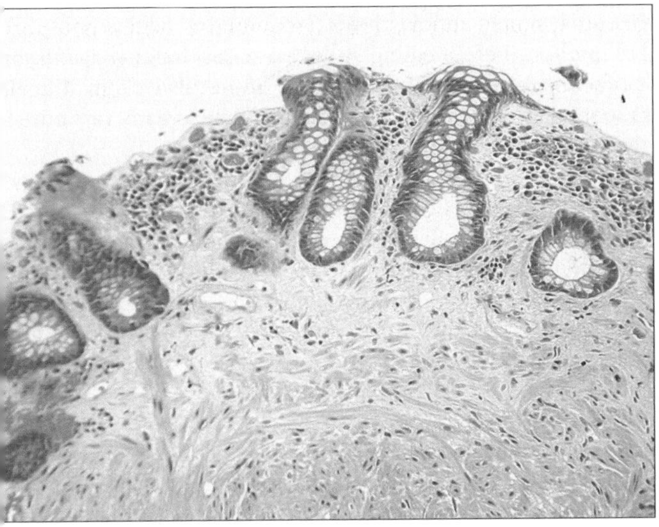

ig. 113.1 **Chronic irradiation proctitis.** Rectal biopsy with chronic radiation proctitis showing crypt architectural distortion, lamina ropria fibrosis, vascular ectasia, and mild focal chronic inflammation. ourtesy of Dr Bryan Warren, John Radcliffe Hospital.

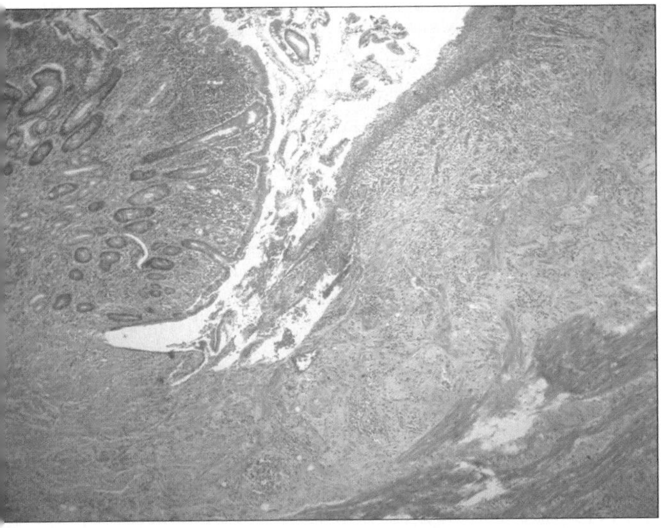

ig. 113.2 **Acute or chronic ischemia of small bowel.** Small bowel vith acute or chronic ischemia showing ulceration, fibrosis, and ascular ectasia. Courtesy of Dr Bryan Warren, John Radcliffe Hospital.

CLINICAL PRESENTATION
Presentation depends on which part of the gastrointestinal tract is affected and also on the presence or absence of complications • Mouth: loss of taste, mucositis • Esophagus: esophagitis, dysmotility • Stomach: gastritis, peptic ulceration • Small bowel: diarrhea, malnutrition, strictures, adhesions, perforation, dysmotility • Large bowel: diarrhea, strictures, adhesions, rectal bleeding, perforation, dysmotility • Anorectum: diarrhea, rectal bleeding, incontinence • Complications: malnutrition bowel obstruction rectal bleeding perforation secondary malignancy

a high index of suspicion in a patient presenting with symptoms. The differential diagnosis (Table 113.2) depends, in part, on the anatomical location of the damage and also what, if any, complications have occurred.

Where diarrhea is related to radiotherapy, there is a large number of potential mechanisms,[4] as illustrated in Table 113.3.

Diagnostic methods

The key to making the diagnosis of radiation-induced bowel injury is to have a high index of suspicion in a patient who has previously received radiotherapy. Nevertheless, patients with symptoms who have previously received radiotherapy should be thoroughly investigated as their symptoms commonly arise from unrelated pathology. The diagnosis is usually made endoscopically or radiologically. Colonoscopic appearances will show changes of mucosal or transmural inflammation such as ulceration, inflamed mucosa, telangectasia, fistulae, or stricturing. Biopsies may be inconclusive. Barium investigations may be normal or show ulceration, submucosal thickening, single or multiple strictures, adhesions or fistulae, or simply a loss of the normal haustral pattern.[5] Mucosal changes can be seen at capsule endoscopy.

Treatment

There is a paucity of good-quality randomized controlled trials (RCTs) on therapies for radiation-induced gastrointestinal tract damage. As discussed above, the symptoms attributable to radiation may be due to complications such as stricturing or perforation (see 'Complications and their management'). Some patients may become malnourished and nutritional assessment and support may be necessary (see Chapter 139).

TABLE 113.2 DIFFERENTIAL DIAGNOSIS OF RADIATION ENTERITIS
• Small bowel enteritis • Any cause of small bowel inflammation or malabsorption • Crohn's disease • NSAID enteropathy • Celiac disease • Small bowel lymphoma • Chronic pancreatitis • Bacterial overgrowth • Lactase deficiency • Amyloidosis • Infection • Giardia • Strongyloides stercoralis • Whipple's disease • Radiation colitis • Any cause of colitis or diarrhea including: – Inflammatory bowel disease – Acute self-limiting colitis (infective) – Pseudomembranous colitis – Drug-induced colitis – Ischemic colitis – Microscopic colitis – Irritable bowel syndrome – Chronic pancreatitis – Malabsorption – Bacterial overgrowth

TABLE 113.3 MECHANISMS OF DIARRHEA IN PATIENTS UNDERGOING RADIOTHERAPY
• Bile salt malabsorption (1–50%) • Colonic strictures (3–15%) • Bacterial overgrowth (8–45%) • Diverticular disease (8–22%) • Relapse or new neoplasia (4–10%) • Pelvic sepsis (4%) • Drug related (5%) • Inflammatory bowel disease (4%) • Stricturing disease • Crohn's disease • Carcinoma • Diverticulitis • Adhesions • Hemorrhage • Carcinoma • Anal fissure • Hemorrhoids • Diverticular disease • Ulcerative colitis • Perforating disease • Carcinoma • Diverticular disease

DIFFERENTIAL DIAGNOSIS

This will, in part, depend on the part of the gastrointestinal tract that is affected

SMALL BOWEL
- Irritable bowel syndrome
- Crohn's disease
- NSAID enteropathy
- Celiac disease
- Small bowel lymphoma

COLON
- Any cause of colitis or diarrhea including:
  - irritable bowel syndrome
  - inflammatory bowel disease
  - acute self-limiting colitis (infective)
  - pseudomembranous colitis
  - drug-induced colitis

Diarrhea

Opiate antagonists such as loperamide or codeine phosphate have been shown to be effective for the treatment of diarrhea in randomized controlled trials.[6] Case reports have suggested that anticholinergic (e.g., hyoscine butylbromide or atropine sulfate) therapies may be affective for radiation-induced diarrheal symptoms. Stercula (Normacol) is anecdotally a very effective treatment for diarrhea and an RCT is currently in progress. Bacterial overgrowth is a common complication of gastrointestinal radiation injury and will usually respond well to an empiric course of metronidazole or ciprofloxacin (see Chapter 46).

Fecal incontinence

There have been no published studies on the treatment of fecal incontinence following radiotherapy. Anecdotal evidence suggests that simple antidiarrheals (loperamide, codeine phosphat half an hour before eating, toilet exercises, bulking agents, ar biofeedback may all be effective. Some also claim dramat responses from topical phenylephidirine cream (an adren receptor agonist).

Abdominal pain

Again, there are few published data relating to the treatme of abdominal pain. It is important to exclude constipation ar fecal loading as the cause of pain. Low-dose antidepressant fentanyl patches, and gabapentin have all, anecdotally, show benefit in some patients.

Bleeding mucosa

Rectal bleeding in patients with suspected radiation-induce GI disease should always be investigated, as the cause is n related to the previous radiotherapy in 25–65% of these patient Sucralfate enemas and oral metronidazole are of proven efficac (RCTs) in rectal bleeding.[7] Treatments that may be of benef include salicylate and corticosteroid enemas (not as efficacio as sucralfate enemas). An RCT demonstrated no benefit fc short-chain fatty acid enemas and a case series suggests th approximately two-thirds of patients will respond to hype baric oxygen therapy.[8] Anecdotal reports suggest that the ant oxidants vitamin C and E and the antitumor necrosis factor-(TNF-α) antibody, infliximab, may all be effective. Bleedin mucosal lesions that fail to respond to medical therapy may b treated with direct endoscopic ablative therapy (laser, heate probe, or argon plasma beamer). A minority of patients suff from recurrent or intractable bleeding requiring multip transfusions.

Fibrosis

There is anecdotal evidence that liposomal copper/zinc supe oxide dismutase, the anti-TNF-α agent pentoxifylline in th presence of high-dose vitamin E and even hyperbaric oxyge may be effective in the treatment of fibrosis. However, fibros leading to stenosis that is symptomatic usually requires surger The symptoms of obstruction seen with small bowel stenos may benefit from a low residue/fiber diet. There is considerab animal model research into potential moderators of fibros including the use of ACE inhibitors, colchicines, endothelin antagonists, and integrin antagonists.

Complications and their management

Complications of radiation damage include:
- Bleeding.
- Fibrosis.
- Stenosis.
- Secondary malignancy.
- Fistulae or extensive small bowel inflammation, which ca lead to nutritional failure. Enteral or even parenteral supplementary feeding may be needed in addition to simple salt, fluid, and vitamin replacement. Fistulae may require surgery (see Chapter 54) if symptomatic.
- Bacterial overgrowth: anywhere between 8% and 45% of patients with diarrhea following radiation damage to the gastrointestinal tract have bacterial overgrowth and should respond well to a simple course of metronidazole or ciprofloxacin. Some patients will be prone to recurren attacks and may need a 'rolling' course of antibiotics

TREATMENT AND PREVENTION

MEDICAL
- Diarrhea: antidiarrheals (codeine phosphate, immodium), normacol
- Bacterial overgrowth: broad-spectrum antibiotics
- Fecal incontinence: simple antidiarrheals, toilet exercises, bulking agents, biofeedback, phenylephidirine cream
- Abdominal pain: low-dose antidepressants, fentanyl patches, gabapentin
- Bleeding: sucralfate enemas, oral metronidazole, salicylate enemas, corticosteroid enemas, hyperbaric oxygen therapy, vitamin C and E, antitumur necrosis factor-α (TNF-α) antibody, endoscopic laser therapy
- Liposomal copper/zinc superoxide dismutase, pentoxyfiline, hyperbaric oxygen.

ENDOSCOPIC
- Direct ablation of bleeding telangectasia

SURGERY
- Resection occasionally needed for fistulae, stenosis, or recurrent bleeding

(e.g., a week of metronidazole, followed by weeks of clarithromycin and then doxycycline).
Disaccharidase deficiency: radiation damage can also cause damage to the gastrointestinal brush border resulting in lactase deficiency and lactose intolerance; a trial of dairy exclusion may be beneficial.

Surgery for complications may be problematic as radiation injury often associated with intra-abdominal adhesions. Furthermore, anastomoses at diseased sites are prone to leaking and surgeons may opt to choose bypass or diversion therapy though this may precipitate any tendency to short bowel syndrome.[9] Topical formaldehyde during examination under anesthetic has been used for radiation proctitis but carries a risk of perianal burning due to spillage and causing colitis.

Prognosis with and without treatment

There are few data about the long-term prognosis in radiation colitis. However, for the vast majority the outlook is good and treatment is symptomatic. Some patients will require surgery for fistulae or stenotic lesions but should do well after surgery. The few patients who have extensive small bowel disease or multiple fistulae have a more uncertain future. They may face the problems associated with nutritional deficiency and intestinal failure and possibly the need for long-term home total parenteral nutrition or even small bowel transplantation (see Chapter 139).

What to tell patients

Patients should be told that on the whole the outlook is good. They should be encouraged to report symptoms as treatment is largely symptomatically based. Since most of the treatment options are based on anecdote, patients should be warned that there might be an element of 'trial and error' in finding the most effective treatment for their particular symptoms. Patients should also be encouraged to report their symptoms and, in particular, to not assume that any change in their symptoms are due to their previous radiation exposure because of the significant comorbidity identified in the published studies. Finally, patients should be informed that there has been relatively little research into this condition in the past but that current research into pathogenesis and potential therapies promises a better outlook for patients in the not too distant future.

Current controversies

Researchers have begun to recognize the importance of this condition and current and future research is focusing on the molecular pathogenesis of radiation damage to the gut as well as on potential therapeutic interventions. An increased understanding of the molecular cascades involved in these processes may lead to the development of more specific molecular therapies. There is no doubt that the significant progress currently being made in the development of molecular and biological therapies for the treatment of inflammatory bowel disease may well have some benefits for patients with radiation damage. One area of concern in trying to fill the evidence-based void is that gastroenterologists will usually have perhaps just one or two patients with this condition under their care and recruitment for therapeutic trials may therefore be difficult.

Sources of advice

A good source of information for patients is: www.nci.nih.gov/cancerinfo/pdq/supportivecare/radiationenteritis/patient The same website, but with 'healthcare' instead of 'patient' at the end of the address, is a good source of information for the clinician.

PHYSICOCHEMICAL INJURY TO THE GUT

Introduction

Millions of foreign bodies (see Chapter 115) are introduced to the gut (both orally and anally) each year and in the vast majority of cases no clinical problems result. Foreign bodies can affect any part of the gut whereas corrosive or chemical injury (including that caused by medication) is usually confined to the oropharynx, esophagus, or stomach. Coins are the most commonly ingested foreign body (though any emergency room doctor will be able to tell tales of children swallowing amazing household objects) and chemical and corrosive injuries are most often caused by medication or household cleaning fluids (strong alkali solutions).

KEY POINTS

- Foreign body ingestion is a common and largely 'benign' clinical problem
- The vast majority occur in children or 'vulnerable' people
- The minority of foreign bodies pass through the tract without sequelae
- Approximately 10–20% of patients will require endoscopic or surgical intervention
- Serious consequences can occur after ingestion of caustic agents
- Caustic agent ingestion treatment should be managed with:
  - resuscitation
  - avoidance of emesis
  - timely endoscopy
  - consideration of corticosteroids and antibiotics
  - sequential dilatations to prevent esophageal stricturing

Epidemiology

More than 2500 people die each year in the US as a result of ingesting a foreign body and more than 25 000 are treated each year following the ingestion of caustic agents. Children are at most risk (more than 80% of all corrosive ingestions occur in children ingesting household cleaning agents), although almost all anally introduced foreign bodies occur in an older population. Other groups at particular risk include: psychiatric patients (corrosives and foreign bodies); prisoners (foreign bodies); elderly patients with dementia (foreign bodies, including dentures); the immobile and infirm (chemical injuries from medication); and people with anatomical malformations, stenosis, strictures, or dysmotility (foreign bodies and chemical injuries from medication) within the gastrointestinal tract.

Causes, risk factors

The larger the foreign body the more likely it is to become 'stuck.' NSAIDs, doxycycline, tetracyclines, quinidine, and phenytoin[10] are among the drugs that particularly cause damage to the esophagus , including 'pill esophagitis.' There are a number of sites at which these pills may become stuck including the upper esophageal sphincter, at the level of the aortic arch, left main bronchus, and left atrium (especially with a dilated left atrium secondary to cardiac disease), and the lower esophageal sphincter. Ingestion of alcohol and taking the tablets last thing at night (with minimal water and just before adopting a prolonged supine position) also increase the risk of esophageal damage.

The most dangerous caustic agents appear to be the strong alkaline cleansing agents that are found in the home including ammonia, sodium hydroxide, and potassium hydroxide. Other agents include hydrochloric acid (cleansing agents), sulfuric acid (batteries), and sodium hypochlorite (bleach).

Pathogenesis

Macroscopically, bolus obstructions can cause inflammation, necrosis, and even perforation. Harmful medications may cause acute, deep, eroding ulceration that can be transmural and hence these injuries can present with anything from discomfort through to signs and symptoms of perforation, mediastinitis, and even death by exsanguinations. Alkaline agents cause an acute necrosis with cell membrane rupture, protein denaturing, and thrombosis. Alkaline agents can cause a relatively acute transmural necrosis and can present with signs of perforation, etc., as above.

Clinical presentation

Children who have swallowed a foreign body often present perfectly well to the emergency room with an extremely worried parent. In the vast majority of cases there is nothing to find on examination. Large object ingestion may present with respiratory distress (tachypnea, stridor, respiratory distress) if the object has caused obstruction in the pharynx or trachea. Obstruction in the esophagus may present with dysphagia, drooling (inability to swallow saliva), retrosternal discomfort, or even signs of perforation (fever, shock, surgical emphysema, etc). Obstruction further down the gastrointestinal tract may present with symptoms of acute bowel obstruction such as colicky abdominal pain, distention, lack of flatus, and vomiting (see Chapter 62). Parents are usually particularly worried about sharp objects but the gastrointestinal tract is remarkably resistant to damage by such objects (more than 70% pass through without incident) although perforation can occur (presenting with peritonism (s Chapter 98).

In cases of pill-induced damage to the esophagus there m be a classical history of retro-sternal discomfort that comes soon after ingesting tablets and adopting a supine posture. However, patients may present with dysphagia or, in extreme cas symptoms of perforation or upper gastrointestinal hemorrhag

Ingestion of corrosive agents may present acutely: with or pharyngeal burns, wheeze, stridor, dyspnea, or hoarseness if t larynx is affected; dyspnoea and respiratory distress if there h been aspiration; or chest pain, odynophagia, vomiting, droolin hematemesis, mediastinitis, or peritonitis if the esophagus the chief site of damage.

CLINICAL PRESENTATION

- History of ingestion of foreign body or caustic agent
- Patients are usually asymptomatic
- Patients may present with:
  - upper respiratory symptoms if oropharynx affected (respiratory distress, stridor)
  - obstruction in the esophagus (dysphagia, drooling, retro-sternal discomfort, or even signs of perforation)
  - obstruction further down the gastrointestinal tract – symptoms of acute bowel obstruction (colicky abdominal pain, distention, lack of flatus, and vomiting)
  - retro-sternal discomfort, upper gastrointestinal bleeding, or perforation in cases of erosive pill damage
  - oro-pharyngeal burns, wheeze, stridor, dyspnea, or hoarseness (laryngeal damage); dyspnea and respiratory distress (aspiration); chest pain, odynophagia, vomiting, drooling, hematemesis, mediastinitis, or peritonitis esophageal damage) following caustic injury

Differential diagnosis

Recurrent childhood attendances to hospital with ingested forei bodies should alert the physician to the possibility of Munchaus by proxy. The differential diagnosis of foreign bodies presenti as obstruction include malignancy, adhesions, inflammato bowel disease, and diverticular disease (see Chapter 62) a presenting with perforation include malignancy, peptic ulceratio diverticular disease, and ischemia. Corrosive damage to t upper gastrointestinal tract can mimic gastroesophageal reflu hematemesis, peptic ulcer disease, ischemic heart disease, musc loskeletal pain, cholecystitis, ruptured esophagus (Boerhaave syndrome), or even pancreatitis. The key to making the corre diagnosis is in obtaining the history of ingestion of the harmf agent or foreign body, and suspecting the diagnosis in the fi place.

Diagnostic methods

Plain radiographs can often show a radiolucent foreign bo and this can be helpful in not only confirming the diagnosis b also in identifying the anatomical position of the foreign bod A chest radiograph may confirm the presence of intramec astinal air or surgical emphysema suggesting esophageal pe foration and an erect chest film may show free air under t diaphragm in a perforation occurring below the diaphrag Barium or gastrografin swallows can be useful in diagnosis

DIFFERENTIAL DIAGNOSIS
Munchausen by proxy Foreign bodies presenting as obstruction: malignancy adhesions inflammatory bowel disease diverticular disease Presenting with perforation: peptic ulceration diverticular disease ischemia Corrosive damage to the upper gastrointestinal tract can mimic: gastroesophageal reflux peptic ulcer disease ischemic heart disease musculoskeletal pain cholecystitis ruptured esophagus (Boerhaave's syndrome) pancreatitis

ute upper gastrointestinal obstruction (e.g., food bolus impaction the esophagus), especially if the endoscopist is unhappy to doscope a patient with acute dysphagia. Endoscopy can be eful in confirming diagnosis if the test is performed soon ter ingestion as the foreign body may be within reach of a ope, although the main role for endoscopy is in treatment e below). The presence of discrete esophageal ulceration ccasionally with the presence of tablet remnants within the cer base) with normal surrounding mucosa seen at endoscopy suggestive of pill-induced damage. The history of corrosive gestion and confluent ulceration and mucosal sloughing seen endoscopy confirms the diagnosis of corrosive damage.

eatment and prevention

rtunately most instances of foreign body ingestion require treatment save reassurance.[11] Watch batteries are extremely rrosive to the esophagus (but safely neutralized in the gastric idic contents) and if radiographs suggest that these are caught the esophagus then urgent endoscopy is indicated.[12] Food lus obstruction can be alleviated by endoscopy either by very utiously 'pushing' the bolus through or by piecemeal removal. me clinicians recommend a trial of smooth muscle relaxants lucagon 1 mg intravenously) or the ingestion of 'fizzy' soda inks in bolus obstruction as carbon dioxide in the drinks can metimes cause esophageal distention and aid the passing of e bolus. Sharp objects within reach of the endoscope can be moved with the aid of an over-tube thereby preventing further mage and airway obstruction. Anesthetic assistance should sought. Retrieval devices are available such as rat's tooth rceps and roth nets.

Some clinicians advocate the use of a Foley catheter (to 'pull') a bougienage method (to 'push') for esophageal foreign dies, especially in children. These should be performed, usually der fluoroscopic guidance, in healthy children who have gested a 'blunt' foreign body within the previous 24 h.

Patients who have ingested corrosive agents should be resustated as necessary and if respiratory compromise is apparent ay even require intubation. The exact nature of the ingested bstance is vital and appropriate advice from a poisons' center should be sought. Emesis should not be induced and the role of gastric lavage via a nasogastric tube remains controversial as this may induce vomiting or even cause perforation. Neutralization of the acid or alkali should not be performed as this can often cause thermal injury. Endoscopy should be performed when the patient is stable though the initial (within 24 h) findings may be minimal. Some clinicians believe that in patients with circumferential erosions, high-dose (more than 1 mg/kg/day) corticosteroids should be given. This regimen is supported by data from animal studies suggesting that corticosteroids may reduce the development of strictures but may increase the risk of septicemia. The only published randomized controlled trial in humans showed no benefit on stricture formation but there were less esophagectomies in the treated group, although the number of patients studied was very small.[13] Corticosteroids should be used in patients with respiratory compromise. There is no evidence regarding the role of broad-spectrum antibiotics in this setting but they are widely used.

To help prevent pill-induced damage patients should be encouraged to ingest tablets at least an hour before going to bed and tablets should be taken with a suitable amount of water. Health education programs should encourage the safe storage of caustic agents in the home.

TREATMENT AND PREVENTION

- Majority of foreign body ingestions require no treatment
- Food bolus obstruction can be alleviated by endoscopy after a trial of smooth muscle relaxants or the ingestion of 'fizzy' soda drinks
- Sharp objects within reach of the endoscope can be removed with the aid of an over-tube
- Management of corrosive agents requires:
  - resuscitation
  - emesis prevention
  - controversy remains over the role of gastric lavage via a nasogastric tube, corticosteroids, and antibiotics
  - timely endoscopy
  - sequential endoscopies and dilatations to prevent esophageal stricturing
- Prevention:
  - foreign body ingestion – education
  - corrosive agents – education and appropriate storing of household cleaning agents
  - pill-induced damage – advice to take pills with plenty of liquid and not just prior to going to sleep

Complications and their management

Perforation or obstruction from foreign bodies not amenable to endoscopic intervention will require surgical intervention. Pills can cause deep erosions leading to aorto-enteric fistula, perforation, and mediastinitis. Mild to moderate hemorrhage from ulcers may be successfully treated endoscopically but aorto-enteric fistulae are likely to cause death by exsanguination.

Up to 30% of patients who have ingested corrosive agents will develop esophageal strictures from 2 weeks to many months after exposure. Prophylactic radiological or endoscopic dilatation or stenting (more controversial) starting at week 3 after exposure has been advocated as a means of preventing stricture development.

Prognosis

Between 10% and 20% of people who have ingested foreign bodies will require some sort of intervention (usually endoscopic) and less than 1% will require surgical intervention, while the outlook for the vast majority (whether they require intervention or not) is excellent.[11] In contrast, the outlook for individuals who have ingested caustic agents is more complicated and studies have suggested that the mortality in this situation is as high as 3%. Other data have suggested that up to 7% of patients with esophageal cancer have had a history of caustic agent ingestion.

What to tell patients

Patients who have ingested foreign bodies should be reassured that, in the vast majority of cases, the item will pass through the gastrointestinal tract without problems. A few will requ intervention depending on the nature of the ingested item a patients should be advised to seek medical help if they devel severe abdominal pain. Patients who have ingested caustic age should be warned that they face a more difficult future that m require several endoscopic or surgical interventions. All patie should be advised to avoid repeating the ingestion and, in t case of parents, there should be more careful storage of hou hold caustic agents.

Sources of advice

A good source of information for both patients and clinicians (p marily aimed at the latter) can be found at: www.asge.org/g resources/manual/uge_ingested.asp and www.emedicine.co emerg/topic379.htm

REFERENCES

1. Yeoh EK, Horowitz M. Radiation enteritis. Surg Gynecol Obstet 1987; 165:373–379.
2. Haddak GK, Grodsinsky C, Allen H. The spectrum of radiation enteritis. Dis Colon Rectum 1983; 26:590–594.
3. Nguyen NP, Antoine JE, Dutta S, Karlsson U, Sallah S. Current concepts in radiation enteritis and implications for future clinical trials. Cancer 2002; 95:1151–1162.
4. Ludgate SM, Merrick MV. The pathogenesis of post-irradiation chronic diarrhoea: measurement of SeHCAT and B12 absorption for differential diagnosis determines treatment. Clin Radiol 1985; 36:275–278.
5. Mendelson RM, Nolan DJ. The radiological features of chronic radiation enteritis. Clin Radiol 1985; 36:141–148.
6. Yeoh EK, Horowitz M, Russo A, Muecke T, Robb T, Chatterton BE. Gastrointestinal function in chronic radiation enteritis – effects of loperamide-N-oxide. Gut 1993; 34:476–482.
7. Denton A, Forbes A, Andreyev J, Maher EJ. Non-surgical interventions for late radiation proctitis in patients who have received radical radiotherapy to the pelvis. Cochrane Database Syst Rev 2002; CD003455.
8. Gouello JP, Bouachour G, Person B, Ronceray J, Cellier P, Alquier P. The role of hyperbaric oxygen therapy in radiation-induced digestive disorders. 36 cases. Presse Med 1999; 28:1579.
9. Wobbes T, Vershueren RC, Lubbers EJ et al. Surgical aspects of radiation enteritis. Dis Colon Rectum 1984; 27:89–92.
10. Semble EL, Wu WC, Castell DO. Nonsteroi antiinflammatory drugs and esophageal injury. Semin Arthritis Rheum 1989; 19:99–109.
11. Vizcarrondo FJ, Brady PG, Nord HJ. Foreig bodies of the upper gastrointestinal tract. Gastrointest Endosc 1983; 29:208–210.
12. Litovitz TL, Schmitz BF. Ingestions of cylindrical and button batteries: analysis of 2382 cases. Pediatrics 1992; 89:747–757.
13. Anderson KD, Rouse TM, Randolph JG. A controlled trial of corticosteroids in children with corrosive injury of the oesophagus. N Engl J Med 1990; 323:10.

Chapter 114

Systemic amyloidosis

P N Hawkins

KEY POINTS

- Amyloidosis is a multisystem disease caused by the deposition of various proteins in a characteristic abnormal fibrillar form in many tissues throughout the body
- Amyloid fibrils bind the dye Congo red producing diagnostic histology
- 1 in 1000 individuals in the UK die of systemic amyloidosis
- Acquired AA and AL amyloidosis occur in about 2% of patients with chronic inflammatory diseases and monoclonal gammopathies, respectively
- Hereditary systemic amyloidosis accounts for 5% of all cases, and is frequently misdiagnosed as AL type

TRODUCTION

ıyloidosis is a disorder of protein folding in which normally ıble proteins are deposited as abnormal, insoluble fibrils t progressively disrupt tissue structure and function and reby cause disease.[1] Amyloid fibrils are principally defined their distinctive staining properties with the dye Congo red ɪ subsequent appearance under light microscopy. They also ve a characteristic ultrastructural appearance on electron croscopy, and the uniform ability to bind the normal plasma tein serum amyloid P component. Some 25 different unrelated teins can form amyloid *in vivo*, and clinical amyloidosis is ssified according to the fibril protein type, as well as by ether it is acquired or inherited. In systemic amyloidosis, deposits can occur in all tissues except within the brain, and present to some extent in blood vessels throughout the body.

IDEMIOLOGY

cise data on the epidemiology of amyloid are not available, systemic amyloidosis is thought to be the cause of death in out 1 in 1000 individuals in the western world. Acquired temic AL (monoclonal immunoglobulin light chain) amyloi- sis is the most common form of the disease and outnumbers es of systemic AA (reactive secondary) amyloidosis by about fold in the UK. AA amyloidosis has a lifetime incidence of 5% among patients with chronic inflammatory diseases such rheumatoid arthritis and inflammatory bowel disease, and amyloidosis occurs in about 2% of individuals with mono- nal gammopathies.[2] It has lately been discovered that hered- ry forms of systemic amyloidosis are much more common n previously thought, and account for about 5% of all cases.[3] reditary amyloidosis is transmitted in an autosomal dominant manner, but penetrance of many forms is low accounting for the frequent absence of a family history.

CAUSES, RISK FACTORS, DISEASE ASSOCIATIONS

AL amyloid fibrils are derived from monoclonal light chains, which have unique structure in each patient, accounting for the extremely heterogeneous spectrum of clinical features in this form of the disease. Almost any dyscrasia of cells of the B lymphocyte lineage, including multiple myeloma, malignant lymphomas and macroglobulinemia, may be complicated AL amyloidosis, but well over 80% of cases are associated with low-grade and otherwise 'benign' monoclonal gammopathy.

AA amyloidosis occurs in association with any kind of chronic inflammatory disorder that can generate an acute phase response for a sustained period. In western Europe and the US the most frequent predisposing conditions are idiopathic rheumatic diseases. Tuberculosis and other chronic infections remain important causes of AA amyloidosis in some parts of the world. About 6% of patients with AA amyloidosis do not have a clinically overt chronic inflammatory disease, and these patients are prone to being misdiagnosed as having AL amyloidosis. The commonest underlying pathology in such cases in our series has been Castleman's disease tumors of the solitary plasma cell type, located in either the mediastinum or gut mesentery.

Hereditary amyloidosis is caused by heterozygous point mutations in the genes for various proteins notably including those of transthyretin, apolipoprotein AI, apolipoprotein AII, lysozyme, and fibrinogen A α-chain.[4] These mutations are usually inherited but may also occur *de novo*.

PATHOGENESIS AND PATHOLOGY

Amyloidogenesis involves substantial refolding of the native structures of the various amyloid precursor proteins, which enables them to autoaggregate in a highly ordered manner to form fibrils with a characteristic β-sheet structure (Fig. 114.1).[5] Amyloid deposition occurs under several conditions:

- firstly, when a normal protein is present for sufficient time at an abnormally high concentration, for example serum amyloid A protein (SAA) during chronic inflammation;
- secondly, in the presence of an ordinary concentration of a normal, but inherently weakly amyloidogenic protein over a very prolonged period, such as in the case of wild-type transthyretin in senile cardiac amyloidosis; and
- thirdly, when there is an acquired or inherited variant protein with abnormal amyloidogenic structure, such as

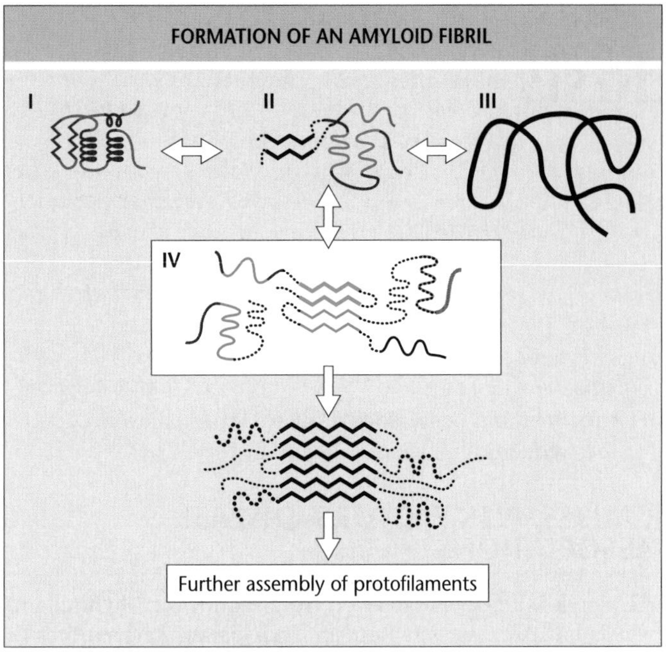

Fig. 114.1 Formation of an amyloid fibril. Cartoon depicting a generic, potentially amyloidogenic protein molecule (I) populating a partly unfolded intermediate state (II) that enables exposed β-sheet structure of like molecules to autoaggregate in an ordered manner to form the earliest nidus of an amyloid fibril. Alternatively, partly unfolded proteins may be cleared away (III). These protofilaments (IV) become lodged in the tissues and may propagate to form mature amyloid fibrils, which associate with glycosaminoglycans and serum amyloid P component.

some monoclonal immunoglobulin light chains or variants of transthyretin, lysozyme, apolipoprotein AI, fibrinogen A a-chain, etc.

All types of amyloid fibril associate with certain glycosaminoglycans and bind serum amyloid P component (SAP), both of which contribute to their formation, stability or persistence.

Amyloidotic organs have a distinctive waxy, lardaceous macroscopic appearance, and deposits in affected tissues show characteristic red-green birefringence when stained with Congo red and viewed in the light microscope under cross-polarized light. Amyloid fibrils have a diameter of 8–10 nm and a rigid nonbranching appearance on electron microscopy (Fig. 114.2).

The symptoms of amyloidosis are caused by progressive disruption of the structure and function of various tissues, and may eventually cause single or multiple organ failure.

CLINICAL PRESENTATION

Systemic amyloidosis is a multisystem disease that may cause an almost limitless range and permutation of organ symptoms. Early symptoms include fatigue and nonspecific deterioration in general well being, the significance of which is often missed. Symptoms include:

- Skin and other visible signs – bruises, especially around the eyes, and enlarged tongue.
- Renal – edema, proteinuria, fatigue with renal failure.
- Cardiac – exertional dyspnea, fatigue and edema associated with restrictive cardiomyopathy.
- Liver – discomfort associated with hepatomegaly and rarely jaundice with liver failure.
- Peripheral neuropathy – paresthesia, numbness, carpal tunnel syndrome, weakness.
- Autonomic neuropathy – low blood pressure, impaired gut motility and bladder emptying.
- Gastrointestinal – poor appetite, bloating, vomiting, diarrhea, constipation, blood loss.
- Adrenal axis – hypoadrenalism.
- Lymphoreticular system – enlarged spleen, enlarged lym nodes.

More than 90% of patients with AA amyloidosis present w nonselective proteinuria, and nephrotic syndrome may deve before progression to end-stage renal failure. Kidney size is u ally normal, but may be enlarged or, in advanced cases, reduc End-stage chronic renal failure is the cause of death in 40–60 of cases. Other presentations include hepatosplenomegaly occasionally thyroid goiter, and gastrointestinal dysfunct including bleeding is common in advanced disease. Neuropa and cardiac involvement are extremely rare.

The heart is affected pathologically in up to 90% of patients, in 30% of whom restrictive cardiomyopathy i presenting feature and in up to half of whom it is fatal. Re AL amyloid has the same manifestations as renal AA amylo but the prognosis is worse. Gut involvement is frequent a may cause motility disturbances (often secondary to autono neuropathy), malabsorption, perforation, hemorrhage, or obstr tion. Macroglossia occurs rarely but is almost pathognomo of AL amyloid. A sensory polyneuropathy, with early loss pain and temperature sensation followed later by motor defic is seen in 10–20% of cases and carpal tunnel syndrome 20%. Autonomic neuropathy leading to orthostatic hypotensi impotence, and gastrointestinal disturbances may occur alo or together with the peripheral neuropathy, and has a v poor prognosis. Skin involvement takes the form of bruisi papules, nodules, and plaques.

Hereditary transthyretin (TTR) amyloidosis presents w progressive and disabling peripheral and autonomic neuropat and/or varying degrees of cardiac involvement, and is of known as familial amyloidotic polyneuropathy (FAP). Depo within the vitreous of the eye occur in a proportion of ca and are very characteristic. Hereditary amyloidosis associa with mutations in the genes for lysosyme, apolipoprotein and fibrinogen A alpha chain usually presents with re dysfunction without neuropathy, but may also variably invo the heart, liver, and other organs.

DIFFERENTIAL DIAGNOSIS

Since amyloidosis is a disease that may affect multiple or systems, the differential diagnosis is extremely wide. It is of not possible to distinguish AA, AL, and hereditary forms of disease clinically, and the presence of a potentially amyloi genic chronic inflammatory disorder, monoclonal gammo thy, or gene mutation can be misleading. Once a histologi diagnosis of amyloidosis has been established, it is vital determine the amyloid fibril type immunohistochemically by analyses of isolated fibril preparations.

DIAGNOSTIC METHODS

The diagnosis of amyloidosis generally requires histologi confirmation. The pathognomonic tinctorial property yloidotic tissue is apple green/red birefringence when stained h Congo red dye and viewed under intense cross-polarized t. 'Screening' biopsies of the rectum and abdominal fat, , are diagnostic in around 50–80% of patients with systemic yloidosis, whereas direct biopsy of an affected organ yields itive histology in close to 100% of cases.

nmunohistochemical staining of amyloid-containing tissue tions is the most accessible method for characterizing the yloid fibril protein type. Radiolabeled SAP scintigraphy is alternative specific, noninvasive, *in vivo* diagnostic method t also enables quantitative monitoring of amyloid deposits ;. 114.3), but which is only available in a few specialized ters.[6,7] Echocardiography is a vital tool for evaluating the trictive diastolic impairment in cardiac amyloidosis.

TREATMENT AND PREVENTION

In the absence of any treatment that specifically causes regression of amyloid deposits, the aim of therapy is to reduce the supply of amyloid fibril precursor proteins in the hope that progression of the disease will be slowed down or halted (Table 114.1). However, few clinical trials have been performed and the approach to treatment remains somewhat empirical. Relatively radical approaches may be justified when the prognosis is otherwise poor, and significant clinical benefits can be obtained including the preservation and restoration of vital organ function along with improved survival. Speculation that amyloid deposits may regress under these circumstances has now been systematically confirmed using serial SAP scintigraphy,[7]

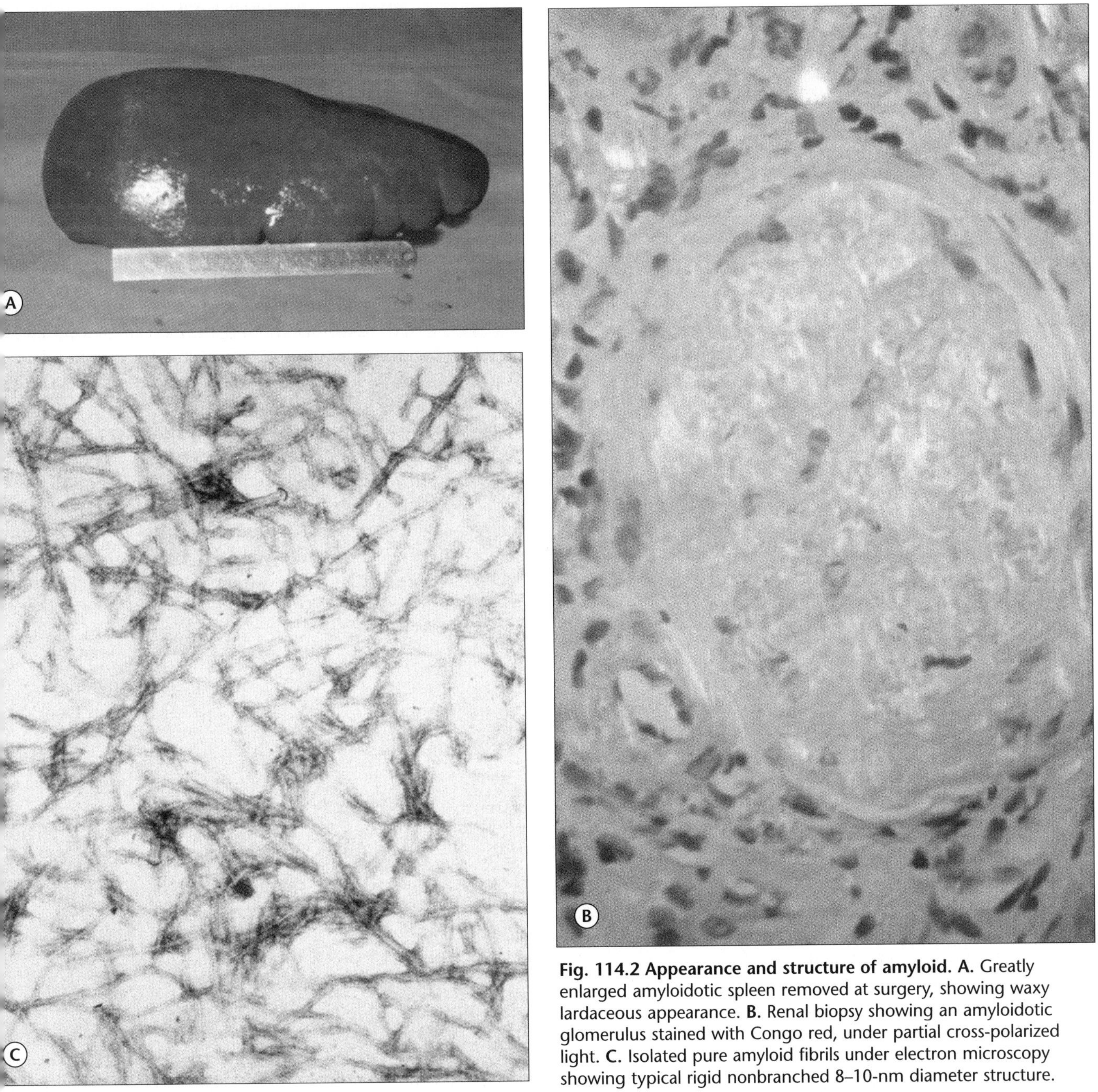

Fig. 114.2 Appearance and structure of amyloid. A. Greatly enlarged amyloidotic spleen removed at surgery, showing waxy lardaceous appearance. **B.** Renal biopsy showing an amyloidotic glomerulus stained with Congo red, under partial cross-polarized light. **C.** Isolated pure amyloid fibrils under electron microscopy showing typical rigid nonbranched 8–10-nm diameter structure.

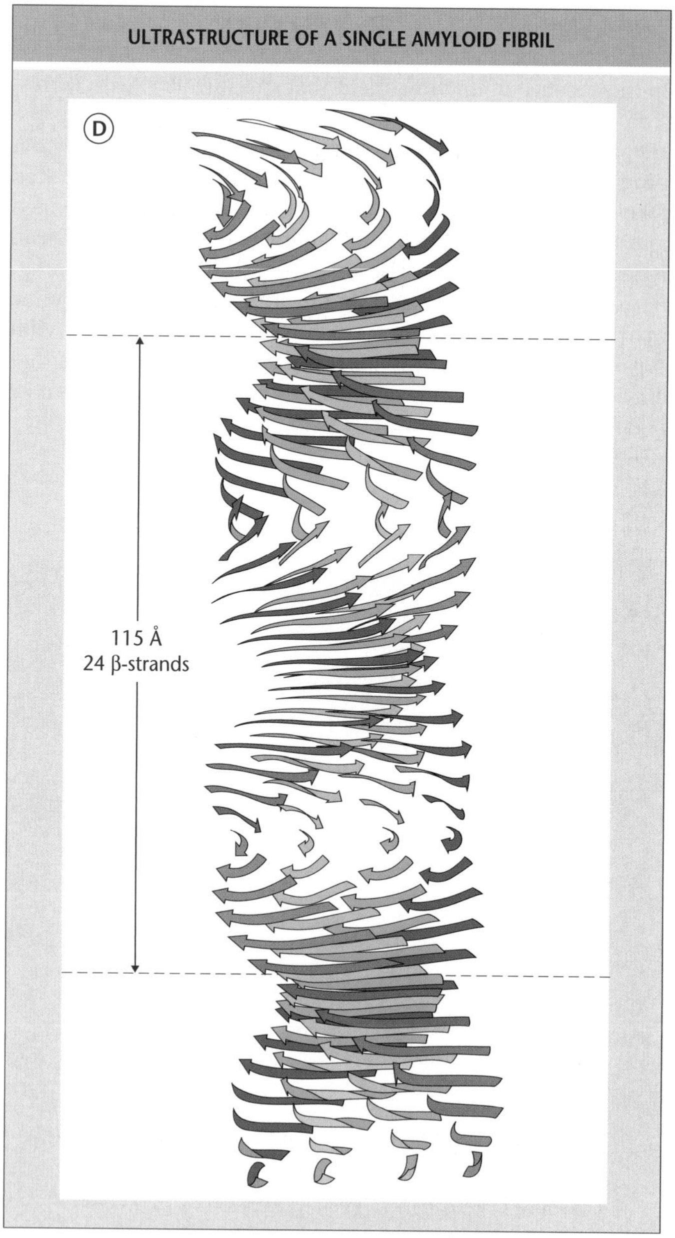

Fig. 114.2—cont'd D. Cartoon depicting the antiparallel twisted β-pleated sheet ultrastructure of a single amyloid fibril.

but it is important to appreciate that clinically signific regression of amyloid may not be evident for months or ye after the supply of the fibril precursor has been reduced.

In **AA amyloidosis** the aim of treatment is to suppress completely as possible the inflammatory process responsi for sustained overproduction of SAA. Extremely good res have been obtained in patients with rheumatoid arthritis trea with oral chlorambucil and more latterly with TNF neutralizi drugs. Follow-up studies have demonstrated that when S values are restored to normal values of less than 10 mg amyloid deposition is halted in all patients, and partial or co plete regression occurs in more than half of cases.[8] Frequ monitoring of the plasma SAA concentration is therefore essential guide to treatment.

In **AL amyloidosis** the goal of treatment is to suppress t B cell clone producing the amyloidogenic monoclo immunoglobulin light chain, using chemotherapy regim based on those used in multiple myeloma. These range fr prolonged low-dose oral therapy, to cyclical infusions, to aut ogous stem cell transplantation.[9] All such treatments are h ardous in this particular setting, and stem cell transplantati carries a substantial procedural mortality that overall excee 15% of cases. Intermediate dose infusional chemothera regimens are favored as first line management in the U guided by serial quantitative measurements of serum-fr immunoglobulin light chain concentration.[10]

In **familial amyloid polyneuropathy** associated wi transthyretin mutations, orthotopic liver transplantation c halt amyloid deposition since the variant amyloidogenic prote is produced mainly in the liver. Successful liver transplantati has been reported in hundreds of cases and, although t peripheral neuropathy usually only stabilizes, autonomic fu tion may improve and the associated visceral amyloid depos regress in many cases. However, cardiac involvement m paradoxically progress after liver transplantation due to depo tion of wild-type TTR on the 'template' of variant TTR am loid.[11] Fibrinogen is synthesized solely by the liver and hepa transplantation is therefore also potentially curative in fibrin gen A a-chain amyloidosis,[12] and has also been demonstrat to be beneficial in hereditary apolipoprotein AI amyloido in which only 50% of the variant amyloidogenic protein produced by the liver.[13]

TABLE 114.1 PRINCIPLES OF TREATMENT IN SYSTEMIC AMYLOIDOSIS

Disease	Aim of treatment	Example of treatment
AA amyloidosis	Suppress acute phase response, thereby reducing SAA production	Anti-TNF in rheumatoid arthritis, colchicine in FMF
AL amyloidosis	Suppress production of monoclonal light chains	Chemotherapy for myeloma and monoclonal gammopathy
Hereditary amyloidosis	Reduce/eliminate production of genetically variant amyloidogenic protein	Orthotopic liver transplantation for variant transthyretin-associated FAP, and selected cases of fibrinogen A α-chain and apolipoprotein AI amyloidosis

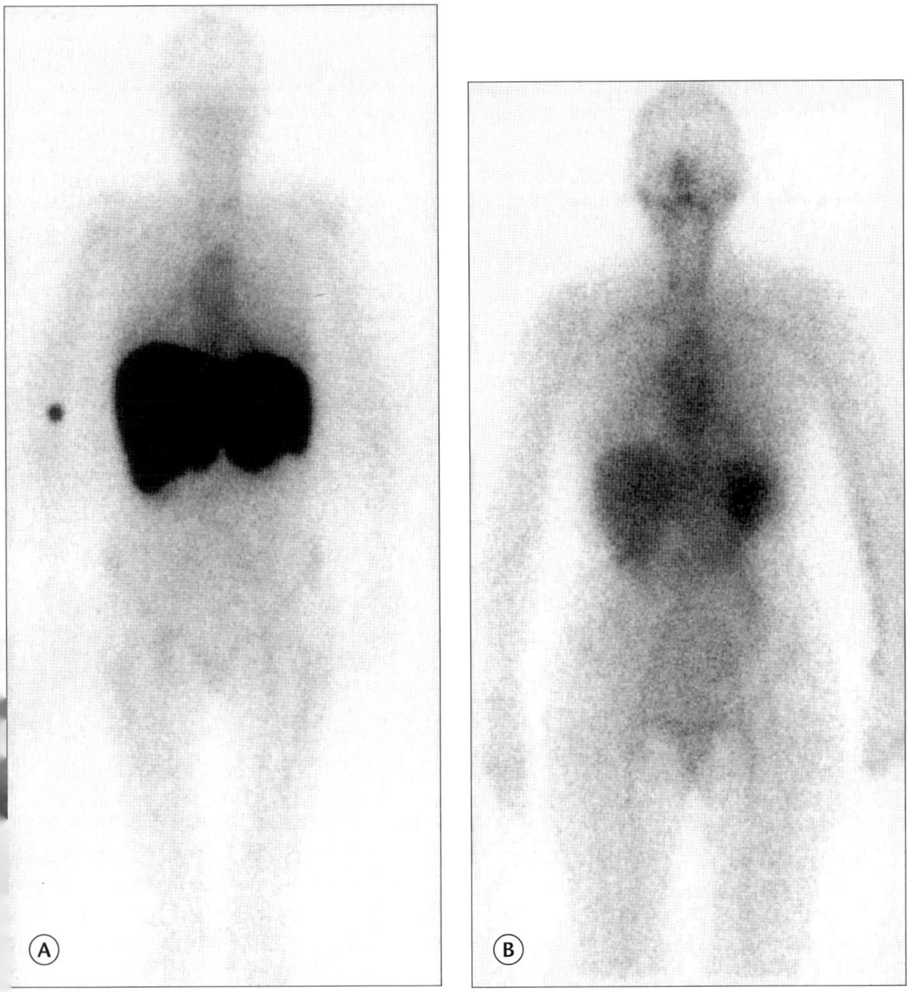

Fig. 114.3 Anterior whole body radiolabeled SAP scan. A. Anterior whole body radiolabeled SAP scan at presentation of a patient with AL amyloidosis, showing abnormal tracer uptake into amyloid deposits within the liver, spleen, kidneys, and bone marrow. **B.** Repeat study 2 years later indicates that substantial regression of the amyloid has occurred following suppression of the patient's underlying plasma cell dyscrasia by chemotherapy; most of the tracer is now confined to the normal blood pool.

Supportive therapy remains a critical component of manage-nent, with the potential for delaying target organ failure, naintaining quality of life, and prolonging survival whilst herapy directed against the underlying metabolic defect can e instituted. Replacement of vital organ function, notably vith renal dialysis, may be necessary, and cardiac and other ransplant procedures have a role in selected cases. Rigorous ontrol of hypertension is vital in renal amyloidosis. Surgical esection of amyloidotic tissue is occasionally beneficial but, in eneral, a conservative approach to surgery, anesthesia, and ther invasive procedures is best. Should any such procedure e undertaken, meticulous attention to blood pressure and fluid alance is essential, especially in patients with renal and/or ardiac involvement. Amyloidotic tissues may heal poorly and re liable to hemorrhage. Diuretics and vasoactive drugs should e used cautiously in cardiac amyloidosis because they can educe cardiac output substantially. Dysrhythmias may respond conventional pharmacological therapy or to pacing.

Prevention of amyloidosis is sometimes possible. Deposition f AA amyloid can be almost completely inhibited in familial lediterranean fever (FMF) by the long-term prophylactic use f colchicine. Mutant genes associated with hereditary forms of nyloidosis can now be identified *in utero*, giving the option f elective termination, and orthotopic hepatic transplantation potentially curative in some forms of hereditary amyloidosis.

PROGNOSIS WITH AND WITHOUT TREATMENT

The prognosis of systemic amyloidosis without treatment is generally very poor. Most such patients with AA amyloidosis die within 5–10 years and in AL type in less than 2 years. Hereditary forms of amyloidosis often have a better prognosis, but in all types life expectancy is greatly increased by therapy that adequately reduces production of the respective amyloid fibril precursor protein.

SOURCES OF INFORMATION FOR PATIENTS AND DOCTORS

The National Amyloidosis Centre in the Royal Free Hospital, London provides specialist clinical evaluation and treatment advice for patients with amyloidosis, and written information: www.ucl.ac.uk/medicine/amyloidosis/nac/index.html

The UK Myeloma Forum has drawn up consensus guidelines on the management of AL amyloidosis, which will be available on: www.ukmf.org.uk/guidelines.htm

The Amyloidosis Support Network provides many international links for patients with physicians, including an email-based patient support network: www.amyloidosis.org

http://www.patient.co.uk/showdoc/1033/

REFERENCES

1. Pepys MB, Hawkins PN. Amyloidosis. In: Warrell DA, Cox TM, Firth JD, Benz EJ Jr, eds. Oxford textbook of medicine, 4th edn. Oxford: Oxford University Press; 2003:162–173.
2. Kyle RA, Therneau TM, Rajkumar SV et al. A long-term study of prognosis in monoclonal gammopathy of undetermined significance. N Engl J Med 2002; 346:564–569.
3. Lachmann HJ, Booth DR, Booth SE et al. Misdiagnosis of hereditary amyloidosis as AL (primary) amyloidosis. N Engl J Med 2002; 346:1786–1791.
4. Lachmann HJ, Hawkins PN. Amyloidosis, familial renal. eMed J 2004:www.emedicine.com/med/topic3379.htm
5. Sunde M, Serpell LC, Bartlam M et al. Common core structure of amyloid fibrils by synchrotron X-ray diffraction. J Mol Biol 1997; 273:729–739.
6. Hawkins PN, Lavender JP, Pepys MB. Evaluation of systemic amyloidosis by scintigraphy with ^{123}I-labeled serum amyloid P component. N Engl J Med 1990; 323:508–513.
7. Hawkins PN. Serum amyloid P component scintigraphy for diagnosis and monitoring amyloidosis. Curr Opin Nephrol Hypertens 2002; 11:649–655.
8. Gillmore JD, Lovat LB, Persey MR, Pepys MB, Hawkins PN. Amyloid load and clinical outcome in AA amyloidosis in relation to circulating concentration of serum amyloid A protein. Lancet 2001; 358:24–29.
9. Comenzo RL, Gertz MA. Autologous stem cell transplantation for primary systemic amyloidosis. Blood 2002; 99:4276–4282.
10. Lachmann HJ, Gallimore R, Gillmore JD et al. Outcome in systemic AL amyloidosis in relation to changes in concentration of circulating free immunoglobulin light chains following chemotherapy. Br J Haematol 2003; 122:78–84.
11. Stangou AJ, Hawkins PN, Heaton ND et al. Progressive cardiac amyloidosis following liver transplantation for familial amyloid polyneuropathy: implications for amyloid fibrillogenesis. Transplantation 1998; 66:229–233.
12. Gillmore JD, Booth DR, Rela M et al. Curative hepatorenal transplantation in systemic amyloidosis caused by the Glu526Val fibrinogen a-chain variant in an English family. Q J Med 2000; 93:269–275.
13. Gillmore JD, Stangou AJ, Tennent GA et al. Clinical and biochemical outcome of hepatorenal transplantation for hereditary systemic amyloidosis associated with apolipoprotein AI Gly26Arg. Transplantation 2001; 71:986–992.

Chapter 115

Foreign bodies

Patrick R Pfau and Gregory G Ginsberg

KEY POINTS

- Gastrointestinal foreign bodies include esophageal food impactions, true foreign bodies (non-food), and bezoars
- Foreign bodies are the second most common endoscopic emergency after gastrointestinal bleeding
- Flexible endoscopy is the diagnostic and therapeutic modality of choice for foreign bodies

NTRODUCTION

;astrointestinal (GI) foreign bodies include food impactions, nimal and fish bones, non-food foreign bodies ingested orally r inserted per rectum, and bezoars (collections of indigestible naterial that accumulate in the GI tract). Foreign bodies of the ;I tract are very common but usually do not result in serious linical morbidity.[1]

The frequency of food bolus impactions, foreign body inges-ions requiring medical attention, and mortality related to oreign bodies is unknown. The oft-quoted annual rate of 1500 o 2750 deaths related to foreign body ingestion in the United tates is likely overstated.[2–4] Recent large series have reported o deaths among 852 adults and one death among 2206 hildren as a result of foreign body ingestion.[5–11] Although the utcome associated with GI foreign bodies is generally benign, vithout proper management potentially fatal sequellae exist. 'or this reason it is important to understand which patients are t risk, proper methods of diagnosis, and the safest, most ffective, methods of treatment.

PIDEMIOLOGY

'ood: Esophageal food impaction is the most common foreign ody with an incidence of 16 per 100 000,[12] occurring rimarily in adults in their fourth decade and above. Most food mpactions occur with pre-existing esophageal pathology, ncluding: benign strictures, webs, rings, diverticuli, surgical :hanges (e.g., fundoplication, anastomoses), motility disorders, nd rarely esophageal cancer.

Other foreign bodies: The early pediatric population, aged rom 6 months to 3 years, accounts for 80% of all non-food oreign bodies.[13] Altered oral tactile sensation and swallowing ontrol may lead to accidental ingestion of non-food foreign bodies, uch as oral prostheses in adults. Non-food foreign bodies are lso more frequent in conditions causing altered judgment such s dementia, intoxication, and psychiatric illness. Intentional ingestion of objects may occur in individuals with psychiatric illness. These patients frequently are multiple ingestors of complex foreign objects (Fig. 115.1). Rectal foreign bodies are usually related to sexual activity and, less frequently, to sexual assault.

Bezoars: The most common types of bezoar are phytobezoars made of vegetable matter, trichobezoars composed of hair, and medication bezoars (Fig. 115.2). Phytobezoars develop with the ingestion of poorly digested foods such as persimmon, celery, prunes, or raisins. Trichobezoars develop classically in young females with a psychiatric disorder that leads to ingestion of hair, clothing, or carpet fibers. Bezoars are commonly associated with prior gastric surgery and gastroparesis.

PATHOGENESIS AND PATHOPHYSIOLOGY

Some 80–90% of foreign bodies pass uneventfully.[14] Ten to twenty per cent of GI foreign bodies produce symptoms requiring intervention. In 1%, operative intervention may be needed. Perforation and obstruction are the most serious complications of foreign bodies and occur most frequently at anatomic sphincters, areas of angulation, or surgical anastomoses (Fig. 115.3).

Esophageal foreign bodies result in the most substantial morbidity and mortality rates. They may cause perforation, fistulae, mediastinitis, and aspiration. An esophageal food bolus or foreign body should not be left in the esophagus for more than 24 h, as the complication rate is directly proportional to the time for which the object resides in the esophagus. The esophagus has four areas of natural narrowing where impaction may occur: the upper esophageal sphincter, level of the aortic arch, crossing of the main stem bronchus, and lower esophageal sphincter. These areas are 23 mm or less in diameter in adults.[15] Further, 75% or more of patients with esophageal impaction have esophageal pathology or disordered motility.

Stomach and intestine: Upon reaching the stomach, most objects pass through the GI tract in 1–2 weeks and can be safely managed with observation. Exceptions are sharp, large, and long objects. Sharp or pointed objects have an associated perforation rate of up to 35%.[16] Objects greater than 2 cm in diameter have difficulty passing through the pylorus, and objects longer than 5 cm have difficulty negotiating the pylorus and duodenal sweep. The fixed angulation of the ligament of Treitz and the ileocecal valve are sites of small bowel impaction for objects that have uneventfully exited the stomach.

Rectum: Foreign bodies in the rectum may cause obstruction, perforation, or bleeding. The sacral curve and valves of Houston impede spontaneous passage after forceful insertion. The internal and external anal sphincters can become tonically contracted and swollen after foreign body insertion.

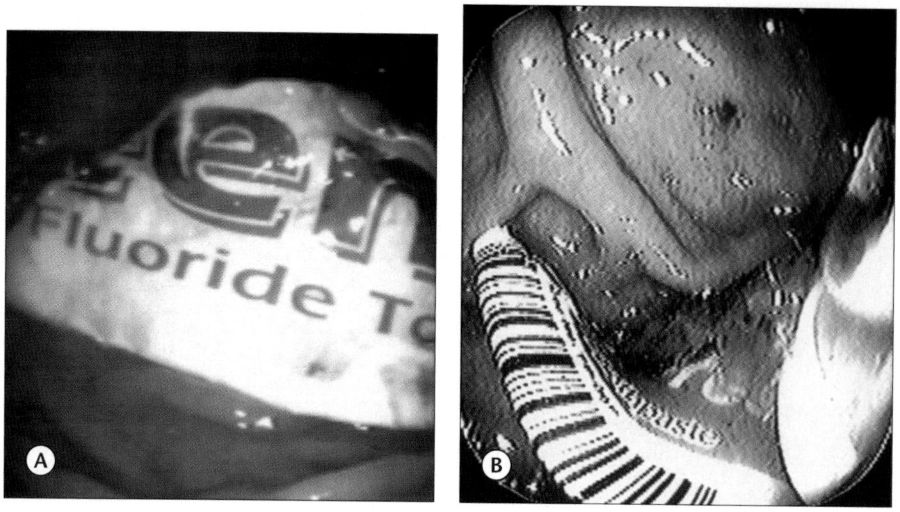

Fig. 115.1 Foreign body in the stomach. **A.** A tube of toothpaste within the stomach. **B.** Second tube of toothpaste (note different toothpaste brand) ingested by the same patient approximately 12 months later.

CLINICAL PRESENTATION

Clinical presentation in children may be subtle. In 40% of cases the patient is asymptomatic, and neither patient nor caregiver gives a history of ingestion.[17] Symptoms of foreign bodies in children include drooling, poor feeding, failure to thrive, and occasionally aspiration. In adults, esophageal obstruction, particularly secondary to food impaction, is nearly always symptomatic with partial obstruction causing substernal chest pain, dysphonia, dysphagia, gagging, or a sense of choking. More complete obstruction leads to drooling and inability to handle secretions. Foreign bodies in the stomach, small intestine, or colon infrequently cause symptoms unless there are complications. Large gastric bezoars may present with vague abdominal discomfort, nausea, vomiting, early satiety, or weight loss.[18] Small bowel bezoars may present with obstructive symptoms.

DIAGNOSTIC METHODS

History is crucial in the diagnosis of foreign bodies as the majority of adults can directly identify the timing and type of ingestion. Past medical history may reveal risk factors for foreign

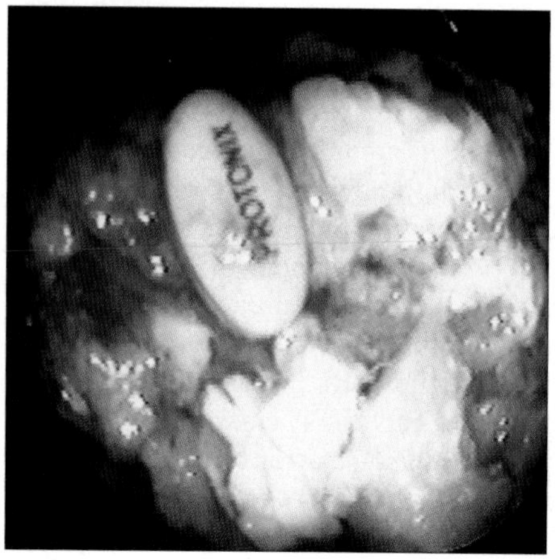

Fig. 115.2 Combination gastric phytobezoar and medication bezoar.

AREAS OF NARROWING AND ANGULATION

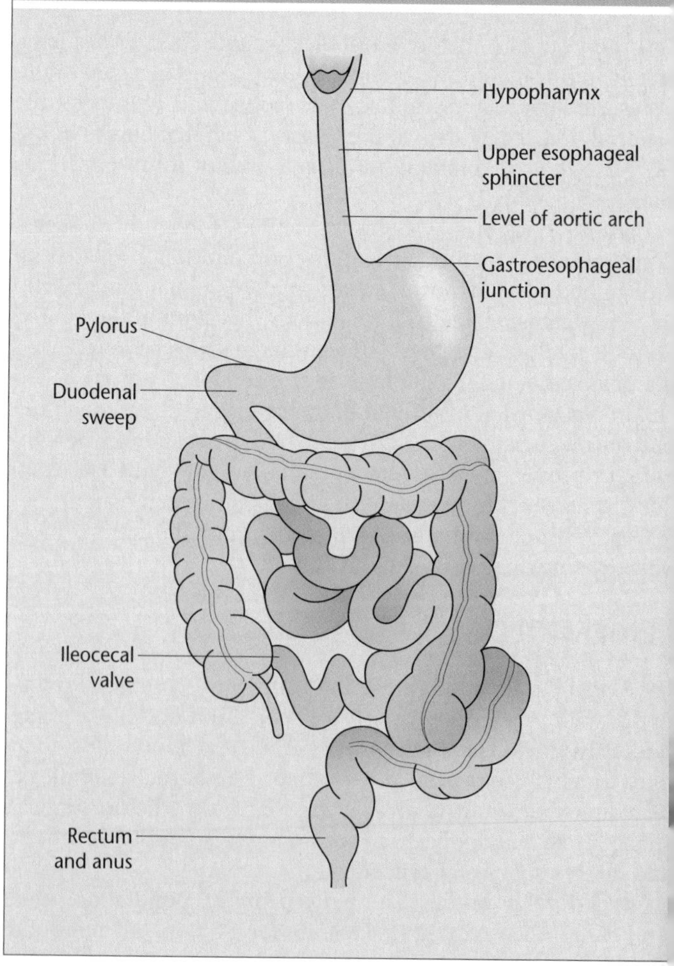

Fig. 115.3 Areas of narrowing and angulation. Gastrointestinal areas of lumenal narrowing and angulation that predispose to foreign body impaction and obstruction. Reproduced from Gastrointestinal and Liver Disease. Pathophysiology, Diagnosis and Management, 7th edn, with permission from Elsevier Ltd.

CLINICAL PRESENTATION

- Some 40% of children are asymptomatic or have a subtle clinical presentation.
- Food impaction or esophageal obstruction is nearly always symptomatic.
- Esophageal food impaction or foreign bodies can result in chest pain, dysphagia, drooling, and inability to handle secretions.
- Foreign bodies of the stomach, small, and large intestine present with symptoms only if a complication of bleeding, obstruction, or perforation occurs.
- The majority of patients with foreign bodies are asymptomatic, presenting only with a history of ingestion or insertion.
- Gastric bezoars are asymptomatic or present with vague nausea, early satiety, or weight loss.

body impaction or potential complications. The physical examination is important to identify any complications related to a foreign body – signs of aspiration or wheezing. The neck and chest may show signs of perforation resulting in crepitus, swelling, or erythema. The abdominal examination may suggest perforation or obstruction.

Radiology: Anteroposterior and lateral radiography of the chest, abdomen, and sometimes neck should be the initial diagnostic test. Radiographs aid in identifying the presence, type, and location of a foreign body as well as potential perforation or subcutaneous emphysema.[6] In children, a mouth-to-anus radiologic evaluation has been advocated because of the difficulty of obtaining an adequate history in the pediatric population. Plain films have obvious diagnostic limitations in patients with food impactions and ingested objects that are not radio-opaque.[19] Barium studies should be avoided because of the risk of aspiration with esophageal obstruction, and barium may interfere with subsequent therapeutic endoscopy.

Endoscopy is the most accurate diagnostic modality for esophageal and gastric foreign bodies, with an accuracy of near 100%. Endoscopy can also identify coexistent pathology such as esophageal stricture or mucosal laceration or ulceration. Endoscopy is contraindicated if there is evidence of a perforation or an obstruction beyond the ligament of Treitz.

DIAGNOSTIC METHODS

- History and physical examination.
- Plain film chest, abdominal, and occasionally neck X-rays – anteroposterior and lateral.
- Endoscopy has near 100% success rate in identifying the type and site of foreign body, and allows identification of coexisting pathology.
- If X-rays are negative and suspicion of foreign body is still present, endoscopy should be performed.

TREATMENT

Treatment of foreign bodies should be performed with the knowledge that 80–90% of foreign bodies will pass spontaneously without complications.[5] The need to intervene is based on symptoms, size and type of foreign body, and location in the GI tract.

Glucagon, a smooth muscle relaxant that reduces lower esophageal sphincter pressure, has achieved success rates of 12–58% in treating food impactions and esophageal foreign bodies.[20] Glucagon may cause nausea and vomiting, and is not effective when a fixed obstruction exists in the esophagus. The use of other muscle relaxants including nitroglycerin and nifedepine, gas-forming agents, and emetics should be avoided because of lack of efficacy and higher complication rates. Papain, a meat tenderizer, is contraindicated because of the risk of aspiration, esophageal necrosis, and perforation. Cellulase has been used for chemical dissolution of small gastric bezoars. A prokinetic agent plus a low-residue or liquid diet may also be beneficial in treating gastric bezoars.

Flexible endoscopy is the treatment of choice for esophageal foreign bodies, with success rates of 95–100% and minimal to no complications.[21] Intervention is indicated for all esophageal foreign bodies within 24 h. In the stomach and proximal small intestine, retrieval is indicated for sharp objects because of the increased risk of perforation, and for objects longer than 5 cm or with a diameter greater than 2 cm that are unlikely to pass through the pylorus or the duodenal sweep. Factors that decrease the chance of successful endoscopic treatment are poor patient cooperation and ingestion of multiple complex objects.[16]

The equipment for successful and safe retrieval of foreign bodies is listed in Table 115.1. Overtubes of both standard length that bypass the upper esophageal sphincter and longer 45–60-cm tubes that extend into the stomach should be available. Overtubes can protect the esophageal mucosa when retrieving sharp objects, allow multiple passes of the endoscope, and protect the airway during retrieval. Alternatively, a latex protector hood attached to the end of the endoscope can protect both the airway and the mucosa, when an object is grasped and pulled tightly against the scope during withdrawal.

Prior to endoscopy, knowledge of the type of object and its location can allow an ex vivo practice 'dry run' to allow proper equipment selection and improve outcome.[5] For complex foreign bodies it may be appropriate to refer to tertiary centers with more experience with foreign body retrieval.

Intravenous conscious sedation is sufficient for the majority of adults. General anesthesia with endotracheal intubation should be considered in the majority of pediatric patients, as well as in uncooperative patients.

Food impactions should be treated endoscopically on an urgent basis if the patient has clinical signs of obstruction, including

TABLE 115.1 EQUIPMENT FOR TREATMENT AND REMOVAL OF GASTROINTESTINAL FOREIGN BODIES AND FOOD IMPACTIONS

Endoscopes	Overtubes	Accessory equipment
Flexible endoscope	Standard esophageal overtube	Retrieval net
Rigid endoscope	45–60-cm foreign body overtube	Alligator or rat tooth forceps
Laryngoscope		Dormia basket
Kelly or McGill forceps		Polypectomy snare
		Three-pronged grabber
		Magnetic extractor
		Steigmann-Goff variceal ligator cap
		Latex protector hood

the inability to handle secretions. The primary endoscopic technique to treat food boluses is the 'push technique.' The endoscope should first be steered around the food impaction into the stomach, if possible, to detect potential physical obstruction beyond the food bolus. The endoscope is then pulled back and the food is pushed carefully into the stomach. Even if the scope cannot be passed around the food impaction, a trial of gently pushing the food bolus can safely be attempted. Forceful pushing increases the perforation risk.[1,16] The push technique has a success rate of 95%, with a near 0% complication rate.[22] If the push technique fails, food may be broken apart with forceps, snares, or baskets, allowing the pieces to be pushed into the stomach or retrieved through the mouth. An overtube can be particularly useful for foods that break apart easily and require multiple endoscopic passes. A Roth retrieval net or a Steigmann-Goff endoscopic variceal ligator can be used to retrieve or suction large pieces of food in one endoscopic pass.

Up to 75–100% of patients with food impaction have associated esophageal pathology, primarily strictures or esophageal narrowing from conditions such as the ringed esophagus (Fig. 115.4). It is generally safe to perform endoscopic dilatation immediately after removal of the food bolus. However, if extensive mucosal injury or mucosal tears are present, the patient should be placed on potent acid suppression, instructed to avoid bulky food that might impact again, and have an esophageal dilatation in the near future.

Sharp foreign bodies within the reach of the endoscope should be removed, if possible. Attempts should be made to remove sharp objects with the sharp end trailing distally away from the endoscope to lessen the chance of perforation or mucosal tear. If a sharp object points proximally in the esophagus, it should be pushed into the stomach, rotated, and removed with the blunt end leading. Snares and rat tooth or alligator forceps allow the greatest control in removing sharp objects (Fig. 115.5), and overtubes or protector hoods should be employed to protect the esophagus and oropharynx. Sharp objects that are beyond the reach of the endoscope or cannot be removed may be observed with serial clinical examinations and radiographs. Surgery should be considered if the object does not progress over approximately 3 days,[4] and obviously if there are signs of perforation, obstruction, or bleeding.

Long foreign bodies such as pens or pencils, toothbrushes, or cutlery may not pass through the duodenal sweep and can be difficult to remove in a retrograde direction through the lower and upper esophageal sphincters. Long objects should be grasped with a basket or snare at the tip of the object, and pulled through

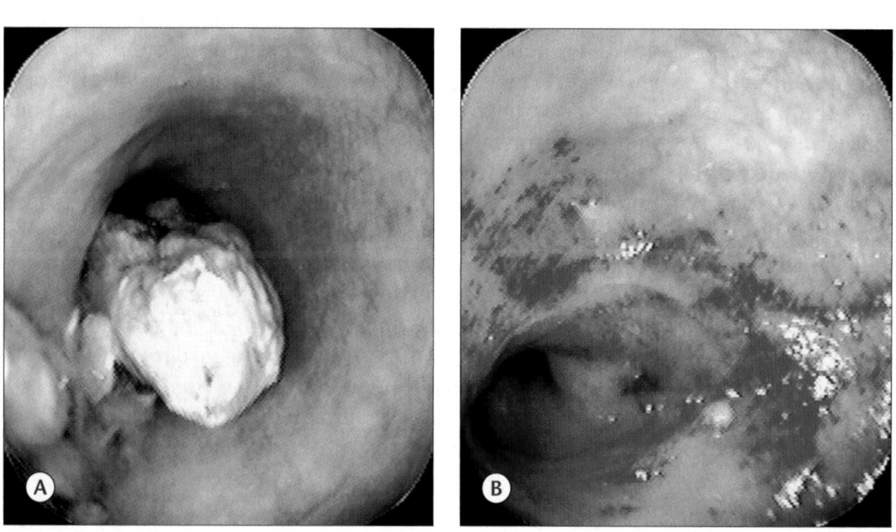

Fig. 115.4 Food impaction. A. Poultry causing acute obstructive symptoms in a patient with a history of dysphagia. **B.** After the food impaction has been pushed into the stomach, evidence of a peptic stricture can be seen.

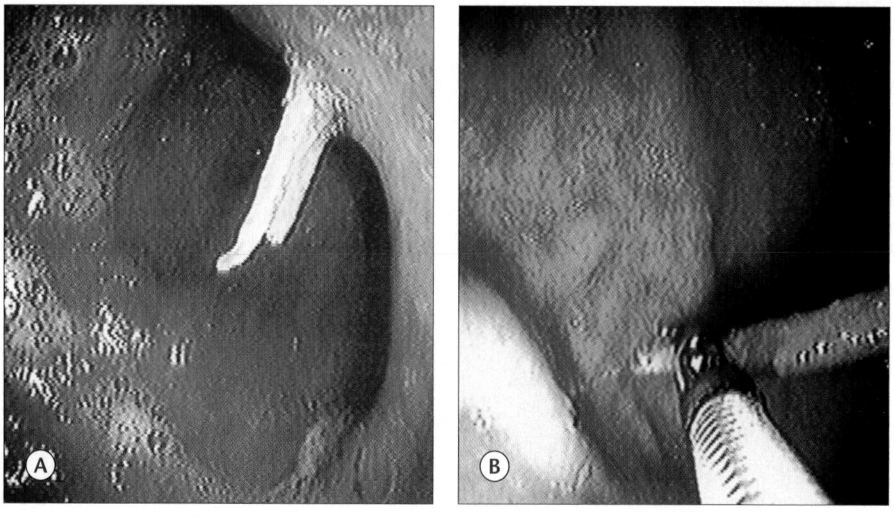

Fig. 115.5 Ingested toothpick. A. Ingested toothpick imbedded in the stomach wall. **B.** Successful removal with a rat tooth forceps.

e esophagus and mouth maintaining the object in a straight ertical plane. Grasping the object closer to the center causes e object to shift to a horizontal plane, prohibiting removal rough the esophageal sphincters. Alternatively, a long foreign ody may be pulled into a longer overtube that extends past e gastroesophageal junction after being snared with the ndoscope. The object, overtube, and endoscope can then be moved as a single unit.

Coins and button batteries lodged in the esophagus can lead pressure necrosis and perforation. Button batteries can cause pid liquefaction necrosis of the esophageal tissue.[5] Prior to moval the airway is protected with an overtube, or with ndotracheal intubation and general anesthesia in children. ne Roth retrieval net permits control of the object during ithdrawal. Once in the stomach, almost all coins except silver half dollars will pass without complications; batteries in the omach rarely cause problems – 85% pass through the GI act within 72 h.[23]

Bezoars: The majority (85–90%) can be treated successfully ith endoscopic mechanical disruption. The bezoar is simply roken into smaller pieces and allowed to pass, or is retrieved trograde with the endoscope through the mouth. An overtube helpful to allow multiple endoscopic passes. More complex ndoscopic techniques such as mechanical or electrohydraulic thotripsy, laser, or pulsed water jet have been employed for ifficult-to-treat bezoars. Surgery is occasionally required with ezoars, usually with a small gastrotomy or enterotomy.[16] epending on the associated clinical circumstances after ezoar removal, the patient may be instructed to take a lower esidue diet and add a prokinetic drug to help avoid ecurrence.

Rectal foreign bodies: Most can be removed manually or with the aid of a flexible or rigid scope with sedation. A latex protector hood attached to the end of the scope or an overtube can be used when removing sharp objects to reduce trauma and overcome the anal sphincters' natural tendency to contract during removal of objects (Fig. 115.6). Larger and more complex objects may require extraction under general anesthesia, with associated sphincter dilatation.[24] Surgery is reserved for complications and failure of above therapies.

COMPLICATIONS

The complication rate in the treatment of foreign bodies ranges from zero to less than 2%.[21] Perforation is the most notable complication associated with either conservative observation of a foreign body or its attempted removal. Risk factors for perforation at the time of endoscopic treatment include an uncooperative patient, extraction of multiple objects, and removal of sharp or pointed objects. Cardiopulmonary complications, aspiration, and GI bleeding occur at a rate similar to that found in standard upper and lower endoscopy.

PROGNOSIS AND FUTURE TRENDS

Endoscopy provides a greater than 95% treatment success rate with negligible complications. Almost all data on the management of foreign bodies are based on retrospective series and reviews. Future challenges are to collect data on the management of foreign bodies in a prospective fashion so that optimal treatment guidelines can be universally provided for patients with this common problem.

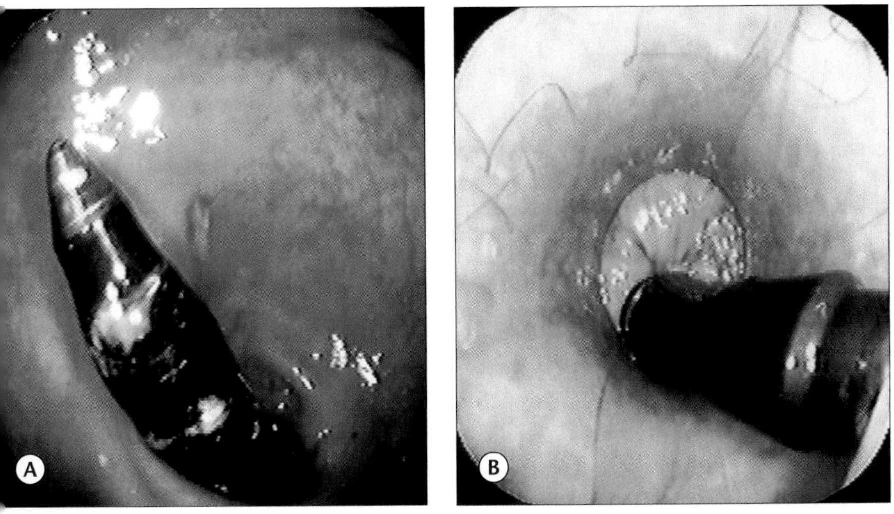

Fig. 115.6 Rectal foreign body. A. Ballpoint pen in the rectum with associated mucosal ulceration. **B.** Successful endoscopic removal with use of snare and overtube.

REFERENCES

1. Eisen GM, Baron TH, Dominitz JA et al. Guideline for the management of ingested foreign bodies. Gastrointest Endosc 2002; 55:802–806.
2. Lyons MF, Tsuchida AM. Foreign bodies of the gastrointestinal tract. Med Clin North Am 1993; 77:1101–1114.
3. Clerf LH. Historical aspects of foreign bodies in the food and air passages. South Med J 1975; 68:1449–1454.
4. Devanesan J, Pisani A, Sharman P et al. Metallic foreign bodies in the stomach. Arch Surg 1977; 112:664–665.
5. Webb WA. Management of foreign bodies of the upper gastrointestinal tract: update. Gastrointest Endosc 1995; 41:39–51.
6. Cheng W, Tam PKH. Foreign-body ingestion in children: experience with 1265 cases. J Pediatr Surg 1999; 34:1472–1476.
7. Chu KM, Choi HK, Tuen HH, Law SYK, Branicki FJ, Wong J. A prospective randomized trial comparing the use of the flexible gastroscope versus the bronchoscope in the management of foreign body ingestion. Gastrointest Endosc 1998; 47:23–27.
8. Velitchkov NG, Grigorov GI, Losanoff JE, Kjossev KT. Ingested foreign bodies of the gastrointestinal tract: retrospective analysis of 542 cases. World J Surg 1996; 20:1001–1005.
9. Kim JK, Kim SS, Kim JI et al. Management of foreign bodies in the gastrointestinal tract: an analysis of 104 cases in children. Endoscopy 1999; 31:302–304.
10. Hachimi-Idrissi S, Corne L, Vandenplas Y. Management of ingested foreign bodies in childhood: our experience and review of the literature. Eur J Emerg Med 1998; 5:319–323.
11. Panieri E, Bass DH. The management of ingested foreign bodies in children – a review of 663 cases. Eur J Emerg Med 1995; 2:83–87.
12. Longstreth GF, Longstreth KJ, Yao JF. Esophageal food impaction: epidemiology and therapy. A retrospective, observational study. Gastrointest Endosc 2001; 53:193–198.
13. Webb WA. Management of foreign bodies in the upper gastrointestinal tract. Gastroenterology 1988; 94:204–216.
14. Schwartz GF, Polsky HS. Ingested foreign bodies of the gastrointestinal tract. Am Surg 1976; 42:236–238.
15. Bloom RR, Nakano PH, Gray SW et al. Foreign bodies of the gastrointestinal tract. Am Surg 1986; 10:618–621.
16. Pfau PR, Ginsberg GG. Foreign bodies and bezoars. In: Feldman M, Friedman LS, Schleisenger MH, eds. Schleisenger & Fordtran's gastrointestinal and liver disease. Pathophysiology/diagnosis/management. Philadelphia: WB Saunders; 2002:386–398
17. Muniz AE, Joffe MD. Foreign bodies, ingest and inhaled. JAAPA 1999; 12:23–46.
18. Dietrich NA, Gau FC. Postgastrectomy phytobezoars: endoscopic diagnosis and treatment. Arch Surg 1985; 120:432–435.
19. Shaffer HA, de Lange EE. Gastrointestinal foreign bodies and strictures: radiologic interventions. Curr Probl Diagn Radiol 199 23:205–249.
20. Trenker SW, Maglinte DT, Lehman G et al. Esophageal food impaction: treatment with glucagon. Radiology 1983; 149:401–403.
21. Pfau PR. Ingested foreign objects and food bolus impactions. In: Ginsberg GG, Gousto CJ, Kochman ML, Norton I, eds. Clinical gastrointestinal endoscopy. London: Elsevie Science; in press.
22. Vicari JJ, Johanson JF, Frakes JT. Outcomes of acute esophageal food impaction: succes of the push technique. Gastrointest Endosc 2001; 53:178–181.
23. Litovitz TL. Battery ingestions: product accessibility and clinical course. Pediatrics 1985; 75:469–476.
24. Kourkalis G, Misiakos E, Dovas N et al. Management of foreign bodies of the rectu report of 21 cases. J R Coll Surg Edinb 199 42:246–247.

Chapter 116

Porphyria

Jean-Charles Deybach and Hervé Puy

KEY POINTS

- Caused by specific deficiencies in one of the enzymes of heme synthesis
- Acute attacks are precipitated by increased demands for heme synthesis (stress, fasting, infection, drugs)
- Glucose and hematin are specific therapeutics for acute attacks
- Opiates can be used for pain relief, chlorpromazine for acute anxiety
- Phlebotomy and avoidance of sunlight are the treatments of choice for porphyria cutanea tarda

INTRODUCTION

The porphyrias are a group of disorders of heme biosynthesis in which specific patterns of overproduction of heme precursors are associated with the following characteristic clinical features:[1]

- acute neurovisceral attacks (acute intermittent porphyria (AIP) and the rare 5-aminolevulinic acid (ALA) dehydratase deficiency[2] porphyria (ADP));
- skin lesions (porphyria cutanea tarda (PCT), congenital erythropoietic porphyria (CEP), and erythropoietic protoporphyria (EPP)); or
- both of the above (variegate porphyria (VP)[3] and hereditary coproporphyria (HC)).

Each type of porphyria is the result of a specific decrease in the activity of one of the enzymes in heme biosynthesis (Fig. 116.1).

Heme is synthetized from succinyl CoA and glycine in all tissues, but mostly in liver and bone marrow, for the synthesis of hemoproteins such as hemoglobin, myoglobin, cytochromes, catalase, peroxidase, nitric oxide synthase, and tryptophan pyrrolase. The mechanisms for the control of heme biosynthesis differ between the liver and the bone marrow. The first step enzyme 5-aminolevulinic acid (ALA) synthase is coded for by two genes: one erythroid specific (ALA synthase-2 on chromosome X) and one ubiquitous (ALA synthase-1 on chromosome 3).

In the erythroid cell, erythropoietin and iron are involved in the control of the enzymes participating in the formation of heme. In the liver, the hemoproteins formed, including cytochrome P450s, are rapidly turned over in response to current metabolic needs.[2] The free cellular heme pool retroinhibits ALA synthase-1 activity via a negative feedback regulation.

Enzyme defect will give rise to a characteristic biochemical profile of porphyrins and porphyrin precursors, ALA and porphobilinogen (PBG), which accumulate in urine, feces, plasma and/or erythrocytes. This allows the type of porphyria to be accurately identified in patients (Table 116.1). Enzyme or DNA analysis must be used for family studies.[3]

CLINICAL CLASSIFICATION OF PORPHYRIAS

Three broad types of porphyric syndromes are recognized: acute hepatic porphyrias characterized by acute neurovisceral attacks with or without cutaneous manifestations; the nonacute hepatic porphyria cutanea tarda characterized by photosensitivity; and erythropoietic porphyrias, which are also characterized by photosensitivity. Porphyrias can be classified as either erythropoietic or hepatic, depending on the primary organ in which excess production of porphyrins or precursors takes place (Fig. 116.1).

ACUTE HEPATIC PORPHYRIAS

Introduction

Acute attacks are identical in four of the hepatic porphyrias: acute intermittent porphyria (AIP), hereditary coproporphyria (HC), variegate porphyria (VP), and ALA dehydratase deficiency porphyria (ADP). With the exception of ADP, an autosomal recessive disorder, the acute hepatic porphyrias are all autosomal dominant conditions in which a 50% reduction in enzyme activity is brought about by a mutation in one of the alleles of the corresponding gene. The penetrance is low and about 90% of affected individuals never experience an acute attack. VP and HC can also be associated with skin lesions, which may be the only manifestation of the condition in 60% of VP patients. In most countries, AIP is the commonest of the acute porphyrias.[4]

Clinical presentation

Acute attacks are precipitated by events that increase the demand for heme synthesis. These include hormonal fluctuations, stress, fasting, infection, and exposure to porphyrinogenic drugs. Most drugs that exacerbate porphyria have the capacity to induce Ala-synthase 1, which is closely associated with induction of cytochrome P450 enzymes, a process that increases the demand for heme synthesis in the liver. Acute attacks are rare before puberty (except in ADP) and after the menopause, with a peak occurrence in the third and fourth decades of life; women are five times more likely to be affected than men. Most patients suffer one or possibly two acute attacks and are then symptom free for the rest of their lives. A few have recurrent acute attacks, which may require a special treatment regimen (see below).

The acute porphyrias may present with a sudden life-threatening crisis characterized by severe abdominal pain, neuropsychiatric

CLASSIFICATION OF MAJOR HUMAN PORPHYRIAS

Enzyme

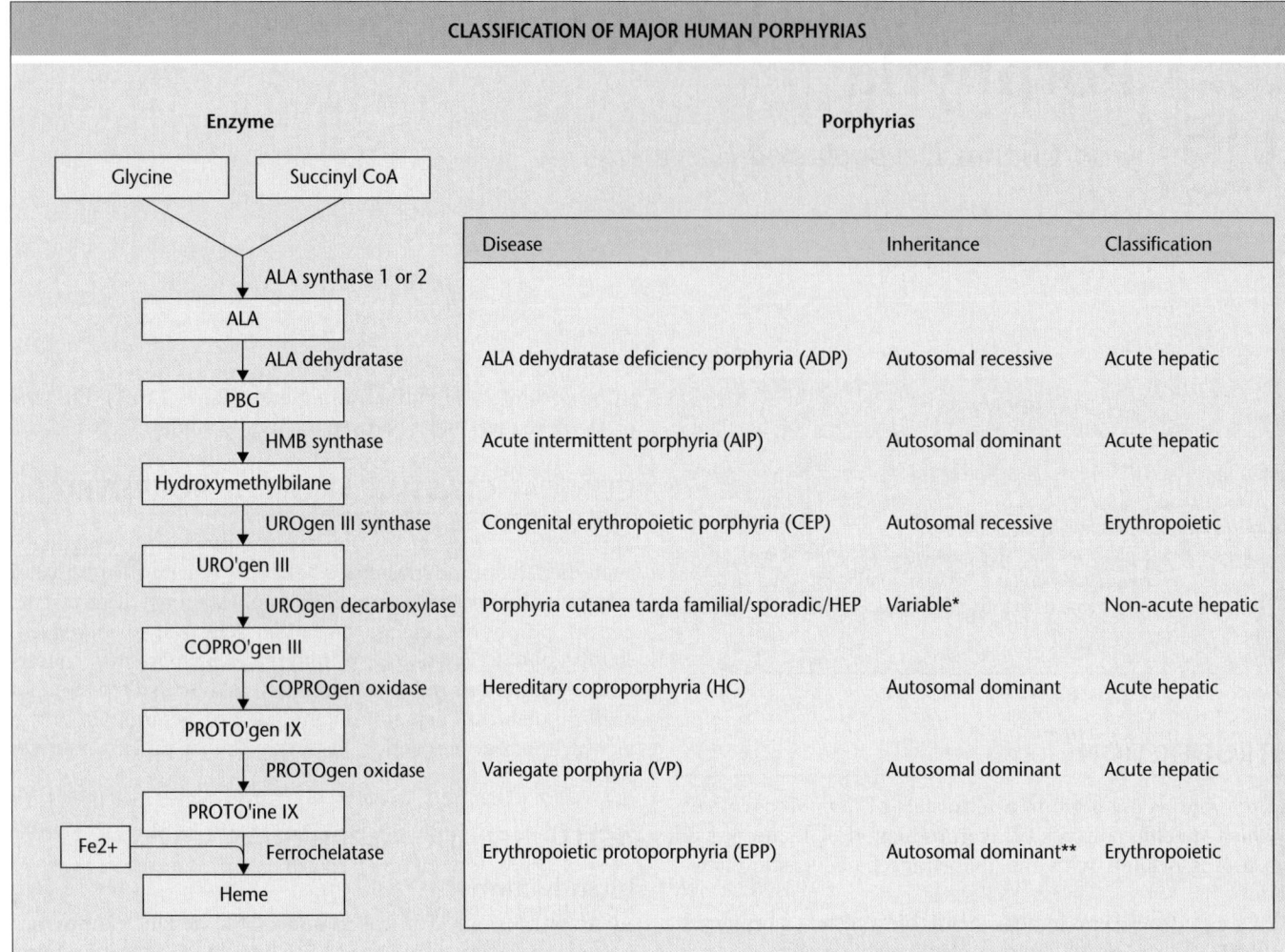

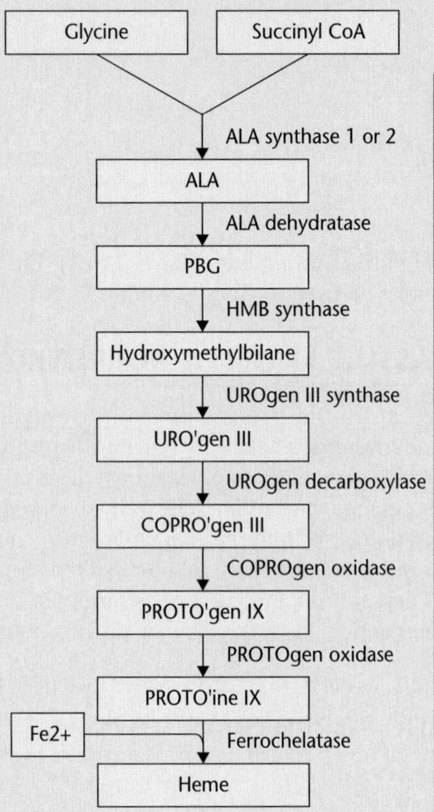

Porphyrias

Disease	Inheritance	Classification
ALA dehydratase deficiency porphyria (ADP)	Autosomal recessive	Acute hepatic
Acute intermittent porphyria (AIP)	Autosomal dominant	Acute hepatic
Congenital erythropoietic porphyria (CEP)	Autosomal recessive	Erythropoietic
Porphyria cutanea tarda familial/sporadic/HEP	Variable*	Non-acute hepatic
Hereditary coproporphyria (HC)	Autosomal dominant	Acute hepatic
Variegate porphyria (VP)	Autosomal dominant	Acute hepatic
Erythropoietic protoporphyria (EPP)	Autosomal dominant**	Erythropoietic

Fig. 116.1 Classification of the major human porphyrias. ALA, 5-aminolevulinic acid; PBG, porphobilinogen; HEP, hepatoerythroporphyria; URO'gen, uroporphyrinogen; COPRO'gen, coproporphyrinogen; PROTO'gen, protoporphyrinogen; PROTO'ine, protoporphyrine; III or IX, typ isomers. * Autosomal dominant inheritance has been documented in familial porphyria cutanea tarda and recessive inheritance has been documented in HEP. ** Erythropoietic protoporphyria is mainly related to the coinheritance of both a ferrochelatase gene mutation and a wea normal ferrochelatase allele; autosomal recessive inheritance has also been reported in a few families.

symptoms, autonomic neuropathy, and electrolyte disturbances (Table 116.2). All these clinical features of an acute attack can be explained by lesions of the nervous system.

Pathogenic mechanism

The skin photosensitivity in cutaneous porphyrias can be ascribed to accumulation of porphyrins in the skin, which absorb light with the formation of destructive free radicals. The mechanism of neural damage in these disorders is poorly understood. Various hypotheses that are not mutually exclusive have been proposed. The leading hypothesis is that ALA and/or PBG overproduced by the liver is neurotoxic. Conversely, formation of hemoproteins may be compromised due to the inherited enzyme deficiency.

Acute attacks usually begin with generalized abdominal pain. Constipation, nausea, vomiting and insomnia may precede and accompany the abdominal crisis. Examination does not show signs of peritoneal irritation; radiographic films of the abdomen usually disclose a normal pattern of bowel gas. Tachycardia, excess sweating, and hypertension are often associated with abdominal pain. Occasionally, the occurrence of red or dark-colored urine may help the physicians in their investigations.

In 20–30% of patients, signs of mental disturbance such a anxiety, depression, disorientation, hallucinations, paranoia, c confused states are observed. Abdominal pain may disappea within a few days, generally when no harmful drug has bee used. When acute attacks last several days, the gastrointestin manifestations frequently lead to weight loss while prolonge vomiting may cause oliguria and hyperazotemia.

Porphyric neuropathy often occurs when harmful drugs hav not been avoided during an acute attack; however, neurologic manifestations are also a problem in differential diagnosis an treatment when the type of porphyria is not known.

Neuropathy is primarily motor: in the early stages, pain i the extremities is very common ('muscle pain'); weakne often begins in the proximal muscles, more commonly in th arms than in the legs. Paresis in the extremities may occur an can also be strikingly local. Muscle weakness may progress an eventuate in tetraplegia with respiratory and bulbar paralys and death. After a severe attack, complete or partial muscl function can improve over a period of months. Recovery fro paralysis may be incomplete, with sequelae mostly o extremities. The central nervous system is seldom involve pyramidal signs, cerebellar syndrome, transitory blindness, c

TABLE 116.1 TREATMENT AND BIOCHEMICAL DIAGNOSIS IN SYMPTOMATIC PORPHYRIC PATIENTS

Porphyria	Diagnosis in symptomatic patients				Treatment
	Urine	Stool	RBC*	Plasma**	
ACUTE HEPATIC					
ALA dehydratase porphyria	**ALA**, Copro III	–	Zn-Proto	–	**Supportive treatment:** avoidance of precipitating factor opiates and chlorpromazine adequate fluid intake
Acute intermittent porphyria	**ALA, PBG**, URO III	–	–	615–620	
Hereditary coproporphyria	**ALA, PBG**, Copro III	Copro III	–	615–620	**Specific treatment:**
Variegate porphyria	**ALA, PBG**, Copro III	Proto Copro	–	624–627	Carbohydrates, heme arginate
NONACUTE HEPATIC					**Supportive treatment:** restriction of sunlight avoidance of precipitating factor
Porphyria cutanea tarda	Uro III, Hepta***	Isocopro, Hepta	–	615–620	**Specific treatment:** Phlebotomy, low-dose chloroquine
ERYTHROPOIETIC					
Congenital erythropoietic porphyria	Uro I, Copro I	Copro I	Uro I, Copro I	615–620	Skin protection/blood transfusion/ bone marrow transplantation
Erythropoietic protoporphyria	–	Proto	Free Proto	626–634	Skin protection/oral beta-carotene liver transplantation

ALA, δ-aminolevulinic acid; PBG, porphobilinogen; Uro, uroporphyrin; Copro, coproporphyrin; Proto, protoporphyrin; Isocopro, isocoproporphyrin; I or III: Type isomers; *, red blood cell; **, fluorescence emission peak in nm; ***, heptacarboxyl-porphyrin.

altered level of consciousness can occur. The cerebrospinal fluid (CSF) is usually normal. In general, neuropathy is now far less common than in the past.

During acute attacks, dehydration and electrolyte imbalance occur frequently. Hyponatremia occurs in 40% and, when severe, can lead to convulsions.

AHP patients are at increased risk of hepatocellular carcinoma and chronic renal failure with progressive tubulo interstitial nephropathy. Clinical manifestations are usually nonspecific, even in the presence of cutaneous lesions. Only biological data allow precise diagnosis of the type of acute hepatic porphyria.

TABLE 116.2 CLINICAL AND BIOLOGICAL SIGNS OF HIGH DIAGNOSTIC VALUE AND TREATMENT IN ACUTE ATTACKS OF HEPATIC PORPHYRIA: ACUTE INTERMITTENT PORPHYRIA, HEREDITARY COPROPORPHYRIA, VARIEGATE PORPHYRIA

SIGNS OF HIGH DIAGNOSTIC VALUE

Clinical symptoms

- Severe abdominal pain / back and thigh pain
- Vomiting, constipation
- Other signs of autonomic neuropathy (muscle weakness, hypertension, tachycardia, etc.)
- Mental symptoms

Biology

- Increased ALA and PBG in the urine
- ± Hyponatremia

MANAGEMENT

- Admission to hospital
- Withdrawal of all common precipitants (drugs, alcohol, fasting, infection, etc.)
- Opiates and chlorpromazine
- Carbohydrates (400 g/day)
- Early heme arginate infusion Normosang® (250 mg/day x 4)

Diagnostic methods

Acute porphyria attacks are characterized by increased excretion of urinary ALA and/or PBG (20–200-fold higher); in ADP, the overexcretion is restricted to ALA. Treatment can be instituted immediately, while further laboratory investigations establish the porphyria type by analyzing porphyrin excretion patterns in urine, feces, and plasma (Table 116.1).

Urinary uro- and coproporphyrin may be secondarily increased in acutely ill patients or in several other conditions as hepatobiliary disease, alcohol abuse, infections, and excess urinary porphyrin excretion alone lack diagnostic specificity. A high level of precursors (ALA and mostly PBG) is the most important diagnostic tool in symptomatic patients. The limited sensitivity of excretion analyses prevents their use in screening individuals without symptoms of acute porphyria.[5]

Acute intermittent porphyria

Acute intermittent porphyria is the most significant hepatic porphyria with respect to its incidence and clinical severity and has been reported in many populations. It is an autosomal dominant disorder due to deficient activity of hydroxymethylbilane synthase (HMBS) or PBG deaminase or uroporphyrinogen I synthase (EC 4.3.1.8). Most of the approximations of AIP prevalence were established by screening populations for urinary porphyrin precursors and are therefore underestimated; erythrocyte HMBS activity provides a better way to screen individuals and healthy populations for latent AIP.

The enzyme deficiency is usually 50% of normal in all somatic cells studied in those who inherit the genetic trait. Measurement in erythrocytes is now widely used to detect clinically latent individuals who often do not show evidence of overproduction of heme precursors.

The 10 kb HMBS gene is located at chromosome 11q24.1-24.2 and contains 15 exons. It encodes erythroid-specific and ubiquitous isoforms of HMBS that are generated by the use of separate promoters and alternative splicing of the two primary transcripts. The genetic heterogeneity of AIP is already well known (Human Gene Mutation Database: www.hgmd.org). A few families showed subjects with the usual phenotypic expression of the disease but with normal HMBS activity in erythrocytes. In these cases, HMBS mutations, which have been identified as the cause of this nonerythroid form of AIP, affect mainly the exon 1 of the gene responsible for the specific ubiquitous isoforms of HMBS.

In the classical or typical AIP, more than 200 mutations of the HMBS gene have been described to date, indicating that the molecular defect in this disorder is highly heterogeneous. Very few unrelated homozygous cases of AIP have been described over the last 50 years.[6] Homozygous variants of AIP, usually present in childhood, have phenotypes of variable severity. The clinical picture is completely different from that of AIP: these children are severely ill and characterized by porencephaly, severe retardation in development, neurological defects, cataracts, and psychomotor retardation.

ALA dehydratase deficiency porphyria (ADP; Doss porphyria)

ADP, the autosomal recessive acute hepatic porphyria, is the most rare form of porphyria. ALA dehydratase activity is dramatically decreased in erythrocytes and bone marrow cells as would be expected for homozygotes with a decrease of approximately 50% in the activities found in parents. ADP is characterized by hugely increased excretion of ALA and coproporphyrin (mainly isomer type III) in urine. Porphobilinogen is only moderately elevated; fecal excretion of porphyrins is normal, but the porphyrin (especially protoporphyrin) content of the erythrocytes is raised as in all forms of homozygous porphyria. The human enzyme is a homo-octamer with a subunit size of 36 kDa, encoded by a gene localized at chromosome 9q34, and is highly sensitive to inhibition by lead. In ADP, the pattern of overproduction of heme precursors closely resembles that of severe lead poisoning and tyrosinemia. However, some features allow us to refute this diagnosis; these include normal urinary and blood levels of lead, or the activity of ALA dehydratase, which is not restored by dithiothreitol. Glucose infusion and heme therapy are effective in some but not all cases. Avoidance of drugs that are harmful in other hepatic porphyrias is also recommended.[7]

Variegate porphyria

Variegate porphyria is a low penetrance, autosomal dominant hepatic porphyria due to the deficient activity of protoporphyrinogen oxidase (PPOX) caused by mutations. VP is common in South Africa, where an estimated 20 000 descendants of a Dutch couple have inherited the same mutation in the PPOX gene.[8] The disease is increasingly recognized, as confusion with PCT is resolved by application of more precise diagnostic methods. Plasma porphyrin peak, more frequently abnormal in adult VP carriers, should be used to screen general populations.

The PPOX gene contains one noncoding and 12 coding exons. It spans 5 kb and is assigned to chromosome 1. More than 100 disease-specific mutations have been identified in VP (Human Gene Mutation Database: www.hgmd.org). The pattern of clinical presentation is not influenced by the type of mutation in the heterozygous form of VP. Eleven homozygous cases of VP have been described.[9] During acute attacks of VP, urinary profiles are rather similar to those in AIP and HC. Carriers with only chronic cutaneous manifestations or without symptoms often show a slight increase of the precursor ALA while PBG is only present in half the carriers. The differentiation of VP and HC is usually possible following fecal porphyrin analysis. In VP, the characteristic finding is elevated fecal protoporphyrin and to a lesser degree coproporphyrin (predominantly type III). HPLC of fecal porphyrins usually shows a peak of protoporphyrin as prominent as the coproporphyrin III peak and protoporphyrin concentrations are about twofold greater than coproporphyrin. A plasma fluorescence emission maximal at 624–628 nm is the most valuable diagnostic marker in adult VP patients. In patients with only cutaneous manifestations, it is usually sufficient for differentiation of PCT from PV (see 'Porphyria cutanea tarda').

Hereditary coproporphyria

Hereditary coproporphyria is an autosomal dominant hepatic porphyria due to the reduced activity of coproporphyrinogen oxidase (CPO; EC 1.3.3.3.). Clinically expressed HC is much less common than other acute hepatic porphyrias. The incidence of HC was estimated at two cases per million but latent HC gene carriers are being recognized with greater accuracy.

Skin photosensitivity occurs in a minority of cases (Fig. 116.2). CPO is decreased to around 50% of the normal level in liver, fibroblasts, lymphocytes, and leukocytes.

In rare homozygous variants, enzyme activity is usually <10%. Two different types of homozygous cases have been described: in the first type, patients were very small, showed skin photosensitivity, and had neurological symptoms with several acute attacks from the age of 5 years. Their feces and urine contained a huge amount of coproporphyrin. The other type of homozygous coproporphyria was found in three children with intense jaundice and hemolytic anemia at birth. The pattern of fecal porphyrin excretion was atypical for coproporphyria because the major porphyrin was harderoporphyrin: this variant was called 'harderoporphyria.'

Human CPO cDNA has an open reading frame of 1062 bp, encoding a protein of 354 amino acid residues. The mature enzyme consists of a homodimer of 323 amino acid residues with a leader peptide of 100 amino acid residues. The gene has been mapped to chromosome 3q12 and spans about 14 kb, consisting of seven exons.

There is a high degree of allelic heterogeneity of the disease (Human Gene Mutation Database: www.hgmd.org) and the severity of the phenotype in heterozygous HC does not correlate with the degree of inactivation by CPO mutation. Only two missense mutations in exon 6 (R401W and K404E) were associated with the harderoporphyria phenotype.

During acute attacks of HC, the profile of urine porphyrins and precursors is similar to those in AIP, although coproporphyrin is almost always dramatically increased. Stool porphyrins usually allow the type of porphyria to be established, the characteristic abnormality being a huge excess of coproporphyrin (predominantly type III) compared with normal protoporphyrin.[10]

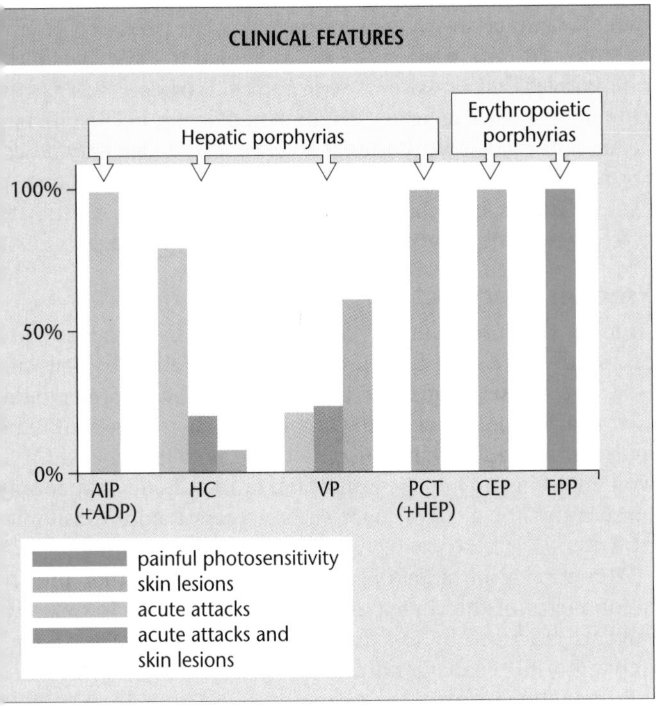

g. 116.2 **Clinical features.** In erythropoietic porphyrias :EP, congenital erythropoietic porphyria or Günther disease; ᵖP, erythropoietic protoporphyria) and in hepatic porphyrias ADP, ALA dehydratase deficiency porphyria; AIP, acute intermittent orphyria; HC, hereditary coproporphyria; VP, variegate porphyria; CT, familial and sporadic porphyria cutanea tarda; HEP, hepato-ythropoietic porphyria).

Ianagement of acute attacks

. European network for acute porphyrias, the European orphyria Initiative (EPI), has been set up and a website roposes guidelines and a consensus for therapeutic care of atients (www.porphyria-europe.com).

upportive treatment

careful search should be made for any precipitating factor, specially drugs (including oral contraceptives), underlying afection, and hypocaloric diet. These precipitants should be vithdrawn as soon as possible. Analgesia is a major compo-ent of supportive treatment. Opiates are usually required, ften in high doses, together with an antiemetic and a pheno-hiazine such as chlorpromazine for anxiety, restlessness, and o decrease the analgesic requirement. Danger of addiction (in atients who experience frequent attacks) must always be onsidered. Adequate fluid intake is essential with regular nonitoring of electrolyte status. Attention should also be paid o calorie intake. Other complications such as persistent hyper-ension and tachycardia, severe motor neuropathy, and seizures hould be treated as they occur using drugs recommended rom a safe drugs list (www.porphyria-europe.com).

pecific treatment

wo specific therapies are mainly used: glucose and hematin.

Before heme became available, carbohydrate loading was he only treatment for an acute attack. An adequate supple-nent (100–300 g per day) should be administered, usually by low intravenous infusion; to minimize the danger of precipitating hyponatremia. Hypotonic solutions should be avoided, and electrolytes measured at least daily.

Treatment of a porphyric attack has been greatly improved by the introduction of hematin. In the USA, the form of lyophilized heme (Panhematin®) is available whereas a more stable preparation of human hemin (heme arginate, Normosang®) is widely available. Heme arginate is supplied as a concentrated stock solution that requires dilution in normal saline immediately before use. This solution should be infused at a dose of 3–4 mg/kg body weight/24 h over 20 min, and usually for 4 days. In practice, adults usually receive the entire contents of a single vial for each dose (Table 116.2). An increased incidence of thrombophlebitis at the infusion site has been reported. It is recommended to resite the intravenous canule each day and flush thoroughly with saline following administration. 5% human serum albumin may be included in the solution. Other side effects are rare and heme arginate has been used successfully during pregnancy.

All the treatments described above must be used early in the attack before any nervous or respiratory complication develops. Neither carbohydrate loading nor intravenous heme will reverse an established peripheral neuropathy.[11]

Recurrent acute attacks

A minority of patients has repeated acute attacks. Women with cyclical premenstrual attack may respond to suppression of ovulation with gonadotropin-releasing hormone (Gn-RH) analogs. If this is successful, this treatment can be continued for up to 2 years before attempting withdrawal. Otherwise, management of repeated attacks severe enough to require hospitalization is difficult. It may be possible to abort the development of an attack by prompt administration of heme arginate without the need of a full course: regular once weekly administration of a single dose may help control the disease. Such patients are likely to require permanent indwelling venous catheters with all their attendant complications. A few patients have now received very large cumulative doses of heme arginate without serious side effects, although hepatic iron overload has been observed.

Prevention

Symptomatic patients and those who are diagnosed by family screening should avoid drugs, alcohol, fasting, or hormones that are known to precipitate acute attacks. Benefit versus risk should always be considered in conjunction with the severity of the disorder requiring treatment and the disease activity of the porphyria. Where difficult decisions on treatment have to be made, consideration should be given to contacting a national center with expertise in managing porphyria for advice.

NONACUTE HEPATIC PORPHYRIAS

Introduction

These cutaneous porphyrias present with photosensitivity, with skin fragility and blisters in sun-exposed skin. The skin lesions of PCT, HC, and VP are quite similar.

Porphyria cutanea tarda

Porphyria cutanea tarda (PCT) is the most common form of porphyria. Cutaneous photosensitivity is the predominating clinical feature; acute attacks with abdominal pain, psychiatric, and/or neurological manifestations are never observed. PCT is a heterogeneous group including at least three types:[12]

1. The sporadic type (75%; sPCT) is more often observed in male patients without a family history of the disease. It can be triggered by alcohol, estrogens, iron overload, or hepatitis C virus. In this sporadic type, uroporphyrinogen decarboxylase (UROD) activity is deficient only in liver during overt disease.
2. The familial type (25%; fPCT) has an earlier onset and is observed equally in both genders. Relatives of the patient may have overt PCT; in fPCT, there is a 50% reduction of activity in all tissues and this defect is inherited in an autosomal dominant pattern.
3. Hepatoerythropoietic porphyria (HEP) is the very rare homozygous form of fPCT. It is characterized by a severe photosensitivity, usually beginning in early infancy, and results from a dramatic defect in UROD activity. Only five different UROD mutations were found both in HEP and in fPCT.

Clinical presentation

The lesions of photosensitivity affect areas exposed to light such as the backs of hands, face, neck, and, in women, the legs and backs of the feet. Skin fragility is perhaps the most specific feature: a minimal trauma is followed by a superficial erosion, soon covered by a crust. Bullae or vesicles usually appear after exposure to sun and take several weeks to heal, leaving hypo- or hyperpigmented atrophic scars (Fig. 116.3). White papules (milia) may develop in areas of bullae, particularly on the backs of the hands. Hypertrichosis is often seen on the upper cheeks (malar area) and sometimes on ears and arms. Increased uniform pigmentation of sun-exposed areas is common. Alopecia and hypopigmented scleroderma-like lesions of the skin are less common.

Variable degrees of liver dysfunction are common among patients with PCT, particularly in association with excessive alcoholic intake. However, it is not clear to what extent liver cell injury is important in the expression of the syndrome. It is well known that in patients with typical cirrhosis PCT is very rare; it has been suggested that in patients with PCT there may be an underlying constitutional abnormality, which may predispose the liver to the development of PCT; uroporphyrin needle-like inclusions have been found in the cytoplasm of hepatocytes, which could promote progressive liver damage.

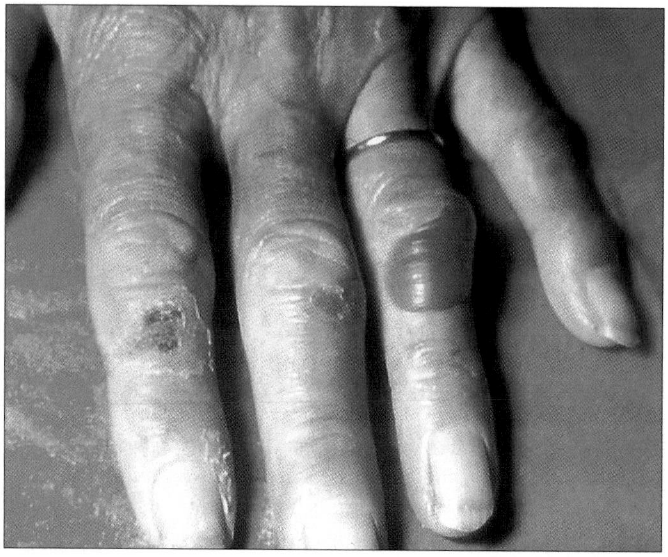

Fig. 116.3 Cutaneous symptoms (bullous) found in porphyria cutanea tarda, variegate porphyria, and hereditary coproporphyria.

Precipitating factors

Among the precipitating factors, alcohol, estrogens, iron overload, HCV, and to a lesser extent hepatitis B virus and HIV, are most frequently incriminated. These precipitating factors act either alone or in combination. Estrogen-containing oral contraceptives have increased the prevalence of PCT in women; as in any hepatic porphyria, most patients may receive these drugs (or alcohol) over several years before developing PCT.

Abnormal iron metabolism appears to be another precipitation factor of the clinical onset probably related to oxidative radicals produced by reactive intracellular iron. Serum iron is frequently 60% above normal levels in patients with PCT. A mild hepatic siderosis has been described in at least 80% of patients. Mutations of the HFE gene associated with hemochromatosis are found in fPCT and sPCT more commonly than in control populations, indicating that genetic factors unrelated to the heme biosynthesis pathway can predispose to PCT. The C282Y mutation seems to be more common in North European countries, USA, and Australia whereas H63D is the most frequent allele linked to PCT in the Mediterranean.

The activity of the cytochrome P4501A2 appears to be another important etiological factor in PCT. A strong association has been found between HCV and PCT in several countries. Hepatitis B virus and HIV are not as closely associated with PCT as HCV; antibodies to HCV should be evaluated in each patient with this porphyria at the time of diagnosis.

Diagnostic methods

Urine contains increased concentrations of uroporphyrin and 7-carboxy-porphyrin. Both precursors, ALA and PBG, are usually normal but the accompanying liver disease may cause a minor increase of ALA excretion (Table 116.1).

In the feces, the specific porphyrin excreted is isocoproporphyrin. During clinical remission total porphyrin excretion decreases progressively and measurement of urinary porphyrins and ferritin are one of the best methods for following the effects of treatment. After a few months, urinary porphyrin levels appear normal but in the feces copro- and isocoproporphyrin may remain increased for a long period. The same porphyrins are also found in plasma exhibiting fluorescence at 620 nm.

Uroporphyrinogen decarboxylase (UROD) is decreased in the liver of all patients with PCT. The human UROD is a 42-kDa polypeptide encoded by a single gene mapped to chromosome 1p34, containing 10 exons within a 4 kb piece of DNA. The enzyme functions as a homodimer. In the familial type, it has been found to be decreased by 50% in all tissues, including erythrocytes, whereas sPCT acts as an acquired disorder. So far, more than 45 different mutations causing fPCT have been reported. A liver-specific mutation for sPCT does not seem plausible and additional factors may in some fashion inactivate the hepatic UROD. Mutations at some other locus predisposing individuals to develop PCT in response to acquired factors (such as alcohol, drugs, iron, HCV) are likely.

Management

General supportive treatment of cutaneous porphyrias

Avoidance of sunlight and wearing appropriate clothing to cover the skin decreases skin symptoms. Absorbent sunscreens are of little help as they are designed to block UV A and B radiations. Reflectant sunscreens containing zinc oxide or titanium dioxide are more effective but their use is limited because they are cosmetically unappealing.[11]

Specific treatment

All patients with PCT should first be advised to treat any infectious disease (e.g., hepatitis C virus, human immunodeficiency virus), and to avoid precipitating factors (e.g., alcohol, pills, porphyrinogenic drugs) and exposure to sunlight until clinical and biological remission has been obtained by treatment. Phlebotomy is at present the treatment of choice, even when serum iron or ferritin levels are not increased. There are variations in protocols for venesection: usually venesections of 300 mL are performed at 10- to 12-day intervals and are continued for 2 months until the ferritin level is reduced to the lower limit of normal. Urine porphyrin levels are monitored every 3 months: clinical and biological remissions are usually obtained within 6 months.

When phlebotomy is contraindicated (anemia, cardiac, or pulmonary disorders, age) low-dose chloroquine therapy (200 mg weekly), which complexes with porphyrin and slowly mobilizes it from the liver, is the favored alternative (Table 116.1). Duration of treatment and relapse rate are only marginally greater than with venesection. High-dose treatment must be avoided because it causes a hepatitis-like syndrome in patients with PCT. In severe cases, combined phlebotomy and chloroquine therapy is often used with good results.[11]

ERYTHROPOIETIC PORPHYRIAS

Congenital erythropoietic porphyria (Günther disease)

Congenital erythropoietic porphyria (CEP) is a rare autosomal recessive disorder resulting from a marked deficiency of uroporphyrinogen III synthase activity (Fig. 116.1). Skin blisters are observed in the neonatal period or in early infancy both in CEP and in HEP, the rare homozygous form of type II PCT. Both are serious, chronic progressive, and mutilating disorders associated with hemolytic anemia (Fig. 116.4). Urine has a reddish brown color from the first day of life and exhibits a purple fluorescence under long UV light. The diagnosis is confirmed by a characteristic porphyrin pattern in urine (isomer I), plasma, and feces (Table 116.1). Treatment of HEP and CEP involves skin protection and blood transfusions to maintain the hemoglobin concentration. Allogenic bone marrow transplantation has been successful in several patients with moderate to severe disease.

Erythropoietic protoporphyria: a painful photosensitive porphyria

Erythropoietic protoporphyria (EPP) results from decreased activity of the final enzyme in the heme synthetic pathway, ferrochelatase (Fig. 116.1). It is an autosomal dominant disorder, with variable penetrance. The variable penetrance is

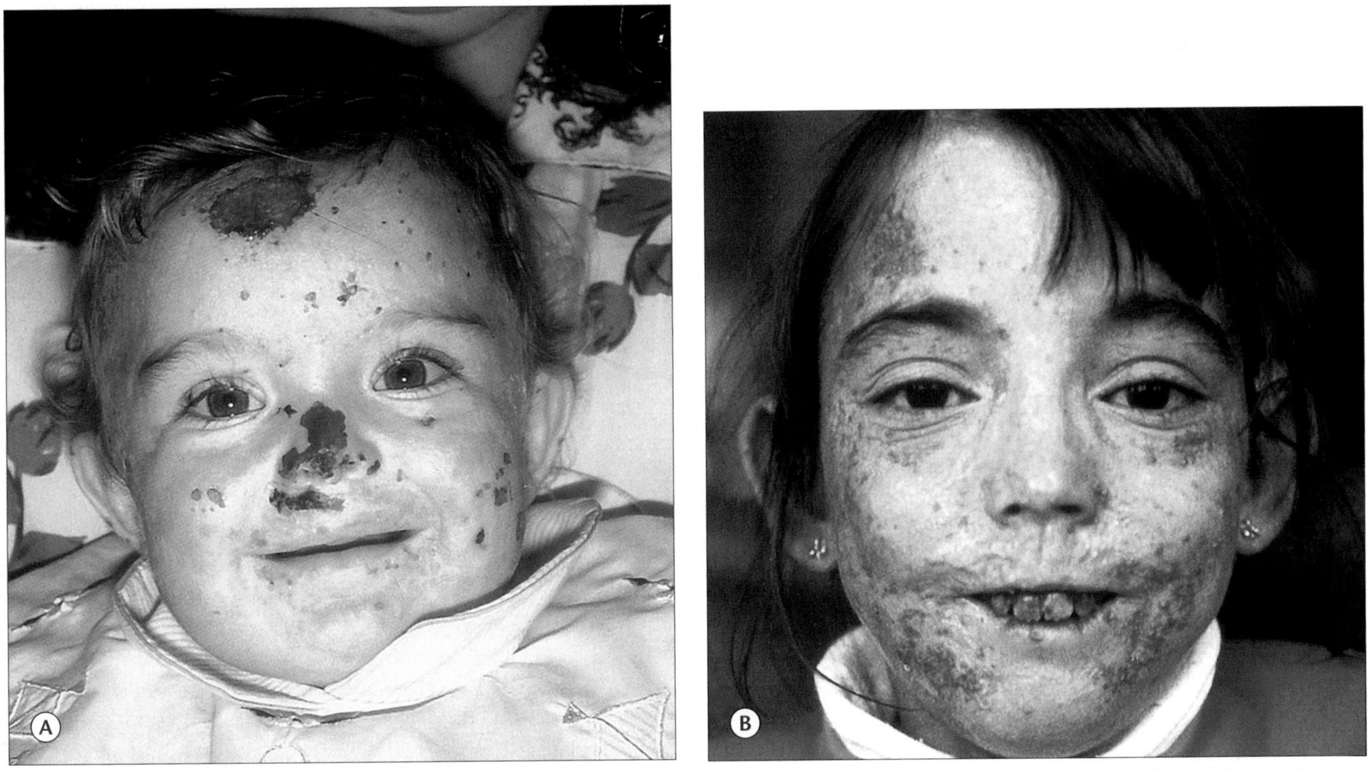

Fig. 116.4 Congenital erythropoietic porphyria. Clinical presentation of congenital erythropoietic porphyria (Günther disease) in an infant **(A)** and an adult **(B)**.

mainly due to the coinheritance of a low expression allele, which in addition to the abnormal allele, results in decreased ferrochelatase activity below the 50% threshold.[13] Clinical manifestation of EPP begins in childhood with acute and severely painful photosensitivity and a history of burning in areas of skin exposed to sunlight. Pain is usually followed by edema, erythema, and swelling. Repeated exposures lead to chronic changes giving the skin a waxy, thickened appearance with faint linear scars.

Urine porphyrin levels are normal; the diagnosis is based on increased free protoporphyrin levels in erythrocytes and in plasma, which has a characteristic fluorescent emission peak (Table 116.1). Patients often exhibit a slight microcytic, hypochromic anemia. Liver dysfunction has been reported in up to 20% of EPP patients and hepatic failure in less than 5%. The liver dysfunction is caused by the accumulation of protoporphyrin in hepatocytes resulting in cell damage, cholestasis and further retention of protoporphyrin. EPP patients may develop gallstones formed from protoporphyrin and are at increased risk of cholelithiasis.

Acute burning pain is ameliorated by application of cold water. Avoidance of sunlight is the mainstay of management. Oral beta-carotene (75–200mg per day; optimal blood concentration of 11–15μmol/L), which acts as a singlet oxygen trap, improves light tolerance in about one-third of patients. It is impossible to predict those patients who will develop severe liver disease, and management should include annual biochemical assessment of liver function. When liver dysfunction appears, treatment with cholestyramine, which depletes hepatic protoporphyrin, or activated charcoal, which binds protoporphyrin in the gut, interrupting the enterohepatic circulation, should be attempted but their efficacy is not proved. Once liver failure is advanced, transplantation is usually the only treatment likely to ensure survival (Table 116.1).

SOURCES OF INFORMATION FOR PATIENTS AND DOCTORS

Advice for patients and doctors can be obtained from the following websites:
Europe: www.porphyria-europe.com and www.hgmd.org
USA: www.enterprise.net/apf/index.html
South Africa: www.uct.ac.za/depts/liver/porphpts.htm
http://www.patient.co.uk/showdoc/502/
http://www.ncchem.com/safe-arbor/porphyri.htm

REFERENCES

1. Anderson KE, Sassa S, Bishop DF, Desnick RJ. The porphyrias. In: Scriver CR, Beaudet AL, Sly WS, Valle D, eds. The metabolic basis of inherited disease, vol. 1, 8th edn. New York: McGraw-Hill; 2001:2991–3062.
2. Ponka P. Cell biology of heme. Am J Med Sci 1999; 318:241–256.
3. Sassa S, Kappas A. Molecular aspects of the inherited porphyrias. J Intern Med 2000; 247:169–178.
4. Elder GH, Hift RJ, Meissner PN. The acute porphyrias. Lancet 1997; 349:1613–1617.
5. Thunell S, Harper P, Brock A, Petersen NE. Porphyrins, porphyrin metabolism and porphyrias. II. Diagnosis and monitoring in the acute porphyrias. Scand J Clin Lab Invest 2000; 60:541–560.
6. Astrin KH, Desnick RJ. Molecular basis of acute intermittent porphyria: mutations and polymorphisms in the human hydroxymethylbilane synthase gene. Hum Mutat 1994; 4:243–252.
7. Maruno M, Furuyama K, Akagi R et al. Highly heterogeneous nature of delta-aminolevulinate dehydratase deficiencies in ALAD porphyria. Blood 2001; 97:2972–2978.
8. Meissner PN, Dailey TA, Hift RJ et al. A R59W mutation in human protoporphyrinogen oxidase results in decreased enzyme activity and is prevalent in South Africans with variegate porphyria. Nat Genet 1996; 13:95–97.
9. Kauppinen R, Timonen K, Fraunberg M et al. Homozygous variegate porphyria: 20 y follow-up and characterization of molecular defect. J Invest Dermatol 2001; 116:610–613.
10. Martasek P. Hereditary coproporphyria. Semin Liv Dis 1998; 18:25–32.
11. Badminton MN, Elder GH. Management of acute and cutaneous porphyrias. Int J Clin Pract 2002; 56:272–278.
12. Bulaj ZJ, Philips JD, Ajioka RS et al. Hemochromatosis genes and other factors contributing to the pathogenesis of porphyria cutanea tarda. Blood 2000; 95:1565–1571.
13. Gouya L, Puy H, Robreau AM et al. How the phenotype of a dominant Mendelian disorder is modulated through the wild-type allele expression level. Nature Genet 2002; 30:27–28.

Chapter 117

Abscesses and other intra-abdominal diseases

Juliane Bingener, Melanie L Richards, and Kenneth R Sirinek

KEY POINTS

- 50% of all serious intra-abdominal infections are found after surgery
- 2% of all laparotomies are followed by an intra-abdominal infection
- Risk factors for increasing mortality from intra-abdominal infections are: older age, severe underlying disease, and malnutrition
- The microbes involved are usually three to five different ones, justifying initial empiric antibiotic treatment in most cases

NTRODUCTION AND DEFINITION

ıe word abscess developed in the mid-sixteenth century from e Latin *abscedere* which means 'to go away'. It refers to 'bodily ımors going away in the pus'. The term was not uniformly used r abdominal infections until much later. The pathogenesis of hat Melier described as 'purulent iliac tumor' in 1827 was ɔt understood until about the mid-nineteenth century.

Abdominal abscesses can be described either by location .g., pelvic) or more specifically by source (e.g., appendiceal). ıey can originate from two principal sources: a perforated ɔllow viscus or a solid organ infection.

PIDEMIOLOGY

ɔday, about half of all intra-abdominal infections and abscesses e found after surgery, although only a small proportion of parotomies (2%) are followed by an abdominal abscess. ifferent mechanisms of abscess formation present in different ɔpulations.

bscesses from hollow viscus perforation

bscesses from hollow viscus perforation, such as perforated ɔpendicitis and diverticulitis, are more frequent in urban dustrialized areas than in nations with a basic diet high in ber.[1]

Appendiceal perforation with abscess formation occurs in one f every three patients presenting with appendicitis. Patients with ɔpendicitis are usually less than 30 years old. Appendicitis is re in older patients and therefore frequently misdiagnosed. he incidence of appendicitis ranges between 6% and 14%. rban industrialized areas have a higher incidence than third orld populations. White children in South Africa are affected 0 times more often than their black neighbors.[2]

Patients with diverticulosis have a 10–25% risk of developing iverticulitis and a 5% risk of complications such as perforaon (Fig. 117.1) and abdominal infection. Diverticular abscesses usually affect patients between 50 and 65 years of age; in the southwestern United States the average age at presentation is 35–40 years (see Chapter 65).

Crohn's disease: Abscesses secondary to perforated Crohn's disease are more frequent in young affluent white populations but are rarely seen in the southwestern United States. About 10% of patients with Crohn's disease are affected by abdominal abscess formation. (see Chapters 53–59).

Solid organ abscess

The bacteriology of solid organ abscesses (liver, spleen) shows geographic variation. Liver abscesses in the United States and other industrialized countries are found most frequently in immunosuppressed patients with biliary disease, whereas amebiasis is a more common cause in Latin America. In urban North America the spleen is the commonest site of abscess formation from hematogenous seeding from endocarditis. In areas with a high incidence of hematologic disorders (e.g., sickle cell disease), splenic abscesses are seen secondary to infarction. Splenic abscesses secondary to brucellosis can be seen where unpasteurized sheep milk products are used (e.g., southeastern Europe). This disease is extremely rare in the United States and northern Europe.

CAUSES, RISK FACTORS, DISEASE ASSOCIATIONS

Advanced age, malnutrition, and severe underlying disease predispose to abdominal abscess formation and predict increased mortality. Infections usually result from hollow organ perforation: perforated appendicitis, perforated diverticulitis, other intestinal perforation secondary to obstruction and neoplasm. In both appendicitis and diverticulitis, luminal obstruction and inflammation lead to perforation. Other mechanisms that disrupt wall integrity include iatrogenic trauma (e.g., endoscopy) or an anastomotic leak.

Appendicitis: Delay in diagnosis is a risk factor for perforation and abscess formation. It is rarer in families where a previous member has had appendicitis as symptoms may be recognized and treatment sought earlier.

Ten per cent of patients with Crohn's disease are affected.

Perforated cholecystitis is usually found in the setting of gangrenous cholecystitis. Risk factors are male sex, older age, and pre-existing cardiovascular disease. Diabetes has been suspected as a risk factor for some time, but no study data have conclusively confirmed this. (See Chapter 76.)

Solid organ infections are frequently caused by hematogenous seeding (e.g., splenic abscess from endocarditis). Abscess

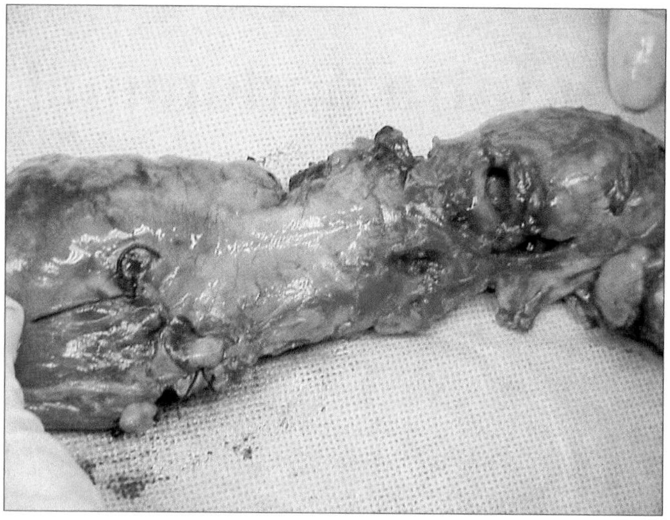

Fig. 117.1 Perforated colon.

formation can also occur in continuity (e.g., hepatic abscess from perforated gangrenous gallbladder). A further mechanism is transgression of bacteria from the intestine to devitalized tissue (necrosis after pancreatitis) or areas of decreased lymphatic clearance (postoperative hematoma).

Pyogenic liver abscesses are rare, occurring in about 0.01% of patients admitted to hospital. Most patients are immunosuppressed. The biliary tree is the commonest source (ascending cholangitis), followed by transmission through the portal vein (appendicitis, diverticulitis), the hepatic artery (systemic bacteremia), and neighboring organs (perforated gallbladder).

Although most splenic abscesses follow bacteremia, they can also be seen in the post-traumatic setting (17%). These usually have a delayed presentation, days or months after nonoperative treatment or splenic repair. Some 12% of splenic abscesses are secondary to infected infarcts in the setting of hematologic disease, and a small proportion are caused by direct extension.

Tuberculosis is a rare cause of intra-abdominal abscess in the industrialized world, although the rate is slowly increasing in patients with immunosuppression (e.g., AIDS).

PATHOGENESIS

Abdominal abscess formation begins when an epithelial barrier (e.g., colonic wall) is breached and microorganisms reach sterile tissues (e.g., peritoneal cavity). The body attempts to contain the contamination with fibrin deposits and omental migration, forming a 'rind.' Vascular permeability increases and protein-rich fluid arrives (Fig. 117.2). The complement and coagulation cascades are activated. Neutrophils and macrophages appear rapidly through enlarged vascular pores. Toxins and proteolytic enzymes from dying macrophages and bacteria cause local irritation. The abscess content becomes liquified. This increases the osmotic pressure, causing more fluid inflow. The result is swelling, pressure, and pain.

The release of proinflammatory cytokines from the activated macrophage–monophage system (tumor necrosis factor, interleukin-1, etc.) can lead to the systemic inflammatory response syndrome (SIRS) with fever (>38°C) or hypothermia (<36°C), tachycardia, tachypnea, and leukocytosis or leucopenia.[3]

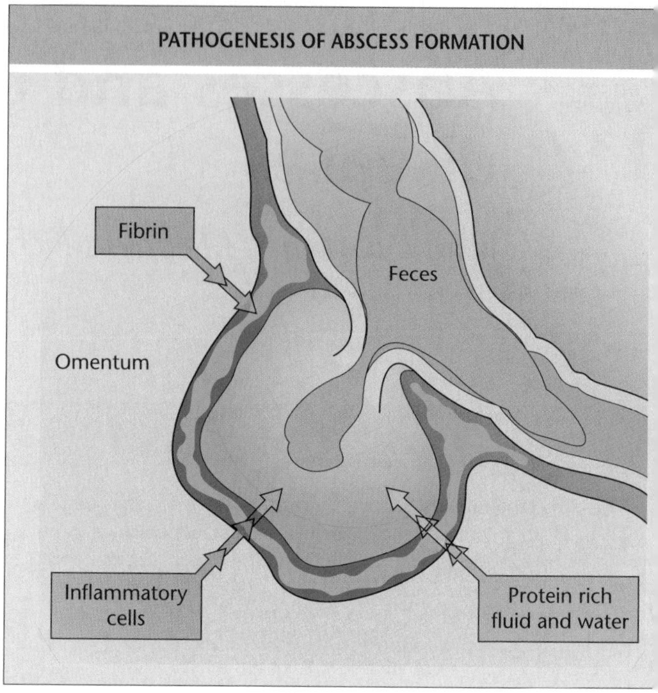

Fig. 117.2 Pathogenesis of abscess formation.

If left untreated, the abdominal infection can cause significar fluid shifts, progressing to hypotension, altered mental statu and significant catabolism. Hypoxemia and local acidosis decreas the effectiveness of the host defense system and th penetration of antibiotics.[4]

The most frequently encountered bacteria in abdomin infections are *Escherichia coli*, *Klebsiella* spp., *Bacterium fragili*, *Pseudomonas*, *Streptococcus*, and *Enterobacter*. Aerobic an anaerobic microbes may work synergistically in peritoniti producing a more severe infection than each microbe alon The mechanism is not fully understood.

CLINICAL PRESENTATION

The interaction between the amount of contamination an host defenses determines the intensity of the infection an inflammatory reaction, leading to variation in presentatior Typically patients complain of fever, abdominal pain, anorexi and occasional nausea and vomiting. This can progress to septic picture with hypotension, tachycardia, and oliguri indicating severe fluid shifts and hypovolemia. Abscesses ca perforate into neighboring organs (bladder, vagina, adjacen bowel loops), leading to fistulization (colovesical, colovagina enteroenteric).

Pain is steadily progressive, and a lull may indicate the tim of perforation (e.g., appendicitis). Pain may be absent, howeve or not particularly pronounced in the morbidly obese. Dependin on the location of the abscess, the patient may have a variet of associated symptoms (Table 117.1).

Right lower quadrant pain is frequently associated with appen dicitis, although a long sigmoid colon can be found in the supra pubic or right lower quadrant position. Left lower quadrant pai is often associated with diverticulitis and its complications although the tip of a long appendix can perforate into the le lower quadrant. Splenic and hepatic abscesses usually presen with a dull, poorly localized, left or right upper quadrant or flan

TABLE 117.1 SYMPTOMS ACCORDING TO ABSCESS LOCATION

Symptom	Possibly due to	Can be associated with
Constipation	Bowel obstruction, ileus	Diverticulitis, colonic cancer, appendicitis
Urge to defecate but not able to	Abscess in pouch of Douglas, vesicorectal recess	Appendiceal abscess, abscess after appendectomy for perforated appendicitis
Pain during sexual intercourse	Motion tenderness	Tubo-ovarian abscess
Singultus (hiccups)	Diaphragmatic irritation	Subphrenic abscess, after recent splenectomy

pain. Chest pain, hepatomegaly or splenomegaly, dullness in the lung bases, or rales may also be present.

Vague complaints: Special attention is needed in the extremes of age and in immunocompromised patients as the symptoms are frequently very subtle and may not be well verbalized. Altered mental status, failure to thrive, or hypothermia may be the presenting symptoms of an abdominal abscess.[5]

CLINICAL PRESENTATION

- Pain
- Fever
- Tachycardia
- Ileus (anorexia, nausea, vomiting)
- Catabolic response, weight loss
- Fluid shift (decreasing urine output, intra-abdominal tissue edema)
- Hypotension, systemic inflammatory response syndrome

DIFFERENTIAL DIAGNOSIS

The differential diagnosis for a patient with an abdominal abscess includes most causes of abdominal pain.

Once the abscess is confirmed, it is important to identify the underlying disease for an effective treatment strategy (see Differential Diagnosis box). A patient with Crohn's disease will require a different therapeutic approach to a patient with a perforated colonic cancer. If the primary source of solid organ infections remains unclear, the chance of recurrence or treatment failure is high.

Patients with nonspecific symptoms may undergo abdominal computed tomography (CT) and be found to have an intra-abdominal fluid collection. The confirmation or exclusion of an abscess can be difficult. Small amounts of intra-abdominal fluid can be physiologic. Typical features on CT will help to differentiate the fluid origin (hematoma, postoperative fluid collection, ascitis, ruptured ovarian cyst, etc.).

DIFFERENTIAL DIAGNOSIS

PELVIC OR INTRAPERITONEAL ABSCESS

- Postoperative: infected hematoma or fluid collection; anastomotic leak
- Appendicitis
- Diverticulitis
- Tubo-ovarian abscess
- Perforated intestine from neoplasm, ulcer or trauma
- Crohn's disease
- Perforated cholecystitis
- Infected pancreatic necrosis or pseudocyst
- Granulomatous disease
- Infectious enteritis (*Shigella*, *Yersinia*)

LIVER ABSCESS

- Amebiasis
- Echinococcal cyst
- Liver neoplasm
- Pyogenic abscess – ascending cholangitis, appendicitis, diverticulitis, gallbladder bacteremia

SPLENIC ABSCESS

- Septic embolus (e.g., cardiac source)
- Infected post-traumatic cyst or infarct (e.g., after embolization)
- Infected infarct in hematologic disorder
- Direct extension from adjacent organ infection
- Brucellosis

DIAGNOSTIC METHODS

The **history** and **physical examination** of the patient will reveal the pattern of pain, associated symptoms and diseases, the travel history, and whether the patient is clinically stable.

The **laboratory analysis** will typically show an increased white blood cell (WBC) count, left shift, or bandemia. These signs may be missing, especially in the immunocompromised patient.

Urine analysis may show a leukocyturia, which points to either a primary urologic infection, an infectious process in proximity to the bladder (e.g., perforated appendicitis), or an infectious process with fistulization (e.g., colovesical fistula in perforated diverticulitis). Electrolyte abnormalities may indicate fluid shifts. A decreased albumin level may be caused by a longstanding infectious process (catabolism), or by malnutrition and other underlying diseases. An albumin level lower than 20 mg/L is a predictor of increased patient mortality for any operative interventions. Liver function tests and coagulation profile are helpful to assess the severity of the infectious disease and important if a hepatic abscess is encountered. Hyperbilirubinemia and dissemination intravascular coagulation (DIC), as well as hypoalbuminemia, serve as predictors of mortality risk in that setting.

Acute abdominal radiography: Sentinel small bowel loops can be seen as a sign of ileus; free air indicates a perforated viscus or recent surgical intervention. A pleural effusion, lower lobe atelectasis, or pneumonia may be indirect indication of a subdiaphragmatic collection. However, less than one-third of all patients will have findings on the acute abdominal radiography that are suggestive of intra-abdominal disease.[6]

CT is currently the most effective diagnostic method. Adequate hydration of the patient should be attempted prior to administration of intravenous, oral, and possibly rectal contrast, to avoid renal injury. A ring-enhancing fluid collection within a solid organ or next to the intestines usually indicates the presence of an abscess.

Abdominal ultrasonography may also demonstrate fluid collections, especially in thin patients. It remains operator dependent and is not often used as primary method in the USA. This investigation is noninvasive and can be a very useful diagnostic tool in children.

If the quality of the fluid collection is still unclear, CT or ultrasonographically guided fine-needle fluid aspiration can be performed. This can be especially helpful in postoperative situations when differentiation between an expected postoperative fluid collection and an infected collection can be difficult. Another use is for the diagnosis of an infected pancreatic necrosis, if operative intervention is being considered.

Leukocyte scan: This can be obtained if the diagnosis remains unclear or CT is precluded. The patient's leukocytes are tagged with a radiotracer and then readministered. The leukocytes gather at the site of infection or inflammation, which is recorded as an area of increased radioactivity. Unfortunately, the results are often not very specific and may be difficult to interpret.

Diagnostic laparoscopy or laparotomy can be considered if the patient's condition is not improving or is deteriorating and no other diagnostic method has been helpful in determining the underlying condition.[7] This procedure is fairly invasive and may or may not indicate the cause of the patient's condition. However, if the cause is encountered at operation, a definitive treatment can frequently be administered.

TREATMENT

- Cardiorespiratory support, fluid resuscitation
- Antibiotic therapy
- Drainage (percutaneous or surgical)
- Treatment of underlying disease.

Intra-abdominal infections can cause significant fluid shifts and generalized sepsis, and lead to multisystem organ failure and death. Fluid resuscitation should be implemented to stabilize the patient while antibiotic therapy is initiated.

The antibiotic regimen should begin with empiric coverage of the 'usual suspects' for a given disease process. Gram-negative bacteria and anaerobes should be adequately covered. Once sensitivities have been obtained, the antibiotic coverage can be adjusted.

For most abscesses, drainage should be pursued. Percutaneous drainage is now often used as it is less invasive than laparotomy and has a high success rate. Limitations include difficult access (e.g., between bowel loops), an uncorrected coagulopathy, and the need for abdominal surgery for other reasons.

The morphology of an abscess on radiographic images (e.g., simple, loculated) predicts the probability of success with percutaneous drainage (Table 117.2).

TABLE 117.2 LIKELY SUCCESS OF PERCUTANEOUS DRAINAGE ACCORDING TO ABSCESS MORPHOLOGY

Radiographic morphology	Success rate
Unilocular or discrete abscess	>90%
Medium complexity abscess (with communication to GI tract)	80–90%
Complicated collections (intermixed pancreatic abscess or necrosis, infected tumor, organized empyema)	30–50%

Postoperative infection

When the infection is due to anastomotic leakage or inadvertent serosal injury, or is secondary to a hematoma or previously sterile fluid collection, the appropriate therapy in a stable patient is percutaneous drainage, antibiotics, and supportive care. If there is peritonitis or the abscess is inaccessible, operative intervention is necessary.

Perforated appendicitis

There are two principal approaches:

- Fluids, antibiotics, urgent surgery with appendectomy and drainage, irrigation, either open or laparoscopic; *or*
- If the abscess is amenable to percutaneous drainage, the patient is otherwise stable, and the abdomen is benign, the process can be localized – fluids, intravenous antibiotics, and percutaneous drainage with interval appendectomy after about 6 weeks. Prior to interval appendectomy a colonoscopy should be performed, especially in older patients.[8]

Diverticular abscess

Patients with abscesses that are not amenable to CT-guided percutaneous drainage or in whom clinical symptoms persist after percutaneous drainage should undergo laparotomy. Usually resection of the diseased segment (rather than drainage and fecal diversion) is performed. If adequate bowel preparation is possible and substantial contamination is not present, a primary anastomosis may be performed, with or without a proximal stoma. Alternatively, Hartmann's resection is the most appropriate procedure.[9] Some recent data suggest that laparoscopic abscess drainage may be a useful temporizing measure or even definitive treatment. These techniques are new and require further study. An algorithm for management is shown in Figure 117.3.

Abscess from Crohn's disease

The three management options are (1) medical alone, (2) antibiotics plus percutaneous drainage, and (3) antibiotics plus surgical intervention. When these three options were compared in a retrospective fashion,[9] the recurrent abscess rate was found to be 50% in the medical group, 67% in the percutaneous group, and 12% in the surgical group. Surgery included abscess drainage and bowel resection. Medical management will obviate surgery in up to 50% of patients treated with antibiotics and steroids; percutaneous drainage can be successful in 20–70% and may be an option for patients with conditions that limit the benefit of the surgical approach.

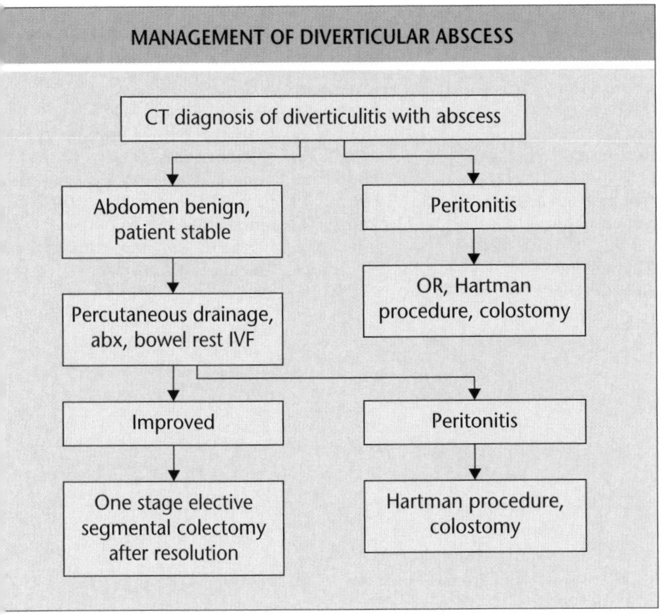

Fig. 117.3 Algorithm for the management of diverticular abscess.

Perforated cholecystitis

The most frequently encountered microbes are *E. coli*, *Klebsiella*, *Pseudomonas*, streptococci (*Enterococcus*), *Staphylococcus* spp., *Bacteroides*, and *Clostridium*.

In long-term critically ill patients *Candida albicans* cholecystitis may be encountered, and in patients infected with the human immunodeficiency virus cholecystitis with *Cryptosporidium* and cytomegalovirus has been described. The treatment strategy will depend on the clinical situation. If the patient is stable, cholecystectomy should be considered, taking into account a high likelihood of an open procedure. If the abscess is amenable to initial percutaneous drainage this would be preferred, especially in patients with severe underlying disease. Cholecystectomy can then be deferred and a laparoscopic cholecystectomy may be possible at a later date. The occurrence of a postoperative abscess is rare.

Liver abscess

When a pyogenic liver abscess is suspected, the first line of treatment is antibiotic therapy. The most frequent bacteria are *E. coli*, *Bacteroides*, and streptococci. The antibiotics should provide a broad Gram-negative and anaerobic coverage for (historically) 6 weeks. Metronidazole is often included as it also covers amebae until the titers return.[10]

If many smaller abscesses (<2 cm) are encountered, it has been recommended that one fluid collection be aspirated for culture and sensitivity. If the abscess is large (Fig. 117.4), percutaneous drainage should be attempted. A 90% success rate has been reported for percutaneous drainage; the complication rate is about 20% and complications include catheter dislodgement, empyema, bacteremia, and hepaticobronchial fistula. Percutaneous drainage should not be attempted in a patient with an uncorrected coagulopathy or need for laparotomy for

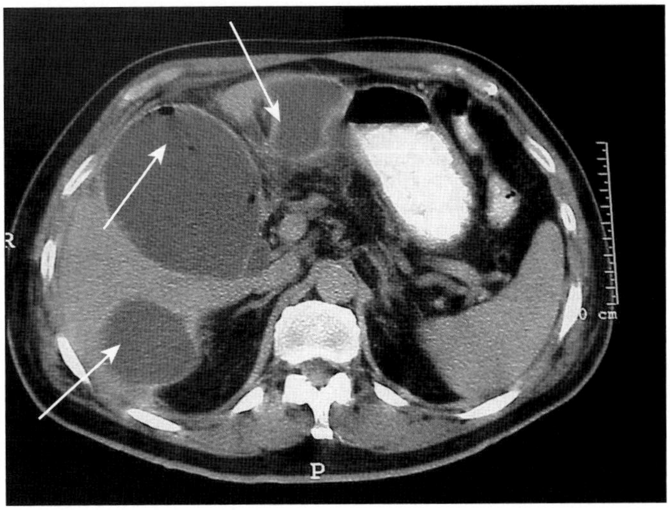

Fig. 117.4 Multiple pyogenic liver abscesses. Arrows indicate multiple liver abscesses.

other reasons. If no improvement is seen in the patient's condition after 72 h of antibiotic treatment and percutaneous drainage, surgical unroofing should be considered. It is important to continue the antibiotics and treatment of the underlying condition.

The mortality rate for a treated hepatic abscess is 12–17%, depending on the patient population. Septic shock, jaundice, hypoalbuminemia, adult respiratory distress syndrome, DIC, and diabetes are predictors of poor outcome.

Splenic abscess

The primary therapy for splenic abscess is antibiotic treatment. The fragile architecture of an infected spleen is important if percutaneous drainage is being considered. If splenectomy becomes necessary, vaccination for encapsulated bacteria should be performed.

Abscess complicating acute pancreatitis

It is difficult to make a clear distinction between abscess, infected necrosis, and initial pseudocyst in the setting of acute necrotizing pancreatitis. About 50% of pancreatic infections are monomicrobial; 36% are polymicrobial.

The most frequently encountered organisms are *E. coli*, *Enterococcus*, *Enterobacter*, *Streptococcus*, *Klebsiella*, *Staphylococcus*, *Proteus*, *Bacteroides*, *Candida*, *Pseudomonas*, and *Serratia*.

Once the diagnosis has been made, therapeutic options are percutaneous drainage and operative debridement. Several authors find percutaneous drainage to be sufficient and less invasive in a patient with severe systemic disease. Others suggest that the infected necrotic material contributing to the severe illness is unlikely to be sufficiently addressed by small percutaneous drains. Mixed results have been reported from both sides.

An abscess complicating acute pancreatitis is usually a severe infection with systemic illness; the mortality rate is up to 100%, or 40% with surgical intervention. For patients with an infected pseudocyst the mortality rate is 12%, or 20% for an abscess.[11]

REFERENCES

1. Telford GL. Diverticulitis. In: Fry DE, ed. Surgical infections. 1st edition. Boston: Little, Brown; 1995:265–271.
2. Bennion RS, Thompson JE. Appendicitis. In Fry DE, ed. Surgical infections. 1st edition. Boston: Little Brown; 1995:241–250.
3. Tchervenkov JI, Meakins JL. Altered host defense mechanisms in septic patients. In: Fry DE, ed. Surgcal infections, 1st edition. Boston: Little Brown: 1995:19–41.
4. Rotstein OD, Brisseau GF. The microenvironment of infection. In: Fry DE, ed. Surgical infections, 1st edition. Boston: Little Brown; 1995:43–51.
5. Podnos YD, Jimenez JC, Wilson SE, Intra-abdominal sepsis in elderly persons. Clin Infect Dis 2002; 35:62–68.
6. Fry DE. Peritonitis. In: Fry DE, ed. Surgical infections. 1st edition. Boston: Little Brown; 1995:227–239.
7. Van Goor V. Interventional management of abdominal sepsis: when and how. Langenbecks Arch Surg 2002; 387:191–120.
8. Klempa I. Zeitgemässe Therapie der komplizierten Appendizitis. Chirurg 2002; 73:799–804.
9. Garcia JC, Persky SE, Bonis PAL, Topazian M. Abscess in Crohn's disease. J Clin Gastroenterol 2001; 32:409–412.
10. Bowers ED, Doberneck RC. Pyogenic liver abscess and splenic abscess. In: Fry DE, ed. Surgical infections, 1st edition. Boston: Little Brown; 1995:297–301.
11. Martin DT. Pancreatitis and secondary infections. In: Fry DE, ed. Surgical infections 1st edition. Boston: Little Brown; 1995:279–284.

Chapter
118

Hernia

James Bourke

KEY POINTS

- Paraumbilical, femoral, indirect inguinal, and trocar hernias are at risk of strangulation
- Surgical hernias are commoner with vertical midline incisions
- The lifetime risk of inguinal hernia is 27% for men and 3% for women
- 45% of femoral hernias strangulate at 20 months vs 4.5% of inguinal hernias over 2 years
- Mesh repair has a lower recurrence rate than suture repair in nonspecialized centers
- Laparoscopic hernia repair can paradoxically lead to post operative trocar-associated hernias

INTRODUCTION AND DEFINITION

The function of the abdominal wall is:

- To provide protection and support for the intra-abdominal contents
- To promote bipedal living and activity
- To permit elimination of some intra-abdominal objects by micturition, defecation, vomiting and childbirth.

A hernia is a protrusion of an organ or tissue through an abnormal opening (most commonly, and in the case of this chapter, through the abdominal wall).[1-3] Hernias occur because of congenital defects in the abdominal wall (often early in life),[4] potential defects that are weakened by rises in intra-abdominal pressure, or defects acquired as a result of trauma or surgery. Uncomplicated hernias are important as a common cause of discomfort. When complicated by incarceration and bowel obstruction, they are potentially life threatening,

Development of the abdominal wall

Developmentally, the gastrointestinal tract begins as a long tube of endoderm comprising the foregut and the ventral bud, the midgut and the hindgut. Initially growth and development occurs outside the abdominal cavity and within the amniotic sac (physiologic exomphalos or omphalocele), but rotation of the gut occurs and the differentiating tube returns to the abdominal cavity; the liver and biliary tract are in the right upper quadrant, the small intestine is in the central abdomen, and the large intestine is draped around the right side, across the upper abdomen and down the left side of the abdominal cavity. This is followed by the migration of mesoderm from the right and left sides to form the muscle of the anterior abdominal wall. Anteriorly, right and left rectus abdominis muscles are formed. The formation of the anterior abdominal wall is completed by the fusion of the linea alba around the umbilicus.

TYPES OF HERNIA

Neonatal hernias

Occasionally, after birth, there is a small persistent defect at the umbilicus – an *infantile umbilical hernia*. The majority close spontaneously and only rarely require surgical treatment. Fusion of the linea alba is not always perfect and a defect or defects may be present. These can develop into potential hernial spaces that in the adult are typically found around the umbilicus and predispose to *paraumbilical hernias* (Fig. 118.1).

Rarely, the anterior abdominal wall does not develop satisfactorily; the intestines do not return to the abdominal cavity and the baby is born with external viscera covered by a membranous sac (but not skin). Such persistent *exomphalos* (omphalocele)[4] (Fig. 118.2) is graded as:

- Minor exomphalos – defect less than 5 cm and containing only gut
- Major exomphalos – defect more than 5 cm and containing gut and liver.

SITES OF HERNIAS

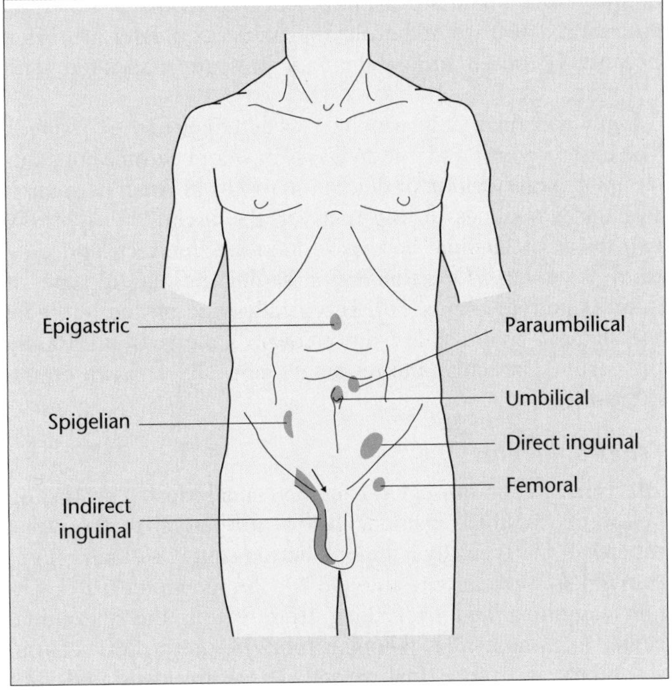

Fig. 118.1 Common sites of anatomically derived hernias.

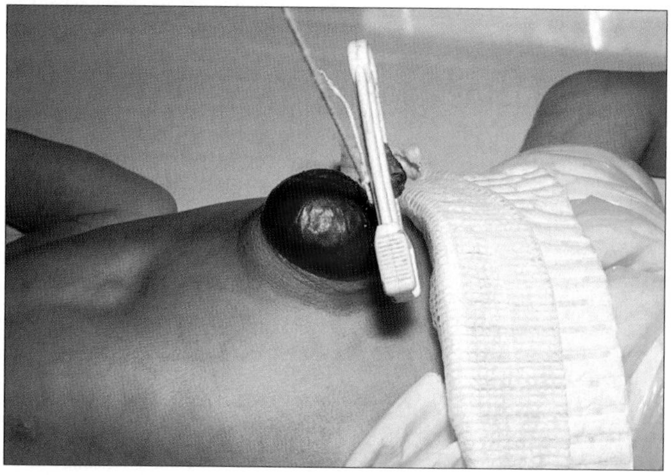

Fig. 118.2 Exomphalos.

Gastroschisis[4] is protrusion of intestines from the abdominal cavity through a defect to the right of the umbilicus. There is no covering membrane and the prolapsed midgut is often edematous and covered by exudate. It may be that gastroschisis is a ruptured exomphalos. Emergency treatment is required to return the intestinal contents to the abdominal cavity.

Adult hernias: anatomically derived

Inguinal hernias

In the male in utero the testis develops on the posterior abdominal wall and migrates through the inguinal canal via a patent processus vaginalis to lie in the scrotum, where the temperature of 35°C permits effective spermatogenesis. Following testicular descent, obliteration of the processus vaginalis should occur at parturition. If this fails to occur, the persistent processus vaginalis allows a *true congenital inguinal hernia* to occur. In addition the anatomic arrangement represents a potential structural defect where herniation can occur in later life, often because of raised intra-abdominal pressure associated with exertion.

Inguinal hernias may be indirect (as described above) or direct. The latter occur in older individuals in whom chronic cough or straining at micturition or defecation results in direct herniation through a weakness in the transversalis fascia.[1–3,5,6] Typically two-thirds of inguinal hernias in men are 'indirect' and one-third is 'direct.' Occasionally, a sliding hernia (a type of indirect hernia) occurs. This is typically seen on the left side; the sigmoid colon 'slides' down towards the scrotum. Rarely the cecum, appendix, and terminal ileum 'slides' down on the right side.

Femoral hernias

This is herniation through the femoral canal causing protrusion below the inguinal ligament, below and lateral to the pubic tubercle.[1–3,5,6] Typically a femoral hernia contains either omentum (45%) or small intestine (45%). The remaining 10% contains anything and everything from within the abdominal cavity (e.g., appendix, fallopian tube, Meckel's diverticulum, secondary gastrointestinal cancer). These are associated with eponymous names that serve no useful purpose.

Paraumbilical hernias

In contrast to findings in children, in adults most hernias in the umbilical region are paraumbilical. They occur in obese patients and can strangulate (Fig. 118.3).

Epigastric hernias

These are small but often painful protrusions, usually of extraperitoneal fat through the linea alba, between the umbilicus and xiphisternum.

Spigelian hernias[7] occurs as a protrusion of fat and peritoneum through the semilunar line, which is formed by the aponeurosis of the internal oblique muscle at its point of division to enclose the rectus muscle, typically between the umbilicus and the symphysis pubis. It presents as a painful swelling along the lateral edge of the rectus sheath.

Rare abdominal wall hernias

Herniation may occur in the lumbar area between the erector spinae muscle posteriorly and external oblique anteriorly, or between external oblique muscle anteriorly and latissimus dorsi posteriorly. Herniation can also occur through the obturator foramen and where the abdominal fascia is penetrated by the sciatic, posterior cutaneous, and pudendal nerves.

Acquired abdominal wall hernias

Any external injury to the abdominal wall, including surgery, can result in its rupture. Herniation can occur through any surgical incision and may be multiple (Fig. 118.4) and/or massive (Fig. 118.5). The risk is increased with every successive abdominal surgical procedure. *Wound sepsis* is the most important etiologic factor.[1–3] Additional associated etiologic factors include:

- Use of a drain through the surgical incision
- Steroid therapy
- Immunosuppression
- Obesity
- Intercurrent medical disease
- Operation through a previous incision
- Wound dehiscence in the early postoperative period
- Surgical materials
- Surgical technique.

The type of incision made is also an important factor. Herniation is more common after vertical midline incisions. Oblique and transverse incisions are associated with the lowest rate of occurrence of herniation.

Herniation through trocar puncture sites

Puncture of the abdominal wall during laparoscopy, surgical drainage, and procedures such as peritoneal dialysis create a defect through which herniation can occur.[5,8] The increasing use of such procedures has substantially altered the spectrum of conditions associated with hernia. Likewise an end stoma – colostomy or ileostomy – may be the site at which a hernia develops. The stoma itself may prolapse, or other intestinal contents may herniate around the site of the defect in the anterior abdominal wall.

Partial enterocele (Richter's hernia)[9]

This occurs when the antemesenteric circumference becomes constricted in the neck of a hernial sac without causing complete intestinal obstruction. It is most frequently associated

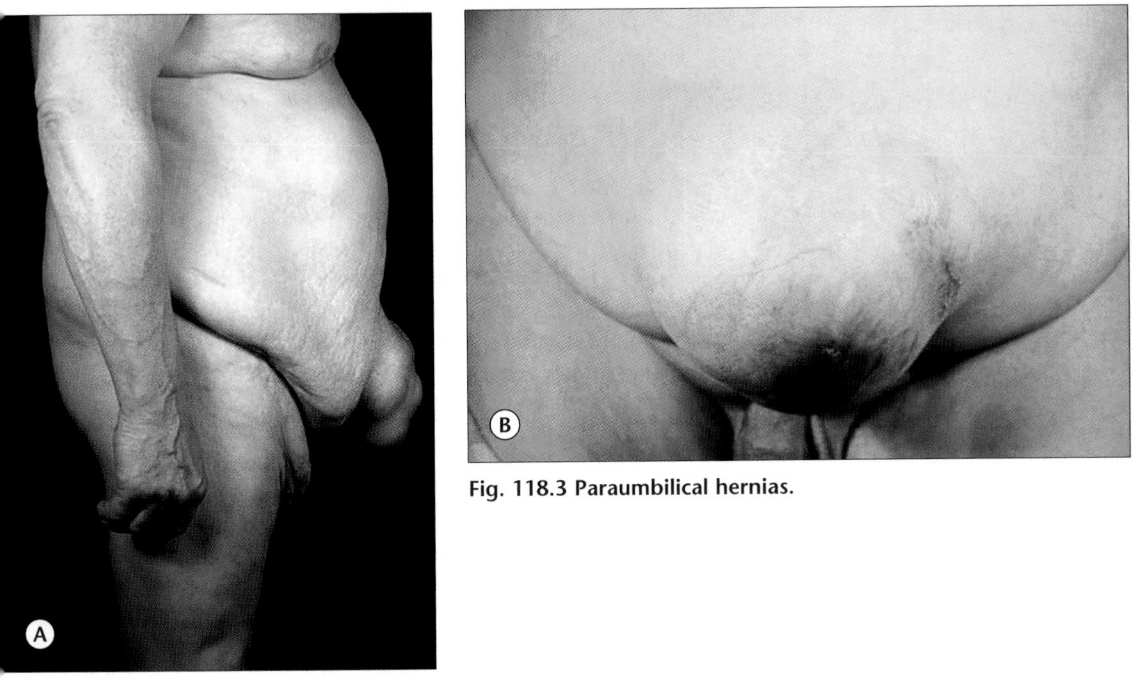

Fig. 118.3 Paraumbilical hernias.

with a femoral hernia, but also increasingly with hernias at the site of previous trocar puncture.

EPIDEMIOLOGY

The lifetime risk of inguinal hernia has been estimated at 27% for men and 3% for women.[1–3,5] Some 1–3 per 1000 people undergo repair each year, resulting in more than 20 million hernia repairs annually (about 100 000 in the UK and 500 000 in the USA).[1–3,5] Hernias, particularly femoral and trocar puncture site hernias, are an important cause of morbidity and mortality. The risk of inguinal hernia strangulation has been estimated at 4.5% over 2 years, and that of femoral hernia strangulation as 45% over 21 months. The death rate increases 10-fold when surgery is performed on complicated versus uncomplicated hernias. For the developmental reasons outlined above, inguinal hernias are more common in men than in women. Because the femoral canal is larger in the female than in the male, owing to the gyne-anthropoid pelvis developed for parturition, femoral hernias are more common in women than in men. Nevertheless (direct) inguinal hernias are the most common groin hernia in women.

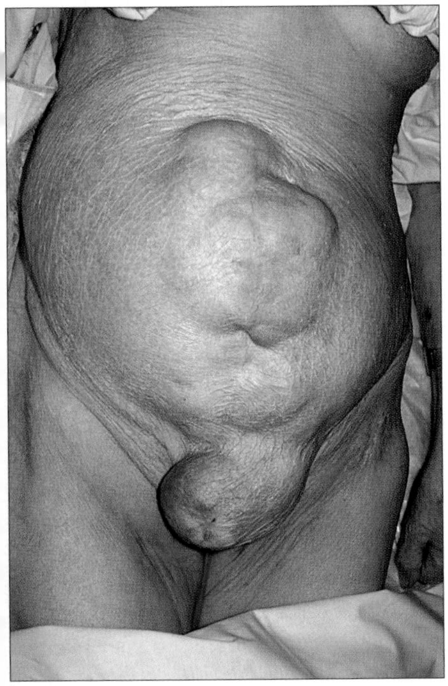

Fig. 118.4 Multiple incisional hernias.

CLINICAL PRESENTATION

Symptoms

Uncomplicated hernias

Most uncomplicated hernias present as a lump that bulges on straining or as a scrotal mass (indirect inguinal hernias[6]) (Fig. 118.6). Hernias may cause a variable amount of discomfort or pain.

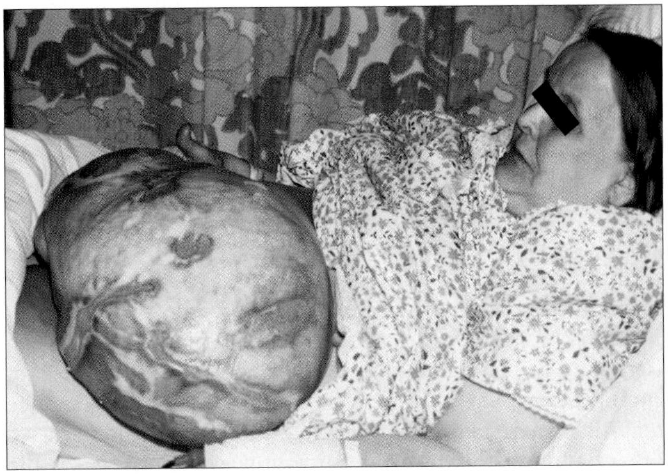

Fig. 118.5 Massive ulcerated incisional hernia.

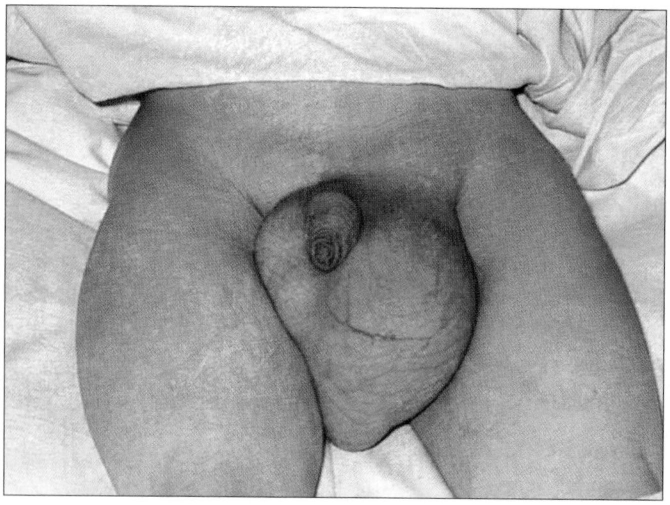

Fig. 118.6 Inguinal hernia inter-scrotum.

Complicated hernias

Pain increases if the hernia becomes irreducible and incarcerated, when symptoms of small bowel obstruction (colicky abdominal pain, nausea, and vomiting) may be superimposed. Obstruction is more likely with narrow-necked hernias (e.g., femoral hernia, indirect inguinal hernia, or hernia at the site of previous trocar puncture of the abdominal wall), and strangulation and gangrene may accompany obstruction.

Examination

A reducible lump with a cough impulse is present with uncomplicated hernias.[6] When the hernia becomes irreducible, the cough impulse goes and pain increases.

Femoral hernias occur below and lateral to the pubic tubercle, whereas inguinal hernias are above and medial. Direct inguinal hernias protrude directly outwards (through Hasselbach's triangle, medial to the inferior epigastric artery) with coughing and straining. With indirect inguinal hernias, the origin of the hernial sac is lateral to the inguinal artery, the protrusion is obliquely downward (see Fig. 118.1), and, once reduced, the hernia can be controlled by pressure over the internal inguinal ring.

DIAGNOSTIC METHODS

Diagnosis is largely clinical. In cases of doubt, ultrasonographic evaluation aids distinction from other lesions, such as lymph nodes, hydrocele, or testicular tumors.[6]

TREATMENT AND PREVENTION

All hernias may cause symptoms of pain and discomfort, and all carry the risk of incarceration, irreducibility, and strangulation, with or without intestinal obstruction. The risks of the complication are greater with narrow-necked hernias. For inguinal hernias, the mortality rate has fallen over the past 50 years,[1,2–4,10] and this has occurred when practice has been to repair inguinal hernias electively before the development of complications. Operative repair should be the norm for the majority of hernias. Additionally, local compression trusses offer symptom control while surgery is awaited or where the patient's condition means that surgery is too risky.

Urgent operative repair is mandatory for:

- Irreducible or strangulated hernias, and with intestinal obstruction in the emergency situation
- Femoral hernias
- Exomphalos and gastroschisis.

Irreducible inguinal hernias and patients presenting with a short history should also be repaired without an undue wait.

Surgical techniques

Many types of hernia, such as inguinal, femoral, and paraumbilical, can be operated on using local infiltrative or regional anesthesia; general anesthesia may not be needed. Currently, there are two main choices with regard to technique.

1 Suture repair versus use of mesh

Traditional hernia repair has involved meticulous suturing of all four layers of the abdominal wall (the Shouldice operation). In specialist units, the 10-year recurrence rate is less than 1%, but it is much higher in nonspecialist units. For these, placement of mesh to achieve a tension-free hernioplasty such as a Lichtenstein operation (Fig. 118.7B) is more appropriate[1,3,5,10–13] because recurrence rates in unselected units are 1.4% versus 4.4% for suturing. Alternative mesh techniques have been applied, and may be supplemented by the placement of a three-dimensional cone-shaped polypropylene plug, although the latter is associated with unacceptable rates of postoperative pain (up to 8%).[3]

Mesh can be placed in the abdominal wall or behind it in the extraperitoneal space. More than 80% of hernia operations carried out in the USA in the 1990s involved the use of a mesh prosthesis and were performed on an outpatient basis.[5]

2 Open versus laparoscopic repair

Although laparoscopic hernia repair was described in 1982, only a few surgeons have adopted it into routine surgical practice because of the greater difficulty, longer duration of surgery, and initial costs of the operation compared with open repair.[14,15] Laparoscopic repair can be totally extraperitoneal (TEP) or the transabdominal preperitoneal procedure (TAPP). It is generally restricted to bilateral or recurrent inguinal hernia repair, where it has advantages.

Antibiotic prophylaxis

Systematic reviews have revealed no benefit for antibiotic prophylaxis in uncomplicated hernia surgery.[3,16]

Outcomes

Patients want to avoid:

- Recurrence
- Long-term postoperative morbidity.

Recurrence

Primary repair of an inguinal hernia should be achieved with a recurrence (defined as a further groin hernia that requires an operation or the provision of a truss) rate of 1%.[3,10] However, rates of 10% are still being reported.[3,10] One-third of recurrences occur within a year of the primary operation and a further third within 5 years of surgery. Recurrence rates of 1% can be achieved by use of open suture (Shouldice) in skilled specialist centers, and by use of mesh in nonspecialized centers.[3,10]

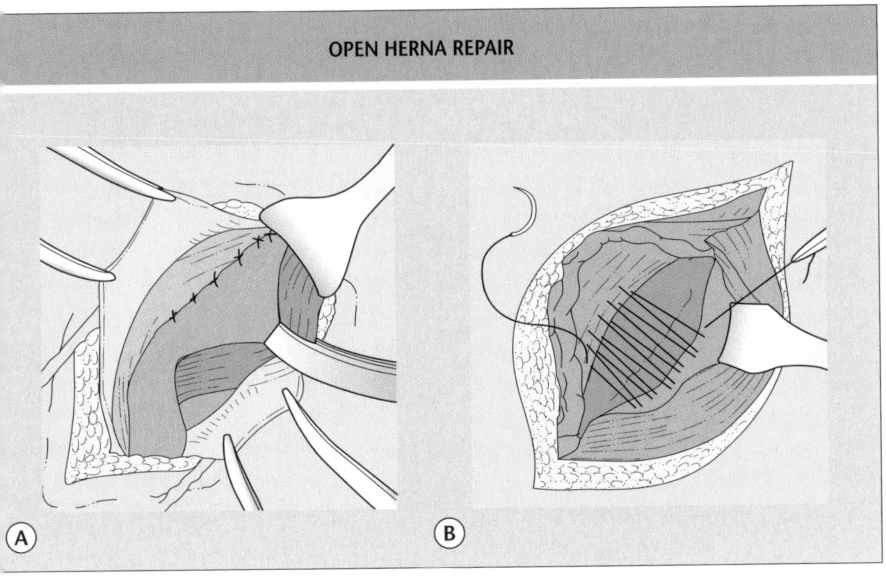

Fig. 118.7 Open hernia repair. A. Four-layer sutured Shouldice repair. **B.** Flat patch Lichtenstein operation. Adapted from Marsden.[2]

omplications

possible disadvantage of mesh hernia repair, particularly hen combined with plugs, is an increased frequency of local ain and paresthesia due to ilioinguinal neuropathy. It remains be seen whether neuropathy occurs with similar frequency hen the laparoscopic technique is used.

OURCES OF INFORMATION FOR PATIENTS ND DOCTORS

ttp://www.nlm.nih.gov/medlineplus/hernia.html
ttp://www.patient.co.uk/showdoc/23068760/
ttp://www.hernia.org/manjava.html (with music!)

CONCLUSION

Hernias are so common that their management and treatment will continue to occupy much surgical time. A new spectrum of hernias has followed the introduction of minimally invasive laparoscopic surgery, which has increased the frequency of hernias related to previous trocar puncture of the abdominal wall.

EFERENCES

1. Devlin HB, Kingsnorth A. Management of Abdominal Hernias. London: Chapman & Hall Medical; 1998.
2. Marsden AJ. Inguinal hernia: a three year review of two thousand cases. Br J Surg 1962; 49:384–391.
3. Kingsnorth A. LeBlanc K. Hernias: inguinal and incisional. Lancet 2003; 362:1561–1571.
4. Molenaar JC, Tibboel D. Gastroschisis and omphalocele. World J Surg 1993; 17:337–341.
5. Rutkow IM. Epidemiologic, economic, and sociologic aspects of hernia surgery in the United States in the 1990s. Surg Clin North Am 1998; 78:941–951, v–vi.
6. Rubenstein RA, Dogra VS, Seftel AD, Resnick MI. Benign intrascrotal lesions. J Urol 2004;171:1765–1772.
7. Montes IS, Deysine M. Spigelian and other uncommon hernia repairs. Surg Clin North Am 2003; 83:1235–1253, viii.
8. Brook NR, White SA, Waller JR, Nicholson ML. The surgical management of peritoneal dialysis catheters. Ann R Coll Surg Engl 2004; 86:190–195.
9. Boughey JC, Nottingham JM, Walls AC. Richter's hernia in the laparoscopic era: four case reports and review of the literature. Surg Laparosc Endosc Percutan Tech 2003; 13:55–58.
10. Royal College of Surgeons of England. Clinical Guidelines for the Management of Groin Hernias in Adults. London: RCS; 1993.
11. EU Hernia Trialists Collaboration. Mesh compared with non-mesh methods of open groin hernia repair: systemic review of randomized controlled trials. Br J Surg 2000; 87:854–859.
12. Luijendick RW, Hop WJC, Van Den Tol MP et al. A comparison of suture repair with mesh repair for incisional hernia. N Engl J Med 2000; 343:392–398.
13. Parra JA, Revuelta S, Gallego T, Bueno J, Berrio JI, Farinas MC. Prosthetic mesh used for inguinal and ventral hernia repair: normal appearance and complications in ultrasound and CT. Br J Radiol 2004; 77:261–265.
14. Roth JS, Johnson J, Hazey J, Pofahl W. Current laparoscopic inguinal hernia repair. Curr Surg 2004; 61:53–56.
15. Neumayer L, Giobbie A, Jonasson O et al. Open mesh versus laparoscopic mesh repair of inguinal hernia. N Engl J Med 2004; 350:1819–1827.
16. Sanchez-Manuel FJ, Seco-Gil JL. Antibiotic prophylaxis for hernia repair. Cochrane Database Syst Rev 2003; (2)CD003769.

Chapter 119

Upper gastrointestinal endoscopy and mucosal biopsy

Krish Ragunath and Paul J Fortun

KEY POINTS

- Currently the gold standard for visualizing the esophagus, stomach, and duodenum
- Can be performed as an outpatient procedure with or without sedation
- A safe and rapid test for investigating upper gastrointestinal disorders
- Mucosal sampling can be diagnostic
- Computerized reporting and digital endoscopic images can be archived
- Therapeutic potential includes hemostasis, stricture dilatation, stent insertion, and management of early and advanced cancer

NTRODUCTION AND SCIENTIFIC BASIS

he introduction of flexible fiberoptic endoscopy by Basil Iirschowitz in 1957[1] opened the floodgates to view the gut with ease and redefine gastrointestinal pathology. The fiberscope was based on optical viewing bundles transmitting light focused onto the face of each fiber by repeated internal reflections. The image reconstructed at the top of the bundle is transmitted to the eye via a focusing lens. Although the fibers are closely packed, there is always some space between them, resulting in a 'packing fraction' that is responsible for the fine mesh-like effect frequently apparent in fiberoptic images.

Videoendoscopy is the current standard. It is based on the charged coupled device (CCD). Essentially a CCD 'chip' is an array of several thousand individual photo cells known as picture elements (pixels) that receive photons reflected back from the mucosal surface and produce electrons in proportion to light eceived. The variable levels of charge are sent electronically to a video processor, which transposes this analog information into digital data, which in turn is processed to produce an image on a television monitor.

DESCRIPTION OF TECHNIQUE

Equipment

The videoendoscopy system consists of the flexible endoscope, electronic processor, light source, and television monitor (Fig. 119.1). The endoscope has a control head and a flexible shaft with a maneuverable tip. The head is connected to a light source via an umbilical cord, through which pass other tubes transmitting air, water, and suction. On the right side of the handle is the control unit, with a wheel for left and right deflection and a wheel for up and down deflection. Inside the vinyl-covered shaft are the to and fro wiring and supporting electronics to the CCD 'chip' mounted at the distal end. The vinyl-covered shaft also houses the light guide for providing illumination at the distal tip, control wires for maneuvering the distal tip, a channel for suction that also accepts a variety of accessory devices, and a channel for insufflation of air and water. The flat tip of the distal end unit has the CCD, lens system, openings for the accessory channel, and the light guide for providing illumination (Fig. 119.2). Endoscopes with a zoom option operate by having a zoom lens attached to the distal tip that can magnify the image up to 115 times when viewed on a 20-inch monitor (Fig. 119.3). The zoom lens can be controlled by a lever in the control head. The zoom facility allows detailed examination of the mucosa, especially to detect epithelial pit pattern and early cancers.

The video processor is connected to the television, wherein the final image is transmitted and viewed. The working length of the scope is about 110 cm, with an insertion tube of external diameter ranging from 5 to 12.5 mm. The angle of the viewing field varies from 80° to 100°, and the depth of the field is in the 3–100-mm range. Deflection of the tip should allow movement of 210° up and 90° down, and 100° to the left and right. The inside diameter of the working channel may range from 2.8 to 3.8 mm depending on instrument design. The suction channel is used for the passage of diagnostic tools via a side port (e.g., biopsy forceps).

Patient preparation and monitoring

This involves assessment of the patient's fitness for the procedure, identifying co-morbidity and at-risk patients, a detailed explanation to the patient of what to expect of the procedure, benefits, risks, alternative investigations, and possible complications, thus leading on to a fully informed consent.[2] Taking a drug history, especially warfarin or other anticoagulation, is essential. A history of metallic cardiac prosthetic valves or recent vascular grafts may necessitate prophylactic antibiotics before the procedure.[3,4] Elective upper GI endoscopy or esophagogastroduodenoscopy (EGD) should be done only after at least 6 h of fasting. Sips of water, especially for essential medications, can be taken up to 4 h before the procedure. Dentures, eye-glasses, and contact lenses should be removed and intravenous access in the form of an indwelling cannula should be inserted in all patients requiring sedation and in all at-risk patients. Blood pressure and heart rate are monitored, a supplemental nasal oxygen cannula attached, and a mouth guard is kept in place. Some patients are able to tolerate EGD under local anesthetic spray to the pharynx (2% lidocaine). Conscious sedation usually includes a benzodiazepine drug, diazepam or midazolam, and sometimes meperidine or pethidine.[5,6] See Chapter 141 for further details of conscious sedation.

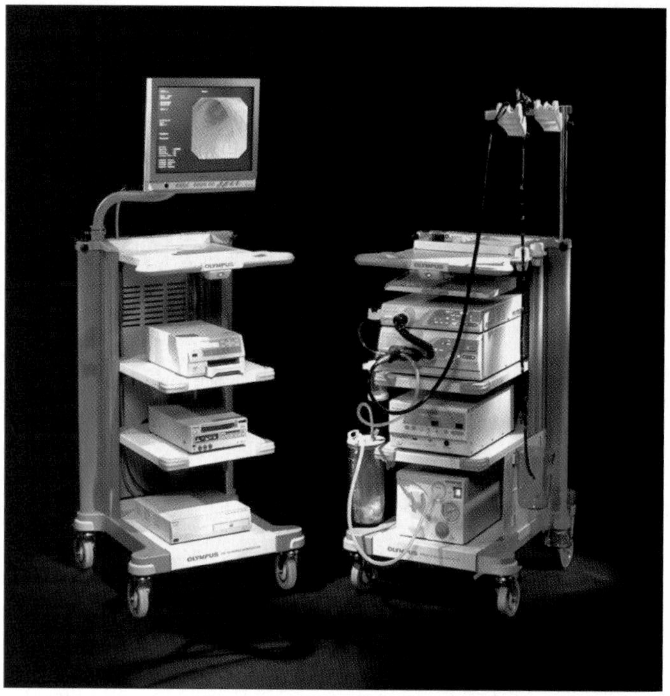

Fig. 119.1 A complete Olympus videoendoscopy system. The cart on the left is fitted with a flat screen monitor, digital video recorder, and printer. The cart on the right contains the gastroscope, light source, processor, and diathermy unit. By permission of Olympus.

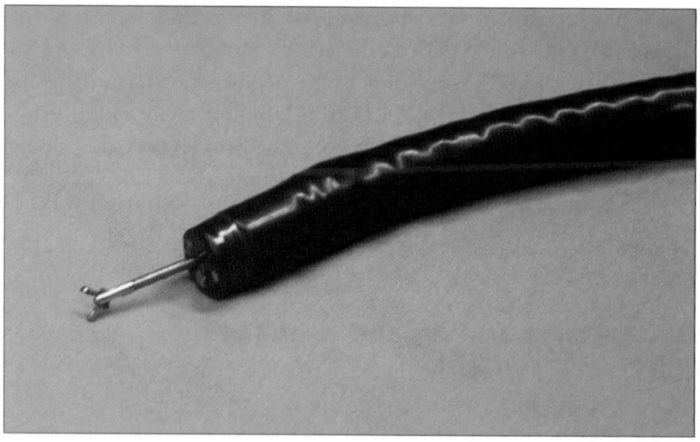

Fig. 119.2 The tip of a gastroscope with a biopsy forceps passed through the accessory channel. The optical lens and two light guides are behind the forceps.

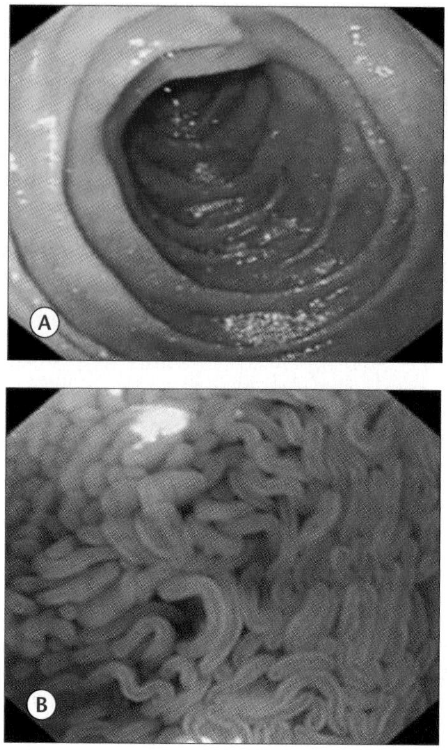

Fig. 119.3 Endoscopi views of the second part of duodenum. **A.** Normal view. **B.** Indigocarmine dye spray and magnification view with an Olympus gastroscope (GIF Q240Z), clearly showing a normal villus pattern.

Procedure

The endoscope should be held in the left hand with the head of the endoscope in the palm of the left hand, gripped between the fourth and fifth fingers and the base of the thumb. The thumb controls the up and down control and right and left knob. The first finger controls the air/water and suction button. The right hand is free to lock the controls in appropriate position, move the shaft to advance or withdraw, or torque the instrument. Acute rotation of the instrument should be effected by rotating the hand, not by rotating the instrument in the hand. Before inserting the endoscope it is important to check for proper functioning of the equipment and to lubricate the distal 10–20 cm of the shaft with a lubricant jelly. In applying lubricant, care should be taken not to cover the lens. The endoscope should be positioned before insertion so that the tip moves in the correct longitudinal axis with the natural contour of the back of the tongue. After inserting the mouth guard between the patient's teeth or gums, the endoscope tip is inserted into the mouth, sliding over the tongue and keeping to the midline to reach the pharynx. The uvula is often seen transiently, projected upwards in the lower part of the view. Then, as the tip advances the epiglottis and, finally, the cricoarytenoid cartilage and vocal cords are visible. The tip should be deflected down to pass below the cricoarytenoid cartilage on either side. At this juncture instructing the patient to 'swallow' allows the tip to slide into the esophagus. This is essentially blinded when the patient swallows. Forceful advancement of the endoscope should be avoided, especially when the patient is gagging, to minimize the risk of a tear or perforation. It is important to talk through the procedure with the patient to ensure maximum cooperation. Sedating the patient lightly or administering pharyngeal anesthesia helps intubation by preventing excess gagging.

Examination of the esophagus

Once the instrument is passed through the cricopharyngeal sphincter, the examination is done under direct vision. The two important 'golden' rules are:

- Do not advance if the lumen is not seen.
- If in doubt, pull back, inflate, and reassess the lumen ahead.

The normal esophagus is an unremarkable tubular lumen with a pale squamous mucosal lining. The landmarks include the indentation of the left main bronchus, left atrial pulsations in the middle third (may not always be seen), and the esophagogastric junction (EGJ), usually seen at about 40 cm. Here the pale pink squamous lining of the esophagus meets the red columnar lining of the stomach, forming the 'Z' line (Fig. 119.4A); it is also the starting point of the gastric mucosal folds. In patients with Barrett's esophagus, the squamocolumnar junction wil

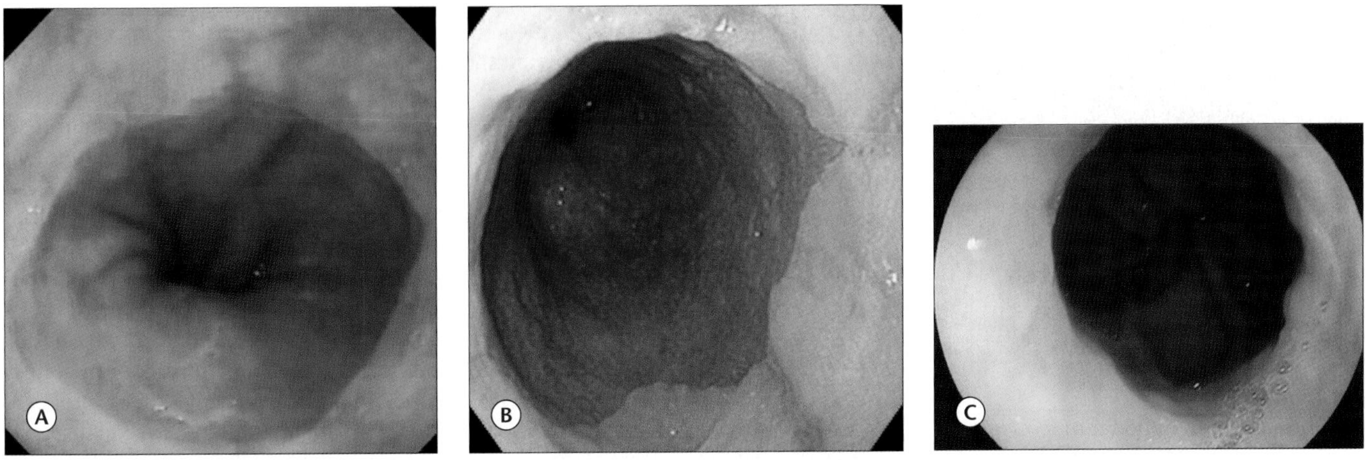

Fig. 119.4 Endoscopic appearance of the esophagus. A. Normal gastroesophageal junction. **B.** Barrett's esophagus with columnar epithelium creeping into the lower esophagus and displacing the squamocolumnar junction proximally. **C.** Hiatus hernia sac seen as 'lumen within a lumen.'

be displaced proximally to varying extents (Fig. 119.4B). Hence the true esophagogastric junction is the end of the tubular esophagus and the beginning of the gastric folds. The diaphragm normally clasps at or just below (<1 cm) the EGJ. This is highlighted if the patient sniffs or takes in deep breaths. Hiatus hernia can be diagnosed when the EGJ is more than 2 cm above the diaphragmatic impression, and can be seen as a sac (Fig. 119.4C).

The proximal third of the esophagus is often overlooked. This is where the ringed esophagus is often most readily appreciated. For those who like to find inlet patches (gastric heterotopia of the upper esophagus), a slow withdrawal on extubation from 5 cm below the upper esophageal sphincter cephalad will expose these curious lesions.

Examination of the stomach

Unless the cardia is unduly lax, the lumen can be lost temporarily as the tip of the endoscope is passed through with a gentle push into the stomach. Insufflation of air distends the stomach to observe the lesser curve on the right and the greater curve on the left. The gastric folds on the anterior and posterior wall can be seen, and there may be some bile-stained gastric secretions, which can be aspirated to avoid pulmonary aspiration. Food debris should not be seen unless the patient is not fasted, or has delayed emptying or gastric outlet obstruction. The distended stomach is 'J' shaped. The instrument is then advanced along the lesser curve with a clockwise twist to visualize the gastric body. If unsuspected retained food is present to any extent, the procedure should be aborted to avoid the risk of aspiration. If it is essential to perform the procedure at that session, removal of the retained tube can be done with an overtube in place to protect the airway.

In teaching upper endoscopy, some stress that it is important to visualize regions before the endoscope passes over them. This refers to examination of the gastric fundus and body on turnaround view. Others inspect this area on withdrawal by pulling the endoscope back into the antrum once the duodenal inspection is complete. The fundus is visualized by retroflexion or the 'J' maneuver (Fig. 119.5). This is done by 180° upward angulation with simultaneous forward push in a fully distended stomach, beginning in the proximal to mid antrum. The retroflexed shaft can be rotated through 360° to visualize the entire fundus and gastric body, thus visualizing all potential blind areas that are not as easily seen end on. By pushing the endoscope forwards, it will paradoxically move distally. By doing this slowly and rotating the endoscope, the whole gastric body can be examined from a turnaround perspective. The endoscope can be straightened when the angularis is visualized on turnaround. Sometimes the angularis is not seen from this angle, but if the endoscope is advanced into the proximal antrum and then a partial turnaround performed, the angularis can be seen as a distinct fold. Finally the scope can be withdrawn with gentle suction to deflate the stomach.

Examining the antrum is straightforward. If peristalsis is active, the advancing peristaltic wave can be followed from about 1–2 cm behind and the total mucosa is exposed right to pylorus. This sometimes reveals subtle lesions.

The pyloric orifice can be seen opening and closing with the peristalsis (Fig. 119.6). When the pylorus is very tight, especially to passage of larger channel endoscopes ('therapeutic endoscopes'), some experienced endoscopists gingerly pass a closed biopsy forceps through the pylorus and then advance the endoscope over it, pulling back on the forceps in gradations as the endoscope advances in order to avoid traumatizing the duodenal bulb wall, which is opposite the pylorus.

Examination of the duodenum

After the tip is passed through the pyloric orifice, the first part of duodenum or the duodenal bulb comes into view. This is a

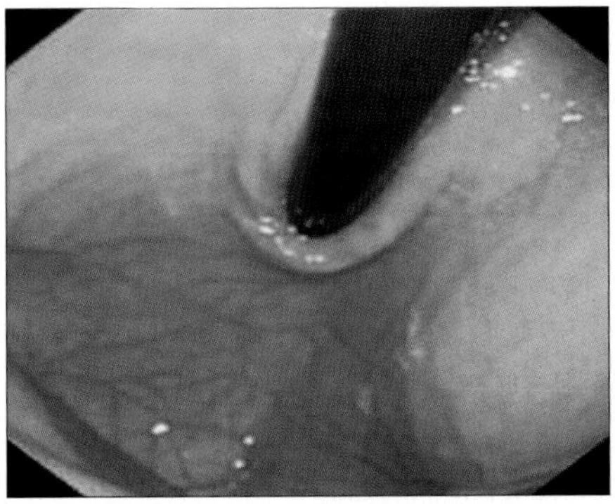

Fig. 119.5 The 'J' maneuver looking back at the gastroesophageal junction and the fundus.

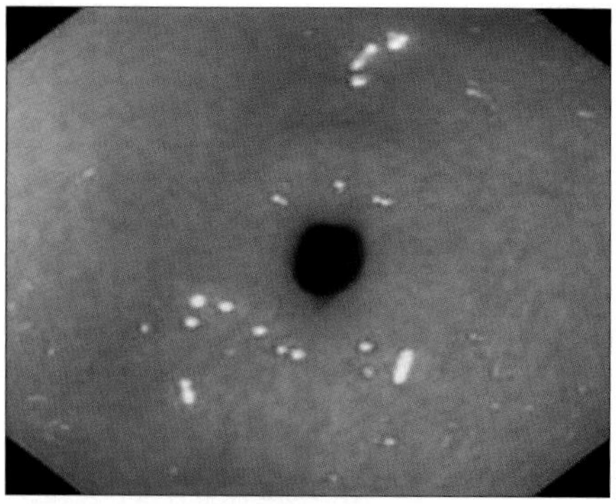

Fig. 119.6 Normal pyloric orifice.

common site for duodenal ulcers and hence careful observation is required (Fig. 119.7). The inferior and posterior wall is difficult to visualize unless the tip is deflected down and towards the right. The second part of the duodenum can be visualized when the scope is advanced further with a clockwise twist, downward flick of the tip followed by gentle withdrawing of the scope; the second part of duodenum then springs into view (see Fig. 119.3). Withdrawal of the scope straightens the loop in the stomach, and the descending duodenum with the papilla in it can be reached with only 50–60 cm endoscope insertion. If one wants to advance beyond the distal second part of the duodenum when the first pass has not accomplished this, the endoscope can be straightened, an assistant can then apply pressure over the left upper quadrant subcostal margin (spleen area) and the scope can be readvanced. This helps to prevent formation of an anchoring loop of endoscope in the fundus.

Mucosal biopsy and tissue sampling

Tissue sampling is done when an abnormality is encountered while performing endoscopy, to detect *Helicobacter pylori* infection, or as a planned procedure when, for example, duodenal biopsies are needed to confirm celiac disease.[7] The most common method is by taking a mucosal biopsy using cupped biopsy forceps passed through the accessories channel (see Fig. 119.2). The lesion should be approached face on, so that firm and direct pressure is applied with the widely open cups. The assistant then gently closes the cup, and the forceps should be withdrawn with a quick 'snappy' motion. Approaching the mucosa *en face*, for esophageal biopsy, is challenging. The 'turn and suction' technique is particularly useful in acquiring larger biopsy samples from the tubular esophagus, and when Barrett's surveillance biopsies are taken.[8] With this technique, the biopsy forceps is advanced out of the biopsy channel of the endoscope and opened. The forceps is then drawn back until almost flush with the endoscope tip and turned into the esophageal wall. Air is then suctioned from the lumen to collapse the mucosa into the forceps cup, which is then advanced slightly until resistance is appreciated. The forceps is then closed while maintaining suction, and the endoscope tip is straightened followed by withdrawal of the biopsy forceps to avulse the mucosal sample.

Ulcers should be biopsied at the edges and it is wise to take several samples from the same site when sampling tumors so that the superficial necrotic area can be penetrated to obtain good-quality tumor tissue. The samples are then placed directly in formalin (see Chapter 135).

Detection of *Helicobacter pylori* infection is done by placing one or two gastric biopsy specimens into a container from a commercially available rapid urease kit, which changes color within a few minutes (yellow to red) if *H. pylori* is present. Traditionally antral biopsies have been used, but in patients taking proton pump inhibitors the gastric antrum can be devoid of organisms in up to 50% of cases, although less so in the gastric body. In these patients, either gastric body biopsies alone or one antral and one gastric body can be used. Gastric body biopsies are best taken from the mid-body greater curve where the oxyntic glands are the thickest.

Tissue sampling using cytology brushes is done less frequently – usually when biopsy specimens are not adequate, especially in strictures or endoscopically difficult places to reach with the biopsy forceps. A combination of biopsy and cytology can improve the diagnostic yield, especially when previous biopsies have been inconclusive. Cytology specimens are taken using a sleeved brush. The head of the brush is advanced out of its sleeve and rubbed repeatedly across the surface of the lesion. It is then withdrawn back into the sleeve and the whole unit is taken out. It is then pushed out of the sleeve and wiped over glass slides and fixed with a fixation spray.

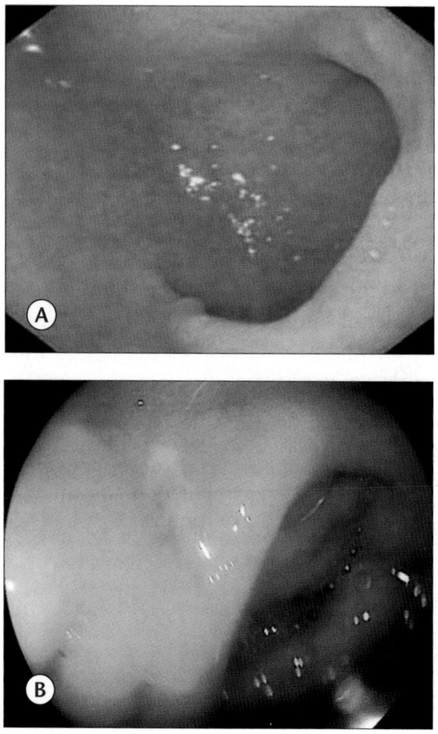

Fig. 119.7 Endoscopic views of the duodenal bulb. **A.** Normal duodenal bulb. **B.** Ulcer in the duodenal bulb.

Endoscopy reporting

Endoscopic findings should be reported accurately using precise simple language.[9,10] Impressions such as 'gastritis' should be relegated to the endoscopic impression and should not substitute for what was actually seen. Some reporting software programs can also incorporate endoscopic images captured during the procedure. Every report should include the following minimum information:

- Indication(s)
- Endoscopist(s) and assistants
- Endoscope used
- Sedation including route and dose, and any reversal agent used

- Supplemental oxygen delivered
- Exact findings in the esophagus, stomach, and duodenum
- Procedures performed (biopsy, etc.)
- Specimens obtained
- Complications encountered
- Treatment, further investigations, follow-up plan, and any specific comments.

ALTERNATIVES TO UPPER GI ENDOSCOPY

Barium studies are now used only for investigation of motility disorders and to provide roadmaps of strictures or gross morphology prior to complex surgery. The most recent technologic advance in endoscopy is the wireless video capsule endoscope (see Chapter 123).[11] After swallowing, the 'video capsule' generates images of the gut by a complementary metal oxide silicon chip camera. This is increasingly being used to investigate the small bowel. However, imaging of the esophagus and stomach is brief and incomplete. Future video capsule designs may emerge with mucosal sampling and controlled movement, which in turn may expand the indications.

INDICATIONS/CONTRAINDICATIONS

INDICATIONS/CONTRAINDICATIONS

INDICATIONS FOR UPPER GI ENDOSCOPY

Diagnostic

- To evaluate upper abdominal symptoms (e.g., dysphagia)
- For surveillance of a known condition (e.g., Barrett's esophagus)
- To obtain tissue samples (e.g., duodenal biopsy for celiac disease)
- Screening for malignancy (e.g., familial adenomatous polyposis)

Therapeutic

- Hemostasis (e.g., variceal banding, ulcer treatment)
- Dilatation (e.g., esophageal stricture)
- Stent insertion (e.g., inoperable esophageal cancer)
- Tumor ablation (e.g., laser, argon beam treatment)
- Polypectomy or endoscopic mucosal resection
- Foreign body removal
- Percutaneous endoscopic gastrostomy insertion

RELATIVE CONTRAINDICATIONS

- Hemodynamically unstable patient
- Recent myocardial infarction or pulmonary embolism
- Acute abdomen (e.g., peritonitis)
- Severe uncorrected coagulopathy
- Anatomic abnormalities in the upper esophagus (e.g., Zenker's diverticulum)

The most common indication for performing EGD is persistent symptoms related to the upper GI tract. Emergency EGD may be necessary in cases of upper GI bleeding to diagnose and treat the bleeding source. It is also done for screening esophagogastric cancers (China and Japan) and Barrett's esophagus surveillance. EGD forms part of other GI investigations in investigating anemia, weight loss, and occult malignancy, and also to obtain duodenal biopsies in patients with suspected celiac disease and other malabsorptive conditions. Endoscopy may be performed following abnormal barium or computed tomography studies for confirmation of diagnosis and tissue sampling. EGD is done to perform a variety of therapeutic procedures including hemostasis of bleeding lesions (varices, ulcers, angiodysplasia) (see Chapter 142), stricture dilatation, stent insertion (see Chapter 146), and management of early and advanced cancer (see Chapters 143 and 145), as described in detail in the therapeutic endoscopy section. The American Society for Gastrointestinal Endoscopy has produced guidelines on the appropriate use of endoscopy.[12] EGD, if performed for appropriate indications, has a high yield of detecting clinically relevant lesions in the upper GI tract.[13]

In the setting of an appropriate indication, in a fit patient who can give informed consent and is able to cooperate with conscious sedation, there is virtually no contraindication to performing EGD. However, the risks are increased in systemically ill patients, anticoagulated patients, and those who have had a recent myocardial infarction or surgery. Occasionally anatomic abnormalities in the esophagus such as Zenker's diverticulum or a high esophageal stricture can render the procedure hazardous. In such cases the benefit of the procedure should be weighed against the therapeutic benefits to be gained by a specific diagnosis. EGD without or without mucosal biopsy is not contraindicated in patients taking warfarin or other anticoagulants, provided the international normalized ratio (INR) is within a reasonable therapeutic range. Neither are aspirin and other antiplatelet medications a contraindication.[14]

COMPLICATIONS AND THEIR MANAGEMENT

COMPLICATIONS AND CONTROVERSIES

COMPLICATIONS OF UPPER GI ENDOSCOPY

- Bleeding
- Perforation
- Aspiration
- Respiratory failure
- Arrhythmias
- Transmission of infection
- Medication allergy

Upper GI endoscopy is a relatively safe procedure, but there are many potential dangers. Large surveys suggest that there is a 1 in 1000 risk of a significant complication, and a 1 in 10 000 risk of death. Problems are more likely to be encountered in elderly frail patients with other co-morbidities, and in emergency situations. Operator experience is also important. All endoscopy units should have a regular update on safety issues, procedure protocols, and resuscitation training, and maintain a log of critical incidents and near-miss incidents as part of quality control. Possible complications are described below.

Bleeding

Bleeding is uncommon after a diagnostic endoscopy. Minor self-limiting bleeding from a biopsy site is common and can be ignored. However, excessive brisk bleeding obscuring vision may occur in patients with impaired coagulation and liver disease or in over-anticoagulated patients. This can be controlled with a 1:10 000 injection of epinephrine and/or diathermy cauterization. It is important to check clotting parameters as part of the pre-endoscopy evaluation in anticoagulated patients.[14]

Perforation

This can happen at all sites, but is more common in the upper esophagus where the endoscope is passed blindly – hence, the dictum, "Do not push, but ask the patient to 'swallow'." The appearance of surgical emphysema in the neck or unexplained chest or abdominal pain should alert the endoscopist. Immediate recognition and prompt involvement of the surgical team is important for further management.

Respiratory complications

These include oxygen desaturation, aspiration, and respiratory arrest. Identifying high-risk patients, close monitoring using pulse oximetry, safe sedation practice, oxygen supplementation, and adequate throat suction by the assistant in case of fluid regurgitation can all help in preventing these complications.

Arrhythmias

Occasionally EGD, especially in the presence of hypoxia, can provoke atrial or ventricular arrhythmias. Pulse and cardiac monitoring identify these. Resuscitation equipment should always be available in the endoscopy suite.

Infection

Bacteremia can occur after endoscopy; the organisms involved are usually the commensals in the throat. This does not have any bearing on the patient unless he or she has valvular heart disease, prosthetic valves, vascular graft, or previous endocarditis; in these cases, prophylactic antibiotics should be administered for higher-risk procedures (sclerotherapy, stent placement).[3,4] High standards of cleaning and disinfection procedures should be followed to prevent transmission of infections such as viral hepatitis, human immunodeficiency virus, etc. If current disinfection protocols are followed, the possibility of transmission of any infection is negligible.[15,16]

Medication reaction

Allergy to local anesthetic is not uncommon and a thorough pre-endoscopy check should be done to avoid drugs to which the patient is known to be allergic. Methemoglobinemia has been reported following lidocaine throat spray. Anticholinergics will not affect treated glaucoma, but may precipitate an attack in occult chronic glaucoma, and thus a diagnosis can be made; there is therefore no ocular contraindications to the use of anticholinergic medications. See Chapter 141 for further details of conscious sedation and its complications.

COSTS AND BENEFITS

The cost-effectiveness of a diagnostic test must be compared with that of a competing test or strategy to produce meaningful information. EGD is now the standard of care for undisputed indications (e.g., hematemesis, melena, dysphagia) in almost any healthcare system. Radiologic investigations such as barium tests are now used only in specific conditions (e.g., motility disorders) or to complement EGD and aid in therapeutic procedures. Symptomatic treatment of young dyspeptic patients (aged less than 45 years) with no alarm symptoms (e.g., dysphagia, anemia, weight loss) is more cost-effective. The diagnostic yield is greater with increasing age, so that EGD will be more cost-effective.

NEW MODALITIES IN ENDOSCOPIC IMAGING

Standard video endoscopes have a focal distance between 1 and 2 cm from the tip of the endoscope and use less than 200 000 pixels to construct an image. Advanced methods are being developed to enhance the endoscopic image. This has been through technical innovation in the resolution and magnification of the endoscope itself, as well as utilizing properties of light beyond the current spectrum, through spectroscopy, fluoroscopy and enhancement with contrasts and dyes. The improved image enhancement has lead to the possibility of diagnosis by the optical properties of a tissue without biopsy for histologic assessment – the 'optical biopsy'. Presently their role is largely confined to the research setting, but this may soon expand into the mainstream. An overview is given below.

Magnification and resolution

Current magnifying or 'zoom' endoscopes enlarge the image up to 170 fold, using a mechanically or electronically movable lens controlled by a lever at the head of the endoscope. Eventually, image quality is lost because for each step of enlargement the image will contain fewer pixels. This distinguishes magnification from high resolution, which is the ability to discriminate between two points; in an electronic image, this is a function of pixel density. High resolution endoscopes can therefore improve the non-magnified image and make it suitable for high magnification without loss of resolution. High resolution endoscopes with high quality CCD chips giving high resolution (>850 000 pixels) and variable focal distance are now commercially available.

Chromoendoscopy

The use of special stains in combination with magnification endoscopy enhances the mucosal detail seen at endoscopy, with characteristic mucosal appearances such as pit patterns in the esophagus, stomach and duodenum (see Fig. 119.3) that can allow targeted biopsy. This has facilitated an improved histologic yield of specialized intestinal metaplasia and dysplasia in Barrett's esophagus, for example. Vital stains such as methylene blue,[17] acetic acid[18], and non-absorbed stains such as indigo carmine[19] (Fig. 119.8) have all been used to target the Barrett's mucosa with increased sensitivity for the detection of specialized intestinal metaplasia.

Although chromoendoscopy is appealing as a relatively low-tech accessible method in, for example, Barrett's surveillance, there have been concerns with methylene blue. Photosensitization of methylene blue with white light can induce formation of reactive oxygen species, causing single-strand breaks and generation of oxidative alterations within the DNA[20]. This has the theoretical risk of accelerating malignant change, although the duration of the effect may be short-lived.

Fluorescent spectroscopy

Tissue spectroscopy relies on the variation in emission and reflection of light between tissues. In laser-induced fluorescence

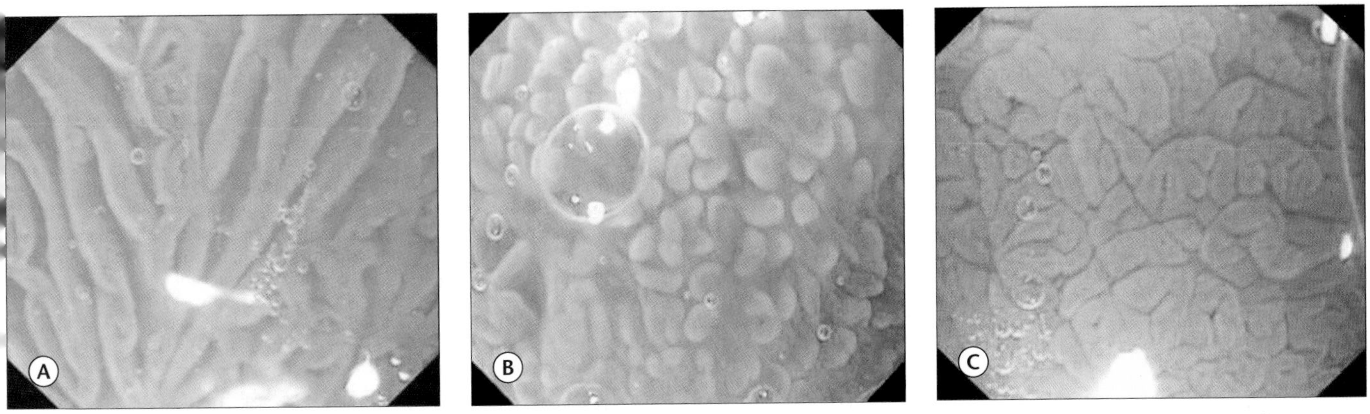

Fig. 119.8 Enhanced magnification with acetic acid showing linear (A), villous (B) and nodular (C) pit patterns within Barrett's mucosa.

endoscopy (LIFE), laser energy is used to excite natural fluorophores (e.g. collagen, NADH, porphyrins) in tissues. This has been applied to esophageal and colonic dysplasia with promising results in terms of discrimination between normal, dysplastic and malignant tissue.[21–23] In point spectroscopy, a fiberoptic probe is passed down the biopsy channel, however only a small surface area can be surveyed at any one time. Newer LIFE plus endoscopy techniques incorporate separate red and green fluorescence imaging channels, and allow real time fluoroscopy and switching to the conventional white light endoscopic image.

Light scattering spectroscopy (LSS)

This technique distinguishes tissues according to their absorption and scattering of light. Absorption is in turn determined by the relative concentrations of hemoglobin, whilst scattering is affected by the size and density of tissue components such as collagen. Crowding of nuclei in Barrett's dysplasia is reflected by characteristic changes in LSS.[24]

Optical coherence tomography (OCT)

OCT provides two dimensional images by detecting the degree of interference that a tissue causes to a split light beam in the near infrared range: one directed directly to the tissue, the other via a mirror at differing positions, and then measuring the backscattered light. Application to Barrett's esophagus diagnosis has again been proposed.[25–26]

Raman spectroscopy

This technique produces a molecular fingerprint for different tissue types based on their emitted resonance spectrum (vibration, rotation) induced by light in the ultraviolet/infrared range. The Raman effect is the inelastic scattering of light by molecules, so that light scattered by tissues is shifted to a lower frequency (i.e. longer wavelength). The resulting emission spectrum is analyzed by a spectral analyzer, to produce a bond signature specific to that tissue sample. In contrast to fluorescence spectroscopy or LSS, molecular changes that occur in proteins, lipids and nucleic acids during malignant transformation produce characteristic signals. Raman spectroscopy has the advantage of high molecular specificity, which may in the future translate into more specific tissue diagnosis. Clinical application to the GI tract is now underway.[27–28]

Confocal microscopy

The laser scanning confocal microscope has been combined with endoscopic delivery to allow *in vivo* microscopic examination of the GI tract,[29] creating the possibility of *in vivo* or 'virtual' histopathology. As with OCT, this will require either the presence of or telelink with a pathologist, or expansion of the gastroenterologist's diagnostic acumen into the field of histopathology.

Narrow band imaging (NBI)

NBI has a standard white light image composed of sequential imaging through a red, green, and blue band pass filter giving a high resolution image, and an NBI mode in which the bandwidths of these three filters have been narrowed and the relative contribution of the blue filter has been increased, resulting in improved mucosal contrast and detail. The endoscopist can switch between the high resolution mode and the NBI mode.

Adaptive index of hemoglobin (IHb)

The degree of redness in mucosal epithelium is correlated with the mucosal content of hemoglobin, so that the degree of redness can be quantified by an index of hemoglobin.[30] Calculations based on the red and green image signals are processed to form a distribution image which gives a measure of mucosal blood flow, which is abnormal in malignant tissues such as gastric cancer.[31]

The fine microvascular detail can be seen in the image below from normal duodenal villi (Fig. 119.9).

SOURCES OF INFORMATION FOR PATIENTS AND DOCTORS

http://www.gastro.org/generalPublic.html

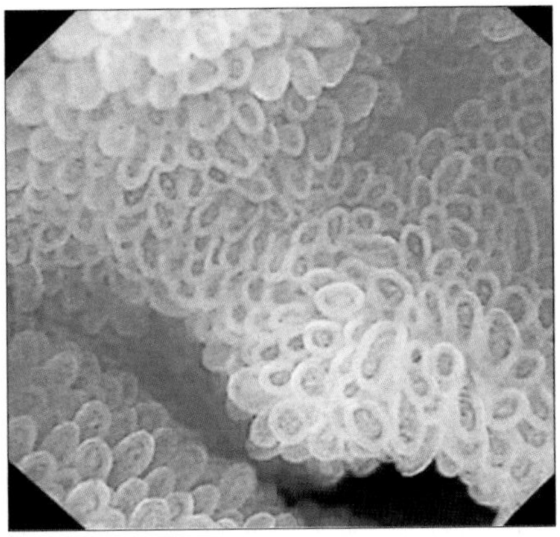

Fig. 119.9 Magnified (X115) high resolution view of duodenal mucosa revealing capillaries within villi.

REFERENCES

1. Hirschowitz B, Peters CW, Curtis LE. Preliminary report on a long fibrescope for examination of stomach and duodenum. Mich Med Bull 1957; 23:178–180.
2. British Society of Gastroenterology. Guideline for the informed consent for endoscopic procedures. London: British Society of Gastroenterology; 1999.
3. British Society of Gastroenterology. Antibiotic prophylaxis in gastrointestinal endoscopy. London: British Society of Gastroenterology; 2001.
4. Guideline for antibiotic prophylaxis for GI endoscopy. Gastrointest Endosc 2003; 58:475–482.
5. Guideline for conscious sedation and monitoring during gastrointestinal endoscopy. Gastrointest Endosc 2003; 58:317–322.
6. British Society of Gastroenterology. Safety and sedation during endoscopic procedures. London: British Society of Gastroenterology; 2003.
7. American Society for Gastrointestinal Endoscopy. Tissue sampling and analysis. Gastrointest Endosc 2003; 57:811–816.
8. Levine DS, Reid BJ. Endoscopic biopsy technique for acquiring larger mucosal samples. Gastrointest Endosc 1991; 37:332–337.
9. European Society for Gastrointestinal Endoscopy. Recommendations for quality control in gastrointestinal endoscopy: guidelines for image documentation in upper and lower GI endoscopy. Endoscopy 2001; 33:901–903.
10. American Society for Gastrointestinal Endoscopy. Computerised endoscopic medical record system. Gastrointest Endosc 2000; 51:793–796.
11. Iddan G, Meron G, Glukhovsky A, Swain P. Wireless capsule endoscopy. Nature 2000; 405:725–729.
12. American Society for Gastrointestinal Endoscopy. Appropriate use of GI endoscopy. Manchester, MA: American Society for Gastrointestinal Endoscopy;1992.
13. Frohlich F, Repond C, Mullhaupt B et al. Is the diagnostic yield of upper GI endoscopy improved by the use of explicit panel based appropriateness criteria? Gastrointest Endosc 2000; 52:333–341.
14. Guideline on the management of anticoagulation and antiplatelet therapy for endoscopic procedures. Gastrointest Endosc 1998; 48:672–675.
15. American Society for Gastrointestinal Endoscopy. Transmission of infection by gastrointestinal endoscopy. Gastrointest Endosc 2001; 54:824–828.
16. Guidelines for decontamination of equipment for gastrointestinal endoscopy. London: British Society of Gastroenterology Endoscopy Committee; 2003.
17. Canto MI, Setrakian S, Willis J, et al. Methylene blue-directed biopsies improve detection of intestinal metaplasia and dysplasia in Barrett's oesophagus. Gastrointest Endosc 2000;51:560–568.
18. Guelrud M, Herrera I, Essenfeld H, Castro J. Enhanced magnification endoscopy: a new technique to identify specialized intestinal metaplasia in Barrett's esophagus. Gastrointest Endosc 2001;53:559–565.
19. Sharma P, Weston AP, Topalovski M, et al. Magnification chromendoscopy for the detection of intestinal metaplasia and dysplasia in Barrett's oesophagus. Gut 2003;52:24-27.
20. Olliver JR, Wild CP, Sahay P, et al. Chromoendoscopy with methylene blue and associated DNA damage in Barrett's oesophagus. Lancet 2003;362:373–374.
21. Kapadia C, Cutruzzola FW, O'Brien KM, et al. Laser-induced fluorescence spectroscopy of human colonic mucosa. Gastroenterology 1990;99:150–157.
22. Cothren RM, Richards-Kortum R, Sivak MV, et al. Gastrointestinal tissue diagnosis by laser-induced fluorescence spectroscopy at endoscopy. Gastrointest Endosc 1996;36:105–111.
23. Panjehpour M, Overholt BF, Vo-Dinh T, et al. Endoscopic fluorescence detection of high-grade dysplasia in Barrett's oesophagus. Gastroenterology 1996;111:93–101.
24. Wallace MB, Perelman LT, Backman V, et al. Endoscopic detection of dysplasia in Barrett's oesophagus using light-scattering spectroscopy. Gastroenterology 2000;119:677–682.
25. Kobayashi K, Izatt JA, Kulkarni MD, et al. High resolution cross-sectional imaging of the gastrointestinal tract using optical coherence tomography. Gastrointest Endosc 1998;47:515–523.
26. Li XD, Boppart SA, Van Dam J, et al. Optical coherence tomography: advanced techniques for endoscopic imaging of Barrett's oesophagus. Endoscopy 2000;32:921–930.
27. Shim MG, Wilson BC, Marple E, et al. Raman spectroscopic system for diagnostic applications. J Raman Spectrosc. 1997;28:131–142.
28. DaCosta RS, Wilson BC, Marcon NE. Optical techniques for the endoscopic detection of dysplastic colonic lesions. Curr Opin Gastroenterol 2005;21(1):70–79.
29. Inoue H, Igari T, Nishikage T, et al. A novel method of virtual histopathology using laser-scanning confocal microscopy in vitro with untreated fresh specimens from the gastrointestinal mucosa. Endoscopy 2000;32:439–443.
30. Tsuji S, Kawano S, Hayashi S, et al. Analysis of mucosal blood hemoglobin distribution in gastric ulcers by computerised color display on electronic endoscopy. Endoscopy 1991;23:321–324.
31. Yao K, Yao T, Matsui T, et al. Hemoglobin content in intramucosal gastric carcinoma as a marker of histologic differentiation: a clinical application of quantitative electronic endoscopy. Gastrointest Endosc 2000;52(2):241–245.

Further reading:

For a concise overview with insight into the complex technical issues, see Van Dam J. Novel methods of enhanced endoscopic imaging. Gut 2003; 52 (Suppl IV):iv12-16.

Chapter 120

Lower GI endoscopy and biopsy

Jerome D Waye

KEY POINTS FOR COLONOSCOPY

- Considered the 'gold standard.'
- Sedation is usually given for the examination for colonic visualization.
- The colon must be well prepared.
- There is a high probability (over 95%) for a complete examination.
- Intubation is accomplished by:
  Rotation of the instrument shaft
  Adding or removing air
  Turning knobs for tip deflection
  Push/pull of shaft.
- Biopsies can be performed at any site.

INTRODUCTION

Video-colonoscopy is currently the best modality for evaluation of the large bowel. The 11–13-mm diameter instrument can be passed through the entire length of the large bowel in a reasonable period of time (less than 30 min) in more than 95% of patients having screening examinations.[1,2] Every surface of the colonic mucosa can be inspected and biopsies may be taken from any portion of the large bowel, or from the distal portion of the terminal ileum. Therapeutic maneuvers are performed utilizing an auxiliary (accessory or instrument) channel. The field of view varies with different instrument manufacturers from 120° to 140°.

DESCRIPTION OF TECHNIQUE

Preparation of the colon

Complete visualization of the colonic mucosa requires a colon devoid of solid fecal material. This can be accomplished with a liquid diet for 24 h and a potent cathartic, usually a 4-L balanced electrolyte solution or a phospho soda purgative.[3] Enemas are not frequently used because of the efficiency of these cathartics. The balanced electrolyte solution is so constituted that there is no net flux of water or electrolytes across the mucous membranes, making this an ideal preparation for patients who have fluid retention syndromes such as congestive heart failure, ascites, or renal disease. The solution is salty and oily, and the large volume required is difficult for some patients to ingest. The sodium phosphate cathartic requires two small doses (45 mL each) along with a 1-day liquid diet. Besides its unpleasant taste, the high sodium and phosphate load may be detrimental to persons with certain conditions, especially renal disease. Tablets of dehydrated sodium phosphate are available.

Equipment

Besides the flexible video-colonoscope (11–13 mm in diameter), a light source and image processor are necessary. Two colonoscope lengths are available; the 168-cm instrument is preferred by physicians in the United States, whereas in Europe the most commonly used instrument is 133 cm in length. The video-colonoscope has a lens system (and miniature camera) at the tip that transmits information to the processor to reconstitute the image on a video monitor. An older and less expensive system is available with the image transmitted via optical glass fibers (fiberoptic) to an eyepiece on the instrument head. Because fluid in the colon from the preparation may not be evacuated completely, a suction apparatus is necessary to permit aspiration of liquid contents through the accessory/instrument channel. Along with the basic instrument (including light source and image processor), biopsy forceps, snares to remove polyps, and an electrosurgical unit should be available whenever colonoscopy is performed.

Procedure

Most colonoscopic examinations are performed with the patient in the left lateral position using a one-person technique, although it is possible to perform the procedure with a two-person team. The performance of colonoscopy requires a combination of several maneuvers using a limited number of available options. The options that can be used during colonoscopy are: inflate with air, deflate with suction, torque (twist) the instrument to the right or to the left, use angulation control knobs to manipulate the tip up/down or right/left, push the instrument in or withdraw it, change the patient's position, or use abdominal pressure. These are the only maneuvers that can be used. The difference between a swift and a slow procedure depends upon the skill and rapidity with which the operator uses combinations of the various options.

Insertion: After sedation, the instrument is inserted into the rectum following a digital rectal examination. The operator's left hand controls the up/down angulation knob to provide adjustments of the instrument tip and also uses buttons that provide suction or air insufflation. The right hand is used to torque (twist) the instrument to provide directional changes while insertion or withdrawal of the shaft is performed simultaneously. Movement of the right/left angulation knob can be performed with either hand. Because of the spiral S-shape configuration of the sigmoid mesocolon, the instrument always tends to loop as it is being advanced through the sigmoid and into the descending colon. Frequent attempts must be made at straightening the instrument by withdrawal, usually in a clockwise fashion, to remove the obligatory loop caused by the mesenteric attachments. The colon can be pleated on to the instrument shaft by jiggling the scope with rapid in-and-out motions during intubation, usually with clockwise torque. The colonoscope is advanced under direct vision, never blindly, and is pushed in only after the direction of the lumen has been identified visually. There is a greater than 95% possibility of reaching the cecum by a trained endoscopist, but persons who have not been taught the specific techniques have a much lower probability of cecal intubation. The ileocecal valve can often be intubated during colonoscopy using various techniques of torque and tip deflection simultaneously after reaching the cecal caput. More detailed descriptions of technique are available.[4]

Landmarks: There are several intraluminal landmarks by which the position of the instrument can be estimated, but these are relatively gross approximations, with the rectum and cecum being the only absolute positional markers. The length of instrument inserted into the rectum is a poor method of tip location, as the entire instrument may be coiled in a long sigmoid colon, but after straightening maneuvers the cecum may be intubated using only 60 cm of the shaft. Each colonic segment has its own identifying anatomic characteristics. A network of thin interlacing vessels can be observed throughout the entire colon (Fig. 120.1), but is most pronounced in the capacious rectum (Fig. 120.2). The sigmoid colon is noted for its tortuosity with thick folds and a relatively narrow lumen. With the patient lying in the left lateral position, the spleni flexure contains a large amount of fluid and is reached at abou 50–70 cm during intubation, and 40–50 cm during withdrawa from the cecum when the instrument is straightened and al loops removed. The air-distended transverse colon is triangula in configuration (Fig. 120.3) because of the three tenia coli a each angle of the equilateral triangle. The hepatic flexure ha a sharply defined blue hue (Fig. 120.4) and the ileocecal valv is seen as a thickened fold having a notch with a yellowis color owing to fat. The cecal pole contains the convergence o the tenia coli and the appendix usually has a slit-like appearance (Fig. 120.5). The ileum can often be intubated and vil visualized (Fig. 120.6). Modern endoscopists use fluoroscop only rarely during the course of colonoscopy. A positionin device is available that relies on electromagnets within a speciall built colonoscope to create a computer-generated image of th instrument shaft on a dedicated monitor. This 'scope guide provides an extremely accurate picture of the location an configuration of the shaft and can be utilized as an aid durin difficult colonoscopy, as well as for teaching purposes.[4]

Marking lesions: The endoscopist is often unable to localiz a specific lesion precisely in the colon because the intralumina landmarks are relatively soft markers. This lack of localizatio and the increasing popularity of laparoscopic colonic operations (along with the inability to palpate the bowel durin

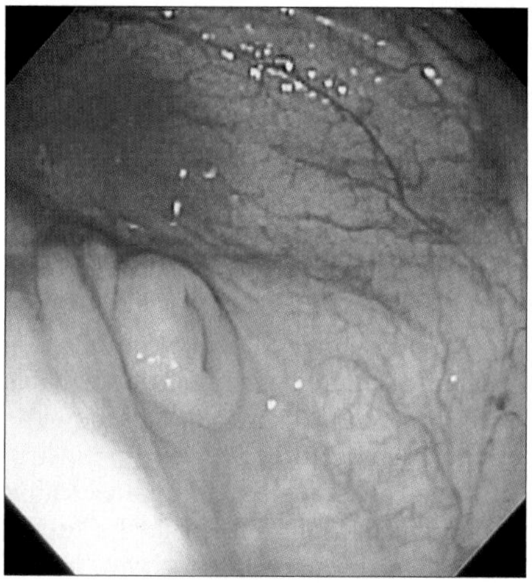

Fig. 120.1 Interlacing blood vessels seen in the area of the cecum adjacent to a partially inverted appendix.

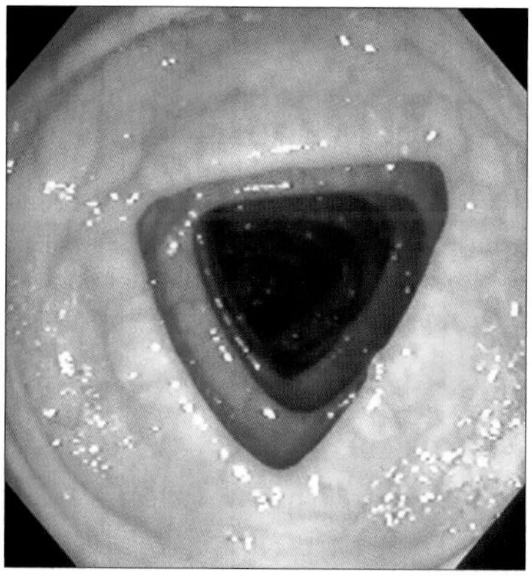

Fig. 120.3 The transverse colon is triangular in appearance.

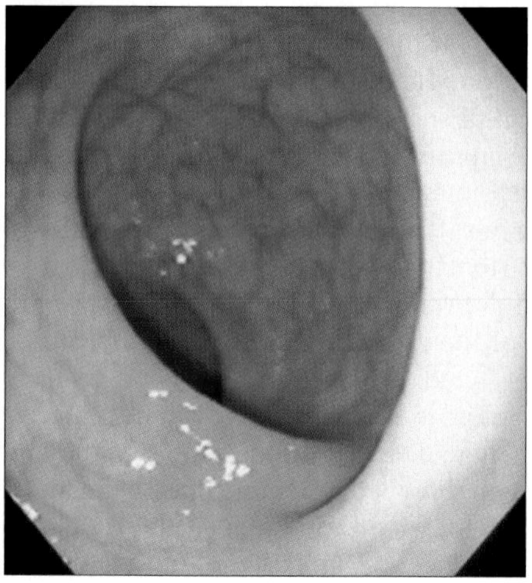

Fig. 120.2 The three valves of Houston can be identified in the air-distended rectum.

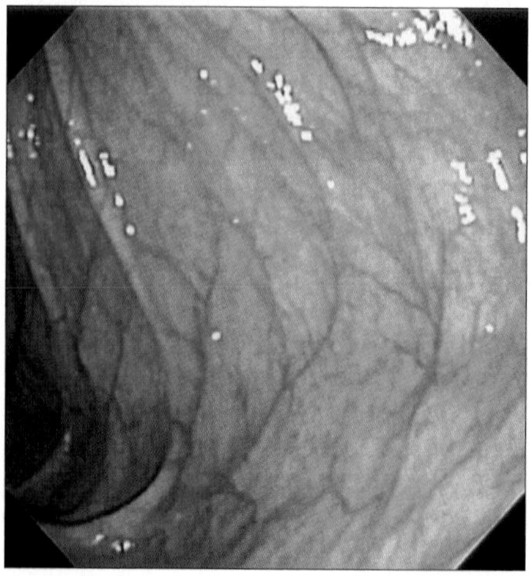

Fig. 120.4 The liver is seen through the colonic wall as a blue hue.

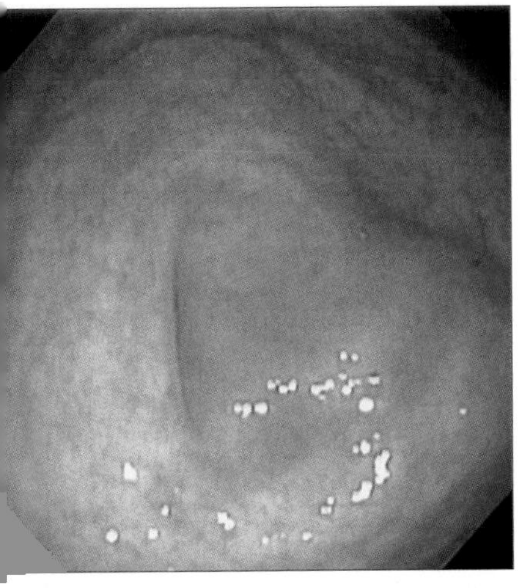

Fig. 120.5 The appendiceal orifice usually has a slit-like configuration but may change in appearance (see Fig. 120.1).

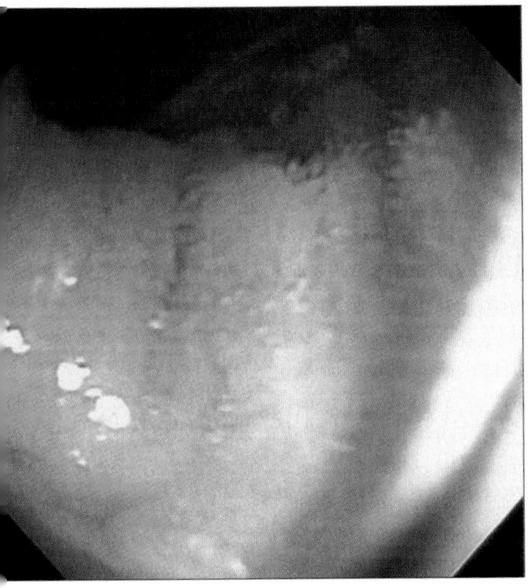

Fig. 120.6 The tiny villi of the normal ileum can often be identified through the colonoscope.

urgery) results in the need for the endoscopist to place a ›ermanent marker in the colon wall at the site of a tumor that nay require subsequent surgery. A permanent marker can ılso be useful when an area requires subsequent colonoscopic dentification, such as for follow-up of a polypectomy. This can ›e accomplished by injecting a solution of carbon particles nto the submucosa at the desired location, resulting in a life-ong black stain that may be visualized readily from both the nucosal and serosal aspects of the bowel. For purely mucosal agging for subsequent follow-up evaluation of a resected lesion, or example, one can focus on producing a more superficial ›leb. Mucosal marking can be accomplished with dilute solu-ions of sterilized drawing ink, but is now available in commer-ial form as a sterile and premeasured aliquot of pure carbon n suspension.[5]

Withdrawal: Once the cecum has been intubated, withdrawal s the most important phase of the examination,[6] as the straightened instrument provides the ability easily to torque he instrument right or left; in concert with manipulation of he up/down angulation control wheel, this makes it possible o visualize the entire mucosal surface of the large bowel. A U-turn maneuver can frequently be accomplished in the capa-cious right colon (Fig. 120.7), often in the transverse colon, but arely in the narrow left colon. Retroversion allows inspection of the proximal surface of folds that may not be seen on direct forward view. A retroflexion maneuver in the rectum should always be performed to visualize completely the distal most portions of the rectal ampulla. The dentate line can be seen during the 'U-turn' maneuver in the rectum (Fig. 120.8).

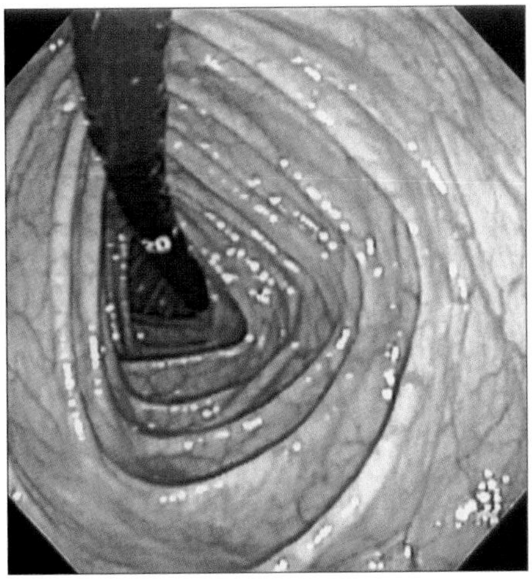

Fig. 120.7 A retroversion in the ascending colon can frequently be performed in the ascending or transverse colon. This provides a view behind interhaustral folds during the examination.

Colonoscopic biopsy

Single or multiple biopsies can be obtained at any site in the large bowel. Biopsies are obtained by passing a long flexible forceps with pincer-type jaws through the accessory channel. The open jaws are gently pushed against the colonic mucosa and closed. Upon withdrawal of the forceps, the mucosa is pulled up to the faceplate of the instrument and, as the forceps is further withdrawn into the accessory/instrument channel, the portion within the jaws of the forceps is actually torn off (avulsed) from the mucosal surface. Significant bleeding does not occur from biopsy sites.

Handling tissue specimens

The best way to remove biopsies from the forceps is to use a blunt dental probe, a toothpick, or dissecting needle, and to scoop it out from the bottom of the opened forceps cups and place the specimen on a support material (lens paper, gel foam, mesh). Routine orientation of biopsies in the endoscopy unit is difficult to maintain at a high level, and is not necessary. A common practice is to shake the opened biopsy forceps in the formalin fixative solution until it floats out, but this has the potential of traumatic detachment of the surface epithelium.

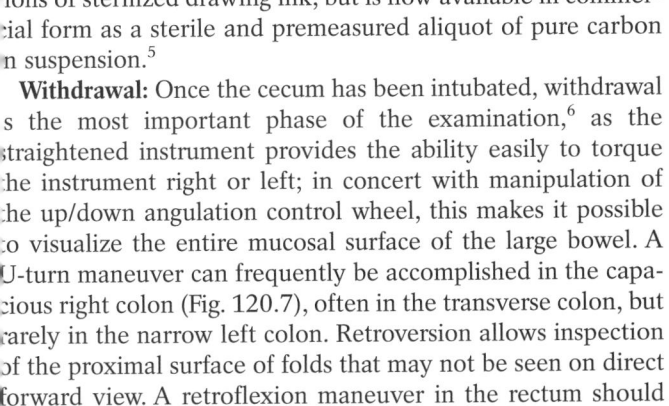

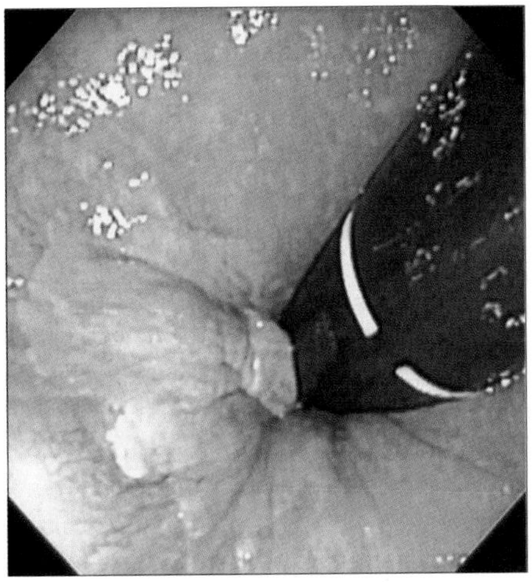

Fig. 120.8 The dentate line is the border between the transitional mucosa of the anal canal and the columnar mucosa of the rectum. The endoscope shaft can be identified as it enters the rectum (retroversion view).

A focused and intelligent differential diagnosis can be obtained by providing the pathologist with some information about the patient's history and requesting specific answers from the pathologist.[7] The key information required by the pathologist is the 'gross pathology' (i.e., what was seen, labeling biopsy sites as normal or abnormal, and brief historic information). For example, in patients with chronic diarrhea (assuming infection is ruled out) and a normal endoscopic appearance, both bits of information should be transmitted: reason for the examination (diarrhea) and the finding of normality. Here, the request for the pathologist is to 'exclude microscopic (collagenous, lymphocytic) colitis or other causes of diarrhea.' Other findings in diarrhea with a normal endoscopy include amyloidosis and melanosis coli where the pigment is not dense enough to be seen endoscopically.

ALTERNATIVES TO COLONOSCOPY

The alternatives to colonoscopic examination of the large intestine are the barium enema and 'virtual colonography.' Before the colonoscope was introduced, the only method of evaluation of the large bowel was through a rigid sigmoidoscope that inspected the lowermost 16–25 cm of mucosa, with barium enema. The air contrast barium enema examination often misses small polyps and bleeding sites throughout the colon (see Chapter 125). Protruding mass lesions are usually discovered with the barium enema, but flat lesions may be undetected.[8]

Virtual colography (VC) is a more recently introduced examination, wherein software programs align the images from helical computed tomography or magnetic resonance imaging in a sequential fashion, creating visual images of a simulated tubular passageway that depict a reconstituted 'virtual' tour of the colon (see Chapter 129).[2,9] The VC procedure is preferred over colonoscopy by most patients. In comparison with colonoscopy, the sensitivity of VC for adenomas larger than 1 cm (in a screening population) ranges from 32% to 73%, and may be higher.[2] Populations with a high prevalence for pathology, including patients with gastrointestinal bleeding and positive screening tests, are best and most cost-effectively evaluated by conventional colonoscopy. Bleeding sites cannot be seen, nor can color changes be evaluated on VC. Flat lesions are often missed with VC, and if any lesion is seen colonoscopy with biopsy or polypectomy is subsequently necessary.[10]

INDICATIONS/CONTRAINDICATIONS

The two major categories of indications for colonoscopic examination of the colon are diagnostic and therapeutic.[11]

Diagnostic

- Screening for colorectal neoplasia – this is the most common indication for colonoscopy.
- Symptom evaluation:
  Bleeding, occult or gross, minimal or severe
  Change in bowel habit such as new-onset constipation or unexplained chronic diarrhea.
- Preoperative or postoperative evaluation of patients with colonic cancer.
- Abnormal barium enema examination.
- Surveillance for neoplasia in high-risk patients:
  Ulcerative colitis or Crohn's disease of longstanding duration that affects a significant portion of the colon
  Family history of polyps or cancer
  Polyposis syndromes such as familial adenomatous polyposis or hereditary nonpolyposis colonic cancer
  Persons over 50 years of age.

Therapeutic

- Polypectomy – the most frequent therapeutic intervention during colonoscopy
- Hemostasis for bleeding lesions
- Stricture dilation
- Removal of foreign bodies
- Decompression (Ogilvie's syndrome or volvulus).

Absolute contraindications

- Peritonitis with or without bowel perforation
- Acute diverticulitis
- Recent myocardial infarction or pulmonary embolus
- Fulminant colitis.

Relative contraindications

- Torrential colonic bleeding
- Cardiopulmonary instability
- Poor bowel preparation
- Uncooperative patient

INDICATIONS/CONTRAINDICATIONS

DIAGNOSTIC
- Screening for colonic cancer
- Symptom evaluation
- Abnormal radiographic findings
- Surveillance of high-risk population

THERAPEUTIC
- Polyp removal
- Hemostasis
- Stricture dilation
- Foreign body removal

CONTRAINDICATIONS
- Peritonitis
- Acute diverticulitis or colitis
- Recent myocardial infarction or pulmonary embolism

COMPLICATIONS AND THEIR MANAGEMENT

The most common complications during colonoscopic examinations involve the cardiopulmonary systems as a result of medication given for the examination. Hypotension and bradycardia may be caused by loop formation and stretch of the mesenteric attachments that provoke a vagus nerve-mediated response. More serious complications such as perforation occur in fewer than 2 per 1000 diagnostic examinations. The incidence of perforation is approximately doubled during therapeutic applications of colonoscopy.[12]

Perforations during diagnostic colonoscopy are caused primarily by loop formation, stretching of the mesentery resulting in a linear 'split' of the colon, most often in the sigmoid region rforations are infrequently caused by pneumatic pressure, or actually pushing the tip of the endoscope through the bowel all during intubation attempts. Almost all traumatic perforations occurring during the course of diagnostic colonoscopic examinations will require surgery for repair. Laparoscopic surgery has been reported to be successful in the closure of ese perforations, most of which occur in the sigmoid colon cause of looping in that segment.

COSTS, COMPLICATIONS, CONTROVERSIES

- Approximate instrument cost $55 000
- Complications:
  Cardiovascular disturbances
  Perforation
  Hemorrhage
- Cost-effectiveness of screening colonoscopy:
  Similar to annual mammography screening
  Better than cervical pap smear every 3 years
  Screening saves lives

Bleeding is an uncommon complication of diagnostic olonoscopy and rarely presents a clinical problem. Bleeding is ore common following removal of polyps. Post-polypectomy leeding may require a repeat colonoscopic examination (usually the unprepped patient) during which the bleeding site may e injected with diluted epinephrine solution to cause vasoonstriction, with or without cautery with a thermal device or lip application.[13]

Missed lesions: Even though colonoscopy is the best way of valuating the mucosal surfaces of the colon, it is possible to verlook lesions during the examination. This may be due to inadequate preparation, inability to reach the cecal pole, hasty withdrawal of the instrument, or lesions hidden behind folds of the colon. Reports of tandem colonoscopies have demonstrated that 24% of lesions may be missed during routine colonoscopic examinations, but most of these are relatively small lesions, in the size range of 1–4 mm in diameter. It is unusual to overlook any lesion of 1 cm or more in diameter.[14]

COSTS AND BENEFITS

The cost for a video-colonoscope instrument is approximately $25 000, a light source $10 000, and an image processor $20 000. All instruments must be disinfected after use,[18] and this can be accomplished with a relatively low-cost handwashing and soak disinfection, or with more expensive automated machinery.

All tests that screen for colorectal cancer in adults at average risk have been shown to be more effective in reducing colorectal cancer incidence and mortality rates as compared with no screening. The US Preventive Services Task Force[15] determined that no single strategy could be recommended at the time of the systematic review. Cost-effective analyses for various procedures for the prevention of colorectal cancer have shown, with modeling, that a single colonoscopy at the age of 65 years is the most cost-effective means of cancer prevention in the general population.[16] Other analyses have stated that the cost-effectiveness ratio is similar to that of breast cancer screening with annual mammography, and is more cost effective than cervical cancer screening with pap smears administered every 3 years.[17]

SOURCES OF INFORMATION FOR PATIENTS AND DOCTORS

http://www.gastro.org/generalPublic.html

REFERENCES

1. Lieberman DA, Weiss DG, Bond JH, Ahnen DJ, Garewal H, Chejfec G. Use of colonoscopy to screen asymptomatic adults for colorectal cancer. N Engl J Med 2000; 343:162–168.
2. Pickhardt PJ, Choi JR, Hwang I et al. Computerized tomographic virtual colonoscopy to screen for colorectal neoplasia in asymptomatic adults. N Engl J Med 2003; 349:2191–2200.
3. Toledo TK, DiPalma JA. Colon cleansing preparation for gastrointestinal procedures. Aliment Pharmacol Ther 2001; 15:605–611.
4. Williams CB. Insertion technique. In: Waye JD, Rex DK, Williams CB, eds. Colonoscopy: principles and practice. London: Blackwell Publishing; 2003:318–338.
5. Askin MP, Waye JD, Fiedler L, Harpaz N. Tattoo of colonic neoplasms in 113 patients with a new sterile carbon compound. Gastrointest Endosc 2002; 56:339–342.
6. Rex DK. Colonoscopic withdrawal technique is associated with adenoma miss rates. Gastrointest Endosc 2000; 51:33–36.
7. Weinstein WM. Mucosal biopsy techniques and interaction with the pathologist. Gastrointest Endosc Clin N Am 2000; 10:555–572.
8. Winawer SJ, Stewart ET, Zauber AG et al. A comparison of colonoscopy and double-contrast barium enema for surveillance after polypectomy. N Engl J Med 2000; 342:1766–1772.
9. Johnson CD, Toledano AY, Herman BA et al. Computerized tomographic colonography: performance evaluation in a retrospective multicenter setting. Gastroenterology 2003; 125:688–695.
10. Rex DK. Is virtual colonoscopy ready for widespread application? Gastroenterology 2003; 125:608–614.
11. Habr-Gama A, Alves PRA, Rex DK. Indications and contraindications. In: Waye JD, Rex DK, Williams CB, eds. Colonoscopy: principles and practice. London: Blackwell Publishing; 2003:102–110.
12. Korman LY, Overholt BF, Box T, Winker CK. Perforation during colonoscopy in endoscopic ambulatory centers. Gastrointest Endosc 2003; 58:554–557.
13. Rex DK, Lewis BS, Waye JD. Colonoscopy and endoscopic therapy for delayed post-polypectomy hemorrhage. Gastrointest Endosc 1992; 38:127–129.
14. Rex DK. Colonoscopic withdrawal technique is associated with adenoma miss rates. Gastrointest Endosc 2000; 51:33–36.
15. Pignone M, Saha S, Hoerger T, Mandelblatt J. Cost-effectiveness analyses of colorectal cancer screening: a systematic review for the US Preventive Services Task Force. Ann Intern Med 2002; 137:96–104.
16. Sonnenberg A. Cost-effectiveness in the prevention of colorectal cancer. Gastroenterol Clin North Am 2002; 31:1069–1091.
17. Provenzale D. Cost-effectiveness of screening the average-risk population for colorectal cancer. Gastrointest Endosc Clin N Am 2002; 12:93–109.
18. Greenwald DA. Cleaning and disinfection. In: Waye JD, Rex DK, Williams CB, eds. Colonoscopy: principles and practice. London: Blackwell Publishing; 2003: 309–317.

Chapter 121

Endoscopic ultrasonography

Jason B Klapman and Kenneth J Chang

KEY POINTS

- Endoscopic ultrasonography uses a combination of endoscopy and high-frequency ultrasound
- Endoscopic ultrasonography is performed with radial and linear echoendoscopes or catheter-based ultrasound probes
- Radial echoendoscopes give up to a 360° ultrasonographic image perpendicular to the axis of the echoendoscope
- Linear echoendoscopes give up to a 180° image parallel to the axis of the echoendoscope, and are capable of performing Doppler imaging, color-flow mapping, and fine-needle aspiration or injection
- Catheter-based ultrasonographic probes are useful for imaging small mucosal or submucosal lesions and can be passed through the accessory channel of a standard endoscope
- Ultrasonographic imaging is facilitated by water filling a balloon around the acoustic tip of echoendoscope, a process called acoustic coupling
- Imaging a lesion requires very fine scope tip movements and repeated back and forth scanning
- Successful performance of endoscopic ultrasonography requires a dedicated team of physicians, nurses, and technical assistants

INTRODUCTION AND SCIENTIFIC BASIS

Endoscopic ultrasonography (EUS) was originally developed in the early 1980s as an alternative diagnostic imaging modality to address the inherent limitations of transcutaneous ultrasonography, such as limited depth of penetration and image interference from intra-abdominal gas and bony structures.[1] With the development of linear-array echoendoscopes and the incorporation of fine-needle aspiration (FNA) and color flow and Doppler data, the field has moved from a diagnostic to an interventional procedure. The principles of EUS are based on the development and interpretation of ultrasound waves. High-frequency ultrasound waves are transmitted from the transducer at the tip of the echoendoscope to the target tissue. For optimal imaging, a balloon surrounding the transducer is inflated with water to improve ultrasound transmission. This process is known as acoustic coupling. Images are constructed from the reflective properties of the tissue components and utilize real-time imaging techniques similar to a B-mode (brightness modulation) display format. The brightness is dependent on the amount reflected. Intensely reflected areas appear white (hyperechoic), whereas areas of low reflection appear dark (hypoechoic). This allows for high-resolution imaging of the five histologic layers of the gastrointestinal wall and the surrounding structures. EUS and EUS-guided FNA are highly accurate procedures in the diagnosis and treatment of many gastrointestinal diseases.

DESCRIPTION OF TECHNIQUE

Equipment and setup

Ultrasonographic endoscopes have become smaller and lighter, and have been coupled with better image resolution. Currently available equipment is listed in Table 121.1.

Radial echoendoscopes

This scope is oblique viewing, similar to a duodenoscope. Radial instruments utilize either a mechanical or an electronic rotating transducer that allows a 360° (270° for electronic) ultrasonographic image that is perpendicular to the axis plane of the echoendoscope (Fig. 121.1). In the esophagus, this gives a spatial orientation of the image similar to that obtained with computed tomography (CT). Current radial echoendoscopes have the ability to switch frequencies from 5 MHz up to 20 MHz to optimize imaging. The depth of penetration and image resolution are inversely proportional and dependent on the frequency of ultrasound wave transmission. High-frequency ultrasound (20 MHz) has a tissue penetration of only 2 cm and is useful for mucosal and submucosal imaging, as opposed to lower frequency (5–7.5 MHz) transmission that has a tissue penetration depth of 8 cm and is useful for imaging extraluminal surrounding structures. The main limitation of the radial echoendoscope is its inability to perform safely FNA because the needle path cannot be tracked accurately.

Linear echoendoscopes

Linear-array echoendoscopes permit the performance of FNA. The ultrasound transducer generates a 100–180° image that is parallel to the shaft of the echoendoscope. The anatomic orientation is at an angle of 90° to the radial anatomy. Linear echoendoscopes have a frequency range of 5–10 MHz. The needle for FNA can be tracked in its entirety from exiting the biopsy channel to entering and aspirating the target lesion (Fig. 121.2). Linear echoendoscopes provide the ability for color flow and Doppler imaging to choose a FNA needle path that avoids vascular structures. The linear-array echoendoscopes allow for simultaneous real-time ultrasonography and Doppler ability.

Probes

Catheter-based ultrasonography probes are used for high-frequency ultrasonographic imaging of lesions that are within 2 cm of the transducer. The probes (12–30 MHz) are easily

TABLE 121.1 CURRENTLY AVAILABLE EUS ECHOENDOSCOPES

Echoendoscope	Scanning frequency (MHz)	Channel diameter (mm)	Scanning range (degrees)	Processor
OLYMPUS				
Radial				
GF-UM160	5–20	2.2	360	EU-M60
GF-UM130	7.5, 12	2.2	360	EU-M60, EU-M30
GF-UMQ130	7.5, 20	2.2	360	EU-M60, EU-M30
Linear				
GF-UC140P	5–10	2.8	180	SSD-5000 Aloka
GF-UCT140	5–10	3.7	180	SSD-5000 Aloka
GF-UC160P	5–10	2.8	150	EU-C60
GF-UCT160	5–10	3.7	150	EU-C60
PENTAX				
Radial				
FG-3630UR	5–10	2.4	270	Hitachi 6000, 6500
Linear				
EG-3630U	5–10	2.4	100	Hitachi 6000, 6500
EG-3830UT	5–10	3.8	120	Hitachi 6000, 6500
FG-36UX	5–10	2.4	100	Hitachi 6000, 6500
FG-38UX (no elevator)	5–10	3.2	100	Hitachi 6000, 6500

passed through the biopsy channel of a standard upper endoscope and give a 360° image in a plane similar to that of radial echoendoscopes. Imaging with the probe is accomplished either by filling the lumen of the target lesion with water or, in areas such as the esophagus, by imaging through a water-filled latex condom attached to the endoscope. Another option in this setting is to use a catheter probe prefitted with a balloon sheath that can be insufflated with water. Other types of probe available include rigid rectal probes to evaluate internal and extern sphincter defects or guidewire probes to evaluate obstructi lesions. Newer-generation probes also have the capability two- and three-dimensional reconstruction of images.

Room setup and nursing personnel

Depending on the volume of the procedure unit, a dedicate room may or may not be necessary. Having two monitors si

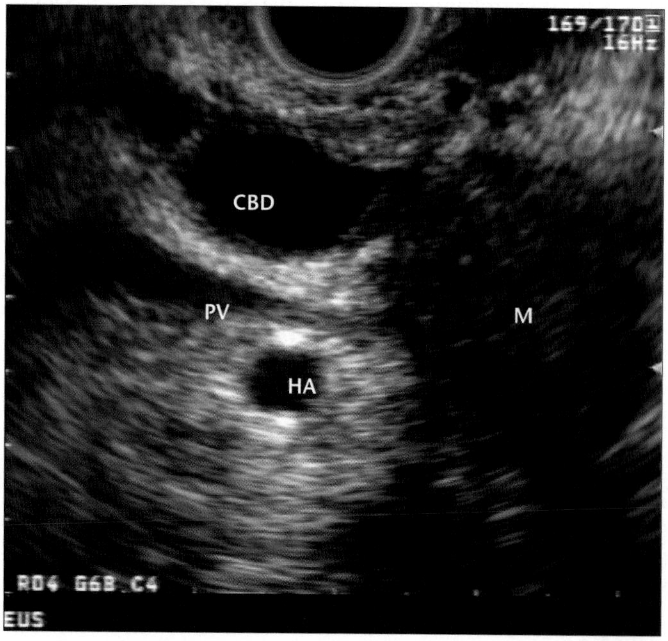

Fig. 121.1 EUS of pancreatic cancer. Linear image of a T3 pancreatic cancer (M) with invasion of common bile duct (CBD) and portal vein (PV). HA, hepatic artery.

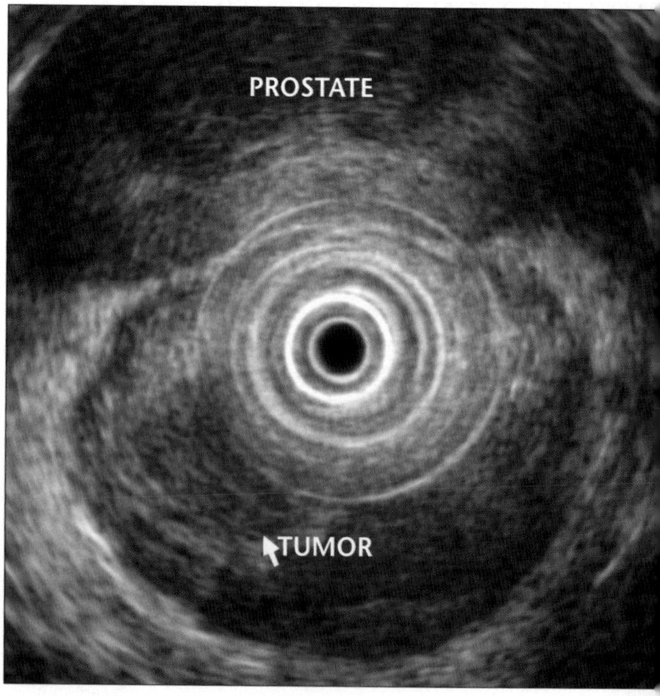

Fig. 121.2 EUS of rectal cancer. Radial image of a T3 rectal cancer without invasion of the prostate.

side to display the endoscopic and ultrasonographic images nultaneously is ideal. In general, the processor console should within comfortable finger distance of the endosonographer allow for optimized picture capturing, labeling, resolution, d Doppler usage.

EUS is performed under conscious sedation. Nurses with ecial skills in assisting with the EUS procedures are required. 'hen the procedure involves FNA, a second nurse or techcal assistant who is knowledgable about the procedure and ocessing of the tissue samples is required.

echnique

e endosonographer must be able to recognize the key anatomic ndmarks. The first important step is to secure a balloon ound the transducer at the tip of the endoscope. The balloon inflated and deflated with water to check for leaks and to iminate air bubbles to maximize acoustic coupling. Intubaon with the oblique-viewing instrument is necessarily perrmed semi-blind. In the esophagus the balloon is reinflated ith water. Constant intermittent suctioning and removal of traluminal air is necessary because air is relatively impeneable to ultrasound waves and causes imaging artifacts. When e lesion of focus is found, the echoendoscope is passed back d forth over the lesion; changing ultrasound frequencies elps to achieve maximal resolution.

For superficial lesions it is important not to compress the sion with the ultrasound balloon as this may cause incorrect naging or staging. The easiest structures to image initially e the esophagus and rectum because of the minimal scope anipulation required to maintain orientation. The major strucres seen corresponding to the scope position are reviewed in able 121.2.

erforming FNA

NA, guided by EUS, has brought the technique to the foreont in the diagnosis and staging of gastrointestinal maligancies. FNA is especially challenging for pancreatic masses. laximization of FNA yield is dependent on prioritizing the equence of FNA with multiple lesions, optimizing needle echnique, onsite cytopathologic interpretation, and avoidance f complications.

The technique of EUS-guided FNA has been described preiously.[2] The most commonly used needle size is 22-gauge. 19-gauge needle may be more appropriate sometimes, for xample for smooth muscle tumors. The lesion to be biopsied placed in the center or just left of center of the imaging field. there is a question about surrounding vascular structures,)oppler imaging can be used to define surrounding vascular ructures; this may necessitate finding a different needleack. The needle advanced through the biopsy channel is seen xiting the biopsy channel into the lesion under real-time ltrasonography. Once in position, the central stylet is removed nd a 10-mL syringe is attached to the hub of the needle and uction is applied as to and fro movements are made within e lesion. Suction is then released and the needle withdrawn. 'he cytologic specimen is then processed and sprayed on glass lides, and can be immediately reviewed by a cytopathology echnician or cytopathologist if available, or placed in formalin, vhich is then processed into a cell block for review. Ideally, naximal procedural yield is obtained with the presence of nsite cytopathology to determine specimen adequacy and to obtain a preliminary diagnosis.[3] If the first few passes reveal necrotic tissue, aiming for the periphery of the lesion may be necessary to obtain a diagnosis.

TABLE 121.2 SCOPE POSITION AND CORRESPONDING MAJOR STRUCTURES

Location	Structures
Proximal esophagus	Spine, trachea, carotid artery, thyroid, aortic arch, subclavian artery
Mid-esophagus	Trachea, carina, main bronchi, spine, SVC, descending aorta, azygous, thoracic duct, PV
Distal esophagus	Left atrium, left ventricle, right atrium, left atrium, liver, IVC, spine, descending aorta
Gastric fundus	Pancreatic tail, spleen, splenic artery, splenic vein, left kidney, left adrena
Gastric body	Pancreatic body, splenic vein, splenic artery, celiac axis, hepatic artery, SMA
Gastric antrum	Pancreatic neck, gallbladder, liver, splenic vein, confluence
Duodenal bulb	Pancreatic head, splenic vein, portal vein, confluence, CBD, gallbladder, liver, hepatic artery
Second portion of duodenum	Pancreatic head, CBD, IVC, confluence, SMA, ampulla, uncinate
Third portion of duodenum	Pancreatic body, IVC, descending aorta
Anal canal	Internal and external sphincters
Rectum (male)	Prostate, bladder, seminal vesicles, urethra
Rectum (female)	Uterus, vagina, bladder, urethra
Sigmoid colon	Iliac vessels

SVC, superior vena cava; PV, pulmonary vessels; IVC, inferior vena cava; SMA, superior mesenteric artery; CBD, common bile duct.

The optimal technique for advancing the needle is dependent on three factors: (1) the consistency of the gastrointestinal wall (wall parameter); (2) the size and consistency of the lesion targeted (lesion parameter); and (3) the proximity of surrounding vessels (vessel parameter). Needle advancement techniques are individualized according to these parameters for a given region or organ.

When there is more than one lesion to biopsy in a patient, the prioritization of lesions becomes important to avoid specimen contamination and improve procedural efficiency. For example, if when staging a pancreatic cancer ascites or a liver lesion is found, this should be biopsied first because it will give the most advanced stage information. In addition, biopsy of a liver lesion is more efficient because it requires one or two passes,[4] compared with a pancreatic mass which on average requires three to five passes to obtain a diagnosis.[5]

INDICATIONS/CONTRAINDICATIONS

Tumor diagnosis and staging

Table 121.3 gives the current tumor node metastasis (TNM) classification of tumors.

Esophagus

Accurate staging of esophageal cancer is important because of the multimodality treatment approach (see Chapter 32). EUS is the most accurate imaging modality for determining the extent of local and regional spread. The diagnostic accuracy by

TABLE 121.3 THE TNM CLASSIFICATION

PRIMARY TUMOR (T)	
TX	Primary tumor cannot be assessed
T0	No evidence of primary tumor
Tis	Carcinoma in situ
T1, T2, T3, T4	Increasing size and/or local extent of primary tumor
REGIONAL LYMPH NODES (N)	
Nx	Regional lymph nodes cannot be assessed
N0	No regional lymph node metastasis
N1, N2, N3	Increasing involvement of regional lymph nodes
DISTANT METASTASIS (M)	
Mx	Distant metastasis cannot be assessed
M0	No distant metastasis
M1	Distant metastasis

EUS alone is 85% for T and 75% for N stage. The addition of FNA increases the N staging accuracy to greater than 90%.[6] Obstructing esophageal tumors that preclude the passage of an echoendoscope are most likely T3 or T4 lesions; however, if information on tumor length, gastric pathology, or presence or absence of celiac nodes is desired, then endoscopic dilatation can be performed. This is best carried out over two to three sessions to lessen the risk of perforation. Alternatively, passage of an EUS probe over a guidewire may provide similar information. With increased use of neoadjuvant treatment in patients with local or regional advanced esophageal cancer, EUS has been employed to restage patients prior to surgical therapy. One of the limitations of EUS here is in differentiating residual cancer from posttreatment inflammation or fibrosis. FNA may help to make the distinction. It appears that assessing residual tumor volume instead of T and N stages may be more accurate and predictive of response to treatment.

EUS has an increasing role in the evaluation of patients with Barrett's esophagus (see Chapter 31) and high-grade dysplasia with or without superficial esophageal cancer, primarily to detect invasion into the submucosa or beyond.[7] The absence of deeper invasion may offer nonsurgical options such as mucosectomy or ablation for the frail and for those who refuse esophagectomy.

Lung

EUS-FNA is an attractive option for staging compared to transbronchial needle aspiration because of the relative safety and minimal invasiveness. The accuracy of EUS-guided FNA of lymph nodes in the setting of lung cancer is 94–100%.[8] EUS in this setting is limited to imaging the posterior mediastinum and is specifically helpful for accessing lymph nodes in the subcarinal, paraesophageal, and aortopulmonary regions.

Stomach

EUS is highly accurate in staging gastric adenocarcinoma and lymphoma, and in the evaluation of thickened gastric folds (see Chapters 37–39). Using a combination of EUS and catheter-based ultrasonography, the accuracy for T stage is approximately 80% and that for N stage 70%. This approach may define a subgroup of patients with early gastric cancer confined to the mucosa or submucosa that may be treated nonoperatively with removal by endoscopic mucosal resection[9] (see Chapter 145).

Tumors that obstruct or bleed require surgical resection palliation regardless of preoperative staging. In these situatio EUS findings would probably not alter management. In ca without bleeding or obstruction, EUS can significantly imp the patient's clinical course (such as finding ascites or tum extension into the liver or pancreas).

Pancreas

EUS-guided FNA is the most accurate diagnostic modality assessing pancreatic masses. In 185 patients with pancrea masses and negative tissue sampling by endoscopic retrogra cholangiopancreatography (ERCP) or negative CT-guided FN EUS-guided FNA had a sensitivity of 94% and accuracy 92% for detecting malignant disease in patients with negati ERCP tissue sampling, and 90% sensitivity and 84% accura in patients with negative CT-guided biopsy.[10] EUS-guided celi plexus neurolysis can be done for poorly controlled pancrea cancer pain at the same session. It is safer and more effecti than traditional approaches.[11] EUS-assisted cyst aspiration a fluid analysis for cytology and estimation of amylase and c cinoembryonic antigen levels can help differentiate betwee benign pseudocyst and a cystic neoplasm (see Chapter 74).

Rectum

EUS appears to have an important potential role in the stagi of rectal cancer to determine surgical approach and neoadjuva adjuvant therapy. The accuracy of rectal cancer staging approach 80–85% for T stage and 70–80% for N stage.[12]

Bile duct and ampulla

EUS is more accurate than CT and transabdominal ultrasono raphy for local staging of cholangiocarcinoma and ampulla cancers. Intraductal ultrasonography (IDUS) can improve t staging of T1 cholangiocarcinomas and distinguish betwe benign and malignant biliary strictures.[13]

Benign disease

Pancreatitis

One of the more common referral indications for EUS is diagnose chronic pancreatitis (see Chapter 72) in patients wi unexplained chronic upper abdominal pain. EUS is most hel ful when the pancreas is completely normal or greatly abnc mal with more than five or six abnormal EUS criteria, t most strongly predictive EUS criteria being calcifications.[14]

Bile duct stones

In patients with intermediate probability for stone diseas EUS is extremely accurate, sensitive, and specific in diagnosi choledocholithiasis.[15] Use of EUS as the initial diagnostic te limits the risk of complications associated with more invasi tests (ERCP) in patients who have documented disease (s Chapter 76). ERCP can be performed during the same proc dure setting in those patients with common bile duct ston detected on EUS.

Submucosal lesions

EUS is an excellent modality for evaluation of the array submucosal lesions found during routine endoscopy. EUS c characterize the shape, size, echotexture, and layer of origi the most commonly identified lesion is a gastrointestinal strom tumor (GIST; see Chapter 39). EUS-guided FNA cannot differe

INDICATIONS/CONTRAINDICATIONS

NDICATIONS
- Staging of esophageal cancer
- Restaging esophageal cancer
- Staging of lung cancer
- Staging of gastric cancer (in selected cases)
- Detection, diagnosis, and staging of pancreatic cancer
- Staging of rectal cancer
- Evaluation of submucosal masses
- Assessment of anal sphincter integrity
- Evaluation of benign pancreatic and biliary disease
- Pancreatic pseudocyst drainage

ONTRAINDICATIONS

bsolute contraindications:
- Lack of patient cooperation
- Known or suspected perforated viscus
- Acute diverticulitis
- Fulminant colitis

elative contraindications include:
- High-grade esophageal stricture
- Unstable cardiac or pulmonary conditions

elative contraindications to FNA:
- Vascular structures in needle path
- Coagulopathy

ate benign from malignant stromal tumors. Hypoechoic lesions eater than 3 cm with heterogeneous architecture and irregu- r borders arising from the muscularis propria have a higher alignant potential and should be resected surgically.[16]

ectum

sing either rigid probes or conventional radial echoendo- opes, EUS can detect structural abnormalities of the internal ad external anal sphincters in patients with fecal inconti- ence (see Chapter 70). This can be performed easily without e need for sedation.

nterventional EUS

urrent interventional procedures commonly performed include US-guided celiac plexus neurolysis and EUS-guided botu- num toxin injection. The success of these procedures has pened the door to more advanced interventional procedures ncluding EUS-guided pseudocyst drainage and EUS-guided nolangiopancreatography. The most exciting and potential pplication is the use of EUS-guided fine-needle injection to eliver antitumor agents in patients with locally advanced ancer. The present authors demonstrated the feasibility and afety of performing antitumor injection therapy by EUS guid- nce in patients with locally advanced pancreatic cancer.[17] urther trials are under way for locally advanced pancreatic nd esophageal cancer.

ontraindications

he contraindications to performing EUS are similar to those f conventional endoscopy and the preps are similar. Because f the longer procedure time and increased sedation requirement, some patients (e.g., those with sleep apnea, neurologic disorders) should have the procedure performed by an anesthesiologist, administering either conscious sedation or general anesthesia.

COMPLICATIONS AND THEIR MANAGEMENT

The overall complication rate of performing diagnostic EUS is similar to that of standard endoscopy.[18] One complication with a slightly higher frequency than standard endoscopy is hypopharyngeal–cervical perforation during intubation. This is most likely due to the longer rigid tip of the EUS scope. The major complications of the EUS occur when FNA is performed, especially of cystic lesions; the overall rate of complications is 1.6–2%.[19–21] The most common complications include hemorrhage, infection, perforation, and pancreatitis.

Antibiotic prophylaxis and treatment for 3–5 days afterwards should be given for FNA of cystic lesions of the pancreas or of perirectal or pericolonic masses.[20] Avoidance of vascular structures has been mentioned previously. Complications secondary to EUS-guided FNA generally occur within the first 24 h. Submucosal hemorrhage or a hemorrhagic FNA should prompt intensive care unit monitoring and early surgical consultation.

COSTS, COMPLICATIONS, CONTROVERSIES

COMPLICATIONS
- Diagnostic EUS has similar complication rates to standard upper endoscopy.
- The most common complications from FNA are hemorrhage and infection.
- Prophylactic antibiotics are given to prevent infection when biopsing perirectal masses and pancreatic cystic lesions.

COSTS
- EUS with FNA is the most cost-effective approach for evaluating a pancreatic mass by providing a tissue diagnosis and staging in one session.
- EUS is the most cost-effective imaging modality in determining resectability in esophageal cancer.
- When used in combination with CT, EUS is cost-effective in staging rectal cancer.
- EUS is the most cost-effective approach when evaluating patients with suspected choledocholithiasis.

RELATIVE COST

Many studies show that EUS incorporated into a diagnostic algorithm is cost-effective, because of lower costs and fewer procedure-related complications. Cost-effectiveness of EUS has been demonstrated in the evaluation of esophageal, proximal rectal, and pancreatic cancers.[22,23] In each case, when EUS with FNA was incorporated into the diagnostic algorithm in place of CT, magnetic resonance imaging, or surgery, or used in conjunction with CT in patients with rectal cancer, it was the least costly staging strategy. EUS has also been shown to be cost-effective when used in place of ERCP in patients with suspected choledocholithiasis.[24]

REFERENCES

1. Dimagno EP, Buxton JL, Regan PT et al. Ultrasonic endoscope. Lancet 1980; i:629–631.
2. Chang KJ, Katz KD, Durbin TE et al. Endoscopic ultrasound-guided fine-needle aspiration. Gastrointest Endosc 1994; 40:694–699.
3. Klapman JB, Logrono R, Dye CE et al. Clinical impact of on-site cytopathology interpretation on endoscopic ultrasound-guided fine needle aspiration. Am J Gastroenterol 2003; 98:1289–1294.
4. Nguyen P, Feng JC, Chang KJ. Endoscopic ultrasound (EUS) and EUS-guided fine-needle aspiration (FNA) of liver lesions. Gastrointest Endosc 1999; 50:357–361.
5. Eloubeidi MA, Jhala D, Chhieng DC et al. Yield of endoscopic ultrasound-guided fine-needle aspiration biopsy in patients with suspected pancreatic carcinoma. Cancer 2003; 99:285–292.
6. Vazquez-Sequerios E, Norton ID, Clain JE et al. Impact of EUS-guided fine needle aspiration on lymph node staging in patients with esophageal carcinoma. Gastrointest Endosc 2001; 53:751–757.
7. Scotiniotis IA, Kochman ML, Lewis JD et al. Accuracy of EUS in the evaluation of Barrett's esophagus and high-grade dysplasia or intramucosal carcinoma. Gastrointest Endosc 2001; 54:689–696.
8. Fritscher-Ravens A. Endoscopic ultrasound evaluation in the diagnosis and staging of lung cancer. Lung Cancer 2003; 41:259–267.
9. Ohashi S, Segewa K, Okamura S et al. The utility of endoscopic ultrasonography and endoscopy in the endoscopic mucosal resection of early gastric cancer. Gut 1999; 45:599–604.
10. Harewood GC, Wiersema MJ. Endosonography-guided fine-needle aspiration biopsy in the evaluation of pancreatic masses. Am J Gastroenterol 2002; 97:1386–1391.
11. Gunaratnam NT, Saram AV, Norton ID et al. A prospective study of EUS-guided celiac plexus neurolysis for pancreatic cancer pain. Gastrointest Endosc 2001; 54:316–324.
12. Savides TJ, Master SS. EUS in rectal cancer. Gastrointest Endosc 2002; 56:S12–S18.
13. Farrell RJ, Agarwal B, Brandwein SL et al. Intraductal ultrasound is a useful adjunct to ERCP for distinguishing malignant from benign biliary strictures. Gastrointest Endosc 2002; 56:681–687.
14. Sahai AV, Zimmerman M, Aabakken L et al. Prospective assessment of the ability of endoscopic ultrasound to diagnose, exclude, or establish the severity of chronic pancreatitis found by endoscopic retrograde cholangiopancreatography. Gastrointest Endosc 1998; 48:18–25.
15. Canto MI, Chak A, Stellato T et al. Endoscopic ultrasonography versus cholangiography for the diagnosis of choledocholithiasis. Gastrointest Endosc 1998; 47:439–448.
16. Palazzo L, Landi B, Cellier C et al. Endosonographic features predictive of benign and malignant gastrointestinal stromal tumours. Gut 2000; 46:88–102.
17. Chang KJ, Nguyen PT, Thompson JA et al. Phase 1 clinical trial of allogeneic mixed lymphocyte culture (cytoimplant) delivered by endoscopic ultrasound-guided fine needle-injection in patients with advanced pancreatic carcinoma. Cancer 2000; 88:1325–1335.
18. Levy MJ, Norton ID, Wiersema MJ et al. Prospective risk of bacteremia and other infectious complications in patients undergoir EUS-guided FNA. Gastrointest Endosc 200 57:672–678.
19. O'Toole D, Palazzo L, Arotcarena R et al. Assessment of complications of EUS-guided aspiration. Gastrointest Endosc 2001; 53:470–474.
20. Wiersema MJ, Vilmann P, Giovannini M et a Endosonography-guided fine-needle aspiratio diagnostic accuracy and complication assessment. Gastroenterology 1997; 112:1087–1095.
21. Gress F, Michael H, Gelrud D et al. EUS-guided fine-needle aspiration of the pancrea evaluation of pancreatitis as a complication. Gastrointest Endosc 2002; 56:864–867.
22. Shumaker DA, de Garmo P, Faigel DO. Potential impact of preoperative EUS on esophageal cancer management and cost. Gastrointest Endosc 2002; 56:391–396.
23. Chang KJ, Soetikno RM, Bastas D et al. Impact of endoscopic ultrasound combined with fine-needle aspiration biopsy in the management of esophageal cancer. Endoscop 2003; 35:962–966.
24. Buscarini E, Tansini P, Vallisa D et al. EUS fo suspected choledocholithiasis: do benefits outweigh costs? A prospective, controlled study. Gastrointest Endosc 2003; 57:510–51

Chapter 122

Diagnostic and interventional endoscopic retrograde cholangiopancreatography (ERCP)

George J M Webster and Stephen P Pereira

KEY POINTS

- Diagnostic endoscopic retrograde cholangiopancreatography (ERCP) in a patient with pain alone and a nondilated common bile duct on ultrasound is associated with a high risk/benefit ratio
- For patients with biliary-type pain and a low probability of choledocholithiasis, less invasive diagnostic modalities than ERCP (i.e. MRI/MRCP or endoscopic ultrasound) are indicated
- There is no evidence from meta-analysis to support routine administration of antibiotics
- Procedure-related complications occur in 10–15% of patients – avoidance of unnecessary ERCP is the best way to avoid post-ERCP pancreatitis
- ERCP is the treatment of choice for patients presenting with pain, abnormal liver function tests and duct dilatation due to choledocholithiasis
- With experienced operators, laparoscopic common bile duct exploration is comparable to postoperative ERCP in terms of safety and stone clearance rates
- Early ERCP is of benefit in severe acute biliary pancreatitis with concomitant cholangitis
- ERCP is used for both diagnosis and decompression of the biliary tree by stenting in patients with suspected pancreaticobiliary malignancy

INTRODUCTION

The development of side-viewing duodenoscopes in the early 1970s allowed endoscopic visualization of the papilla of Vater (point of entry of the bile and pancreatic ducts) and, when combined with radiography, high-quality visualization of the bile and pancreatic ducts – endoscopic retrograde cholangiopancreatography (ERCP). For many years ERCP was the gold standard for investigating pancreatic and biliary disorders, but with improvement in other imaging modalities, including ultrasonography (transabdominal and endoscopic), multislice helical computed tomography (CT), magnetic resonance imaging/cholangiopancreatography (MRI/MRCP), and intraoperative cholangiography, the need for diagnostic ERCP has declined.[1] Consequently, ERCP has evolved into a predominantly therapeutic modality, used for the removal of bile and pancreatic duct stones, the treatment of biliary strictures, and the palliation of malignancy. However, ERCP still has a diagnostic role in patients with suspected pancreaticobiliary malignancy in whom noninvasive imaging is normal or equivocal, and it also allows tissue to be obtained for diagnosis by endobiliary brush cytology, needle aspiration, and biopsy.

DESCRIPTION OF TECHNIQUE

Equipment and staff

Endoscope: To view and cannulate the duodenal papilla, sited on the medial wall of the duodenum, it is necessary to use a side-viewing endoscope. A range of video-duodenoscopes are available. The supporting video image processing system is the same as for gastroscopy and colonoscopy. Duodenoscopes have a working shaft of approximately 1.2 m, with an external diameter ranging from 10.5 to 13.5 mm, and a working channel of 2.2–4.8 mm. Control wheels allow 90–120° up/down angulation, 90–110° right–left angulation, and a variable elevator to alter the angle at which accessories leave the duodenoscope. The smaller-diameter duodenoscopes allow greater maneuverability, and the narrower bridge provides greater catheter stability, but the larger scopes have a working channel that allows the passage of 10-Fr (i.e., 3.3 mm external diameter) plastic stents, metal stents, and large mechanical lithotripters (Fig. 122.1).

Cannulae: A range of instruments is available for biliary cannulation, including Teflon-coated 5-Fr (1.7 mm) catheters and bow-string sphincterotomes with a variable number of lumens, external diameter, length of leading cannula, and length of exposed wire. In addition to biliary sphincterotomy, sphincterotomes are also useful in the setting of altered papillary anatomy or a difficult duodenal position. X-ray imaging is a central component of ERCP, and the procedure is performed on an X-ray table, with imaging provided by standard fluoroscopy or using a digital C-arm unit with hard copy facilities. The minimum staffing requirements for ERCP are the endoscopist, one assisting nurse to manage the patient's airway and mouthguard, another to assist with endoscopic accessories, and a radiographer/radiologist.

The patient

It is essential that the indication, risks and benefits, and intended outcomes of ERCP are discussed in advance, allowing the patient to provide informed written consent. Procedure-related complications occur in 5–10% of patients, and include acute pancreatitis, bleeding, and perforation, as discussed below. It should be noted that this complication rate is derived mainly from large multicenter studies performed in specialist units.[2] Ideally, units or individuals should be able to provide their own data for complications, thus improving the extent to which consent is truly informed.[3] Clinicians and their patients should also be fully aware of the situations in which the risks of ERCP are increased (see Table 122.1).

Contraindications to ERCP are generally similar to those for other types of endoscopy performed under conscious sedation,

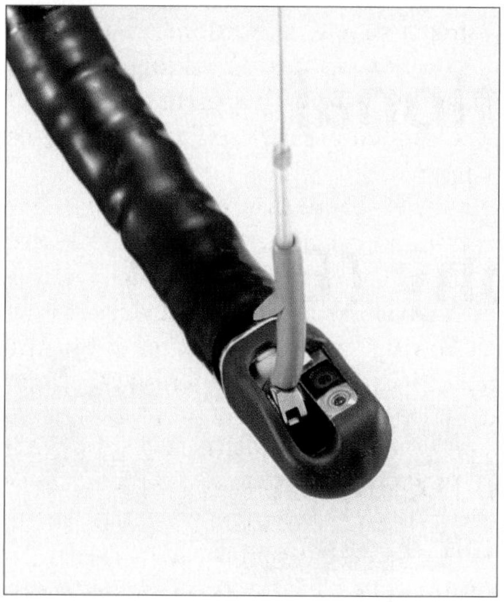

Fig. 122.1 Example of a side-viewing duodenoscope, showing the elevator used for controlling the insertion of accessories. A 10-Fr polyethylene stent is seen passing out of the duodenoscope, over a guiding catheter and guidewire. (Olympus Keymed, UK)

including lack of informed consent and significant cardiorespiratory disease. Most contraindications to ERCP are relative, and it is vital to weigh up the potential risks and benefits for the individual patient. For example, ERCP in a jaundiced patient with gallstone pancreatitis and systemic inflammatory response syndrome may be high risk, but is potentially life-saving. In contrast, solely diagnostic ERCP in a patient with pain alone and a normal pancreaticobiliary tree on noninvasive imaging is associated with a high risk:benefit ratio.

Special situations: When indicated, therapeutic ERCP in pregnancy is safe provided appropriate pelvic lead shielding is used. The risk of sphincterotomy bleeding is increased in patients taking anticoagulants, and is probably also increased in patients with deranged clotting as a result of underlying disease. In the authors' unit, a prothrombin time prolongation of less than 3 s and platelet count greater than 50×10^9/L is required before the procedure, with intravenous vitamin K, fresh frozen plasma, and platelet infusions given as appropriate, but there are few expert guidelines in this area.[4] Despite the widespread use of prophylactic antibiotics for ERCP, a meta-analysis concluded that there was no clinical benefit to their routine administration.[5] The risk of cholangitis is very low unless adequate biliary drainage is not achieved at ERCP. Prophylaxis is certainly indicated where there is a risk of contrast injection into poorly draining intrahepatic ducts or a communicating pancreatic pseudocyst at the time of ERCP, but many units use prophylaxis for all ERCPs.

Patient positioning for the procedure under sedation affects the ease with which ERCP is performed. The patient lies on their front, with the left arm extended behind the body, the right arm flexed, with the hand near to the face, and the head turned to the right, so that the left side of the face lies flat on the pillow. The appearance is that of the 'freestyle' swimming position. In some units, the right leg is flexed initially, allowing the right side of the body to be lifted a little from the bed to aid intubation of the pylorus. Oxygen is delivered at 2–4 L/min via nasal cannulae, and pulse rate and arterial oxygen saturation are monitored continuously using a standard finger probe. Intravenous opiate (e.g., fentanyl 50–100 μg or pethidine 25–50 mg) analgesia followed by a benzodiazepine (e.g., midazolam 2.5–5 mg) is given, with the dose titrated to achieve adequate conscious sedation. Higher levels may be required than for upper gastrointestinal endoscopy or colonoscopy. Alternatively, some centers use deep sedation with propofol and/or general anesthesia for ERCP. Intravenous hyoscine butylbromide 20–40 mg or glucagon 0.5–1 mg may also be given to reduce duodenal and biliary sphincter contractions.

Technique

Esophageal intubation with the duodenoscope is similar to that for standard endoscopy. Examination of the upper gastrointestinal tract is also possible but, because the scope is side-viewing, the scope tip needs to be angled down in order to gain a luminal view. After identifying the pylorus the tip is angled up (producing a 'setting sun' view of the pylorus), so allowing duodenal intubation. In order to identify the major papilla, a complex series of maneuvers of sharp angulation of the scope tip to the right, right torque on the shaft, and pulling back, is performed. As with most aspects of ERCP, this procedure is reliably performed only after close supervision and training.

Optimal duodenal position: This is the prerequisite of successful papillary cannulation. The duodenoscope is positioned just below the major papilla (Fig. 122.2). On viewing the papilla *en face*, pancreatic duct cannulation is often achieved by cannula insertion into the middle of the papilla, with common bile duct cannulation achieved by insertion in an upwards direction, from below the papilla, aimed at 11 o'clock, and following the line of the bulge of the intramural bile duct. Before ERCP, it is

TABLE 122.1 RISK FACTORS FOR POST-ERCP PANCREATITIS
• Young age
• Female sex
• Suspected sphincter of Oddi dysfunction
• Normal serum bilirubin level
• Previous ERCP-related pancreatitis
• Recurrent pancreatitis
• Difficult bile duct cannulation
• Pancreatic duct filling
• Precut (needle-knife) sphincterotomy
• Pancreatic sphincterotomy
• Balloon sphincter dilatation
• Pain during ERCP

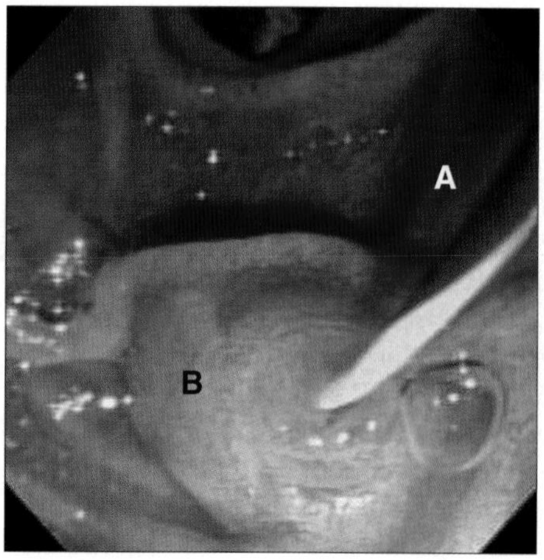

Fig. 122.2 Normal major papilla as seen with the duodenoscope in position within the duodenum. A 0.035-inch guidewire (A) is seen within the papilla (B).

ıportant to decide which anatomy needs to be defined. ıncreatic duct cannulation should not be performed unless of inical relevance, as repeated attempts at pancreatic duct nnulation are an important cause of procedure-related ıncreatitis. Once deep cannulation of the desired duct has en obtained, the need for further instrumentation will pend on the indications and findings on cholangiography or ıncreatography. Insertion of a 0.018–0.035-inch guidewire rough the cannula and into the duct helps to maintain endo-opic position, and allows the cannula to be exchanged for her ERCP accessories as required.

Biliary sphincterotomy may be indicated for a variety of asons, including stone extraction, papillary stenosis, and ent insertion (Fig. 122.3). The sphincterotome is connected to standard electrosurgical unit, as used for polypectomy, which ıs 'cut' and 'coagulate' settings. The optimal contribution of ıch during sphincterotomy is debated, with excessive coagu-tion implicated in thermal damage to the pancreatic sphinc-r and pancreatitis, and 'pure cut' carrying a possible increased sk of sphincterotomy bleeding. Microprocessor-controlled ectrocautery generators use a combined cut and coagulation, ıd may reduce the risk of an uncontrolled ('zipper') cut recipitating bleeding or perforation. Balloon dilatation of the liary sphincter is an alternative to sphincterotomy for the ktraction of bile duct stones, although there are conflicting ata on its safety compared with standard sphincterotomy.[6,7]

Difficulties: Bile duct cannulation may be difficult for a range f reasons, such as the papilla being sited within a duodenal iverticulum or the presence of papillary pathology (e.g., impacted one, ampullary tumor). Repeated attempts at cannulation may ad to edema around the papilla, making cannulation even ıore difficult. The use of a sphincterotome allows the angle of ınnulation to be altered, as may moving from a 'short' to a ong' scope position. A needle-knife precut sphincterotomy ıay facilitate deep cannulation, but in multicenter studies has een shown to carry a greater risk of complications than stan-ard bow-string sphincterotomy, particularly when the bile duct not dilated. In experienced hands, placement of a pancreatic ent before precutting may increase immediate bile duct access ıccess rates and reduce the risk of pancreatitis.[8] Where endo-copic bile duct cannulation or stent insertion has proved impos-ble, a percutaneous transhepatic approach and drain insertion ıay be necessary. Endoscopic access and intervention may ıen be achieved by a combined ('rendezvous') procedure, with the radiologist passing a guidewire down the transhepatic biliary drain and out of the papilla into the duodenum. The endoscopist can then grasp the wire with a snare and bring it out through the scope to facilitate stent, sphincterotome, or balloon insertion, as required.

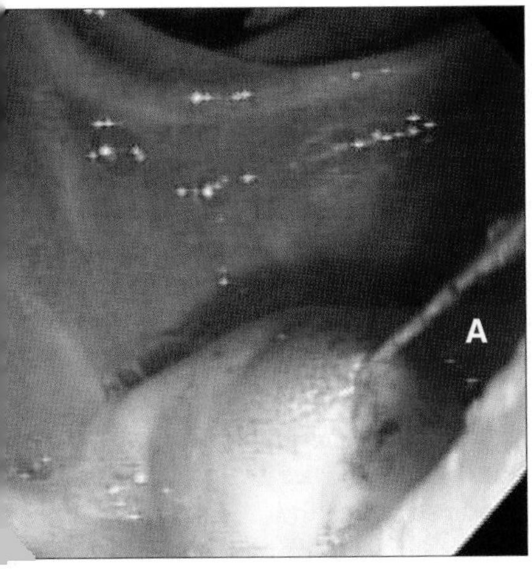

Fig. 122.3 Biliary sphincterotomy using bow-string sphincterotome (A).

Endoscopic stone extraction: There are several approaches to endoscopic stone extraction, including balloon or basket extraction, or mechanical lithotripsy. Stone removal using a balloon extraction catheter has the advantage that it may be performed over a wire, allowing easy recannulation of the bile duct (Fig. 122.4). Its main disadvantages are that small stones within a dilated bile duct may 'skip past' the balloon as the bile duct is trawled, and larger stones may become impacted at the ampulla. Standard baskets allow the extraction of most stones smaller than 1 cm, but carry the risk of not being able to deliver larger stones through the ampulla, or to disengage the stone from the basket within the bile duct, requiring the use of a reel mechanism to crush the stone or snap the basket, thus allowing disengagement. An alternative to either of these techniques is the use of a mechanical lithotripter, which is similar to a standard basket but has a metal sleeve that may be advanced over the closed basket, thereby crushing the stone (Fig. 122.5). Although the mechanical lithotripter is bulkier and more difficult to maneuver than the standard basket, it avoids the risk of stone impaction.

Three main types of biliary endoscopic stent are in use:

- **Straight polyethylene stents** – available in a range of lengths, with external diameters of 7 Fr and 10 Fr being used most commonly. The stents are slightly curved and have a flange approximately 1 cm short of each end, which helps to prevent slippage above or below a stricture. 10-Fr stents generally last longer and provide

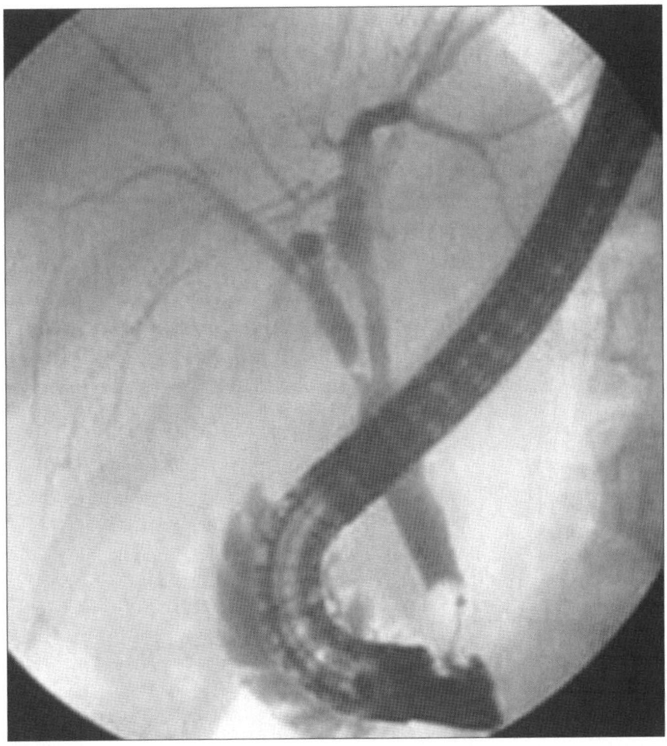

Fig. 122.4 Balloon occlusion cholangiogram following successful removal of stones within the common bile duct. Note the right hepatic duct stricture related to previous bile duct injury at open cholecystectomy.

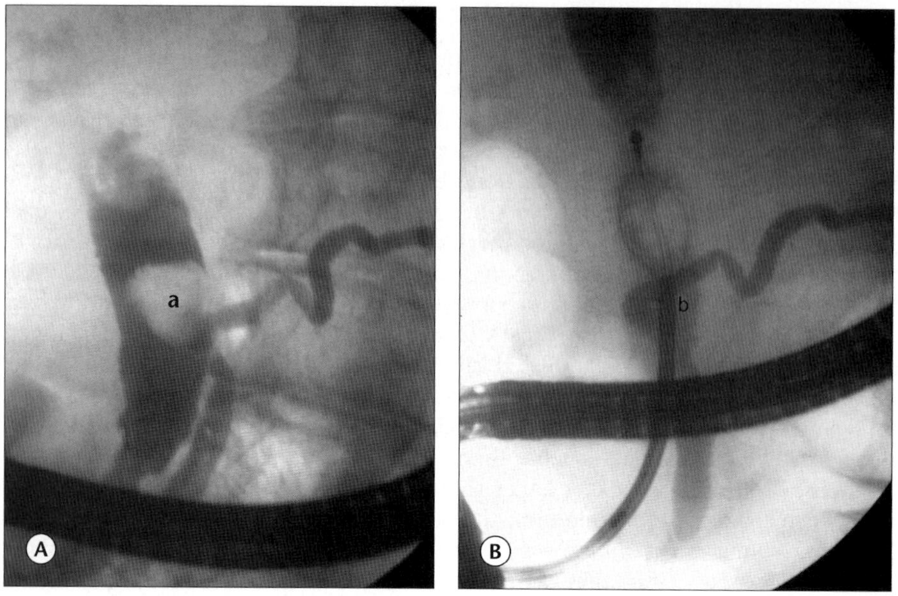

Fig. 122.5 Mechanical lithotripsy. At ERCP, a large 1.5-cm stone is seen within the mid common bile duct **(A)**. This was crushed, fragmented, and removed using a mechanica lithotripter, with the metal sheath advanced over the basket holding the stone **(B)**.

better drainage than 7-Fr stents, but there is little advantage in more unwieldy stents larger than 10 Fr.

- **7-Fr double pigtail stents** – generally used when straight stents might become displaced, such as after sphincterotomy and incomplete stone extraction from a dilated bile duct. 7-Fr stents are inserted directly over an 0.035-inch wire, whereas a 6–7-Fr guiding catheter is first inserted over the guidewire when a 10-Fr stent is used, because of the larger internal stent diameter. With the wire and guiding catheter placed into the proximal biliary tree, the stent is pushed into place using a pushing tube.
- **A range of self-expanding metal biliary stents**, compressed within the tip of a continuous 7.5–10-Fr delivery catheter, can also be inserted endoscopically. On withdrawal of the compressing sleeve, the stent is deployed, expanding up to a maximum diameter of 10 mm (Fig. 122.6).

Stent occlusion: At least one-third of patients with pancreatic cancer will survive long enough for a polyethylene stent to become occluded, in which case a further procedure is performed to remove the blocked stent and replace it with a new one. In patients who are expected to survive longer than 6 months, metal stents play an important role in the palliation of malignant biliary strictures. These stents are approximately 20 times more expensive than polyethylene stents, but the 1 cm expanded

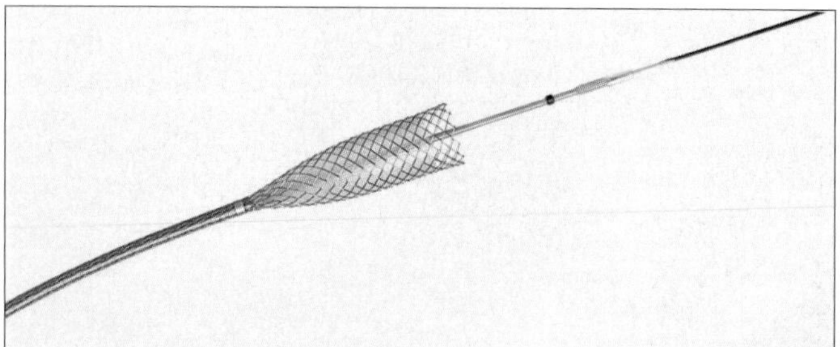

Fig. 122.6 Insertion mechanism for a biliary Wallstent. The 8.5-Fr introducing system is inserted across the stricture over a 0.035-inch wire. The plastic sheath is then drawn back, allowing deployment of the stent. (Boston Scientific Corp, USA.)

lumen remains patent for a median of 4–9 months compare with the 3–4 months seen with plastic stents.[9] However, tissu ingrowth through the mesh may lead to further obstructio necessitating insertion of further metal stents (or more usuall plastic stents) inside the lumen of the metal stent. In dist malignant biliary obstruction, polyurethane-covered sel expandable metal stents remain patent for longer than uncovere metal stents, but are more expensive and may be associate with a slightly higher risk of acute cholecystitis, pancreatiti and stent migration.[10]

INDICATIONS FOR ERCP

A National Institutes of Health State-of-the-Science conferenc on ERCP for diagnosis and therapy in 2002[11,12] examined th current state of knowledge regarding the indications for ERC in clinical practice.

Gallstone disease

Common bile duct stones can be removed by preoperativ ERCP, laparoscopic common bile duct exploration, or pos operative ERCP. The endoscopic removal of common bile duc stones at the time of ERCP is the treatment of choice fc patients presenting with pain, abnormal liver function, an duct dilatation. ERCP with sphincterotomy is also the primar treatment for patients with cholangitis resulting from commo bile duct stones, with urgent (within 24 h) ERCP indicated fo those who do not respond promptly to immediate resuscita tion with intravenous fluids and antibiotics.

Alternatives: For patients with biliary-type pain and a lov probability of choledocholithiasis, less invasive diagnostic modal ities than ERCP (i.e., MRI/MRCP or endoscopic ultrasonography are indicated, or alternatively operative cholangiography at th time of laparoscopic cholecystectomy is performed to demon strate the presence or absence of common bile duct stones. I surgical expertise in the technique is available, laparoscopi common bile duct exploration is comparable to postoperativ ERCP in terms of safety and stone clearance rates, and associate with lower hospital stay and use of healthcare resources.[13] Other wise, postoperative ERCP is indicated for patients with retaine ones, as well as for the diagnosis and endoscopic therapy of ıost postcholecystectomy bile duct injuries (Fig. 122.7).

In selected patients at prohibitive operative risk, ERCP with one clearance, but without cholecystectomy, may be definive therapy, as may repeated endoscopic stenting beside very ırge bile duct stones to facilitate biliary drainage. However, in ontrolled studies the latter approach was associated with an ıcreased burden of biliary symptoms compared with complete one clearance.[14]

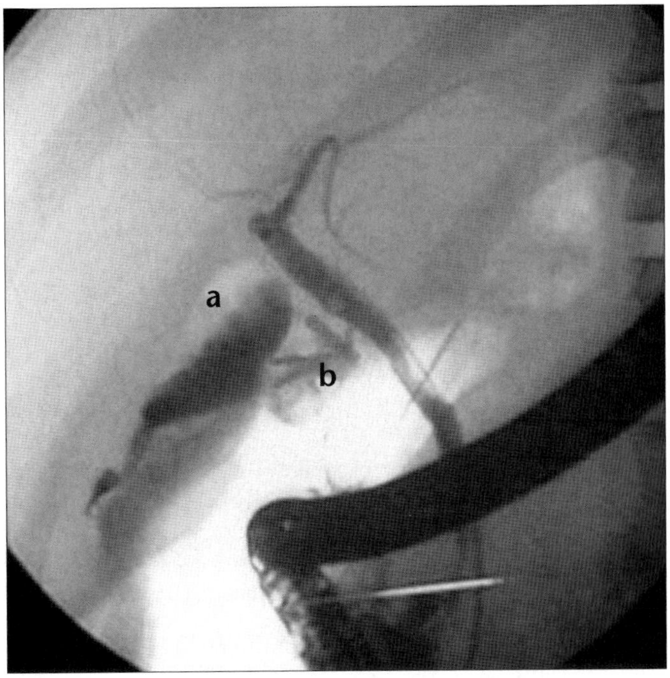

Fig. 122.7 Leakage after cholecystectomy. ERCP in a patient 1 week after laparoscopic cholecystectomy, showing contrast leak into the gallbladder bed (a), due to displacement of clips from the cystic duct stump (b).

ıcute and chronic pancreatitis

RCP has been used for both the diagnosis and treatment of cute, recurrent, and chronic pancreatitis (Fig. 122.8).

Diagnosis: In patients who present with the typical findings f acute pancreatitis (abdominal pain and raised levels of ancreatic enzymes), ERCP has little role except in the setting f severe acute biliary pancreatitis with concomitant cholangitis, ı which case randomized trials comparing urgent versus delayed RCP show a benefit for early intervention.[15]

In patients with recurrent pancreatitis, when the etiology of ecurrent pancreatitis has not been defined by history, laboatory tests, and noninvasive pancreaticobiliary imaging (CT nd MRI/MRCP), further evaluation by endoscopic ultrasonoraphy (see Chapter 121) or ERCP with or without sphincter f Oddi manometry (see Chapter 77) may be considered. 'otential causes include biliary stones, microlithiasis, pancreas ivisum, small neoplasms or benign pancreatic strictures, or phincter of Oddi dysfunction. Occasionally, recurrent or chronic ancreatitis may result from the effects of an intraductal apillary mucinous tumor, which may have a typical endoscopic ppearance (Fig. 122.9).

Treatment: In patients with acute, relapsing, or chronic panreatitis, a variety of endoscopic therapies have been described. After pancreatic sphincterotomy, stones can be removed from he pancreatic duct, strictures can be stented or balloon-dilated, nd drainage of the dorsal duct in pancreas divisum can be nproved by a combination of accessory papilla sphincterotomy nd stent placement, with uncontrolled studies suggesting that oth immediate- and long-term pain relief are possible. Peripancreatic fluid collections and pseudocysts can also be managed by pancreatic duct drainage or direct endoscopic cystenterostomy and stenting techniques, with the results of several studies suggesting that ERCP provides a similar rate of pain relief and pseudocyst resolution as surgery, with equivalent or reduced mortality.[16,17] However, there have been no formal randomized comparisons of these ERCP techniques with interventional radiology or surgery.

Benign and malignant bile duct strictures

Postoperative anastomotic strictures or those following bile duct damage at the time of cholecystectomy can initially be

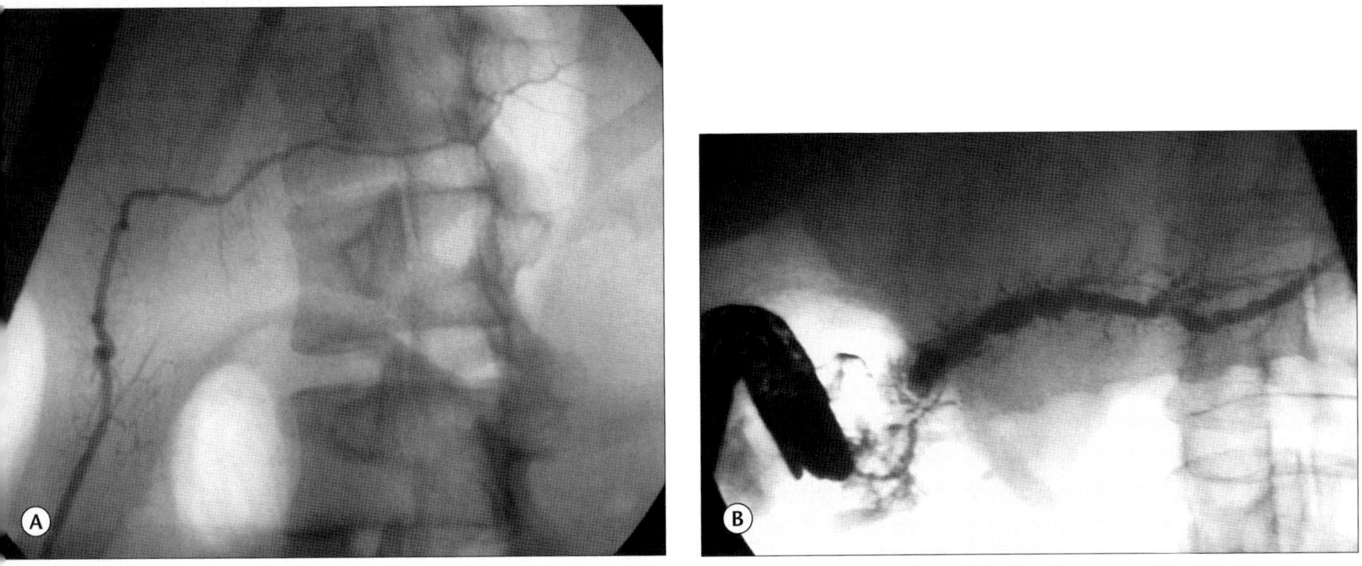

ig. 122.8 Chronic pancreatitis. Comparison of a normal pancreatogram (A) with that in a patient with chronic pancreatitis (B), showing a ilated, irregular main pancreatic duct with side-branch dilatation.

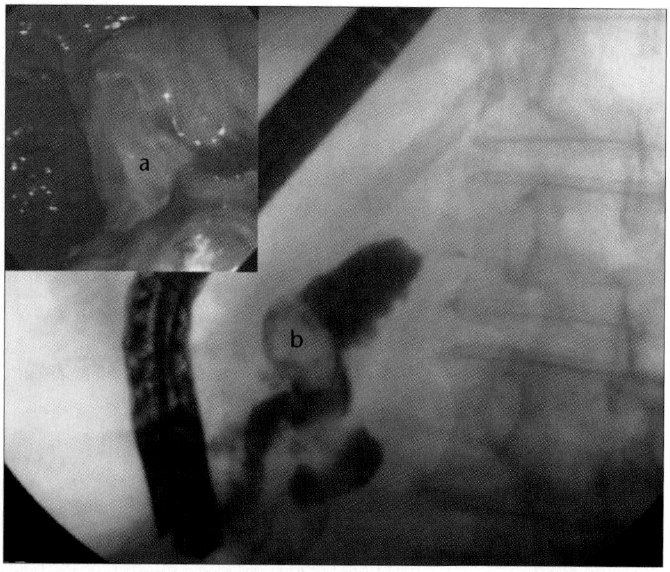

Fig. 122.9 Typical appearances of an intraductal papillary mucinous tumor. At ERCP, mucus was seen to be extruding from a patulous papilla (a), with pancreatography showing a filling defect within a dilated duct in the head of pancreas (b).

managed with intermittent biliary balloon dilatation or endoscopic stent placement at the time of ERCP, with surgical reconstruction of the bile duct reserved for patients in whom endoscopic treatment has not led to resolution of the stricture. In patients with primary sclerosing cholangitis, uncontrolled studies suggest that endoscopic balloon dilatation or stenting of dominant biliary strictures may prolong survival or time to transplantation, but there is also an increased risk of cholangiocarcinoma development during long-term follow-up[18] (Fig. 122.10). Pancreatic and biliary tract cancer (cholangiocarcinoma, gallbladder cancer, and ampullary cancer) can all produce stricturing of the biliary tree at different levels (Fig. 122.11). ERCP is used for both diagnosis and decompression of the biliary tree by endoscopic stenting in patients known or suspected to have pancreaticobiliary malignancy.

Tissue diagnosis may be achieved at ERCP by using needle aspiration, brush cytology, and forceps biopsy. Individually, the diagnostic yield from these techniques is low, but their combination improves the ability to establish a tissue diagnosis[19] (Fig. 122.12). However, ERCP is generally unnecessary for the diagnosis of cancer in a patient presenting with a localized pancreatic mass initially seen on CT if the patient is a candidate for surgery. The use of preoperative stent placement and staging by ERCP in such cases is not supported by evidence from clinical trials, and it may complicate or even preclude surgical intervention.

Unfortunately, most cases of pancreatic or biliary tract cancer are not detected at a curable stage, so only palliation can be offered. Palliative intervention for malignant biliary obstruction may involve ERCP with stent placement or surgical bypass (Fig. 122.13). The available evidence does not indicate a major advantage to either alternative, with the choice depending on the performance status of the patient and local expertise.[20]

Pancreaticobiliary-type pain

ERCP is a commonly used technique for the evaluation and management of patients with anatomic evidence of pancreatic or bile duct obstruction. The role of ERCP in patients wit pancreaticobiliary-type pain in the absence of obvious obstruc tive disorders of the pancreatic or bile duct, often referred t as suspected sphincter of Oddi dysfunction, is less well define The use of ERCP and sphincter of Oddi manometry in the assess ment and treatment of such patients is discussed in Chapter 7

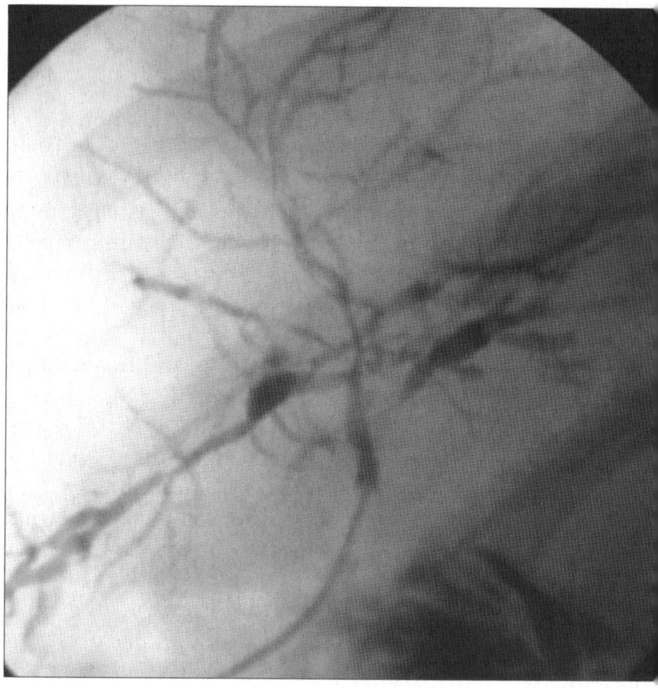

Fig. 122.10 Primary sclerosing cholangitis. Cholangiogram showin intrahepatic duct beading and stricturing consistent with primary sclerosing cholangitis.

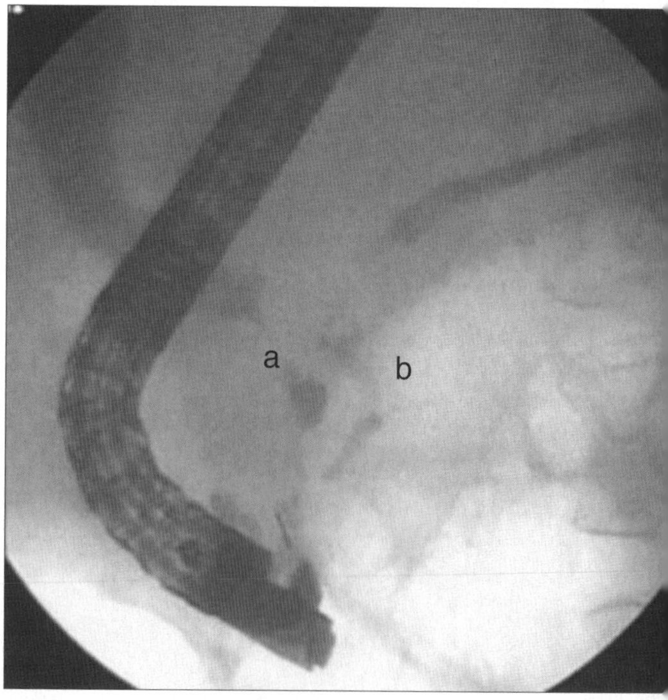

Fig. 122.11 Carcinoma of the head of the pancreas. ERCP shows 'double duct sign' of strictures of the distal common bile duct (a) and pancreatic duct (b), with associated proximal duct dilatation. This pattern is classically seen in carcinoma of the head of the pancreas.

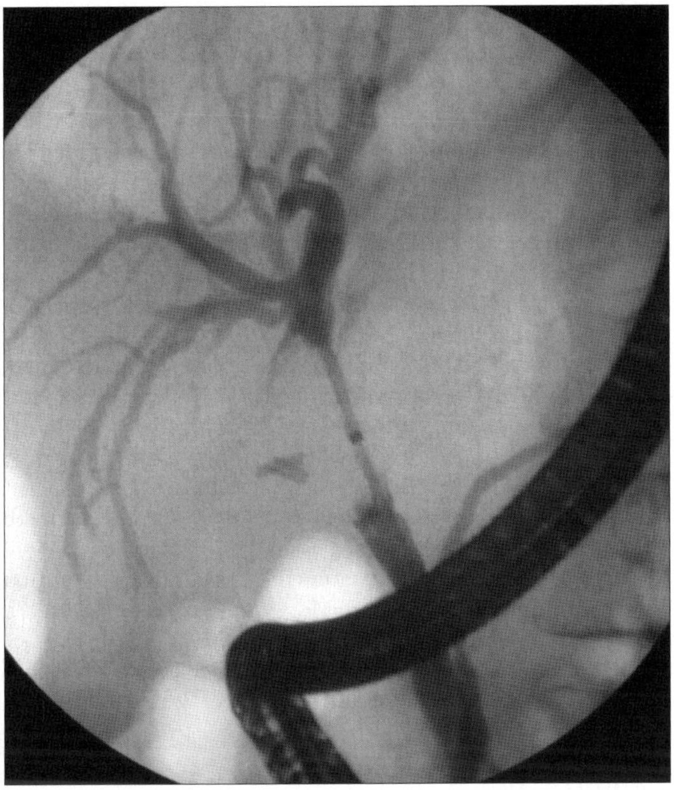

Fig. 122.12 **Cholangiocarcinoma.** ERCP shows a stricture of the common hepatic duct in a patient with painless obstructive jaundice. Endoscopic biopsies confirmed cholangiocarcinoma. Clips from a previous cholecystectomy can also be seen.

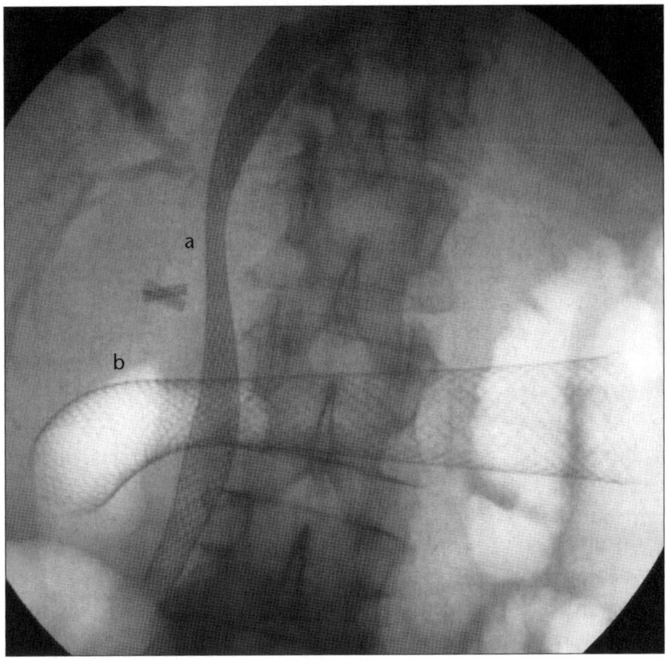

Fig. 122.13 **Pancreatic carcinoma.** An endoscopically placed mesh metal biliary stent (a) and duodenal stent (b) in a patient with obstructive jaundice and duodenal obstruction due to pancreatic carcinoma.

COMPLICATIONS AND THEIR MANAGEMENT

A number of specific complications are associated with ERCP. Large multicenter studies have reported rates of procedure-related complications of approximately 5–10%, due mainly to pancreatitis and sphincterotomy-associated problems. In general, those doing fewer ERCPs have higher complication rates, although no consistent correlation has been found with rates of post-ERCP pancreatitis – due in part to high-volume endoscopists attempting higher-risk cases.[21] Most complications occur within 12h, although delayed sphincterotomy-related bleeding may occur several days after the procedure, and late complications such as sphincter stenosis have been reported in up to 5% of patients after sphincterotomy.[22] The mortality rate from diagnostic ERCP is approximately 0.2%, with double the risk for therapeutic ERCP.[23] However, these

ERCP COMPLICATIONS AND SEVERITY GRADING

Complication	Mild	Moderate	Severe
Pancreatitis	Amylase more than three times normal level more than 24h after ERCP, with hospital stay extended by 2–3 days	Hospitalization for 4–10 days	Hospitalization for >10 days, or hemorrhagic pancreatitis, phlegmon, pseudocyst, or intervention (percutaneous or surgical)
Retroperitoneal perforation	Possible, or only very slight leak, with <4 days of treatment required	Proven perforation treated medically for 4–10 days	Medical treatment for >10 days, or intervention (percutaneous or surgical)
Bleeding	Clinical evidence of bleeding, but hemoglobin level falls <3g/dL, and no transfusion required	Transfusion required, but <5 units, and no angiographic or surgical intervention	>4 units transfused, or angiographic/surgical intervention
Cholangitis	Temperature >38°C for 24–48h	Septic illness requiring >3 days of hospital treatment, or endoscopic/radiographic intervention	Septic shock or need for surgery
Stone impaction in basket	Basket released spontaneously or by repeat endoscopy	Percutaneous intervention	Surgery

Any intensive care unit admission after procedure grades the complication as severe.
From Reference 24.

values must be considered in the context of the potential consequences of not performing an interventional ERCP when necessary.

Pancreatitis

Pancreatitis is the most common complication of ERCP, with prospective studies reporting this in approximately 7% of cases,[25,26] although there is a wide range, related in part to differing criteria for diagnosis. One consensus definition is that of new or worsened abdominal pain and a serum amylase level that is three or more times the upper limit of normal 24 h after the procedure, necessitating at least 2 days in hospital.[24] More than 90% of episodes of pancreatitis are self-limiting, with a severe course in 4.5–7% of cases.[25,26]

Severe pancreatitis may be associated with extensive pancreatic necrosis, sepsis, and multiorgan failure, with an overall mortality rate from ERCP-induced pancreatitis of approximately 0.5%. The experience of the endoscopist influences the rate of pancreatitis, but patient- and intervention-related factors add to the risk (Table 122.1). For example, a young woman with abdominal pain, normal bilirubin, a nondilated common bile duct, and difficult biliary cannulation at ERCP may have a 20–40% chance of developing pancreatitis, irrespective of any intervention. Overall, the risk of pancreatitis is similar for diagnostic and therapeutic ERCP. A pancreatitis risk of approximately 3% in patients requiring fewer than five attempts at biliary cannulation increases to 15% when more than 20 attempts are made.[25] The avoidance of unnecessary ERCP is the single best strategy for avoiding post-ERCP pancreatitis.

Prevention: A range of approaches has been studied to reduce ERCP-related pancreatitis. In advanced centers, temporary pancreatic stent placement reduces the risk of pancreatitis in patients undergoing ERCP for suspected sphincter of Oddi dysfunction,[27] although failed attempts to insert a stent may be associated with an even higher risk of pancreatitis.[21]

With regard to drug treatments, although a meta-analysis suggested that both somatostatin and gabexate (which inhibits proteolytic activity), given as continuous infusions, reduced the rate of ERCP pancreatitis,[28] a subsequent multicenter randomized placebo-controlled trial showed no benefit with either gabexate or octreotide (a somatostatin analog).[29] However, a recent single-center study reported a benefit in giving a single bolus of somatostatin immediately after ERCP.[30] Agents shown not to be consistently effective include interleukin-10, glyceryl trinitrate, nifedipine, allopurinol, corticosteroids, platelet-activating factor inhibitors, and the use of nonionic contrast.[31] A recent trial reported a benefit for rectal diclofenac over placebo,[32] but the experience of previous pharmacologic approaches re-emphasizes the fact that careful patient selection and consideration of noninvasive alternatives to diagnostic ERCP are likely to have the greatest effect on the burden of ERCP-related pancreatitis.

Other complications include:

- Perforation
- Hemorrhage
- Cholangitis
- Cholecystitis
- Stent-related complications
- Cardiopulmonary complications.

Perforation

Perforation may be retroperitoneal because of extension of a sphincterotomy incision beyond the intramural portion of the bile or pancreatic duct, intraperitoneal as a result of perforation of the bowel wall by the endoscope, or occur at any location because of extramural passage or migration of guidewires or stents. Risk factors for sphincterotomy perforation include a long incision, papillary stenosis, Billroth II anatomy, and needle-knife precut techniques. Clinically important perforation is reported in less than 1% of endoscopic sphincterotomies, but its overall frequency is probably significantly underdiagnosed, as the symptoms and radiologic appearances may be difficult to recognize. The development of surgical emphysema following sphincterotomy is indicative of retroperitoneal perforation, but the development of abdominal pain in the absence of a significant rise in serum amylase concentration may also provide a diagnostic clue. In those patients in whom the diagnosis cannot be made by plain abdominal radiography, CT is sensitive in documenting air extravasation into the retroperitoneal space. More than 90% of cases settle with intravenous antibiotics and a strict 'nil by mouth' policy, but the development of retroperitoneal collections may require percutaneous or surgical drainage. Bowel wall perforations usually require surgery.

Hemorrhage

Although minor ooze following a sphincterotomy is common, significant bleeding is a rare (0.2–2% of sphincterotomies[33]), but potentially serious, complication. Bleeding is more common in those with abnormalities of hemostasis (e.g., cirrhosis, chronic renal failure) or ongoing sepsis, in the setting of papillary stenosis, and in patients treated with anticoagulants within 72 h after the sphincterotomy. Arterial bleeds may result from cutting the retroduodenal artery as it runs within the transverse duodenal fold, often in association with a long, uncontrolled sphincterotomy. Bleeding that is noted at the time of sphincterotomy and that does not settle spontaneously can be controlled endoscopically, using either epinephrine (e.g., 1:10,000) injected into the cut surfaces of the sphincterotomy, or occasionally a hemoclip placed over the bleeding point. Ongoing bleeding may require angiographic embolization of the feeding artery, or surgery.

Cholangitis and cholecystitis

These complications occur in approximately 1% of patients after ERCP.[34] Although ERCP may introduce bacteria into a previously sterile biliary tree, clinical cholangitis is rare if effective biliary drainage is obtained. Cholangitis is a particular risk if the intrahepatic ducts are overfilled and cannot be drained adequately because of segmental obstruction. In case–control studies of patients with complex hilar strictures opacified with contrast at ERCP, bilateral intrahepatic duct stenting is associated with a lower rate of cholangitis than unilateral stenting.[35,36]

Stent-related complications

Long-term sequelae of endoscopic biliary sphincterotomy and stent placement include recurrent stone formation, as a result of sphincterotomy stenosis or bacteriobilia caused by duodenal–biliary reflux, and recurrent pancreatitis, presumably ecause of thermal injury to the pancreatic sphincter. The long-rm effects of pancreatic sphincterotomy are largely unknown. ancreatic stents have the potential to cause ductal injury with enosis, especially in patients with a normal pancreas.

ardiopulmonary complications

lthough uncommonly related to ERCP, cardiopulmonary complications are the leading cause of death from ERCP and, as expected, occur in older, sicker patients at high anesthetic risk.

SOURCES OF INFORMATION FOR PATIENTS AND DOCTORS

http://www.gastro.org/generalPublic.html

EFERENCES

1. Kaltenthaler E, Vergel YB, Chilcott J et al. A systematic review and economic evaluation of magnetic resonance cholangiopancreatography compared with diagnostic endoscopic retrograde cholangiopancreatography. Health Technol Assess 2004; 8:1–89.
2. Freeman ML. Adverse outcomes of ERCP. Gastrointest Endosc 2002; 56:S273–S282.
3. Cotton PB. ERCP is most dangerous for people who need it least. Gastrointest Endosc 2001; 54:535–536.
4. Eisen GM, Baron TH, Dominitz JA et al. Guideline on the management of anticoagulation and antiplatelet therapy for endoscopic procedures. Gastrointest Endosc 2002; 55:775–779.
5. Harris A, Chan AC, Torres-Viera C, Hammett R, Carr-Locke D. Meta-analysis of antibiotic prophylaxis in endoscopic retrograde cholangiopancreatography (ERCP). Endoscopy 1999; 31:718–724.
6. Bergman JJ, Rauws EA, Fockens P et al. Randomised trial of endoscopic balloon dilation versus endoscopic sphincterotomy for removal of bileduct stones. Lancet 1997; 349:1124–1129.
7. Vlavianos P, Chopra K, Mandalia S, Anderson M, Thompson J, Westaby D. Endoscopic balloon dilatation versus endoscopic sphincterotomy for the removal of bile duct stones: a prospective randomised trial. Gut 2003; 52:1165–1169.
8. Tarnasky PR. Mechanical prevention of post-ERCP pancreatitis by pancreatic stents: results, techniques, and indications. JOP 2003; 4:58–67.
9. Flamm CR, Mark DH, Aronson N. Evidence-based assessment of ERCP approaches to managing pancreaticobiliary malignancies. Gastrointest Endosc 2002; 56:S218–S225.
0. Isayama H, Komatsu Y, Tsujino T et al. A prospective randomised study of "covered" versus "uncovered" diamond stents for the management of distal malignant biliary obstruction. Gut 2004; 53:729–734.
1. National Institutes of Health State-of-the-Science Statement on endoscopic retrograde cholangiopancreatography (ERCP) for diagnosis and therapy. NIH Consens State Sci Statements 2002; 19:1–26.
2. Cohen S, Bacon BR, Berlin JA et al. National Institutes of Health State-of-the-Science Conference Statement: ERCP for diagnosis and therapy, January 14–16, 2002. Gastrointest Endosc 2002; 56:803–809.
3. Rhodes M, Sussman L, Cohen L, Lewis MP. Randomised trial of laparoscopic exploration of common bile duct versus postoperative endoscopic retrograde cholangiography for common bile duct stones. Lancet 1998; 351:159–161.
14. Tham TC, Carr-Locke DL. Endoscopic treatment of bile duct stones in elderly people. BMJ 1999; 318:617–618.
15. Sharma VK, Howden CW. Metaanalysis of randomized controlled trials of endoscopic retrograde cholangiography and endoscopic sphincterotomy for the treatment of acute biliary pancreatitis. Am J Gastroenterol 1999; 94:3211–3214.
16. Mark DH, Lefevre F, Flamm CR, Aronson N. Evidence-based assessment of ERCP in the treatment of pancreatitis. Gastrointest Endosc 2002; 56:S249–S254.
17. Lehman GA. Role of ERCP and other endoscopic modalities in chronic pancreatitis. Gastrointest Endosc 2002; 56:S237–S240.
18. Stiehl A, Rudolph G, Kloters-Plachky P, Sauer P, Walker S. Development of dominant bile duct stenoses in patients with primary sclerosing cholangitis treated with ursodeoxycholic acid: outcome after endoscopic treatment. J Hepatol 2002; 36:151–156.
19. Khan SA, Davidson BR, Goldin R et al. Guidelines for the diagnosis and treatment of cholangiocarcinoma: consensus document. Gut 2002; 51(Suppl VI):vi1–vi9.
20. Strasberg SM. ERCP and surgical intervention in pancreatic and biliary malignancies. Gastrointest Endosc 2002; 56:S213–S217.
21. Freeman ML, Guda NM. Prevention of post-ERCP pancreatitis: a comprehensive review. Gastrointest Endosc 2004; 59:845–864.
22. Rabenstein T, Schneider HT, Hahn EG, Ell C. 25 years of endoscopic sphincterotomy in Erlangen: assessment of the experience in 3498 patients. Endoscopy 1998; 30:A194–A201.
23. Loperfido S, Angelini G, Benedetti G et al. Major early complications from diagnostic and therapeutic ERCP: a prospective multicenter study. Gastrointest Endosc 1998; 48:1–10.
24. Cotton PB, Lehman G, Vennes J et al. Endoscopic sphincterotomy complications and their management: an attempt at consensus. Gastrointest Endosc 1991; 37:383–393.
25. Vandervoort J, Soetikno RM, Tham TC et al. Risk factors for complications after performance of ERCP. Gastrointest Endosc 2002; 56:652–656.
26. Freeman ML, DiSario JA, Nelson DB et al. Risk factors for post-ERCP pancreatitis: a prospective, multicenter study. Gastrointest Endosc 2001; 54:425–434.
27. Tarnasky PR, Palesch YY, Cunningham JT, Mauldin PD, Cotton PB, Hawes RH. Pancreatic stenting prevents pancreatitis after biliary sphincterotomy in patients with sphincter of Oddi dysfunction. Gastroenterology 1998; 115:1518–1524.
28. Andriulli A, Leandro G, Niro G et al. Pharmacologic treatment can prevent pancreatic injury after ERCP: a meta-analysis. Gastrointest Endosc 2000; 51:1–7.
29. Andriulli A, Clemente R, Solmi L et al. Gabexate or somatostatin administration before ERCP in patients at high risk for post-ERCP pancreatitis: a multicenter, placebo-controlled, randomized clinical trial. Gastrointest Endosc 2002; 56:488–495.
30. Poon RT, Yeung C, Liu CL et al. Intravenous bolus somatostatin after diagnostic cholangiopancreatography reduces the incidence of pancreatitis associated with therapeutic endoscopic retrograde cholangiopancreatography procedures: a randomised controlled trial. Gut 2003; 52:1768–1773.
31. Mallery JS, Baron TH, Dominitz JA et al. Complications of ERCP. Gastrointest Endosc 2003; 57:633–638.
32. Murray B, Carter R, Imrie C, Evans S, O'Suilleabhain C. Diclofenac reduces the incidence of acute pancreatitis after endoscopic retrograde cholangiopancreatography. Gastroenterology 2003; 124:1786–1791.
33. Masci E, Toti G, Mariani A et al. Complications of diagnostic and therapeutic ERCP: a prospective multicenter study. Am J Gastroenterol 2001; 96:417–423.
34. Freeman ML, Nelson DB, Sherman S et al. Complications of endoscopic biliary sphincterotomy. N Engl J Med 1996; 335:909–918.
35. De Palma GD, Galloro G, Siciliano S, Iovino P, Catanzano C. Unilateral versus bilateral endoscopic hepatic duct drainage in patients with malignant hilar biliary obstruction: results of a prospective, randomized, and controlled study. Gastrointest Endosc 2001; 53:547–553.
36. Chang WH, Kortan P, Haber GB. Outcome in patients with bifurcation tumors who undergo unilateral versus bilateral hepatic duct drainage. Gastrointest Endosc 1998; 47:354–362.

Chapter 123

Capsule endoscopy

Paul J Fortun and C Paul Swain

KEY POINTS
• The main indication for capsule endoscopy is for the investigation of obscure gastrointestinal bleeding • Capsule endoscopy is superior to enteroscopy and small bowel radiology in the detection of small intestinal bleeding, but lacks therapeutic options • Abnormalities such as erosions and arteriovenous malformations are found in asymptomatic healthy volunteers. These findings in patients must therefore be interpreted cautiously and in the clinical context • The presence of an intestinal stricture is a contraindication to the procedure

INTRODUCTION

Capsule endoscopy in its current form arose from innovative technological developments in optics and integrated circuits that allowed the creation of a radiotelemetry capsule endoscope small enough to pass through the small bowel.[1,2] Wireless capsule video-endoscopy was first used in humans in 1999.[2] The capsule provides optical, colored, moving images from the mucosa of the entire small intestine. The small intestine accounts for three-quarters of the total length of the gastrointestinal tract and has a median length of 5.7 m in adults at autopsy. Although push enteroscopy can image the proximal small intestine to a variable extent beyond the ligament of Trietz, and ileoscopy via the colon examines a short length of ileum, most of the small intestine was previously imaged only indirectly by barium studies, or incompletely by push enteroscopy.

Capsule endoscopy allows the investigation of patients with suspected small intestinal disease, especially obscure gastrointestinal bleeding. The procedure, indications, contraindications, and limitations are discussed below.

DESCRIPTION OF TECHNIQUE

The capsule

The capsule (M2A; GivenImaging, Yoqneam, Israel) contains a video-imager, transmitter, light source, antenna, and batteries in a rounded cylindrical plastic container measuring 11×26 mm (Fig. 123.1). There is a clear optical dome-shaped window that allows the intestine to be illuminated by an array of six (formerly four) white light-emitting diodes (Fig. 123.2). Light passes through the dome, and the colored image is acquired as the light returns through the dome. The image is focused through a lens of short focal length with a wide angle on to the imager CMOS (complementary metal oxide silicon) chip as the optical window of the capsule sweeps past the gut wall, without requiring air inflation of the gut lumen. The video images are transmitted using radiotelemetry (operating in UHF at 432 MHz) to an array of eight aerials attached to the body, which allow image capture and are also used to calculate and indicate the position of the capsule in the body (Fig. 123.3). The aerials are similar to leads worn by patients undergoing electrocardiography or Holter evaluation. The capsule transmits images at a rate of two frames per second for more than 7 h, allowing the acquisition of over 50 000 images.

The procedure

Consent should specifically include an explanation that the capsule may become stuck in the small intestine, occasionally requiring surgical removal. Additionally, in approximately 15% of patients capsule endoscopy does not image the entire small intestine as the battery life may expire before the cecum is reached. Plain abdominal radiography may be performed within a few days if colonic images are seen and the capsule has not been seen to pass by the patient. Magnetic resonance imaging (MRI) should not be done until the capsule has been confirmed to have passed. The patient is nil by mouth for 12 h prior to ingesting the capsule.

Preparation: Colonoscopic bowel preparation may improve the quality of images in the ileum, which can appear rather dark (Fig. 123.4). However, there are few data to support one regimen versus another. The only exception is when capsule endoscopy is required to visualize the right colon; in this situation a colonic preparation is strongly recommended in order to maximize visualization potential. It is easiest to attach the eight aerial leads to the patient in the supine position. The aerial cable should be attached securely to the recorder and placed in the belt. The capsule is partially embedded in a small case containing a magnet, which inhibits capsule activation. Once removed from its case, the capsule is activated by the release of an internal magnetic switch. At this point the white light-emitting diodes starts to flash and the capsule begins to transmit images. It is helpful to check that a green light on the recorder is flashing in synchrony with the capsule prior to ingestion. Some investigators hold the capsule in front of the patient for several seconds so that the recorder may acquire a visual image that can further identify the patient if other records should become lost or incorrectly recorded.

Procedure: The patient can then swallow the capsule, usually with a few sips of water. Once the capsule is ingested, the patient should periodically check the flashing light on the recorder as well as the connection between the aerial and the recorder. The patient should report back immediately if the recorder stops flashing. Patients can ingest clear liquids immediately; however, they are asked *not to eat solids for 3 h* after swallowing the

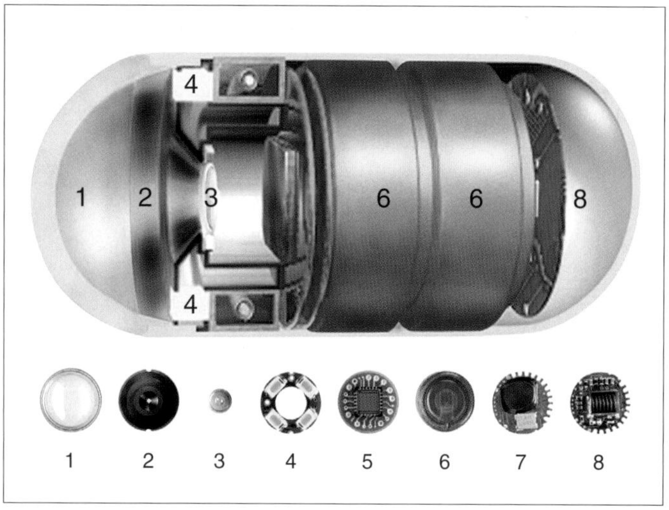

Fig. 123.1 Inside the capsule. 1, Optical dome; 2, lens holder; 3, lens; 4, illuminating light-emitting diodes (LEDs); 5, complementary metal oxide semiconductor (CMOS) imager; 6, battery; 7, applicator specific integrated circuit (ASIC) transmitter; 8, antenna. Courtesy of GivenImaging, Yoqneam, Israel.

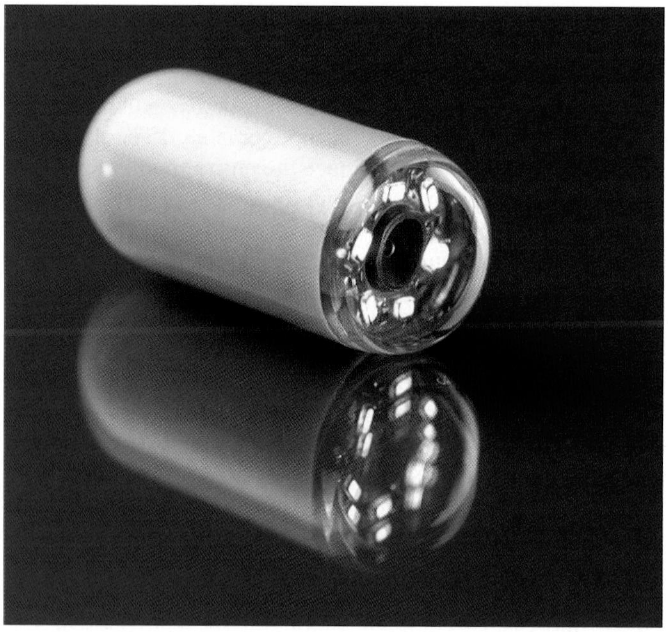

Fig. 123.2 The capsule. Courtesy of GivenImaging, Yoqneam, Israel.

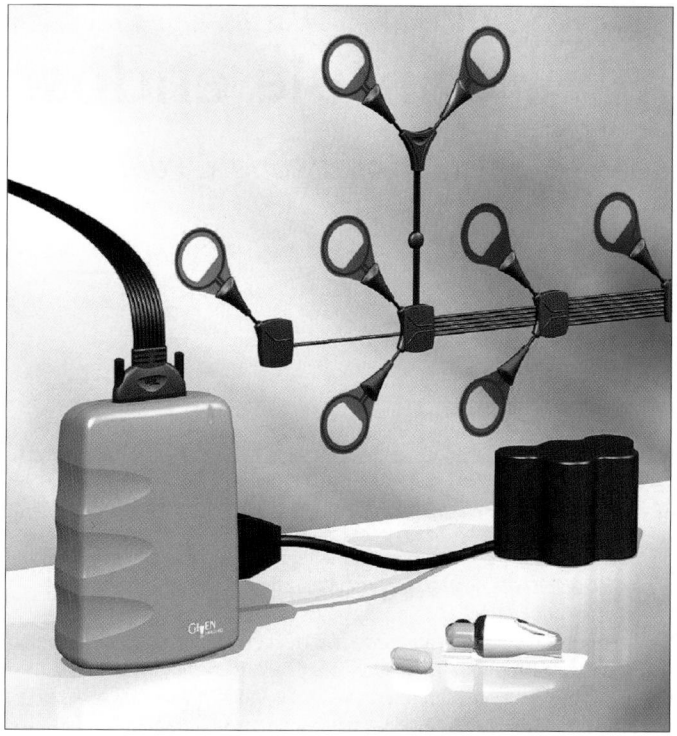

Fig. 123.3 Sensor array. Courtesy of GivenImaging, Yoqneam, Israel.

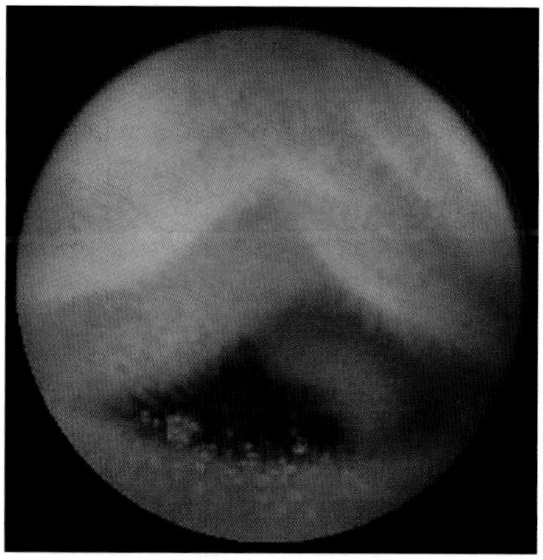

Fig. 123.4 Normal ileum.

capsule. They can remove the belt and aerial 8 h after swallowing the capsule, or when the recorder has stopped flashing. The recorder and its attached aerials are returned to the physician's office, but not the capsule itself, which is disposable.

Analysis: The images on the recorder are downloaded and processed prior to interpretation. Image analysis requires between 30 to 60 min. It is probably unwise to read all the images at the fastest of the three available speeds. It is helpful to save any unusual images as well as definite abnormalities as 'thumbnails' for more careful subsequent review. The points of entry into the stomach, duodenum and cecum are marked to enable the localization software to image the passage of the capsule inside the abdomen. Particular attention to abnormalities detected as blood (by the blood sensing algorithm) is required, and some investigators choose to start their evaluation at these sites. Others do not activate this software option until an entire viewing of the video has been completed, to avoid interpretation bias. Newer software places two adjacent images side by side to allow faster image analysis.

INDICATIONS

The capsule's main clinical application is in the investigation of obscure gastrointestinal bleeding.[3–5] Comparative prospective evaluations to other accepted modalities have been performed. Capsule endoscopy has been demonstrated to be superior to enteroscopy,[4–7] as well as small bowel radiologic studies.[8–10] Comparative studies with enteroscopy are summarized in Table 123.1.

Additionally, other studies have now demonstrated the value of capsule endoscopy compared to other imaging modalities in

TABLE 123.1 COMPARISON OF THE DIAGNOSTIC YIELD OF CAPSULE ENDOSCOPY AND PUSH ENTEROSCOPY IN THE DIAGNOSIS OF GASTROINTESTINAL BLEEDING

	Capsule endoscopy	Push enteroscopy
Mata et al. (2003)[11]	66%	19%
Mylonaki et al. (2003)[12]	68%	32%
Saurin et al. (2003)[13]	69%	38%
Lewis & Swain (2002)[14]	55%	30%
Ell et al. (2002)[15]	66%	28%

areas of Crohn's disease.[16] Capsule endoscopy has also proved useful in assessment of the extent of celiac disease, especially in nonresponsive cases. Other areas of interest to which capsule endoscopy has been applied are listed below:

- Nonsteroidal anti-inflammatory drug (NSAID) mucosal damage[17]
- Small intestinal polyposis due, for example, to Peutz-Jeghers disease
- Graft versus host disease
- Human immunodeficiency virus enteropathy
- Small bowel infections[18–20]
- Assessment of Meckel's diverticulum.[21]

Capsule endoscopy has proved highly effective in the diagnosis of small intestinal tumors and has altered the decisions about surgery for many patients. The advent of capsule endoscopy has altered the perception that endoscopy was fixed forever as a flexible tube-based technology that would remain an uncomfortable examination usually requiring sedation, performed mostly by doctors in hospitals and requiring substantial hand–eye control skills.

INDICATIONS/CONTRAINDICATIONS

ABSOLUTE INDICATIONS
- Recurrent or continued gastrointestinal bleeding in patients with negative gastroscopy, colonoscopy, and push enteroscopy findings.

STRONG INDICATIONS
- Recurrent or continued gastrointestinal bleeding in patients with negative gastroscopy and colonoscopy findings, especially if one or both of these examinations has been repeated by an experienced endoscopist.

EMERGING INDICATIONS REQUIRING FURTHER ASSESSMENT
- Symptoms or inflammatory markers suggesting Crohn's disease with negative imaging
- Investigation of unresponsive celiac disease
- Whipple's disease
- Graft versus host disease, HIV, intestinal parasitosis
- Peutz-Jeghers polyposis
- Small intestinal abnormalities on barium follow-through, enteroclysis, or CT
- Assessment of NSAID small intestinal damage

CONTRAINDICATIONS
- Presence of an intestinal stricture
- Small children

ROLE OF CAPSULE ENDOSCOPY IN OBSCURE GI BLEEDING

Obscure gastrointestinal bleeding is defined as recurrent or persistent iron deficiency anemia in which there is no visible bleeding and no source is found at a gastroscopy and colonoscopy. The adequacy of these examinations should be reviewed. In female patients a menstrual history is mandatory. Consider a gynecologic opinion, including pelvic ultrasonography and fecal occult blood testing prior to intensive investigation of the small intestine.

Repeat gastroscopy should be considered before any further investigations. One study evaluating push enteroscopy found that a significant proportion of patients (42%) referred for enteroscopy had lesions in the stomach or proximal duodenum that were missed at diagnostic endoscopy.[22]

Case review: The clinical history and any other investigations should be reviewed for hints about the possible location of the obscure bleeding. A list of the possible causes of small bowel bleeding is shown in Table 123.2. Age, location of any discomfort, length of history, color of blood seen by patient, presence of skin abnormalities, unexplained abnormal blood tests, weight loss, and previous history of malignancy (e.g., melanoma) should be used to focus the search (see Fig. 123.11). Investigation pathways can be constructed based on the age and symptoms of the patient.

Young male patients (10–25 years): A Meckel's scan should be performed. If positive, surgery should be undertaken without further imaging. Because the scans are frequently negative in such patients and bleeding from a Meckel's diverticulum accounts for bleeding in two-thirds of this group of patients, capsule examination could be the next step to look for this and other causes of bleeding, such as Crohn's disease. If the capsule examination is negative, an early laparoscopy should still be considered.

Older patients: Specific questioning about aspirin or NSAID use, site of abdominal pain if any, history of previous treatment for malignancy (e.g., melanoma), duration of symptoms, and time since last bleed should influence the choice and order of investigations. If aged between 40 and 65 years, with a short history of recurrent anemia, continuous bleeding or transfusion requirement, or weight loss and raised inflammatory markers, a more intensive investigational algorithm should be followed with early push enteroscopy or capsule examination. Once again, the need for repeat gastroscopy and/or colonoscopy should be considered. Capsule endoscopy is likely to find a source of bleeding if there is a short history and the anemia is transfusion dependent (see Figs 123.5 and 123.6).

LIMITATIONS AND COMPLICATIONS

Quality of data: The images from the esophagus, stomach, and colon are not as good as those acquired during conventional endoscopy, but may occasionally show pathology in these areas. An esophageal capsule (with two imagers, back and front) is due to be released. The images from the small intestine are inferior to video push enteroscopic views because the capsule cannot wash, be pulled back to re-examine a possible abnormality, take biopsies, or deliver therapy. With its current acquisition time of 7–8 h, the capsule fails to provide images from the cecum about 15% of the time. In consequence, an indeterminate length of small intestine remains unexamined.

TABLE 123.2 POSSIBLE CAUSES OF SMALL BOWEL BLEEDING

- Angiodysplasia and vascular malformations (Fig. 123.5)
- NSAID enteropathy (Fig. 123.6)
- Erosive jejunitis
- Diverticula
- Crohn's disease (Fig. 123.7)
- Jejunal or ileal ulceration – idiopathic, NSAID-induced, etc. (Fig. 123.8)
- Intussusception
- Small intestinal tumors (Fig. 123.9)
- Ischemic enteropathy
- Graft versus host disease
- Cytomegalovirus infection
- Aortoenteric fistula
- Blue rubber bleb syndrome (Fig. 123.10)

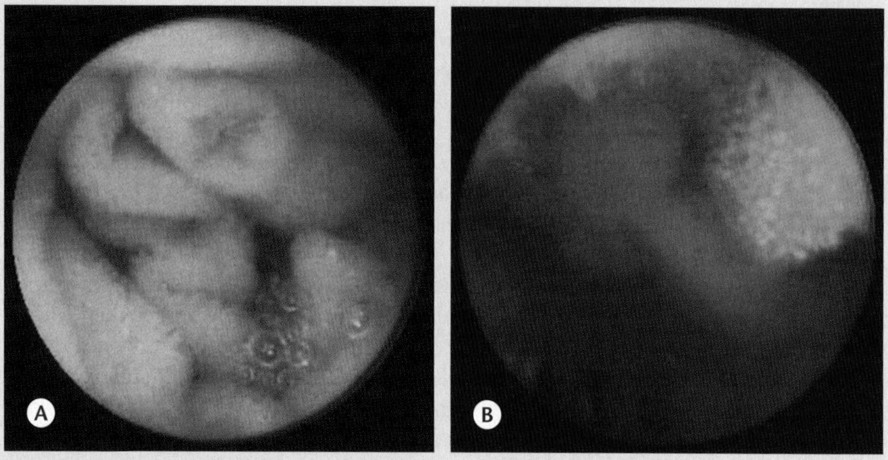

Fig. 123.5 A. Ileal angiodysplasia. B. Active small bowel bleeding.

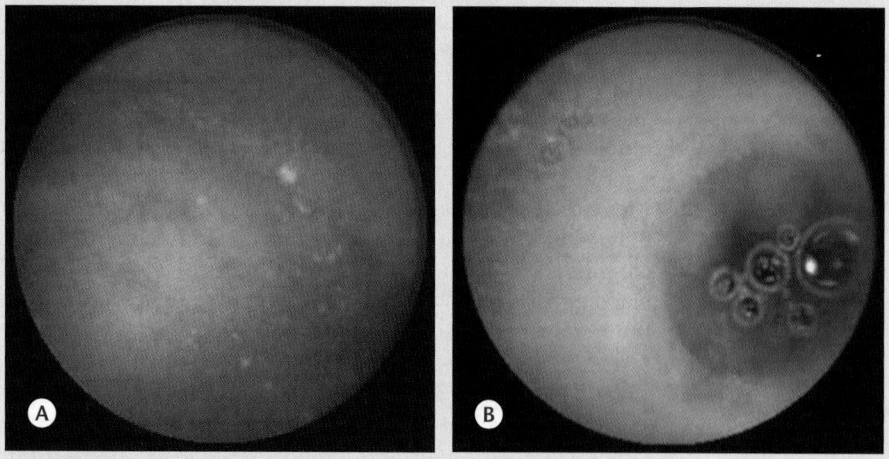

Fig. 123.6 A. Ileal erosions secondary to aspirin. B. NSAID-associated stricture.

TABLE 123.2 POSSIBLE CAUSES OF SMALL BOWEL BLEEDING—cont'd

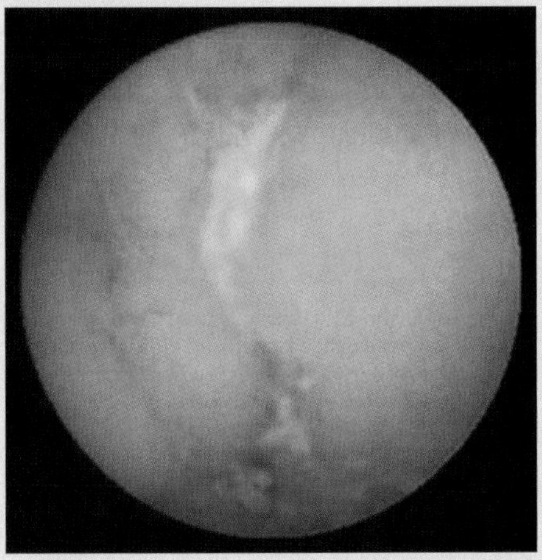

Fig. 123.7 Crohn's disease.

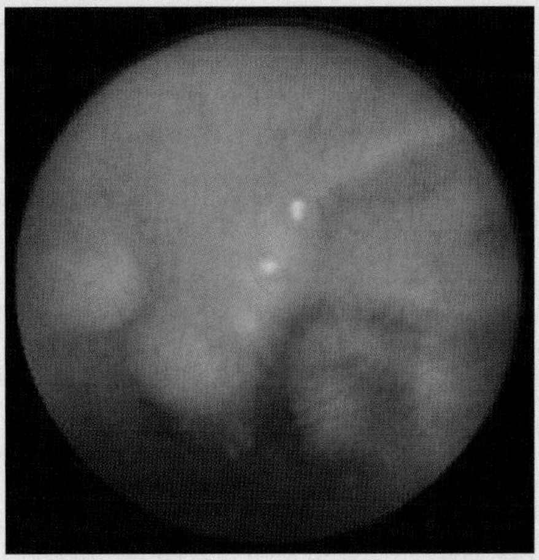

Fig. 123.9 Small bowel polyps in a patient with familial adenomatous polyposis.

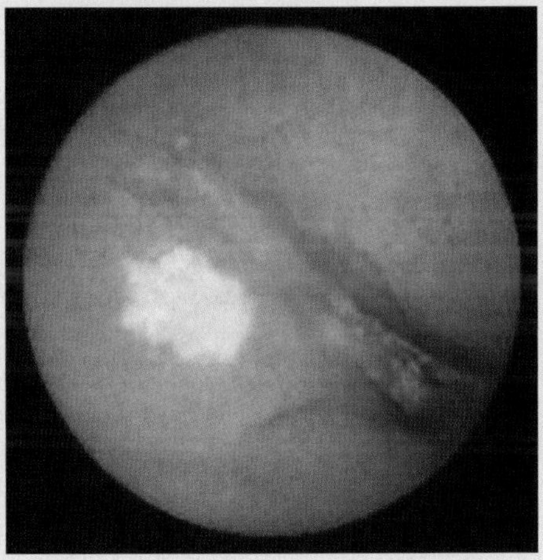

Fig. 123.8 Ileal ulceration.

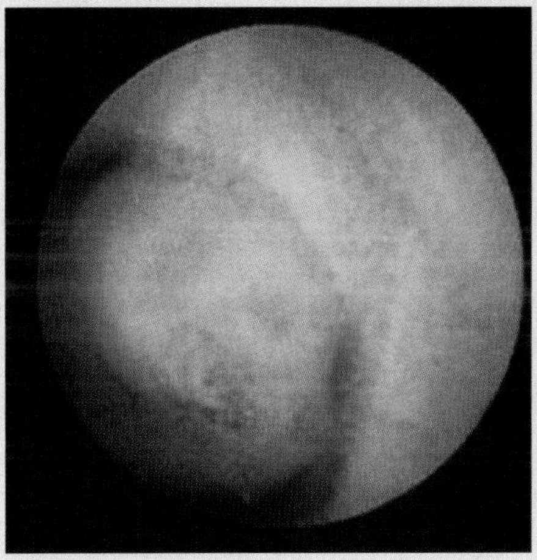

Fig. 123.10 Blue rubber bleb syndrome.

Practical limitations: A few patients, especially children, have difficulty swallowing the capsule. Occasionally patients retain it for prolonged periods in the stomach, as there is a very wide range of 'normal' gastric emptying times. Images may be poor in patients with morbid obesity. It may take a long time to interpret the images; skill and experience are required.

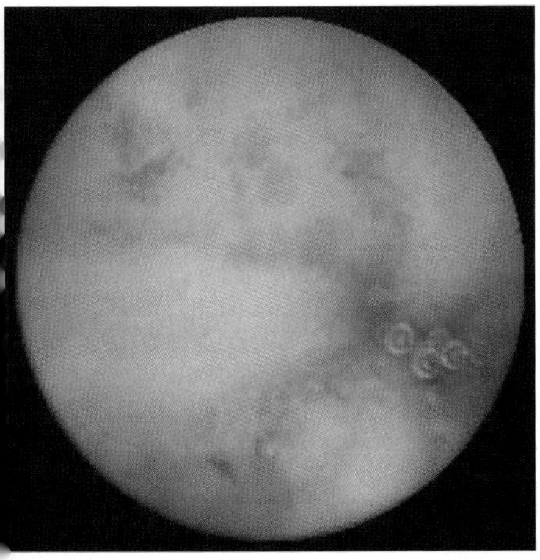

Fig. 123.11 Small bowel changes after radiotherapy for lymphoma.

Interpretation: Many of the findings may be of unknown significance, or their relevance to the etiology of obscure gastrointestinal bleeding, for example, uncertain. Researchers[23] have found a high incidence in patients with obscure bleeding, especially older patients (57% in those aged under 40 years; 51% in those over 40 years old), but a large number of such lesions are also found in controls (30% in subjects under 40 years; 51% in those over 40 years). Similarly, a large number of background small bowel lesions were seen in healthy volunteers (13.8%) prior to evaluating the effects of NSAID and cyclo-oxygenase-2-specific inhibitors.[24]

Pathology may be seen on only a single frame. As the capsule may travel looking forwards or backwards, it may not observe pathology in an expected direction. Images in lower small intestine are often rather dark. The recurring cost of the capsule as a disposable item and the relatively lengthy examination times require specific funding and organizational strategies.

Impaction: The main complication is that the capsule may become impacted in strictures[25] or diverticula.[26] Most commonly, capsule impaction is symptomless. Sometimes capsule impaction may be a good outcome, leading to the identification of diverticula or strictures, which can be resected. If the capsule can be reached by an endoscope, a snare with a net is the most useful retrieval tool, as the capsule is more difficult to grasp with a stone basket or simple snare. Inadvertent MRI might cause complications because the capsule will respond to a magnetic field. If a capsule examination does not provide colonic images and the patient does not see the capsule in the toilet, it might be sensible to perform plain abdominal radiography to check for passage. Pacemakers are probably not a contraindication. Capsule endoscopy has been approved by the US Food and Drug Administration for use in children aged over 10 years.

SOURCES OF INFORMATION FOR PATIENTS AND DOCTORS

http://www.acg.gi.org/patients/gihealth/smallbowel.asp

REFERENCES

1. Gong F, Mills TN, Swain CP. Wireless endoscopy. Gastrointest Endosc 2000; 51:725–729.
2. Iddan G, Meron G, Glukovsky, Swain P. Wireless capsule endoscopy. Nature 2000; 405:417.
3. Appleyard M, Fireman Z, Glukhovsky A et al. A randomized trial comparing wireless capsule endoscopy with push enteroscopy for the detection of small-bowel lesions. Gastroenterology 2000; 119:1431–1438.
4. Lewis BS, Swain P. Capsule endoscopy in the evaluation of patients with suspected small intestinal bleeding: Results of a pilot study (comment). Gastrointest Endosc 2002; 56:349–353.
5. Ell C, Remke S, May A, Helou L, Henrich R, Mayer G. The first prospective controlled trial comparing wireless capsule endoscopy with push enteroscopy in chronic gastrointestinal bleeding. Endoscopy 2002; 34:685–689.
6. Mylonaki M, Fritscher-Ravens A, Swain P. Wireless capsule endoscopy: a comparison with push enteroscopy in patients with gastroscopy and colonoscopy negative gastrointestinal bleeding. Gut 2003; 52:1122–1126.
7. Pennazio M, Santucci R, Rondonotti E et al. Outcome of patients with obscure gastrointestinal bleeding after capsule endoscopy: report of 100 consecutive cases. Gastroenterology 2004; 216:643–653.
8. Liangpunsakul S, Chadalawada V, Rex DK, Maglinte D, Lappas J. Wireless capsule endoscopy detects small bowel ulcers in patients with normal results from state of the art enteroclysis. Am J Gastroenterol 2003; 98:1295–1298.
9. Scapa E, Jacob H, Lewkowicz S et al. Initial experience of wireless-capsule endoscopy for evaluating occult gastrointestinal bleeding and suspected small bowel pathology. Am J Gastroenterol 2002; 97:2776–2779.
10. Costamagna G, Shah SK, Riccioni ME et al. A prospective trial comparing small bowel radiographs and video capsule endoscopy for suspected small bowel disease (comment). Gastroenterology 2002; 123:999–1005.
11. Mata A, Llach J, Bordas JM et al. Role of capsule endoscopy in patients with obscure digestive bleeding. Gastroenterol Hepatol 2003; 26:619–623.
12. Mylonaki M, Fritscher-Ravens A, Swain P. Wireless capsule endoscopy: a comparison with push enteroscopy in patients with gastroscopy and colonoscopy negative gastrointestinal bleeding. Gut 2003; 52:1122–1126.
13. Saurin JC, Delvaux M, Gaudin JL et al. Diagnostic value of endoscopic capsule in patients with obscure digestive bleeding: blinded comparison with push enteroscopy. Endoscopy 2003; 35:576–584.
14. Lewis BS, Swain P. Capsule endoscopy in the evaluation of patients with suspected small intestinal bleeding: results of a pilot study. Gastrointest Endosc 2002; 56:349–353.
15. Ell C, Remke S, May A et al. The first prospective controlled trial comparing wireless capsule endoscopy with push enteroscopy in chronic gastrointestinal bleeding. Endoscopy 2002; 34:685–689.
16. Fireman Z, Mahajna E, Broide E et al. Diagnosing small bowel Crohn's disease with wireless capsule endoscopy (comment). Gut 2003; 52:390–392.
17. Chutkan R, Toubia N. Effect of nonsteroidal anti-inflammatory drugs on the gastrointestinal tract: diagnosis by wireless capsule endoscopy. Gastrointest Endosc Clin N Am 2004; 14:67–85.
18. Appleyard M, Glukhovsky A, Swain P. Wireless-capsule diagnostic endoscopy for recurrent small-bowel bleeding. N Engl J Med 2001; 344:232–233.
19. Reddy DN, Sriram PV, Rao GV, Reddy DB. Capsule endoscopy appearances of small-bowel tuberculosis. Endoscopy 2003; 35:99.
20. Soares J, Lopes L, Villas-Boas G, Pinho C. Ascariasis observed by wireless-capsule endoscopy. Endoscopy 2003; 35:194.
21. Mylonaki M, MacLean D, Fritscher-Ravens A, Swain P. Wireless capsule endoscopic detection of Meckel's diverticulum after nondiagnostic surgery. Endoscopy 2002; 34:1018–1020.
22. Hayat M, Axon AT, O'Mahony S. Diagnostic yield and effect on clinical outcomes of push enteroscopy in suspected small-bowel bleeding. Endoscopy 2000; 32:369–372.
23. Mascarenhas-Saraiva MN, Lopes LM, Villas-Boas G. Small bowel arteriovenous malformations seen by wireless capsule endoscopy. Differences in their prevalence between bleeders and non-bleeders. Gut 2003; 52:A97.
24. Goldstein JL, Eisen G, Lewis B et al. Celecoxib is associated with fewer small bowel lesions than naproxen plus omeprazole in healthy subjects as determined by capsule endoscopy. Gut 2003; (Suppl VI):A16.
25. Jonnalagadda S, Prakesh C. Intestinal strictures can impede wireless capsule enteroscopy. Gastrointest Endosc 2003; 57:418–420.
26. Van Gossum A, Hittelet A, Schmit A et al. A prospective comparative study of push and wireless capsule enteroscopy in patients with obscure digestive bleeding. Acta Gastroenterol Belg 2003; 66:199–205.

Chapter 124

Percutaneous ultrasound

William Lees

KEY POINTS

- Technological advances have improved image resolution and reduced operator dependence
- Doppler ultrasound is more sensitive than CT or MRI in examining portal blood flow
- Hemangiomas and cysts can be reliably confirmed on ultrasound; fibrosis without cirrhosis is not detectable
- Contrast-enhanced ultrasound is at least as sensitive as CT or MRI in detection of colorectal liver metastases and Klatskin tumors
- Doppler ultrasound is helpful in staging pancreatic tumors whereas endoscopic ultrasound is useful in visualizing small tumors (e.g., ampullary tumors or cholangiocarcinoma)
- Doppler ultrasound is of value in detecting active inflammatory bowel disease

INTRODUCTION

Like the other major imaging techniques, ultrasound has developed very rapidly in the past few years, resulting in ultrasound machines that are much easier to use and produce clearer, artifact-free images that can be obtained by almost anyone. This has greatly reduced the operator dependence that has always limited the use of the technology. Today, a perfect image is available at the touch of a button.

Ultrasound is harmless, portable, and can be performed at the patient's bedside (Fig. 124.1). This means that it is often the first test to be applied to patients with abdominal symptoms. Whilst it may lack the diagnostic power of computed tomography (CT) or magnetic resonance imaging (MRI), it will usually clarify the clinical questions and point the way to an accurate diagnosis. A normal ultrasound of good quality is rarely wrong and can be relied upon to exclude major disease.[1–4]

RECENT ADVANCES IN ULTRASOUND TECHNOLOGY

All of radiology has been driven by technology in the past 20 years. Computing power has doubled every 18 months over this period. The number of active channels in an imaging system (the number of measurements going into a scan reconstruction) has doubled every 3 years (Fig. 124.2). This applies to ultrasound, CT, and MRI and is one reason why there has been progress on all imaging fronts.

Ultrasound has developed in several ways:

- More channels in a system with more computing power means better image resolution and less artifact.
- The cost per channel has diminished as the channel number has increased. Thus, it is possible to build a basic ultrasound system very cheaply; hand-held machines with excellent image quality are now available and have the possibility to spread the availability of ultrasound to every physician and surgeon. Ultrasound as the stethoscope of the future has finally arrived.
- The other major advance is the development of ultrasound contrast agents.[5] Currently, microbubbles of a stable gas such as a perfluorocarbon are used, which are injected intravenously and stay within the blood pool. They are typically 2–5 μm in diameter and resonate strongly in an ultrasound beam. Physical analysis of their properties has shown that their response to insonation is nonlinear.[6,7] That is, insonated at 2 MHz they produce a signal response at harmonic frequencies of 4 MHz and above.

By tuning the ultrasound system it is possible to amplify this nonlinear response selectively to gain signals from the contrast agent only and to suppress the normal tissue signal.[8] Very high-contrast ratios can be obtained in this way and a fortuitous observation has been that the microbubbles are trapped in the sinusoids and Kupfer cells of the liver for up to 1 h to produce a very high signal from normal liver with virtually no signal from the tumor.[6,9]

Modern transducers have sufficient sensitivity and bandwidth to exploit the nonlinear physics of ultrasound in tissue. The massive increase in available computing power has also enabled intelligence within the machine, greatly reducing operator dependence. A good ultrasound image is now available at the touch of a button.

ULTRASOUND OF THE LIVER

Chronic liver disease

The presence of fat, iron, or collagen within the liver alters its acoustic properties, particularly the echogenicity of the parenchyma and the attenuation of the ultrasound pulse. This can be recognized by comparing the liver signal to the spleen or renal cortex.

Fibrosis without cirrhosis is not detectable, but ultrasound is sensitive to established cirrhosis using relative echogenicity, increased attenuation, and visualization of regenerative nodules.[10] This is best seen using a small parts high-frequency probe to study the surface of the liver. New techniques such as spatial compounding show the real structure of the liver, not just a random speckle pattern (Figs 124.3–124.6). Diagnosis of different types of cirrhosis is generally not possible, although some causes such as schistosomiasis produce characteristic patterns.

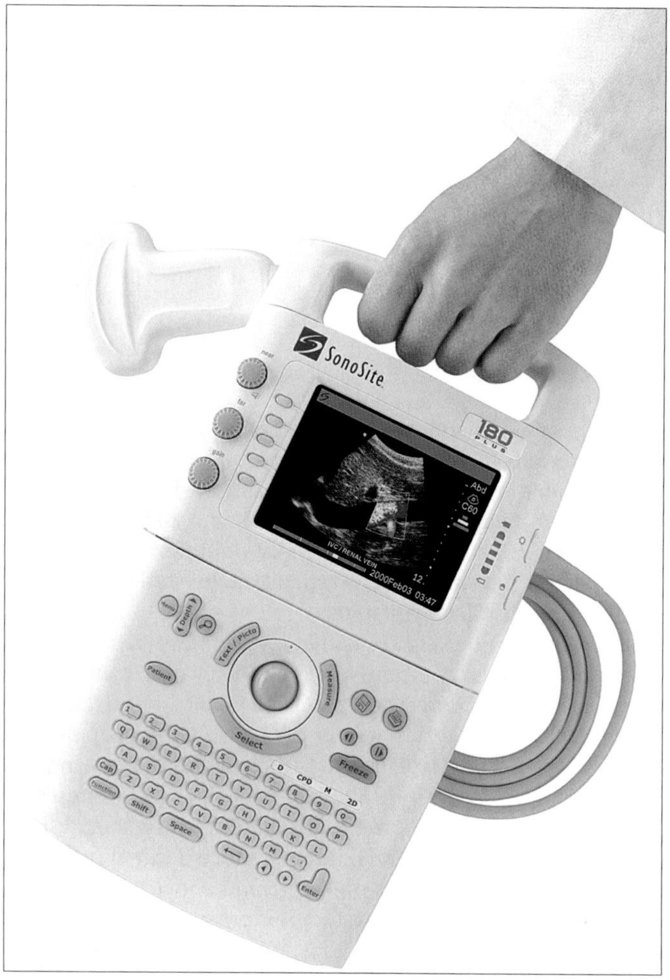

Fig. 124.1 Hand-held ultrasound machine. A hand-held ultrasound machine of the type in use at the Middlesex Hospital. Courtesy of SonoSite.

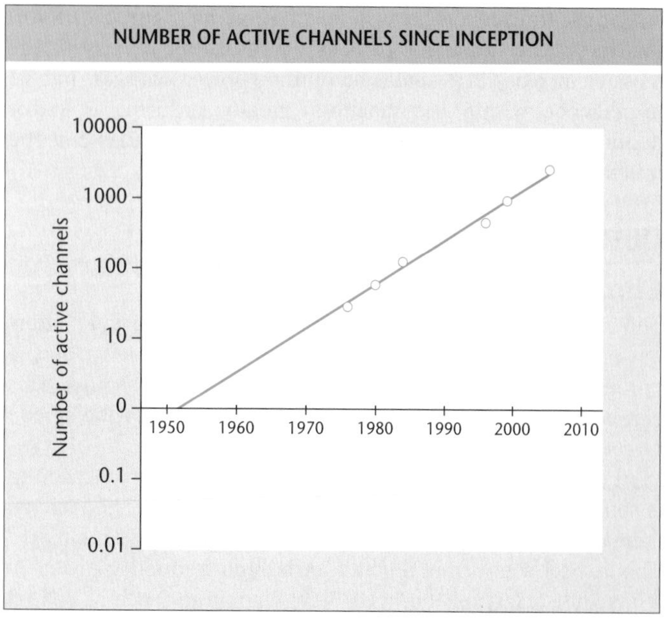

Fig. 124.2 Number of active channels since inception. A log plot of the number of active measurement channels in typical ultrasound systems since the inception of clinical ultrasound in 1952.

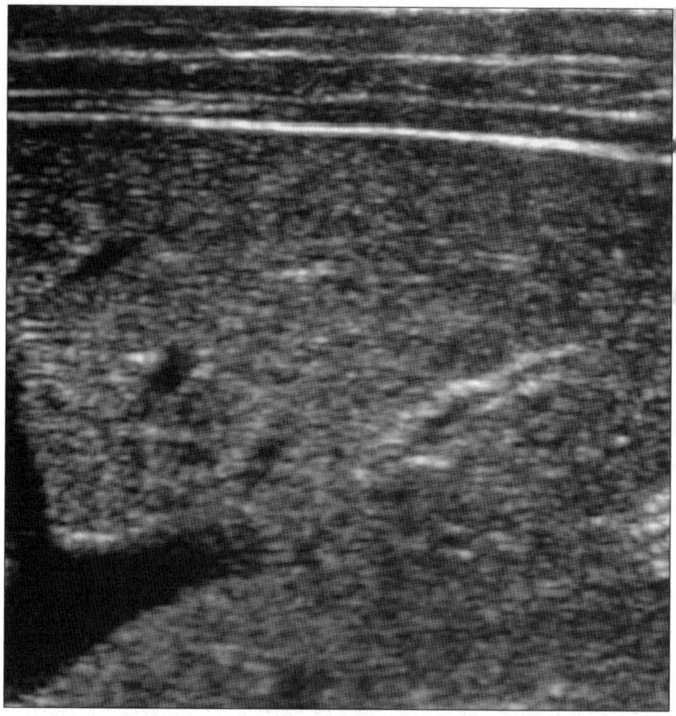

Fig. 124.3 Ultrasound scan of the normal liver with spatial compounding. This development reduces speckle noise in the image and shows much more real structure.

Using Doppler imaging, the blood flow in the hepatic and portal veins and in the hepatic arteries can be characterized.[11] Many attempts to quantify hepatic blood flow with ultrasound have ended in failure and confusion largely because flow values without pressure measurements are not very useful.[12]

Doppler studies of the portal vein show flow direction with greater sensitivity than CT or MRI, and even where the forward

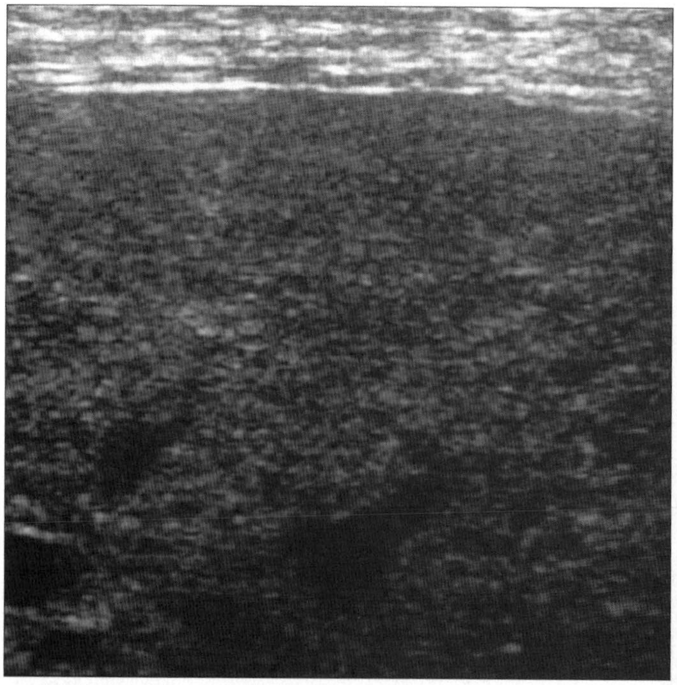

Fig. 124.4 Spatial compounding. A micronodular cirrhosis imaged using spatial compounding.

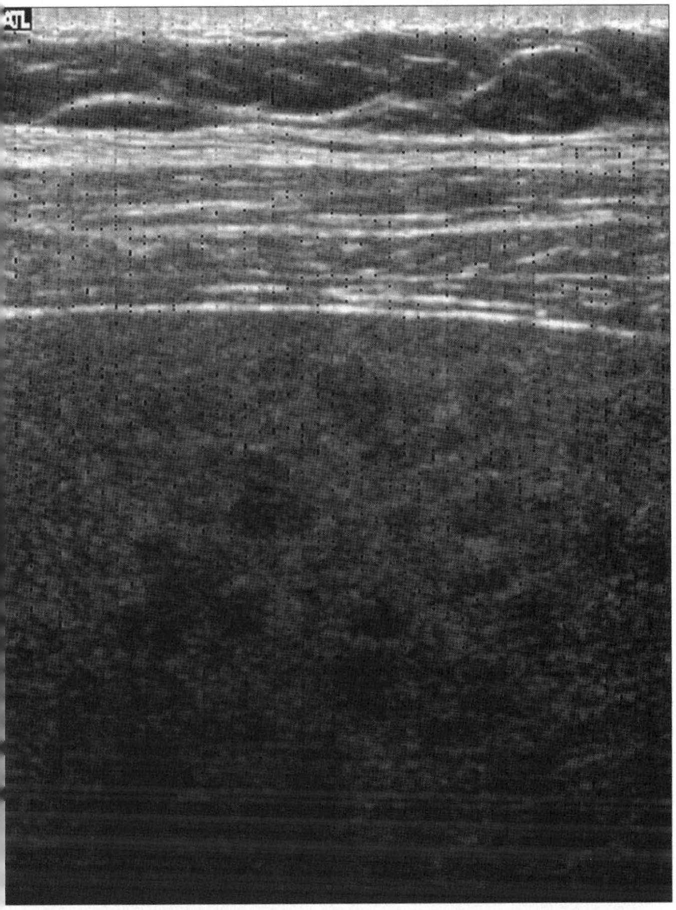

Fig. 124.5 Nodular regeneration seen with spatial compounding.

flow in the portal vein is zero Doppler ultrasound shows flow variation with respiration, thus distinguishing low flow from thrombosis. A combination of Doppler methods and ultrasound contrast agents (see below) are very effective in diagnosing Budd-Chiari syndrome. Ultrasound contrast agents can also be used to measure hepatic transit times, which promises to be highly sensitive to early cirrhosis.

Varices can be seen at the porta hepatis and in relation to the spleen and pancreas. After transjugular portosystemic shunt (TIPS) Doppler studies can show stent patency and by measuring the velocity gradient along the TIPS give an idea of the degree of portosystemic shunting. After hepatic transplantation Doppler imaging is vital in showing vessel patency but is not good at showing acute rejection.

Acute hepatitis

The ultrasound features of an active hepatitis are:

- liver swelling with attenuation of the hepatic veins;
- reduced parenchymal echogenicity; and
- edema of the gallbladder wall.

None of these signs are specific but can be useful in a clinical context.[13,14]

Focal liver disease

Hepatocellular carcinoma

Early hepatocellular carcinoma (HCC) can now be effectively treated in a number of ways, but early detection is key to effective treatment. Patients with cirrhosis need to be evaluated at 3- to 6-monthly intervals and the only economical way to do this is with ultrasound even though CT or MRI may be technically better.

Ultrasound is very reliable in picking up HCC bigger than 2 cm in diameter. Smaller lesions are detected frequently but are difficult to distinguish from regenerative nodules (Fig. 124.7 and Fig. 124.8). Color or power Doppler techniques are not sensitive enough in small lesions to make the distinction but ultrasound contrast can be used in a manner analogous to CT contrast to image arterial and portal venous phases. Early arterial phase enhancement with washout in the portal venous phase is indicative of malignancy (see Fig. 124.6). A number of studies have shown that contrast-enhanced ultrasound yields results similar to multislice CT.[15]

It is still debated whether ultrasound contrast should be used in routine screening studies for HCC.[16] In my institution we routinely scan all HCV cirrhotics every 6 months using ultrasound contrast. Two years into this study we have picked up four HCCs on contrast-enhanced scans that were not visible on the unenhanced scans (Fig. 124.9 and Fig. 124.10). This increased sensitivity has been obtained at the expense of some false positives and an increase in our biopsy rates. A similar study recently performed at the Hammersmith Hospital (London, UK) has shown no significant benefit in screening with contrast.

Other liver tumors

Hemangiomas and cysts are so common as to be an everyday occurrence in the ultrasound department. An experienced radiologist should be able to diagnose them with near complete confidence from their characteristic appearances (Fig. 124.11). The only problems arise with hemangiomas larger than 5 cm, which may appear very heterogeneous or in patients with known neuroendocrine tumors whose metastases can look very similar to hemangiomas.[17] A dynamic study with ultrasound contrast will show diagnostic 'blobby' peripheral enhancement in the arterial phase as in CT.

Focal nodular hyperplasia (FNH) is the second most common liver tumor and is thought to be an overgrowth of normal liver tissue in response to an underlying arteriovenous (A-V) malformation. Sometimes, guided liver biopsies of very large FNH can come back as normal liver tissue to the embarrassment of the radiologist. The ultrasound characteristics are a subcapsular mass with mass effect but with normal liver echogenicity. The key to the diagnosis is the increased blood supply usually by a

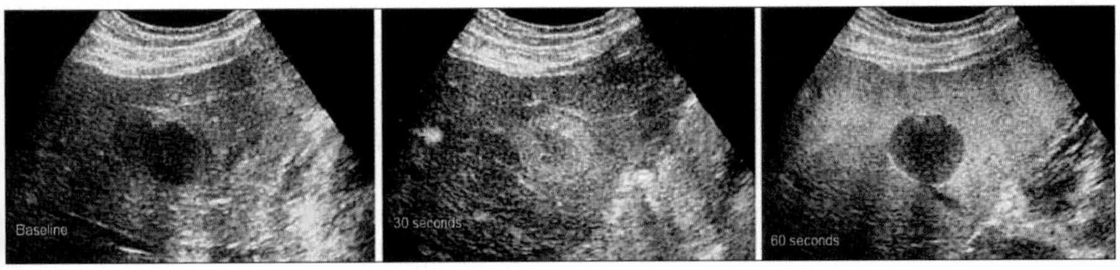

Fig. 124.6 An HCC enhanced with ultrasound contrast. There is strong enhancement in the arterial phase with early washout.

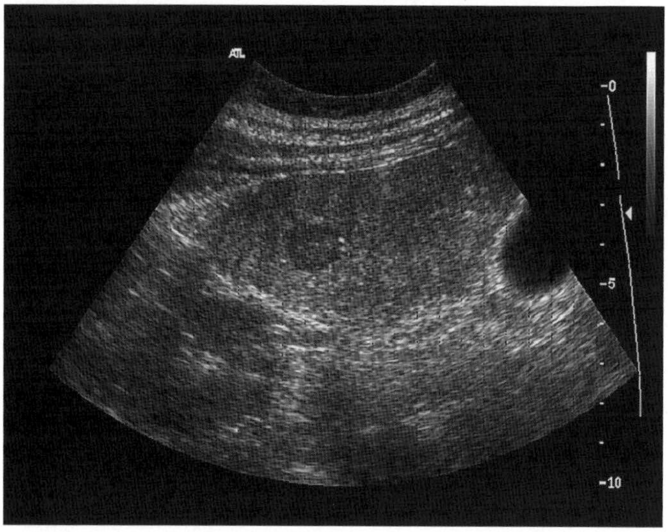

Fig. 124.7 Detection of HCC. A small screen detected HCC; seen only after administration of ultrasound contrast.

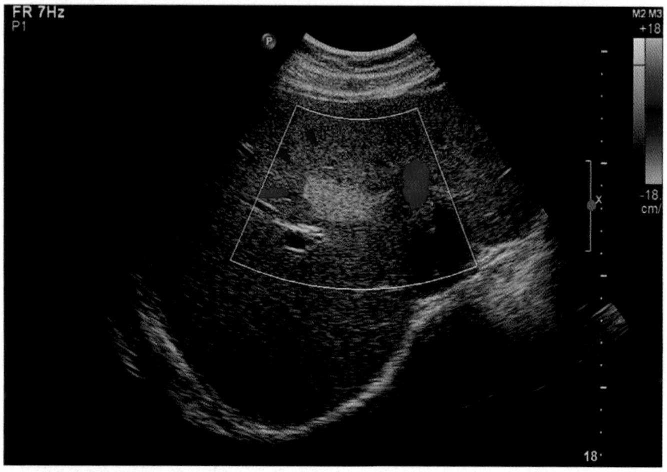

Fig. 124.8 A typical small hemangioma.

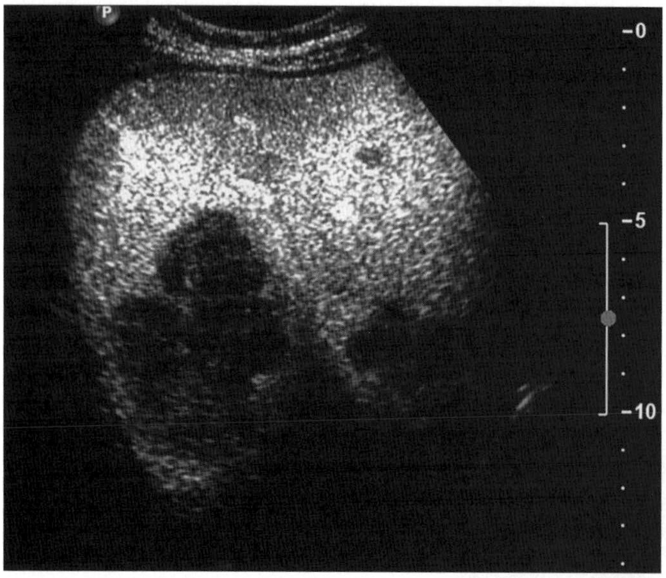

Fig. 124.9 Delayed pulse inversion imaging. Contrast-enhanced colorectal cancer liver metastases seen with delayed pulse inversion imaging at low mechanical index.

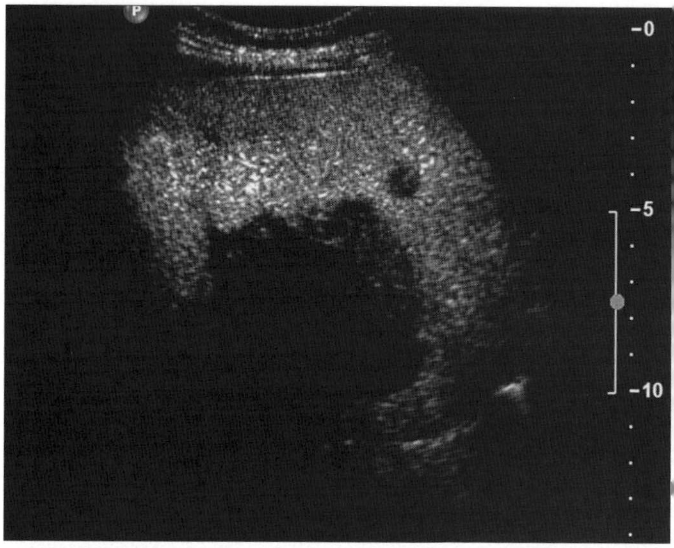

Fig. 124.10 Satellite nodule. Same study as Fig. 124.9 showing a typical satellite nodule.

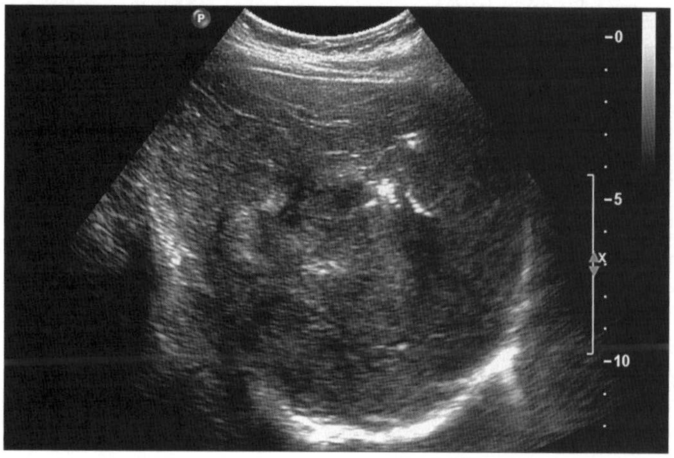

Fig. 124.11 A hemangioma. Ultrasound contrast shows typical peripheral arterial phases enhancement.

single large vessel radiating spokes to the periphery. This is in contrast to a hepatic adenoma or HCC where the blood supply is from the periphery to the center. The central scar is difficult to identify without the use of ultrasound contrast. Unfortunately, only half of FNH show the characteristic features; the central scar is always present but may be less than 1 mm thick on histology. Where doubt remains, corroboration with MRI is needed.

Liver metastases from most primary tumors are poorly echogenic and show a halo of even lower echogenicity. This appearance is almost pathognomonic for metastases and biopsy confirmation is rarely required.[18] Some metastases are hyperechoic, typically neuroendocrine metastases (Fig. 124.12). Ultrasound is exquisitely sensitive to these and may demonstrate dozens of tumors whereas CT and MRI show only a few. Hemangiomas are rarely present in such numbers and moreover look different.

Metastases from colorectal cancer have presented the most difficulty for ultrasound hitherto. The literature reports a sensitivity of 60–80% compared with 80–90% for MRI. The lesions can be isoechoic with normal liver and often have very ill-defined margins with small satellite lesions around the periphery. Demonstration of all lesions and their positions is essential to manage-

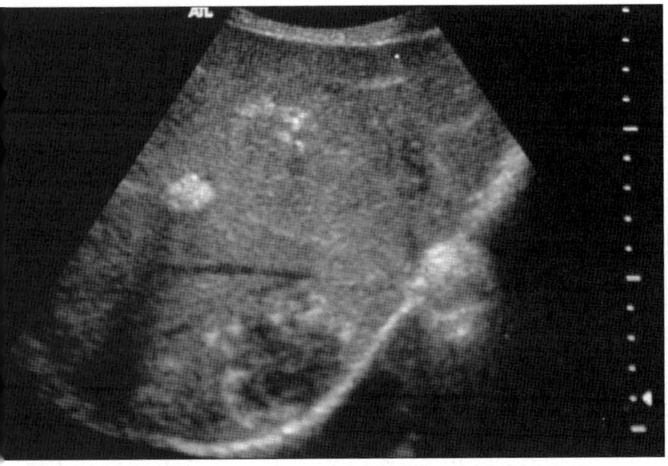

Fig. 124.12 **Large liver tumor.** A large liver tumor scanned with spatial compounding and speckle-reducing image processing.

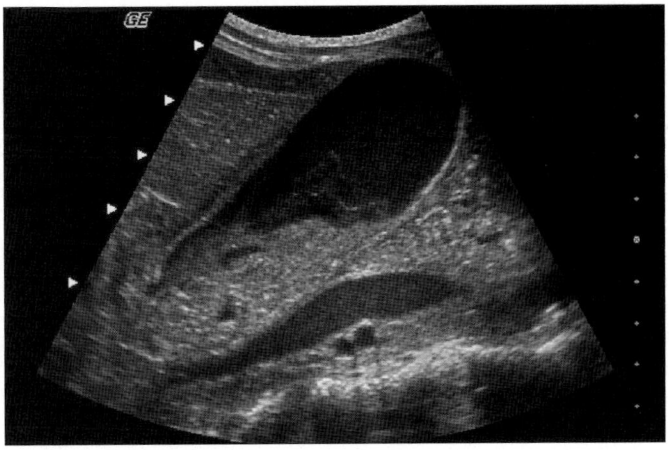

Fig. 124.13 **CBD stone.**

ment and ultrasound previously has simply not been good enough. In our cancer network the protocol calls for a CT scan every 6 months for 2 years after primary resection. Analysis of our data has shown that over 90% of patients with colorectal cancer who ultimately develop liver metastases will present within 2 years.

Contrast-enhanced ultrasound

The situation has changed dramatically with the advent of ultrasound contrast and the new imaging modes. Contrast-enhanced ultrasound is at least as sensitive as CT and MRI and is often more so. Ultrasound contrast has transformed the situation but a poor ultrasound subject remains difficult. Some areas of the liver can be hard to access and contrast does not change this. We still maintain a 6-monthly CT as the basis of our follow-up but every patient should receive an ultrasound contrast study prior to therapy either by resection or RF ablation.

ULTRASOUND OF THE BILIARY SYSTEM

Ultrasound is very sensitive to the presence of fluid and hence dilated bile ducts are obvious within the liver.[19] The extrahepatic biliary tree can be more difficult to visualize particularly at the ampulla of Vater. An experienced operator can use oral fluid loads and careful positioning to displace gas from the duodenum to visualize the distal common bile duct but this only emphasizes the operator dependence of ultrasound as only experts can achieve an 80–90% detection rate for CBD stones.[20,21] Demonstration of biliary dilatation is by measurement and thus inherently reliable (Fig. 124.13).

Klatskin tumors present a difficult challenge.[22] The tumor may be small and may infiltrate along the bile duct wall with no significant mass effect (Fig. 124.14). We have recently performed a study using contrast-enhanced ultrasound to delineate Klatskin tumors. This proved to be significantly better than CT and equal to MRI in showing the tumor mass and better than both techniques for showing liver parenchymal involvement, a vital feature in planning surgery (Fig. 124.15).

The gallbladder is readily accessible to ultrasound and clinicians should expect 100% accuracy in the diagnosis of gallstones, characterized by echogenic lesions that cast an acoustic shadow,[23,24] and an accuracy of >95% in the diagnosis of acute cholecystitis[25–27] (see Fig. 124.16 and Fig. 124.17). Gallbladder polyps are very common and of no clinical significance.[28,29] Most are small and composed of cholesterol and are easy to diagnose. Adenomatous polyps are larger and show internal blood flow on Doppler ultrasound. They are significant, carrying a similar risk of malignancy to colonic polyps.[30] The introduction of laparoscopic cholecystectomy presented some challenges to the preop ultrasound assessment.[30] However, we now know that a normal caliber common bile duct on ultrasound combined with normal liver function tests (LFTs) carries a near zero risk of CBD stones being present.

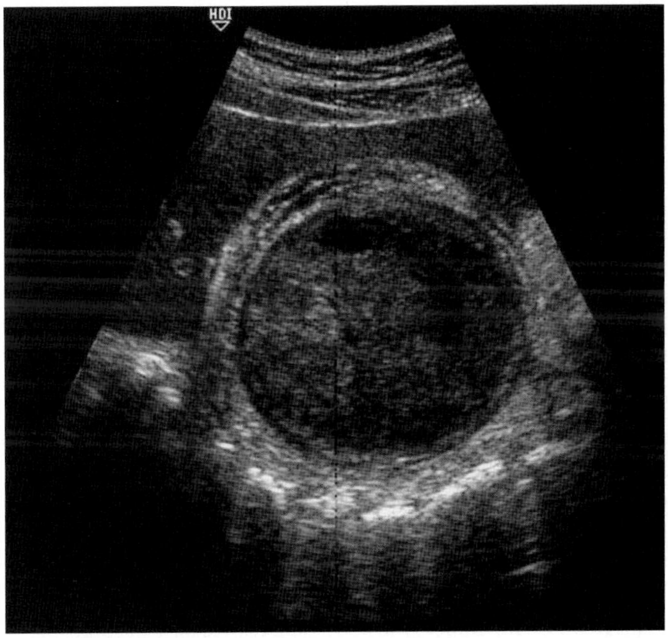

Fig. 124.14 **Klatskin tumor.** Note the linear infiltration along the wall of the bile duct and the absence of a mass effect.

ULTRASOUND OF THE PANCREAS

Pancreatic ultrasound is overshadowed by CT and MRI but is much underrated. Very often all the information we need to manage the patient is to be found on the ultrasound scan. Which,

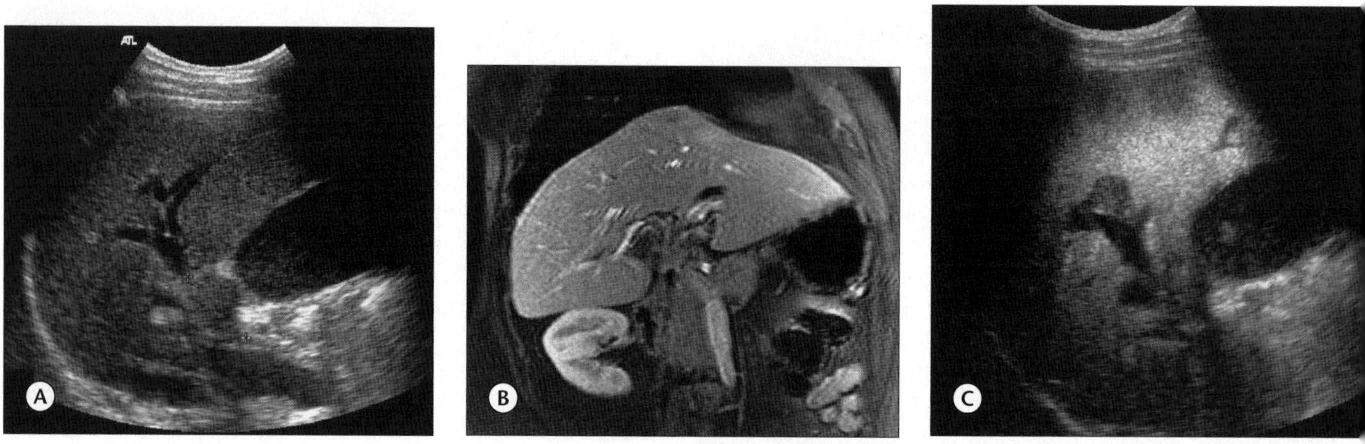

Fig. 124.15 A hilar cholangiocarcinoma. A. Baseline ultrasound of a small hilar cholangiocarcinoma. **B.** T1-weighted MRI with fat saturation shows the tumor but fails to accurately delineate its boundaries. **C.** Contrast-enhanced ultrasound shows tumor infiltrating the liver parenchyma.

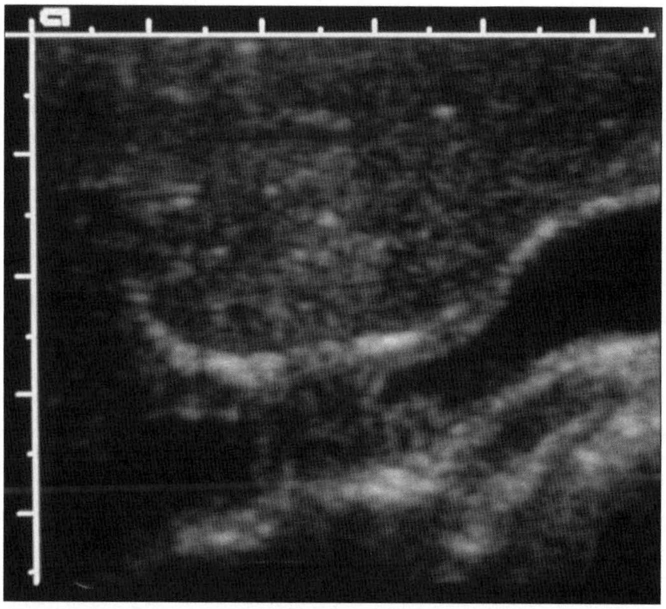

Fig. 124.16 Acute cholecystitis. Longitudinal section of acute cholecystitis.

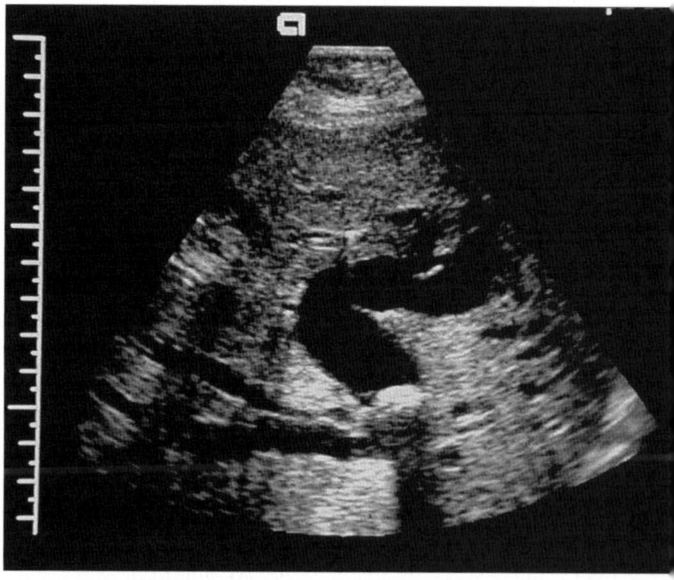

Fig. 124.17 Acute cholecystitis cross-section. Note wall thickening, separation of the layers of the wall, and fluid in the hepatocholecystic space.

then, is the best modality for investigating the pancreas? Ultrasound, CT, and MRI are each best roughly one-third of the time. Usually, all three techniques are done since it is hard to predict which method will provide the most information in individual patients.[31,32]

Pancreatic ductal adenocarcinoma is usually poorly echogenic and easily seen in most patients, particularly in the head of the pancreas where most tumors arise (Fig. 124.18).[33] The use of positioning and oral fluid loads distinguishes the expert scanner from the ordinary.

Ultrasound is not as good as CT or MRI in distinguishing ductal adenocarcinoma from other types of pancreatic tumor, but odd-looking tumors by any modality are usually not ductal adenocarcinomas.[34,35] Doppler ultrasound is very helpful is staging pancreatic tumors preoperatively and is improved by ultrasound contrast studies.[36,37] Ultrasound is of use in the follow-up of acute and chronic pancreatitis but is not as definitive as CT or MRI.[38]

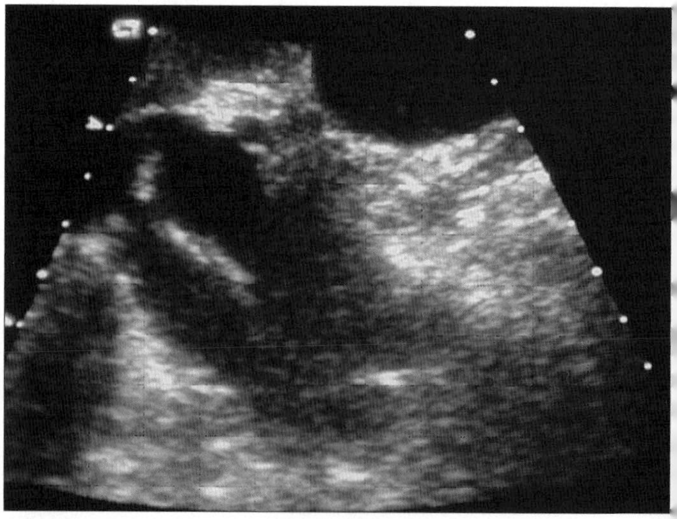

Fig. 124.18 A small ductal adenocarcinoma of the pancreas. The tumor mass is poorly echogenic, sharply marginated, and infiltrative.

PERCUTANEOUS VERSUS ENDOSCOPIC ULTRASOUND

The closer that we bring the ultrasound probe to the target, the better the images. This is the principle behind endoscopic ultrasound. There is no doubt that the highest resolution images we can obtain from the human body are gained by endoscopic ultrasound. This is offset by the fact that the tissue properties are the same with both methods. A hypoechoic tumor on ultrasound remains a hypoechoic tumor on endoscopic ultrasound, for example. Thus, the extraspatial resolution gains us very little. The best use of endoscopic ultrasound is to image the very small, such as ampullary tumors and cholangiocarcinomas.[39]

We now have over 20 years of experience of endoscopic ultrasound at the Middlesex Hospital and it remains a limited technique. It has undoubtedly been oversold in the gastroenterology community and recent reports from early enthusiasts have cast doubt on its effectiveness.

Endoscopic ultrasound-guided fine needle aspiration holds some promise.[40] We have had a policy for almost 20 years of diagnosing all pancreatic tumors by ultrasound or CT-guided trucut biopsy using a 1.2 mm needle.[41] This yields a sensitivity for the diagnosis of malignancy of approximately 94% for pancreatic cancer.[42] The small sample volume of endoscopic ultrasound biopsy needles does not yield such good results and has not significantly reduced the numbers of percutaneous biopsies that we perform.

ULTRASOUND AND THE GUT

The gas-filled bowel has long been thought of as a no go area for ultrasound. This is not true.[43–45] With careful scanning most of the bowel can be accessed by ultrasound and wall thickening, inflammation, and perforation can all be diagnosed.[46–48] Doppler ultrasound is very powerful in inflammatory bowel disease and can show disease activity. Unfortunately, it is hard to quantify compared with similar perfusion measurements in CT or MRI but is still useful in clinical practice. The literature shows that ultrasound is not as effective as low-dose CT in diagnosing acute appendicitis but the younger the patient the better the scan, and mesenteric adenitis is easily distinguished from appendicitis.[2,49,50] With conditions such as diverticulitis ultrasound does not perform as well as CT but may still identify the nature of the problem to allow a better CT protocol to be used.[51,52]

ULTRASOUND-GUIDED INTERVENTION

Diagnosis: We have been using ultrasound to guide biopsy needles for over 25 years. Many years ago we abandoned cytology-based FNA in favor of core biopsy using a powered cutting needle.[53] With this technique we can obtain complete tumor typing with sensitivities of 98% in the liver, 94% in the pancreas, and 97% elsewhere in the abdomen.[54] Biopsy is now as much a part of imaging as are the scans. The maxim, 'if you don't know what it is needle it' is practiced in nearly every ultrasound department today.[55] In my own department 95% of all abdominal biopsies are performed with ultrasound guidance with CT reserved for repeat biopsies or the obviously difficult case. The risks of needle biopsy are very small but do undoubtedly increase with needle size.[53] For pancreatic core biopsy we have a rate of acute pancreatitis of approximately 1% (about the same as endoscopic retrograde cholangiopancreatography) with a fatality rate of 1 in 5000. We believe that this is an acceptable complication rate given the quality of the resulting data.

Therapy: The potential of image guidance has expanded from diagnosis to therapy. Ethanol ablation of HCC was developed over 20 years ago and has been shown to have results comparable to surgical resection.[56] Although we still use ethanol and acetic acid to ablate HCC in high-risk cases this has been displaced by radiofrequency ablation, which has greater efficiency in tumor destruction. Primary and secondary liver tumors up to 5 cm in diameter can reliably be ablated using radiofrequency ablation. Recent survival figures from Italy on the ablation of small HCC are comparable to transplantation.

Our own practice of liver tumor ablation focuses mainly on colorectal liver metastases and delivers a 5-year survival in inoperable patients of 30% comparable to the surgical median of 32%.[57] Our techniques are constantly improving and with lower cost and morbidity are a great threat to surgical practice.[58,59]

However therapeutic innovation is littered with techniques that never made it such as percutaneous cholecystolithotomy and the rotary lithotrite in the gallbladder.[60,61]

CONCLUSION

Despite the power and effectiveness of CT and MRI in gastrointestinal imaging ultrasound still has a major role to play. It is cheaper, faster, and easier and has the enormous advantage that the radiologist interacts directly with the patient. The concept of ultrasound as an enhanced clinical examination is very strong. Miniaturization of ultrasound systems means that a US$20 000 hand-held machine has the performance of a large radiology system of only 5 years ago. In my opinion every gastroenterologist should have his own machine and be trained in its use. Ultrasound has been described as the stethoscope of the future for the last 20 years.[62] The technology is now available to make this come true.[63]

REFERENCES

1. Marincek B. Nontraumatic abdominal emergencies: acute abdominal pain: diagnostic strategies. Eur Radiol 2002; 12:2136–2150.
2. Puylaert JB. Ultrasound of acute GI tract conditions. Eur Radiol 2001; 11:1867–1877.
3. Shuman WP, Ralls PW, Balfe DM et al. Imaging evaluation of patients with acute abdominal pain and fever. American College of Radiology. ACR Appropriateness Criteria. Radiology 2000; 215 (Suppl):209–212.
4. Vasavada P. Ultrasound evaluation of acute abdominal emergencies in infants and children. Radiol Clin North Am 2004; 42:445–456.
5. Giuseppetti GM, Argalia G, Abbattista T. Liver cirrhosis: evaluation of haemodynamic changes using an ultrasound contrast agent. Eur J Radiol 2004; 51:27–33.
6. Leen E. The role of contrast-enhanced ultrasound in the characterisation of focal liver lesions. Eur Radiol 2001; 11 (Suppl 3):E27–E34.
7. Wilson SR, Burns PN. Liver mass evaluation with ultrasound: the impact of microbubble contrast agents and pulse inversion imaging. Semin Liver Dis 2001; 21:147–159.
8. Foster FS, Burns PN, Simpson DH et al. Ultrasound for the visualization and

quantification of tumor microcirculation. Cancer Metastasis Rev 2000; 19:131–138.
9. Solbiati L, Tonolini M, Cova L, Goldberg SN. The role of contrast-enhanced ultrasound in the detection of focal liver lesions. Eur Radiol 2001; 11 (Suppl 3):E15–E26.
10. Nicolau C, Bianchi L, Vilana R. Gray-scale ultrasound in hepatic cirrhosis and chronic hepatitis: diagnosis, screening, and intervention. Semin Ultrasound CT MR 2002; 23:3–18.
11. Michielsen PP, Duysburgh IK, Pelckmans PA. Ultrasound and duplex-Doppler in the diagnosis and follow-up of portal hypertension. Acta Gastroenterol Belg 1995; 58:409–421.
12. O'Donohue J, Ng C, Catnach S, Farrant P, Williams R. Diagnostic value of Doppler assessment of the hepatic and portal vessels and ultrasound of the spleen in liver disease. Eur J Gastroenterol Hepatol 2004; 16:147–155.
13. Ralls PW, Wren SM, Radin R, Stain SC, Yang J, Parekh D. Color flow sonography in evaluating the resectability of periampullary and pancreatic tumors. J Ultrasound Med 1997; 16:131–140.
14. Tchelepi H, Ralls PW, Radin R, Grant E. Sonography of diffuse liver disease. J Ultrasound Med 2002; 21:1023–1032.
15. von Herbay A, Donner A, Jung G, Vogt C, Haussinger D. Contrast-enhanced sonography using Levovist is decisive for staging and therapeutic schedule in hepatocellular carcinoma. Med Klin (Munich) 2004; 99:89–92.
16. Saab S, Ly D, Nieto J et al. Hepatocellular carcinoma screening in patients waiting for liver transplantation: a decision analytic model. Liver Transpl 2003; 9:672–681.
17. Elvin A, Wilander E, Oberg K, Eriksson B, Lindgren PG. Ultrasound-guided biopsies of neuroendocrine metastases. Comparison of 0.9 and 1.2 mm biopsy-gun needle biopsies. Acta Radiol 1993; 34:474–477.
18. Caturelli E, Ghittoni G, Roselli P, De Palo M, Anti M. Fine needle biopsy of focal liver lesions: the hepatologist's point of view. Liver Transpl 2004; 10 (Suppl 1):S26–S29.
19. Sharma MP, Ahuja V. Aetiological spectrum of obstructive jaundice and diagnostic ability of ultrasonography: a clinician's perspective. Trop Gastroenterol 1999; 20:167–169.
20. Laing FC, Jeffrey RB, Wing VW. Improved visualization of choledocholithiasis by sonography. Am J Roentgenol 1984; 143:949–952.
21. Varghese JC, Liddell RP, Farrell MA et al. The diagnostic accuracy of magnetic resonance cholangiopancreatography and ultrasound compared with direct cholangiography in the detection of choledocholithiasis. Clin Radiol 1999; 54:604–614.
22. Bloom CM, Langer B, Wilson SR. Role of US in the detection, characterization, and staging of cholangiocarcinoma. Radiographics 1999; 19:1199–1218.
23. Walker J, Chalmers RT, Allan PL. An audit of ultrasound diagnosis of gallbladder calculi. Br J Radiol 1992; 65:581–584.
24. Kalimi R, Gecelter GR, Caplin D et al. Diagnosis of acute cholecystitis: sensitivity of sonography, cholescintigraphy, and combined sonography-cholescintigraphy. J Am Coll Surg 2001; 193:609–613.
25. Brakel K, Lameris JS, Nijs HG, Ginai AZ, Terpstra OT. Accuracy of ultrasound and oral cholecystography in assessing the number and size of gallstones: implications for non-surgical therapy. Br J Radiol 1992; 65:779–783.
26. Laing FC. Diagnostic evaluation of patients with suspected cholecystitis. Surg Clin North Am 1984; 64:3–22.
27. Sood BP, Kalra N, Gupta S et al. Role of sonography in the diagnosis of gallbladder perforation. J Clin Ultrasound 2002; 30:270–274.
28. Gouma DJ. When are gallbladder polyps malignant? HPB Surg 2000; 11:428–430.
29. Myers RP, Shaffer EA, Beck PL. Gallbladder polyps: epidemiology, natural history and management. Can J Gastroenterol 2002; 16:187–194.
30. Lee CL, Wu CH, Chen TK et al. Prospective study of abdominal ultrasonography before laparoscopic cholecystectomy. J Clin Gastroenterol 1993; 16:113–116.
31. Fishman EK, Horton KM. Imaging pancreatic cancer: the role of multidetector CT with three-dimensional CT angiography. Pancreatology 2001; 1:610–624.
32. Pasanen P, Partanen K, Pikkarainen P et al. Diagnostic accuracy of ultrasound, computed tomography and endoscopic retrograde cholangiopancreatography in the detection of pancreatic cancer in patients with jaundice or cholestasis. In Vivo 1992; 6:297–301.
33. Tanaka S, Kitamra T, Yamamoto K et al. Evaluation of routine sonography for early detection of pancreatic cancer. Jpn J Clin Oncol 1996; 26:422–427.
34. Kiely JM, Nakeeb A, Komorowski RA, Wilson SD, Pitt HA. Cystic pancreatic neoplasms: enucleate or resect? J Gastrointest Surg 2003; 7:890–897.
35. Oberg K, Eriksson B, Lundqvist M. Neuroendocrine tumours of the upper gastrointestinal tract and pancreas. Acta Chir Scand Suppl 1988; 541:76–85.
36. Wren SM, Ralls PW, Stain SC, Kasiraman A, Carpenter CL, Parekh D. Assessment of resectability of pancreatic head and periampullary tumors by color flow Doppler sonography. Arch Surg 1996; 131:812–817.
37. Yoshimori M, Tajiri H, Nakamura K, Ozaki H, Kishi K. Diagnosis of small carcinoma of the pancreas: importance of ultrasound scanning and endoscopic retrograde cholangiopancreatography (ERCP). Jpn J Clin Oncol 1984; 14:359–367.
38. Jeffrey RB Jr, Laing FC, Wing VW. Extrapancreatic spread of acute pancreatitis: new observations with real-time US. Radiology 1986; 159:707–711.
39. Rosch T. Staging of pancreatic cancer. Analysis of literature results. Gastrointest Endosc Clin N Am 1995; 5:735–739.
40. Agarwal B, Abu-Hamda E, Molke KL, Correa AM, Ho L. Endoscopic ultrasound-guided fine needle aspiration and multidetector spiral CT in the diagnosis of pancreatic cancer. Am J Gastroenterol 2004; 99:844–850.
41. Jennings PE, Donald JJ, Coral A, Rode J, Lees WR. Ultrasound-guided core biopsy. Lancet 1989; 1:1369–1371.
42. Balen FG, Little A, Smith AC et al. Biopsy of inoperable pancreatic tumors does not adversely influence patient survival time. Radiology 1994; 193:753–755.
43. Sarrazin J, Wilson SR. Manifestations of Crohn disease at US. Radiographics 1996; 16:499–520.
44. O'Malley ME, Wilson SR. US of gastrointestinal tract abnormalities with CT correlation. Radiographics 2003; 23:59–72.
45. Parente F, Greco S, Molteni M et al. Role of early ultrasound in detecting inflammatory intestinal disorders and identifying their anatomical location within the bowel. Aliment Pharmacol Ther 2003; 18:1009–1016.
46. Hanbidge AE, Lynch D, Wilson SR. US of the peritoneum. Radiographics 2003; 23:663–684.
47. Hogan MJ. Appendiceal abscess drainage. Tech Vasc Interv Radiol 2003; 6:205–214.
48. Jeffrey RB Jr, Laing FC, Townsend RR. Acute appendicitis: sonographic criteria based on 250 cases. Radiology 1988; 167:327–329.
49. Kessler N, Cyteval C, Gallix B et al. Appendicitis: evaluation of sensitivity, specificity, and predictive values of US, Doppler US, and laboratory findings. Radiology 2004; 230:472–478.
50. Taylor GA. Suspected appendicitis in children: in search of the single best diagnostic test. Radiology 2004; 231:293–295.
51. Bruel JM. Acute colonic diverticulitis: CT or ultrasound? Eur Radiol 2003; 13:2557–2559.
52. Chou YH, Chiou HJ, Tiu CM et al. Sonography of acute right side colonic diverticulitis. Am J Surg 2001; 181:122–127.
53. Smith BC, Desmond PV. Outpatient liver biopsy using ultrasound guidance and the Biopsy gun is safe and cost effective. Aust N Z J Med 1995; 25:209–211.
54. Wotherspoon AC, Norton AJ, Lees WR, Shaw P, Isaacson PG. Diagnostic fine needle core biopsy of deep lymph nodes for the diagnosis of lymphoma in patients unfit for surgery. J Pathol 1989; 158:115–121.
55. O'Connell MJ, Paulson EK, Jaffe TA, Ho LM. Percutaneous biopsy of periarterial soft tissue cuffs in the diagnosis of pancreatic carcinoma. Abdom Imag 2004; 29:115–119.
56. Livraghi T, Meloni F, Morabito A, Vettori C. Multimodal image-guided tailored therapy of early and intermediate hepatocellular carcinoma: long-term survival in the experience of a single radiologic referral center. Liver Transpl 2004; 10 (Suppl 1):S98–106.
57. Gillams AR, Lees WR. Radio-frequency ablation of colorectal liver metastases in 167 patients. Eur Radiol 2004; 14:2261–2267.
58. Bown SG, Rogowska AZ, Whitelaw DE et al. Photodynamic therapy for cancer of the pancreas. Gut 2002; 50:549–557.
59. Cinat ME, Wilson SE, Din AM. Determinants for successful percutaneous image-guided drainage of intra-abdominal abscess. Arch Surg 2002; 137:845–849.
60. Donald JJ, Cheslyn-Curtis S, Gillams AR, Russell RC, Lees WR. Percutaneous cholecystolithotomy: is gall stone recurrence inevitable? Gut 1994; 35:692–695.
61. Gillams A, Donald JJ, Russell RC, Hatfield AR, Lees WR. The percutaneous rotary lithotrite: a new approach to the treatment of symptomatic cholecystolithiasis. Gut 1993; 34:837–842.
62. Filly RA. Ultrasound: the stethoscope of the future, alas. Radiology 1988; 167:400.
63. Roelandt JR. A personal ultrasound imager (ultrasound stethoscope). A revolution in the physical cardiac diagnosis! Eur Heart J 2002; 23:523–527.

Chapter 125

Barium radiology

Simon A Jackson and Bruce M Fox

KEY POINTS

- Contrast radiology offers a readily available and cost-effective gastrointestinal assessment that complements other imaging modalities
- Effective contrast examinations require optimal patient preparation, good technique, and meticulous interpretation
- Double contrast radiology provides the best mucosal detail
- Water-soluble contrast agents should be used if there is a risk of perforation or aspiration

INTRODUCTION

The development of modern barium radiology resulted from improvements in technical apparatus and the development of barium suspensions that heralded the introduction of single and double contrast techniques to diagnose gastrointestinal tract pathology.

Single contrast examinations are performed using a low-density barium suspension. Bowel distention with contrast enables the visualization of such findings as filling defects or alterations in normal contour of the bowel wall. The technique, however, has a number of limitations including the degree of luminal distention and limited quality of mucosal coating.

Double contrast studies, on the other hand, use gas to distend the bowel combined with mucosal coating by a thin layer of high-density barium suspension. The technique allows the demonstration of fine mucosal detail and subtle pathology. In addition, the radiation dose is reduced both due to a reduction in fluoroscopic screening time and radiographic exposure settings. For these reasons a well-performed double contrast study is usually regarded as the examination of choice.

The number of barium examinations performed world-wide has significantly decreased due to the introduction of alternative techniques, especially endoscopy, and also the cross-sectional imaging modalities of computed tomography (CT), magnetic resonance imaging (MRI), and ultrasound. Despite this, contrast examinations still remain cost-effective investigations and high-quality barium studies continue to play an important role in the diagnosis of gastrointestinal disorders.

THE PHARYNX – MODIFIED BARIUM SWALLOW OR VIDEO FLUOROSCOPY

The normal swallowing mechanism is a complex but orderly sequence of neuromuscular events, which can be divided into two main components: oropharyngeal and esophageal (see Chapter 3). Disorders of the oropharyngeal component are increasingly recognized in routine clinical practice and are associated with significant morbidity and mortality, particularly in the elderly population. The development of digital fluoroscopy and, in particular, the ability to video record the study has contributed to the development of the modified barium swallow (MBS) or video fluoroscopic examination.

Description of technique

The study is performed as a multidisciplinary examination in the fluoroscopy suite and is usually undertaken in the presence of a speech therapist and/or ENT surgeon. This functional assessment examination complements fiber-optic examination of the pharynx to exclude mucosal pathology (see Chapter 132). Video recording of the examination is used to enable slow-motion review of the patient's swallowing mechanism and help reduce overall radiation exposure.[1,2] The patient is seated in specially designed chairs to aid support and positioning during the study. Clinical status and relevant medical history are reviewed prior to the study. Swallowing movements are recorded in the lateral position using barium as the contrast agent. Barium is mixed into varying consistencies ranging from thin liquid to solid food boluses. Initial bolus size is restricted to small volumes in order to assess the presence or absence of aspiration.

The study includes assessment of all phases of the oropharyngeal swallow mechanism with particular emphasis on the presence of vocal cord penetration and aspiration. The strength of the patient's cough reflex when aspiration occurs is also noted. Maneuvers such as chin tucking or head turning can also be performed and assessed with regard to their efficacy in improving the patient's swallowing mechanism. The complete examination should include an assessment of the esophagus in order to exclude associated pathology.

Indications/contraindications

The examination is performed in patients with oropharangeal swallowing dysfunction and in many cases symptoms of high dysphagia. The majority of these cases are elderly and include patients with a medical history of cerebrovascular event or neuromuscular disease (see Chapter 3). A further group consists of patients with a previous history of head and neck malignancy with radiation therapy or surgical resection leading to swallowing problems.

A diagnostic examination requires sufficient patient mobility and awareness to understand instructions and thus is contraindicated in the severely incapacitated subject. Significant aspiration of contrast occurring during the study is a relative contraindication to a complete assessment and chest physiotherapy should be performed after the examination.

KEY POINTS
VIDEOFLUOROSCOPY
• Provides a functional, dynamic examination of the pharynx • Principally indicated for the investigation of oropharyngeal swallowing dysfunction and high dysphagia • Complex examination performed with multiple contrast consistencies

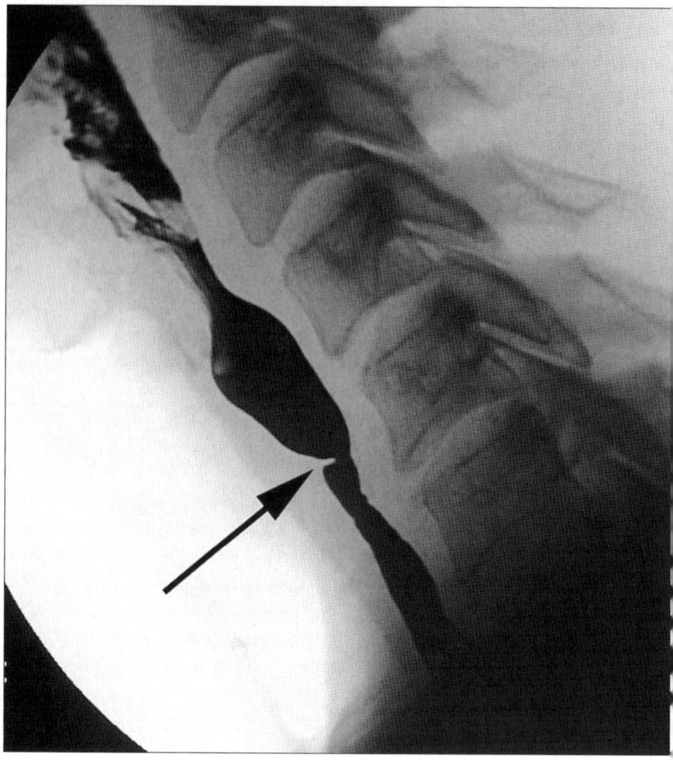

Fig. 125.1 Single contrast barium swallow. Single contrast barium swallow demonstrating a pharyngeal web (arrow).

THE UPPER GASTROINTESTINAL TRACT – ESOPHAGRAM AND UPPER GASTROINTESTINAL SERIES

The double contrast study has facilitated the accurate assessment of mucosal pathology. The modern contrast examination of the upper gastrointestinal tract combines the advantages of the two techniques (single and double contrast) and in many radiology departments is performed as a biphasic examination.[3]

Endoscopy may comprise the initial examination, but contrast imaging may demonstrate other clinically significant pathology.[4] This is especially true in the assessment of dysphagia and odynophagia (see Chapter 3) and for upper gastrointestinal motility in general.

Description of technique

The standard upper gastrointestinal contrast study should be performed as a biphasic examination allowing the combination of both double contrast and single contrast views to maximize the sensitivity of the test.[3] All examinations must be performed with meticulous attention to technique and interpretation in order to maximize diagnostic accuracy.

Double contrast images rely on initial gaseous distention of the bowel lumen after the ingestion of effervescent granules followed by the even coating of the mucosa by a thin layer of high-density barium suspension. Residual fluid or food results in reduced mucosal detail and thus sensitivity of the examination. The patient is therefore fasted for at least 6h prior to the study. The quality of the examination is improved by the injection of smooth muscle relaxants to cause gastric hypotonia and increase distention. The radiologist uses intermittent fluoroscopy throughout the examination to aid in patient positioning and confirm adequate luminal distention/mucosal coating. Single contrast views are also obtained during and after ingestion of a low-density barium suspension for further assessment of the esophagus, stomach, and duodenum. The modern examination is tailored to the patient's symptoms. An esophagram is performed in patients with suspected esophageal pathology whereas an upper gastrointestinal series is tailored to suspected abnormalities within the stomach and duodenum.

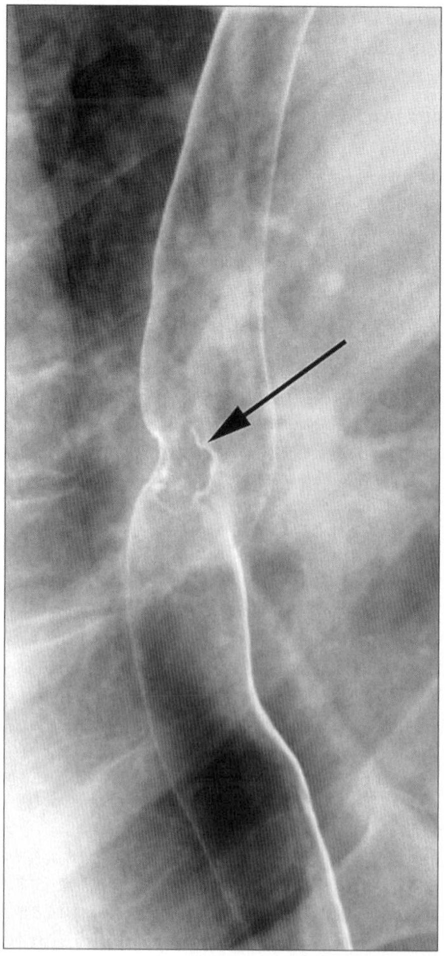

Fig. 125.2 Double contrast barium swallow. Double contrast barium swallow showing an early esophageal carcinoma (arrow).

Indications

Esophagus

Dysphagia remains a recognized indication for undertaking a barium examination of the esophagus (Fig. 125.1 and Fig. 125.2), in particular if the symptom is related to a motility disturbance (see Chapters 3 and 40).

Barium studies are also sensitive for the diagnosis of certain features in patients presenting with reflux symptoms, especially if they are atypical. An examination can confirm the presence of a hiatus hernia and gastroesophageal reflux as well as detecting morphological changes secondary to the reflux such as erosive esophagitis, esophageal rings, and peptic strictures. The esophagram is invaluable in the assessment of the integrity of a fundoplication and after pneumatic dilatation or surgery for achalasia (see Chapters 29, 30, 31, and 32).

Stomach and duodenum

Upper gastrointestinal endoscopy has largely replaced barium studies as the primary diagnostic investigation for patients presenting with possible gastric or duodenal pathology (see Chapter 119). However, if endoscopy is contraindicated or unavailable a well-performed barium examination is the next most sensitive diagnostic modality.[5] Occult strictures and fistulae can be identified as well as extrinsic or submucosal disease distorting the bowel lumen. In addition, a double contrast barium examination demonstrates the morphology of the stomach and duodenum in patients with a suspected volvulus or gastric outlet obstruction (see Chapter 62) (Fig. 125.3). Opacification of the distal duodenum also allows the potential visualization of pathology that may be missed during upper gastrointestinal endoscopy.

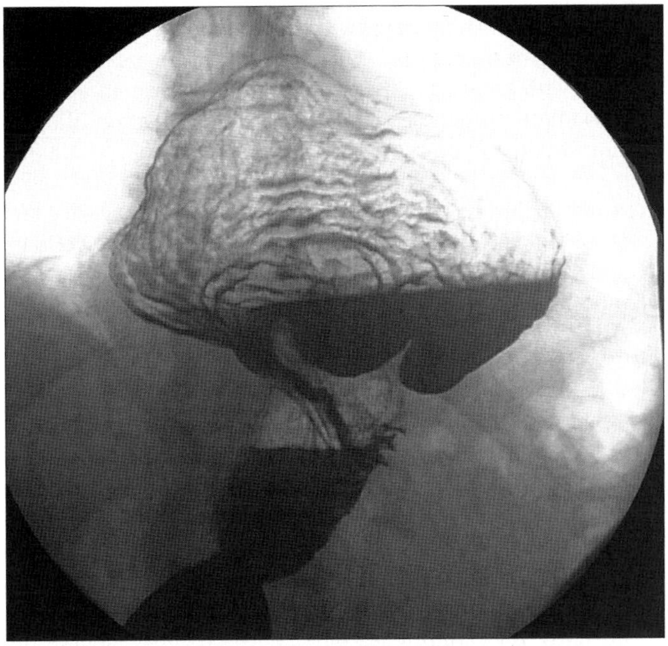

Fig. 125.3 Water-soluble upper gastrointestinal series. Water-soluble upper gastrointestinal series demonstrating a gastric volvulus.

Contraindications

Similar to other areas of the gastrointestinal tract, a barium examination is contraindicated in patients with possible perforation. If a perforation is suspected, a water-soluble contrast study should be performed. In addition, patients with high-grade gastric outlet obstruction should also undergo a water-soluble examination, to avoid the risk of barium impaction. Immobile patients are only able to undergo a limited study of reduced accuracy.

KEY POINTS
ESOPHAGRAM AND UPPER GASTROINTESTINAL SERIES
• Commonly performed as a biphasic examination utilizing both single and double contrast techniques • Esophagram provides a rapid assessment of dysphagia and motility disorders complimenting endoscopy • A contrast examination is a useful investigation for assessment of the upper gastrointestinal tract following local gastrointestinal surgery

THE BARIUM FOLLOW-THROUGH AND ENTEROCLYSIS

Description of technique

Barium follow-through (small bowel meal)

Patients fast for at least 6–8h prior to the procedure. They drink approximately 500mL of a low-density barium suspension. Unless contraindicated, metoclopramide (10–20mg) is also taken orally by the patient to accelerate passage of contrast through the gastrointestinal tract. A sequence of plain abdominal films is then obtained to evaluate the progress of the barium contrast through small bowel loops. Following demonstration of either significant small bowel pathology and/or passage of the contrast through to the colon, a dedicated fluoroscopic examination is performed. This is used to provide a detailed assessment of the small bowel and, in particular, the terminal ileum using compression techniques. Where the terminal ileum is poorly demonstrated, gas can be introduced per rectum to provide double contrast views of the region.

Enteroclysis

This more invasive technique is performed entirely in the fluoroscopy suite. A specifically designed catheter is introduced nasally and manipulated under fluoroscopic guidance through the stomach and duodenum to the proximal jejunum. Contrast is then introduced via the catheter to directly opacify the small bowel using either a single contrast or double contrast technique. Whilst the single contrast examination allows the distention and assessment of small bowel loops, demonstration of fine mucosal detail is limited.

Images are obtained after initial introduction of approximately 200mL of high-density barium suspension immediately followed by an infusion of 1000–2000mL of a 0.5% solution of methylcellulose to provide a double contrast appearance. In many departments contrast infusion is achieved by the use of a dedicated contrast delivery pump.

During the examination the radiologist performs intermittent fluoroscopy accompanied by graded compression to assess the passage of contrast through small bowel loops and look for abnormalities along the way.

Indications

Barium follow-through

The main advantages of barium follow-through when compared to enteroclysis include the less invasive nature of the examination (reduced patient discomfort) and shorter fluoroscopic screening times with a lower radiation dose to the patient. The examination is widely used for the assessment of patients with known or suspected Crohn's disease. In addition barium follow-through can be used for the evaluation of other small bowel pathologies (Fig. 125.4) that compromise luminal diameter such as ischemia and radiation enteritis. Traditionally, the examination has also been used to assess the severity and level of small bowel obstruction; however, cross-sectional imaging techniques and, in particular, CT have been shown to be more accurate[6,7] (see Chapter 126).

Enteroclysis

Enteroclysis provides better luminal distention and mucosal detail than a barium follow-through. Thus, more accurate assessment of subtle mucosal pathology and changes in fold pattern can be evaluated. This has led some authors to suggest that enteroclysis should comprise the initial method of small bowel imaging[8–10] although there is general acceptance that both types of examination currently play a role in the diagnosis of small bowel pathology (see Chapters 15 and 54).

Currently, the main indications for enteroclysis include the assessment of patients with chronic or recurrent small bowel obstruction, patients with Crohn's disease in order to establish the extent and severity of disease and related complications prior to surgery, and diagnosis of small bowel pathology in patients with malabsorption states. In celiac disease, for example, a 'malabsorption pattern' is absent in more than 50% of cases. The main value of enteroclysis or barium follow-through in malabsorption is for radiologically diagnosable or highly suggestive causes of malabsorption such as jejunal diverticulosis or the featureless 'toothpaste pattern' of amyloidosis. Studies are also sensitive for the diagnosis of small bowel tumors and Meckel's diverticulum. Importantly, contrast studies remain complementary to other radiological investigations such as CT/MRI/ultrasound and radionuclide examinations. The place of both capsule and fiber-optic endoscopy in the triage of patients is continuing to evolve (see Chapters 119 and 123).

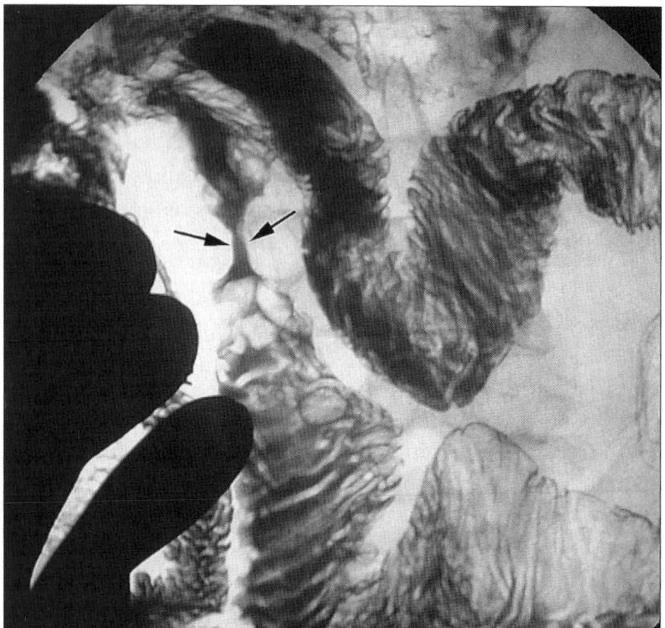

Fig. 125.4 Barium follow-through. Compression view from a small bowel follow-through showing an adenocarcinoma of the jejunum (arrows) in a patient with occult anemia.

KEY POINTS
SMALL BOWEL FOLLOW-THROUGH AND ENTEROCLYSIS
• Contrast examination remains the principal imaging investigation of small bowel pathology • Although more invasive, the enteroclysis provides mucosal detail not provided by the small bowel meal

THE COLON – BARIUM ENEMA

Description of technique

The large bowel can be studied using either a single or double contrast technique although the single contrast barium enema examination plays a limited role. In similarity to other double contrast studies, the examination also uses a limited volume of high-density barium suspension to coat the colonic mucosa followed by luminal distention with either air or carbon dioxide. Importantly, the double contrast bowel enema (DCBE) enables the demonstration of mucosal lesions, which may be missed during a single contrast study (Figs. 125.5 and 125.6).[11]

Patient preparation prior to a DCBE remains fundamental to the accuracy of a successful study. The patient must be able to understand and comply with preprocedure colonic cleansing instructions as well as physically able to roll during the study in order to obtain the necessary images. Whilst a number of bowel preparation regimes can be used, the majority of these combine a low-residue diet prior to the study with a preparation that stimulates colonic peristalsis and keeps the bowel contents semi liquid. It is important that patients are encouraged to drink sufficient quantities of liquid to prevent dehydration during the period of the bowel preparation.

As for all contrast examinations, the physician requesting the examination must provide relevant clinical details on the request form. Relevant current or past medical/surgical history should be included as well as information on recent endoscopic procedures. This latter information is particularly important because of the increased risk of colonic perforation if a DCBE is performed less than 7 days following a therapeutic endoscopic procedure such as snare polypectomy or deep forceps biopsy via a rigid sigmoidoscope.[12] Standard biopsies obtained during colonoscopy or flexible sigmoidoscopy do not contraindicate a DCBE during the same bowel preparation.

Alternative imaging techniques

Colonoscopy is more accurate than the barium enema for the demonstration of small mucosal lesions (<1 cm).[13] Although colonoscopy is more expensive with a higher complication rate when compared to a DCBE examination[14] it is currently recognized as the procedure of choice when screening for colorectal neoplasia.

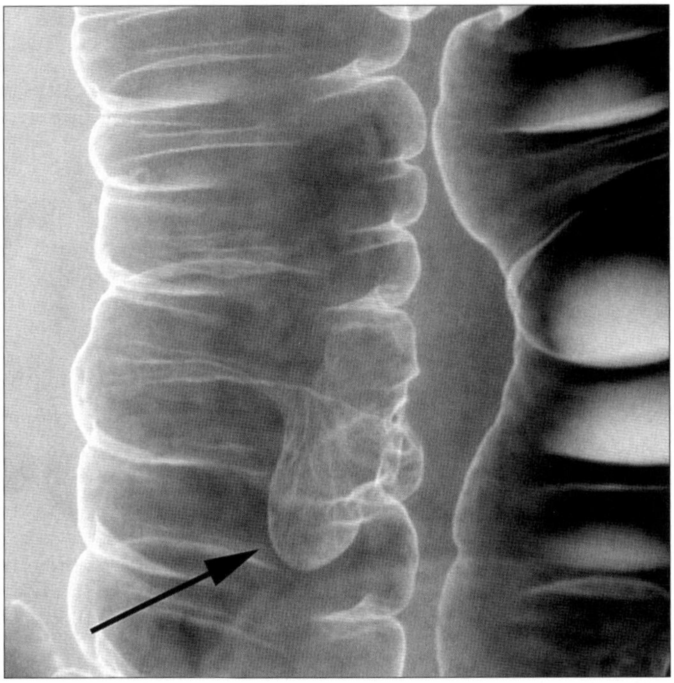

Fig. 125.5 Double contrast barium enema. Double contrast barium enema demonstrating a colonic lipoma (arrow).

Cross-sectional imaging techniques including CT, MRI, and ultrasound can also be used as alternative imaging techniques to visualize the large bowel. The main alternative evolving technique is CT colonography (CTC) or virtual colonoscopy (see Chapter 129). This technique not only assesses colonic mucosal abnormalities with a greater sensitivity than the DCBE but can also evaluate the presence of extracolonic pathology. The DCBE or CT colonography are done if the colonoscopy procedure cannot be completed.

Indications

In many parts of the world barium enema is less frequently used for the detection of colorectal cancer and polyps. Other indications for a double contrast barium enema include the diagnosis of diverticular disease and its complications as well as the assessment of extrinsic pathology involving the colon (see Chapters 11, 60A–D, and 65). The routine use of the barium enema to assess the extent and severity of inflammatory bowel disease (IBD) has now largely been replaced by colonoscopy. However, the barium enema plays a critical role in the assessment of patients with colonic strictures secondary to IBD, which do not allow the passage of an endoscope. In addition, contrast studies can assess the position and nature of fistulae and play a role in the assessment of patients with indeterminate colitis (see Chapter 55).

Contraindications

Whilst the DCBE is a very safe examination with a mortality rate of approximately 1 in 56 000[16] a number of important contraindications exist. In particular, where there is suspicion of a colonic perforation an examination should be undertaken using water-soluble contrast media. This is because the inadvertent introduction of barium into the peritoneal cavity is associated with a significant morbidity and mortality. In addition pathology such as toxic megacolon and ischemic colitis, which increase the risk of bowel perforation, provide a relative contraindication to DCBE. As previously described, DCBE should be delayed for a week in patients who have undergone a deep mucosal biopsy or snare polypectomy.

KEY POINTS

BARIUM ENEMA

- Optimal mucosal assessment requires double contrast examination of a clean colon
- Meticulous attention must be paid to the acquisition and interpretation of images
- Colonoscopy remains the gold standard investigation for the colon
- Barium enema can be used as an alternative to CT colonography for a complete colonic examination in cases of failed colonoscopy

COMPLICATIONS AND THEIR MANAGEMENT

In the context of contrast examination of the upper gastrointestinal tract, barium aspiration can occur. This may result in a pneumonitis or pneumonia and should be managed (unless very mild) by physiotherapy and postural drainage. Where there is any suspicion of a risk of aspiration prior to an examination, an iso-osmolar water-soluble contrast agent should be used.

Whilst extremely rare, the most significant complication of any barium examination is perforation. Within the abdomen this may be intra- or retroperitoneal. Intraperitoneal extravasation of contrast is diagnosed by the visualization of contrast outlining bowel loops and/or the appearance of a pneumoperitoneum. When identified, the treatment in most cases is operative although conservative management using antibiotic therapy and intravenous fluid replacement may be successful.

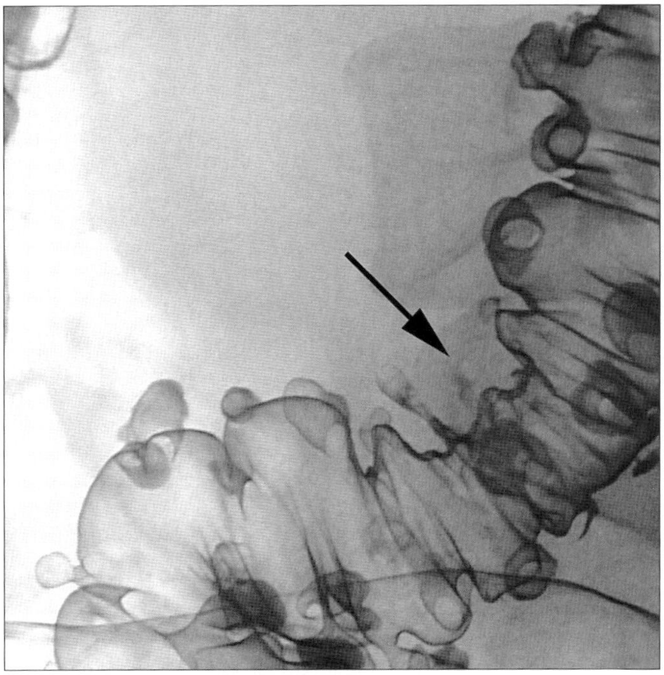

Fig. 125.6 Double contrast barium enema. Focal colonic diverticulitis on a double contrast barium enema (arrow).

Retroperitoneal perforation has been reported during DCBE examinations in patients with rectal pathology (for example proctitis), following inadvertent laceration of the rectum during introduction of the enema tip or inflation of a retention balloon. Rectal pathology should thus be excluded by sigmoidoscopy performed during initial clinical consultation, with the result included on the radiology request form.

In addition, when a contrast study is used to investigate the obstructed gastrointestinal tract, water-soluble contrast agents should be used to avoid the risk of barium impaction.

SOURCES OF INFORMATION FOR PATIENTS AND DOCTORS

http://www.goingfora.com/radiology/barium_room.html
http://www.patient.co.uk/showdoc/27000480/
http://www.patient.co.uk/showdoc/27000478/
http://www.radiologyinfo.org/content/lower_gi.htm
http://www.radiologyinfo.org/content/upper_gi.htm

REFERENCES

1. Ekberg O, Pokieser P. Radiologic evaluation of the dysphagic patient. Eur Radiol 1997; 7:1285–1295.
2. Ekberg O, Wahlgren L. Dysfunction of pharyngeal swallowing. A cineradiographic investigation in 854 dysphagia patients. Acta Radiol Diagn 1985; 26:389–395.
3. Levine MS, Rubesin SE, Herlinger H, Laufer I. Double contrast upper gastrointestinal examination: technique and interpretation. Radiology 1988; 168:593–602.
4. Levine MS, Chu P, Furth EE et al. Carcinoma of the esophagus and esophagogastric junction: sensitivity of radiographic diagnosis. Am J Roentgenol 1997; 168:1423–1426.
5. Low VH, Levine MS, Rubesin SE et al. Diagnosis of gastric carcinoma: sensitivity of double contrast barium studies. Am J Roentgenol 1994; 162:329–334.
6. Maglinte DDT, Kelvin FM, Rowe MG et al. Small bowel obstruction: optimising radiologic investigation and nonsurgical management. Radiology 2001; 218:39–46.
7. Maglinte DDT, Balthazar EJ, Kelvin FM, Megibow AJ. The role of radiology in the diagnosis of small bowel obstruction. Am J Roentgenol 1997; 168:1171–1180.
8. Nolan DJ. Enteroclysis of non neoplastic disorders of the small intestine. Eur Radiol 2000; 10:342–353.
9. Dixon PM, Roulston ME, Nolan DJ. The small bowel enema: a ten year review. Clin Radiol 1993; 47:26–28.
10. Maglinte DDT, Kelvin FM, O'Connor K et al. Current status of small bowel radiography. Abdom Imaging 1996; 21:247–257.
11. Rubesin SE, Levine MS, Laufer I, Herlinger H. Double contrast barium enema examination technique. Radiology 2000; 215:642–650.
12. Harned RK, Consigny PM, Cooper NB et al. Barium enema examination following biopsy of the rectum or colon. Radiology 1982; 145:11–16.
13. Winawer SJ, Stewart ET, Zauber AG et al. A comparison of colonoscopy and double contrast barium enema for surveillance after polypectomy. National polyp study work group. N Engl J Med 2000; 342:1766–1772.
14. de Zwart IM, Griffioen G, Shaw MP et al. Barium enema and endoscopy for the detection of colorectal neoplasia: sensitivity, specificity, complications and its determinants. Clin Radiol 2001; 56:401–409.
15. Chong A, Shah JN, Levine MS et al. Diagnostic yield of barium enema examination after incomplete colonoscopy. Radiology 2002; 223:620–624.
16. Blakeborough A, Sheridan MB, Chapman AH. Complications of barium enema examinations: a survey of UK Consultant Radiologists 1992 to 1994. Clin Radiol 1997; 52:142–148.

Chapter 126

Computed tomography

Paula Hidalgo, Koenraad J Mortele, and Pablo R Ros

KEY POINTS

- High resolution 3D-reconstruction allows CT colonography and angiography
- Different contrast phases (arterial, portal venous, hepatic) allow for discrimination between hypovascular and hypervascular lesions, and perfusion anomalies
- Multiphase MDCT is useful in staging pancreatic cancer
- CT colonography allows for safe, reliable screening of polyps >10 mm in size
- The small bowel can now be examined by CT enterography

INTRODUCTION

Multidetector-row computed tomography (MDCT), initially introduced in 1998, has rapidly become a part of clinical imaging practice. High speed is combined with thin image thickness to create data best suited for workstation analysis in two-dimensional axial display, multiplanar reformations, or three-dimensional imaging.[1] In addition to technical advances, such as shorter scanning times, multiplanar imaging, and improved ability to perform true multiphasic contrast-enhanced studies, advances in postacquisition data processing techniques have made MDCT a powerful imaging tool in abdominal visceral imaging.

DESCRIPTION OF TECHNIQUE

Acquisition

MDCT imaging uses a new detector array with multiple rows in the Z-axis.[2] The improved spatial resolution reduces certain artifacts, such as partial-volume averaging (providing exaggeration of small lesions),[3] allows improved spatial resolution in nonaxial planes, and improves the ability to perform true multiphasic contrast-enhanced studies.[4] One of the remaining disadvantages is the probable increased radiation dose because of an increased usage of CT, more phases per patient, narrower collimation, and the cone beam effect.

Volume and rate of contrast administration are two very important and interdependent variables to maximize lesion detection.[5–6] A software package (Smart-Prep) allows scanning to be initiated at the optimal point during intravenous injection of contrast during the early and late arterial phase, portal venous phase, or maximum parenchymal enhancement phase.[7] The software eliminates the guesswork involved in timing delays to correct for anticipated slow transit times in patients with varying degrees of cardiac output, lung disease, or other conditions that affect circulation time.

CLINICAL APPLICATIONS

In solid organs, MDCT allows improved lesion detection because: (1) thinner sections are routinely obtained; (2) motion artifacts are reduced; and (3) enhancement can now be multiphasic, with three phases of enhancement routinely acquired.

High-resolution three-dimensional reconstructions are possible and routinely available, providing the basis for CT colonography, CT angiography (both arteriography and venography), models for surgical planning, and CT enterography.

Hepatobiliary imaging

The liver has complex circulatory dynamics. Approximately 80% of the hepatic blood supply is derived from the portal venous system and 20% from the hepatic artery. The injected bolus of contrast material initially enhances the liver via inflow through hepatic arteries (pure arterial phase) and is followed by a second 'late arterial/portal venous inflow phase' that reflects arterial inflow with a substantial component secondary to splanchnic venous inflow of contrast material into the portal vein and hepatic parenchyma. The phase of maximum hepatic parenchymal enhancement and hepatic venous opacification occurs 45 s after the beginning of the pure early arterial phase (hepatic phase).

Hypervascular lesions

Typical examples of hypervascular lesions include hemangioma, focal nodular hyperplasia, hepatocellular adenoma/carcinoma, and hypervascular metastases (neuroendocrine, breast, melanoma, renal cell carcinoma, thyroid carcinoma, sarcomas). Clinical imaging trials have demonstrated that hypervascular lesions are best demonstrated during the late arterial/portal venous inflow phase[8] (Fig. 126.1). Therefore, imaging is performed as a triple-phase study with imaging 25 s, 40 s, and 70 s after intravenous administration of 100 mL nonionic contrast material injection and water as oral contrast agent.[8–9]

Hypovascular lesions

Examples are hypovascular metastases (colorectal, pancreas, gastrointestinal), lymphoma, and cystic lesions (bile duct cyst, biliary cystadenoma, abscess, hydatid disease). These are best evaluated by using conventional portal venous phase or hepatic phase imaging with 100 mL nonionic contrast material injection and a scan delay of 70 s. Barium sulfate is routinely used as oral contrast agent.[9]

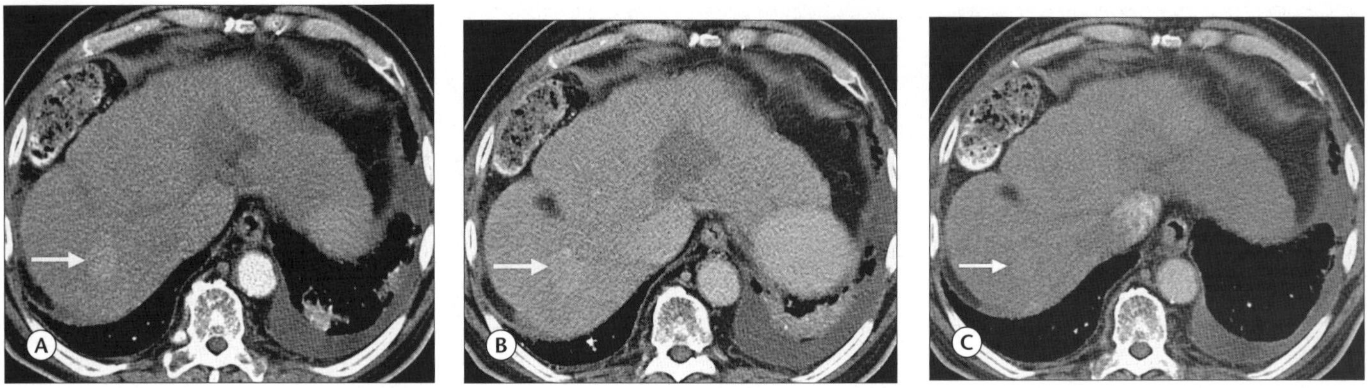

Fig. 126.1 Triphasic contrast-enhanced CT scan for hypervascular lesion. Early **(A)** and late **(B)** arterial phase contrast-enhanced CT images show a hypervascular lesion (hepatocellular carcinoma; arrow) in segment 7 of the right hepatic lobe, which is better appreciated on the late arterial phase image. **C.** On the portal venous phase image, the lesion is hardly appreciated due to the rapid washout of contrast material and enhancement of the surrounding liver parenchyma.

Diffuse liver disease

Examples include cirrhosis, confluent fibrosis, hemochromatosis, and steatosis. The utility of CT is most apparent in the evaluation of patients with underlying cirrhosis who are at risk for hepatocellular carcinoma. The appropriate CT technique is a combination of late arterial/portal venous inflow phase and hepatic phase imaging.[9]

Presurgical planning

Prior to hepatic resection, orthotopic liver transplantation (OLT), living related donor transplantation (LRDT), cryoablation, and chemoembolization it is mandatory to evaluate the vascular structures supplying and draining the liver (Fig. 126.2). The addition of early arterial phase imaging allows for production of a CT arteriogram and CT portal venogram, which can help define important anatomic vascular variants and stenosis or thrombosis of the extrahepatic portal venous system.[7]

Perfusion anomalies

Perfusion anomalies occur in patients with focal interruptions to the liver blood supply and venous drainage and in patients with vascular hepatic neoplasms, both before and after ablative therapy. Perfusion anomalies are most pronounced during the arterial phase. In patients with lobar or segmental portal vein stenosis or thrombosis there may be compensatory increased hepatic arterial inflow to the affected segments or lobes.

In patients with vascular hepatic neoplasms, the surrounding normal hepatic parenchyma may be relatively hyperenhanced during the late arterial phase of imaging because the liver tumor produces increased hepatic arterial inflow in a segmental or lobar distribution to supply both the tumor and adjacent normal parenchyma (Fig. 126.3).

Arterioportal fistulae occur in vascularized hepatic tumors with neocirculation and after penetrating trauma such as percutaneous biopsy leading to hyperenhancement of adjacent hepatic parenchyma.

Biliary disease

Thin-section imaging performed before the administration of contrast material may be useful in detecting partially calcified ductal stones.[10] Postcontrast imaging is useful in defining the

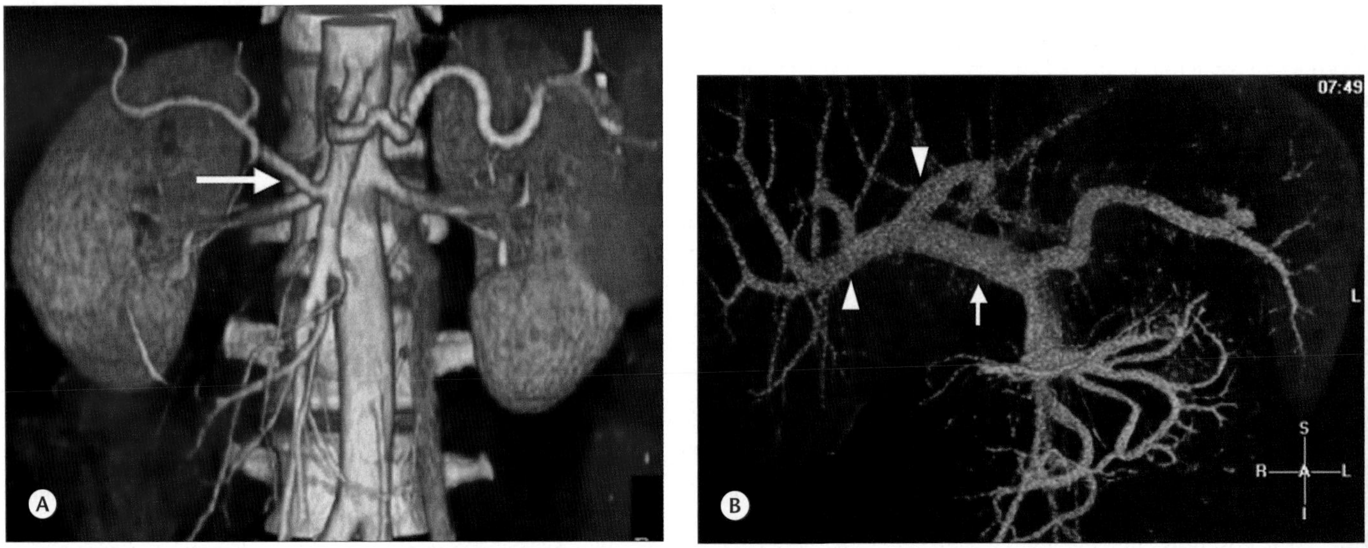

Fig. 126.2 Use of multiplanar reconstruction prior to liver transplantation. A. Three-dimensional volume-rendered CT image shows arterial system supplying the liver. Note replaced common hepatic artery originating from superior mesenteric artery (arrow). **B.** Three-dimensional volume-rendered image shows normal intrahepatic (arrowheads) and extrahepatic (arrow) portal venous anatomy.

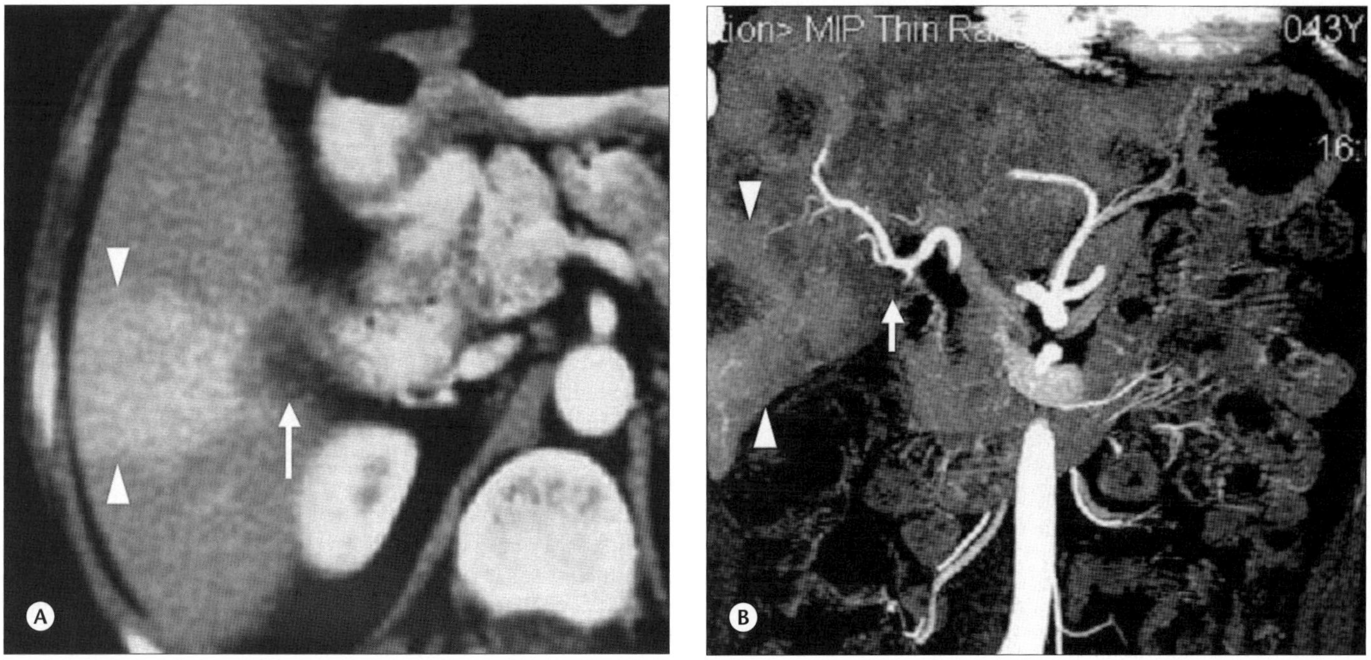

Fig. 126.3 Perfusion anomalies. A. Late arterial phase contrast-enhanced CT shows a liver metastasis in segment 6 of the right hepatic lobe (arrow) with associated wedge-shaped enhancement of the peripheral hepatic parenchyma due to segmental portal vein obstruction (arrowheads). **B.** Coronal maximum intensity projection (MIP) image of an arterial phase contrast-enhanced CT demonstrates the hepatic artery supplying the tumor (arrow) and hyperemia of the adjacent parenchyma (arrowheads) due to the 'sump' effect.

site and extent of biliary tract obstruction and, in cases of malignant duct obstruction, the location and size of lymphadenopathy and hepatic metastasis. CT cholangiography is a novel technique that provides high-resolution images of the biliary tree based on thin-section MDCT after the intravenous administration of a biliary contrast agent.

Pancreatic imaging

A triple phase imaging technique that includes an early arterial phase, pancreatic phase (or late arterial phase), and hepatic phase is routinely employed. The early arterial phase is used in patients with suspected pancreatic carcinoma who are potential candidates for surgery and it can be used to produce a CT angiogram for a vascular road map. Neoplasms, focal pancreatitis, and intrapancreatic pseudocyst are best delineated in the pancreatic phase. Thin-section technique (1 mm in the early arterial phase and 2.5 mm in the pancreatic phase) and rapid coverage are used in conjunction with rapid intravenous bolus injection of 100 mL nonionic contrast agent. Water is used as enteric contrast material in patients with suspected pancreatic carcinoma.[11]

Pancreatic adenocarcinoma

Multiplanar reformations including curved planar reformations optimize display of pancreatic tumors and local metastases by providing high-resolution images of the whole organ in planes other than the axial plane, with a better demonstration of peripancreatic tumor extension, vascular invasion, and lymphadenopathy (Fig. 126.4).

Other pancreatic neoplasms

A major advantage of thin-section MDCT in cystic pancreatic neoplasms is duct visualization to detect the extent of ductectatic tumor or intraductal papillary mucinous tumor. The relationships of neoplasms to surrounding vessels and adjacent organs can be well displayed[12] (Fig. 126.5).

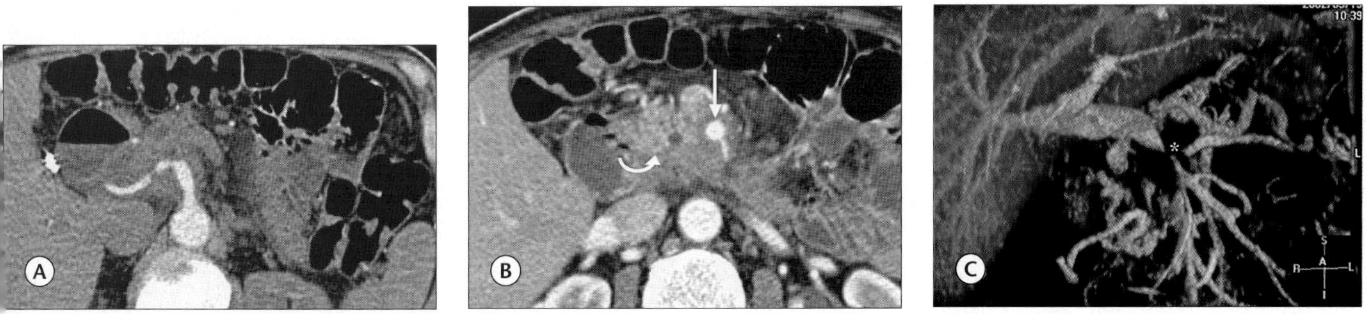

Fig. 126.4 Pancreatic head carcinoma involving the hepatic artery. Early **(A)** and late **(B)** arterial phase contrast-enhanced CT images show encasement of the hepatic artery (arrow) and, more caudally, the superior mesenteric artery (arrow). Note the nice contrast between enhancing normal pancreatic parenchyma and tumor (curved arrow). **C.** Three-dimensional volume-rendered CT image shows thrombosis of the venous system at the level of the confluence of the superior mesenteric vein, portal vein, and splenic vein (asterisk).

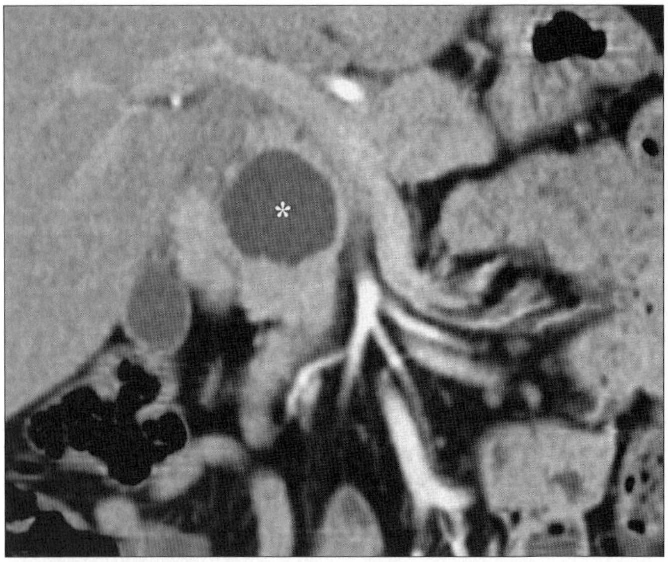

Fig. 126.5 Multiplanar coronal reformatted CT image. Multiplanar coronal reformatted CT image from the pancreatic phase data demonstrates a cystic neoplasm (asterisk) in the head of the pancreas and its relation to the surrounding vessels.

Regarding hypervascular islet cell tumors, the advantage of multiphasic MDCT is the detection and localization of the lesions and vascular hepatic metastases. These are optimally detected in the late arterial/portal venous inflow phase.

Pancreatitis

In patients with acute pancreatitis, a single phase (40s after injection) technique is performed using barium sulfate as oral contrast agent. Coronal reformatted images are used to evaluate the extent, severity, and associated complications of pancreatitis[13] (Fig. 126.6).

Digestive tract

CT colonography (CTC)

CTC is a promising method for colorectal screening providing a full structural evaluation of the entire colon (see Chapter 129). It is gaining in popularity due to a safety profile that is superior to that of conventional colonography, a low rate of complications, and high patient acceptance. The basic principles are: cleansing the colon using a standard barium enema or colonoscopy bowel preparation; colonic insufflation with room air or carbon dioxide; and thin-section MDCT of the abdomen and pelvis in both the supine and prone position followed by off-line computer manipulation of the CT dataset to facilitate inspection of the colonic wall (Fig. 126.7). Use of intravenously administered contrast material is recommended in patients with symptoms of colorectal disease or those with known colorectal cancer.

The most important measure of CTC as a colorectal screening test is its accuracy in detecting adenomatous polyps and other precursor lesions. Polyp size has a major impact on accuracy. Diagnostic performance and interobserver agreement are high (>90%) for large polyps (10mm) but more variable for smaller ones. Other indications for CTC are the preoperative assessment, the colon proximal to an occlusive tumor, and detection of extracolonic findings that can be considered clinically important when applied to an asymptomatic screening population.[11]

CT enterography (CTE)

CTE is a method of examining the small intestine that combines the advantages of enteral evaluation by cross-sectional imaging and depiction of extraintestinal manifestations of the disease.[14] Adequate opacification of the small intestine using oral contrast agents is essential for accurate CT scanning. The use of intravenous contrast is necessary for the evaluation of inflammatory and neoplastic diseases of the small bowel.

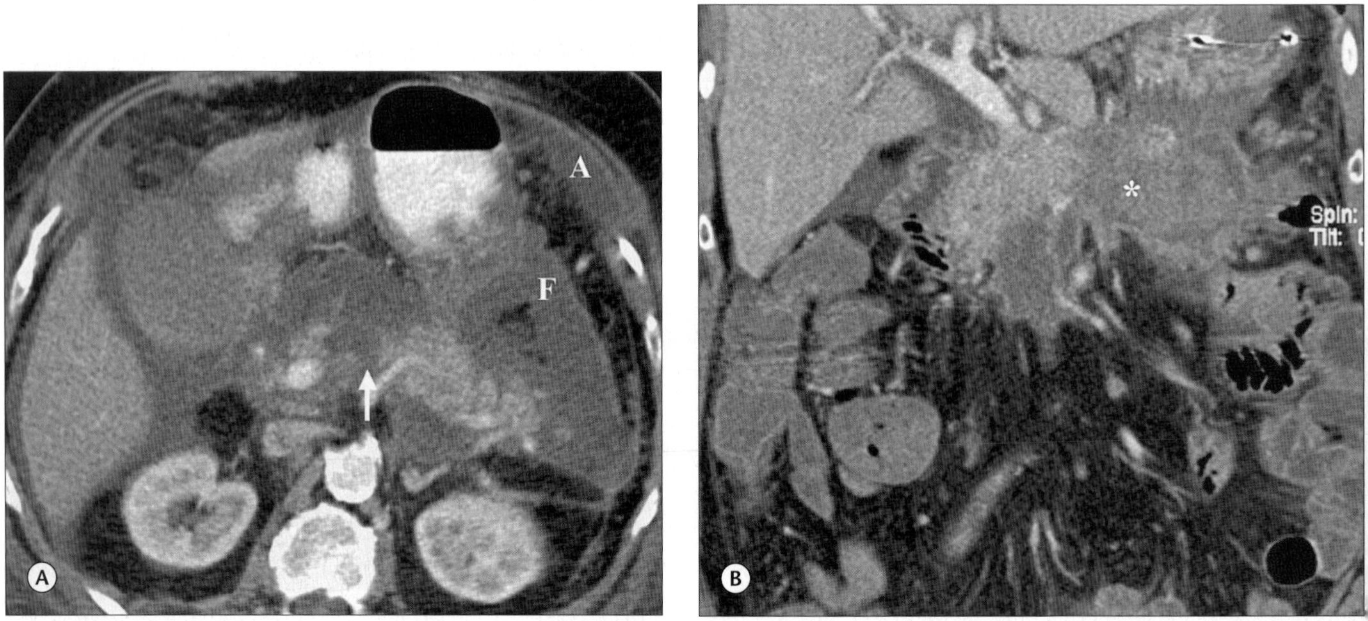

Fig. 126.6. Acute pancreatitis. A. Late arterial phase contrast-enhanced CT image shows an area of necrosis (arrow) in the neck and body of the pancreas associated with peripancreatic fluid (F) accumulation and ascites (A). **B.** Multiplanar coronal reformatted CT image better illustrates the peripancreatic vasculature and extent of peripancreatic inflammation (asterisk).

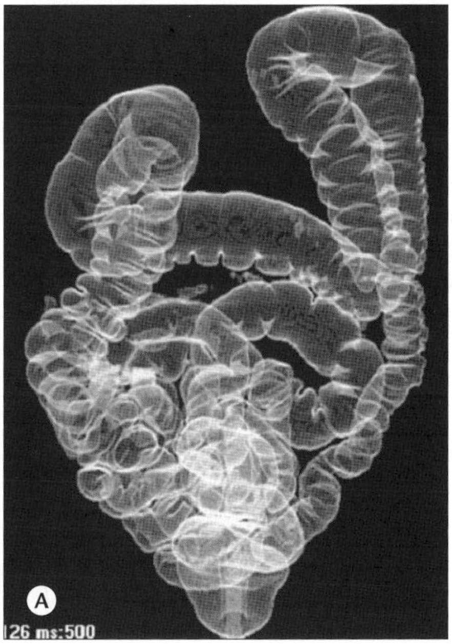

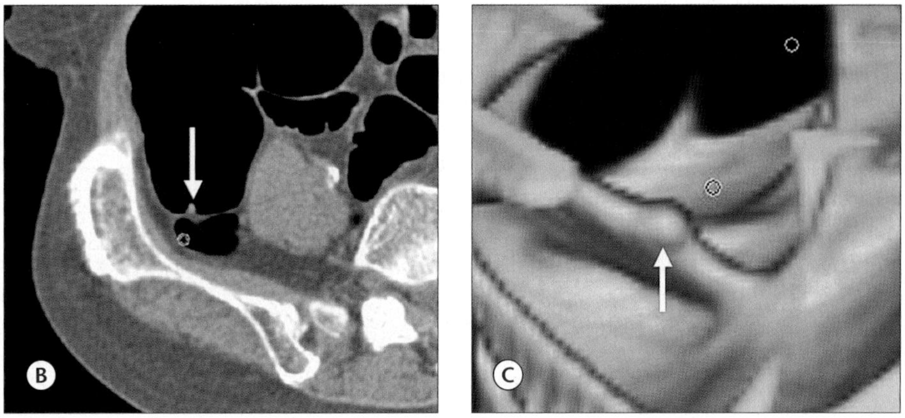

Fig. 126.7 CT colonography. A. Three-dimensional volume-rendered extraluminal CT image of the normal colon. **B.** Two-dimensional axial CT image with the patient in supine position demonstrates a polyp on a fold in the ascending colon (arrow). **C.** Three-dimensional volume-rendered endoluminal image in the same patient shows the polyp (arrow).

Many conditions, such as mesenteric ischemia, Crohn's disease, small bowel obstruction, and neoplasms that would traditionally be imaged with other modalities, are now routinely imaged with CTE (Fig. 126.8). The development of MDCT and improvements in three-dimensional imaging systems has greatly improved the ability to examine the small bowel and mesenteric vasculature.[15]

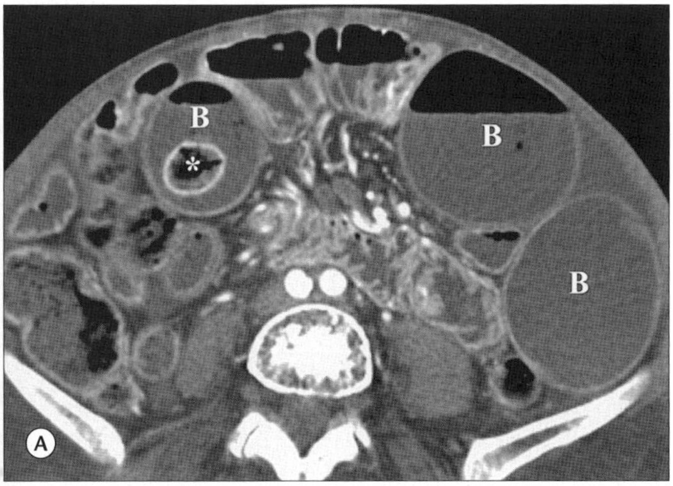

Fig. 126.8 CT enterography. Axial contrast-enhanced MDCT enterography image **(A)** and coronal multiplanar reconstruction **(B)** demonstrates dilatation of the small bowel loops (B) and 'enterolith' (asterisk) due to chronic obstruction as a result of an adhesive band.

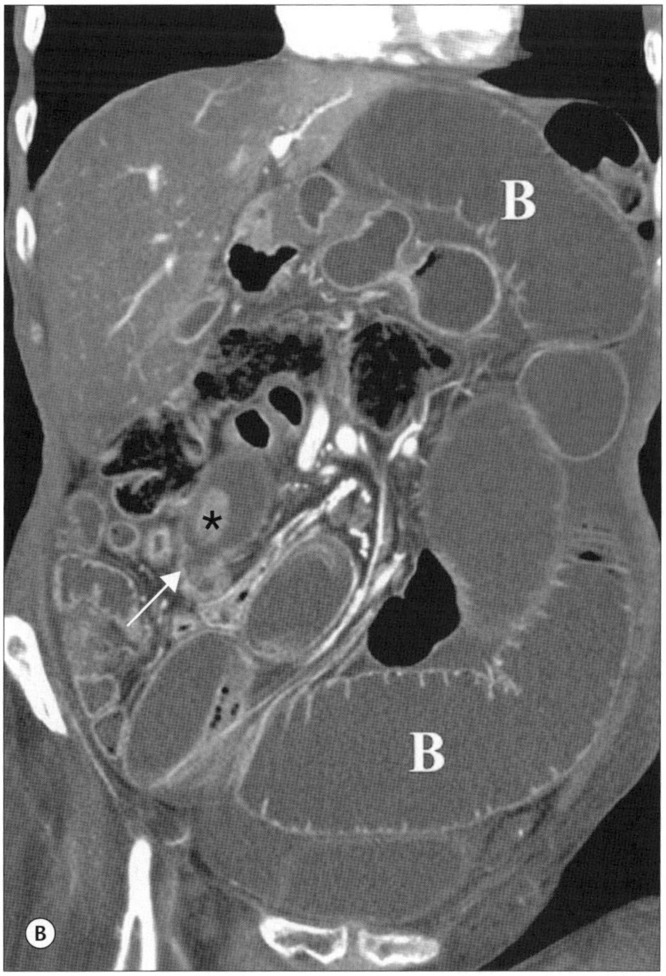

SOURCES OF INFORMATION FOR PATIENTS AND DOCTORS

http://www.patient.co.uk/showdoc/27000478/
http://www.radiologyinfo.org/content/ct-abdomen.htm

REFERENCES

1. Hu H, He HD, Foley WD, Fox SH. Four multidetector-row helical CT; image quality and volume coverage speed. Radiology 2000; 215:55–62.
2. Ji H, McTavish JD, Mortele KJ, Wiesner W, Ros PR. Hepatic imaging with Multidetector CT. Radiographics 2001; 21:71–80.
3. Klingenbeck-Regn K, Schaller S, Flohr T et al. Subsecond multi-slice computed tomography: basics and applications. Eur J Radiol 1999; 31:110–124.
4. Rubin GD, Shiau MC, Schmidth AJ et al. Computed tomographic angiography: Historical perspective and new state-of-the-art using multidetector-row helical computed tomography. J Comp Assist Tomogr 1999; 23 (Suppl 1): 83–90.
5. Chambers TP, Baron RL, Lush RM et al: Hepatic CT enhancement: Comparison of ionic and non-ionic contrast agents in the same patients. Radiology 1994; 193: 513–517.
6. Chambers TP, Baron RL, Lush RM. Hepatic CT enhancement: II. Alterations in contrast material volume and rate of injection within the same patients. Radiology 1994; 193:518–522.
7. Mortele KJ, McTavish S, Ros PR. Current techniques of computed tomography: Helical CT, multidetector CT, and 3D reconstruction. Clin Liv Dis 2002; 6:29–52.
8. McCollough CH, Zink FE. Performance evaluation of a multi-slice CT system. Med Phys 1999; 26:2223–2230.
9. Foley WD, Mallisee TA, Hohenwalter MD et al. Multiphase hepatic CT with a multi-row detector CT scanner. Am Roentgenol 2000; 175:679–685.
10. Neitlich JD, Topazian M, Smith RC et al. Detection of choledocholithiasis: comparison of unenhanced helical CT and endoscopic retrograde cholangiopancreatography. Radiology 1997; 203:753–757.
11. Ji H, Rolnick JA, Haker S, Barish MA. Multislice CT colonography: current status and limitations. Eur J Radiol 2003; 47:123–134.
12. Procacci C, Megibow AJ, Carbognin G et al. Intraductal papillary mucinous tumor of the pancreas: a pictorial essay. Radiographics 1999; 19:1447–1463.
13. Robinson PJA, Sheridan MB. Pancreatic computed tomography and magnetic resonance imaging. Eur Radiol 2000; 10:401–408.
14. Maglinte DT, Bender GN, Heitkamp DE, Lappas JC, Kelvin FM. Multidetector-row helical enteroclysis. Radiol Clin North Am 2003; 41:249–262.
15. Maglinte DT, Lappas JC, Heitkamp DE, Bender GN, Kelvin FM. Technical refinements in enteroclysis. Radiol Clin North Am 2003; 41:213–229.

Chapter 127

Magnetic resonance imaging

M Raquel Oliva, Koenraad J Mortele, and Pablo R Ros

KEY POINTS

- The use of magnetic resonance imaging (MRI) in the gastrointestinal tract is expanding
- MRI is the modality of choice in staging rectal cancer, but is limited in detection of lymph node metastases
- MRI has a major role in assessment of perianal fistulae e.g. in Crohn's disease
- Contrast enhancement with gadolinium is particularly useful in characterizing focal hepatic and pancreatic lesions
- T2W images are useful in differentiating benign and malignant focal liver lesions
- MRI is less sensitive than spiral CT in assessment of pancreatic cancers vs pancreatitis
- MR enterography and colonography show future promise

INTRODUCTION AND SCIENTIFIC BASIS

In magnetic resonance imaging (MRI), the body or a part of it is placed in a magnetic field, generated by a large whole-body or smaller surface multicoil magnet. Radiofrequency pulses are applied intermittently, resulting in the realignment of molecules within the magnetic field. The patterns by which stored energy is released, when the radiofrequency pulse is turned off, provide data that are converted into images by the use of a Fourier transform.

Hitherto, the use of MRI in patients with abdominal diseases has been limited compared with the use of computed tomography (CT) (see Chapter 126), because of limitations, particularly the time needed to acquire the required data. However, technical improvements, such as the development of phased-array multicoils, enhanced gradients, and methods to reduce motion-related artefacts, are expanding its use. In many diseases, MRI provides both a more accurate delineation of the extent of disease and improved disease characterization compared with CT and ultrasonography. Evaluation can be optimized by using contrast-enhanced dynamic MRI for MR angiography (MRA), which visualizes the vessels, and MR cholangiopancreatography (MRCP), which depicts the biliopancreatic ductal system. At present, MRI is particularly valuable in evaluating the liver, pancreas, and biliary tree. Currently, the indications for MRI of the gastrointestinal tract are limited to staging of rectal cancer and assessing the extent of perianal fistulae and anal sphincter tears, but the potential roles of MR colonography, MR enteroclysis, and MRI of appendicitis are under extensive evaluation.

DESCRIPTION OF TECHNIQUE

Theoretical considerations

Protons in a magnetic field become aligned along that field. Exposure to specific (Larmor) radiofrequencies causes nuclei to jump into a higher energy state, so that the net magnetization factor rotates to lie in a transverse plane. T1 relaxation is based upon the rate of return to the original alignment when the radiofrequency pulse is switched off. T2 relaxation is based upon loss of transverse magnetization. T1 and T2 relaxation can be made dominant by varying the echo time and repetition time of the radiofrequency wave. The theoretical basis of commonly used protocols such as spin echo (SE), gradient echo (GRE), fast SE and turbo SE protocols, chemical shift methods for fat suppression, half-Fourier acquisition single-shot turbo spin echo (HASTE), and thick-section rapid acquisition with relaxation enhancement (RARE) are discussed in Runge et al[1] and Heuck and Reiser.[2]

Use of multiple signals

To detect and characterize abdominal pathology accurately, the use of multiple-pulse sequences providing complementary information is required and, in general, a combination of T1-weighted (T1W) and T2-weighted (T2W) sequences is obtained. In the ideal MRI sequence, the spatial resolution is maximized within a short acquisition time while the signal to noise ratio is maintained sufficiently high. The development of surface coils oriented to image a specific volume of the body (phased-array surface multicoil system or torso coil) proved to be an important tool in improving the diagnostic value of individual pulse sequences and in producing higher-resolution images compared with the whole-volume body coil.[3]

T1W images using conventional spin-echo (SE) technique require significant image time and are no longer routinely performed.[4] Instead, breath-hold T1W spoiled gradient-echo (GRE) images are used.[5,6] These sequences generate an echo by gradient reversal, allowing a short echo time (TE) and consequently a much faster sequence.[4]

T2W imaging is performed with a longer repetition time (TR) and TE compared with the T1W sequences, and is achieved by conventional SE, fast SE, or GRE imaging. Images obtained with conventional SE pulse sequences take longer and are sensitive for motion artefacts; thus supplementary techniques such as fat suppression are mandatory.[7] In contrast to conventional SE technique, fast SE (FSE) or turbo SE (TSE) imaging can be performed in significantly less time, in one or two breath-holds, and compares favorably to conventional SE sequences for lesion detection and characterization.[8,9]

Fat-suppressed images

The so-called 'chemical shift method' for fat suppression uses a frequency selection 90° pulse on the fat proton frequency and crusher gradient to suppress fat prior to imaging. Resonance frequency differences can also be used to generate in-phase and opposed-phase images.[4,10] This is the most commonly used method, and exploits the difference in resonance between triglyceride protons and water.[4] By careful selection of echo time, voxels containing both fat and water will exhibit a high signal when in phase, and a signal cancellation while in opposed phase.

Contrast-enhanced images

These are a special adjunct in the abdominal examination, using intravenous gadolinium. Contrast enhancement is particularly useful in characterizing focal hepatic and pancreatic lesions, and in defining a variety of other intra-abdominal processes. Theoretically, it is desirable to acquire images before and after contrast administration utilizing the same technique. Typically, these are T1W images, which may be obtained with SE or, preferentially, fat-suppressed GRE techniques, as described above.[11] Preferably, postgadolinium imaging is performed in different phases of perfusion.

MRCP typically employs 'heavily' T2W images of the biliary tree and pancreatic duct, in which bile, pancreatic juices, and other stationary or slowly moving fluids appear hyperintense relative to other abdominal tissues. Two different MRCP 'snapshot' techniques are usually applied: thin-section HASTE and thick-section RARE. MRCP has the following advantages over endoscopic retrograde cholangiopancreatography (ERCP):[12]

- It is noninvasive, requiring no anesthesia, medication, or ionizing radiation.
- There is no increased risk of pancreatitis.
- It can be performed on patients with altered pancreaticobiliary system morphology following prior surgery.
- In patients with complete obstruction of the ducts, MRCP can demonstrate the upstream anatomy and periductal abnormalities.

General considerations

Before the examination, the patient should be screened for contraindications to MRI such as presence of certain metals in critical regions such as the eyes, spinal cord, or brain, and metal devices such as cardiac pacemaker, implantable defibrillator, and cerebral aneurysm surgical clips. Claustrophobic subjects do not tolerate the examination and may require conscious sedation. The presence of hip prostheses is not normally regarded a contraindication to MRI, but does impede a complete analysis of the rectum and sigmoid colon.

LIVER IMAGING

The normal liver demonstrates a higher signal intensity to that of the spleen on T1W images owing to the presence of larger amount of free water binding protein within hepatocytes.[13] Most focal hepatic lesions (metastases, cysts, and hemangiomas) have a long T1 and thus have lower signal intensity compared with surrounding normal hepatic tissue. However, lesions originating from hepatocellular tissue, such as adenoma, focal nodular hyperplasia, regenerative nodule, and well differentiated hepatocellular carcinoma (HCC), are isointense or even hyperintense compared with liver parenchyma. Such hyperintense signal intensity within a liver mass is suggestive, but not specific, for a lesion of hepatocellular origin.

To detect focal liver lesions and help differentiate benign from malignant conditions, T2W images are extremely important.[14] As most hepatic neoplasms have a longer T2 than liver, they demonstrate a high signal intensity on T2W images. Breath-hold FSE T2W sequences with a long TE are helpful in differentiating benign cysts and hemangiomas from other hepatic neoplasms.[15] In general, on these 'heavily' T2W images, malignancies show signal intensity similar to spleen, whereas cysts and hemangiomas demonstrate a very high signal intensity.

Several types of contrast agent have been clinically investigated for MRI of the liver. According to their biodistribution pattern, four major categories can be recognized.[16,17]

Extracellular agents

Gadolinium (Gd) chelates initially distribute in the intravascular space but are then rapidly filtered into the extracellular or interstitial space of normal and abnormal tissues. They are the most frequently used MRI contrast and have an important role in tissue characterization because many different enhancement and washout patterns are characteristic of a variety of lesions.

Reticuloendothelial agents

Superparamagnetic iron oxides particles (SPIOs), or ferumoxides, are taken up specifically by the Kupffer cells of the liver. Most focal hepatic lesions, especially metastases, are devoid of reticuloendothelial cells and contrast sharply with the adjacent normal liver parenchyma, which is darkened by iron oxide phagocytosis on T2W images, improving lesion detection.[18] Lesion characterization is also enhanced as most focal nodular hyperplasia and adenomas, and some well differentiated HCCs, show uptake of ferumoxides due to the presence of Kupffer cells; thus establishing a decrease of signal intensity on postcontrast T2W images.

Hepatobiliary-specific agents

Several soluble paramagnetic molecules (Gd-BOPTA, Gd-EOB-DPTA and Mn-DPDP) are taken up by the hepatocytes and excreted into bile.[17] They predominantly affect T1 contrast, increasing signal in normal liver tissue without enhancement of nonhepatocellular lesions (metastases, lymphoma, intrahepatic cholangiocarcinoma) and, therefore, increase lesion detection on T1W images.[16] The specific biliary excretion of hepatobiliary contrasts agents has the potential to improve delineation of the biliary tree, which may be helpful in the diagnosis of biliary invasion by hepatic lesions, and to increase the diagnostic accuracy in patients with associated biliary diseases.

Intravascular agents

Dextran-coated ultra-small superparamagnetic iron oxide particles (USPIOs) (AMI-227) contrast with all other contrast agents discussed above, as they are molecules with a long half-time in blood and thus very suitable to be used as intravascular (blood pool) agents. Because of differences in blood volume between normal liver and solid hepatic tumors, improved detection of focal liver lesions can be achieved. Furthermore, as USPIO particles generate a fairly strong T1 and T2 relativity these contrast agents can be used as either negative (on T2W images) or positive (on T1W images) agents.[17]

:haracteristics of individual pathologies

-lepatic adenoma (see Chapter 102)

-lepatic adenoma is an important diagnosis because of its isk of life-threatening hemorrhage.[19] MRI classically shows a eterogeneous (93%) mass, with predominantly hyperintense ignal intensity on T2W images (47–75%), and variable signal ntensity on T1W images due to fatty change (25%), hemorhage (38%), and necrosis (16%).[19] On dynamic gadolinium-nhanced T1W images, 86% of adenomas show early arterial nhancement, secondary to their hepatic arterial blood supply.[19]

-lepatocellular carcinoma (see Chapter 102)

-ICC commonly arises in the setting of underlying cirrhosis.[20] Typically T2W images demonstrate a mild hyperintensity relative o normal liver, with T1W signal intensity varying with the presence or absence of steatosis or hemorrhage.[21] High signal intensity n T2W helps differentiation from dysplastic nodules, which ypically have a low T2W intensity, due to accumulation of iron.[20] After intravenous administration of gadolinium, smaller lesions end to be hypervascular. Larger lesions are more hypovascular nd reveal a mosaic-like enhancement pattern. Signs of vascular nvasion and arterial–portal shunting are frequently present.

ntrahepatic cholangiocarcinomas (see Chapter 102)

'eripheral intrahepatic cholangiocarcinomas are homogeneously ypointense on T1W images (100%), and heterogeneous but enerally high in signal on T2W images.[22] Tumors characteristically have minimal or moderate rim enhancement on dynamic MR studies (75%) and delayed persistent enhancement is ommon.[22] A combination of features is common. Other MRI eatures are dilatation of peripheral bile ducts with focal tricturing due to tumor obstruction, capsular retraction, and ncasement without invasion of the portal veins.

Metastases

Aetastases often have a nonspecific appearance. They usually lemonstrate a lower signal intensity than liver on T1W images, nd a higher signal intensity on T2W images, both generally sointense to the spleen.[23] After administration of gadolinium, im enhancement, heterogeneous diffuse enhancement, and eripheral washout on equilibrium phase images may be seen.[23]

Cavernous hemangioma[17]

Compared with normal liver tissue, a hemangioma shows decreased and markedly increased signal intensity on T1W images and T2W images, respectively,[20,24,25] usually sufficient to characterize this lesion.[15] Dynamic T1W imaging obtained following intravenous administration of gadopentate dimeglumine classically shows a peripheral nodular centripetal enhancement pattern progressing to homogeneity[25] (Fig. 127.1).

Hepatic bile duct cysts

These are typically round, ovoid, and well delineated,[26] with very low pre- and post-contrast T1W signal intensity and a very high signal intensity on T2W images. 'Heavily' T2W images show very high signal intensity, comparable to that of cerebrospinal fluid, sufficient to differentiate benign cysts from both hemangiomas and solid liver lesions.

Focal nodular hyperplasia

These lesions are usually homogeneous and isointense on T1W (35%) and/or T2W (69%) images. They may have central scars that are hyperintense on T2W images due to vascular and biliary components,[19] and may be highlighted by SPIOs.

Diffuse liver disease

Cirrhosis (see Chapter 95)

Typical findings include surface nodularity and morphologic changes, as well as extrahepatic signs such as splenomegaly, portosystemic collateral vessels, ascites, small bowel edema, and gallbladder wall thickening.[27] Enlargement of the hilar periportal space has been described as a helpful sign in the diagnosis of early cirrhosis.[28] More pronounced lobar or segmental changes of hepatic morphology, such as atrophy of the right hepatic lobe and left medial segment, enlargement of the caudate lobe and left lateral segment, and the expanded gallbladder fossa sign are seen in advanced cirrhosis.[28] MR angiography provides useful information regarding the location and flow pattern in portosystemic shunts that is useful for diagnosis (e.g., detection of varices) and treatment planning (e.g., prior to TIPS placement, shunt surgery).

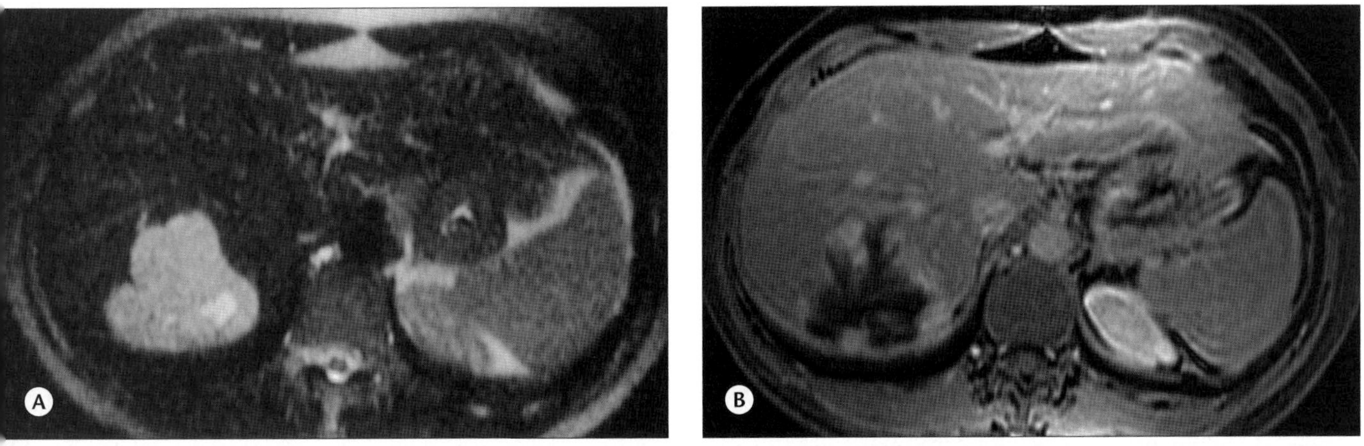

-ig. 127.1 Hepatic hemangioma. A. 'Heavily' T2-weighted MR image shows a focal hepatic lesion with markedly increased signal intensity :ompared with surrounding normal hepatic tissue. **B.** Peripheral nodular incomplete enhancement on a late arterial phase gadolinium-enhanced T1-weighted image. Both the signal intensity and enhancement pattern are consistent with hepatic hemangioma.

Nodules in the cirrhotic liver

MRI is the most specific imaging technique for differentiating regenerative from dysplastic or malignant nodules in cirrhosis.

Regenerative nodules are usually isointense with other background nodules on both T1W and T2W images, and show no predominant enhancement pattern following gadolinium administration, reflecting their predominantly portal venous blood supply.[28] Unlike the majority of HCCs, regenerative nodules are almost never hyperintense on T2W images.

Dysplastic nodules are typically smaller than 3 cm, with no capsule; they show homogeneous hyperintensity on T1W images and hypointensity on T2W images.[28] The main blood supply is from the portal venous system, but some cases may demonstrate hypervascular lesions on contrast-enhanced MRI study because of the hepatic artery supply, especially those with high-grade dysplasia.

Foci of HCC in dysplastic nodules

Classically, a high-signal intensity focus within a low signal intensity dysplastic nodule is seen on T2W images ('nodule within a nodule').[27]

Hepatic steatosis (see Chapter 88)

Steatosis is most sensitively detected using GRE MR pulse sequences.[28] By varying the echo time to image water and fat in and out of phase, chemical shifts between water and lipid protons can be demonstrated. Areas with a significant amount of intracellular fat show a characteristic lower signal intensity on out-of-phase images compared with the corresponding in-phase images.[29] Typical features of focal fatty change include the typical periligamentous and periportal location, lack of mass effect, sharply angulated boundaries of the area, nonspherical shape, absence of vascular displacement or distortion, and lobar or segmental distribution.[28]

Hereditary or primary hemochromatosis (see Chapter 89)

MRI is more specific than any other imaging modality for the characterization of iron overload because of the unique magnetic susceptibility effect of iron.[30] The superparamagnetic effect of accumulated iron in the hepatocytes results in a significant reduction of signal intensity of the liver parenchyma on T2W images, particularly T2*W GRE sequences.[28] The paraspinal musculature, which is normally less intense than liver, provides a useful internal control.[28]

Hemosiderosis or siderosis

In transfusional iron overload states or dyserythropoiesis, the excessive iron is processed and accumulates in organs containing reticuloendothelial cells.[29] Consequently, low signal intensity changes are seen in liver, as in primary hemochromatosis, but also in the spleen and bone marrow.[31]

PANCREATOBILIARY IMAGING

The normal pancreas has higher signal intensity on T1W images than the liver; this has been attributed to a larger amount of manganese within the pancreatic acini. The most common exocrine pancreatic diseases (i.e., pancreatitis, pancreatic adenocarcinoma) have longer T1 values because of increased free water protons and, therefore, have lower signal intensity compared with surrounding normal pancreatic parenchyma.[3] Pancreatic tumors and the delineation of the pancreas from surrounding fat are best established on fat-suppressed T1W images.[32]

Normal pancreatic parenchyma has a short T2 value compared with liver and spleen; consequently the signal is low to intermediate on T2W images, with higher values in both liver and spleen, but also most pancreatic lesions.[32] Heavily T2W images are breath-hold 'fast' sequences with an extended TE used to characterize pancreatic cysts or hypervascular lesions. Dynamic gadolinium contrast-enhanced T1W imaging accentuates differences between normal pancreas and usually less vascular neoplastic or necrotic tissue and hypervascular pancreatic masses that may simulate cystic lesions on noncontrast scans.

Gadolinium-enhanced MRI is also useful in evaluating pancreatitis, especially detection of necrosis and evaluation of pseudocysts. Currently, three-dimensional gadolinium-enhanced MR angiography (3D-Gd-MRA) is the best technique for evaluating the peripancreatic vessels, especially in patients with pancreatic neoplasm, to exclude arterial or venous invasion. Some specific MR contrast media are currently under investigation, such as manganese dipyridoxyl diphosphate (Mn-DPDP), which enhances the normal pancreas on T1W images[3] and monocrystalline iron oxide labeled with cholecystokinin targeted at pancreatic receptors.

Characteristics of individual pathologies

Pancreatic adenocarcinoma (see Chapter 73)

Detection is based on noncontrast T1W fat-suppressed images and immediate post-gadolinium T1W spoiled GRE images. On T1W fat-suppressed SE images, pancreatic cancer appears as a mass of low signal intensity, and is clearly separated from normal pancreatic tissue, which is high in signal intensity. On T1W images after intravenous administration of gadolineum, normal pancreatic tissue becomes hyperintense and unenhanced pancreatic adenocarcinoma can be delineated from normal pancreas[34] (Fig. 127.2). Although this seems to be especially useful in the diagnosis of smaller tumors and in the differentiation between pancreatic carcinomas and chronic pancreatitis, studies have shown that Mn-DPDP-enhanced MRI seems to be less sensitive than spiral CT for these purposes.[34,35]

Serous cystic tumor (see Chapter 74)

This well circumscribed hypervascular benign tumor is often lobulated and contains a central, stellate, calcified scar in addition to multiple small cysts divided by thin septations.[36] Imaging studies commonly show a cystic mass with multiple small cysts, although the tumor may appear homogeneously solid. Six or more small cysts favor a serous rather than mucinous cystic neoplasm.[36] Serous cystic tumors are usually markedly hyperintense on T2W MR images, although fibrous scars may yield some central areas of low signal intensity.[37] On T1W MR images, the tumor is of low signal intensity, except where hemorrhage is present.[37]

Mucinous cystic tumors (see Chapter 74)

These range from tumors with malignant potential to frankly malignant cystadenocarcinomas. Most typically, these hypovascular tumors are multilocular with individual cysts measuring ore than 2 cm in size; they are typically located in the tail or ɔdy of the pancreas.[38] They contain mucin and usually have thick wall, internal septations, solid papillary excretions, and, casionally, peripheral calcifications.[36] MR images show the ɔntents of these cystic masses to be variable in signal intenty; this variability is related to internal hemorrhage or the oteinaceous nature of the fluid.[38]

traductal papillary mucinous tumor

ɪis is a relatively new and increasingly reported entity typilly presenting on MRI as a dilated main pancreatic duct comned with a unilocular or multilocular cystic lesion.[39] Commucation between the main pancreatic duct and the cystic lesion ay be depicted.[39]

ndocrine tumors (see Chapter 109)

ɪese are benign or malignant neoplasms with endocrine cell fferentiation. MRI plays a role in their detection and evaluaon. Typically these tumors give a low signal intensity on T1W ıd a high signal intensity on T2W imaging.[37,40,41] Following travenous gadolinium–DTPA, ring-like enhancement in ıe periphery of the tumor is typically seen because of ypervascularity, whereas the center may remain hypointense condary to fibrosis.

cute pancreatitis (see Chapter 71)

IRI can depict the presence and extent of necrosis and periancreatic fluid collections. A routine pancreas protocol includg T2W, fat-suppressed T1W, and a series of T1W GRE quences before and immediately after gadolinium adminisation, is a reliable method for staging acute pancreatitis and aching a prognosis.[42] In severe acute pancreatitis, gadoliniumɪhanced MRI is particularly useful for assessing pancreatic arenchymal perfusion and detecting necrosis. Parenchymal dema is better shown on unenhanced T1W images. T2W quences are the most sensitive in demonstrating fluid collections. Additionally MRCP or MRA enables the diagnosis of underlying etiologies, such as choledocholithiasis, or the detection of vascular complications.

Chronic pancreatitis (see Chapter 72)

The role of MRCP in chronic pancreatitis is still controversial. Comparisons between MRCP and ERCP in cases of chronic pancreatitis have revealed agreement of 83–100% for identification of ductal dilatation, 70–92% for identification of narrowing, and 92–100% for identification of filling defects.[43] MRI should include T1W and T2W images and MR cholangiography. Several centers have investigated functional MR evaluation and shown improved visualization of the pancreatic duct and its side branches following intravenous secretin administration.[44] Furthermore, the volume of effluent into the duodenum can be used for functional evaluation of relative estimate exocrine reserve.[44]

Focal pancreatitis versus pancreatic adenocarcinoma

In contrast to some earlier reports, a recent study showed that MRI could not reliably differentiate these two conditions.[45] Mn-DPDP may have potential, but further studies are necessary.

Extrahepatic cholestasis

MRI has an increasing role here. MRI can visualize the bile ducts both above and below a stricture or obstruction, and avoids inherent complications of ERCP or percutaneous transhepatic cholangiography (PTC).[46]

Stone in the common bile duct

This is the most common cause of biliary obstruction; MRI is highly accurate in its detection and characterization.[47] Usually common bile duct stones are hypointense on both T1W and T2W images, and are typically surrounded by bile[47] (Fig. 127.3) in a dependent position (compared with pneumobilia air bubbles, which float, and bile flow artefacts, which are typically central in location).[47]

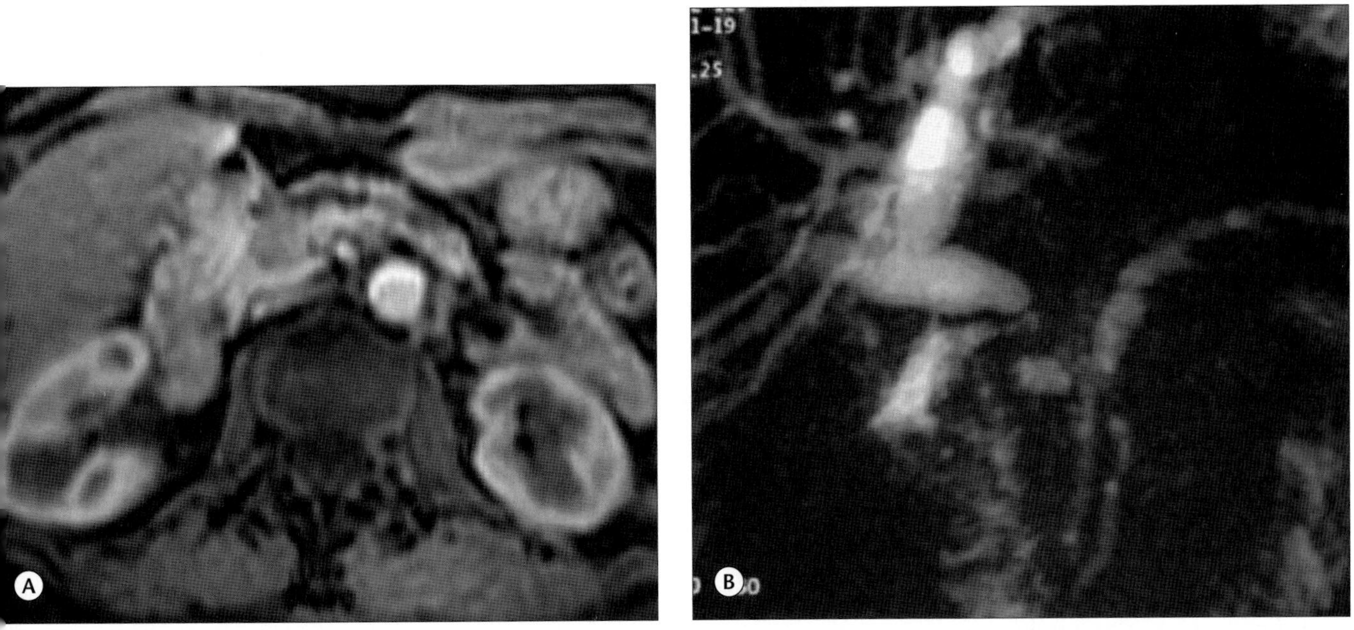

ig. 127.2 **Pancreatic ductal adenocarcinoma. A.** Fat-suppressed gadolinium-enhanced axial T1-weighted MR image shows a hypointense ass that is clearly delineated from normal hyperintense pancreatic parenchyma. **B.** Projective oblique–coronal MRCP image demonstrates latation of the common bile duct and pancreatic duct ('double duct sign').

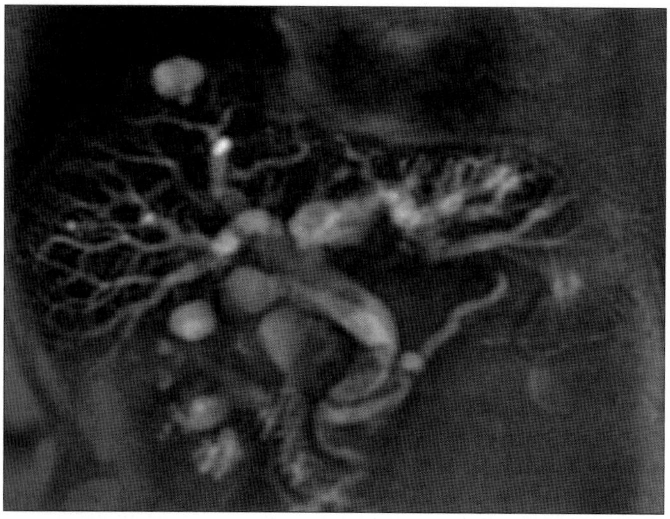

Fig. 127.3 Common bile duct stones. Projective oblique–coronal MRCP image shows multiple filling defects compatible with stones in the distal common bile duct with proximal dilatation of the duct.

Primary sclerosing cholangitis (see Chapter 78)

On MRI, the characteristic appearance is marked by presence of multiple stenoses,[48] minor dilatation of the proximal segments (due to periductal fibrosis), beaded appearance of intrahepatic bile ducts, the presence of sacculations resembling diverticula, and intrahepatic lithiasis.

Extrahepatic cholangiocarcinoma (see Chapter 79)

Extrahepatic cholangiocarcinomas include biliary adenocarcinomas located at the bifurcation or proximal hepatic duct (Klatskin tumors) and the distal duct types.[49] On MRI, they typically present as a mass located at the liver hilum causing biliary dilatation and are usually hypointense on T1W and slightly hyperintense on T2W images. Enhancement following gadolinium administration is variable.[49] Less frequently, vascular involvement, lobar atrophy, and lymph node involvement is seen.[49] MRCP typically reveals a stenotic lesion at the bifurcation with proximal biliary dilatation; nodular intraductal tumor components are seen occasionally.[49]

DIGESTIVE TRACT IMAGING

Currently, the indications for MRI of the gastrointestinal tract are limited to staging of rectal cancer and assessing the extent of perianal fistulae and anal sphincter tears. Technical improvements, including development of pelvic surface phased-array coils, endorectal coils, and thin-section scanning, allow high-resolution imaging of the pelvic organs with exquisite detail of the rectal wall. The potential role of MR enterography, MR colonography, and MRI of appendicitis has been researched extensively. Recent studies have shown that procedural refinements, especially the application of oral contrast agents, have increased the ability of MRI to provide data that supplement clinical and endoscopic findings of the digestive tract.[50]

Rectal cancer (see Chapter 60)

MRI is used increasingly because it gives more information for preoperative staging than any other diagnostic method.[51] It can

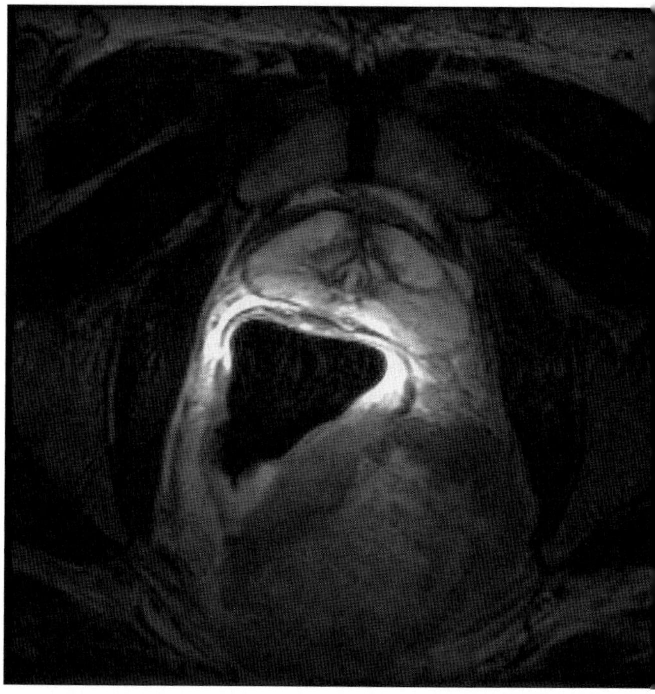

Fig. 127.4 Adenocarcinoma. Axial T2-weighted MR image shows a large rectal mass extending beyond the muscularis propria (T3) into the mesorectal fat.

show the relationship between the rectal cancer and the rectal wall and any adjacent pelvic organ, the lateral pelvic lymph node status, involvement of pelvic floor muscles beyond the reach of transrectal ultrasonography, and invasion of sphincters or surrounding structures, thereby helping in the selection of patients for sphincter preservation.[51] In the authors' experience, the optimal imaging sequences for endoluminal MRI are multiplanar T2W TSE and axial T1W SE MR sequences. The T2W images clearly demonstrate normal anal anatomy and allow differentiation of the rectal wall layers. T1W imaging is particularly helpful in determining the extent of the lesion in the mesorectal fat. Intravenous gadolinium helps to determine tumor extent and differentiate T2 from T3 tumors (Fig. 127.4). A drawback of the endorectal MRI technique is that insertion of the coil can be difficult or impossible in patients with stenosing rectal tumors. The major limitation of endoluminal MRI remains its limited ability to detect lymph node metastasis.[52]

Perianal fistulae (see Chapters 54 and 70)

Clinical history and physical examination are often sufficient for the diagnosis of perianal fistulae. MRI has a major role in establishing the extent of the fistula and its relation to the anal sphincter and perirectal structures. MRI assessment of perianal fistula includes dynamic contrast-enhanced MRI and axial fat-saturated T2W sequences, and provides the anatomic and pathologic information required to guide surgical management[5 (Fig. 127.5).

Fecal incontinence (see Chapter 10)

Recently, MRI using an endoanal coil has been shown to be capable of visualizing the external anal sphincter muscle and pelvic floor muscles, and to detect muscle atrophy and tears. Definition of its role in fecal incontinence is evolving.

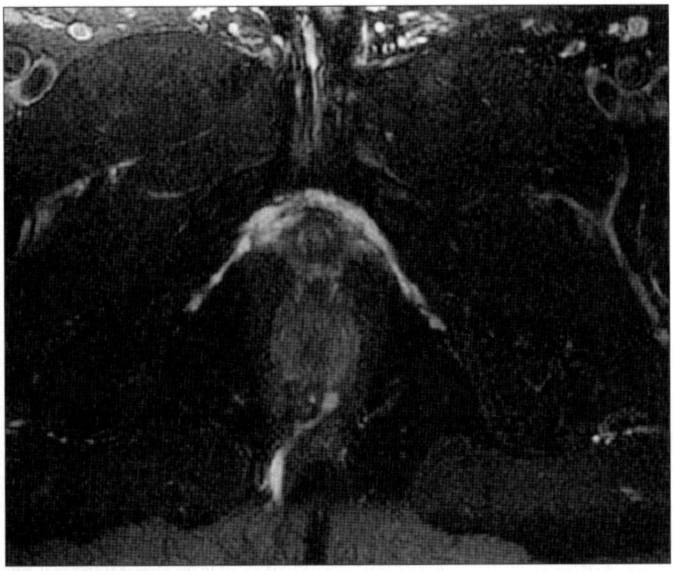

Fig. 127.5 Perianal fistula. Axial fat-saturated T2-weighted MR image shows a perianal fistula extending from the anal canal through both the internal and external sphincter into the ischioanal fat.

MR enterography

Detection of small bowel disease by MR enteroclysis depends on visualization of circumscribed areas of thickening of the intestinal wall, caused by malignant or inflammatory small bowel disease, that have been shown to correlate with changes identified at pathologic and histologic examination.[50]

MR enterography is performed almost exclusively after application of oral contrast medium, including commercially available gadolinium chelates as well as iron oxide particles, manganese chloride, iron phytate, and some foods. Oral contrast media are categorized as positive or negative, based on their ability to increase or decrease signal intensity on T1W images. Positive oral contrast media result in good contrast between the hypointense bowel wall and the high signal intensity of the intraluminal fluid content and intra-abdominal adipose tissue in T1W sequences.[50] Intravenous gadolinium chelate enhances signal from inflamed bowel segments, resulting in a reduction of this contrast. The use of fat suppression does not significantly improve image quality because, although the contrast between the intestinal wall and mesenteric adipose tissue is enhanced, that between the intestinal lumen and intestinal wall is not.

MR colonography

MR colonography is similarly performed using positive or negative luminal contrast media.[55] Gadolinium-containing enemas are used for positive ('bright lumen') MR colonography, which shows lesions as filling defects. A tap-water enema and intravenous gadolinium are used for negative ('dark lumen') MR colonography, which allows direct analysis of the bowel wall by comparison of signal intensities on precontrast and postcontrast images to detect lesions such as polyps, which are more enhanced than normal bowel mucosa. Dark-lumen MR colonography can be used for subsequent virtual colonographic viewing. Other advantages include reduced examination and post-processing times.

SOURCES OF INFORMATION FOR PATIENTS AND DOCTORS

Having an MRI can be a noisy and/or claustrophobic experience. Good sources of information can be found at:
http://www.hitachimed.com/openmri/
http://www.healthsystem.virginia.edu/internet/radiology/mri/mri-patient-info.cfm

Theoretical and training information is at:
http://www.cis.rit.edu/htbooks/mri/
http://www.howstuffworks.com/mri.htm
http://www.mrieducation.com/

REFERENCES

1. Runge VM, Nitz WR, Schmeets SH et al. The physics of clinical MR taught through images. New York: Thieme; 2005.
2. Heuck A, Reiser M, eds. Abdominal and pelvic MRI. Berlin: Springer; 1998.
3. Gauger J, Holzknecht NG, Lackenbauer CA et al. Breathhold imaging of the upper abdomen using a circular polarized-array coil: comparison with standard body coil imaging. MAGMA 1996; 4:93–104.
4. Soyer P, Bluemke DA, Rymer R. MR imaging of the liver: technique. Magn Reson Imaging Clin N Am 1997; 5:205–221.
5. Martin J, Sentis M, Puig J et al. Comparison of in-phase and opposed-phase GRE and conventional SE MR pulse sequences in T1-weighted imaging of liver lesions. J Comput Assist Tomogr 1996; 20:890–897.
6. Yamashita Y, Yamamoto H, Tomohiro N et al. Phased-array breath-hold versus non-breath-hold MR imaging of focal liver lesions: a prospective comparative study. J Magn Reson Imaging 1997; 7:292–297.
7. Felmlee JP, Ehman RL. Spatial presaturation: a method for suppressing flow artifacts and improving depiction of vascular anatomy in MR imaging. Radiology 1987; 164:559–564.
8. Mitchell DG, Stolpen AH, Siegelman ES et al. Fatty tissue on opposed-phase MR images: paradoxical suppression of signal intensity by paramagnetic contrast agents. Radiology 1996; 198:351–357.
9. Siewert B, Müller MF, Foley M et al. Fast MR imaging of the liver: qualitative comparison of techniques. Radiology 1994; 193:37–42.
10. Mitchell DG, Kim I, Chang TS et al. Chemical shift phase-difference and suppression magnetic resonance imaging techniques in animals, phantoms, and humans: fatty liver. Invest Radiol 1991; 26:1041–1052.
11. Semelka RC, Cumming MJ, Shoenut JP et al. Islet cell tumors: comparison of dynamic contrast-enhanced CT and MR imaging with dynamic gadolinium enhancement and fat suppression. Radiology 1993; 186:799–802.
12. Robinson PJA, Sheridan MB. Pancreatitis: computed tomography and magnetic resonance imaging. Eur Radiol 2000; 10:401–408.
13. Cameron IL, Ord VA, Fullerton GD. Characterization of proton NMR relation times in normal and pathological tissues by correlation with other tissue parameters. Magn Reson Imaging 1984; 2:97–106.
14. Li KC, Glazer GM, Quint LE et al. Distinction of hepatic cavernous hemangioma from hepatic metastases with MR imaging. Radiology 1988; 169:409–415.
15. McFarland EG, Mayo-Smith WW, Saini S et al. Hepatic hemangiomas and malignant tumors: improved differentiation with heavily T2-weighted conventional spin-echo MR imaging. Radiology 1994; 193:43–47.
16. Hahn PF, Saini S. Liver-specific MR imaging contrast agents. Radiol Clin N Am 1998; 36:287–297.
17. Mahfouz A-E, Hamm B. MR imaging of the liver. Contrast agents. Magn Reson Imaging Clin N Am 1997; 5:223–240.
18. Ros PR, Freeny PC, Harms SE et al. Hepatic MR imaging with ferumoxides: a multicenter clinical trial of the safety and efficacy in the detection of focal hepatic lesions. Radiology 1995; 196:481–488.
19. Chung KY, Mayo-Smith W, Saini S et al. Hepatocellular adenoma: MR imaging features with pathologic correlation. AJR Am J Roentgenol 1995; 165:303–308.
20. Powers C, Ros PR, Stoupis C et al. Primary liver neoplasms: MR imaging with pathologic correlation. Radiographics 1994; 14:459–482.

21. Kadoya M, Matsui O, Takashima T, Nonumura A. Hepatocellular carcinoma: correlation of MR imaging and histopathologic findings. Radiology 1992; 183:819–825.
22. Hamrick-Turner J, Abbitt PL, Ros PR. Intrahepatic cholangiocarcinoma: MR appearance. AJR Am J Roentgenol 1992; 158:77–79.
23. Siegelman ES, Outwater EK. Magnetic resonance imaging of focal and diffuse hepatic disease. Semin Ultrasound CT MR 1998; 19:2–34.
24. Bree RL, Schwab RE, Glazer GM, Fink-Bennett D. The varied appearances of hepatic cavernous hemangiomas with sonography, computed tomography, magnetic resonance imaging and scintigraphy. Radiographics 1987; 7:1153–1175.
25. Semelka RC, Sofka CM. Hepatic hemangiomas. Magnet Reson Imaging Clin N Am 1997; 5:241–253.
26. Mortele KJ, Ros PR. Benign liver neoplasms. Clin Liver Dis 2002; 6:119–145.
27. Brown JJ, Naylor MJ, Yagan N. Imaging of hepatic cirrhosis. Radiology 1997; 202:1–16.
28. Ros PR, Mortele KJ. Diffuse liver disease. Clin Liver Dis 2002; 6:181–201.
29. Siegelman ES, Outwater EK, Vinitski S et al. Fat suppression by saturation/opposed-phase hybrid technique: spin echo versus gradient echo imaging. Magn Reson Imaging 1995; 13:545–548.
30. Siegelman ES, Mitchell DG, Semelka RC. Abdominal iron deposition: metabolism, MR findings, and clinical importance. Radiology 1996; 199:13–22.
31. Siegelman ES, Mitchell DG, Rubin R et al. Parenchymal versus reticuloendothelial iron overload in the liver: distinction with MR imaging. Radiology 1991; 179:361–366.
32. Semelka RC, Kroeker MA, Shoenut JP, Kroeker R, Yaffe CS, Micflikier AB. Pancreatic disease: prospective comparison of CT, ERCP, and 1.5-T MR imaging with dynamic gadolinium enhancement and fat suppression. Radiology 1991; 181:785–791.
33. Kettritz U, Warschauer D, Brown E, Schlund J, Eisenberg L, Semelka R. Enhancement of the normal pancreas: comparison of manganese–DPDP and gadolinium chelate. Eur Radiol 1996; 6:14–18.
34. Mayosmith WW, Scima W, Saini S et al. Pancreatic enhancement and pulse sequence analysis using low-dose mangafodipir trisodium. AJR Am J Roentgenol 1998; 170:649–652.
35. Rieber A, Tomczak R, Nussle K et al. MRI with mangafodipir trisodium in the detection of pancreatic tumours: comparison with helical CT. B J Radiol 2000; 73:1165–1169.
36. Ros PR, Hamrick-Turner JE, Chiechi MV et al. Cystic masses of the pancreas. Radiographics 1992; 12:673–686.
37. Mergo PJ, Helmberger TK, Buetow PC, Helmberger RC, Ros PR. Pancreatic neoplasms: MR imaging and pathologic correlation. Radiographics 1997; 17:281–301.
38. Scott J, Martin I, Redhead D et al. Mucinous cystic neoplasms of the pancreas: imaging features and diagnostic difficulties. Clin Radiol 2000; 55:187–192.
39. Sugiyama M, Atomi Y, Hachiya J. Intraductal papillary tumors of the pancreas: evaluation with magnetic resonance cholangiopancreatography. Am J Gastroenterol 1998; 93:156–159.
40. Chung MJ, Choi BI, Han JK et al. Functioning islet cell tumor of the pancreas: localization with dynamic spiral CT. Acta Radiol 1997; 38:135–138.
41. Mortele KJ, Oei A, Bauters W et al. Dynamic gadolinium-enhanced MR imaging of pancreatic VIPoma in a patient with Verner-Morrison syndrome. Eur Radiol 2001, 11:1952–1955.
42. Lecesne R, Tourel P, Bret PM et al. Acute pancreatitis: interobserver agreement and correlation of CT and MR cholangiopancreatography with outcome. Radiology 1999; 211:727–735.
43. Soto JA, Barish MA, Yücel EK et al. Pancreatic duct: MR cholangiography with a three-dimentional fast spin echo technique. Radiology 1995; 196:459–464.
44. Matos C, Metens T, Deviere J et al. Pancreatic duct: morphologic and functional evaluation with dynamic MR pancreatography after secretin stimulation. Radiology 1997; 203:435–441.
45. Johnson PT, Outwater EK. Pancreatic carcinoma versus chronic pancreatitis: dynamic MR imaging. Radiology 1999; 212:213–218.
46. Mortele KJ, Wiesner W, Cantisani V, Silverman SG, Ros PR. Usual and unusual causes of extrahepatic cholestasis: assessment with magnetic resonance cholangiography and fast MRI. Abdom Imaging 2004; 29:87–99.
47. Reinhold C, Bret PM. Current status of MR cholangiopancreatography. AJR Am J Roentgenol 1996; 166:1285–1295.
48. Majoie CBLM, Reeders JW, Sanders JB et al. Primary sclerosing cholangitis: a modified classification of cholangiographic findings. AJR Am J Roentgenol 1991; 157:495–497.
49. Mortele KJ, Ji H, Ros PR. CT and magnetic resonance imaging in pancreatic and biliary tract malignancies. Gastrointest Endosc 2002; 56(6 Suppl):S206–S212.
50. Rieber A, Nussle K, Reinshagen M, Brambs HJ, Gabelmann A. MRI of the abdomen with positive oral contrast agents for the diagnosis of inflammatory small bowel disease. Abdom Imaging 2002; 27:394–399.
51. Kim NK, Kim MJ, Park JK, Park SI, Min JS. Preoperative staging of rectal cancer with MRI: accuracy and clinical usefulness. Ann Surg Oncol 2000; 7:732–737.
52. Matsuoka H, Nakamura A, Masaki T et al. Comparison between endorectal coil and pelvic phased-array coil magnetic resonance imaging in patients with anorectal tumor. Am J Surg 2003; 185:328–332.
53. Spencer JA, Ward J, Beckingham IJ, Adams C, Ambrose NS. Dynamic contrast-enhanced MR imaging of perianal fistulas. AJR Am J Roentgenol 1996; 167:735–741.
54. deSouza NM, Puni R, Zbar A, Gilderdale DJ, Coutts GA, Krausz T. MR imaging of the anal sphincter in multiparous women using an endoanal coil: correlation with in vitro anatomy and appearances in fecal incontinence. AJR Am J Roentgenol 1996; 167:1465–1471.
55. Debatin JF, Lauenstein TC. Virtual magnetic resonance colonography. Gut 2003; 52(Suppl 4):iv17–22.

Chapter 128

Magnetic resonance cholangiopancreatography

Maria Sheridan

> **KEY POINTS**
>
> Static fluid is high signal on heavily T2-weighted sequences
> Background signal is suppressed
> Overall view is obtained with 'thick slab' technique
> Detail obtained with thin multi-slice technique
> Multiplanar capability
> No biliary contrast medium required
> Examination completed in 15 min

ITRODUCTION AND SCIENTIFIC BASIS

ıgnetic resonance cholangiopancreatography (MRCP) has en available for over 10 years and is a well accepted method evaluating the bile ducts, gallbladder, and pancreatic duct.[1,2] e magnetic resonance (MR) techniques used for MRCP exploit inherent contrast between static fluids and the adjacent id structures. The T2 relaxation time of static fluid is extremely ıg compared with that of the liver and pancreas. On heavily -weighted images, therefore, the signal from static fluid is ;h (white) and the signal from solid organs is suppressed ırk). This allows the production of an image that is very nilar to the conventional images obtained at endoscopic rograde cholangiopancreatography (ERCP) or percutaneous nshepatic cholangiography (PTC).

ESCRIPTION OF TECHNIQUE

RCP sequences are available on all modern MR scanners.[3] e total room time for a MRCP examination is 15–20 minutes. eally the patient should be fasted, as this reduces the amount fluid in the stomach and duodenum. Modern MRCP techques allow a very short acquisition time, which reduces the tential artifact from respiratory and peristaltic motion. The awback of faster acquisitions is a lower signal to noise ratio. compensate for this and to produce good quality images, it essential to use a phased-array body coil. These faster sequences e performed in a single breathhold, usually at the end of piration. The best quality images are obtained if the operator kes a few moments before the examination to coach the tient in breathholding. If the patient is unable to suspend spiration, respiratory gating can be used, where the patient n breathe quietly. This is not successful, however, in patients ıo have an erratic breathing pattern.

Bile and pancreatic ducts: Different sequences are required for l examination of the bile and pancreatic ducts. Initially the biliary tree and pancreatic ducts are localized using a thick-slab technique applied in the coronal plane. The slab can be up to 5–7 cm in thickness and a single acquisition taking about 4 s is often sufficient to encompass the region of interest. This can be repeated at varying degrees of obliquity to take account of overlapping ducts or other structures. This produces an image similar to the conventional ERCP image. After this, two- and three-dimensional single-shot fast-spin echo sequences are used to produce multiple thin slices (slice thickness 2–5 mm). This requires breathholding for 15–20 s, or respiratory gating. The slices can be obtained in multiple planes, but are most commonly acquired in an axial and a coronal oblique plane (chosen after evaluating the thick-slab images).

The thick-slab acquisition produces an image that is similar to the conventional ERCP image, but with inferior spatial resolution. The multislice technique produces images with much higher spatial resolution and therefore greater detail. It is essential, therefore, to use both techniques.

Special techniques: For some indications, for instance tumor detection and staging, it is appropriate to combine the MRCP techniques with conventional MR imaging to demonstrate the parenchyma of adjacent organs. Dynamic MR techniques, using intravenous contrast, have been shown to yield the maximum diagnostic information in this setting.

There has been interest in MRCP following intravenous administration of secretin. This has two potential uses. First, it may allow a more accurate depiction of pancreatic duct strictures in chronic pancreatitis.[4] Second, it has been suggested that exocrine functional information can be obtained by acquiring thick-slab images before and at 30-s intervals after intravenous secretin administration. A visual assessment is made of the filling of the duodenum with pancreatic secretions.[5]

INDICATIONS/CONTRAINDICATIONS

Suspected bile duct stones are a common indication for MRCP. A large number of patients with suspected bile duct stones fall into a low or intermediate probability category following clinical, biochemical, and ultrasonographic assessment. It is inappropriate for all of these patients to undergo ERCP, and the development of a noninvasive reproducible test has been extremely helpful, allowing ERCP to be reserved for therapy only (Figs 128.1 and 128.2). In a recent meta-analysis of the performance of MRCP, the overall sensitivity for the diagnosis of bile duct stones was 92% with a specificity of 97%.[6] Some studies, however, suggest that the sensitivity for detecting stones smaller than 3 mm may be as low as 64%.[7]

Strictures: MRCP is accurate in demonstrating the presence and level of bile duct strictures. The spatial resolution of MRCP

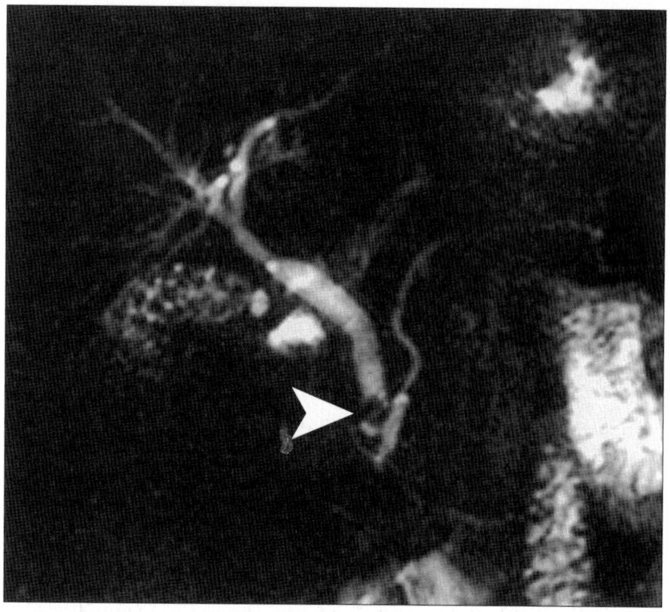

Fig. 128.1 Stones in the common bile duct. Thick-slab MRCP shows two small stones in the distal common bile duct (arrowhead). Note multiple stones in the gallbladder. The pancreatic duct is normal.

is not as good as the resolution of conventional ERCP or PTC, and therefore detail of stricture contour (irregular, shouldered or smooth and tapering) is limited. Despite this, MRCP does compare well with diagnostic ERCP in the diagnosis of pancreatic and biliary malignancy.

In one study the sensitivity and specificity of MRCP for the diagnosis of pancreatic malignancy were 84% and 97% respectively, compared with 70% and 94% for ERCP.[8] In a meta-analysis the sensitivity and specificity for malignant bilia obstruction were 88% and 95%.[6] If conventional MR imagi of the liver and pancreas are added to MRCP, the diagnos accuracy improves further. In the setting of malignant disea this full examination allows complete preoperative assessme (Fig. 128.3). In patients with hilar cholangiocarcinoma, MR can be extremely helpful in assessing biliary anatomy to info decision-making about endoscopic or percutaneous drainag

Chronic pancreatitis: The main use of MRCP is as a nc invasive method of demonstrating the anatomy of the bile a pancreatic ducts prior to surgical or endoscopic interventi in patients with advanced disease. The length and site of pa creatic duct, and associated bile duct strictures, are well sho (Fig. 128.4). Additional complications, such as intralumi stones or concretions, are also demonstrated. Several ca reports describe the use of MRCP to identify the commu cation of pancreatic pseudocysts with pancreatic ducts and t demonstration of complex pancreatic fistulae (Fig. 128.5), su as pancreaticopleural fistula. Because of the limited spat resolution, however, MRCP cannot show the early duct chang in mild disease.[2]

Secretin stimulation: There has been considerable interest MRCP following intravenous administration of secretin patients with chronic pancreatitis. The diameter of the ma pancreatic duct increases in the 1–2 min following intraveno secretin and returns to its normal baseline diameter with 10–15 min. It has been suggested that in patients with chror pancreatitis the baseline duct diameter is increased and t degree of variability of the diameter is reduced. There has al been interest in secretin-stimulated MRCP for assessment pancreatic exocrine function. Further research is needed establish the clinical use of these techniques.

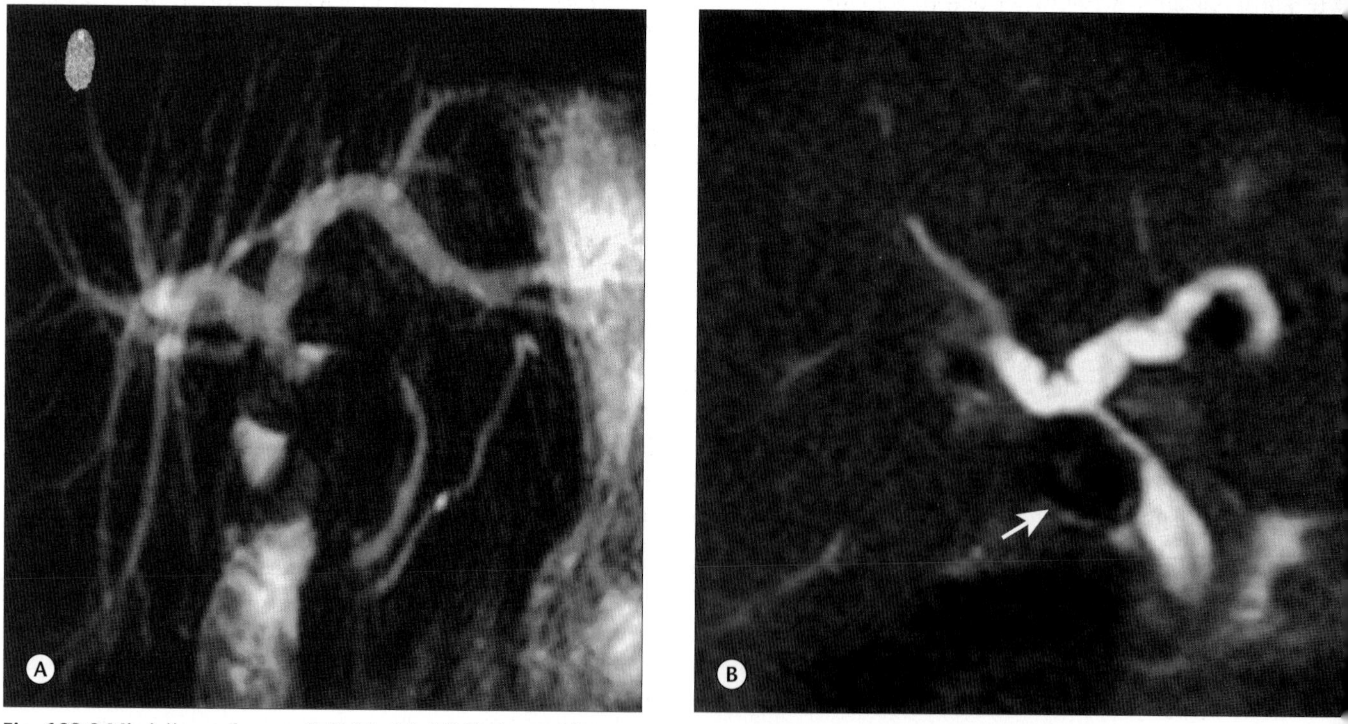

Fig. 128.2 Mirrizi's syndrome. A. Thick-slab MRCP shows a large stone in the neck of the gallbladder, compressing the common bile duct at this point. Note dilated intrahepatic and proximal common hepatic duct and collapsed distal common duct. **B.** Detail of the stone is better appreciated on the thin slice (arrow).

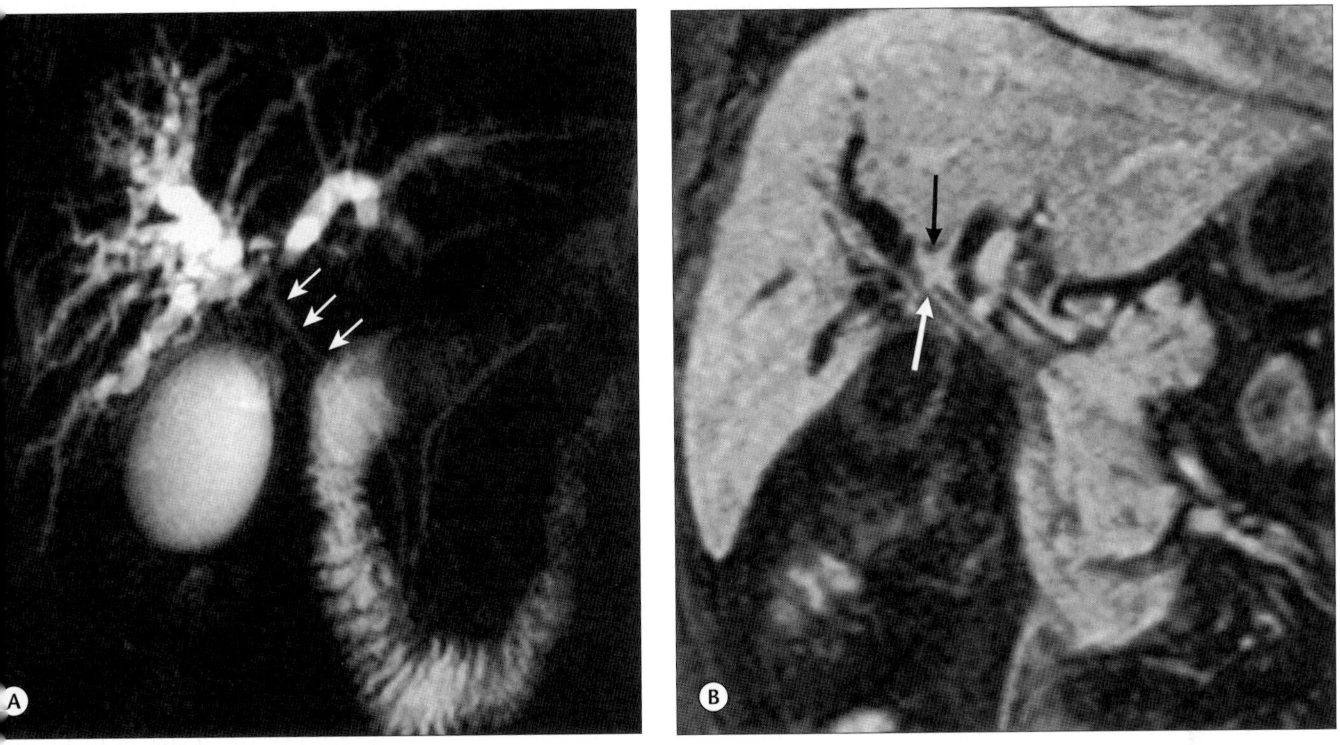

. **128.3 Intrahepatic duct dilatation. A.** Thick-slab MRCP shows intrahepatic duct dilatation with a collapsed extrahepatic duct. The dynamic postcontrast MR image shows the cause as a 1.0-cm tumor at the hilum of the liver (arrow). Note that on postcontrast ıging the bile ducts are of low signal (black) and the vessels are high signal (white).

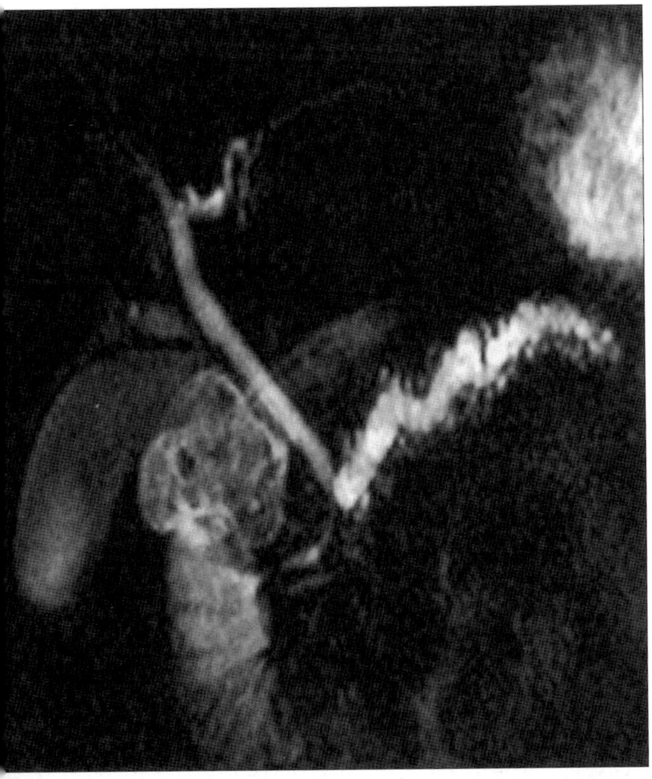

ȷ. **128.4 Dilatation of the main pancreatic duct.** Thick-slab MRCP ows dilatation of the main pancreatic duct in the body and tail, oximal to a high-grade stricture.

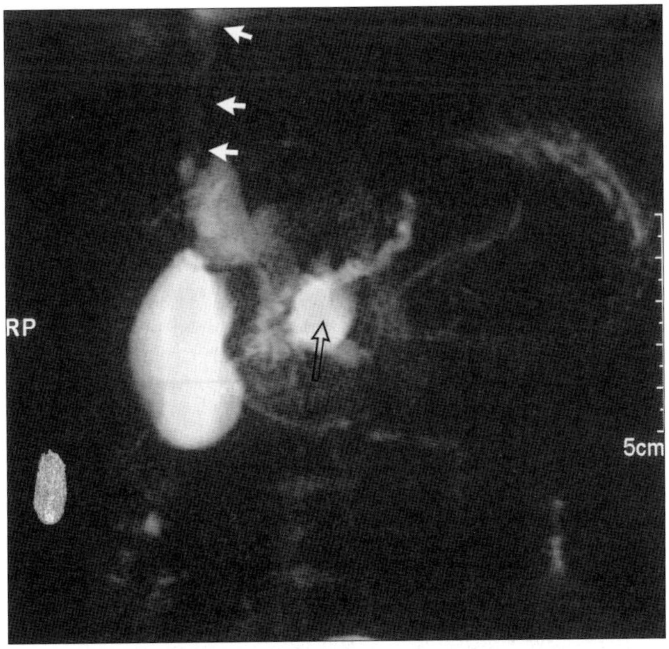

Fig. 128.5 Pancreatic pseudocyst and fistula. Thick-slab MRCP shows a dilated pancreatic duct with a pseudocyst (arrow) and a complex fistula extending up into the pleural cavity (arrowheads).

Bile duct injury: When this is suspected following surgery (e.g., laparoscopic cholecystectomy, liver transplantation, or bilioenteric anastomosis), accurate imaging of the biliary tree is crucial. MRCP has the potential to assess the biliary tree fully, including those cases where endoscopic access is limited. It also demonstrates the bile duct both above and below a stricture, and multiple strictures (e.g., ischemic strictures following liver transplantation). The number of such studies is small, but they suggest that MRCP is sufficiently accurate to inform decision-making about the most appropriate therapy.[10]

Sclerosing cholangitis: Studies on the use of MRCP are limited. Although advanced changes can be well shown, it is not yet clear whether the spatial resolution of MRCP is sufficient confidently to exclude early duct changes. The technique cannot be recommended for making the initial diagnosis, but it may be useful in the follow-up of patients with an established diagnosis[11] (Fig. 128.6).

Many case reports and small case series suggest that MRCP is useful in a variety of congenital abnormalities of the biliary tree such as choledochoceles and choledochochal cysts. The numbers are too small to draw conclusions, but it is clear that in some cases MRCP can be extremely helpful.[2]

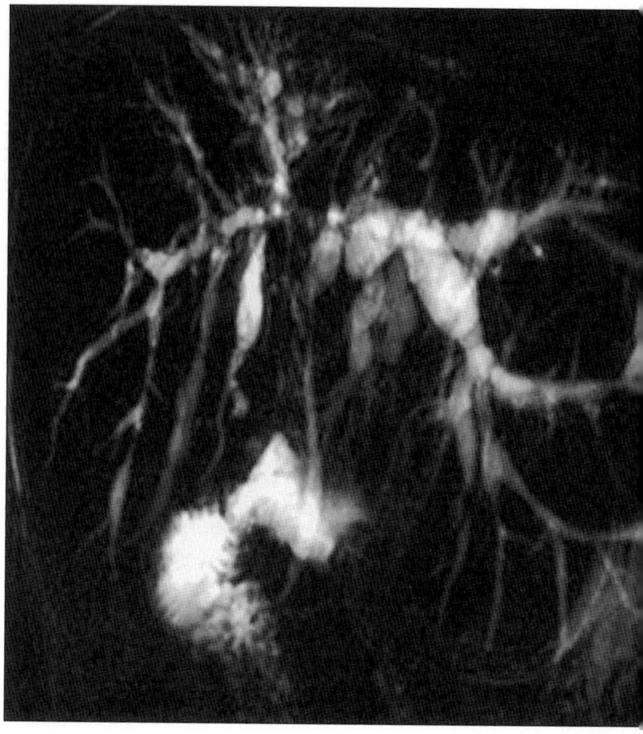

Fig. 128.6 Multiple intrahepatic structures. Thick-slab MRCP sho multiple areas of intrahepatic stricturing in primary sclerosing cholangitis.

INDICATIONS/CONTRAINDICATIONS

INDICATIONS
- Suspected bile duct stones
- Suspected malignant bile duct obstruction
- Chronic pancreatitis
- Evaluation of postoperative bile duct complications

CONTRAINDICATIONS
- Cardiac pacemaker
- Some metallic implants
- Claustrophobia

Contraindications: There are very few absolute contraindications to MRCP. Patients with cardiac pacemakers are excluded from the examination, as are those with some types of metallic implant (e.g., aneurysm clips). Not all implants are an absolute contraindication, however, and further information about the nature of the metal should be sought. Patients who are claustrophobic may find the confines of the MR machine intolerable, although the incidence of inadequate or failed MRCP examination appears to be lower than that of failed ERCP.

PITFALLS IN INTERPRETATION

There are a number of potential pitfalls in the interpretation of MRCP images.[12] In the distal common bile duct, a central filling defect of 1–2 mm in diameter, simulating a small stone, is commonly seen and is due to a flow artifact. It is seen o in axial images and is not visible in thin-slice coronal imag Filling defects may also be seen on the thick-slab images caus by mucosal folds in the bile duct; again this is clarified on t thin slices. Extrinsic compression of the bile duct by adjac arteries can produce a signal void simulating a stricture. This seen most commonly at the bifurcation of the common hepa duct into the right and left duct, where the right hepatic arte may compress the common hepatic duct.

RELATIVE COST

To date there have been few studies regarding the co effectiveness of MRCP. There are potential cost savings in t avoidance of ERCP and PTC and their complications. It likely, however, that there will be more referrals for MR than there have been for diagnostic ERCP because it is a nc invasive test. Some patients who have MRCP will go on to ha therapeutic ERCP in any case. A health technology assessme report recently suggested that cost savings of approximat £149 could be made by the avoidance of unnecessary ERCP

REFERENCES

1. Hartman EM, Barish MA. MR Cholangiography. Magn Reson Imaging Clin N Am 2001; 9: 841–855.
2. Fulcher AS, Turner MA. MR cholangiopancreatography. Radiol Clin N Am 2002; 40:1229–1242.
3. Morrin MM, Rofsky NM. Techniques for liver imaging. Magn Reson Imaging Clin N Am 2001; 9:675–696.
4. Matos C, Winant C, Deviere J. Magnetic resonance pancreatography. Abdom Imaging 2001; 26:243–253.
5. Fukukura Y, Fujiyoshi F, Sasaki M et al. Pancreatic duct: morphological evaluation with MR cholangiopancreatography after secretin stimulation. Radiology 2002; 222:674–680.
6. Matos C, Metens T, Deviere J et al. Pancreatic duct: morphological and functional evaluation with dynamic MR pancreatography after secretin stimulation. Radiology 1997; 2003:435–441.
7. Romagnuolo J, Bardou M, Rahme E et al. Magnetic resonance cholangiopancreatography: a meta-analysis of test performance in suspected biliary disease. Ann Intern Med 2003; 139:547–557.
8. Adamek HE, Albert J, Weitz M et al. A prospective evaluation of magnetic resonance cholangiopancreatography in patients with suspected bile duct obstruction. Gut 1998; 43:680–683.
9. Adamek HE, Albert J, Breer H et al. Pancreatic cancer detection with magnetic resonance cholangiopancreatography and endoscopic retrograde cholangiopancreatography: a prospective controlled study. Lancet 2000; 356:190–193.
10. Kim MJ, Mitchell DJ, Ito K. Biliary dilatation: differentiation of benign from malignant causes: value of adding conventional MR imaging to MR cholangiopancreatography. Radiology 2000; 214:173–181.
11. Ward J, Sheridan MB, Guthrie JA et al. Bile duct strictures after hepatobiliary surgery: assessment with MR cholangiography. Radiology 2004; 231:101–108.
12. Angulo P, Pearce DH, Johnson CD et al. Magnetic resonance cholangiography in patients with biliary disease: its role in primary sclerosing cholangitis. J Hepatol 2000; 33:520–527.
13. Vivek D, Reinhold C, Hochman M et al. Pitfalls in the interpretation of MR cholangiopancreatography. AJR Am J Roentgenol 1998; 170:1055–1059.

Chapter 129

Virtual endoscopy imaging

Abraham H Dachman and Hiroyuki Yoshida

KEY POINTS

- Virtual colonoscopy (VC) is a new minimally invasive technique to detect colorectal polyps and masses that avoids the need for sedation and can be done in an outpatient setting
- VC is the best test for patients who have an incomplete optical colonoscopy or who cannot undergo or refuse optical colonoscopy
- VC for colorectal cancer screening is still controversial, but is offered by several centers
- VC can be performed after colon cleansing, but is adaptable to less vigorous cleansing strategies as compared to optical colonoscopy because it can be done with oral contrast to 'tag' stool and residual fluid
- VC interpretation requires significant training and experience
- Specialized software for 2D multiplanar and 3D image generation is commercially available, ideally with an automated 3D fly-through of the colon
- MRI is a rapidly evolving alternative technique to CT VC and avoids the need for radiation
- Rapid advance in computer-aided detection (computer software that automatically finds polyps and masses) will help radiologists achieve accurate and confident interpretations

INTRODUCTION AND SCIENTIFIC BASIS

Colorectal cancer is the second most common cause of cancer deaths in the US. Compliance with current screening strategies by the population is poor,[1] so any minimally invasive alternative would be very attractive. Virtual colonoscopy (VC), which is also known as computed tomographic colonography (CTC), has emerged as a potential viable alternative to colonoscopy.

The test typically requires supine and prone CT of the cleansed colon, after mechanical or manual insufflation of the colon with air or carbon dioxide within patient tolerance, which is interpreted with specialized software using both 2-dimensional (2D) and endoluminal 3-dimensional (3D) imaging.[2] Virtual colonoscopy, where available, is often the investigation of choice for patients who have undergone an incomplete colonoscopy or who cannot undergo conventional colonoscopy. Its use for mass population screening for colorectal cancer has not yet been fully endorsed. One large multicentre trial has shown it to compare well with optical colonoscopy[3] and other published data[4,5] are supportive of its use (Figs 129.1–129.4). Consequently, several community CT screening centers now offer VC for colorectal cancer screening.[1] Because the goal of screening is to detect premalignant adenomas from which more than 80% of colorectal carcinomas arise, the technique must be sensitive enough to pick up lesions 10 mm or larger and preferably as small as 6 mm.

Terminology

Some technical terms used in describing VC interpretation are defined here. The source images are the axial 2D images. Multiplanar reconstructions (MPR) can be viewed in standard coronal and sagittal planes or in a variable or 'oblique' plane. Comparison of various MPR views can be helpful in understanding the complex winding anatomy of the colon and in differentiating polyps from folds located at the inside of a bend in the colon. The 2D views are also critical in finding the flat lesions, which may be missed on 3D images.

The 3D views, which are less fatiguing to read than 2D views, can be created by the computer using either:

- Surface rendering, which shows the interface of two densities such as the colon wall outlined by gas. In surface-rendered images, the proper 'threshold' must be selected to make the wall opaque and lighting/contrast can be adjusted as well.
- Volume rendering. Here, 3D views retain all voxel data and require optimization of upper-lower threshold, shape of the rendering curve, and opacity level. The view can be adjusted to look similar in opacity to a surface-rendered view or can be made transparent to mimic the appearance of a barium enema. A typical VC 3D view shows the colon from an endoluminal perspective mimicking the appearance of a conventional colonoscopy. Novel 3-dimensional views can artificially 'cut the colon open' and lay it out flat like a piece of paper. Artificial 'color' can be added to either surface or volume-rendered.

DESCRIPTION OF TECHNIQUE

Bowel preparation

Because retained fluid can hide masses, the bowel should be prepared using a relatively 'dry prep' laxative (magnesium citrate or sodium phosphate), given the day prior to the procedure. A bisacodyl suppository on the morning of the examination helps evacuate residual fluid.

Radiologists prescribing colon cleansing should note that sodium phosphate laxatives are contraindicated in patients with renal failure and are relatively contraindicated in patients with known electrolyte abnormalities, congestive heart failure, ascites, and ileus. It should be noted that most published data comparing VC and optical colonoscopy have been on patients undergoing both examinations on the same day after a 'wet prep' (polyethylene glycol), which is not optimal for virtual colonoscopy.

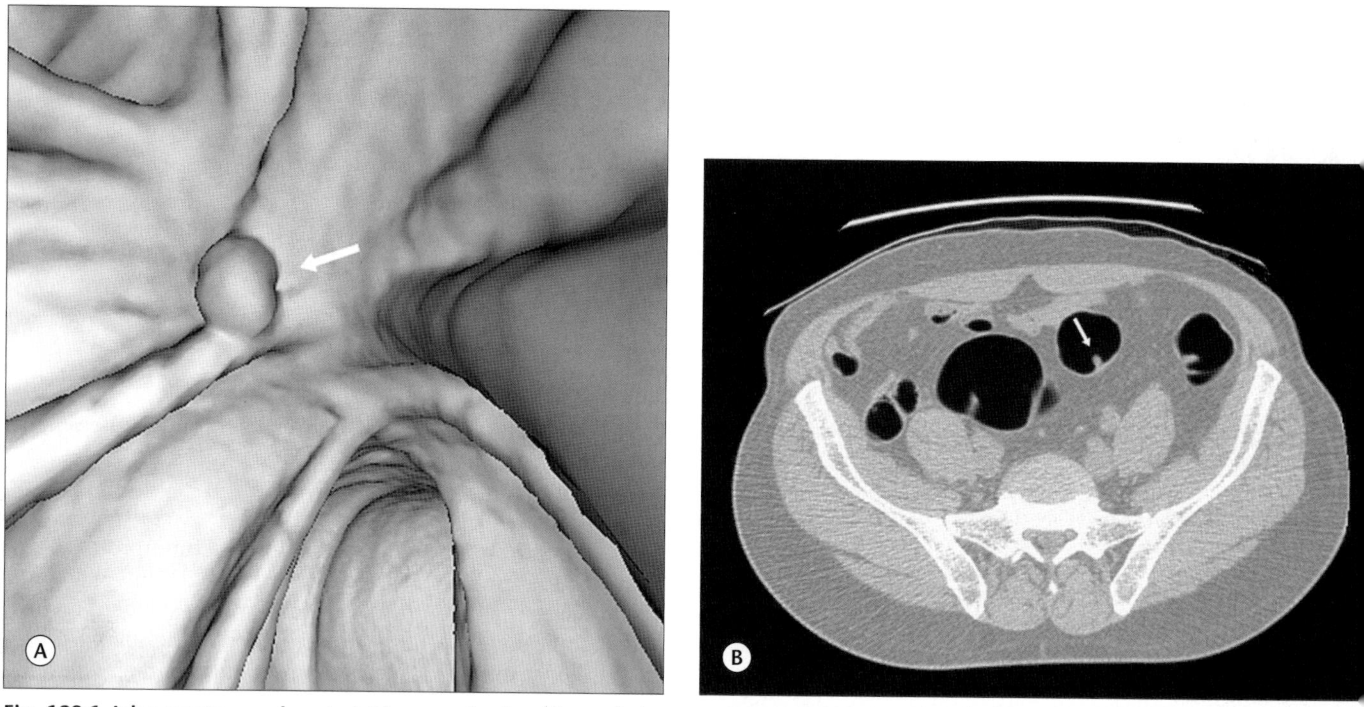

Fig. 129.1 Adenomatous polyp. A. A 15-mm polyp is well seen in between folds on the 3D endoluminal view. **B.** Corresponding prone axial image shows the polyp (arrow) on the posterior, nondependent surface of a redundant transverse colon dipping into the patient's pelvis. From Dachman AH et al. Progress in Oncology, 2003: Jones and Bartlett Publishers, Sudbury, MA. www.jbpub.com. Reprinted with permission.

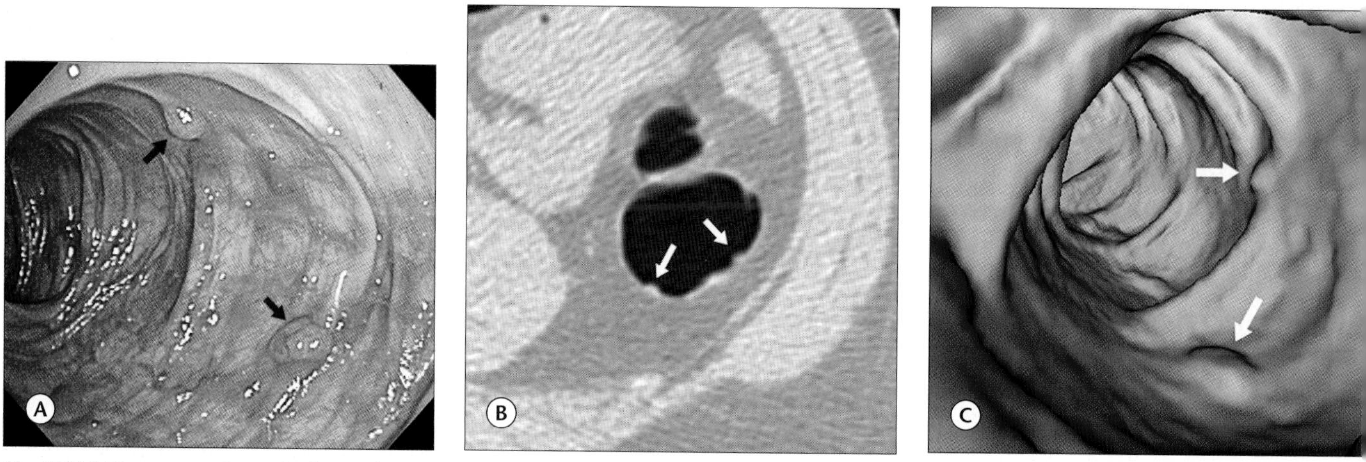

Fig. 129.2 Demonstration of sub-centimeter polyps. A. Conventional colonoscopy shows two sub-centimeter sessile polyps (arrows). **B.** Magnified axial 2D supine view of the descending colon shows two small sessile lesions (arrows) corresponding to the polyps seen on conventional colonoscopy. These lesions did not move on the prone image (not shown) and did not contain any internal air. These findings suggest that these lesions are true polyps. **C.** 3D endoluminal view of the corresponding lesions, which are shown by the arrows. Additional apparent lesions seen in this image represented stool. Reproduced with permission from Dachman et al. CT colonography and colon cancer screening. Semin Roentgenol 2003; 38:54–64.

Stool and fluid opacification

These are under investigation as alternatives to bowel preparation.[6] Both barium and a water-soluble oral contrast medium can be administered with each meal on the day prior to the examination or on the morning of the examination. The resultant images can be read as 2D or 3D. Electronic subtraction (also termed 'digital bowel cleansing') of stool and fluid is a further strategy that may help make the exam easier to interpret and more amenable to a primary 3D read.[2,7]

Colonic insufflation method and role of antispasmodics

Antispasmodics are often used because VC requires insufflation to an extent that causes patient discomfort. Scopolamine butylbromide or glucagon 1 mg subcutaneously 10 min prior to the scan can be used. There is some recent controversial evidence that use of antispasmodics may improve the diagnostic quality of the examination, but it probably does make patients more comfortable.

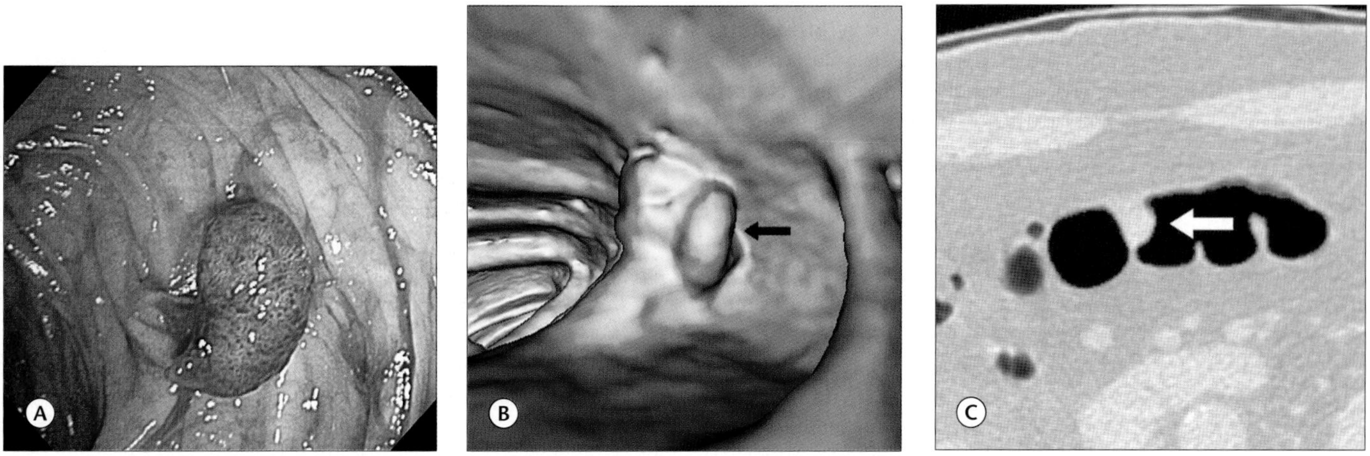

Fig. 129.3 Sessile polyp in the transverse colon. Conventional colonoscopy shows a 15-mm sessile polyp **(A)**, which is seen on the endoluminal view **(B)** and the prone axial view **(C)** as indicated by arrows. The polyp abuts a fold on the ventral wall of the transverse colon. Although relatively dependent in location, it is solid with no internal gas and is thus most consistent with a polyp rather than stool. (Reproduced with permission from Dachman AH, Yoshida H. Virtual colonography: past, present and future. Radiologic Clin North Am 2003; 41:377–393.)

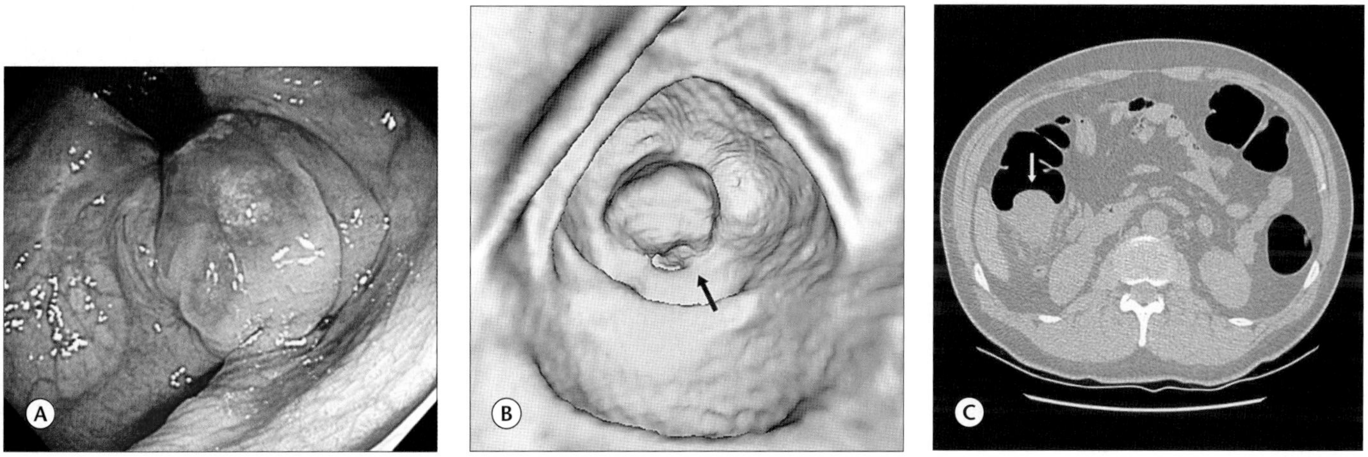

Fig. 129.4 Right-sided adenocarcinoma. A. Colonoscopy showed a lobulated right-sided mass, which prevented evaluation of the cecum. **B.** Endoluminal perspective view shows the same mass (arrow). **C.** Supine axial image from a virtual colonoscopy showing the mass (arrow). B and C from Dachman AH et al. Progress in Oncology, 2003: Jones and Bartlett Publishers, Sudbury, MA. www.jbpub.com. Reprinted with permission

Insufflation and scanning

A rectal examination should be done before proceeding to VC (by either the referring physician or the radiologist), because lesions in the anal canal or near the anal verge may be missed on VC. A rectal tube with or without a retention cuff is introduced. Patients with painful hemorrhoids may benefit from use of lidocane jelly and a small caliber catheter. Insufflation can be accomplished with either room air or carbon dioxide. The latter may have the benefit of rapid absorption making the patient more comfortable after the examination. A mechanical pump designed specifically for VC is now available and may permit a technologist to work quickly to both insufflate and to perform the CT.

When insufflation has caused moderate patient discomfort, a scout view is performed in deep inspiration to judge the adequacy of colonic distention. Once adequate insufflation is seen, the patient should hyperventilate to minimize respiratory movement on the subsequent scan. (Newer volume scanners that are fast enough to scan the entire abdomen and pelvis in 10s or less may permit scanning in expiration to 'stretch out' the flexures). The supine scan is usually performed first. The patient is then turned to a prone position and the scout view is repeated before doing the prone scan. If distention is inadequate on one view, or there is a large amount of retained fluid, an additional decubitus view may be performed or further manual insufflation may be attempted with or without use of an antispasmodic. With the use of fast 16-slice CT scanners or higher (40- and 64-slice are now on the market) respiratory motion is rare, but elderly patients can benefit from supplemental nasal oxygen to ensure an adequate breath hold.

CT data acquisition protocol

A multidetector scanner should be used with collimation of 3 mm or less. Reconstruction should be approximately 30–50% of the collimation (e.g., 1.5 mm) to permit high-quality 3D endoluminal images. There are advocates of thin collimation <1 mm, to improve the quality of the multiplanar (axial, coronal, and sagittal) reformatted views, making them potentially as reliable as the axial source images and to give better resolution 3D endoluminal views. This is likely to improve the detection of small polyps, flat lesions, and to help with differentiation of stool, but the ideal parameters remain to be proved. The trade-off is a longer breath hold, a noisier image, possibly decreased specificity due to visualization of small lesions, and possibly a higher radiation dose. The tube current is usually 50–100 mA for 0.8-s and 1.0-s helical scanners. Even lower radiation doses have been successful as well. A standard algorithm is used; however, we have evidence to suggest that a soft algorithm is better. The pitch (standard definition) should be kept under 2.

Image display: how to read a virtual colonoscopy

Software

Any software package used for the interpretation of VC must permit both 2D and 3D evaluation of the colon.[2] Ideally, both styles of interpretation should be used in every case but one of two initial approaches are: a 'primary 2D read with 3D problem solving'[8] and a 'primary 3D read with 2D problem solving.' In this context, a 3D view refers to an endoluminal perspective view optimized to viewing the colon, regardless of whether it is a surface- or volume-rendered view. The 2D and 3D views should be seamlessly integrated. The 3D view should offer both manual navigation and an automated centerline fly-through navigation of the lumen. The 2D view should offer simultaneous viewing of sagittal and coronal views and ideally should permit simultaneous synchronized paging through the supine and prone views.

Interpretation of VC

Skillful reading of VC requires reading an adequate number of proven cases with a sufficient number of true polyps and pitfalls. These authors suggest that 20–50 proven cases (with a substantial number of abnormal cases included) are read under supervision with the reader achieving a reasonable sensitivity for polyps 10 mm or larger. Several publications deal with methods and pitfalls of interpretation.[3,9] In a 3D approach, each view (supine and prone) is read twice, once with a forward and once with a backward fly-through. Lesions are characterized as stool, polyps, or lipomas by viewing of 2D images. 'Wide soft-tissue' windows can be used to search the 2D images for flat lesions. Care must be taken not to skip segments of the colon that might be excluded from an automated centerline fly-through. In a primary 2D read, magnified axial images are used to page through the scan and meticulously evaluate each loop (Fig. 129.5). 3D images can be used to help differentiate normal folds from polyps. Flat lesions must be searched for as well, particularly on the 2D views using a wide soft tissue window setting. Generally, polyps greater than 5 mm or 10 mm are reported. Foci 5 mm or smaller usually represent stool or hyperplastic polyps (Fig. 129.6).

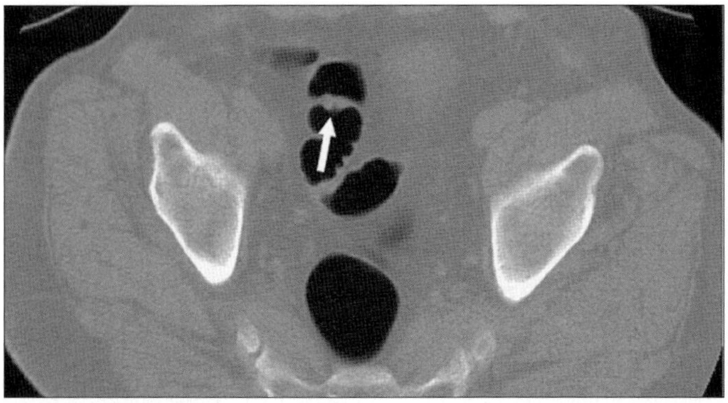

Fig. 129.5 Kissing folds. Two kissing bulbous ridges of normal colonic folds are shown abutting each other on this 2D axial view of the sigmoid colon. Muscular hypertrophy is commonly present in this portion of the colon, creating areas of colonic folds mimicking a polyp. As demonstrated here, such abutting folds can be potentially mistaken as a polyp. Reproduced with permission from Dachman AH et al. CT colonography and colon cancer screening. Semin Roentgenol 2003; 38:54–64.

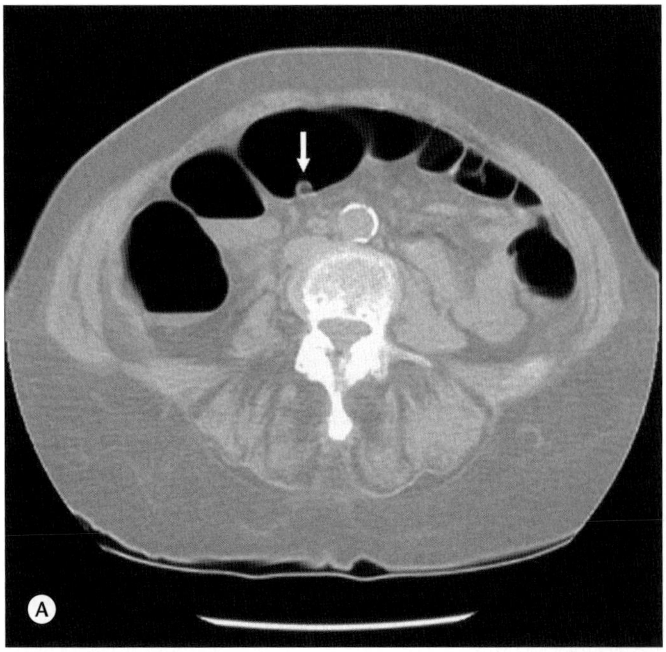

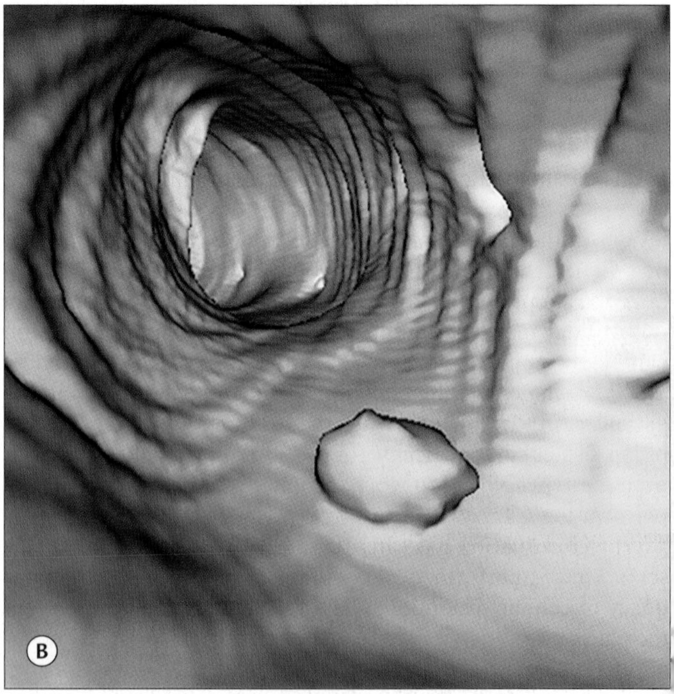

Fig. 129.6 Stool. A. 2D axial view of the lesion corresponding to the stool in A shows an internal air bubble (arrow), further suggesting that this finding probably represents a retained stool sample. **B.** A small collection of stool resembles a polyp in this 3D endoluminal view. Irregular edges of this apparent lesion suggest that this may represent a retained stool rather than a true polyp. Reproduced with permission from Dachman AH et al. CT colonography and colon cancer screening. Semin Roentgenol 2003; 38:54–64.

Stool is characterized by mottle seen on lung or soft tissue indow setting; thus, active adjustment of window/level set-ngs during the interpretation is necessary. For stool lacking mottled pattern, comparison of supine and prone views will elp to show the mobility characteristic of stool. A pitfall is obility of a polyp on a long stalk or mobility of the colon self.[9]

lternative and novel views

he segmented colon can be shown in a volume-rendered emitransparent view, similar to a double-contrast enema (Fig. 29.7A). A similar view can be created using surface rendering. This view is ideally suited to display the location of the lesion visually for documentation, for comparison with follow-up CT examinations, endoscopy, or surgical planning and measuring the distance of the lesion from the anus with greater accuracy than is achieved by conventional colonoscopy.

Other novel views hold promise for a more user-friendly primary read. In particular, views that open the colon for display as a flat object (Fig. 129.7B; 'virtual pathology' or 'virtual dissection' and 'endo 3D unfolded' are some terms used to describe this view) would permit viewing of the entire colonic mucosa and avoid nearly all of the blind spots associated with an endoluminal fly-through view.

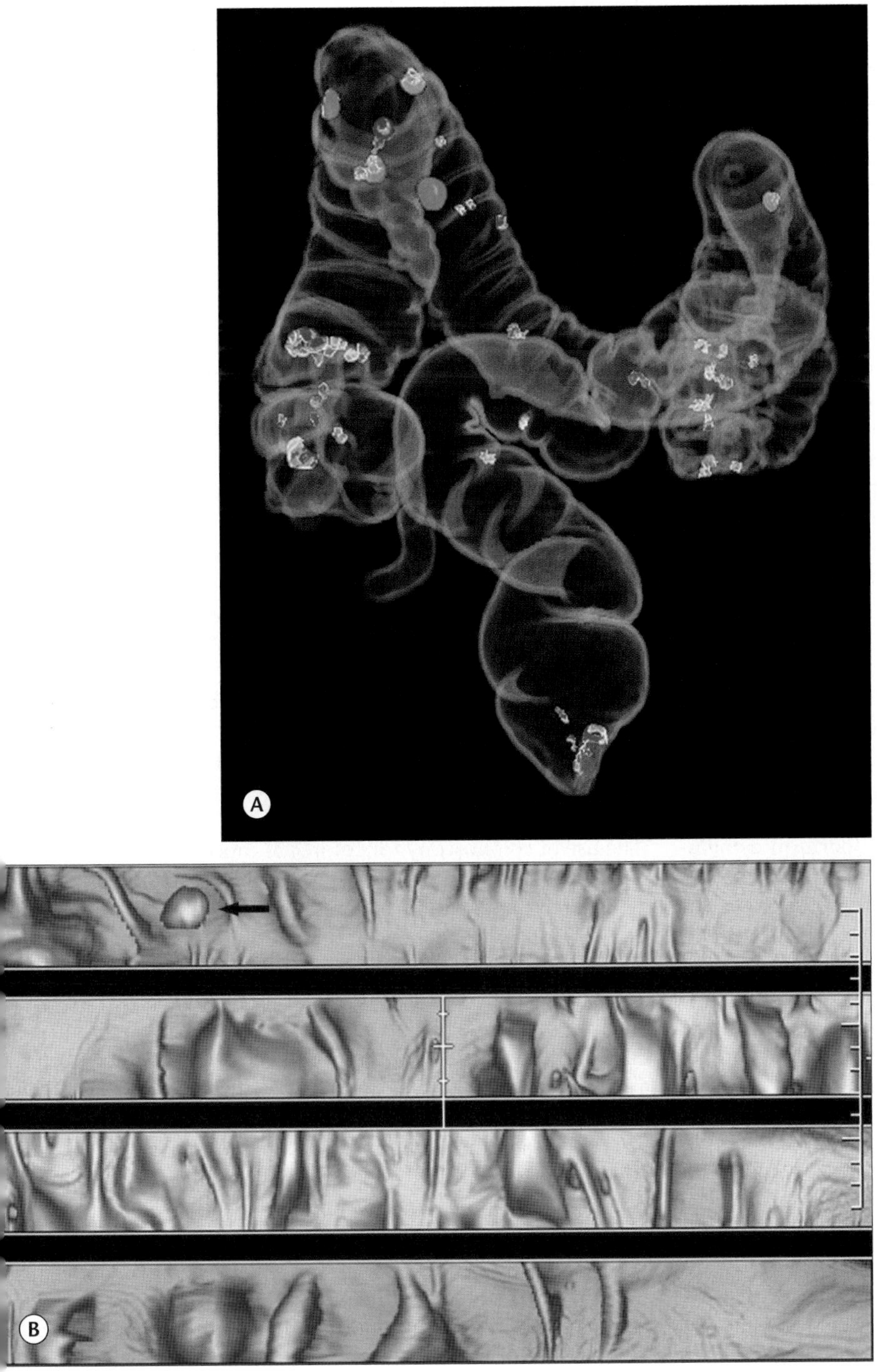

Fig. 129.7 Alternate and novel views.
A. A transparent view indicating the locations of polyps with green and mass with red.
B. A virtual dissection view (GE Medical Systems). A polyp is indicated by an arrow.

Extracolonic findings

If VC is performed with a sufficient radiation dose, CT will be able to detect and characterize incidental lesions in the kidney as solid (possible renal cell carcinoma) or cystic. Other significant abnormalities such as an abdominal aortic aneurysm, ovarian masses, lung lesions, and adenopathy can be detected. Many authors report a 12% incidence of significant extracolonic findings on VC.[10]

Virtual MRI colonoscopy

Magnetic resonance imaging (MRI) in virtual colonoscopy has been studied, particularly by European investigators, in order to avoid the use of ionizing radiation, particularly in an asymptomatic screening population. Most protocols involve the use of a liquid gadolinium enema for distending the colon and providing a high-contrast interface with the colonic mucosa. Distending the colon with air or carbon dioxide has met with limited success due to artifacts. Although sensitivity and specificity rates have been good in the hands of experts, widespread use of MRI virtual colonoscopy is limited by the lower resolution of MRI as compared to CT. Efforts are underway to study MR virtual colonoscopy in larger cohorts and to develop new protocols that would permit a good-quality examination while using gaseous distention of the colon.

Computer-aided detection of polyps

Computer-aided detection (CAD) offers the possibility of a double reading of VC images by the combination of a radiologist and a computer (Fig. 129.8).[11] A CAD system automatically detects polyps and masses from VC data and provides the locations of suspicious polyps for radiologists. If CAD is sufficiently sensitive and specific, the 'second opinion' it offers has the potential to increase the radiologist's diagnostic performance in the detection of polyps and masses and to reduce the variable detection performance among readers because of the difference in their interpretation skill.

Several prototype CAD systems have been proposed for VC.[12,13] To date, most of the CAD systems for VC consist of the following three steps: extraction of the colonic wall from 3D volume generated from axial VC images, detection of polyp candidates in the extracted colon, and removal of false positives from the polyp candidates. The performance of these systems has been evaluated on VC cases that were collected retrospectively at a single institution. It is difficult to perform a meta-analysis on the performance of CAD systems because databases used for evaluation of these systems and the methods for evaluation of the detection performance differ greatly among studies. However, it appears that the best performance can reach up to a 100% by-patient sensitivity with 1.3 false positives per patient[14] for polyps >5 mm, and the performance of many CAD systems ranges between 80 and 100% sensitivity with 2–8 false positives per patient. When this performance is compared with that of human readers, it appears that the performance, especially the sensitivity, of CAD is approaching that of a human reader.

It should be noted that CAD does not have to be as accurate as human readers to improve the detection performance of the latter. Computers make detection errors, as do human beings. However, together, they can improve the diagnostic performance, as demonstrated in clinical studies in which CAD for mammography was shown to reduce human errors and, as a result, to improve the diagnostic accuracy of radiologists.

INDICATIONS/CONTRAINDICATIONS

Screening for colorectal cancer

Alternatives

There currently are several proposed screening choices for colorectal cancer,[15] including fecal occult blood testing, flexible sigmoidoscopy, a combination of the two, double-contrast barium enema, and colonoscopy. Two additional tests under investigation include virtual colonoscopy and the testing of stool for genetic markers.

The **fecal occult blood test** (which can be administered in several forms and methods) is inexpensive and readily applied at the mass level. However, it is insensitive to the detection of adenomatous polyps, and a single application has only fair sensitivity for colorectal cancer and requires repeat testing. **Flexible sigmoidoscopy** visualizes about one-third of the bowel but a protocol of performing colonoscopy after an adenoma is detected improves the sensitivity to approximately 75% for detection of neoplasms. Although flexible sigmoidoscopy is much safer and less expensive than colonoscopy and does not require sedation, a significant portion of lesions will be missed because of their location in the proximal colon. The double-contrast barium enema is relatively inexpensive and safe. As with colonoscopy, it requires colonic cleansing, while usually associated with mild to moderate discomfort. Observational studies suggest that this test can detect up to 80–90% of large adenomas and 85–95% of cancers but a randomized controlled trial versus colonoscopy reported a detection rate of only 50% of large adenomas.

Colonoscopy is considered the definitive procedure for evaluating the colon because it directly visualizes the mucosa and can be used both for diagnosis and for therapy because polyps can be removed if they are small or pedunculated and can be biopsied for histologic diagnosis. Although the risks of perforation and hemorrhage are relatively low, they are higher than with any of the screening alternatives. Unlike sigmoidoscopy, colonoscopy also requires more intensive preparation, which many patients find to be the most difficult aspect of the test. The completion rate for colonoscopy ranges from 75% to 99% and the national average completion rate for colonoscopy is about 90%.

Colonoscopy vs VC

The use of colonoscopy for colorectal cancer screening has been recommended by several gastroenterology organizations. The widespread application of screening with optical colonoscopy is hindered by an increasing recognition that the waiting time for optical colonoscopy is often many months and, in some locations, more than a year. Also, there is evidence based on back-to-back colonoscopies that 6% of polyps less than 1 cm in diameter may be missed. The recent VC multicenter trial reported by Pickhardt et al.,[3] used a 'segmental unblinding' strategy to test the effectiveness of the colonoscopy. They found VC to be superior to optical colonoscopy for the detection of 8–10-mm polyps,[3] thus presenting a new challenge to colonoscopy as the 'gold standard.'

VC and colon cancer

VC has been advocated for:

1. evaluating the colon proximal to an obstructing colonic mass or stricture;

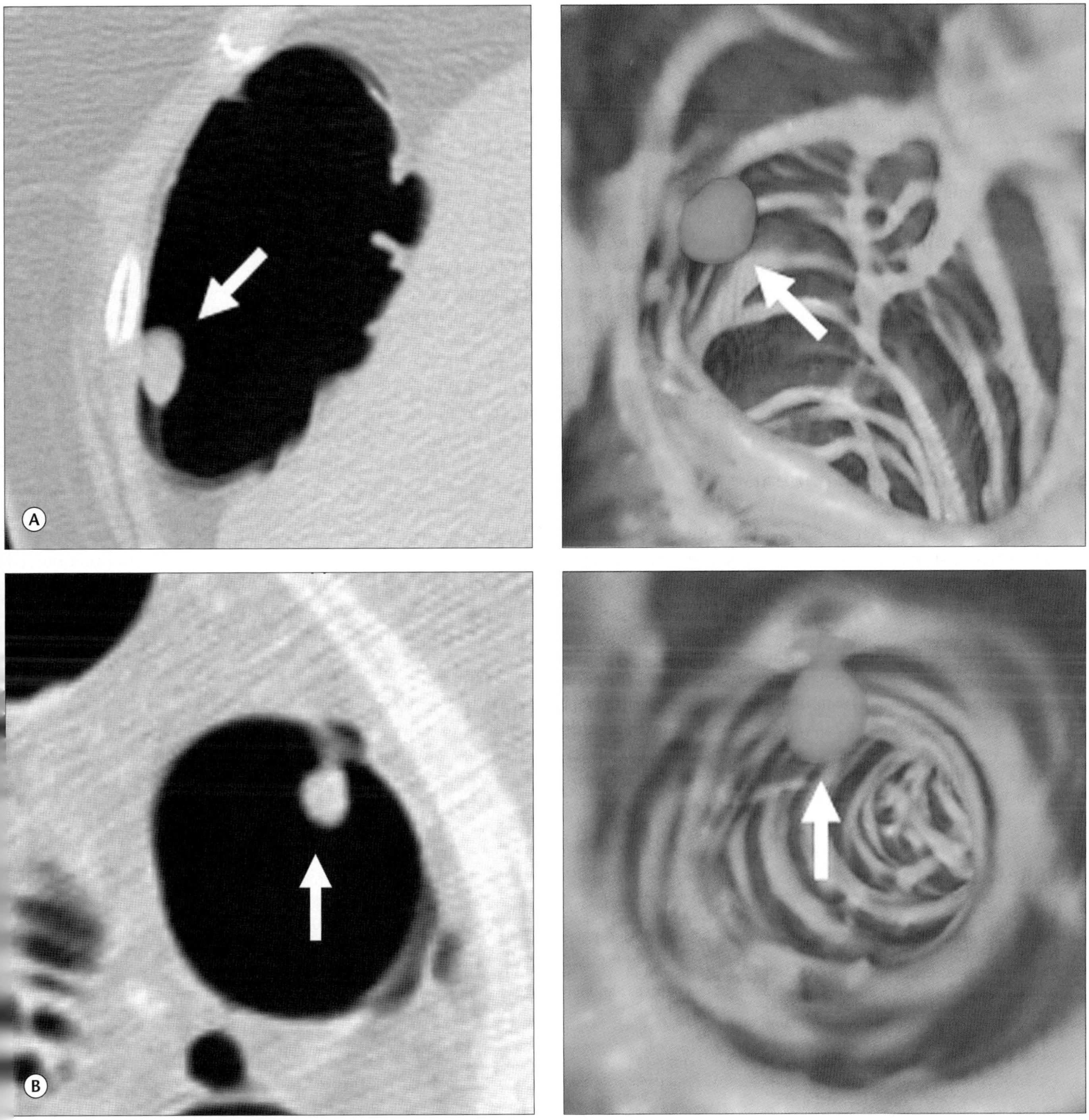

ig. 129.8 Polyps detected by computer-aided detection (CAD). A. 12-mm sessile polyp at the hepatic flexture. Left image reproduced with ermission from Dachman AH, Yoshida H. Virtual colonography: past, present and future. The Radiologic Clinics of North America 41: 377-393, 003 **B.** 10-mm pedunculated polyp in the splenic flexure. In each figure, left and right images show axial CT images containing polyps arrows) and the 3D endoscopic views of the polyps, respectively. The CAD color coding delineates the regions corresponding to the polyp, olds, and colonic wall by green, pink, and brown, respectively. The color coding is based on the shape analysis of the colonic structures erformed during the process of automated detection of polyps by CAD.

- completing the colonic examination after an incomplete optical colonoscopy;
- searching for polyps or masses in above average colorectal cancer risk patients who refuse optical colonoscopy or whose physician prefers VC because of the risk of sedation or bleeding (e.g., for patients on anticoagulation); and
- screening informed, average risk patients for colorectal cancer.

Obstructing cancer and incomplete colonoscopy

Virtual colonoscopy has achieved a significant role in the evaluation of patients with incomplete colonoscopy. The patient who is already prepared and has undergone an incomplete colonoscopy can be accommodated for a same-day, unscheduled VC examination, thus obviating the need for a return visit and repeat preparation. Morrin et al.[16] studied 40 patients using CT within 2 h of an incomplete colonoscopy. Their study showed the portion of the colon that was not visualized by endoscopy in more than 90% of patients, and found a probable cause for the obstruction in 74% of patients. Fenlon et al.[17] showed that CT depicted all 29 occlusive carcinomas, and they also fully evaluated the proximal colon in 26 out of 29 patients. CT also demonstrated two synchronous cancers and 24 polyps in the proximal colon, many of which were subsequently confirmed by endoscopy, although none could be palpated at surgery. Identification of the synchronous cancers in two patients altered the surgical plan. CT was also more accurate than colonoscopy in localizing the cancers; this may be helpful in preoperative planning. Neri et al. studied 34 patients with CT, pre and post intravenous contrast injection.[18] In 29 patients, surgery showed 30 cancers (including three synchronous cancers). Colonoscopy missed 10 cancers and three synchronous cancers, all of which were detected with CT. The use of intravenous contrast also permitted a definitive search for metastatic disease with a single CT examination.

Screening average risk patients

The use of VC for screening of average risk patients is still controversial. It is important to differentiate between by-patient and by-polyp sensitivities.[19] For patient triage to colonoscopy, only the by-patient results are relevant. The sensitivity of VC to date is based on cohorts with mixed indications and is often weighted towards above average risk increase of the prevalence of polyps in the cohort. In one meta-analysis of 1324 patients, the pooled per-patient sensitivity for polyps 10 mm or larger was 88%, and for 6–9-mm polyps, the sensitivity was 84%. The specificity remained high. In a recent trial by Pickhardt et al., the by-patient sensitivity for adenomas 8 mm or larger was 93.9% with 92.2% specificity, and the by-polyp sensitivity for adenomas 8 mm or larger was 92.6%.[3]

COMPLICATIONS AND THEIR MANAGEMENT

No serious complications have been reported from VC. Patients may experience some bloating and cramping from the gaseous distention of the colon and small bowel. Small bowel reflux is expected, particularly if an antispasmodic is used, which may make the ileocecal valve incompetent. The use of carbon dioxide rather than room air is thought to reduce postprocedural cramping.

RELATIVE COST

One of the arguments for the use of VC is the limited availability of optical colonoscopy, suggesting that gastroenterologists' resources should be reserved for a prescreened cohort with a high prevalence of disease. This may be a more cost-effective use of resources, because every positive VC must be referred to optical colonoscopy. The cost-effectiveness of VC will depend on the charges, and on the interval at which a normal exam needs to be repeated. Very few insurance companies have started reimbursing for this test at the time of this writing. In the US new category III CPT billing codes have been created for VC; however, this category code is typically not reimbursed by insurers. There is a slow but steady increased recognition of the value of VC by insurers and the utilization of VC in general radiology practice is likely to grow.

SOURCES OF INFORMATION FOR PATIENTS AND DOCTORS

http://www.medical.siemens.com/siemens/en_INT/gg_ct_FBAs/files/brochures/CT_Patient_Information.pdf

REFERENCES

1. Johnson CD, Dachman AH. CT colonography: The next colon screening examination. Radiology 2000; 216:331–341.
2. McFarland EG. Reader strategies for CT colonography. Abdom Imaging 2002; 27:275.
3. Pickhardt PJ, Choi R, Hwang I et al. Computed tomographic virtual colonoscopy to screen for colorectal neoplasia in asymptomatic adults. New Engl J Med 2003; 349:2191–2200.
4. Dachman AH. Diagnostic performance of virtual colonoscopy. Abdom Imaging 2002; 27:260–267.
5. Sosna J, Morrrin MM, Kruskal JB et al. CT colonography of colorectal polyps: A meta analysis. Am J Roentgenol 2003; 181:1593–1598.
6. Callstrom MR, Johnson CD, Fletcher JG et al. CT colonography without cathartic preparation: feasibility study. Radiology 2001; 219:693–698.
7. Zalis ME, Perumpillichira J, Del Frate C et al. CT colonography: digital subtraction bowel cleansing with mucosal reconstruction initial observations. Radiology 2003; 226:911–917.
8. Dachman AH, Kuniyoshi JK, Boyle CM et al. CT colonography with three-dimensional problem solving for detection of colonic polyps. Am J Roentgenol 1998; 171:989–995.
9. Dachman (ed) Atlas of Virtual Colonoscopy, New York, NY: Springer-Verlag, 2003.
10. Gleucker TM, Johnson CD, Wilson LA et al. Extracolonic findings at CT colonography: evaluation of prevalence and cost in a screening population. Gastroenterology 2003; 124:911–916.
11. Summers R, Yoshida H. Future directions of CT colonography: computer-aided diagnosis. In: Dachman AH, ed. Atlas of virtual colonoscopy. New York, NY: Springer-Verlag; 2002:55–62.
12. Summers RM, Johnson CD, Pusanik LM et al. Automated polyp detection at CT colonography: feasibility assessment in a human population. Radiology 2001; 219:51–59.
13. Yoshida H, Masutani Y, MacEneaney P et al. Computerized detection of colonic polyps at CT colonography on the basis of volumetric features: pilot study. Radiology 2002; 222:327–336.
14. Näppi J, Yoshida H. Feature-guided analysis for reduction of false positives in CAD of polyps for computed tomographic colonography. Med Phys 2003; 30:1592–1601.
15. Byers T, Levin B, Rothenberger D et al. American Cancer Society guidelines for screening and surveillance for early detection of colorectal polyps and cancer: update 1997. CA Cancer J Clin 1997; 47:154–160.
16. Morrin MM, Kruskal JB, Farrell RJ et al. Endoluminal CT colonography after an incomplete endoscopic colonoscopy. Am J Roentgenol 1999; 172:913–918.
17. Fenlon HM, MacEneaney DB, Nunes DP et al. Occlusive colon carcinoma: virtual colonoscopy in the preoperative evaluation of the proximal colon. Radiology 1999; 210:423–428.
18. Neri E, Giusti P, Battolla L et al. Colorectal cancer: role of CT colonography in preoperative evaluation after incomplete colonoscopy. Radiology 2002; 223:615–619.
19. Dachman AH, Zalis ME. Quality and consistency in CT colonography and research reporting. Radiology 2003; 230:319–323.

Chapter 130

Positron emission tomography

Michael S Kipper

KEY POINTS

- Positron emission tomography (PET) scans highlight tumors which preferentially metabolize glucose
- Glucose analogs such as FDG are also taken up by tumors with inflammation or infection
- Interpretation requires corroboration with other recent imaging studies
- In colorectal cancer, PET is useful for assessing recurrence and hepatic staging to select candidates for resection of isolated metastases
- PET is useful in upstaging esophageal cancer, but of less certain utility in gastric and pancreatic cancer

NTRODUCTION

ositron emission tomography (PET) is a rapidly evolving techology with increasing applicability in gastrointestinal disorders. iagnostic images display the *in vivo* distribution of molecules beled with positron emitting radioisotopes. The majority of inical studies are performed for the investigation of cancer, sing the glucose analog 2-deoxy-2 [^{18}F] fluoro-D-glucose DG). It has been recognized for decades that tumor cells referentially utilize glucose as a metabolic substrate. PET takes dvantage of this fact, depicting areas of increased glucose etabolism as ‘hot spots’ on images. Substantial data support e unique as well as incremental value of PET for staging, estaging, and monitoring therapy. PET has shown high sensivity, specificity, and accuracy in most malignancies, including olorectal, esophageal, and pancreatic. This chapter details the urrent indications, supporting data, methodology, and potenal pitfalls of PET imaging in gastrointestinal disease.

DESCRIPTION OF TECHNIQUE

ET uses radiopharmaceuticals labeled with positron-emitting adionuclides. The emitted positrons collide with electrons and, a process termed annihilation radiation, produce two highnergy photons, which travel at approximately 180 degrees rom each other (Fig. 130.1). Dedicated PET scanners are able o detect annihilation radiation and determine positional inforation. Current PET scanners routinely identify lesions >1 cm. recent major innovation in PET cameras is the development nd dissemination of PET computed tomography (CT) integrated ystems. A dedicated PET scanner and multi-slice CT scanner re mounted on a single support system using the same imaging able. CT and PET data are acquired and reconstructed to produce fusion images of anatomy and metabolism. The end result is a high-quality transmission scan, diagnostic quality CT, excellent registration of PET plus CT data, and a significant reduction in scan time. These combination systems may add more than 1 million $US to the cost and require additional space.

RADIOPHARMACEUTICALS

The number of biological molecules that can be labeled with positron emitting radioisotopes is nearly limitless. Radionuclides used in PET are summarized in Table 130.1. Very short-lived radionuclides can be difficult to use due to limited time to perform a diagnostic study. Fortunately, the vast majority of clinical studies are performed with fluorine-18, which has a half-life of ~110 min. The current radiopharmaceutical of choice for clinical PET is FDG. This glucose analog is transported intracellularly and phosphorylated by hexokinase to FDG-6-PO_4. Owing to a decreased intracellular level of glucose-6-phosphatase in malignant cells, FDG-6-PO_4 is trapped, resulting in a detectable increase in nearly all cancers. Most FDG-PET studies are performed for cancer; however, nonmalignant processes (especially inflammation/infection) can show enhanced FDG uptake. While this may provide an opportunity to investigate other diseases, it results in one of PET's major pitfalls, i.e., reduced specificity.

TABLE 130.1 RADIONUCLIDES USED IN PET

Radionuclide	Radioactive half-life	Applications
Fluorine-18	110 min	Measure of metabolic rate in tissues (e.g., tumors, inflammation, infection); assess myocardial viability
Carbon-11	20 min	Measure of metabolic activity (tumor, cardiac); receptor binding
Nitrogen-13	10 min	Blood-flow tracer (myocardial perfusion studies); protein synthesis; cell proliferation
Oxygen-15	2 min	Labeling of gases, such as oxygen, carbon dioxide and carbon monoxide, and water (permits measurements of blood flow, blood volume, and oxygen consumption)
Rubidium-82	76 s	Utilized to measure myocardial blood flow

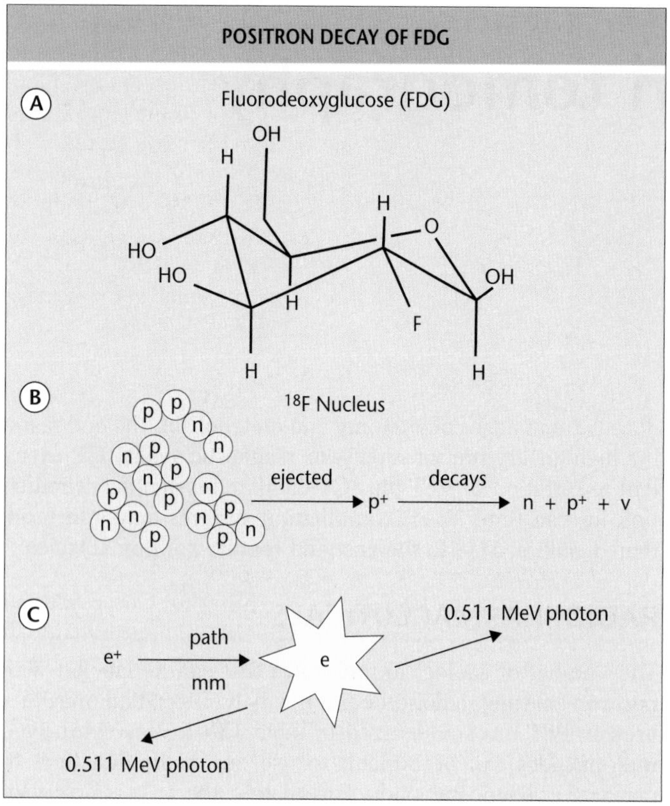

Fig. 130.1 Positron decay of FDG. Positron decay of FDG resulting in production of measurable radiation. **A.** Chemical structure of FDG. **B.** Positron decay of fluorine-18 (^{18}F) nucleus (n, neutron; p, proton; e^+, positron; v, neutrino). **C.** Production of photons by annihilation (e^-, electron).

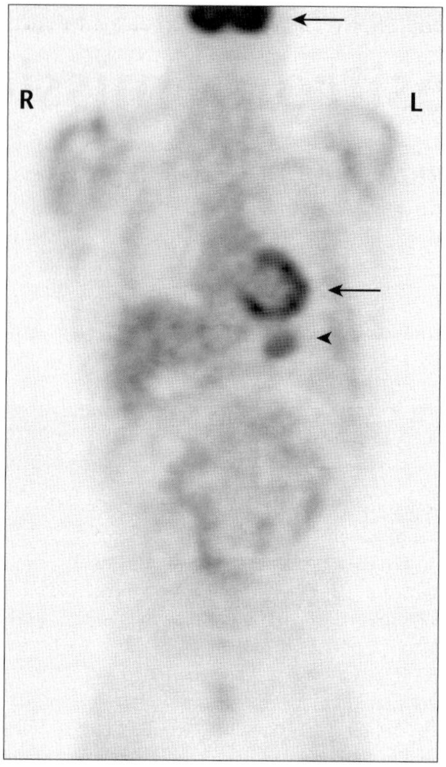

Fig. 130.2 Normal PET scan. Note expected concentration of FD in brain and heart (arrows) as well as activity in the stomach (arrowhea R = right, L = left.

PERFORMANCE OF A PET SCAN

While PET scanning has demonstrated efficacy in both neurological and cardiac disorders (e.g., localization of seizure focus, evaluation of dementia, movement disorders, identification of myocardial viability), >90% of clinical studies are for cancer. Therefore, the method presented is directed at evaluation of the cancer patient. The patient is fasted for a minimum of 4–6h prior to the study. Water and regular medications are permitted. Endogenous glucose competes with injected FDG, lowering study sensitivity, affecting quantitation of data, and may result in false-negative examinations. Most centers measure serum glucose prior to administration of FDG. Values >200mg/dL necessitate rescheduling the patient. Following the intravenous injection of FDG, the patient rests quietly for 45–60min (uptake phase). There is emerging data that some cancers may be better detected by increasing the uptake phase to 2h. During the uptake phase patients are asked to remain sedentary as well as relatively quiet, minimizing FDG localization to skeletal muscle (including laryngeal muscles secondary to talking). Imaging is then performed in a supine position for 20–60min.

FDG will normally concentrate in brain, heart, the genitourinary system, the tonsils, and mildly in the liver and spleen. Variable uptake is seen in the thyroid, stomach, and gastrointestinal tract (Fig. 130.2). Accurate scan interpretation is based on many factors: patient history, review of clinical data, familiarity with specific disease patterns, temporal relationship of scan to therapies (especially radiation), and knowledge of normal variants (Fig. 130.3). A crucial factor in interpretatic is comparison of PET data to recent anatomical imagi studies. Interpretive accuracy is significantly improved b comparing all imaging studies.[1]

INDICATIONS FOR PET IN GASTROINTESTINAL MALIGNANCIES

FDG-PET has demonstrated variable utility in colorecta esophageal/gastric, pancreatic, and hepatobiliary cancers. Stagin restaging, localization of recurrence, determination of operabilit

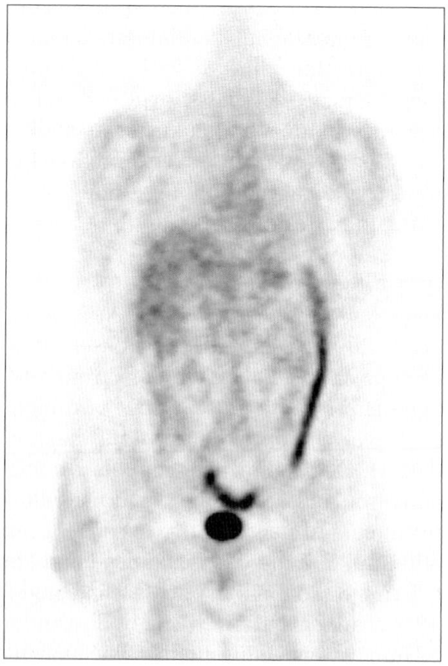

Fig. 130.3 Normal, nonpathologic bowel activity. This pattern is unlikely to represent malignanc although inflammatory bowel disease is not excluded. Note absence of cardiac and gastric activity (see Fig. 130.2).

discrimination between tumor recurrence and treatment-related changes, and response to therapy are all areas of potential applicability. Conventional anatomical imaging modalities such as CT, magnetic resonance imaging (MRI), and ultrasound (US) remain critical for evaluation of the size and shape of normal organs and pathological sites, as well as their relationship to other structures. However, these methods may not accurately separate benign from malignant lymph nodes based on size alone, may not be able to differentiate tumor recurrence from treatment-related abnormalities, and may remain normal for months after metabolic changes produce a positive PET scan. Additionally, PET offers the advantage of a whole body search at low radiation exposure and without contrast agents.

INDICATIONS

- Colorectal cancer: restaging/evaluation for recurrence (especially useful with elevated or rising CEA and negative conventional work-up), determination of resectability or recurrence, monitoring response to therapy
- Esophageal cancer: evaluation for distant metastases, possible monitoring response to therapy
- Gastric cancer: probable indication for monitoring response to therapy in gastrointestinal stromal tumors
- Pancreatic cancer: helpful in differentiating local recurrence from changes due to surgery or radiation, or in patients with elevated serum tumor markers and negative conventional work-ups
- Hepatobiliary cancer: PET has shown low sensitivity in primary hepatocellular carcinoma. PET is very sensitive in detecting hepatic metastases with a greater sensitivity than CT, ultrasound, or MRI in most gastrointestinal cancers.

COLORECTAL CANCER

PET has demonstrated efficacy in staging, detection of recurrence, differentiating tumor recurrence from post-treatment changes, and has shown encouraging preliminary results in monitoring response to therapy. While primary lesions are almost always seen with PET, at present PET is not indicated for screening or evaluation of the primary site. With respect to screening, the detection rate for adenomatous polyps that were 5–30 mm in size was only 24% in a recent prospective study.[2] The authors did demonstrate an improved sensitivity for lesions >13 mm but there was a 5.5% false-positive rate (probably due to FDG uptake in normal bowel as well as localized areas of inflammation). In contrast to screening and primary site evaluation, PET has proven very useful for assessing recurrence and selecting patients who may benefit from curative-intent surgery for isolated metastases. A meta-analysis by Huebner and colleagues found a sensitivity of 97% and a specificity of 76% for FDG-PET detecting recurrent colorectal cancer throughout the whole body.[3] Situations where FDG-PET has shown strong value are evaluation of recurrent disease, including those patients with an elevated or rising CEA and negative conventional diagnostic work-up, separation of true recurrence from changes due to surgery or radiation, assessing the whole body for distant metastases (note that CT is more sensitive than PET in the chest), and accurate hepatic staging.

One particular area where PET can play a major role is in assessing the patient suspected of having recurrent but resectable disease. A significant percentage of these patients will have their treatment plan altered as a result of PET, most being upstaged and thereby avoiding noncurative, potentially morbid surgery. In a large prospective study (>100 patients) PET directly influenced management in 59% of patients.[4] Since resection of isolated hepatic metastases may have a cure rate as high as 40%, careful preoperative evaluation of these patients is critical to select appropriate candidates for curative-intent surgery (Fig. 130.4).

GASTROESOPHAGEAL CANCER

In esophageal cancer PET is most valuable for assessing distant metastases and in the evaluation of suspected recurrence. Although PET has shown a sensitivity of >90% for primary site detection it offers no advantage over more established modalities (e.g., CT, endoscopic ultrasonography (EU)). PET is insensitive in assessing regional lymph node basins adjacent to the primary due to intense uptake at the primary site. The diagnostic accuracy for detecting distant metastases is higher with PET than with conventional imaging methods (Fig. 130.5). Based on one study the accuracy for detecting distant nodal metastases is 86% for PET versus 62% for the combined use of CT and EU.[5] FDG-PET is useful for detection of recurrence in previously treated patients. An important question yet to be answered is the impact on survival in this poor prognostic group. Preliminary data on the role for PET in monitoring response to neoadjuvant chemotherapy have been encouraging. The use of PET for monitoring response in patients with esophageal cancer is still considered investigational.

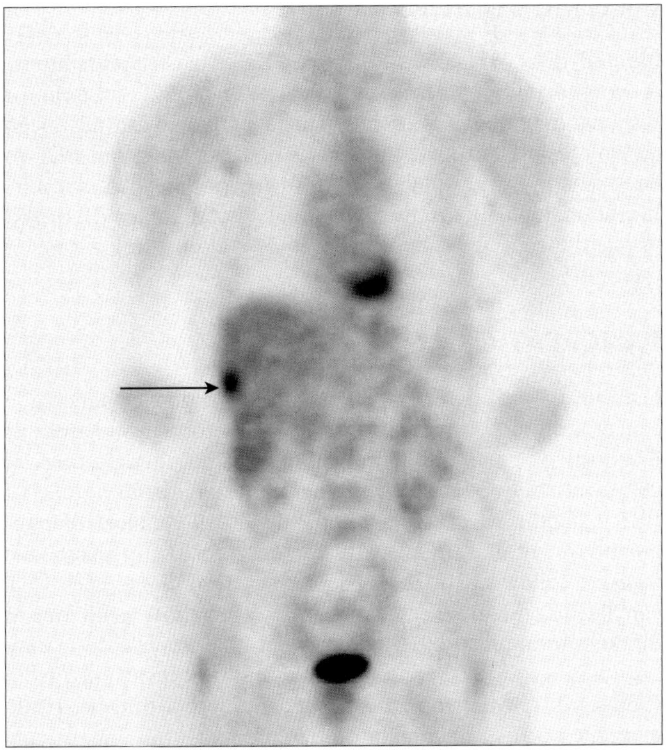

Fig. 130.4 Solitary hepatic metastasis (arrow). Patient considered to be operative candidate.

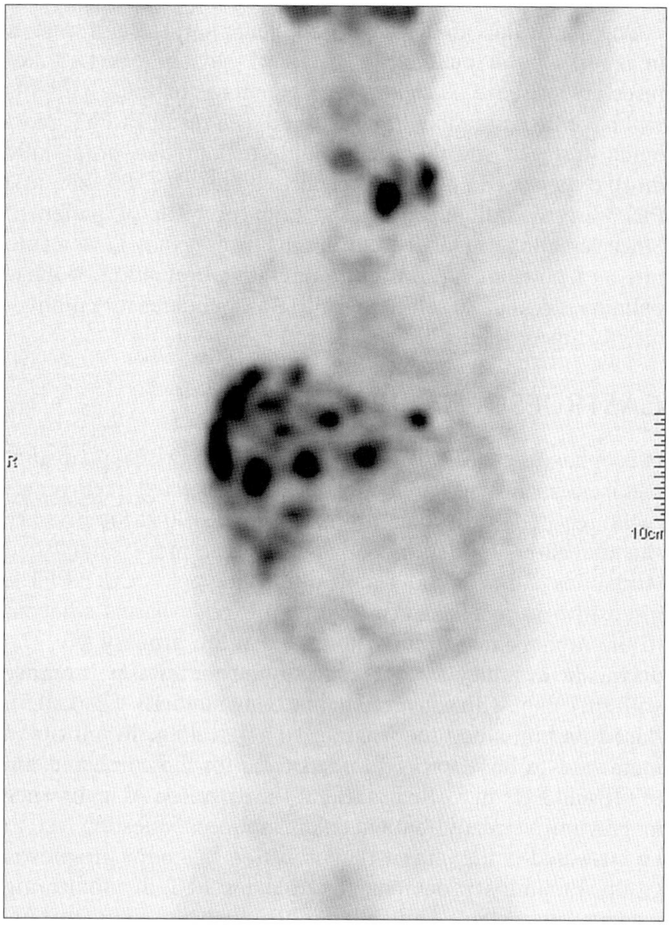

Fig. 130.5 Metastatic adenocarcinoma of the esophagus. Multiple hypermetabolic foci consistent with metastases are identified in the liver and left neck.

GASTRIC TUMORS

Limited data exist on the use of PET in gastric carcinoma. A very exciting area is the use of FDG-PET to monitor response to therapy with imatinib in patients with advanced gastrointestinal stromal tumors. Demetri et al. found PET to be a sensitive and reliable indicator of resistance to imatinib. In responding patients, the FDG uptake in the tumor decreased markedly from baseline as early as 24 h after a single dose of imatinib.[6]

PANCREATIC CANCER

Data on the use of FDG-PET in the evaluation of pancreatic cancer are both preliminary and contradictory. In the areas of diagnosis, staging, follow-up, and monitoring therapy there is consensus only in recommending against the routine use of PET. Chapter 73 presents an update on the subject of pancreatic cancer and underscores the need for better diagnostic tools. In follow-up, or the evaluation of recurrence, FDG-PET can be helpful in selected patients, often those with tumor marker elevation and negative conventional studies. There may also be a role for PET in differentiating local recurrence from changes due to postoperative or postradiation fibrosis. However, the results rarely lead to an improvement in patient outcome. Lastly, some reports document the ability of PET to assess response to neoadjuvant chemoradiation. CT has proven unreliable in this setting, and if further studies with PET support the current preliminary findings, PET may ultimately play a role in improving the resectability rate of pancreatic cancer and in selecting alternative chemoradiation protocols.

HEPATOBILIARY CANCER

This category can be divided into primary hepatocellular carcinoma (HCC), hepatic metastases, and primary biliary cancer. PET has performed poorly in HCC. Sensitivity is relatively low (~60–70%). Thus, the use of PET for diagnosis or preoperative staging of HCC is not recommended.

For hepatic metastases PET has proven to be very reliable. Kinkel et al. performed a meta-analysis comparing US, CT, MR, and FDG-PET. Selecting a specificity cutoff of 85% they found a mean weighted sensitivity of 55% for US, 72% for

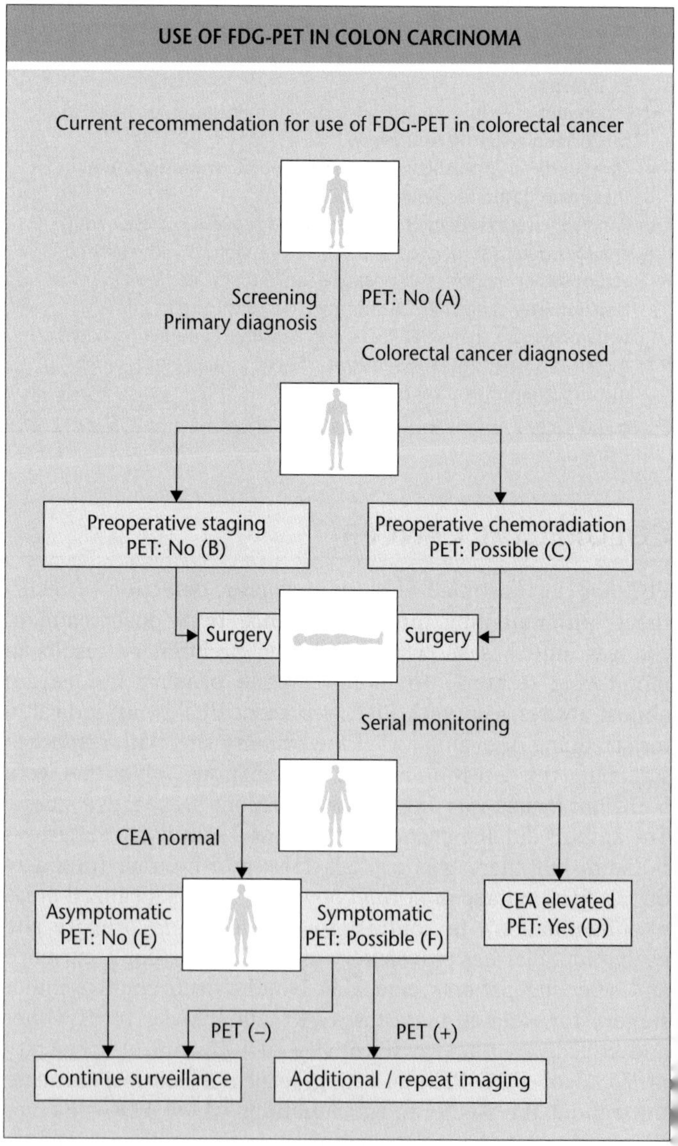

Fig. 130.6 Algorithm for use of FDG-PET in patients with colon carcinoma. (A) No advantage over conventional testing. (B) Low sensitivity. (C) May separate responders from nonresponders with prognostic value. (D) Superb sensitivity for identifying site(s) of recurrence. (E) Expense not justified. (F) Modest success in this subset with low probability of recurrence.

CT, 76% for MRI, and 90% for PET.[7] They concluded that at equivalent specificity, FDG-PET is the most sensitive noninvasive imaging modality for the diagnosis of hepatic metastases from colorectal, gastric, and esophageal cancers. In cholangiocarcinoma the data suggest that the use of FDG-PET should still be considered experimental.

COST EFFECTIVENESS

Reliable data on cost effectiveness exist for recurrent colorectal cancer. Based on Medicare reimbursement of $US1800 for a PET scan, the potential savings per patient ranged from $US220 to $US3003.[8] The major reason for these cost savings was the reduction in noncurative surgeries for recurrences shown to be nonresectable. An algorithm for the use of PET in colorectal cancer is suggested in Fig. 130.6. In 2000 the Health Care Financing Administration approved reimbursement for PET in esophageal cancer (colorectal cancer was approved in 1999) but to date has not approved PET for pancreatic, gastric, or hepatobiliary cancer.

COSTS, COMPLICATIONS, AND CONTROVERSIES

- Cost effectiveness: demonstrated for colorectal and esophageal cancer, primarily based upon savings resulting from the elimination of noncurative surgeries; not proven for gastroesophageal, pancreatic, or hepatobiliary malignancies
- Effect on patient outcome or prolongation of patient survival: thus far demonstrated only in colorectal cancer
- FDG localization is not cancer specific; areas of inflammation, infection, postradiation, and normal physiological uptake may reduce study specificity
- Sensitivity limitation: lesion detectability inversely related to size and directly related to metabolic rate (i.e., low-grade or low metabolic rate tumors may be PET negative)
- Unresolved issues include: when to image following radiation therapy to maximize specificity; the level of change of FDG uptake in tumor sites indicative of meaningful response to therapy; and the incremental value of combined PET-CT scanners versus PET only systems

SUMMARY

PET has now become an indispensable tool in the evaluation of selected patients with gastrointestinal malignancies. Data are strongest for colorectal and esophageal cancer, with more limited indications for gastric, hepatic, and pancreatic cancers.

The future promises technical advances including improved resolution and broader use of combination PET-CT scanners, the development of new radiotracers, which will significantly expand the role of PET in molecular imaging, and a clearer delineation for the use of PET in gastrointestinal malignancies as well as benign disease.

REFERENCES

1. Kipper MS, Tartar M. Clinical atlas of PET with imaging correlation. Philadelphia: Saunders; 2004:5–74.
2. Yasuda S, Fujii H, Nakahara T et al. 18F-FDG PET detection of colonic adenomas. J Nucl Med 2001; 42:989–992.
3. Huebner RH, Park KC, Shepherd JE et al. A meta-analysis of the literature for whole-body FDG-PET detection of recurrent colorectal cancer. J Nucl Med 2000; 41:1177–1189.
4. Kalff V, Hicks RJ, Ware RE et al. The clinical impact of (18) F-FDG PET in patients with suspected or confirmed recurrence of colorectal cancer: a prospective study. J Nucl Med 2002; 43:492–499.
5. Lerut T, Flamen P, Ectors N et al. Histopathologic validation of lymph node staging with FDG-PET scan in cancer of the esophagus and gastroesophageal junction: a prospective study based on primary surgery with extensive lymphadenectomy. Ann Surg 2000; 232:743–752.
6. Demetri GD, von Mehren M, Blanke CD et al. Efficacy and safety of imatinib mesylate in advanced gastrointestinal stromal tumors. New Engl J Med 2002; 347:472–480.
7. Kinkel K, Lu Y, Both M et al. Detection of hepatic metastases from cancers of the gastrointestinal tract by using noninvasive imaging methods (US, CT, MR imaging, PET): a meta-analysis. Radiology 2002; 224: 748–756.
8. Wahl RL. Principles and practice of positron emission tomography. Philadelphia: Lippincott Williams & Wilkins; 2002:48–64.

Chapter 131

Functional evaluation of the gastrointestinal tract

Malcolm Bateson

KEY POINTS

- Many gastrointestinal symptoms arise by dysfunction
- Motility and secretory studies are important functional tests
- Acid secretion studies are less commonly performed than previously but when needed should be performed to an orthodox protocol
- Breath testing is a useful evaluation of small bowel motility, digestive/absorptive function and of small bowel overgrowth
- Pancreatic function can also be tested by tubeless methods
- There are two secretin tests – for pancreatic function and for diagnosis of gastrinoma (some cases)
- Dynamic tests of liver function are of limited applicability compared to biochemical or histological assessment

:SOPHAGUS

•H studies (Fig. 131.1 and Fig. 131.2)

'he most useful test in functional evaluation of the esophagus ; 24-h esophageal pH monitoring. The electrode is positioned cm proximal to the high-pressure zone. If manometry is not vailable the pH step on withdrawing the probe from the stom-ch to the esophagus locates the high-pressure zone to within cm. Continuous monitoring over 24 h allows recording of :flux episodes, defined as any fall in pH of 2 units or more. he length of time during which esophageal pH is below 4 is :corded and should be less than 6% of the time supine and 0.5% of the time erect in normal adults. Generally, the total xposure to a pH less than 4 will be less than 5% in adults, ıough in children the cut-off is much higher at a total acid xposure of 18% or less.

/lanometry (Fig. 131.3)

. multichannel tube is used either with lateral orifices or balloon ps. Pressure changes are transmitted via transducers or a multi-hannel direct recorder and multiple recordings are taken in ıe stomach, at the gastroesophageal junction, and at various :vels of the esophagus both during and between swallowing. 'he level of the high-pressure zone can be accurately located sing a pull-through technique. Normal swallowing shows a ormal procession of peristaltic waves sweeping down the sophagus with relaxation of the high-pressure zone. In acha-ısia there is no peristalsis and the lower esophageal sphincter oes not relax during swallowing. Diffuse spasm can be recog-ized by incoordinate contractions in the lower part of the sophagus. The presence of a hiatus hernia will change recordings nd it is important that this is known to assist in interpretation.

Isotope swallow

This is more physiological than a barium swallow though results are equivalent. The fasted patient lies under a gamma camera and swallows a small volume of water containing technetium 99m colloid, which is injected into the mouth through a small flexible tube. Normally, 90% of the activity should have left the esophagus in 15 s. The test is repeated to ensure reproducibility and can be extended by allowing the patient to sit up and swallow 300 mL of 0.1 mol/L hydrochloric acid flavored with orange juice and repeating distal esophageal scanning to see if spontaneous reflux occurs.

Empiric proton pump inhibitor (PPI) test

Where symptoms are suspected to be caused by acid reflux disease the use of double dose PPI therapy such as omeprazole 40 mg twice daily for a week can be used as a diagnostic test. If such treatment completely abolishes symptoms they can safely be ascribed to acid reflux disease (see Chapter 29).

NASOGASTRIC INTUBATION

The passage of a nasogastric or orogastric tube allows collection of gastric, pancreatic and duodenal juices, and also bile. The main use of this procedure is in collection of gastric acid and sampling duodenal and jejunal contents for bacterial culture.

STOMACH

Gastric acid secretion

A nasogastric tube is passed and the aspiration ports are positioned under the surface of the pool of gastric juice with the patient positioned on the left side. This may be checked by bubbling air through or by aspiration of gastric juice and testing the pH. Fluoroscopy may sometimes be required to locate the tube in the correct position. The stomach is aspirated and the overnight secretion discarded after an overnight fast. Pentagastrin (6 μg/kg) is then given subcutaneously or intramuscularly. Aspiration for 10 min is conducted and this collection discarded, and then all the gastric secretions over a 10–30-min period are collected and saved. The volume and hydrogen ion are measured to give peak acid output. Normal peak acid output is 10–30 mmol/h for women and 15–40 mmol/h for men. Values are higher in duodenal ulcer but fall to normal after vagotomy. There is achlorhydria in pernicious anemia, and low values exclude duodenal ulcer.

Where gastrinoma is suspected, the spontaneous gastric secretion over a 1-h period is collected and its volume and acidity measured, which is then compared with peak acid

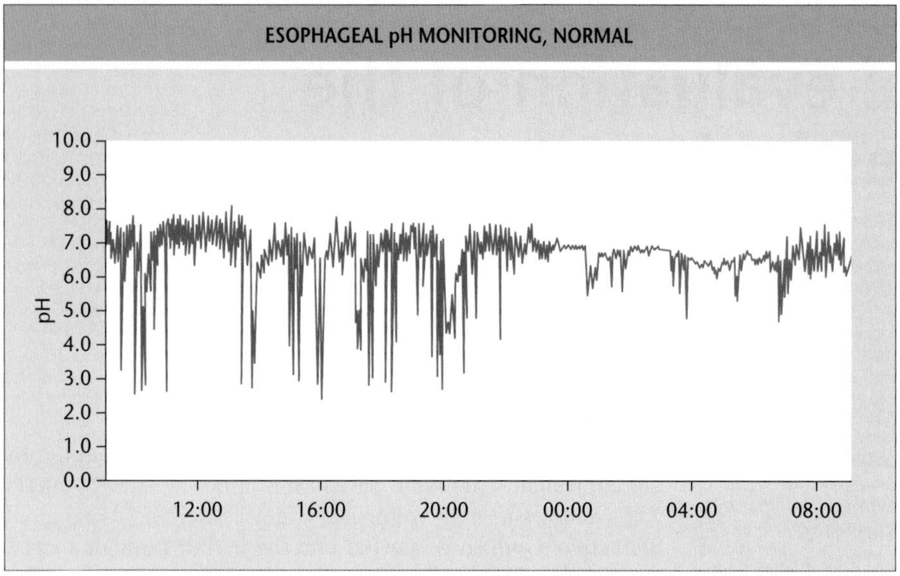

Fig. 131.1 Esophageal pH monitoring. Normal.

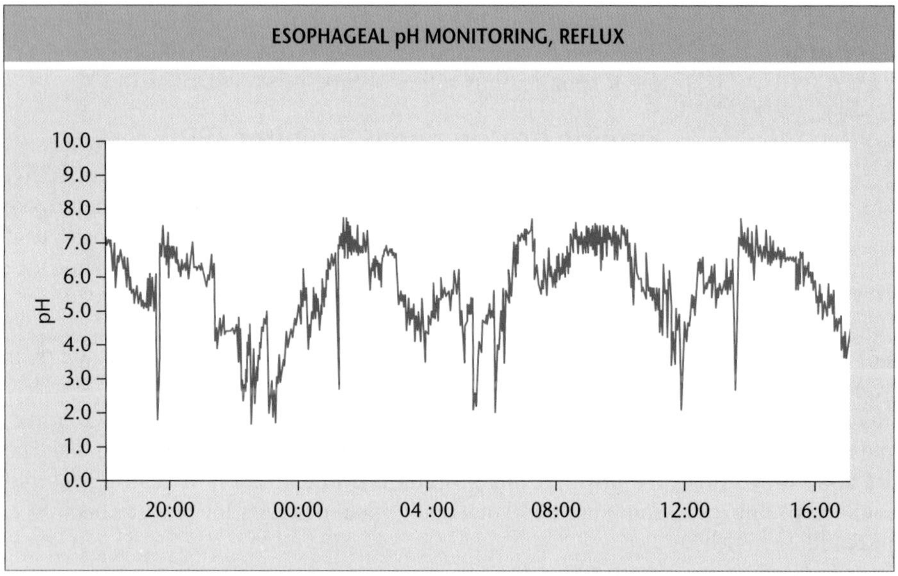

Fig. 131.2 Esophageal pH monitoring. Reflux.

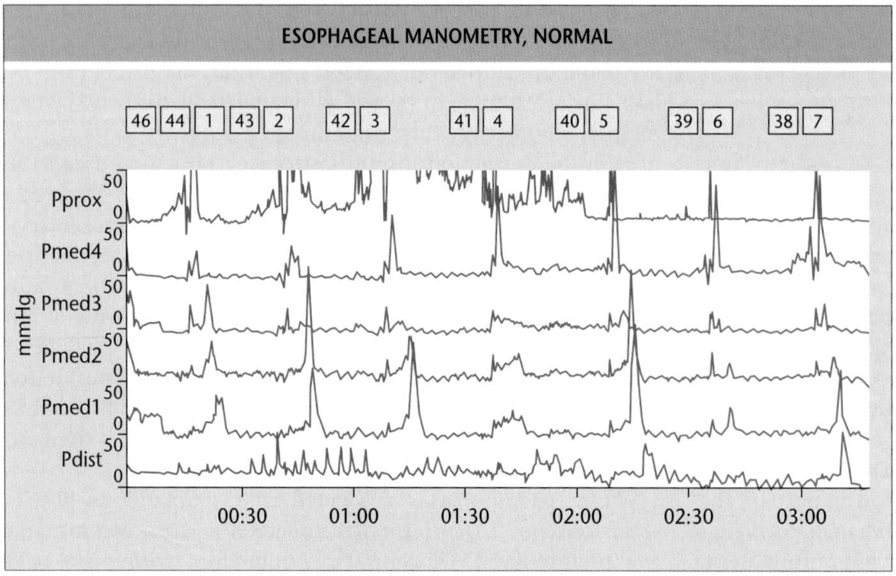

Fig. 131.3 Esophageal manometry. Normal.

PENTAGASTRIN GASTRIC ACID SECRETION TEST
1. Cease antacids day before test 2. Cease H_2-receptor antagonists, proton pump inhibitors, tricyclic antidepressants 1 week prior to test 3. Overnight fast 4. Pass nasogastric tube 5. Position patient in left lateral position and encourage them to spit out saliva 6. Aspirate stomach and discard secretion 7. Pentagastrin 6µg/kg s.c. or i.m. 8. Aspirate at 10 min and discard 9. Aspirate at 30 min and save (i.e., 10–30 min collection) 10. Send for volume, pH, titratable acidity (titrated against 0.01 mol/L NaOH to pH 7)
NORMAL VALUES Male: 15–40 mmol/h Female: 10–30 mmol/h pH 1–3, achlorhydria 7–8 Low volume in achlorhydria High volume in duodenal ulcer, hypercalcemia; very high in gastrinoma

output. With gastric overstimulation the basal acid output is at least 60% of the peak acid output and the two values may be the same.

Alternatively, a secretin test can be performed.

Fasting serum gastrin over 100 pmol/L is seen in gastrinoma and also in pernicious anemia and after vagotomy. When doubtful values occur intravenous secretin can be used as a provocative test and will cause a rise in serum gastrin, with an increase in levels of greater than 50% in gastrinoma.

Gastric emptying can be studied by ultrasonography and also by dual label isotopes, with different labeling of liquids and solids, but this is generally a research technique only.

In pernicious anemia the diagnosis is confirmed by low serum vitamin B_{12} levels, and the presence of intrinsic factor and gastric antibodies. This diagnosis is important because it establishes the presence of achlorhydria and makes benign spontaneous peptic ulcer disease an impossibility.

Helicobacter pylori (see also Chapter 34)

This organism is important in causation of duodenal ulcer and gastric cancer. The urea breath test measures *H. pylori* urease activity. Samples are collected over 30 min from fasting patients not receiving antacids or antibiotics, after the administration by mouth of urea labeled with carbon 13 or carbon 14 breath. In active *H. pylori* infection the excretion of radiolabeled CO_2 is increased (Fig. 131.4). Serology for anti-*H. pylori* IgG by ELISA is useful in screening surveys and where patients have not been given anti-*Helicobacter* therapy; it is not useful is assessing the effect of anti-*Helicobacter* therapy. *Helicobacter pylori* stool antigen testing has been developed as a useful non-invasive technique for active infection and is reliable except in cirrhosis.

SMALL BOWEL AND ABSORPTION

In celiac disease (see Chapter 44) endomysial antibody testing is usually positive (tissue transglutaminase is a more refined

SECRETIN TEST IN THE DIAGNOSIS OF GASTRINOMA (ZOLLINGER-ELLISON SYNDROME)
1. Overnight fast as above 2. Cease PPIs 30 h prior to test 3. Site intravenous cannula 4. Serum [gastrin] at t-15, t-1, t 2, 5, 10, 15, 20, 30 min 5. Secretin 2 units/kg i.v. over 2 min in 20 mL normal saline

Over 95% of gastrinoma patients respond to secretin infusion with a significant elevation (>50%) of gastrin levels above basal levels with a rise to at least 100 pmol/L

version of this test under development). Patients are often anemic with low serum folate and ferritin levels. In pancreatic and terminal ileal disease vitamin B_{12} levels may be low because of malabsorption.

A useful way of measuring absorption is the triolein breath test, based on the administration by mouth of radiolabeled triolein and cumulative measurement of breath excretion of radiolabeled CO_2, which is low in malabsorption (Fig. 131.5).

Direct collection of stools over 24 h and measurement of fecal fat is still sometimes employed. This will directly quantitate over-excretion of fat, but many hospitals prefer to avoid this test.

Measurement of breath hydrogen can be used in several ways. Following ingestion of lactulose by mouth, the time taken to a rise in breath hydrogen excretion will indicate transit time to the cecum. After lactose by mouth, patients with lactase deficiency will secrete much higher levels of hydrogen in the breath than normal. Sugar breath tests can also detect small bowel bacterial overgrowth (see Chapter 9): both glucose and lactose can be used for this purpose. Radiolabeled glycocholate breath tests have been used to assess bacterial overgrowth and radiolabeled SEHCAT testing is a technique for assessing bile acid malabsorption.

In obscure diarrhea a panel of hormone tests on fasting blood may be helpful, including glucagon, vasoactive intestinal peptide, and gastrin. In addition urine analysis for hydroxyindoles in carcinoid syndrome and catecholamines in pheochromocytoma can sometimes be helpful.

Radio capsule enteroscopy has recently been introduced and is under evaluation. It allows examination of the small bowel, and may help in diagnoses of Crohn's disease, angiodysplasia, and small bowel tumors. It does not permit biopsy or therapy and establishing the exact location of the capsule may be difficult. The test itself and analysis can be very prolonged (see Chapter 123).

Small bowel permeability tests such as chromium-51 labeled EDTA can provide useful information on the functional integrity of the intestinal mucosa. Intestinal permeability is increased in inflammatory bowel disease, celiac disease, chronic alcoholic liver disease, and by bacterial toxins and nonsteroidal anti-inflammatory drugs (NSAIDs).

White cell scanning: A sample of the patient's blood is labeled with Technetium 99m and reinjected. Abdominal scanning allows localization of inflammation by increased uptake. This is particularly useful in assessing the extent of involvement and activity of Crohn's disease.

Food allergy: Objective evidence may be obtained by measuring the level of serum IgE, which is usually elevated, and serum radio-allergosorbent testing (RAST) for specific suspect allergens

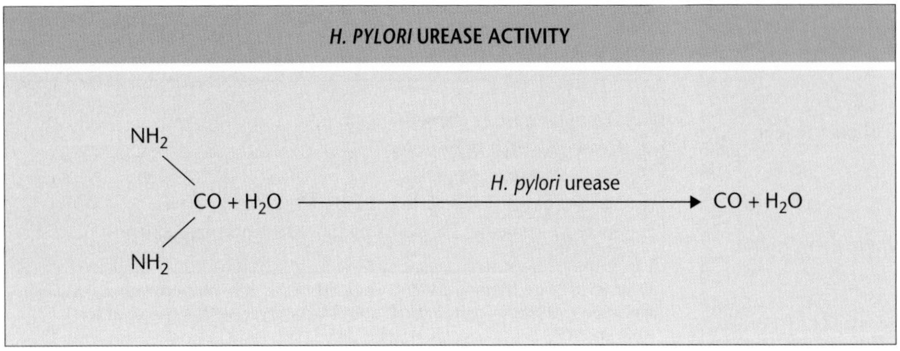

Fig. 131.4 ***Helicobacter pylori*** **urease activity.**

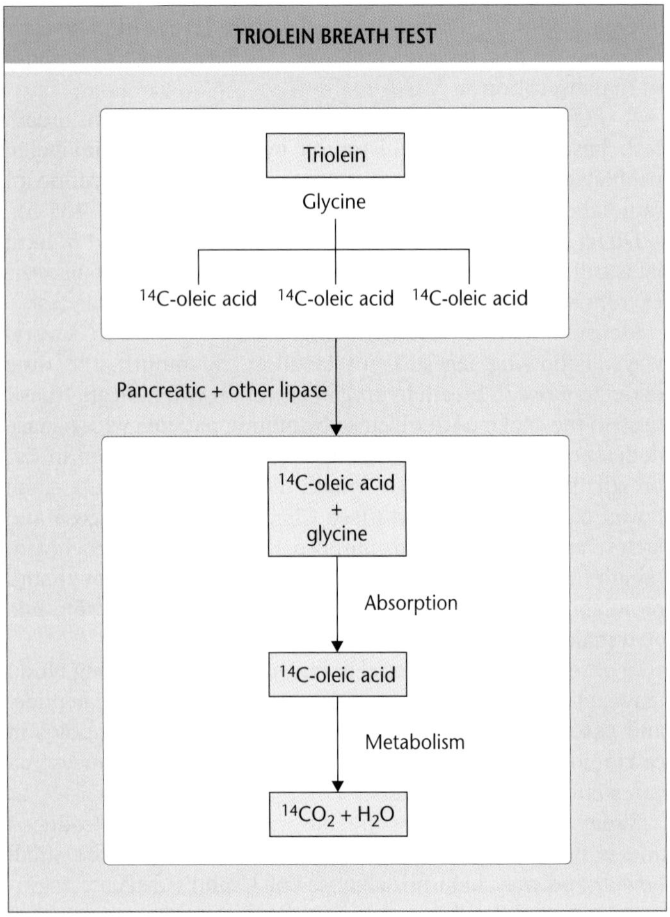

Fig. 131.5 Triolein breath test.

CAPSULE ENDOSCOPY

1. 12-h fast
2. Day procedure 08.00 to 16.00
3. Simethicone orally prior to ingestion of capsule with small volume of water
4. Fit template, sensor array, recorder, and battery pack
5. Avoid MRI
6. Can eat and take medications after 4 h
7. Remove sensors after 8 h
8. Patient is asked to note passage of the capsule in stool, but retrieval is not necessary

SMALL BOWEL PERMEABILITY

CHROMIUM-51 LABELED EDTA

1. Overnight fast
2. Void first morning urine
3. Drink 100 μCi ^{51}Cr-EDTA followed by 125 mL of water
4. Strict 24-h urine collection
5. Measure urine volume
6. Send 3 x 5-ml aliquots for gamma scintillation counter

Patients can eat and drink 2 h after ^{51}Cr-EDTA drink (no alcohol)

such as wheat, chocolate, and milk. These tests are not perfect and sometimes more useful information is obtained by dietary exclusion testing in individuals, particularly in those at high risk such as patients with atopy.

PANCREAS (see Chapter 72)

Functional evidence of pancreatic disease may be derived by indirect methods. In pancreatic steatorrhea fecal fat is elevated, and diarrhea and fecal fat excretion is reduced by administration of full-dose enzyme therapy such as with pancreatin 25 000 units three times daily with meals.

Pancreatic exocrine function can be assessed using the secretin test.

Tubeless pancreatic function testing: A readily available and reasonably accurate technique is the Pancreolauryl test (Fig. 131.6), which measures fluorescein excretion in the urine. A baseline is established by administering fluorescein by mouth, which is avidly absorbed. The test consists of administering fluorescein dilaurate by mouth. This is not absorbed unless it is cleaved by pancreatic esterase and in pancreatic insufficiency fluorescein excretion will be much reduced. An alternative, the bentiromide/PABA test, has practical difficulties, because bentiromide is not always readily available. This test is based on measurement of PABA in the urine. Bentiromide, which is administered by mouth, is cleaved by pancreatic chymotrypsin resulting in the liberation of PABA, which is absorbed and excreted in the urine. A more recent test of pancreatic function by estimation of fecal elastase I in stool samples appears to give more reliable results than the Pancreolauryl and bentiromide tests.

PANCREATIC SECRETION TEST

- Overnight fast
- Pass double-lumen gastroduodenal tube (or separate nasogastric and nasojejunal tube)
- Confirm position in antrum and distal duodenum by fluoroscopy
- Position patient in left lateral position
- Continuous suction on tubes (–5 to –10 mmHg), and manual aspiration to ensure patency
- Discard gastric aspirate (to avoid contaminating duodenal collection)
- Basal duodenal aspirate for 10–30 min (pH should be >7.5)
- Intravenous injection of 1 unit secretin/kg in 20 mL normal saline over 2 min (warn the patient they may experience flushing)
- Continuous duodenal aspirate for 60 min (also aspirate and discard gastric secretions)
- Duodenal aspirate in iced containers – record volume
- Mix aliquot of sample with equal volume glycerol
- Analyze for [bicarbonate], [amylase], (trypsin in children)

NORMAL RESULTS

Volume >2 mL/kg
[Bicarbonate] >90 mmol/L, average 108 mmol/L
[Amylase] >6 units/kg, average 14 units/kg
Chronic pancreatitis: low volume and concentration of bicarbonate (in cases of exocrine pancreatic failure, bicarbonate secretion is lost early and enzyme secretion lost later)
Cancer of pancreas: low volume, normal concentration (normal in cancer of tail)

Simple blood tests can be useful in acute pancreatitis where serum amylase, lipase, and immunoreactive trypsin will be markedly elevated. In pancreatic carcinoma serum carbohydrate antigen CA 19-9 is a more specific test, although CA125 and carcinoma embryonic antigen (CEA) may also be elevated.

Cystic fibrosis: A simple and reliable test in infants is the direct measurement of chloride levels in sweat, with values over 70 mmol/L reliably establishing the diagnosis; however, this test is much less reliable in adults. Gene testing is also very useful. The specific CFTR (cystic fibrosis transmembrane conductance regulator) gene is a useful marker of this condition.

Where 90% of pancreatic function is lost patients are usually diabetic and this can be established by measurement of fasting blood glucose or, where this gives a negative result, by formal glucose tolerance testing after a 75-g glucose load.

FLUOROSCEIN DILAURATE TEST

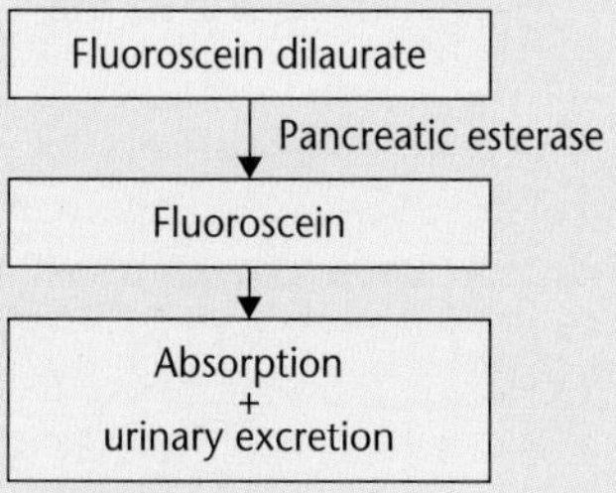

Fig. 131.6 Fluorescein dilaurate test.

COLON

Stool culture and microscopy are invaluable in diarrheal illnesses, where salmonella, *Campylobacter*, and *Shigella* may be directly cultured. Microscopy will also demonstrate the presence of ameba and cysts. Worms might be directly visible. In pseudomembranous colitis *Campylobacter difficile* enterotoxin can be demonstrated in stool even when culture is not successful (see Chapter 58).

In carcinoma of the large bowel CEA levels may be elevated, but this is most useful in serial assessment of metastatic disease or recurrence after resection.

GASTROINTESTINAL BLEEDING (see Chapter 24)

Where active bleeding continues from obscure sites not identified by endoscopic evaluation radioscanning using technetium colloid or labeled red blood cells may locate specific bleeding sources. Angiography can also be useful in identifying active bleeding and also vascular malformation between bleeding episodes.

Where Meckel's diverticulum is the site of active gastric metaplasia and ulceration simple pertechnetate scanning will locate a hot spot, usually in the lower right quadrant.

GALLBLADDER (see Chapter 76)

Most information on the gallbladder is derived from ultrasonography, but radio-scintigraphy using hepatic iminodiacetic acid scanning can be useful where there is doubt about the origin of symptoms. In biliary colic gallbladder function is temporarily lost; the isotope is taken up by the liver and excreted in the biliary system but the gallbladder is not outlined.

ASCITES (see Chapter 20, 95 and 96)

Often the origin of ascites is obvious but where there is doubt, or where spontaneous bacterial peritonitis is suspected, then aspiration is a very helpful technique. In infection there will be increased numbers of leukocytes and sometimes positive culture. In malignant disease high protein levels are seen (exudates) and cytology may demonstrate the presence of malignant cells.

Laparoscopy is a very useful technique that allows direct visualization and biopsy of the peritoneum and liver. This should be a reliable way of identifying the presence of malignant disease and cirrhosis.

LIVER

Serum biochemistry is the first line investigation in liver disease though none of the tests performed is specific to the liver. Raised serum bilirubin may indicate intra- or extrahepatic obstruction to bile flow but it may also be seen in hemolysis. Elevated alkaline phosphatase and glutamyl transferase are typically seen in diseases of the biliary epithelium such as gallstone disease and extrahepatic obstruction, but are also frequently a marker for malignant disease, especially metastatic. Serum albumin and also urea are markers of liver synthesis and may be low in cirrhosis, but renal and intestinal disease may also affect levels. Serum globulin may be markedly elevated in autoimmune liver disease, particularly IgG in autoimmune hepatitis and IgM in primary biliary cirrhosis. Serum transaminase elevation is seen in various forms of hepatitis, e.g. viral, autoimmune and alcoholic.

Autoantibodies give valuable information about the liver. In autoimmune hepatitis type I there is characteristic elevation of nuclear and smooth muscle antibodies. In autoimmune hepatitis type II these are absent but liver and kidney microsomal antibodies are present. The presence of a soluble liver antigen has been postulated in type III autoimmune hepatitis but this is contentious. In primary biliary cirrhosis almost all patients carry mitochondrial antibody and its specific subfraction M2.

Viral serology can be used as a screen in acute and chronic liver disease (see Chapters 82A-C). Most useful tests are hepatitis A IgM, anti-hepatitis C viral antibodies, and hepatitis B surface antigen. Other antibodies to Epstein-Barr virus and cytomegalovirus can also sometimes be helpful. It may be necessary to do repeated tests in acute hepatitis to pick up positive results.

For monitoring the progress of liver disease and its treatment HBV DNA viral copy counts, and hepatitis B surface antibody, hepatitis B e antigen and antibody are all useful. Similarly, hepatitis C antibody titers and hepatitis C RNA viral counts can be used to monitor progress.

Dynamic tests of liver function: Several have been proposed over the years including clearance of aminopyrine, indocyanine green, bromsulfthalein, ammonia, and caffeine. These have not been used much outside the super-specialist centers for monitoring the progress of disease. The simpler clinical measures, such as the presence of ascites and serial measurement of serum albumin and bilirubin, furnish most of the information necessary to decide on progress of liver disease and suitability of liver transplantation.

Hemochromatosis: Serum ferritin is characteristically very high and the iron-binding capacity completely saturated. Search for the HFE gene will identify most cases, but the simplest way of proving the diagnosis is by liver biopsy with staining for iron deposits, which is very reliable (see Chapter 89).

Wilson's disease may be screened using serum ceruloplasmin but again liver biopsy with copper stains is usually required to prove diagnosis (see Chapter 91).

Urine and blood porphyrins can be estimated; however, often patients with porphyria do not have overt liver disease but rather abdominal pain, neuropathy, and skin rashes.

Liver biopsy is often necessary to establish diagnosis unequivocally. This should always be preceded by liver imaging such as ultrasonography, but in parenchymal disease percutaneous unguided biopsy yields results that are as good as those from ultrasound- or computed tomography-guided biopsies. Where focal lesions are detected and are suspicious of metastatic carcinoma or hepatoma then ultrasonically or radiologically guided biopsy is useful in establishing the diagnosis, but is often avoided nowadays to obtain better results after surgery. Where liver biopsy cannot be safely performed percutaneously because of bleeding tendencies, techniques of transvenous biopsy and laparoscopic biopsy will allow safer acquisition of tissue.

Metastatic bowel carcinoma characteristically gives very raised CEA levels and primary hepatocellular carcinoma will often be associated with very elevated levels of alpha fetoprotein, but neither of these is completely reliable.

Developments in radiology have largely displaced technetium 99m colloid liver scanning but this technique is still useful where there is portal hypertension in cirrhosis (small cool liver and large hot spleen with diversion to outline the bone marrow). Dynamic liver scanning can yield semiquantitative information about portal blood flow.

Chapter 132

Motility testing

George Triadafilopoulos

KEY POINTS

- Esophageal motility studies are useful in the diagnosis of achalasia, diffuse esophageal spasm, and motor abnormalities associated with systemic diseases
- Motility studies are important in assessment prior to anti-reflux surgery
- Gastroduodenal motility studies differentiate between neuropathy or myopathy and partial small bowel obstruction, and can be a useful adjunctive investigation for non-specific postprandial symptoms
- Sphincter of Oddi motility testing carries a 5–10% risk of pancreatitis
- Anorectal manometry studies are used in the evaluation of patients with constipation or fecal incontinence, and prior to stoma reversal

ESOPHAGEAL MOTILITY STUDY

Introduction

The performance of an esophageal motility study accurately defines esophageal motor activity and is the procedure of choice for the diagnosis of esophageal motility disorders. It can be complemented by endoscopy, barium swallow radiography, video-fluorography and esophageal scintigraphy.

Indications/contraindications

An esophageal motility study should be performed when an esophageal motor disorder (i.e., achalasia or diffuse esophageal spasm) is suspected (see example in Fig. 132.1). It may be indicated for detecting esophageal motor abnormalities associated with systemic diseases (e.g., connective tissue diseases) if their detection would contribute to establishing a multisystem diagnosis or to other aspects of management. It is also valuable in patients with dysphagia or chest pain when other studies have failed to reach a diagnosis. An esophageal motility study is useful to define the degree of esophageal motor function in gastroesophageal reflux disease (GERD) prior to anti-reflux surgery, particularly if uncertainty remains regarding the correct diagnosis. Esophageal motility is performed prior to placement of an intraluminal pH-monitoring probe when positioning is dependent on the relationship to functional landmarks, such as the lower esophageal sphincter (LES).[1] Esophageal motility is not indicated for making or confirming a suspected diagnosis of GERD, and should not be routinely used as the initial test for chest pain or other esophageal symptoms because of the low specificity of the findings and the low likelihood of detecting a clinically significant motility disorder.[2]

Description of technique

Esophageal motility is usually performed using a perfused motility catheter 3–4 mm in diameter containing eight individual lumens that terminate in side-hole orifices positioned at 5-cm intervals along its length. Each lumen is connected to an external pressure transducer and perfused with distilled water at 0.5 mL/min by a low-compliance pneumo-hydraulic perfusion pump. Occlusion of the side-holes by esophageal contractility increases the pressure within the lumen of the catheter; the pressure is sensed by the transducer and is converted to an electrical signal that is digitally transformed and displayed on a computer screen using commercial software. Simultaneous recording of pressure at several sites allows assessment of coordination of the esophageal motor activity. As the catheter traverses the upper or lower esophageal sphincters measurement of the sphincter pressure profile is performed using the slow pull-through technique along the length of the sphincter.

The procedure is performed without sedation under local pharyngeal anesthesia and lasts approximately 20 min. Normal values are shown in Table 132.1 and a typical tracing is shown in Fig. 132.1A. The motility catheter is passed through the nose or the mouth into the stomach and then slowly withdrawn at 1-cm intervals while recording of the intragastric, intrasphincteric, and intraesophageal pressure profiles is performed. During the procedure, the patient remains supine and receives 5 cm^3 water boluses to stimulate esophageal body peristalsis and sphincter relaxation.

Lower esophageal sphincters: By slowly withdrawing the catheter or using the sleeve, the basal lower esophageal sphincter (LES) pressure is measured at end-expiration and referenced to the baseline intragastric pressure. The LES pressure profile has typically two components, an intra-abdominal component and an intrathoracic one. Transition from one to the other occurs as the catheter crosses the diaphragmatic hiatus and is noted by the reversal of the phasic activity induced by respiration (respiratory inversion point). LES relaxation is evaluated during swallows. Upon swallowing, the LES relaxes and remains relaxed for 5–10 s until the esophageal body peristaltic wave reaches the sphincter.

Esophageal body peristaltic function is measured simultaneously by the side-hole sensors, which span the entire length of the esophagus, and is assessed using at least 10 5-cm^3 water swallows. Such swallows evoke a propagating contraction sequence that sweeps the esophageal body uninterruptedly. The contraction wave moves fastest in the pharynx and proximal esophagus and slows distally. Esophageal contractions are typically single-peaked. Multiphasic, repetitive, simultaneous, spontaneous, or retrograde contractions are abnormal. Diffuse

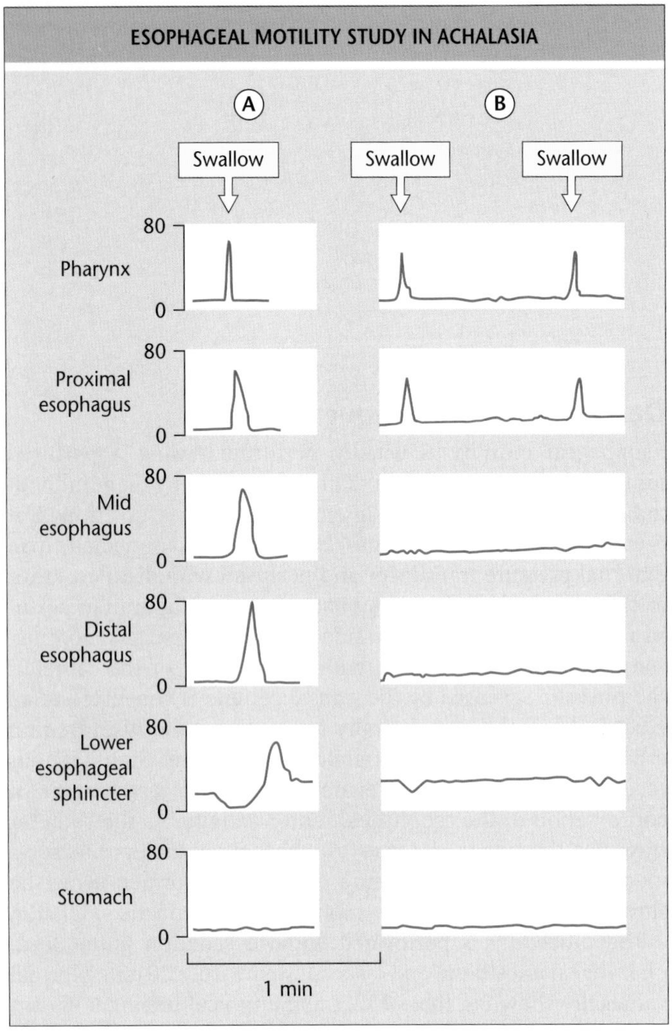

Fig. 132.1 Esophageal motility study in achalasia. Esophageal motor response to swallowing in a normal subject **(A)** and a patient with achalasia **(B)**.

TABLE 132.1 NORMAL VALUES FOR ESOPHAGEAL MOTILITY STUDY[a]

STOMACH

- Baseline intragastric pressure: 0–15 mmHg (reference)

LOWER ESOPHAGEAL SPHINCTER (LES)

- Location: variable
- Intra-abdominal length: >1 cm
- Intrathoracic length: 1–3 cm
- Basal resting LES pressure: 10–30 mmHg
- LES relaxation: >90%, 5–10 s in duration
- Residual pressure: 3–5 mmHg

ESOPHAGEAL BODY

- Baseline intraesophageal pressure: 1–3 mmHg lower than baseline intragastric pressure
- Mean amplitude of contractions: 50–100 mmHg
- Mean duration of contractions: 3–5 s
- Mean speed of peristalsis: 2–5 cm/s
- Simultaneous contractions: none
- Repetitive contractions: none
- Multiphasic contractions: none
- Spontaneous contractions: none
- Retrograde contractions: none
- Segmental lack of peristalsis: none

UPPER ESOPHAGEAL SPHINCTER (UES)

- Location: variable
- UES length: 1 cm
- Basal resting UES pressure: 60–100 mmHg
- Relaxation: >90%, 5 s in duration
- Residual pressure: 3–5 mmHg

[a] Values established at Stanford Motility Center, Stanford, California, USA using the low-compliance pneumo-hydraulic perfusion pump (Arndorfer) and the slow pull-through technique.

or segmental lack of peristalsis in response to water swallows is also abnormal (failed peristalsis).

Pharynx and upper esophageal sphincter (UES): At this level, the perfusion recording system becomes less accurate but the occurrence and timing of contractions and the degree of pharyngeal-upper esophageal coordination can be adequately assessed. Solid-state intraluminal transducers are preferable at this level. Because of the short (~1 cm) UES length, a sleeve sensor should be used to record accurately the basal pressure and the onset and completeness of the UES relaxation. Upon swallowing, the UES relaxes abruptly and remains relaxed until the pharyngeal peristaltic wave reaches the sphincter.

Costs and benefits

The procedure is safe and inexpensive but requires detailed expert interpretation that is time consuming.

GASTRODUODENAL MOTILITY STUDY

Introduction and scientific basis

The performance of a gastroduodenal motility study accurately defines antral and small intestinal motor activity and coordination, thus distinguishing neuropathy or myopathy from partial small bowel obstruction.[3] It may be complemented by endoscopy, small bowel follow-through radiography, and gastric and intestinal scintigraphy.

Indications/contraindications

Gastroduodenal motility is indicated when gastric and small intestinal neuropathy or myopathy are suspected, and when the possibility of partial small bowel obstruction is entertained. It is useful in the evaluation of many nonspecific symptoms, such as postprandial bloating, nausea and vomiting, diarrhea, and postprandial, crampy, periumbilical or diffuse abdominal pain, associated with weight loss and malabsorption.[4] The procedure is also important in identifying concomitant small bowel involvement in cases of severe constipation due to colonic inertia and in the differentiation of functional from organic disorders. Other indications include recurrent or refractory small intestinal bacterial overgrowth syndrome, gastroparesis, and assessment of postoperative small intestinal motility or effectiveness of prokinetic therapy. There are no contraindications for the procedure.[5]

Description of technique

A gastroduodenal motility study is usually performed using a perfused motility catheter 3–4 mm in diameter containing eight individual lumens that terminate in side-hole orifices, the distal four of which are positioned at 10-cm intervals along its distal length and the proximal four are positioned at 1-cm intervals. Each lumen is connected to an external pressure transducer and perfused with distilled water at 0.5 mL/min by a low-compliance pneumo-hydraulic perfusion pump. Occlusion of the side-holes by antral, pyloric, or duodenal contractility increases the pressure within the lumen of the catheter, the pressure is sensed by the transducer and is converted to an electrical signal that is digitally transformed and displayed on a computer screen using commercial software. Simultaneous recording of pressure at several sites allows assessment of coordination of the motor activity along the distal stomach and proximal intestine.

The procedure is performed in two stages. During the first stage, an endoscopy is performed under intravenous sedation and local pharyngeal anesthesia. Under a combined endoscopic/fluoroscopic visualization, a stiff 500-cm guidewire is placed beyond the ligament of Treitz and the scope is removed. A long motility catheter is then threaded over the wire and positioned along the C-loop of the duodenum with its distal tip beyond the ligament of Treitz. The proximal end of the motility catheter is then connected to the recording system. During the second stage of the procedure, a continuous recording of the intragastric (antral and pyloric) and intraduodenal pressure profiles is performed while the patient remains in the supine position for 5 h. During the first 3 h of recording, the patient remains fasting, then a standard meal is administered and a fed-state recording is performed for an additional 2 h. The peristaltic function of the distal stomach and proximal duodenum is measured simultaneously by the side-hole sensors, which span the entire length of the catheter. Many centers use a 24-h ambulatory study using pressure transducers instead of hydraulic perfusion catheters; others use provocation with prokinetic agents, such as erythromycin or octreotide in addition to a baseline recording.

The main feature of a gastroduodenal motility study is the identification of the migratory motor complex (MMC) consisting of three phases (I–III) that originates in the antrum and spreads through the small intestine in a propagating fashion during fasting (Fig. 132.2). Phase I, usually lasting 90 min, is a period of quiescence. Phase II, lasting 30–60 min, is characterized by intermittent phasic contractions of variable amplitude and frequency. Phase III, lasting 5–15 min, is the 'housekeeper' activity that clears the small intestine from food and cellular debris and consists of high-frequency contractions. In contrast to this characteristic appearance of the MMC during fasting, the fed state is associated with irregular contractions of variable frequency and amplitude simulating phase II and lasting for at least 90 min after the meal (Fig. 132.3). Poorly coordinated activity of normal amplitude suggests a small intestinal

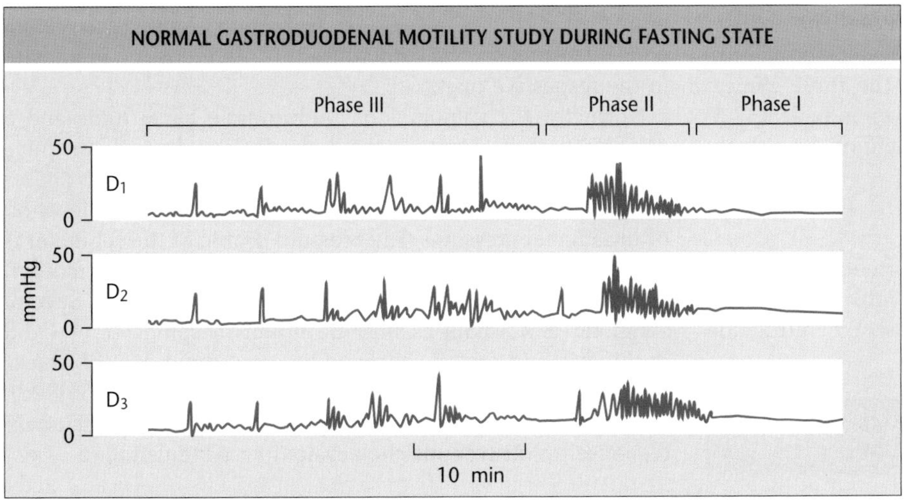

Fig. 132.2 Normal gastroduodenal motility study during the fasting state. D_1–D_3, duodenal recording sites 10 cm apart.

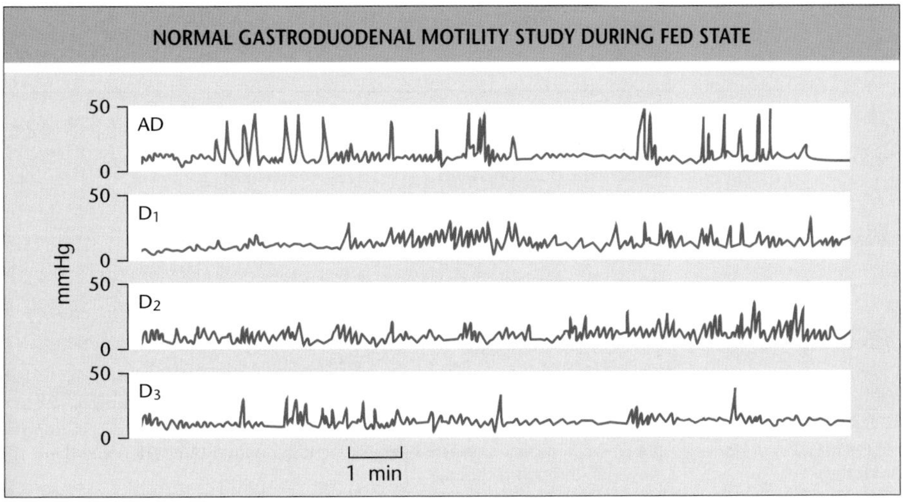

Fig. 132.3 Normal gastroduodenal motility study during the fed state. AD, antroduodenal junction recording site; D_1–D_3, duodenal recording sites 10 cm apart.

neuropathy. In contrast, no- or low-pressure activity and little (if any) contractile response postprandially are seen in myopathy. Patterns that need to be assessed on gastroduodenal motility study are shown in Table 132.2.

Costs and benefits

The procedure is safe. It requires a hospital stay of at least 5 h and detailed interpretation that is time consuming and expensive. The procedure is limited by occasional technical failures with placement of catheter and by false-positive patterns that can be found in normal controls.

SPHINCTER OF ODDI MOTILITY

Introduction and scientific basis

The performance of a sphincter of Oddi motility study accurately defines myopathic or neuropathic dysfunction of the sphincter of Oddi. It is complemented by endoscopic visualization of the ampulla of Vater, radiological visualization of the biliary and pancreatic ducts, provocative ultrasound with fatty meal stimulation, and functional biliary scintigraphy.

Indications/contraindications

A sphincter of Oddi motility study is indicated when a nonmechanical, functional process involving the sphincter of Oddi is suspected. Such sphincter dyskinesia may present clinically with episodes of postprandial right upper quadrant or upper abdominal pain without demonstrable hepatobiliary disease, with or without liver function and pancreatic test abnormalities, or with recurrent idiopathic pancreatitis.[6,7] The three clinical types of sphincter of Oddi dyskinesia are shown in Table 132.3. Such classification is important because it defines the risk-to-benefit ratio of therapeutic sphincterotomy.

Description of technique

A sphincter of Oddi motility study is performed after placement of a special water-perfused catheter into the bile and pancreatic ducts during a diagnostic endoscopic retrograde cholangiopancreatography (ERCP). The catheter records pressures in the bile duct, the pancreatic duct, the sphincter of Oddi, and the duodenum. Normal values are shown in Table 132.4. During the study, it is important to maintain the patient in the semi-prone position, sedated without using narcotics, and to obtain at least two readings for each sphincter evaluation using the slow-perfusion pneumo-hydraulic system connected to a special catheter that is placed over a guidewire in the respective duct.

Normally, the sphincter of Oddi muscle has a tonic and a phasic action that controls the flow of bile and pancreatic juice into the duodenum, coordinates this flow with the various phases of digestion, and protects against duodenal reflux and elevation of intraductal pressures. The pressure profile of the sphincter is influenced by gastrointestinal peptides (cholecystokinin, motilin) as well as by local autonomic nervous system reflexes. Several sphincter abnormalities may be noted in sphincter of Oddi dyskinesia and include tachyoddia, or a rapid rate of phasic contractility, elevated basal pressure of the sphincter of Oddi, and paradoxical elevation of sphincter of Oddi pressure in response to intravenous cholecystokinin administration.

TABLE 132.2 NORMAL FEATURES TO BE ASSESSED IN GASTRODUODENAL MOTILITY STUDY[a]

STOMACH
- Antral contractions at baseline that increase postprandially

SMALL INTESTINE

Fasting
- Propagating MMC with sequencial phases I–III
- Absence of simultaneous or retrograde contractions
- Lack of baseline (tonic) elevation (>30 mmHg and >3 min duration)
- Absence of bursts of nonpropagating contractile activity (>20 mmHg and >10/min)
- Lack of isolated and sustained (>30 min) pressure activity

Fed state
- Absence of early (<90 min) appearance of phase III
- Lack of appearance of fed state (phase II-like) contractions
- Absence of low-amplitude contractions
- Lack of nonpropagating, multiphasic contractions (minute contractions)

[a] Values established at Stanford Motility Center, Stanford, California, USA using the low-compliance pneumo-hydraulic perfusion pump (Arndorfer).

TABLE 132.3 CLINICAL TYPES OF SPHINCTER OF ODDI DYSKINESIA[a]

TYPE I: BILIARY OR PANCREATIC PAIN
- Abnormal liver function tests (total bilirubin, alkaline phosphatase, aminotransferases 1.5–2 x N)
- Abnormal pancreatic tests (amylase, lipase 1.5–2 x N)
- Dilated bile duct (>12 mm) or pancreatic duct (head >6 mm, body >5 mm)
- Delayed drainage of bile duct (>12 min) or pancreatic duct (>9 min)

TYPE II: BILIARY OR PANCREATIC PAIN
- One or two of above criteria

TYPE III: BILIARY OR PANCREATIC PAIN WITHOUT ANY LABORATORY OR RADIOLOGICAL ABNORMALITIES

[a] According to Hogan and Geenen, modified by Sherman in: Sherman S. What is the role of ERCP in the setting of abdominal pain of pancreatic or biliary origin (suspected sphincter of Oddi dysfunction)? Gastrointest Endosc 2002; 56:S258–266.

TABLE 132.4 NORMAL VALUES FOR SPHINCTER OF ODDI MOTILITY STUDY[a]

Intraduodenal pressure:	0–5 mmHg
Bile duct pressure:	3–10 mmHg
Pancreatic duct pressure:	8–15 mmHg
Basal sphincter of Oddi pressure:	15–25 mmHg
Amplitude of phasic contractions:	120–200 mmHg
Frequency of phasic contractions:	5–7 per min
Duration of phasic contractions:	3–5 s
Retrograde waves:	<15%
CCK administration:	Reduction in basal sphincter of Oddi pressure

[a] Values established at Stanford Motility Center, Stanford, California, USA using the low-compliance pneumo-hydraulic perfusion pump (Arndorfer) and the slow pull-through technique.

Complications

Even if performed in expert centers, sphincter of Oddi motility has a 5–10% risk for pancreatitis. This risk may be reduced but not eliminated by not cannulating the pancreatic duct and by using an aspirating catheter.

Costs and benefits

The procedure is invasive, costly, and requires significant endoscopic expertise, as well as careful and time-consuming analysis of recordings. Clinical correlation is imperative prior to therapeutic decision making.

ANORECTAL MOTILITY STUDY

Introduction and scientific basis

An anorectal motility study is useful in the evaluation of a patient with constipation or fecal incontinence. It is also used to evaluate patients who are about to have a stoma closure to ensure that continence will be preserved. The test determines the anal sphincter pressure profile, which sphincter is responsible for the problem, whether rectal sensation is intact, and the anorectal coordination.[8] The procedure may be complemented by anoscopy, sigmoidoscopy, barium enema, anal ultrasonography, a colonic transit time study, and defecography.

Indications/contraindications

In patients with chronic constipation or pelvic dyssynergia, anorectal motility studies may be used to measure internal anal sphincter (IAS) relaxation in response to rectal distention, as well as rectal and sphincter pressure changes during simulated defecation.[9] Lack of IAS relaxation to rectal balloon distention, particularly in children, is suggestive of Hirschsprung's disease. When evaluating fecal incontinence, anal canal pressures do not correlate well with continence due to the wide range of normal pressures. Maximum squeeze pressure rather than resting pressure has better correlation with clinical symptoms. Additionally, other factors may influence fecal incontinence in the absence of decreased anal canal pressures. Nevertheless, anorectal motility is useful in the biofeedback training of patients with fecal incontinence since normalization or reduction of the threshold correlates with therapeutic success, and poor or absent sensation makes a good response unlikely.[10] Assessment of the maximum tolerable balloon volume evaluates for the presence of visceral hypersensitivity, poor rectal compliance, or rectal irritability.[11]

Description of technique

An anorectal motility study is usually performed using a perfused motility catheter 3–4 mm in diameter containing four individual lumens that terminate in side-hole orifices positioned at 1-cm intervals along its distal length. At the end of the catheter, an inflatable balloon is used to elicit responses of rectal sensation and anorectal coordination. Within the catheter, each lumen is connected to an external pressure transducer and perfused with distilled water at 0.5 mL/min by a low-compliance pneumo-hydraulic perfusion pump. Occlusion of the side-holes by sphincteric contractility or tone increases the pressure within the lumens of the catheter, the pressure is sensed by the transducer and is converted to an electrical signal that is digitally transformed and displayed on a computer screen using commercial software. Simultaneous recording of pressure at several sites allows assessment of coordination of the anorectal motor activity. As the catheter traverses the anal sphincter, measurement of the sphincter pressure profile is performed using the slow pull-through technique along the length of the sphincter. The procedure is performed with the unsedated patient in the left lateral position, hips flexed 90 degrees, and lasts approximately 15 min. Normal values are shown in Table 132.5 and a typical tracing is shown in Fig. 132.4. The motility catheter is passed through the anus into the rectum and then slowly with-

TABLE 132.5 NORMAL VALUES FOR ANORECTAL MOTILITY STUDY[a]

RECTUM
- Baseline intrarectal pressure: 0–15 mmHg (reference)

INTERNAL ANAL SPHINCTER (IAS)
- Location: variable
- Length: 2–3 cm
- Basal resting IAS pressure: 20–50 mmHg
- IAS relaxation: >90%, 5–10 s in duration
- Residual pressure: 3–5 mmHg

EXTERNAL ANAL SPHINCTER (EAS)
- Location: variable
- Length: 2–3 cm
- Squeeze (EAS) pressure: 100–200 mmHg

BALLOON DISTENTION
- Threshold to balloon sensation: 15 cm^3
- Anorectal inhibitory reflex: present
- Balloon expulsion: 50 cm^3

[a] Values established at Stanford Motility Center, Stanford, California, USA using the low-compliance pneumo-hydraulic perfusion pump (Arndorfer) and the slow pull-through technique.

NORMAL ANORECTAL MOTILITY STUDY

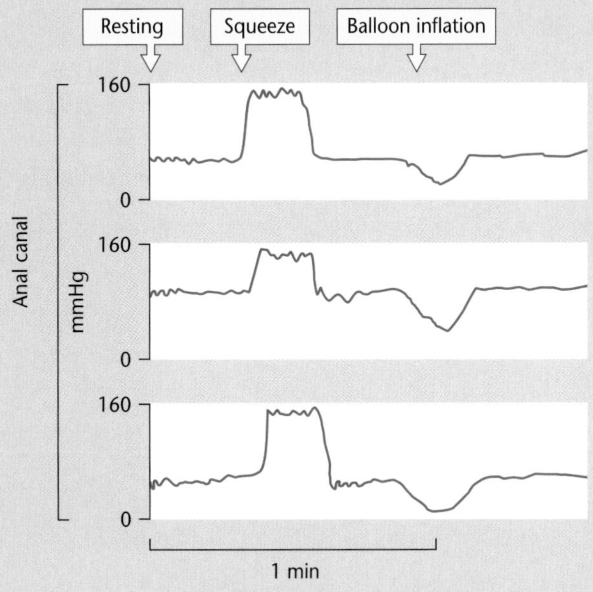

Fig. 132.4 Normal anorectal motility study. Recording of anal canal pressure at rest, upon voluntary squeeze, and balloon inflation in the rectum.

drawn at 0.5- to 1-cm intervals while recording the intrarectal and intrasphincteric pressure profiles. During the procedure, the patient is asked to squeeze and induce external anal sphincter (EAS) contraction and to relax in order to assess for internal anal sphincter (IAS) tone. By slowly withdrawing the catheter, both the external and internal sphincter pressures are measured and referenced to the baseline intrarectal pressure. Balloon inflation normally elicits a sensory perception and evokes the anorectal inhibitory reflex, that is, the relaxation of the internal anal sphincter upon balloon distention. Balloon expulsion is measured by asking the patient to expel the water-filled balloon.

Costs and benefits

The procedure is safe and inexpensive but requires expert interpretation.

REFERENCES

1. American Gastroenterological Association. Medical position statement: Guidelines on use of esophageal pH recording. Clinical esophageal pH recording: A technical review for practice guideline development. Gastroenterology 1996; 110:1981–1996.
2. American Gastroenterological Association. Medical position statement on the clinical use of esophageal manometry. AGA technical review on the clinical use of esophageal manometry. Gastroenterology 1994; 107:1865–1884.
3. Parkman HP, Harris AD, Krevsky B et al. Gastroduodenal motility and dysmotility: An update on techniques available for evaluation. Am J Gastroenterol 1995; 90:869–892.
4. American Gastroenterological Association. Medical position statement: Nausea and vomiting. AGA technical review on nausea and vomiting. Gastroenterology 2001; 120:263–286.
5. Soffer E, Thongsawat S. Clinical value of duodeno-jejunal manometry. Dig Dis Sci 1996; 41:859–863.
6. Petersen BT. An evidence-based review of sphincter of Oddi dysfunction: part I, presentations with "objective" biliary findings (types I and II). Gastrointest Endosc 2004; 59:525–534.
7. Petersen BT. Sphincter of Oddi dysfunction, part 2: Evidence-based review of the presentations, with "objective" pancreatic findings (types I and II) and of presumptive type III. Gastrointest Endosc 2004; 59:670–687.
8. American Gastroenterological Association. Medical position statement on anorectal testing techniques. AGA technical review on anorectal testing techniques. Gastroenterology 1999; 116:732–760.
9. Rao SSC, Patel RS. How useful are manometric tests of anorectal function in the management of defecation disorders? Am J Gastroenterol 1997; 92:469–475.
10. Rao SSC. Technical aspects of biofeedback therapy for defecation disorders. The Gastroenterologist 1998; 6:96–103.
11. Rao SSC, Azpiroz F, Diamant N et al. Minimum standards for anorectal manometry. Neurogastroenterol Motil 2002; 14:553–560.

Chapter 133

Measurement of portal pressure

Juan Carlos García-Pagán, Juan Turnes, and Jaime Bosch

KEY POINTS

- Portal pressure should be expressed as the pressure gradient between the portal vein and the inferior vena cava, which represents the perfusion pressure within the portal-hepatic circulation (portal pressure gradient or PPG)
- Direct measurements of portal pressure are invasive investigations based on the surgical, percutaneous transhepatic, or transvenous (transjugular) catheterization of the portal vein
- Hepatic vein catheterization, with measurements of the wedged and free hepatic venous pressures (WHVP and FHVP, respectively) and determination of the hepatic venous pressure gradient or HVPG (WHVP minus FHVP), is an indirect, safe, and reproducible technique and is therefore the preferred method to estimate portal pressure
- WHVP is measured by occluding the hepatic vein, either by inflating a balloon or by advancing the catheter until it becomes 'wedged' into a small branch of a hepatic vein. The balloon occlusion technique is preferred since it reflects the pressure of a greater hepatic area than the 'manual occlusion' technique
- WHVP is a measurement of the hepatic sinusoidal pressure and not of portal pressure itself. However, many studies have shown that WHVP is equal to portal pressure in alcoholic and hepatitis C-related cirrhosis
- A limitation of HVPG is that it does not reflect the PPG in diseases where the increased resistance is located at presinusoidal sites
- The main applications of measurements of HVPG are:
  classification of portal hypertension
  evaluation of portal hypertension and assessment of the response to pharmacological therapy
  prognostic evaluation during variceal bleeding
  preoperative evaluation of resection risk in patients with small hepatocellular carcinoma
  evaluation of progression of chronic liver disease, especially in severe chronic hepatitis C and in alcoholic hepatitis

INTRODUCTION AND SCIENTIFIC BASIS

Measurement of portal pressure is the single most important hemodynamic measurement in portal hypertension. In 1951, Myers and Taylor developed the measurement of wedge hepatic venous pressure (WHVP), which assesses hepatic sinusoidal pressure and is an index of portal venous pressure.[1] The scientific basis is the same as the measurement of the wedged pulmonary arterial pressure, an index of left atrial pressure. When blood flow in a hepatic vein is stopped by a 'wedged' catheter, the static column of blood transmits the pressure from the preceding communicated vascular territory, in this case, the hepatic sinusoids. Thus, WHVP is a measurement of the hepatic sinusoidal pressure and not of portal pressure itself. However, many studies have demonstrated that WHVP is equal to portal pressure in alcoholic liver disease ('sinusoidal' portal hypertension). It is important to remark that WHVP adequately reflects portal pressure in hepatitis C- and hepatitis B-related cirrhosis. These entities are, by far, the most frequent etiologies of chronic liver disease in developed countries.

In the following years, the technique was improved introducing new tools, such as the balloon catheter,[2] that enhanced the reliability and accuracy of the measurements. It was soon evident that hepatic vein catheterization constituted a safe and relatively simple technique to perform accurate measurements of portal pressure in patients with liver disease.[3–5] However, it took five decades of extensive experience with the technique before hepatic vein pressure measurements were recognized as a useful tool in the clinical management of patients with cirrhosis and portal hypertension.

Portal pressure should be expressed in terms of the pressure gradient with the inferior vena cava (the portal pressure gradient or PPG), which represents the perfusion pressure within the portal-hepatic circulation. The normal PPG value is up to 5 mmHg. Expressing portal pressure as the PPG has the advantage of not being modified by changes in intra-abdominal pressure. Increased intra-abdominal pressure will increase both the portal pressure and the inferior vena cava (IVC) pressure, but will not significantly modify the PPG (except in the case of marked changes in intra-abdominal pressure, which are associated with changes in splanchnic and systemic hemodynamics).

DESCRIPTION OF TECHNIQUE

Although, as mentioned above, WHVP is the most commonly utilized method to assess portal pressure, in this section we also describe other methods to assess portal pressure; these can be divided into direct and indirect techniques.

Direct measurement of portal pressure

Direct measurements of portal pressure are invasive investigations based on the surgical, percutaneous transhepatic, or transvenous (transjugular) catheterization of the portal vein. In these techniques, except for the transjugular approach, the measurement of IVC pressure requires the additional, simultaneous puncture of a hepatic vein in order to determine the PPG. Because of this inconvenience and of the risk of intraperitoneal bleeding, direct measurements of portal pressure are rarely used. When required, as in presinusoidal portal hypertension, the percutaneous transhepatic approach or the transjugular catheterization of the portal vein are the preferred techniques. The safety of the percutaneous transhepatic or transjugular catheterization of the portal vein are increased by performing the procedures under ultrasonographic guidance. The risk of intraperitoneal bleeding is greater in the percutaneous procedure, which precludes its use in patients with impaired coagulation. This can be partly overcome by using a thin needle, which allows the measurement of portal pressure, but not to the performance of portal venography.

Indirect measurement of portal pressure

As mentioned previously, the indirect and safe approach of hepatic vein catheterization, with measurements of the wedged and free hepatic venous pressure (WHVP and FHVP, respectively), is the preferred technique to estimate portal pressure.[2] Under local anesthesia, a venous introducer is placed in the right jugular or femoral vein using the Seldinger technique. Under fluoroscopic control, a 5F or 7F balloon-tipped catheter (Fig. 133.1) is advanced into a hepatic vein to measure WHVP and FHVP. The FHVP is measured by maintaining the tip of the catheter 'free' in the hepatic vein. FHVP is close to the IVC pressure (the difference between both should be less than 2 mmHg). WHVP is measured by occluding the hepatic vein, either by inflating a balloon at the tip of the catheter (Fig. 133.2), or by advancing the catheter until it becomes 'wedged' into a small branch of a hepatic vein. The 'balloon occlusion' technique is preferred due to the fact that it reflects the pressure of a greater hepatic area than the 'manual occlusion' technique. With the balloon inflated, a slow injection of 5 mL of contrast dye should show the typical 'wedged' pattern, without reflux of contrast or wash-out through communications with other hepatic veins (Fig. 133.3). The catheter should be carefully rinsed with 5% dextrose before measuring pressures. At hepatic vein catheterization, the PPG is expressed as the hepatic venous pressure gradient (HVPG; the gradient between WHVP and FHVP). All measurements are performed at least in duplicate and permanent tracings are recorded on a multichannel recorder (Fig. 133.4).

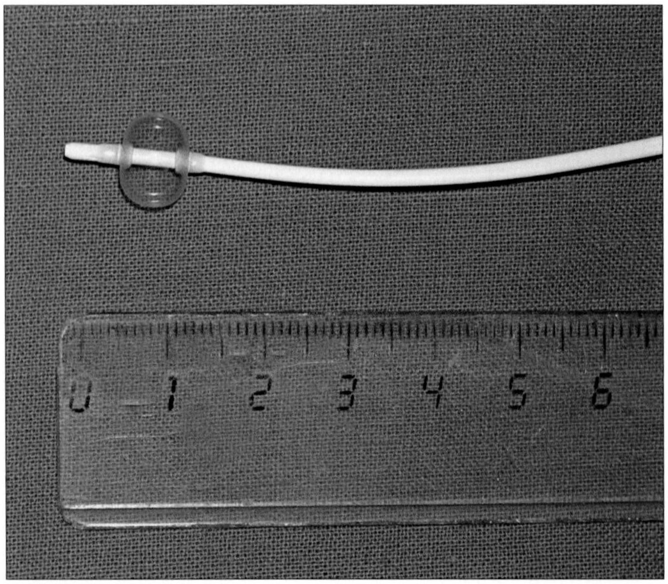

Fig. 133.1 Balloon-tipped catheter. The balloon-tipped catheter has an inflatable balloon placed 1 cm proximal to the distal end hole to ensure a good occlusion of the hepatic vein without obstructing the end hole.

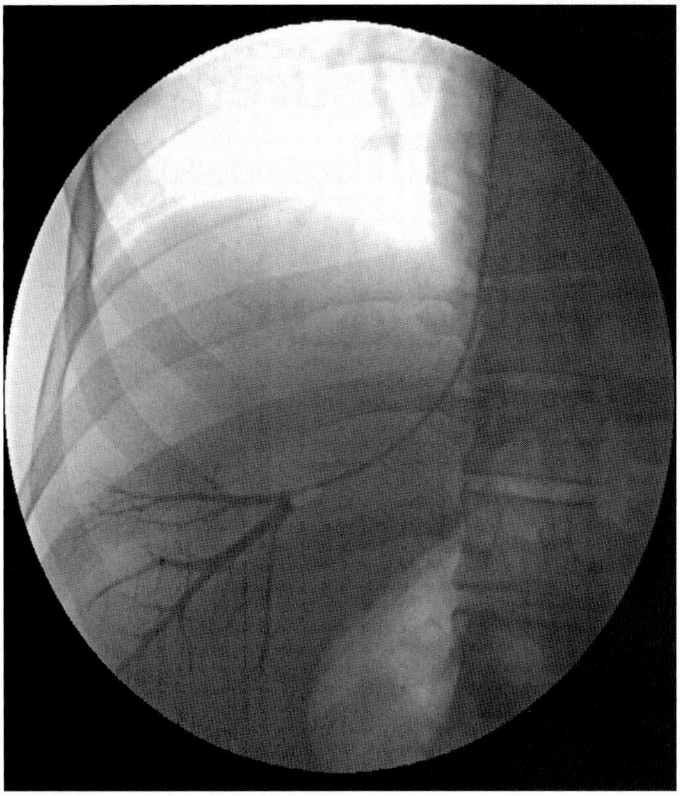

Fig. 133.2 Occlusion balloon catheter. Occlusion balloon catheter located in the main right hepatic vein. Wedged hepatic vein pressure (WHVP) is measured after occluding the hepatic vein by inflating a balloon at the tip of the catheter. When the balloon stops blood flow, the static column of blood transmits the pressure existing in the preceding communicated vascular territory (the hepatic sinusoids). Thus, WHVP is a measurement of the hepatic sinusoidal pressure and not of portal pressure itself. Free hepatic vein pressure (FHVP) is measured after releasing the balloon, and should be very similar to the inferior vena cava pressure.

HVPG is the parameter most commonly used to report portal pressure in the medical literature. In the older literature, HVPG was frequently referred to as 'corrected' WHVP or 'corrected' sinusoidal pressure. Although it is easy and simple to perform, accurate measurements require specific training, since the procedure differs from those used at heart catheterization laboratories and intensive care units. The following are a few useful tips to ensure adequate measurements:

1. An appropriate scale able to detect small changes (i.e., from –5 to 40 mmHg) must be used. Scales used for arterial pressure measurements are not adequate. The scale should be set at 1 mmHg = 1 mm of paper.
2. Venous pressures should be allowed to stabilize over a period of at least 1 min for WHVP and 15 seconds for FHVP (some patients may require longer). A slow paper speed (<5 mm/s) should be used in the recorder.
3. Digital readings on a monitor screen are usually not reliable. Paper recordings should be used, allowing for the independent review of pressure tracings.
4. The transducer should be calibrated against known external pressures before starting measurements (e.g., 13.6 cm H_2O should read 10 mmHg, 27.2 cm H_2O should read 20 mmHg, and 40.8 cm H_2O should read 30 mmHg). Transducers that do not calibrate exactly should be discarded.

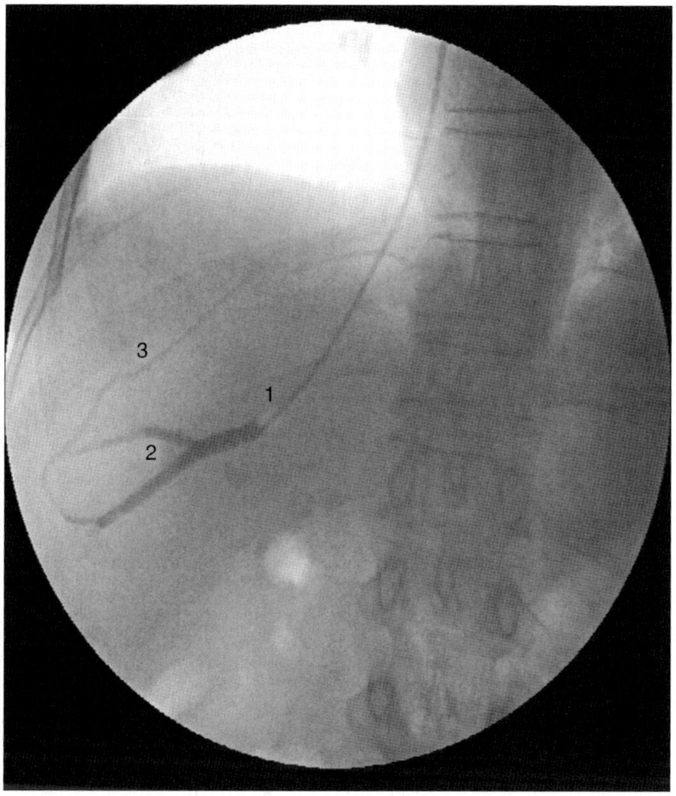

Fig. 133.3. After occluding the suprahepatic blood flow with the balloon catheter (1) the distal branches of the suprahepatic vein are shown (2), but a communicating vein between the distal and proximal suprahepatic vein can also be observed (3). In this case, the WHVP is underestimated and another suprahepatic vein should be catheterized in order to obtain accurate measurements.

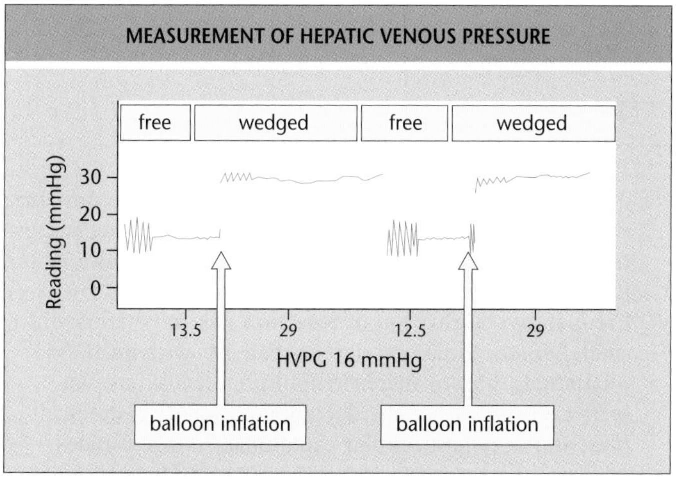

Fig. 133.4 Measurement of hepatic venous pressure. Measurements are recorded (on paper or computer) to assess accurately the values of hepatic venous pressure before (FHVP) and after balloon inflation (WHVP).

5. The transducer should be placed at the level of the right atrium (mid-axillary line) and the 'zero' pressure (the atmospheric pressure with the transducer open to air) should correspond with the 'zero' line in the pressure tracing.
6. FHVP should be measured with the catheter tip less than 5 cm in the hepatic vein. FHVP should not be more than 2 mmHg different from the IVC pressure, measured at the level of the hepatic veins. If the difference is greater, a hepatic outflow problem should be investigated.
7. Any event that may cause an artifact, such as coughing or moving, should be noted.

HVPG does not reflect the PPG in diseases where the increased resistance is located at presinusoidal sites, such as portal vein thrombosis or liver diseases affecting predominantly the portal tracts, such as schistosomiasis, initial stages of primary biliary cirrhosis, or idiopathic portal hypertension. In these cases, a direct measurement of portal pressure is indicated.

In addition to pressure measurements, hepatic vein catheterization allows for the performance of a wedged hepatic retrograde portography using CO_2 as a contrast agent (Fig. 133.5). This will demonstrate the portal vein in most instances. In fact, inability to demonstrate the portal vein on CO_2 retrograde portography strongly suggests the presence of presinusoidal portal hypertension.[6]

Hepatic vein catheterization also allows for the performance of a transjugular liver biopsy, which adds very little time, discomfort, and risk to the procedure and can be done on a day-hospital basis. Furthermore, at hepatic vein catheterization it is also possible to measure the hepatic blood flow using indocyanine green (ICG) as the indicator, as well as the intrinsic clearance of ICG, a quantitative liver function test that assesses the overall hepatic metabolic activity.

INDICATIONS

The main applications of measurements of HVPG are:

1. Classification of portal hypertension. Findings at hepatic vein catheterization may help to identify the cause of portal hypertension (Table 133.1) except in diseases causing an hepatic outflow block, classified as 'postsinusoidal' or 'posthepatic' portal hypertension, in which both WHVP and FHVP are increased with normal HVPG.
2. Evaluation of portal hypertension and assessment of the response to pharmacological therapy. The HVPG needs to

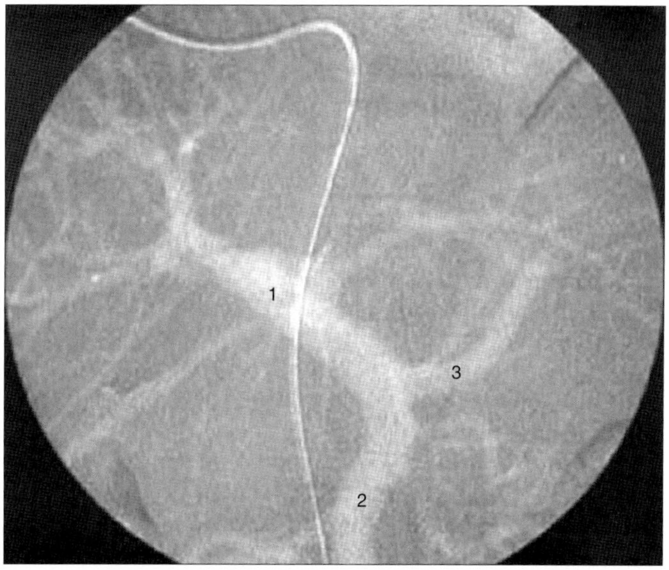

Fig. 133.5 Wedged retrograde portography. Wedged retrograde portography using CO_2 as a contrast agent showing a patent portal (1), mesenteric (2), and splenic (3) vein in a patient with HCV-related cirrhosis.

TABLE 133.1 PORTAL HYPERTENSION: CLASSIFICATION OF MAIN DISEASES ACCORDING TO HVPG MEASUREMENTS

PRESINUSOIDAL	**Prehepatic:** • Thrombosis of the porto-splenic axis • Congenital stenosis of the portal vein • Arteriovenous fistulae (splenic, aortomesenteric, aortoportal, and hepatic artery-portal vein)	• PP increased • WHVP normal • FHVP normal
	Intrahepatic: • Partial nodular transformation • Nodular regenerative hyperplasia • Congenital hepatic fibrosis • Peliosis hepatis • Polycystic liver disease • Idiopathic portal hypertension • Hypervitaminosis A • Arsenic, copper sulfate, and vinyl chloride monomer poisoning • Sarcoidosis • Tuberculosis • Primary biliary cirrhosis • Schistosomiasis • Amyloidosis • Acute fatty liver of pregnancy	• PP increased • WHVP normal • FHVP normal
SINUSOIDAL	• Alcoholic liver cirrhosis • Liver cirrhosis from viral etiology	• PP and WHVP increased • FHVP normal
POSTSINUSOIDAL	**Intrahepatic** • Budd-Chiari syndrome • Veno-occlusive disease[a]	• PP, WHVP and FHVP increased • IVC pressure normal
	Posthepatic • Congenital malformations and thrombosis of the inferior vena cava • Constrictive pericarditis • Tricuspid valve diseases	• PP, WHVP, and FHVP increased • IVC pressure increased

[a] In veno-occlusive disease FHVP is normal but PP and WHVP are both increased.
PP, portal pressure; WHVP, wedge hepatic venous pressure; FHVP, free hepatic venous pressure; IVC, inferior vena cava.

increase above a critical threshold value for the complications of portal hypertension to develop. The threshold value of HVPG for the formation of varices is 10 mmHg, and 12 mmHg for the appearance of other complications, such as variceal bleeding, ascites and portal hypertensive gastropathy.[7,8] Therefore, patients with a HVPG below 10 mmHg are at negligible or null risk of experiencing portal hypertension-related complications. Importantly, prospective studies have demonstrated that variceal hemorrhage does not occur if HVPG is reduced, either spontaneously or pharmacologically, to levels below 12 mmHg[8–10] or by over 20% from baseline values[11] (this is extensively discussed in Chapter 96).

3. Prognostic evaluation during variceal bleeding. Early measurement of HVPG in cirrhotic patients during acute variceal bleeding provides useful prognostic information on the evolution of the bleeding episode and long-term survival. Patients admitted because of variceal hemorrhage with an HVPG >20 mmHg are 5 times more likely to experience failure to control acute variceal bleeding or early rebleeding. These patients also require significantly more blood transfusions and days in the intensive care unit and have a higher mortality on follow-up. This suggests that the pharmacological reduction of HVPG may improve the outcome of acute variceal bleeding.[12]
4. Preoperative evaluation of resection risk in patients with small hepatocellular carcinoma. Patients with an HVPG >10 mmHg, and/or increased bilirubin levels have an increased risk of hepatic decompensation after surgical resection of hepatocellular carcinoma,[13] even in cases with well-preserved liver function (Child-Pugh A). In a recent study, more than 50% of patients with Child-Pugh class A had hepatic decompensation after surgery. This decompensation not only affected quality of life but was also associated with reduced long-term survival.[13] Surgical resection should therefore be restricted to patients with an HVPG below 10 mmHg.
5. Evaluation of progression of chronic liver disease, especially in severe chronic hepatitis C and in alcoholic hepatitis. In these situations, HVPG measurements may be a good index to assess the evolution and the response to therapy.[14,15] HVPG could be considered a dynamic marker of disease progression.[15]

CONTRAINDICATIONS

Past episodes of allergic reaction to radiographic contrast medium constitutes the only major contraindication to hepatic vein catheterization. Coagulation disorders are usually seen in cirrhotic patients, but the evidence of complications associated with severe thrombocytopenia or low prothrombin time is limited.

COMPLICATIONS

The main advantages of the hepatic vein catheterization technique are its simplicity, reproducibility, and safety. We have observed no fatalities in over 10000 studies. Major complications have been limited to local injury of the femoral or jugular veins (arteriovenous fistulae, leakage, or rupture of venous introducers). These complications are greatly reduced by performing the venous puncture under Doppler ultrasonography guidance. The procedure carries very little discomfort. Performed under slight conscious sedation (midazolam 0.2 mg/kg i.v.), its acceptability is comparable to that of upper gastrointestinal endoscopy[16] and the cost is similar to that of a conventional venography. Because of the many clinical applications, hepatic vein catheterization is becoming a routine test in many hospitals.

REFERENCES

1. Myers JD, Taylor WJ. An estimation of portal venous pressure by occlusive catheterization of an hepatic venule. J Clin Invest 1951; 30:662.
2. Groszmann RJ, Glickman M, Blei AT, Storer E, Conn HO. Wedged and free hepatic venous pressure measured with a balloon catheter. Gastroenterology 1979; 76:253–258.
3. Reynolds TB, Geller HM, Kuzma OT, Redeker AG. Spontaneous decrease in portal pressure with clinical improvement in cirrhosis. N Engl J Med 1960; 263:734–739.
4. Viallet A, Joly JG, Marleau D, Lavoie P. Comparison of free portal venous pressure and wedged hepatic venous pressure in patients with cirrhosis of the liver. Gastroenterology 1970; 59:372–375.
5. Boyer TD, Triger DR, Horisawa M, Redeker AG, Reynolds TB. Direct transhepatic measurement of portal vein pressure using a thin needle. Comparison with wedged hepatic vein pressure. Gastroenterology 1977; 72:584–589.
6. Debernardi-Venon W, Bandi JC, Garcia-Pagan JC et al. CO(2) wedged hepatic venography in the evaluation of portal hypertension. Gut 2000; 46:856–860.
7. Garcia-Tsao G, Groszmann RJ, Fisher RL et al. Portal pressure, presence of gastroesophageal varices and variceal bleeding. Hepatology 1985; 5:419–424.
8. Casado M, Bosch J, Garcia-Pagan JC et al. Clinical events after transjugular intrahepatic portosystemic shunt: correlation with hemodynamic findings. Gastroenterology 1998; 114:1296–1303.
9. Vorobioff J, Groszmann RJ, Picabea E et al. Prognostic value of hepatic venous pressure gradient measurements in alcoholic cirrhosis: a 10-year prospective study. Gastroenterology 1996; 111:701–709.
10. Groszmann RJ, Bosch J, Grace ND et al. Hemodynamic events in a prospective randomized trial of propranolol versus placebo in the prevention of a first variceal hemorrhage [see comments]. Gastroenterology 1990; 99: 1401–1407.
11. Feu F, Garcia-Pagan JC, Bosch J et al. Relation between portal pressure response to pharmacotherapy and risk of recurrent variceal haemorrhage in patients with cirrhosis. Lancet 1995; 346:1056–1059.
12. Moitinho E, Escorsell A, Bandi JC et al. Prognostic value of early measurements of portal pressure in acute variceal bleeding. Gastroenterology 1999; 117:626–631.
13. Bruix J, Castells A, Bosch J et al. Surgical resection of hepatocellular carcinoma in cirrhotic patients: prognostic value of preoperative portal pressure. Gastroenterology 1996; 111:1018–1022.
14. Groszmann RJ. The hepatic venous pressure gradient: has the time arrived for its application in clinical practice? Hepatology 1996; 24:739–741.
15. Burroughs AK, Groszmann R, Bosch J et al. Assessment of therapeutic benefit of antiviral therapy in chronic hepatitis C: is hepatic venous pressure gradient a better end point? Gut 2002; 50:425–427.
16. Steinlauf AF, Garcia-Tsao G, Zakko MF. Low-dose midazolam sedation: an option for patients undergoing serial hepatic venous pressure measurements. Hepatology 1999; 29:1070–1073.

Chapter 134

Liver biopsy

David Patch

KEY POINTS

- Liver biopsy remains a key diagnostic tool in the management of liver diseases
- The risk of liver biopsy is reduced by a careful technique and pre-biopsy work-out, including ultrasound and coagulation profile
- Guided liver biopsy (during real-time imaging) allows accurate sampling of focal liver lesions
- Spring-loaded needles for transjugular liver biopsy allow the physician to obtain samples as adequate as transparietal biopsies in patients with significant coagulation abnormalities

INTRODUCTION

Histology has been a lynch pin in diagnosis and management. It is hard if not impossible to envisage management of patients without recourse to liver biopsy, and yet it is a procedure that is often feared by patients, and when done incorrectly can have devastating complications. There is, however, a significant volume of evidence to guide the clinician with respect to technique, complications, and contraindications, and these are examined below.

Erlich is credited with the first liver aspiration in 1883 and subsequently the first percutaneous liver biopsy for diagnostic purposes was reported in 1923.[1] Lack of serum markers that predict the presence of fibrosis and the advent of liver transplantation as well as the burden of hepatitis C and NASH have all resulted in a continued demand for this procedure.

THE BIOPSY PROCEDURE

Hematological investigations

All patients undergoing percutaneous liver biopsy should be grouped and the serum saved, and compatible blood should be readily available. The prothrombin time (or international normalized ratio, INR) and platelet count should be checked prior to the biopsy.

Vitamin K, fresh frozen plasma (FFP), and platelet transfusion

Vitamin K, fresh frozen plasma, and platelet support is in wide use for the correction of coagulation abnormalities prior to liver biopsy. Vitamin K should be given parenterally at least 48h prior to the biopsy, and is usually only effective where the disturbance in coagulation is due to biliary obstruction or malabsorption. (NB. Factor VII levels may be returned to normal within 24h of vitamin K administration, but the levels of other factors may take longer, and any deficiency will not be reflected in an INR measurement.) If this does not work then fresh frozen plasma given immediately prior to the biopsy at a dose of 12–15mL/kg body weight may correct the prothrombin time in the majority of cases.[2] Platelet transfusion prior to percutaneous liver biopsy in thrombocytopenic patients has been used widely, although post-transfusion platelet increments do not necessarily correlate with decreased risk of bleeding.[3]

The high cost of recombinant factor VII and early recourse to transjugular biopsies limits the use of this agent except when a targeted biopsy is required.

Prebiopsy ultrasound

All patients being considered for liver biopsy should undergo a prebiopsy ultrasound. Prebiopsy ultrasound aims to rule out anatomical variation (e.g., the presence of an intrahepatic gallbladder or Chilaiditi syndrome, where bowel lies between a shrunken liver and the abdominal wall), thereby avoiding inadvertent puncture of an adjacent viscus.[4] Ultrasound also permits the detection of focal lesions such as hemangioma, which may be asymptomatic and may or may not have been suspected.

Informed consent

Informed consent should be obtained in writing prior to the biopsy procedure in accordance with individual hospital policies.

Sedation

Patients should be given the opportunity to have midazolam sedation for the biopsy procedure if there is no contraindication.

Percutaneous liver biopsy

This may be classified according to the site of entry of the biopsy needle, whether the biopsy is performed in a blind or guided manner, and/or whether the biopsy track is plugged after the procedure.

Transthoracic (transparietal) and subcostal liver biopsy

Technique

The patient lies supine. The borders of the liver are delineated by percussion or visualized by ultrasound. The liver may be higher than expected (particularly in transplant patients) or lower, such as in patients with chronic lung disease. This author recommends the use of ultrasound and, although the routine use of ultrasound is not recommended in the UK, no longer carries out biopsies without it.

The usual site for biopsy is between the 10th and 12th ribs in the mid-axillary line.

The site of biopsy should be infiltrated with local anesthetic and a small incision made through the dermis. It is vital that the anesthetic is injected all the way into the liver, as inadequate anesthesia of the capsule will result in pain. The liver itself will often feel 'gritty' on the end of the hypodermic needle, and safe placement of the needle may be confirmed by asking the patient to take a very gentle breath in, when the syringe plunger will move cranially as the liver moves caudally. This is also a good time to ensure the patient clearly understands the sequence of breathing, as they must be able to hold their breath in expiration.

The biopsy needle should be advanced into the intercostal space, but not into the liver. This author's technique is to then clearly command 'breathe in, breathe out, HOLD IT, one, two, three, four, five, and breathe away.' The biopsy is taken during the counting phase when the biopsy needle is advanced into the parenchyma, and the biopsy taken. The subsequent procedure for taking the biopsy varies according to whether the biopsy needle is of the aspiration (e.g., Menghini needle) or cutting type (e.g., Tru-cut needle).

Menghini needle: This employs a suction technique. As the needle is advanced into the parenchyma, the plunger on a 10-ml syringe attached to the end of the needle is pulled back. Therefore, the needle cuts the parenchyma, and the syringe sucks the specimen into the barrel. This technique has the advantage in that it is very quick and involves only one movement.[5] This allows less time for the patient to move, thereby minimizing the potential for tearing the capsule. However, it is less reliable at obtaining good cores of tissue from cirrhotic patients, where the hard liver may 'bounce' away from the tip. Samples obtained from cirrhotic livers may also be fragmented.

The Tru-cut needle involves a three-stage process, requiring greater operator skill and patient compliance. The needle is advanced into the parenchyma. The needle tip is then extended, followed by the cutting bevel. To avoid a scissoring action, there needs to be a slight forward force, so that the cutting bevel actually moves forward, slicing liver, as opposed to pushing the needle tip back. This needle has the advantage of reliable specimens even in hard cirrhotic livers.

Comparisons: When comparing the two needle types, the largest series[6] has shown the Tru-cut to have the greater morbidity (3.5/1000 vs 1/1000) and mortality. Death, serious hemorrhagic complications, pneumothorax, and biliary peritonitis all occurred more frequently with the Tru-cut needle when compared to the Menghini needle, while puncture of other viscera and sepsis were more frequent with the Menghini needle. No studies have compared the newer (but more expensive) spring-loaded Trucut needles with the Menghini needle.

The gauge of the biopsy needle and its effect on post biopsy bleeding has only been investigated for suction needles. A recent study reported similar results with respect to staging the degree of inflammation and fibrosis in biopsies taken from patients with chronic viral hepatitis using either a 20G or a 17G needle.[7]

Number of passes

It has been demonstrated that taking more than one core of liver at biopsy can increase the diagnostic yield,[8] but it is self evident that making more passes increases the incidence of complications. It is the author's recommendation that if an adequate specimen is not obtained after two passes, an alternative approach/needle/operator should be employed, after a suitable period of observation.

Postbiopsy observation/analgesia

Factors dictating time spent in hospital include the likely time period in which complications are going to occur, distance from hospital, whether the patient lives alone, ease of the procedure, and the time at which the biopsy was taken in the day. Delayed hemorrhage can occur up to 15 days after percutaneous liver biopsy in patients who develop a coagulopathy post biopsy.[9] The economic drive to perform outpatient biopsies prompted studies showing that the majority of complications occurred in the first 3 h after liver biopsy.[10] It was therefore recommended that patients should be kept in hospital for 6 h after the procedure; a later paper described 61% of complications after liver biopsy occurring in the first 2 h, 82% occurring in the first 10 h, and 96% occurring in the first 24 h.[6]

Outpatient percutaneous liver biopsy has been performed in many centers in the US since the early 1970s. In 1989 the American Gastroenterological Association published a consensus statement on outpatient percutaneous liver biopsy, recommending that patients undergoing this procedure should have no conditions that might increase the risk of the biopsy including: encephalopathy, ascites, hepatic failure with severe jaundice or evidence of significant extrahepatic biliary obstruction, significant coagulopathies, serious diseases involving other organs such as severe congestive heart failure, or advanced age. The consensus statement also recommends that the place where the biopsy is performed should have easy access to a laboratory, blood bank, and inpatient facilities should the need arise, and there should be staff available to observe the patients for 6 h. The patient should be hospitalized if there is any significant complication including pain requiring more than one dose of analgesic in the 4 h post liver biopsy. The patient should also be able to return easily to the hospital where the biopsy was undertaken within 30 min, and should have a reliable individual to stay with on the first post biopsy night. If the above criteria cannot be met, then the patient should not be biopsied as an outpatient.

Observations: This author's policy is to recommend quarter hourly observation for 2 h, half hourly observation for the next 2 h, and hourly observation for the following 2 h. Suitable analgesia is written up at the time of the procedure, including tramadol and pethidine. If the procedure is planned as a day case, the biopsy should be performed in the first half of the morning, allowing time for complications to occur in hospital, as opposed to at home. This author prefers the patients to lie on their right-hand side post procedure for 2 h in order to tamponade the liver. There is no evidence for this practice.

Indicators of biopsy complications: These are usually severe pain (either shoulder tip or abdominal), unrelieved by a single injection of pethidine, hypotension, and tachycardia. The presence of all or some of the signs should prompt the physician to recommend the patient is observed overnight and, if ongoing, investigate and treat. These are not patients who can be 'left until the next morning' – a liver biopsy bleed may be a life-threatening event, particularly if left undetected.

Blind and guided liver biopsies

A blind liver biopsy is taken without imaging of the liver immediately prior to taking the biopsy.

A guided biopsy can be defined as a liver biopsy that is undertaken during real-time imaging of the liver whether that imaging modality be ultrasound, computed tomography (CT), or magnetic resonance imaging (MRI). Guided biopsies should give access to thicker hepatic parenchyma, should avoid the puncture of adjacent organs, and should allow the accurate biopsy of focal hepatic lesions where appropriate.

There is lack of agreement whether previous identification of the optimal site for liver biopsy by ultrasound examination counts as 'blind' or 'ultrasound guided.' It has been postulated that ultrasound-guided biopsy should reduce complications. Studies comparing blind and ultrasound-guided liver biopsies[11,12] show that the latter are more efficient and associated with fewer major and minor complications than blind biopsies.

Clearly, focal lesions will require real-time image guidance. The use of ultrasound guidance in percutaneous liver biopsy for diffuse liver disease may reduce some of the complications and therefore cost and inconvenience to a small number of patients. The cost of mobile ultrasound equipment has fallen dramatically and would be recouped with the avoidance of just one major complication.

Plugged liver biopsy

Plugged liver biopsy is a modification of the percutaneous approach, which was first described in 1984.[13] It has been advocated as an alternative method for obtaining liver tissue in patients with impaired coagulation where transjugular biopsy is not available.

In this technique a biopsy is taken with a Tru-cut needle in the conventional manner but only the obturator containing the specimen is removed leaving the outer cutting sheath within the liver substance. A prefilled syringe containing gelfoam is then placed into the external end of the sheath, and gelfoam injected as the sheath is withdrawn and while the breath is still held in expiration. The procedure is safe and well tolerated, but does require a prolonged breath-hold in expiration. The specimens also tend to be small as the needle is usually 18F, and multiple passes are obviously not appropriate.

Transvenous liver biopsy

Where there is significant disturbance of clotting conventional practice is to avoid percutaneous liver biopsy because of the risk of bleeding and to opt for a transjugular approach. Transjugular liver biopsy was first described in 1964. It is performed in a vascular catheterization laboratory with video-fluoroscopy equipment and cardiac monitoring because of the risk of cardiac arrhythmias as the catheter passes through the right atrium.[14] Until recently, the transjugular needle relied on a suction technique, and samples, particularly in cirrhotic patients, were small, as the liver would 'bounce' away from the needle. However, the introduction of spring-loaded Tru-cut-type devices has greatly improved the ease of the procedure, as well as the reliability of obtaining enough histological material.

The technique is straightforward. The internal jugular vein is cannulated under ultrasound guidance on the right side (usually) and a 45-cm-long 7F sheath is then guided under fluoroscopic control through the right side of the heart to the inferior vena cava. A 5F cobra catheter allows access into the hepatic vein, and with a wire and catheter in the hepatic vein, the sheath is advanced into the hepatic vein and position checked by injection of contrast medium (Fig. 134.1). The catheter and wire are removed, and the biopsy needle passed down the sheath and the tip advanced outside of the sheath (Fig. 134.2). The patient briefly holds their breath and the needle is advanced further and then fired. The needle is then withdrawn, with the sheath remaining in the hepatic vein. This allows easy re-access so that multiple biopsies may be quickly taken, ensuring adequate material is available for histology. A small quantity of contrast is injected to ensure there is no evidence of a capsular breach. If found, the tract should be plugged with 1–2 coils. Specimens taken by the transjugular route tend to be shorter than those taken by the percutaneous route but are usually adequate for diagnostic purposes.[15]

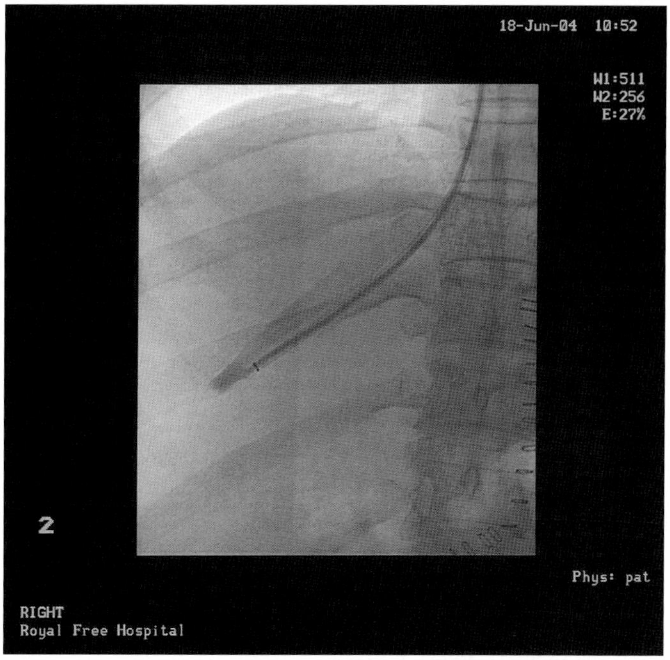

Fig. 134.1 A 7F catheter advanced into the hepatic vein prior to insertion of biopsy needle.

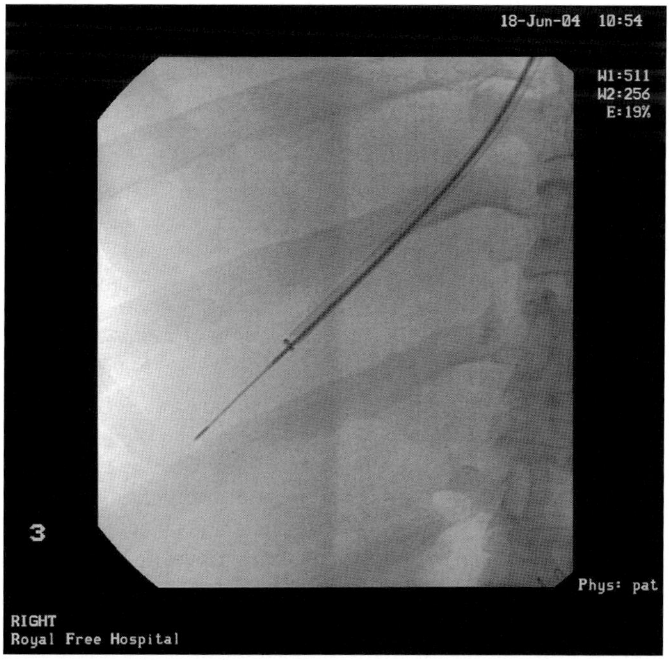

Fig. 134.2 A spring-loaded transjugular needle extended into the hepatic parenchyma prior to firing.

The post biopsy observations are for 4h, lending this technique as an excellent day case procedure, as it is well tolerated. Furthermore, it allows simultaneous carbon dioxide portography as well as measurement of hepatic wedge pressure gradient.[16] This author particularly favors this technique for patients who may require multiple biopsies over time. The procedure takes possibly less time from start to finish than a percutaneous biopsy, and it is this author's policy not to correct coagulation in patients undergoing this procedure, as the use of ultrasound-guided internal jugular puncture has been shown to significantly reduce the complications associated with this approach. Its principal disadvantage is greater up-front costs although this is partly offset by the more efficient use of hospital beds.

Sometimes, a transjugular approach is not possible and a transfemoral route may be used instead.[17] The biopsy technique involves pinch-type crocodile forceps, as the angle of the hepatic vein from the femoral approach is invariably acute. As a consequence the specimens are crushed and small. This author does not recommend this technique.

Laparoscopic liver biopsy

This technique is well established and its use varies widely between centers. It has also been used in centers where access to transjugular liver biopsy is not available, for patients with abnormal clotting parameters, and also in patients who have a combination of a focal liver lesion and a coagulopathy where a histological diagnosis is essential in the management of that patient. Since laparoscopic biopsy allows for biopsy under direct vision, it is possible to apply hemostatic techniques where there is early bleeding. Some US centers are performing laparoscopic liver biopsy on an outpatient basis and in some Japanese centers more than 50% of liver biopsies are performed laparoscopically.[18]

The complications in laparoscopic liver biopsy include those of laparoscopy itself.

Mortality

A generally accepted mortality rate in standard textbooks is between 0.1% and 0.01%,[19] but does vary.[6] The main cause of mortality after percutaneous liver biopsy is intraperitoneal hemorrhage[6] and is usually in patients with cirrhosis or malignant disease, both of which are risk factors for bleeding. Puncture of the gallbladder followed by biliary peritonitis is also a recognized cause of death.

Hemorrhage should be suspected when there is ongoing pain (due to liver capsular distention by an expanding hematoma), as well as shock. Urgent imaging should be performed immediately to confirm the presence of a hematoma or free intra-abdominal blood, and in the presence of ongoing bleeding our approach is to then proceed to angiography, when a spurting vessel can be embolized. If no single vessel is seen to be bleeding, the options are to either do nothing, assuming that a proportion of patients will continue to bleed and require either laparotomy or further angiography, or blindly embolize the right lobe of the liver, with the risk of a significant deterioration in liver function. In transplant patients, the latter is not an option, and early recourse to laparotomy and evacuation of hematoma is recommended.

Patients with suspected biliary peritonitis should have an early laparotomy.

Morbidity

Percutaneous liver biopsy

Pain occurs in up to 30% with moderate and severe pain occurring in 3% and 1.5%, respectively. Hypotension and vasovagal episodes are common accompaniments to pain, occurring in approximately 3% of liver biopsies and vasovagal episodes occasionally require the administration of atropine.

Significant hemorrhage (indicated by a drop in hemoglobin of >2 g/dL) occurs in 0.35–0.5% of all procedures.[10] Hemobilia occurs in 0.05% of patients who present with biliary pain, jaundice, and melena, and arterial embolization may rarely be required.

Puncture of other viscera occur infrequently with an incidence of between 0.01% and 0.1%.[6] The puncture of lung, colon, kidney, and gallbladder together with pneumothorax, pleural effusion, and subcutaneous emphysema are well-recognized complications, which rarely require intervention.[12]

Other recognized complications include sepsis, reaction to the anesthetic, breakage of the biopsy needle,[20] and intrahepatic arteriovenous fistulae.[21]

Transjugular liver biopsy

The complications from transjugular liver biopsy range from 1.3% to 20% and the mortality up to 0.5%. A true comparison with percutaneous biopsy is not appropriate since the methods are complimentary rather than alternatives. Complications include neck hematoma, puncture of the neck and/or intrathoracic arteries, transient Horner's syndrome, transient dysphonia, pneumothorax, cardiac arrhythmias, fever and infection, perforation of the liver capsule, and rarely fistula from hepatic artery to either portal vein or biliary radicles.

Contraindications

Whilst some of the contraindications appear to be common sense, many of them have been quoted as dogma in medical texts with very little evidence to support them.

The uncooperative patient

If the patient remains uncooperative despite midazolam and the benefit of obtaining liver histology outweighs the risk to the patient, general anesthesia should be considered.

Extrahepatic biliary obstruction

Extrahepatic biliary obstruction is frequently quoted as a contraindication to liver biopsy and may be complicated by pain, biliary peritonitis, septicemic shock, and death.[22]

Bacterial cholangitis

The risk of inducing peritonitis and septic shock after liver biopsy has made cholangitis a relative contraindication. However, if a liver biopsy is performed when a biliary system is infected then culture of a piece of liver can give useful bacteriological information especially in the context of investigation of tuberculosis or a PUO. Bacteremia after percutaneous biopsy of a normal liver is a well-recognized phenomenon[23] that occurs in up to 14% of biopsies. These findings confirm the risks of disseminating infection at the time of liver biopsy.

Abnormal coagulation indices

If the prothrombin time is prolonged by 4 s or more (or INR > 1.4) alternative strategies should be employed.[24]

The level of the platelet count at which a percutaneous liver biopsy should not be done is as controversial. The author recommends a platelet count above 80 000/mm^3 for a percutaneous biopsy, in the absence of hematological disease or renal failure.

Ascites

Percutaneous biopsy of the liver in the presence of tense ascites is considered a contraindication in many texts. The reasons for this vary from the high likelihood of not obtaining a biopsy specimen because of the distance between the abdominal wall and the liver to the risk of uncontrollable bleeding into the ascites. Whilst these reasons appear sensible they are not substantiated in randomized controlled clinical trials. It seems logical that if a liver biopsy is clinically indicated in a patient with tense ascites then there are several alternatives, including performing a total paracentesis prior to performing the percutaneous biopsy, and transjugular liver biopsy.

Cystic lesions

Modern imaging techniques can often identify benign cystic lesions of the liver as such thereby eliminating the need for biopsy in many cases. Cystic lesions within the liver may communicate with several structures including the biliary tree and therefore run the risk of biliary peritonitis after biopsy.

Amyloidosis

Reports of hemorrhage and death after liver biopsy in patients with amyloid have led to the inclusion of amyloid liver disease in the list of contraindications to percutaneous liver biopsy. If a diagnosis of amyloidosis had already been made or is strongly suspected then one would need a good indication for performing a percutaneous liver biopsy rather than for performing a more benign procedure such as a rectal biopsy.

Malignancy

Patients with a strong suspicion of malignancy should not be biopsied as an outpatient because they have a 6–10 times higher risk of hemorrhage compared to patients without cancer.[25]

Obesity

In the obese patient, it may be difficult to identify the liver by percussion. The biopsy should be done under ultrasound control, or via the transjugular route.

Sickle cell disease

There is an increased risk of bleeding in patients with sickle cell disease undergoing percutaneous liver biopsy for hepatic complications of the condition.[26] A transjugular route is the obvious choice.

Valvular heart disease

Bacteremia associated with liver biopsy has been well documented.[23] Therefore, prophylactic antibiotics should be used in the context of valvular heart disease.

The current data on the use of prophylactic antibiotics is inconclusive but for patients in whom biliary sepsis is suspected or likely to be present (such as with a Roux-en-Y anastomosis) prophylactic antibiotic use would be prudent.[17]

CONCLUSION

Liver biopsy will remain a vital tool for the assessment of liver disease for many years to come. It is this author's opinion that the development of spring-loaded Tru-cut transjugular needles has meant that there are very few people who cannot be biopsied safely and without discomfort, and that the use of this method of biopsy will continue to increase.

SOURCES OF INFORMATION FOR PATIENTS AND DOCTORS

http://www.patient.co.uk/showdoc/27000462/
http://www.patient.co.uk/showdoc/907/
http://www.gicare.com/pated/epdlv27.htm

REFERENCES

1. Bingel A. Ueber die parenchympunktion der leber. Verh Dtsch Ges Inn Med 1923; 35:210–212.
2. Contreras M, Ala FA, Greaves M et al. Guidelines in the use of fresh frozen plasma. Transfus Med 1992; 2:57–63.
3. Kristensen J, Eriksson L, Olsson K et al. Functional capacity of transfused platelets estimated by the Thrombostat 4000/2. Eur J Haematol 1993; 5:152–155.
4. Dixon AK, Nunez DJ, Bradley JR et al. Failure of percutaneous liver biopsy: anatomical variation. Lancet 1987; 2:437–439.
5. Menghini G. One-second biopsy of the liver – problems of its clinical application. N Engl J Med 1970; 283:582–585.
6. Piccininio F, Sagnelli E, Pasquale G et al. Complications following percutaneous liver biopsy. J Hepatol 1986; 2:165–173.
7. Petz D, Klauck S, Rohl FW, et al. Feasibility of histological grading and staging of chronic viral hepatitis using specimens obtained by thin-needle biopsy. Virchows Arch 2003; 442(3):238–244.
8. Maharaj B, Leary WP, Naran AD et al. sampling variability and its influence on the diagnostic yield of percutaneous needle biopsy of the liver. Lancet 1986; 1:523–525.
9. Reichert CM, Wiesenthal LM, Klein HG. Delayed haemorrhage after percutaneous liver biopsy. J Clin Gastroenterol 1983; 5:263–266.
10. Knauer MC. Percutaneous biopsy of the liver as a procedure for outpatients. Gastroenterology 1978; 74:101–102.
11. Caturelli E, Giacobbe A, Facciorusio D et al. Percutaneous biopsy in diffuse liver disease: Increasing diagnostic yield and decreasing complication rate by routine ultrasound assessment of puncture site. Am J Gastroenterol 1996; 91:1318–1321.
12. Stotland BR, Lichtensrein GR. Liver biopsy complications and routine ultrasound. Am J Gastroenterol 1996; 91:1295–1296.
13. Riley SA, Ellis WR, Irving HC et al. Percutaneous liver biopsy with plugging of the needle tract: a safe method for use in patients with impaired coagulation. Lancet 1984; 2:436.
14. Dotter CT. Catheter biopsy. Experimental technique for transvenous liver biopsy. Radiology 2004; 82:312–314.
15. Papatheodoridis GV, Patch D, Watkinson A, Tibballs J, Burroughs AK. Transjugular liver biopsy in the 1990s: A 2-year audit. Aliment Pharmacol Ther 1999; 13:603–608.
16. Vlachogiannakos J, Patch D, Watkinson A, Tibballs J, Burroughs AK. Carbon-dioxide portography: an expanding role? Lancet 2000; 355:987–988.
17. Blubak ME, Porayko MK, Krom RAF et al. Complications of liver biopsy in liver transplant patients: increased sepsis associated with choledochojejunostomy. Hepatology 1991; 14:1603–1605.
18. Sue M, Caldwell SH, Dickson RC et al. Variation between centres in technique and guidelines for liver biopsy. Liver 1996; 16:267–270.
19. Sherlock S, Dooley J. Diseases of the liver and biliary system, 10th edn. London: Blackwell Scientific; 1997.
20. Lazar H. Fractured liver biopsy needles. Gastroenterology 1978; 74:801.

21. Okuda K, Musha H, Nakajima Y et al. Frequency of intrahepatic arteriovenous fistula as a sequelae to percutaneous needle puncture of the liver. Gastroenterology 1978; 74:1204–1207.
22. Caturelli E, Giacobbe A, Facciorusio D et al. Percutaneous biopsy in diffuse liver disease: Increasing diagnostic yield and decreasing complication rate by routine ultrasound assessment of puncture site. Am J Gastroenterol 1996; 91:1318–1321.
23. Le Frock JL, Ellis CA, Turchik JB et al. Transient bacteraemia associated with percutaneous liver biopsy. J Infect Dis 1975; 131:S104–107.
24. Grant A, Neuberger J. Guidelines on the use of liver biopsy in clinical practice. British Society of Gastroenterology. GUT 1999; 45:Suppl 4: IVI-IVII.
25. McGill DB, Rakela J, Zinsmeister AR et al. A 21-year experience with major haemorrhage after percutaneous liver biopsy. Gastroenterology 1990; 99:1396–1400.
26. Zakaria N, Knisely A, Portmann B et al. Acute sickle cell hepatopathy represents a potential contraindication for percutaneous liver biopsy. Blood 2003; 101:101–103.

Chapter 135

Histopathology primer for gastroenterologists and hepatologists

Robert M Genta and Laura Rubbia-Brandt

KEY POINTS

- The histologist's conclusion is shaped by the clinical information provided
- Biopsies from endoscopically normal mucosa can yield unexpected findings
- Biopsy of normal and abnormal mucosa can be vital in distinguishing ulcerative colitis from Crohn's disease
- Endoscopic pictures can aid histological interpretation
- Marked ascites, obesity and right pleural cavity infection are relative contraindications to percutaneous liver biopsy
- Liver biopsy is useful in conditions (e.g. chronic hepatitis C, alcoholic liver disease, nonalcoholic steatohepatitis) where there is poor correlation between symptoms, liver function tests and histologic findings

INTRODUCTION

The histopathologic examination of tissue samples is one of the central steps in the investigation and management of patients with gastrointestinal and hepatologic disorders. Although no-one disagrees with the notion that many lesions and abnormalities seen during an endoscopic examination should be biopsied, the view that biopsy specimens should be obtained from the normal-looking mucosa of the digestive tract in selected circumstances is not as pervasive as it should be. Crucial information is often obtained by submitting to the pathologist tissue samples from areas that appear entirely normal. Table 135.1 provides a list of the most common situations in which biopsy specimens from endoscopically unremarkable mucosa may either reveal unexpected and otherwise undetectable pathologic processes or, when combined with samples from abnormal areas, make a decisive contribution to the diagnostic process.

Despite the recent development of serologic tests and non-invasive imaging techniques that have modified its indications, needle liver biopsy commonly remains the gold standard against which many other diagnostic modalities are evaluated. It is also an indispensable tool for monitoring the effectiveness of treatment and estimating prognosis.

The purpose of this brief primer is twofold: to explain the diagnostic process of mucosal and hepatic biopsy specimens from the viewpoint of the pathologist, and to present guidelines for the optimal biopsy sampling of each organ in different conditions. This chapter is intended to answer the clinician's questions: 'What can I expect from my pathologist?' and 'What should I give the pathologist to get the best answers?'

The references at the end of this chapter are annotated in order to provide perspective for the reader concerning their content.

MUCOSAL BIOPSY OF THE DIGESTIVE TRACT

A trip into the pathologist's mind: approach to the mucosal biopsy

Histopathologic diagnoses result from a combination of three categories of informational elements: those contained in the histologic structure of the specimen itself (the 'histologic elements'); those that accompany the specimen (demographic and clinical history, previous pathologic diagnoses); and those that derive from the knowledge, experience, and attitude of the pathologist and the institution in which he or she works. The latter two can be termed 'suprahistologic.'

The diagnostic process begins with a systematic analysis and description of the histologic characteristics, followed by a comparison with the entities known to the observer. A set of diagnostic hypotheses is then formulated and checked for plausibility against clinical information provided, until a rank of possible diagnoses is generated. Experienced pathologists usually skip some or all of the above steps and make diagnoses based on pattern recognition. They automatically match the histologic features of the case under examination with a pattern known to be associated with one or more nosologic entities, then stop considering other factors and generate a diagnosis. Some pathologists prefer to assess the histological findings first, without the clinical information, and others approach the histologic examination in the same way as a clinician does a physical examination (i.e., targeted towards the unique and relevant information derived from the history).

The shortcut process is what separates 'easy' cases from 'difficult' ones – a distinction related to each pathologist's bank of recognizable patterns, that is, his or her knowledge and experience.

To illustrate the diagnostic process we can use the schematic representation of a colonic mucosal biopsy depicted in Figure 135.1. The first area the observer examines is the luminal surface, which should normally be either completely devoid of any substance or contain small amounts of mucus. The surface is clean in panel A (normal mucosa), but shows several small round corpuscles attached to the surface in B, which represent *Cryptosporidium*. The normal epithelium (panel A), both on the surface and the crypts, is composed by regularly arranged populations of mucin-containing cells interspersed with absorptive cells. In panel B (evolving mucosal inflammation), there are fewer mucin-containing cells, the cells are in disarray, and the epithelium is infiltrated by polymorphonuclear

TABLE 135.1 BIOPSY APPROACHES TO THE EVALUATION OF THE DIGESTIVE TRACT ACCORDING TO VARIOUS SUSPECTED OR UNSUSPECTED DISORDERS

Organ and condition or endoscopic appearance	Location of biopsies	Diagnostic benefits
Esophagus (Barrett's)	Four quadrant every 2 cm from LES region to the top of the apparent Barrett's zone	Precise determination of extension of Barrett's metaplasia and detection of dysplasia
Esophagus (reflux-like symptoms in children)	Distal and mid-portions	Distinction between reflux and eosinophilic esophagitis
Stomach (normal)	Two from antrum, one from angularis, two from body (corpus) greater curve (Updated Sydney System)	Phenotypic and topographic classification of gastritis Detection of *Helicobacter pylori* Detection of intestinal metaplasia and dysplasia
Stomach (patchy inflammation)	Several specimens from both normal and inflamed areas	For surrogate evidence of Crohn's disease when diagnosis is suspected but elusive Phenotypic and topographic classification of gastritis Detection of *H. pylori*
Stomach (atrophy gastric body)	Multiple specimens from normal antrum and atrophic gastric body	Confirmation of body-restricted autoimmune gastritis Determination of *H. pylori* status Detection of ECL cell hyperplasia and microcarcinoids
Stomach (ulcer)	Normal mucosa surrounding ulcer; samples as per Updated Sydney System	Help distinguish between ulcers caused by *H. pylori* and ulcers caused by chemical injury (NSAIDs) Phenotypic and topographic classification of gastritis
Stomach (polyp or cancer)	Normal mucosa surrounding polyp or tumor; samples as per Updated Sydney System	Detection of submucosal invasion Phenotypic and topographic classification of gastritis; detection of unsuspected atrophic body gastritis which might reflect need for vitamin B_{12} therapy now or in future
Stomach (MALT lymphoma)	Samples as per Updated Sydney System, more extensive if feasible	Detection of multifocality Phenotypic and topographic classification of gastritis
Duodenum (normal)	Third or fourth portion	Detection of borderline or mild lesions (e.g., mild villus atrophy and epithelial lymphocytosis; Marsh 1, 2 lesions) Diagnosis of rare conditions (e.g., Whipple disease) Detection of unusual infections (e.g., *Giardia*, cryptosporidiosis, atypical mycobacteria)
Terminal ileum (IBD in colon)	Several centimeters proximal to ileocecal valve	Detection of "backwash ileitis" Distinction between ulcerative colitis and Crohn's disease
Colon (normal)	One or two specimens from each anatomic portion of the colon from cecum to rectum	Detection of lymphocytic or collagenous colitis Detection of unusual infections (e.g., cryptosporidiosis, spirochetosis)
Colon (inflamed distally)	Several specimens from all segments proximal to inflamed area	Determination of extension of ulcerative colitis Detection of "skip lesions" or granulomas (Crohn's disease)
Colon (patchy inflammation)	Sampling each anatomic area as for normal colon above, both endoscopically normal and abnormal areas	Distinction between ulcerative colitis and Crohn's disease
Colon (UC for follow-up)	Four-quadrant sampling each 10 cm or according to anatomic landmarks (30–40 biopsies in total)	Detection of dysplasia

ECL, enterochromaffin-like; IBD, inflammatory bowel disease; LES, lower esophageal sphincter; MALT, mucosa-associated lymphoid tissue; NSAID, nonsteroidal anti-inflammatory drug; UC, ulcerative colitis.

Details of the Updated Sydney System can be found in Chapter 36.

neutrophils (PMNs), which are also abundant in the lamina propria. In panel C (chronic active inflammation) PMNs have accumulated at the bottom of a crypt, causing a microscopic crypt abscess. The normal lamina propria (panel A) contains scattered lymphocytes, plasma cells, and rare eosinophils; in contrast, in acute inflammation (panel B, left) it is almost obliterated by infiltrating PMNs; as the inflammation continues over a period of a few weeks (panel B, center) increasing numbers of lymphocytes and plasma cells join the PMNs, until they become the predominant cells in the chronic phase, several months into the process (panel B, right). Longstanding chronic inflammation causes destruction of the epithelium and crypts, which regenerate in an irregular fashion, often resulting in a profound rearrangement and distortion of the mucosal architecture, depicted in C. Observation of the muscularis mucosae may give useful information as to the chronicity of a process (when fibrosis may develop) and to its extent (i.e., whether it is limited to the mucosa or reached the deeper portion of the intestinal wall).

When the pathologist cannot visualize all the features by examining the slides stained with the traditional hematoxylin and eosin stain, a wide range of techniques is available to enhance the visibility of certain normal and abnormal structures. A number of special stains, so named because in most

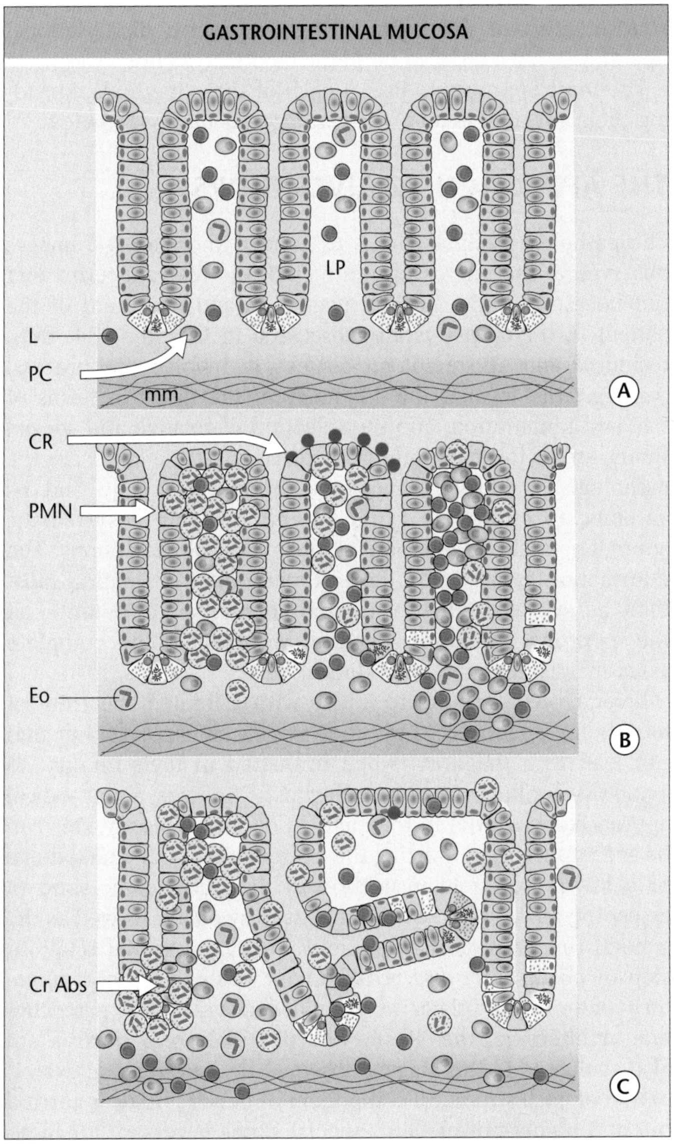

Fig. 135.1 Schematic representation of the gastrointestinal mucosa. A. Normal. **B.** Evolution from acute (left) to subacute (center) and chronic inflammation (right). **C.** Chronic active inflammation with the architectural disarray characteristic of longstanding destructive–regenerative processes. L, lymphocyte; LP, lamina propria; PC, plasma cell; mm, muscularis mucosae; Cr, *Cryptosporidium;* PMN, polymorphonuclear neutrophil; Eo, eosinophil; Cr Abs, crypt abscess.

laboratories they are not part of routine processing, can be used to detect fibrous tissue, better to demonstrate the brush border, or to visualize bacteria and parasites. When even more specific elements need to be assessed, immunohistochemical techniques can be used. For example, determining the subtype of lymphocytes infiltrating the epithelium of a small intestinal biopsy is useful to diagnose the potential very early stages (latent) of celiac disease and to differentiate them from other causes of villus atrophy (e.g., tropical sprue); information on the distribution of vascular and lymphatic channels can be obtained by applying antibodies that react selectively with their endothelial components; the evaluation of gastrin-producing cell hyperplasia in the gastric antrum (a feature of severe atrophic gastritis) can be achieved by selectively staining these cells with specific antibodies.

For the pathologist who examines the specimen before fitting in the history, demographics, etc., the histologic data so acquired will allow the observer either to make a diagnosis or to place the specimen into a holding category (e.g., chronic colitis with architectural disarray, ischemic injury, acute inflammation with normal architecture), until the clinical information is incorporated.

HOW TO GET THE BEST ANSWERS FROM A MUCOSAL BIOPSY

The keys to a successful mucosal biopsy, that is, one that yields clinically useful answers, are in the hands of the gastroenterologist. They can be summarized in the following sequence: acquisition, handling, and information.

Acquisition

The most appropriate locations for biopsy depend on the organ, its lesions or absence thereof, and the clinical suspicion. Some lesions encountered are not considered relevant or necessary in the endoscopist's experience and hence are rarely if ever biopsied. These include tiny innocuous-looking antral bumps, patchy erythema, or streaks in the esophagus and gastric antrum. However, if the lesion has potential relevance or is something that the endoscopist has never seen before, the visible abnormalities and adjacent, and even distant, areas should be biopsied. Adjacent refers to normal-looking mucosa to within 1 cm of the lesion. A classic example is the distinction between ulcerative colitis and Crohn's disease, which can be made only if samplings from both inflamed and apparently normal colon are examined and macroscopically unaffected areas ('skip lesions') are confirmed to be normal.

Table 135.1 summarizes the most commonly recommended biopsy protocols for the optimal histopathologic evaluation of certain esophageal, gastric, duodenal, and colonic conditions. This list, which is neither exhaustive nor absolute, is intended mostly to stimulate clinicians to become aware of the fact that for many conditions and suspected conditions there is an optimal way to obtain satisfactory answers from pathological examination. Like many 'best ways,' these too are subject to change as knowledge evolves. Clinicians should share relevant new information, which commonly appears in nonpathology journals, with the pathologist. The idea is to strive continually to work as a maximally informed team.

Handling

Just as a map without points of reference is useless for navigation, even the most thorough biopsy protocol is futile if the location of each specimen is not known to the pathologist. Thus, each mucosal sample must be placed into a container that indicates its location. Endoscopists should as a rule furnish pathologists with narrative and diagrammatic summaries of the patient's findings and biopsy sites. In many centers, a set of endoscopic pictures with indications of the biopsy locations and other key features is routinely forwarded to the pathologist. Modern digital endoscopy set-ups have printout options that include drawings of the organ with topographic references for the images. If such a device is not available, a simple drawing of the organ can be used to mark the location from which each sample was obtained.

It is now rare for endoscopy centers to have assistants trained to remove the mucosal sample from the forceps and orient it flat (with the mucosal surface facing up) on a piece of absorbent paper, a fine mesh (plastic or cloth), or a slice of organic material. Properly performed, this technique greatly facilitates the orientation of the sample in the histology laboratory; however, if the specimen is overly stretched or crushed, the resulting artifacts will hamper its microscopic evaluation. Thus, unless the endoscopy unit makes it a special mission with highly trained assistants, the safest way to remove the specimen from the forceps is to shake it gently in the fixative until it detaches. In buffered formalin the biopsy will quickly curl up on the side of the muscularis mucosae and histotechnologists will be able to embed it on edge and cut well-oriented sections (Fig. 135.2).

Information

One of the questions most frequently heard at the microscope during the signing-out of biopsies is: 'Why was this patient scoped and what is the question for us?' The pathologist can describe the histologic features of a specimen – and initially, to avoid bias, can do so 'blind' to the clinical history, if so desired. However, a proper interpretation is impossible without the aid of clinical information, at the core of which lies a succinct pertinent clinical history ending with specific questions for the pathologist.

THE LIVER BIOPSY

Liver biopsy first began to become a widely used procedure in 1958, when Menghini's technique was introduced. New core needle devices, such as the Tru-cut biopsy and biopsy guns, have been added recently to the hepatologist's equipment. Transjugular catheterization of the hepatic veins has been expanded to include the potential for liver biopsy; as such, it has broadened considerably the spectrum of patients on which a biopsy may be performed. Fine-needle aspiration biopsy (most often performed under the guidance of radiologic imaging) permits safe access to space-occupying lesions.

Wedge biopsy consists of the surgical excision of a small portion of hepatic tissue (usually measuring around 1 cm); this procedure is occasionally performed by surgeons who notice abnormalities in the liver during the course of abdominal operations, but may also be performed electively.

The most appropriate use of each of these methods, including their advantages and disadvantages, is discussed below.

THE APPROACH TO LIVER BIOPSY

The pathologist's first goal is to convert morphologic images observed at the microscope into clinically relevant terms that can be used for the further evaluation and treatment of the patient. Liver biopsy is also discussed in Chapter 134. Both technical and epistemologic issues are involved in process. Amongst the former, the adequacy of the tissue in terms of size and preparation, and the selection of fixative and special stains, are of foremost importance. Amongst the latter are the pathologist's ability to recognize normal histology and its variants, to appreciate artifacts, and to apply a systematic approach to the evaluation of the morphologic lesions. The information gathered by the histopathologic evaluation must then be synthesized into a comprehensive interpretation of the specimen. The conclusion will be based on this complete assessment integrated with clinical data.

Liver tissues respond to injury with a limited spectrum of morphologic features, often individually nonspecific, but that can lead to a diagnosis when evaluated in their totality. To avoid overlooking significant diagnostic findings, a methodical approach is essential in the analysis of a liver biopsy. This can be accomplished by starting the examination with a naked-eye or a low-power field inspection of the microscopic slide to assess the amount and quality of tissue available, as well as the general topography of the lesions. Next, the spatial relationship of portal tract and centrilobular veins and the arrangement of the hepatic plates are examined to evaluate the parenchymal architecture; the degree and distribution of fibrosis are also evaluated at this stage. Subsequently, a systematic examination of each structural component of hepatic tissue is carried out at a higher-power field. Special stains necessary for identification of specific histologic features are routinely prepared and help complete the analysis.

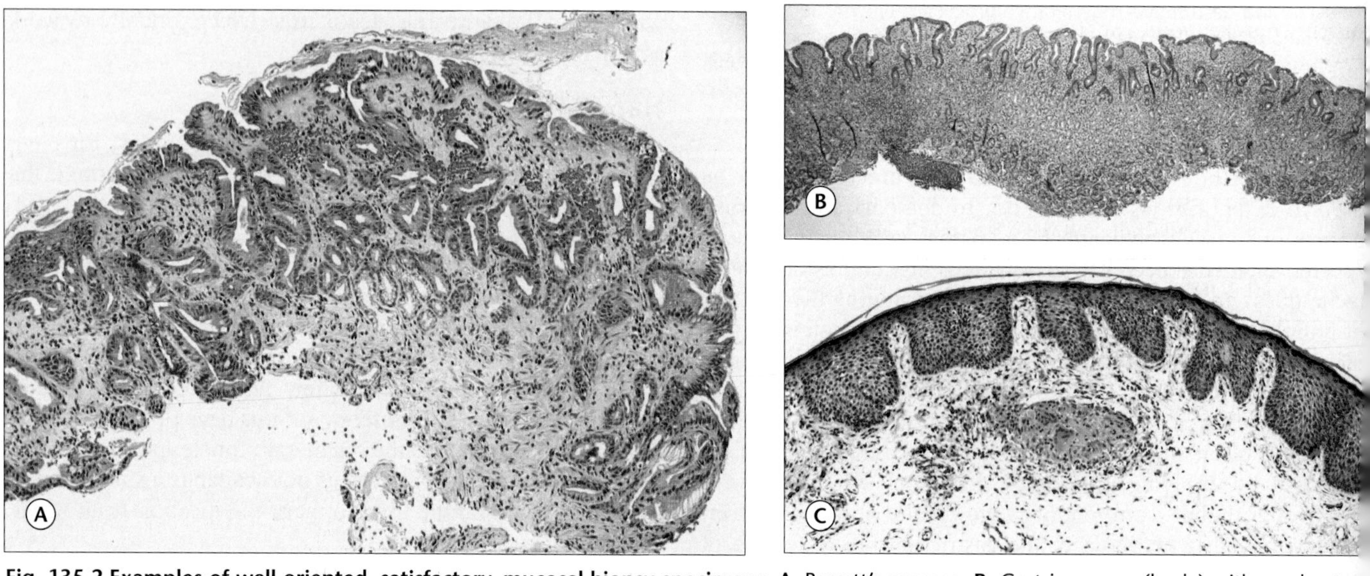

Fig. 135.2 Examples of well oriented, satisfactory, mucosal biopsy specimens. A. Barrett's mucosa. **B.** Gastric corpus (body) with moderate chronic gastritis. **C.** Anal mucosa with a granuloma.

As the histologic features of many hepatic conditions are not pathognomonic of a unique etiology, the identification of their origin requires integration with clinical and laboratory data. Many pathologists advocate examining each case unaware of any patient's clinical data and clinicians' provisional diagnoses in order to avoid interpretive bias. The argument is that a pathologist who reads biopsies with the conscious or unconscious aim of confirming the clinical suspicions betrays his or her role of an independent observer and may eventually fail the patients. Clinicians used to encourage pathologists to do this, but are now less inclined to do so. Part of the reason is that when they interpret images in their own domain (e.g., at endoscopy) they find that the most relevant observations come from knowing what special features should be sought, again like doing a physical examination armed with the focus of the history.

DIFFERENT TYPES OF LIVER BIOPSY

See also Chapter 134.

Percutaneous liver biopsy

Percutaneous biopsy is usually carried out transthoracically, but if necessary can be performed subcostally or in the epigastrum. Various permanent or disposable needle devices are currently available with a range in external diameter from 0.1 to 0.2 cm; they also differ according to their mechanisms, with suction needles (Menghini needle, Klatskin needle, Jamshidi needle), cutting needles (Vim-Silverman needle, Tru-cut needle), or spring-loaded cutting needles available. If cirrhosis is suspected clinically, a cutting needle should be preferred over a suction needle because fibrotic tissue tends to fragment with the use of the latter.

A good overall performance is obtained and the liver biopsy techniques are safe procedures and reliable in experienced hands. Guidelines in different countries are available for what constitutes sufficient training to achieve a threshold for competence. In most settings no mandated minimum number of annual liver biopsies is set out. The size of the biopsy specimen varies between 1 and 3 cm in length and between 0.12 and 0.2 cm in diameter. Although the liver has a rich vascular supply, complications associated with percutaneous liver biopsy are rare (Fig. 135.3). There are some clinical situations in which percutaneous liver biopsy is definitely contraindicated and other situations in which this procedure should be performed under exceptional circumstances.

INDICATIONS/CONTRAINDICATIONS

CONTRAINDICATIONS FOR PERCUTANEOUS LIVER BIOPSY

Absolute	**Relative**
Bleeding diathesis/Anticoagulation	Severe ascites
Dilatation of intrahepatic bile ducts	Severe obesity
Cholangitis	Right pleural cavity infection
Cystic lesions	
Uncooperative patient	
Vascular tumors	
Hepatic amyloidosis	
Unavailability of blood for transfusion	

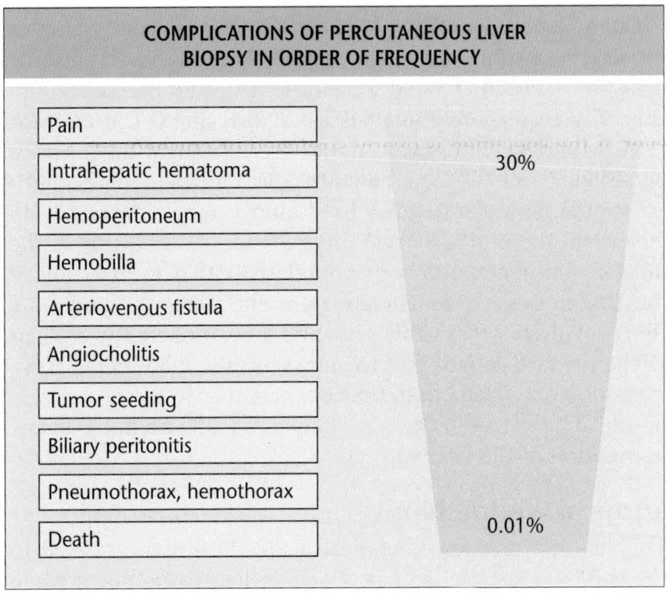
COMPLICATIONS OF PERCUTANEOUS LIVER BIOPSY IN ORDER OF FREQUENCY
Pain
Intrahepatic hematoma
Hemoperitoneum
Hemobilla
Arteriovenous fistula
Angiocholitis
Tumor seeding
Biliary peritonitis
Pneumothorax, hemothorax
Death
30%
0.01%

Fig. 135.3 Complications of percutaneous liver biopsy in order of frequency.

Transjugular biopsy

In this technique, liver tissue is obtained through a catheter inserted through transjugular and passed into superior vena cava. The tissue is obtained within the vascular system and the risk of bleeding into the liver parenchyma or the peritoneal cavity is virtually eliminated. Transjugular liver biopsy is an acceptable substitute for a transcutaneous biopsy when the latter is not feasible because of existing contraindications, but a biopsy is essential for the patient's management. In some situations the transjugular procedure is specifically indicated because of the additional information it can yield or because it is performed at the same time as hemodynamic studies (Table 135.2).

INDICATIONS/CONTRAINDICATIONS

INDICATIONS FOR TRANSJUGULAR LIVER BIOPSY

- Prothrombin <50%; platelets <60 000 g/L; partial thromboplastin time >1.5N; Ivy bleeding time >10 min (normal range 4–10 min)
- Clinically massive ascites
- Pulmonary emphysema
- Myeloproliferative syndromes
- Hemorrhagic telangiectasia, congestive liver, peliosis
- Amyloidosis
- Severe obesity
- Failure of percutaneous liver biopsy

TABLE 135.2 SPECIFIC INFORMATION MORE LIKELY TO BE OBTAINED DURING TRANSJUGULAR LIVER BIOPSY

- Hepatic venous pressure gradient (HVPG) measurement
- Hemodynamic study (e.g. pre-orthoptic liver transplant)
- Morphologic study of hepatic veins
- Transjugular intrahepatic portosystemic shunt (TIPS) assessment

The main disadvantage of this technique is that the samples obtained are small and fragmented. Tissue specimens usually measure between 0.3 and 2 cm in length, and the procedure generally requires multiple passes. In specialized centers with large experience, adequate tissue for histologic diagnosis is obtained in 80–97% of patients. The rate of complications associated with transjugular liver biopsy ranges from 1% to 20%, and the mortality rate ranges from 0.1% to 0.5%. The most common complications are related either to insertion of the catheter (neck hematoma, transient Horner's syndrome, transient dysphonia, cardiac arrhythmias, pneumothorax) or to the damage caused by the biopsy needle (abdominal pain, formation of a fistula from the hepatic artery to the portal vein or the biliary tree, and, especially in small, cirrhotic livers, perforation of the liver capsule).

Surgical wedge biopsy

The main advantages of surgical wedge biopsy are related to the ability to sample large portions of liver tissue taken while the operator has a view of the macroscopic appearance of the organ. Thus, a better sampling of tissue, particularly bile ducts and vessels from areas that are judged to be affected by a pathologic process, can be obtained.

This advantage is partly offset by subcapsular fibrosis, which is particularly common in the inferior margin of the liver and may be misinterpreted as cirrhosis (Fig. 135.4). Major complications include perforation of a viscus, bleeding, hemobilia, laceration of the spleen, leakage of ascitic fluid, abdominal wall hematoma, vasovagal reaction, prolonged abdominal pain, and seizures.

Fine-needle aspiration biopsy

Fine-needle aspiration biopsy of the liver is performed under ultrasonographic or computed tomography guidance, and is used mostly to obtain samples from a liver mass suspected of being malignant. The diagnostic accuracy ranges from 80% to 95% and is strongly related to the expertise of the cytopathologist. It is important to remember that a negative finding does not necessarily rule out a malignant tumor, which may have been missed by the aspiration. Fine-needle aspiration biopsy is generally a very safe procedure, even in patients with hemangiomas and echinococcal cysts. In patients with malignant tumors, however, there a small risk of seeding the needle tract with neoplastic cells.

Indications for liver biopsy

See also Chapter 134.

Liver biopsy is an invasive procedure associated with rare but significant risks of complications. Consequently, controversy persists regarding its use and there is no universally accepted consensus about its precise indications, as there is no consensus regarding contraindications, optimal technique, and training requirements. The most important criterion in the decision to perform a liver biopsy must be a clear diagnostic need, and the histopathologic results must be expected to have substantial impact in the patient's management. Consequently, it is clear that the indications are largely dependent on what we know about liver disease, and will change as this knowledge evolves. Once the decision has been made that a biopsy is needed, its goals will help determine the method to be used. The most common indications for liver biopsy are shown in the box.

INDICATIONS/CONTRAINDICATIONS

INDICATIONS FOR LIVER BIOPSY

- Evaluation, grading, and staging of chronic hepatitis
- Diagnosis, grading, and staging of alcoholic liver diseases and non-alcohol-induced steatohepatitis (NASH)
- Evaluation, grading, and staging of cholestatic liver disease
- Diagnosis of suspected cirrhosis
- Identification of systemic inflammatory or granulomatous disorders
- Evaluation of fever of unknown origin
- Identification of the type and extent of drug-induced liver injury
- Diagnosis of the nature of intrahepatic masses
- Diagnosis of multisystem infiltrative disorders
- Evaluation of abnormal liver biochemical tests and hepatomegaly
- Screening relatives of patients with familial diseases
- Identification of a metabolic or storage disease
- Obtaining tissue to culture infectious agents
- Obtaining tissue for quantitative estimation of copper or iron levels
- Diagnosis of vascular disease
- Evaluation of donor liver before transplantation
- Diagnosis of liver test abnormalities following transplantation
- Evaluation of effectiveness of therapies for liver disease

Clinical information and laboratory tests are pivotal means of establishing an etiologic diagnosis in several situations; however, liver biopsy can yield valuable information concerning the nature and extent of hepatic injury (grading), the degree of fibrosis (staging), and the presence of additional lesions. This body of information gathered from a biopsy may be relevant to the diagnosis, prognosis, and response to treatment. For example, in patients with chronic hepatitis C, alcoholic liver disease, and nonalcoholic steatohepatitis there is a poor correlation between symptoms, hepatic function test results (e.g., serum levels of alanine aminotransferase), and histologic features of the liver: patients with normal levels of liver enzymes may be found to have significant fibrosis or cirrhosis. Other conditions in which liver histology is crucial to determining the diagnosis, staging, and ultimately the patient's prognosis are drug-induced injury, primary sclerosing cholangitis, primary biliary cirrhosis, and the presence of an overlap syndrome. When combined with special detection techniques, liver biopsy may permit the quantification of iron in patients with hemochromatosis and of copper in patients with Wilson's disease.

Liver biopsy provides an accurate diagnosis in approximately 90% of patients with unexplained liver function test abnormalities; in this respect, its role is particularly critical in recipients of a liver transplantation. In these patients even minor alterations of liver function may herald rejection, and the performance of rapidly processed liver biopsies is pivotal to their follow-up and management. In the pretransplantation phase, liver biopsy is the method of choice for the evaluation of a donor graft.

Systemic disorders with protean and often nonspecific manifestations, such as sarcoidosis, lymphoma, acquired immune deficiency syndrome, and amyloidosis, are occasionally suggested or diagnosed by a liver biopsy.

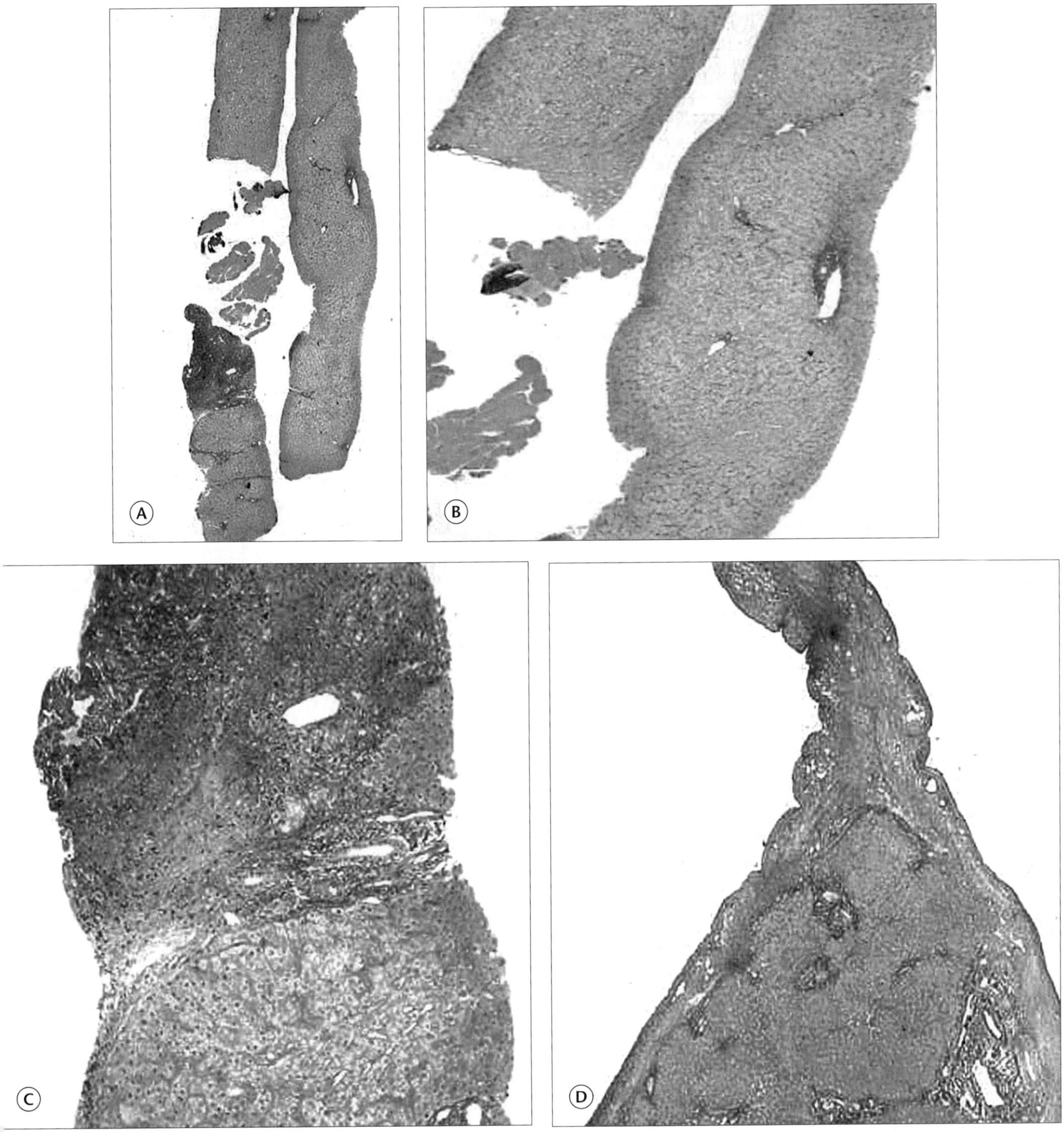

ig. 135.4 Capsular fibrous tissue in a needle liver biopsy mimicking a fibrous septum in cirrhosis. A. At low power this needle biopsy of ne liver shows a heterogeneous blue staining (trichrome stain) collagen content. **B.** At higher power in the deeper area of the biopsy the liver ; normal with no evidence of fibrosis. **C.** High-power field: the fibrous capsule is included at the end of a needle biopsy and may be nisinterpreted as significant fibrosis. **D.** The subcapsular region of a wedge biopsy of a nonfibrotic liver. Note the apparent band of fibrosis nmediately beneath the capsule, whereas the deeper portions of the parenchyma are normal.

In certain conditions that are generally well characterized by ither laboratory tests or noninvasive imaging techniques the isks of a liver biopsy may outweigh the relevance of the infornation it can provide. These conditions include acute viral epatitis; metastatic lesions of known origin; a suspicion of epatocellular carcinoma with established cirrhosis and an x-fetoprotein level above 400 ng/mL or vascular invasion; a genetically proven hemochromatosis with *HFE*$^{+/+}$ and ferritin levels lower than 1000 ng/mL; and benign liver tumors.

TISSUE SAMPLING

An average needle liver biopsy specimen represents approximately 1/50 000 of the total mass of the organ. It is clear that the potential for sampling error, particularly in conditions with an uneven distribution of the lesions, may be a major problem.

Experience indicates that the number of portal tracts present in the specimen is one of the major indicators of appropriate sampling. Most pathologists consider the presence of five to ten portal tracts to be adequate for the evaluation of drug-induced hepatitis, chronic hepatitis, and alcoholic liver disease; 10 to 20 portal tracts are often needed to assess lesions of small bile ducts (primary biliary cirrhosis, the vanishing bile duct syndrome, graft rejection). Liver biopsy is generally inadequate to diagnose the Budd-Chiari syndrome or large bile duct pathology; in these situations, examination of the entire liver (clearly not a clinically viable option) is necessary.

The number of portal tracts is related to the length of the specimen; although the ideal length is around 2.5 cm, a minimum length of 1.5 cm may be considered acceptable for the evaluation of diffuse liver disease. With current techniques, experienced operators usually provide adequate specimens irrespective of the needle used. The exception is the transjugular procedure, as several passages are often needed to obtain a satisfactory amount of material.

HANDLING, PROCESSING, AND STAINING OF TISSUE

High-quality histologic preparations depend on the rapid fixation of fresh tissues. The longer a specimen remains exposed to the air or in a nonfixative medium (e.g., saline solution), the more likely that drying or autolysis artifacts will affect its morphology and ultimately the histopathologic interpretation. Before being immersed in the fixative liquid, the biopsy core should not be touched; particular care should be exerted to avoid squeezing, which may give the specimen a nodular aspect that affects the assessment of its architecture.

In most centers the decision of which media to use for the fixation of liver biopsy specimens is made by the histopathologist. This decision is based on both individual preferences and the stains most commonly used in each laboratory. Special diagnostic questions may determine the usage of different fixatives that are better suited for the subsequent performance of special stains or immunohistochemical techniques.

The most widely use fixative is 10% neutral buffered formali a stable and inexpensive solution that yields excellent mo phologic detail when sections are stained with tradition stains, while allowing the subsequent performance of mo immunohistochemical and molecular biologic techniques.

When special diagnostic questions are anticipated, a pr portion of fresh material may be snap-frozen for the staini of lipids (which are dissolved during routine processing), vir quantification, molecular biology, or for storage in tissue bank Dry tissue is necessary for iron and copper quantitative assay Glutaraldehyde fixative is used when electron microscopy to be performed; this is essential for the diagnosis of sever mitochondrial and metabolic diseases, some cholestatic diseas in children, and for the detection of viral particles.

No one stain can demonstrate all the morphologic featur that need to be evaluated for the interpretation of a liver biops The choice of stains is often a matter of each pathologist personal preference and experience. Most experts recommen the inclusion of stains for different collagens of the connectiv tissue (Masson trichrome and reticulin); a reliable iron sta such as Prussian Blue, periodic acid–Schiff stain with diastas digestion (D-PAS), is useful for the detection of cytoplasm deposits of lipofuscin within Kupffer cells signaling rece foci of hepatocellular death, or of globules in α_1-antitrypsi deficiency.

CONCLUSIONS

Both mucosal and liver biopsies have become essential too in the diagnosis and management of digestive condition Clinicians, however, should keep in mind that, unlike auto matically generated chemical and hematologic laborator tests, histopathology is not an exact science. Pathologists bas their diagnoses on visual observations, biased knowledge, inte pretations, and opinions, and are subject to errors of judg ment, just like other physicians. Only the development of team in which clinicians and pathologists communicate an learn to speak the same language can bring results that a useful, as accurate as human opinion can be, and ultimatel useful to the patient.

FURTHER READING

Mucosal biopsy of the gastrointestinal tract

Carpenter HA, Talley NJ. Gastroscopy is incomplete without biopsy: clinical relevance of distinguishing gastropathy from gastritis. Gastroenterology 1995; 108: 917–924.
This review argues for the practice of taking mucosal biopsies from the stomach during every gastroscopy, even if no endoscopic abnormalities are visualized.

Carpenter HA, Talley NJ. The importance of clinicopathological correlation in the diagnosis of inflammatory conditions of the colon: histological patterns with clinical implications. Am J Gastroenterol 2000; 95:878–896.
Histological reaction patterns within the colon are not disease-specific but reflect mechanisms of injury and duration of disease. By correlating these patterns with known causes of colonic inflammation, the authors provide guidelines to enhance the diagnostic value of colonoscopic samples. Difficulties in differential diagnosis are underscored, and biopsy strategies are suggested.

Dixon MF, Genta RM, Yardley JH, Correa P. Classification and grading of gastritis. The Updated Sydney System. International Workshop on the Histopathology of Gastritis, Houston 1994. Am J Surg Pathol 1996; 20:1161–1181.
The Updated Sydney System, with recommendations for the acquisition of topographically defined gastric biopsies that can yield the maximum diagnostic information in the recognition of different types of gastritis and gastropathy.

Govindarajan S, Bonacini M. Liver biopsy and histopathological diagnosis. In: Yamada T, ed. Textbook of gastroenterology. Philadelphia: Lippincott Williams & Wilkins; 2003: 2947–2974.
A highly informative book chapter that discusses the technical and histopathologic aspects of liver biopsy.

Levine DS, Blount PL, Rudolph RE, Reid BJ. Safety of a systematic endoscopic biopsy protocol in patients with Barrett's esophagus Am J Gastroenterol 2000; 95:1152–1157.
A rigorous, systematic endoscopic biopsy protocol in patients with Barrett's esophagu does not produce esophageal perforation or bleeding when performed by an experience team of physicians, nurses, and technicians.

Rubin CE, Bronner MP. Endoscopic mucosal biopsy – a memorial to Rodger C. Haggitt, MD. In: Yamada T, ed. Textbook of gastroenterology. Philadelphia: Lippincott Williams & Wilkins; 2003:2893–2946.
In this book chapter the extraordinary experience of the gastrointestinal mucosa

histopathology laboratory at the University of Washington, Seattle, is transmitted in the form of practical suggestions and innumerable useful tips. It will benefit both gastroenterologists and pathologists.

'einstein WM. Mucosal biopsy techniques and interaction with the pathologist. Gastrointest Endosc Clin N Am 2000; 10:555–572.
This article illustrates how gastrointestinal biopsy and other practices can be improved so that patients benefit more than they might otherwise. It focuses on forceps biopsy technique and on dialog with the pathologist.

.iver biopsy

edossa P, Dargere D, Paradis V. Sampling variability of liver fibrosis in chronic hepatitis C Hepatology 2003; 38:1449–1457.
A recent carefully conducted study relating biopsy length to the variability of fibrosis as measured by image analysis. It determines the minimum cylinder length giving acceptable representative measurement.

Cadranel JF, Rufat P, Degos F. Practices of liver biopsy in France: results of a prospective nationwide survey. Hepatology 2000; 32:477–481.
A nationwide prospective study that evaluates practice, perception, and patient tolerance of biopsy procedures.

Crawford AR, Lin XZ, Crawford JM.The normal adult human liver biopsy: a quantitative reference standard. Hepatology 1998; 28:323–331.
This reference standard for adult human liver histology has great practical value and may assist in the histopathologic assessment of liver biopsies, particularly those performed for disease conditions featuring loss of intrahepatic bile ducts.

Grant A, Neuberger J. Guidelines on the use of liver biopsy in clinical practice. British Society of Gastroenterology. Gut 1999; 45(Suppl 4):IV1–IV11.
A nationwide British study on the use of liver biopsy in clinical practice.

Van Leeuwen DJ, Wilson L, Crowe DR. Liver biopsy in the mid-1990s: questions and answers. Semin Liver Dis 1995; 15:340–359.
A review of the changing indications and the usefulness of liver biopsy over the course of the last decades.

Chapter 136

Drugs used in gastrointestinal and liver disease

R N Cunliffe

KEY POINTS

- Proton pump inhibitors are more potent in suppressing acid than H2 antagonists
- Inhibition of cytochrome P450 by cimetidine can result in clinically important accumulation of warfarin, theophylline and phenytoin
- Aminosalicylates can cause photosensitivity
- Chronic opiates (e.g. for terminal pain relief) should normally be accompanied by a laxative
- Corticosteroids are widely used in gastroenterology
- Azathioprine/6-mercaptopurine is useful maintenance treatment for inflammatory conditions, but individuals deficient in the TPMT enzyme are at risk of bone marrow depression
- Cyclosporine, tacrolimus and methotrexate act more quickly than azathioprine/6-mecaptopurine
- Infliximab is only useful in a proportion of patients with Crohn's disease: prediction is uncertain
- All drugs should be used with caution in pregnancy
- Ribavirin is contraindicated as it has proven teratogenicity
- Patients with esophageal spasm may respond to nitrates and calcium channel blockers leading to a fallacious diagnosis of angina
- Such smooth muscle antagonists given before meals can help swallowing in achalasia

INTRODUCTION

This chapter provides an outline of established drugs used in the treatment of gastrointestinal and liver diseases. Details of drug pharmacology, indications for use, adverse effects, and important drug interactions are provided. Summary tables for many drug categories give details of routes of administration, standard dosages, and pharmacokinetics where appropriate, in order to aid rational prescribing. Further details on the drug treatment of specific conditions is given in preceding chapters.

Information provided and abbreviations used in the tables

Administration: available routes for administration of the drug; oral (po); intravenous (iv); intramuscular (im); subcutaneous (sc); topical (top; e.g., enema or suppository formulation).
Dose: typical dose regimen by stated route of administration (od, once daily; bd, twice daily; tds, three times daily; qds, four times daily).
Oral bioavailability: percentage of the oral dose that reaches arterial blood.
Time to peak concentration (T_{max}): time required for the drug to reach maximal concentration in the blood (after an oral dose).
Half-life ($T_{1/2}$): time required for the concentration of drug in the blood to decline by one half.
Urinary excretion (%): percentage of drug that is excreted unchanged in the urine.
Dose reduction: drug dose reduction may be required to prevent accumulation in significant renal (R) or liver (L) disease.
Abbreviations: u, unknown; n/a, not applicable (e.g., when drug has a local rather than systemic effect).
Drug dosages: all dosages quoted are those for use in adults.

DRUGS USED IN INTESTINAL MOTILITY DISORDERS

Antispasmodic agents (Table 136.1)

Pharmacology

The muscarinic antagonist drugs atropine, dicylomine, hyoscine, and propantheline competitively inhibit binding of acetylcholine to smooth muscle muscarinic receptors, thus resulting in smooth muscle relaxation and reduced gastrointestinal motility. Alverine and mebeverine have a direct smooth muscle relaxant effect.

Indications for use

- Relief and prevention of painful smooth muscle spasm in irritable bowel syndrome (see Chapter 64)[1]
- Hyoscine may be used intravenously (20 mg) to reduce bowel spasm during endoscopic and radiologic procedures.

Side effects

Common side effects of antimuscarinic agents include constipation, urinary retention, blurred vision, and dry mouth. The muscle relaxants alverine and mebeverine are well tolerated

TABLE 136.1 ANTISPASMODIC AGENTS

	Dicyclomine	Hyoscine	Propantheline	Alverine	Mebeverine
Administration	po	po, iv, im	po	po	po
Oral dose	20 mg tds	10–20 mg qds	15–30 mg qds	60–120 mg tds	135–270 mg tds
Dose reduction	–	–	–	–	–

with no serious side effects. Antispasmodics should not be used in paralytic ileus. Limited data are available on their use in pregnancy.

Additional information

Tricyclic and monoamine oxygenase inhibitor antidepressants, and antihistamines, potentiate the side effects of antimuscarinic drugs.

Miscellaneous smooth muscle relaxants

(Table 136.2)

Peppermint oil

Peppermint oil is believed to have a direct smooth muscle relaxant action and may be used to relieve painful intestinal spasm and bloating in irritable bowel syndrome (see Chapter 64). It is less constipating than the antimuscarinic antispasmodic agents, but may cause heartburn.

Calcium channel antagonists

Dihydropyridine calcium channel antagonists, such as nifedipine, and isosorbide dinitrate reduce smooth muscle tone. They may be useful in the management of esophageal spasm, and occasionally for short-term relief of achalasia prior to more definitive management. Both commonly cause headache, which may diminish on dose reduction.

Botulinum toxin

Botulinum toxin inhibits release of acetylcholine from cholinergic nerve terminals at the neuromuscular junction, resulting in muscular paralysis. Achalasia may be treated by local injection of botulinum toxin A (Botox; 100 units) into the lower esophageal sphincter at endoscopy, using a sclerotherapy needle.[2] Sphincter paralysis results in resolution of dysphagia (see Chapter 3) lasting for up to 4 months, after which further injections may be administered periodically.

TABLE 136.2 MISCELLANEOUS SMOOTH MUSCLE RELAXANTS

Drug	Dosage
Peppermint oil	1–2 capsules po tds
Calcium antagonists, e.g., nifedipine	5–10 mg po before meals
Nitrates, e.g., isosorbide dinitrate	5–10 mg po before meals
Botulinum toxin	100 IU intrasphincteric at endoscopy

Prokinetic agents (Table 136.3)

Prokinetic agents stimulate gastric emptying and intestinal transit. A variety of drug classes are used.

Pharmacology

Dopaminergic neurons have an inhibitory effect on cholinergic myenteric motor neurons and reduce gastrointestinal motility. Domperidone, a dopamine receptor antagonist, therefore prevents this inhibition and results in a prokinetic effect. Excitatory neurons with 5-hydroxytryptamine type 4 (5-HT_4) receptors also synapse with cholinergic neurons in the myenteric plexus. Metoclopramide acts predominantly as an agonist at 5-HT_4 receptors, stimulating intestinal motility. It also has a minor antagonist effect at the inhibitory dopamine receptors. Motilin is a peptide hormone produced by M cells and enterochromaffin cells in the gastrointestinal tract. It acts on specific receptors on intestinal smooth muscle cells resulting in amplification of the migrating motor complex and a prokinetic effect. Erythromycin acts as a motilin receptor agonist. Neostigmine is an acetylcholinesterase inhibitor and thus allows acetylcholine to accumulate at its sites of release, including the neuromuscular junction in the myenteric plexus, with a resultant prokinetic effect.

Indications

- Nonulcer dyspepsia (domperidone) (see Chapter 5)
- Gastroparesis
- Delayed gastric emptying (see Chapter 41) after surgery
- Acute intestinal pseudo-obstruction (see Chapter 62) (erythromycin and neostigmine[3]).

Side effects

Domperidone and metoclopramide are generally well tolerated. Rarely they may cause serious extrapyramidal side effects including dystonic reactions, particularly in young people. They can also raise prolactin levels and cause galactorrhea. Rare side effects of erythromycin include allergic reactions, cholestatic jaundice, and reversible hearing loss. Side effects associated with the use of neostigmine for pseudo-obstruction include abdominal pain, salivation, and vomiting.

Additional information

Prokinetic agents should not be used when mechanical intestinal obstruction is suspected. Rectal suppository formulations of domperidone are available. Metoclopramide can raise plasma ciclosporin levels. Erythromycin inhibits the CYP3A enzyme system and thus has important interactions with drugs metab-

TABLE 136.3 PROKINETIC AGENTS

	Domperidone	Metoclopramide	Erythromycin	Neostigmine
Administration	po, top	po, iv, im	po, iv	iv
Oral dose	10–20 mg tds	10 mg tds	250 mg qds	2 mg once only
Oral bioavailability (%)	17	76	35	–
T_{max} (h)	0.5	1	2	–
$T_{1/2}$ (h)	7	5	1.6	1.3
Urinary excretion (%)	31	20	12	67
Dose reduction	–	L, R	R	R

olized by it (including ciclosporin), often resulting in increased plasma levels. Limited data are available on use of domperidone, metoclopramide, and neostigmine in pregnancy, but they should be avoided unless essential. Erythromycin is not contraindicated in pregnancy.

DRUGS USED IN ACID/PEPTIC DISORDERS

Proton pump inhibitors (Table 136.4)

Pharmacology

Proton pump inhibitors (PPIs) are highly effective at inhibiting gastric acid secretion and work by irreversibly binding to the hydrogen potassium ATPase (proton pump) of the gastric parietal cell. They are the first-line treatment for acid/peptic related disorders. At standard oral doses for 7 days, production of gastric acid is reduced by more than 95%. After discontinuation of these drugs, production of acid resumes only once new proton pump molecules have been generated, and the duration of action is not directly related to the drug plasma half-life.

Indications for use

- Gastroesophageal reflux disease (GERD; see Chapter 29) – standard dose may be doubled in severe and complicated cases, or halved where long-term maintenance is required
- Acid-related dyspepsia and nonulcer dyspepsia (see Chapter 5)
- Healing of nonsteroidal anti-inflammatory drug (NSAID)-induced gastroduodenal ulceration and erosions (see Chapter 35)
- Maintenance of peptic ulcer healing and prevention of ulceration in selected groups of patients, including those who require continued NSAID treatment (see Chapters 25 and 35)
- Healing of benign gastric and duodenal ulcer, not due to NSAIDs; standard dose may be doubled in severe cases. *Helicobacter pylori* eradication is now the primary preferred approach in such patients
- *H. pylori* eradication regimens (see below; see also Chapter 34)
- Reduction of intestinal secretory output in management of short bowel (see Chapter 45) and high-output jejunostomy[4]
- Reduction of gastric acid production during general anesthesia
- Zollinger-Ellison syndrome (high doses often required).

Side effects

The most common side effects of PPIs are diarrhea, headache, and skin rashes. Other reported side effects are abdominal pain, flatulence, and constipation.

Additional information

PPIs are metabolized by the hepatic cytochrome P450 enzyme system. High-dosage regimens may result in drug accumulation in severe liver disease and standard doses only are recommended. PPIs inhibit some hepatic cytochrome P450 enzymes and may reduce the clearance of warfarin and phenytoin; this effect is less of a problem with lansoprazole. Omeprazole and pantoprazole may be used intravenously in the treatment of peptic ulcers complicated by acute bleeding, where rapid reduction of gastric acid output promotes blood clot formation and stability, and reduces the chance of rebleeding.[5] Very little information is available on the use of PPIs in pregnancy and, although there is no evidence of significant teratogenicity, they should be given only when considered essential.

Histamine H_2 receptor antagonists (Table 136.5)

Pharmacology

H_2 receptor antagonists (H2RAs) competitively inhibit binding of histamine to H_2 receptors on the basolateral membrane of gastric parietal cells. Resultant decreased levels of intracellular cyclic adenosine monophosphate (cAMP) lead to reduced activation of the hydrogen potassium ATPase, and reduced acid secretion.

Indications for use

The indications for H2RA use are the same as those for PPI use listed above. PPIs are considered superior to H2RAs, with faster healing of ulceration and relief of acid-related symptoms. H2RAs are not effective in healing or preventing the recurrence of gastric ulceration associated with continued NSAID use (see Chapters 25 and 35). H2RAs are not used in *H. pylori* eradication regimens (see Chapter 34). They may be used in a 'step-down' approach to symptom relief in GERD (see Chapter 29) and acid-related dyspepsia (see Chapter 5). In the setting of critical illness, intravenous H2RAs may be used for prophylaxis of gastroduodenal stress ulceration (see Chapter 35); this indication may become superseded now that intravenous PPIs are available.

TABLE 136.4 PROTON PUMP INHIBITORS

	Omeprazole	Esomeprazole	Lansoprazole	Rabeprazole	Pantoprazole
Administration	po, iv	po	po	po	po, iv
Standard oral dose (PU and GERD)	20 mg od	40 mg od	30 mg od	20 mg od	40 mg od
Oral bioavailability (%)	60	89	81	52	77
T_{max} (h)	1–4	1.5	1.3	4	2.5
$T_{1/2}$ (h)	0.7	1.3	0.9	1.3	1
Urinary excretion (%)	<1	<1	<1	<1	<1
Dose reduction	L	L	L	–	–

PU, peptic ulcer; GERD, gastroesophageal reflux disease.

TABLE 136.5 H_2 RECEPTOR ANTAGONIST DRUGS

	Cimetidine	Ranitidine	Famotidine	Nizatidine
Administration	po, iv, im	po, iv, im	po	po, iv
Standard oral dose (PU and GERD)	400 mg bd or 800 mg nocte	150 mg bd or 300 mg nocte	40 mg nocte	150 mg bd or 300 mg nocte
Oral bioavailability (%)	60	52	40	70
T_{max} (h)	0.5	2.1	1	0.5
$T_{1/2}$ (h)	2.0	2.1	2.5	1
Urinary excretion (%)	62	69	30	60
Dose reduction	L, R	L, R	R	R

PU, peptic ulcer; GERD, gastroesophageal reflux disease

Side effects

H2RAs are well tolerated and side effects are rare. Recognized minor side effects include diarrhea, constipation, headache, and altered liver chemistry. Confusion, hallucinations, pancreatitis, cardiac dysrhythmias, gynecomastia in men, and blood disorders have been reported.

Additional information

Cimetidine inhibits cytochrome P450 and this can result in clinically relevant increased levels of some drugs metabolized by this enzyme (e.g., warfarin, theophyllines, and phenytoin). Limited data are available on the use of H2RAs in pregnancy, and they should be avoided unless considered essential.

Misoprostol (Table 136.6)

Pharmacology

Misoprostol is a synthetic analog of prostaglandin E1. By binding to prostanoid receptors on parietal cells it results in reduced levels of cAMP and subsequent inhibition of acid production. It also has a gastric mucosal cytoprotective effect, stimulating mucin and bicarbonate secretion from gastric mucosal cells, and increasing mucosal blood flow.

Indications[6]

- Healing of NSAID-induced gastric (see Chapters 25 and 35) and duodenal ulceration
- Prevention of NSAID-induced gastroduodenal ulceration
- Healing of benign gastric and duodenal ulcer (rarely used for this purpose).

Side effects

Diarrhea is reported in up to 30% of patients and may be sufficiently severe to require misoprostol withdrawal. This effect is dose dependent and may resolve upon dose reduction.

Additional information

Misoprostol increases uterine contractility and can cause abortion; its use should be avoided in women of childbearing potential, unless adequate contraceptive measures are taken.

Sucralfate (Table 136.6)

Pharmacology

Sucralfate is a complex of aluminum hydroxide and sulfated sucrose. Its pharmacologic action is due to local rather than systemic effects. In the acidic gastric environment it polymerizes to form a viscous gel that adheres to gastric epithelial cells and ulcer craters. Pepsin-mediated hydrolysis of mucosal proteins is inhibited, which has a mucosal protectant effect. Sucralfate may also stimulate local production of prostaglandins and epidermal growth factor, to promote ulcer healing.

TABLE 136.6 MISCELLANEOUS ULCER HEALING DRUGS

	Misoprostol	Sucralfate
Administration	po	po
Oral dose (peptic ulcer)	200 μg qds	1 g qds
Oral bioavailability (%)	80	n/a
T_{max} (h)	0.4	n/a
$T_{1/2}$ (h)	0.5	n/a
Urinary excretion (%)	<1	n/a
Dose reduction	–	R

Indications for use

- Prophylaxis of stress ulceration in critically ill patients (1 g six times daily)[7]
- Healing of benign gastric and duodenal ulceration (see Chapter 35).

Side effects

The most common side effect is constipation, occurring in 2% of patients.

Additional information

Small amounts of aluminum may be absorbed from sucralfate which should be used cautiously in patients with renal failure who are prone to aluminum overload.

Antacids and alginates

A wide variety of aluminum- and magnesium-containing compounds (e.g., aluminum hydroxide and magnesium trisilicate) have been used historically and are still available as acid-neutralizing agents for relief of dyspeptic symptoms. They may be combined with alginate compounds to reduce symptoms due to gastroesophageal reflux.

Helicobacter pylori eradication regimens

Gastric and duodenal ulcers associated with *H. pylori* infection can usually be healed by eradicating the organism. After sucessful eradication, recurrence of an ulcer is unlikely. Typical *I. pylori* eradication regimens are shown in Table 136.7 and onsist of standard dose of PPI combined with two of the antiiotics amoxicillin, clarithromycin, and metronidazole (triple ierapy), taken twice daily for 1 week. Using such a regimen, *I. pylori* will be eradicated in 90% of cases. For resistant infecons, an alternative 2-week regimen (quadruple therapy) may e given, as shown in Table 136.7.

TABLE 136.7 TRIPLE- AND QUADRUPLE-THERAPY REGIMENS FOR ERADICATION OF *HELICOBACTER PYLORI*

7-DAY TRIPLE-THERAPY REGIMEN
Standard-dose PPI twice daily, *plus*
Two of: amoxicillin 1 g, clarithromycin 500 mg, or metronidazole 500 mg, all twice daily

14-DAY QUADRUPLE-THERAPY REGIMEN FOLLOWING TRIPLE-THERAPY FAILURE
Double-dose PPI twice daily, *plus*
Bismuth subsalicylate or subcitrate tablet four times daily
Tetracycline hydrochloride 500 mg four times daily
Metronidazole 500 mg three times daily

AMINOSALICYLATES AND OTHER ANTIDIARRHEAL AGENTS

Aminosalicylates (Table 136.8)

Pharmacology

Aminosalicylate drugs are used predominantly for the treatment of inflammatory bowel disease (IBD). Mesalazine (5-aminosalicylic acid) is the active component of these drugs and is believed to act locally at the intestinal mucosal surface. The mechanism of action of mesalazine is unknown, but reduction of inflammatory mediator production via inhibition of cyclooxygenase and 5-lipoxygenase pathways, free radical scavenging, and abrogation of interferon expression may be important. Sulfasalazine, olsalazine, and balsalazide all incorporate an azo bond requiring metabolism by colonic bacteria to release mesalazine in the colon. Other preparations consist of mesalazine contained within an inert coating that allows release of the drug in a time- or pH-dependent manner within the small bowel and colon (Pentasa) or colon (Asacol, Salofalk).

Indications

- Induction of remission of mild–moderate active IBD (see Chapters 53–59)
- Maintenance of remission in IBD (dose may be reduced)
- Treatment of microscopic colitis (see Chapter 56) (limited evidence of benefit).

Side effects

Dose-related side effects of sulfasalazine, such as nausea, abdominal pain, and headache, are common (up to 50% of patients). These side effects are reduced with alternative mesalazine preparations which are much better tolerated and are now more popular because the sulphapyridine component of sulphasalazine causes serious side effects (Stephens Johnson syndrome, agranulocytosis and acute hemolysis). Use of sulphasalazine should be restricted to patients already established on it. Rare side effects of other aminosalicylates include blood dyscrasias, hypersensitivity reactions (avoid in salicylate hypersensitivity), interstitial nephritis, diarrhea, and a paradoxical exacerbation of colitis. Interstitial nephritis is serious and potentially irreversible, so periodic monitoring of serum creatinine may be prudent. Diarrhea is particularly common with olsalazine (20%). Salicylates increase photosensitivity.

Additional information

Enema and suppository formulations of most of these agents are also available for use in left-sided colitis and proctitis. Aminosalicylates may influence the metabolism of azathioprine and 6-mercaptopurine, and increase the risk of leukopenia.[8] Aminosalicylates are not contraindicated in pregnancy.

Other antidiarrheal agents (Table 136.9)

Colestyramine

Colestyramine is an anion exchange resin that binds bile salts; it may be useful in patients with bile salt malabsorption-associated diarrhea. In patients with idiopathic bile salt malabsorption (see Chapter 47), or terminal ileal disease or resection, excessive concentrations of bile salts reach the colon and stimulate salt and water secretion with resultant diarrhea. Colestyramine may bind medications and reduce their absorption, and so should be given separately, at least 1 h later.

Opioids

Loperamide and co-phenotrope (diphenoxylate and atropine) bind opioid receptors on myenteric neurons, resulting in hyperpolarization and reduction of acetylcholine release, with resultant

TABLE 136.8 AMINOSALICYLATE DRUGS

	Sulfasalazine	Balsalazide	Olsalazine	Mesalazine: Pentasa	Mesalazine: Asacol	Mesalazine: Salofalk
Administration	po, topical	po	po	po, topical	po, topical	po, topical
Oral dose	1–2 g qds	2.25 g tds	1 g tds	2 g bd	800 mg tds	500 mg tds
Oral bioavailability (%)	3	u	2.4	30	28	u
T_{max} (h)	6	1	1	4	4	u
$T_{1/2}$ (h)	7.6	u	0.9	u	2	1.4
Urinary excretion (%)	37	<1	<1	29	<1	<1
Dose reduction	–	–	–	–	–	–

Note that pharmacokinetic data for the delayed-release mesalazine preparations do not reflect that drug continues to be absorbed and eliminated over several hours. This is not clinically relevant as aminosalicylate drugs act topically.

TABLE 136.9 ANTIDIARRHEAL DRUGS

Drug	Dosage
Colestyramine	8 g qds; titrate down with response
Loperamide	4 mg qds; titrate down
Co-phenotrope	2 tablets qds; titrate down
Codeine	30 mg tds or qds
Bulk laxative, e.g., isphagula	3.5 g tds
Kaolin mixture	10–20 ml every 4 h
Octreotide	50–100 μg bd, sc

See text for further details on indications for use of individual drugs.

reduced bowel motility. Intestinal transit time is reduced and these drugs are useful in control of symptoms in acute and chronic diarrheal illnesses. CNS penetration is minimal, particularly with loperamide, and side effects are rare. Codeine may also be used, but the potential for dependence and abuse is greater. Opioid drugs should be avoided in active inflammatory colitides (see Chapters 53–55), where their antimotility action may precipitate the development of toxic megacolon, and in liver disease because of the risk of promoting encephalopathy.

Miscellaneous agents

Laxative bulk-forming agents such as bran and isphagula husk may be useful in chronic diarrhea (see Chapter 9), particularly that due to diverticular disease (see Chapter 65), by increasing stool bulk.

Kaolin is a hydrated aluminum silicate that binds water avidly and may be used to reduce diarrhea; it is used infrequently now.

The somatostatin analog octreotide inhibits the release of a variety of intestinal hormones and may be used to treat secretory diarrheas seen in carcinoid syndrome (see Chapter 110); it has also been used with success in other refractory diarrheas.[9]

LAXATIVES (Table 136.10)

Laxative agents may be classified according to their mode of action as bulk forming, osmotic, fecal softening, and stimulant. There may be a degree of overlap between these categories for some agents (e.g., docusate sodium has fecal softening and stimulant properties).

Pharmacology

Bulk laxatives are composed of fiber which passes undigested to the colon and attracts water, thereby increasing stool bulk and softness, and stimulating peristalsis. Osmotic laxatives are poorly or not absorbed, and bring about net water accumulation which stimulates peristalsis. Fecal softeners promote easier defecation; docusate acts as a surfactant, and liquid paraffin penetrates and softens hard stool. Stimulant laxatives probably produce a mild inflammatory reaction in the mucosa which results in the accumulation of water in the colonic lumen and stimulates intestinal motility.

Indications

- Constipation (see Chapter 63)
- Treatment and prophylaxis of opiate-induced constipation
- Fecal impaction (see Chapter 66) (Movicol)
- Hepatic encephalopathy (see Chapter 100) (lactulose).

TABLE 136.10 LAXATIVES

Category	Agent	Dose
Bulk forming	Bran	1–2 tablespoons daily
	Isphagula	Fybogel 3.5 g bd
	Methylcellulose	Celevac 1 g bd
	Stercula	Normacol 7 g bd
Osmotic	Lactulose	Lactulose 15 mL bd
	Polyethylene glycols	Movicol 1 sachet tds
	Magnesium salts	Magnesium sulfate 5 g od
Fecal softening	Liquid paraffin	10 mL nocte
Stimulant	Biscaodyl	10 mg nocte
	Dantron	Co-danthramer 2 capsules nocte
	Docusate	200 mg bd
	Anthraquinone	Senna 15 mg nocte

A wide variety of preparations of each agent are available, and dosages may vary.

Side effects

Bloating, flatulence, and abdominal pain are common with bulk forming laxatives and lactulose. Magnesium-containing preparations should be used with caution in patients with renal impairment, in whom magnesium may accumulate. Long-term use of anthraquinone laxatives may cause melanosis coli. Prolonged use of stimulant laxatives may result in a dilated atonic colon. There is danger of lipoid pneumonia with liquid paraffin.

Additional information

Laxatives should be avoided if there is a suspicion of intestinal obstruction (see Chapter 62). Dantron is a potential carcinogen and should be used to treat constipation only in terminally ill patients. Enema preparations of a variety of osmotically active and stimulant preparations are also available. Osmotic laxative based bowel cleansing solutions are used to provide an empty colon for surgical, endoscopic, and radiologic procedures. Laxatives are not known to be harmful in pregnancy.

CORTICOSTEROIDS

Prednisolone, budesonide, and hydrocortisone (intravenous) are corticosteroid preparations used frequently in gastroenterology and hepatology. Prescribing and pharmacokinetic data for prednisolone and budesonide are shown in Table 136.11.

Pharmacology

Corticosteroids have potent anti-inflammatory and immunosuppressant actions. Multiple actions result in inhibition of pro-inflammatory cytokine production and inhibition of leukocyte function.

Indications

- Induction of remission in moderately and severely active IBD (see Chapters 53–59)
- Induction and maintenance of remission in autoimmune hepatitis (see Chapter 86)
- Severe alcoholic hepatitis[10] (controversial; see Chapter 87)
- Refractory celiac disease (see Chapter 44).

TABLE 136.11 CORTICOSTEROIDS			
	Prednisolone	Budesonide	Hydrocortisone
Administration	po, top	po, top	iv, top
Starting oral/iv dose	40 mg od	9 mg od	100 mg qds
Oral bioavailability (%)	82	9	n/a
T_{max} (h)	1.5	0.5–10	n/a
$T_{1/2}$ (h)	2.2	2	1.5
Urinary excretion (%)	26	<1	<1
Dose reduction	–	L	–

Side effects

Corticosteroid preparations are generally fairly well tolerated, but many important side effects do occur, particularly with medium- to long-term use. These include mood changes, infections, hypertension, glucose intolerance, adrenal suppression, osteonecrosis, and weight gain. Patients requiring prolonged treatment with corticosteroids are at risk of osteoporosis; concurrent vitamin D and calcium supplements, or bisphosphonate treatment if the patient is elderly and/or osteopenic, should be considered. Budesonide is a novel synthetic corticosteroid with high first-pass hepatic metabolism, designed to minimize the systemic side effects associated with corticosteroid use. Corticosteroid withdrawal should be graded in order to prevent acute adrenal insufficiency.

Additional information

A variety of topical (suppository and enema) formulations of corticosteroids are available for the treatment of proctitis and distal colitis. Corticosteroid therapy may mask symptoms and clinical signs of complications such as peritonitis in severely ill patients. Corticosteroids can be given in pregnancy when their use is important for disease management, but have been associated with hair lip and cleft palate.

IMMUNOMODULATING AGENTS

Immunomodulating drugs are used widely in gastroenterology and hepatology, for a variety of indications. The main agents in current use are shown in Table 136.12.

Azathioprine/6-mercaptopurine

Pharmacology

Azathioprine is a pro-drug that is metabolized to 6-mercaptopurine. 6-Thioguanine purine analogs are the major active metabolites of these drugs. The mechanism of action is unclear, but is probably largely through a T cell-suppressant effect.

Indications

- Induction of remission in chronically active and corticosteroid refractory IBD (see Chapters 53–59)
- Maintenance of remission in IBD
- Maintenance of remission in autoimmune hepatitis (see Chapter 86)
- Prevention of rejection in liver transplantation (see Chapter 106).

Side effects

Some 5–10% of patients experience side effects such as nausea, vomiting, malaise, diarrhea, and arthralgia. Pancreatitis occurs in 3% of patients, and abnormal liver chemistry in 2%. Bone marrow suppression with leukopenia may occur in up to 4% of patients, usually within the first few weeks of treatment, but sometimes much later. Individuals deficient in thiopurine methyltransferase, an enzyme involved in 6-mercaptopurine metabolism whose activity is genetically determined, are particularly at risk of profound bone marrow depression. Regular monitoring of the full blood count should take place to detect development of leukopenia.

TABLE 136.12 IMMUNOMODULATING DRUGS						
	Azathioprine	6-Mercaptopurine	Ciclosporin	Tacrolimus	Mycophenolate	Methotrexate
Administration	po	po	po, iv	po, iv	po, iv	po, im, sc
Daily oral dose (IBD)[a]	2.5 mg/kg	1.5 mg/kg	5 mg/kg	0.2 mg/kg	20 mg/kg	Given weekly[b]
Oral bioavailability (%)	60	12	28	25	94	70
T_{max} (h)	1–2	2.4	1.5	1.4	1–2	0.9
$T_{1/2}$ (h)	0.16	1	10.7	12	16	7.2
Urinary excretion (%)	<2	22	<1	<1	<1	81
Dose reduction	R, L	R, L	R, L	L	–	R

[a] Dosages given are for use in inflammatory bowel disease (IBD); dosages in transplantation may be higher.
[b] Methotrexate is given at a dosage of 15–25 mg *once weekly*; intramuscular administration may be superior to oral.

Additional information

These agents have a delayed onset of action, and 2–4 months of treatment are required before their full effect is achieved. Xanthine oxidase is also involved in the metabolism of 6-mercaptopurine to inactive metabolites. Allopurinol, which is an inhibitor of this enzyme, should not be co-prescribed with azathioprine/6-mercaptopurine. Azathioprine and 6-mercaptopurine are not contraindicated in pregnancy.

Mycophenolate mofetil

Pharmacology

Mycophenolate is rapidly hydrolyzed to the active metabolite mycophenolic acid, which inhibits inosine monophosphate dehydrogenase. This enzyme is particularly important in purine nucleotide synthesis for T- and B-cell proliferation, and treatment with mycophenolate results in a lymphocyte suppressant effect.

Indications

- Prevention of rejection in liver transplantation (see Chapter 106)
- Treatment of chronically active IBD (see Chapters 53–59) (emerging treatment).[11]

Side effects

Diarrhea, constipation, nausea, arthralgia, pancreatitis, and abnormal liver chemistry have all been reported. As with azathioprine, bone marrow suppression and leukopenia is a serious side effect and regular monitoring of the full blood count should be undertaken. Severe drug-induced colitis has also been reported.

Additional information

Mycophenolate absorption is reduced by cholestyramine, so co-prescription should be avoided. Mycophenolate may increase plasma levels of acyclovir and ganciclovir. It is contraindicated in pregnancy.

Ciclosporin

Pharmacology

Ciclosporin is a peptide calcineurin inhibitor which prevents transcription of interleukin 2 and inhibits T-cell activation.

Indications

- Induction of remission in severely active, corticosteroid refractory, ulcerative colitis (see Chapter 53) (usually initiated +/– corticosteroids intravenously at a dose of 2–4 mg/kg)
- Prevention of rejection in liver transplantation (see Chapter 106).

Side effects

Headache, nausea, gingival hyperplasia, hypertrichosis, paresthesias, and tremors all occur commonly. Potentially serious side effects occur in about 10%, and include hypertension, electrolyte abnormalities (usually hyperkalemia), renal impairment, and abnormal liver chemistry. Careful clinical and laboratory monitoring is required. These effects usually resolve on dose reduction or drug withdrawal. Seizures may occur; patients with hypocholesterolemia (cholesterol level <3.1 mmol/L) and hypomagnesemia are at particular risk.

Additional information

Ciclosporin is metabolized in the liver by the cytochrome P450 3A (CYP3A) enzymes. Consequently ciclosporin has a number of important interactions with other drugs that influence the activity of this enzyme system. Calcium channel antagonists (diltiazem, verapamil), antifungal agents (ketoconazole, fluconazole), antibiotics (erythromycin, doxycycline) methylprednisolone, omeprazole, and grapefruit juice all can increase ciclosporin plasma concentrations. Anticonvulsants (phenytoin, carbamazepine, phenobarbital), and rifampin can reduce ciclosporin plasma concentrations. Close laboratory monitoring of ciclosporin levels is therefore required. Other potentially nephrotoxic agents, such as NSAIDs should be used with caution in patients on ciclosporin. On balance ciclosporin is not contraindicated in pregnancy.

Tacrolimus (FK506)

Pharmacology

Tacrolimus is a calcineurin inhibitor with a mechanism of action very similar to that of ciclosporin.

Indications

- Prevention of rejection in liver transplantation (see Chapter 106)
- Treatment of chronically active IBD (see Chapters 53–59) (emerging treatment).[12]

Side effects

Gastrointestinal disturbances, headache, paresthesia, and tremors may all occur. As with ciclosporin, hypertension, hyperkalemia, nephrotoxicity, and seizures are important limiting side effects. Tacrolimus has an inhibitory effect on pancreatic beta-cells, and glucose intolerance and diabetes may develop.

Additional information

Like ciclosporin, tacrolimus is extensively metabolized by the CYP3A enzyme system in the liver, and the potential for drug interactions is great. It is necessary to monitor tacrolimus blood levels closely to prevent toxicity and optimize therapeutic efficacy. Tacrolimus is contraindicated in pregnancy.

Methotrexate

Pharmacology

Methotrexate is a dihydrofolate reductase inhibitor and inhibits folate-dependent metabolic pathways. An immunosuppressant effect is found as a result of reduced DNA synthesis, leukocyte proliferation, and pro-inflammatory cytokine synthesis.

Indications

- Chronically active, steroid refractory Crohn's disease (see Chapter 56).

Side effects

Nausea, abdominal pain, diarrhea, and mucositis may occur in up to 10% of patients. Weekly dosing and daily folic acid supplementation on the six days that methotrexate is not given reduce the risk of these side effects. Bone marrow suppression and leukopenia occurs in up to 1%, and the full blood count should be monitored. Methotrexate-induced hepatic toxicity is important. Liver chemistry should be monitored; abnormalities are seen in 6% of patients at some stage during therapy, and may be transient. Liver fibrosis or cirrhosis may develop with long-term use and there may be a role for periodic liver biopsy. Methotrexate treatment should probably be avoided in patients with underlying liver disease, or in those at risk of liver disease (e.g., alcohol excess, diabetes, obesity). Hypersensitivity pneumonitis occurs in up to 2% and should be suspected if cough and dyspnea develop.

Additional information

Concurrent use of other drugs that inhibit folate metabolism (e.g., sulfonamides, trimethoprim) will potentiate the effect of methotrexate and should be avoided. Methotrexate is abortifacient, and is contraindicated in pregnancy.

BIOLOGIC AGENTS: INFLIXIMAB

A variety of biologic agents are currently under investigation as gastrointestinal therapeutics. The value of infliximab is now well established, and it is in widespread use.

Pharmacology

Infliximab is a mouse–human chimeric IgG_1 monoclonal antibody directed against tumor necrosis factor (TNF). It acts by neutralization of soluble and membrane-bound TNF, and thus inhibits amplification of the inflammatory cytokine cascade seen in inflammatory diseases such as rheumatoid arthritis and Crohn's disease. It may also result in the destruction of TNF-producing cells by complement fixation, antibody-dependent cytotoxicity, and induction of apoptosis.

Indications and dosing

Infliximab is administered as an intravenous infusion at a dose of 5–10 mg/kg.

- Induction of remission in severely active Crohn's disease (see Chapter 56) refractory to corticosteroid treatment
- Maintenance of remission in Crohn's disease (if treatment with conventional immunomodulators fails)
- Fistulating Crohn's disease.

Side effects

Infliximab treatment is generally well tolerated, but a variety of important side effects are now recognized.[13] These include infusion reactions (urticaria, dyspnea, hypotension), delayed hypersensitivity reactions (rash, fever, arthralgia, myalgia, facial swelling), lupus-like syndrome, and serious infections, including reactivation of latent tuberculosis. Congestive heart failure is made worse by infliximab and is a contraindication to treatment.

Additional information

Infliximab is contraindicated in pregnancy.

ANTIVIRAL AGENTS USED IN VIRAL HEPATITIS

Antiviral drugs are used to treat chronic hepatitis B virus (HBV) and hepatitis C virus (HCV) infection. Agents in current use are shown in Table 136.13.

Interferon-α

Pharmacology

Interferons are natural cytokines with antiviral and immunomodulatory actions. Recombinant preparations are used therapeutically. Interferons bind to specific cellular receptors and, via a signal transduction pathway, result in the synthesis of a variety of proteins that inhibit viral replication. Mechanisms include inhibition of translation of viral proteins, inhibition of virus particle maturation, and prevention of membrane budding. Conjugation of interferon to inert polyethylene glycol (PEG–interferon) prolongs the plasma half-life and increases therapeutic efficacy.

Indications

- Chronic HBV infection (see Chapter 82A)
- Chronic HCV infection (see Chapter 82B) (ideally in combination with ribavirin).

Side effects

Common dose-related side effects include influenza-like symptoms such as headache, myalgia, arthralgia, fever, and lethargy, and also depression and insomnia. Myelosuppression with minor leukopenia and thrombocytopenia also occurs, and the blood count should be monitored. Rarer serious side effects include neuropsychiatric disturbances with psychosis and suicidal ideation, and autoimmune disorders including hepatitis.

TABLE 136.13 ANTIVIRAL AGENTS USED IN CHRONIC VIRAL HEPATITIS

	Interferon-α	PEG–interferon-α 2a	Lamivudine	Adefovir dipivoxil	Ribavirin
Administration	sc	sc	po	po	po
Dosage	HBV: 10 MU three times weekly HCV: 3 MU three times weekly	1.5 μg/kg weekly	100 mg od	10 mg od	<75 kg: 1000 mg od >75 kg: 1200 mg od
Bioavailability (%)	80–90	84	86	59	45
T_{max} (h)	7	80	0.5–1.5	1.75	3
$T_{1/2}$ (h)	0.7	77	9	7.5	28
Urinary excretion (%)	–	–	71	45	35
Dose reduction	–	–	R	R	–

HBV, hepatitis B virus; HCV, hepatitis C virus; MU, million units.

Additional information

Interferon can inhibit metabolism of theophylline by the cytochrome P450 system, resulting in significantly enhanced levels. Interferon should be used with great caution in patients with decompensated liver disease, and is contraindicated in immunosuppressed patients. Data are not available on the use of interferon in pregnancy.

Lamivudine

Pharmacology

Lamivudine is a cytidine nucleoside analog that inhibits HBV DNA polymerase and prevents viral replication.

Indications

- Chronic HBV infection (see Chapter 82A).

Side effects

Lamivudine is well tolerated, but headache, nausea, fatigue, and insomnia can all occur. Severe cases (including death) of lactic acidosis with severe hepatomegaly and steatosis have been reported with the use of antiviral nucleoside analogs, including lamivudine. Patients should be monitored closely and have their liver chemistry checked regularly.

Additional information

Co-trimoxazole and trimethoprim can increase lamivudine plasma levels. There are no data on the use of lamivudine in pregnancy.

Adefovir dipivoxil

Pharmacology

Adefovir is an adenosine nucleotide analog that inhibits HBV DNA polymerase and prevents replication. It is active against lamivudine-resistant strains.

Indications

- Chronic HBV infection (see Chapter 82A).

Side effects

Nausea, abdominal pain, headache, and diarrhea can all occur. Nephrotoxicity is a serious side effect that may occur after several months' treatment, particularly at higher doses. Hepatotoxicity and hepatic steatosis with hepatomegaly and lactic acidosis have also been reported. Patients should have their renal and liver function monitored carefully.

Additional information

Adefovir is contraindicated in pregnancy.

Ribavirin

Pharmacology

Ribavirin is a purine nucleoside analog that inhibits viral messenger RNA synthesis and prevents HCV replication.

Indications

- Chronic HCV infection (see Chapter 82B) (in combination with interferon).

Side effects

Common side effects are fatigue, depression, insomnia, and nausea. Dose-related hemolytic anemia is the major serious side effect, occurring in about 8% of patients. Ribavirin should not be used in patients with decompensated chronic liver disease, renal impairment, or severe cardiovascular disease.

Additional information

Ribavirin is teratogenic. It is contraindicated in pregnancy; effective contraception should be continued for 6 months after cessation of ribavirin treatment.

VASOACTIVE AGENTS USED FOR VARICEAL HEMORRHAGE

Vasoactive agents are useful adjuncts to endoscopic therapy in the control of esophageal variceal hemorrhage. Octreotide and terlipressin are the two agents in most frequent use; vasopressin is infrequently used now owing to its significant side effect of cardiac ischemia. Octreotide and terlipressin have other indications for use in gastroenterology and hepatology (see below).

Octreotide

Pharmacology

Octreotide is a synthetic analog of the hypothalamic release inhibiting peptide hormone somatostatin. It has a direct action on vascular smooth muscle that brings about splanchnic arteriolar vasoconstriction and so reduces portal blood flow.

Indications

- Control of esophageal variceal hemorrhage (see Chapter 23) (50 μg/h intravenous infusion)
- Symptomatic treatment of carcinoid syndrome (see Chapter 110) and VIPoma (50–100 μg subcutaneously three times daily).
- Refractory diarrhea
- Gastric dumping syndrome.

Side effects

Octreotide is well tolerated but can cause nausea and bloating. Both hyperglycemia and hypoglycemia have been reported.

Additional information

Long-acting octreotide preparations are available with monthly intramuscular dosing for the treatment of symptoms associated with carcinoid tumors and VIPomas. Long-term octreotide therapy can cause gallstone formation.

Terlipressin

Pharmacology

Terlipressin is a synthetic derivative of vasopressin. It is a V_1 receptor agonist that causes splanchnic arteriolar vasoconstriction and so reduces portal blood flow.

Indications

- Control of esophageal variceal hemorrhage (see Chapter 23) (2 mg intravenously every 4–6 h)
- Adjunct for the treatment of hepatorenal failure.

Side effects

Terlipressin is usually well tolerated, but dose-related tremor, sweating, nausea, vomiting, and abdominal cramps can all occur. Coronary artery constriction precipitating angina may also occur, and terlipressin should be avoided in patients with ischemic heart disease.

ANCREATIC ENZYME SUPPLEMENTS

harmacology

ancreatic enzyme supplements contain protease, lipase, and mylase enzymes. A variety of different preparations at variable trengths, mainly of porcine origin, are available. Dosage is itrated according to clinical response, but a typical requirement s 1200 units protease and 20 000 units lipase with each meal; mylase is least important as salivary amylase is still produced.

ndications

- Malabsorption due to pancreatic exocrine sufficiency in chronic pancreatitis (see Chapter 72), cystic fibrosis, and following pancreatectomy
- Treatment of pain in chronic pancreatitis.

ide effects

ancreatic enzyme preparations are well tolerated. Nausea and bdominal discomfort can occur.

Additional information

ancreatic enzyme supplements should be taken with meals as he enzymes are inactivated by gastric acid; most preparations re also enteric-coated. There have been reports of colonic stricure formation in children with cystic fibrosis following the use of high-strength pancreatic enzyme preparations. High doses an also cause perianal irritation.

URSODEOXYCHOLIC ACID

Pharmacology

Ursodeoxycholic acid is a hydrophilic dehydroxylated bile acid that naturally forms 1–3% of the total bile acid pool in humans. Administration of ursodeoxycholic acid alters the bile acid composition of bile, decreases biliary lipid excretion, and reduces the biliary cholesterol content. It also alters plasma bile acid composition and may have a cytoprotective effect on hepatocytes.

Indications

- Treatment of cholestatic liver diseases, including primary biliary cirrhosis (see Chapter 85) and primary sclerosing cholangitis (see Chapter 78) (10–15 mg/kg daily in two to four divided doses)
- Symptomatic relief of pruritus in cholestasis.

Side effects

Ursodeoxycholic acid can cause nausea, vomiting, and diarrhea, and may sometimes exacerbate pruritus.

Additional information

Ursodeoxycholic acid was originally used with limited success for the dissolution of gallstones. With the advent of laparoscopic surgical and endoscopic techniques, it is rarely used for this indication now.

EFERENCES

1. Poynard T, Naveau S, Mory B, Chaput JC. Meta-analysis of smooth muscle relaxants in the treatment of irritable bowel syndrome. Aliment Pharmacol Ther 1994; 8:499–510.
2. Pasricha PJ, Ravich WJ, Hendrix TR, Sostre S, Jones B, Kalloo AN. Intrasphincteric injection of botulinum toxin for the treatment of achalasia. N Engl J Med 1995; 332:774–778.
3. Ponec RJ, Saunders MD, Kimmey MB. Neostigmine for the treatment of acute colonic pseudo-obstruction. N Engl J Med 1999; 341:137–141.
4. Nightingale JMD, Walker ER, Farthing MJG, Lennard Jones JE. Effect of omeprazole on intestinal output in short bowel syndrome. Aliment Pharmacol Ther 1991; 5:405–412.
5. Lau JY, Sung JJ, Lee KK et al. Effect of intravenous omeprazole on recurrent bleeding after endoscopic treatment of bleeding peptic ulcers. N Engl J Med 2000; 343:310–316.
6. Walt RP. Misoprostol for the treatment of peptic ulcer and antiinflammatory-drug-induced gastroduodenal ulceration. N Engl J Med 1992; 327:1575–1580.
7. Cook D, Guyatt G, Marshall J et al. A comparison of sucralfate and ranitidine for the prevention of upper gastrointestinal bleeding in patients requiring mechanical ventilation. Canadian Critical Care Trials Group. N Engl J Med 1998; 338:791–797.
8. Lowry PW, Franklin CL, Weaver AL et al. Leucopenia resulting from a drug interaction between azathioprine or 6-mercaptopurine and mesalamine, sulphasalazine, or balsalazide. Gut 2001; 49:656–664.
9. Szilagyi A, Shrier I. The use of somatostatin or octreotide in refractory diarrhoea. Aliment Pharmacol Ther 2001; 15:1889–1897.
10. Ramond MJ, Poynard T, Rueff B. A randomised trial of prednisolone in patients with severe alcoholic hepatitis. N Engl J Med 1992; 326:507–512.
11. Ford AC, Towler RJ, Moayyedi P, Chalmers DM, Axon ATR. Mycophenolate mofetil in refractory inflammatory bowel disease. Aliment Pharmacol Ther 2003; 17:1365–1369.
12. Sandborn WJ, Present DH, Isaacs KL et al. Tacrolimus for the treatment of fistulas in patients with Crohn's disease: a randomised placebo controlled trial. Gastroenterology 2003; 125:380–388.
13. Colombel J, Loftus EV, Tremaine WJ et al. The safety profile of infliximab in patients with Crohn's disease: the Mayo Clinic experience in 500 patients. Gastroenterology 2004; 126:19–31.

Chapter 137

Drug prescription in liver disease

Stefan Russmann and Jürg Reichen

KEY POINTS

- No liver test reliably predicts pharmacokinetics and pharmacodynamics in individual patients with liver disease
- For an estimation of pharmacokinetic changes, consider probable changes in physiologic parameters associated with liver disease, and the main mechanism of elimination, hepatic extraction ratio, and mode of application of the drug. Generally avoid drugs with a high first-pass metabolism in cirrhosis
- Pre-existing liver disease does not necessarily imply an increased risk of hepatotoxicity, although the capacity to compensate for an additional drug-induced damage may be impaired
- Closely monitor drug effects and, if indicated, plasma concentrations, and adjust the dose accordingly rather than using a standard dose ('start low, go slow')

INTRODUCTION

Most drugs undergo extensive metabolism in the liver, which therefore represents the central organ for drug elimination, and the liver may also become a major determinant of bioavailability after oral administration of a drug. Liver disease may modify the effect of a drug independently of its pharmacokinetics, and may also increase the risk or be the target of adverse drug effects. Pharmacotherapy in patients with liver disease consequently raises three major issues:[1]

1. Are pharmacokinetics altered?
2. Are pharmacodynamics altered?
3. Is there an increased risk of adverse reactions including hepatotoxicity?

PHARMACOKINETICS IN LIVER DISEASE

From the pharmacokinetic point of view, the physiologic processes that may be primarily altered in liver disease are:

- Hepatic circulation, particularly portosystemic shunting
- Intrahepatic diffusion processes (fibrosis of the space of Disse and loss of fenestrae with consequent functional impairment of sinusoidal exchange)
- Amount of functional liver cell and enzyme mass with consequent changes in metabolic capacity
- Biliary excretion
- Body fluid distribution (ascites)
- Low plasma albumin levels leading to a decrease in plasma protein binding of drugs.

Pharmacokinetic alterations in liver disease that will ultimately lead to changes in a drug's plasma concentration over time may be predicted by integrating physiologic alterations with basic pharmacokinetic principles. Physiologic alterations result mainly from the effect of liver disease on:

- Drug distribution
- Liver perfusion
- Intrinsic hepatic drug clearance.

Organ clearance: The most important step for this integration is the application of the organ clearance concept.[2] Clearance is generally defined as the proportionality factor between drug concentration (C) and rate of elimination ($Rate_{eli}$). If clearance is related to a specific organ, in this case the liver (CL_h), this relation can be expressed as:

$$Rate_{eli} = CL_h * C \qquad [1]$$

This equation implies that more drug is eliminated per unit of time as its plasma concentration increases. This concept is valid as long as drug removal in the range of the usual therapeutic concentrations is dependent on hepatic enzymes, which follow Michaelis-Menten kinetics. Hepatic clearance is therefore a measure of the liver's capacity to eliminate a drug, independent of its plasma concentration.

Extraction ratio: From the physiologic point of view, the drawback of this equation is that only the actual 'intrinsic' hepatic metabolic capacity is a function of enzyme mass and activity, and that other factors such as diffusion processes and hepatic perfusion are not considered. The issue of hepatic perfusion can be addressed if the concept of the extraction ratio of an eliminating organ is introduced. The extraction ratio (E) is defined as the fraction of drug in the incoming blood supply of the liver (i.e., portal vein and hepatic artery) that is removed during one passage through the liver:

$$E = \frac{(\text{Concentration in inflow tract} - \text{Concentration in outflow tract})}{\text{Concentration in inflow tract}} \qquad [2]$$

Hepatic clearance can now be expressed as the product of hepatic blood flow (Q) and extraction ratio:

$$CL_h = Q * E \qquad [3]$$

For example, if the extraction ratio of a drug is 0.1 and the liver blood flow is 1.3 L/min, then 0.13 L blood are cleared from the drug per minute by the liver (eqn [3]). Further, if the average concentration in the hepatic artery and the portal vein were, for example, 10 mg/L, the rate of elimination from blood would be 1.3 mg/min (eqn [1]). Like hepatic clearance, the extraction ratio is a measure of the rate of elimination that is independent of concentration, but is also independent of liver blood flow. Therefore it directly reflects the functional metabolic capacity of the liver, i.e., the intrinsic hepatic clearance. Some examples of drugs with low and high extraction ratios are presented in Table 137.1.

Hepatic blood flow and clearance: Equation [3] now also allows a quantification of the impact of a drug's extraction ratio and therefore its intrinsic hepatic clearance on total hepatic clearance when liver perfusion is altered. This relation between hepatic blood flow and clearance is presented in Figure 137.1. This figure demonstrates the important difference between flow-limited and enzyme-limited hepatic drug clearance, which is further discussed below and is exemplified in Figure 137.2. In this context it is important to realize that liver disease usually does not decrease metabolic capacity sufficiently to turn a high extraction drug into one with a low extraction ratio. The effect of changes in metabolic capacity, portosystemic shunting, and plasma protein binding for drugs with high and low extractions on the most important parameters are summarized in Table 137.2, in which the role of the route of administration is also considered. All changes are based on the discussed concepts, equations [1] to [3], and the following basic pharmacokinetic equations:

$$\text{Half-life} = \frac{0.693 * \text{volume of distribution}}{\text{CL}} \quad [4]$$

$$\text{Concentration steady state} = \frac{\text{drug input rate}}{\text{CL}} \quad [5]$$

$$\text{AUC} = \frac{\text{dose} * \text{bioavailability}}{\text{CL}} \quad [6]$$

(AUC stands for area under the concentration-versus-time curve.)

The following section briefly presents the typical therapeutic situations in liver disease and the associated physiologic and pharmacokinetic processes, with particular emphasis on the impact of extraction ratio and the route of administration on pharmacokinetics.

Effect of decreased metabolic activity and portosystemic shunting on drugs with a high extraction ratio

If a drug's extraction ratio approaches 1 (100%), its hepatic first-pass metabolism is almost complete. Equation [3] shows that in this situation hepatic clearance equals hepatic perfusion, and a decrease in flow will also proportionally decrease the hepatic clearance. Further, portosystemic shunting can have a dramatic effect, as it may increase bioavailability and therefore peak concentration and total drug exposure (as reflected

TABLE 137.1 DRUGS WITH LOW AND HIGH HEPATIC EXTRACTION RATIOS (ONLY A FEW DRUGS HAVE AN INTERMEDIATE EXTRACTION RATIO)

Low extraction ratio (<0.3)	High extraction ratio (>0.7)
Carbamazepine	Diltiazem
Diazepam	Ergot alkaloids
Phenobarbital	Lidocaine
Phenprocoumon (coumarin)	Metoprolol
Phenytoin	Morphine
Salicylic acid	Nitroglycerin
Theophylline	Propranolol
Valproate	Verapamil
Warfarin	

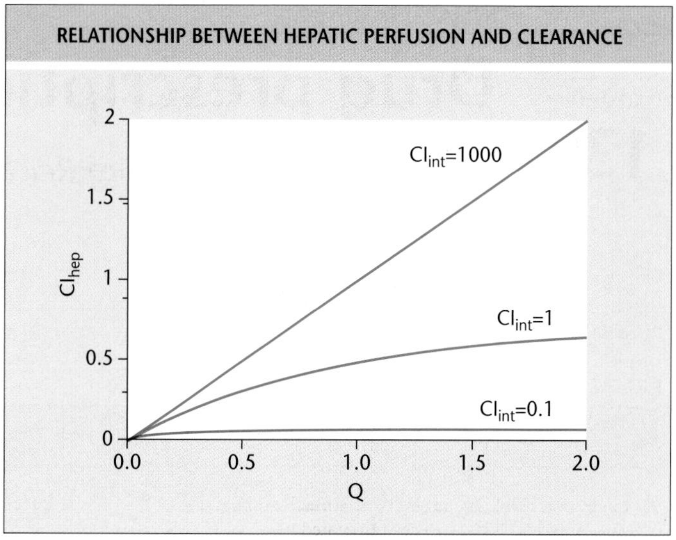

Fig. 137.1 Relationship between hepatic perfusion and clearance. Illustration showing the effect of a drug's intrinsic hepatic clearance (Cl_{int}) on the relationship between total hepatic clearance (Cl_{hep}) and hepatic perfusion (Q). When the intrinsic hepatic clearance is very high, the hepatic extraction is close to 100%. In this case the total hepatic clearance equals hepatic blood flow and is thus described as 'flow limited.' In contrast, when intrinsic hepatic clearance is very low, changes in hepatic blood flow will have no effect on total hepatic clearance, which is then said to be 'enzyme limited.'

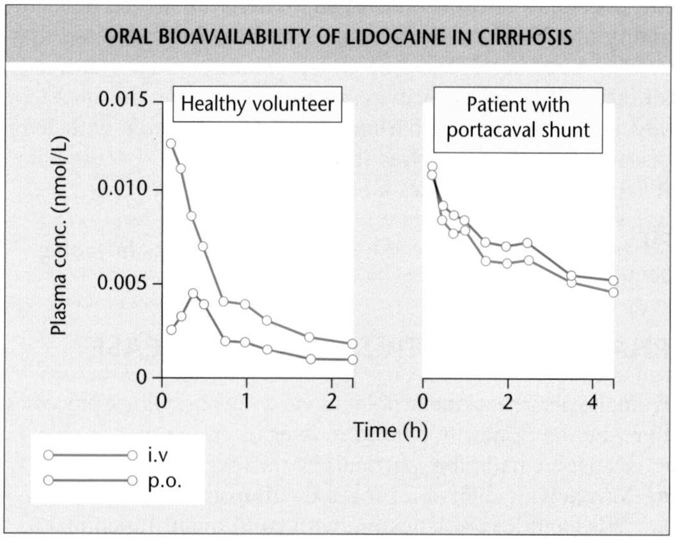

Fig. 137.2 Oral bioavailability of lidocaine in cirrhosis. This figure exemplifies the effect of liver disease on a compound with a high extraction ratio. In a healthy control subject, plasma concentrations after oral administration are lower compared with those following intravenous administration, and oral bioavailability is about 30%. In a cirrhotic patient with a surgical portacaval shunt, the plasma concentration–time curve is almost identical for both modes of administration, and oral bioavailability approaches 100%. Adapted from Karlaganis G, Bircher J. Biomed Environ Mass Spectrom 1987; 14:513–516.

TABLE 137.2 EFFECTS ON PHARMACOKINETICS OF ALTERED PHYSIOLOGIC PARAMETERS ASSOCIATED WITH LIVER DISEASE

	Decreased plasma protein binding				Decreased metabolic activity or intrahepatic diffusion				Portosystemic shunting			
	Extraction ratio				Extraction ratio				Extraction ratio			
	Low		High		Low		High[a]		Low		High	
	i.v.	*p.o.*	*i.v.*	*p.o.*	*i.v.*	*p.o.*	*i.v.*	*p.o.*	*i.v.*	*p.o.*	*i.v.*	*p.o.*
Bioavailability	–	⇔	–	⇓	–	⇔	–	⇑	–	⇔	–	⇑⇑
Apparent volume of distribution	⇑	⇑	⇑	⇑	–	–	–	–	–	–	–	–
Total hepatic clearance	⇑	⇑	⇔	⇔	⇓	⇓	⇔	⇔	⇔	⇔	⇔	⇔
Hepatic clearance of unbound fraction	⇔	⇔	⇓	⇓	–	–	–	–	–	–	–	–
Half-life	⇔	⇔	⇑	⇑	⇑	⇑	⇔	⇔	⇔	⇔	⇔	⇔
Total steady-state concentration	⇓	⇓	⇔	⇓	⇑	⇑	⇔	⇑	⇔	⇔	⇔	⇑⇑
Free steady-state free concentration	⇔	⇔	⇑	⇔[c]	–	–	–	–	–	–	–	–
AUC[b]	⇓	⇓	⇔	⇓	⇑	⇑	⇔	⇑	⇔	⇔	⇔	⇑⇑

Effects are valid for drugs that are eliminated mainly via the liver. Note that both extraction ratio category and route of administration are essential factors in predicting pharmacokinetic changes. Pharmacodynamic consequences may additionally be dependent on the presence of active metabolites.
AUC, area under concentration–time curve.
The symbol ⇔ indicates minor and usually irrelevant changes.
[a] It is assumed that the decrease in metabolism is not sufficient to transform high-extraction into low-extraction drugs.
[b] Volume of distribution and AUC are based on total plasma drug concentration.
[c] The decrease in bioavailability is assumed to compensate for the decrease in clearance of the unbound fraction.

by the AUC of the concentration–time curve) many fold. In contrast, a moderate decrease in the functioning liver cell mass will hardly influence the hepatic clearance because the 'normal' intrinsic clearance, and therefore the functional metabolic reserve, must be very high. Most of the drug will still be removed when blood passes through the liver. High extraction drugs (E>0.7) therefore have a *flow-limited hepatic clearance*. Beta-blockers with a high extraction ratio are a clinically relevant example as they are prescribed for the prophylaxis of variceal bleeding in cirrhosis, which is a consequence of portosystemic shunting. In this case, controlled-release formulations can avoid the extremely high peak concentrations that occur in preparations with fast absorption. Similarly cirrhosis with portosystemic shunting may increase the bioavailability of oral lidocaine from 30% to almost 100%, as shown in Figure 137.2.

Effect of decreased metabolic activity and portosystemic shunting on drugs with a low extraction ratio

If the intrinsic hepatic clearance for a certain drug is low (i.e., E approaches zero), hepatic clearance is limited by the metabolizing hepatic enzymes, and low extraction drugs (E<0.3) therefore have an *enzyme-limited hepatic clearance*. Given a very low hepatic first-pass extraction, portosystemic shunting will have a negligible impact on bioavailability. For example, a decrease in functioning liver cell mass or drug transport from the blood to the site of metabolism of 50% may decrease the extraction ratio from a normal value of 0.1 to 0.05. Bioavailability, defined as 1-E, would then only increase from 90% to 95%, which is clinically irrelevant. However, in contrast to a high extraction drug, according to equation [3], this alteration will be associated with a 50% reduction in total hepatic clearance and therefore require a 50% reduction of the maintenance dose or, alternatively, a doubling of the dosing interval.

Effect of hypoalbuminemia on low extraction ratio drugs

Low plasma albumin concentration will result in an increased fraction of unbound (f_u) drug in plasma. For a drug such as phenprocoumon, which is normally 99% bound to plasma proteins, a relatively minor change in plasma binding to 98% will in fact double f_u. It may now be tempting to conclude that

PHARMACODYNAMIC EFFECTS OF FUROSEMIDE IN LIVER CIRRHOSIS

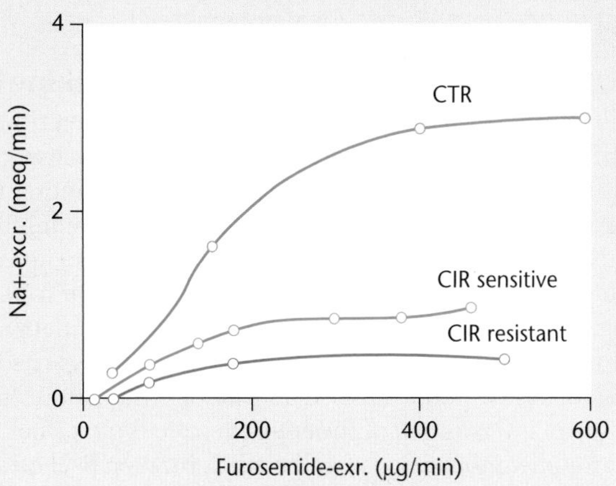

Fig. 137.3 Pharmacodynamic effects of furosemide in liver cirrhosis. The relationship between renal furosemide and sodium excretion demonstrates that the pharmaco*dynamic* response to furosemide is altered in cirrhosis. There is much less sodium excretion per drug excreted in cirrhotics responsive to furosemide (CIR sensitive) compared with that in healthy control subjects (CTR). In patients with ascites resistant to diuretic therapy (CIR resistant), the response is further blunted. Adapted from Villeneuve JP et al. Clin Pharmacol Ther 1986; 40:14–20.

the free concentration will also double and therefore produce a pronounced increase in prothrombin time. However, phenprocoumon has a low extraction ratio, and from equation [1], in which rate of elimination and not hepatic clearance is the dependent variable for a low extraction drug, it follows that in the resulting steady state the rate of elimination will increase, leading to a lower total but unchanged free drug concentration. Therefore, its maintenance dose is independent of f_u.

Effect of hypoalbuminemia on high extraction ratio drugs

For a high extraction drug such as lidocaine, the rate of elimination is not dependent on plasma protein binding because the equilibration processes are fast enough to allow almost complete drug removal upon one passage through the liver. Decreased protein binding will therefore lead to an unchanged total and increased free concentration. Fortunately higher free concentrations will occur only when drugs are given as a constant intravenous infusion, because the bioavailability of a high extraction drug is expected to decrease with an increase in f_u and thus compensate for the lower unbound clearance.

Although changes in the plasma protein binding of drugs with either a high or a low extraction ratio usually do not require oral dose adjustment, they must be considered when interpreting total plasma concentrations in relation to the usual therapeutic range. The clinician can easily be misled if looking only at the laboratory determination of a total concentration: if f_u is increased, therapeutic free concentrations will be accompanied by lower total concentrations than usual, and this may lead to unjustified dosage increases (Table 137.2).

Effect of ascites on drug pharmacokinetics

If a drug is distributed primarily in body water, ascites will increase its volume of distribution. In this case the clearance, reflecting metabolic capacity, will be unchanged in a low extraction drug. According to equation [4] the half-life and thus the time to reach steady state will increase, whereas the steady-state plasma concentration, which depends only on clearance and input rate (eqn [5]), will remain unaltered.

Effect of cholestasis on drug pharmacokinetics

Although bile flow is less than 1 mL/min, biliary excretion may be a major pathway for drug elimination due to active transport processes, and resulting bile to plasma concentration ratios may exceed 100. Obstructive cholestasis or selective inhibition of active drug transport into bile can therefore significantly limit elimination. However, if there is extensive enterohepatic cycling, and elimination occurs mainly through liver metabolism or through the kidney, biliary excretion must be regarded as a process of distribution rather than one of elimination. In this situation an interruption of the enterohepatic cycle, as has been shown for phenprocoumon after the administration of cholestyramine, will increase hepatic clearance, whereas a decrease in biliary excretion will merely result in a functional decrease in the volume of distribution.

Finally, the clinical relevance of pharmacokinetic alterations and the resulting changes in plasma concentration will depend on the therapeutic range of the individual drug. Further, for the prediction of pharmacodynamic effects, it must be considered that metabolites may also demonstrate pharmacologic activity. So-called pro-drugs, where the actual drug is pharmacologically inactive and only its metabolite is responsible for the desired effect, represent an extreme example of this situation.

PHARMACODYNAMICS IN LIVER DISEASE

Not only pharmacokinetics but also susceptibility to drugs and the risk of adverse reactions may be altered in patients with liver disease. In contrast to pharmacokinetic changes, these are related to the numerous mechanisms of drugs and therefore do not share general common principles. However, the most frequent and clinically relevant changes occur in a limited number of drug classes.

The *pharmacokinetics of loop diuretics* are unaltered in liver disease; however, as sodium excretion is decreased in cirrhosis, it is not surprising that their natriuretic response may be decreased (Fig. 137.3). Similarly, an increased sensitivity to *oral anticoagulants* (warfarin, phenprocoumon) in liver disease may not be due to altered pharmacokinetics, but to decreased synthesis of coagulation factors. Nonselective as well as COX2-selective *cyclooxygenase inhibitors* (nonsteroidal anti-inflammatory drugs; NSAIDs) reduce the synthesis of renal prostaglandins that regulate the maintenance of an adequate glomerular perfusion pressure. NSAIDs may therefore precipitate renal failure, even in patients without ascites. Further examples of altered pharmacodynamics or a higher susceptibility to develop adverse reactions may be found with *benzodiazepines* and other sedative agents, which may even precipitate hepatic encephalopathy, an increased response to vasoconstrictors in cirrhotic patients, who may also have a higher risk of developing neutropenia with β-lactam antibiotics and a higher risk of developing nephrotoxicity with aminoglycosides in obstructive cholestasis. In these latter cases the exact mechanism for increased response or adverse reactions remains to be determined.

HEPATOTOXICITY AND PRE-EXISTING LIVER DISEASE

Physicians are often concerned about prescribing potentially hepatotoxic drugs to patients with liver disease. Although most drugs may potentially be hepatotoxic, and great caution is often recommended by the manufacturer when prescribed to patients with liver disease, a closer look at the mechanisms of hepatotoxicity suggests that the risk of hepatotoxicity is not necessarily higher in patients with pre-existing liver disease. In fact, only in rare instances is this concern supported by convincing physiologic or clinical evidence. If the liver is responsible for the toxic activation of a drug, the risk of hepatotoxicity from this drug may theoretically be even lower in a patient with liver disease. Examples of the few drugs for which pre-existing liver disease has been identified as a risk factor for drug-induced liver disease are acetaminophen (paracetamol) in alcoholic cirrhosis, and tuberculostatic and antiretroviral therapy in patients with concomitant viral hepatitis (see also Chapter 92). Nevertheless, it should be considered that even if the risk of hepatotoxicity is unchanged in a patient with pre-existing liver disease, this patient may have an impaired ability to compensate for additional injury, which therefore justifies more frequent clinical and laboratory monitoring of symptoms and signs of hepatotoxicity, and should lower the threshold for discontinuation of therapy.

CLINICAL GUIDELINES FOR PHARMACOTHERAPY IN LIVER DISEASE

Fortunately, changes in drug effects that result from liver disease are often not clinically relevant. However, dramatic changes may occur in certain situations, of which some examples have been shown. Although quantitative tests of liver function with probe substances such as erythromycin, galactose, or indocyanine green are available, a correlation of their results with pharmacokinetic or pharmacodynamic parameters of specific drugs has not been validated in clinical practice. In contrast to what occurs in renal dysfunction, where rational dose adjustment can be calculated according to creatinine clearance and fraction of renal elimination, liver tests do not allow a quantification of liver function with subsequent prediction of individual pharmacokinetic parameters. Pharmacokinetic modeling is difficult in liver disease and the results of clinical studies evaluating drug pharmacokinetics in patients with liver disease may not be easily extrapolated to individual patients. However, application of the principles discussed in this chapter allows for more rational drug prescription in the presence of liver disease. In some patients, dose adjustment can be further supported by therapeutic plasma drug monitoring, if the therapeutic effect of the drug involved cannot be monitored sufficiently and the plasma concentration therapeutic range is well defined.

REFERENCES

1. Reichen J. Prescribing in liver disease. J Hepatol 1997; 26(Suppl 1):36–40.
2. Rowland M, Tozer TN. Elimination and integration with kinetics. In: Clinical pharmacokinetics – concepts and applications, 3rd edn. Media, PA: Williams & Wilkins; 1995:156–200.

Chapter 138

An approach to nutritional assessment

T E Bowling

KEY POINTS

- Undernutrition affects 5% of western populations as a whole, 10% of the elderly, and up to 40% of hospitalized patients
- Causes are multifactorial, but often reflect socioeconomic circumstances as well as the presence of disease
- Undernutrition increases morbidity and mortality rates, and the cost of care
- All patients should be screened, with an appropriate care plan commenced if nutritionally at risk
- Nutritional assessment should include clinical and social history, patient examination, weight and weight loss±body mass index. Anthropometry and measurement of plasma protein levels are not essential, and should be interpreted with caution
- All practising clinicians should have at least a rudimentary knowledge of energy and nutrient requirements

INTRODUCTION

Malnutrition and undernutrition are terms often used interchangeably. Although there is no universally agreed definition of either term, malnutrition is commonly taken as a nutritional status that deviates from normal. This can be due to either overnutrition (obesity) or undernutrition. This chapter deals only with adult undernutrition, which can be defined as an inadequate intake of energy (and sometimes termed 'protein energy malnutrition').

PREVALENCE

Undernutrition is a major global problem, with a prevalence cited in the USA and many European countries of approximately 5% of the population as a whole. Up to 10% of free-living elderly are undernourished, with a further 14% at risk of becoming so. These figures rise dramatically with illness.

In hospitalized patients the situation is even more pronounced. The quoted prevalence of undernutrition ranges from 5 to 50% (body mass index (BMI) $<20\,kg/m^2$), but within clinical subgroups these figures are much higher: cancer (5–80%), elderly (0–85%), HIV/AIDS (8–98%), gastroenterologic disease (3–100%). Furthermore, most patients will lose weight in hospital through a combination of their illness, its investigation and treatment, and poor-quality food provision.[1–3]

CAUSES OF UNDERNUTRITION

These are shown in Table 138.1.

TABLE 138.1 CAUSES OF UNDERNUTRITION

FACTORS DECREASING DIETARY INTAKE

- Difficulties with acquisition or preparation of food – poverty, limited mobility, lack of cooking skills
- Lack of interest in food – bereavement, isolation, mental illness
- Loss of appetite – illness, anxiety, depression
- Difficulties feeding or chewing – ill-fitting dentures, arthritis, dry mouth
- Symptoms associated with illness or treatment – nausea, vomiting, sore mouth, taste disturbance
- Altered consciousness
- Nil by mouth – after surgery, investigations

INCREASED NUTRITIONAL REQUIREMENTS

- Metabolic stress – critical care, after surgery, infection
- Increased gut losses – vomiting, diarrhea, fistula

IMPAIRED ABILITY TO ABSORB OR UTILIZE NUTRIENTS

- Gastrointestinal disease – malabsorption, motility disorder, bacterial overgrowth
- Intestinal resection
- Gastric stasis and ileus – critical illness, following surgery, metabolic disturbance

CONSEQUENCES OF UNDERNUTRITION

The clinical consequences of undernutrition in hospital are demonstrated in Figure 138.1. Overall there is an undeniable increase in both morbidity and mortality for the undernourished patient compared to the normally nourished one, and this leads to longer lengths of hospital stay and increased costs of care.[4] Recent estimations have calculated that it costs four times as much to look after an undernourished surgical patient than a well nourished one. There can therefore be no doubt that undernutrition and its consequences, both clinical and financial, put a very considerable pressure on healthcare economies.

DIAGNOSIS

Undernutrition is seen in all areas of hospital and community-based medicine, but often goes unrecognized and untreated. The responsibility for identifying patients either with established undernutrition or at risk of developing it usually lies with ward-based clinical and nursing staff.[5] Such patients suitably identified can then be referred on to dietitians, multidisciplinary nutrition teams, or other professionals with a specialist nutrition interest and experience for appropriate input and advice.

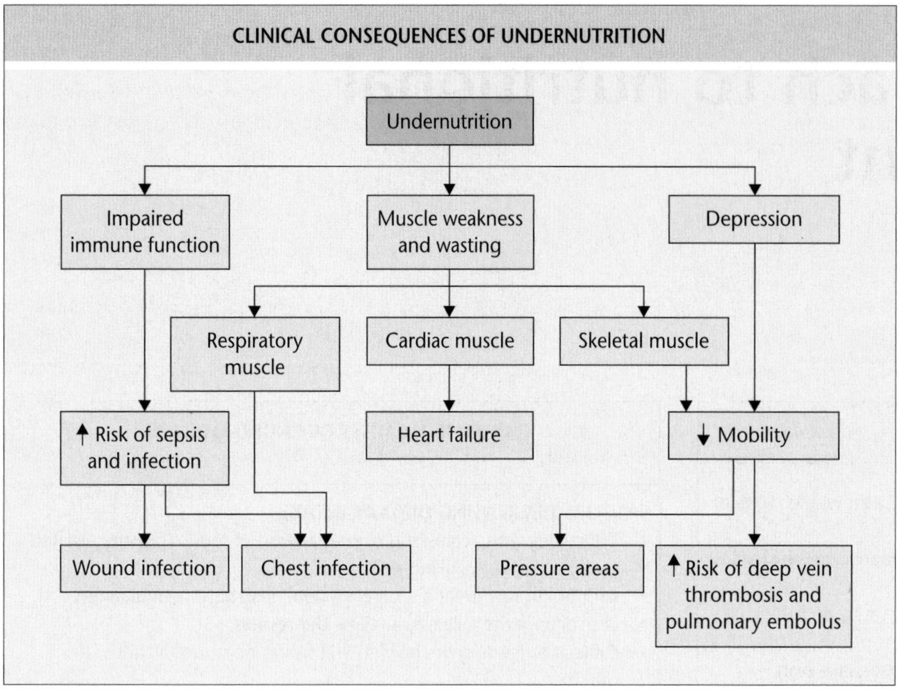

Fig. 138.1 Clinical consequences of undernutrition.

Assessment

Assessing a patient's nutritional status should be a fundamental part of the medical and nursing admission process.[6,7] However, it is sadly often neglected or overlooked. This is partly because attention is mainly directed at the primary clinical presentation, and partly because there is an undoubted lack of awareness of the importance of nutrition and nutritional status amongst many healthcare professionals. Weight loss, BMI, anthropometry, biochemical measurements, history, and examination are all important.

Weight loss

This is a very useful parameter and, as a guide, more than 10% of unintentional weight loss over 6 months is likely to be clinically significant and to reflect a situation of nutritional risk. Often, though, patients are unable to quantify how much weight they may have lost, or what their baseline weight may have been. In such situations clinical impression, for example observation of how well clothes or rings fit, and views from family members or carers may be useful. It must be remembered that a 10% unintentional weight loss in an obese patient is as relevant as in a normally nourished patient. Edematous patients, or those with ascites, will have increased weight and this needs to be accounted for (Table 138.2). Overall, weight loss can be regarded as a marker of risk, but on its own, nothing more.

TABLE 138.2 GUIDELINES FOR ESTIMATING FLUID WEIGHT IN PATIENTS WITH ASCITES AND EDEMA

	Edema	Ascites
FLUID WEIGHT (kg)		
Minimal	1.0	2.0
Moderate	5.0	6.0
Severe	10.0	14.0

Body mass index (BMI)

BMI is an extension of weight calculated as weight in kg divided by height in meters squared. Conventionally, a BMI of less than 20 kg/m^2 indicates undernutrition, and over 30 kg/m^2 indicates obesity. Patients, especially the elderly, are notoriously unreliable at recalling their height accurately. However, if reasonably accurate height measurements are obtainable, then BMI is a universally recognized measurement of nutritional status. It is, however, not the perfect tool as it does not reflect loss of height in the elderly, and therefore artificially increases readings in this group.[8] There are alternative methods to eliminate this factor, such as using demispan (sternal notch to finger webs), but on the whole these are not widely used.

Anthropometry

This is the measurement of body composition. A number of different measures are used:

- Triceps skinfold thickness (TSF) – fat
- Mid upper arm circumference (MAC) – muscle mass[9]
- Mean arm muscle circumference (MAMC) – skeletal muscle mass. This is a composite of TSF and MAC ($MAMC = MAC - 3.14 \times TSF$)
- Bioimpedance analysis assesses body composition
- Grip strength – not, strictly speaking, an anthropometric measurement, but an assessment of muscle function. It uses a dynamometer and relies on patient motivation and compliance.

The place of anthropometry in day-to-day clinical practice lies mainly in the ongoing follow-up of at-risk patients. Serial measurements done by the same (experienced) professional – as there is a great deal of interindividual variation – are a useful way of monitoring a patient's nutritional status. However, as one-off measurements, anthropometry is not helpful. Overall, these are used more in the research setting than in day-to-day practice.

Biochemical measurements

There remains a great deal of mythology about the use of biochemical measurements in nutritional assessment.[10]

- Albumin – in protein energy malnutrition albumin synthesis is low but, as albumin has a half-life of 21 days, falls due to poor nutrition are slow. Much more commonly, changes in albumin are due to alterations in hydration, for example dilution secondary to intravenous fluids, and catabolism or sepsis. On its own, albumin is not a reliable marker of undernutrition.
- Transferrin – half-life of 8–10 days. Main function is to bind and transport iron, so it is affected by iron status and the acute-phase response.
- Pre-albumin – more sensitive to protein depletion (with a half-life of 2–3 days), but also extremely sensitive to changes in metabolic stress and disease.
- Retinal binding protein – short half-life of 12 h with similar indications to pre-albumin; however, it is technically very difficult to measure, and so this measurement is not widely available.

Estimation of the level of plasma proteins, therefore, may be useful, but the limitations as described above need to be appreciated, and plasma protein levels should never be used in isolation as a marker of nutritional status.

History

- Medical history – the primary disease process and any co-morbidity may be relevant. Disease instability and catabolism from inflammation or sepsis are important, as are any symptoms that may affect food intake or nutrient absorption, such as difficulties chewing or swallowing, anorexia, vomiting, and diarrhea (see Table 138.1).
- Social history – mobility, depression, ability to obtain and prepare food, and underlying poverty may all influence nutritional state.

Examination

The appearance of a patient is very important in nutritional assessment. Generalized muscle wasting and cachexia, hydration, appearances of apathy, and abnormalities of gait and mobility due to lower limb weakness are all signs of nutritional compromise. In addition, the various trace element and micronutrient deficiencies that may coexist have their own individual clinical signs (Table 138.3).

Nutrition screening

The methods of assessment described above will give a very good picture as to whether a patient is undernourished and whether they would benefit from nutritional support and advice. However, many of these parameters, if taken individually, do not fulfill the essential criteria of being a good and reproducible assessment tool for nutritional risk, because the initial assessment of patients is often carried out by nurses or doctors who may lack expertise. As this has implications for clinical risk and patient care, many hospitals are now introducing nutrition screening tools in an attempt to ensure consistency and reliability.

Nutrition screening tools need to be rapid and simple, and able to identify all patients being admitted to hospital or other institutions who are undernourished or at risk of becoming so.

There are hundreds of screening tools, many designed by individual hospitals, and usually including a combination of the various methods of assessment described above.[11] Recently, the British Association for Parenteral and Enteral Nutrition and the European Society of Parenteral and Enteral Nutrition (ESPEN) have both proposed tools in an attempt to achieve consistency in practice. The one proposed by ESPEN[12] is shown to illustrate an example (Table 138.4).

Care plans

In addition to the screening process itself, it is essential that there are defined courses of action dependent on the outcome of the screening. In other words, each healthcare setting in which patients are being screened must have an established 'care plan,' as mentioned in Table 138.4, to progress patients' nutritional management. For example:

- The patient is adequately nourished and not at risk. Screening should be repeated at regular intervals throughout admission (at least weekly).
- The patient is adequately nourished, but at risk of becoming undernourished either because of their underlying disease process or because of the treatment of it (e.g., complex surgery).
- The patient has established undernutrition.

Patients in the latter two groups would then need referral to appropriate professionals with the necessary expertise in nutrition and nutritional support, such as dietitians, nutrition nurses/clinicians, or multidisciplinary nutrition teams. The various ways of providing optimal nutritional support are considered in Chapter 139.

NUTRITIONAL REQUIREMENTS

Part of nutritional assessment is the determination of nutritional requirements. The detail of this is in the remit of dietitians or clinicians/nurses with a specialist interest in nutrition, but it is necessary for all practicing clinicians – and certainly gastroenterologists – to have a rudimentary knowledge of nutritional requirements.

Energy requirements

Energy expenditure consists of three components:

- Resting energy expenditure (REE)
- Metabolic requirements
- Thermic effects of food (i.e., the energy required to utilize nutrients).

The hospitalized patient tends to eat little, and therefore energy expenditure is primarily the REE and metabolic requirements.[13]

Energy supply is mainly from the three macronutrients – fat, carbohydrate, and protein. The supply of too little energy leads to tissue breakdown; the supply of too much to excess storage of glycogen and fat. Neither is desirable, and the aim therefore is for energy balance, where intake roughly equates to expenditure.

Calculation of energy requirements

The calculation of energy requirements is therefore very important. *Indirect calorimetry* is the most accurate method, but the cost of the equipment and time involved make this impractical.

There are several 'mathematical' calculations with which to determine requirements, the most common being the Harris-Benedict equation. This estimates basal energy expenditure

TABLE 138.3 ELECTROLYTES, TRACE ELEMENTS AND VITAMINS – THEIR FUNCTIONS AND DEFICIENCY SYNDROMES

Element	Function	Deficiency
ELECTROLYTES		
Calcium	Forms teeth and bones, muscle contraction	Muscle aches, pain, twitching, spasm, cramps, tetany, and loose teeth/gum infection
Phosphate	Bone development, release energy from food	Anorexia, lethargy, bone pain, calcification of soft tissue
Magnesium	Bone development, muscle and nerve conduction, metabolism, DNA synthesis	Neuromuscular abnormalities, loss of appetite, nausea, vomiting, premenstrual syndrome, diarrhea, numbness, tingling, dizziness, hypertension
Sodium	Maintenance of extracellular fluid volume	Muscle cramps, vertigo, nausea, apathy, reduced appetite
Potassium	Acid–base balance, nerve, muscle function	Muscle weakness/paralysis, cardiac arrest
TRACE ELEMENTS		
Iron	Blood formation	Fatigue, pallor, headache, dizziness, sore tongue/mouth, concave brittle nails
Zinc	Metabolism, cell membranes	Poor growth, wound healing, eczema, psoriasis, acne, poor hair growth, increased risk of infection, delayed puberty, low sperm count, loss of smell, diarrhea
Copper	Healthy skin, hair, and red blood cells	Metabolic and muscle problems
Iodine	Metabolic rate maintenance, thyroid function	Lethargy, thyroid goiter, brittle course hair, weight gain, hypothyroidism
Manganese	Bone and tendon growth, synthesis of carbohydrates and proteins	Depression, weakness, leg cramps
Fluoride	Prevention of dental caries	Tooth decay, soft bones
Chromium	Energy metabolism and effective insulin action	Inability to metabolize glucose
Selenium	Antioxidant	Muscle weakness, cardiomyopathy
Molybdenum	Part of enzymes	Rare
VITAMINS		
Vitamin A	Vision, bone and teeth formation, growth and tissue repair	Night blindness, keratomalacia, dry scaly skin, joint pain, fatigue, impaired growth and development in children
B_1 (thiamine)	Energy metabolism, appetite, and nervous system function	Neurologic disorders, confusion, cardiac irregularity, loss appetite, fatigue, wet or dry beri-beri
B_2 (riboflavin)	Cell respiration, normal vision, and skin	Lesions on mucocutaneous surfaces of mouth, skin rash, vascularization of cornea
B_6 (pyridoxine)	Protein metabolism and sensory function	Glossitis, dermatitis, convulsions, muscle weakness, anemia
B_{12}	Cell synthesis, nerve myelination	Megaloblastic anemia, fatigue, brain degeneration
Niacin	Energy metabolism, healthy skin, nervous system and GI tract	Pellagra, fatigue, confusion
Pantothenic acid	Release of energy from foods	Headache, dizziness, cramps, weakness, GI disturbance
Biotin	Lipogenesis, gluconeogenesis, and protein metabolism	Nausea, vomiting, depression, hair loss, dermatitis, mental and physical retardation in child development
Folate	Cell growth	GI disorders, macrocytic anemia, neural tube defects in newborns
Vitamin C (ascorbic acid)	Immunity, collagen formation, and wound healing	Bleeding gums, scurvy, poor wound healing, bruising or hemorrhaging, fatigue, depression, muscle degeneration
Vitamin D	Development of bones and teeth, enhances absorption of calcium	Rickets in children, osteomalacia in adults, reduced teeth and bone development
Vitamin E	Antioxidant	Hemolytic anemia, muscle wasting, reproductive failure, nerve damage
Vitamin K	Blood clotting	Prolonged blood clotting time

(BEE), i.e., the energy expended by a fasting person at rest in a thermoneutral environment.

Estimation of BEE is calculated as follows:

$$\text{Males (kcal/24 h)} = 66.5 + (13.8W) + (5H) - (6.8A)$$
$$\text{Females (kcal/24 h)} = 655 + (9.6W) + (1.8H) - (4.7A)$$

where W is weight in kg, H is height in meters, and A is age in years.

To convert BEE to a more realistic measure of TEE, various multiples need to be added to account for the types of stress factors seen in the hospitalized patient:[13,14]

Postoperative (no complications)	1.0
Peritonitis or sepsis	1.1–1.3
Severe infection or multiple trauma	1.2–1.4
Burns	1.2–2.0

Rule of thumb

However, for the busy clinician, these types of calculations are not very practical, and the so-called 'rule of thumb' is a very good, albeit crude, estimation of energy requirements:

- Energy requirements should lie between 25 and 35 kcal/kg/day
- 25 kcal/kg/day – bedbound, but not catabolic (i.e., apyrexial, nonsurgical)
- 30 kcal/kg/day – pyrexial or postoperative
- 35 kcal/kg/day – pyrexial and postoperative, multiple trauma
- If weight gain is required, add approximately 200 kcal to total daily requirements
- If weight loss is required, subtract approximately 200 kcal from total daily requirements.

TABLE 138.4 NUTRITION RISK SCREENING TOOL (AFTER KONDRUP ET AL. CLIN NUTR 2003; 22:415–421, WITH PERMISSION)

INITIAL SCREENING

		Yes	No
1	Is BMI <20.5?		
2	Has patient lost weight within last 3 months?		
3	Has the patient had a reduced dietary intake in the last week?		
4	Is the patient severely ill (e.g., in intensive care)?		

Yes: Is the answer is 'yes' to any question, the screening below is performed
No: If the answer is 'no' to all questions, the patient is rescreened at weekly intervals.
If it is anticipated that the patient is likely to eat inadequately (e.g., scheduled for major surgery), a preventive nutritional care plan can be considered.

FINAL SCREENING

	Impaired nutritional status			**Severity of disease**	
Absent	**Score 0**	Normal nutritional status	Absent	**Score 0**	Normal nutritional requirements
Mild	**Score 1**	Weight loss >5% in 3 months *or* food intake below 50–75% of normal requirements in preceding week	Mild	**Score 1**	Chronic patients with acute complications (e.g., chronic airway disease, cirrhosis, diabetes, cancer)
Moderate	**Score 2**	Weight loss >5% in 2 months *or* BMI 18.5–20.5 plus impaired general condition *or* food intake 25–60% of normal requirements in preceding week	Moderate	**Score 2**	Major abdominal surgery, stroke, severe pneumonia, hematologic malignancy
Severe	**Score 3**	Weight loss >5% in 1 month *or* BMI <18.5 plus impaired general condition *or* food intake 0–25% of normal requirements in preceding week	Severe	**Score 3**	Head injury, intensive care, bone marrow transplantation
Score		+	**Score**		**= Total score**
Age: If ≥70 years add one to total score					**= Age-adjusted total score**

Score ≥3: Patient nutritionally at risk. Care plan to be initiated
Score <3: Weekly rescreening
If it is anticipated that the patient is likely to eat inadequately (e.g., scheduled for major surgery), a preventive nutritional care plan can be considered.

In obese people, the use of actual bodyweight to calculate energy (and macronutrient) requirements would overestimate needs. For those with a BMI >30 kg/m^2, requirements are determined by using either 75% of actual bodyweight or 130% of ideal bodyweight.

Macronutrients

These are shown in Table 138.5.

Micronutrients

- Vitamins
- Minerals
- Trace elements.

These are listed in Table 138.3. They are all essential for metabolism, tissue structure, enzyme systems, fluid balance, and cellular function.

There are no definitive guidelines as to how much of each micronutrient may be required in an individual patient. The dietary reference values often referred to in the literature are only relevant to the needs of healthy adults, and are not therefore always appropriate for the needs of hospitalized patients. On the whole, manufactured diets, both enteral and parenteral, contain reasonable quantities of the various micronutrients, and it is therefore unusual for a patient to have problems with deficiency or excess unless they are on prolonged nutritional support. Appropriate monitoring (see Chapter 139) should prevent this.

CONCLUSION

Undernutrition is a major cause of morbidity and drain on healthcare resources worldwide. Its recognition is a fundamental part of patient assessment, and only if this is done correctly will appropriate management be possible.

TABLE 138.5 MACRONUTRIENTS

	Protein	Fat	Carbohydrate
Energy density	1 g=4 kcal energy	1 g=9 kcal energy	1 g = 4 kcal energy
Function	Provision of amino acids essential for growth and continuous replacement of body tissue and enzymes. Protein plays only a small role in energy metabolism – this is supplied primarily by fat and carbohydrate	More concentrated form of energy than protein or carbohydrate. Tissues that can utilize fatty acids as an energy source include liver, kidney, heart, and skeletal muscle	Source of glucose, the most readily available source of energy to the body
Requirements	The intake requirements for protein in a healthy adult are 0.75 g/kg/day. However, metabolic stresses increase requirements, and to account for these the following intakes are recommended: 'Normal' (no catabolic illness): 0.8–1.0 g/kg/day Postoperative (no complications): 1.0–1.2 g/kg/day Postoperative + septic complications: 1.2–1.4 g/kg/day Severe sepsis, multiple organ failure, or burns: 1.4–2.0 g/kg/day Overall protein should supply 15–25% of total dietary energy	1.0–1.5 g/kg/day 30–50% total energy Imbalance in the provision of fat and carbohydrate can lead to significant metabolic and clinical complications Excess fat leads directly to fat deposition in liver and adipose tissue, and the relative lack of carbohydrate can result in glucose (and therefore energy) coming from alternative sources, e.g., fat, lactate, and protein (gluconeogenesis), with the risk of ketosis and lactic acidosis Excess carbohydrate is stored as glycogen or converted into fatty acids. In addition there is an increase in insulin release and this inhibits lipolysis, producing an increase in tissue fat deposition	4–5 g/kg/day 40–60% total energy

REFERENCES

1. McWhirter JP, Pennington CR. Incidence and recognition of malnutrition in hospital. BMJ 1994; 308:945–958.
2. Kondrup J, Johansen N, Plum L et al. Incidence of nutritional risk and causes of inadequate nutritional care in hospitals. Clin Nutr 2002; 21:461–468.
3. Gallagher-Allred CR, Voss AC, Finn SC et al. Malnutrition and clinical outcomes: the case for medical nutrition therapy. J Am Diet Assoc 1996; 96:361–369.
4. Correia MI, Waitzberg DL. The impact of malnutrition, morbidity, length of hospital stay and costs evaluated through a multivariate model analysis. Clin Nutr 2003; 22:235–239.
5. Omran ML, Salem P. Diagnosing undernutrition. Clin Geriatr Med 2002; 18:719–736.
6. Jeejeebhoy KN. Nutritional assessment. Gastroenterol Clin North Am 1998; 27:347–369.
7. Hensrud DD. Nutrition screening and assessment. Med Clin North Am 1999; 83:1525–1546.
8. Beck A, Ovesen L. At which body mass index and degree of weight loss should hospitalized elderly patients be considered at nutritional risk? Clin Nutr 1998; 17:195–198.
9. Powell-Tuck J, Hennessy EM. A comparison of mid upper arm circumference, body mass index and weight loss as indices of undernutrition in acutely hospitalised patients. Clin Nutr 2003; 22:307–312.
10. Selberg O, Sel S. The adjunctive value of routine biochemistry in nutritional assessment of hospitalized patients. Clin Nutr 2001; 20:477–485.
11. Arrowsmith H. A critical evaluation of the use of nutrition screening tools by nurses. Br J Nurs 1999; 8:1483–1490.
12. Kondrup J, Allison SP, Elia M et al. ESPEN guidelines for nutrition screening 2002. Clin Nutr 2003; 22:415–421.
13. Pellett PL. Food energy requirements in humans. Am J Clin Nutr 1990; 51:711–722.
14. Barak N, Wall-Alonso E, Sitrin MD. Evaluation of stress factors and body weight adjustments currently used to estimate energy expenditure in hospitalized patients. J Parenter Enteral Nutr 2002; 26:231–238.

Chapter 139

Nutritional support

T E Bowling

KEY POINTS

- If a patient requires nutritional support, always consider optimizing oral intake before more interventional methods
- For long-term feeding, gastrostomy access is preferred to nasogastric tubes, and often insisted upon by community-based care facilities
- Gastrostomy feeding is not without risks, and needs careful consideration against the background of co-morbidity and the appropriateness of ongoing nutritional support
- As a general principle, enteral feeding is favoured over parenteral feeding because of lower complication rates and costs. Whether using the gut leads to better functional and nutritional outcomes remains open to debate
- The major complication of parenteral feeding is catheter sepsis. Anything short of meticulous attention to line care and handling is unacceptable

INTRODUCTION

Once a patient has been assessed and deemed in need of nutritional support (see Chapter 138), the next step is to determine the most appropriate method of feeding.[1] Figure 139.1 illustrates the decision-making pathway and demonstrates that simpler methods should always be considered first.

The options for providing nutritional support are:

- Oral feeding: food, nutritional supplements
- Enteral (tube) feeding
- Parenteral (intravenous) feeding.

ORAL NUTRITIONAL SUPPORT

Food

Food should always be considered as the first option.[2] Strategies to increase nutritional intake from food include:

- Providing high-energy/high-protein choices on the hospital menu
- Fortifying foods, for example by adding cream, skimmed milk powder, or cheese
- Attention to presentation, availability, and appropriate assistance.

Oral nutritional supplements

Oral nutritional supplements, for those unable to meet nutritional requirements from food and drink, come as liquids, semi-solids, or powders in many different flavors. They can be nutritionally complete (i.e., are appropriate as a sole source of intake) or can contain different concentrations of calories, fat, fiber, or electrolytes for specific needs (e.g., low-electrolyte preparations in renal failure).

It is therefore usually sensible to involve a dietitian or other suitably trained professional to advise on an oral nutritional supplement that is appropriate to the clinical condition(s) and that complements the patient's dietary intake.

ENTERAL FEEDING

If a patient is unable to eat or cannot adequately meet nutritional requirements with food ± oral nutritional supplements, and has a functioning and accessible gastrointestinal tract, enteral feeding is indicated.[3–6] The options are:

- Gastric feeding:
  Nasogastric (NG) tube
  Percutaneous endoscopic gastrostomy (PEG)
- Postpyloric feeding:
  Nasojejunal (NJ) tube
  Percutaneous endoscopic gastrojejunostomy (PEGJ)
  Percutaneous endoscopic jejunostomy (PEJ)
  Surgically placed jejunostomy.

Indications and contraindications of the various routes of feeding along with their complications are shown in Tables 139.1 and 139.2.

Routes for enteral feeding

Nasogastric (NG) tube

There are two main types of NG tube: fine bore and wide bore (e.g., Ryles). Wide-bore tubes should not be sited specifically for enteral feeding, because they are more uncomfortable and can cause complications such as ulceration of the esophagus and nasal passages.

Tube insertion

NG tubes should be passed by individuals (usually nursing staff) with appropriate training. Tube position should be verified either by pH testing (gastric pH <4, unless on acid-suppressing medication) or chest X-ray after tube insertion, following vomiting or violent coughing, if the tube is accidentally dislodged, or if the patient complains of discomfort.

Nasojejunal (NJ) tube

Specifically designed NJ tubes such as the Bengmark tube (Nutricia, UK) will cross the pylorus in 70–80% of patients with normal gastroduodenal motility, especially with a concurrent intravenous bolus of metoclopramide 10 mg. If the stomach is atonic, NJ tubes usually require endoscopic placement. The distal end must be placed beyond the duodenojejunal flexure

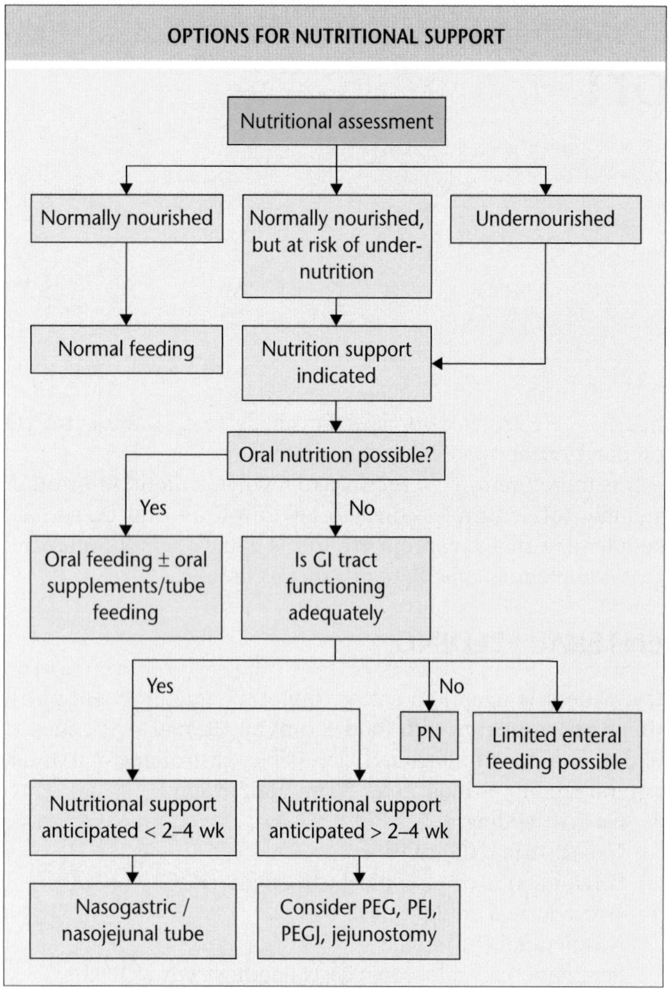

Fig. 139.1 Options for nutritional support.

(Fig. 139.2) or the tube will almost invariably pass retrogradely back into the stomach. Weighted tubes have no advantage over unweighted tubes and are seldom indicated. Plain abdominal radiography is required to verify placement, unless placed under screening.

Percutaneous endoscopic gastrostomy (PEG)

What tube?

There are a number of different types of PEG tube in terms of size (9–24 Fr), internal fixator (flange, balloon), and material,

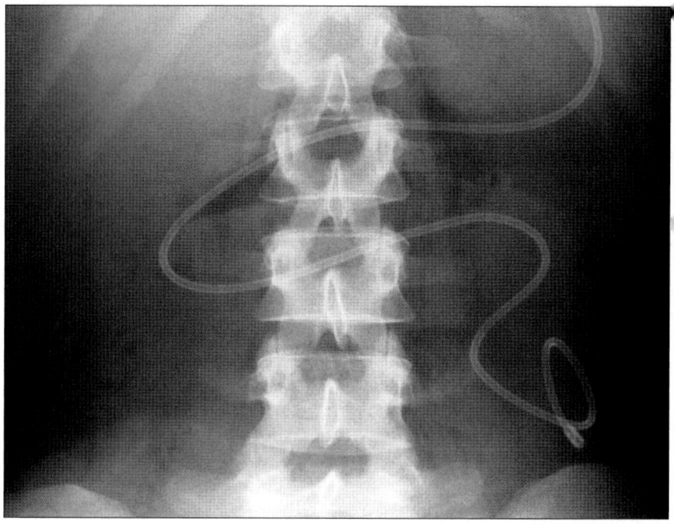

Fig. 139.2 Nasojejunal tube in situ.

including more cosmetically acceptable 'button' gastrostomies (Fig. 139.3).

PEG tube insertion

This is now a standard endoscopic procedure, and details of insertion technique are not included here. Although not a sterile procedure, many guidelines recommend antibiotic prophylaxis, e.g., cefotaxime 2 g or co-amoxiclav 2.2 g 30 min prior to the procedure.[7]

PEG tube removal

If the PEG tube is removed within 2–3 weeks of insertion, a formal tract will not have formed, with consequent risk of leakage of gastric contents into the peritoneal cavity leading to peritonitis. This also means that it will not be possible to reinsert a feeding tube down the same tract as it will not find its way into the gastric lumen. Therefore, if the PEG tube does come out in the first few weeks of insertion – whether at the hand of the patient or some other mishap – the stoma site should be covered, antibiotic cover instituted, and, if nutritional support is still required, an alternative access (e.g., NG tube) used until the wound has healed.

After 2–3 weeks, removal presents little risk of peritonitis or sepsis. However, closure is rapid, so replacement is required within 4–6 h using a fresh PEG or, temporarily, a balloon gastrostomy or Foley catheter.

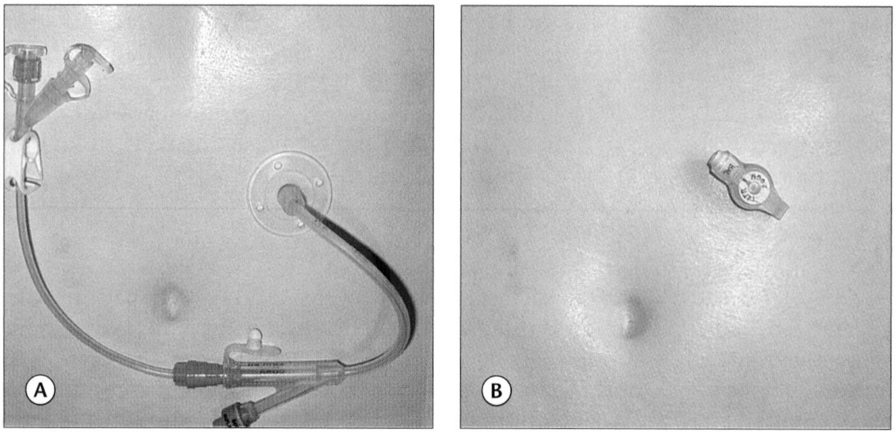

Fig. 139.3 Percutaneous endoscopic gastrostomy. A. PEG tube. **B.** Button gastrostomy.

TABLE 139.1 INDICATIONS AND CONTRAINDICATIONS OF ENTERAL FEEDING

INDICATIONS – GASTRIC FEEDING

- Patients with a functioning stomach and with no vomiting or aspiration:
  Impaired swallow (e.g., stroke, motor neuron disease, Parkinson's disease)
  Altered level of consciousness making oral feeding impossible
  Ventilated patients with tracheostomy
  Dysphagia without complete oropharyngeal or esophageal obstruction (i.e., head and neck, and esophageal cancer).
- Supplement inadequate oral intake:
  Cystic fibrosis
  Hypercatabolic states (e.g., burn injury, decompensated liver disease)
  Facial injury
  HIV wasting
  Psychologic or psychiatric reasons (e.g., anorexia nervosa)
- For short-term feeding (i.e., <4 weeks, a NG tube is usually the most appropriate. For longer-term feeding, PEG is preferable.

INDICATIONS – POSTPYLORIC FEEDING

- Feeding a functioning gastrointestinal tract when the stomach needs to be bypassed, i.e., where there is a gastric outflow obstruction (see NG tube contraindications below)
- Pancreatitis
- Risk of aspiration with intragastric feeding

The four different methods of delivering postpyloric feeding (i.e., NJ, PEJ, PEGJ, and surgical jejunostomy) all have similar indications. For short-term feeding, NJ would be the route of choice; for longer-term feeding the other three options could all be considered.

CONTRAINDICATIONS – GASTRIC FEEDING

NG tube

- Obstructive pathology in oropharynx or esophagus preventing passage of tube
- Gastric outflow obstruction:
  Mechanical (e.g., pyloric ulceration or stricture, tumor)
  Functional gastroparesis
- Intestinal obstruction:
  Mechanical intestinal obstruction (e.g., tumor)
  Functional intestinal obstruction (i.e., ileus).
- Intestinal perforation
- Proximal gastrointestinal tract fistula
- Facial injury

PEG

Absolute

- Inability to pass endoscope due to obstructing pathology in oropharynx or esophagus[a]
- Obstructing gastric outflow pathology

Relative

- Severe obesity (due to technical difficulties accessing the stomach)[a]
- Uncorrected coagulopathy
- Portal hypertension or ascites
- Active gastric ulceration or malignancy
- Gastroparesis
- Gastrectomy (total or partial)[a]
- Severe kyphoscoliosis (may be difficult to access stomach)[a]
- Current peritoneal dialysis

CONTRAINDICATIONS – POSTPYLORIC FEEDING

NJ

As per NG tube.

PEJ

As per PEG.

TABLE 139.1 INDICATIONS AND CONTRAINDICATIONS OF ENTERAL FEEDING—CONT'D

PEGJ

As per PEG.

Surgical jejunostomy

Absolute

- Jejunal disease (e.g., Crohn's disease or radiation enteritis at insertion site)
- Obstructing distal pathology.

Relative

- Ascites
- Portal hypertension
- Peritoneal dialysis

[a] May be achievable if done under radiologic guidance to locate stomach.

Elective removal is usually done endoscopically. Alternatively, the tube can be cut close to the skin, allowing the internal fixator to pass spontaneously through the gastrointestinal tract. There are no reported incidents of obstruction (e.g., at the ileocecal junction), and this method is probably safe.

Jejunal extension to PEG (PEGJ) and percutaneous endoscopically placed jejunostomy (PEJ)

PEGJ are 'extensions' that attach to a PEG and can be passed endoscopically beyond the duodenojejunal flexure. PEJ is similar to PEG, but requires a direct puncture into the small intestine. Insertion techniques are not straightforward and, on the whole, there is probably no advantage over a surgically placed jejunostomy for postpyloric feeding, except in a patient who is too unfit to have a general anesthetic.

Removal of PEGJ/PEJ is similar to that for PEG.

Surgical jejunostomy

Needle jejunostomies inserted using a wide-bore needle tunneled subserosally to reduce the risk of leakage are used most commonly but tend to be fine-bore and prone to block if poorly managed. Other tubes such as Foley catheters can be used but are not ideal because of leakage and difficulties in connecting with feeding equipment.

Increasingly, jejunostomies are inserted preoperatively to allow for early postoperative feeding. Although complications can occur, the advantages of improved postoperative nutrition usually outweigh the risks.

Enteral feeds

There are many different enteral feeds available. Broadly speaking they can be divided into the following groups.

Polymeric feeds

Polymeric feeds contain whole protein, carbohydrate, and fat, and can be used as a sole source of nutrition for those with no special nutrient requirements. The standard concentration is 1 kcal/mL, but feeds can be more or less energy dense (0.8–2.0 kcal/ml) and can also contain fiber, which may improve bowel function if this is problematic.

TABLE 139.2 TUBE-RELATED COMPLICATIONS OF ENTERAL FEEDING

GASTRIC FEEDING

NG tube

- **Removal by patient:**
  Purposeful – consider patient withdrawal of consent
  Confused – may need to be resited, or if repeated removal consider either means of restraint or alternative means of nutritional support (e.g., PEG)
- Esophageal ulceration or strictures – now uncommon if fine-bore tubes are used for the short term
- Malposition into lungs can lead to infection, effusion, and empyema. Occasionally tube may be malpositioned intracranially. With appropriate means of verification, this should not happen.
- **Blockage** – all types of enteral feeding tubes may become blocked; fine-bore tubes are particularly at risk. This problem is avoidable if the tube is flushed with water before starting and after completion of a feed, every 4–6h throughout feeding, and before and after medication, as residue can quickly build up. All types of tube can be unblocked using either soda water or pancreatic enzymes, which break down the coagulated protein. Acidic fizzy drinks, such as cola, can coagulate protein in the tube and exacerbate the problem, and should therefore not be used.

PEG

Early complications

- **Pain:**
  Usually within first 24h
  Treat with simple analgesia
  If severe, exclude peritonitis or tube displacement into anterior abdominal wall
- Hemorrhage – unusual if clotting screen within normal limits. As malnutrition can lead to vitamin K deficiency, the prothrombin time or international normalized ratio (INR) should always be checked prior to procedure
- Peritonitis
- Pneumoperitoneum – it should be noted that there will always be some free after PEG insertion
- Gastrocolic fistula – due to interposition of colon between anterior abdominal wall and stomach

Late complications

- **Stoma infection:**
  Attention to proper stoma care
  Take swabs from stoma
  Course of appropriate antibiotics (e.g., flucloxacillin)
  Not necessary to remove PEG or stop feeding unless severe ulceration or wound breakdown occurs
- **Tube blockage** – always flush with water before and after each feed/medication (see NG tube)
- **Aspiration** – can be minimized by feeding for no more than 20h per day at an elevation of at least 30°
- Buried bumper – internal fixator migrates into gastric or anterior abdominal wall leading to tube blockage; surgery is usually required for removal
- Tumor tract seeding – there are a few case reports of PEGs inserted in esophageal or oropharyngeal tumors developing neoplastic seeding in stoma tracts. Where the PEG is inserted as part of palliative care, this is unlikely to be of relevance in the patient's lifetime
- Overgranuation – can occur at stoma site; may bleed or become painful. Steroid cream or silver nitrate can usually deal with it.

POSTPYLORIC FEEDING

NJ

As per NG tube.

PEJ

As per PEG.

TABLE 139.2 TUBE-RELATED COMPLICATIONS OF ENTERAL FEEDING—CONT'D

PEGJ

As per PEG.

Surgical jejunostomy

Early complications

- Pain – usually not separable from pain of the definitive procedure. Treat with appropriate analgesia. Care should be taken to exclude other postoperative problems
- Hemorrhage – rarely the site of postoperative hemorrhage, both intraperitoneal and intraluminal
- Peritonitis – leakage around site of luminal contents or feed may lead to peritonitis

Late complications

- Entry site infection – as for PEG
- Tube blockage – as for NG tube

Common complications are shown in bold type.

Elemental feeds

Elemental feeds contain protein in amino acid form, and carbohydrate as glucose or maltodextrins. Fat content is very low. These feeds are used primarily in situations of malabsorption or (by some) as a primary treatment for Crohn's disease. Because of their high osmolality they should not be used in short bowel syndrome.

Disease-specific feeds

Certain clinical situations require alterations in diet. For example, there are high-energy, low-electrolyte feeds designed for patients on dialysis, and low-carbohydrate, high-fat diets for those with carbon dioxide retention, such as patients on ventilators (carbohydrate has a higher respiratory quotient than fat or protein and leads to more carbon dioxide production).

Immune-modulating feeds

These feeds contain extra substrates that may alter the immune and inflammatory responses. The commonly used substrates are glutamine, arginine, RNA, omega-3 fatty acids, and antioxidants. Evidence is gathering for the use of these products in certain surgical, trauma, critically ill, and cancer patients, but their exact place and indications for use have yet to be fully agreed.

Administration of tube feeds

- Ideally at 30–45°C
- Tube feeds can be delivered by:
  (i) continuous pump feeding over 16–18h a day, allowing some 'freedom' away from the pump
  (ii) intermittent administration of 50–250-mL boluses over 30min by syringe. Concerns that this method results in more complications, including aspiration, have not been adequately tested in clinical trials.

Complications of enteral feeding

On the whole, enteral feeding is safe and complications are not usually serious. They can be divided into those due to the tubes and routes of feeding (see Table 139.2), and those due to the feeding itself. The latter group include the following.

Diarrhea

This is the commonest complication, with quoted rates between 5% and 60%. It is most frequently associated with antibiotics, laxative use, contaminated feeds, and hypoalbuminemia. Management is first to exclude other explanations (e.g., *Clostridium difficile*, colitis, and malabsorption). Concomitant medications should be rationalized if causing diarrhea, especially antibiotics. Antidiarrheal medication (loperamide and/or codeine phosphate) is often successful, and fiber can help, although evidence is lacking.

Constipation

This is usually due to a combination of inadequate fluid, dehydration, poor mobility, and drugs (e.g., opiates). If colonic pathology is excluded or unlikely, management is by laxatives, suppositories, and fiber feeds.

Vomiting, aspiration, and reflux

Both nasogastric and PEG feeding can increase the risk of aspiration. Both can interfere with gastroesophageal sphincter function, and wide-bore nasogastric tubes do so more than fine-bore tubes. Where possible patients should be fed at an angle of 30–45°. Standard antiemetics and prokinetic agents are usually effective. Alternative or additional management options include alteration of feed delivery (change from bolus to continuous feeding), or changing the diet to a more energy dense one, with smaller volumes delivering equivalent calories. Occasionally postpyloric feeding is required.

Metabolic complications

Both underhydration and overhydration can be avoided by rigorous fluid balance control (1000 mL enteral feed delivers approximately 900 mL free fluid).

Overfeeding

Overfeeding – giving calories in excess of requirements – can cause serious or even fatal metabolic complications, especially in critically ill patients.

- Hyperglycemia – this is especially important in critically ill patients where it has been found that controlling blood glucose levels within 4–6 mmol/l reduces mortality.[8,9]
- Hypercapnia – nutrient metabolism requires oxygen and produces carbon dioxide. Overfeeding should be avoided as greater amounts of carbon dioxide are produced; this can delay weaning from a ventilator or cause problems for patients with significant respiratory disease.
- Azotemia – catabolism and excessive protein intake contribute to this.
- Hypertonic dehydration – this can be due to excessive protein intake combined with inability to excrete nitrogenous waste effectively. This occurs with patients who are dehydrated.

Overfeeding is usually caused by a combination of inaccurate nutritional assessments and by not taking into consideration energy from nonfood sources (e.g., propofol and glucose-containing dialysate solutions).

Refeeding syndrome

Refeeding syndrome can be defined as severe fluid and electrolyte shifts and related metabolic implications in malnourished patients undergoing refeeding.[10] Excess carbohydrate stimulates insulin release leading to substantial cellular uptake of phosphate, magnesium, and potassium, and a consequent fall in their serum levels. This may lead to dangerous cardiac arrhythmias and neurologic events, and can be fatal. Emaciated patients must *never* be fed beyond appropriate requirements. In such patients initial feeding should be 20 kcal/kg (600 kcal/day for a 30-kg patient). Phosphate, magnesium, and potassium supplements should be monitored daily, and supplemented if necessary.

Vitamin and trace element deficiencies

These are rare as most commercially available feeds are now nutritionally complete. Patients receiving small volumes of feed over a prolonged period of time may be at risk. See Table 138.3 details of clinical syndromes. Appropriate monitoring should avoid problems.

PARENTERAL (INTRAVENOUS) FEEDING

Parenteral feeding is the administration of nutrient solutions via a central or peripheral vein.[11] It is an expensive way to feed patients and is associated with a greater and more serious risk of complications than enteral feeding. Furthermore, it is not more effective then enteral feeding and, therefore, should be used only when the gut is either not working or is inaccessible. The indications are listed in Table 139.3, and complications in Tables 138.4 and 138.5.

Routes for parenteral nutrition

Parenteral nutrition should be administered through a dedicated feeding line. The following routes are available for short-term feeding (less than 28 days).

Central line

This enables use of the widest range of feeds without local complications such as phlebitis. However, insertion complication rates are higher than for peripheral lines. The most common complication is line sepsis, which can be reduced by use of single-lumen tubes, by a preference for the subclavian route

TABLE 139.3 INDICATIONS FOR PARENTERAL FEEDING
SHORT-TERM FEEDING (<28 DAYS)
• Nonfunctioning gastrointestinal tract (e.g., prolonged ileus, intra-abdominal malignancy)
• Proximal gut fistula
• Before surgery only if severely undernourished (e.g., BMI <17 kg/m^2) and enteral feeding not possible
• Postoperatively only when enteral feeding is contraindicated[12]
• Where requirements cannot be fully met enterally (e.g., multiorgan failure, major trauma, burns)
• Postchemotherapy mucositis
LONG-TERM FEEDING (>28 DAYS)
• Following extensive bowel resection (e.g., Crohn's disease, gut infarction)
• Extensive Crohn's disease with malabsorption
• High-output fistula
• Radiation enteritis
• Motility disorders (e.g., pseudo-obstruction, visceral myopathy or neuropathy)

TABLE 139.4 COMPLICATIONS OF PARENTERAL FEEDING: INSERTION RELATED

Failure to insert
Malposition
Pneumothorax[a]
Hemothorax[a]
Arterial puncture
Air embolism
Hemopericardium or tamponade[a]
Arrhythmias[a]
Central venous thrombosis[a]
Nerve injury, phrenic, vagus, brachial plexus[a]
Thoracic duct injury or chylothorax[a]

[a] Central lines only.

over jugular or femoral routes, and by meticulous care. In critical cases multi-lumen lines may be needed. One lumen should be reserved exclusively for nutrition, but there is a greater risk of line sepsis than with single-lumen lines.

Peripherally inserted central catheter

A catheter approximately 60 cm long is inserted into an antecubital vein and advanced to lie in the central veins so that hyperosmolar solutions can be used. This technique requires veins of good size, aseptic technique, and skill, but such lines can last for many months and are preferred by some authorities to central lines. Major complications are phlebitis (5–15%), malposition (8%), and catheter failure or leakage (4%).

Peripherally inserted catheter

These are shorter catheters, typically 20 cm long, also inserted into antecubital veins. As the proximal end is only in the axil-

TABLE 139.5 COMPLICATIONS OF PARENTERAL FEEDING: LINE AND FEEDING RELATED

Complication	Management[a]
LINE RELATED	
Exit site infection	Swab, clean, and appropriate antibiotics (e.g., flucloxacillin)
Tunnel infection (tunnelled lines only)	Swab exit site, take peripheral and central blood cultures Commence systemic antibiotics and consider removing line
Catheter-related sepsis (CRS)[13]	Consider if pyrexial, leukocytosis, and no other explanation (urine, chest) Stop parenteral nutrition and lock line with heparin Swab exit site, take peripheral and central blood cultures If CRS confirmed on cultures, lock line with vancomycin and systemic antibiotics, and observe closely. If sepsis persists, line will need to be removed. Alternatively line can be removed straight away with systemic antibiotics If cultures indicate *Staphylococcus aureus* or *Candida albicans*, line must be removed If cultures negative, reuse line and observe (and look for other sources). If doubt, remove line
Thrombophlebitis (peripheral lines)	Stop feed and remove line Care of inflamed site with appropriate dressings and cleansing
Catheter occlusion	Due to fibrin or lipid sludge Lipid occlusion takes a while to build up, so early occlusion (<7–14 days) is likely to be due to fibrin, and late occlusion (>14 days) more likely to be due to lipid Fibrin can usually be dislodged with urokinase or concentrated alcohol; lipid with alcohol
FEEDING RELATED	
Deficiency or excess of any electrolyte, vitamin, or trace element can occur	Adequate monitoring should prevent this – hospital will have policies to refer to
Hepatobiliary	Cholestasis, cholelithiasis, liver steatosis, and cirrhosis can all occur, but usually only with longer-term feeding. For an appropriate review, see reference 14
Bone disease	Metabolic bone disease and osteoporosis. For an appropriate review, see reference 15

[a] A brief description of the management of line-related complications is given here. Local hospital policy should be referred to for detailed management.

lary vein, hyperosmolar feeds are avoided because of the risk of thrombophlebitis. There is little, if anything, to recommend peripherally inserted short catheters over peripherally inserted central catheters.

Peripheral cannula

Low osmolality feeds can be administered through peripheral cannulae. They are easy to insert for short-term use, and with meticulous care can be maintained for several weeks.

To optimize efficacy, a fine-bore (22- or 24-Fr polyurethane cannula) should be inserted into a large forearm vein and a glyceryl trinitrate patch placed over the vein distal to cannula. The line should be changed regularly (every 48 h). Only low osmolality feed can be used, making this route unsuitable for patients either with high nutritional requirements or those requiring longer-term feeding.

For long-term feeding (>28 days) tunneled central lines with a Dacron cuff (e.g., Hickman or Broviac catheters), or an implantable venous access disk, will be required.

Discontinuing parenteral nutrition

Parenteral nutrition should never be stopped abruptly before alternative methods of feeding have been established, as rebound hypoglycemia may occur. Once oral or enteral feeding has begun, the patient can be weaned off parenteral nutrition gradually over 1–2 days. If parenteral nutrition does need to stop suddenly (e.g., line problems), a dextrose infusion should be administered.

NUTRITIONAL SUPPORT IN SPECIFIC GASTROINTESTINAL CONDITIONS

Inflammatory bowel disease[16] (see Chapters 53–59)

Nutrition is used for both nutritional support in an acute illness and as primary therapy in Crohn's disease.

In both acute ulcerative colitis and Crohn's disease, patients are unwell and catabolic, and may have malabsorption and weight loss. Unless there is clinical concern regarding imminent surgery (e.g., toxic dilatation), the patient should eat normally with or without administration of oral supplements if necessary – there is no evidence to support the concept of 'gut rest.' Parenteral nutrition is necessary only when enteral feeding is contraindicated, for instance in patients with proximal fistulae.

Both elemental and polymeric diets (see Chapter 138) are used as primary treatment for acute Crohn's disease. Response rates similar to those seen with steroids can be achieved, without steroidal side effects. However, the diet has to be the sole source of nutrition (over 6–8 weeks) for maximal efficacy; many patients find this difficult.

- Colonic Crohn's disease is probably less responsive to dietary therapy than small intestinal disease.
- There is no difference in the efficacy of elemental and polymeric diets, but polymeric diets are more palatable and compliance is generally better where taken orally (as opposed to via a feeding tube).
- There is probably a higher relapse rate after dietary treatment than after steroids.
- It is still unclear what 'ingredient or ingredients' (if any) in the diets are effective.

The evidence in favor of diet is more consistent in children than in adults. Many gastroenterologists, however, use diet as an adjunct to steroids in adults with difficult cases or as sole therapy where steroids are contraindicated or refused.

Acute pancreatitis[17] (see Chapter 69)

Traditionally 'gut rest' has been used in acute pancreatitis but there is now good evidence, in severe acute pancreatitis, that early feeding (within 24–48 h of onset) decreases the incidence of nosocomial infections, systemic inflammatory response syndrome, and overall disease severity. Enteral feeding should be provided via a tube placed distal to the ampulla of Vater. Parenteral nutrition can be used as a supplement when enteral feeding is inadequate to meet requirements, or is not possible because of toleration or contraindications.

In mild to moderate pancreatitis there is no evidence that either enteral or parenteral nutrition has a beneficial effect on clinical outcome, and nutritional support is not usually required unless complications occur.

Liver disease[18] (see Section 4)

Some 20–40% of patients with compensated cirrhosis and 80–100% with decompensated cirrhosis are undernourished because of anorexia, nausea, vomiting, and satiety due to ascites and/or unpalatable dietary restrictions; repeated hospital admissions often with prolong periods of 'nil by mouth.'

Patients with decompensated cirrhosis are hypercatabolic, and intensive nutritional support is essential to meet requirements. Although protein restriction was used previously, this worsens encephalopathy, diminishes skeletal and respiratory muscle function, delays mobilization, and increases the incidence of chest infections.[18] Protein requirements are, therefore, similar to those with an acute catabolic illness.[19] Sodium restriction and fluid management are essential on an individually tailored basis.

The place for branched-chain amino acid (BCAA) diets remains controversial. The rationale is that there is an excess of aromatic amino acids over BCAAs in patients with liver failure, which can be reversed using a diet that is rich in BCAAs. Animal studies have shown good benefit, but the findings have not been reproduced consistently in human studies. Currently the European Society of Parenteral and Enteral Nutrition recommend that BCAA diets should be used only in the few patients who are intolerant (i.e., encephalopathic) of standard protein intake.[19]

Many patients require tube feeding if they are unable or unwilling to eat enough to meet nutritional requirements. Passing a fine-bore tube in the presence of varices carries negligible risk, and parenteral nutrition should be reserved for those not prepared to cooperate with oral or tube feeding.

REFERENCES

1. American Dietetic Association. Position of the American Dietetic Association: food fortification and dietary supplements. J Am Diet Assoc 2001; 101:115–125.
2. Green CJ. Existence, causes and consequences of disease-related malnutrition in the hospital and community, and clinical and financial benefits of nutritional intervention. Clin Nutr 1999; 18(Suppl 2): 3–28.
3. DiSario J, Baskin W, Brown R et al. Endoscopic approaches to enteral nutritional support. Gastrointest Endosc 2002; 55:901–908.
4. Kirby DF, Delegge MH, Fleming CR. American Gastroenterological Association technical review on tube feeding for enteral nutrition. Gastroenterology 1995; 108:1282–1301.
5. Pearce CB, Duncan HD. Enteral feeding. Nasogastric, nasojejunal, percutaneous endoscopic gastrostomy, or jejunostomy: its indications and limitations. Postgrad Med J 2002; 78:198–204.
6. Dormann AJ, Huchzermeyer H. Endoscopic techniques for enteral nutrition: standards and innovations. Dig Dis 2002; 20:145–153.
7. Sharma V, Howden C. Meta-analysis of randomized, controlled trials of antibiotic prophylaxis before percutaneous endoscopic gastrostomy. Am J Gastroenterol 2000; 95:3133–3136.
8. Klein CJ, Stanek GS, Wiles CE. Overfeeding macronutrients to critically ill adults: metabolic complications. J Am Diet Assoc 1998; 98:795–806.
9. Van Den Berghe G, Wouters P, Weekers F et al. Intensive insulin therapy in critically ill patients. N Engl J Med 2001; 345:1359–1367.
10. Cook Ma, Hally V, Panteli JV. The importance of refeeding syndrome. Nutrition 2001; 17:632–637.
11. American Gastroenterological Association. AGA technical review on parenteral nutrition. Gastroenterology 2001; 121:970–1001.
12. Lewis SJ, Egger M, Sylvester PA et al. Early enteral feeding versus "nil by mouth" after gastrointestinal surgery: systematic review and meta-analysis of controlled trials. BMJ 2001; 323:773–776.
13. Department of Health. Guidelines for preventing infections associated with the insertion and maintenance of central venous catheters. J Hosp Infect 2001; 47(Suppl): S47–S67.
14. Buchman A. Total parenteral nutrition-associated liver disease. JPEN J Parenter Enteral Nutr 2002; 26:S43–S48.
15. Seidner DL. Parenteral nutrition-associated metabolic bone disease. JPEN J Parenter Enteral Nutr 2002; 26:S37–S42.
16. Goh J, O'Morain. Nutrition and adult inflammatory bowel disease. Aliment Pharmacol Ther 2003; 17:307–320.
17. Meiier R, Beglinger C, Layer P et al. ESPEN guidelines on nutrition in acute pancreatitis. Clin Nutr 2002; 21:173–183.
18. Florez DA, Aranda-Michel J. Nutritional management of acute and chronic liver disease. Semin Gastrointest Dis 2002; 13:169–178.
19. Plauth M, Merli M, Kondrup J et al. Consensus statement: ESPEN guidelines for nutrition in liver disease and transplantation. Clin Nutr 1997; 16:43–55.

Chapter 140

Complementary medicine for irritable and inflammatory bowel

George Thomas Lewith

> **KEY POINTS**
>
> - Patients with GI symptoms commonly try complementary and alternative medicine (CAM)
> - There is a lack of rigorous scientific trials on the efficacy of CAM in IBS and IBD
> - Single randomized controlled trials shows the benefit of acupuncture and Chinese herbal medicine in IBS
> - There is strong evidence for the efficacy of hypnotherapy in IBS
> - Interventions for food intolerance face problems with diagnosis and compliance
> - Dietary manipulation is a useful therapy in Crohn's disease
> - It is possible that *Candida albicans* may have a pathogenic role in IBS

INTRODUCTION AND SCIENTIFIC BASIS

Complementary and alternative medicine (CAM) is used by a growing number of patients with gastrointestinal (GI) diseases. This chapter will focus particularly on the use of herbal medicine, homeopathy, mind body therapies, acupuncture, specific dietary exclusion, food intolerance diets, and the use of nutritional supplements in irritable bowel syndrome (IBS) and inflammatory bowel disease (IBD). Gastrointestinal candidiasis is a well-developed concept in CAM and the evidence for gastrointestinal candidiasis as a cause of ill health is also discussed.

WHO USES CAM?

Use of CAM doubled in the USA in the 1990s[1] and now accounts for approximately US$30billion (Fig. 140.1). In the UK, 10% of the population use some form of CAM each year.

The use of CAM is common in gastrointestinal disease, having being tried by 43% of patients attending GI outpatient clinics. CAM use is more common in the young, urban dwellers, those in the higher income bracket, and those reporting poor quality of life or dissatisfied with conventional therapy. Many CAM users view hospitals as dangerous and do not disclose their use of CAM to orthodox physicians.[2]

Verhoef et al. have demonstrated that over 80% of CAM therapists in Canada (chiropractors, herbalists, and health food store employees) regularly see patients with inflammatory bowel disease using a wide range of unproven treatments. Giese's study involved a variety of GI disorders and indicated that 43% of patients had used some form of CAM over the previous 2 years, the majority of whom had found these approaches beneficial. Younger people were more likely to use CAM than the retired. Langmead et al. studied 239 patients with inflammatory bowel disease attending a UK hospital gastroenterology clinic and found that 26% had used some form of CAM, mainly herbal remedies; 53 of the CAM users reported significant benefit as a consequence. Poor quality of life correlated positively with increased CAM use in this group of patients. Rawsthorne et al. reported CAM use in four national centers for the treatment of inflammatory bowel disease (Stockholm, Cork, Los Angeles, and Winnipeg). Fifty-one per cent of patients attending these centers had used CAM, numbers being highest in North America. Perceived benefit among CAM users was not reported in this study.

It seems essential that conventional physicians should ask about CAM use. They also should be aware of its high prevalence and have some knowledge of the possible benefits and potential dangers of common CAM treatments.

SPECIFIC TREATMENTS

Complementary and alternative medicine covers a wide range of treatments. One feature that characterizes many of them and differs from orthodox medicine is that treatments are 'individualized' for each patient.

Herbal medicines

Herbal medicines have been widely used in Europe, China, and in indigenous North American populations. Traditional Chinese medicine, Ayurveda, and indigenous North American herbal traditions possessed vast herbal pharmacopeias.

Herbal medicine has diverse origins. There is a strong traditional European history of herbal medicine involving specific remedies for particular conditions such as the use of foxglove or digitalis for dropsy (heart failure), as well as the use of herbal mixtures defined on an individual basis through consultation. The methods used to prescribe herbal remedies are usually based on 'whole systems' of diagnosis and treatment that differ from conventional medicine, involving individualized prescriptions of herbal mixtures.

Irritable bowel syndrome

Herbal medicines have been widely used in the treatment of the irritable bowel syndrome, but, to date, there is very little strong scientific evidence to sustain this use. However, Isphagula and peppermint oil have achieved a place in orthodox medical treatment. Three randomized controlled trials involving Isphagula present overall positive data for its use in IBS with two trials involving 122 patients showing clear benefits while the third 80-patient study showed no specific treatment effect.[3] Similarly, a meta-analysis of the use of peppermint oil in IBS involving

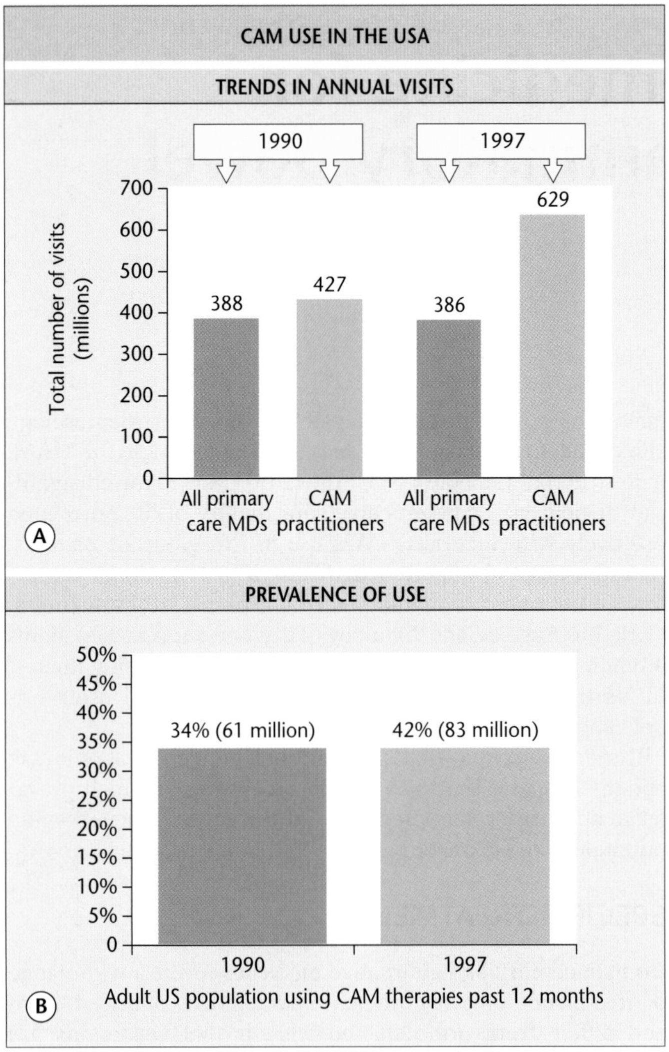

Fig. 140.1 CAM use in the USA. A. Trends in annual visits. **B.** Prevalence of use. Reproduced with permission from Eisenberg DM et al. JAMA 1998; 280:1569–1575.

eight studies suggested benefit with an odds ratio of 0.20 (95% confidence intervals of 0.04–0.89) for symptom reduction over placebo. However, the design of some of these studies has been criticized.[3]

Chinese herbal remedies

A recent rigorous, randomized, double-blind, controlled trial of the use of traditional Chinese herbal remedies over 2 years as treatment for IBS showed that such remedies are safe and effective.[4] Chinese herbs were given either in a standardized or an individualized way (as is traditional in China). Both approaches were successful, but only the individualized treatment group maintained improvement 14 weeks after treatment completion. Appital, a herbal mixture, showed no effect over placebo in an 8-week, double-blind, randomized, controlled trial involving 59 patients. Asafoetida extract combined with Nux Vomica shows some marginal benefit in IBS. Artichoke leaf extract may also be of value in IBS, although current evidence is flimsy.

Homeopathy

Samuel Hahnemann, a German physician, developed homeopathy some 200 years ago. It involves the use of very weak or ultramolecular dilutions (below the Avogadro number) of animal, mineral, or vegetable products. In normal clinical practice, these are usually prescribed after a long and involved homeopathic consultation and each prescription is individualized to the patient's presenting symptoms. Therefore, there is no 'standard' remedy for IBS or IBD, so these conditions may be treated with any one of perhaps 100 remedies.

Homeopathy in IBS

Three randomized controlled trials of homeopathy suggest benefit in patients with IBS. One trial involved absinthium and two involved the use of asafoetida.

However, a recent systematic review of homeopathy suggested that while all these trials were positive for homeopathy and suggested some effect on irritable bowel, their scientific quality was poor.[5] Conversely, because treatment was not individualized, the studies may not have tested the homeopathic approach fully.

Homeopathy in IBD

There are no existing trials evaluating the use of individualized homeopathy in IBD. Therefore, we must conclude that the evidence base for homeopathy in GI disease is very limited and largely anecdotal, while being aware that almost no rigorous studies are available on which to base an informed opinion.

Acupuncture

Acupuncture literally means 'to puncture with a needle.' Its practice is a central pillar of traditional Chinese medicine. Traditional Chinese medicine is based on the assumption that the body's own energy or 'qi' moves around the 12 main acupuncture meridians. A traditional Chinese diagnosis is made after listening to the patient's symptoms, feeling their pulse, and looking at their tongue. This is an individually based diagnosis and part of the whole system of traditional Chinese medicine, so there is no specific acupuncture point for a particular condition. Within the traditional Chinese model of illness, points are then selected to normalize the flow of qi and expel the appropriate 'pathogen' so that the body will return to a more normal state of 'balance.' In the West, acupuncture is frequently used for treatment of pain. This type of treatment is frequently based on examining the patient to define 'tender trigger points' and therapy is often based on needling these local painful areas rather than a traditional Chinese approach.

Effects of acupuncture on GI function and disease

Acupuncture is commonly used for GI disease in China and elsewhere.[6] Although there are quality issues for existing data, animal and human studies demonstrated that acupuncture has certain regulatory functions on GI motility and gastric acid secretion. Acupuncture promotes gastric peristalsis in subjects with low initial gastric motility and suppresses peristalsis in those with active initial motility. One controlled study also demonstrated that acupuncture significantly reduced basal acid output, albeit briefly.

Acupuncture in IBS

In a randomized controlled crossover trial, 25 patients showed a significantly greater improvement for all IBS symptoms after receiving one real compared to one sham acupuncture treatment. The study may have underestimated the effects of acupuncture, which normally involves much more intensive treatment than was used in this case.

Acupuncture in IBD

There is only one study evaluating the effect of acupuncture in IBD, which involves a Chinese diagnosis of 'chronic colitis.' The study is of very poor quality, but suggests that acupuncture may be of value.

Mind and body techniques

It has been suggested that various relaxation techniques such as yoga, autogenic training, and hypnosis can be used to manage IBS.

Hypnosis and IBS

In 'gut directed hypnosis,' pioneered by Whorwell et al., patients are given a simple account of how the gut works and, subsequently, during a fairly light hypnotic session, they are asked to modify their own GI function towards a more normal model. Given over 16 weeks this therapy results overall in an 80% individual improvement rate, affecting the symptoms of general well-being, pain, distention, and bowel habit. This benefit is maintained for 6 months or more post treatment. There is also a decrease in the colonic motility index and resting pulse rate. Overall, treatment has a profound effect on the patient's quality of life. Other researchers have been able to confirm Whorwell et al.'s observations using a variety of other relaxation techniques. Spanier and colleagues reviewed hypnotherapy, psychotherapy, behavioral therapy, and multicomponent therapy concluding that all were effective in IBS.[7] Although hypnosis is rarely used by conventional gastroenterologists[7,8] one must ask why, in our current evidence-based culture, as it appears to be effective.

Nutritional and dietary approaches

These approaches encompass the use of specific food exclusion diets (food intolerance) or the addition of a variety of nutritional supplements to a daily medication regime. Food exclusion diets are dependent on diagnosing food intolerance and encouraging compliance with subsequent prolonged food avoidance. Unfortunately, there are no 'gold standard diagnostic techniques' for unmasking food intolerance. Furthermore, there are problems with compliance when suggesting prolonged dietary intervention. This has generated considerable debate about the very existence of food intolerance as a viable diagnosis. However, there is some evidence for specific and individualized food avoidance diets in both IBS and IBD.

As reported in Chapter 42, Hunter and his colleagues have suggested that identification of specific food triggers was possible with symptomatic improvement from food exclusion in 50% of patients or more.[9] The foods reported to be most likely to trigger IBS are shown in Table 140.1. Many patients react to several foods, with two-thirds reporting six or more trigger foods.

Hunter's group has demonstrated triggering of IBS by double-blind food challenge of 44 double-blind tests in 11 patients, using active and placebo foods – 41 were correctly identified. In their experience, 70% of patients with IBS can be successfully managed in this way: on follow-up 2–3 years later, 90% of those who improved with food exclusion continued to be well. Most were still keeping to their diets but a quarter did not need to. A 50% success rate was achieved in another study[9] in patients resistant to conventional treatment, even though only one diet was employed, and those who did not improve were told that foods were not their problem.

TABLE 140.1 INTOLERANCE TO PARTICULAR FOODS IN A GROUP OF 122 PATIENTS WITH IBS

Food	%	Food	%
CEREALS		**VEGETABLES**	
Wheat	60	Onions	22
Corn	44	Potatoes	20
Oats	34	Cabbage	19
Rye	30	Sprouts	18
Barley	24	Peas	17
Rice	15	Carrots	15
DAIRY PRODUCTS	44	Lettuce	15
Milk	39	Leeks	15
Cheese	25	Broccoli	14
Butter	24	Soybeans	13
Yoghurt	10	Spinach	13
FISH	10	Mushrooms	12
White fish	7	Parsnips	12
Shellfish	16	Tomatoes	11
Smoked fish	14	Cauliflower	11
MEAT	13	Celery	11
Beef	11	Green beans	10
Pork	8	Cucumber	10
Chicken	24	Turnip/swede	10
Lamb	12	Marrow	8
Turkey	12	Beetroot	8
FRUIT	11	Peppers	6
Citrus	8	**MISCELLANEOUS**	33
Apples	8	Coffee	26
Rhubarb	8	Eggs	25
Banana	7	Tea	22
Strawberries	5	Chocolate	22
Pineapple	5	Nuts	20
Pears	4	Preservatives	12
Grapes		Yeast	12
Melon		Sugar beet	12
Avocado pear		Sugar cane	12
Raspberries		Alcohol	10
		Tap water	9
		Saccharin	2
		Honey	

Reproduced with permission from Alum Jones V, Hunter JO. Irritable bowel syndrome and Crohn's disease. In: Brostoff J, Challacombe SJ, eds. Food allergy and intolerance. Eastbourne: Baillière Tindall; 1987.

There is clearly positive evidence for the use of food exclusion diets and nutritional supplements in Crohn's disease.[10] Following the first demonstration that significant and prolonged periods of disease remission can be achieved with specific food exclusion diets compared to unrefined carbohydrate-rich diets (see Chapters 42 and 54). However, a low fiber diet may achieve the same improvement as individualized food exclusion. King and colleagues provide an excellent review of the literature in relation to dietary intervention for Crohn's, which suggests that dietary intervention should be considered as a serious evidence-based and viable alternative to the prescription of powerful disease-modifying agents. In spite of this evidence, dietary manipulation seems to be used very infrequently by conventional gastroenterologists.

Ulcerative colitis (see Chapters 42 and and 53)

As many as 20% of patients with ulcerative colitis have been reported to improve symptomatically with milk exclusion. Enzyme-potentiated desensitization (EPD), a food desensitizing technique designed to neutralize local reactions triggered by food intolerance also appeared to be effective. In a controlled study of 81 patients, EPD was associated with improvement in 13 patients compared to 2 controls with fewer subsequent acute exacerbations and overall a reduced steroid use.

Conclusions

The evidence for dietary exclusion having beneficial effects in Crohn's and IBS, while not definitive, is certainly strong and worthy of further study. The suggestion is frequently made to patients that food exclusion is of limited or no value in these conditions, a statement that is entirely unsupported by the evidence available. The addition of fish oil supplements may also prevent relapses in Crohn's[11,12] and there is some evidence that the same may be true in colitis.

GASTROINTESTINAL CANDIDA – MYTH OR REALITY?

It is well recognized by primary care and hospital physicians alike that investigation and examination of more than half of polysymptomatic patients fails to elucidate a unifying disease process. These patients commonly complain of chronic fatigue, poor concentration, impaired memory, respiratory tract symptoms, gastrointestinal distress (usually indicative of IBS), pain in muscles and joints, skin problems, and urogenital symptoms. Such patients are commonly found to be anxious or depressed, prompting a belief that their illness is psychologically based.

In 1978, Dr Orian Truss first suggested that in such patients there might be a separate condition identified by response to the combined treatment effects of a low-sugar diet, yeast- and mold-containing foods, and antifungal drug therapy. He proposed that the symptoms relate to diffuse hypersensitivity effects of the reservoir of candida and other yeasts present in the GI tract and suggested that the natural history of disease had become aggravated greatly by the increased use of antibiotics, oral contraceptives, immunosuppressant (including corticosteroid) agents, and highly refined carbohydrate diets.

Since this original description there have been many reports of patients experiencing remarkable and unexpected improvements in a wide array of symptoms (including chronic fatigue, psoriasis, eczema, headache, premenstrual syndrome, and psychoneurological disturbances) when treated with antifungal drugs alone or together with a diet low in sugars and yeasts.

Attempts to verify these findings have yielded conflicting data. In a primary care study, volunteers were recruited who had answered a magazine advertisement and displayed symptoms that appeared to be predictive of gastrointestinal candida defined by questionnaire. The study involved 116 Norwegian subjects who elected to follow either a normal diet or one low in sugars, food yeasts, and molds. They underwent block randomization to nystatin or placebo, which ensured an even distribution of dieters and nondieters in each drug group. Patients treated with nystatin, irrespective of diet, experienced a significantly greater reduction in overall symptom score than those who had received placebo ($p < 0.003$).[13]

Conversely, there was no effect of combined oral and vaginal nystatin compared to placebo in a group of women with vaginitis who complained also of depression, PMS, or other symptoms. However, this study has been heavily criticized because of the lack of any associated diet therapy and choice of a crossover model without wash-out period for a treatment potentially likely to have a carry-over effect. The patient selection was also at variance with the hypothesis, and some relevant outcomes were not recorded.

Mechanisms

Gut fermentation

Many patients with a suggestive clinical history show elevated blood alcohol 1 h after a postfasting 1 g glucose load, which is not seen after successful treatment. However, fecal cultures from a patient suspected of suffering from gastrointestinal candida and who had pre-existing ileostomy failed to demonstrate growth of any yeast including *Candida albicans.*[14] Laboratory studies show that subjects who have a positive gut fermentation test also have defective absorption of B vitamins, zinc, and magnesium, as well as increased gut permeability. They also show reduced urinary excretion of histidine (a marker for increased histamine demand) when compared to controls, but not when compared to subjects with atopic allergy suggesting the presence of immune activation.

Immune activation

Truss' original hypothesis of an immune mechanism is plausible since *Candida albicans* contains many distinct antigens and glycoproteins, which by triggering histamine release and provoking atopy, could favor the growth of candida. Sensitization is common and starts early in life. Patients with systemic candida infection show predominantly anti-candida IgG whilst in recurrent vaginal candidiasis the main antibody response has been reported as consisting mainly of secretory IgA.

Assessment

The evidence for gastrointestinal candida as a cause of this polysymptomatic condition that certainly includes IBS is far from definitive but, at the same time, there is certainly preliminary evidence to suggest that it is also far from being a myth.

CONCLUSION

The common CAM approaches to GI disease have been reviewed and present some provocative arguments about the existence of the 'candida syndrome.' While there is limited evidence and limited research for many of the CAM approaches in GI disease, use of diet in Crohn's disease and hypnosis and herbal remedies in IBS are treatment options that many gastroenterologists should consider. Further research into the 'candida syndrome' is essential, but there is some clear evidence to support the argument that it may be a viable diagnosis.

ACKNOWLEDGMENTS

I am very grateful to Dr Michael Radcliffe, Research Fellow in the Department of Medicine at the University of Southampton, for his help with this chapter, in particular in relation to the section on GI disease and the candida syndrome.

REFERENCES

1. Eisenberg DM, Davis RB, Ettner SL. Trends in alternative medicine use in the United States. JAMA 1998; 280:246–252.
2. Langmead L, Chitnis M, Rampton D. Use of complementary therapies by patients with IBD may indicate psychosocial distress. Inflamm Bowel Dis 2002; 8:175–179.
3. Ernst E, ed. The desktop guide to complementary and alternative medicine. Edinburgh: Mosby; 2001:300.
4. Bensoussan A, Talley NJ, Hing M et al. Treatment of irritable bowel syndrome with Chinese herbal medicine. JAMA 1998; 280: 1585–1589.
5. Linde K, Clausius N, Ramirez G et al. Are the clinical effects of homeopathy placebo effects? A meta-analysis of placebo-controlled trials. Lancet 1997; 350:834–843.
6. Diehl DL. Acupuncture for gastrointestinal and hepatobiliary disorders. J Alternat Complement Med 1999; 5:27–45.
7. Spanier JA, Howden CW, Jones MP. A systematic review of alternative therapies in the irritable bowel syndrome. Arch Intern Med 2003; 163:265–274.
8. Galovski TE, Blanchard EB. The treatment of irritable bowel syndrome with hypnotherapy. Appl Psychophysiol Biofeed 1998; 23:219–232.
9. Nanda R, James R, Smith H et al. Food intolerance and the irritable bowel syndrome. Gut 1989; 30:1099–1104.
10. King TS, Woolner JT, Hunter JO. Review article: the dietary management of Crohn's disease. Aliment Pharmacol Ther 1997; 11:17–31.
11. Belluzzi A, Brignola C, Campieri M et al. Effect of an enteric-coated fish-oil preparation on relapses in Crohn's disease. N Engl J Med 1996; 334:1557–1560.
12. Lorenz-Meyer H, Bauer P, Nicolay C et al. Omega-3 fatty acids and low carbohydrate diet for maintenance of remission in Crohn's disease. A randomized controlled multicenter trial. Study Group Members (German Crohn's Disease Study Group). Scand J Gastroenterol 1996; 31:778–785.
13. Santelmann H, Laerum E, Roennevig J, Fagertun HE. Effectiveness of nystatin in polysymptomatic patients. A randomized, double-blind trial with nystatin versus placebo in general practice. Family Practice 2001; 18:258–265.
14. Eaton KK. Do yeasts play any part in 'Candida' (fungal-type dysbiosis)? Discussion paper. J Nutr Environ Med 1998; 8:247–255.

Chapter 141

Conscious sedation

Sandeep C Patel and John J Vargo

KEY POINTS

- With conscious sedation, the patient should be able to make meaningful verbal responses, whilst maintaining ventilatory and cardiovascular function
- Benzodiazepine-narcotic combinations potentiate the risk of oversedation
- Droperidol is associated with fatal arrhythmia
- Use of propofol requires specific training in administration, monitoring and airway management
- Capnography is superior to oximetry in detection of hypoventilation
- When in doubt, ask for an anesthetic opinion

INTRODUCTION AND SCIENTIFIC BASIS

Sedation and analgesia represents a continuum from minimal sedation or anxiolysis through to general anesthesia. The American Society of Anesthesiologists' Task Force on Sedation and Analgesia by Non-Anesthesiologists has issued practice guidelines for sedation and analgesia by nonanesthesiologists[1] (Table 141.1). Most endoscopic procedures are performed under moderate sedation and analgesia, which is known as 'conscious sedation.' At this level of sedation, the patient is able to make a purposeful response to verbal and tactile stimulation, and both ventilatory and cardiovascular function are maintained. With deep sedation, patient responsiveness involves purposeful responses to painful stimuli. Airway support may be required. At a level of general anesthesia, the patient is unarousable, even to painful stimuli. Airway support is frequently required and cardiovascular function may be impaired. At all times, the endoscopy team must be able to recognize the various levels of sedation and analgesia, and rescue a patient who exhibits loss of responsiveness, airway protection, spontaneous respiration, or cardiovascular function.

The level of sedation should be titrated to achieve a safe, comfortable, and technically successful procedure. The purpose of sedation and analgesia is to relieve anxiety, discomfort, or pain, and to reduce recall for the procedure. Cardiopulmonary complications that may arise from sedation and analgesia include aspiration, oversedation, hypoventilation, vasovagal episodes, and airway obstruction.

The risk of cardiovascular complications is related to both the procedure being performed and the patient's general health status. Very old patients and those with co-morbidities, including cardiovascular, pulmonary, renal, hepatic, metabolic, and neurologic disorders, or morbid obesity may be at increased risk from sedation. These patients, as well as patients who are chronic users of narcotics and benzodiazepines, alcoholics, drug addicts, and those with neuropsychiatric disorders, may require more intense monitoring during endoscopic procedures.

SEDATIVES AND ANALGESICS FOR ENDOSCOPY

The choice of sedative is largely operator dependent, but generally consists of benzodiazepines used either alone or in combination with an opiate.[2] The most common benzodiazepines are midazolam and diazepam. Although similar in efficacy, most endoscopists prefer midazolam for its rapid onset of action, short duration of action, and high amnesic properties. Narcotics, such as meperidine or fentanyl, provide analgesia and sedation. Fentanyl has a rapid onset of action and clearance, and a reduced incidence of nausea compared with meperidine. Morphine is usually avoided because of concern about stimulating smooth

TABLE 141.1 CONTINUUM OF SEDATION AND ANALGESIA

	Minimal sedation	Moderate sedation	Deep sedation	General anesthesia
Responsiveness	Normal response to verbal stimulation	Purposeful response to verbal and tactile stimulation	Purposeful response after repeated or painful stimulation	Unarousable, even with painful stimulation
Airway	Unaffected	No intervention required	Intervention may be required	Intervention often required
Spontaneous ventilation	Unaffected	Adequate	May be inadequate	Frequently inadequate
Cardiovascular function	Unaffected	Usually maintained	Usually maintained	May be impaired

From American Society of Anesthesiologists Task Force on Sedation and Analgesia by Non-Anesthesiologists. Practice guidelines for sedation and analgesia by non-anesthesiologists. Anesthesiology 2002; 96:1005.

muscle contraction and inducing spasm of the sphincter of Oddi during endoscopic retrograde cholangiopancreatography. Combinations of benzodiazepine and opioid agents are commonly used for moderate to deep sedation. However, their potentiated effect of sedation may increase the risk of desaturation and cardiopulmonary complications.

Adjuncts to the benzodiazepine–narcotic combination include diphenhydramine, promethazine, and droperidol. They potentiate the action by achieving a deeper level of sedation. Droperidol is a neuroleptic agent that is efficacious in difficult to sedate patients undergoing therapeutic endoscopy. However, it is associated with potentially life-threatening cardiac arrhythmia (torsade de pointes) and therefore guidelines have been established for its use in endoscopic procedures.

Anesthetic agents that have been used during endoscopic procedures include inhalation agents (nitrous oxide, enflurane, isoflurane, and sevoflurane) and propofol. Although inhalation agents are rarely used now, propofol is increasingly becoming administered during endoscopic procedures.[3] Propofol is an ultrashort-acting hypnotic agent that provides amnesia but minimal levels of analgesia. Propofol has a rapid onset of action, which causes rapid depression of level of consciousness and cardiopulmonary function, requiring ventilatory support. Personnel specifically trained in the administration of propofol with expertise in emergency airway management must independently monitor sedation during endoscopic procedures.

PRE-PROCEDURAL MONITORING

Patients undergoing endoscopic procedures require pre-procedural evaluation to assess their risk and to help manage problems related to pre-existing medical conditions. A thorough pre-procedural assessment includes a careful history and physical examination, review of current medications and drug allergies, and assessment of cardiopulmonary status at the time of the procedure.

It is very useful for endoscopy units to keep an updated list of drug interactions that might occur with the drugs commonly used for conscious sedation. Some, such as monoamine oxidase inhibitors, may result in serious complications. In addition, some specific associated disorders (e.g., systemic mastocytosis, pheochromocytoma) should represent indications to arrange for an anesthesiologist to administer the conscious sedation.

STANDARD AND EXTENDED MONITORING DURING PROCEDURES

Patients undergoing endoscopic procedures should have continuous monitoring before, during, and after the administration of sedatives. Standard monitoring of sedated patients undergoing gastrointestinal procedures includes recording the heart rate, blood pressure, respiratory rate, and oxygen saturation. Although not conclusively seen in controlled trials, continuous electrocardiographic monitoring is reasonable for high-risk patients; those with a history of significant cardiac arrhythmia or cardiac dysfunction, elderly patients, and those undergoing prolonged procedures. Supplemental oxygen administration has been shown to reduce the magnitude of oxygen desaturation when given during endoscopic procedures. Its use should be considered in high-risk patients, those with impairment of pulmonary function or significant pre-sedation desaturation, and those in whom prolonged or complex procedures are anticipated.

Extended monitoring by means of transcutaneous and end-tidal carbon dioxide monitoring are noninvasive methods of measuring respiratory activity. Capnography has become a favored mode of extended monitoring, and is based on the principle that carbon dioxide absorbs light in the infrared region of the electromagnetic spectrum. Quantification of the absorption leads to the generation of a curve that represents a real-time display of the patient's respiratory activity (Fig. 141.1). Capnography more readily identifies episodes of apnea and periods of hypoventilation. It is a superior way to evaluate ventilation, compared with pulse oximetry, which assesses oxygenation.[4]

Bispectral (BIS) monitoring is a technology that has potential to prevent oversedation during endoscopic procedures. BIS monitoring uses continuous EEG recordings to generate an objective assessment of degree of sedation. A value on a linear scale from 100 (fully awake) to 0 (flat-line EEG) is generated during a procedure to reflect brainwave activity and level of sedation (Fig. 141.2). BIS values seem to correlate with the Modified Observer's Assessment of Alertness/Sedation (MOAA/S) scale, a subjective sedation assessment scale.[5]

CAPNOGRAPHY FINDINGS IN NORMAL AND APNEIC PATIENTS

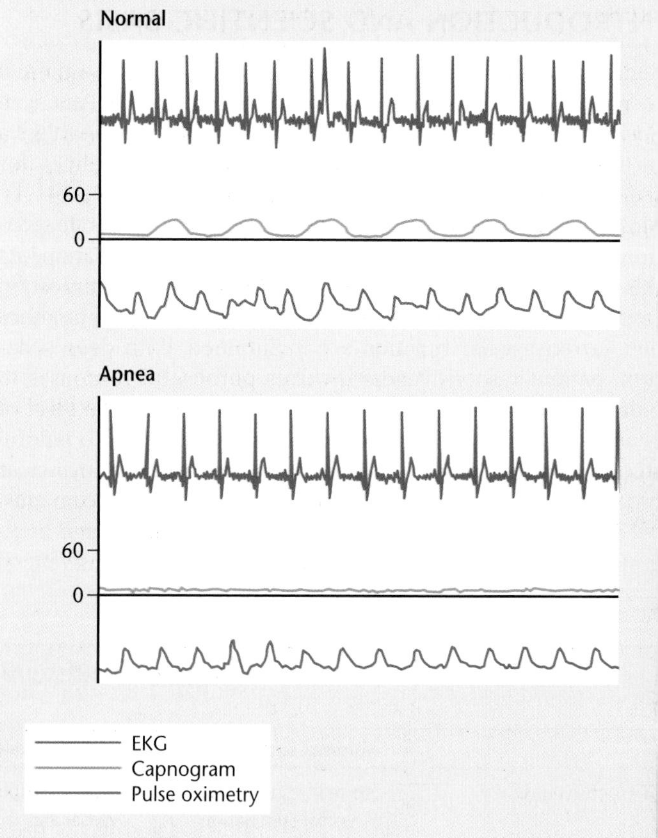

Fig. 141.1 Capnography findings in normal and apneic patients. Normal (top panel): (Red) Normal electrocardiogram. (Green) Capnograph – the peaks of the curve signify end-expiration; the abrupt trough in the curve represents inspiration. (Purple) Normal pulse oximetry curve. **Apnea (lower panel):** (Red) Normal electrocardiogram. (Green) Capnograph – representation of apnea; there is no evidence of respiratory activity. (Purple) Note that the pulse oximetry curve remains normal in the setting of apnea.

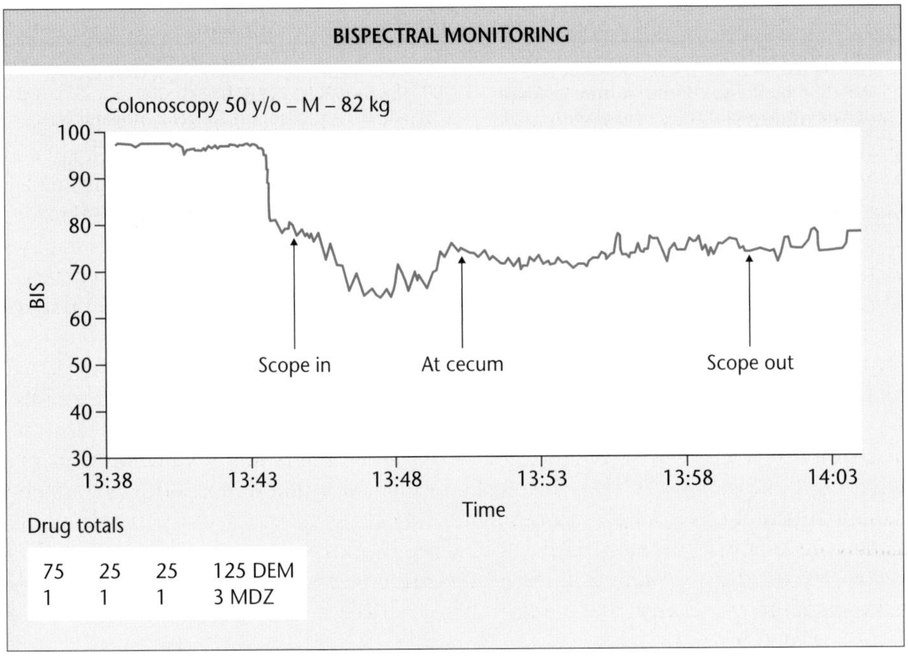

Fig. 141.2 Bispectral monitoring. The Bispectral Index (BIS) value as a function of time during a colonoscopy with meperidine (DEM) and midazolam (MDZ). Note that repeated boluses of medication were necessary to achieve a state of moderate sedation and analgesia throughout the procedure.

POST-PROCEDURAL MONITORING

On completion of endoscopic procedures, patients should be observed for adverse effects from either instrumentation or sedation, and may be discharged from the post-procedure recovery area or endoscopy unit once vital signs are stable and an appropriate level of consciousness is reached. The Aldrete score is a post-anesthesia recovery score that takes into account a patient's level of consciousness, activity, respiration, circulation, and oxygen saturation (Table 141.2), and guides clinicians when optimal conditions are met for safe patient discharge.[6]

SUMMARY

Some complications of conscious sedation are idiosyncratic. Others may be prevented by paying careful attention to the patient's general health condition, the drugs they are taking, and their co-morbidities. If there is doubt about the safety of the planned conscious sedation or the need for other drugs such as propofol, then a useful rule is: *when in doubt ask the anesthesiologist to administer the conscious sedation.*

TABLE 141.2 POST-ANESTHESIA RECOVERY SCORE (ALDRETE SCORE)

Category	Description	Score
Consciousness	Fully awake and oriented (name, place, date)	2
	Arousable on calling	1
	Not responding	0
Activity	Moves all four extremities voluntarily or on command	2
	Moves two extremities	1
	Unable to move extremities	0
Respiration	Breathes deeply and coughs freely	2
	Dyspnea, limited breathing, or tachypnea	1
	Apneic or on mechanical ventilation	0
Circulation	Blood pressure ±20% of preanesthetic level	2
	Blood pressure ±20–49% of preanesthetic level	1
	Blood pressure ±50% of preanesthetic level	0
Oxygen saturation	spO_2 >92% on room air	2
	Supplemental oxygen required to maintain spO_2 >90%	1
	spO_2 >92% with oxygen supplementation	0
Maximum score		10

Modified from Aldrete JA, Kroulik D. A postanesthetic recovery score. Anesth Analg 1970; 49:924–349.

REFERENCES

1. Gross JB, Bailey PL, Connis RT et al. Practice guidelines for sedation and analgesia by non-anesthesiologists. Anesthesiology 2002; 96:1004–1017.
2 Faigel DO, Baron TH, Goldstein JL et al. ASGE: guidelines for the use of deep sedation and general anesthesia for GI endoscopy. Gastrointest Endosc 2002; 56:613–617.
3. Nelson DB, Barkun AN, Block KP et al. ASGE: propofol use during gastrointestinal endoscopy. Gastrointest Endosc 2000; 53:876–878.
4. Vargo JJ, Zuccaro G, Dumot JA, Conwell DL, Morrow JB, Shay SS. Automated graphic assessment of respiratory activity is superior to pulse oximetry and visual assessment for detection of respiratory activity during therapeutic upper endoscopy. Gastrointest Endosc 2002; 55:826–831.
5. Bower AL, Ripepi A, Dilger J, Boparai N, Brody FJ, Ponsky JL. Bispectral index monitoring of sedation during endoscopy. Gastrointest Endosc 2000; 52:192–196.
6. Aldrete JA, Kroulik D. A post-anesthetic recovery score. Anesth Analg 1970; 49:924–934.

Chapter 142

Sclerotherapy, banding, and other hemostatic techniques for varices and other lesions

James Y W Lau and S C Sydney Chung

KEY POINTS

- Upper gastrointestinal bleeding still carries a 10% mortality
- Esophageal banding should start distally (and usually only the lower 5 cm)
- EVL is preferable to EIS/EVL+EIS in terms of reduced local complications, recurrent bleeding and mortality
- Gastric varices are treated with histoacryl glue
- Thermal devices consistently seal arteries up to 2mm in diameter in upper gastrointestinal bleeding
- Beware large ulcers in the posterior wall of the duodenal bulb (gastroduodenal artery)
- Combined modalities (e.g. adrenaline injection and heater probe) are preferable to adrenaline injection alone in upper gastrointestinal bleeding

NTRODUCTION AND SCIENTIFIC BASIS

pper gastrointestinal bleeding remains a common medical nergency and a cause for hospital admissions. In an aging opulation, mortality from upper gastrointestinal bleeding is excess of 10% despite improvement in the medical care. arious endoscopic methods are proven in their efficacy in the ntrol of upper gastrointestinal bleeding. Endoscopic therapy often the first treatment modality in the management algorithm combination with medical therapy. For practical purposes, uses of upper gastrointestinal bleeding can be categorized to variceal and nonvariceal in origin. This chapter discusses e use of endoscopic therapy in variceal and nonvariceal hemor-age, and includes their diverse prognosis and the different odes of endoscopic intervention. Because of their diverse ognosis, management of variceal and nonvariceal bleeding e discussed separately.

ARICEAL HEMORRHAGE

ndoscopic variceal ligation (EVL)

he concept of variceal ligation was derived from band ligation r hemorrhoids. The basic principle of variceal banding volves placement of elastic 'O' ring ligatures around varices. he assembly consists of a friction-fit adaptor on the end of e scope, an inner ligation cylinder with an elastic 'O' ring, nd a trip wire.

The varix is aspirated into the inner cylinder. This produces red-out appearance in the endoscopic view. The trip wire is ulled to release the 'O' rubber ring. Strong suction is required nd complete red-out of the endoscopic view is mandatory efore firing the rubber band (Fig. 142.1).

Treatment begins with ligation of most distal variceal columns in the esophagus just above the esophagogastric junction. Larger varices should have additional bands cephalad to the first band. In the treatment of actively bleeding varices or varices with stigmata of bleeding, the bleeding point can be aspirated directly into the drum and a band can then be applied. In situations where the exact bleeding point cannot be seen, it is recommended the scope be first passed into the stomach and variceal columns banded at their most distal portions, usually just caudal or at the esophagogastric junction.

Multifire band ligation devices are now available and are quicker, more comfortable for the patient, safer, and more convenient to use than the original single band device. This requires passage of an overtube (Fig. 142.2) across the crico-pharyngeus, but this could cause esophageal laceration, perforation, and pinch injury of the esophageal wall.

Endoscopic injection sclerotherapy (EIS)

In many parts of the world, injection sclerotherapy remains the primary treatment for bleeding esophagogastric varices. The technique is used both in the control of acute bleeding and the elective obliteration of varices.

Sclerosants are either chemical irritants such as the fatty acids (e.g., ethanolamine oleate, polidocanol) or dehydrating agents (e.g., ethanol, hypertonic glucose, and phenol), which cause an acute inflammatory reaction and thrombosis of venous channels. Choice largely reflects personal preference and availability.

Injection often starts from the esophagogastric junction using a flexible tip sclerotherapy needle (Fig. 142.3). Depending on the size of the varix, 1–2-mL aliquots are injected into each column at the esophagogastric junction, then 2.5 and 5 cm cephalad. Injections may be intravariceal (directed into the veins) or paravariceal. Most endoscopists use a free hand method injecting sclerosant into the bleeding varix or variceal column that shows stigmata of bleeding such as a fibrin clot.

Depending on the type of sclerosant used, we restrict its total volume to 20 mL per session. Weekly injection is then continued until eradication. In the event that bleeding is provoked during injection, the therapeutic endoscope can be passed into the stomach so that the body of the equipment compresses on the bleeding spots. Bleeding usually stops within 1–2 min and more sclerosant can then be injected.

Band ligation versus EIS

Evidence from the literature suggests that band ligation is preferred over sclerotherapy in the treatment of esophageal varices. In the original Denver trial of 129 patients, band ligation required fewer treatment sessions to achieve eradication,

BAND LIGATION OF ESOPHAGEAL VARICES

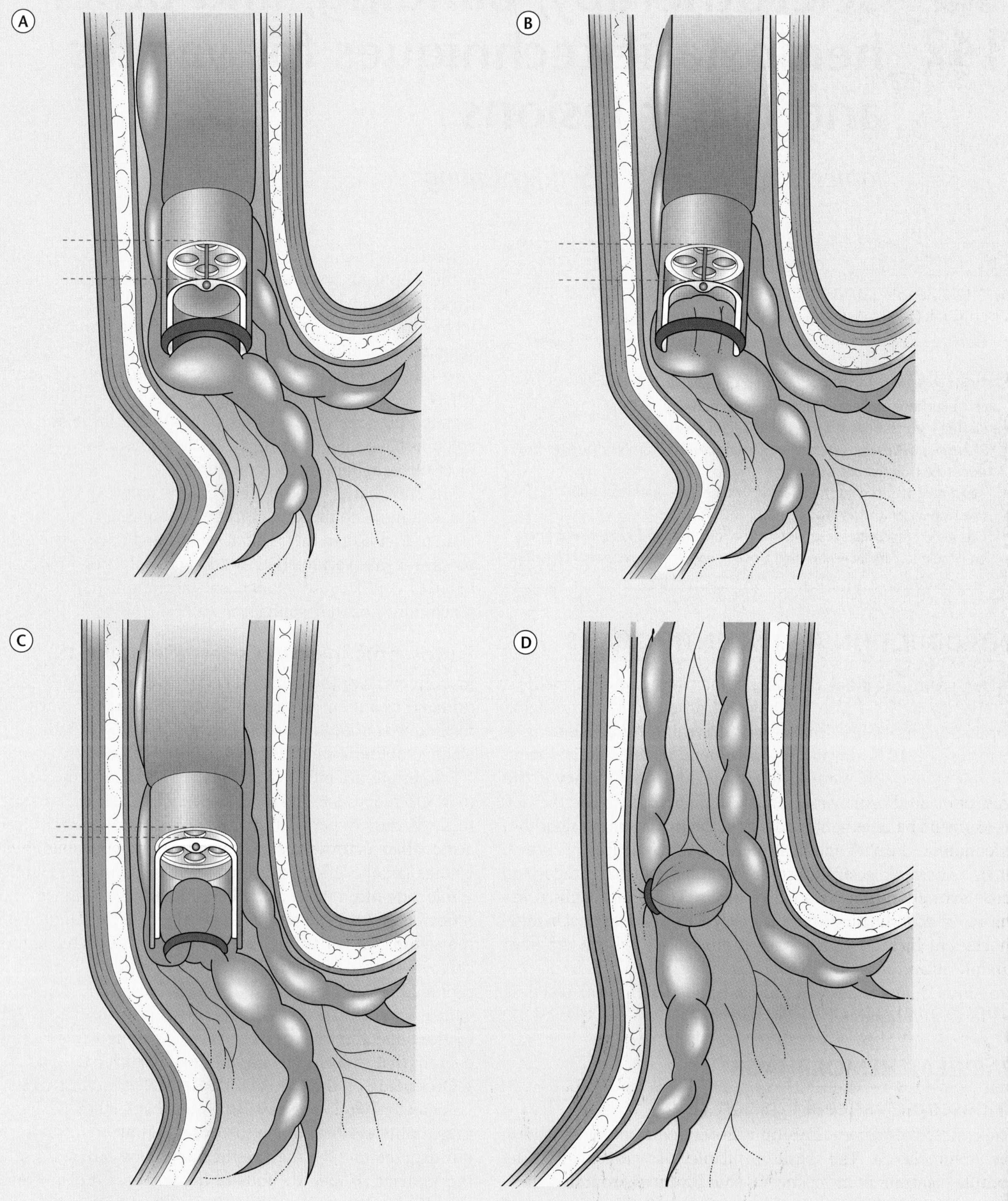

Fig. 142.1 Band ligation. Band ligation of esophageal varices. Reproduced from Stiegmann GV. Endoscopic management of esophageal varices. Adv Surg 1994; 27:209–231 with permission from Chicago Mosby Year Book, 1994 Elsevier, Health Sciences Division.

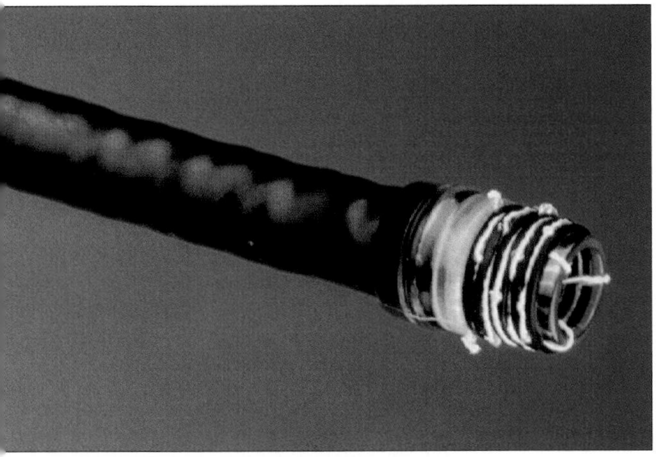

g. 142.2 **Banding device.** A multifire banding device, Six-shooter, ilson Cook (Salem, Winston, USA).

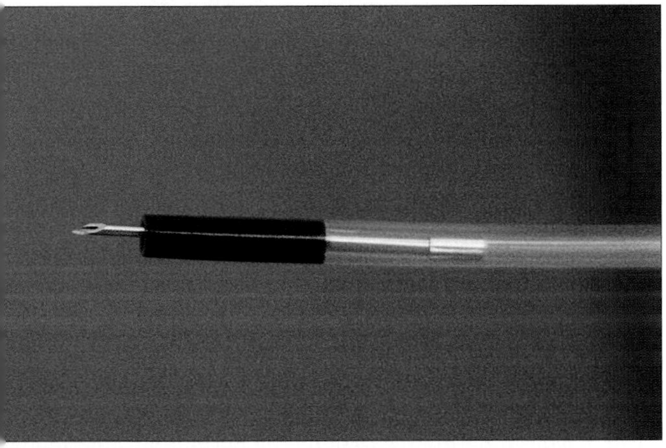

g. 142.3 A Marcon-Haber 23G sclerotherapy injection syringe with short bevel.

SCLEROTHERAPY INTO LIGATED VARIX

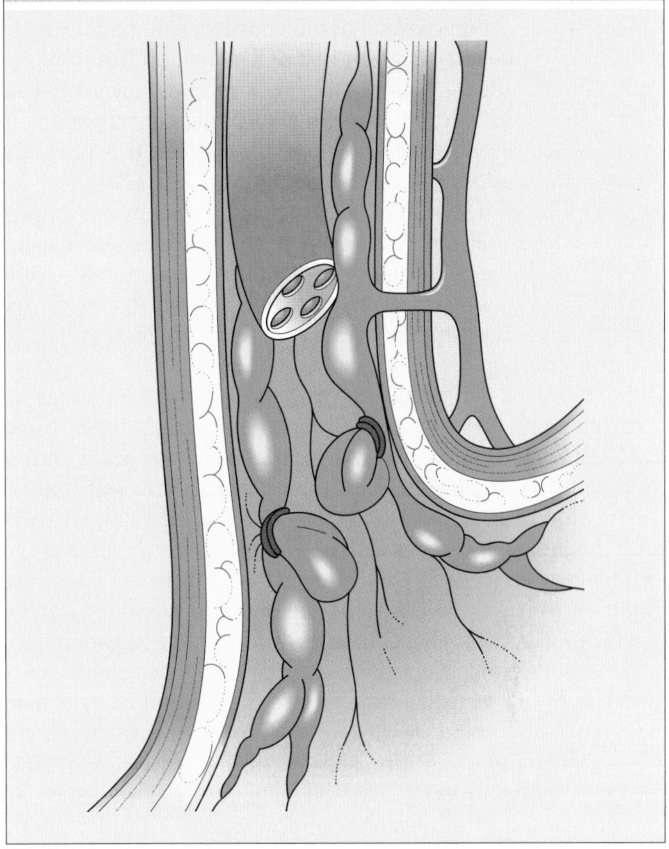

Fig. 142.4 Sclerotherapy into a ligated varix. Combined low-volume sclerotherapy into a ligated varix. Reproduced from Stiegmann GV. Endoscopic management of esophageal varices. Adv Surg 1994; 27:209–231 with permission from Chicago Mosby Year Book, 1994 Elsevier, Health Sciences Division.

as associated with less recurrent bleeding, fewer complica- ons (principally esophageal strictures, pneumonia, and other fections, 2 v 22%) and, in patients with Child-Pugh grades A r B, a survival benefit.[1] A subsequent meta-analysis of seven ials showed banding was superior to sclerotherapy in reduc- g recurrent bleeding as well as bleeding related and overall ortality.[2] Band ligation was also associated with fewer local omplications, principally esophageal strictures.

ombining banding ligation and sclerotherapy the treatment of esophageal varices

s an attempt to hasten eradication of varices, many use com- ined low-volume sclerotherapy proximal to bands (Fig. 142.4). his synchronous approach theoretically lessens the volume of lerosants used and hence associated local side effects. Venous asis induced by band ligation enhances the effect of a scle- osant. Ligation of individual esophageal varices is first done ear the gastroesophageal junction. Intravariceal injection then performed cephalad to the site of ligation. Alterna- vely, some endoscopists apply two bands above and below varix and inject sclerosant intravariceally between the two ands. In a meta-analysis of trials comparing combined ligation/ lerotherapy to band ligation alone, a higher rate of compli- ation, notably esophageal stricture formation, was noted with ynchronous band ligation and scleroinjection.[3]

A metachronous approach using band ligation initially to reduce varices to a small size followed by injection of residual varices may however be worthwhile. In practice, band ligation is less effective in smaller varices and in particular when there is fibrosis induced by previous banding or sclerotherapy. This renders suction of residual varices difficult. Lo et al. tested this staged approach in a randomized study and found that it reduced both recurrence of varices and recurrent bleeding with a median follow-up of 2 years.[4]

Tissue adhesives

N-butyl-2-cyanoacrylate (Histoacryl glue, Braun, Melsungen, Germany) is a watery substance that polymerizes and hardens instantaneously when in contact with blood. This unique property is useful in the obliteration of varices. To slow down clotting and to allow fluoroscopic monitoring of the injection, cyanoacrylate is mixed with radiological contrast (Lipoidol®) prior to injection. Before its injection, the working channel of the endoscope and the injector catheter are flushed with 0.5–1 mL of Lipoidol® to prevent channel blockage. The varix is then punctured and a histoacryl/Lipoidol® (0.5 mL/0.7 mL) mixture injected. When seen on fluoroscopy, a serpentine structure confirms successful intravariceal injection. Before retraction of the needle, the remaining glue is pushed into the varix with another 2 mL of Lipoidol®. The needle is then rinsed with distilled water on retraction. Suction aspiration via the endoscope should be avoided at this time to avoid glue clogging the suction channel of the endoscope and adhering to the lenses of the endoscope. A cast will slough off from the site of injection within 1–2 weeks leaving a mucosal ulcer behind. Cyanoacrylate is very effective in controlling actively spurting variceal hemorrhage in esophagogastric varices. It is probably superior to sclerosant in the acute control of bleeding.

The repeated injection of such histoacryl glue in esophageal varices can cause significant dysphagia, strictures, and ulcerations. There have been reports of distal embolization into pulmonary and cerebral vasculatures. In esophageal varices, we reserve histoacryl glue as a rescue when band ligation fails to control bleeding.

Sarin et al. classified gastric varices into four types based on their anatomic location: gastroesophageal varices types 1 and 2 (GOV1 and 2) and isolated gastric varices types 1 and 2 (IGV1 and 2) (Fig. 142.5).[5] Gastroesophageal varices are gastric varices found in association with esophageal varices, whereas isolated gastric varices are those occurring in the absence of esophageal varices. GOV1 extend along the lesser curvature into the stomach whereas GOV2 extend into the fundus of the stomach. Gastroesophageal varices are treated as esophageal varices with band ligation close to the esophagogastric junction. IGV1 are located in the gastric fundus and carry a high risk of bleeding and death (Fig. 142.6). In the treatment of IGV1, histoacryl glue is probably the only effective endoscopic treatment in controlling acute bleeding and was shown to be better than ligation in one clinical trial.[6] Ectopic gastric varices or IGV2 are uncommon and occur in any part of the stomach.

Complications of endoscopic therapy

When compared to EST, EVL has been associated with fewer complications. This is related to the fact that EVL produces

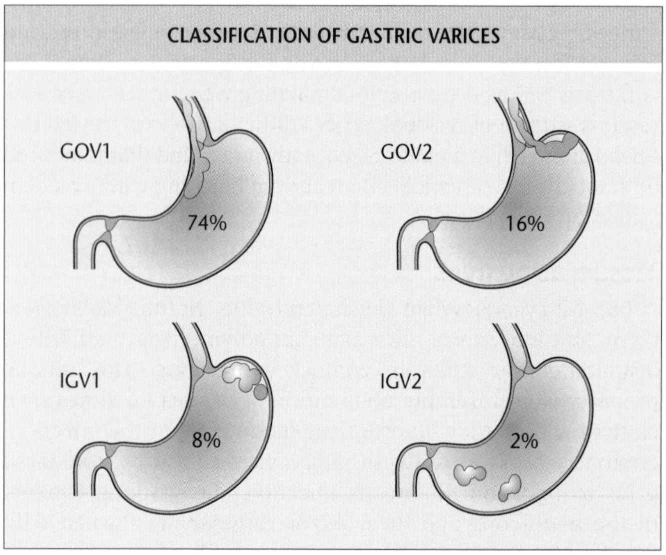

Fig. 142.5 Classification of gastric varices. Reproduced from Sarin SK et al. Prevalence, classification and natural history of gastric varices: a long-term follow-up study in 568 portal hypertension patients. Hepatology 1992; 16:1343–1349, Copyright © 1992 Wiley-Liss, Inc. reprinted with permission of Wiley-Liss Inc., a subsidiary of John Wiley & Sons, Inc.

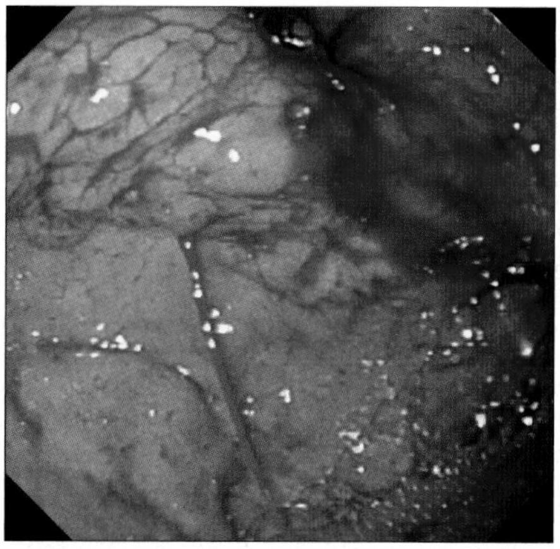

Fig. 142.6 Gastric varix. A bleeding gastric varix.

only mechanical strangulation of varices without much tissu inflammation and injury. Small ulcers are produced after th 'O' ring and the strangulated varix sloughs off from th esophageal wall. The ulcers are usually superficial and almo never produce stricture of esophagus. Complications associate with chemical irritation are also uncommon. The only seriou complication associated with EVL is related to the use of a over-tube. Esophageal laceration, perforation, and pinchin injury of the esophageal wall in the gap between over-tube an the endoscope have been described. The use of multiban devices has eliminated such injuries.

Conversely, EST causes significant complications in abou 20% of patients. These vary from minor transient complicatio such as chest pain, temporary dysphagia, and fever to mo serious complications such as recurrent bleeding from esophage ulcer, bacterial peritonitis, esophageal perforation, and media tinitis. Aspiration pneumonia is not uncommon in agitate patients with active bleeding and can potentially be avoided b endotracheal intubation before EST. Severe esophageal ulcer tions heal with extensive fibrosis and esophageal strictur Portal vein thrombosis, brain abscess, spinal cord paralysi and pericarditis have been reported but are rare complication

NONVARICEAL HEMORRHAGE

Injection therapy

Soehendra first described endoscopic injection in the trea ment of nonvariceal hemorrhage. Polidocanol was injected int a bleeding gastric ulcer.[7] Owing to the limited volume of pol docanol that could be injected, the technique was subsequent modified. Diluted adrenaline (epinephrine) was first injecte around the vessel to stop bleeding followed by its targete injection of a sclerosant to induce thrombosis. Injection therap has become the most widely practiced form of endoscop hemostasis. An array of agents is used in injection therap including diluted adrenaline, sclerosants, absolute alcoho thrombin, and recently fibrin sealant.

Submucosal injection of diluted adrenaline (1:10 000) work by a combination of volume tamponade and local vasocor striction. Because adrenaline is nontissue damaging, a large volume of 10–20 mL can be injected submucosally. The live rapidly metabolizes systemically absorbed adrenaline. Fe complications are observed following submucosal injection c adrenaline other than transient tachycardia. Submucosal inje on of adrenaline is generally safe except in patients with arginal hepatic reserve.

Injection therapy is simple to perform. A disposable 23- or 5-gauge sclerotherapy needle with a short bevel is used. The eedle protrudes about 5 mm beyond the sheath. The use of dual channeled endoscope allows simultaneous delivery of ierapy and suctioning. An additional channel also provides an lternative angle of access. Aliquots of 0.5–1 mL are injected round the bleeding vessel. In actively bleeding ulcers, cessaon of bleeding signifies a treatment end-point (Fig. 142.7). ucosal edema and blanching are observed following adrenane injection. In nonbleeding visible vessels (defined as a proberant discoloration), the treatment end-point is less distinct. ften, a volume of up to 10 mL is injected around the vessel. any consider injection of adrenaline alone inadequate because f its mode of action. Most endoscopists would apply a second odality to induce vessel thrombosis.

Polidocanol, ethanolamine, and sodium tetradecyl sulfate STD) were widely used sclerosants. In clinical trials, adding a clerosant to diluted adrenaline injection failed to improve utcome when compared to adrenaline injection alone. There ave been reports in the literature of fatal gastric necrosis and erforation. For this reason and the lack of evidence suggestng added benefit of combined treatment, the use of sclerosants is probably not advised.

Thrombin is a component of the clotting cascade and represents the most physiologic agent of injection therapy. When econstituted, thrombin is watery and can be injected with a tandard injection catheter. In earlier studies, bovine thrombin vas used. A group from Scotland added human thrombin to drenaline injection and compared this combination treatment o adrenaline alone.[8] Human thrombin was derived from pooled lasma supplied by the local blood transfusion service and vas administered in a high dose with a median of 3.5 mL 500–1000 IU). The authors treated 140 patients with arterial leeding or a nonbleeding visible vessel and demonstrated a ignificantly lower rate of recurrent bleeding, transfusion requirement, and mortality.

Fibrin sealant is commercially available and consists of the wo components fibrinogen and thrombin. A dual channel njection catheter is required for its injection. The channels are f different sizes. Because of the higher viscosity of fibrinogen, one of the channels is wider for its injection. Some of the injector heads are color coded to ensure the correct solution goes into the respective channel. Mixing of the two components occurs at the tip of the injection catheter deep in submucosal tissue. Clogging of the needle is a frequent problem.

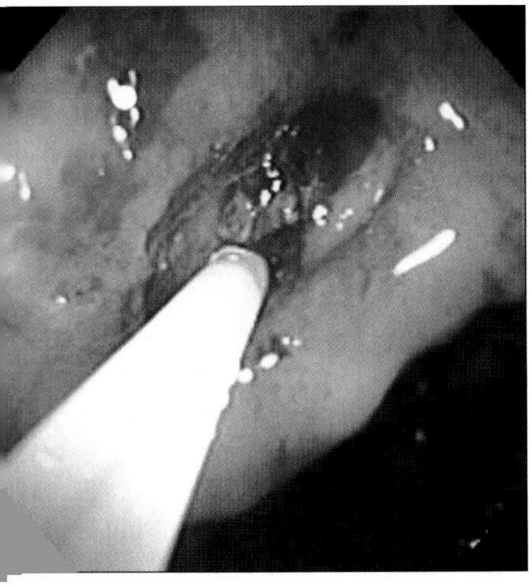

Fig. 142.7 Adrenaline injection. Injection of diluted adrenaline into a gastric ulcer.

In ulcers with active bleeding, preinjection with adrenaline is required. Considerable abutment is required to advance the needle sufficiently deep in the submucosa. The bleeding point is injected at its four quadrants, each with 0.5 mL of fibrinogen and thrombin (added to 1 mL fibrin sealant). After each injection with the needle remaining in the tissue, the reconstituted sealant is immediately followed by 1–1.5 mL of normal saline in order to drive the sealant submucosally. Following four-quadrant injection, the point of bleeding is then injected. As the sealant is being injected, the needle is slowly withdrawn, leaving a central fibrin plug.

Both thrombin and fibrin are derived from pooled human plasma. There is a theoretical concern of transmission of viral agent, anaphylaxis, especially with the use of the bovine type, and intra-arterial injection causing systemic thrombosis.

In a large European multicenter trial, patients with actively bleeding ulcers and ulcers with nonbleeding visible vessels were randomized into three groups (polidocanol alone, single adrenaline and fibrin treatment, and daily adrenaline and fibrin treatment) until complete fading of bleeding stigmata from ulcer floors.[9] Recurrent bleeding was seen less in the single and repeated fibrin treatment group when compared to polidocanol injection alone. Statistically, fibrin injection was superior to polidocanol injection only when injected repeatedly. It was unclear whether the superiority of fibrin injections was a consequence of tight surveillance of daily endoscopy and injection or the fibrin sealant itself. Prophylactic retreatment with fibrin sealant is costly and can be uncomfortable to patients. A more selective approach based on the severity of index bleeding and local characteristics of ulcers seems more rational. The cost of using fibrin sealant is also substantial.

Contact thermal device: heater probe

Thermal devices can be divided into contact devices, such as heater probe and multipolar probe, and noncontact methods such as neodymium:yttrium-aluminum-garnet (YAG) laser and, recently, argon plasma coagulation (Fig. 142.8). In canine mesenteric arteries, Johnston and coworkers studied the effect of different thermal devices on arterial coagulation and emphasized the importance of vascular compression and tamponade and the concept of coaptive coagulation (Fig. 142.9) and the use of a hemostat to tamponade blood flow and coapt the vessel walls, followed by the application of cautery to thermally seal the vessel.[10] Contact thermal devices such as the heater probe are more effective than laser electrocoagulation in coagulating medium size arteries and can consistently seal arteries of up to 2 mm in diameter. In these *in vitro* experiments, laser was effective only for direct coagulation of 0.25-mm exposed arteries. Without mechanical compression, the 'heat-sink' effect from flowing arterial blood leads to dissipation of thermal energy. In clinical practice, laser units are no longer used, as they are bulky and not readily portable.

The heater probe consists of a heat coil inside a Teflon-coated copper tip. The probe is heated to 250 °C and can be programed to deliver a fixed amount of energy. There are three irrigation ports to the side 1 cm from the probe tip. This enables

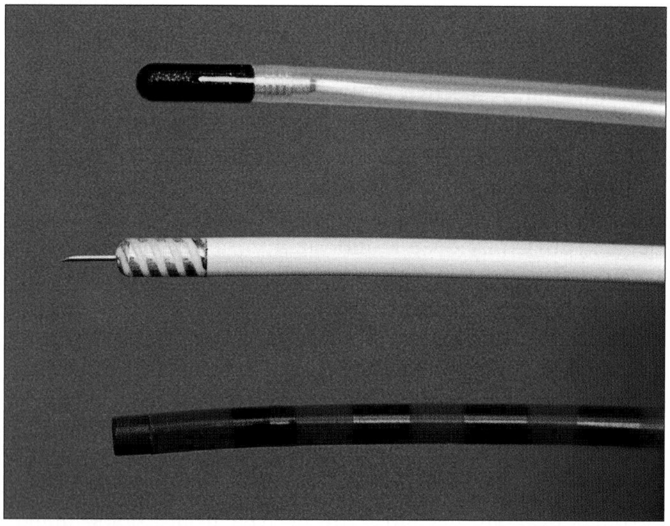

Fig. 142.8 Thermal devices for hemostasis. From top to bottom: a heat probe, an injector (gold probe), and a catheter for argon plasma coagulation.

simultaneous washing with the probe tip in contact with tissue. Irrigation of the ulcer bed washes off clots and debris allowing accurate positioning of the probe. After vessel coagulation, activation of the irrigation ports floats the probe off the tissue bed and thereby avoids lifting of coagulum and provoking bleeding. Coagulation of arteries was found to be ineffective if only light touch was applied. We prefer the use of a larger 3.2-mm probe in securing hemostasis. The following settings are generally recommended for the treatment of bleeding peptic ulcers: (1) firm tamponade; (2) four continuous 30-joule pulses given per tamponade station before repositioning. In actively bleeding ulcers, we preinject with diluted adrenaline for initial hemostasis. This allows a clear view of the vessel for application of heat probe thermocoagulation to the vessel itself. In a clinical trial, we demonstrated a marginal reduction in the need for surgery in patients with spurting bleeding.

Hemoclips

Clips of different sizes are available for different purposes. Th clip can now be rotated by torque into the desired axis befor its final deployment. Clipping is conceptually an ideal metho for achieving hemostasis. The method promises definitive hemo stasis and is nontissue damaging. In real-life situations, cli deployment tangentially or with an endoscope in a retroflexe position can be difficult, for example, in the treatment of a ulcer in the posterior wall of the duodenal bulb or in the lesse curve. Clip retention rate is uncertain. Its deployment onto fibrotic ulcer base can be difficult.

The use of hemoclips is yet to be proven in both anima experiments and clinical trials. Hepworth and coworkers com pared the use of hemoclips to other endoscopic treatment o canine mesenteric arteries.[11] Similar to injection sclerotherapy hemoclips were ineffective in stopping bleeding in mediur size arteries (1–2 mm).

Limits of endoscopic therapy

Swain et al. studied bleeding arteries in gastrectomy specimen of recurrent bleeding gastric ulcers and in postmortem exami nations of patients who had succumbed to bleeding pepti ulcers.[12] In surgical specimens, the mean external diamete of the bleeding artery was 0.7 mm (range 0.1–1.8 mm). Serosa arteries were significantly larger than submucosal arterie (mean 0.88 mm vs. 0.50 mm) (Fig. 142.10). In patients wh died of exsanguination from bleeding ulcers, the artery was a large as 3.85 mm in external diameter. Results from *in vitro* experiments suggested that arteries greater than 2 mm in siz could not be controlled by contact thermal probes. In a clinica setting, conditions are less ideal and it has been suggested tha bleeding from arteries greater than 1 mm in size is difficult t control endoscopically. The main trunk of the gastroduodena artery, for instance, is estimated to be 3–6 mm in size. Large deep ulcers in the posterior wall of the duodenal bulb or th lesser curve should alert one to such a possibility. Erosion into major arteries are not amenable to endoscopic therapy Immediate surgery should be considered in such cases.

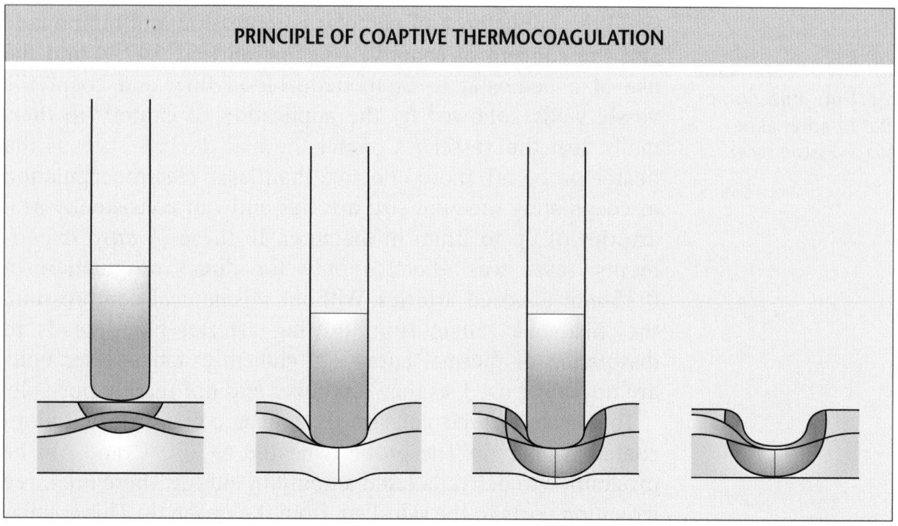

Fig. 142.9 Thermocoagulation. Principle of coaptive thermocoagulation. Reproduced from Johnston JH et al. Experimental comparison of endoscopic yttrium-aluminum-garnet laser, electrosurgery and heater probe for canine gu arterial coagulation. Gastroenterology 1987; 92:1101–1108, Copyright © 1987, with permission from the American Gasteroenterological Association.

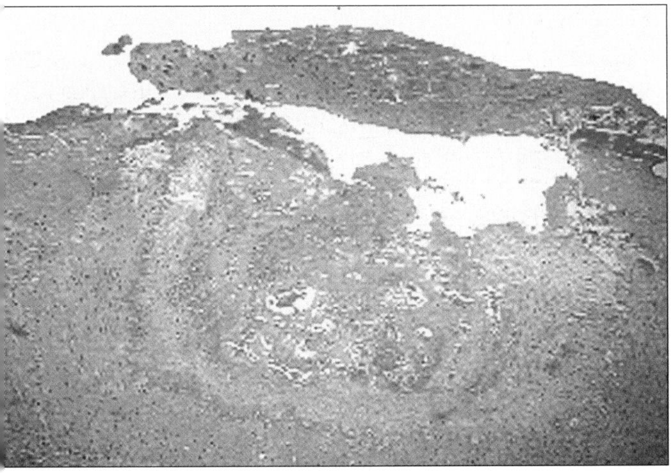

Fig. 142.10 A histological formalin-fixed specimen of a bleeding artery in a gastric ulcer resected during surgery. The artery measures 8 mm in size in the fixed specimen.

REFERENCES

1. Stiegmann GV, Goff JS, Michaletz-Onody PA et al. Endoscopic sclerotherapy as compared with endoscopic ligation for bleeding esophageal varices. N Engl J Med 1992; 326:1527–1532.
2. Laine L, Cook D. Endoscopic ligation compared with sclerotherapy for treatment of esophageal variceal bleeding. A meta-analysis. Ann Intern Med 1995; 123:280–287.
3. Singh P, Pooran N, Indaram A, Bank S. Combined ligation and sclerotherapy versus ligation alone for secondary prophylaxis of esophageal variceal bleeding: a meta-analysis. Am J Gastroenterol 2002; 97:623–629.
4. Lo GH, Lai KH, Cheng JS et al. The additive effect of sclerotherapy to patients receiving repeated endoscopic variceal ligation: a prospective, randomized trial. Hepatology 1998; 28:391–395.
5. Sarin SK, Lahoti D, Saxena SP, Murthy NS, Makwana UK. Prevalence, classification, and natural history of gastric varices: a long-term follow-up study in 568 portal hypertension patients. Hepatology 1992; 16:1343–1349.
6. Lo GH, Lai KH, Cheng JS, Chen MH, Chiang HT. A prospective, randomized trial of butyl cyanoacrylate injection versus band ligation in the management of bleeding gastric varices. Hepatology 2001; 33:1060–1064.
7. Soehendra N, Grimm H, Stenzel M. Injection of nonvariceal bleeding lesions of the upper gastrointestinal tract. Endoscopy 1985; 17: 129–132.
8. Kubba KA, Murphy W, Palmer KR. Endoscopic injection for bleeding peptic ulcer: a comparison of adrenaline alone with adrenaline plus human thrombin. Gastroenterology 1996; 111:623–628.
9. Rutgeerts P, Rauws E, Wara P et al. Randomised trial of single and repeated fibrin glue compared with injection of polidocanol in treatment of bleeding peptic ulcer. Lancet 1997; 350:692–696.
10. Johnston JH, Jensen DM, Mautner W. Comparison of endoscopic electrocoagulation and laser photocoagulation of bleeding canine gastric ulcers. Gastroenterology 1982; 82:904–910.
11. Hepworth CC, Kadirkamanathan, Gong F, Swain CP. A randomised controlled comparison of injection, thermal, and mechanical endoscopic methods of haemostasis on mesenteric vessels. Gut 1998; 42:462–469.
12. Swain CP, Storey D, Bown S et al. Nature of the bleeding vessel in recurrently bleeding gastric ulcers. Gastroenterology 1986; 90: 595–608.

Chapter 143

Photodynamic therapy in the gastrointestinal tract

Kenneth K Wang and Vivek Mittal

KEY POINTS

ESOPHAGUS
- Palliation of esophageal cancer – FDA approved
- Curative therapy for early esophageal cancer – promising in squamous and in Barrett's cancers
- May provide cure of localized lesions when combined with endoscopic mucosal resection
- Therapy for Barrett's esophagus with high-grade dysplasia – FDA approved

STOMACH
- Appears to be limited to superficial gastric cancers in patients who are not candidates for surgery

BILIARY TRACT
- Promising in cholangiocarcinoma – technically difficult

AMPULLA AND DUODENUM
- For palliation of ampullary cancers

PANCREAS AND COLON
- No proven role for PDT at this time

INTRODUCTION

Photodynamic therapy (PDT) has been applied to a wide variety of gastrointestinal, pulmonary, urological, dermatologic, and ophthalmologic disorders. In the gastrointestinal tract, the treatment can be applied to the mucosa without the need to target a specific lesion. This advantage allows this treatment to be applied to any area where light can be delivered. The treatment involves the use of a drug that must be given prior to the application of light. This therapy is well suited for gastrointestinal tract because of the use of the fibers, which can deliver the light perpendicular to the axis of the endoscope. The treatment is currently approved in the US by the FDA to be used in the gastrointestinal tract for palliation of esophageal cancer and for the treatment of Barrett's esophagus with high-grade dysplasia. Other applications have been to treat early cancers in the esophagus, gastric cancers, duodenal adenomas, colon cancer, and cholangiocarcinoma.

BACKGROUND

Early work on PDT established that the components needed to create the photodynamic effect were a photosensitizing drug, light, and oxygen. These early observations are consistent with what is known about PDT today. Photosensitizers are generally large complex molecules that can absorb light. Drugs that are used as photosensitizers are generally derivatives of chlorophyll or hemoglobin.[1] The current generation of photosensitizers are derivatives of porphyrins. The commercialized porphyrin photosensitizer is referred to as sodium porfimer. These porphyrin-derived photosensitizers are activated by light of around 630 nm wavelength, which is a visible red light. Another photosensitizer is aminolevulinic acid (ALA), a prodrug. It is primarily used in Europe where it is administered orally 4 h prior to photoradiation. This drug is converted inside the cell to protoporphyrin IX, which serves as the actual photosensitizer. This drug is not commercially available in the United States for use in the gastrointestinal tract.

MECHANISM OF ACTION OF PDT

The photodynamic effect requires an interaction between light and the photosensitizer (Fig. 143.1). The photosensitizer must be present in adequate concentrations within the target tissue prior to light irradiation.

In tissues that do not absorb the drug, very little necrosis will occur. Light must also be of a certain concentration to activate the drug. With too little light, there is not enough drug interaction to produce a photodynamic effect. With too much light, the drug is destroyed by the light instead of being activated by it. The dosimetry for PDT requires careful attention to the geometry of the area to be treated, the power of the light available, and the total energy of light that will be needed to produce tissue necrosis. In addition, the light must be of an appropriate wavelength for the tissues to absorb it. It is typical to use the longest wavelength of light that can still activate the drug since it has the greatest depth of tissue penetration. The best absorption for photodynamic effect is actually in the shorter wavelength of light such as in ultraviolet light but there is very little depth of tissue penetration with this type of light due to absorption from hemoglobin (Fig. 143.2).

Finally, oxygen must be present in the tissue. If the tissue is compressed or lacks oxygen flow, there will be no PDT. This must be carefully considered when using balloon photoradiating systems since they can compress the tissue.

Once the drug is activated, it in turn interacts with surrounding molecular oxygen creating singlet oxygen that mediates cell damage. Since singlet oxygen only persists a few picoseconds after activation, the damage is limited to the area of tissue that has been photoradiated.

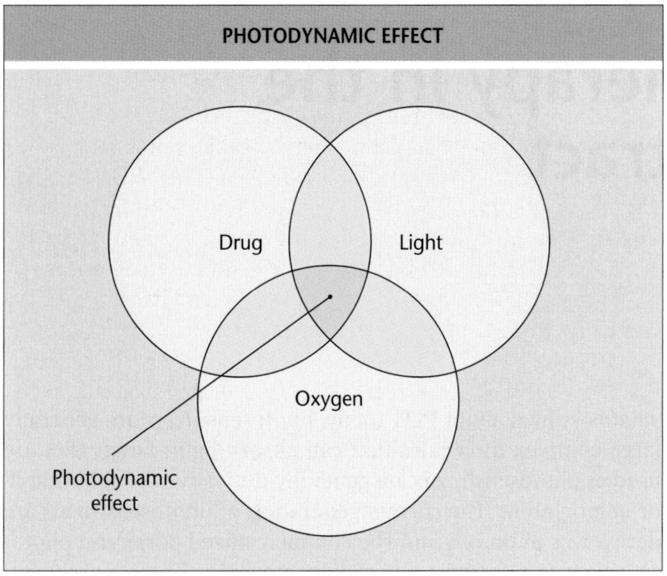

Fig. 143.1 Photodynamic effect. The photodynamic effect is contingent on the presence of adequate concentrations of photosensitizing drug, light, and oxygen.

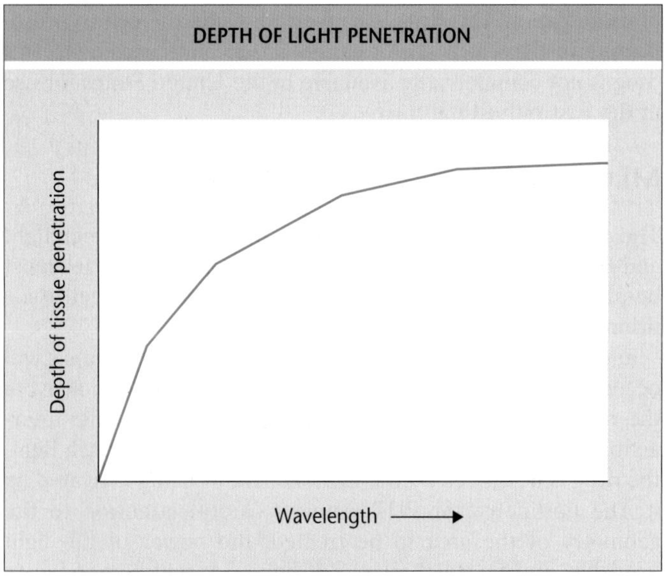

Fig. 143.2 Depth of light penetration. As the wavelength of light gets longer, the depth of tissue penetration also increases. Red light is used in PDT since it has the longest wavelength.

CLINICAL USES OF PDT IN THE GASTROINTESTINAL TRACT

The photosensitizer sodium porfimer photosensitizer is administered intravenously 48h prior to photoradiation. The light is provided by a laser, which can be of several different types. The most compact and technologically advanced of these is a diode laser, which is a solid-state laser that is generally reliable and can be made compactly. The earlier laser types were tunable dye lasers that used a laser of one wavelength to activate a dye that could emit laser energy of longer wavelength. Photoradiation is performed in the gastrointestinal tract through the use of a photoradiating device that can be a fiber or a balloon photoradiator. The fiber is generally a cylindrical photoradiator since this can disperse light.

Esophagus

- Palliation of esophageal cancer
- Curative therapy for early esophageal cancer
- Therapy for Barrett's esophagus with high-grade dysplasia

Palliation therapy of esophageal cancer

The first approved application for PDT therapy in the US was for the palliation of esophageal cancer. Esophageal cancer is diagnosed in more than 12000 persons each year in the US with most of these patients diagnosed late in their disease course with symptoms of dysphagia. The traditional approach has been to place a stent to relieve these symptoms. However, stents have a number of deficiencies in regards to efficacy and durability.[2] PDT appears to be more easily applied than traditional laser palliation devices.

A cylindrical diffusing fiber is easily inserted through all but the most completely obstructing tumors (Fig. 143.3). The light energy can then be delivered directly to the tumor surface. A multicenter randomized control trial compared PDT with sodium profimer (110 patients) and Nd:YAG laser therapy (108 patients) for the palliation of esophageal cancer.[3] Symptomatic improvement of dysphagia was similar in both groups. Nine patients had complete tumor responses after PDT compared with two after Nd:YAG. Nineteen per cent of the PDT patients experienced sunburn and 1% had perforations; Nd:YAG patients had a higher perforation rate (7%). Efficacy of PDT was similar to that of Nd:YAG but there were fewer significant complications.

A large single-center retrospective study of 215 patients who underwent palliative therapy with PDT for esophageal cancer found that it was most effective in patients who had obstructing luminal tumors.[4] This patient group underwent 318 courses of therapy for obstruction and for hemorrhage. Eighty-five per cent of the patients had improvement in their dysphagia with a mean period of dysphagia-free time of 66 days. About a third (30%) of patients on nutritional supplementation were able to come off this after PDT. Complications reported in this series included perforation in 2%, strictures in 2%, pleural effusions in 4%, and sunburn in 6%. The procedure related mortality rate was 1.8% with a median survival of 5 months.

The use of PDT in esophageal cancer for palliation of dysphagia may provide an improvement in symptoms for a duration of around 2 months.

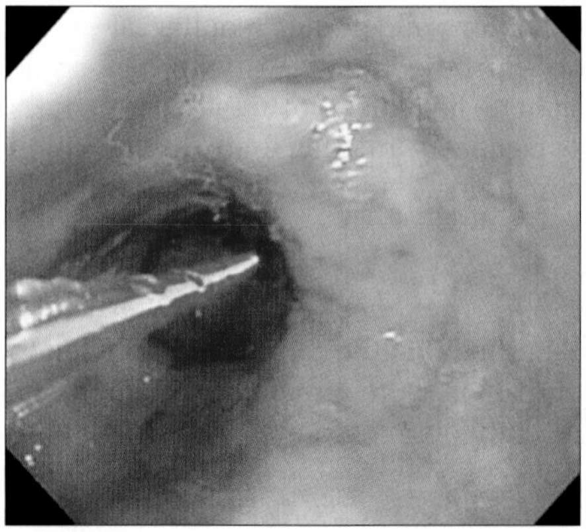

Fig. 143.3 Cylindrical diffusing fiber. A 5-cm cylindrical diffusing fiber positioned in the central lumen of the esophagus. The light is distributed to the mucosal surface that is parallel to the fiber.

Curative therapy for superficial esophageal cancer

A more intriguing application of PDT in the esophagus has been its use in the treatment of superficial cancers. In one of the larger studies reported, PDT was used to treat 123 patients with esophageal cancer: 104 squamous cell carcinomas and 19 adenocarcinomas.[5] Although these cancers were thought to be superficial, at least 27 were staged T2 by endoscopic ultrasound. This study used a hematoporphyrin derivative as a photosensitizer. A complete response was found in 87% of the patients at 6 months. The 5-year survival rate was 25% but the 5-year disease-specific survival rate was 74%. This study certainly pointed out the possibility of using PDT as a curative treatment for superficial cancers.

Treatment of superficial cancers related to Barrett's esophagus has been reported using a combination of PDT and endoscopic mucosal resection. A major problem with endoscopic therapy of esophageal cancers can be the inaccuracy of EUS staging for esophageal cancers.[6,7] The technique of endoscopic mucosal resection (EMR) resolves this issue since tumor extent can be assessed with histology (see Fig. 143.4).

Combination therapy using PDT and mucosal resection for early cancers has been reported with a 94% initial response rate in 17 patients.[8] Compared with esophagectomy for early cancer, this approach has significantly fewer complications.[9]

PDT with aminolevulinic acid for treatment of superficial cancer of the esophagus is much less effective, probably because of the more superficial uptake of aminolevulinic acid by the mucosa.[10] Porphyrin-based photosensitizers have a much greater depth of penetration, although they also have greater toxicities.

Barrett's esophagus with high-grade dysplasia

PDT may be used in Barrett's esophagus with high-grade dysplasia as an alternative to surgical therapy. The FDA approval of the technique for use in this setting was based upon a multicenter prospective randomized trial of 208 patients randomized 2:1 to PDT and omeprazole versus a control group on omeprazole alone.[11] The study used a unique balloon diffusing system that allowed the endoscopist to treat up to 7 cm of Barrett's esophagus at a time (Fig. 143.5).[11]

At 24 months there was a significant (50%) reduction in cancer in the treatment group. Twenty-eight per cent of the controls developed cancer versus 13% in the PDT-treated patients. In addition, the number of patients with high-grade dysplasia also decreased significantly in the treatment group from 77% in the control group to 39% in the treated group. Longer-term data beyond 24 months is required in such studies as in the treatment of any 'early' neoplastic process. Strictures occurred in a third of the PDT-treated patients and cutaneous photosensitivity occurred in two-thirds of the patients (see 'Adverse effects' below). The role of PDT in relation to other therapies for Barrett's-associated high-grade dysplasia is discussed in Chapter 31.

Stomach

Treatment of superficial gastric cancers

PDT has been approved for use in the treatment of gastric cancers in Japan but there has not been a randomized controlled trial using this therapy in gastric cancers. It appears that PDT's role in the treatment of superficial gastric cancer is for frail patients with high risks of mortality with gastric surgery. More than 133 cases of gastric cancers have been reported that have been treated with PDT.[12] Over 90% of these cancers were early staged and all of these cancers had an initial complete response to PDT. However, there was a 22% recurrence rate. The depth of invasion definitely affects the response rate.[13] A number of other retrospective reports have been reported in the literature with small numbers of patients.[14–16] The overall success rates of treatment using PDT for gastric cancers range from 100% to 50%. PDT appears to be most effective for the treatment of type I, IIa, and IIb gastric cancers that are less than 2 cm in diameter. In a European series, the typical dose of 2 mg/kg of sodium porfimer and light dose of 15–300 J/cm of

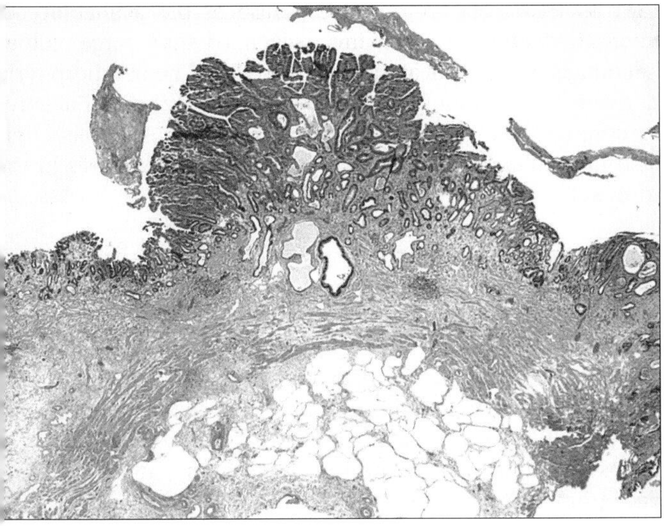

Fig. 143.4 Endoscopic mucosal resection. Histological section of an endoscopic mucosal resection of a small nodule. The resection allows the accurate assessment of the depth of penetration of this early cancer.

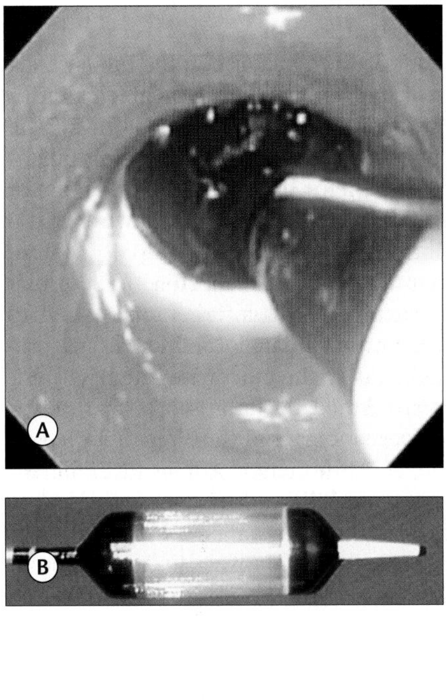

Fig. 143.5 Balloon system. A balloon system has been created specifically for the application of PDT to Barrett's esophagus. The balloon has an optical window in the center of the balloon that can treat up to 3–7 cm of tissue. Image B courtesy of Axcan Pharma.

fiber led to a cure in 82% of patients.[15] Thirteen of 16 (80%) early intestinal type gastric cancers responded to meso-tetrahydroxyphenyl-chlorin (mTHPC) as a photosensitizer.[14]

The use of PDT in the stomach appears to be limited to superficial gastric cancers in patients who are not candidates for surgery, with the intestinal type responding better than the diffuse type of gastric cancer.

The palliation of advanced gastric cancer appears to have little advantage over alternative laser or thermal methods.[15] The adverse effects (strictures, perforation) of PDT therapy in the stomach are comparatively minimal compared with PDT therapy in the esophagus.

Pancreas

There are no current approvals for the use of PDT in the pancreas. Porphyrin-derived photosensitizers have been found to concentrate in pancreatic tumors.[17] PDT therapy was reported in 16 patients with locally unresectable pancreatic cancer.[18] Sodium porfimer was given intravenously 72 h prior to photoradiation, administered with CT-placed diffusing fibers. Patients had a median survival time of 9.5 months after treatment. Treatment complications included strictures of the duodenum in three patients and gastrointestinal bleeding in two. No pancreatitis was reported.

Currently there is no evidence to support PDT therapy for pancreatic cancer.

Biliary tract

PDT has been applied to cholangiocarcinomas with considerable success although it is not approved for use in this setting. The primary problem has been in securing light delivery systems that can be placed into the bile duct without fracturing. The diffusing fibers require special catheters and very careful placement in the biliary tract.[19] The first small case series was described in 1998.[20] A prospective randomized trial was reported in which 39 patients received either a stent alone or a stent with PDT.[21] Specially designed flexible diffusing fiber systems were developed for use in the study. The patients who received PDT had a significantly prolonged survival of 493 days versus only 98 days in the control population. Although there are methodological problems with this study, this degree of survival benefit was significant and may be important in the treatment of these cancers.

The photoradiation is difficult to perform in the biliary tract because of the rigidity of the commercially available cylindrical diffusing fibers. To overcome this problem, a 1.0- or 2.5-cm cylindrical diffusing fiber can be preloaded into an 8F biliary catheter (Fig. 143.6). This catheter has a 0.038-inch diameter hole to accommodate a 0.035-inch diameter guidewire. Endoscopic retrograde cholangiopancreatography (ERCP) is preformed and the cholangiocarcinoma is localized with the proximal and distal margins recorded. This information is used to pass the guidewire through the cholangiocarcinoma. The preloaded catheter is advanced over the guidewire after the position of the catheter is confirmed by fluoroscopy. The power used to treat the cholangiocarcinoma is 400 mW/cm fiber length for a total dose of 180 J/cm^2. After therapy, 10F or 11.5F biliary catheters are placed to ensure biliary drainage after therapy. Cholangitis is a possible complication of this therapy. Although it has not been proven, cutaneous photosensitivity may be of greater magnitude than PDT of the esophagus. This may be because the porphyrins may be retained in an obstructed biliary system.

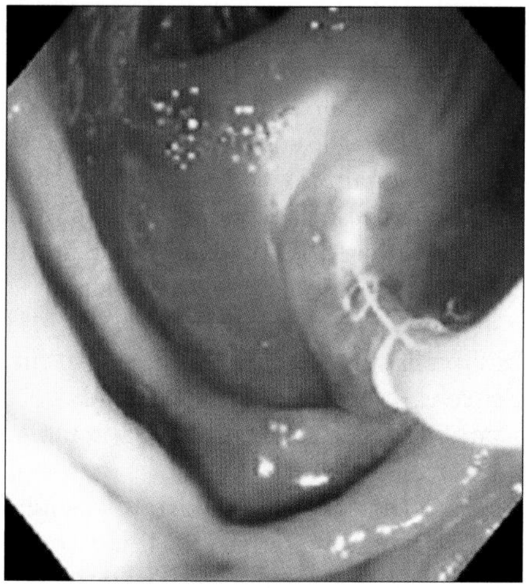

Fig. 143.6 PDT diffusing fiber. A PDT diffusing fiber is inserted through a catheter, which is positioned in the common bile duct. During photoradiation the bile duct 'glows' from the laser energy diffusing in the bile duct.

Duodenum and ampulla

Small case series have been reported for the use of PDT in ampullary lesions. Ampullary carcinomas were treated in one pilot series of 10 nonsurgical candidates.[22] All were treated with a hematoporphyrin derivative at a dose of 4 mg/kg, which is similar to a dose of 2 mg/kg of the currently available photosensitizer, sodium porfimer. Cutaneous photosensitivity occurred in three of the ten patients. Seven of the ten patients had a response to the therapy with a decrease in tumor size while three had no response. Smaller tumors appeared to respond completely although all recurred. PDT of three cases of ampullary adenomas (1–1.5 cm) demonstrated a decrease in size but no destruction of the lesions.[23]

Overall, the potential role of PDT in the treatment of ampullary lesions is for palliation rather than cure.

Colon and rectum

There has been little enthusiasm, and few studies, about using PDT to treat colonic tumors, because of the availability of alternative effective therapies. Seven of nine large villous adenomas were eradicated with PDT with a hematoporphyrin derivative or sodium porfimer after failure of thermal ablative techniques such as Nd:YAG laser therapy.[24] Aminolevulinic acid in familial polyposis adenomas produced necrosis in the most superficial portions of the polyps.[25]

ADVERSE EFFECTS

The adverse effects of PDT are primarily related to its mechanism of action and the photosensitivity.[26] Immediate effects are those of cutaneous photosensitivity, which can occur within hours of injection of the photosensitizer. Patients need to be carefully instructed regarding the need to avoid sunlight exposure. The rates of photosensitivity with sodium porfimer vary from 30% reported in previous studies to the 60% noted in a recent FDA approval trial. Most of these events are mild and do not require therapy, although severe cases may involve full-thickness skin injury. This cutaneous photosensitivity can persist for from 30 to 90 days after injection. Patients should e cautioned that sunscreen is of little benefit as it only protects gainst ultraviolet light and not visible light. Sun protection nust be in the form of light-proof clothing and gloves, large vide-brimmed hats, and sunglasses.

With PDT of the esophagus, odynophagia and chest pain are ommon in the first 2 weeks after photoradiation and are treated vith narcotic analgesics. Nausea and vomiting may occur in the irst 2–3 days following photoradiation and require anti-emetics.

Stricture formation is relatively common after PDT of the sophagus and can occur in between 16% and 40% of treated atients, forming about 3–4 weeks after photoradiation. These trictures can be very fibrotic and require repeated dilatation.

SUMMARY

PDT has several natural advantages for use in the gastrointestinal tract. The treatment does not require targeting by the hysician for a specific lesion, which allows the therapy to be pplied to areas outside of the visual range of the endoscope uch as the biliary system where its use has been shown to dramatically improve life expectancy in patients with cholangiocarcinoma. This treatment also allows rapid therapy of large amounts of mucosal area, which should be beneficial in Barrett's esophagus-associated dysplasia. Newer agents are being developed that will hopefully decrease the frequency and severity of potential adverse events. Overall, with indications for esophageal cancer, Barrett's esophagus, and high-grade dysplasia, as well as other nongastrointestinal tumors, the potential for PDT is bright.

SOURCES OF INFORMATION FOR PATIENTS AND DOCTORS

http://omlc.ogi.edu/pdt/ptinfo/esophca/esophtreatment.html

ACKNOWLEDGMENTS

The authors would like to acknowledge the support of NIH grants CA85992-01 and R01CA097048-01 and the Mayo Foundation.

REFERENCES

1. Dougherty TJ, Gomer CJ, Henderson BW et al. PDT. J Nat Cancer Instit 1998; 90:889–905.
2. Lightdale CJ. Role of PDT in the management of advanced esophageal cancer. Gastrointest Endosc Clin North Am 2000; 10:397–408.
3. Lightdale CJ, Heier SK, Marcon NE et al. PDT with porfimer sodium versus thermal ablation therapy with Nd:YAG laser for palliation of esophageal cancer: a multicenter randomized trial. Gastrointestinal Endoscopy 1995; 42:507–512.
4. Litle VR, Luketich JD, Christie NA et al. PDT as palliation for esophageal cancer: experience in 215 patients. Ann Thorac Surg 2003; 76:1687–1692.
5. Sibille A, Lambert R, Souquet JC, Sabben G, Descos F. Long-term survival after PDT for esophageal cancer. Gastroenterology 1995; 108:337–344.
6. Grimm H, Binmoeller KF, Hamper K et al. Endosonography for preoperative locoregional staging of esophageal and gastric cancer. Endoscopy 1993; 25:224–230.
7. Siemsen M, Svendsen LB, Knigge U et al. A prospective randomized comparison of curved array and radial echoendoscopy in patients with esophageal cancer. Gastrointestinal Endoscopy 2003; 58:671–676.
8. Buttar NS, Wang KK, Lutzke LS, Krishnadath KK, Anderson MA. Combined endoscopic mucosal resection and PDT for esophageal neoplasia within Barrett's esophagus. Gastrointest Endosc 2001; 54:682–688.
9. Pacifico RJ, Wang KK, WongKeeSong LM, Buttar NS, Lutzke LS. Combined endoscopic mucosal resection and PDT versus esophagectomy for management of early adenocarcinoma in Barrett's esophagus. Clin Gastroenterol Hepatol 2003; 1:252–257.
10. Gossner L, Stolte M, Sroka R et al. PDT of early squamous epithelial carcinomas and severe squamous epithelial dysplasias of the esophagus with 5-aminolevulinic acid. Z Gastroenterol 1998; 36:19–26.
11. Overholt BF, DeNovo RC, Panjehpour M, Petersen MG. A centering balloon for PDT of esophageal cancer tested in a canine model. Gastrointest Endosc 1993; 39:782–787.
12. Kato H, Kito T, Furuse K et al. PDT in the early treatment of cancer. Review 10 refs Japanese. Gan to Kagaku Ryoho [Japanese Journal of Cancer & Chemotherapy] 1990; 17:1833–1838.
13. Mimura S, Ichii M, Imanishi K, Otani T, Okuda S. Indications for and limitations of HpD PDT for esophageal cancer and gastric cancer. Gan to Kagaku Ryoho [Japanese Journal of Cancer & Chemotherapy] 1988; 15:1440–1444.
14. Ell C, Gossner L, May A et al. Photodynamic ablation of early cancers of the stomach by means of mTHPC and laser irradiation: preliminary clinical experience. Gut 1998; 43:345–349.
15. Gossner L, Ell C. PDT of gastric cancer. Gastrointest Endosc Clin N Am 2000; 10:461–480.
16. Vonarx V, Eleouet S, Carre J et al. Potential efficacy of a delta 5-aminolevulinic acid bioadhesive gel formulation for the photodynamic treatment of lesions of the gastrointestinal tract in mice. J Pharm Pharmacol 1997; 49:652–656.
17. Schroder T, Chen IW, Sperling M et al. Hematoporphyrin derivative uptake and PDT in pancreatic carcinoma. J Surg Oncol 1988; 38:4–9.
18. Bown SG, Rogowska AZ, Whitelaw DE et al. PDT for cancer of the pancreas. Gut 2002; 50:549–557.
19. Rumalla A, Baron TH, Wang KK et al. Endoscopic application of PDT for cholangiocarcinoma. Gastrointest Endosc 2001; 53:500–504.
20. Ortner MA, Liebetruth J, Schreiber S et al. PDT of nonresectable cholangiocarcinoma. Gastroenterology 1998; 114:536–542.
21. Ortner ME, Caca K, Berr F et al. Successful PDT for nonresectable cholangiocarcinoma: a randomized prospective study. Gastroenterology 2003; 125:1355–1363.
22. Abulafi AM, Allardice JT, Williams NS et al. PDT for malignant tumours of the ampulla of Vater. Gut 1995; 36:853–856.
23. Mlkvy P, Messmann H, Regula J et al. PDT for gastrointestinal tumors using three photosensitizers – ALA induced PPIX, Photofrin and MTHPC. A pilot study. Neoplasma 1998; 45:157–161.
24. Loh CS, Bliss P, Bown SG, Krasner N. PDT for villous adenomas of the colon and rectum. Endoscopy 1994; 26:243–246.
25. Mlkvy P, Messmann H, Debinski H et al. PDT for polyps in familial adenomatous polyposis – a pilot study. Eur J Cancer 1995; 31A:1160–1165.
26. Wang KK, Nijhawan PK. Complications of PDT in gastrointestinal disease. Gastrointest Endosc Clin N Am 2000; 10:487–495.

Chapter 144

Percutaneous endoscopic gastrostomy and jejunostomy

Jeffrey L Ponsky

KEY POINTS
SUMMARY OF TECHNIQUE OF PEG

- Define point of optimal contact using finger pressure
- Employ the 'safe tract' method of entry
- Capture suture in snare, and pull from patient's mouth
- Attach suture to end of gastrostomy tube and pull tube into esophagus
- Follow tube with endoscope to assure proper final position of tube
- Apply outer crossbar several millimeters from the skin, avoiding tension

INTRODUCTION AND SCIENTIFIC BASIS OF PEG

For generations, surgeons have fixed the stomach and other hollow viscera to the skin with tubes in order to create fistulous tracts used for feeding or decompression. In 1980, the first description of such a fistula, produced endoscopically, was published.[1] The principle of percutaneous endoscopic gastrostomy (PEG) has now been established with widespread clinical experience. In addition, fixation of the jejunum[2] for feeding, and of the cecum[3] for decompression, have been also shown to be safe and effective.

Initially, the serosal surface of the viscus is held in apposition to the peritoneal wall by the endoscopically guided tube. After approximately 1 week, an adhesive connection forms that serves to maintain the surfaces in more permanent contact. Once the adhesive connection has been established, the tube may be removed or changed. Should the tube be removed and not immediately replaced, the fistulous tract is likely to close within a few hours.

The two surfaces need not be tightly opposed to assure tract formation.[4] Extreme tension applied to the outer fixating crossbar to assure close approximation of the gastric and abdominal walls is unnecessary, and may be harmful by producing ischemia of the interposed tissue.

DESCRIPTION OF THE PEG TECHNIQUE

The 'pull' technique is employed most commonly.[5] A single dose of an intravenous antibiotic (usually a cephalosporin) is given as the procedure is commenced. Conscious sedation is usually done, but general anesthesia may be required for some patients and in children may be the optimal approach. The abdomen should be cleansed with an antiseptic solution and sterilely draped.

Upper endoscopic examination is performed to rule out significant unsuspected lesions. The endoscope is then pulled back into the gastric body and full inflation of the stomach commenced. The assistant, working at the abdominal site, then probes the abdomen with a finger, beginning at the subxiphoid region and proceeding down the left costal margin. While this is occurring, the endoscopist looks for a point of clear and prominent indentation of the gastric wall when finger pressure is applied (Fig. 144.1). This is a crucial point in the procedure, and extra time spent at this juncture is well rewarded.

When such a site is agreed upon, the assistant will introduce a syringe half filled with local anesthetic, and fitted with a small-caliber needle, while pulling back upon the syringe barrel to create negative pressure. The needle is slowly advanced into the abdominal wall and into the gastric lumen. The endoscopist carefully looks for the needle's entry into the stomach while the assistant's attention is focused on the barrel of the syringe. The endoscopist calls out when the needle enters the gastric lumen and the assistant calls out if air bubbles into the syringe barrel (Fig. 144.2). Should air bubble into the syringe barrel before the needle has appeared in the gastric lumen, there is a high likelihood that another air-containing viscus (small bowel or colon) has been entered. In such a case the needle is withdrawn and an alternate site of entry selected. This latter method, named the 'safe tract' technique, has greatly added to the safety of percutaneous enteral access.[6]

Grasping the suture: Once the site has been so identified, the endoscopist opens a polypectomy snare over that area of the gastric wall and the assistant injects a small amount of local anesthetic in the skin at the proposed site of entry. A scalpel is used to make a 0.5-cm skin incision, and a larger sheathed needle is thrust through the opposed gastric and abdominal walls and into the waiting snare loop. The snare is then closed about the needle sheath and the needle withdrawn or pulled back. A long suture or wire is then threaded through the sheath and into the gastric lumen. The snare is then open slightly, the sheath sheath withdrawn slightly, and the snare retightened around the suture itself. The endoscope and suture are then pulled from the patient's mouth.

Tube placement: The suture exiting the patient's mouth is affixed to the tapered end of the gastrostomy tube and the assistant begins pulling at the abdominal site. The second passage of the endoscope may be facilitated by grasping half the head of the gastrostomy tube with the snare passed through the channel of the endoscope (Fig. 144.3). The tube is well lubricated, pulled down the esophagus, and should be followed by the endoscope to ensure that its tip comes to lie in proper position (Fig. 144.4). The endoscope then closely follows the tube into the esophagus

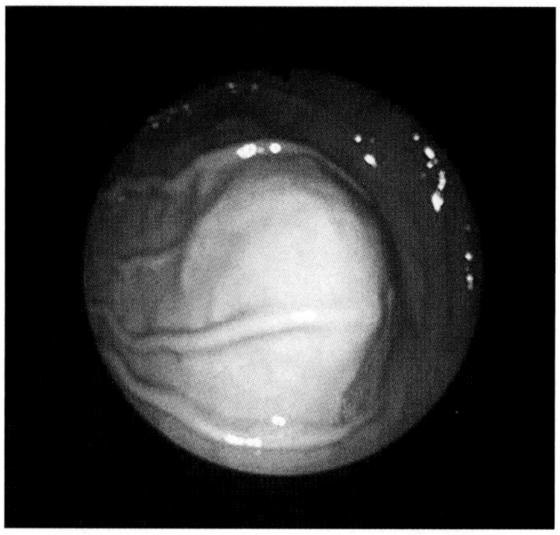

Fig. 144.1 The PEG technique. Clear indentation of the gastric wall should be noted at the optimal site for PEG placement.

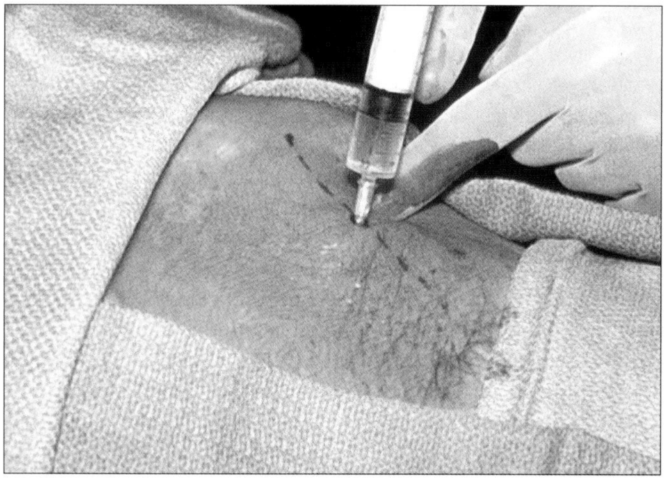

Fig. 144.2 The PEG technique. Using the 'safe tract' method, air should not enter the syringe barrel until the needle is seen in the gastric lumen.

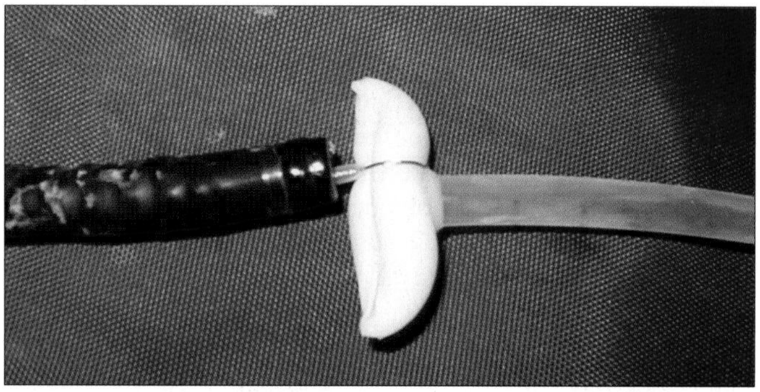

Fig. 144.3 The PEG technique. Half of the head of the tube is grasped with a snare through the scope so that it may lead the second passage of the scope easily into the esophagus.

and is gently pushed as the tube is pulled. The snare is opened to release the gastrostomy tube about halfway down the esophagus. The head of the tube should come to lie in loose approximation to the gastric mucosa (Fig. 144.5). The endoscope is then removed.

Fixation: Attention is then turned to the abdominal exit point of the tube. The tube is cleansed of any remaining lubricant and trimmed to the desired length. The outer crossbar or retention disk is applied and brought down to within several millimeters of the skin (Fig. 144.6). It is *not* desirable for the crossbar or retention disk to meet the skin as this may produce undue tension with resultant ischemia and necrosis of the

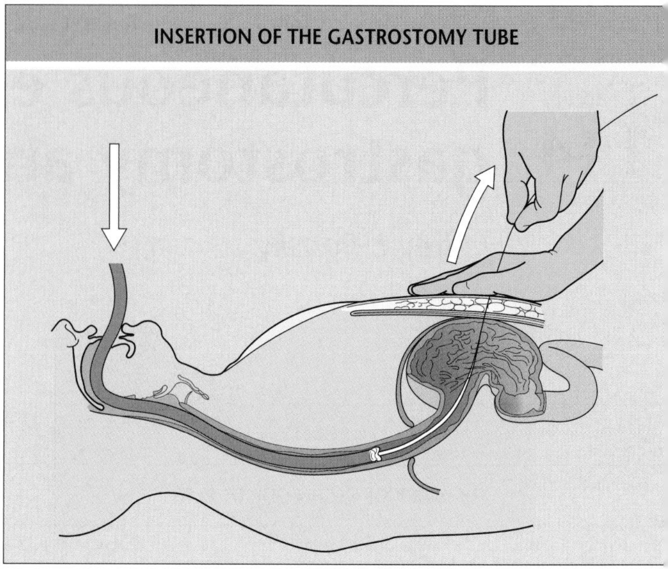

Fig. 144.4 Insertion of the gastrostomy tube. The endoscope–gastrostomy tube combination is passed down the esophagus. Halfway down the esophagus, the gastrostomy tube is released and pulled into the stomach as the endoscopist observes its position.

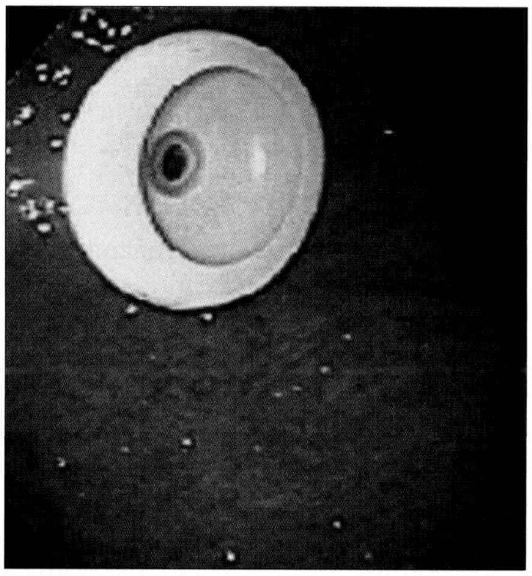

Fig. 144.5 Position of the gastrostomy tube. The head of the gastrostomy tube should come to lie in loose contact with the gastric mucosa.

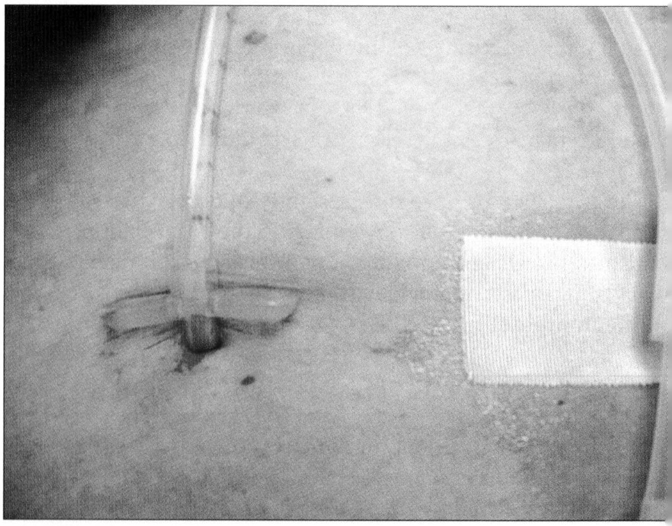

Fig. 144.6 Position of the outer crossbar. The outer crossbar should be applied several millimeters from the skin to avoid producing ischemia of the underlying tissue.

abdominal walls. The crossbar should be positioned several millimeters from the skin; after 1 week the crossbar can be moved 2–3 cm from the skin. Once the tract is mature the only purpose of the crossbar is to prevent migration of the tube's head distally to the pylorus, where it may cause obstruction.

The redundant tube is taped to the abdominal wall. Occlusive dressings are not required. The tube may be used for feeding immediately after the procedure.

INDICATIONS/CONTRAINDICATIONS FOR PEG

Percutaneous enteral access should not be performed in patients with overwhelming sepsis, multiorgan failure, or severe malnutrition. Nasogastric feedings should be employed in such patients until such time as these problems are resolved. Should the need for long-term enteral alimentation or decompression continue, percutaneous enteral access may be considered. Massive ascites and bleeding diatheses are relative contraindications. Severe gastroesophageal reflux may actually be exacerbated by gastrostomy, causing more frequent aspiration. Patients with a life expectancy of less than 30 days have a very high mortality rate associated with the procedure.[7]

Percutaneous gastrostomy is of value in providing long-term enteral access in patients who are unable to swallow but have a functional gastrointestinal tract. Such patients include those with oropharyngeal tumors, facial trauma, and neurologic impairment. The method has also been used with success in providing supplemental feedings in those with inflammatory bowel disease and for the delivery of unpalatable medications in children. It has been used as a means of recycling bile in some cases of biliary obstruction where internal drainage cannot be achieved.[8]

Patients with chronic, surgically irremediable, intestinal obstruction secondary to gastric or intestinal atony, malignancy, adhesions, or radiation may be candidates for decompressive gastrostomy.

INDICATIONS/CONTRAINDICATIONS

INDICATIONS FOR PEG
- Inability to swallow due to neurologic impairment
- Oropharyngeal tumors
- Need for long-term gastrointestinal decompression
- Need for supplemental feedings
- Facial trauma

CONTRAINDICATIONS TO PEG
- Sepsis
- Multiorgan failure
- Massive ascites
- Severe malnutrition
- Severe gastroesophageal reflux
- Life expectancy < 30 days

PERCUTANEOUS ENDOSCOPIC JEJUNOSTOMY

First described in 1984, the original method involved placement of an enteral feeding tube alongside a PEG tube with the latter used for decompression.[9] High failure rates were reported as a result of tube dysfunction and frequent tube manipulation.

Direct percutaneous endoscopic jejunostomy (PEJ) utilizes the same technique and principles as percutaneous gastrostomy, but in the small bowel. An enteroscope or pediatric colonoscope is employed to intubate the small bowel deeply, distal to the ligament of Treitz. Finger pressure is used to assess the best probable site for puncture. The use of fluoroscopy may also be helpful in assessing the position of the tip of the endoscope (Fig. 144.7). Once the site of proposed puncture has been selected, the 'safe tract' method is used to minimize the potential of inadvertent puncture of adjacent bowel. A useful method is to place the 'finder' needle on the end of the syringe and advance this until it successfully enters the visible lumen ahead of the endoscope. The endoscopist may now grasp this needle with a snare. The syringe is removed from the 'finder' needle and attached to the larger sheathed needle required for the procedure and this is then passed immediately beside and parallel to the 'finder' needle. When the large sheathed needle enters the visible lumen, the snare is transferred to grasp the sheath, and both needles are removed. The rest of the method is identical to that of PEG (Fig. 144.8). Again, tension is to be avoided in the application of the outer crossbar.

KEY POINTS

SUMMARY OF TECHNIQUE OF PEJ

AS EXTENSION OF PEG
- Place PEG in usual fashion
- Guide small-caliber feeding tube through or alongside PEG tube and into small bowel

AS DIRECT PEJ
- Pass enteroscope or pediatric colonoscope beyond ligament of Treitz
- Verify position of scope's tip with finger pressure or fluoroscopy
- Utilize 'safe tract' method to assure adjacent bowel is not punctured
- Perform in same fashion as PEG

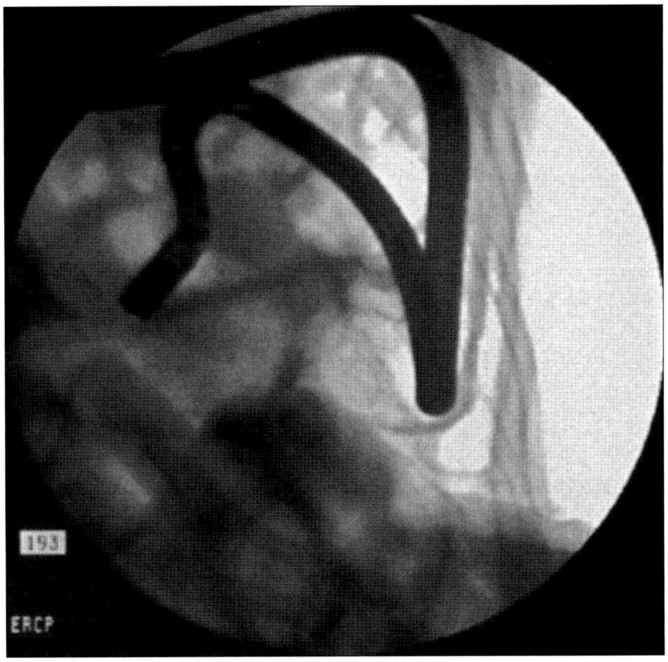

Fig. 144.7 Percutaneous endoscopic jejunostomy. Fluoroscopy is useful in assessing the position of the scope in the abdomen and selecting the best site for puncture.

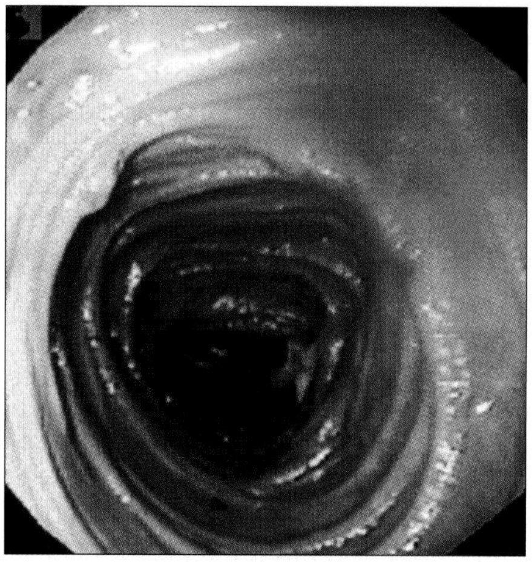

Fig. 144.8 Position of the PEJ tube. The PEJ tube should come to lie in loose contact with the jejunal wall. A tube of up to 20 Fr may be used without compromising the intestinal lumen.

INDICATIONS/CONTRAINDICATIONS
INDICATIONS FOR PEJ • Severe gastroesophageal reflux in a patient requiring long-term enteral feedings • Gastric atony **CONTRAINDICATIONS TO PEJ** • Massive ascites • Bleeding diatheses • Intestinal obstruction

COMPLICATIONS AND THEIR MANAGEMENT

Infections have become much less common with the use of the single-dose antibiotic as described. Many of the earlier severe infections were the result of excessive tension applied to the outer crossbar with resultant ischemia and necrotizing infection. The tube site should be inspected each day after performing the procedure. Infection should be suspected if redness, erythema, or induration develops. If a local, peritubal, abscess is suspected, drainage with local anesthesia and incision of the indurated site followed by antibiotic therapy may allow for uncomplicated resolution. If the site continues to worsen, surgical consultation must be sought.

Leakage around the tube is a common complaint. Most often this represents a small amount of drainage, which is a foreign body reaction to the tube. Good hygiene with frequent cleansing usually suffices. Granulation tissue may develop in response to the tube and may cause exudation or bleeding. Use of silver nitrate to cauterize this tissue is often helpful. When true leakage of gastric contents occurs around the tube, one must be concerned about gastric outlet obstruction or tubal obstruction.

Migration of the head of the catheter out of the stomach and into the abdominal wall may present in this way. In such cases, injection of water-soluble contrast into the tube may more clearly demonstrate the location of the tube's head and help to assess the effectiveness of gastric emptying. Migration into the abdominal wall may occur secondary to excessive tension on the outer crossbar. This may be avoided as discussed above.

Gastrocolic fistula is an infrequent but well recognized complication of gastrostomy. It results from puncturing the colon on the way to the stomach. This complication usually goes unnoticed for long periods of time, becoming apparent only when the tube is changed and the new tube comes to lie in the first lumen it reaches, the colon. The patient then will develop severe diarrhea after feedings. Injection of water-soluble contrast through the tube, contrast enema, computed tomography or colonoscopy may also make the diagnosis. If the problem is discovered long after the initial gastrostomy (i.e., more than 6 weeks), it can usually be resolved by simple removal of the tube by traction. The colonic fistula usually closes spontaneously within a week or two. When the fistula is discovered acutely because of patient deterioration, surgical intervention to remove the tube, close the colonic hole, and re-establish the gastrostomy is indicated. Use of the 'safe tract' method in performing the gastrostomy is the best approach to minimizing, if not preventing, the occurrence of this complication.

COSTS AND CONTROVERSIES

Economic, moral, and ethical issues have been raised with the expanded use of this technique.[9] Although PEG is clearly less costly than surgical gastrostomy, its ease of performance has increased total costs to society by increasing the total number of gastrostomies performed and perhaps by extending the lives, and resultant costs, of patients who would otherwise die more quickly. The selection of patients for percutaneous enteral access is clearly important and controversial.[10] Conflict regarding prolonged feeding in end-of-life decisions is now commonly recognized in society at large. The procedure offers little to patients with a short life expectancy. Beyond that, the physician must carefully consult with the patient and/or their family to assure that all involved understand the implications of placement of the tube. Percutaneous enteral access has greatly facilitated the care of patients in a minimally invasive way. It has been of great value to physicians and their patients, but must be applied with great care both technically and ethically.[11]

COSTS, COMPLICATIONS, CONTROVERSIES
• More cost-effective than surgical gastrostomy • Complications include: Infection Tube leakage Tube dislodgment Gastrocolic fistula • Controversies: Short-term advantages versus nasoenteric tubes End-of-life issues

SOURCES OF INFORMATION FOR PATIENTS AND DOCTORS

http://www.patient.co.uk/showdoc/40024638/
http://www.rcr.ac.uk/crplg15.doc

REFERENCES

1. Gauderer M, Ponsky JL, Izant RJ Jr. Gastrostomy without laparotomy: a percutaneous endoscopic technique. J Pediatr Surg 1980; 15:872–875.
2. Fan AC, Baron TH, Rumalla A, Harewood GC. Comparison of direct percutaneous endoscopic jejunostomy and PEG with jejunal extension. Gastrointest Endosc 2002; 56:890–894.
3. Ponsky JL, Aszodi A, Perse D. Percutaneous endoscopic cecostomy: a new approach to nonobstructive colonic dilation. Gastrointest Endosc 1986; 32:108–111.
4. Mellinger JD, Simon IB, Schlechter B, Lash RH, Ponsky JL. Tract formation following percutaneous endoscopic gastrostomy (PEG) in an animal model. Surg Endosc 1991; 5:189–191.
5. Ponsky JL, Gauderer M. Percutaneous endoscopic gastrostomy: a nonoperative technique for feeding gastrostomy. Gastrointest Endosc 1981; 27:9–11.
6. Foutch PG, Talbert GA, Waring JP et al. Percutaneous endoscopic gastrostomy in patients with prior abdominal surgery: virtues of the safe tract. Am J Gastroenterol 1988; 83:147–150.
7. Bumpers HL, Collure DW, Best IM et al. Unusual complications of long-term percutaneous gastrostomy tubes. J Gastrointest Surg 2003; 7:917–920.
8. Ponsky JL, Aszodi A. External biliary–gastric fistula: a simple method for recycling bile. Am J Gastroenterol 1982; 77:939–940.
9. Angus F, Burakoff R. The percutaneous endoscopic gastrostomy tube, medical and ethical issues in placement. Am J Gastroenterol 2003; 98:1904.
10. Kruse A, Misiewicz JJ, Rokkas T et al. Recommendations of the ESGE workshop on the ethics of percutaneous endoscopic gastrostomy placement for nutritional support. First European symposium on ethics in gastroenterology and digestive endoscopy, Kos, Greece, June 2003. Endoscopy 2003; 35:778–780.
11. Klose J, Heldwein W, Rafferzeder M et al. Nutrition life in patients with percutaneous endoscopic gastrostomy (PEG) in practice: prospective one-year follow-up. Dig Dis Sci 2003; 48:2057–2063.

Chapter 145

Endoscopic mucosal resection of neoplasms in the gastrointestinal tract

Haruhiro Inoue

KEY POINTS

- Mucosal lesions with a low risk of vascular or lymphatic spread and at least moderately differentiated histology are suitable for endoscopic mucosal resection
- The submucosal connection between mucosa and muscularis propria is easily separated by injection of saline
- Submucosal elevation must be sustained to reduce the risk of perforation
- Chromoendoscopy is useful in defining the lateral margins of tumors
- Endoscopic mucosal dissection (ESD) allows en bloc mucosal resection of tumors >2–3 cm in diameter

INTRODUCTION

Surgical resection of gastrointestinal cancers is often associated with significant morbidity and mortality. Therefore methods for endoscopic cancer resection have been sought. With adequate staging techniques, endoscopic resection of early lesions looks promising.[1–6] In surgically resected specimens, intramucosal cancer generally has an extremely small risk of lymph node metastasis. Therefore endoscopic resection of mucosal cancer can be done without lymph node dissection. Endoscopic mucosal resection (EMR) is a technique of local excision of neoplastic lesions confined to the mucosal layer. In this chapter the use of EMR is discussed, with a focus on current techniques.

BASIC PRINCIPLES OF ENDOSCOPIC MUCOSAL RESECTION

The mucosa and muscularis propria are, in a sense, attached to each other by the loose connective tissue of the submucosa, and can be easily separated by injection of saline. This allows resection of the mucosa alone, leaving the muscularis propria layer intact. Saline injection into the submucosal layer is the easiest and most cost-effective technique for separating both layers. Lifting of the mucosal surface can be achieved after correct submucosal injection in any part of the gastrointestinal tract. After a sufficient volume of saline has been injected, the mucosa, including the target lesion, can be safely captured and resected by electrocautery.

Choosing the appropriate lesions

Only mucosal lesions with a low risk of vascular or lymphatic spread are appropriate for EMR. Endoscopic ultrasonography is often used in conjunction with conventional or magnification endoscopy to assess lesion depth. Biopsy and review of the lesion's histology prior to resection should be a routine because poorly differentiated tumors are more likely to have metastases. In general, well or moderately differentiated mucosal lesions are considered acceptable targets for EMR.

Defining the lesion endoscopically

Chromoendoscopy may be a very useful aid in defining the lesion prior to EMR. The edges of tumor extension may be ill defined, particularly with flat lesions. In the esophagus Lugol's solution can be used to delineate the boundary between normal squamous mucosa (positive-staining, brown-green-black) and regions of dysplasia, Barrett's, or carcinoma (negative staining). Elsewhere in the gastrointestinal tract indigo carmine can be used as a 'highlighter' to increase contrast at the interface between normal mucosa and neoplastic lesions.

Once fully visualized, it is useful to mark the edges of the lesions prior to removal. This can be accomplished with cautery from a snare tip a few millimeters outside the lesion's border. The presence of cautery markings may be helpful in reorienting the tissue once it is removed.

EMR TECHNIQUES

Endoscopic mucosal resection using a 'cap'-fitted endoscope (EMR-C)

The EMR 'cap' technique[7] is fast, easy to perform, and can be applied to relatively small lesions (<1 cm). 'Cap' here refers to an attachment on the distal tip of the forward-viewing endoscope that is made from a transparent plastic material (Fig. 145.1). The steps involved in EMR-C technique follow.

Step 1: Preparation

In preparation for the EMR-C procedure, a cap is attached to the tip of the forward-viewing endoscope and is fixed tightly with an adhesive tape. For the initial session of EMR in the esophagus and stomach, an obliquely cut, large-capacity cap with a rim (Olympus MAJ297) (Fig. 145.1A) is most commonly used by fixing it on to the tip of the standard-size endoscope in order to obtain a larger sample. For trimming a residual lesion, a straight-cut medium-sized cap with a rim (Olympus MH595) (Fig. 145.1B) is appropriate. All of the items needed for the EMR-C procedure are commercially available in an EMR-Kit (Olympus).

Step 2: Markings

The mucosal surface that surrounds the margin of the lesion is carefully marked with cautery using the tip of the snare wire.

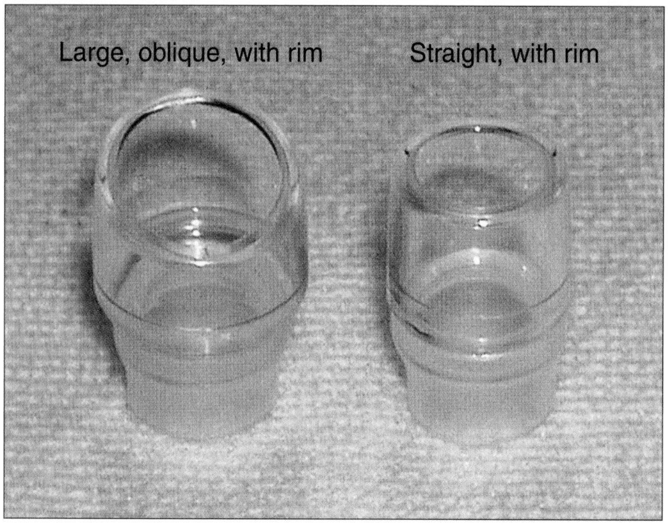

Fig. 145.1 Distal attachment caps. *Left:* Large, oblique with rim; 16.5-mm outer diameter. This large-cap is applied to a first capture during EMR-C procedure; 2–3 cm mucosa can be resected. *Right:* Straight, with rim; 13.5-mm outer diameter. This cap is used for trimming the lesion; approximately 1–2 cm mucosa can be removed.

Markings are positioned 2 mm away from the actual lesion margin. The color enhancement produced by chromoendoscopy disappears within a couple of minutes, and marking by electrocoagulation is therefore essential, especially for a flat lesion.

Step 3: Injection

A diluted epinephrine–saline solution (0.5 mL 0.1% epinephrine solution in 100 mL normal saline) is injected into the submucosa with an injection needle (23-gauge, tip length 4 mm). Puncturing the target mucosa at a sharp angle is important to avoid transmural penetration of the needle tip. The total volume of injected saline depends on the size of the lesion, *but it is necessary to inject enough saline to lift up the entire lesion.* Usually, more than 20 mL is injected. When saline is accurately injected into the submucosal layer, lifting of the mucosa or its bulging is observed (Fig. 145.2A).

Step 4: Prelooping of the snare wire

A specially designed small-diameter snare (with an outer diameter of 1.8 mm; Olympus SD-7P) is essential for the 'prelooping' process. The snare wire is fixed along the rim of the EMR-C cap. To create prelooping conditions, moderate suction is first applied to the normal mucosa to seal the outlet of the cap, and the snare wire that passes through the endoscope instrument channel is then opened. The opened snare wire is fixed along the rim of the cap, and the snare's outer sheath sticks up to the rim of the cap. This completes the prelooping process for the snare wire.

Step 5: Suction of the target mucosa

With the prelooping position maintained, the lesion is fully captured inside the cap and strangulated by simple closing of the prelooped snare wire. At this moment, the strangulated mucosa looks like a snared polypoid lesion (Fig. 145.2B and C).

Step 6: Resection

The pseudo-polyp of the strangulated mucosa is cut using blended-current electrocautery (Fig. 145.2C). The resected specimen can be easily taken out by keeping it inside the cap, without using any grasping forceps. The smooth surface of the muscularis propria layer will be exposed at the bottom of the EMR-induced ulcer.

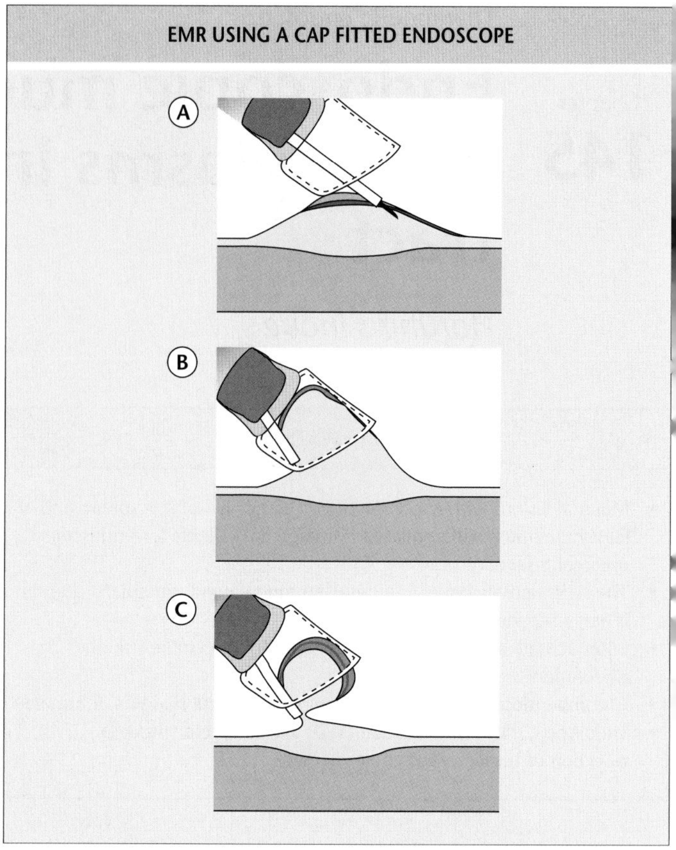

Fig. 145.2 EMR using a cap-fitted endoscope (EMR-C). A. Submucosa injection of epinephrine–saline solution. The distal part of the lesion is punctured first to ensure that the lesion is always kept in view. **B.** Prelooping of the snare wire and drawing up the target mucosa. Full suction draws the lifted mucosa into the cap. Use of a large volume of saline–epinephrine solution avoids resection of muscularis propria. **C.** Target mucosa is captured as a pseudo-polyp. The snare-entrapped strangulated mucosa is resected by electrocautery. Coagulation current is the best to achieve complete hemostasis.

Step 7: Additional resection

If additional resection is necessary to remove the residual lesion completely, all of the procedures, including saline injection, should be repeated step by step. The injected saline usually infiltrates and disappears within a few minutes at the initial injection site, so that it no longer acts as a cushion between the mucosa and muscle layer. Repeated saline injection is therefore necessary to reduce the risk of perforation.[8]

Endoscopic submucosal dissection (ESD)

EMR is a technique originally based on snare polypectomy. The size of the specimen resected by EMR is limited to around 2–3 cm. Endoscopic submucosal dissection (ESD) is a novel technique of EMR that enables one-piece resection, even for a superficially spreading tumor. In ESD, first described by Ono et al,[9] a knife activated by electrocautery is used both to cut margins and for submucosal dissection beneath isolated mucosa. Devices designed for ESD include the insulation-tip knife, hook knife, flex knife, and triangle-tip knife (Fig. 145.3).[9–12]

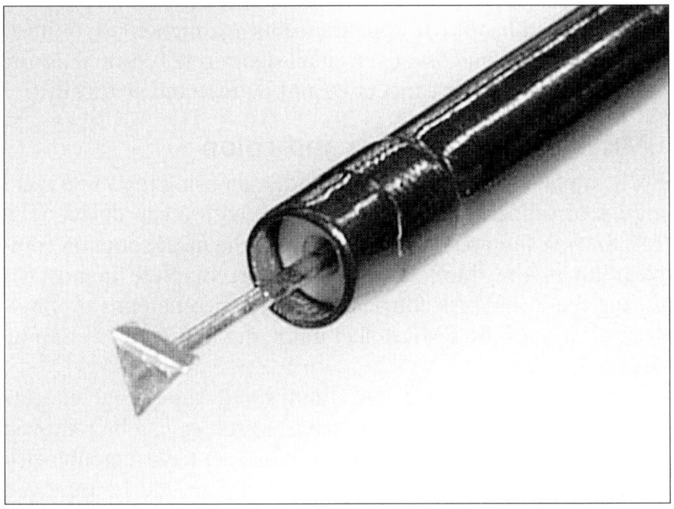

Fig. 145.3 The triangle-tip knife. The outer diameter of the device is 1.8 mm. The tip is made of metal so that the electric current passes through it.

Triangle-tip knife procedure

The ESD technique using a triangle-tip knife[13] allows removal of the lesion in a single specimen, even for an extended lesion (Fig. 145.3). The triangle-tip knife works as a multipurpose device (Figs 145.4 and 145.5) that can be utilized for marking, cutting, dissecting, and even hemostasis. Using an edge of the triangle-tip knife, markings are put on to the normal mucosa around the lesion. Injection with high-viscosity solution is mandatory for this procedure because it maintains mucosal lifting for longer duration. The authors utilize hyaluronic acid for injection. The energy source is an important factor in performing safe ESD. Swift coagulation (ERBE; Vaio) is now considered to be the best electrocautery device for the triangle-tip knife. Marginal cutting about 5 mm outside the markings is the next step. The triangle-tip knife hooks the mucosal edge and pulls up the target mucosa away from the surface of the muscle layer, and then cuts it by electrocautery. By repeating the process, circumferential incision around the lesion is completed. Submucosal dissection using the tip of a triangle-tip knife is subsequently carried out. A hood mounted on the tip of the endoscope creates a working space beneath the mucosa, and provides counter-traction to the tissue in the submucosa. After removal of the mobilized mucosa, complete hemostasis is achieved by a coagulation forceps.

ENDOSCOPIC SUBMUCOSAL DISSECTION USING TRIANGLE-TIP KNIFE

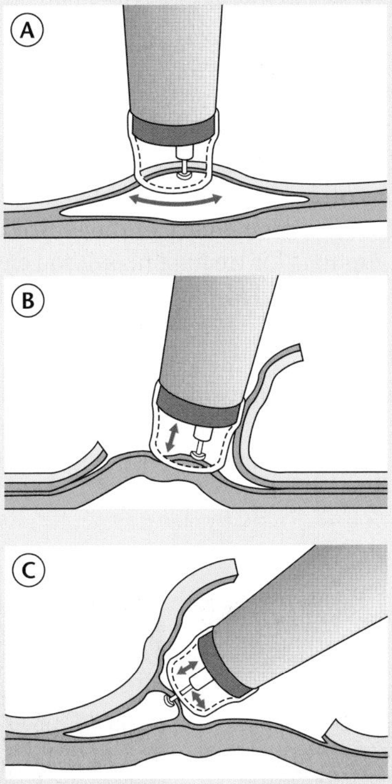

Fig. 145.4 Endoscopic submucosal dissection (ESD) using the triangle-tip knife. A. After submucosal injection, mucosal dissection is carried out using a triangle-tip knife. The energy source is swift coagulation, 60 W, effect 4 (ERBE). **B.** Bleeding from the ulcer bed is controlled by coagulation using the bottom of the triangle tip. **C.** Submucosal dissection is completed by electrosurgical cauterization, using the triangle tip. Fibers in the submucosa are hooked and cut step by step.

WHICH PROCEDURE SHOULD BE APPLIED?

Generally, small lesions can be easily excised by EMR-C procedure. In the esophagus, lesions smaller than 2 cm can be resected

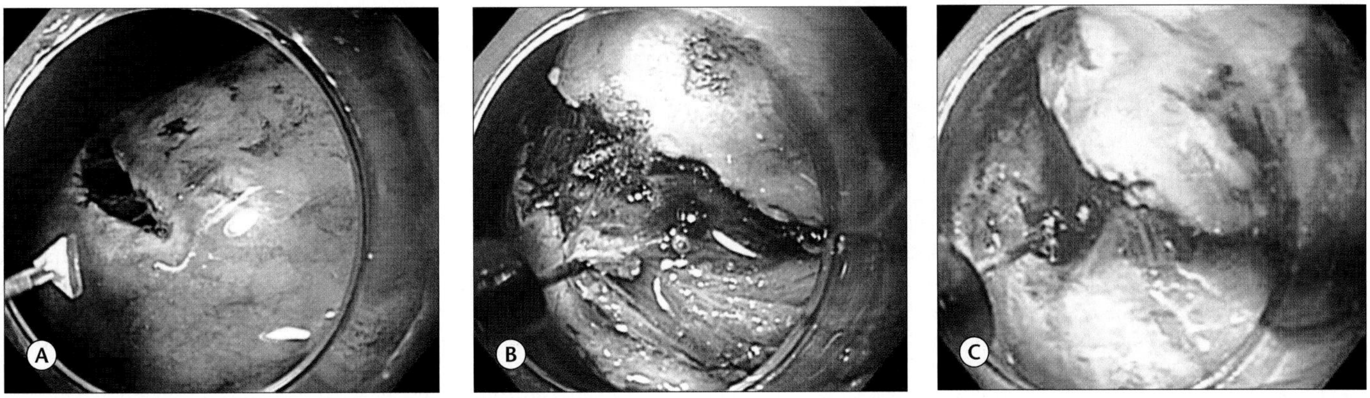

Fig. 145.5 Endoscopic view during ESD using the triangle-tip knife. A. Mucosal cutting – marginal mucosa surrounding the lesion is dissected circumferentially. **B.** Submucosal dissection – submucosal fibers are cut by hooking them with a triangle-tip knife. **C.** Hemostasis – bleeding from the ulcer bed is controlled by coagulation with the bottom of triangle-tip knife.

by one session of EMR-C. In the stomach lesions less than 1 cm can be resected in one piece. The triangle-tip knife procedure is used for larger lesions, with the intent of performing en bloc mucosal resections in the stomach.

EMR in the esophagus

Squamous cell carcinomas without extension past the lamina propria can be removed by EMR with a very low risk of distal spread (Fig. 145.6) Lesions of 2–3 cm can be resected, although those that encompass a greater circumference of the lumen carry a higher risk of stricture. Options for treating neoplastic change in Barrett's esophagus are discussed at the end of this chapter.

EMR in the stomach

Mucosal adenocarcinomas of 1–2 cm can be removed by EMR (Fig. 145.7) with a low risk of invasion, with the following caveats. Lesions with ulceration or ulcer scar and those with a poorly differentiated histologic appearance have a higher risk of invasion beyond the mucosa. Even small signet-ring type and poorly differentiated gastric cancers should be resected surgically.[14]

EMR in the duodenum and colon

EMR can be carried out in the duodenum using the same techniques of saline injection and cautery with a cap device (Fig. 145.8). Post-therapeutic bleeding poses the most common complication in the duodenum, even after complete hemostasis during the initial procedure. The author recommends prophylactic closure of the EMR defect in the duodenum by a clipping device.

Large adenomatous polyps and small superficial cancers with moderate or well differentiated histology can be removed with EMR. Colonic cancers larger than 1 cm have a greater risk of lymphatic or submucosal invasion and should be removed surgically.

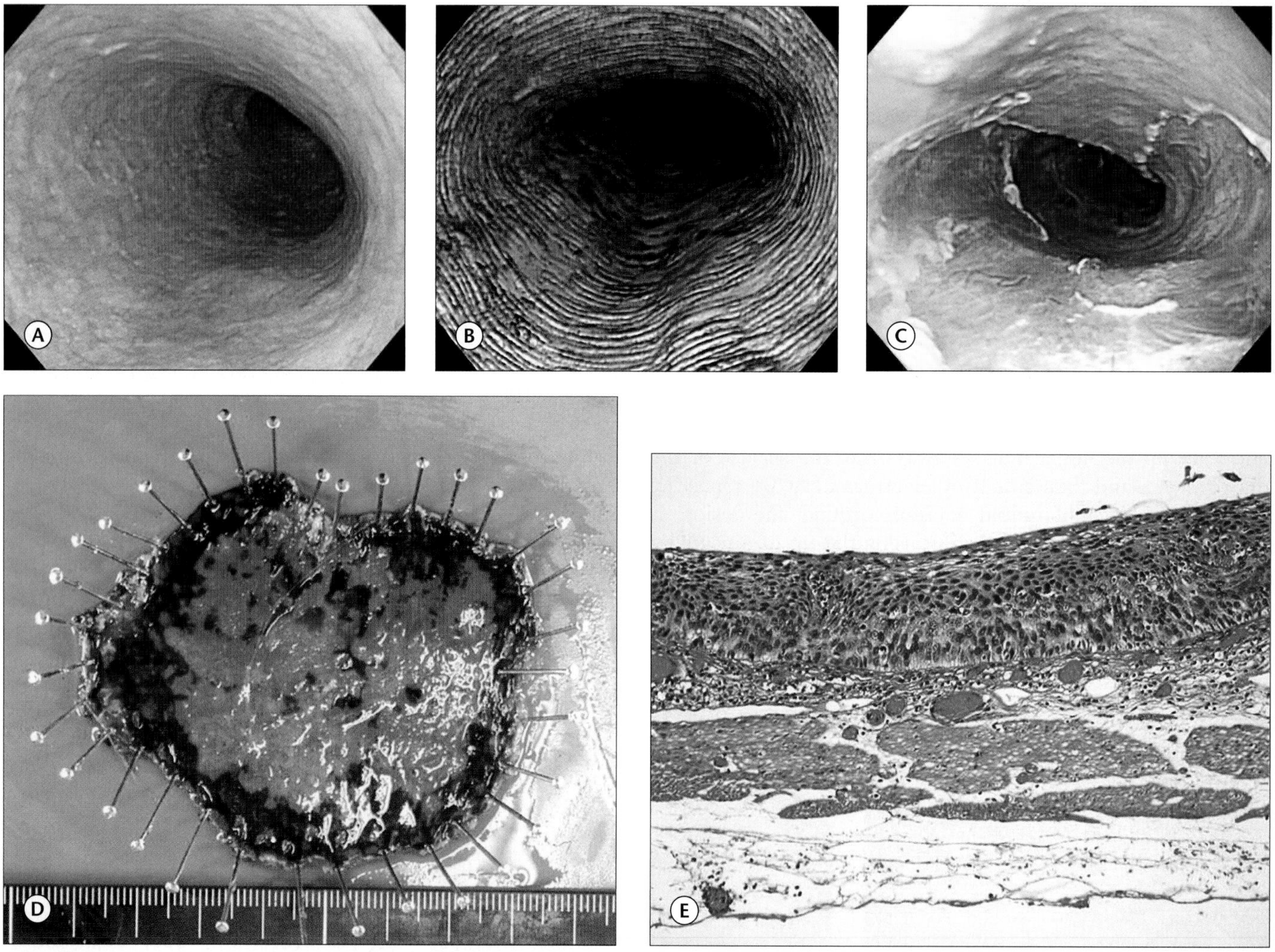

Fig. 145.6 ESD using the triangle-tip knife. Squamous cell carcinoma in the esophagus; mucosal cancer. **A.** Routine endoscopic view. Superficial erosion is recognized in the 6 o'clock direction. Protrusion of mucosa as a result of compression by the spine is also observed distal to the erosion. **B.** Large unstained area with Lugol's iodine staining. Regularly arranged 'fernization' or wrinkling of the mucosa was maintained, so the lesion was diagnosed as m1. **C.** An artificial ulcer induced by triangle-tip knife EMR, three-quarters circumferential. The muscularis propria surface is covered with a thin connective tissue layer. **D.** Resected mucosal specimen. Large unstained area surrounded by positive-staining margins indicates a successful single-specimen en bloc removal. **E.** Microscopic image of the resected specimen; hematoxylin and eosin staining. Carcinoma in situ (high-grade dysplasia) is present. The dark area in the bottom third of the squamous mucosa highlights the neoplastic change.

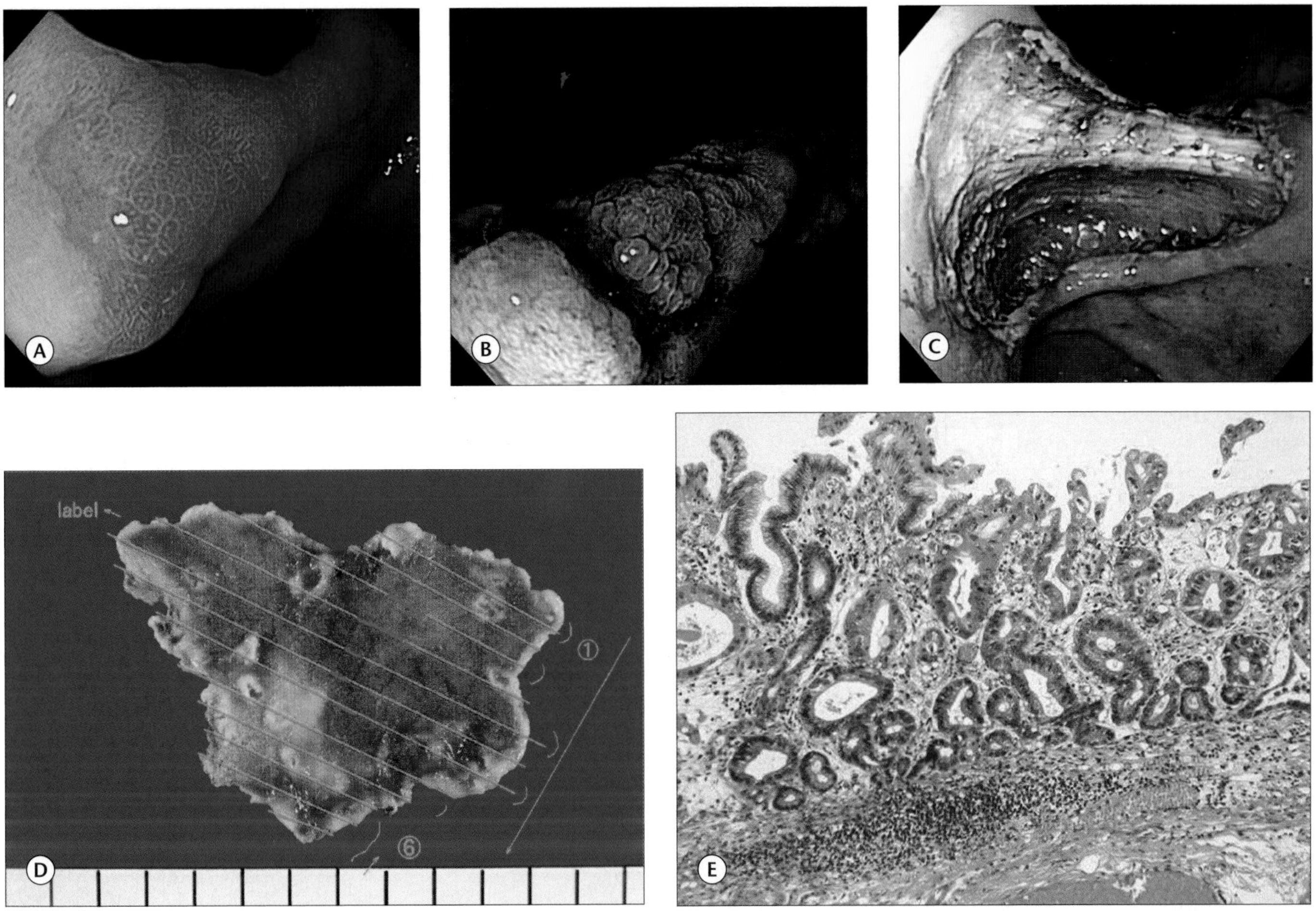

Fig. 145.7 ESD using the triangle-tip knife. Differentiated adenocarcinoma in the stomach; mucosal cancer. **A.** Routine endoscopic view. Superficial slightly depressed lesion (IIc) with erosion was observed at the anterior wall of the gastric angularis. **B.** Chromoendoscopic view. IIc depressive lesion was well demonstrated with indigo carmine staining. **C.** Artificial ulcer induced by ESD. The smooth surface of the muscle layer was exposed. The lower horizontal edge of the green-stained ulcer shows swollen submucosa because of the hyaluronic acid injection. **D.** Histologic mapping of the resected specimen. For the histologic examination, the resected specimen was cut into 2-mm strips (green lines). The distribution of the cancer was demonstrated as red lines. **E.** Histology – well differentiated adenocarcinoma.

COMPLICATIONS OF EMR

Potential complications include bleeding, perforation, and stricture. Bleeding can generally be managed with standard hemostasis techniques, including the use of endoclips. Perforation is rare and is treated by surgery, endoscopic clipping, or conservative management depending on the size and location of the perforation. In a series of 412 patients the present author's group have used the EMR-C procedure for 222 lesions in the esophagus and 190 in the stomach.[8] ESD with the triangle-tip knife was used in an additional 78 patients (13 in the esophagus, 65 in the stomach). Perforation occurred in the esophagus in one patient and in the stomach in seven. The perforation in the esophagus was treated conservatively. In all cases of gastric perforation, the perforated wound was closed using a hemostatic clip. There was no procedure-related mortality in 490 cases of EMR or ESD.

FUTURE DIRECTIONS

EMR of neoplastic change (high-grade dysplasia, intramucosal cancer) in Barrett's esophagus is an appealing strategy. Satodate et al[15] performed a total of eight cases of EMR for superficial carcinoma arising in Barrett's esophagus using the EMR-C procedure. All patients were successfully treated solely with EMR, with no major complications. One-piece resection with ESD for focal adenocarcinoma arising on long-segment Barrett's esophagus was carried out in three cases (Fig. 145.9).

A large series of patients has been reported in which local endoscopic therapy was used for intraepithelial high-grade dysplasia and early adenocarcinoma in Barrett's esophagus.[16] The overall complication rate was 9.5%, and the calculated 3-year survival rate 88%. On the basis of the results, local endoscopic therapy may be an effective and safe alternative to esophagectomy for high-grade dysplasia and early adenocarcinoma. It is not unusual to have to repeat EMR in these patients, presumably because their residual Barrett's mucosa is more subject to neoplastic change or because endoscopically invisible synchronous lesions were present at the time of the original treatment.

Ablative therapy, for instance with photodynamic therapy,[17] has also been used as an alternative to surgical therapy, but there may be several limitations to ablative therapy compared with EMR. Adenocarcinoma may appear beneath re-

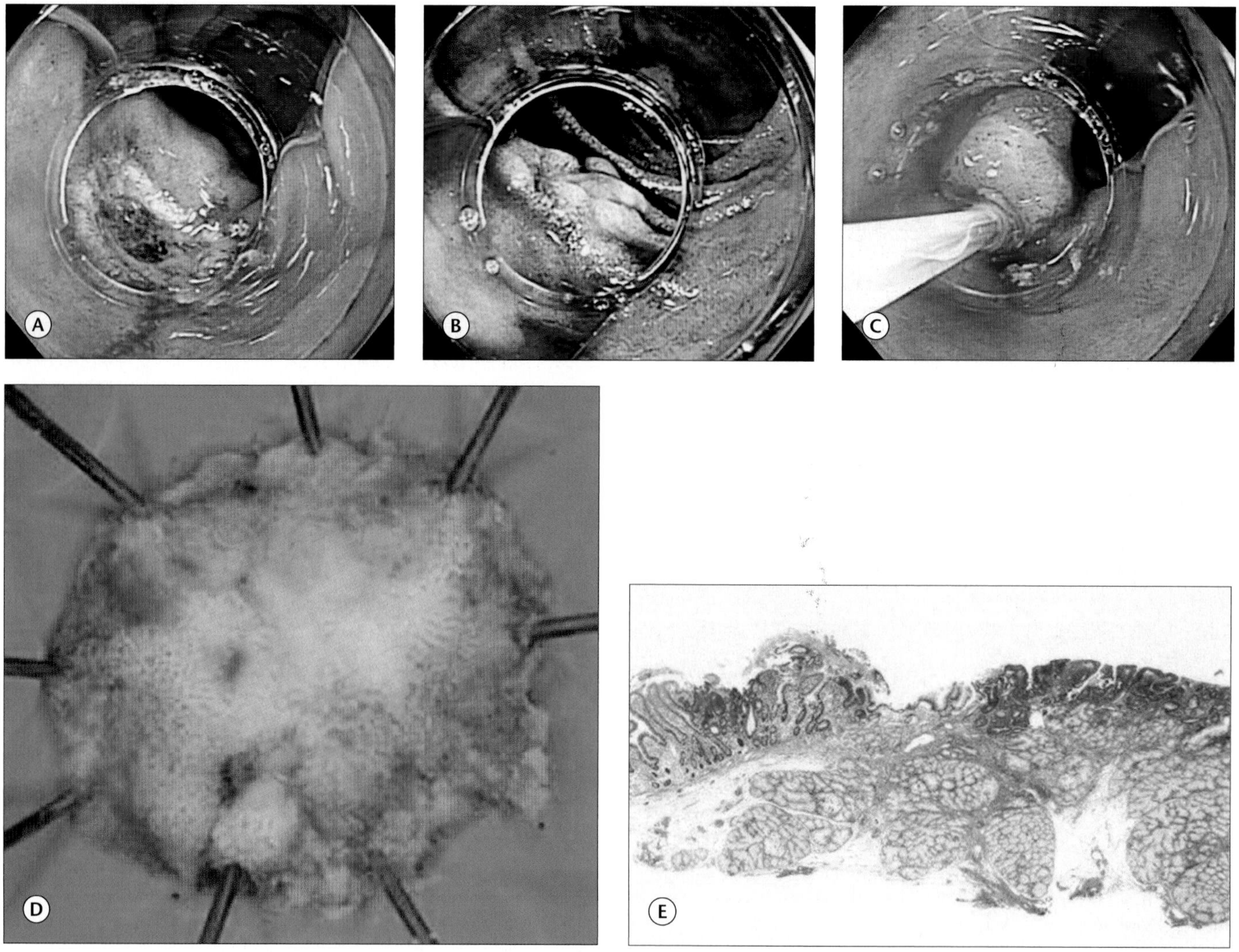

Fig. 145.8 Adenomatous neoplasia of the duodenum. A. Incidentally discovered small erosion surrounded by swollen irregular mucosa. **B.** After indigo carmine staining. **C.** Snare around the lesion after injection and suction into cap. **D.** Base of resection zone. **E.** Histology showing neoplastic/dysplastic lesion. Most of the right half of the figure shows the dark-staining superficial neoplastic change. There is a smaller area of dark-staining mucosa on the left of the depressed center of the lesion.

epithelialized squamous epithelial tissue.[18] In addition, EMR permits staging of the neoplastic change, because it allows detection of occult carcinoma or areas of invasion not suspected on the basis of endoscopic biopsy and endoscopic ultrasonography.

It has been proposed that EMR should be limited to within three-quarters of the circumference of the esophagus, and that near-total or total mucosal resection should be avoided owing to refractory stenosis after healing of the resulting ulcer.[19] Possible approaches may include a two-stage full-circumference resection at an interval of 8 weeks[20] or photodynamic therapy after EMR. When circumferential mucosal resection is performed with this technique on long-segment Barrett's esophagus, multiple specimens[9–20] are obtained, making precise reconstruction of the resected specimens extremely difficult. This may be theoretically averted by using a triangle-tip knife to acquire one-piece specimens for better histologic analysis.

SUMMARY

In the elderly and/or frail patients with early neoplastic disease of the gastrointestinal tract, the need for less invasive procedures becomes more compelling. EMR affords a unique and exciting treatment mode. For some of the techniques described here, the availability of endoscopic ultrasonography is invaluable. It is likely that in the future many of these procedures will be done in specialized centers.

The standards and expectations for EMR should be similar to those of conventional oncologic surgery. That is, we need long-term outcome data that include survival data, complications, and the need for retreatment, especially for diseases such as gastric cancer and Barrett's esophagus where a diffuse preneoplastic 'field defect' may be involved.

SOURCES OF INFORMATION FOR PATIENTS AND DOCTORS

http://personalweb.sunset.net/~mansell/polyp.htm

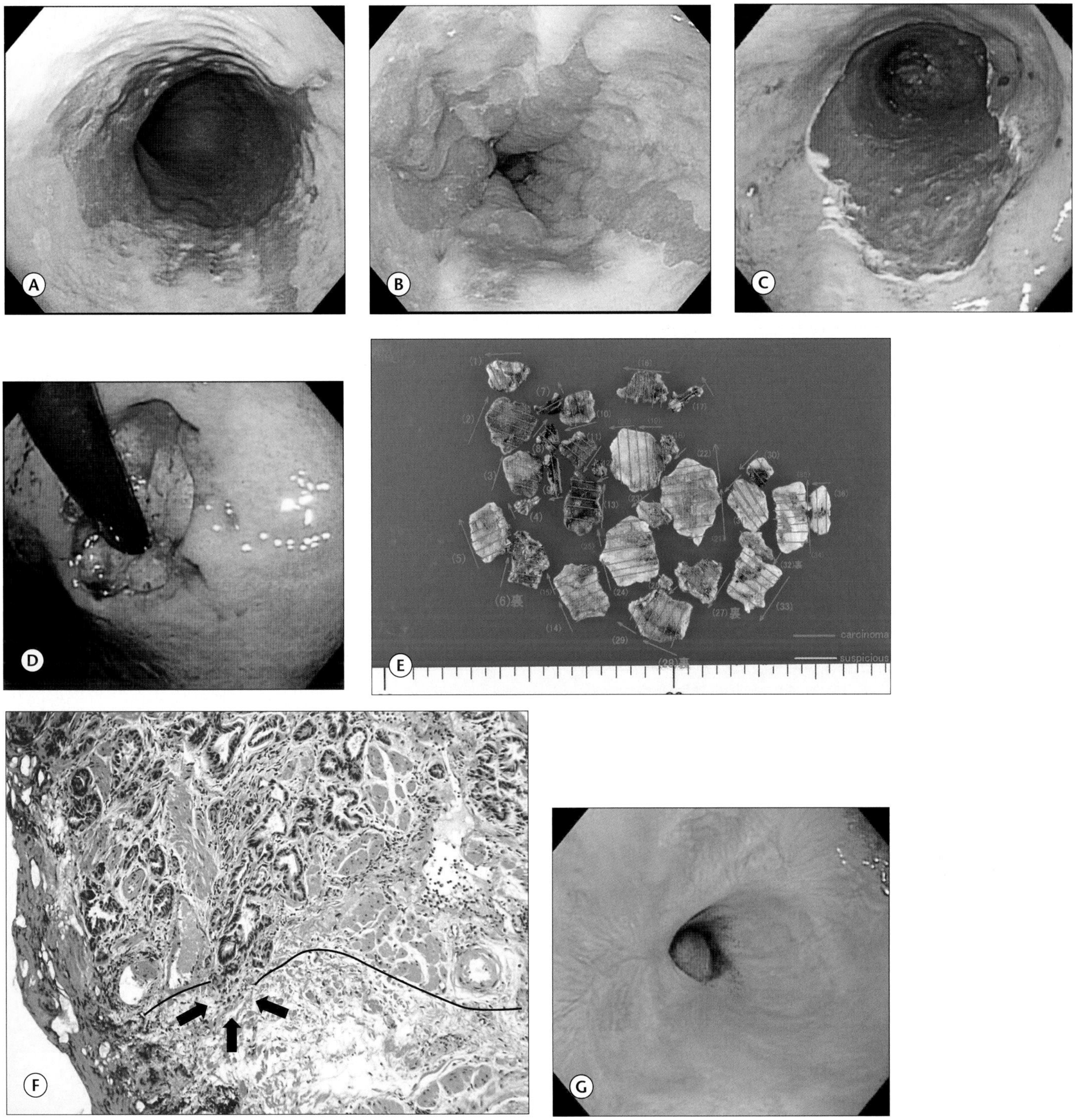

Fig. 145.9 Circumferential EMR for Barrett's cancer. A. Endoscopic photograph shows long-segment Barrett's esophagus. Reddish, irregular 'tongues' of columnar epithelium extend more than 5 cm above the gastroesophageal junction. **B.** With partial deflation, swollen linear folds become evident in the Barrett's zone. There are residual adjacent 'flat' areas of red-staining Barrett's mucosa. Multiple four-quadrant biopsies revealed well differentiated adenocarcinoma. **C.** Barrett's esophageal mucosa was completely excised circumferentially. **D.** Turnaround view in the stomach showing the proximal gastric mucosa (cardia region). A 2-cm long circumferential zone was also resected. **E.** Resected specimens (30 pieces in all), including small trimmings at the edge. There was multifocal intramucosal carcinoma. **F.** One section showed slight invasion (10 μm) into the submucosal layer (indicated by arrows). The black line shows lower border of muscularis mucosae. The pathologic diagnosis was suspicious of invasive carcinoma, Vienna classification category 4.3. **G.** Three months after circumferential EMR. Normal 'neosquamous' epithelium with slight scarring radiating to a central point at the 9 o'clock location.

REFERENCES

1. Maku-uchi H. Endoscopic mucosal resection for early esophageal cancer. Dig Endosc 1996; 8:175–179.
2. Monma K, Sakaki N, Yoshida M. Endoscopic mucosectomy for precise evaluation and treatment of esophageal intraepithelial cancer. Endosc Dig 1990; 2:447–452.
3. Inoue H, Endo M. Endoscopic esophageal mucosal resection using a transparent tube. Surg Endosc 1990; 4:198–201.
4. Inoue H. Endoscopic mucosal resection for gastrointestinal mucosal cancers. In: Classen M, Tytgat GNJ, Lightdale C, eds. Gastroenterological endoscopy. Stuttgart: Thieme; 2000:322–333.
5. Endo M, Takeshita K, Yoshida M. How can we diagnose the early stage of esophageal cancer? Endoscopy 1986; 18:11–18.
6. Lambert R. Diagnosis of esophagogastric tumors. Endoscopy 2004; 36:110–119.
7. Inoue H, Takeshita K, Hori H et al. Endoscopic mucosal resection with a cap-fitted panendoscope for esophagus, stomach, and colon mucosal lesions. Gastrointest Endosc 1993; 39:58–62.
8. Inoue H, Kawano T, Tani M et al. Endoscopic mucosal resection using a cap: technique for use and preventing perforation. Can J Gastroenterol 1999; 13:477–480.
9. Ono H, Kondo H, Gotoda T et al. Endoscopic mucosal resection for treatment of early gastric cancer. Gut 2001; 48:225–229.
10. Yamamoto H, Yube T, Isoda N et al. A novel method of endoscopic mucosal resection using sodium hyaluronate. Gastrointest Endosc 1999; 50:251–256.
11. Oyama T, Kikuchi Y. Aggressive endoscopic mucosal resection in the upper GI tract – Hook knife EMR method. Minim Invas Ther Allied Technol 2002; 11:291–295.
12. Yahagi N, Fujishiro M, Iguchi M et al. Theoretical and technical requirements to expand EMR indications. Dig Endosc 2003; 15:S19–S21.
13. Inoue H, Satoh Y, Kazawa T et al. Endoscopic submucosal dissection using a newly developed triangle-tip knife. Stomach Intest 2004; 39:73–75.
14. Soetikno RM, Gotoda T, Nakanishi Y, Soehendra N. Endoscopic mucosal resection. Gastrointest Endosc 2003; 57:567–579.
15. Satodate H, Inoue H, Yoshida T et al. Circumferential EMR of carcinoma arising in Barrett's esophagus: case report. Gastrointest Endosc 2003; 58:288–289.
16. May A, Gossner L, Pech O et al. Local endoscopic therapy for intraepithelial high-grade neoplasia and early adenocarcinoma in Barrett's esophagus: acute-phase and long-term results of new treatment approach. Eur J Gastroenterol Hepatol 2002; 14:1085–1091.
17. Overholt BF, Panjehpour M, Haydek JM. Photodynamic therapy for Barrett's esophagus: follow-up in 100 patients. Gastrointest Endosc 1999; 49:1–7.
18. Sampliner RE, Fass R. Partial regression of Barrett's esophagus: an inadequate endpoint. Am J Gastroenterol 1993; 88:2092–2094.
19. Inoue H, Kudo S. Endoscopic mucosal resection for gastrointestinal mucosal cancer. In: Meinhard C, Guido NJ, Charles JL, eds. Gastroenterological endoscopy. Stuttgart: Thieme; 2002:322–333.
20. Makuuchi H. Endoscopic mucosal resection for early esophageal cancer, indication and technique. Dig Endosc 1996; 8:175–179.

Chapter 146

Dilation and stenting of the gastrointestinal tract

Drew Schembre

Introduction

Dilation stands as one of the oldest interventions performed on the digestive tract. Esophageal dilation had been performed for centuries with wax candles and other tapered, rigid devices. Although esophageal dilation has evolved into a more precise procedure, the principle of stretching or fracturing benign and malignant strictures with gradual, radial force has not changed. Dilation creates longitudinal tears in the visceral wall, disrupting circular collagen and even shearing smooth muscle, but leaves more compliant tissues intact. Repair over this lattice of intact tissue usually results in restored tissue integrity and a widened lumen.[1] The safety, reach and durability of dilatations have improved dramatically. Esophageal dilation can be accomplished with tapered dilators or through-the-scope (TTS) hydrostatic inflatable balloons. The use of guidewires in conjunction with endoscopic and fluoroscopic guidance, along with the concept of incremental dilation, has made perforations unusual.

While many strictures resolve with simple dilation, malignant constrictions and, very rarely, tenacious benign strictures, may benefit from placement of a stent. While earlier stents were composed of rigid materials, self-expanding metal stents (SEMS) have proven to be safer and easier to place and have quickly replaced rigid stents for treating esophageal malignancies (Fig. 146.1). SEMS have been increasingly used to palliate malignant obstructions of the gastric outlet, duodenum, colon, and rectum. This chapter will describe the techniques of dilation and stenting as well as the indications and limitations of these methods. Unfortunately, few good studies exist comparing various dilation and stenting technologies. Fewer studies have compared stenting to surgical or other palliative therapies. Therefore, discussion of these topics will rely on the available literature along with the opinions of experts.

ESOPHAGEAL DILATION

Indications: Chapter 30 reviews the management of benign peptic and caustic strictures. All types of esophageal strictures or other lesions causing dysphagia are reviewed in this chapter.

Dilation can improve dysphagia caused by Schatzki's rings, esophageal webs, peptic and caustic strictures, and postsurgical and postradiation strictures, as well as provide temporary relief of dysphagia caused by malignancies. Forceful dilation can be used to treat achalasia, and simple dilation can sometimes improve dysphagia caused by other types of esophageal dysmotility.[2] Food obstruction caused by esophageal strictures represents one of the most common endoscopic emergencies and can usually be treated with immediate, gentle dilation.[3]

KEY POINTS

ESOPHAGEAL DILATION

- Not all strictures are the same
- The approximate length and diameter of any stricture should be known before attempting dilation
- Fluoroscopy should be employed whenever there is doubt about anatomy beyond the stricture or if the stricture has not been traversed endoscopically
- A guidewire should be used in all but the simplest strictures
- The 'rule of threes' should be followed when dilating malignant or complex esophageal strictures
- Large dilators may safely be used to treat webs and simple inflammatory strictures
- Injecting steroid into inflammatory or anastomotic strictures at the time of dilation may reduce restricturing and delay recurrent dysphagia

The success and durability of any esophageal dilation depends less on the type or size of dilator used than on the etiology and characteristics of the stricture. Simple webs and congenital and peptic rings will often resolve with a single dilation of 16–18 mm.[4] Dysphagia caused by carcinoma or a long caustic stricture may improve after dilation for only a few days, if at all. Dysphagia caused by extrinsic compression, such as malignant mediastinal adenopathy, generally does not respond to dilation.

Preparation: Before undertaking dilation, the physician should know the location, length, and character of the stricture. Contrast radiographs can define the location, size, and length of a stricture. Esophagoscopy additionally provides the ability (with biopsy) to differentiate benign from malignant strictures. Blind passage of dilators should be avoided as the initial means of treatment because of the higher risk of perforation.[5] Fluoroscopic guidance during endoscopy can aid dilation, especially if the stricture does not allow passage of the endoscope.

Procedure: Even mildly suspicious strictures should be biopsied. Collection of pinch biopsies prior to dilation does not appear to increase the risk of perforation or bleeding.[6] For very simple strictures with openings greater than 10 mm and without esophageal angulation or the presence of pseudodiverticuli or shelves, a non-wire-guided Maloney dilator can be used. In most cases, however, it is safer to use a guidewire. If the endoscope can pass through the stricture a guidewire can be left in the stomach as the endoscope is removed. Alternatively, a TTS balloon can be placed across the stricture under direct endoscopic and/or fluoroscopic visualization. If the stricture will not permit passage of an endoscope, a wire or a balloon can still be placed safely if

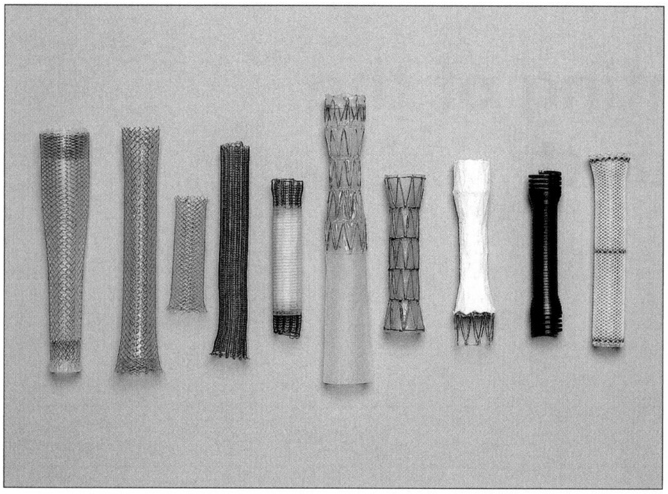

Fig. 146.1 Self-expanding metal stents. From left to right: Flamingo stent, Esophageal Wallstent, Enteral Wallstent, Uncovered Ultraflex, partially covered Ultraflex, Z-stent with Dua antireflux system, covered Z-stent, Z-stent with SIS (small intestinal submucosa) covering (not currently available), EsophaCoil, and Polyflex stent.

the stricture appears to be short and offers no resistance. If the wire or balloon will not pass easily, or if there is any concern about the length or angulation of the stricture or of the anatomy beyond the stricture, fluoroscopy should be used to guide placement.

Dilators can be grouped as blind bougies, wire-guided, tapered bougies, and polyethylene balloons. When choosing bougies (rigid dilators), the initial diameter should be equal to or slightly greater than the estimated diameter of the stricture. Sequentially larger dilators can then be used until resistance is felt. The 'rule of threes' states that once resistance is felt, no more than three additional dilators, at 1-mm-diameter increments, should be used (see Chapter 30).[7] Others have suggested monitoring mucosal damage endoscopically between dilators and stopping when deep mucosal tears first appear.[8] Webs and Schatzki's rings represent an exception, in that these simple strictures can usually be safely dilated with passage of one 16–18-mm dilator. At the other extreme, small increments should be used when dilating stenoses in patients with eosinophilic esophagitis, as they may be at higher risk for perforation due to the brittle nature of the chronically inflamed esophagus.[9]

TTS polyethylene balloons are designed to be inflated with water or radiopaque contrast medium to specified pressure. Inflation to this pressure expands the balloon to a specified diameter. During inflation, the presence of a radiographic 'waist' on fluoroscopy confirms the correct position and its disappearance at full inflation signals a successful dilation. Balloons can be used without fluoroscopy in short, well defined strictures. Constant radial expansion (CRE) balloons expand in a stepwise fashion to multiple diameters (usually three stages at 1- or 1.5-mm increments) depending on the inflation pressure, thus eliminating the need to pass multiple balloons. Newer balloons are also more transparent, enabling visualization of the stricture (and mucosal tears) through the balloon as it expands.

Both rigid dilators and TTS balloons effectively relieve dysphagia caused by peptic strictures in over 85% of patients.[8] Most individuals will experience lasting improvement after one dilation. Others will improve only temporarily, because the fractured stricture constricts during healing. Intralesional injection of steroids, such as triamcinolone (50 mg divided in four quadrants), has been shown to increase the duration of luminal patency and decrease the frequency of subsequent dilations in a subgroup of individuals with tenacious strictures such as those caused by caustic ingestion.[10] The application of cautery to difficult strictures has its advocates, but this has been associated with perforations.[11] With some particularly recalcitrant strictures such as those caused by radiation, surgery, or endoscopic ablative methods, self-dilation can be taught to motivated individuals and provide an effective, low-cost treatment.[12]

Indications/contraindications

Endoscopic esophageal dilation is indicated for almost any symptomatic stricture. The only absolute contraindications are a suspected or recent perforation or ill health that precludes safe endoscopy. Relative contraindications include bleeding disorders, recent myocardial infarction, recent esophageal or abdominal surgery, severe pulmonary disease, severe pharyngeal deformity, history of endocarditis, and large thoracic aortic aneurysm.[8]

INDICATIONS/CONTRAINDICATIONS

- Dilation should be tried as an initial therapy in most gastrointestinal strictures
- Absolute contraindications are suspected or recent perforation and ill health that precludes endoscopy

Costs, complications, and controversies

Dilation alone, either with a TTS balloon or via wire-guided bougienage, offers an inexpensive and effective therapy for dysphagia caused by benign esophageal strictures. Unfortunately, relief from malignant dysphagia tends to be short-lived. Furthermore, dilation carries the risk of tumor fracture, which can cause perforation, bleeding, or fistula formation. The risk of complications associated with dilating malignant strictures may be as high as 10%.[13] In contrast, complications from dilation of benign strictures are quite rare (<1%) and seem to be largely related to attempts at blind dilation with Maloney-type dilators (2%).[5] Balloon dilation has not been convincingly shown to reduce complications.[14] An exception is in patients with epidermolysis bullosa, a condition associated with very fragile esophageal mucosa, which leads to severe stricturing where balloon dilation is preferred.

Esophageal perforations traditionally require urgent surgical treatment. However, some perforations, especially those that occur during palliation of malignant disease, can be treated conservatively if recognized immediately. Placement of a covered expandable mesh stent, combined with nasogastric suction and broad-spectrum antibiotics, can often control the leak before significant soiling of the mediastinum occurs.[15] Immediate closure of the defect can also be accomplished with endoscopically placed clips although this is technically more difficult.[16]

Bleeding following dilation may be difficult to control, especially in patients with coagulopathies or with portal hypertension. Bacteremia following dilation may be as high as 50%.[17] Antibacterial prophylaxis is recommended in cases of prosthetic cardiac valves, recent endoluminal prosthetic grafts or stents, or in patients with significant valvular damage or previous endocarditis.[18]

Balloon dilation may, at times, be faster and more comfortable for the patient than wire-guided bougienage, but it is certainly more expensive. Wire-guided dilators can last for years and require only high-level decontamination between uses. TTS balloons are sold as single-use devices and are difficult to reprocess. In addition, CRE balloons lose their ability to inflate to sequential diameters after one use and cost up to $US300 each.

COSTS, COMPLICATIONS, AND CONTROVERSIES
• Over-the-wire rigid dilators are as safe and effective for esophageal strictures as balloon dilation, but are much less expensive • Perforation is a risk of dilation and increases in the setting of bulky tumors and after radiation therapy • Bleeding and bacteremia can result from esophageal dilation • Teaching self-dilation to some patients can be an effective approach to certain tenacious esophageal strictures

KEY POINTS
SELF-EXPANDING METAL STENTS
• Self-expanding metal stents (SEMSs) have essentially replaced rigid stents in industrialized countries because of easier placement, better tolerance and fewer immediate complications • A variety of stents exist; new stent designs appear frequently; it is imperative to understand the uses and limitations of each major stent design and to choose the appropriate stent for a given stricture • Stents should be placed under fluoroscopic guidance, but can also be placed safely under endoscopic guidance only or under radiographic guidance without endoscopy in certain situations • With SEMSs, aggressive predilation is not usually necessary • Proximal and distal margins of the stricture should be clearly defined and identified with radiopaque markers prior to stent deployment • SEMSs should be deployed slowly and carefully to avoid improper placement • Some stents can be safely manipulated and even removed after deployment; those with exposed barbs cannot • Coated esophageal stents can be used to treat limited esophageal perforations and fistulae in high-risk patients • Stents with antireflux devices should be employed when tumors extend to the gastroesophageal junction

SELF-EXPANDING MESH STENTS (SEMSs)

Introduction

Rigid stents require stricture dilation up to 18 mm before placement. Heavy sedation is frequently necessary and perforation rates have been reported to be 8% or higher.[19] SEMSs have virtually replaced rigid stents. SEMSs can be placed through narrow strictures, often without dilation. Once deployed, constant radial expansion forces open the lumen and, in conjunction with flared ends, hold the stent within the stricture (Fig. 146.2). The exposed wires in SEMSs quickly become incorporated into the esophageal wall and become covered with a layer of reactive collagenous tissue.[20] Ultimately, SEMSs appear to provide increased survival and higher quality of life than rigid stents.[21] SEMS can be divided into coated versus uncoated, nitinol versus surgical steel versus plastic, and two-way patency versus anti-reflux construction.

Insertion

In order to choose the correct stent length, the endoscopist must be familiar with the degree to which the stent will shorten during deployment, which varies widely. The deployed stent should extend about 2 cm above the proximal margin and about 2–3 cm below the distal margin of the tumor in order for the flanges to seat properly and to delay obstruction from tumor growing around the ends of the stent. With partially covered stents, the total covered length should be at least 2 cm longer than the tumor and extend beyond the tumor by a centimeter or more at each end. An exception is if the tumor is in the proximal esophagus, in which case the proximal extent of the stent should not reach within 2 cm of the upper esophageal sphincter. If a tumor extends to the esophagogastric junction, the stent should extend at least 1 cm into the stomach. If the stent extends too far it risks abutting the greater curvature of the stomach. For tumors extending to the esophagogastric junction, or in those individuals in whom tumor invasion has affected the vagus nerve and created free gastroesophageal reflux, an antireflux stent should be seriously considered (Fig. 146.3). Reflux following stent placement can lead to aspiration of gastric contents.[22]

Preparation: Prior to SEMS insertion, the length and margins of the tumor should be clearly identified. This is usually accomplished at endoscopy and may require gentle dilation to allow passage of a gastroscope. In patients with particularly tight strictures or those at high risk for perforation (post chemo/radiotherapy), injection of contrast solution through a cannulation catheter under fluoroscopy can provide some of the same

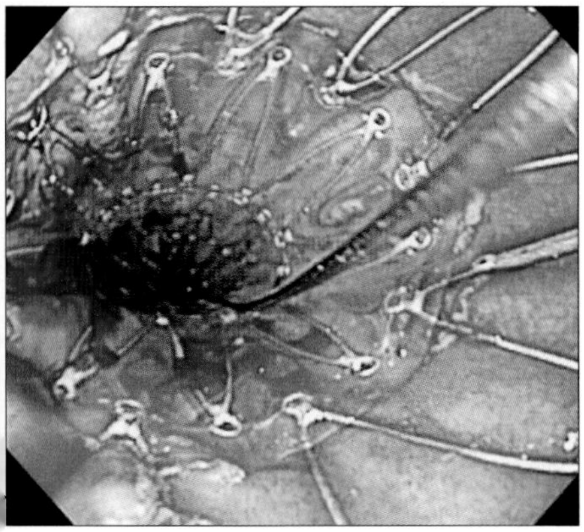

Fig. 146.2 Z-Stent with the Dua antireflux device. Fluoroscopic image of Z-Stent with the Dua antireflux device in position across the esophagogastric junction. Antireflux valve is in the gastric fundus.

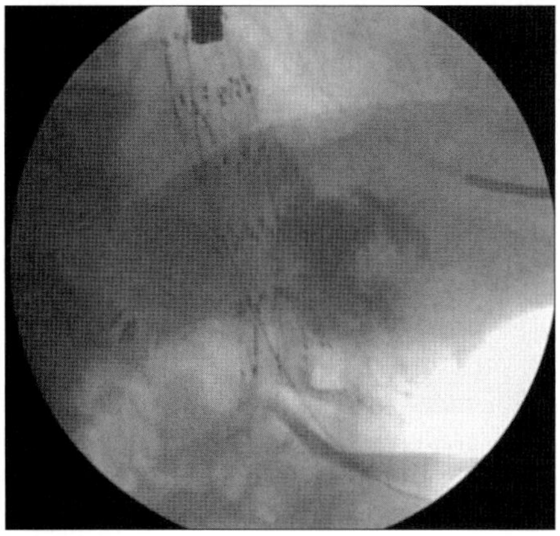

Fig. 146.3 Z-stent. Z-stent just after deployment in the mid-esophagus, before delivery device has been withdrawn.

information. If available, a narrow profile gastroscope (<6 mm) can often pass through tight strictures.

Marking: The proximal and distal extent of the tumor should be marked for fluoroscopy. A submucosal injection of 1–2 ml of contrast medium is common. This will tend to dissipate after several minutes unless an oil-soluble contrast agent is used. External markers such as paperclips can be taped to the patient's chest. Endoscopically placed clips can also be used, although these are expensive and could hinder stent placement. A stiff piano-style guidewire should be placed into the stomach under direct visualization or under fluoroscopy, after which the endoscope is removed.

Placement: While dilation is usually necessary for placement of rigid stents, the tapered delivery systems of SEMS can usually pass through all but the tightest strictures without dilation. Occasionally, gentle dilation up to about 27F may be necessary.

The delivery device should then be passed over the guidewire. Lubrication of the wire with water or silicone may be helpful and lubricating the outside of the stent may allow it to pass through the stricture more easily. Some stents need to be preloaded prior to insertion. The endoscopist should become familiar with loading the stent before beginning the actual procedure.

Deployment of a SEMS is initiated once the stent is confirmed to be in the correct position. Fluoroscopy should follow the entire deployment process, as it only takes an instant for the position to change. Some endoscopists choose to place the endoscope into the proximal esophagus to add an additional view of the deployment. In the absence of available fluoroscopy, endoscopic visualization alone can suffice.[23] Conversely, in many institutions, radiologists place a SEMS without endoscopic guidance. This appears to be safe and is probably equally effective.[24]

Confirming accurate positioning: Once the stent has been deployed, the wire and delivery device can usually be withdrawn. Gentle pressure may be necessary to pull the tip; however, fluoroscopy should be checked to ensure that the stent does not move. Rarely, passage of a balloon dilator into the stent may be necessary to remove the dilator tip. Routine postdeployment balloon dilation is not recommended, as the stent will continue to expand over several hours. Postdeployment endoscopy is useful to ensure that the proximal end of the stent remains above the tumor, but passing the endoscope through the stent immediately after deployment is unwise, as this may displace it. Occasionally, if the stent does not extend far enough proximally, rat's tooth forceps can be used to grasp the proximal edge of the stent and pull it cephalad. If the esophagus remains occluded distally, a second stent should be inserted. A barium swallow should be obtained after 24 h to ensure stent patency and that it has not migrated.

Indications/contraindications

SEMSs are indicated for palliation of dysphagia resulting from unresectable esophageal cancer. Containing acute esophageal perforations and chronic esophageal fistulae in high-surgical-risk patients represents an additional indication (Fig. 146.4A–C). **The main contraindication** for esophageal stent placement is poor performance status with life expectancy of less than 4 weeks. Stent placement in tumors of the upper esophagus may displace or compress the trachea. If this is a possibility, an 18-mm balloon should be inflated within the stricture for

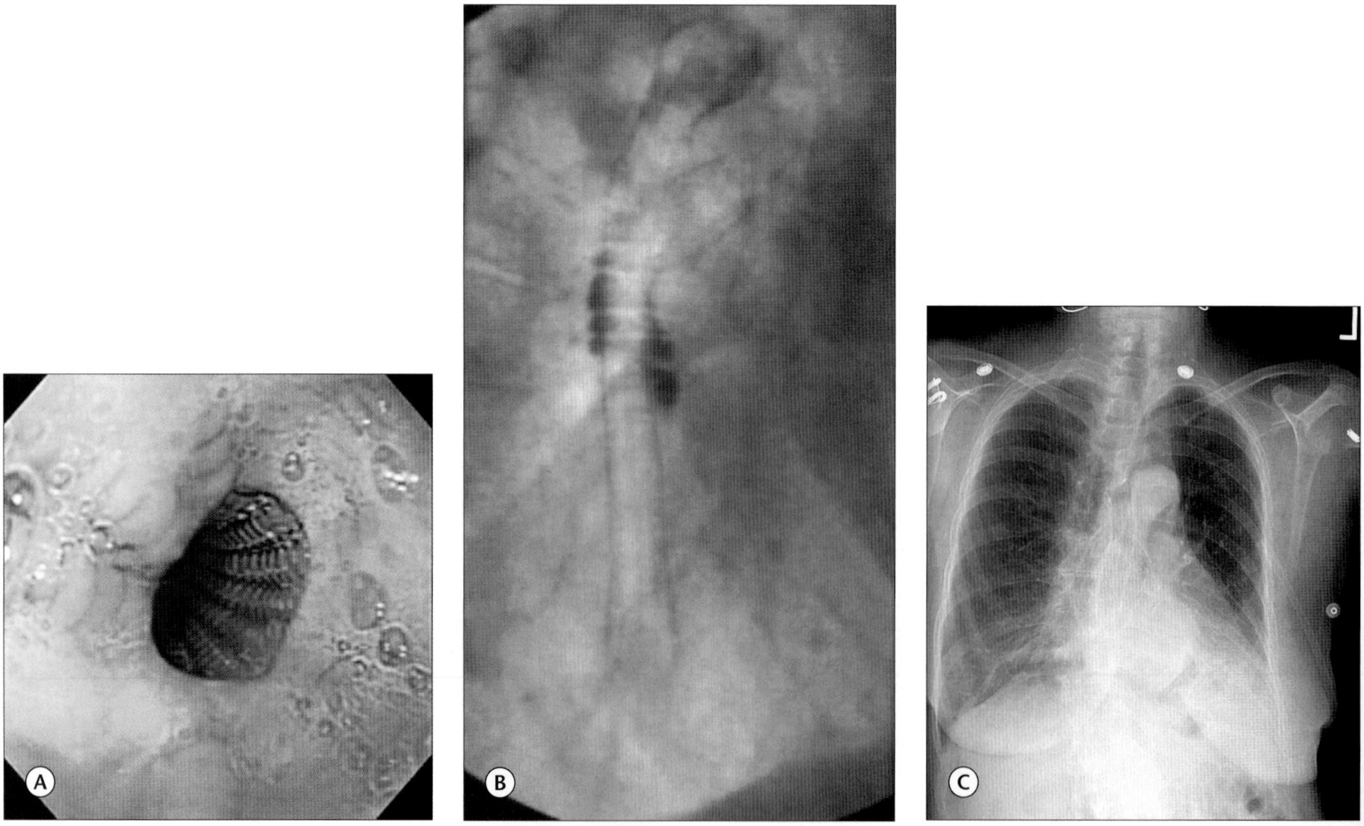

Fig. 146.4 Bilateral bronchial stents. Bronchoesophageal fistula resulting from erosion of a bronchial SEMS in a patient with bilateral bronchial stents for advanced squamous cell cancer. **A.** An Ultraflex esophageal stent was placed to close the fistula. **B.** Fluoroscopic view after stent deployment. Contrast has been injected at the level of the fistula. **C.** Chest X-ray showing one esophageal and two bronchial stents.

several minutes while the patient is monitored for stridor and desaturation. Stents should not be placed in patients undergoing or planning to undergo chemo- or radiotherapy, as tumor shrinkage may lead to stent migration.

Relative contraindications include tumors within 2 cm of the upper esophageal sphincter, uncorrectable coagulopathy, or tumor invasion of the aorta. Previous stent migration is not a contraindication, but does signal a need to try a larger or different type of stent or use a securing device. Endoscopically placed clips can temporarily anchor a stent and give it time to incorporate into the esophageal wall (Fig. 146.5). Placement of SEMSs in benign strictures had been considered a contraindication by many until the advent of the Polyflex® stent, which can be removed up to 4 or more weeks after placement. Covered metal stents can also be removed days or even weeks after placement, although this can be difficult and can cause significant tissue trauma.

INDICATIONS/CONTRAINDICATIONS
• Esophageal stents are appropriate for palliation of malignant dysphagia • Permanent stents should not be used to treat nonmalignant diseases • Stents should not be routinely placed in the proximal esophagus • Stents should not be placed in individuals with life expectancies of less than 4 weeks

Costs, complications, and controversies

Complications remain an unavoidable part of palliating esophageal cancer. Kozarek et al. described the propensity for the development of late problems from SEMS in 1992[25] and numerous other articles since then have documented a broad array of potential complications, including chest pain, stent migration, perforation, obstruction, hemorrhage, epidural abscess, aspiration, and stent fracture.[26–29] Stent placement following chemo- and radiation therapy is associated with an increased risk of complications, probably due to the increased fibrosis and fragility of the post-treatment stricture.[30]

It appears that all available SEMSs effectively control dysphagia and none are free from complications. In general, coated stents delay tumor ingrowth, but are at increased risk of migration. SEMSs with larger flanges and greater radial force tend to migrate less frequently, but may increase the risk of post-deployment pain and eventual erosion. The choice of stent depends in large part on the characteristics of the stricture.

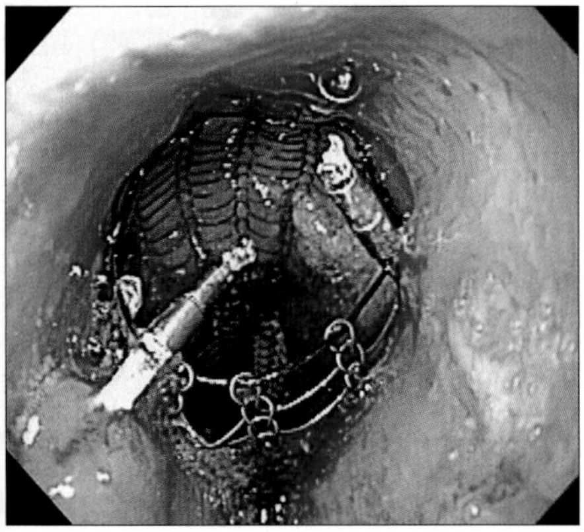

Fig. 146.5 Hemoclips®. Three Hemoclips® have been applied to the proximal edge of the stent to reduce the risk of migration.

Broad strictures resulting from extraluminal compression may be best treated with an uncoated stent. An eccentric mid-esophageal mass may demand a partially covered, widely flaring stent. Tumors that extend across the EG junction are probably best treated with antireflux stents.[22] Covered stents with greater diameters should be used to treat perforations and fistulae. Removable plastic stents may be ideal for this purpose, especially in the setting of benign disease.

Stent occlusion can be treated with heater probe, Nd:YAG laser, argon plasma coagulation, or even photodynamic therapy. Thermal modalities may take several sessions and it is often easier and equally effective to place a second, longer stent within the first. Migrated stents can rarely be manipulated into position if identified immediately; however, most will need to be removed. This is usually accomplished with a snare and an overtube, and several removal techniques have been described.[33,34]

SEMSs cost over ten times the price of rigid prostheses, but the actual stent cost represents a small portion of the expense of caring for patients with esophageal cancer. While rigid plastic stents may be less expensive to purchase than SEMSs, this benefit is often lost beyond 4 weeks because of the need for more frequent interventions with rigid stents.[21] Few studies have compared the cost of treating esophageal cancer with SEMSs with other modalities. A preliminary study by Canto et al. suggested that treatment of malignant dysphagia with SEMS cost about a third of treatment with photodynamic therapy.[35] A trial of thermal ablation versus SEMSs suggested lower cost but reduced quality of life in the SEMS group.[36] A new study suggests that single-dose brachytherapy may be more effective and associated with fewer complications than placement of a SEMS.[37]

COSTS, COMPLICATIONS, AND CONTROVERSIES
• Expandable stents cost substantially more than rigid stents • Costs associated with rigid stents quickly exceed the difference in stent price • In many cases, stenting may be more cost-effective than other modalities for palliating malignant dysphagia • Numerous early and late complications can result from stent placement in the esophagus, ranging from mild to fatal • Refinements in stent design continue to improve performance and reduce complications

DILATION OF STOMACH AND INTESTINES

Introduction

Until about 20 years ago, treating benign strictures of the duodenum and colon fell to the surgeon. With the advent of TTS balloons, any stricture approachable by an endoscope has become at least theoretically treatable by balloon dilation. Newer, CRE balloons have made the dilation process easier as one balloon can be used to dilate over a 3-mm diameter range. Colonic strictures can be dilated with TTS balloons in a manner similar to esophageal or duodenal strictures. Some very distal strictures can be dilated with wire-guided, tapered dilators.

As with esophageal strictures, before the endoscopist attempts to treat a duodenal or colonic stricture its cause should be known. Avoidance of nonsteroidal anti-inflammatory drugs (NSAIDs), control of acid secretion, and, in the case of Crohn's disease, aggressive immunosuppression remain important for control and prevention of certain types of benign strictures. Pyloric or duodenal stenosis may result from peptic ulcer disease, which in turn may have come from NSAID use or *Helicobacter pylori* infection, or from a duodenal or pancreatic neoplasm. In rare cases, a gastric outlet obstruction may result from fibrosis within an annular pancreas. Gaining additional information from biopsies, CT scans, and endoscopic ultrasound may be necessary before attempting to treat a gastric outlet or duodenal stricture. Similarly, while many strictures of the colon may result from inflammatory bowel disease (IBD), ischemia, diverticulitis, or scarred anastamoses, many also develop in the setting of luminal malignancies as well as extrinsic cancers such as ovarian, renal and other metastatic processes.

Technique

The technique of enteral dilation is similar to esophageal dilation. Advancing the balloon through the endoscope can be difficult in a tortuous colon or duodenum. Therefore, using a large-channel endoscope may facilitate balloon passage and withdrawal. Because most strictures are not traversable by the endoscope before dilation, fluoroscopy is often helpful to define the anatomy of the stricture. A waist should be visible during balloon inflation. Resolution of the waist usually indicates successful dilation. Although some experts suggest leaving the balloon inflated for up to 2 min, there is little evidence that this is more effective than inflation for 10–15 s (Fig. 146.6).

KEY POINTS

- Benign enteral strictures must be differentiated from malignant strictures
- Benign strictures can often be dilated while malignant strictures will remain patent only after stenting
- Dilation can be performed anywhere reachable by an endoscope
- Enteral dilation is generally performed with TTS balloons

Indications/contraindications

An attempt at dilation is indicated for most endoscopically approachable benign, fibrotic strictures of the gastric outlet, duodenum, terminal ileum, and colon. Attempts at dilation are not generally recommended for malignant processes, except to allow stenting, and should not be considered in patients with uncontrolled coagulopathy, known perforation, recent surgery, active, untreated inflammatory bowel disease, or inability to tolerate endoscopy.

INDICATIONS/CONTRAINDICATIONS

- Dilation is indicated as primary treatment of nonmalignant, fibrotic strictures of the gastric outlet, duodenum and colon
- Strictures resulting from Crohn's disease, which have failed treatment with anti-inflammatory medications, may be appropriate for endoscopic dilation
- Dilation in the setting of recent surgery, suspected perforation, or uncontrolled coagulopathy is contraindicated

Costs, controversies, and complications

Duodenal webs, anastomotic strictures, and short (<5 cm) Crohn's strictures can usually be safely dilated to 15–20 mm and may result in long-term patency. Pyloric stenoses and longer stenoses resulting from radiation, ischemia and Crohn's disease may be more difficult to treat. These often require multiple sequential dilations over several weeks or months. Reported success and complication rates for treatment of pyloric stenosis vary, but a recent series suggesting a 70% long-term success rate with a 2% complication rate (perforation or bleeding) is probably accurate.[38] Injecting long-acting steroids in four quadrants of the pylorus may improve results. A small series reported that adding two or three radial electrocautery incisions at the pylorus before dilation improves long-term patency in difficult to treat postvagotomy stenoses.[39] Ultimately, balloon dilation for pyloric strictures is unsuccessful in a quarter or more of patients who may require either surgical pyloroplasty or antrectomy and vagotomy.

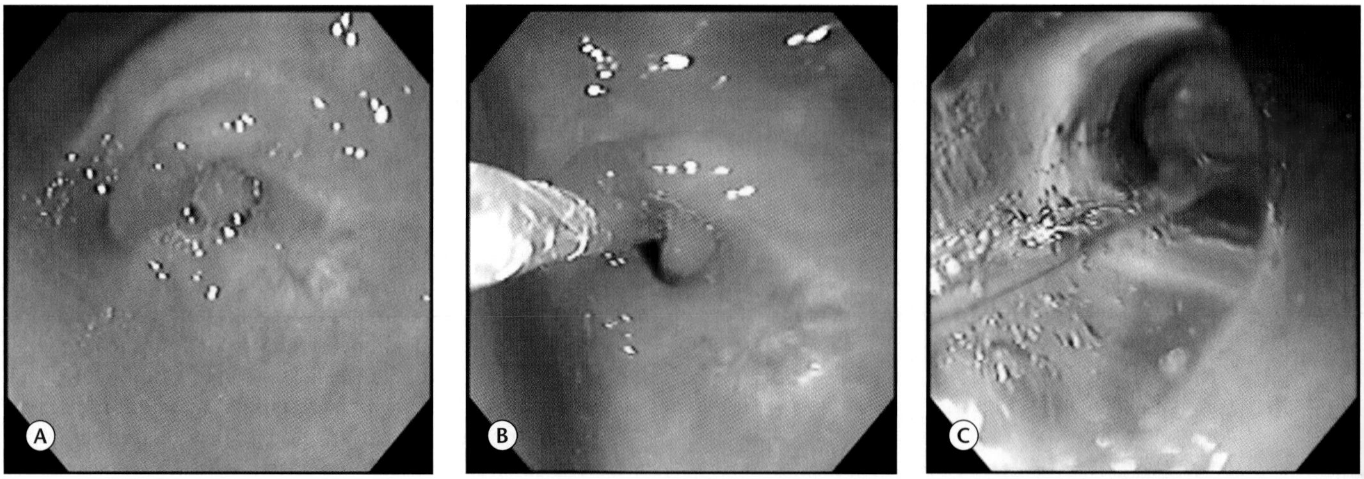

Fig. 146.6 Use of constant radial expansion balloon. A. Pyloric channel stricture resulting from chronic NSAID use. **B.** A CRE balloon in position across the pylorus. **C.** Balloon dilation of the pylorus. Note that the blanching mucosa can be visualized through the balloon.

COSTS, COMPLICATIONS, AND CONTROVERSIES

- Dilation of gastric outlet obstruction is effective in over half of cases and should be tried before surgery
- Bleeding and perforation remain the most serious complications of enteral dilation

ENTERAL STENTING

Gastric and duodenal stenting

Gastric and duodenal stenting differs from esophageal stenting in that delivery devices designed for esophageal stenting are not easily deployable beyond the proximal stomach. Enteral stents are best deployed through an endoscope and, currently, only the enteral Wallstent® (Microvasive, Inc., Natick, MA) is approved for this by the US Food and Drug Administration. This stent is uncoated and available in various lengths and diameters. Its 10F profile allows it to pass through a 3.7-mm working channel. Withdrawing a plastic sleeve while keeping the introducer in a fixed position deploys the stent.

Technique: Prior to deploying an enteral stent, dilation of the stricture is often necessary. Traversing the stricture with an endoscope after dilation is often more difficult than in the esophagus, due to loss of mechanical advantage from the endoscope looping in the stomach. Contrast should be injected into the submucosa at the proximal end of untraversable strictures, and at both margins of others. If the endoscope cannot be passed through the stricture, a biliary catheter can be used to inject contrast beyond the stricture to define its length as well as to pass a stiff, 0.03-inch hydrophilic guidewire well beyond the stricture. The stent is then passed over the wire leaving 2–3 cm of stent on either side of the stricture. Stent position should be confirmed fluoroscopically and endoscopically. The stent is then deployed slowly by pulling back the restraining sheath. Full expansion may take several hours. The stent cannot be re-positioned once it is deployed because manipulation can lead to perforation by exposed barbs. A second stent is sometimes necessary in longer strictures or if the stent shifts during deployment.

Stent deployment is technically successful in 90–95% of cases and will allow resumption of intake of soft food and liquids in the majority of cases. Median survival after enteral stent placement is usually less than 4 months, often due to extensive underlying disease.[40]

Colonic stenting

Traditionally, operating on a colon that has not been prepared requires creation of a diverting colostomy at the time of tumor resection and a second surgery for re-anastomosis several weeks or months later. Endoscopic stenting of a colonic obstruction due to malignancy can decompress the colon and allow for proper colon cleansing in preparation for a one-stage resection of the tumor and primary anastomosis. Stenting can also help improve a patient's nutrition status, correct metabolic problems and allow a more elective surgery. In cases where a patient has widespread disease or is not a surgical candidate, stenting can serve as the primary palliation. In a recent series, colonic stent placement was successful in 66 of 71 (93%) patients with colon cancer, allowing 65 to undergo resection and primary anastomosis soon after.[41]

Techniques: While some esophageal-type stents can be deployed in the rectum and left colon, stents with covered designs and distal tapering are generally inappropriate for colon use. Covered stents tend to migrate in the colon and esophageal stents designed to reduce reflux end up positioned backward when placed in the colon. Greater radial force and wider expansion is often preferable in the colon. In some cases, extensive tumor involvement of the colon may lead to severe angulation and prevent passage of a rigid delivery system or even an endoscope.

Actual deployment of colonic stents is much like deployment of esophageal and duodenal stents. This can be accomplished without fluoroscopy if the stent can be traversed by the endoscope, but should in most cases be performed with fluoroscopic guidance to minimize the chance of mal-deployment. The amount of air used for insufflation should be limited as air may accumulate proximal to the stricture and further distend an already dilated colon, leading to perforation. As in the upper gastrointestinal tract, stent deployment should be slow and controlled, with stent overlapping the stricture by 2–3 cm at both ends. If there is not an immediate rush of fluid and stool after full deployment, or if the stent does not fully expand at either end, a second, overlapping stent may be necessary (Fig. 146.7).

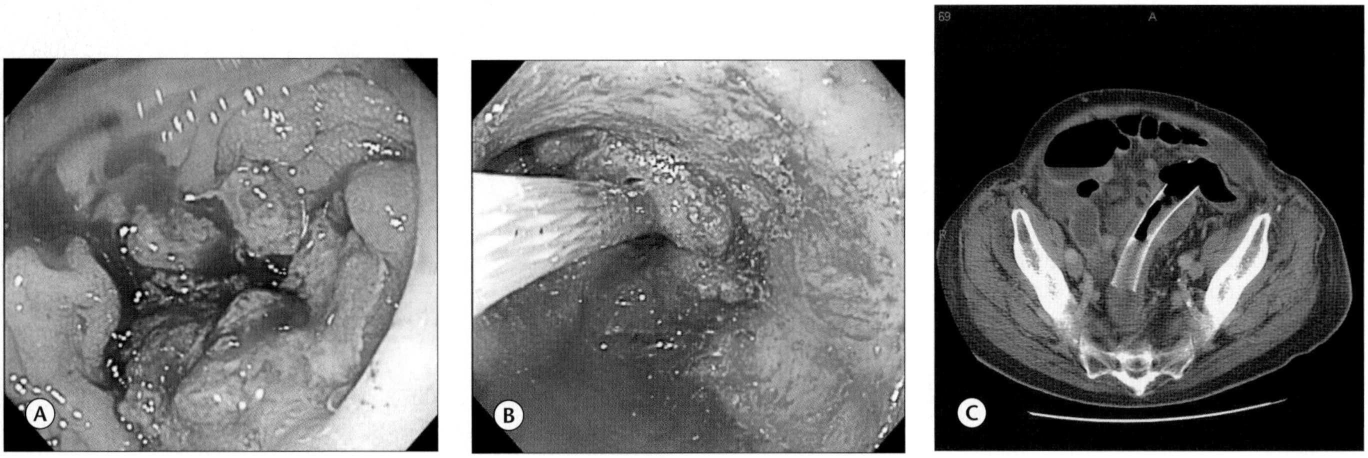

Fig. 146.7 Use of colonic stent. A. Obstructing mass at the rectosigmoid junction. **B.** Undeployed colonic stent in position across a malignant obstruction at the rectosigmoid junction. **C.** CT scan confirms position and patency.

KEY POINTS

- Stents can be deployed anywhere reachable by an endoscope
- Stenting can palliate intrinsic and extrinsic obstructions of the stomach, duodenum, and colon
- Colonic stents can facilitate one-step definitive surgery by allowing bowel cleansing

Indications/contraindications

Enteral stent placement is indicated for malignant gastric outlet obstruction in nonsurgical patients and can be offered as an option to patients who are capable of tolerating surgical bypass. Stents are indicated for relieving colonic obstruction due to malignancy as a bridge-to-surgery in surgical candidates and as primary palliation in those who are not candidates.

Contraindications to enteral stent placement include active perforation with peritonitis, uncorrectable coagulopathy, and multiple malignant stenoses. Functional class IV patients in whom stent placement is unlikely to produce significant benefit or in whom life expectancy is less than 2 weeks represent a group who should not undergo enteral stenting. In cases of concurrent biliary obstruction, biliary tree decompression should take place before stenting the duodenum. Enteral mesh stents provide at least the theoretical possibility of accessing the bile duct after placement.

Relative contraindications include tumor extending to within 1 cm of the anal verge, as these patients often experience tenesmus, pain, and incontinence. Individuals with friable, bleeding rectal cancers may be better treated with thermal ablative methods or local irradiation. As a rule, benign strictures should not be permanently stented; however, temporary placement of a covered stent or a Polyflex® stent may be useful for difficult strictures, as long as the stent is removed within 2–3 weeks.

INDICATIONS AND CONTRAINDICATIONS

- Enteral stents should be considered for malignant obstructions of the pylorus, duodenum, or colon in patients not willing or able to undergo surgical bypass
- Permanent stents should not be used to treat nonmalignant diseases
- Stents should not be placed in patients with carcinomatosis or multiple strictures where relief of obstruction is unlikely
- Stents should not be placed in the distal rectum

Costs, controversies, and complications

Reported complications of enteral and colonic stents are similar. Stent occlusion, bleeding, migration, and perforation have been reported in both locations. Total complication rates range from 9% to 30% with perforations occurring in 4% of colonic and 3% of duodenal stent placements.[40,42] Perforations can be particularly disastrous during enteral and colonic stent placement, especially if detection is delayed, because of patients' already weakened conditions and limited surgical options. Dilation prior to stent placement appears to increase the risk of perforation, at least in the colon (10% vs 2%).[42] Regular use of coated stents may increase stent migration, which has been reported in over a quarter of cases in which covered stents were used to treat malignant gastric outlet obstruction[43] (Fig. 146.8).

Although purchase prices vary, enteral stents cost about as much as esophageal stents ($US 1000–2000). This can be misleading, however, since a third of enteral strictures will require placement of two or more stents.[44] Debate exists regarding the benefits of enteral stenting versus surgery. Studies comparing cost and efficacy of endoscopic thermal therapies versus stenting for colon and rectal cancers have not been published.

COSTS, COMPLICATIONS, AND CONTROVERSIES

- In many cases, stenting may be more cost-effective than other modalities for palliating malignant bowel obstruction
- Stent occlusion and migration continue to be problems
- Stent erosion and perforation are uncommon but potentially fatal complications
- Studies comparing enteral stents to surgery or other endoscopic ablations are lacking

CONCLUSIONS

When performed carefully, esophageal and enteral dilation and stenting can be safe and effective and provide significant symptom relief in a relatively noninvasive manner. An increasing number of endoscopists employ expandable metal stents for treatment of malignant dysphagia and other gastrointestinal obstructions caused by cancer. Improvements in dilators and SEMSs have made treatment of benign and malignant

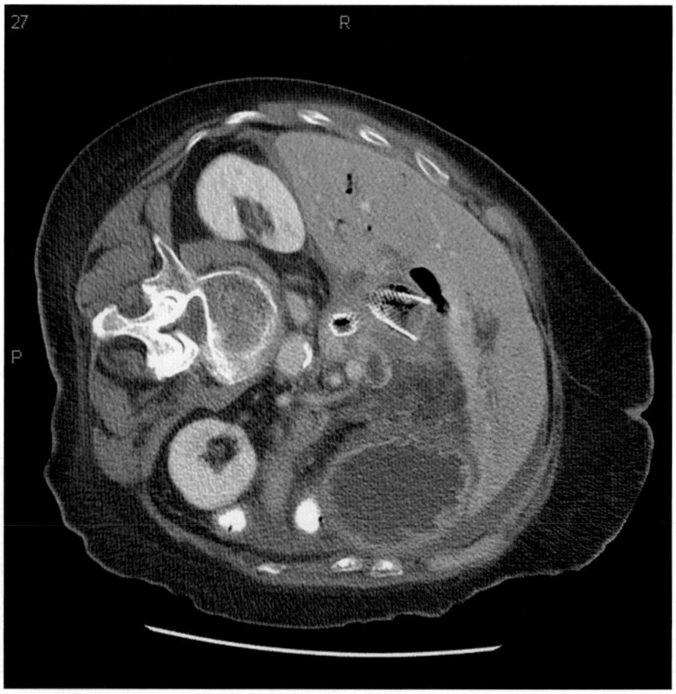

Fig. 146.8 Enteral Wallstent. Periduodenal air adjacent to an Enteral Wallstent, which caused the perforation. Courtesy of Richard Kozarek.

strictures below the esophagus not only possible but also relatively simple and highly successful. Complications do exist and should be carefully weighed against anticipated benefits, just as stent placement itself should be weighed against other options. Newer innovations in dilator and stent designs will probably reduce complications and improve outcomes. Prospective randomized studies comparing enteral stenting with surgery as well as other endoscopic therapies are greatly needed.

SOURCES OF INFORMATION FOR PATIENTS AND DOCTOR

http://www.rcr.ac.uk/crplg6.doc
http://www.healthsystem.virginia.edu/internet/radiology/angio/angio-pted-stents.cfm

REFERENCES

1. Aste H, Munizzi F, Saccomanno S, Pugliese V. "Splitting" and stretching dilation of esophageal strictures. Endoscopy 1983; 5:41.
2. Marshall JB, Chowdhury TA. Does empiric esophageal dilation benefit dysphagia when endoscopy is normal? Dig Dis Sci 1996; 41:1099–1101.
3. Vicari J, Johanson JF, Frakes JT. Outcomes of acute esophageal food impaction: Success of the push technique. Gastrointest Endosc 2001; 53:178–181
4. Harrison ME, Sanowski RA. Mercury dilation of benign strictures. Hepatogastroenterology 1992; 39:497.
5. Hernandez LJ, Jacobson JW, Harris MS. Comparison among the perforation rates of Maloney, balloon, and Savary dilation of esophageal strictures. Gastrointest Endosc 2000; 51:460–462.
6. Barkin JS, Taub S, Rogers AI. The safety of combined endoscopy, biopsy, and dilation in esophageal strictures. Am J Gastroenterol 1981; 76:23–26.
7. Tulman AB, Boyce HW. Complications of esophageal dilation and guidelines for their prevention. Gastrointest Endosc 1981; 27:229–234.
8. Anonymous. Esophageal dilation. Gastrointest Endosc 1998; 48:702–704.
9. Croese J, Fairley SK, Masson JW et al. Clinical and endoscopic features of eosinophilic esophagitis in adults. Gastrointest Endosc 2003; 58:516–522.
10. Kochhar R, Ray JD, Sriram PV, Kumar S, Singh K. Intralesional steroids augment the effects of endoscopic dilation in corrosive esophageal strictures. Gastrointest Endosc 1999; 49:509–513.
11. Disario J, Pedersen P, Bichis-Canoutas C et al. Incision of recurrent distal esophageal (Schatzki) ring after dilation. Gastrointest Endosc 2002; 56:244–248.
12. Grobe JL, Kozarek RA, Sanowski RA. Self-bougienage in the treatment of benign esophageal stricture. J Clin Gastroenterol 1984; 6:109–112.
13. Van Dam J, Rice TW, Catalano MF et al. High-grade malignant stricture is predictive of esophageal tumor stage. Cancer 1993; 71:2910–2917.
14. Reed CE. Pitfalls and complications of esophageal prosthesis, laser therapy, and dilation. Chest Surg Clin N Am 1997; 7:623–637.
15. Siersema PD, Homs M, Haringsma J et al. Use of large-diameter metallic stents to seal traumatic nonmalignant perforations of the esophagus. Gastrointest Endosc 2003; 58:356–361.
16. Abe N, Sugiyama M, Hashimoto Y et al. Endoscopic nasomediastinal drainage followed by clip application for treatment of delayed esophageal perforation with mediastinitis. Gastroint Endosc 2001; 54:646–648.
17. Schembre D. Infectious complications associated with gastrointestinal endoscopy. Gastrointest Endosc Clin N Am 2000; 10:215–232.
18. Hirota WK, Petersen K, Baron TH et al. Guidelines for antibiotic prophylaxis for GI endoscopy. Gastrointest Endosc 2003; 58:475–482.
19. Tytgat GJN, Tytgat S. Esophageal endoprostheses in malignant strictures. J Gastroenterol 1994; 29 (Suppl VII):80–84.
20. Bethge N, Somer A, Grosss U, von Kleist D, Vakil N. Human tissue reponses to metal stents implanted in vivo for the palliation of malignant stenoses. Gastrointest Endosc 1996; 43:596–602.
21. O'Donnell CA, Fullarton GM, Watt E et al. Randomized clinical trial comparing self-expanding metallic stents with plastic endoprostheses in the palliation of oesophageal cancer. Br J Surg 2002; 89:985–992.
22. Dua KS, Kozarek R, Kim J et al. Self expanding metal esophageal stent with anti-reflux mechanism. Gastrointest Endosc 2001; 53:603–613.
23. Austin AS, Khan Z, Cole AT, Freeman JG. Placement of esophageal self-expanding metallic stents without fluoroscopy. Gastrointest Endosc 2001; 54:357–359.
24. Laasch HU, Martin DF, Do YS et al. Interventional radiology for the management of inoperable carcinoma of the oesophagus. Endoscopy 2003; 35:1060–1068.
25. Kozarek RA, Ball TJ, Patterson DJ. Metallic self-expanding stent applications in the upper gastrointestinal tract: caveats and concerns. Gastrointest Endosc 1992; 38:1–6.
26. Dirks K, Schulz T, Schellmann B et al. Fatal hemorrhage following perforation of the aorta by a barb of the Gianturco-Rosch esophageal stent. Z Gastroenterol 2002; 40:81–84.
27. Mersol J, Kozarek R. Spine complications of stent placement. Gastrointest Endosc 2002; 55:241.
28. Binkert C, Petersen B. Two fatal complications after parallel tracheal-esophageal stenting. Cardiovasc Intervent Radiol 2002; 25:144–147.
29. Baron TH: A practical guide for choosing an expandable metal stent for GI malignancies: Is a stent by any other name still a stent? Gastrointest Endosc 2001; 54:269–271.
30. Kinsman KJ, DeGregorio BT, Katon RM et al. Prior radiation and chemotherapy increase the risk of life-threatening complications after insertion of metallic stents for esophagogastric malignancy. Gastrointest Endosc 1996; 43:196–203.
31. Siersema PD, Hop WCJ, van Blankenstein M et al. A comparison of 3 types of covered metal stents for the palliation of patients with dysphagia caused by esophagogastric carcinoma: a prospective, randomized study. Gastrointest Endosc 2001; 54:145–153.
32. Wang MQ, Sze DY, Wand ZP et al. Delayed complications after esophageal stent placement for treatment of malignant esophageal obstructions and esophagorespiratory fistulas. J Vasc Intervent Radiol 2001; 21:465–474.
33. Farkas PS, Farkas JD, Koenigs KP. An easier method to remove migrated esophageal Z-stents. Gastrointest Endosc 1999; 50:277–279.
34. Low DE, Kozarek R. Removal of esophageal expandable metal stents: description of technique and review of potential applications. Surg Endosc 2003; 17:990–996.
35. Canto MI, Smith C, McClelland L et al. Randomized trial of PDT vs. stent for palliation of malignant dysphagia: cost-effectiveness and quality of life. Gastrointest Endosc 2002; 55:AB100.
36. Dallal HJ, Smith GD, Grieve DC et al. A randomized trial of thermal ablative therapy versus expandable metal stents in the palliative treatment of patients with esophageal carcinoma. Gastrointest Endosc 2001; 54:549–557.
37. Homs M, Steyeberg EW, Eijkenboom W et al. Single dose brachytherapy versus metal stent placement for the palliation of obstructive oesophageal cancer: a randomized trial. Lancet 2004; 364:1497–504.
38. Solt V, Bayer J, Szabo ÖM, Horvath G. Long-term results of balloon catheter dilation for benign gastric outlet stenosis. Endoscopy 2003; 35:490–495.
39. Hagiwara A, Sonoyama Y, Togawa T et al. Combined use of electrosurgical incisions and balloon dilation for the treatment of refractory postoperative pyloric stenosis. Gastrointest Endosc 2001; 53:504–508.
40. Nassif T, Prat B, Meduri J et al. Endoscopic palliation of malignant gastric outlet obstruction using self-expandable stents: results of a multicenter study. Endoscopy 2003; 36:483–489.
41. Mainar A, De Gregorio A, Tejero E et al. Acute colorectal obstruction: treatment with self-expandable metallic stents before scheduled surgery – results of a multicenter study. Radiology 1999; 210:65–69.
42. Khot UP, Lang AW, Murali K, Parker MC. Systematic review of the efficacy and safety of colorectal stents. Br J Surg 2002; 89:1096–1102.
43. Jung GS, Song HY, Kang SG et al. Malignant gastroduodenal obstructions: treatment by means of a covered expandable metallic stent – initial experience. Radiology 2000; 216:758–763.
44 Mosler P, Mergener KD, Brandabur J et al. Palliation of gastric outlet obstruction and proximal small bowel obstruction with self-expandable metal stents – a single center series. Gastrointest Endosc (in press).
43. Yim HB, Jacobson BC, Saltzman JR et al. Clinical outcome of the use of enteral stents for palliation of patients with malignant upper GI obstruction. Gastrointest Endosc 2001; 53:329–332.
44. Saida Y, Sumiyama Y, Nagao J, Uramatsu M. Long-term prognosis of preoperative "bridge to surgery" expandable metallic stent insertion for obstructive colorectal cancer: comparison with emergency operation. Dis Colon Rectum 2003; 46:S44–49.

Chapter 147

The transjugular intrahepatic portosystemic shunt (TIPS)

Martin Rössle

INTRODUCTION AND SCIENTIFIC BASIS

The transjugular intrahepatic portosystemic shunt (TIPS) is a communication between a central hepatic vein and an intrahepatic branch of the portal vein. Its hemodynamic characteristics are comparable to that of the surgical small-caliber portocaval side-to-side shunt. In contrast to end-to-side shunts in which the portal blood flow is completely and definitely deviated, side-to-side shunts may result in absent, prograde, or retrograde portal perfusion of the liver depending on the diameter of the shunt. In patients with markedly reduced liver function, a smaller shunt diameter providing some residual portal perfusion may be chosen to prevent decompensation. In general, a cautious approach with smaller shunts, e.g., 8–10 mm in diameter, is recommended because later enlargement of the TIPS is certainly easier than its reduction.

The data and interpretations given in this review are almost exclusively based on studies using bare stents. The recently marketed PTFE-covered stent (Viatorr) may reduce most of the technical complications and improve clinical outcome variables including mortality.[1] Additional technical and randomized clinical studies are, however, required.

TECHNIQUE

The key points of the technique and the materials used in our institution are summarized in the box and in Fig. 147.1. The most difficult step is the puncture of the portal vein, which can be facilitated by three-dimensional sonography. This is of particular importance in patients (about 10%) where the puncture has to be directed backward and not to the ventral plane as usual. The puncture of the portal vein must be at least 2 cm away from the bifurcation since it is located extrahepatically in 47% of patients.[2] After successful access to the portal system an angiography should be performed from the splenic hilum to opacify all varices. If large varices are seen, they may be occluded by bucrylate or ethanol injection or coils. This may be indicated when bleeding occurs at low pressure gradients, e.g., <15 mmHg. The TIPS procedure is continued by dilatation of the tissue tract and implantation of a stent.

Self-expandable nitinol-stents have now gained priority. Their physical characteristics are improved to provide sufficient radial force combined with high flexibility and little axial recoil. In most patients, a stent with an inner diameter of 10 mm will be selected and dilated to 8–10 mm to reach a sufficient pressure reduction to 10–12 mmHg or 50% of the baseline pressure gradient. The need for a greater shunt (e.g., 10 mm) is likely in patients with a large portal vein diameter (>1.6 cm). In patients with an increased risk of shunt-induced complications (age >60 years, previous episodes of hepatic encephalopathy, bilirubin concentration of >3 mg/dL) a smaller shunt and lower pressure reduction may be preferred. A final pressure measurement and angiography is then performed to document shunt patency, absence of variceal flow, and the intrahepatic portal flow pattern.

The TIPS cannot be performed in patients with cavernoma of the portal vein. Patients with cardiac insufficiency with an ejection fraction of <30% or with insufficient perfusion of the hepatic artery should be excluded because of the lack of adequate hepatic perfusion after a TIPS.

KEY POINTS

- Ultrasonographic marcation of portal bifurcation (transverse plane). Sedoanalgesia (50 mg pethidine, 2–5 mg midazolam), monitoring of oxygen saturation and ECG. Puncture of right internal jugular vein, if occluded use right external or left internal jugular vein
- Introduce/advance J-wire (0.035 i, 150 cm) into inferior caval vein (IVC). Introduce sheath (11 F, 12 cm, St. Jude Medical)
- Introduce/advance transjugular guiding catheter (9 F, 45 cm, Cook) into IVC inferior to hepatic veins. Introduce TIPS puncture needle (1.8-mm diameter, 60 degrees, Optimed, Bard-Angiomed, or Cook) and advance under fluoroscopic control until close to end of guiding catheter
- Remove needle/catheter assembly (tip shows to the right) slowly until change of resistance indicates entrance to hepatic vein. Advance J-wire into hepatic vein and follow with needle/catheter assembly
- Inject contrast through needle to verify hepatic vein. Release needle completely. Start with puncture close to IVC by turning the needle counterclockwise (approx. 60–90 degrees)
- Puncture towards the skin marker. Inject small amounts of diluted contrast to verify intrahepatic position. Use three-dimensional ultrasound guidance routinely. Stay away from bifurcation! If blood can be aspirated and the portal vein verified by contrast insert guidewire through needle (Terumo stiff, bend tip, 180 cm, or Kayac stiff 180 cm, 0.035 i, Boston Scientific)
- Push guiding catheter over the needle into stem of portal vein. Remove needle and insert angiographic catheter (pigtail 5 F, 70 cm, 0.035 i) through the guiding catheter. Perform angiography (25 degrees right oblique position of tube) from splenic hilum and pressure measurement
- Insert stiff guidewire (Amplatz super stiff 0.035, 180 cm, Boston Scientific/Medi-tech). Remove catheters, insert 8–10-mm balloon catheter (PTA catheter 7 F, 8–10/40 mm, 75 cm, 0.035 i), and dilate parenchymal tract. Add additional analgesia (e.g., disoprivan) before
- Introduce, release, and dilate the appropriate stent (e.g., Luminexx, Baard-Angiomed; Sinus-Superflex, Optimed; Smart, Cordis; or Viatorr, Gore). Perform final angiography and pressure measurements

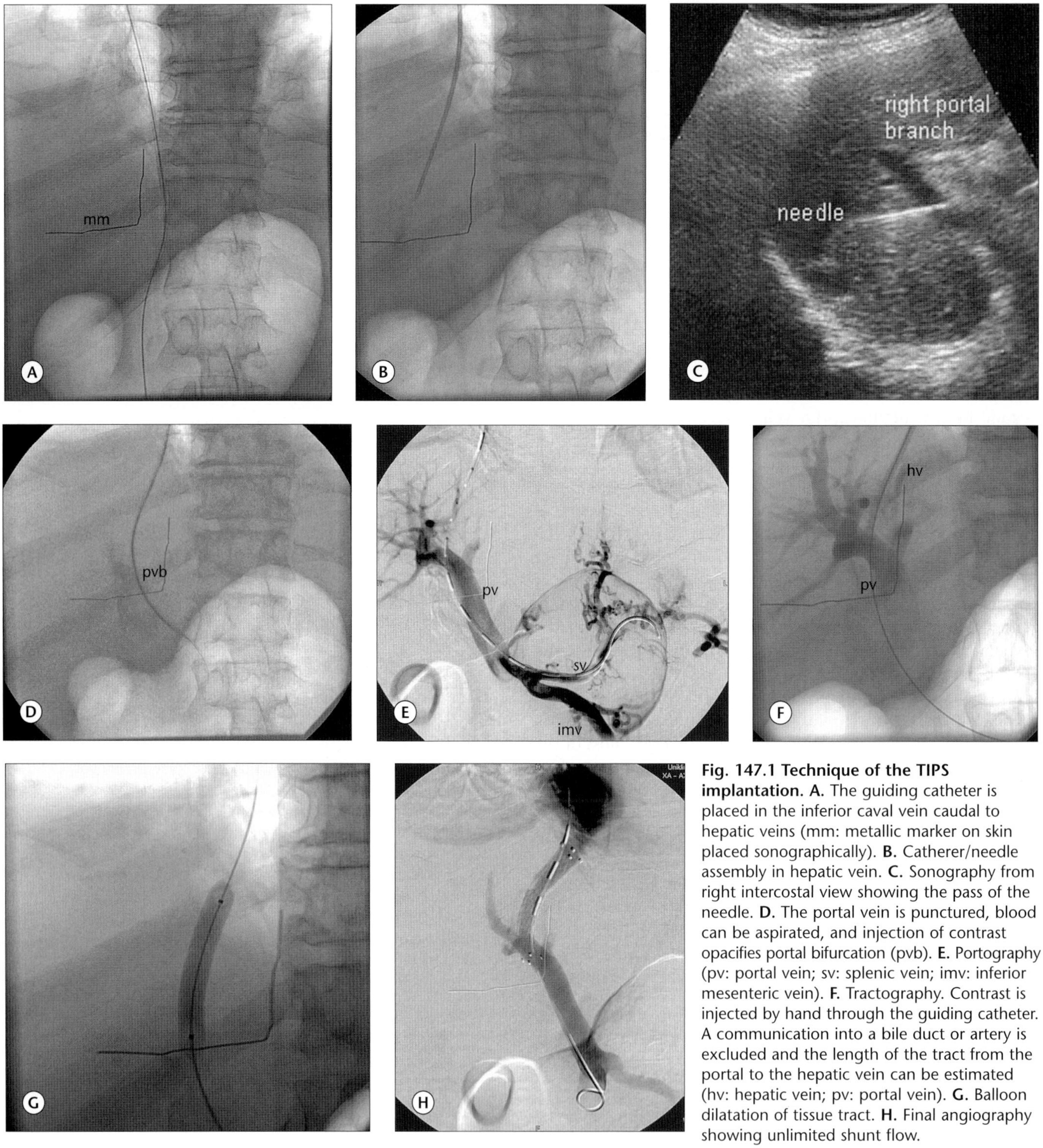

Fig. 147.1 Technique of the TIPS implantation. A. The guiding catheter is placed in the inferior caval vein caudal to hepatic veins (mm: metallic marker on skin placed sonographically). **B.** Catherer/needle assembly in hepatic vein. **C.** Sonography from right intercostal view showing the pass of the needle. **D.** The portal vein is punctured, blood can be aspirated, and injection of contrast opacifies portal bifurcation (pvb). **E.** Portography (pv: portal vein; sv: splenic vein; imv: inferior mesenteric vein). **F.** Tractography. Contrast is injected by hand through the guiding catheter. A communication into a bile duct or artery is excluded and the length of the tract from the portal to the hepatic vein can be estimated (hv: hepatic vein; pv: portal vein). **G.** Balloon dilatation of tissue tract. **H.** Final angiography showing unlimited shunt flow.

Follow-up, shunt insufficiency

Duplex-sonography at 3- to 6-month intervals detects shunt insufficiency with a high sensitivity of 82%. The measurement of the flow velocity in the extrahepatic portal vein may be the most reliable single parameter to detect shunt dysfunction. Its decrease by more than 50% of the gain achieved by the TIPS or a decrease to <28 cm/s indicates significant malfunction and need for revision. Shunt angiography with measurement of the portal-venous pressure gradient is the gold standard. It is indicated when the duplex-sonography is not diagnostic or when the shunt did not lead to a clear improvement or recurrence of the clinical index symptom.

Shunt insufficiency may occur early (within 30 days) or late during follow-up. Early, thrombotic shunt occlusion was found in 0–15%. Studies using prophylactic heparin had a lower incidence of shunt occlusion (0–3%) compared with studies not using peri-interventional anticoagulation (10–15%).[3] Late shunt insufficiency seen in 31–80% (cumulative 1-year probability) is due to intimal proliferation within the stent or in the hepatic vein. It may be caused by a communication between a bile duct with the shunt or by shear stress produced by the high flow in the draining hepatic vein or the axial recoil of the stent. Redilatation, restenting, parallel stenting, and/or local thrombolytic treatment of occluded shunts result in a 2-year secondary patency rate of 80–90%. Shunt insufficiency does not necessarily indicate the need for shunt revision. Since the shunt is a symptomatic treatment it should be reestablished only when symptoms do not improve or recur. Therefore, in patients with variceal bleeding, endoscopic evaluation is required to decide whether radiological intervention is indicated or not.

INDICATIONS/CONTRAINDICATIONS

The indications and contraindications for the TIPS are given in Table 147.1. Only the major indications, variceal bleeding and refractory ascites, are discussed below. The other indications are briefly commented on in Table 147.1.

Variceal bleeding

Acute variceal bleeding

The TIPS has become accepted as a rescue if standard treatment of acute variceal bleeding fails. Thus, a recent assessment of the management of acute variceal bleeding in the USA found that 6.6% of patients with first variceal bleeding and 15.2% with recurrent bleeding received a TIPS.[4] In comparison, only 0.7% and 3.3% of patients received a surgical shunt. The use of a TIPS as a rescue treatment is based upon the results of 11 studies including 383 patients.[3] They demonstrate that the emergency TIPS stopped the refractory, active bleeding in over 90% of cases. The early rebleeding rate was 16–30% and the early mortality rate 17–55%. Similar results were obtained for ectopic variceal bleeding with a hemostasis rate of 90% together with a very low hospital rebleeding rate and mortality of 14% and 25%, respectively. Additional embolization, which was not performed in most of the studies, may improve the early rebleeding rate.

TABLE 147.1 TIPS INDICATIONS AND CONTRAINDICATIONS

Indication	Comment and contraindications	Evidence, no. of studies & patients
BLEEDINGS		
Acute variceal bleeding	TIPS rescue (significant rebleeding within 48 h); disregard patients ventilated, comatose, infected, and in multiorgan failure	II, 11 studies, 383 pts
Prevention of recurrent variceal bleeding	Similar mortality between TIPS and endoscopy; TIPS is second-line treatment (consensus) after failure of medical therapy (2 or more rebleedings); disregard patients with bilirubin >3 mg/dL, overt encephalopathy, or MELD >1.8	I, 2 meta-analyses, 14 RCTs, 966 pts,
Gastric varices	TIPS useful, no consensus on timing; hemostasis rate 90%, early rebleeding 14–25%; embolization of varices during TIPS procedure is recommended	II, 4 studies, 97 pts
Ectopic varices	Good rationale but limited experience (case reports). Transjugular embolization of 'distant' varices may be recommended	III
Hypertensive gastropathy (PHG)	Positive results with 89–100% response in severe PHG, no effect on GAVE	II
Gastric antral vasc. ectasia (GAVE)		4 studies, 144 pts
Stomal/conduit bleeding, vascular colopathy	Good results but limited experience (case reports)	III
ASCITES AND RELATED COMPLICATIONS		
Refractory ascites	Good response to TIPS, survival advantage possible; avoid patients with bilirubin >3 mg/dL or MELD >1.8	I, 16 studies, 5 RCTs 531 pts
–hydrothorax	Response in 75%, survival similar to refractory ascites	II, 2 studies, 61 pts
–hepatorenal syndrome (HRS)	Good response in type 2, exceptional treatment for type 1 HRS; TIPS is recommended as a bridge to transplantation	II, 2 studies, 59 pts
–spontaneous bacterial peritonitis	Diminished after TIPS	II, 1 RCT
OTHER INDICATIONS		
Budd-Chiari syndrome (BCS)	Good results in acute and fulminant disease with rapid recovery of hepatic and renal function.	II, 36 studies/case reports, 117 pts
Fresh portal vein thrombosis	Potential of complete resolution in noncavernoma; right intrahepatic portal branch should be patent (puncture site)	III
Hypersplenism	Only minor effect on platelet count; improves pain if present	III
To facilitate major abdominal surgery	Three positive reports on the experience of surgeons	III 3 reports, 9 pts
Before liver transplantation	No benefit, no harm; use of covered stent avoids problems with stent protrusion into inferior caval vein	II

For further information see Rossle M. TIPS: an update. Best Pract Res Clin Gastroenterol 2004; 18:99–123 and Russo et al. Transjuglular intrahepatic portosystemic shunt for refactory ascites: an analysis of the literature on efficacy, morbidity, and mortality. Am J Gastroenterol 2003; 98:2521–2527.
Rating of quality of evidence: I: Evidence from multiple well-designed randomized controlled trials each involving a number of participants to be of sufficient statistical power. II: Evidence from at least one large well-designed clinical trial with or without randomization, from cohort or case–control analytic studies, or well-designed meta-analysis. III: Evidence based on clinical experience, descriptive studies, or reports of expert committees.
Abbreviations: RCT, randomized controlled trial; pts, patients; MELD, model for end-stage liver disease.

Once the general decision to use a rescue TIPS has been made, the patient should then be assessed for suitability to avoid futile interventions. It could be demonstrated that patients who are ventilated after aspiration and require more than 50% oxygen, inotropic support, have renal dysfunction, and features of sepsis should not be accepted for the TIPS treatment since they may have a hospital mortality (after a TIPS) approaching 100%.[3]

Prevention of rebleeding

The 1-year estimated rebleeding rate of about 40% demonstrates that drugs or ligation have a limited efficacy indicating the need for a more effective treatment. A meta-analysis of the results of 13 randomized studies on TIPS versus endoscopic treatment with or without additional drug treatment[5] shows that TIPS had a lower rebleeding rate (19% versus 47%, odds ratio, OR: 3.8; 95% confidence interval, CI: 2.5–5.2; $p < 0.001$), a higher incidence of hepatic encephalopathy (34% versus 19%, OR: 0.43; 95% CI: 0.30–0.60; $p < 0.001$), and similar mortality (OR: 0.97; 95% CI: 0.71–1.34). TIPS was not regarded as a first-line treatment since the higher rate of encephalopathy after a TIPS was considered to be a greater disadvantage than the higher rate of rebleeding after endoscopic treatment.

Timing: The accepted use of a TIPS as a second-line treatment leads to the question when should standard treatment be stopped and a TIPS offered? Most centers demand two clinically significant rebleedings before switching from standard treatment to a TIPS. Such an arrangement requires the TIPS in 20% of patients treated endoscopically. In these elective candidates, the risk factors for a poor outcome after a TIPS need strict consideration. It was demonstrated that a bilirubin concentration of >3 mg/dL was closely correlated with mortality (relative risk, RR: 5.4; 95% CI: 1.4–10.2). This was confirmed by the finding that an elevated pre-TIPS bilirubin level is a powerful independent predictor of 30-day mortality after TIPS creation, with a 40% increased risk of death for each 1 mg/dL increase above 3.0 mg/dL.[3]

Recently, using data from 231 patients receiving TIPS for variceal bleeding or refractory ascites, a mathematical model for end-stage liver disease (MELD) including serum creatinine, bilirubin, and international normalized ratio (INR) has been developed and validated. It predicts 3-month mortality after a TIPS with a positive predictive value of 80–90%, which is superior to the Child-Pugh score (70%). However, its superiority for predicting long-term mortality is questionable.

Refractory ascites and related complications

An analysis of the literature on TIPS for refractory ascites including 16 studies showed a complete response in 51%, a partial response not requiring paracenteses in 68%, encephalopathy in 30%, and mortality in 34% of the patients included in prospective studies.[6] The results of five randomized studies[3] comparing TIPS with paracentesis are summarized in Figure 147.2. Overall, the TIPS arm showed a better response, slightly increased incidence of hepatic encephalopathy, and a trend towards improved survival. In addition, the TIPS improved renal function and other ascites-related complications. Although the results are favorable, until additional studies are available, TIPS should be used as a second-line treatment in patients not responding to paracentesis or developing ascites-related complications such as hepatic hydrothorax, hepatorenal syndrome, or recurrent spontaneous bacterial peritonitis.

COMPLICATIONS, COSTS, QUALITY OF LIFE

Procedural complications, technical quality assessment

Prospective studies investigating procedural complications of the TIPS intervention are not available. Complications with a potential of death are rare including perforations of anatomical vascular structures such as cardiac perforation, caval, and portal laceration. More frequently, the liver capsule is perforated leading to intraperitoneal bleeding. Fortunately, severe bleeding requiring surgical rescue is rare (<1%). Mispunctures

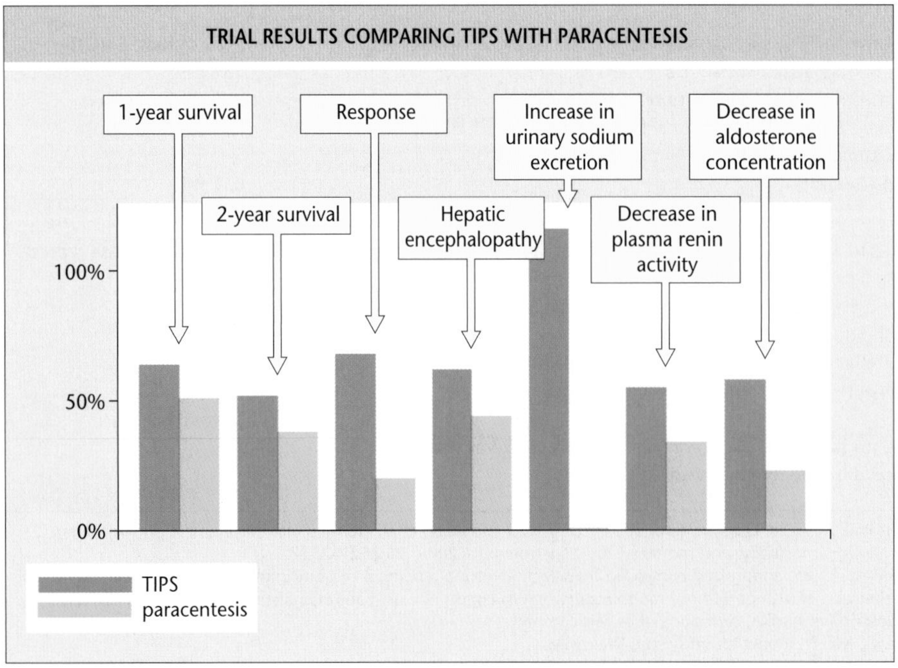

Fig. 147.2 Trial results comparing the TIPS with paracentesis. Pooled estimates of the results of randomized controlled trials comparing the TIPS with paracentesis. One small trial was disregarded because of insufficient statistical power (only 10 successful TIPS-implantations). The 1- and 2-year survival rates, the response to treatment, and the incidence of hepatic encephalopathy are the means of intention-to-treat results of four studies. The urinary sodium excretion (1 study, 6 months of follow-up), plasma renin activity (2 studies, 6 months of follow-up and 1 study, 3 months of follow-up), and aldosterone concentration (2 studies, 6 months of follow-up) are expressed as mean percentage changes (increases or decreases) obtained by the respective treatment.

into the biliary ducts or hepatic artery are not uncommon during the procedure. However, the occurrence of a fistula requiring radiological occlusion is exceptional. The repeated reports of radiodermatitis after the TIPS procedure clearly shows that adequate training is not always guaranteed. The assessment of the following quality parameters by an independent board would help to improve the performance of the intervention: technical success rate (aim: >97%), duration of the procedure (aim: 60 min, range 30–120 min), radiation time (aim: 10 min, range 5–30 min), area dose of radiation (aim: 6000 cGy × cm^2). In addition, septicemia, severe intra-abdominal bleeding requiring transfusions, or death from any technical complication should not exceed 2%, 2%, and 1%, respectively.

Shunt-related complications

The most important clinical complications related to the shunt are deterioration of liver function and worsening of hepatic encephalopathy. Both are related to the shunt diameter and the degree of reduction of the portosystemic pressure gradient. As demonstrated recently, 25 of 27 patients who developed hepatic encephalopathy after the TIPS implantation had a pressure gradient of <12 mmHg.[7] Thus, pressure gradients below 10–12 mmHg should be avoided whenever possible. Apart from the reduction of the pressure gradient the incidence of postshunt hepatic encephalopathy depends on age, Child-Pugh class, and the presence of encephalopathy before the shunt but not on hemodynamic variables such as the incremental increase of the arterial liver perfusion by the TIPS or the absence or presence of portal liver perfusion before the TIPS. If liver function or hepatic encephalopathy deteriorate progressively, immediate shunt reduction or occlusion is necessary to stabilize liver function until transplantation. Fortunately, the need for shunt reduction is rare amounting to just 3%.[3]

Costs

The TIPS implantation or revision is relatively inexpensive amounting to about €2000 (bare stent: €600; guidewires, catheters, needle: €600; two interventionalists and two assistants for 2 h: €480; miscellaneous: €320). The charges (not the resources) for the TIPS treatment including follow-up in comparison to the respective alternative treatments are assessed in six trials on variceal bleeding and one on ascites.[8] The costs for the TIPS were reported to be higher, similar, or less than for the endoscopic therapy. In a cost-effectiveness analysis, the total annual costs in the USA per patient for sclerotherapy, ligation, and TIPS were similar amounting to US$23 459, US$23 111, and US$26 275, respectively. With respect to ascites, higher costs for the patients treated with a TIPS (US$ 9125) compared to those receiving paracentesis (US$ 6333) have been reported.

Quality of life, nutritional status

A significant improvement of the quality of life was shown in three out of four nonrandomized, longitudinal TIPS studies.[3] In the randomized North American study on refractory ascites, TIPS and paracentesis showed similar improvements in physical and mental scores.

Three studies focused on the effect of the TIPS on body weight and nutrition. Their uniform findings were a significant improvement in dry weight, total body nitrogen, total body fat, and total body protein.

SUMMARY AND OUTLOOK

Advances in technical development and improved skills have made the TIPS procedure safe and little invasive. The TIPS seems to be the rescue treatment of choice when standard treatment fails to stop acute bleeding or prevent recurrent bleeding. More randomized studies on refractory ascites comparing a TIPS with paracentesis are needed to confirm the present trend towards improved survival by use of the TIPS.

Apart from the indications mentioned above the TIPS has been applied successfully for a number of rare diseases such as Budd-Chiari syndrome, ectopic variceal or mucosal portal hypertensive bleeding, or to facilitate major abdominal surgery. The TIPS probably has no value in the treatment of veno-occlusive disease and does not facilitate liver transplantation.

The major drawback of the TIPS with bare stent is its high failure rate. This may be solved by the use of a self-expanding stent covered with polytetrafluoroethylene (PTFE) (Viatorr®, Gore-Medical), which was licensed recently in Europe for the TIPS procedure and shows a patency rate of about 90%.[1] Since the covered stent does not develop narrowing with time by proliferation of the neo-intima, it opens up the possibility of inserting custom-made thin-lumen shunts from the start. The high patency rate together with a smaller stent diameter may reduce both the risk of rebleeding and the incidence of hepatic encephalopathy.[1] This concept may, however, not be applied to ascites patients where a larger shunt with a greater pressure reduction is needed to achieve a good response.

SOURCES OF INFORMATION FOR PATIENTS AND DOCTORS

http://glenlivet.mph.ed.ac.uk/endo/general/tipss.htm

REFERENCES

1. Bureau C, Garcia-Pagan JC, Otal P et al. Improved clinical outcome using polytetrafluoroethylene-coated stents for TIPS: results of a randomized study. Gastroenterology 2004; 126:469–475.
2. Kwock PC, Ng WF, Lam CS, Tsui PP, Faruqi A. Anatomy of the portal vein bifurcation: Implication for transjugular intrahepatic portosystemic shunts. Cardiovasc Intervent Radiol 2003; 26:261–264.
3. Rössle M. TIPS: an update. Best Pract Res Clin Gastroenterol 2004; 18:99–123.
4. Sorbi D, Gostout CJ, Peura D et al. An assessment of the management of acute bleeding varices: A multicenter prospective member-based study. Am J Gastroenterol 2003; 98: 2424–2434.
5. Burroughs AK, Vangeli M. Transjugular intrahepatic portosystemic shunt versus endoscopic therapy: Randomized trials for secondary prophylaxis of variceal bleeding: an updated meta-analysis. Scand J Gastroenterol 2002; 37:249–252.
6. Russo MW, Sood A, Jacobson IM, Brown RB. Transjugular intrahepatic portosystemic shunt for refractory ascites: an analysis of the literature on efficacy, morbidity, and mortality. Am J Gastroenterol 2003; 98:2521–2527.
7. Casado M, Bosch J, Garcia-Pagan JC et al. Clinical events after transjugular intrahepatic portosystemic shunt: correlation with hemodynamic findings. Gastroenterology 1998; 114:1296–1303.
8. Rosado B, Kamath PS. Transjugular intrahepatic portosystemic shunts: an update. Liver Transplant 2003; 9:207–217.

Chapter 148

Interventional radiology

Michael Darcy

KEY POINTS

- Interventional radiology offers enteral access where endoscopic access is not possible
- Percutaneous transhepatic cholangiography and percutaneous transhepatic biliary drainage are more difficult in nondilated systems
- In biliary stricture dilatation the complication rate can be as high as 25%
- Biliary stenting is possible for the lesions of the CBD, hilar lesions and left or right hepatic ducts
- Duodenal stents can be placed via the transhepatic tract
- Cholecystostomy offers decompression of the inflamed gallbladder for patients who are not surgical candidates

INTRODUCTION

Interventional radiology techniques address many gastrointestinal and hepatobiliary pathologic problems, often providing less invasive solutions through image-guided procedures. A discussion of all the uses of interventional radiology in this context is not possible here because of space constraints and the main purpose of this textbook. Topics that are not discussed include management of gastrointestinal bleeding, duodenal stenting, transjugular intrahepatic portosystemic shunting (TIPS), liver biopsy, hepatic abscess drainage, and treatment of hepatic malignancies; many of these techniques are discussed in other chapters.

GASTROSTOMY AND GASTROJEJUNOSTOMY

Introduction

Interventional radiology techniques can provide several forms of fluoroscopically assisted enteral access. Compared with endoscopic techniques in general, interventional radiology techniques have fewer complications, and require less sedation and less postprocedure narcotic analgesia. Technical success rates are excellent. Overlying bowel or prior surgical changes may prevent placement in up to 4% of patients.[1,2] Chapter 144 contains a detailed discussion of endoscopically placed gastrostomy and jejunostomy.

Description of technique

First a nasogastric (NG) tube is placed. An angiographic catheter can usually be passed even when nasopharyngeal or esophageal pathology prevents endoscope passage. In rare cases when a catheter cannot be passed, the stomach can be punctured percutaneously with a 22-gauge Chiba needle to allow air instillation. Glucagon is given to help retain air injected via the NG tube to distend the stomach. Rotational fluoroscopy is done to detect the presence of overlying bowel loops. An 18-gauge needle is directed under fluoroscopic guidance through the mid-body of the stomach. After passing a 0.038-inch wire into the stomach, the tract is dilated with serial dilators. T-fasteners (suture anchors) are useful for special situations (placement of large tubes, or patients with ascites or on steroids), but their routine use is debatable. Cope loop and balloon fixation catheters may be inserted in this manner. Mushroom peroral pull-type gastrostomies can also be inserted using fluoroscopic control to direct the percutaneous transgastric wire up the esophagus and out the mouth.[3]

The placement of gastrojejunal (GJ) tubes (Fig. 148.1) requires a few modifications. The tract into the stomach should be angled slightly towards the antrum. Once the stomach is accessed, directional catheters are used to steer the guidewire out into the distal duodenum before advancing the definitive GJ catheter over the wire.

Indications/contraindications

See also Chapter 144.

Gastrostomy and GJ tubes are indicated for patients needing long-term enteral nutrition and/or delivery of medications requiring enteral absorption. Radiologic techniques are especially useful for patients with nasopharyngeal and esophageal pathology that prevents endoscope passage, or when gastric transillumination is not possible. Gastrostomy tubes are easiest to manage and should be used when possible. GJ tubes are indicated for patients with gastric outlet obstruction, gastric dysmotility, gastroesophageal reflux, or significant respiratory compromise when any aspiration would be disastrous.

Gastrostomy may be used for long-term decompression in patients with malignant bowel obstruction. Rarely, gastrostomy creation is indicated to provide access for other procedures such as duodenal stenting.[4]

Contraindications primarily include uncorrectable coagulopathy and lack of safe access. Safe access may be precluded by overlying bowel loops. If colon is in the way, a rectal tube may be used to decompress the colon, allowing safe passage to the stomach. The stomach may be inaccessible if it is positioned high under the ribs. Postoperative stomachs may be more challenging to access because of the small size of the gastric remnant and altered outflow, but prior surgery is not an absolute contraindication unless the patient has had a total gastrectomy.

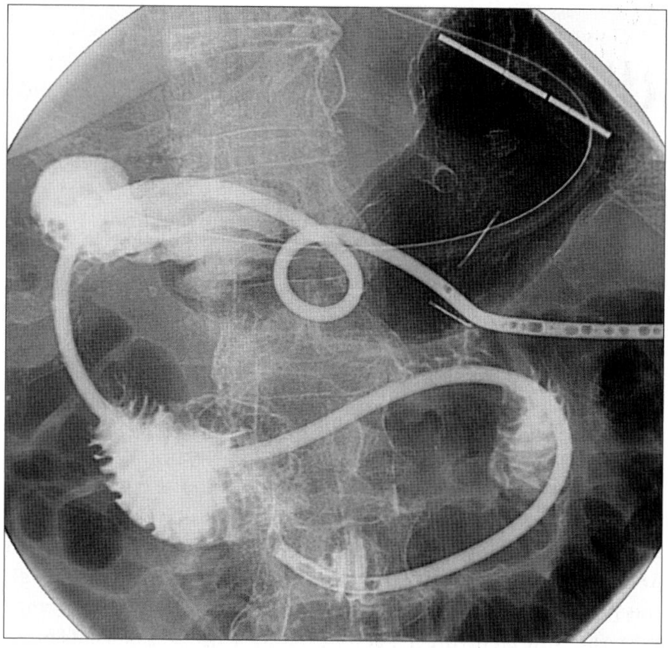

Fig. 148.1 Percutaneous single-lumen gastrojejunostomy catheter. Two T-fasteners are seen at the entry into the stomach. The catheter tip is in the proximal jejunum.

Complications and their management

Major complications are uncommon (0.5–1.4%) and minor complications occur in around 5% of patients.[1,3] Mild peritonitis from spillage of gastric contents may be managed conservatively with antibiotics. Localized perigastric abscesses can be drained percutaneously. Although rare, acute displacement of the tube from the stomach or improper extragastric placement may lead to peritonitis requiring surgical intervention. If symptoms are mild, conservative management with nasogastric suction and antibiotic therapy may suffice. A randomized prospective comparison between radiologic and endoscopic techniques yielded a slightly higher complication rate in the endoscopy group as a result of pneumonia in this group.[2]

Delayed complications are more common. Pericatheter infection will typically clear with aggressive wound cleansing and antibiotics. Leakage around the tube may require upsizing of the catheter to obturate the hole. Catheter occlusion is more common with smaller tubes (14–16 Fr) and is managed by catheter exchange and upsizing. If the tube is inadvertently pulled out, the tract is usually easily recanalized if there is a mature tract. See also Chapter 144 for a discussion of the complications.

DIRECT JEJUNOSTOMY

Introduction

Direct jejunostomy is used primarily in patients with postoperative changes that preclude accessing the stomach. This differs from gastric access in that the jejunum is smaller, more mobile, and does not distend as readily. These differences lead to both a lower technical success rate (85–88%)[5] and higher complication rates. Technical success is improved in patients who have previously had a surgical jejunostomy. At surgery, the bowel is typically sutured to the anterior abdominal wall; thus going through the old jejunostomy scar enhances the ease of dilating the percutaneous tract into the jejunum.

Chapter 144 discusses endoscopic placement of jejunostomy tubes.

Description of technique

An NG tube is passed, and air and contrast are instilled to opacify the jejunum and distend the loops to aid puncture. A 90–100-cm angiographic catheter can be directed out into the duodenum or proximal jejunum for optimal opacification and distention. Alternatively ultrasonography can be used to localize an anterior bowel loop and guide the needle puncture into the bowel.[5] The increased mobility of jejunum requires a different approach compared with gastrostomy. Although it is possible to dilate a tract into an air-distended stomach without any gastropexy, fixation is essential in jejunal access. Thus the initial puncture is best done with the needle containing the T-fastener, which is deployed to hold the jejunal loop against the abdominal wall while the tract is dilated. A 12–14-Fr Cope loop catheter is often used because larger tubes are difficult to pass into the compliant jejunum and catheters with balloon fixation can obstruct the jejunal loop.

Indications/contraindications

Direct jejunostomy is indicated when the stomach is absent (postgastric resection) or inaccessible (located high behind ribs, intrathoracic, or after esophageal resection with gastric pull-up). Tumor involvement of the stomach is another indication for direct jejunal access, because of increased potential for bleeding and pericatheter leakage around a catheter traversing a gastric malignancy.

Uncorrectable coagulopathy is the primary contraindication. Inability to identify a ventrally positioned jejunal loop also precludes this procedure. Ascites is a relative contraindication, as it increases the difficulty of tract dilatation and may lead to pericatheter leakage of ascites. Also there is a risk of contaminating the ascites with bowel contents that spill during tract dilatation.

Complications and their management

Major complications occur in about 13% of cases.[5] Pericatheter leakage is most common, likely due to the thinner jejunal wall. Minor cases of peritonitis can be treated with antibiotics, analgesics, and hydration. Significant leakage is heralded by persistent or increasing pain coupled with fever and signs of peritonitis. This typically requires surgical correction. Fever or leukocytosis without peritoneal signs may indicate a walled-off peritoneal abscess, which can be diagnosed by computed tomography and may be drained percutaneously. Inadvertent puncture of colon instead of jejunum can occur. A tube placed into the colon by mistake can be left in place for 2–4 weeks until a tract has matured, at which time tube removal is possible.

PERCUTANEOUS TRANSHEPATIC CHOLANGIOGRAPHY AND PERCUTANEOUS TRANSHEPATIC BILIARY DRAINAGE

Introduction

Percutaneous transhepatic cholangiography (PTC) provides opacification and visualization of the bile ducts and related pathology. Technical failure to access a duct may occur when the ducts are not dilated, as in patients with iatrogenic biliary leak or an obstructed anastomosis in liver transplant patients where the liver is too stiff to permit the ducts to dilate. Percutaneous transhepatic biliary drainage (PTBD) can be used to provide definitive drainage or access for future procedures such as biopsy, cholangioplasty, stone removal, or stenting. Technical success can be achieved in more than 90% of patients, even those with nondilated systems; however, significant experience and judgment is required to determine when and how many catheters to place. This is particularly true when the pathology is in the hilar region causing separate obstructions of branch ducts. When PTBD access is used as a conduit for common duct stone removal, stones can be cleared in 93% of cases.[6]

Description of technique

The patient must be assessed for signs of cholangitis as this may alter the magnitude of the procedure (i.e., simple external drainage versus trying to cross the obstruction). Preprocedure computed tomography is useful to assess the liver morphology, determine the degree and distribution of dilated ducts, and exclude the presence of interposed structures (bowel loops, tumors, etc.).

The traditional entry site for PTC is the right mid-axillary line. A starting point two-thirds of the way down the lateral margin of the liver is chosen fluoroscopically. A 22-gauge Chiba needle is passed medially, parallel to the inferior margin of the liver. Contrast is injected while slowly withdrawing the needle under fluoroscopic guidance. If a duct is not entered, the needle is redirected and the process repeated. Upon entering a duct, contrast is injected to opacify the ducts. Just enough contrast is injected to obtain the desired diagnostic information. Overinjection increases the risk of bacteremia and sepsis. While opacifying the ducts, images should be obtained in multiple projections to assess the extent of lesions fully.

Drainage is initiated by fluoroscopically selecting a duct that provides smooth access to the common duct. A peripheral part of the duct is chosen to avoid major vascular structures and to allow a long segment of catheter within the duct to maximize drainage. A 15–20-cm needle is advanced into the target duct. When ducts are significantly dilated, a peripheral left anterior segmental duct can be punctured with ultrasonographic guidance via a subxiphoid approach. Once the duct has been entered and a guidewire inserted, the needle is exchanged for a directional catheter used to steer the wire across the common duct to the bowel. The tract is dilated and an internal/external drain is placed. If the patient is septic, the manipulation should be minimized and an external drain can be placed above the obstruction.

Indications/contraindications

PTC is indicated for diagnosis of pathology and extent of abnormality in the biliary tree. This includes both obstructing lesions (malignancy, benign stricture, and calculi) as well as leaks (e.g., postoperative duct transections). PTC may also be requested for the evaluation of jaundice, liver function test abnormalities, symptoms of cholangitis, or pain. It is especially useful when tight obstructing lesions or postsurgical anatomy (e.g., a Roux-en-Y loop) prevent endoscopic access to the bile ducts. PTC can also be used to opacify the ducts to guide PTBD.

PTBD is indicated to provide relief of pain or relief from cholangitis due to biliary obstruction. It can provide access for dilatation or stenting of benign and malignant strictures respectively. Drainage may be used before surgery to restore normal liver function and reduce infection prior to resection of obstructing malignancies or surgical repair of duct injuries. PTBD can also provide access for intraductal procedures such as biopsy of strictures, endoscopic evaluation of masses, or stone removal (Fig. 148.2).

Uncorrectable coagulopathy and thrombocytopenia are the major contraindications. Significant ascites increases the risk of capsular hemorrhage as well as catheter displacement from the liver. Multiple lesions making effective drainage impossible is a relative contraindication to drainage. This should be considered in patients with sclerosing cholangitis or hilar malignancy where multiple catheters would be required to drain all of the liver.

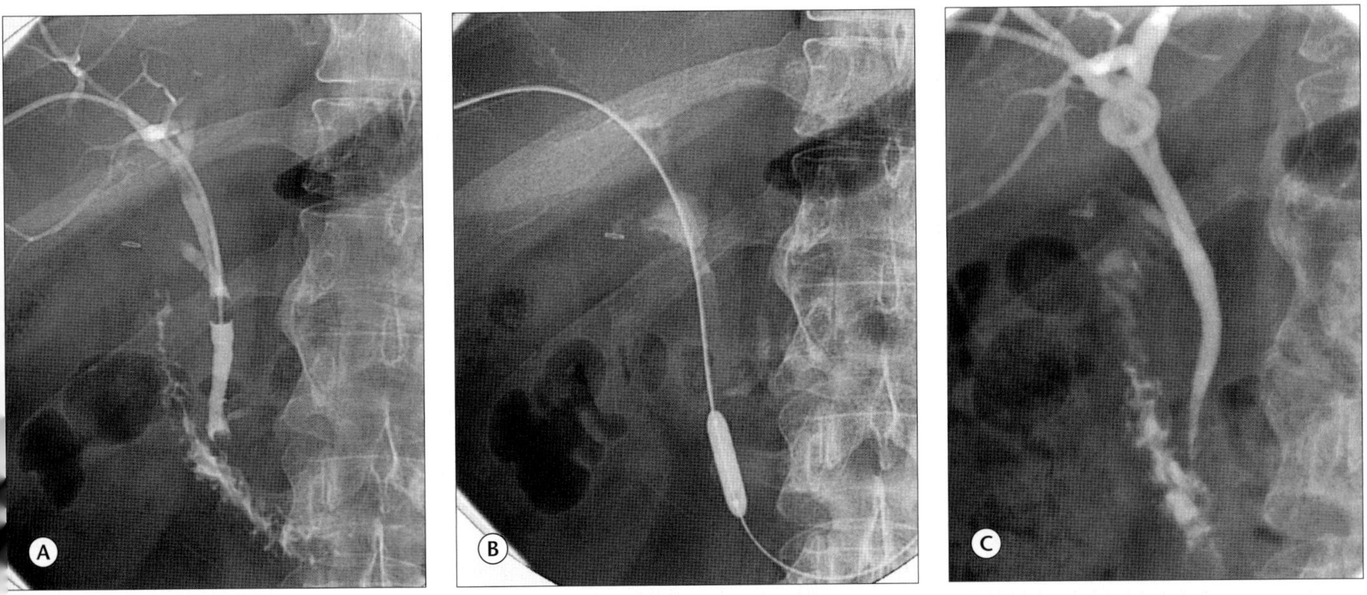

Fig. 148.2 Use of PTBD for intraductal stone removal. A. Cholangiogram done with a balloon occlusion catheter showing a stone just above the ampulla. The study was performed via transhepatic access after several days of external drainage. **B.** Balloon sphincteroplasty of the ampulla using a 6-mm angioplasty balloon. The balloon occlusion catheter was then used to push the stone into the duodenum. **C.** Final cholangiogram shows good antegrade drainage and no residual stone.

Complications and their management

The incidence of major complications is 3–6%, with bacteremia and sepsis being most common. Although rare, sepsis or hemorrhage can be severe enough to be fatal. After ensuring adequate biliary drainage, therapy must include antibiotics plus supportive measures such as adequate hydration, pressors, and ventilatory support. Hemorrhage may be intraperitoneal or into bile ducts (hemobilia). Bleeding is usually venous in origin and catheter tamponade of the tract typically resolves the problem. Persistent bleeding may indicate a hepatic arterial injury that may require superselective arterial embolization. Arterial injury may rarely cause an arteriovenous fistula. Persistent bleeding into the drainage catheter can indicate catheter malposition with a side hole in the parenchyma, and is managed by repositioning the catheter.

As right-sided PTBD always uses an intercostal approach, pleural complications may occur. Pleural complications may include pneumothorax, a biliary–pleural fistula, and empyema. These can be minimized by avoiding punctures that are too cephalad. When these complications occur, chest tube drainage may be required.

BILIARY STRICTURE DILATATION

Introduction

Benign strictures may result from operative complications (e.g., postlaparoscopic cholecystectomy), fibrosis at anastomoses (e.g., posttransplant), or inflammatory conditions. Attempts at nonoperative management may be justified given the difficulty and risks of surgical correction. Transhepatic balloon dilatation offers a less invasive approach but requires a prolonged course of therapy that entails multiple dilatations and long-term stenting. The success for dilatation of strictures ranges from 67% to 90%.[7,8]

Description of technique

Dilatation of strictures follows PTBD in a staged fashion as obstructed bile ducts often have bacterial colonization. Excessive manipulation prior to adequate drainage increases the risk of sepsis. Cholangiography is done to define the length of the stricture and the ductal diameter. High-pressure balloons are required owing to the fibrotic nature of these strictures. Repeated dilatation (three to four sessions spread over several weeks) yields better results than single dilatation procedures. Dilatation is quite painful, so moderate conscious sedation or general anesthesia is needed.

An internal/external catheter is placed as a stent to hold open the stricture so that, as scarring occurs, the duct should stay open to the diameter of the stent. Large-diameter catheters (12–16 Fr) are recommended. Long-term stenting (6 months or more) is commonly advocated.[7]

Indications/contraindications

Dilatation is indicated for benign strictures including iatrogenic duct injuries, anastomotic fibrotic scarring, and inflammatory strictures such as those caused by pancreatitis, stones, or sclerosing cholangitis. Inflammatory strictures are less likely to respond. Simple common ductal strictures are more amenable than complex strictures involving several branches in the hilum or multiple intrahepatic strictures.

Because of the risk of sepsis, ongoing cholangitis must be treated before a biliary dilatation procedure is done. Strictures caused by pathology extrinsic to the duct (e.g., pancreatic cancer or nodal compression) will not respond to dilatation and should be treated with other techniques.

Complications and their management

Overall complications (major and minor) occur in as many as 25% of patients.[8] Some reported complications (e.g., pleural complications) relate to the initial biliary access. Dilatation adds several complications beyond that of basic PTBD. Dilatation can cause bleeding, which is usually self-limiting but clots can obstruct the drainage catheter left in to stent the stricture open. As clots lyze spontaneously in bile, maintaining tube patency with flushing is often all that is required. Duct disruption with periductal leakage is rare and extravasation is generally well contained by the dense surrounding fibrosis. The provision of good biliary drainage is the only therapy needed.

INTERNAL BILIARY STENTING

Introduction

Internal stenting is utilized mostly in patients with malignant obstruction who have a limited life expectancy. The problem is not technical success, which ranges from 75%[9] to 100%;[10,11] it is limited patency. Even with larger self-expanding metallic stents, patency at 6 months is only around 60–70%. Newer polytetrafluoroethylene (PTFE) covered stents have a more encouraging patency rate of 76–77% at 12 months.[10,11]

Description of technique

Typically patients first have an internal/external drain placed to allow time for bleeding and sepsis to resolve before stenting. If there are no signs of cholangitis and aspirated bile is clear, internal stents can be placed during the initial procedure. Cholangiography is done to determine the length of stent needed and appropriate position for the stent. Self-expanding metal stents are preferred owing to their greater flexibility. Balloon dilatation is not usually needed to get a stent across the obstruction. After stent deployment, balloon dilatation of the stent is done cautiously to avoid causing bleeding. After confirming good stent position, a small catheter is typically left behind to tamponade the tract and decrease bleeding, and to allow follow-up cholangiography. It is possible to remove the external catheter immediately after stent placement, however it is recommended to occlude the hepatic parenchymal tract with Gelfoam pledgets to prevent bleeding or bile leakage.

Indications/contraindiations

The primary indication is relief of malignant obstruction of the bile ducts. Lesions of the common duct (e.g., pancreatic cancer) are most amenable, but hilar lesions (e.g., cholangiocarcinoma) can also be stented with dual stents, extending up separately into the left and right ducts (Fig. 183.3).

Patients with benign disease or low-grade cancers who cannot tolerate an external tube may benefit from internal stenting. In this setting, plastic internal stents that can be exchanged may be of benefit, provided there is close coordination with an endoscopist who can change or remove the stents.

Internal stents are usually contraindicated in patients with benign strictures because the patient will outlive the patency of the stent. The stent can also complicate future operative

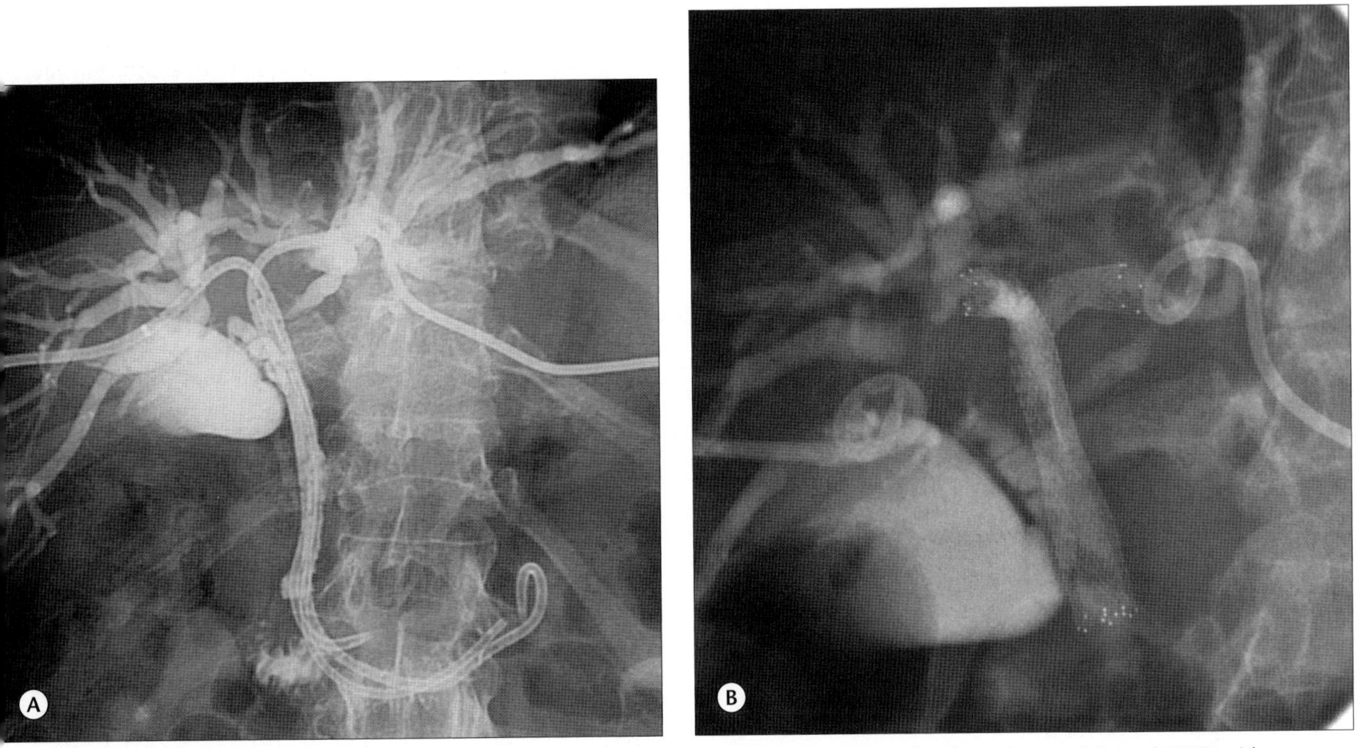

ig. 148.3 **Bilateral internal biliary stenting. A.** Patient with cholangiocarcinoma who had previously undergone bilateral PTBD with lacement of internal/external drains. The hilar strictures are evident by the lack of contrast around the biliary drains. **B.** Bilateral selfxpanding metallic internal stents. External catheters were left above the internal stents for a few days and later removed.

epair. Coagulopathy and ongoing sepsis must be resolved efore placing an internal stent. Concurrent duodenal or roximal jejunal obstructions are relative contraindications nless the bowel obstruction is dealt with. Placing a biliary tent above an unresolved duodenal obstruction can lead to ecurrent cholangitis and ineffective biliary drainage. Duodenal stents can be placed via the transhepatic tract to esolve the obstruction (Fig. 183.4).

Complications and their management

Complications occur in 5–19% of patients. Sepsis and bleeding are the most common. Bile leakage along the percutaneous ract can cause biloma formation or bile peritonitis. If a biloma does develop, percutaneous drainage is indicated. Acute cholecystitis can be caused by the stent occluding the cystic duct. The eported incidence with the PTFE-covered stent is 7–12%.[10,11] Cholecystitis is managed by cholecystostomy or cholecystectomy. Stent migration can occur with self-expanding stents, and restenting of the common duct as well as retrieval of the migrated stent may be required.

CHOLECYSTOSTOMY

Introduction

In some cases of cholecystitis the gallbladder may be too inflamed to allow cholecystectomy, or the patient may be too ill to tolerate surgery. In these settings, percutaneous drainage can be used to decompress the gallbladder. In patients who are not surgical candidates, the cholecystostomy tract can be used as a pathway for percutaneous removal of the stones. With acalculous cholecystitis, drainage may provide the definitive therapy. Once the inflammation has resolved and cystic duct patency has been restored, the catheter can often be removed after confirming a mature tract has formed around the catheter.

A catheter can be successfully placed in 97–100% of patients.[12,13] Extreme wall thickening and a small contracted lumen predispose to technical failure. Only 73–80% of patients have an appropriate clinical response, although the chance of clinical success is improved if the patients selected have typical clinical right upper quadrant pain and tenderness, and ultrasonographic findings of pericholecystic fluid. Simple aspiration of the gallbladder has been proposed,[13] but has lower technical success rates and also lesser clinical responses (90% versus 61%).

Description of technique

Ultrasonography or computed tomography is used to localize the gallbladder and guide the needle into it. A transhepatic tract is often recommended to stabilize the drainage catheter and prevent bile leakage around the tube into the peritoneum, although puncture of the gallbladder too close to its neck may be required. In this case a transperitoneal approach is used. Fluoroscopic evaluation is useful to exclude the presence of bowel interposed along the access tract. Stones can subsequently be removed via the percutaneous tract.

In patients who are not surgical candidates, stones can subsequently be removed via the percutaneous tract. The tract is dilated to accept an 18-Fr biliary sheath. Through this sheath stones can be basketed under fluoroscopic guidance. Alternatively a choledochoscope can be inserted to guide basketing, or electrohydraulic lithotripsy used to break up larger stones (Fig. 148.5).

Indications/contraindications

Patients with suspected acalculous cholecystitis are candidates for drainage if they have a dilated gallbladder with wall thickening

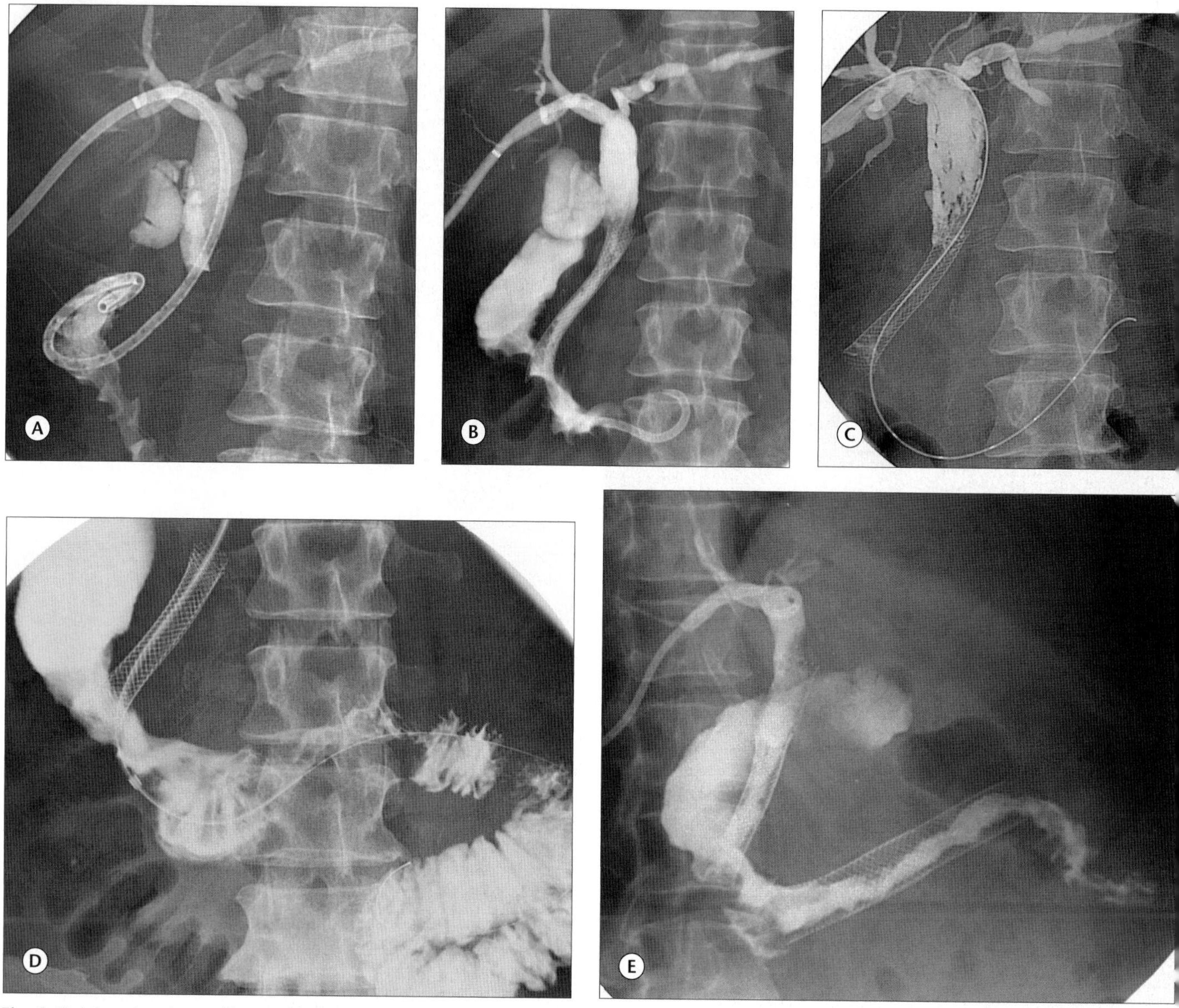

Fig. 148.4 Duodenal stenting. **A.** Cholangiogram through a percutaneous biliary drainage catheter placed across a common duct stricture caused by pancreatic cancer. **B.** Cholangiogram showing a Wallstent placed for internal stenting. **C.** The patient had recurring problems with stent obstruction. This cholangiogram shows the obstructed stent but also increased ductal dilatation with considerable debris in the duct. **D.** Injection of contrast into the duodenum revealed an obstruction of the fourth portion of the duodenum. After negotiating a catheter across the obstruction, contrast injection into the jejunum shows more normal bowel beyond the obstruction. A 20-mm Wallstent was passed through the transhepatic access and deployed across the duodenal obstruction. **E.** Cholangiogram a week after stenting the duodenum shows the duct has returned to normal caliber and both the biliary and duodenal stents are patent. The patient also had relief of persistent nausea experienced before duodenal stenting.

or pericholecystic fluid and appropriate clinical signs of infection (fever, leukocytosis, pain). Nonvisualization by hepatoiminodiacetic acid (HIDA) scanning can confirm the diagnosis. Patients with calculous cholecystitis who are not candidates for cholecystectomy but have persistent pain or infections can be drained as a prelude to percutaneous stone removal.

Contraindications include uncorrectable coagulopathy, lack of safe access (i.e., overlying bowel loops), or a small contracted gallbladder (particularly if filled with stones) which would make tube placement technically impossible.

Complications and their management

Complications of simple drainage occur in the range of 3–10% of patients. A common but infrequently reported complication is severe pain that occurs after dilator/catheter exchanges and probably relates to peritoneal irritation from spilled bile. This resolves within an hour and the patient should be maintained with adequate analgesia until it passes. Sepsis may be exacerbated. Bile leakage around the catheter may cause bile peritonitis and can be treated by upsizing the cholecystostomy catheter. Bleeding is uncommon and usually self-limiting. Catheter dislodgement before a mature tract has formed can cause bile to spill into the peritoneum and may require cholecystectomy. Puncture of overlying colon is rare but is managed by reaccessing the gallbladder through a different tract and removal of the initial catheter. Waiting until a mature tract has formed around the colonic catheter may be advisable.

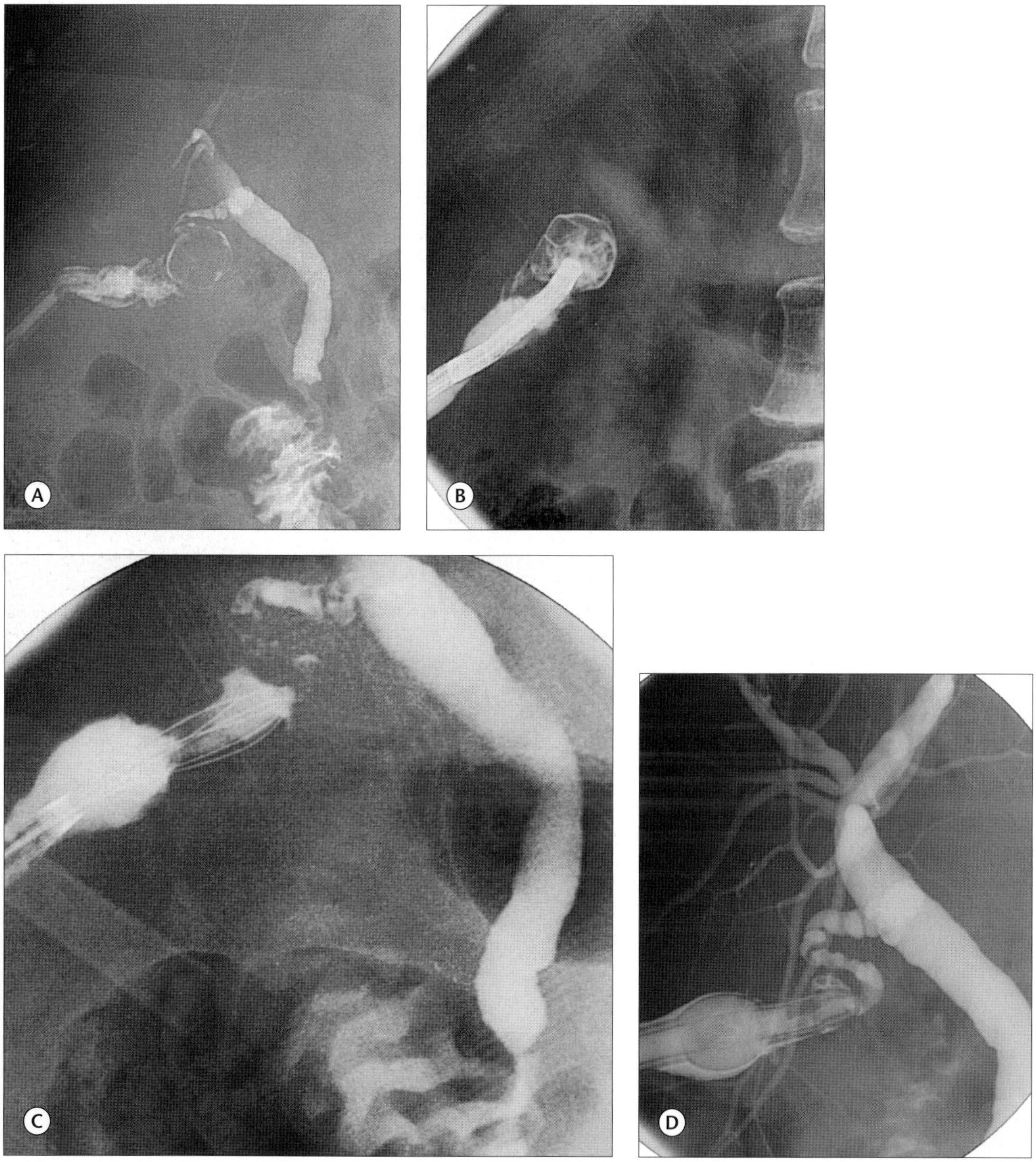

Fig. 148.5 Percutaneous stone removal. A. Cholangiogram done after percutaneous cholecystostomy in a patient with a large gallstone in the neck of the gallbladder. The study was performed after draining the patient until she was afebrile. **B.** As the patients was not a surgical candidate, percutaneous stone removal was performed. This image shows the choledochoscope through which an electrohydraulic lithotripsy probe was used to break up the stone. The stone is partially fragmented in this image. **C.** A stone basket introduced through the percutaneous tract is being used to remove stone fragments. **D.** Final cholangiogram showed a patent biliary system with no residual stone fragments. The tube was removed soon afterwards.

REFERENCES

1. Dewald CL, Hiette PO, Sewall LE, Fredenberg PG, Palestrant AM. Percutaneous gastrostomy and gastrojejunostomy with gastropexy: experience in 701 procedures. Radiology 1999; 211:651–656.
2. Hoffer EK, Cosgrove JM, Levin DQ, Herskowitz MM, Sclafani SJ. Radiologic gastrojejunostomy and percutaneous endoscopic gastrostomy: a prospective, randomized comparison. J Vasc Interv Radiol 1999; 10:413–420.
3. Yip D, Vanasco M, Funaki B. Complication rates and patency of radiologically guided mushroom gastrostomy, balloon gastrostomy, and gastrojejunostomy: a review of 250 procedures. Cardiovasc Intervent Radiol 2004; 27:3–8.
4. Pinto Pabon IT, Diaz LP, Ruiz De Adana JC, Lopez Herrero J. Gastric and duodenal stents: follow-up and complications. Cardiovasc Intervent Radiol 2001; 24:147–153.
5. van Overhagen H, Ludviksson MA, Lameris JS et al. US and fluoroscopic-guided percutaneous jejunostomy: experience in 49 patients. J Vasc Interv Radiol 2000; 11:101–106.
6. Garcia-Garcia L, Lanciego C. Percutaneous treatment of biliary stones: sphincteroplasty and occlusion balloon for the clearance of bile duct calculi. AJR Am J Roentgenol 2004; 182:663–670.
7. Venbrux AC, Osterman FA Jr. Percutaneous management of benign biliary strictures. Tech Vasc Interv Radiol 2001; 4:141–146.

8. Laasch HU, Martin DF. Management of benign biliary strictures. Cardiovasc Intervent Radiol 2002; 25:457–466.
9. Pinol V, Castells A, Bordas JM et al. Percutaneous self-expanding metal stents versus endoscopic polyethylene endoprostheses for treating malignant biliary obstruction: randomized clinical trial. Radiology 2002; 225:27–34.
10. Bezzi M, Zolovkins A, Cantisani V et al. New ePTFE/FEP-covered stent in the palliative treatment of malignant biliary obstruction. J Vasc Interv Radiol 2002; 13:581–589.
11. Schoder M, Rossi P, Uflacker R et al. Malignant biliary obstruction: treatment with ePTFE–FEP-covered endoprostheses – initial technical and clinical experiences in a multicenter trial. Radiology 2002; 225:35–42.
12. England RE, McDermott VG, Smith TP, Suhocki PV, Payne CS, Newman GE. Percutaneous cholecystostomy: who responds? AJR Am J Roentgenol 1997; 168:1247–1251.
13. Ito K, Fujita N, Noda Y et al. Percutaneous cholecystostomy versus gallbladder aspiration for acute cholecystitis: a prospective randomized controlled trial. AJR Am J Roentgenol 2004; 183:193–196.

Chapter 149

Paracentesis

Andrés Cárdenas, Mónica Guevara, and Pere Ginès

KEY POINTS

- Usually performed in the right or left lower abdominal quadrant with patient lying supine
- Ultrasound guidance is not required but may be helpful in cases where the patient is obese or has surgical scars
- Should be performed under strict sterile conditions
- After the skin, subcutaneous tissue, and peritoneum are infiltrated with local anesthetic, the presence of ascites is confirmed by performing intermittent aspiration with a needle or cannula
- The use of specially designed paracentesis cannulas (14–16 gauge) is preferred to large angiocath needles
- Once inside the abdominal cavity, the inner cannula is connected to either suction bottles (1–2-L capacity) with the aid of noncollapsible tubing or to a large-capacity suction pump
- The physician or nurse should remain at the bedside during the entire procedure
- Paracentesis is terminated when ascitic fluid flow from the cannula becomes intermittent despite gentle mobilization of the cannula within the abdominal cavity and turning the patient on to the left side
- After removal of the cannula, patients should be asked to recline for 2–3 h on the side opposite to paracentesis

INTRODUCTION AND SCIENTIFIC BASIS

Paracentesis was the first technique to be used for the treatment of ascites. It was described in the time of Hippocrates; however, the first detailed description of a therapeutic paracentesis has been ascribed to Aulus Cornelius Celsus (30 BC–50 AD).[1] In the mid 1500s, Sanctorius, a surgeon from the University of Padua, designed the first trocar for paracentesis.[1] This form of therapy whereby several liters of fluid were removed every other week from patients with cirrhosis and ascites gained widespread use by the first half of the 20th century. By then the practice of paracentesis was accepted as the first-line therapy for ascites. After the introduction of diuretics in the 1950s the use of large-volume paracentesis for therapy of ascites began to decline due to the ease of diuretic administration and their apparent lack of significant side effects. Additionally, other factors such as patient discomfort and the fact that it was a time-consuming procedure for both patients and doctors, along with some reports of significant deleterious hemodynamic effects of large-volume drainage, led to the abandonment of therapeutic paracentesis.[2] It was not until the mid 1980s that this form of therapy was reevaluated showing that it was a safe and effective therapy for patients with a large amount of ascites.[3]

DESCRIPTION OF TECHNIQUE

Ascites can be removed in one tap or repeated taps of 4–6 L/day associated with intravenous albumin (6–8 g per liter tapped) to prevent postparacentesis circulatory dysfunction (a circulatory derangement with marked activation of the renin-angiotensin system that occurs in most patients treated with large-volume taps).[4] Therapeutic paracentesis is a quick, effective therapy that is associated with fewer side effects than diuretics.[5]

Paracentesis: Although large-volume paracentesis is a simple procedure, several precautions should be taken to avoid complications. Paracentesis is usually performed in the left lower abdominal quadrant, approximately 5 cm cephalad and 5 cm medial to the anterior superior iliac crest. Before starting the procedure, the presence of ascitic fluid at the selected puncture site should be documented by demonstrating shifting dullness. Ultrasound guidance is not required but may be helpful in cases where the patient is obese or has surgical scars. Puncture of surgical scars and visible abdominal collaterals should be avoided. This procedure should be performed under strict sterile conditions. The abdominal wall should be cleansed, disinfected with an iodine solution, and draped in a sterile fashion. The practitioner should wear a sterile gown, gloves, mask, and cap during the entire procedure. Once the skin, subcutaneous tissue, and peritoneum are infiltrated with local anesthetic (1% lidocaine), the presence of ascites is confirmed by performing intermittent aspiration with a needle or cannula.

Cannulas: There are several specially designed paracentesis cannulas, which should be preferred to large angiocath needles (14–16 gauge) for venous access. All paracentesis cannulas have an inside needle which is removed after the abdominal wall has been punctured. The cannulas are between 14 and 18 gauge and have several side holes and a distal hole. In addition, and contrary to angiocath needles, paracentesis cannulas are blunt ended. These characteristics seem to reduce the risk of injuring intra-abdominal organs and prevent the interruption of flow frequently seen with angiocath needles due to occlusion of the distal hole by peritoneal fat or bending of the needle. We use a modified Kuss needle, a sharp-pointed, blind, metal needle with a 7-cm long, and 17 gauge blunt-edged cannula with side holes. Once inside the abdominal cavity, the inner cannula is connected to either suction bottles (1–2-L capacity) with the aid of noncollapsible tubing or to a large capacity suction pump. This allows for a faster elimination of the ascitic fluid as compared to the relatively slow free flow of ascitic fluid.

The physician or nurse should remain at the bedside during the entire procedure. After there is good flow of fluid, the needle needs to be held in place throughout the procedure to avoid displacement secondary to respiratory or other movements. If displacement occurs, the needle can be reinserted very slowly (with the suction turned off) until fluid is aspirated again. If the flow becomes sluggish it usually indicates that the omentum is obstructing and in this case the patient should be asked to slightly turn on his left side as this sometimes allows for more drainage.

Cannula removal: Paracentesis is finished when ascitic fluid flow from the cannula becomes intermittent despite gentle mobilization of the cannula within the abdominal cavity and turning the patient on to the left side. The duration of the whole procedure ranges from 30 to 90 min depending on the amount of ascitic fluid to be removed and the intensity of suction. When the cannula has been removed, patients should be asked to recline for 2–3 h on the opposite side to the paracentesis site to facilitate the closure of the puncture hole and prevent leakage of ascitic fluid. Factors associated with a high risk of leakage are the presence of edema in the abdominal wall and small-volume paracentesis where a large volume of ascitic fluid is left behind. Therefore, the elimination of most of the ascitic fluid is recommended to prevent leakage, particularly in patients with edema of the abdominal wall. The effectiveness of the so-called 'Z-tracking' for abdominal puncture in the prevention of ascites leakage after large-volume paracentesis has not been proven and may increase the risk of laceration of vessels of the abdominal wall. Albumin (6–8 g per liter tapped) is infused after the procedure and patients may be discharged from the hospital the same day if treated on an outpatient basis.

INDICATIONS/CONTRAINDICATIONS

Indications: Therapeutic paracentesis is the treatment of choice in the management of patients with cirrhosis and large ascites. Patients with mild and moderate ascites are best managed with a low-sodium diet and diuretics. Therapeutic paracentesis is also the first-line therapy for patients with refractory ascites.[6]

Contraindications: There are few contraindications to paracentesis. There has been a lot of controversy surrounding coagulopathy; nonetheless, most authors agree that the typical coagulopathy seen in advanced cirrhosis is not considered a contraindication to diagnostic or therapeutic paracentesis unless it is very severe (see later). Bleeding into the ascitic fluid is extremely rare with a risk of 1/1000.[7] Complications such as an abdominal wall hematoma may occur in approximately 2% of cases. Infection such as spontaneous bacterial peritonitis has been considered a relative contraindication for performing therapeutic paracentesis. Although large-volume paracentesis may have a theoretical beneficial effect by removing cytokines and vasoactive mediators in the infected fluid that possibly contribute to circulatory dysfunction and renal failure, this procedure could cause a detrimental effect on the already compromised circulatory function present in these patients. Owing to the lack of data addressing these points it is recommended that large paracentesis be performed only after the infection has been cured.

COMPLICATIONS

With the technique described above, the rate of local complications is very low. Complications other than leakage, such as bleeding, infection, or intestinal perforation, are exceedingly rare after large-volume paracentesis. Intraperitoneal bleeding or large abdominal wall hematomas are very uncommon.[8] Nevertheless, because most of the studies assessing the use of large-volume paracentesis in patients with cirrhosis and ascites have excluded patients with a prothrombin time over 21 s (prothrombin ratio of less than 40% or international normalized ratio (INR) greater than 1.6) and significant thrombocytopenia (less than 50 000 platelets per mm^3), the occurrence of bleeding complications after large-volume paracentesis in patients with severe coagulation disturbances is not known.

Management: If bowel perforation after therapeutic paracentesis is suspected, the patient should be kept fasting, placed on intravenous broad-spectrum antibiotics, and abdominal imaging with a computed tomography (CT) scan and surgical consultation should be sought. Some patients respond well to conservative measures, but given that a majority has advanced liver disease, further decompensation with sepsis and multiorgan failure is a distinct possibility. The decision to intervene surgically must be carefully evaluated because most are Child Class C cirrhotic patients, in whom surgical intervention is associated with high mortality rates in the order of 80%. Leakage of ascitic fluid through the skin after a paracentesis most commonly occurs with small-volume taps. In these cases, an attempt should be made to extract all the ascitic fluid from a different abdominal site and keep the patient on relatively high doses of diuretics if tolerated. In patients with grossly hemorrhagic ascites, paracentesis should be attempted at a different site to exclude local trauma of the vessel. If bloody nontraumatic ascites is confirmed, abdominal imaging should be performed with an abdominal CT scan. In cases of traumatic paracentesis, patients should be carefully observed with strict monitoring of vital signs, complete blood count, and coagulation studies. In patients with underlying coagulopathy, fresh frozen plasma and platelets should be administered to keep the INR near 1.0 and platelet count over 50 000. If patients continue to show signs of ongoing blood loss, an angiogram and surgical consultation should be sought.

CONTROVERSIAL ISSUES

There are two controversial issues surrounding therapeutic paracentesis.

Paracentesis vs diuretics: The first regards the use of large-volume paracentesis with plasma expansion as front-line therapy in all patients with large ascites versus the use of diuretics only. Although there was some initial skepticism, a large controlled study demonstrated that paracentesis was an effective, safe and fast therapy that was associated with fewer side effects, such as hepatic encephalopathy and renal dysfunction, compared to diuretics.[5] Although the use of a plasma expander (albumin) may be expensive in some countries, therapeutic paracentesis with albumin is more cost effective and reduces the period of hospitalization when compared with diuretics alone.[8] In cases of refractory ascites, in which patients do not respond to high doses of diuretics or have significant side effects that preclude their use, therapeutic paracentesis with albumin administration is also the preferred initial treatment.[9,10]

Plasma expander: The second controversy is regarding the concomitant use of plasma expansion with albumin after large volume paracentesis. The removal of large volumes of ascitic fluid without the use of concomitant plasma expanders is associated with a circulatory dysfunction characterized by a reduction in effective arterial blood volume with subsequent activation of vasoconstrictor and antinatriuretic factors.[4] This circulatory dysfunction and the mechanisms activated to maintain circulatory homeostasis are detrimental to cirrhotic patients. First, circulatory dysfunction is associated with rapid reaccumulation of ascites.[11] Second, approximately 20% of patients treated with large-volume paracentesis develop renal impairment and/or water retention leading to dilutional hyponatremia.[11,12] Third, portal pressure increases in patients developing circulatory dysfunction after large-volume paracentesis, probably owing to an increased intrahepatic resistance due to the action of vasoconstrictor systems on the hepatic vascular bed.[4] Finally, the development of circulatory dysfunction is associated with a shortened survival.[11]

Currently, the only effective method to prevent circulatory dysfunction after large-volume paracentesis is the administration of plasma expanders. Albumin is more effective than other plasma expanders (dextran-70, polygeline) probably owing to its longer persistence in the intravascular compartment.[12]

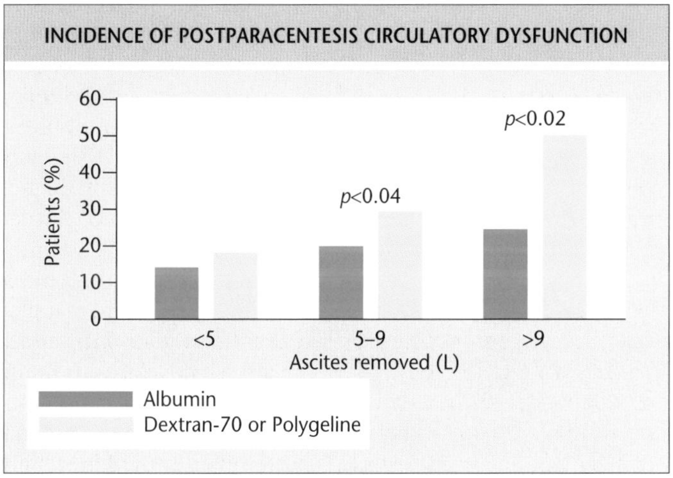

Fig. 149.1 Incidence of postparacentesis circulatory dysfunction. Incidence of postparacentesis circulatory dysfunction, as defined by marked activation of the renin-angiotensin system, according to the plasma expander used and the amount of ascites fluid removed. *$p=0.04$ and **$p=0.02$ with respect to patients receiving albumin. Modified from Ginès A et al. Randomized trial comparing albumin, dextran-70 and polygelin in cirrhotic patients with ascites treated by paracentesis. Gastroenterology 1996; 111:1002–1110, Copyright 1996, with permission from the American Gastroenterological Association.

When less than 5 L of ascites are removed, dextran-70, polygeline, or saline show a similar efficacy compared with albumin. However, albumin is more effective than these artificial plasma expanders when more than 5 L of ascites are removed[11,12] (Fig. 149.1). Despite this greater efficacy, randomized comparative studies have shown no differences in survival of patients treated with albumin compared with that of patients treated with other plasma expanders.[11,12] Larger trials would be required to demonstrate that the greater protective efficacy of albumin on circulatory function compared with other plasma expanders results in a survival benefit. Although no significant differences in survival have been demonstrated, preventing hyponatremia and hepatorenal syndrome and diminishing the recurrence of ascites provides better care for patients by decreasing their morbidity. Taken together, the currently available data indicate that circulatory dysfunction after large-volume paracentesis should be prevented because it is potentially harmful to patients with cirrhosis. Intravenous albumin appears to be the best plasma expander when more than 5 L of ascitic fluid are removed and is administered at a dose of 6–8 g/L of ascites removed.[11]

RELATIVE COST

There are no specific studies examining the cost of therapeutic paracentesis for ascites. In the initial studies comparing therapeutic paracentesis with diuretics, it was found that paracentesis was more effective, safer, and associated with less side effects than diuretics.[5] In addition, patients treated with paracentesis had a shorter stay in hospital than those treated with diuretics. Although a cost analysis was not performed, the fact that patients treated with paracentesis were discharged earlier translates into a cheaper treatment strategy. Although albumin administration has been a matter of controversy due to its high cost, no studies on cost effectiveness have shown that giving albumin increases cost when compared to diuretics. A preliminary report specifically addressing the question of cost effectiveness in the treatment of ascites concluded that the cost of treatment per patient with large ascites was lower for large-volume paracentesis than for diuretics.[13] The current cost of albumin in the USA is nearly US$1.50 per gram; so if a large tap of 8 L is performed the cost of albumin alone is around US$100. Although other plasma expanders may be cheaper, none have proven to be as good or better than albumin in preventing postparacentesis circulatory dysfunction when more than 5 L of fluid are removed.

REFERENCES

1. Dawson A. Historical notes on ascites. Gastroenterology 1960; 39:790–791.
2. Reynolds TB. Renaissance of paracentesis in the treatment of ascites. Adv Intern Med 1990; 35:365–373.
3. Quintero E, Ginès P, Arroyo V et al. Paracentesis versus diuretics in the treatment of cirrhotics with tense ascites. Lancet 1985; 1: 611–612.
4. Ruiz-del-Arbol L, Monescillo A, Jiménez W et al. Paracentesis-induced circulatory dysfunction: mechanism and effect on hepatic hemodynamics in cirrhosis. Gastroenterology 1997; 113:579–186.
5. Gines P, Arroyo V, Quintero E et al. Comparison of paracentesis and diuretics in the treatment of cirrhotics with tense ascites. Results of a randomized study. Gastroenterology 1987; 93:234–241.
6. Moore KP, Wong F, Ginès P et al. The management of ascites in cirrhosis: report on the consensus conference of the International Ascites Club. Hepatology 2003; 38:258–266.
7. McVay PA, Toy PT. Lack of increased bleeding after paracentesis and thoracentesis in patients with mild coagulation abnormalities. Transfusion 1991; 31:164–171.
8. Ginès P, Tito L, Arroyo V et al. Randomized comparative study of therapeutic paracentesis with and without intravenous albumin in cirrhosis. Gastroenterology 1988; 94:1493–1502.
9. Ginès P, Uriz J, Calahorra B et al. Transjugular intrahepatic portosystemic shunting versus paracentesis plus albumin for refractory ascites in cirrhosis. Gastroenterology 2002; 123:1839–1847.
10. Sanyal AJ, Genning C, Reddy KR et al. The North American Study for the Treatment of Refractory Ascites. Gastroenterology 2003; 124:634–641.
11. Ginès A, Fernandez-Esparrach G, Monescillo A et al. Randomized trial comparing albumin, dextran 70, and polygeline in cirrhotic patients with ascites treated by paracentesis. Gastroenterology 1996; 111:1002–1010.
12. Ginès P, Guevara M, De Las Heras D, Arroyo V. Review article: albumin for circulatory support in patients with cirrhosis. Aliment Pharmacol Ther 2002; 16 (Suppl 5):24–31.
13. Ginès P, Uriz J, Trilla A et al. Treatment of ascites in patients with cirrhosis; a cost-effective analysis. Hepatology 2001; 34:1509A.

Chapter 150

Liver operations

J Michael Henderson

KEY POINTS
• Accurate preoperative anatomical definition by imaging techniques and assessment of liver function is crucial to reduce the morbimortality from liver operations • Liver resection is increasingly used to remove primary and secondary tumors affecting the liver • Liver ablation by percutaneous ethanol injection or by radiofrequency ablation are less invasive ways to treat small, well-circumscribed tumors, especially in patients with significant comorbidities

INTRODUCTION AND SCIENTIFIC BASIS

The surgeon plays a role as one of the team members taking care of patients with various liver diseases. Many authors refer to the need for surgery, so the aim of this chapter is to bring together the types of operations that are used in taking care of the clinical problems described elsewhere in this book. The broad categories are:

- liver resections and/or ablation;
- biliary procedures;
- operations for portal hypertension; and
- liver transplantation.

The surgeon should not work in isolation, but is heavily interdependent on the team of hepatologists, radiologists, pathologists, anesthesiologists, and support personnel. This chapter will not focus on the detail of operative procedures, but rather on the broad concepts of the indications for surgery, evaluation methods to reach decisions, the types of procedures available, and overall management strategies from a surgeon's perspective.

Evaluation methods

The patient's history and physical examination play an important part in reaching a decision on which patients require surgery, for example: surgery may be indicated for resection of benign liver tumors if they are symptomatic; resection of metastatic liver tumors is indicated only for certain types of primary tumors; surgical intervention for variceal bleeding is only indicated when the first-line treatment options have been exhausted; and components of the patient history are a critical part of the evaluation for liver transplant.

Laboratory studies including liver chemistries, hematology, and coagulation profiles are essential for all patients being considered for liver surgery. In some patients, liver biopsy may be indicated either to define a specific tumor, or more frequently to define underlying liver disease such as cirrhosis. The decision to operate or not may be based on the activity and the degree of fibrosis in the liver, rather than on the tumor pathology.

Imaging studies play an important role in evaluation of all patients considered for liver surgery, biliary operations, or transplant. The increasing sophistication of radiologic imaging is one of the major factors that have improved the selection and outcome of patients being considered for liver surgery.

Liver function[1] is assessed by a combination of physical findings, laboratory studies, and in certain circumstances more sophisticated liver function testing. The broad goal is to address the ability of the liver to tolerate an operative procedure without precipitating liver failure. The two main scoring systems in current use are the Child-Pugh score (Table 150.1) and the model for end-stage liver disease (MELD) score (Table 150.2).[2]

Anatomy[3]

Liver structure must be clearly understood by the surgeon, both from the evaluation and treatment perspective. The segmental anatomy of the liver (Fig. 150.1) using Couinaud's classification is based on the eight liver segments that have their own hepatic arterial and portal venous blood supply, biliary drainage, and hepatic venous drainage. It is this segmental anatomy that dictates the ability to perform liver resections based upon these segments of the liver.

An accurate knowledge of the portal and hepatic venous system is critical to the liver surgeon. This can be defined or verified with intraoperative ultrasound. The variability of extra-

TABLE 150.1 CHILD-PUGH CLASSIFICATION

Parameter	1 Point	2 Points	3 Points
Serum bilirubin (mg/dL)	<2	2–3	<3
Albumin (g/dL)	>3.5	2.8–3.5	<2.8
Prothrombin time (↑, s)	1–3	4–6	>6
Ascites	None	Slight	Moderate
Encephalopathy	None	1–2	3–4

Grades: A, 5 to 6 points; B, 7 to 9 points; C, 10 to 15 points.

TABLE 150.2 MELD SCORE FOR SEVERITY OF CIRRHOSIS

$$\text{MELD score} = 0.957 \times \log_e \text{creatinine} + 0.378 \times \log_e \text{bilirubin} + 1.120 \times \log_e \text{protime}$$

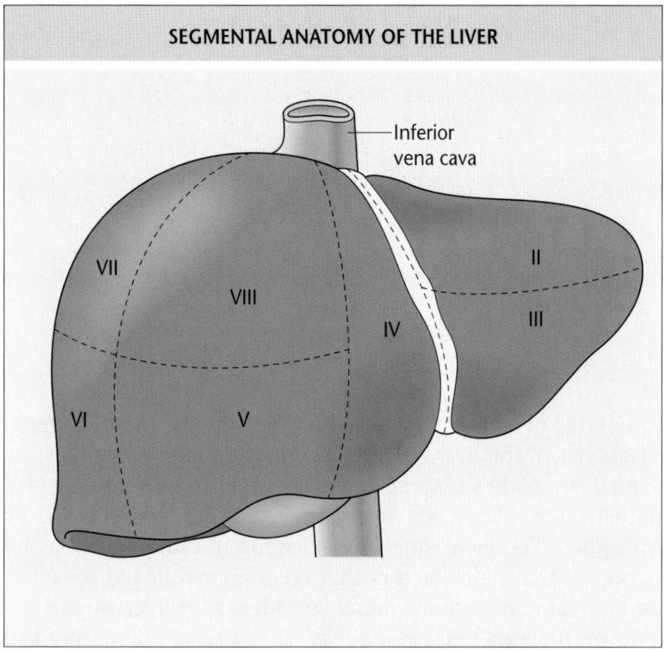

Fig. 150.1 Anatomy of liver. Segmental anatomy of the liver according to Couinaud; each of the eight liver segments has its own blood supply and biliary drainage. From Meyers WC. Atlas of biliary surgery. In: Bell RH, Rikkers LF, Mulholland MW, eds. Digestive tract surgery; 1996:499–600. Reproduced with permission from Lippincott Williams & Wilkins.

hepatic arterial anatomy may be seen on some imaging studies, but should be assessed at the time of surgery. The most common variations are replaced or accessory arteries to the right liver from the superior mesenteric artery and the left liver from the left gastric artery.

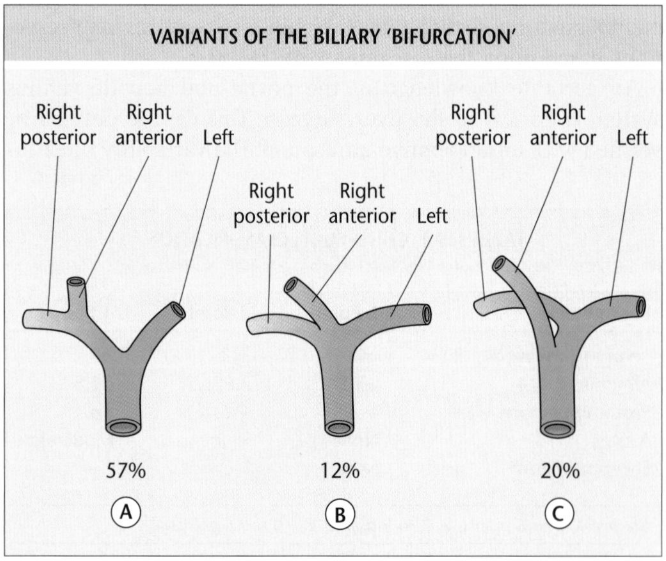

Fig. 150.2 Biliary bifurcation. The most common variants of the biliary 'bifurcation.' **A.** A true bifurcation with intrahepatic right anterior and posterior ducts. **B.** A trifurcation occurs in 12% with the right anterior and posterior ducts meeting at the same point as the left duct. **C.** In 20%, one of the right ducts (usually posterior) crosses to enter the left duct. From Meyers WC. Atlas of biliary surgery. In: Bell RH, Rikkers LF, Mulholland MW, eds. Digestive tract surgery; 1996:499–600. Reproduced with permission from Lippincott Williams & Wilkins.

The biliary anatomy is also very variable. The experienced surgeon will usually define the biliary anatomy by preoperative or intraoperative cholangiography. The major questions for a surgeon are around the hilus; Fig. 150.2 illustrates the most common variants.

The hilar plate is the fusion of the liver capsule over the portal vein, hepatic artery, and bile duct at the liver hilus. Opening of this capsular plane below segment IV allows elevation of the hilar plate and greatly facilitates dissection of the hilar structures.

Management

When patients undergo surgery to treat liver conditions or patients with liver disease require a surgical procedure, the surgeon is the captain of the team and must assume responsibility for overall patient management. Preoperative preparation should be done in conjunction with the hepatologist to optimize the patient's liver condition. Perioperative management must be planned with the anesthesiologist (for example, low central venous pressure for liver resection). In patients with cirrhosis requiring an operation, overall fluid and nutritional management are critical. Defined protocols for management of each of these phases will lead to overall better patient care and has become the standard in most major liver surgery centers.

LIVER RESECTIONS (see also Chapters 79 and 102)

Introduction

Liver resections are indicated for removal of benign or malignant neoplasms. Some benign lesions, such as giant hemangiomas, form pseudocapsules and can be enucleated. Malignant tumors are resected with the goal of at least a 1-cm margin. The extent of resection is determined by liver anatomy (Fig. 150.1) with either segmental or lobar resections.

Technique

The essential technical steps for successful liver resections are: (1) exposure; (2) mobilization; (3) definition of anatomy (visual and ultrasound); (4) determination of resection planes; (5) division of main vascular pedicles; (6) parenchymal transection; (7) confirmation of margins; and (8) check liver remnant.[4]

Incisions, exposure, and mobilization of the liver have been aided by transplant experience and technology. Most liver resections can be accomplished using an abdominal approach, but occasionally a combined thoraco-abdominal incision (right sided) may be needed. Fixed retractor systems aid and maintain exposure. Left and right sides of the liver can be mobilized by dividing the triangular ligaments, and the liver fully mobilized off the inferior vena cava up to the hepatic veins if needed (Fig. 150.3A,B).

Anatomic definition may require careful hilar dissection of the arteries, portal vein, and bile ducts when anatomic lobar resection is being done. Intrahepatic anatomic definition, in particular localizing the hepatic and portal veins, is done with intraoperative ultrasound. Concurrently, tumor extent is defined by palpation and ultrasound. These maneuvers allow for planning of the resection plane.

Transection of the parenchyma can be done in many ways, including crush and clamp, ultrasonic dissection (Fig. 150.4), and water pick dissection; all define the vessels for ligation or clipping by clearing away the hepatocytes. The second component to this phase is achieving hemostasis, which can again be done in many ways: ligatures, clips, diathermy, argon diathermy,

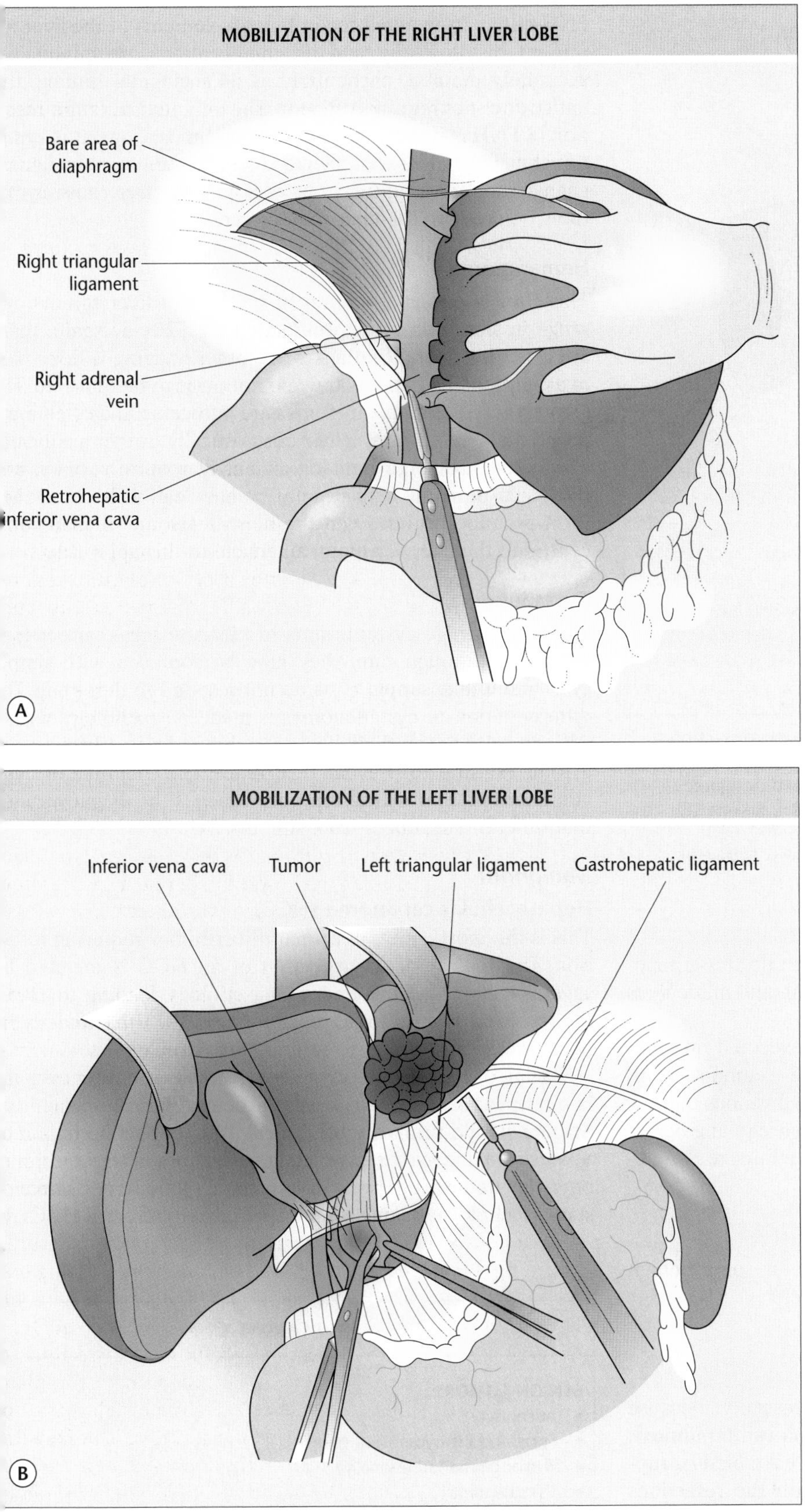

Fig. 150.3 Mobilization. A. Mobilization of the right lobe of the liver by diversion of the right triangular ligament. This goes right back to the inferior vena cava (IVC) and may include ligation of retrohepatic veins draining into the IVC. **B.** Mobilization of the left lobe of the liver requires diversion of the left triangular ligament, the gastrohepatic ligament, and the peritoneum on the left side of the IVC. These three lines come together superiorly at the left posterior side of the suprahepatic IVC. From Meyers WC. Atlas of biliary surgery. In: Bell RH, Rikkers LF, Mulholland MW, eds. Digestive tract surgery; 1996:499–600. Reproduced with permission from Lippincott Williams & Wilkins.

LIVER PARENCHYMAL TRANSECTION

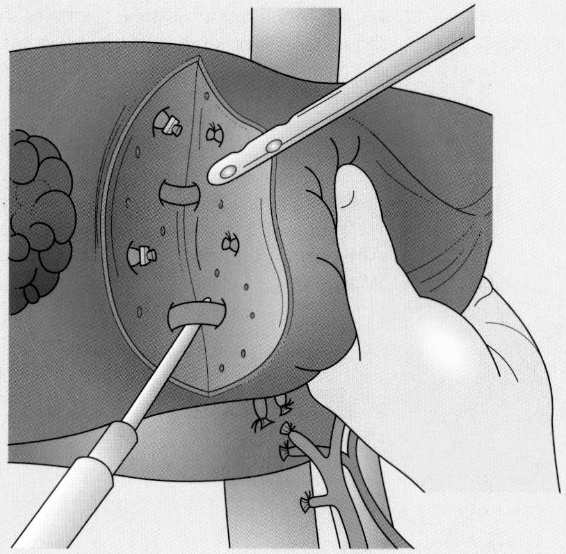

Fig. 150.4 Liver parenchymal transection. Ultrasonic dissection (as illustrated) is one method of defining the vessels and bile ducts in the plane of transection, which used to be clipped or ligated. From Meyers WC. Atlas of biliary surgery. In: Bell RH, Rikkers LF, Mulholland MW, eds. Digestive tract surgery; 1996:499–600. Reproduced with permission from Lippincott Williams & Wilkins.

and TissueLink. There is no one 'right' way to do this component of a liver resection, but attention to detail and meticulous technique are important.

If the resection is properly planned and executed, margins should be satisfactory. Inspection of the remnant liver, checking the inflow vessels, ensuring there is no venous outflow obstruction, and possibly doing a completion cholangiogram if dissection has been at the bifurcation will minimize complications.

Indications

Liver resection may be a treatment option for some benign and malignant liver tumors.

Benign

Adenoma

As a general rule, liver adenomas require resection because of their risk of rupture or bleeding. Resection can be limited, usually to a segmentectomy. Adenomas that have bled or ruptured require urgent/emergency surgery, with the resections largely being a debridement. Debate continues about surgery for patients with small adenomas (<4 cm) or multiple adenomas – observation is probably justified.

Focal nodular hyperplasia (FNH)

This benign condition is a common finding now that more patients have incidental imaging of the liver by ultrasound. FNH differs from adenoma in that all elements of the liver are present histologically and its complications are minimal. If accurately defined, particularly as an incidental finding, this entity does not require resection. The only indication for resection of FNH is if there is doubt as to diagnosis, or if it is symptomatic. FNH does not bleed, does not undergo malignant change, does not rupture, but occasionally may cause symptoms by pressure on adjacent structures.

Hemangioma

These are the most common of the benign liver tumors and range in size from a few millimeters to >20 cm. Again, these are often incidental findings when other imaging is done, and in asymptomatic patients they do not need to be removed. The greatest risks with hemangiomas are iatrogenic and often inappropriate interventions, either diagnostically or therapeutically. The occasional large hemangioma may require surgery, and these can be dealt with usually by enucleation because they form pseudocapsules. Even the most 'fearsome' hemangioma central in the liver is usually amenable to this approach.

Cystadenomas

These are benign cystic tumors of biliary origin that occur in the liver. Although rare, they may be confused with simple cysts and unlike simple cysts do not respond to deroofing. The differentiation of cystadenomas is made on pathology with a defined cuboidal epithelial lining to these tumors. They require a total excision to prevent recurrence. The majority of cystadenomas present with symptoms, which is the diagnostic clue that differentiates them from simple cysts.

Malignant

Hepatocellular carcinoma (HCC)

This is the most common primary liver tumor requiring resection. The indication for resection of an HCC is dictated by several factors: (1) the underlying etiology leading to HCC; (2) technical factors for resectability; and (3) the underlying liver disease and ability to tolerate resection.

Staging of HCC has received considerable attention over the last few years and plays a role in determining resectability. Staging should primarily be clinical using either the Italian or Spanish staging systems, which consider tumor size, morphology, the underlying liver disease, and patient performance status. Pathologic staging is only applicable to resected HCCs. In

INDICATIONS

BENIGN TUMORS
- Adenoma
- Focal nodular hyperplasia (rarely)
- Hemangioma (occasionally)
- Cystadenoma

MALIGNANT TUMORS
- Hepatocarcinoma (1 nodule <5 cm + good liver function)
- Cholangiocarcinoma
- Liver metastasis from:
  colorectal carcinoma
  neuroendocrine tumors

patients with advanced liver disease, development of HCC may become an indication for higher priority for liver transplantation.

Resection for HCC has acceptable outcomes for small (<5 cm) tumors in patients with well-preserved liver function (Child's Class A). Thus, patients without cirrhosis, or early cirrhosis with small tumor, may be managed by surgical resection. Intermediate staged tumors (>5 cm or >1 nodule) and patients with more advanced liver disease (portal hypertension and Child's Class B+) are poorer candidates for resection. Adverse prognostic factors are tumor size and vascular invasion (macro- or microscopic). In patients who have resection for HCC, approximately 50% have further intrahepatic HCC within 5 years.[6]

Cholangiocarcinoma

Intrahepatic cholangiocarcinoma may require liver resection. These tumors histologically are adenocarcinomas with either pathologic features suggestive of biliary origin, or determined by exclusion of other primary sites for adenocarcinoma. Resection is the optimal treatment for such cancers, but technical issues may limit the indication for resection. As some of these tumors occur in patients with primary sclerosing cholangitis, as with HCC the status of the underlying liver is important in making a decision to resect.

Secondary liver tumors

The indications for resection of secondary tumors in the liver are relatively limited, but are the most common reason for liver resection.[7] Colorectal carcinoma metastatic to the liver is the main indication to consider a resection. Neuroendocrine metastatic tumors also may be managed by resection. There are very few other primary cancers with metastases to the liver that warrant a liver resection, the exception being solitary metastasis, which has been present for a documented time interval.

Indications for both colorectal and neuroendocrine metastasis resection have expanded over the last 10 years, with a general guideline of 'if it is resectable, it probably should be resected.' The ability to resect such metastases with adequate margins, but at the same time preserve liver mass, has led to the above approach. For colorectal metastases, large single metastasis or multiple metastases confined to one lobe are the most common indications for resection. However, 'cherry picking' of individual lesions in the right and left liver may now be justified if such resection renders the patient visibly tumor free. The ability to do this has been greatly enhanced with improved intraoperative ultrasound. Resection may also be combined with ablation of residual disease (see below).

Contraindications

In general terms, contraindications to liver resection are either due to technical issues that make resection not feasible, or contraindications to liver resection based on underlying liver disease and poor liver function.

Technical contraindications are largely determined by burden of disease in the liver, involvement of major vascular structures, or the natural history of the underlying tumor.

Poor liver function as a contraindication to liver resection is seen primarily in patients with HCC and underlying cirrhosis. Liver resection may be appropriate and have satisfactory outcomes in HCC in Child's Class A patients, but is rarely indicated in patients with more advanced liver disease.

LIVER ABLATION

Introduction

Ablation of liver tumors is complementary to rather than competitive with liver resection. Ablation attempts to locally control a liver tumor by direct tissue destruction of the tumor and a rim of surrounding normal tissue. Ablation is more likely to be effective with well-circumscribed tumors rather than diffusely infiltrating liver tumors. Ablation may be indicated for primary and secondary malignant tumors in the liver, but is probably not indicated for any of the benign tumors.

Technique

Techniques of liver ablation have evolved over the last 20 years from direct tumor injection with absolute alcohol, to cryoablation, and currently radiofrequency ablation (Fig. 150.5). This technology will continue to evolve with other methods of tumor destruction. The key elements are the ability to focally destroy tissue, monitor the extent of destruction, and leave surrounding normal tissue undamaged.[8]

Placement of probes into tumors to deliver the modality being used for tissue destruction may be achieved percutaneously, at laparoscopy, or by open operation. All of the techniques require accurate imaging to define placement of probes, to monitor the extent of tissue destruction, and to avoid damage to surrounding vital structures, such as blood vessels or bile ducts. The technique used varies from center to center and at the present time is largely a factor of local expertise.

Indications

The indication for ablation of liver tumors is similar to that with resection of malignant tumors given above. Ablation may be considered instead of resection in patients with other significant comorbidities in whom a major resection is contraindicated. The complementary nature of ablation to resection extends the ability to reduce tumor burden in a liver that has too much disease to be con-

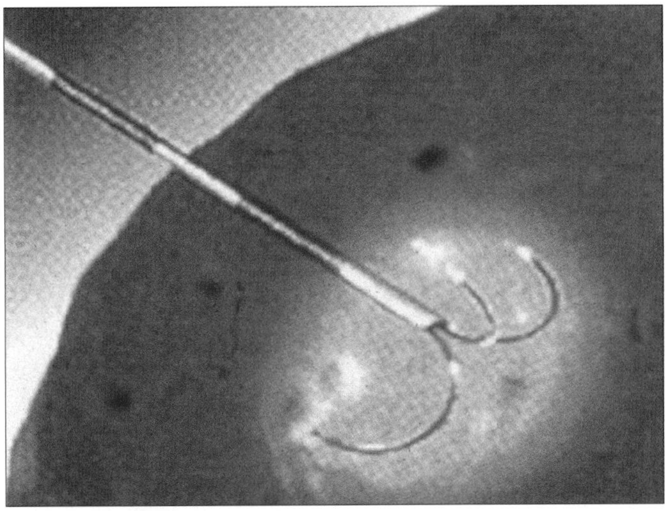

Fig. 150.5 Radiofrequency ablation of a liver tumor. The probe is placed into the tumor, opened, and an energy source applied sufficient to destroy the tumor and a rim of surrounding tissue. The ablation zone is monitored by ultrasound. From Meyers WC. Atlas of biliary surgery. In: Bell RH, Rikkers LF, Mulholland MW, eds. Digestive tract surgery; 1996:499–600. Reproduced with permission from Lippincott Williams & Wilkins.

sidered for resection. Thus, depending on the type of tumor, up to 10 foci of tumor within a liver may be ablated at a single setting.

Complications

The major local complications from ablation are bleeding and abscess formation. These occur with relatively low frequency (<10%) in experienced hands. The major late complication of ablation is tumor recurrence.

Outcomes

The results of surgical approaches to liver tumor ablations are variable with no controlled trials. Local recurrences, particularly in proximity to major vessels, occurs in 15–50% of cases, and de novo tumor appearance is a manifestation of the natural history of the tumors being treated. At the present time, the data appear to indicate that radiofrequency ablation is associated with fewer systemic or local side effects compared to cryoablation. This is probably the currently preferred treatment modality.

BILIARY PROCEDURES

Introduction

Operations on the bile duct may be done for benign or malignant conditions. Benign conditions requiring surgery are biliary strictures or injuries. The incidence of bile duct injuries in the laparoscopic cholecystectomy era has increased 2- to 3-fold and encompasses leaks, transections, and strictures.[9,10]

Technique

There are common themes to the surgical techniques for all biliary procedures:[12]

- Accurate definition of the anatomy is essential to make sure all the major segments of the liver are appropriately drained at the completion of the procedure (Fig. 150.2).
- Anastomoses of bile ducts to the GI tract require mucosa-to-mucosa apposition with normal tissues to avoid subsequent stricture (Fig. 150.6).
- All biliary procedures require close collaboration with a multidisciplinary team, including an endoscopist and an interventional radiologist to define and assist in managing bile duct pathology.
- Benign strictures do not require resection – normal duct, above the stricture, must be defined for anastomosis. Malignant tumors should be resected with surrounding nodes and lymphatics as illustrated in Fig. 150.7A,B.

When pathology includes the biliary bifurcation, be it tumor or stricture, it is helpful to the surgeon to have a transhepatic stent in place to define anatomy prior to exploration and help identify the bile duct by palpation at the operation. Prior to completing any biliary anastomosis, it is good practice to take intraoperative cholangiograms of the bile ducts being anastomosed to be certain all the main liver segments are drained. Anastomoses should be formed with absorbable sutures (PDS works well), ensuring apposition of mucosa from the Roux Y limb to a normal bile duct mucosa. Leaving stents across the anastomosis has the benefit of reducing the risk of an immediate biliary leak and allowing study of the anastomosis in the few weeks following the procedure. The anastomotic site should be drained for several days immediately following the procedure in case there is any bile leak. The transhepatic stent, if used, can be removed in 4–6 weeks.

Indications

The indications for biliary operations are either for benign or malignant conditions.

Benign biliary pathology requiring surgery includes primarily strictures and biliary leaks. The majority of patients are seen following cholecystectomy; there has been an approximately

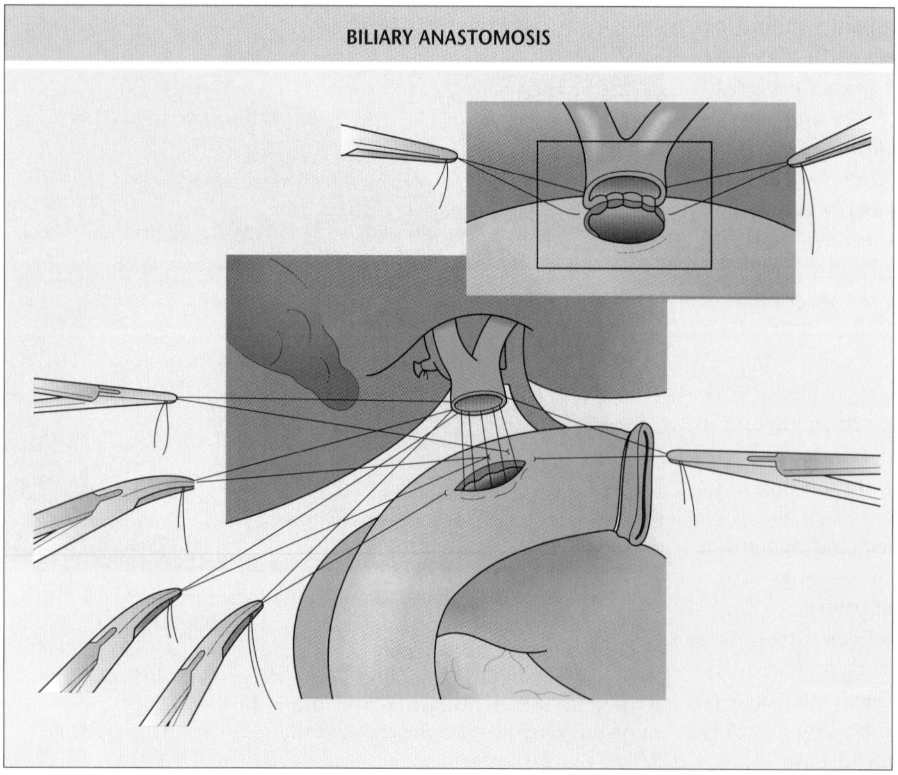

Fig. 150.6 Biliary anastomosis. Hepaticojejunostomy is fashioned with mucosa-to-mucosa opposition with interrupted absorbable suture. Decision to stent needs to be individualized. From Meyers WC. Atlas of biliary surgery. In: Bell RH, Rikkers LF, Mulholland MW, eds. Digestive tract surgery; 1996:499–600. Reproduced with permission from Lippincott Williams & Wilkins.

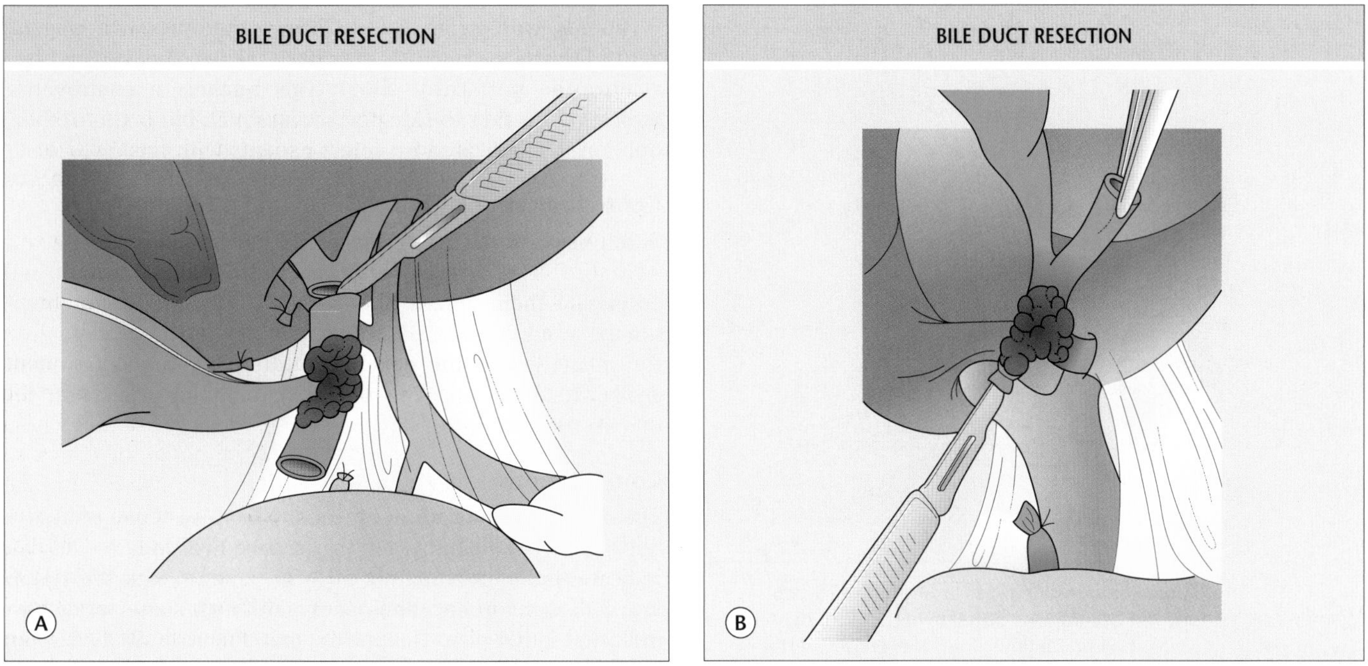

Fig. 150.7 Bile duct resection. A. A mid common duct tumor resected from suprapancreatic to the bifurcation. **B.** A bifurcation cholangiocarcinoma (Klatskin tumor) resected to the right and left intrahepatic ducts. For both tumors, the portal vein and hepatic artery are skeletonized to remove lymph nodes and lymphatics. From Meyers WC. Atlas of biliary surgery. In: Bell RH, Rikkers LF, Mulholland MW, eds. Digestive tract surgery; 1996:499–600. Reproduced with permission from Lippincott Williams & Wilkins.

twofold increase in such injuries in the laparoscopic era. Careful evaluation prior to operating is essential to optimize outcome. Biliary strictures may also occur with other pathology such as sclerosing cholangitis, pancreatitis, or extrinsic compression.

Malignant pathology requiring surgery is primarily bile duct tumors with cholangiocarcinoma being most common.[11] The majority of these patients present with an obstructive jaundice, and imaging studies will define the extent of pathology. The indications for and extent of resection is defined by the tumor. The additional evaluation for these malignancies is assessment of the vessels with either portal vein or hepatic artery involvement being a contraindication to resection.

Complications

Early complications are bile leak and infection. The risk of bile leak is minimized by careful technique as described above with mucosa-to-mucosa apposition. However, the risk increases with high lesions and small ducts, which make for difficult anastomoses. The role of stenting in minimizing leaks is debatable, but may provide a safety margin and can be achieved by either the transhepatic or internal route. The role of drains in anticipation of and for managing biliary leaks is also debatable. Most leaks close spontaneously given time provided there has been good apposition of the duct to the bowel mucosa.

Infection risk increases with an intraperitoneal bile leak, or when there has been an obstructed bile duct that has been stented. The risk is minimized by careful technique, anastomosis of healthy viable tissue, and by the use of perioperative antibiotics.

The main late complication of biliary procedures is an anastomotic stricture. Small bile ducts have greater risk of stricture than large bile ducts, recurrent operations carry a greater risk of stricture than first time operations, and operative repair in an infected field carries a greater risk than repair in a clean field. Monitoring for a recurrent stricture may have some value, and suspicion of recurrent stricture mandates a repeat study, usually a percutaneous transhepatic cholangiogram to define the anastomosis.

Outcomes

Biliary reconstruction gives good results in the hands of experts. Early leaks and anastomotic strictures occur in approximately 10% of primary biliary reconstructions. Results are less good when secondary or tertiary repairs are attempted. The higher the anastomosis and the smaller the bile ducts, the higher the complication rate.

The risk of prolonged biliary obstruction and of recurrent stricture is a secondary biliary cirrhosis and its associated morbidity.

PORTAL HYPERTENSION (see also Chapters 96 and 147)

Surgical intervention for portal hypertension has changed dramatically over the last 2 decades primarily because of widespread use of liver transplantation.[13] Liver transplant has become the definitive management for cirrhosis and portal hypertension and is discussed below. There are a limited number of patients who are eligible for operative shunts for decompression of bleeding varices, or who are candidates for devascularization procedures for variceal bleeding. There are virtually no indications currently for operative procedures for management of ascites, with the exception of patients with Budd-Chiari syndrome.

Technique

Operative shunts for portal hypertension fall into three categories:
- total portal systemic shunts;
- partial portal systemic shunts; and
- selective variceal decompression.

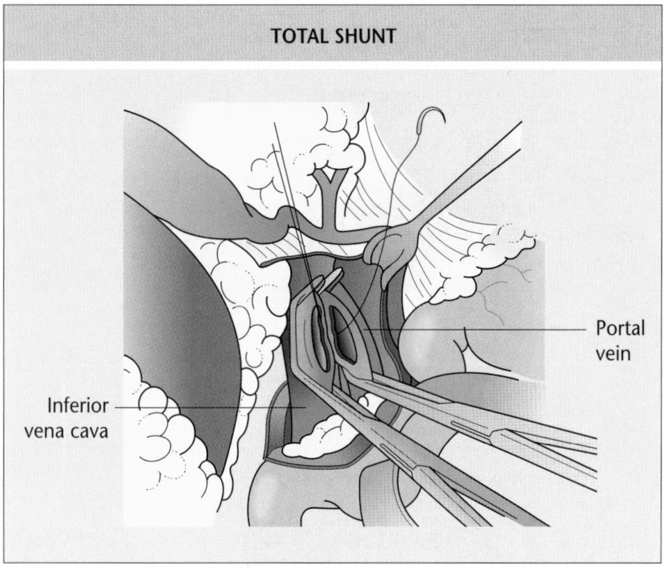

Fig. 150.8 Total shunt. Side-to-side portacaval shunt >10 mm diameter. This shunt will decompress portal hypertension, decompress the sinusoids, and divert all portal flow. From Meyers WC. Atlas of biliary surgery. In: Bell RH, Rikkers LF, Mulholland MW, eds. Digestive tract surgery; 1996:499–600. Reproduced with permission from Lippincott Williams & Wilkins.

Total portal systemic shunts

Total portal systemic shunts[14] are any shunt between the portal vein or one of its main tributaries and the inferior vena cava or one of its main tributaries that are greater than 10 mm in diameter. The classic total portal systemic shunt is a side-to-side portacaval shunt carried out just below the liver hilus. The portal vein and inferior vena cava can be mobilized sufficiently to be approximated in the majority of patients and a direct vein-to-vein anastomosis made between these two relatively robust vessels (Fig. 150.8). The anastomosis is fashioned between these two vessels over 1.5 cm with a direct vein-to-vein apposition. This shunt will decompress all portal hypertension very effectively as well as decompressing the hepatic sinusoids. A total shunt will effectively control variceal bleeding, control ascites, and decompress a congested liver of acute Budd-Chiari syndrome. The disadvantage is that it totally diverts all portal flow away from the liver, and thus has a higher incidence of hepatic encephalopathy than operations that maintain some portal flow. A total shunt at the hilus also makes subsequent transplant technically more difficult because it requires hilar dissection of the same vessels that are required for later transplant.

Indications

Total portal systemic shunts are rarely indicated at present. Their use for ongoing acute variceal bleeding not controlled with medical therapy has largely been replaced by the transjugular intrahepatic portosystemic shunt (TIPS). In some patients with recurrent variceal bleeding who are not candidates for endoscopic therapy or a TIPS, and who are not candidates for liver transplant (such as patients with ongoing active alcoholic liver disease) a side-to-side portacaval shunt will remove the bleeding risk for such patients. This may remain an indication for this operation.

Patients with acute Budd-Chiari syndrome with ongoing active hepatocyte necrosis may have the necrosis stopped by a side-to-side portacaval shunt. This remains a controversial indication for side-to-side portacaval shunt, but in this author's opinion it is indicated for select patients with this disease.

Contraindications

Side-to-side portacaval shunt is not indicated in patients with advanced liver disease and incipient liver failure. It will accelerate their course. Side-to-side portacaval shunt should not be used in patients who are likely to proceed to liver transplant within the next few years. They are better managed with TIPS and the operative field for transplant left undisturbed.

Complications

The major complication of total portal systemic shunts is hepatic encephalopathy and progressive liver failure. Old data indicate that approximately 50% of patients with this operation will develop encephalopathy, although some series have indicated otherwise. It appears that the risk of developing encephalopathy depends on the severity of the underlying liver disease in addition to the total diversion of portal flow. Thus, Child's Class A patients or alcoholics with good liver mass who have stopped drinking may tolerate this procedure reasonably well.

Other total portal systemic shunts that physiologically have the same effect are large-diameter mesocaval or mesorenal shunts that usually require interposition grafts >10 mm in diameter. The same principles as discussed above apply. The details of the operative procedure are beyond the scope of this chapter.

Partial portal systemic shunt and distal splenorenal shunt

Partial portal systemic shunt[15]

Technically, this operation requires the same exposure as a side-to-side total shunt outlined above. The difference is that an 8-mm interposition reinforced PTFE graft is placed between the portal vein and the inferior vena cava (Fig. 150.9). The advantage of this procedure is that, while it decompresses portal hypertension to approximately 10 mmHg, it has also been shown to maintain portal flow in approximately 80% of patients. This is associated with a lower rate of encephalopathy than a total portal systemic shunt.

Distal splenorenal shunt[16]

The operation most commonly used to decompress varices is a selective distal splenorenal shunt. This operation decompresses the varices trans-splenically through the splenic vein to the left renal vein, while at the same time maintaining portal hypertension and portal flow to the cirrhotic liver in the superior mesenteric and portal veins (Fig. 150.10). Over the last 2 decades this has been the most commonly used operation worldwide for management of variceal bleeding. This shunt decompresses the esophagus, stomach, and spleen by taking the splenic vein out of the back of the pancreas and bringing it down to the left renal vein for a comfortable anastomosis. The devascularization component interrupts all collaterals between the portal vein and this low-pressure system; thus, the left gastric and right gastric venous systems, the gastroepiploic, and the veins in the

PARTIAL SHUNT

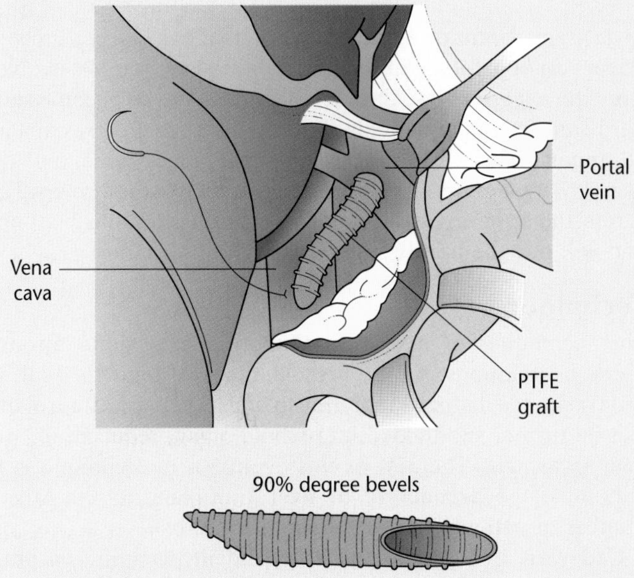

Fig. 150.9 Partial shunt. An 8-mm graft between the portal vein and IVC will decompress portal hypertension enough to control bleeding, but maintain some portal flow to the liver. From Meyers WC. Atlas of biliary surgery. In: Bell RH, Rikkers LF, Mulholland MW, eds. Digestive tract surgery; 1996:499–600. Reproduced with permission from Lippincott Williams & Wilkins.

DISTAL SPLENORENAL SHUNT

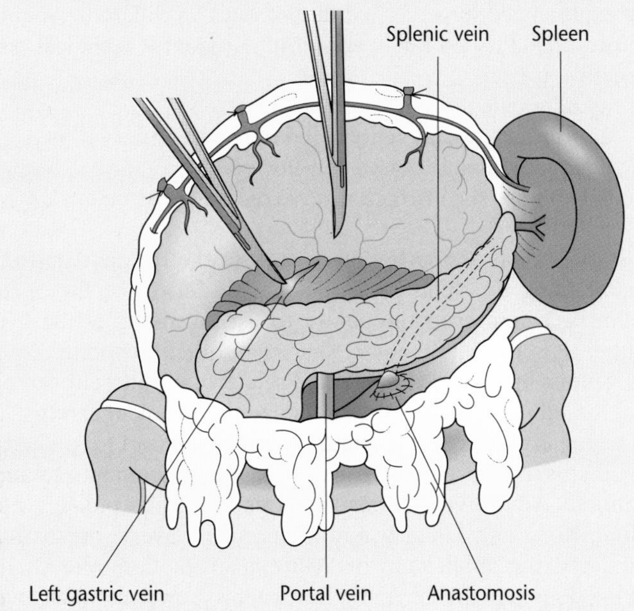

Fig. 150.10 Selective shunt. Distal splenorenal shunt decompresses varices and the spleen, but maintains portal hypertension and portal flow to the liver. From Meyers WC. Atlas of biliary surgery. In: Bell RH, Rikkers LF, Mulholland MW, eds. Digestive tract surgery; 1996:499–600. Reproduced with permission from Lippincott Williams & Wilkins.

mesocolon at the splenic hilus all need to be interrupted. This selective separation of the portal venous from the splenic venous system allows portal perfusion to be initially maintained in all patients. The development of collaterals, however, is more aggressive in patients with alcoholic cirrhosis than nonalcoholic cirrhosis, leading to loss of portal flow in approximately 50% of the alcoholic group. Control of bleeding has been excellent with distal splenorenal shunt and the incidence of encephalopathy lower than with total shunts.

Indications

The indications for both partial and selective variceal decompression are similar, as are the contraindications and complications:

- Variceal bleeding refractory to first-line treatment with pharmacologic and endoscopic therapy.
- Suitable anatomy for the selective shunt procedure. Adequate liver reserve to tolerate the operative procedure (Child's Class A and B patients).

Contraindications

- Advanced liver disease that will not tolerate a major operative procedure.
- Anatomy that is not suitable for surgical decompression.

Outcomes

Control of variceal bleeding with both partial and selective shunts has been greater than 90% in series published in the last two decades. Data on survival in Child's Class A and B patients over this time have shown 90% 1-year and 75% 5-year survival rates. The rate of encephalopathy for both of these procedures has been in the 10–20% range, and is largely a function of the underlying liver disease.

The choice between one of these operative procedures or TIPS remains one of the major controversies in decompression for management of variceal bleeding. A published randomized trial of partial shunt versus TIPS indicates superiority of the operative procedure over the radiologic procedure in terms of bleeding control, need for transplant, and overall complications. There is an ongoing prospective, randomized controlled trial being conducted of DSRS versus TIPS, funded by the National Institute of Health (NIH). This study closed entry in 2002 and data should be presented in 2005.

Complications

The early complications after both partial and selective shunts relate to the operative procedure and its effect on the liver. Liver decompensation can occur, ascites may be worsened, and infection is a risk. Careful attention to detail in patient selection, in operative technique, and in perioperative fluid, nutrition, and antibiotic management will minimize these immediate postoperative complications.

Late complications relate to progression of the liver disease with encephalopathy occurring with progressive disease, liver failure being a risk leading to the need for transplant in some patients.

DEVASCULARIZATION PROCEDURES

Surgical devascularization for management of variceal bleeding has been popular in Japan for several decades, and used

DEVASCULARIZATION

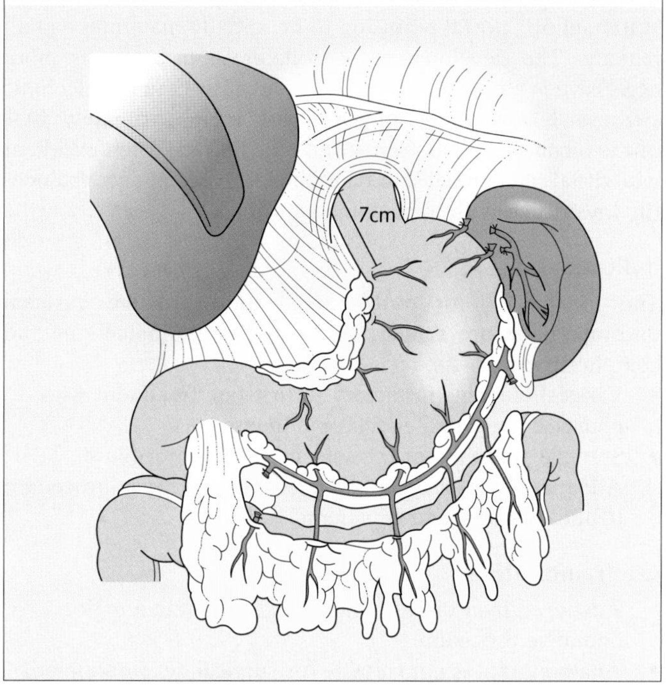

Fig. 150.11 Devascularization. The components of this operation are splenectomy, and gastric and esophageal devascularization. The goal is to reduce blood flow into varices at the gastroesophageal junction. From Meyers WC. Atlas of biliary surgery. In: Bell RH, Rikkers LF, Mulholland MW, eds. Digestive tract surgery; 1996:499–600. Reproduced with permission from Lippincott Williams & Wilkins.

selectively elsewhere. The principle is to reduce inflow to the varices with the operative components of splenectomy, gastric, and esophageal devascularization.

Technique

The operation is illustrated in Fig. 150.11. While initially described by Sugiura as a combined thoracic and abdominal procedure, it is now primarily done as an abdominal operation. The key element is adequate devascularization at the gastroesophageal junction, the most common site of bleeding; the distal 7 cm of the esophagus, the entire greater curvature of the stomach, and the upper two-thirds of the lesser curve should be devascularized. Esophageal transection was initially a component of this operation, but as most patients have had extensive sclerotherapy it is no longer advocated.

Indications

This operation is indicated for persistent variceal bleeding in patients with no shuntable vessels (extensive portal thrombosis).

Contraindications

Advanced liver disease is a contraindication as it increases operative risk.

Outcomes

Devascularization procedures have a higher rebleeding rate than operative shunts. While in Japan this is in <10% of cases, in the USA and Europe it is 20–40% at 3 years. Encephalopathy rates are lower than for shunt procedures.

LIVER TRANSPLANTATION (see also Chapters 106 and 107)

Introduction

Liver transplantation is the operation that has had the greatest impact on hepatology in the past 3 decades.[17, 18] It has evolved from the experimental, through the innovative, to become standard care for many patients. Indications have greatly expanded, organ availability has remained the major issue, and the use of living donors has come of age in the past few years. This is referred to in many other chapters throughout this textbook and will only be briefly summarized in this section.

Technique

The techniques of liver transplantation have gone through different iterations. At the present time we tend to think of cadaveric and living donor transplant. Cadaveric transplants can be further subdivided into whole organ, reduced, or split liver transplant. The aim of this evolution in technique is to maximize the availability of liver transplant to the largest number of patients who will benefit from it.

Cadaveric liver transplant is dependent primarily on brain dead donors, who are maintained on life-support until the time of organ harvest. Livers obtained from organ donors after cardiac death can be used, but have been shown to have poorer overall outcomes. The majority of liver transplants are performed using whole organ grafts, although the increased use of split livers, whereby two recipients are transplanted from one organ donor, has expanded the donor pool.[19] For split livers, it is best if the smaller left lateral segment is used for a pediatric recipient and the larger right segment plus segment 4 is used for an adult recipient. The techniques of implantation have become fairly standardized in terms of vascular anastomoses and biliary reconstruction. Many options and variations exist and are utilized by experienced surgeons in different ways for different patients.

The major issues for liver transplant from a technical perspective are:

- an adequate volume of viable liver;
- appropriate portal venous and hepatic arterial inflow;
- adequate hepatic venous outflow; and
- safe biliary reconstruction to avoid any obstruction or leak.

Preservation of appropriate vessels in the recipient, such as maintaining the vena cava or adequate length of the portal vein, have improved the ability to use segments of the liver rather than the whole organ. The use of other technology, such as venous bypass, is variable and selective in different centers and based upon factors that optimize the recipient safety.

Living donor liver transplant[20] was first utilized for pediatric recipients using segments 2 and 3 for implantation into smaller children. Adult living donor liver transplant was pioneered in Hong Kong and Japan where a lack of cadaveric organs had hindered the application of liver transplantation. The use of living donors in the USA and Europe has grown markedly over the last 5 years where this has become a viable option for some patients. In 2002, 358 pediatric and adult living donor liver transplants were carried out in the USA. Discussion continues as to the optimal graft, be it the whole right lobe or a left lobe graft for the adult population. The major issue that transplant centers face in living donor liver transplant is donor safety. Whichever graft is used, the donor operation is a major procedure in an otherwise totally healthy person and, as such, it inherently carries risk. There is mortality and over the last few years an increasingly documented morbidity to donors of liver grafts. Ongoing study and monitoring of this cohort is a priority.

Indications

The indications for liver transplantation have been dealt with elsewhere in this book (see Chapter 106). In general terms, the indication is end-stage liver disease, but the route by which this is defined varies with different diseases and different populations. Some diseases, such as primary sclerosing cholangitis and primary biliary cirrhosis (PBC), have a very predictable course with much better opportunity to define timing of transplant. Other diseases, such as hepatitis C or alcoholic cirrhosis, may remain 'compensated' until an acute event such as a variceal bleed or spontaneous bacterial peritonitis lead to rapid decompensation. Thus, although it is clear that most chronic liver diseases make patients candidates for transplant, timing remains a major issue. Defining disease severity has been a national priority over the last few years, which has led to the use and implementation of the MELD score for disease severity, and is the current system used for organ allocation.

Contraindications

The contraindications to liver transplantation continue to be defined. In broad terms, these can be thought of in terms of medical contraindications and psychosocial indications. As the criteria of indications for transplant have increased, the contraindications have diminished. Factors such as age, other medical comorbidities, with vascular and renal disease being dominant, and the whole issue of psychosocial contra-indications remain controversial. While standards are set, contraindications often remain.

SOURCES OF INFORMATION FOR PATIENTS AND DOCTORS

http://www.patient.co.uk/showdoc/583/

REFERENCES

1. Zimmermann H, Reichen J. Assessment of liver function in the surgical patient. In: Blumgart H, Fong Y, eds. Surgery of the liver and biliary tract, 3rd edn. Philadelphia: Saunders; 2000:35–63.
2. Malinchoc M, Kamath PS, Gordon FD et al. A model to predict poor survival in patients undergoing transjugular intrahepatic portosystemic shunts. Hepatology 2000; 31:864–871.
3. Bismuth H. Surgical anatomy and anatomical surgery of the liver. World J Surg 1982; 6:2.
4. Blumgart LH, Jarnigan W, Fong Y. Hepatic resection – Section 12. In: Blumgart H, Fong Y, eds. Surgery of the liver and biliary tract, 3rd edn. Philadephia: Saunders; 2000: 1639–1798.
5. Henderson JM, Sherman M, Tavill A et al. AHPBA/AJCC Consensus Conference on Staging of Hepatocellular Carcinoma: consensus statement. HPB 2003; 5:243–250.
6. Fan ST, Lo CM, Liu CL et al. Hepatectomy for hepatocellular carcinoma: towards zero hospital deaths. Ann Surg 1999; 229:322–330.
7. Fong Y, Fortner J, Sun RL et al. Clinical score for predicting recurrence after hepatic resection for metastatic colorectal cancer: analysis of 1001 consecutive cases. Ann Surg 1999; 230:309–318.
8. Helton WS. Minimizing complications with radiofrequency ablation for liver cancer. The importance of properly controlled clinical trials and standardized reporting. Ann Surg 1004; 239:459–463.
9. Melton GB, Lillemoe KD. The current management of postoperative bile duct strictures. Adv Surg 2002; 36:193–221.
10. Chapman WC, Abecassis M, Jarnagin W, Mulvihill S, Strasberg SM. Bile duct injuries 12 years after the introduction of laparoscopic cholecystectomy. J Gastrointest Surg 2003; 7:412–416.
11. Chamberlain RS, Blumgart LH. Hilar cholangiocarcinoma: a review and commentary. Ann Surg Oncol 2000; 7:55–66.
12. Meyers WC. Atlas of biliary surgery. In: Bell RH, Rikkers LF, Mulholland MW, eds. Digestive tract surgery. Philadelphia: Lippincott-Raven; 1996:499–600.
13. Henderson JM, Barnes DS, Geisinger MA. Portal hypertension. Curr Problems Surg 1998; 35:379–452.
14. Orloff JM, Orloff MS, Orloff SL, Rambotti M, Girard B. Three decades of experience with emergency portacaval shunt for acutely bleeding esophageal varices in 400 unselected patients with cirrhosis of the liver [see comments]. J Am College Surg 1995; 180:257–272.
15. Rosemurgy AS, Serofini FM, Zweibal BR et al. TIPS versus small diameter prosthetic H-graft portacaval shunt: extended follow-up of an expanded randomized prospective trial. J Gastrointest Surg 2000; 4:589–597.
16. Henderson JM, Nagle A, Curtas S, Geisinger MA, Barnes D. Surgical shunts and TIPS for variceal decompression in the 1990s. Surgery 2000; 128:540–547.
17. Keefe EB. Liver transplantation at the millennium. Past, present, and future. Clin Liver Dis 2000; 4:241–255.
18. Roberts J. Clinical liver transplantation. Am J Transplant 2001; 1:18–20.
19. Ghobrial RM, Busuttil RW. Future of adult living donor. Liver Transplant 2003; 9: 573–579.
20. Malago M, Hertl M, Testa G, Rogiers X, Broelsch CE. Split-liver transplantation: future use of scarce donor organs. World J Surg 2002; 26:275–282.

Chapter 151

Gastrointestinal operations

Robert J C Steele

KEY POINTS

- Surgery is the only definitive treatment for esophageal and gastric cancer
- Only 30% of patients with esophageal cancer have resectable disease at diagnosis and only 24% of these survive 5 years
- Assessment prior to reflux surgery should include gastroscopy, esophageal manometry, and 24-h pH manometry
- Partial fundoplication reduces the rate of gas bloat syndrome compared to previous operations
- Partial gastrectomy for gastric cancer is feasible if there is 5-cm clearance of tumor
- The extent of lymph node clearance required at gastrectomy for gastric cancer is debated
- The goal of surgery in small bowel Crohn's disease is to conserve as much functional intestine as possible
- Careful mesorectal excision reduces the recurrence rate of rectal cancer

INTRODUCTION

In this chapter the common operations carried out on the gastrointestinal tract are listed according to anatomy and pathology. In addition to a brief description of each operation, the main indications, contraindications, and complications are given, as well as the relative use of open and laparoscopic approaches.

ESOPHAGUS

Cancer (see Chapter 32)

Esophagectomy is the only definitive treatment for the vast majority of squamous and adenocarcinomas of the esophagus and represents the only chance of cure. Unfortunately, only about 30% of esophageal tumors are resectable but the overall 5-year survival rate after resection is 24%. For those in whom esophagectomy is carried out for curative intent the 5-year survival increases to 40%.[1]

The actual procedure carried out will depend largely on the position of the tumor. For adenocarcinoma of the lower third of the esophagus or the gastroesophageal junction a one-stage procedure through a left thoracotomy or left thoracoabdomino incision is commonly performed. Gastrointestinal continuity can be achieved either by using the stomach remnant or by creating a Roux-en-Y loop (Fig. 151.1). For tumors of the mid esophagus it is usual to carry out a two-stage procedure with mobilization of the stomach through a laparotomy incision followed by resection of the esophagus via a right thoracotomy and reconstruction using the mobilized stomach. Alternatively, a three-stage procedure can be carried out, which is similar to the two-stage with the exception that the anastomosis between the mobilized stomach and the esophageal remnant is carried out in the neck. A further alternative is to perform a trans-hiatal esophagectomy. This involves mobilizing the stomach and the esophagus via a laparotomy incision without opening the pleural cavities and then carrying out the anastomosis in the neck. This is preferable for more elderly patients and those with compromised respiratory function, but there are concerns about how radical a resection can be achieved.

The main contraindications to esophagectomy are non-resectability, an advanced tumor, and poor respiratory function. The main complications are respiratory failure after thoracotomy and anastomotic leakage. The mortality rate from esophagectomy, even in specialist centers, is in the region of 5–10%.

Bypass operations for esophageal cancer using segments of colon have now been almost entirely replaced by modern endoscopic stenting techniques but colon may still be used when esophagectomy is necessary following a previous gastrectomy.

Achalasia and other motility disorders

(see Chapter 40)

Surgical treatment of achalasia is indicated in children and young adults where repeated nonsurgical treatments may create morbidity, and after failure of pneumatic dilation or botulinum toxin injection therapy. The operation of choice, Heller's cardiomyotomy, involves anterior division of the muscle at the lower end of the esophagus down to the mucosa. This may be done through the left chest or the abdomen and in recent years a thoracoscopic or laparoscopic approach has become standard practice.[2] There is some debate as to the distal extent and limit of the myotomy but it is agreed that incision should be carried on to the stomach at least far enough to ensure complete division of the lower esophageal muscle layer. The main complication after achalasia (providing care is taken not to breach the mucosa) is gastroesophageal reflux. For this reason some surgeons will add an antireflux procedure (see below) to the cardiomyotomy. Occasionally, in long-standing achalasia with an immotile mega-esophagus, cardiomyotomy is ineffective and subtotal esophagectomy is necessary.

Other esophageal motility disorders (see Chapter 40) may be amenable to surgical treatment and a long esophageal myotomy has been advocated for both diffuse esophageal spasm and nutcracker esophagus. However, whether these are real clinical entities is controversial (see Chapter 40) and the results of treatment are highly variable and they should not be performed

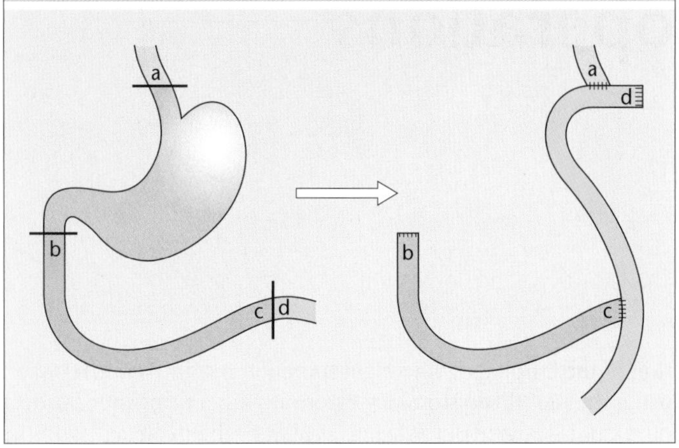

Fig. 151.1 Roux-en-Y reconstruction after total gastrectomy.

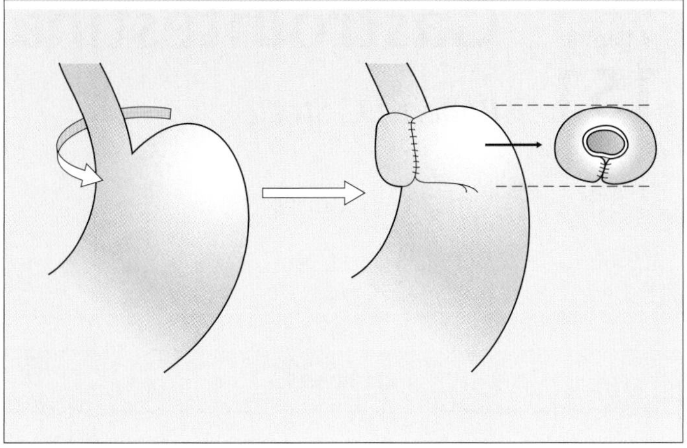

Fig. 151.2 Nissan fundoplication.

until attempts at controlling the symptoms by medical means have been exhausted.

Gastroesophageal reflux (see Chapter 29)

Surgery for gastroesophageal reflux is only appropriate in about 10% of patients with this condition owing to the effectiveness of modern medical management.[3] The indications include failure of medical management (particularly where volume reflux is an important issue), persistence of reflux in children beyond the age of 2 years, alkaline reflux after previous abdominal surgery, and patient preference. This last category is particularly relevant for young patients who do not wish to embark on a lifetime of medication. Prior to surgical intervention it is essential to establish the presence of gastroesophageal reflux beyond doubt and this involves upper gastrointestinal endoscopy, esophageal manometry, and 24-h pH monitoring. Once the decision to operate has been made there are a wide variety of operations; it is beyond the scope of this chapter to describe these but for the purposes of illustration four examples are given below.

Nissan fundoplication

Originally developed in the 1960s, this operation consists of repair of the hiatus hernia that is usually present and a circumferential fundal wrap around the esophagus (Fig. 151.2). This is thought to be effective because it realigns the lower esophagus with the esophageal crus and produces a pinch valve effect such that increased intragastric pressure, which would tend to promote reflux, exerts pressure on the lower esophagus via the wrap. It is important that the wrap is loose otherwise the patient will suffer from postoperative dysphagia. The Nissan fundoplication is highly effective in preventing reflux but approximately 20% of patients will suffer from gas bloat syndrome, which is due to distention of the stomach consequent on the inability to belch and vomit. Although Nissan fundoplication was previously done by open operation, most surgeons now use the laparoscopic approach.

Partial fundoplication

Owing to the problems of gas bloat following the classical Nissan operation, a variety of partial fundoplications have been developed. Perhaps the most common of these is the Toupet partial posterior fundoplication, which involves anchoring the fundus and the upper part of the posterior wall of the stomach to the right and left crura and then carrying out a partial (270 degree) fundoplication by suturing the stomach to the anterior wall of the esophagus. This appears to be associated with good control of reflux but a low incidence of gas bloat syndrome.

Belsey mark 4 repair

This procedure, favored by thoracic surgeons, is performed through a left thoracotomy. Here the stomach is rolled around the lower 3–5 cm of the anterior aspect of the mobilized esophagus by two wraps, the second covering the first and including the diaphragm. By this means the intra-abdominal segment of the esophagus is restored and, because the wrap is not circumferential, gas bloat syndrome is rarely a problem.

Angelchick prosthesis

This procedure has now been discredited owing to the high rate of postoperative dysphagia and migration of the prosthesis, which often required prosthesis removal, but it is mentioned here purely because gastroenterologists may well encounter patients who have had this procedure carried out. It involved the wrapping of a silicon gel split-ring prosthesis around the gastroesophageal junction after limited mobilization of the esophagus. Although control of reflux was good the high rate of complications has led to its abandonment.

STOMACH AND DUODENUM

Cancer (see Chapter 37)

For most adenocarcinomas of the stomach the only treatment that is potentially curative is a gastrectomy. The extent of the gastrectomy will depend upon the position and size of the tumor. Partial gastrectomy is adequate when a 5-cm clearance of the tumor is possible and this is usually the case for cancers of the antrum, but for cancers of the body and the cardia a total gastrectomy is usually necessary. Reconstruction after a distal partial gastrectomy can be achieved using either the Polya or the Billroth I procedure (Fig. 151.3). Although most surgeons prefer to use the Polya gastrectomy for cancer there is probably little to choose between the two operations. Reconstruction after total gastrectomy is usually performed using a Roux-en-Y loop (Fig. 151.1) although some advocate jejunal interpositions with or without pouch construction.

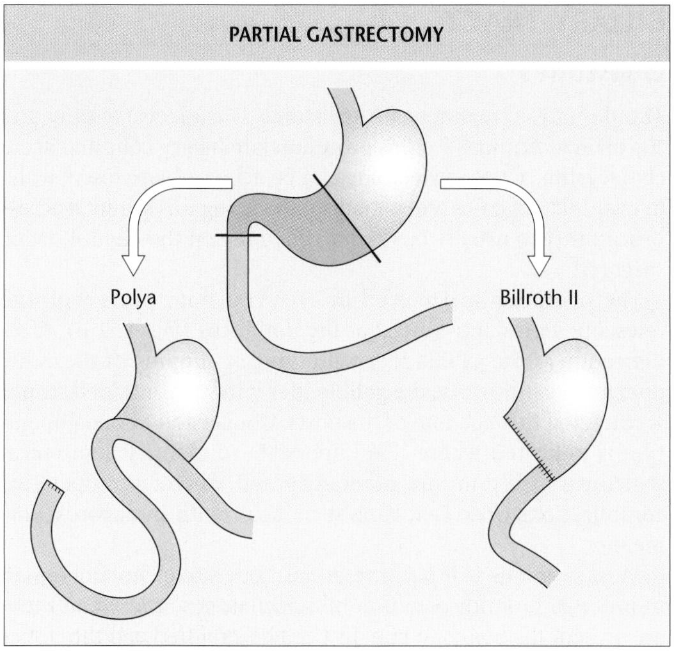

Fig. 151.3 Partial gastrectomy.

The main controversy in the performance of a gastrectomy for cancer is the extent of the lymphadenectomy. Traditionally in the West a D1 operation (removal of lymph nodes immediately adjacent to the part of the stomach being removed) has been the operation of choice, but over many years Japanese surgeons have advocated the use of a D2 or D3 resection, both of which are associated with additional clearance of the lymph nodes around the main arteries. Randomized trials carried out in the Netherlands and in the UK[4,5] have failed to show an advantage for the more radical operations but this may be related to surgical expertise and patient selection.

The main contraindication to gastrectomy in a fit patient is metastatic disease although it may still be appropriate to operate for palliation. The main complications of gastrectomy are anastomotic breakdown, nutritional problems, particularly weight loss, anemia, bone disease, dumping, reactive hypoglycemia, and bile vomiting.

Peptic ulcer disease (see Chapter 35)

Elective surgery

Elective surgery for peptic ulcer disease has almost completely disappeared from surgical gastroenterological practice. However, as there are still large numbers of individuals who have undergone surgical treatment for peptic ulcer in the past, it is important to mention the common operations. For duodenal ulcer the main procedures carried out up until the 1980s were truncal vagotomy and drainage (either pyloroplasty or gastrojejunostomy) or highly selective vagotomy (HSV). Latterly, HSV, which involved denervation of the fundus and the body of the stomach to reduce acid secretion without damaging the motility of the antrum, was the favored procedure.[6] For gastric ulcer a partial gastrectomy was usually favored, particularly as it was often impossible to exclude carcinoma. In the US a Polya type gastrectomy was also commonly used for duodenal ulcer owing to its low rate of recurrent disease.

The main complications arising from truncal vagotomy were dumping and postvagotomy diarrhea, both of which were considerably reduced by the introduction of HSV.

Emergency surgery

Surgery is still occasionally required for perforation, bleeding, and pyloric stenosis caused by peptic ulceration. Perforation (Fig. 151.4) is treated by simple closure of the ulcer whenever possible and thorough peritoneal lavage. This can now be accomplished by laparoscopy in skilled hands. For a bleeding peptic ulcer that has not responded to endoscopic therapy, simple oversewing of the bleeding vessel is recommended. For pyloric stenosis that does not respond to endoscopic dilatation, gastrojejunostomy is usually required. Few surgeons would now advocate adding vagotomy to any of these procedures preferring to rely on postoperative medical management.

Obesity

Antiobesity (or bariatric) surgery has been a growth area in western surgical practice in recent years. Jejunal bypass has been abandoned owing to the high risk of liver failure and currently used procedures depend on bypassing or reducing the capacity of the stomach. The most commonly performed operation is the vertical banded gastroplasty, which involves partitioning the stomach with staples and a band. This operation is effective but the revision rate is high at around 30%. Other operations include a Roux-en-Y gastric bypass, resectional gastric bypass and, most recently, laparoscopic adjustable gastric banding.[7] Contraindications to antiobesity surgery include patients at risk of postoperative cardiac complications, significant lung disease and significant psychological disorders. The main postoperative complications are disruption of staple lines, pouch dilatation, gastroesophageal reflux, and incisional hernia.

LIVER

Cancer (see Chapter 102)

Liver resection for cancer is employed in two main situations: for primary hepatocellular cancer and for limited metastatic disease from colorectal cancer. The liver can be subdivided into segments according to its portal venous blood supply (Fig. 151.5) and resections are carried out using these anatomical subdivisions. With modern techniques specialist surgeons can achieve hepatectomy with an operative mortality of less than 5% and minimal blood loss.[8]

For both primary and secondary liver cancer the aim is to achieve complete resection of all malignancy with a margin of

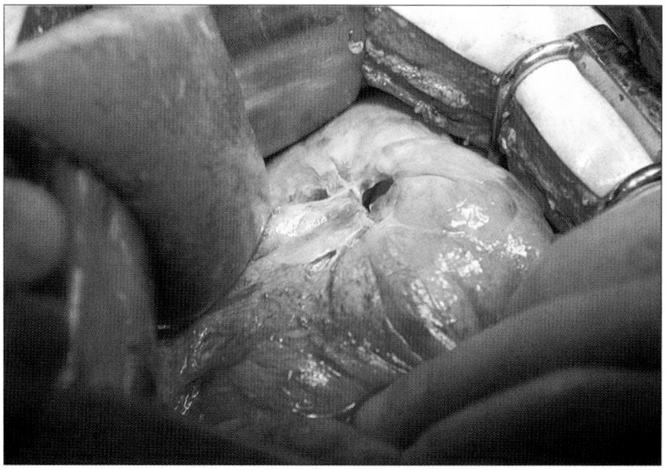

Fig. 151.4 Perforated peptic ulcer.

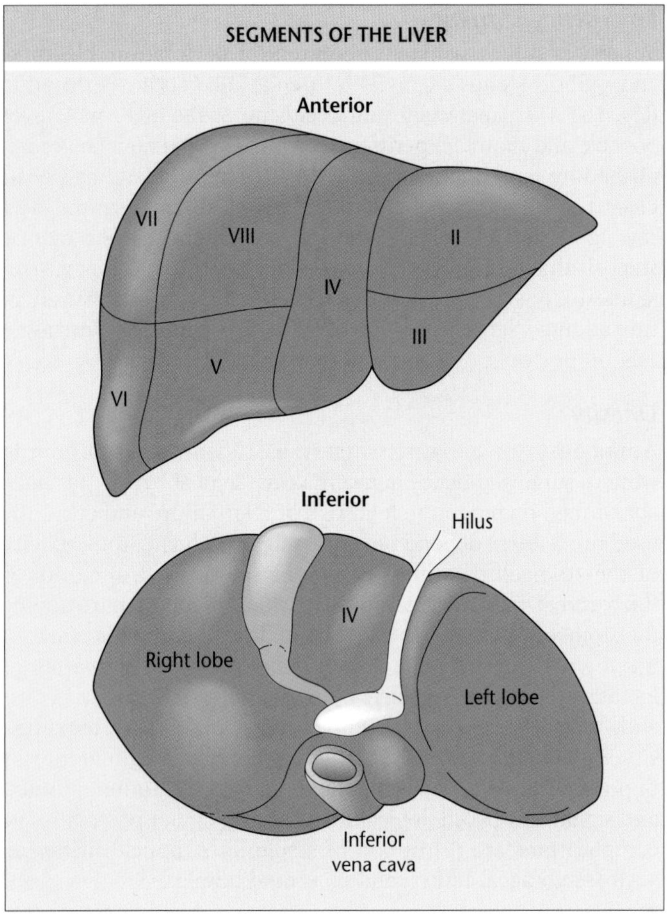

Fig. 151.5 Segments of the liver.

healthy liver tissue of 2 cm or more with sufficient residual liver tissue to sustain adequate liver function. Liver resection is contraindicated where this cannot be achieved and it must be remembered that in patients with cirrhosis (which often accompanies hepatocellular carcinoma) resection may be poorly tolerated. The main complications after a liver resection are hypoglycemia and coagulation defects, which can be treated by intravenous glucose and appropriate use of fresh frozen plasma and vitamin K injections. Hypoalbuminemia is almost inevitable and repeated plasma or albumin infusions may be required. The liver has a remarkable ability to regenerate and this occurs within 3 months if the remaining liver parenchyma is normal.

Transplantation (see Chapter 106)

Liver transplantation is indicated for irreversible hepatic failure and patients with primary biliary cirrhosis, primary sclerosing cholangitis, inborn errors of metabolism, and trauma have the best results with survival rates of around 80% at 5 years. Transplantation may also be used for end-stage cirrhosis and patients with extensive hepatocellular carcinoma confined to the liver. Livers for transplantation may be cadaveric, in which case the whole organ may be used, or from living donors where a liver split has to be employed. At the present time rejection rates are between 10% and 20% with the use of modern immunosuppression including the use of cyclosporin.[9]

BILIARY TRACT

Gallstones

The definitive treatment for gallstones is cholecystectomy and the main indications for this procedure are biliary colic and acute cholecystitis. Cholecystectomy can be achieved laparoscopically in over 90% of cases and patients undergoing this minimal access procedure can usually be discharged home on the day following surgery.[10]

The operation is achieved by means of four ports with the telescope being introduced at the umbilicus (Fig. 151.6). After dissection of the gallbladder with tying or clipping of the cystic duct and cystic artery, the gallbladder with its contained stones is extracted through one of the ports. Conversion to open operation is indicated where it is impossible to identify anatomical structures safely in any other way and where intraoperative complications arise that cannot be dealt with by laparoscopic means.

Most surgeons will perform an intraoperative cholangiogram in order to look for common bile duct stones, and when these are present the common bile duct can be explored and the stones removed. When this is done it is normal to close the common bile duct around a T-tube to provide decompression of the duct. The T-tube is removed at about 2 weeks after surgery. The main complications of cholecystectomy are bile duct stricture consequent on damage to the common bile duct and bile leakage usually after removal of a T-tube.

Bile duct strictures

Bile duct strictures can either be benign (usually postoperative) or malignant (cholangiocarcinoma). In either case the treatment is usually resection of the appropriate section of the bile duct with drainage into the gastrointestinal tract achieved by means of a Roux loop.

PANCREAS

Pancreatic cancer (see Chapter 73)

The most common operation for pancreatic cancer (other than palliative bypass) is the Whipple's operation. This involves removal of the head of the pancreas and the duodenum for either a carcinoma of either the pancreatic head or the ampulla of

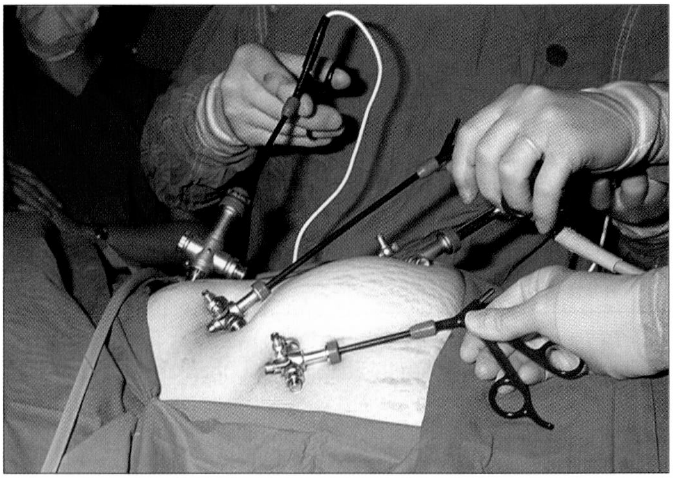

Fig. 151.6 Laparoscopic cholecystectomy. Arrangement of the ports.

Vater. Reconstruction is then achieved by anastomosing the jejunum to the stomach remnant, the common bile duct, and the body of the pancreas (Fig. 151.7). The 5-year survival after Whipple's operation for an ampullary tumor is in the region of 40% whereas this drops to less than 10% with true carcinoma of the head of the pancreas.[11] Carcinoma of the body or the tail of the pancreas is removed by the much simpler operation of distal pancreatic resection usually combined with splenectomy. Pancreatic resection is contraindicated in advanced tumors particularly where the portal vein is involved. The main specific complication following pancreatic resection is the development of a pancreatic fistula.

Chronic pancreatitis (see Chapter 72)

Chronic pancreatitis is particularly unrewarding to treat surgically except where chronic inflammation of the head of the pancreas is causing obstructive jaundice. In this instance a Whipple's operation is indicated and is associated with good results. Occasionally, surgery may be indicated for chronic pain where the main pancreatic duct is alternately strictured and dilated. Here, laying open the pancreatic duct and draining it into a loop of jejunum (Peustow operation) may alleviate the symptoms.[12]

Acute pancreatitis (see Chapter 71)

In a patient with acute pancreatitis complicated by infected pancreatic necrosis, necrosectomy (removal of necrotic pancreatic tissue) may be indicated as a life-saving procedure although the mortality associated with this procedure is in the region of 50%.[13] It is indicated where contrast-enhanced CT scanning in a patient with severe acute pancreatitis demonstrates nonperfusion of the pancreatic gland and subsequent needle aspiration reveals bacterial infection. The other situation in which surgery may be indicated in a patient with acute pancreatitis is for the internal drainage of a pancreatic pseudocyst. It is important to allow the cyst to mature over several weeks before operation and the most commonly performed procedure is a cystogastrostomy allowing the cyst to drain into the stomach. External drainage of large established pseudocysts is rarely successful.

SMALL BOWEL

Crohn's disease (see Chapter 54)

Surgery for small bowel Crohn's disease is usually indicated for obstructive symptoms caused by stricturing. Although small bowel resection may be necessary in these cases the aim is to retain as much functioning intestine as possible and in many instances it may be possible to alleviate obstructive symptoms by means of strictureplasty. The cumulative recurrence rate after small bowel resection for Crohn's disease is 30% at 5 years, 50% at 10 years, and 60% at 15 years.[14]

Other indications for surgery in small bowel Crohn's disease is growth retardation in children, particularly those with ileocecal disease. Here, resection is usually followed by a growth spurt. Surgery is also usually required for Crohn's related abscesses and fistulae and for the rare complication of massive hemorrhage. Unfortunately, operations for Crohn's disease are followed by a high incidence (10%) of postoperative complications including anastomotic leakage and fistula formation, and the operative mortality for reoperation ranges from 2% to 8%. In patients who have undergone extensive resection intestinal failure may develop.

COLON

Cancer (see Chapter 60)

The definitive treatment for colon cancer is resection, and this is associated with an overall 5-year survival in the region of 40–45%. In general terms, tumors of the cecum and ascending colon are treated by right hemicolectomy, those of the transverse colon by extended right hemicolectomy, those of the descending colon by left hemicolectomy, and those in the sigmoid by sigmoid colectomy. Although the majority of these operations are still performed by means of open surgery an increasing number are being carried out laparoscopically. For a number of years it was considered that laparoscopic resection may compromise oncological principles but the emerging results from randomized trials do not substantiate these fears.[15]

After resection anastomosis is achieved either by means of stapling devices or hand suturing (Fig. 151.8) and the anastomotic leakage rate should be less than 5%.[16] The other complications of colectomy are those of any major intra-abdominal operation including hemorrhage, postoperative myocardial infarction, deep vein thrombosis, chest infection, pulmonary embolus, ileus, and wound infection/dehiscence. All patients undergoing colectomy should have antibiotic prophylaxis and measures to prevent deep vein thrombosis (subcutaneous low molecular weight heparin).

Diverticular disease (see Chapter 65)

Surgery for uncomplicated diverticular disease is now very rarely performed and even patients with diverticulitis are usually

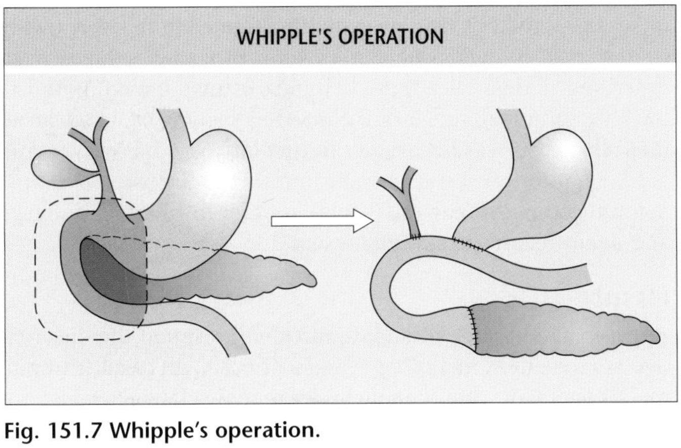

Fig. 151.7 Whipple's operation.

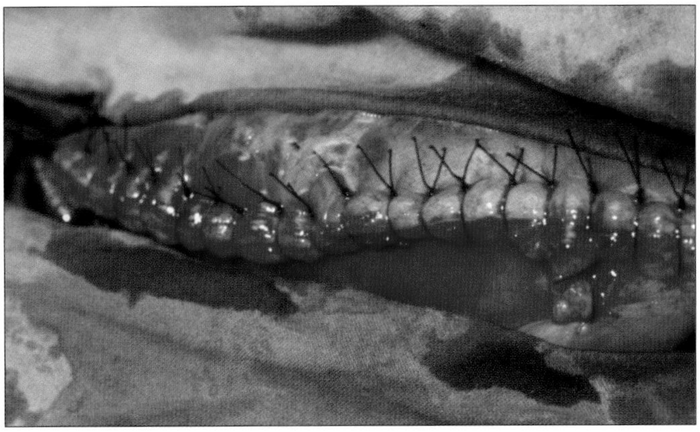

Fig. 151.8 Hand-sewn anastomosis.

treated conservatively. However, in a patient with perforated diverticular disease it is necessary to carry out a colectomy (usually sigmoid) and this is commonly done as a Hartmann's procedure where the proximal colon is brought out as a colostomy and the rectal stump over-sewn. Reanastomosis can be performed at a later stage when all inflammation has resolved. The other main indications for operating for diverticular disease are stricture formation causing obstructive symptoms and massive hemorrhage.

Inflammatory bowel disease

In the patient with ulcerative colitis emergency surgery is indicated for severe disease that fails to respond to medical treatment, perforation, and bleeding. Elective surgical treatment is required for failure of medical management, growth retardation in young patients, and the development of colonic malignancy. The correct surgical treatment for ulcerative colitis is panproctocolectomy with either permanent end ileostomy or reconstruction by means of an ileo-anal pouch.[17] In the emergency situation it is common practice to carry out a subtotal colectomy going on to proctectomy with or without pouch reconstruction at a later stage.

The specific complications of panproctocolectomy are either those of the ileostomy (ileostomy diarrhea, stenosis, retraction, and skin problems associated with ileostomy effluent) or with a pouch (frequency of bowel action and pouchitis). In patients with Crohn's colitis it is usual to avoid ileo-anal pouch formation owing to the risk of small bowel Crohn's disease. In some cases of Crohn's colitis it may be appropriate to carry out a segmental resection according to the distribution of the disease. This is never indicated in patients with ulcerative colitis.

Constipation (see Chapter 63)

A proportion of patients with idiopathic constipation may benefit from colectomy and ileo-rectal anastomosis.[18] This is only indicated, however, if marker studies indicate that there is no evidence of obstructed defecation with confirmation by normal anal manometry, normal electromyography, and normal evacuation proctography. Even then about 25% of patients will still be troubled by constipation and a further 25% will have troublesome diarrhea. In some instances it may be necessary to resort to ileostomy but patients may continue to be troubled by abdominal pain and bloating owing to impaired small bowel motility. Another approach to intractable idiopathic constipation is appendicostomy where the appendix is brought out as a stoma and can be used as a conduit to irrigate the colon on a regular basis.

RECTUM

Cancer (see Chapter 60D)

The standard surgical approach for cancer of the rectum is either anterior resection (with anastomosis between the distal colon and rectal remnant or anal canal) or abdominoperineal resection of the rectum (with permanent end colostomy). The choice between these two operations depends on a combination of the position of the tumor within the rectum and the patient's body habitus, but in general terms tumors of the upper two-thirds of the rectum should be amenable to anterior resection whereas those of the lower third of the rectum usually require abdominoperineal resection.

In both of these procedures the principle of mesorectal excision is now firmly established. This involves careful dissection in the plane immediately outside the fatty tissue surrounding the rectum with careful preservation of the pelvic nerves. Adoption of this procedure has led to a reduction in local recurrence rates after surgery for rectal cancer from around 30% to less than 10%.[19] In addition, taking care to avoid damage to the pelvic nerves minimizes the risk of urinary and sexual dysfunction. Under certain circumstances transanal local excision of early rectal cancer may be possible but is associated with higher risk of locally recurrent disease than radical surgery.

Rectal prolapse (see Chapter 70)

A full-thickness rectal prolapse can only be treated by surgical repair. The most definitive procedure is rectopexy where the rectum is mobilized transabdominally down to the pelvic floor and fixed to the sacrum. This is now commonly combined with a sigmoid resection to eliminate redundant large bowel and reduce the risk of postoperative constipation.[20] Increasingly, this procedure is being carried out laparoscopically. A number of other procedures are available but the most successful alternative to rectopexy is perineal rectosigmoidectomy where the redundant rectum and sigmoid colon are excised through the perineum and continuity is restored by a coloanal anastomosis.

ANAL CANAL

Hemorrhoids (see Chapter 70)

Although there are a number of office procedures available for the treatment of hemorrhoids, patients with symptomatic third or fourth degree hemorrhoids are best treated by a formal hemorrhoidectomy. In modern practice this is carried out with the patient in the prone position using diathermy, and with the use of local anesthesia this may now be performed as a day-case procedure. It is, however, still associated with significant postoperative discomfort and the alternative operation of stapled anopexy is gaining ground. In this procedure a stapling device is used to excise a circular disk of rectal mucosa just above the anal canal restoring continuity with a line of staples. This pulls the anal cushions back up into an anatomical position and randomized trials indicate similar results to conventional hemorrhoidectomy but with less postoperative pain.[21]

Fistula-in-ano

The low-level or intersphincteric fistula may be treated safely by laying open (Fig. 151.9). However, the higher trans-sphincteric or supra-sphincteric fistulae cannot be treated in this way owing to the risk of incontinence. Various procedures have been described to deal with these complex fistulae including fistula track excision with repair of the internal opening by an advancement flap.[22] The results are not particularly good, however, and in many instances it is necessary to resort to the use of a simple Seton (ligature through the fistula) in order to maintain drainage and avoid recurrent perianal sepsis.

Fissure

Approximately 80% of anal fissures will respond to conservative management including the use of 0.2% glyceryl trinitrate (GTN) ointment[23] but the remainder require a lateral sphincterotomy, which involves dividing the fibers of the internal anal

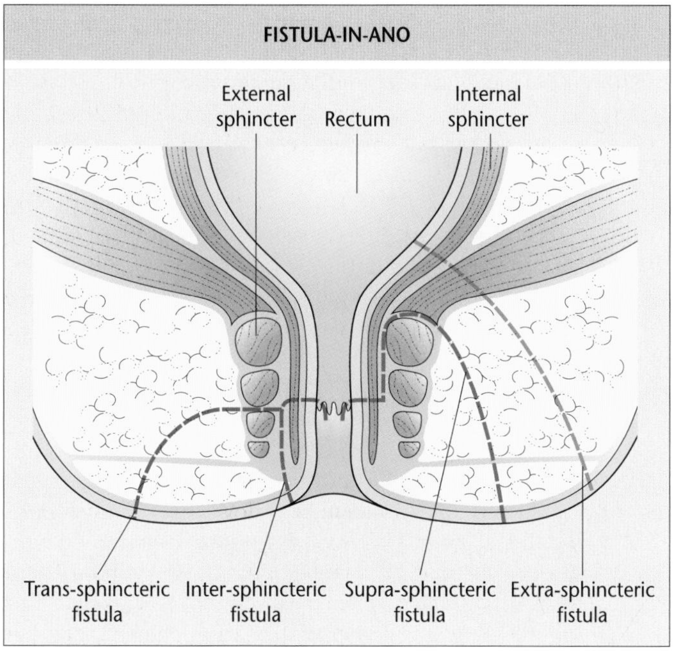

Fig. 151.9 Fistula-in-ano.

sphincter up to the level of the dentate line. This is associated with a high rate of fissure healing but may be complicated by minor degrees of incontinence, particularly to mucus.

Incontinence

Surgery for incontinence is only successful when a defined defect in the external anal sphincter is responsible. This is diagnosed preoperatively by transanal ultrasound and surgical treatment by means of an overlapping repair will improve symptoms in between 60% and 80% of cases. In patients who are not suitable for a straightforward sphincter repair, reconstruction using the gracilis muscle can be attempted but for this to be successful the gracilis muscle requires electrical stimulation.[24] Unfortunately, the failure rate of this procedure is high and this has stimulated interest in a variety of artificial sphincter devices that can be implanted around the anal canal. In a proportion of patients, however, permanent colostomy may be the only solution to the problem.

SOURCES OF INFORMATION FOR PATIENTS AND DOCTORS

http://www.betterhealth.vic.gov.au/bhcv2/bhcarticles.nsf/pages/Anal_fissure?Open
http://www.patient.co.uk/showdoc/583/

REFERENCES

1. Leonard GD, McCaffrey JA, Maher M. Optimal therapy for oesophageal cancer. Cancer Treat Rev 2003; 29:275–282.
2. Balaji NS, Peters JH. Minimally invasive surgery for esophageal motility disorders. Surg Clin North Am 2002; 82:763–782.
3. Tutuian R, Castell DO. Management of gastroesophageal reflux disease. Am J Med Sci 2003; 326:309–318.
4. Bonenkamp JJ, Songun I, Hermans J et al. Randomised comparison of morbidity after D1 and D2 dissection for gastric cancer in 996 Dutch patients. Lancet 1995; 345:745–748.
5. Cuschieri A, Weeden S, Fielding J et al. Patient survival after D1 and D2 resections for gastric cancer: long-term results of the MRC randomised surgical trial. Surgical Co-operative Group. Br J Cancer 1999; 79:1522–1530.
6. Johnston D. Operative technique of highly selective (parietal cell) vagotomy. Acta Chir Scand Suppl 1988; 547:49–53.
7. Fisher BL, Shauer P. Medical and surgical options in the treatment of severe obesity. Am J Surg 2002; 184(6B):9S–16S.
8. Allen PJ, Jarnagin WR. Current status of hepatic resection. Adv Surg 2003; 37:29–49.
9. Nash KL, Gimson AE. Liver transplantation. Hosp Med 2003; 64:200–204.
10. Scott-Conner CE. Laparoscopic gastrointestinal surgery. Med Clin North Am 2002; 86:1401–1422.
11. Yeo CJ. The Whipple operation: is a radical resection of benefit? Adv Surg 2003; 37:1–27.
12. Hartel M, Tempia-Caliera AA, Wente MN et al. Evidence-based surgery in chronic pancreatitis. Langenbecks Arch Surg 2003; 388:132–139.
13. Hartwig W, Werner J, Uhl W, Buchler MW. Management of infection in acute pancreatitis. J Hepatobiliary Pancreat Surg 2002; 9:423–428.
14. Delaney CP, Fazio VW. Crohn's disease of the small bowel. Surg Clin North Am 2001; 81:137–158.
15. Pikarsky AJ. Update on prospective randomised trials of laparoscopic surgery for colorectal cancer. Surg Oncol Clin N Am 2001; 10:639–653.
16. Leslie A, Steele RJC. The serosubmucosal anastomosis – still the gold standard. Colorectal Dis 2003; 5:362–366
17. Sagar PM, Pemberton JH. Ileo-anal pouch function and dysfunction. Dig Dis 1997; 15:172–188.
18. Bharucha AE, Phillips SF. Slow transit constipation. Gastroenterol Clin North Am 2001; 30:77–95.
19. Quirke P. Training and quality assurance for rectal cancer: 20 years of data is enough. Lancet Oncol 2003; 4:695–702.
20. Karulf RE, Madoff RD, Goldberg SM. Rectal prolapse. Curr Probl Surg 2001; 38:771–832.
21. Ashraf S, Srivastava P, Hershman MJ. Stapled haemorrhoidectomy: a novel procedure. Hosp Med 2003; 64:526–529.
22. McLeod RS. Management of fistula-in-ano: 1990 Roussel Lecture. Can J Surg 1991; 34: 581–585.
23. Utzig MJ, Kroesen AJ, Buhr HJ. Concepts of pathogenesis and treatment of chronic anal fissure a review of the literature. Am J Gastroenterol 2003; 98:968–974.
24. Hinninghofen H, Enck P. Fecal incontinence: evaluation and treatment. Gastroenterol Clin North Am 2003; 32:685–706.

Chapter 152

Minimally invasive surgery

Todd A Ponsky and Jeffrey L Ponsky

KEY POINTS

- Laparoscopic surgery has advantages over open surgery in biliary surgery, abdominal hernia and hiatus hernia repair
- The incidence of bile duct injury is 0.6% with an 8% mortality
- Bile duct leak should be suspected in patients with post-operative jaundice, nausea, abdominal pain and/or fever
- Laparoscopy is the treatment of choice for elective splenectomy
- The role of laparoscopic colectomy in oncology is under evaluation
- Laparoscopic antireflux surgery should be considered in gastroesophageal reflux disease patients who are refractory to medical therapy, or unwilling to take long-term medication

GENERAL LAPAROSCOPIC TECHNIQUE

- Cut-down to peritoneal cavity at umbilicus and insertion of 10-mm trocar
- CO_2 insufflation to create tension pneumoperitoneum
- Insertion of camera through 10-mm port
- Placement of subsequent trocars through 5-mm incisions
- Performance of operation by inserting instruments through the trocars
- Removal of trocars and release of CO_2
- Incision closure
- Bowel or vascular injury from trocar insertion may necessitate conversion to open

INTRODUCTION

The first report of laparoscopy was in 1910 when Kelling explored an insufflated abdomen with a cystoscope. Laparoscopy was thereafter utilized primarily within the field of gynecology. The first general surgical application of laparoscopy was a cholecystectomy performed in Germany by Muhe in 1985. Since then, laparoscopic surgery has advanced at an extraordinary pace to the point where almost every surgical operation has undergone some sort of minimally invasive transformation. The decrease in pain, shortened hospital stay, earlier return to work, and improved cosmesis has enhanced its popularity.

For the past 20 years minimally invasive surgery has been synonymous with laparoscopy. However, robotic surgery and therapeutic surgical endoscopy have entered the arena of everyday surgical practice. While endoscopic surgery is still in its infancy, many believe that there is a movement towards ‘incision free’ surgery.

DESCRIPTION OF TECHNIQUE

General laparoscopic technique

The first step of all laparoscopic procedures is entry into the peritoneum. This can be accomplished by either an open, cut-down procedure or by insertion of a needle into the abdomen. Carbon dioxide is slowly pumped into the abdomen to distend the peritoneal cavity and create an open space for operating. A camera is then placed through a small hole in the abdomen, typically at the umbilicus. Subsequent small holes are placed in different locations throughout the abdomen and special ports, called trocars, are placed into these holes. Instruments can be inserted and removed through these ports as needed throughout the operation. Following the operation, all ports are removed and the carbon dioxide is released from the peritoneal space.

COMPLICATIONS AND THEIR MANAGEMENT

Risks of laparoscopy in general include major intra-abdominal vascular or visceral injury during trocar placement. The incidence of bowel injury is approximately 0.05–0.3%.[1] Major vascular injuries may also occur during trocar placement and carry approximately a 15% mortality rate. Minor bleeding or bowel injury may occasionally be repaired laparoscopically. In the face of brisk, uncontrollable bleeding or a significant bowel injury, conversion to an open procedure is necessary.

GALLBLADDER SURGERY

Description of technique

Although there are minor variations to the procedure, most cholecystectomies today are performed through four small incisions measuring from 5 to 10 mm in length at the umbilicus, epigastrium, right upper quadrant, and right lower quadrant. The basic steps of the operation involve dissection of the gallbladder from surrounding adhesions, dissection of the triangle of Calot (Fig. 152.1), identification and ligation of the cystic artery and duct, removal of the gallbladder from the liver bed, and removal of the gallbladder from one of the 10-mm port sites. Once the cystic duct has been identified, a cholangiogram is often performed. This involves making a small incision in the cystic duct, inserting a catheter into the duct and injecting contrast under fluoroscopy. This helps to more clearly assess the biliary anatomy and to evaluate for choledocholithiasis.

Indications/contraindications

The indications for laparoscopic cholecystectomy are the same as for the open technique, and include biliary colic, biliary dyskinesia, and acute cholecystitis (see Chapter 76). The only exception is gallbladder carcinoma, which should be treated with open cholecystectomy to ensure an adequate resection and to eliminate the possibility of port site tumor cell seeding. Liver cirrhosis, pregnancy, morbid obesity, or previous right upper quadrant surgery are not contraindications for laparoscopic cholecystectomy.[2]

Most patients have minimal postoperative pain and usually are discharged to home from the recovery room or are admitted overnight and discharged the following morning. Patients can usually return to work within 1 week.

INDICATIONS/CONTRAINDICATIONS
LAPAROSCOPIC CHOLECYSTECTOMY
INDICATIONS • Biliary colic • Biliary dyskinesia • Acute cholecystitis • Chronic cholecystitis **CONTRAINDICATIONS** • Gallbladder cancer

Complications and their management

The overall complication rate from laparoscopic cholecystectomy is approximately 0.38%.[3]

Bleeding

Intraoperative bleeding may occur during dissection of the gallbladder at the triangle of Calot or from the liver bed. Prudent dissection and identification of the cystic artery with absolute secure ligation is essential. Bleeding may also result from major vascular injury during trocar insertion or in the postoperative period as a result of a slipped clip around the cystic duct, relaxation from a vessel that was in spasm intraoperatively, or from the liver bed. In the face of tachycardia, hypotension, change in mental status, decreased urine output, increased abdominal distention, and/or a drop in hemoglobin the patient should be taken back to the operating room for re-exploration, either laparoscopically or open.

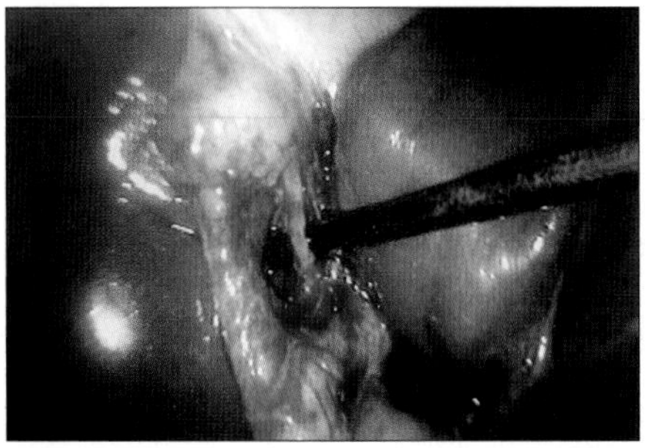

Fig. 152.1 Dissection of triangle of Calot.

Bile duct injury

The most feared complication of a laparoscopic cholecystectomy is bile duct injury. The variable anatomy of the extrahepatic biliary tree, pericholecystic inflammation, and/or inadequate dissection and identification of the triangle of Calot may contribute to injury. Injury may range from a small pinhole to a complete transection.

The incidence of bile duct injury is approximately 0.6% with an 8% mortality rate.[4] Approximately half of bile duct injuries are identified at the time of injury while 30% are discovered postoperatively. Injury carries a high risk of eventual bile duct stricture. Many advocate routine intraoperative cholangiography to help identify extrahepatic biliary anatomy and decrease the chance of misidentification or injury.

Patients presenting with postoperative jaundice, nausea, abdominal pain, and/or fever should be investigated for a bile leak. When a bile leak is suspected the work-up should start with a computed tomography (CT) scan or ultrasound to evaluate for a subhepatic fluid collection. This can be followed by a hepatic indolacetic acid (HIDA) scan or endoscopic retrograde cholangiopancreatography (ERCP). ERCP offers both diagnosis and possible therapy through stent placement and sphincterotomy.

COMPLICATIONS
LAPAROSCOPIC CHOLECYSTECTOMY
• Bleeding • Bile duct injury

VENTRAL HERNIA REPAIR

Introduction

Given the unacceptably high rate of recurrence of ventral hernias, laparoscopic repair of incisional, abdominal wall hernias is growing in popularity (see Chapter 118). Laparoscopic ventral hernia repair provides tension-free closure of the abdominal wall defect. Data suggest that laparoscopic ventral hernia repair has a lower recurrence rate than open repair with mesh.[5–7] The majority of patients are discharged from hospital on the second postoperative day.[6] While many have claimed recurrence rates of less than 5%, others have suggested that with longer follow-up the recurrence rate is closer to 17%.[8]

Description of technique

The operation typically begins with insertion of a 10-mm camera port. The location of this port varies but should be safely away from the suspected hernia defect. Once pneumoperitoneum is attained, two to three subsequent ports are placed under direct vision. Adhesiolysis is performed with blunt and sharp dissection until the entire defect is cleared with a 3–4-cm border of visualized peritoneum. A piece of mesh large enough to cover the entire defect is rolled and placed into the abdomen through a 10-mm trocar. The mesh is unfurled and is attached to the abdominal wall with full-thickness, through and through fascial sutures. The mesh is tacked to the peritoneum and fascia with a tacking device. The trocars are removed and the incisions are closed.

Indications/contraindications

It is generally recommended that midline ventral hernias greater than 3–5 cm in diameter be repaired laparoscopically.[9] Contraindications for laparoscopic repair include any pre-existing intra-abdominal infection, intraoperative enterotomy, open abdominal wound, or poor skin coverage over fascial defect. Noncentral defects or multiple previous abdominal operations are not contraindications to laparoscopic ventral hernia repairs.

INDICATIONS/CONTRAINDICATIONS
VENTRAL HERNIA REPAIR
INDICATIONS • Ventral hernias greater than 3–5 cm in diameter **CONTRAINDICATIONS** • Pre-existing intra-abdominal infection • Intraoperative enterotomy • Open abdominal wound • Poor skin coverage over fascial defect

Complications and their management

Complications of this procedure include mesh/wound infection, hernia recurrence, seroma, and bowel or vascular injury. Patients who present with postoperative fever, leukocytosis, wound erythema and/or fluctuance, and a fluid collection around the mesh on CT scan will probably warrant removal of the mesh through a midline incision with primary closure of the fascia if possible. The presence of a fluid collection in the absence of signs of infection is most likely a seroma and is usually managed expectantly.

While recurrence may occur with this operation, the incidence is lower than in any of the other repair options. Repair of a recurrent hernia after laparoscopic repair presents a challenge especially if the mesh is adherent to the underlying bowel.

COMPLICATIONS
VENTRAL HERNIA REPAIR
• Mesh/wound infection • Hernia recurrence • Seroma • Bowel or vascular injury

INGUINAL HERNIA REPAIR

For years there has been immense debate as to the most effective and symptom-free repair of inguinal hernias. Most surgeons now agree that the most effective repair is a 'tension-free' repair with mesh (see Chapter 118). There has been debate as to which procedure is ideal, laparoscopic or open. Although there is disagreement among many of the studies, most agree that with the laparoscopic repair there is less pain and an earlier return to work but not necessarily a decrease in recurrence.

Description of technique

There are essentially two techniques, the transabdominal preperitoneal repair (TAPP) and the total extraperitoneal repair (TEP). Both techniques ultimately describe placing a piece of mesh into the preperitoneal space. In the TAPP procedure, an incision is made in the peritoneum in order to access the preperitoneal space. In the TEP procedure, the peritoneum is never entered: the entire dissection takes place within the preperitoneal space. Both procedures typically require three trocar site incisions. Once in the preperitoneal space, both procedures involve dissection and exposure of the pubic bone medially (Fig. 152.2), identification of the hernia, reduction of the direct hernia sac, if present, examination for and reduction of an indirect hernia sac, and dissection and identification of the vas deferens and gonadal vessels. Finally, a piece of polypropylene mesh is placed from the pubic bone medially to the internal ring laterally, covering the cord structures and extending into the space of Retzius. Most patients are discharged to home from the recovery room.

Indications/contraindications

Most of the contraindications are relative contraindications including previous lower abdominal or extraperitoneal surgery (retropubic prostatectomy), pelvic radiation, or patients who would not tolerate general anesthesia.[10]

INDICATIONS/CONTRAINDICATIONS
INGUINAL HERNIA REPAIR
INDICATIONS • Presence of an inguinal hernia **CONTRAINDICATIONS** • Would not tolerate general anesthesia **RELATIVE CONTRAINDICATIONS** • Previous lower abdominal or extraperitoneal surgery (retropubic prostatectomy), or pelvic irradiation

Complications and their management

Laparoscopic inguinal hernia repairs are associated with the same complications seen with open repair, with additive risks associated with laparoscopy in general. There is no difference in the complication rate between the laparoscopic and open approaches. The complication rates vary from 3.8% to 13.6% for both open and laparoscopic repairs.[10]

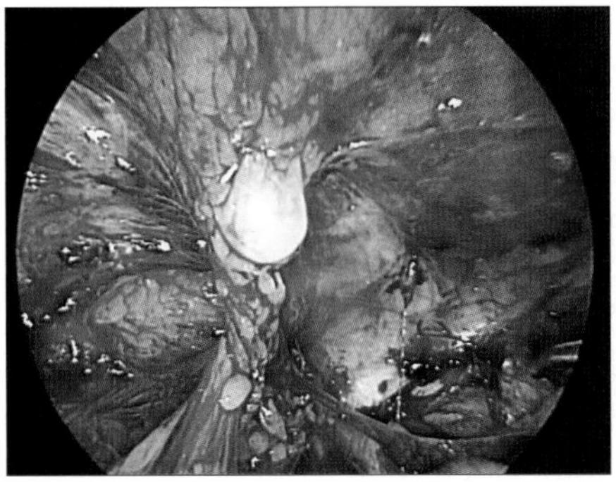

Fig. 152.2 Laparoscopic hernia anatomy.

The most common complications are postoperative urinary retention, hematoma, leg or groin pain from an injured or impinged nerve, seroma, or wound infection. Most of these complications can be managed expectantly. Most wound infections can be managed by simply opening the wound and draining the infection. A complicated wound infection, however, suggested by pus or erythema from the wound accompanied by systemic signs of infection, may require reoperation with removal of the mesh and a primary repair.

COMPLICATIONS
INGUINAL HERNIA REPAIR
• Mesh/wound infection • Hernia recurrence • Postoperative urinary retention • Hematoma • Leg or groin pain from an injured or impinged nerve • Wound infection

SPLENECTOMY

Introduction

Laparoscopic splenectomy is one of the most common laparoscopic solid organ procedures. The laparoscopic technique appears to have decreased blood loss, shorter hospital stay, and faster recovery. It is the procedure of choice for elective splenectomy. As with open splenectomy, patients should undergo pneumococcal vaccination.

Description of technique

The procedure typically involves three trocars. The spleen is freed from the pancreaticosplenic ligament, splenocolic ligament, lienorenal ligament and lienophrenic ligament followed by dissection of the gastrosplenic ligament and short gastric vessels. The splenic artery and vein are typically ligated at the splenic hilum with a laparoscopic stapling device (Fig. 152.3). Careful attention is paid to avoiding injury to the tail of the pancreas, which lies very close to the spleen. Once dissected free, the spleen is placed into an endoscopic bag in which it is morselized and brought out through one of the larger trocar sites.[11]

Indications/contraindications

The elective indications for laparoscopic splenectomy are the same as for open splenectomy and include specific circumstances of immune thrombocytopenic purpura (ITP), sickle cell disease, β-thalassemia, hereditary spherocytosis, Gaucher's disease, lymphoma, angiosarcoma, and occasionally large cysts or abscesses. ITP is the most common indication for elective splenectomy in adults and is indicated if the thrombocytopenia is refractory to medical therapy or relapses after an initial response.[12] The indications and contraindications are currently evolving. While it has been suggested that splenomegaly and trauma are contraindications to laparoscopic splenectomy, others believe that it depends on the experience of the surgeon.

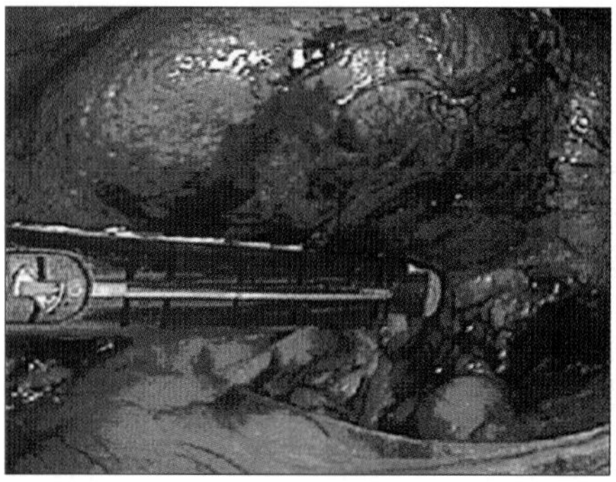

Fig. 152.3 Transection of splenic hilum.

INDICATIONS/CONTRAINDICATIONS
SPLENECTOMY
INDICATIONS • ITP • Sickle cell disease • β-thalassemia • Hereditary spherocytosis • Gaucher's disease • Lymphoma/angiosarcoma • Occasional large cysts or abscesses **CONTRAINDICATIONS** • Splenomegaly • Trauma

Complications and their management

Laparoscopic splenectomy is a relatively safe procedure and may even have fewer complications than the open procedure. Morbidity rates for open splenectomy have ranged from 15% to 61% and mortality rates between 6% and 13%, whereas laparoscopic morbidity and mortality rates range from 0% to 15% and 0% to 5%, respectively. It is difficult, however, to compare these outcomes given that the more critical patients are frequently selected to undergo an open procedure.[13]

Complications include intraoperative and postoperative bleeding, pancreatic injury, postoperative thrombocytopenia from a missed accessory spleen or splenosis, postoperative thrombocytosis, overwhelming postsplenectomy sepsis (OPSS), subphrenic abscess, and pleural effusions.

The most common reasons for intraoperative bleeding are coagulopathy from thrombocytopenia or technical error including vessel injury during dissection or loss of a surgical tie. Bleeding related to coagulopathy can be minimized by administering clotting factors or platelets prior to or during the operation. Platelet transfusion is typically reserved for counts less than 10 000 cells/μL.[14]

COLECTOMY

Introduction

Just when laparoscopy had become accepted as a reasonable alternative to many elective operations, the introduction of laparoscopic colectomy demonstrated the role of laparoscopy in oncologic surgery. While it is clear that this procedure offers a cosmetic benefit to the open procedure, many have questioned whether or not this procedure offered the same survival benefit as its open counterpart.

COMPLICATIONS
SPLENECTOMY
• Bleeding • Pancreatic injury • Postoperative thrombocytopenia from a missed accessory spleen or splenosis • Postoperative thrombocytosis • Overwhelming postsplenectomy sepsis (OPSS) • Subphrenic abscess • Pleural effusions

In 1994, the American Society of Colon and Rectal Surgeons released a policy statement that said until convincing data were published, laparoscopic colectomies should only be performed within clinical trials.[15] In a prospective randomized trial of 219 patients with a 4-year follow-up, patients in the laparoscopic group had a lower morbidity rate, shortened hospital stay, decreased tumor recurrence, and improved cancer-related survival.[16] While these data are intriguing, further studies with larger cohorts are necessary in order to confirm these results.

Description of technique

Laparoscopic colectomy begins with the placement of four trocar ports. The steps of the colectomy are the same as for the open procedure and involve mobilization of the segment of colon to be resected, division of the mesentery, resection of the involved segment of colon, and restoration of continuity or formation of a stoma. Once the colon has been resected and continuity restored, a small midline incision is made just large enough to remove the resected segment of colon.

Indications/contraindications

As stated above, many still consider laparoscopy to be an experimental technique in those patients with potentially curable colon cancer. However, as evidenced by Milsom et al. at the Cleveland Clinic in 2000, laparoscopic colectomy may be beneficial for palliative resection in patients with stage IV colorectal cancer.[17] Other indications for laparoscopic colectomy may be polyps, diverticular disease, colovesicular fistula, phlegmon, chronic constipation, rectal prolapse, ulcerative colitis, fecal incontinence, stoma formation, or any other benign colonic disorder. Relative contraindications may include morbid obesity, multiple previous operations, or bulky or fixed tumors.

INDICATIONS/CONTRAINDICATIONS
LAPAROSCOPIC COLECTOMY
INDICATIONS • Colon cancer (controversial) • Palliative colon resection or stoma formation • Polyps • Any benign colonic disorder requiring operation **RELATIVE CONTRAINDICATIONS** • Morbid obesity • Multiple previous operations • Bulky or fixed tumors

Complications and their management

Intraoperative complications include hemorrhage, inadvertent enterotomy, ureteral injury, and iliac or other major vessel injury.[18] Significant bowel, vessel, or bladder injury usually necessitates conversion to an open procedure. Conversion rates have been reported to range from 1.45% to 48% with the mean conversion rate of approximately 17.5%.[18] Postoperative complications include anastomotic leak or breakdown, urinary incontinence, deep venous thrombosis, delayed bleeding, or delayed identification of ureter injury. Delayed identification of ureter injury may be treated with stent placement or re-exploration and primary repair. The complication rate of laparoscopic colectomy is similar to open colectomy approximating 0% to 12%.[18]

COMPLICATIONS
LAPAROSCOPIC COLECTOMY
INTRAOPERATIVE COMPLICATIONS • Hemorrhage • Inadvertent enterotomy • Ureteral injury • Iliac or other major vessel injury **POSTOPERATIVE COMPLICATIONS** • Anastomotic leak or breakdown • Urinary incontinence • Deep venous thrombosis • Delayed bleeding • Delayed identification of ureteral injury

ANTIREFLUX SURGERY

Introduction

The optimal treatment for gastroesophageal reflux disease (GERD) continues to be debated (see Chapter 29). The Veterans Affairs Cooperative Trial in 2001 performed a prospective randomized trial comparing medication versus surgical therapy for GERD.[19] Sixty-two per cent of patients who had undergone an open Nissen fundoplication reported continued dependency on antisecretory medication. The gastroesophageal reflux disease activity index (GRACI), however, was significantly lower in the surgical group. More recent trials have shown that surgical therapy has a significantly lower failure rate than medical therapy.[20] Dallemagne et al. described the first laparoscopic Nissen in 1991.[21] Since then the procedure has been perfected and has now become the gold standard operation.[2,22,23]

Description of technique

The procedure typically begins with approximately five trocar incisions in the upper abdomen. The dissection begins with mobilization of the esophagus from the surrounding tissue within the diaphragmatic hiatus and the crura are closed (Fig. 152.4). The short gastric vessels are then divided in order to mobilize

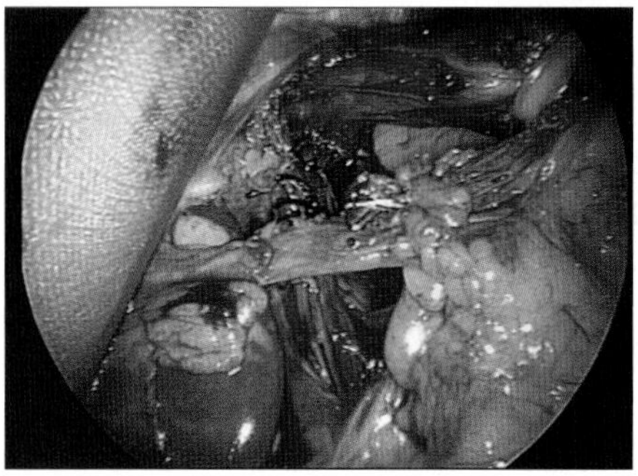

Fig. 152.4 Diaphragmatic hiatus. View of diaphragmatic hiatus with accessory left hepatic artery.

gastric fundus, which is then wrapped loosely around the posterior side of the esophagus and sutured to itself anteriorly. This creates a 360 degree wrap. Partial fundoplications such as the Toupet or Dor may have a decreased incidence of postoperative dysphagia but may not offer the same long-term efficacy.[2]

Indications and contraindications

Because debate still exists regarding surgical versus medical therapy for GERD (see Chapter 29), the decision to operate should be decided on a case-by-case basis. There are, however, certain circumstances that most agree are best treated with surgical therapy. These include intolerance to medical therapy because of side effects, or patients who do not wish to deal with the inconvenience of long-term medical therapy.[24] A poor response to medical therapy is often cited as an indication but one should be cautious in this group of patients. In some their poor response to medical therapy may indicate that they do not have GERD.

Absolute contraindications to surgery include those patients who cannot tolerate general anesthesia or have an uncorrectable coagulopathy. Previous upper abdominal operations as well as chronic reflux with associated esophageal shortening or diminished peristalsis may be relative contraindications to laparoscopic antireflux surgery.[25] While some consider morbid obesity a relative contraindication, others have noted that in experienced hands, morbid obesity has no higher morbidity than other patients.[26]

INDICATIONS/CONTRAINDICATIONS
LAPAROSCOPIC NISSEN
INDICATIONS • Intolerance to medical therapy • Poor response to medical therapy • Patients who do not desire long-term medical therapy • Intractable esophageal ulcer or stricture • Recurrent aspiration **ABSOLUTE CONTRAINDICATIONS** • Inability to tolerate general anesthesia • Uncorrectable coagulopathy **RELATIVE CONTRAINDICATIONS** • Previous upper abdominal operations • Chronic reflux with associated esophageal shortening or diminished peristalsis

Complications and their management

Intraoperative complications include bleeding and esophageal or gastric perforation. Bleeding most often occurs from the short gastric vessels during the mobilization of the gastric fundus. While most bleeding can be controlled laparoscopically, uncontrollable bleeding may warrant conversion to an open procedure. The advent of ultrasonic shears allows a safer dissection of the blood vessels as this device coagulates blood vessels as it divides tissue. While an unrecognized esophageal or gastric perforation may be fatal, early recognition and repair is usually feasible laparoscopically.

Dysphagia: While most surgeons perform the gastric wrap with a calibrated esophageal bougie in place, occasionally the wrap may be too tight leading to postoperative dysphagia. This is the most common postoperative complication and occurs in between 2% and 17% of patients.[2,27] Most cases of postoperative dysphagia resolve; however, about 4% of patients will continue to have long-term symptoms. These patients are typically treated with endoscopic dilatations. It is rare that reoperative surgery is required to treat the dysphagia. Occasionally, patients complain of gas bloat, inability to belch, nausea, dumping symptoms, or diarrhea. Most of these symptoms resolve and can usually be managed conservatively.

Newer therapies: While laparoscopic Nissen is still considered the standard of care for surgical therapy of GERD, newer therapies are under investigation for the treatment of GERD. The Stretta procedure involves trans-oral delivery of radiofrequency energy to the lower esophageal sphincter (LES). This allows scar formation at the LES, which in turn decreases transient LES relaxations. Preliminary results are encouraging but long-term outcome data are required. Recent reports do, however, show encouraging results with this technique.[23,28]

Another technique to reduce GERD symptoms that is currently under investigation is endoscopic suturing. This technique involves plicating the gastric cardia in order to increase the angle of His using an endoscopic suturing device. This modality is still in its infancy and there have been no studies to date that demonstrate convincing efficacy.[23]

COMPLICATIONS
LAPAROSCOPIC NISSEN
INTRAOPERATIVE COMPLICATIONS • Hemorrhage • Esophageal or gastric perforation **POSTOPERATIVE COMPLICATIONS** • Dysphagia • Gas bloat/inability to belch • Nausea • Dumping symptoms • Diarrhea

MORBID OBESITY

Obesity has become an increasingly more prevalent disease in the US; 55% of Americans are obese.[29] With this increase, the demand for weight loss surgery has intensified. The Roux-en-Y gastric bypass (RYGB) operation has become one of the most commonly performed operations with encouraging results. Recently, however, a laparoscopic technique for this operation has been developed and is being adopted universally. The operation has two components: gastric restriction and biliary-pancreatic diversion. By diverting the biliary and pancreatic secretions to the more distal small bowel, ingested food spends less time in contact with the digestive enzymes and absorption is limited.

Debate still exists as to the safety of the laparoscopic RYGB. However, data have shown that in experienced hands laparoscopic RYGB offers lower perioperative morbidity, shorter hospital stay, and quicker recovery compared to open RYGB.[30,31] Given that morbidly obese patients have a particularly high risk of wound complications including infection, dehiscence, and incisional hernia, many advocate that the smaller incisions with the laparoscopic procedure offer a significant advantage. At present both the laparoscopic and the open procedure are accepted as the standard of care.

OTHER LAPAROSCOPIC PROCEDURES

There are many other procedures that are being performed laparoscopically such as appendectomy, pancreatectomy (Fig. 152.5), paraesophageal hernia repair, adrenalectomy, liver thermal ablation, feeding tube placement, small bowel resection, and mesenteric lymph node biopsy. In fact, many of these, such as laparoscopic appendectomy, are slowly becoming the standard of care.

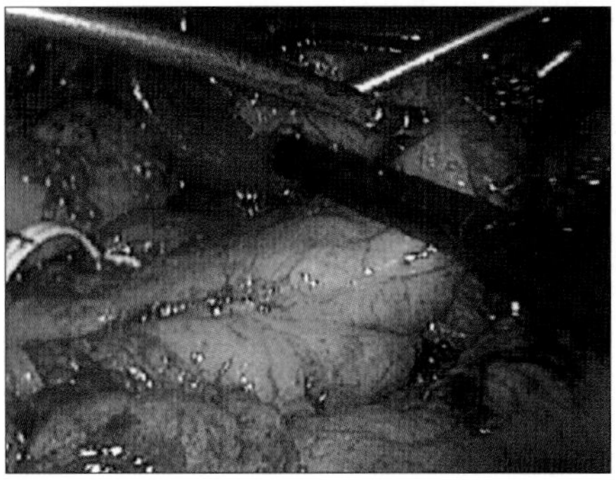

Fig. 152.5 Laparoscopic ultrasound. Laparoscopic ultrasound probe is used to localize a pancreatic lesion.

THE FUTURE

In the current era of surgical training, residents are introduced to laparoscopy from the outset. The next generation of surgeons will be more comfortable and facile with laparoscopy and this will promote further advances within the field. In fact, laparoscopy itself may be replaced by newer, more advanced technology such as robotic surgery. Advocates of robotic surgery note that it offers the surgeon six degrees of freedom versus three with laparoscopy. This offers the surgeon more 'life-like' mobility. Furthermore, with robotics, telesurgery can allow surgeons to perform delicate operations from a remote location. Some suggest that the ultimate in minimally invasive surgery may be endoscopic. Transvisceral surgical applications of endoscopy are currently being investigated and this may be the solution to 'incision-free' surgery.

SOURCES OF INFORMATION FOR PATIENTS AND DOCTORS

http://www.patient.co.uk/showdoc/27000468/

REFERENCES

1. Phillips P, Amaral J. Abdominal access complications in laparoscopic surgery. J Am Coll Surg 2001; 192:525–536.
2. Scott-Conner CE. Laparoscopic gastrointestinal surgery. Med Clin North Am 2002; 86:1401–1422.
3. Ponsky JL. Complications of laparoscopic cholecystectomy. Am J Surg 1991; 161:393–395.
4. Gigot J, Etienne J, Aerts R et al. The dramatic reality of biliary tract injury during laparoscopic cholecystectomy. An anonymous multicenter Belgian survey of 65 patients. Surg Endosc 1997; 11:1171–1178.
5. Cassar K, Munro A. Surgical treatment of incisional hernia. Br J Surg 2002; 89:534–545.
6. Ramshaw BJ, Esartia P, Schwab J et al. Comparison of laparoscopic and open ventral herniorrhaphy. Am Surg 1999; 65:827–831; discussion 831–832.
7. Goodney PP, Birkmeyer CM, Birkmeyer JD. Short-term outcomes of laparoscopic and open ventral hernia repair: a meta-analysis. Arch Surg 2002; 137:1161–1165.
8. Rosen M, Brody F, Ponsky J et al. Recurrence after laparoscopic ventral hernia repair. Surg Endosc 2003; 17:123–128.
9. Dumanian GA, Denham W. Comparison of repair techniques for major incisional hernias. Am J Surg 2003; 185:61–65.
10. Davis CJ, Arregui ME. Laparoscopic repair for groin hernias. Surg Clin North Am 2003; 83:1141–1161.
11. Tan M, Zheng CX, Wu ZM, Chen GT, Chen LH, Zhao ZX. Laparoscopic splenectomy: the latest technical evaluation. World J Gastroenterol 2003; 9:1086–1089.
12. Friedman RL, Fallas MJ, Carroll BJ, Hiatt JR, Phillips EH. Laparoscopic splenectomy for ITP. The gold standard. Surg Endosc 1996; 10:991–995.
13. Friedman R, Phillips E. Laparoscopic splenectomy. In: Ponsky J, ed. Complications of endoscopic and laparoscopic surgery. Philadelphia: Lippincott-Raven Publishers; 1997:159–170.
14. Katkhouda N, Mavor E. Laparoscopic splenectomy. Surg Clin North Am 2000; 80:1285–1297.
15. American Society of Colon and Rectal Surgeons approved statement on laparoscopic colectomy. Dis Colon Rectum 1994; 37: 8–12.
16. Lacy AM, Garcia-Valdecasas JC, Delgado S et al. Laparoscopy-assisted colectomy versus open colectomy for treatment of non-metastatic colon cancer: a randomised trial. Lancet 2002; 359:2224–2229.
17. Milsom JW, Kim SH, Hammerhofer KA, Fazio VW. Laparoscopic colorectal cancer surgery for palliation. Dis Colon Rectum 2000; 43:1512–1516.
18. Hartley JE, Monson JR. The role of laparoscopy in the multimodality treatment of colorectal cancer. Surg Clin North Am 2002; 82: 1019–1033.
19. Spechler SJ, Lee E, Ahnen D et al. Long-term outcome of medical and surgical therapies for gastroesophageal reflux disease – follow-up of a randomized controlled trial. JAMA 2001; 285:2331–2338.
20. Lundell L, Miettinen P, Myrvold HE et al. Continued (5-year) followup of a randomized clinical study comparing antireflux surgery and omeprazole in gastroesophageal reflux disease. J Am Coll Surg 2001; 192:172–179; discussion 179–181.
21. Dallemagne B, Weerts JM, Jehaes C, Markiewicz S, Lombard R. Laparoscopic Nissen fundoplication: preliminary report. Surg Laparosc Endosc 1991; 1:138–143.
22. Peters JH, DeMeester TR, Crookes P et al. The treatment of gastroesophageal reflux disease with laparoscopic Nissen fundoplication: prospective evaluation of 100 patients with "typical" symptoms. Ann Surg 1998; 228:40–50.
23. Oleynikov D, Oelschlager B. New alternatives in the management of gastroesophageal reflux disease. Am J Surg 2003; 186:106–111.

24. Waring JP. Surgical and endoscopic treatment of gastroesophageal reflux disease. Gastroenterol Clin North Am 2002; 31:S89–109.
25. Soper N, Jones D. Laparoscopic Nissen fundoplication. In: Nyhus L, Baker R, Fischer J, eds. Mastery of surgery, vol. 1. Boston: Little, Brown and Company; 1997:763–770.
26. Fraser J, Watson DI, O'Boyle CJ, Jamieson GG. Obesity and its effect on outcome of laparoscopic Nissen fundoplication. Dis Esophagus 2001; 14:50–53.
27. Hogan WJ, Shaker R. Life after antireflux surgery. Am J Med 2000; 108 (Suppl 4a): 181S–191S.
28. Triadafilopoulos G, DiBaise JK, Nostrant TT et al. The Stretta procedure for the treatment of GERD: 6 and 12 month follow-up of the U.S. open label trial. Gastrointest Endosc 2002; 55:149–156.
29. Flegal KM, Carroll MD, Kuczmarski RJ, Johnson CL. Overweight and obesity in the United States: prevalence and trends, 1960–1994. Int J Obes Relat Metab Disord 1998; 22:39–47.
30. Schauer PR. Open and laparoscopic surgical modalities for the management of obesity. J Gastrointest Surg 2003; 7:468–475.
31. Schauer P, Ikramuddin S, Hamad G, Gourash W. The learning curve for laparoscopic Roux-en-Y gastric bypass is 100 cases. Surg Endosc 2003; 17:212–215.

Index

Note
Abbreviations:
ERCP - endoscopic retrograde cholangiopancreatography
GERD - gastro-esophageal reflux disease
HPN - home parenteral nutrition
IBD - inflammatory bowel disease
IBS - irritable bowel syndrome
MRCP - magnetic resonance cholangiopancreatography
MRI - magnetic resonance imaging
PEG - percutaneous endoscopic gastrostomy
PET - positron emission tomography
PTC - percutaneous transhepatic cholangiography
TIPS - transjugular intrahepatic portosystemic shunt
Page numbers in *italics* refer to figures and those in **bold** refer to tables and/or boxed material. *vs* denotes differential diagnosis or comparisons.
This index is in letter-by-letter order whereby spaces and hyphens between words are ignored in the alphabetization e.g. pancreaticoduodenectomy precedes pancreatic pseudocyst

A

D

E

H

M

N

Q

R

T

U